Radiology Review Manual

Fourth Edition

Radiology Review Manual

Fourth Edition

Wolfgang Dähnert, M.D.
Department of Radiology
Good Samaritan Regional Medical Center
Phoenix, Arizona

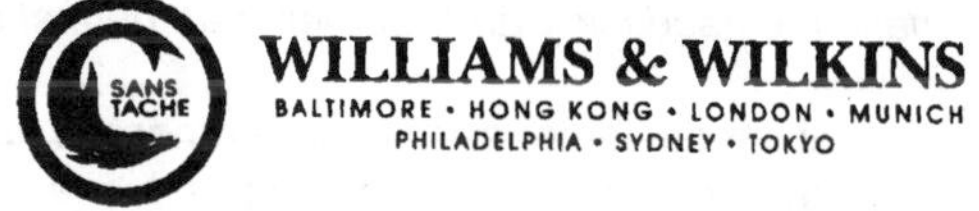

WILLIAMS & WILKINS
BALTIMORE • HONG KONG • LONDON • MUNICH
PHILADELPHIA • SYDNEY • TOKYO

Editor: Charles W. Mitchell
Managing Editor: Grace E. Miller
Marketing Manager: Peter Darcy
Cover Designer: Jeffrey S. Myers

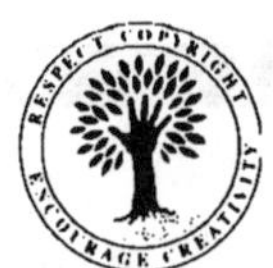

351 West Camden Street
Baltimore, Maryland 21202-2436 USA

Rose Tree Corporate Center
1400 North Providence Road
Building II, Suite 5025
Media, Pennsylvania 19063-2043 USA

Printed in the United States of America

First Edition 1991 Third Edition 1996
Second Edition 1993

Library of Congress Cataloging-in-Publication Data

Dähnert, Wolfgang.
Radiology review manual / Wolfgang Dähnert.—4th ed.
p. cm.
Includes index.
ISBN 0-683-30623-5
1.Radiology, Medical—Outlines, syllabi, etc. 2. Diagnosis, Radioscope—Outlines, syllabi, etc. I. Title.
[DNLM: 1. Radiography outlines. WN 18.2 D131r 1999]
RC78.17.D34 1999
616.07'57—dc21
DNLM / DLC
for Library of Congress

95–27272
CIP

The publishers have made every effort to trace the copyright holders for borrowed material. If they have inadvertently overlooked any, they will be pleased to make the necessary arrangements at the first opportunity.

To purchase additional copies of this book, call our customer service department at **(800) 638-0672** or fax orders to **(800) 447-8438**. For other book services, including chapter reprints and large quantity sales, ask for the Special Sales department.

Canadian customers should call **(800) 665-1148**, or fax **(800) 665-0103**. For all other calls originating outside of the United States, please call **(410) 528-4223** or fax us at **(410) 528-8550**.

Visit Williams & Wilkins on the Internet: **http://www.wwilkins.com** or contact our customer service department at **custserc@wwilkins.com**. Williams & Wilkins customer service representatives are available from 8:30 am to 6:00 pm, EST, Monday through Friday, for telephone access.

98 99 00 01 02
1 2 3 4 5 6 7 8 9 10

"Nothing in the world can take the place of persistence. Talent will not; nothing is more common than unsuccessful men with talent. Genius will not; unrewarded genius is almost a proverb. Education will not; the world is full of educated derelicts. Persistence and determination alone are omnipotent."

Calvin Coolidge 1872–1933
Vice President 1921–1923
President 1923–1929

To my dear wife Sue,
to our children Mathias and Patrick
who mean so much to me

About the Author

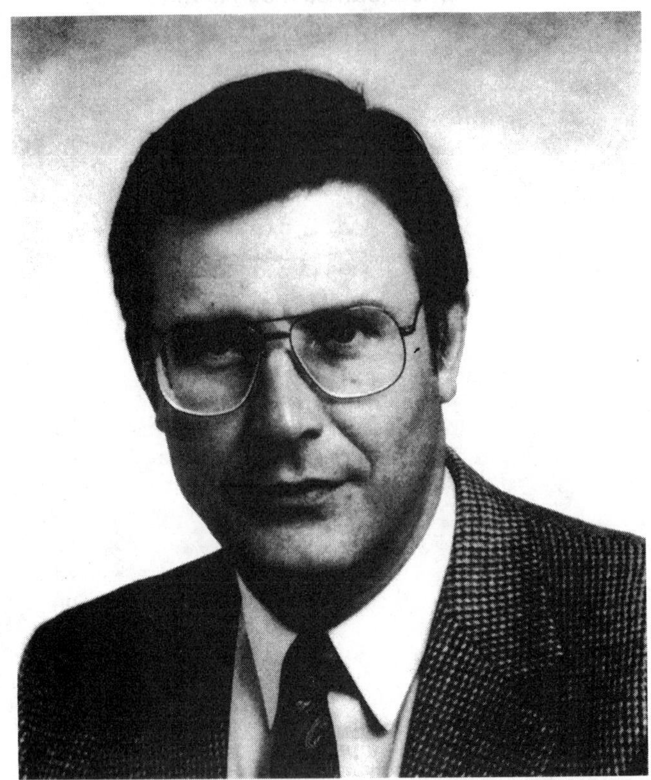

Wolfgang Dähnert, M.D.

Wolfgang Dähnert was born in Hamburg, Germany. He studied medicine at the universities of Düsseldorf and Mainz, where he graduated in 1975. After internship and a short surgical residency he enrolled in a 4-year radiology residency program at the Johannes-Gutenberg University in Mainz and received his German certification for radiology in 1982. In 1984 he started a 2-year fellowship in ultrasound and computed tomography at the Johns Hopkins Hospital in Baltimore and was appointed Clinical Instructor at the same institution in 1986. During his Hopkins years he sat for the FLEX exam, and the radiology specialty exam with the American Board of Radiology. During these three years the foundation of *Radiology Review Manual* was laid. Between 1987 and 1989 he worked as Assistant Professor of Radiology in ultrasound at Thomas Jefferson Hospital in Philadelphia. During these three years *Radiology Review Manual* was taken to fruition. Since December of 1989 he has been associated with Clinical Diagnostic Radiology & Nuclear Medicine, a large subspecialized radiology group practice in Phoenix, Arizona, providing radiology services to Good Samaritan Regional Medical Center, St. Joseph's Hospital and Medical Center, both tertiary care hospitals in Phoenix, Good Samaritan Hospital in Lake Havasu City, and the Children's Hospital of Phoenix.

PREFACE

The depth of medical knowledge and scope of image interpretation expected from an average general radiologist has soared over the last two decades. The emergence of subspecialties within radiology is witness to this development. Books have become available on so many different imaging topics and in such a large number that it is impossible even for the avid reader to consume them all, catalogue them, and have instant access to them. While some radiologists have the luxury to practice exclusively in their area of special interest with impressive expertise, many practice a much broader scope of diagnostic radiology and find themselves occasionally in situations where recollections have become nebulous. I know that I regret my inability to recall many facts or – more frustrating – where to look them up. In a busy practice it is simply not possible to take time out and disappear in the library.

Radiology Review Manual has become my carry-on memory jogger, in an attempt to put into a single reference much of the information that is or could be relevant to my practice. I use it like a dictionary, always available at my workstation. It is published under the assumption that many colleagues practice like I do: trying to do a good job vis-à-vis significant time constraints. This concept has resonated well with the radiologic community. The popularity of the "green giant" or the "green bible", as it has been dubbed by residents, confirms the usefulness of this type of publication. At the time of this writing approximately 28,000 copies have been sold, one half outside the United States of America.

Radiology Review Manual was created in preparation for the specialty exam as the "book under the pillow." I have to credit the idea to publish this material to several residents at the Johns Hopkins Hospital who urged me to do so. Over the years, this material has been changed and expanded. Our voluminous field of diagnostic radiology makes it necessary to use an outline style for the sake of conserving space and thus provides only an extract of information. This may, at times, jeopardize the full meaning of statements when the context is lost. It should be kept in mind that this book is not intended for the novice and that it requires familiarity with the subject of radiology and the background information of major textbooks.

How to use this book:
The organization of this book has caused a major headache as any topic can be looked at from various points of view. I have selected just one of many possibilities to avoid redundancy. The material is presented in a manner that is in keeping with the topics of the current board exam. Unfortunately, this grouping is inconsistent, sectioning off by age (Pediatric Radiology) and image modality (Nuclear Medicine, Ultrasound). In order to avoid repetition, pediatric entities are subsumed within organ systems. Ultrasound and Nuclear Medicine are used from head to heel and consequently are mentioned in all body sections. However, Nuclear Medicine is treated in a separate section when emphasis is on technique and functional aspects not covered elsewhere. The skull and spine, a crossing point of many subspecialties, are dealt with as the first part of the CNS section. A section on eye, ear, nose, and throat topics is placed at the end of the section on CNS disorders. Small chapters on statistics and contrast media are added.

The organization within the individual chapters follows the practical approach of reading films. The initial step of film interpretation is the description of radiologic patterns that serves to identify categories in which they belong. Therefore, radiologic patterns for differential diagnoses are found in the first portion of a chapter. Once the diagnostic possibilities have been reviewed in brief outline, one can look up detailed information about a disease entity in the last segment of a chapter. The disease entities are presented in alphabetical order. Both these segments are separated by a few pages of functional, anatomic, or embryologic aspects. Occasionally, important clinical signs and their differential diagnoses, relevant to the practice of radiology, are included in the first portion of a chapter. Mnemonics (which I personally abhor) have been liberally added by request. Accepted therapies for contrast reactions are printed on the inside of the back cover page for immediate access. A table of contents and abbreviations used throughout the book are found in front. A user-friendly index, which selectively refers to those pages with significant information concludes the manual. Notice that many systemic diseases will be mentioned in more than one chapter with some unavoidable redundancy. However, emphasized are those manifestations of the disease that occur within the organ under which it is listed. The index also includes so-called "buzz words" that are miraculously attached to diseases.

The backbone of the book are disease entities, radiologic symptoms, as well as lists of differential diagnosis. Disease entities are headed by their most commonly used name with other designations listed below. As a radiologic diagnosis should be entertained in context with its probability to be correct, percentages in regard to frequency of signs and symptoms are included liberally, often giving the lowest and the highest number found in the literature. The truth may be somewhere in between for a nonselected patient population, and occasionally a third number is provided between the high and low number as the most frequently cited. Arbitrary choices have been made in situations when different or contradictory results are found in the literature—unfortunately, an occurrence not at all infrequent.

Lists of differential diagnoses can be presented in many fashions. There is no right or wrong way, but there certainly is a chaotic versus an organized approach. An orderly thought process portrays familiarity with a problem. Examinees have always felt that "nailing" the diagnosis is secondary, but including it in one's consideration is paramount to a successful exam. Accordingly, an attempt is made to categorize differential diagnostic considerations or etiologies of certain diseases in a manner digestible for recapitulation. It is a common experience that this is not always possible, logically satisfactory, or complete.

Acknowledgement:
The information contained herein has been gathered over several years and stems from various sources. The most significant ones are the journals dedicated to imaging with brilliant review articles, in particular the practice-oriented publication of Radiographics, ACR syllabi, handouts from various CME courses, hand-written notes taken during lectures, as well as feed-back from candidates having taken the board exam. Anecdotal contributions can no longer be traced. I realize, in retrospect, that this may present a problem when certain statements appear unlikely and their verification has to be left to the user. For my defense, I can only say that I have tried to extract all data as diligently as possible.

The following textbooks have been particularly helpful and deserve mention: Barkovich AJ: *Pediatric Neuroimaging;* Burgener FA, Kormano M: *Differential Diagnosis in Conventional Radiology;* Chapman S, Nakielny R: *Aids to Radiological Differential Diagnosis;* Davidson AJ: *Radiology of the Kidney;* Eideken J: *Roentgen Diagnosis of Diseases of Bone;* Fraser RG, Pare JAP: *Diagnosis of Diseases of the Chest;* Gedgaudas E, Moller JH, Castaneda-Zuniga WR, Amplatz K: *Cardiovascular Radiology;* Harnsberger HR: *Handbooks in Radiology, Head and Neck Imaging;* Kadir S: *Diagnostic Angiography;* Kirks DR: *Practical Pediatric Imaging;* Margulis AR, Burhenne HJ: Alimentary Tract Radiology; Megibow AJ, Balthazar EJ: *Computed Tomography of the Gastrointestinal Tract;* Mittelstaedt CA: *Abdominal Ultrasound;* Newton TH, Hasso AN, Dillon WP: *Computed Tomography of the Head and Neck in Modern Neuroradiology;* Reed JC: *Chest Radiology: Plain Film Patterns and Differential Diagnosis;* Reeder MM, Felson B: *Gamuts in Radiology;* Sanders RC, James AE: *Ultrasonography in Obstetrics and Gynecology;* Resnick D, Niwayama G: *Diagnosis of Bone and Joint Disorders;* Romero R, Pilu G, Jeanty P, Ghidini A, Hobbins JC: *Prenatal Diagnosis of Congenital Anomalies;* Swischuk LE: *Plain Film Interpretation in Congenital Heart Disease;* Tabár L, Dean PB: *Teaching Atlas of Mammography;* Taveras JM, Ferrucci JT: *Radiology – Diagnosis – Imaging – Intervention.*

I would like to acknowledge the input of numerous teachers, residents, and fellows at the Johns Hopkins Hospital in Baltimore, Thomas Jefferson University Hospital in Philadelphia as well as many colleagues that have helped subsequently. I am particularly indebted to the following individuals for reviewing the separate sections of this book: Christopher Canino, Thomas Chang, Adam E. Flanders, Keith Haidet, Charles Intenzo, David Karasick, Stephen Karasick, Alfred B. Kurtz, Esmond M. Mapp, Joel Raichlen, Paul Spirn, Robert M. Steiner, and C. Amy Wilson. My special thanks go to Flavius ("Buddy") Guglielmo, who supplied me with probably the largest collection of mnemonics in existence. While completing his training at Thomas Jefferson University Hospital, he compiled a long list of memory joggers together with Tom Helinek and Les Folio with contributions from Barbara McComb, Barry Tom, and Ron Wachsberg. Thomas S. Chang of Montefiori University Hospital in Pittsburgh has made valuable suggestions for improvement. My thanks also go to my colleague Ross Levatter for his thorough review of the section on nuclear medicine.

Finally, my thanks go to Charles W. Mitchell, senior editor at Williams & Wilkins, and his staff who have been able to reduce the paper weight of this edition and have kept its price reasonable and affordable for residents. They have also created a CD-ROM version, released in October 1997, for those who use computers at their reading stations or love to lug around their portable personal computers.

I sincerely hope that *Radiology Review Manual* will serve you in the same manner it has helped me in preparation for the board exam, in teaching situations, and particularly in my daily work assignments.

Phoenix, September 1998

CONTENTS

ABBREVIATIONS

√	radiologic sign
•	clinical sign, symptom
=	equals, is
@	at anatomic location of
/	or, per
+	and, plus, with
±	with or without
<	less than
>	more than, over
◊	important comment
AAA	abdominal aortic aneurysm
ABC	aneurysmal bone cyst
AC	abdominal circumference
ACA	anterior cerebral artery
ACE	angiotensin I–converting enzyme
ACom	anterior communicating artery
ACTH	adrenocorticotropic hormone
ADEM	acute disseminated encephalo-myelitis
ADH	antidiuretic hormone
AFP	alpha-fetoprotein
AICA	anterior inferior cerebellar artery
AIDS	acquired immune deficiency syndrome
ALL	acute lymphoblastic leukemia
AMA	antimitochondrial antibody
AML	acute myeloblastic leukemia
AML	angiomyolipoma
aML	anterior mitral valve leaflet
ANA	antinuclear antibodies
Angio	angiography
ANT	anterior
Ao	aorta
AP	anteroposterior
APUD	amine precursor uptake and decarboxylation
APVR	anomalous pulmonary venous return
ARA-C	arabinoside C
ARDS	acute respiratory distress syndrome
AS	aortic stenosis
ASA	acetylsalicylic acid
ASD	atrial septal defect
ASH	asymmetric septal hypertrophy
aTL	anterior tricuspid valve leaflet
ATN	acute tubular necrosis
AV	arteriovenous
AV	atrioventricular
AVF	arteriovenous fistula
AVM	arteriovenous malformation
AVN	avascular necrosis
AVNA	atrioventricular node artery

Ba	barium
BCDDP	breast cancer detection demonstration project
BCG	bacille Calmette-Guérin
BE	barium enema
BIDA	butyl iminodiacetic acid
BIH	benign intracranial hypertension
BKG	background
BOOP	Bronchiolitis obliterans organizing pneumonia
BP	blood pressure
BPD	biparietal diameter
BPH	benign prostatic hyperplasia
bpm	beats per minute
BPP	biophysical profile
BSA	body surface area
Bx	biopsy
Ca	calcium
CAD	coronary artery disease
CAM	cystic adenomatoid malformation
CBD	common bile duct
CC	craniocaudad
CCA	common carotid artery
CCAM	congenital cystic adenomatoid malformation
CCK	cholecystokinin
CDC	Center for Disease Control
CECT	contrast-enhanced computed tomography
CEMR	contrast-enhanced MR
CFI	color flow imaging
cGy	centigray = rad
CHD	common hepatic duct; congenital heart defect
CHF	congestive heart failure
CLL	chronic lymphatic leukemia
CMC	carpometacarpal
CML	chronic myelogenous leukemia
CMV	cytomegalovirus
CNS	central nervous system
CO	carbon monoxide
CoA	coarctation of aorta
COPD	chronic obstructive pulmonary disease
CPA	cerebellopontine angle
CPPD	calcium pyrophosphate dihydrate
CPR	cardiopulmonary resuscitation
CRT	cathode ray tube
CSF	cerebrospinal fluid
CST	contraction stress test
CT	cardiothoracic ratio
CT	computed tomography

CVA	cerebrovascular accident
CWP	coal worker's pneumoconiosis
Cx	complication
CXR	chest x-ray
DCIS	ductal carcinoma in situ
DDx	differential diagnosis
DES	diethylstilbestrol
DIC	disseminated intravascular coagulation
DIDA	diethyl iminodiacetic acid
DIL	drug-induced lupus erythematosus
DIP	desquamative interstitial pneumonia
DIP	distal interphalangeal
DISH	diffuse idiopathic skeletal hyperostosis
DISIDA	diisopropyl iminodiacetic acid
DIT	diiodotyrosine
DMSA	dimercaptosuccinic acid
DTPA	diethylenetriamine pentaacetic acid
DVT	deep vein thrombosis
Dx	diagnosis
EAC	external auditory canal
ECA	external carotid artery
ECD	endocardial cushion defect
ECF	extracellular fluid
ECG	electrocardiogram
ECHO	echocardiogram
ED	end-diastole
EDV	end-diastolic volume
EEG	electroencephalogram
EF	ejection fraction
EFW	estimated fetal weight
EG	eosinophilic granuloma
eg	exempli gratia
EHDP	ethylene hydroxydiphosphonate
ERC	endoscopic retrograde cholangiography
ES	end-systole
esp.	especially
ESR	erythrocyte sedimentation rate
ESV	end-systolic volume
F	female
FDA	Federal Drug Administration
FDG	fluorodeoxyglucose
FEV	forced expiratory volume
FIGO	Fédération Internationale de Gynécologie et d'Obstétrique
FISP	fast imaging with steady-state precession

FLASH fast low-angle shot
FN false negative
FNH follicular nodular hyperplasia
FP false positive
FRC functional residual capacity
FS fractional shortening
FSH follicle stimulating hormone
FUO fever of unknown origin
FWHM full-width at half-maximum

GA gestational age
GB gallbladder
GBM glioblastoma multiforme
GBS group B streptococcus
Gd gadolinium
GE gastroesophageal
GER gastroesophageal reflux
GFR glomerular filtration rate
GI gastrointestinal
GIST gastrointestinal stromal tumor
GMRH germinal matrix–related hemorrhage
GN glomerulonephritis
GNRH gonadotropin releasing hormone
GRE gradient refocused echo
GU genitourinary

Hb hemoglobin
HC head circumference
hCG human chorionic gonadotropin
Hct hematocrit
HD Hodgkin disease
HIAA hydroxyindole acetic acid
HIDA hepatic 2,6-dimethyl iminodiacetic acid
HIP health insurance plan
Histo histology
HIV human immunodeficiency virus
HL Hodgkin lymphoma
HOCM hypertrophic obstructive cardiomyopathy; high-osmolarity contrast media
HPT hyperparathyroidism
HRCT high-resolution CT
HSA human serum albumin
HSE herpes simplex encephalitis
HSG hysterosalpingography
HSV herpes simplex virus
HTLV human T-cell lymphotropic virus
HU Hounsfield unit
HWP hepatic wedge pressure
Hx history

IAC internal auditory canal
ICA internal carotid artery
IDA iminodiacetic acid
IDM infant of diabetic mother
IDP iminodiphosphonate
ie id est
IHSS idiopathic hypertrophic subaortic stenosis
IM intramuscular
IMA inferior mesenteric artery
In indium
IPF idiopathic pulmonary fibrosis
IPH idiopathic pulmonary hemosiderosis
IR inversion recovery
IRP international reference preparation
IS ileosacral; international standard
IUD intrauterine device
IUGR intrauterine growth retardation
IV intravenous
IVC inferior vena cava
IVH intraventricular hemorrhage
IVP intravenous pyelogram
IVS intraventricular septum
IVU intravenous urogram

KCC Kulchitzky cell carcinoma
KUB kidney + ureter + bladder on one film

L left
L-DOPA 3-(3,4-dihydroxyphenyl)-levo-alanin
LA left atrium
LAD left anterior descending
LAO left anterior oblique
LAT lateral
LATS long-acting thyroid stimulating
LAV lymphadenopathy-associated virus
LCA left coronary artery
LCIS lobular carcinoma in situ
LCX left circumflex coronary artery
LDH lactate dehydrogenase
LE lupus erythematosus
LES lower esophageal sphincter
LGA large for gestational age
LH luteinizing hormone
LIP lymphocytic interstitial pneumonitis
LL lower lobes
LLL left lower lobe
LLQ left lower quadrant
Lnn lymph nodes
LOCM low-osmolarity contrast media
LPA left pulmonary artery
LPO left posterior oblique
LSD lysergic acid diethylamide
LUL left upper lobe
LUQ left upper quadrant
LV left ventricle
LVET left ventricular ejection time
$LVFT_2$ left ventricular slow filling time
LVOT left ventricular outflow tract
LVT_1 left ventricular fast filling time

M male
MA menstrual age
MAA macroaggregated albumin
MAG mercaptoacetyltriglycine
MAI Mycobacterium avium intracellulare
MCA middle cerebral artery
MCDK multicystic dysplastic kidney
MCK multicystic kidney
MCP metacarpophalangeal
MDP methylene diphosphonate
MEA multiple endocrine adenomas
MEN multiple endocrine neoplasms
MFH malignant fibrous histiocytoma
MIBG metaiodobenzylguanidine
MID multi-infarct dementia
MIT monoiodotyrosine
ML middle lobe
MLCN multilocular cystic nephroma
MLO mediolateral oblique
MMAA mini-microaggregated albumin colloid
MMFR maximal midexpiratory flow rate
MPS mucopolysaccharidosis
MR magnetic resonance
MS-AFP maternal serum α-fetoprotein
MTP metatarsophalangeal
MUGA multiple gated acquisition
MV mitral valve
Myelo myelography

N.B. nota bene
NBS National Bureau of Standards
NEC necrotizing enterocolitis
NECT nonenhanced computed tomography
NHL non-Hodgkin lymphoma
NPH normal pressure hydrocephalus
NPH nucleus pulposus herniation
npl neoplasm
NPO nulla per os
NSAID nonsteroidal anti-inflammatory drug
NST nonstress test
NTD neural tube defect
NUC nuclear medicine

OB-US obstetrical ultrasound
OCG oral cholecystogram
OCVM occult vascular malformation
OHP orthogonal-hole test pattern

OHSS ovarian hyperstimulation syndrome
OIH orthoiodohippurate

P phosphorus
PA posteroanterior
PA pulmonary artery
PAC premature atrial contraction
PAH para-aminohippurate
PAP primary atypical pneumonia
PAP pulmonary alveolar proteinosis
PAPVR partial anomalous pulmonary venous return
PAS periodic acid Schiff
Path pathology
PAVM pulmonary arteriovenous malformation
PBF pulmonary blood flow
PCA posterior cerebral artery
PCAVC persistent complete atrioventricular canal
PCKD polycystic kidney disease
PCom posterior communicating artery
PCP Pneumocystis carinii pneumonia
PCWP pulmonary capillary wedge pressure
PD posterior descending artery
PDA patent ductus arteriosus
PE pulmonary embolism
PEEP positive end expiratory pressure
PEP preejection period
PET positron emission tomography
pHPT primary hyperparathyroidism
PICA posterior inferior cerebellar artery
PIE pulmonary infiltrate with eosinophilia
PIE pulmonary interstitial emphysema
PIOPED prospective investigation of pulmonary embolus detection
PIP proximal interphalangeal
PIPIDA paraisopropyl iminodiacetic acid
PLES parallel-line–equal spacing
PM photomultiplier
PMF progressive massive fibrosis
PML progressive multifocal leukoencephalopathy
pML posterior mitral valve leaflet
PMN polymorphonuclear
PMT photomultiplier tube
PNET primitive neuroectodermal tumor
PO per oral
POST posterior
PPD purified protein derivative
PPG photoplethysmography
PPLO pleuropneumonia-like organism
ppm posterior papillary muscle
PS pulmonary stenosis
PSS progressive systemic sclerosis
PTC percutaneous transhepatic cholangiography
PTH parathyroid hormone
pTL posterior tricuspid valve leaflet
PTU propylthiouracil
PVC polyvinyl chloride
PVE periventricular echogenicity
PVH pulmonary venous hypertension
PVL periventricular leukomalacia
PVNS pigmented villonodular synovitis
PYP pyrophosphate
PVR pulse volume recording; postvoid residual

R right
RA rheumatoid arthritis
RA right atrium
RAO right anterior oblique
RBC red blood cell
RCA right coronary artery
RCC renal cell carcinoma
RDS respiratory distress syndrome
RES reticuloendothelial system
RI resistive index
RIND reversible ischemic neurologic deficit
RISA radioiodine serum albumin
RLL right lower lobe
RLQ right lower quadrant
RML right middle lobe
ROC receiver operating characteristic
ROI region of interest
RPA right pulmonary artery
RPF renal plasma flow
RPO right posterior oblique
RTA renal tubular acidosis
RUL right upper lobe
RV residual volume
RV right ventricle
RVOT right ventricular outflow tract
Rx therapy

S/P status post
SAE subcortical arteriosclerotic encephalopathy
SAG sagittal
SAH subarachnoid hemorrhage
SAM systolic anterior motion of mitral valve
SANA sinoatrial node artery
SBE subacute bacterial endocarditis
SBO salpingo-oophorectomy
SD standard deviation
SE spin echo
SGA small for gestational age
sHPT secondary hyperparathyroidism
SIJ sacroiliac joint
SFA superficial femoral artery
SLE systemic lupus erythematosus
SMA superior mesenteric artery
SMV superior mesenteric vein
Sn stannum
SOB small bowel obstruction
SONK spontaneous osteonecrosis of knee
S/P status post
SPECT single photon emission
SQ subcutaneous
STIR short tau inversion recovery
SV stroke volume
SVC superior vena cava

T1WI T1-weighted image
T2WI T2-weighted image
TAH total abdominal hysterectomy
TAPVR total anomalous pulmonary venous return
TB tuberculosis
TBG thyroxin-binding globulin
TBPA thyroxin-binding prealbumin
TCC transitional cell carcinoma
TDLU terminal ductal lobular unit
TE tracheoesophageal fistula
TGA transposition of great arteries
tHPT tertiary hyperparathyroidism
TIA transitory ischemic attack
TLC total lung capacity
TN true negative
TOF tetralogy of Fallot
TORCH toxoplasmosis, rubella, cytomegalovirus, herpes virus
TP true positive
TR repetition time
TRH thyrotropin-releasing hormone
TRV transverse
TSH thyroid-stimulating hormone
TURP transurethral resection of prostate
TV tidal volume

UGI upper gastrointestinal series
UIP usual interstitial pneumonia
UL upper lobe
UPJ ureteropelvic junction
US ultrasound
USP XX United States Pharmacopoeia, 20th edition
UTI urinary tract infection
UVJ ureterovesical junction

VC vital capacity
VIP vasoactive intestinal peptides
VMA vanillylmandelic acid
V/Q ventilation perfusion

VS interventricular septum
VSD ventricular septal defect
WBC white blood cells
WDHA watery diarrhea, hypokalemia, achlorhydria
WDHH watery diarrhea, hypokalemia, hypochlorhydria
XGP xanthogranulomatous pyelonephritis

ACRONYMS AND MNEMONICS

MUSCULOSKELETAL SYSTEM

DIFFERENTIAL DIAGNOSIS OF MUSCULOSKELETAL DISORDERS

Differential-diagnostic gamut of bone disorders

Conditions to be considered = "dissect bone disease with a DIATTOM"

Dysplasia + **D**ystrophy
Infection
Anomalies of development
Tumor + tumorlike conditions
Trauma
Osteochondritis + ischemic necrosis
Metabolic disease

DYSPLASIA = disturbance of bone growth
DYSTROPHY = disturbance of nutrition

Delayed bone age

A. CONSTITUTIONAL
   1. Familial
   2. IUGR
B. METABOLIC
   1. Hypopituitarism
   2. Hypothyroidism
   3. Hypogonadism (Turner syndrome)
   4. Cushing disease, steroid therapy
   5. Diabetes mellitus
   6. Rickets
   7. Malnutrition
C. SYSTEMIC DISEASE
   1. Congenital heart disease
   2. Renal disease
   3. GI disease: celiac disease, Crohn disease, ulcerative colitis
   4. Anemia
D. SYNDROME
   1. Trisomies
   2. Noonan disease
   3. Cornelia de Lange
   4. Cleidocranial dysplasia
   5. Lesch-Nyhan disease
   6. Metatrophic dwarfism

BONE SCLEROSIS

Diffuse osteosclerosis

mnemonic: "5 M'S To PROoF"

Metastases
Myelofibrosis
Mastocytosis
Melorheostosis
Metabolic: hypervitaminosis D, fluorosis, hypothyroidism, phosphorus poisoning
Sickle cell anemia
Tuberous sclerosis
Pyknodysostosis, **P**aget disease
Renal osteodystrophy
Osteopetrosis
Fluorosis

Constitutional sclerosing bone disease

1. Engelmann-Camurati disease
2. Infantile cortical hyperostosis
3. Melorheostosis
4. Osteopathia striata
5. Osteopetrosis
6. Osteopoikilosis
7. Pachydermoperiostosis
8. Pyknodysostosis
9. Van Buchem disease
10. Williams syndrome

Solitary osteosclerotic lesion

A. DEVELOPMENTAL
   1. Bone island
B. VASCULAR
   1. Old bone infarct
   2. Aseptic / ischemic / avascular necrosis
C. HEALING BONE LESION
   (a) <u>trauma</u>: callus formation
   (b) <u>benign tumor</u>: fibrous cortical defect / nonossifying fibroma, brown tumor; bone cyst
   (c) <u>malignant tumor</u>: lytic metastasis after radiation, chemo-, hormone therapy
D. INFECTION / INFLAMMATION
   (low-grade chronic infection / healing infection)
   1. Osteoid osteoma
   2. Chronic / healed osteomyelitis: bacterial, tuberculous, fungal
   3. Sclerosing osteomyelitis of Garré
   4. Granuloma
   5. Brodie abscess
E. BENIGN TUMOR
   1. Osteoma
   2. Ossifying fibroma
   3. Enchondroma / osteochondroma
   4. Osteoblastoma
F. MALIGNANT TUMOR
   1. Osteoblastic metastasis (prostate, breast)
   2. Lymphoma
   3. Sarcoma: osteo-, chondro-, Ewing sarcoma
G. OTHERS
   1. Sclerotic phase of Paget disease
   2. Fibrous dysplasia

Multiple osteosclerotic lesions

A. FAMILIAL
   1. Osteopoikilosis
   2. Enchondromatosis = Ollier disease
   3. Melorheostosis
   4. Multiple osteomas: associated with Gardner syndrome
   5. Osteopetrosis
   6. Pyknodysostosis
   7. Osteopathia striata

8. Chondrodystrophia calcificans congenita = congenital stippled epiphyses
9. Multiple epiphyseal dysplasia = Fairbank disease

B. SYSTEMIC DISEASE
1. Mastocytosis = urticaria pigmentosa
2. Tuberous sclerosis

Dense metaphyseal bands

mnemonic: "**H**eavy **C**retins **S**ift **S**currilously through **R**ickety **S**ystems"

Heavy metal poisoning (lead, bismuth, phosphorus)
Cretinism
Syphilis, congenital
Scurvy
Rickets (healed)
Systemic illness
also: normal variant; methotrexate therapy

mnemonic: "DENSE LINES"

D-vitamin intoxication
Elemental arsenic, bismuth, phosphorus
Normal variant
Systemic illness
Estrogen to mother during pregnancy
Leukemia, **L**ead poisoning
Infection (TORCH), **I**diopathic hypercalcemia
Never forget rickets
Early hypothyroidism
Scurvy, **S**ickle cell disease

Bone-within-bone appearance

= endosteal new bone formation

1. Normal
   (a) thoracic + lumbar vertebrae (in infants)
   (b) growth recovery lines (after infancy)
2. Infantile cortical hyperostosis (Caffey)
3. Sickle cell disease / thalassemia
4. Congenital syphilis
5. Osteopetrosis / oxalosis
6. Radiation
7. Acromegaly
8. Paget disease

mnemonic: "BLT PLT RSD RSD"

Bismuth ingestion
Lead ingestion
Thorium ingestion
Petrosis (osteopetrosis)
Leukemia
Tuberculosis
Rickets
Scurvy
D toxicity (vitamin D)
RSD (reflex sympathetic dystrophy)

OSTEOPENIA

= decrease in bone density

Categories:

1. Osteoporosis = decreased osteoid production
2. Osteomalacia = undermineralization of osteoid
3. Hyperparathyroidism
4. Multiple myeloma / diffuse metastases

Osteoporosis

= reduced bone mass of normal composition secondary to (a) osteoclastic resorption (85%) (trabecular, endosteal, intracortical, subperiosteal)
(b) osteocytic resorption (15%)

Incidence: 7% of all women between ages 35–40 years; 1 in 3 women > age 65 years

Etiology:

A. CONGENITAL DISORDERS
1. Osteogenesis imperfecta (the only osteoporosis with bending)
2. Homocystinuria

B. IDIOPATHIC (bone loss begins earlier + proceeds more rapidly in women)
1. Juvenile osteoporosis: <20 years
2. Adult osteoporosis: 20–40 years
3. Postmenopausal osteoporosis: >50 years (40–50% lower trabecular bone mineral density in elderly than in young women)
4. Senile osteoporosis: >60 years progressively decreasing bone density at a rate of 8% in females; 3% in males

C. NUTRITIONAL DISTURBANCES
scurvy; protein deficiency (malnutrition, nephrosis, chronic liver disease, alcoholism, anorexia nervosa, kwashiorkor, starvation), calcium deficiency

D. ENDOCRINOPATHY
Cushing disease, hypogonadism (Turner syndrome, eunuchoidism), hyperthyroidism, hyperparathyroidism, acromegaly, Addison disease, diabetes mellitus, pregnancy

E. RENAL OSTEODYSTROPHY
decrease / same / increase in spinal trabecular bone; rapid loss in appendicular skeleton

F. IMMOBILIZATION = disuse osteoporosis

G. COLLAGEN DISEASE, RHEUMATOID ARTHRITIS

H. BONE MARROW REPLACEMENT
infiltration by lymphoma / leukemia, multiple myeloma, diffuse metastases, marrow hyperplasia secondary to hemolytic anemia

I. DRUG THERAPY
heparin (15,000–30,000 U for >6 months), methotrexate, corticosteroids, vitamin A

J. RADIATION THERAPY

K. LOCALIZED OSTEOPOROSIS
Sudeck dystrophy, transient osteoporosis of hip, regional migratory osteoporosis of lower extremities

- serum calcium, phosphorus, alkaline phosphatase frequently normal
- hydroxyproline may be elevated during acute stage

Technique:

(1) <u>Single photon absorptiometry</u>
measures primarily cortical bone of appendicular bones, single-energy I-125 radioisotope source
Site: distal radius (= wrist bone density), os calcis
Dose: 2–3 mrem
Precision: 1–3%

(2) Dual photon absorptiometry
radioactive energy source with two photon peaks; should be reserved for patients <65 years of age because of interference from osteophytosis + vascular calcifications
Site: vertebrae, femoral neck
Dose: 5–10 mrem; Precision: 2–4%

(3) Quantitative computed tomography
high-turnover cancellous bone + low-turnover compact bone can be measured separately
Site: vertebrae L1–L3, other sites
(a) single energy: 300–500 mrem; 6–25% precision
(b) dual energy: 750–800 mrem; 5–10% precision

(4) Dual energy radiography = quantitative digital radiography = dual energy x-ray absorptiometry
x-ray tube produces a two-peak energy spectrum
Site: vertebrae, femoral neck
Dose: <3 mrem; Precision: 1–2%

◊ Radiographs are insensitive prior to bone loss of 25–30%
◊ Bone scans do NOT show a diffuse increase in activity

Location: axial skeleton (lower dorsal + lumbar spine), proximal humerus, neck of femur, wrist, ribs
√ decreased number + thickness of trabeculae
√ cortical thinning (endosteal + intracortical resorption)
√ juxtaarticular osteopenia with trabecular bone predominance
√ delayed fracture healing with poor callus formation (DDx: abundant callus formation in osteogenesis imperfecta + Cushing syndrome)

@ Spine
- √ diminished radiographic density
- √ vertical striations (= marked thinning of transverse trabeculae with relative accentuation of vertical trabeculae along lines of stress)
- √ prominence of endplates
- √ "picture framing" (= accentuation of cortical outline with preservation of external dimensions secondary to endosteal + intracortical resorption)
- √ compression deformities with protrusion of intervertebral disks
  - √ biconcave vertebrae
  - √ Schmorl nodes
  - √ wedging
  - √ decreased height of vertebrae
- √ absence of osteophytes

Cx: (1) Fractures at sites rich in labile trabecular bone (eg, vertebrae, wrist) in postmenopausal osteoporosis
(2) Fractures at sites containing cortical + trabecular bone (eg, hip) in senile osteoporosis

Rx: calcitonin, sodium fluoride, diphosphonates, parathyroid hormone supplements, estrogen replacement

Osteomalacia

= accumulation of excessive amounts of uncalcified osteoid with bone softening + insufficient mineralization of osteoid due to
(a) high remodeling rate: excessive osteoid formation + normal / little mineralization
(b) low remodeling rate: normal osteoid production + diminished mineralization

Etiology:
(1) dietary deficiency of vitamin D_3 + lack of solar irradiation
(2) deficiency of metabolism of vitamin D:
— chronic renal tubular disease
— chronic administration of phenobarbital (alternate liver pathway)
— diphenylhydantoin (interferes with vitamin D action on bowel)
(3) decreased absorption of vitamin D:
— malabsorption syndromes (most common)
— partial gastrectomy (self-restriction of fatty foods)
(4) decreased deposition of calcium in bone
— diphosphonates (for treatment of Paget disease)

Histo: excess of osteoid seams + decreased appositional rate

- bone pain / tenderness; muscular weakness
- serum calcium slightly low / normal
- decreased serum phosphorus
- elevated serum alkaline phosphatase

√ uniform osteopenia
√ fuzzy indistinct trabecular detail of endosteal surface
√ thin cortices of long bone
√ coarsened frayed trabeculae decreased in number + size
√ bone deformity from softening: hourglass thorax, bowing of long bones, buckled / compressed pelvis
√ increased incidence of fractures, biconcave vertebral bodies
√ mottled skull
√ pseudofractures

Localized Osteopenia

1. Disuse atrophy
   Etiology: local immobilization secondary to
   (a) fracture (more pronounced distal to fracture site)
   (b) neural paralysis
   (c) muscular paralysis
2. Reflex sympathetic dystrophy = Sudeck dystrophy
3. Regional migratory osteoporosis, transient osteoporosis of hip
4. Osteolytic tumor
5. Lytic phase of Paget disease
6. Inflammation: rheumatoid arthritis, osteomyelitis, tuberculosis
7. Early phase of bone infarct and hemorrhage
8. Burns + frostbite

Bone Marrow Edema

= hypointensity on T1WI + hyperintensity on T2WI
1. Transient osteoporosis of hip
2. Osteonecrosis = early stage of AVN

3. Trauma
   (a) "bone bruise"
   (b) radiographically occult fracture in elderly women
4. Infection = osteomyelitis
5. Infiltrative neoplasm

Transverse lucent metaphyseal lines

mnemonic: "LINING"

Leukemia
Illness, systemic (rickets, scurvy)
Normal variant
Infection, transplacental (congenital syphilis)
Neuroblastoma metastases
Growth lines

Frayed metaphyses

mnemonic: "CHARMS"

Congenital infections (rubella, syphilis)
Hypophosphatasia
Achondroplasia
Rickets
Metaphyseal dysostosis
Scurvy

PERIOSTEAL REACTION

1. Trauma, hemophilia
2. Infection
3. Inflammatory: arthritis
4. Neoplasm
5. Congenital: physiologic in newborn
6. Metabolic: hypertrophic osteoarthropathy, thyroid acropachy, hypervitaminosis A
7. Vascular: venous stasis

Solid periosteal reaction

= reaction to periosteal irritant
√ even + uniform thickness >1 mm
√ persistent + unchanged for weeks

Patterns:
(a) thin: eosinophilic granuloma, osteoid osteoma
(b) dense undulating: vascular disease
(c) thin undulating: pulmonary osteoarthropathy
(d) dense elliptical: osteoid osteoma; long-standing malignant disease (with destruction)
(e) cloaking: storage disease; chronic infection

Interrupted periosteal reaction

= pleomorphic, rapidly progressing process undergoing constant change
(a) lamellated = "onion skin": acute osteomyelitis; malignant tumor (osteosarcoma, Ewing sarcoma)
(b) perpendicular = "sunburst": osteosarcoma; Ewing sarcoma; chondrosarcoma; fibrosarcoma; leukemia; metastasis; acute osteomyelitis
(c) amorphous: malignancy (deposits may represent extension of tumor / periosteal response); osteosarcoma
(d) Codman triangle: hemorrhage; malignancy (osteosarcoma, Ewing sarcoma); acute osteomyelitis; fracture

Symmetric periosteal reaction in adulthood

1. Vascular insufficiency (lower extremity)
2. Hypertrophic osteoarthropathy
3. Pachydermoperiostosis
4. Thyroid acropachy
5. Fluorosis
6. Rheumatoid arthritis
7. Psoriatic arthritis
8. Reiter syndrome
9. Idiopathic-degenerative

Periosteal reaction in childhood

(a) benign
1. Physiologic (up to 35%): symmetric involvement of diaphyses during first 1–6 months of life
2. Battered child syndrome
3 Infantile cortical hyperostosis <6 months of age
4. Hypervitaminosis A
5. Scurvy
6. Osteogenesis imperfecta
7. Congenital syphilis

(b) malignant
1. Multicentric osteosarcoma
2. Metastases from neuroblastoma + retinoblastoma
3. Acute leukemia

mnemonic: "PERIOSTEAL SOCKS"

Physiologic, **P**rostaglandin
Eosinophilic granuloma
Rickets
Infantile cortical hyperostosis
Osteomyelitis
Scurvy
Trauma
Ewing sarcoma
A-hypervitaminosis
Leukemia + neuroblastoma
Syphilis
Osteosarcoma
Child abuse
Kinky hair syndrome
Sickle cell disease

BONE TUMOR

Assessment of aggressiveness

A. BENIGN
1. Diagnosis certain: no further work-up necessary
2. Asymptomatic lesion with highly probable diagnosis may be followed clinically
3. Symptomatic lesion with highly probable diagnosis may be treated without further work-up

B. CONFUSING LESION
not clearly categorized as benign or malignant; needs staging work-up

C. MALIGNANT
needs staging work-up

Staging work-up:
Bone scan: identifies polyostotic lesions (eg, multiple myeloma, metastatic disease, primary osteosarcoma with bone-forming metastases, histiocytosis, Paget disease)

Chest CT: identifies metastatic deposits + changes further work-up and therapy

Local staging with MR imaging:

(1) Margins: encapsulated / infiltrating
(2) Compartment: intra- / extracompartmental
(3) Intraosseous extent + skip lesions
(4) Soft-tissue extent (DDx: hematoma, edema)
(5) Joint involvement
(6) Neurovascular involvement

Local assessment with CT: matrix / rim calcifications

Age incidence of malignant bone tumors

◊ 80% of bone tumors are correctly determined on the basis of age alone!

Age (years)	Tumor
0.1	Neuroblastoma
0.1–10	Ewing tumor in tubular bones (diaphysis)
10 –30	Osteosarcoma (metaphysis); Ewing tumor in flat bones
30 –40	Reticulum cell sarcoma (similar histology to Ewing tumor); fibrosarcoma; malignant giant cell tumor (similar histology to fibrosarcoma); parosteal sarcoma; lymphoma
>40	Metastatic carcinoma; multiple myeloma; chondrosarcoma

SARCOMAS BY AGE:

mnemonic: "**E**very **O**ther **R**unner **F**eels **C**rampy **P**ain **O**n **M**oving"

Ewing sarcoma	0 –10 years
Osteogenic sarcoma	10–30 years
Reticulum cell sarcoma	20–40 years
Fibrosarcoma	20–40 years
Chondrosarcoma	40–50 years
Parosteal sarcoma	40–50 years
Osteosarcoma	60–70 years
Metastases	60–70 years

ROUND CELL TUMORS:

arise in mid shaft; osteolytic; reactive new bone formation; no tumor new bone

mnemonic: "LEMON"

Leukemia, **L**ymphoma
Ewing sarcoma, **E**osinophilic granuloma
Multiple myeloma
Osteomyelitis
Neuroblastoma

MALIGNANCY WITH SOFT-TISSUE INVOLVEMENT

mnemonic: "**M**y **M**other **E**ats **C**hocolate **F**udge **O**ften"

Metastasis
Myeloma
Ewing sarcoma
Chondrosarcoma
Fibrosarcoma
Osteosarcoma

Tumor matrix of bone tumors

Cartilage-forming bone tumors

A. BENIGN
1. Enchondroma
2. Parosteal chondroma
3. Chondroblastoma
4. Chondromyxoid fibroma
5. Osteochondroma

B. MALIGNANT
1. Chondrosarcoma

√ centrally located ringlike / flocculent / flecklike radiodensities

Bone-forming tumors

A. BENIGN
1. Osteoma
2. Osteoid osteoma
3. Osteoblastoma
4. Ossifying fibroma

B. MALIGNANT
1. Osteogenic sarcoma

√ inhomogeneous / homogeneous radiodense collections of variable size + extent

Fibrous connective tissue tumors

A. BENIGN FIBROUS BONE LESIONS

(a) cortical
1. Benign cortical defect
2. Avulsion cortical irregularity

(b) medullary
1. Herniation pit
2. Nonossifying fibroma
3. Ossifying fibroma
4. Congenital generalized fibromatosis

(c) corticomedullary
1. Nonossifying fibroma
2. Ossifying fibroma
3. Fibrous dysplasia
4. Cherubism
5. Desmoplastic fibroma
6. Fibromyxoma

B. MALIGNANT
1. Fibrosarcoma

Tumors of histiocytic origin

A. LOCALLY AGGRESSIVE
1. Giant cell tumor
2. Benign fibrous histiocytoma

B. MALIGNANT
1. Malignant fibrous histiocytoma

Tumors of fatty tissue origin

A. BENIGN
1. Intraosseous lipoma
2. Parosteal lipoma

B. MALIGNANT
1. Intraosseous liposarcoma

◊ Lipomas follow the signal intensity of subcutaneous fat in all sequences!

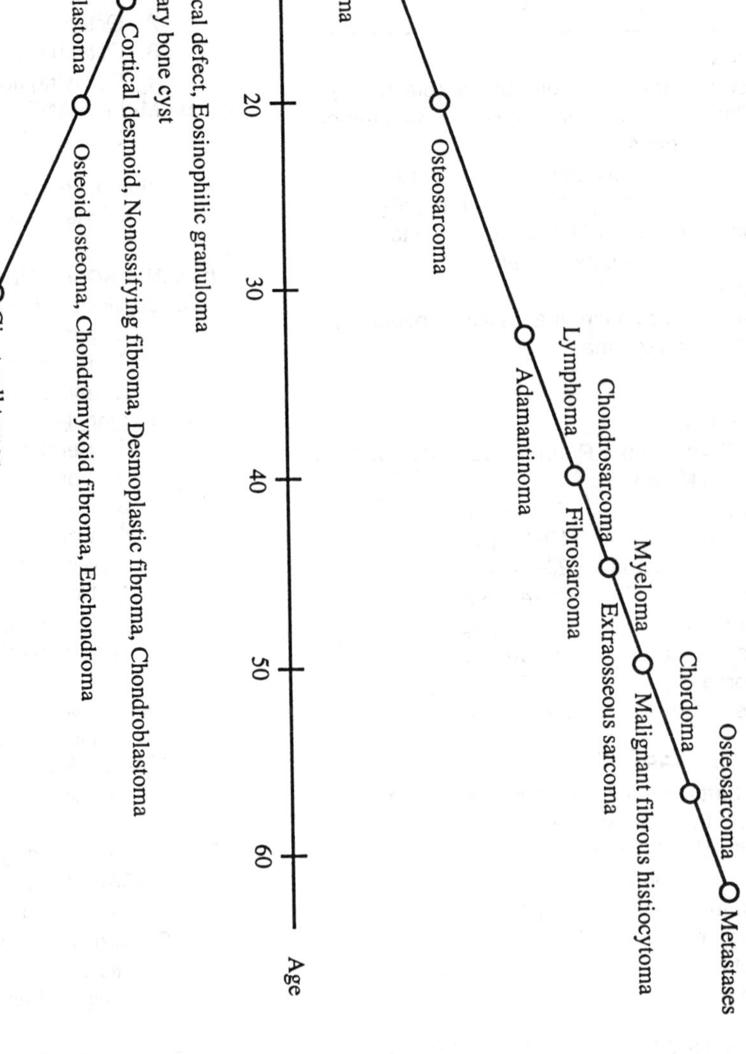

Average Age for Occurrence of Benign and Malignant Bone Tumors

Tumors of vascular origin

<1% of all bone tumors

A. BENIGN
1. Hemangioma
2. Glomus tumor
3. Lymphangioma
4. Cystic angiomatosis
5. Hemangiopericytoma

B. MALIGNANT
1. Malignant hemangiopericytoma
2. Angiosarcoma = hemangioendothelioma
   Metastatic sites: lung, brain, lymph nodes, other bones

Tumors of neural origin

A. BENIGN
1. Solitary neurofibroma
2. Neurilemoma

B. MALIGNANT
1. Neurogenic sarcoma = malignant schwannoma

Pattern of bone destruction

A. GEOGRAPHIC BONE DESTRUCTION
   Indicative of slow-growing usually benign tumor
   √ well-defined smooth / irregular margin
   √ short zone of transition

B. MOTH-EATEN BONE DESTRUCTION
   Indicative of more rapid growth as in malignant bone tumor / osteomyelitis
   √ less well defined / demarcated lesional margin
   √ longer zone of transition
   mnemonic: "H LEMMON"
   Histiocytosis X
   Lymphoma
   Ewing sarcoma
   Metastasis
   Multiple myeloma
   Osteomyelitis
   Neuroblastoma

C. PERMEATIVE BONE DESTRUCTION
   Aggressive bone lesion with rapid growth potential (eg, Ewing sarcoma)
   √ poorly demarcated lesion imperceptibly merging with uninvolved bone
   √ long zone of transition

D. SIZE OF LESION
   Primary malignant tumors are larger than benign tumors

E. ELONGATED LESION
   √ greatest lesional diameter is >1 1/2 times the least diameter
   Ewing sarcoma, reticulum cell sarcoma, chondrosarcoma, angiosarcoma

Tumor position in transverse plane

A. CENTRAL MEDULLARY LESION
1. Enchondroma
2. Solitary bone cyst

B. ECCENTRIC MEDULLARY LESION
1. Giant cell tumor
2. Osteogenic sarcoma, chondrosarcoma, fibrosarcoma
3. Chondromyxoid fibroma

C. CORTICAL LESION
1. Nonossifying fibroma
2. Osteoid osteoma

D. PAROSTEAL / JUXTACORTICAL LESION
1. Juxtacortical chondroma
2. Osteochondroma
3. Parosteal osteogenic sarcoma

Tumor position in longitudinal plane

A. EPIPHYSEAL LESION
1. Chondroblastoma
2. Intraosseous ganglion
3. Giant cell tumor (originating in metaphysis)
   mnemonic: "CAGGIE"
   Chondroblastoma
   Aneurysmal bone cyst
   Giant cell tumor
   Geode
   Infection
   Eosinophilic granuloma
   [after 40 years of age throw out "CEA" and insert metastases / myeloma]

B. METAPHYSEAL LESION
1. Nonossifying fibroma
2. Chondromyxoid fibroma
3. Solitary bone cyst
4. Osteochondroma
5. Brodie abscess
6. Osteogenic sarcoma, chondrosarcoma

C. DIAPHYSEAL LESION
1. Round cell tumor (eg, Ewing sarcoma)
2. Nonossifying fibroma
3. Solitary bone cyst
4. Aneurysmal bone cyst
5. Enchondroma
6. Osteoblastoma
7. Fibrous dysplasia
   mnemonic: "FEMALE"
   Fibrous dysplasia
   Eosinophilic granuloma
   Metastasis
   Adamantinoma
   Leukemia, **L**ymphoma
   Ewing sarcoma

Tumorlike conditions

1. Solitary bone cyst
2. Juxta-articular ("synovial") cyst
3. Aneurysmal bone cyst
4. Nonossifying fibroma; cortical defect; cortical desmoid
5. Eosinophilic granuloma
6. Reparative giant cell granuloma
7. Fibrous dysplasia (monostotic; polyostotic)
8. Myositis ossificans
9. "Brown tumor" of hyperparathyroidism
10. Massive osteolysis

INTRAOSSEOUS LESION

Bubbly bone lesion

mnemonic: "FOG MACHINES"

- **F**ibrous dysplasia, **F**ibrous cortical defect
- **O**steoblastoma
- **G**iant cell tumor
- **M**yeloma (plasmacytoma), **M**etastases from kidney, thyroid, breast
- **A**neurysmal bone cyst / **A**ngioma
- **C**hondromyxoid fibroma, **C**hondroblastoma
- **H**istiocytosis X, **H**yperparathyroid brown tumor, **H**emophilia
- **I**nfection (Brodie abscess, Echinococcus, coccidioidomycosis)
- **N**onossifying fibroma
- **E**nchondroma, **E**pithelial inclusion cyst
- **S**imple unilocular bone cyst

Infectious bubbly lesion

1. Brodie abscess (Staph. aureus)
2. Coccidioidomycosis
3. Echinococcus
4. Atypical mycobacterium
5. Cystic tuberculosis

Blowout lesion

A. METASTASES
   Carcinoma of thyroid, kidney, breast

B. PRIMARY BONE TUMOR
   1. Fibrosarcoma
   2. Multiple myeloma (sometimes)
   3. Aneurysmal bone cyst
   4. Hemophilic pseudotumor

Nonexpansile unilocular well-demarcated bone defect

1. Fibrous cortical defect
2. Nonossifying fibroma
3. Simple unicameral bone cyst
4. Giant cell tumor
5. Brown tumor of HPT
6. Eosinophilic granuloma
7. Enchondroma
8. Epidermoid inclusion cyst
9. Posttraumatic / degenerative cyst
10. Pseudotumor of hemophilia
11. Intraosseous ganglion
12. Histiocytoma
13. Arthritic lesion
14. Endosteal pigmented villonodular synovitis
15. Fibrous dysplasia
16. Infectious lesion

Nonexpansile multilocular well-demarcated bone defect

1. Aneurysmal bone cyst
2. Giant cell tumor
3. Fibrous dysplasia
4. Simple bone cyst

Expansile unilocular well-demarcated osteolysis

1. Simple unicameral bone cyst
2. Enchondroma
3. Aneurysmal bone cyst
4. Juxtacortical chondroma
5. Nonossifying fibroma
6. Eosinophilic granuloma
7. Brown tumor of HPT

Poorly demarcated osteolytic lesion without periosteal reaction

A. NONEXPANSILE
   1. Metastases from any primary neoplasm
   2. Multiple myeloma
   3. Hemangioma

B. EXPANSILE
   1. Chondrosarcoma
   2. Giant cell tumor
   3. Metastasis from kidney / thyroid

Poorly demarcated osteolytic lesion with periosteal reaction

1. Osteomyelitis
2. Ewing sarcoma
3. Osteosarcoma

Mixed sclerotic and lytic lesion

A. WITH SEQUESTRUM: osteomyelitis

B. WITHOUT SEQUESTRUM:
   1. Osteomyelitis
   2. Tuberculosis
   3. Ewing sarcoma
   4. Metastasis
   5. Osteosarcoma

Trabeculated bone lesion

1. Giant cell tumor: delicate thin trabeculae
2. Chondromyxoid fibroma: coarse thick trabeculae
3. Nonossifying fibroma: loculated
4. Aneurysmal bone cyst: delicate, horizontally oriented trabeculae
5. Hemangioma: striated radiating trabeculae

Lytic bone lesion surrounded by marked sclerosis

mnemonic: "BOOST"

- **B**rodie abscess
- **O**steoblastoma
- **O**steoid osteoma
- **S**tress fracture
- **T**uberculosis

Multiple lytic lesions

mnemonic: "FEEMHI"

- **F**ibrous dysplasia
- **E**nchondromas
- **E**osinophilic granuloma
- **M**etastases, **M**ultiple myeloma
- **H**yperparathyroidism (brown tumors), **H**emangiomas
- **I**nfection

Lytic bone lesion in patient <30 years of age

mnemonic: "CAINES"

Chondroblastoma
Aneurysmal bone cyst
Infection
Nonossifying fibroma
Eosinophilic granuloma
Solitary bone cyst

Lytic bone lesion on both sides of joint

mnemonic: "SAC"

Synovioma
Angioma
Chondroid lesion

DWARFISM

Classification:

(1) OSTEOCHONDRODYSPLASIA
= abnormalities of cartilage / bone growth and development
(a) identifiable at birth:
— usually lethal: achondrogenesis, fibrochondrogenesis, thanatophoric dysplasia, short rib syndrome
— usually nonlethal: chondrodysplasia punctata, camptomelic dysplasia, achondroplasia, diastrophic dysplasia, chondroectodermal dysplasia, Jeune syndrome, spondyloepiphyseal dysplasia congenita, mesomelic dysplasia, cleidocranial dysplasia, oto-palato-digital syndrome
(b) identifiable in later life: hypochondroplasia, dyschondrosteosis, spondylometaphyseal dysplasia, acromicric dysplasia
(c) abnormal bone density: osteopetrosis, pyknodysostosis, Melnick-Needles syndrome

(2) DYSOSTOSIS
= malformation of individual bones singly / in combination
(a) with cranial + facial involvement: craniosynostosis, craniofacial dysostosis (Crouzon), acrocephalosyndactyly, acrocephalopolysyndactyly, branchial arch syndromes (Treacher-Collins, Franceschetti, acrofacial dysostosis, oculo-auriculo-vertebral dysostosis, hemifacial microsomia, oculo-mandibulo-facial syndrome
(b) with predominant axial involvement: vertebral segmentation defects (Klippel-Feil), Sprengel anomaly, spondylocostal dysostosis, oculovertebral syndrome
(c) with predominant involvement of extremities: acheiria (= absence of hands), apodia (= absence of feet), polydactyly, syndactyly, camptodactyly, Rubinstein-Taybi syndrome, pancytopenia-dysmelia syndrome (Fanconi), Blackfan-Diamond anemia with thumb anomaly, thrombocytopenia-radial aplasia syndrome, cardiomelic syndromes (Holt-Oram), focal femoral deficiency, multiple synostoses

(3) IDIOPATHIC OSTEOLYSIS
= disorders associated with multifocal resorption of bone

(4) CHROMOSOMAL ABERRATION

(5) PRIMARY METABOLIC DISORDER
(a) calcium / phosphorus: hypophosphatasia
(b) complex carbohydrates: mucopolysaccharidosis

Terminology:

Micromelia = shortening involves entire limb (eg, humerus, radius + ulna, hand)
Rhizomelia = shortening involves proximal segment (eg, humerus)
Mesomelia = shortening involves intermediate segment (eg, radius + ulna)
Acromelia = shortening involves distal segment (eg, hand)

Micromelic dwarfism

= disproportionate shortening of entire leg

A. Mild micromelic dwarfism
1. Jeune syndrome
2. Ellis-van Creveld syndrome = chondroectodermal dysplasia
3. Diastrophic dwarfism

B. Mild bowed micromelic dwarfism
1. Camptomelic dysplasia
2. Osteogenesis imperfecta, type III

C. Severe micromelic dwarfism
1. Thanatophoric dysplasia
2. Osteogenesis imperfecta, type II
3. Homozygous achondroplasia
4. Hypophosphatasia
5. Short-rib polydactyly syndrome
6. Fibrochondrogenesis

Acromelic dwarfism

= distal shortening (hands, feet)
1. Asphyxiating thoracic dysplasia

Rhizomelic dwarfism

= shortening of proximal segments (humerus, femur)

mnemonic: "MA CAT"

Metatrophic dwarfism
Achondrogenesis (most severe shortening)
Chondrodysplasia punctata (autosomal recessive)
Thanatophoric dysplasia
Achondroplasia, heterozygous

Osteochondrodysplasia

A. Failure of
(a) articular cartilage: spondyloepiphyseal dysplasia
(b) ossification center: multiple epiphyseal dysplasia
(c) proliferating cartilage: achondroplasia
(d) spongiosa formation: hypophosphatasia
(e) spongiosa absorption: osteopetrosis
(f) periosteal bone: osteogenesis imperfecta
(g) endosteal bone: idiopathic osteoporosis

B. Excess of
   (a) articular cartilage: dysplasia epiphysealis hemimelica
   (b) hypertrophic cartilage: enchondromatosis
   (c) spongiosa: multiple exostosis
   (d) periosteal bone: progressive diaphyseal dysplasia
   (e) endosteal bone: hyperphosphatemia

Lethal bone dysplasia

in order of frequency

1. Thanatophoric dysplasia
2. Osteogenesis imperfecta type II
3. Achondrogenesis type I + II
4. Jeune syndrome (may be nonlethal)
5. Hypophosphatasia, congenital lethal form
6. Chondroectodermal dysplasia (usually nonlethal)
7. Chondrodysplasia punctata, rhizomelic type
8. Camptomelic dysplasia
9. Short-rib polydactyly syndrome
10. Homozygous achondroplasia

◊ Lethal short-limbed dysplasias typically are manifest on sonograms before 24 weeks MA!

Nonlethal dwarfism

1. Achondroplasia (heterozygous)
2. Asphyxiating thoracic dysplasia
3. Chondroectodermal dysplasia
4. Chondrodysplasia punctata
5. Spondyloepiphyseal dysplasia (congenital)
6. Diastrophic dwarfism
7. Metatrophic dwarfism
8. Hypochondroplasia

Late-onset dwarfism

1. Spondyloepiphyseal dysplasia tarda
2. Multiple epiphyseal dysplasia
3. Pseudoachondroplasia
4. Metaphyseal chondrodysplasia
5. Dyschondrosteosis
6. Cleidocranial dysostosis
7. Progressive diaphyseal dysplasia

Hypomineralization in fetus

A. DIFFUSE
   1. Osteogenesis imperfecta
   2. Hypophosphatasia
B. SPINE
   1. Achondrogenesis

Large head in fetus

1. Achondroplasia
2. Thanatophoric dysplasia

Narrow chest in fetus

1. Short-rib polydactyly syndrome
2. Asphyxiating thoracic dysplasia
3. Chondroectodermal dysplasia
4. Camptomelic dysplasia
5. Thanatophoric dwarfism
6. Homozygous achondroplasia
7. Achondrogenesis
8. Hypophosphatasia

Platyspondyly

1. Thanatophoric dysplasia
2. Osteogenesis imperfecta type II
3. Achondroplasia

Bowed long bones in fetus

1. Campomelic syndrome
2. Osteogenesis imperfecta
3. Thanatophoric dysplasia
4. Hypophosphatasia

Bone fractures in fetus

1. Osteogenesis imperfecta
2. Hypophosphatasia
3. Achondrogenesis

LIMB REDUCTION ANOMALIES

Amelia = absence of limb
Hemimelia = absence of distal parts
Phocomelia = proximal reduction with distal parts attached to trunk

Aplasia / hypoplasia of radius

mnemonic: "The Furry Cat Hit My Dog"
Thrombocytopenia–absent radius syndrome
Fanconi anemia
Cornelia de Lange syndrome
Holt-Oram syndrome
Myositis ossificans progressiva (thumb only)
Diastrophic dwarfism ("hitchhiker's thumb")

Pubic bone maldevelopment

mnemonic: "CHIEF"
Cleidocranial dysostosis
Hypospadia, epispadia
Idiopathic
Exstrophy of bladder
F for syringomyelia

BONE OVERGROWTH

Bone overdevelopment

1. Marfan syndrome
2. Klippel-Trénaunay syndrome
3. Nerve territory-oriented macrodactyly
   (a) Macrodystrophia lipomatosa
   (b) Fibrolipomatous hamartoma with macrodactyly

Erlenmeyer flask deformity

= expansion of distal end of long bones, usually femur

1. Gaucher disease, Niemann-Pick disease
2. Rickets
3. Anemia, eg, thalassemia
4. Fibrous dysplasia
5. Osteopetrosis
6. Heavy metal poisoning

7. Metaphyseal dysplasia = Pyle disease
8. Down syndrome
9. Achondroplasia
10. Rheumatoid arthritis
11. Hypophosphatasia

mnemonic: "TOP DOG"
- **T**halassemia
- **O**steopetrosis
- **P**yle disease
- **D**iaphyseal aclasis
- **O**llier disease
- **G**aucher disease

JOINTS

Approach to arthritis

mnemonic: "ABCDE'S"
- **A**lignment
- **B**one mineralization
- **C**artilage loss
- **D**istribution
- **E**rosion
- **S**oft tissues

Signs of arthritis

Prevalence of arthritis: 15% of population in USA

Conventional x-ray:
- √ narrowing of radiologic joint space
  - (a) uniform = inflammatory arthritis
  - (b) nonuniform = degenerative arthritis
- √ evidence of disease on both sides of joint:
  - √ osteopenia
  - √ subchondral sclerosis
  - √ erosion
  - √ subchondral cyst formation
  - √ malalignment
- √ joint effusion
- √ joint bodies

NUC:
- √ increase in regional blood flow (active disease)
- √ distribution of disease

MR:
- √ irregularity + narrowing of articular cartilage
- √ Gd-DTPA enhancement of synovium (active disease)

Classification of arthritides

A. SEPTIC ARTHRITIS
1. Tuberculous
2. Pyogenic
3. Lyme arthritis
4. Fungal arthritis: Candida, Coccidioides immitis, Blastomyces dermatitidis, Histoplasma capsulatum, Sporothrix schenckii, Cryptococcus neoformans, Aspergillus fumigatus

B. COLLAGEN / COLLAGEN-LIKE DISEASE
1. Rheumatoid arthritis
2. Ankylosing spondylitis
3. Psoriatic arthritis
4. Rheumatic fever
5. Sarcoidosis

C. BIOCHEMICAL ARTHRITIS
1. Gout
2. Chondrocalcinosis
3. Ochronosis
4. Hemophilic arthritis

D. DEGENERATIVE JOINT DISEASE = Osteoarthritis

E. TRAUMATIC
1. Secondary osteoarthritis
2. Neurotrophic arthritis
3. Pigmented villonodular synovitis

F. ENTEROPATHIC ARTHROPATHY
- (a) INFLAMMATORY BOWEL DISEASE
  1. Ulcerative colitis (in 10–20%)
  2. Crohn disease (in 5%): peripheral arthritis increases with colonic disease
  3. Whipple disease (in 60–90% transient intermittent polyarthritis: sacroiliitis, spondylitis)

  ◊ Resection of diseased bowel is associated with regression of arthritic symptomatology!
- (b) INFECTIOUS BOWEL DISEASE

  Infectious agents: Salmonella, Shigella, Yersinia
- (c) after intestinal bypass surgery

SPONDYLARTHRITIS + positive HLA-B 27 HISTOCOMPATIBILITY COMPLEX
1. Ankylosing spondylitis 95%
2. Reiter disease 80%
3. Arthropathy of inflammatory bowel disease 75%
4. Psoriatic spondylitis 70%
5. Normal population 10%

Synovial disease with decreased signal intensity

= hemosiderin deposition
1. Pigmented villonodular synovitis
2. Rheumatoid arthritis
3. Hemophilia

Chondrocalcinosis

mnemonic: "WHIP A DOG"
- **W**ilson disease
- **H**emochromatosis, **H**emophilia, **H**ypothyroidism, 1° **H**yperparathyroidism (15%), **H**ypophosphatasia, Familial **H**ypomagnesemia
- **I**diopathic (aging)
- **P**seudogout (CPPD)
- **A**rthritis (rheumatoid, postinfectious, traumatic, degenerative), **A**myloidosis, **A**cromegaly
- **D**iabetes mellitus
- **O**chronosis
- **G**out

mnemonic: "3 C's"

Crystals	CPPD, sodium urate (gout)
Cations	calcium (any cause of hypercalcemia), copper, iron
Cartilage degeneration	osteoarthritis, acromegaly, ochronosis

Subchondral cyst
= SYNOVIAL CYST = SUBARTICULAR PSEUDOCYST = NECROTIC PSEUDOCYST = GEODES

Etiology: bone necrosis allows pressure-induced intrusion of synovial fluid into subchondral bone; in conditions with synovial inflammation

Cause: (1) Osteoarthritis (2) Rheumatoid arthritis (3) Osteonecrosis (4) CPPD

√ size of cyst usually 2–35 mm
√ may be large + expansile (especially in CPPD)

DDx: (1) Giant cell tumor
(2) Pigmented villonodular synovitis
(3) Metastasis
(4) Intraosseous ganglion
(5) Hemophilia

Loose intraarticular bodies
1. Osteochondrosis dissecans
2. Synovial osteochondromatosis
3. Chip fracture from trauma
4. Severe degenerative joint disease
5. Neuropathic arthropathy

Premature osteoarthritis
mnemonic: "COME CHAT"
Calcium pyrophosphate dihydrate arthropathy
Ochronosis
Marfan syndrome
Epiphyseal dysplasia
Charcot joint = neuroarthropathy
Hemophilic arthropathy
Acromegaly
Trauma

Arthritis with periostitis
1. Juvenile rheumatoid arthritis
2. Psoriatic arthritis
3. Reiter syndrome
4. Infectious arthritis

Arthritis with demineralization
mnemonic: "HORSE"
Hemophilia
Osteomyelitis
Rheumatoid arthritis, **R**eiter disease
Scleroderma
Erythematosus, systemic lupus

Arthritis without demineralization
1. Gout
2. Neuropathic arthropathy
3. Psoriasis
4. Reiter disease
5. Pigmented villonodular synovitis

mnemonic: "PONGS"
Psoriatic arthritis
Osteoarthritis
Neuropathic joint
Gout
Sarcoidosis

Articular disorders of the hand + wrist
1. Osteoarthritis = degenerative joint disease
   = abnormal stress with minor + major traumatic episodes
   Target areas: DIP, PIP, 1st CMC, trapezioscaphoid
   √ sclerosis + osteophytes
2. Erosive osteoarthritis = inflammatory osteoarthritis
   Age: predominantly middle-aged / postmenopausal women
   • acute inflammatory episodes
   Target areas: DIP, PIP, 1st CMC, trapezioscaphoid
   √ subchondral "gull wing" erosions
   √ rare ankylosis
3. Psoriatic arthritis
   = rheumatoid variant / seronegative spondyloarthropathy; peripheral manifestation in monarthritis / asymmetric oligoarthritis / symmetric polyarthritis
   Target areas: all hand + wrist joints (commonly distal)
   √ "mouse ears" marginal erosions
   √ new bone formation
4. Rheumatoid arthritis
   = synovial proliferative granulation tissue = pannus
   Target areas: PIP, MCP, all wrist joints, ulnar styloid
   √ marginal poorly defined erosions
   √ joint deformities
5. Gouty arthritis
   • monosodium urate crystals in synovial fluid
   • asymptomatic periods from months to years
   Target areas: commonly CMC + all hand joints
   √ development of chronic tophaceous gout
   √ well-defined erosions with overhanging edge (often periarticular)
   √ joint space narrowing
6. Calcium pyrophosphate dihydrate crystal deposition disease = CPPD
   Target areas: MCP, radiocarpal
   √ chondrocalcinosis
   √ "degenerative changes" in unusual locations
   √ no erosions
7. SLE
   = myositis, symmetric polyarthritis, deforming nonerosive arthropathy, osteonecrosis
   Target areas: PIP, MCP
   √ reversible deformities
8. Scleroderma = progressive systemic sclerosis (PSS)
   Target areas: DIP, PIP, 1st CMC
   √ tuft resorption
   √ soft-tissue calcifications

Arthritis involving distal interphalangeal joints
mnemonic: "POEM"
Psoriatic arthritis
Osteoarthritis
Erosive osteoarthritis
Multicentric reticulohistiocytosis

Ankylosis of interphalangeal joints

mnemonic: "S - Lesions"

1. P**s**oriatic arthritis
2. Ankylo**s**ing spondylitis
3. Ero**s**ive osteoarthritis
4. **S**till disease

Sacroiliitis

Anatomy:

only anterior inferior aspect of sacroiliac apposition is covered with cartilage (1 mm thick hyalin cartilage on iliac side, 3–5 mm thick fibrous cartilage on sacral side); 2–5 mm normal joint width

Positioning: Ferguson view = AP projection with 23° angulation toward head

A. BILATERAL SYMMETRICAL
   1. Ankylosing spondylitis
      √ small regular erosion = loss of definition of white cortical line on iliac side
      √ ankylosis
      √ ossification of intraosseous ligaments
   2. Rheumatoid arthritis (in late stages)
      √ joint space narrowing without reparation
      √ osteoporosis
      √ ankylosis may occur
   3. Deposition arthropathy: gout, CPPD, ochronosis, acromegaly
      √ slow loss of cartilage
      √ subchondral reparative bone + osteophytes
   4. Enteropathic arthropathy:
B. BILATERAL ASYMMETRICAL
   1. Psoriatic arthritis
      √ large + extensive erosive + reparative process
      √ occasional ankylosis
   2. Reiter syndrome
   3. Juvenile rheumatoid arthritis
C. UNILATERAL
   1. Infection
   2. Osteoarthritis from abnormal mechanical stress
      √ irregular narrowing of joint space with subchondral bone repair
      √ osteophytes at anterosuperior / -inferior aspect of joint (may resemble ankylosis)

DDx: Hyperparathyroidism
   √ subchondral bone resorption on iliac side resembling erosion + widening of joint

Sacroiliac joint widening

mnemonic: "CRAP TRAP"

Colitis
Rheumatoid arthritis
Abscess (infection)
Parathyroid disease
Trauma
Reiter syndrome
Ankylosing spondylitis
Psoriasis

Sacroiliac joint fusion

mnemonic: "CARPI"

Colitic spondylitis
Ankylosing spondylitis
Reiter syndrome
Psoriatic arthritis
Infection (TB)

Widened symphysis pubis

mnemonic: "EPOCH"

Exstrophy of the bladder
Prune belly syndrome
Osteogenesis imperfecta
Cleidocranial dysostosis
Hypothyroidism

Arthritis of interphalangeal joint of great toe

1. Psoriatic arthritis
2. Reiter disease
3. Gout
4. Degenerative joint disease

Enthesopathy

Enthesis = osseous attachment of tendon composed of 4 zones, ie, tendon itself + unmineralized fibrocartilage + mineralized fibrocartilage + bone

Cause:

1. Degenerative disorder
2. Seronegative arthropathies: ankylosing spondylitis, Reiter disease, psoriatic arthritis
3. Diffuse idiopathic skeletal hyperostosis
4. Acromegaly
5. Rheumatoid arthritis (occasionally)

Location: at site of tendon + ligament attachment
√ bone proliferation (enthesophyte)
√ calcification of tendon + ligament
√ erosion

EPIPHYSIS

Epiphyseal / apophyseal lesion

1. Chondroblastoma
2. Brodie abscess
3. Fungal / tuberculous infection
4. Langerhans cell histiocytosis
5. Osteoid osteoma
6. Chondromyxoid fibroma
7. Enchondroma
8. Bone cyst
9. Foreign-body granuloma

Stippled epiphyses

1. Normal variant
2. Avascular necrosis
3. Hypothyroidism
4. Chondrodysplasia punctata
5. Multiple epiphyseal dysplasia
6. Spondyloepiphyseal dysplasia
7. Hypoparathyroidism
8. Down syndrome
9. Trisomy 18

10. Fetal warfarin syndrome
11. Homocystinuria (distal radial + ulnar epiphyses = pathognomonic)
12. Zellweger cerebrohepatorenal syndrome

Epiphyseal overgrowth
1. Juvenile rheumatoid arthritis
2. Hemophilia
3. Healed Legg-Perthes disease
4. Tuberculous arthritis
5. Pyogenic arthritis (chronic)
6. Fungal arthritis
7. Epiphyseal dysplasia hemimelica
8. Fibrous dysplasia of epiphysis
9. Winchester syndrome

Ring epiphysis
1. Severe osteoporosis
2. Healing rickets
3. Scurvy

Epiphyseolysis
= SLIPPED EPIPHYSIS (zone of maturing hypertrophic cartilage affected, not zone of proliferation)
1. Idiopathic / juvenile epiphyseolysis
   Age: 12–15 years (? puberty-related hormonal dysregulation)
   • adiposogenital type; tall stature
2. Renal osteodystrophy
3. Hyperparathyroidism in chronic renal disease
4. Hypothyroidism
5. Radiotherapy

TRAUMA

Childhood fractures
1. Greenstick fracture
   = incomplete fracture of soft growing bone with intact periosteum
2. Bowing fracture
3. Traumatic epiphyseolysis
4. Battered child syndrome
5. Epiphyseal plate injury

Pseudarthrosis in long bones
1. Nonunion of fracture
2. Fibrous dysplasia
3. Neurofibromatosis
4. Osteogenesis imperfecta
5. Congenital: clavicular pseudarthrosis

Exuberant callus formation
1. Steroid therapy / Cushing syndrome
2. Neuropathic arthropathy
3. Osteogenesis imperfecta
4. Congenital insensitivity to pain
5. Paralysis
6. Renal osteodystrophy
7. Multiple myeloma
8. Battered child syndrome

RIBS

Rib lesions
A. BENIGN RIB TUMOR
1. Fibrous dysplasia (most common benign lesion)
   √ predominantly posterior location
2. Eosinophilic granuloma
3. Benign cortical defect
4. Hemangioma of bone
5. Enchondroma: at costochondral / costovertebral junction
6. Osteochondroma: at costochondral / costovertebral junction
7. Giant cell tumor
8. Aneurysmal bone cyst

B. PRIMARY MALIGNANT RIB TUMOR
1. Chondrosarcoma (calcified matrix)
2. Osteosarcoma (rare)
3. Fibrosarcoma

C. SECONDARY MALIGNANT RIB TUMOR
— in adult:
1. Metastasis (most common malignant lesion)
2. Multiple myeloma
3. Desmoid tumor

— in child:
1. Ewing sarcoma
2. Metastatic neuroblastoma

D. TRAUMATIC RIB DISORDER
1. Healing fracture
   (a) cough fractures: 4–9th rib in anterior axillary line
   (b) fatigue fracture: 1st rib (from carrying a heavy back pack)
2. Radiation osteitis

E. Aggressive granulomatous infections
= osteomyelitis

Rib notching on inferior margin
= minimal scalloping to deep ridges along the neurovascular groove
◊ Minor undulations in the inferior ribs are normal!
◊ The medial third of posterior ribs near transverse process of vertebrae may be notched normally!

A. ARTERIAL
Cause: intercostal aa. function as collaterals to descending aorta / lung
(a) Aorta: coarctation, thrombosis
(b) Subclavian artery: Blalock-Taussig shunt
(c) Pulmonary artery: pulmonary stenosis, tetralogy of Fallot, absent pulmonary artery

B. VENOUS
Cause: enlargement of intercostal veins
(a) AV malformation of chest wall
(b) Superior vena cava obstruction

C. NEUROGENIC
1. Intercostal neuroma
2. Neurofibromatosis
3. Poliomyelitis / quadriplegia / paraplegia

D. OSSEOUS
1. Hyperparathyroidism
2. Thalassemia
3. Melnick-Needles syndrome

Rib notching on superior margin
1. Rheumatoid arthritis
2. Scleroderma
3. Systemic lupus erythematosus
4. Hyperparathyroidism
5. Restrictive lung disease
6. Marfan syndrome

Ribbon ribs
1. Osteogenesis imperfecta
2. Neurofibromatosis

Bulbous enlargement of costochondral junction
1. Rachitic rosary
2. Scurvy
3. Achondroplasia

Wide ribs
1. Marrow hyperplasia (anemias)
2. Fibrous dysplasia
3. Paget disease
4. Achondroplasia
5. Mucopolysaccharidoses

Expansile rib lesion
mnemonic: "FEEL THE CLAMP"

Fibrous dysplasia
Eosinophilic granuloma
Enchondroma
Lymphoma
Tuberculosis
Hematopoiesis
Ewing sarcoma
Chondromyxoid fibroma
Leukemia
Aneurysmal bone cyst
Metastases
Plasmacytoma

Short ribs
1. Achondroplasia
2. Achondrogenesis
3. Thanatophoric dysplasia
4. Asphyxiating thoracic dysplasia
5. Mesomelic dwarfism
6. Short rib-polydactyly syndrome
7. Spondyloepiphyseal dysplasia
8. Enchondromatosis
9. Chondroectodermal dysplasia (Ellis-van Creveld)

Dense ribs
1. Osteopetrosis
2. Mastocytosis
3. Fluorosis

Hyperlucent ribs
1. Osteopetrosis
2. Cushing disease
3. Acromegaly
4. Scurvy

CLAVICLE

Absence of outer end of clavicle
1. Rheumatoid arthritis
2. Hyperparathyroidism
3. Posttraumatic osteolysis
4. Metastasis / multiple myeloma
5. Cleidocranial dysplasia

Penciled distal end of clavicle
mnemonic: "SHIRT Pocket"

Scleroderma
Hyperparathyroidism
Infection
Rheumatoid arthritis
Trauma
Progeria

Destruction of medial end of clavicle
mnemonic: "MILERS"

Metastases
Infection
Lymphoma
Eosinophilic granuloma
Rheumatoid arthritis
Sarcoma

WRIST & HAND

Carpal angle
= angle of 130° formed by tangents to proximal row of carpal bones

A. DECREASED CARPAL ANGLE (<124°)
   1. Turner syndrome
   2. Hurler syndrome
   3. Morquio syndrome
   4. Madelung deformity

B. INCREASED CARPAL ANGLE (>139°)
   1. Down syndrome
   2. Arthrogryposis
   3. Bone dysplasia with epiphyseal involvement

Metacarpal sign
= tangent between 4th + 5th metacarpals intersects 3rd metacarpal = shortening of 4th metacarpal
1. Idiopathic
2. Gonadal dysgenesis: Turner syndrome, Klinefelter syndrome
3. Pseudo- and pseudopseudohypoparathyroidism
4. Ectodermal dysplasia = Cornelia de Lange syndrome
5. Hereditary multiple exostoses
6. Peripheral dysostosis
7. Basal cell nevus syndrome
8. Melorheostosis

mnemonic: "**P**ing **P**ong **I**s **T**ough **T**o **T**each"
Pseudohypoparathyroidism
Pseudopseudohypoparathyroidism
Idiopathic
Trauma
Turner syndrome
Trisomy 13–18

Lucent lesion in finger

A. BENIGN TUMOR
1. Giant cell tumor
2. Aneurysmal bone cyst
3. Brown tumor
4. Hemophilic pseudotumor
5. Epidermoid inclusion cyst
6. Glomus tumor
7. Solitary bone cyst
8. Osteoblastoma
9. Enchondroma

B. MALIGNANT TUMOR
1. Osteosarcoma
2. Fibrosarcoma
3. Metastasis from lung, breast, malignant melanoma

mnemonic: "GAMES PAGES"
Glomus tumor
Arthritis (gout, rheumatoid)
Metastasis (lung, breast)
Enchondroma
Simple cyst (inclusion)
Pancreatitis
Aneurysmal bone cyst
Giant cell tumor
Epidermoid
Sarcoid

Resorption of terminal tufts

A. TRAUMA
1. Amputation
2. Burns, electric injury
3. Frostbite
4. Vinyl chloride poisoning

B. NEUROPATHIC
1. Congenital indifference to pain
2. Syringomyelia
3. Myelomeningocele
4. Diabetes mellitus
5. Leprosy

C. COLLAGEN-VASCULAR DISEASE
1. Scleroderma
2. Dermatomyositis
3. Raynaud disease

D. METABOLIC
1. Hyperparathyroidism

E. INHERITED
1. Familial acroosteolysis
2. Pyknodysostosis
3. Progeria = Werner syndrome
4. Pachydermoperiostosis

F. OTHERS
1. Sarcoidosis
2. Psoriatic arthropathy
3. Epidermolysis bullosa

Acroosteolysis

1. Acroosteolysis: (a) acquired, (b) familial
2. Massive osteolysis
3. Essential osteolysis
4. Ainhum disease

Acquired acroosteolysis

mnemonic: "PETER's DIAPER SPLASH"
Psoriasis, **P**orphyria
Ehlers-Danlos syndrome
Thrombangitis obliterans
Ergot therapy
Raynaud disease
Diabetes, **D**ermatomyositis, **D**ilantin therapy
Injury (thermal + electrical burns, frostbite)
Arteriosclerosis obliterans
PVC (polyvinylchloride) worker
Epidermolysis bullosa
Rheumatoid arthritis, **R**eiter syndrome
Scleroderma, **S**arcoidosis
Progeria, **P**yknodysostosis
Leprosy, **L**esch-Nyhan syndrome
Absence of pain
Syringomyelia
Hyperparathyroidism
also in: yaws; Kaposi sarcoma; pachydermoperiostosis

√ lytic destructive process involving distal + middle phalanges
√ NO periosteal reaction
√ epiphyses resist osteolysis until late

Acroosteosclerosis

= focal opaque areas + endosteal thickening
1. Incidental in middle-aged women
2. Rheumatoid arthritis
3. Sarcoidosis
4. Scleroderma
5. Systemic lupus erythematosus
6. Hodgkin disease
7. Hematologic disorders

Fingertip calcifications

1. Scleroderma / CREST syndrome
2. Raynaud disease
3. Systemic lupus erythematosus
4. Dermatomyositis
5. Calcinosis circumscripta universalis
6. Hyperparathyroidism

Syndactyly

= osseous ± cutaneous fusion of digits
1. Apert syndrome
2. Carpenter syndrome
3. Down syndrome

4. Neurofibromatosis
5. Poland syndrome
6. Others

Polydactyly

Frequently associated with:
1. Carpenter syndrome
2. Ellis-van Creveld syndrome
3. Meckel-Gruber syndrome
4. Polysyndactyly syndrome
5. Short rib-polydactyly syndrome
6. Trisomy 13

Clinodactyly

= curvature of finger in mediolateral plane
1. Normal variant
2. Down syndrome
3. Multiple dysplasia
4. Trauma, arthritis, contractures

Brachydactyly

= shortening / broadening of metacarpals ± phalanges
1. Idiopathic
2. Trauma
3. Osteomyelitis
4. Arthritis
5. Turner syndrome
6. Osteochondrodysplasia
7. Pseudohypoparathyroidism, Pseudopseudohypoparathyroidism
8. Mucopolysaccharidoses
9. Cornelia de Lange syndrome
10. Basal cell nevus syndrome
11. Hereditary multiple exostoses

HIP

Snapping hip syndrome

A. INTRAARTICULAR
   1. Osteocartilaginous bodies
B. EXTRA-ARTICULAR = tendon slippage
   1. fascia lata / gluteus maximus over greater trochanter
   2. iliopsoas tendon over iliopectineal eminence
   3. long head of biceps femoris over ischial tuberosity
   4. iliofemoral ligament over anterior portion of hip capsule

Protrusio acetabuli

= acetabular floor bulging into pelvis
√ acetabular line projecting medially to ilioischial line by >3 mm (in males) / >6 mm (in females)
√ crossing of medial + lateral components of pelvic "teardrop" (U-shaped radiodense area medial to hip joint with (a) lateral aspect = acetabular articular surface (b) medial aspect = anteroinferior margin of quadrilateral surface of ilium)

A. UNILATERAL
   1. Tuberculous arthritis
   2. Trauma
   3. Fibrous dysplasia
B. BILATERAL
   1. Rheumatoid arthritis
   2. Paget disease
   3. Osteomalacia

mnemonic: "PROT"
Paget disease
Rheumatoid arthritis
Osteomalacia (HPT)
Trauma

Pain with hip prosthesis

Approximately 120,000 hip arthroplasties per year in USA

1. Heterotopic ossification
2. Trochanteric bursitis
3. Prosthetic fracture / periprosthetic fracture / cement fracture
4. Dislocation
5. Loosening (10–30% after 10 years)
   (a) aseptic loosening (most common)
      Cause: mechanical wear + tear
   (b) septic loosening (1–9%)
      Organism: Staphylococcus epidermidis (50%), Staphylococcus aureus, Peptostreptococcus

Plain film:
√ subsidence of prosthesis
√ area of lucency >2 mm at bone-cement interface
√ focal lytic area (due to foreign body granuloma / abscess)
√ rapid bone resorption (due to particulate debris / infection)
√ extensive periostitis (in infection, but rare)

NUC (83% sensitive, 88% specific):
√ increased uptake of bone agent, gallium-67, indium-111–labeled leukocytes, complementary technetium-labeled sulfur colloid + combinations

Arthrography:
√ irregularity of joint pseudocapsule
√ filling of nonbursal spaces / sinus tracts / abscess cavities

Aspiration of fluid under fluoroscopy (12–93% sensitive, 83–92% specific for infection):
√ injection of contrast material to confirm intraarticular location

Evaluation of total hip arthroplasty

Measurements

Reference line: transischial tuberosity line (R)
1. Leg length = vertical position of acetabular component
   = comparing level of greater / lesser tuberosity (T) with respect to line R

High placement: shorter leg, less effective muscles crossing the hip joint
Low placement: longer leg, muscles stretched to point of spasm with risk of dislocation

2. Vertical center of rotation
   = distance from center of femoral head (C) to line R
3. Horizontal center of rotation
   = distance from center of femoral head (C) to teardrop / other medial landmark
   Lateral position: iliopsoas tendon crosses medial to femoral head center of rotation increasing risk of dislocation
4. Lateral acetabular inclination = horizontal version
   = angle of cup in reference to line R (40° ± 10° desirable)
   Less angulation: stable hip, limited abduction
   Greater angulation: risk of hip dislocation
5. Varus / neutral / valgus stem position
   Varus position: tip of stem rests against medial endosteum, increased risk for loosening
   Valgus position: tip of stem rests against lateral endosteum, not a significant problem
6. Acetabular anteversion (15° ± 10° desirable)
   = lateral radiograph of groin
   Retroversion: risk of hip dislocation
7. Femoral neck anteversion
   works synergistically with acetabular anteversion, true angle assessed by CT

Radiographic findings

A. NORMAL
   √ irregular cement-bone interface
      = normal interdigitation of polymethylmethacrylate (PMMA) with adjacent bone remodeling providing a mechanical interlock
      ◊ PMMA is not a glue!
   √ thin lucent line along cement-bone interface
      = 0.1–1.5 mm thin connective tissue membrane ("demarcation") along cement-bone interface accompanied by thin line of bone sclerosis
B. ABNORMAL
   √ wide lucent zone at cement-bone interface
      = ≥2 mm lucent line along bone-cement interface due to granulomatous membrane
      Cause: component loosening ± reaction to particulate debris (eg, PMMA, polyethylene)
   √ lucent zone at metal-cement interface along proximal lateral aspect of femoral stem
      = suboptimal metal-cement contact at time of surgery / loosening
   √ well-defined area of bone destruction (= histiocytic response, aggressive granulomatous disease)
      Cause: granulomatous reaction as response to particulate debris / infection / tumor
   √ asymmetric positioning of femoral head within acetabular component
      Cause: acetabular wear / dislocation of femoral head / acetabular disruption / liner displacement / deformity
   √ cement fracture
      Cause: loosening

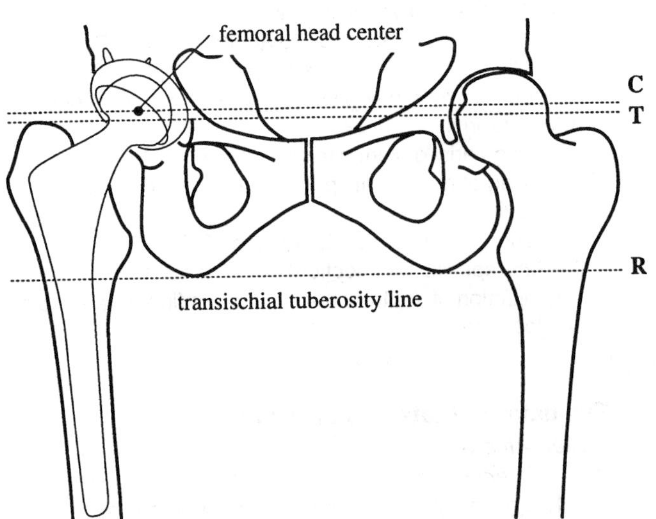

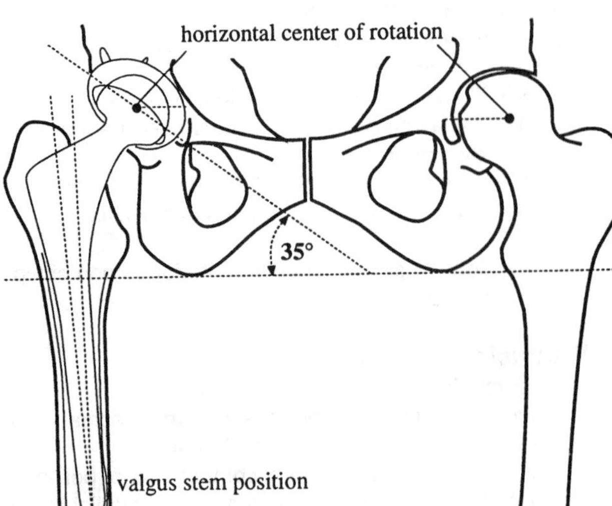

Initial Evaluation Of Total Hip Arthroplasty

Tibiotalar slanting

= downward slanting of medial tibial plafond

1. Hemophilia
2. Still disease
3. Sickle cell disease
4. Epiphyseal dysplasia
5. Trauma

FOOT

Abnormal foot positions

A. FOREFOOT
   1. Varus = adduction
      = axis of 1st metatarsal deviated medially relative to axis of talus
   2. Valgus = abduction
      = axis of 1st metatarsal deviated laterally relative to axis of talus
   3. Inversion = supination
      = inward turning of sole of foot
   4. Eversion = pronation
      = outward turning of sole of foot

B. HINDFOOT
   talipes (talus, pes) = any deformity of the ankle and hindfoot
   1. Equinus
      = hindfoot abnormality with reversal of calcaneal pitch so that the heel cannot touch the ground
   2. Calcaneal foot
      = very high calcaneal pitch so that forefoot cannot touch the ground
   3. Pes planus = flatfoot
      = low calcaneal pitch + (usually) heel valgus + forefoot eversion
   4. Pes cavus
      = high calcaneal pitch (fixed high arch)

Clubfoot = talipes equinovarus

Common severe congenital deformity characterized by
- equinus of heel (reversed calcaneal pitch)
- heel varus (talocalcaneal angle of almost zero on AP view with both bones parallel to each other)
- metatarsus adductus (axis of 1st metatarsal deviated medially relative to axis of talus)

1. Arthrogryposis multiplex congenita
2. Chondrodysplasia punctata
3. Neurofibromatosis
4. Spina bifida
5. Myelomeningocele

Rocker-bottom foot = vertical talus

√ vertically oriented talus with increased talocalcaneal angle on lateral view
√ dorsal navicular dislocation at talonavicular joint
√ heel equinus
√ rigid deformity

Associated with: Arthrogryposis multiplex congenita; spina bifida; trisomy 13–18

Heel pad thickening

= heel pad thickening >25 mm (normal <21 mm)

mnemonic: "MAD COP"

Myxedema
Acromegaly
Dilantin therapy
Callus
Obesity
Peripheral edema

SOFT TISSUES

Histologic classification of soft-tissue lesions

A. FATTY
   1. Lipoma
   2. Angiolipoma
   3. Liposarcoma
B. FIBROUS
   1. Fibroma
   2. Nodular fasciitis
   3. Aggressive fibromatosis / desmoid
   4. Fibrosarcoma
C. MUSCLE
   1. Rhabdomyoma
   2. Leiomyoma
   3. Rhabdomyosarcoma
   4. Leiomyosarcoma
D. VASCULAR
   1. Hemangioma
   2. Hemangiopericytoma
   3. Hemangiosarcoma
E. LYMPH
   1. Lymphangioma
   2. Lymphangiosarcoma
   3. Lymphadenopathy in lymphoma / metastasis
F. SYNOVIAL
   1. Nodular synovitis
   2. Pigmented villonodular synovitis
   3. Synovial sarcoma
G. NEURAL
   1. Neurofibroma
   2. Neurilemoma
   3. Ganglioneuroma
   4. Malignant neuroblastoma
   5. Neurofibrosarcoma
H. CARTILAGE AND BONE
   1. Myositis ossificans
   2. Extraskeletal osteoma
   3. Extraskeletal chondroma
   4. Extraskeletal chondrosarcoma
   5. Extraskeletal osteosarcoma

Fat-containing soft-tissue masses

A. BENIGN LIPOMATOUS TUMORS
   1. Lipoma
   2. Intra- / intermuscular lipoma
   3. Synovial lipoma
   4. Lipoma arborescens = diffuse synovial lipoma
   5. Neural fibrolipoma = fibrolipomatous tumor of nerve
   6. Macrodystrophia lipomatosa

B. LIPOMA VARIANTS
1. Lipoblastoma (exclusively in infancy + early childhood)
2. **Lipomatosis** = diffuse overgrowth of mature adipose tissue infiltrating through the soft tissues of affected extremity / trunk
3. **Hibernoma** = rare benign tumor of brown fat; often in peri- / interscapular region, axilla, thigh, chest wall
√ marked hypervascularity

C. MALIGNANT LIPOMATOUS TUMOR
1. Liposarcoma

D. OTHER FAT-CONTAINING TUMORS
1. Hemangioma
2. Elastofibroma

E. LESIONS MIMICKING FAT-CONTAINING TUMORS
1. Myxoid tumors: intramuscular myxoma, extraskeletal myxoid chondrosarcoma, myxoid malignant fibrous histiocytoma
2. Neural tumors: neurofibroma, neurilemoma, malignant schwannoma
√ 73% have tissue attenuation less than muscle
3. Hemorrhage

Muscle hyperintensity on STIR images

A. INFLAMMATION
1. Polymyositis
2. Dermatomyositis
3. Inclusion body myositis

B. CELLULAR INFILTRATE
1. Lymphoma
2. Bacterial myositis

C. EDEMA

D. RHABDOMYOLYSIS
1. Sport / electric injury
2. Diabetic muscular infarction
3. Focal nodular myositis
4. Metabolic myopathy: eg, phosphofructokinase deficiency, hypokalemia, alcohol overdose
5. Viral myositis

E. TRAUMATIC DENERVATION

Extraskeletal osseous + cartilaginous tumors

A. OSSEOUS SOFT-TISSUE TUMORS
√ cloudlike "cumulus" type of calcification
1. Myositis ossificans
2. Fibrodysplasia ossificans progressiva
3. Soft-tissue osteoma
4. Extraskeletal osteosarcoma
5. Myositis ossificans variants
(a) Panniculitis ossificans
(b) Fasciitis ossificans
(c) Fibro-osseous pseudotumor of digits

B. CARTILAGINOUS SOFT-TISSUE TUMORS
√ arcs and rings, spicules and floccules of calcification
1. Synovial osteochondromatosis
2. Soft-tissue chondroma
3. Extraskeletal chondrosarcoma

DDx:
(1) Synovial sarcoma
(2) Benign mesenchymoma
= lipoma with chondroid / osseous metaplasia
(3) Malignant mesenchymoma
= 2 or more unrelated sarcomatous components
(4) Calcified / ossified tophus of gout
(5) Ossified soft-tissue masses of melorheostosis
(6) **Pilomatricoma** = calcifying epithelioma of Malherbe
• lesion arises from hair matrix cells with slow growth confined to the subcutaneous tissue of the face, neck, upper extremities
√ central sandlike calcifications (84%)
√ peripheral ossification (20%)
(7) Tumoral calcinosis

Soft-tissue calcification

Metastatic calcification

= deposit of calcium salts in previously normal tissue
(1) as a result of elevation of Ca x P product above 60–70
(2) with normal Ca x P product after renal transplant

Location: lung (alveolar septa, bronchial wall, vessel wall), kidney, gastric mucosa, heart, peripheral vessels

Cause:
(a) Skeletal deossification
1. 1° HPT
2. Ectopic HPT production (lung / kidney tumor)
3. Renal osteodystrophy + 2° HPT
4. Hypoparathyroidism

(b) Massive bone destruction
1. Widespread bone metastases
2. Plasma cell myeloma
3. Leukemia

(c) Increased intestinal absorption
1. Hypervitaminosis D
2. Milk-alkali syndrome
3. Excess ingestion / IV administration of calcium salts
4. Prolonged immobilization
5. Sarcoidosis

(d) Idiopathic hypercalcemia

Dystrophic calcification

= in presence of normal serum Ca + P levels secondary to local electrolyte / enzyme alterations in areas of tissue injury

Cause:
(a) Metabolic disorder without hypercalcemia
1. Renal osteodystrophy with 2° HPT
2. Hypoparathyroidism
3. Pseudohypoparathyroidism
4. Pseudopseudohypoparathyroidism
5. Gout
6. Pseudogout = chondrocalcinosis
7. Ochronosis = alkaptonuria
8. Diabetes mellitus

(b) Connective tissue disorder
1. Scleroderma

2. Dermatomyositis
3. Systemic lupus erythematosus

(c) Trauma
1. Neuropathic calcifications
2. Frostbite
3. Myositis ossificans progressiva
4. Calcific tendinitis / bursitis

(d) Infestation
1. Cysticercosis
2. Dracunculosis (guinea worm)
3. Loiasis
4. Bancroft filariasis
5. Hydatid disease
6. Leprosy

(e) Vascular disease
1. Atherosclerosis
2. Media sclerosis (Mönckeberg)
3. Venous calcifications
4. Tissue infarction (eg, myocardial infarction)

(f) Miscellaneous
1. Ehlers-Danlos syndrome
2. Pseudoxanthoma elasticum
3. Werner syndrome = progeria
4. Calcinosis (circumscripta, universalis, tumoral calcinosis)
5. Necrotic tumor

Generalized Calcinosis

(a) Collagen vascular disorders
1. Scleroderma
2. Dermatomyositis

(b) Idiopathic tumoral calcinosis
(c) Idiopathic calcinosis universalis

Interstitial Calcinosis

Calcinosis Circumscripta

1. Acrosclerosis: granular deposits around joints of fingers + toes, fingertips
2. Scleroderma: acrosclerosis + absorption of ends of distal phalanges
3. Dermatomyositis: extensive subcutaneous deposits
4. Varicosities: particularly in calf
5. 1° Hyperparathyroidism: infrequently periarticular calcinosis
6. Renal osteodystrophy with 2° hyperparathyroidism: extensive vascular deposits even in young individuals
7. Hypoparathyroidism: occasionally around joints; symmetrical in basal ganglia
8. Vitamin D intoxication: periarticular in rheumatoid arthritis (puttylike); calcium deposit in tophi

Calcinosis Universalis

Progressive disease of unknown origin

Age: children + young adults

√ plaquelike calcium deposits in skin + subcutaneous tissues; sometimes in tendons + muscles

√ NO true bone formation

Soft-tissue Ossification

= formation of trabecular bone

1. Myositis ossificans progressiva / circumscripta
2. Paraosteoarthropathy
3. Soft-tissue osteosarcoma
4. Parosteal osteosarcoma
5. Posttraumatic periostitis = periosteoma
6. Surgical scar
7. Severely burned patient

Connective Tissue Disease

= CTD = [COLLAGEN VASCULAR DISEASE]

= group of disorders that share a number of clinical + laboratory features

• Features:
(a) relatively specific: arthritis, myositis, Raynaud phenomenon with digital ulceration, tethered skin in extremities + trunk, malar rash sparing nasolabial folds, morning stiffness
(b) relatively nonspecific: polyarthralgias (most common initial symptom), myalgias, mottling of extremities, muscle weakness + tenderness

• Laboratory findings:
(a) relatively specific: ANA in peripheral rim / nucleolar pattern, anti-DNA, elevated muscle enzyme
(b) relatively nonspecific: ANA in homogeneous pattern, anti-single-stranded DNA, positive rheumatoid factor

Types and most distinctive features:

1. Rheumatoid arthritis
positive rheumatoid factor, prominent morning stiffness, symmetric erosive arthritis
2. Systemic lupus erythematosus
malar rash, photosensitivity, serositis, renal disorders with hemolytic anemia, leukopenia, lymphopenia, thrombocytopenia, positive antinuclear antibody (ANA)
3. Sjögren syndrome
dry eyes + mouth, abnormal Schirmer test
4. Scleroderma
Raynaud phenomenon, skin thickening of distal extremities proceeding to include proximal extremities + chest + abdomen, positive ANA in a nucleolar pattern
5. Polymyositis, dermatomyositis
heliotrope rash over eyes, proximal muscle weakness, elevated muscle enzymes, inflammation at muscle biopsy

Mixed Connective Tissue Disease

= disorder that shares distinctive features of ≥2 different connective tissue diseases in same patient (eg, overlapping features of SLE, PSS, polymyositis)

• pulmonary hypertension (due to interstitial pulmonary fibrosis / intimal proliferation of pulmonary arterioles)

FIXATION DEVICES

Internal fixation devices

A. Screws
   1. Cortical screw = threaded over entire length, shallow closely spaced threads, blunt tip
   2. Cancellous screw = wide thread diameter with varying length of smooth shank between head + threads
   3. Malleolar screw = partially threaded
   4. Interference screw = short, fully threaded, cancellous thread pattern, self-tapping tip, recessed head

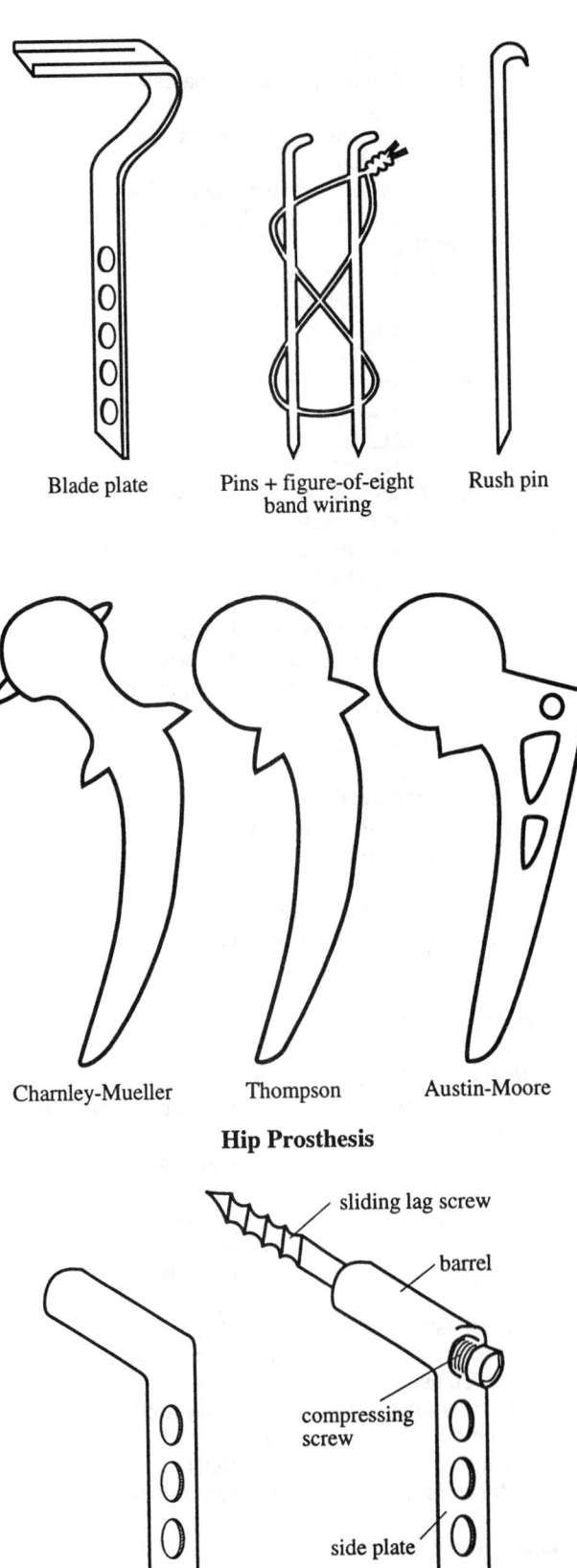

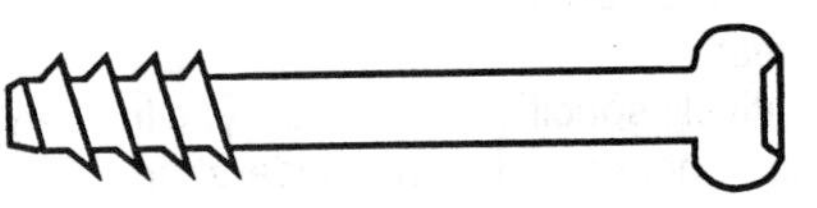
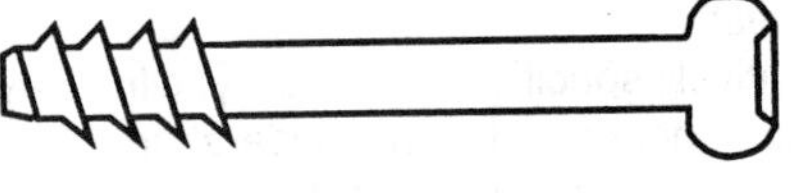
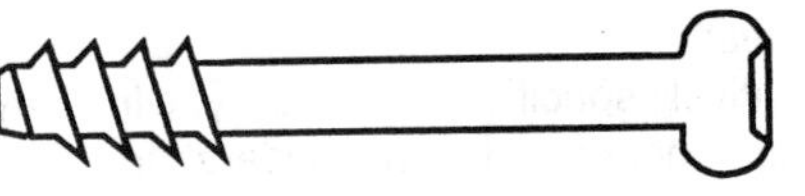
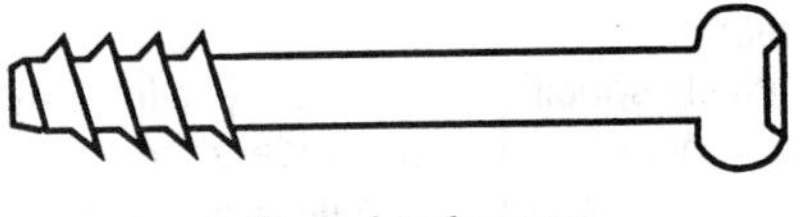

Cannulated screw

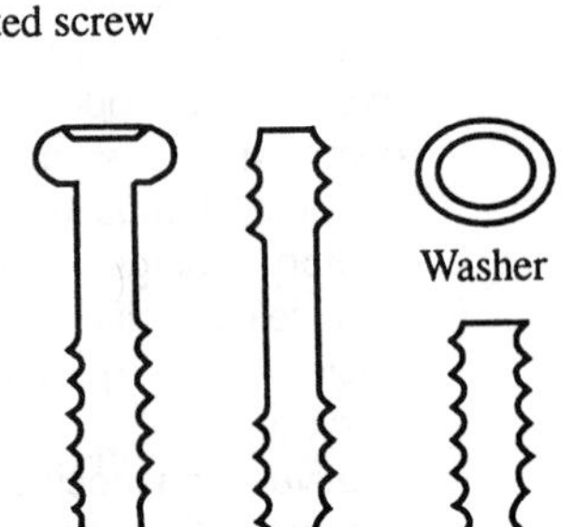

Screws

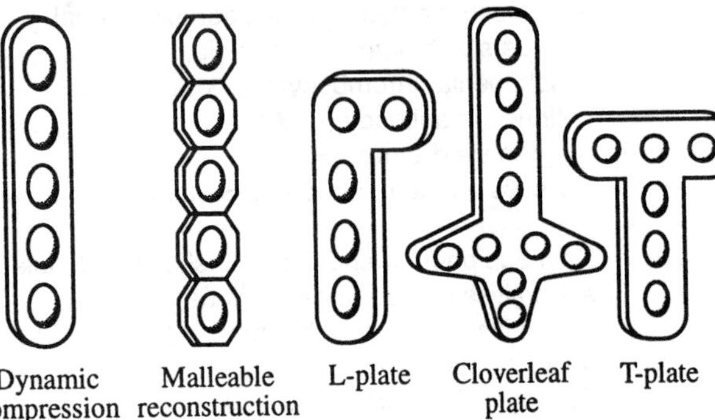

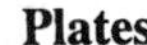

Plates

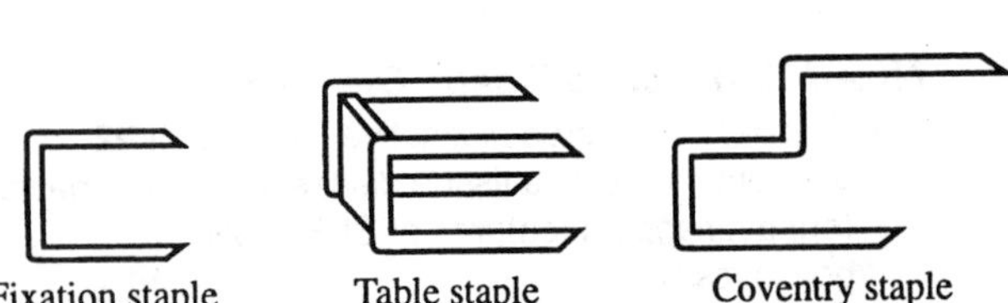

Staples

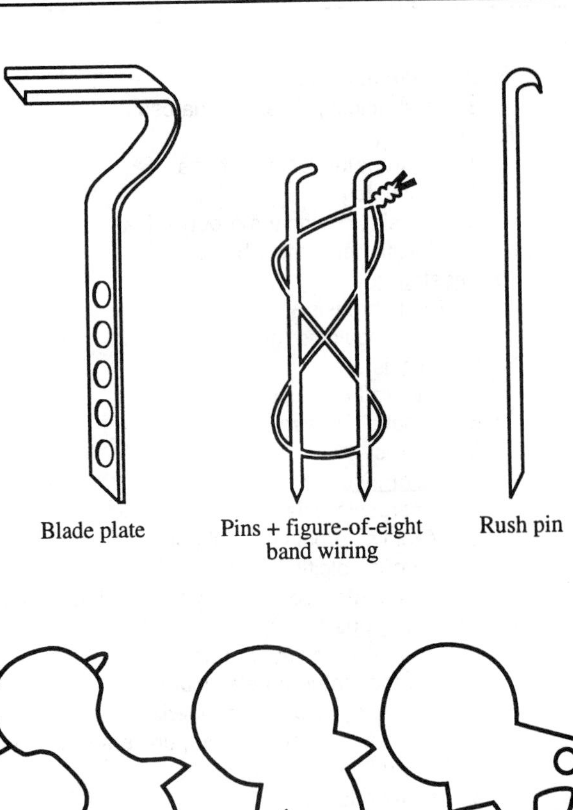

Hip Prosthesis

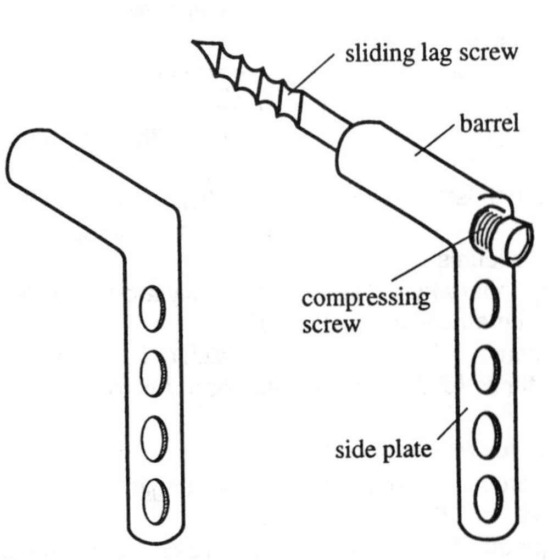

5. Cannulated screw = hollow screw inserted over guide pin
6. Herbert screw = cannulated screw threaded on both ends with different pitches, no screw head

B. Washer
1. Flat washer = increase surface area over which force is distributed
2. Serrated washer = spiked edges used for affixing avulsed ligaments

C. Plates
— Compression plate = used for compression of stable fractures
— Neutralization plate = protects fracture from bending, rotation + axial-loading forces
— Buttress plate = support of unstable fractures in compression / axial loading
1. Straight plate
(a) straight plate with round holes
(b) dynamic compression plate = oval holes
(c) tubular plate = thin pliable plate with concave inner surface
(d) reconstruction plate = thin pliable plate to allow bending, twisting, contouring
2. Special plates
T-shaped, L-shaped, Y-shaped, cloverleaf, spoon, cobra, condylar blade plate, dynamic compression screw system

D. Staples
Fixation = bone = epiphyseal = fracture staples with smooth / barbed surface
— Coventry = stepped osteotomy staple
— stone = table staple

E. Wires
1. K wire = unthreaded segments of extruded wire of variable thickness
2. Cerclage wiring = wire placed around bone
3. Tension band wiring = figure-of-eight wire placed on tension side of bone

External fixation devices

= smooth / threaded pins / wires attached to an external frame
(a) unilateral pin = enters bone only from one side
1. Steinmann pin = large-caliber wire with pointed tip
2. Rush pin = smooth intramedullary pin
3. Schanz screw = pin threaded at one end to engage cortex, smooth at other end to connect to external fixation device
4. Knowles pin (for femoral neck fracture)
(b) transfixing pin = passes through extremity supported by external fixation device on both ends

Intramedullary fixation devices

(a) nail = driven into bone without reaming
(b) rod = solid / hollow device with blunted tip driven into reamed channel
(c) interlocking nail = accessory pins / screws / deployable fins placed to prevent rotation
1. Rush pin = beveled end + hooked end
2. Ender nail = oval in cross section
3. Sampson rod = slightly curved rigid rod with fluted surface
4. Küntscher nail = cloverleaf in cross section with rounded tip

ANATOMY AND METABOLISM OF BONE

BONE MINERALS

Calcium

A. 99% in bone
B. serum calcium
  (a) protein-bound fraction (albumin)
  (b) ionic (pH-dependent) 3% as calcium citrate / phosphate in serum

Absorption: facilitated by vitamin D
Excretion: related to dietary intake; >500 mg/24 hours = hypercalciuria

Phosphorus

Absorption: requires sodium; decreased by aluminum hydroxide gel in gut
Excretion: increased by estrogen, parathormone
decreased by vitamin D, growth hormone, glucocorticoids

HORMONES

Parathormone

Major stimulus: low levels of serum calcium ions (action requires vitamin D presence)
Target organs:
(a) BONE: increase in osteocytic + osteoclastic activity mobilizes calcium + phosphate = bone resorption
(b) KIDNEY: (1) increase in tubular reabsorption of calcium
(2) decrease in tubular reabsorption of phosphate (+ amino acids) = phosphate diuresis
(c) GUT: increased absorption of calcium + phosphorus

Major function:
- increase of serum calcium levels
- increase in serum alkaline phosphatase (50%)

Vitamin D metabolism

required for
(1) adequate calcium absorption from gut
(2) synthesis of calcium-binding protein in intestinal mucosa
(3) parathormone effects (stimulation of osteoclastic + osteocytic resorption of bone)

Biochemistry:
inactive form of vitamin D_3 present through diet / exposure to sunlight; vitamin D_3 is converted into 25-OH-vitamin D_3 by liver and then converted into 1,25-OH vitamin D_3 (= hormone) by kidney
Stimulus for conversion: (1) hypophosphatemia
(2) PTH elevation

Action:
(a) INTESTINE: (1) increased absorption of calcium from bowel
(2) increased absorption of phosphate from distal small bowel
(b) BONE: (1) proper mineralization of osteoid
(2) mobilization of calcium + phosphate (potentiates parathormone action)
(c) KIDNEY: (1) increased absorption of calcium from renal tubule
(2) increased absorption of phosphate from renal tubule

Calcitonin

secreted by parafollicular cells of thyroid
Major stimulus: increase in serum calcium
Target organs:
(a) BONE: (1) inhibits parathormone-induced osteoclasis by reducing number of osteoclasts
(2) enhances deposition of calcium phosphate; responsible for sclerosis in renal osteodystrophy
(b) KIDNEY: inhibits phosphate reabsorption in renal tubule
(c) GUT: increases excretion of sodium + water into gut

Major function: decreases serum calcium + phosphate

PHYSIS

Four distinct zones of cartilage in longitudinal layers
(1) Germinal zone = small cells adjacent to epiphyseal ossification center
(2) Proliferating zone = flattened cells arranged in columns
(3) Hypertrophic zone = swollen vacuolated cells
(4) Zone of provisional calcification

	PTH ACTION	NET EFFECT	
Principal:	(1) phosphate diuresis (2) resorption of Ca + P from bone	(1) Serum:	increase in Ca decrease in P
Secondary:	(3) resorption of Ca from gut (4) reabsorption of Ca from renal tubule	(2) Urine:	increase in Ca increase in P

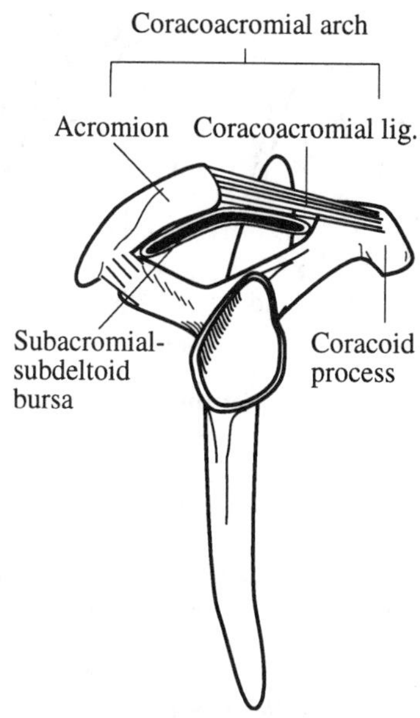

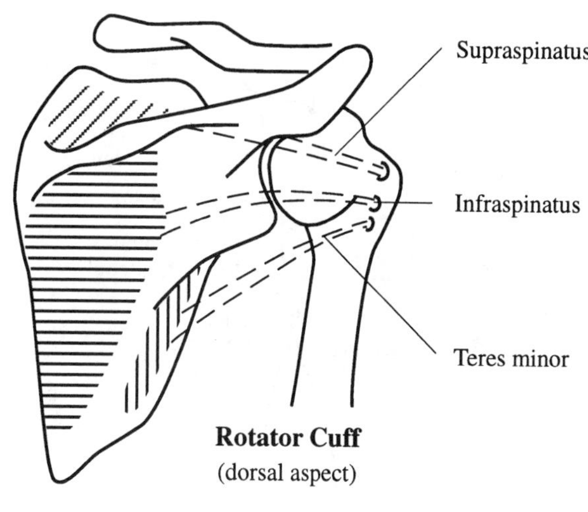

Rotator Cuff
(dorsal aspect)

Rotator cuff muscles

mnemonic: "SITS"

- **S**upraspinatus
- **I**nfraspinatus
- **T**eres minor
- **S**ubscapularis

Muscle Attachments of Shoulder

Name of muscle	*Origin*	*Insertion*
Deltoid	lateral third of clavicle	deltoid tuberosity of humerus
	lateral border of acromion	deltoid tuberosity of humerus
	lower part of spinous process of scapula	deltoid tuberosity of humerus
Subscapularis	medial 2/3 of costal surface of scapula	superior aspect of lesser tubercle of humerus
Pectoralis major		
— clavicular portion	medial half of clavicle	crest of greater tubercle of humerus
— sternocostal portion	manubrium + corpus of sternum	crest of greater tubercle of humerus
— abdominal portion	anterior sheath of rectus abdominis	crest of greater tubercle of humerus
Pectoralis minor	2nd / 3rd–5th ribs	superomedial aspect of coracoid process
Biceps brachii		
– long head	supraglenoid tubercle of scapula	tuberosity of radius
– short head	tip of coracoid process	tuberosity of radius
Coracobrachialis	tip of coracoid process	medial surface of middle third of humerus
Supraspinatus	supraspinatous fossa of scapula	greater tubercle of humerus, highest facet
Infraspinatus	infraspinatous fossa of scapula	greater tubercle of humerus, middle facet
Teres minor	upper 2/3 of lateral border of scapula	greater tubercle of humerus, lower facet
Teres major	dorsum of inferior angle of scapula	inferior crest of lesser tubercle of humerus

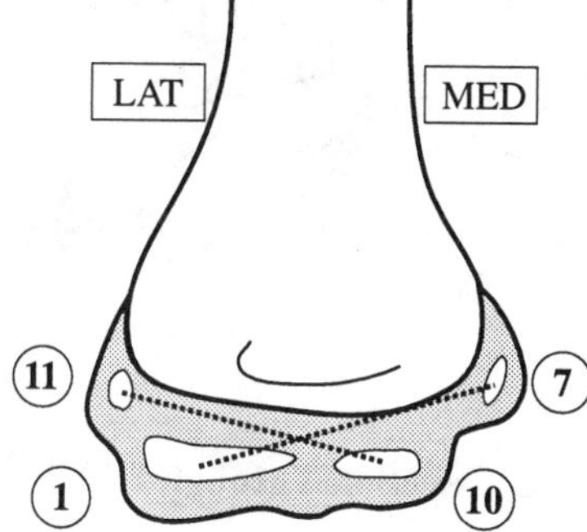

Occurrence of bone centers at elbow

mnemonic: "CRITOE"

Capitellum	1 year	(3–6 months)
Radial head	4 years	(3–6 years)
Internal humeral epicondyle	7 years	(4–6 years, last to fuse)
Trochlea	10 years	(9–10 years)
Olecranon	10 years	(6–10 years)
External humeral epicondyle	11 years	(9–12 years)

mnemonic: "Nelson's X: 1, 7, 10, 11 years"

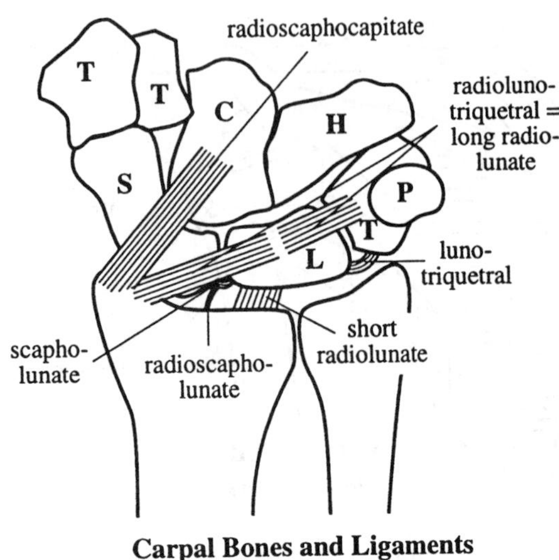

Carpal Bones and Ligaments
(volar aspect)

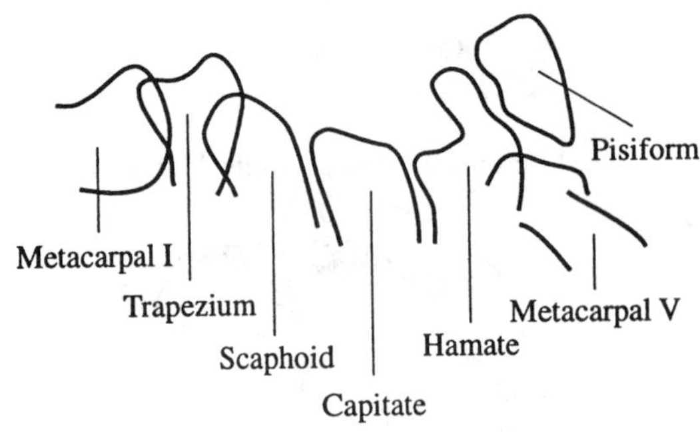

Carpal Tunnel View

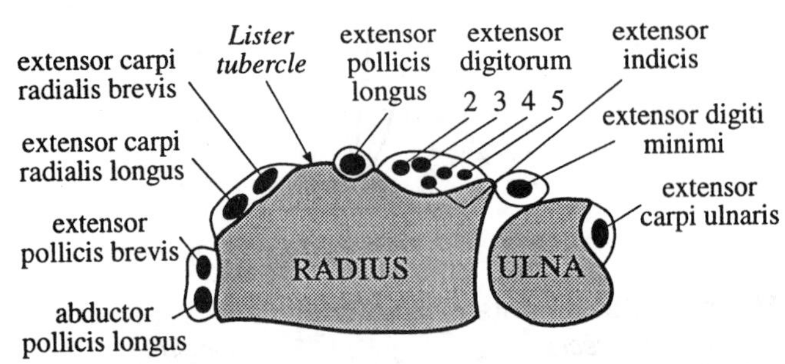

Wrist Cross Section of Distal Radioulnar Joint With the 6 Extensor Compartments

Carpal bones

mnemonic: "**S**ome **L**overs **T**ry **P**ositions **T**hat **T**hey **C**an't **H**andle"

proximal row	distal row
Scaphoid	**T**rapezium
Lunate	**T**rapezoid
Triquetrum	**C**apitate
Pisiform	**H**amate

◊ Remember that trapezium comes before trapezoid in the dictionary as well!

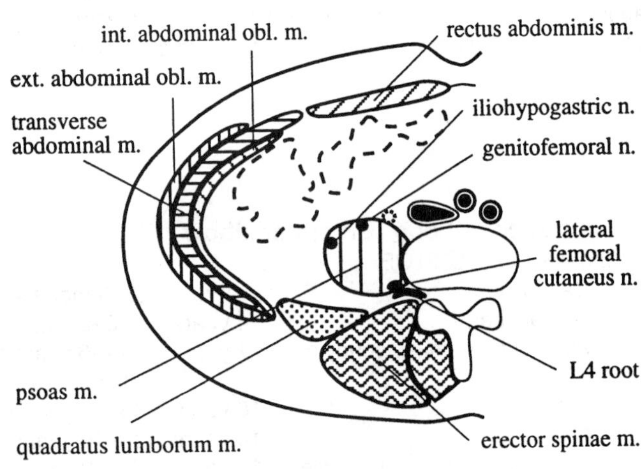

Crossection Through L4-5

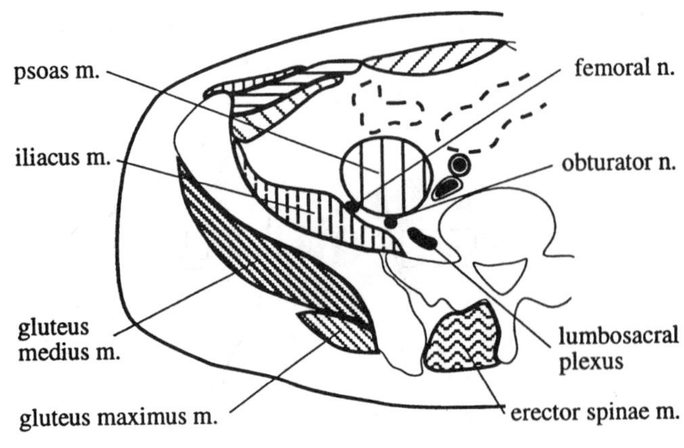

Crossection Through L5-S1

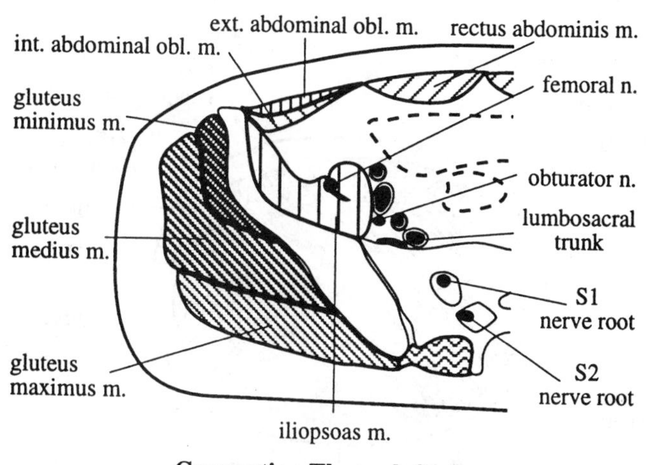

Crossection Through S1-2

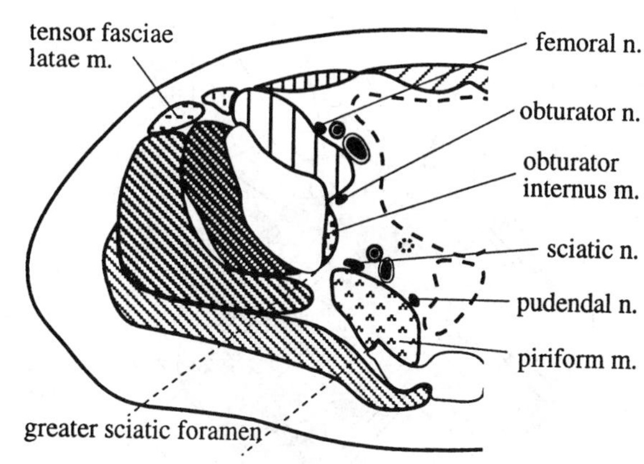

Crossection Through S4

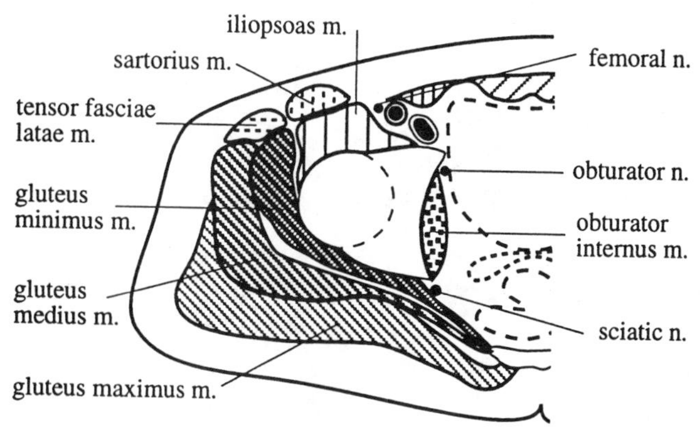

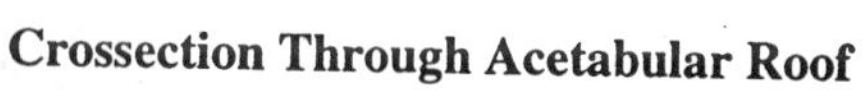

Crossection Through Acetabular Roof

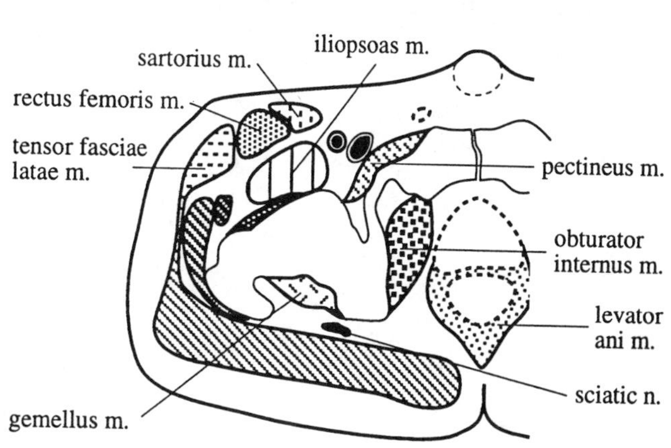

Crossection Through Greater Trochanter

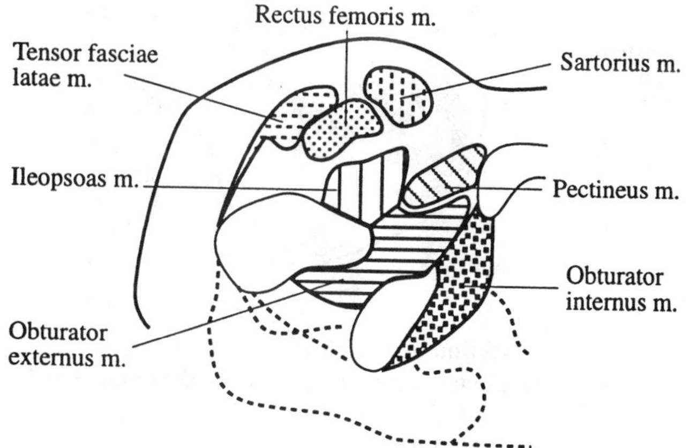

Crossection Through Level of Obturator Foramen

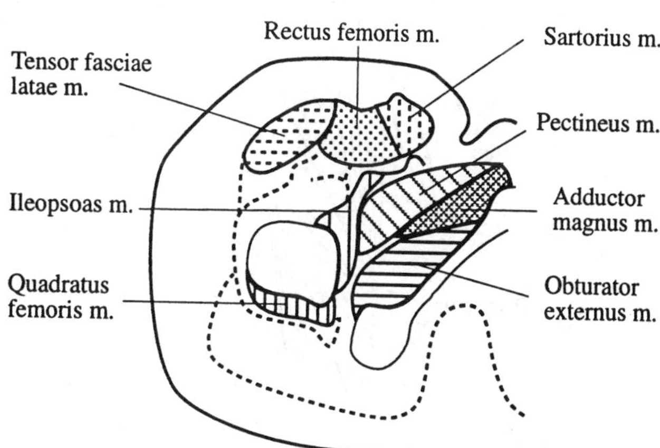

Crossection Through Level of Minor Trochanter

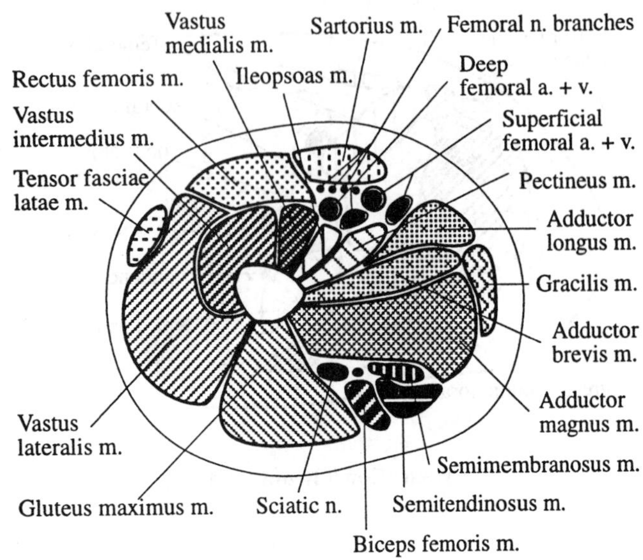

Crossection Through Proximal Thigh

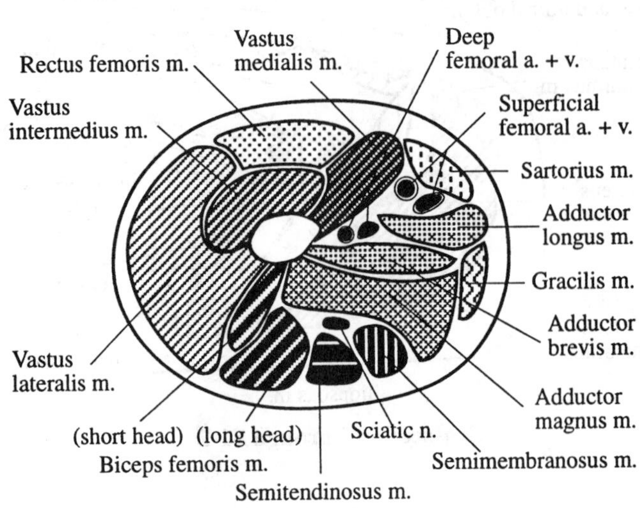

Crossection Through Mid Thigh

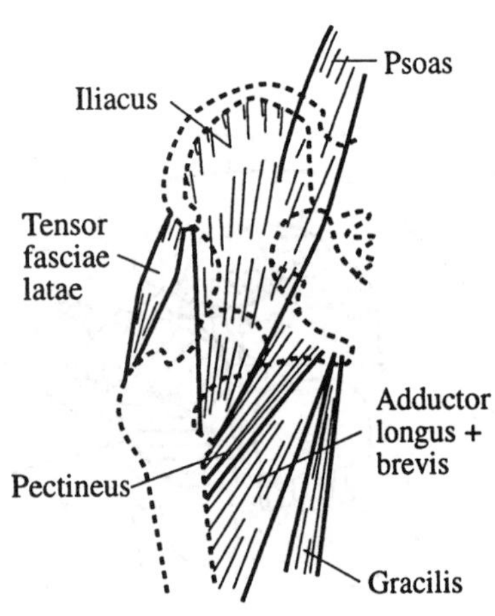

Musculature About the Hip

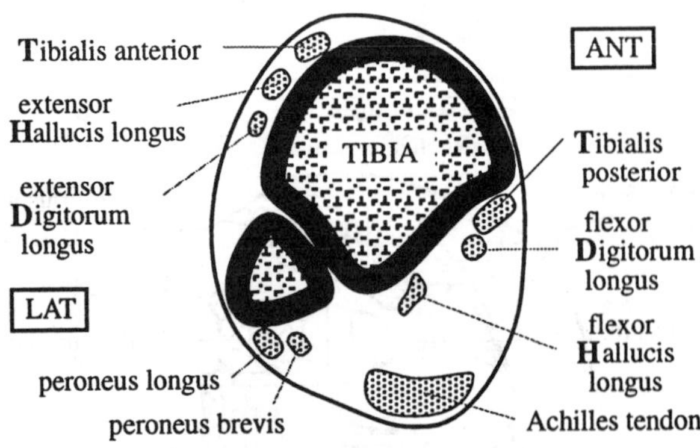

Cross-section Through Distal Right Leg

mnemonic for posterior tendons: "**T**om, **D**ick and **H**arry"

Tibialis posterior
Digitorum longus (flexor)
Hallucis longus (flexor)

Muscle Attachments of Thigh

Name of muscle	*Origin*	*Insertion*
Gracilis	inferior pubic ramus	pes anserinus
Semimembranosus	ischial tuberosity	medial tibial condyle
Semitendinosus	ischial tuberosity	pes anserinus
Biceps femoris		
— long head	ischial tuberosity	fibular head
— short head	lateral linea aspera	fibular head
Adductor		
— longus	superior pubic ramus	medial linea aspera
— magnus	inferior pubic ramus	medial linea aspera
Sartorius	anterior superior iliac spine	pes anserinus
Quadriceps		
— rectus	anterior inferior iliac spine	patellar tendon
— vastus lateralis	greater trochanter	patellar tendon
— vastus medialis	medial intertrochanteric line	patellar tendon
Iliopsoas		
— iliacus	ilium	lesser trochanter
— psoas	lumbar spine	lesser trochanter
Tensor fasciae latae	anterior superior iliac spine	anterolateral tibia

Cruciate ligaments

◊ Both cruciate ligaments are intracapsular but extrasynovial!

A. ANTERIOR CRUCIATE LIGAMENT (ACL)
Origin: inner face of lateral femoral condyle
Insertion: noncartilaginous region of anterior aspect of intercondylar eminence of tibia
Anatomy: several distinct bundles of fibers
(1) posterior bulk = spiraling together at femoral origin
(2) anteromedial bundle diverging at tibial insertion
√ thin solid taut dark band (sagittal MR with knee in extension) almost parallel to intercondylar roof (= Blumensaat line)
√ thin hypointense band parallel to inner aspect of lateral femoral condyle + fanlike configuration toward tibial spine (coronal MR)
√ thin ovoid hypointense band proximally, elliptical configuration distally with higher intensity (axial MR)
√ greater signal intensity than posterior cruciate ligament (due to anatomy)

B. POSTERIOR CRUCIATE LIGAMENT (PCL)
Origin: in a depression posterior to intercondylar region of tibia below joint surface
Insertion: most distal + anterior aspect of inner face of medial femoral condyle
√ thick dark band slightly posteriorly convex (arclike course on sagittal MR with knee in extension)
√ medial to ACL (coronal MR)

Collateral ligaments of knee joint

A. MEDIAL (TIBIAL) COLLATERAL LIGAMENT
Origin: just distal to adductor tubercle of femur
Insertion: anteromedial face of tibiadistal to level of tibial tubercle about 5 cm below joint line
(a) deep portion:
- meniscofemoral ligament
- meniscotibial ligaments

(b) superficial portion
- vertical band from femoral epicondyle to pes anserinus
- posterior oblique ligament = posterior oblique band from femoral epicondyle to semimembranosus tendon

√ deep and superficial dark bands separated by a thin bursa + fatty tissue (on coronal MR)

B. LATERAL (FIBULAR) COLLATERAL LIGAMENT
Origin: lateral aspect of lateral femoral condyle
Insertion: styloid process of fibular head
√ bicipital tendon + iliotibial band join lateral collateral ligament

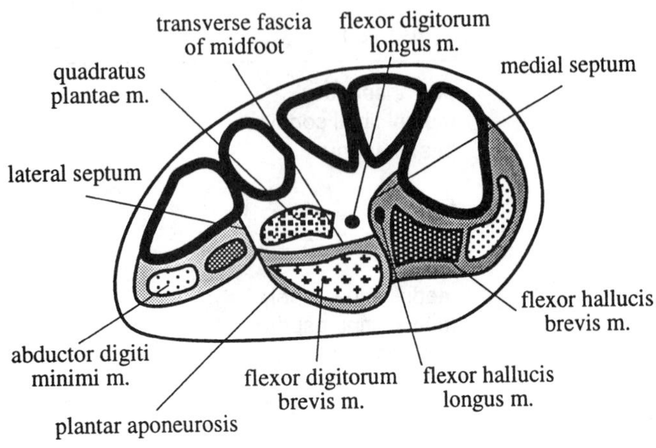

Plantar Compartments of the Midfoot

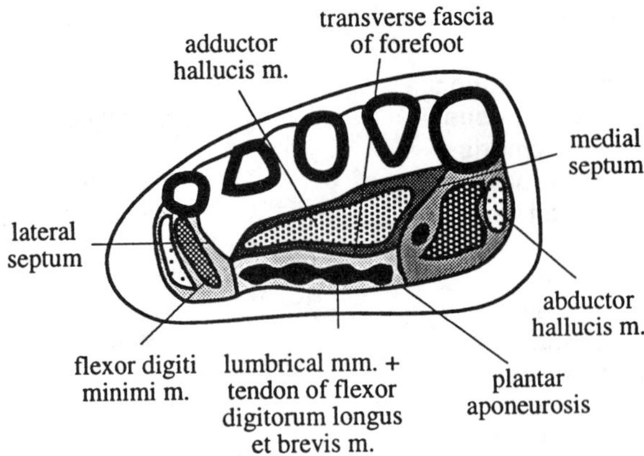

Plantar Compartments of the Forefoot

Medial compartment = bordered by medial septum (extending from plantar aponeurosis to navicular bone, medial cuneiform bone, and lateral border of plantar surface of 1st metatarsal bone);
contains abductor hallucis m. + flexor hallucis brevis m. + flexor hallucis longus tendon

Lateral compartment = bordered by lateral septum (extending from plantar aponeurosis to medial surface of 5th metatarsal bone);
contains abductor m. + short flexor m. + opponens m. of 5th toe

Central compartment = bordered by medial + lateral septa; communicates directly with posterior compartment of calf;
subdivided by horizontal septa: adductor hallucis m. separated from quadratus plantae m.
contains flexor digitorum brevis m. + flexor digitorum longus tendon + quadratus plantae m. + lumbricales mm.. + adductor hallucis m.

Deep subcompartment = bordered by transverse fascia of forefoot; separated from quadratus plantae m.; contains adductor hallucis m.

Accessory Ossicles of the Foot and Ankle

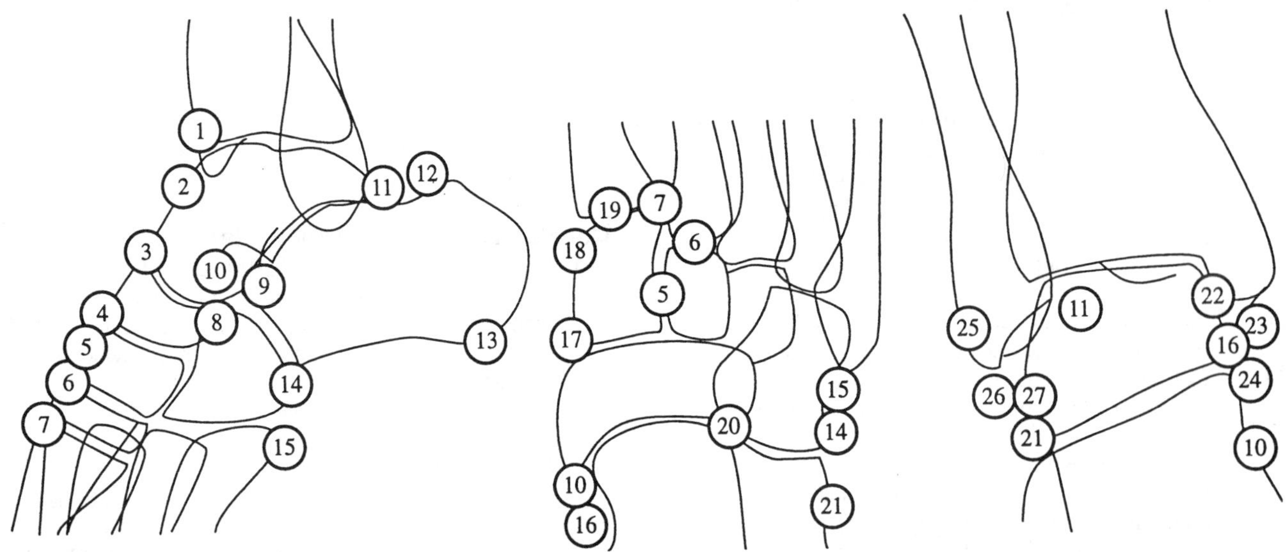

1 Os talotibiale
2 Os supratalare
3 Os supranaviculare
4 Os infranaviculare
5 Os intercuneiforme
6 Os cuneometatarsale II dorsale
7 Os intermetatarsale
8 Secondary cuboid
9 Calcaneus secundarius
10 Os tibiale externum
11 Trigonum
12 Os accessorium supracalcaneum
13 Os subcalcis
14 Os peroneum
15 Os vesalianum
16 Talus accessorius
17 Os cuneonaviculare mediale
18 Sesamum tibiale anterius
19 Os cuneometatarsale I plantare
20 Cuboides secundarium
21 Os trochleare calcanei
22 Sesamoid talus - int. malleolus
23 Os subtibiale
24 Os sustentaculi
25 Os retinaculi
26 Os subfibulare
27 Talus secundarius

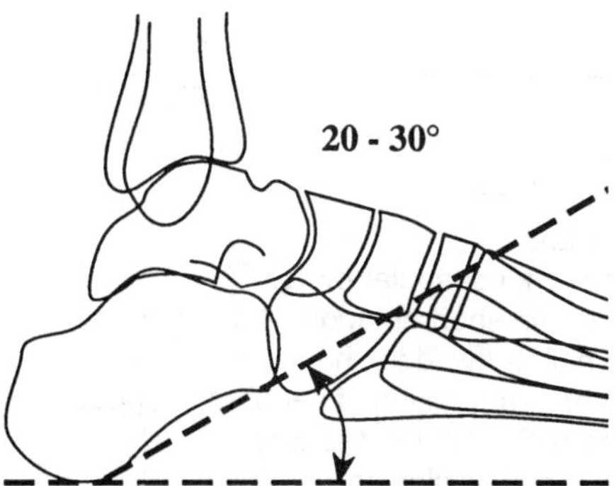

Calcaneal Pitch
= Calcaneal Inclination Angle
= determines longitudinal arch of foot; angle between line drawn along the inferior border of calcaneus connecting the anterior and posterior prominences + line representing the horizontal surface

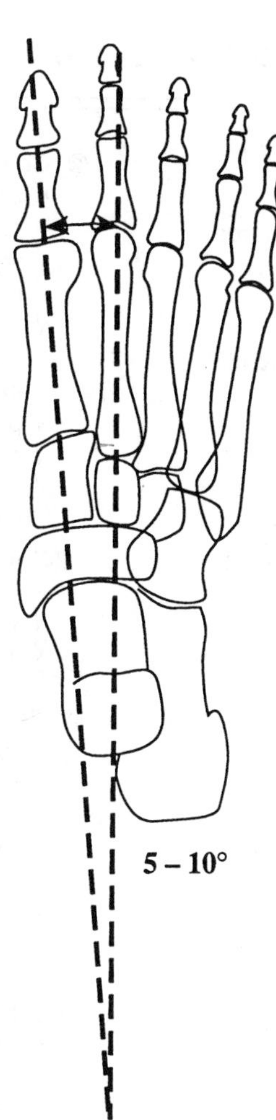

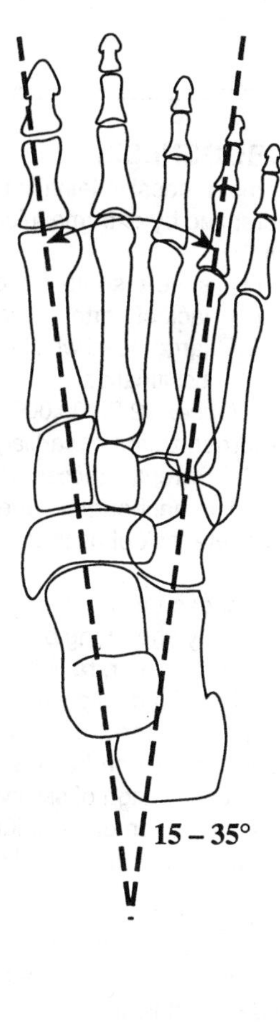

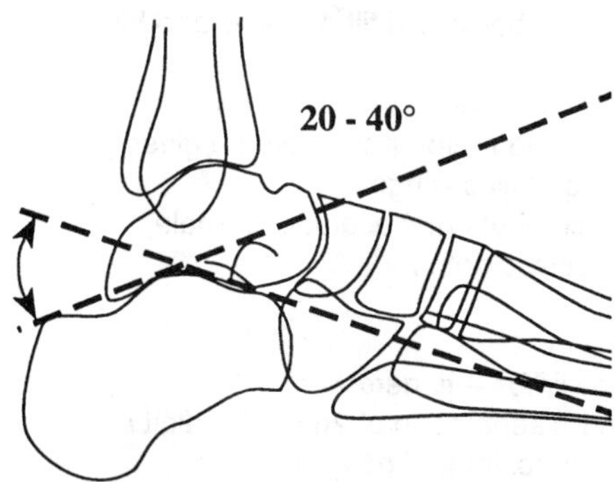

Boehler Angle
= angle between first line drawn from posterosuperior prominence of calcaneus anteriorly to sustentaculum tali + second line drawn from anterosuperior prominence posteriorly to sustentaculum tali; measures integrity of calcaneus

Intermetatarsal Angle
amount that 1st + 2nd metatarsals diverge from each other

Talocalcaneal Angle on AP View
= KITE ANGLE = the midtalar and midcalcaneal lines parallel the 1st + 4th metatarsals; angle is greater in infants

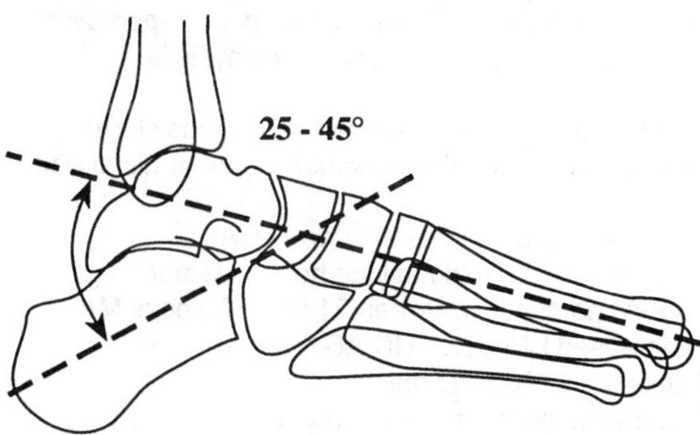

Talocalcaneal Angle on LAT View
= angle between lines drawn through mid-transverse planes of talus + calcaneus; the midtalar line parallels the longitudinal axis of the first metatarsal

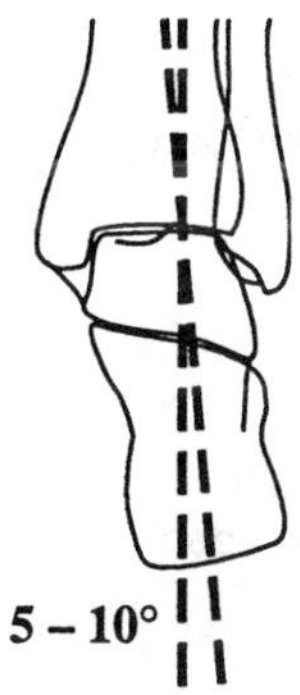

Heel Valgus
cannot be measured directly on radiographs but inferred from the talocalcaneal angle and estimated on coronal CT sections

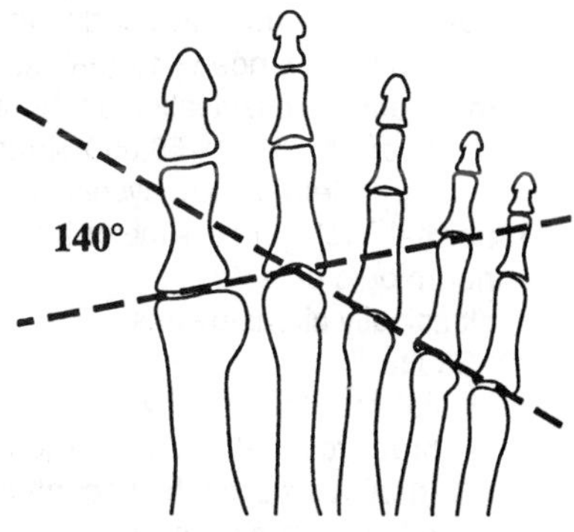

Angle of Metatarsal Heads
= obtuse angle formed by lines tangential to metatarsal heads

BONE AND SOFT-TISSUE DISORDERS

ACHONDROGENESIS
= autosomal recessive lethal chondrodystrophy characterized by extreme micromelia, short trunk, large cranium

TRIAD: (1) severe short-limb dwarfism
(2) lack of vertebral calcification
(3) large head with normal / decreased calvarial ossification

Birth prevalence: 2.3:100,000

Path: disorganization of cartilage

A. TYPE I = Parenti-Fraccaro disease
= defective enchondral + membranous ossification
√ complete lack of ossification of calvarium + spine + pelvis
√ absent sacrum + pubic bone
√ extremely short long bones without bowing, especially femur, radius, ulna
√ thin ribs with multiple fractures (frequent)

B. TYPE II = Langer-Saldino disease
= defective enchondral ossification only
√ good ossification of skull vault
√ nonossification of lower lumbar vertebrae + sacrum
√ short + stubby horizontal ribs without fractures

• often subcutaneous edema
√ irregular flared metaphyses (esp. humerus)
√ short trunk with narrow chest + protruding abdomen
√ redundant soft tissues
√ polyhydramnios (common)
√ increase in HC:AC ratio

Prognosis: lethal often in utero / within few hours or days after birth (respiratory failure)

DDx: often confused with thanatophoric dwarfism

ACHONDROPLASIA
Heterozygous achondroplasia
◊ Prototype of rhizomelic dwarfism!
= autosomal dominant / sporadic (80%) disease with quantitatively defective endochondral bone formation; related to advanced paternal age; epiphyseal maturation + ossification unaffected

Incidence: 1:26,000–66,000 births, most common of lethal bone dysplasias; M < F

• normal intelligence + motor function
• neurologic defects
• classically circus dwarfs

@ Skull
• flat nasal bridge (hypoplastic base of skull)
• brachycephaly with enlarged bulging forehead (nonprogressive hydrocephalus)
• relative prognathism
√ large calvarium with frontal bossing
√ broad mandible
√ shortened base of skull + small foramen magnum
√ communicating hydrocephalus caused by constricted basicranium + foramen magnum (obstruction of basal cisterns + aqueduct)

@ Chest & spine
• protuberant abdomen
• prominent buttocks
√ squaring of inferior scapular margin
√ narrow chest with short anteriorly flared ribs
√ hypoplastic bullet- / wedge-shaped vertebra
= rounded anterior beaking of vertebra in upper lumbar spine (DDx: Hurler disease)
√ posterior vertebral scalloping
√ scoliosis
√ spinal stenosis (ventrodorsal + interpediculate space) in lumbar spine
√ laminar thickening
√ bulging discs
√ wide intervertebral foramina
√ lumbar angular kyphosis (gibbus) + sacral lordosis

@ Pelvis
• rolling gait from backward tilt of pelvis and hip joints
√ square-shaped flattened iliac bones with tombstone configuration ("champagne glass")
√ lack of flaring of iliac wings
√ horizontal acetabula (flat acetabular angle)
√ small sacrosciatic notch

@ Extremities
• short stubby limbs + fingers
• trident hand = separation of 2nd + 3rd digit and inability to approximate 3rd + 4th finger
• limited range of motion of elbow
√ brachydactyly (short tubular bones of hand + feet), especially short proximal + middle phalanges
√ "trumpet" appearance with short long bones and metaphyseal flaring (normal width of metaphysis)
√ predominantly rhizomelic shortness of long bones (femur, humerus)
√ short femoral necks
√ limb bowing
√ "ball-in-socket" epiphysis = broad V-shaped distal femoral metaphysis in which epiphysis is incorporated
√ high position of fibular head (fibula less short)
√ short ulna with thick proximal + slender distal end

OB-US (diagnosable >21–27th week GA):
√ shortening of proximal long bones: femur length <99th percentile between 21 and 27 weeks MA
√ increased BPD, HC, HC:AC ratio
√ decreased FL:BPD ratio
√ normal mineralization, no fractures
√ normal thorax + normal cardiothoracic ratio
√ three-pronged (= trident) hand = 2nd + 3rd + 4th finger of similarly short length without completely approximating each other (= PATHOGNOMONIC)

Cx: (1) Hydrocephalus + syringomyelia (small foramen magnum)

(2) Recurrent ear infection (poorly developed facial bones)
(3) Neurologic complications (compression of spinal cord, lower brain stem, cauda equina, nerve roots): apnea and sudden death
(4) Crowded dentition + malocclusion

Prognosis: long life
DDx: various mucopolysaccharidoses

Homozygous achondroplasia

= hereditary autosomal dominant disease with severe features of achondroplasia (disproportionate limb shortening, more marked proximally than distally)

Risk: marriage of two achondroplasts to each other

√ large cranium with short base + small face
√ flattened nose bridge
√ short ribs with flared ends
√ hypoplastic vertebral bodies
√ decreased interpedicular distance
√ short squared innominate bones
√ flattened acetabular roof
√ small sciatic notch
√ short limb bones with flared metaphyses
√ short, broad, widely spaced tubular bones of hand

Prognosis: often stillborn; lethal in neonatal period (from respiratory failure)
DDx: thanatophoric dysplasia

ACROCEPHALOSYNDACTYLY

= syndrome characterized by
(1) increased height of skull vault due to generalized craniosynostosis (= acrocephaly, oxycephaly)
(2) syndactyly of fingers / toes

Type I : Apert syndrome = acrocephalosyndactyly
Type II : Vogt cephalosyndactyly
Type III : Acrocephalosyndactyly with asymmetry of skull + mild syndactyly
Type IV : Wardenburg type
Type V : Pfeiffer type

ACROOSTEOLYSIS, FAMILIAL

dominant inheritance

Age: onset in 2nd decade; M:F = 3:1

• sensory changes in hands + feet
• destruction of nails
• joint hypermobility
• swelling of plantar of foot with deep wide ulcer + ejection of bone fragments

@ Skull
√ wormian bones
√ craniosynostosis
√ basilar impression
√ protuberant occiput
√ resorption of alveolar processes + loss of teeth

@ Spine
√ spinal osteoporosis ± fracture
√ kyphoscoliosis + progressive decrease in height

ACROMEGALY

Etiology: excess growth hormone due to eosinophilic adenoma / hyperplasia

• gigantism in children (DDx: **Soto syndrome** of cerebral gigantism = large skull, mental retardation, cerebral atrophy, advanced bone age)

√ osseous enlargement (phalangeal tufts, vertebrae)
√ flared ends of long bone
√ cystic changes in carpals, femoral trochanters
√ osteoporosis

@ Hand
• spadelike hand
√ widening of terminal tufts

@ Skull
√ prognathism (= elongation of mandible) in few cases
√ sellar enlargement + erosion
√ enlargement of paranasal sinuses: large frontal sinuses (75%)
√ calvarial hyperostosis (especially inner table)
√ enlarged occipital protuberance

@ Vertebrae
√ posterior scalloping in 30% (secondary to pressure of enlarged soft tissue)
√ anterior new bone
√ loss of disk space (weakening of cartilage)

@ Soft tissue
√ heel pad >25 mm

@ Joints
√ premature osteoarthritis (commonly knees)

ACTINOMYCOSIS

Organism: Actinomyces israelii, Gram-positive anaerobic pleomorphic small bacterium with proteolytic activity, superficially resembling the morphology of a hyphal fungus; closely related to mycobacteria

Histo: mycelial form in tissue; rod-shaped bacterial form normally inhabiting oropharynx (dental caries, gingival margins, tonsillar crypts) + GI tract

Predisposed: individuals with very poor dental hygiene, immunosuppressed patients

Location: mandibulofacial > intestinal > lung

Types:

(1) Mandibulo- / cervicofacial actinomycosis (common)
Cause: poor oral hygiene
• draining cutaneous sinuses
• "sulfur granules" in sputum / exudate = colonies of organisms arranged in circular fashion = mycelial clumps with thin hyphae 1–2 mm in diameter
√ osteomyelitis of mandible (most frequent bone involved) with destruction of mandible around tooth socket
√ no new-bone formation
√ spread to soft tissues at angle of jaw + into neck

(2) Abdominal / ileocecal actinomycosis (60%)
Cause: rupture / surgery of appendix; IUD use
Location: initially localized to cecum / appendix
• fever, leukocytosis, mild anemia
• weight loss, nausea, vomiting, pain
• chronic sinus in groin

√ fold thickening + ulcerations (resembling Crohn disease)
√ rupture of abdominal viscus (usually appendix)
√ fistula formation
√ abscess in liver (15%), retroperitoneum, psoas muscle (containing yellow "sulphur granules" = 1–2 mm colony of gram-positive bacilli)

(3) Pleuropulmonary actinomycosis
Cause: hematogenous spread / inhalation
@ Lung
• draining chest wall sinuses (spread through fascial planes)
√ consolidation extending across interlobar fissures (acute airspace pneumonia rare)
√ cavitary lesion (abscess)
√ pleuritis + empyema
@ Vertebra + ribs
√ destruction of vertebra with preservation of disk + small paravertebral abscess without calcification (DDx to tuberculosis: disk destroyed, large abscess with calcium)
√ thickening of cervical vertebrae around margins
√ destruction / thickening of ribs
@ Tubular bones of hands
√ destructive lesion of mottled permeating type
√ cartilage destruction + subarticular erosive defects in joints (simulating TB)

Rx: surgical débridement + penicillin

ADAMANTINOMA

= (MALIGNANT) ANGIOBLASTOMA = locally aggressive / malignant lesion
Histo: pseudoepithelial cell masses with peripheral columnar cells in a palisade pattern with varying amounts of fibrous stroma; areas of squamous / tubular / alveolar / vessel transformation; prominent vascularity; resembles ameloblastoma of the jaw
Age: 25–50 years, commonest in 3rd–4th decade

• frequently history of trauma
• local swelling ± pain
Location: middle 1/3 of tibia (90%), fibula, ulna, carpals, metacarpals, humerus, shaft of femur
√ eccentric round osteolytic lesion with sclerotic margin, may have additional foci in continuity with major lesion (CHARACTERISTIC)
√ may show mottled density
√ bone expansion frequent
√ often multiple
Prognosis: tendency to recur after local excision; after several recurrences pulmonary metastases may develop
DDx: fibrous dysplasia (possibly related)

AINHUM DISEASE

= DACTYLOLYSIS SPONTANEA
[ainhum = fissure, saw, sword]
Etiology: unknown
Histo: hyperkeratotic epidermis with fibrotic thickening of collagen bundles below; chronic lymphocytic inflammatory reaction may be present; arterial walls may be thickened with narrowed vessel lumina
Incidence: up to 2%
Age: usually in males in 4th + 5th decades; Blacks (West Africa) + their American descendants; M > F
• deep soft-tissue groove forming on medial aspect of plantar surface of proximal phalanx with edema distally
• painful ulceration may develop
Location: mostly 5th / 4th toe (rarely finger); near interphalangeal joint; mostly bilateral
√ sharply demarcated progressive bone resorption of distal / middle phalanx with tapering of proximal phalanx to complete autoamputation (after an average of 5 years)
√ osteoporosis
Rx: early surgical resection of groove with Z plasty
DDx:
(1) Neuropathic disorders (diabetes, leprosy, syphilis)
(2) Trauma (burns, frostbite)
(3) Acroosteolysis from inflammatory arthritis, infection, polyvinyl chloride exposure
(4) Congenitally constricting bands in amniotic band syndrome

AMYLOIDOSIS

= accumulation + infiltration of a chemically diverse group of protein polysaccharides in body tissues; tends to form around capillaries + endothelial cells of larger blood vessels causing ultimately vascular obliteration with infarction
Path: stains with Congo red
• bone pain
• periarticular rubbery soft-tissue swelling + stiffness (shoulders, hips, fingers)
• Bence-Jones protein (without myeloma)
√ periarticular soft-tissue swelling (amyloid deposited in synovium, joint capsule, tendons, ligaments) ± extrinsic osseous erosion
√ subluxation of proximal humerus + femoral neck
√ osteoporosis
√ coarse trabecular pattern (DDx: sarcoidosis)
√ focal medullary lytic lesion with endosteal scalloping (± secondary invasion + erosion of articular bone)
√ pathologic fractures may occur (vertebral fracture)

ANEURYSMAL BONE CYST

= expansile lesion of bone containing thin-walled blood-filled cystic cavities; name derived from roentgen appearance
Etiology:
(a) primary ABC (65–99%)
local circulatory disturbance as a result of trauma
(b) secondary ABC (1–35%)
arising in preexisting bone tumor causing venous obstruction / arteriovenous fistula: giant cell tumor (39%), osteoblastoma, chondroblastoma, angioma, telangiectatic osteosarcoma, solitary bone cyst, fibrous dysplasia, xanthoma, chondromyxoid fibroma, nonossifying fibroma, metastatic carcinoma

Histo: "intraosseous arteriovenous malformation" with honeycombed spaces filled with blood + lined by granulation tissue / osteoid; areas of free hemorrhage; sometimes multinucleated giant cells; solid component predominates in 5–7%

Types:

1. INTRAOSSEOUS ABC
   = primary cystic / telangiectatic tumor of giant cell family, originating in bone marrow cavity, slow expansion of cortex; rarely related to history of trauma
2. EXTRAOSSEOUS ABC
   = posttraumatic hemorrhagic cyst; originating on surface of bones, erosion through cortex into marrow

Age: peak age 16 years (range 10–30 years); in 75% <20 years; F > M

- pain of relatively acute onset with rapid increase of severity over 6–12 weeks
- ± history of trauma
- neurologic signs (radiculopathy to quadriplegia) if in spine

Location: (a) spine (12–30%) with slight predilection for posterior elements; thoracic > lumbar > cervical spine (22%); involvement of vertebral body (40–90%); may involve two contiguous vertebrae (25%)
(b) long bones: eccentric in metaphysis of femur, tibia, humerus, fibula; pelvis

√ purely lytic eccentric radiolucency
√ aggressive expansile ballooning lesion of "soap-bubble" pattern + thin internal trabeculations
√ rapid progression within 6 weeks to 3 months
√ sclerotic inner portion
√ almost invisible thin cortex (CT shows integrity)
√ tumor respects epiphyseal plate
√ no periosteal reaction (except when fractured)

CT:
√ "blood-filled sponge" = fluid-fluid levels due to blood sedimentation (in 10–35%)

MR:
√ multiple cysts of different signal intensity representing different stages of blood by-products
√ low-signal intensity rim = intact thickened periosteal membrane

NUC:
√ "donut sign" = peripheral increased uptake (64%)

Angio:
√ hypervascularity in lesion periphery (in 75%)

Prognosis: 20–30% recurrence rate

Rx: complete resection; embolotherapy; radiation therapy (subsequent sarcoma possible)

Cx: (1) pathologic fracture (frequent)
(2) extradural block with paraplegia

DDx: (1) Giant cell tumor (particularly in spine)
(2) Hemorrhagic cyst (end of bone / epiphysis, not expansile)
(3) Enchondroma
(4) Metastasis (renal cell + thyroid carcinoma)
(5) Plasmacytoma
(6) Chondro- and fibrosarcoma
(7) Fibrous dysplasia
(8) Hemophilic pseudotumor
(9) Hydatid cyst

ANGIOMATOSIS

= diffuse infiltration of bone / soft tissue by hemangiomatous / lymphangiomatous lesions

Age: first 3 decades of life

May be associated with:
chylothorax, chyloperitoneum, lymphedema, hepatosplenomegaly, cystic hygroma

A. OSSEOUS ANGIOMATOSIS (30–40%)
   - indolent course

   Location: femur > ribs > spine > pelvis > humerus > scapula > other long bones > clavicle
   √ osteolysis with honeycomb / latticework ("hole-within-hole") appearance
   √ may occur on both sides of joint
   DDx: solitary osseous hemangioma

B. CYSTIC ANGIOMATOSIS
   = extensive involvement of bone
   Histo: endothelial lined cysts in bone
   Age: peak 10–15 years; range of 3 months to 55 years
   Location: long bones, skull, flat bones
   √ multiple osteolytic metaphyseal lesions of 1–2 mm to several cm with fine sclerotic margins + relative sparing of medullary cavity
   √ may show overgrowth of long bone
   √ endosteal thickening
   √ sometimes associated with soft-tissue mass ± phleboliths
   √ chylous pleural effusion suggests fatal prognosis
   DDx: (other polyostotic diseases as) histiocytosis X, fibrous dysplasia, metastases, Gaucher disease, congenital fibromatosis, Maffucci syndrome, neurofibromatosis, enchondromatosis

C. SOFT-TISSUE ANGIOMATOSIS (60–70%)
   = VISCERAL ANGIOMATOSIS
   - poor prognosis

D. ANGIOMATOUS SYNDROMES
   1. Maffucci syndrome
   2. Osler-Weber-Rendu syndrome
   3. Klippel-Trénaunay-Weber disease
   4. Kasabach-Merritt syndrome
   5. Gorham disease

ANGIOSARCOMA

= aggressive vascular malignancy with frequent local recurrence + distant metastasis

Histo: vascular channels surrounded by hemangiomatous / lymphomatous cellular elements with high degree of anaplasia

Age: M:F = 2:1

Associated with: **Stewart-Treves syndrome**
= angiosarcoma with chronic lymphedema developing in postmastectomy patients

Location: skin (in 33%); soft tissue (in 24%); bone (in 6%): tibia (23%), femur (18%), humerus (13%), pelvis (7%)
DDx: hemangioendothelioma, hemangiopericytoma

ANKYLOSING SPONDYLITIS

= chronic inflammatory disease of unknown etiology primarily affecting spine
Age: 15–35 years; M:F = 4:1–10:1; Caucasians:Blacks = 3:1
Associated with: (1) ulcerative colitis, regional enteritis
(2) iritis in 25%
(3) aortic insufficiency + atrioventricular conduction defect
• HLA-B 27 positive in 96%
• insidious onset of low back pain + stiffness
Location: axial skeleton; HALLMARK is sacroiliac joint involvement; peripheral skeleton (10–20%)
√ temporomandibular joint space narrowing, erosions, osteophytosis
@ Hand (30%)
Target area: MCP, PIP, DIP
√ exuberant osseous proliferation
√ osteoporosis, joint space narrowing, osseous erosions (deformities less striking than in rheumatoid arthritis)
@ Sacroiliac / symphysis pubis
√ initially sclerosis of joint margins primarily on iliac side (bilateral + symmetric late in disease, may be unilateral + asymmetric early in disease)
√ later irregularities + widening of joint (cartilage destruction)
√ bony fusion
@ Spine
√ straightening / squaring of anterior vertebral margins = osteitis of anterior corners
√ reactive sclerosis of corners of vertebral bodies
√ asymmetric erosions of laminar + spinous process at level of lumbar spine
√ marginal syndesmophyte formation = thin vertical radiodense spicules bridging the vertebral bodies = ossification of outer fibers of annulus fibrosus (NOT anterior longitudinal ligament)
√ "trolley-track" sign on AP view = central line of ossification (supraspinous + interspinous ligaments) with two lateral lines of ossification (apophyseal joints)
√ "bamboo" spine on AP view = undulating contour due to syndesmophytes; prone to fracture resulting in pseudarthrosis
√ diskal ballooning ± diskal calcification
√ apophyseal + costovertebral ankylosis
√ periostitic "whiskering": ischial tuberosity, iliac crest, ischiopubic rami, greater femoral trochanter, external occipital protuberance, calcaneus
√ dorsal arachnoid diverticula in lumbar spine with erosion of posterior elements (Cx: cauda equina syndrome)
√ atlantoaxial subluxation
@ Chest
√ bilateral upper lobe pulmonary fibrosis (1%) with upward retraction of hila (DDx: tuberculosis)
@ Cardiovascular
1. Aortitis (5%) of ascending aorta ± aortic valve insufficiency
Prognosis: 20% progress to significant disability; occasionally death from cervical spine fracture / aortitis
DDx: (1) Reiter syndrome (unilateral asymmetric SI joint involvement, paravertebral ossifications)
(2) Psoriatic arthritis (unilateral asymmetric SI joint involvement, paravertebral ossifications)
(3) Inflammatory bowel disease

ANTERIOR TIBIAL BOWING

= WEISMANN-NETTER SYNDROME = congenital painless nonprogressive bilateral anterior leg bowing
Age: beginning in early childhood
• may be accompanied by mental retardation, goiter, anemia
√ anterior bowing of tibia + fibula, bilaterally, symmetrically at middiaphysis
√ thickening of posterior tibial + fibular cortices
√ minor radioulnar bowing
√ kyphoscoliosis
√ extensive dural calcification
DDx: Luetic saber shin (bowing at lower end of tibia + anterior cortical thickening)

APERT SYNDROME

@ Skull
√ oxycephalic skull + flat occiput
√ hypertelorism + bilateral exophthalmos
√ underdeveloped paranasal sinuses
√ underdeveloped maxilla with prognathism
√ high pointed arch of palate
√ prominent vertical crest in middle of forehead (increased intracranial pressure)
√ V-shaped anterior fossa due to elevation of lateral margins of lesser sphenoid
√ sella may be enlarged
√ cervical spine may be fused
@ Hand & feet
√ fusion of distal portions of phalanges, metacarpals / carpals (2nd, 3rd + 4th digit)
√ absence of middle phalanges
√ missing / supernumerary carpal / tarsal bones
√ pseudarthroses

ARTERIOVENOUS FISTULA OF BONE

Etiology: (a) acquired (usually gunshot wound)
(b) congenital
Location: lower extremity most frequent
√ soft-tissue mass
√ presence of large vessels
√ phleboliths (DDx: long-standing varicosity)
√ accelerated bone growth

√ cortical osteolytic defect (= pathway for large vessels into medulla)
√ increased bone density

ARTHROGRYPOSIS

= ARTHROGRYPOSIS MULTIPLEX CONGENITA
= nonprogressive congenital syndrome complex characterized by poorly developed + contracted muscles, deformed joints with thickened periarticular capsule and intact sensory system

Pathophysiology:
congenital / acquired defect of motor unit (anterior horn cells, nerve roots, peripheral nerves, motor endplates, muscle) early in fetal life with immobilization of joints at various stages in their development

Cause: ? neurotropic agents, toxic chemicals, hard drugs, hyperthermia, neuromuscular blocking agents, mytotic abnormalities, mechanical immobilization

Incidence: 0.03% of newborn infants; 5% risk of recurrence in sibling

Path: diminution in size of muscle fibers + fat deposits in fibrous tissue

Associated with:
(1) neurogenic disorders (90%)
(2) myopathic disorders
(3) skeletal dysplasias
(4) intrauterine limitation of movement (myomata, amniotic band, twin, oligohydramnios)
(5) connective tissue disorders

Distribution: all extremities (46%), lower extremities only (43%), upper extremities only (11%); peripheral joints >> proximal joints; symmetrical

• clubfoot
• congenital dislocation of hip
• claw hand
• diminished muscle mass
• skin webs

√ flexion + extension contractures
√ osteopenia ± pathologic fractures
√ congenital dislocation of hip
√ carpal coalition
√ vertical talus
√ calcaneal valgus deformity

ASPHYXIATING THORACIC DYSPLASIA

= JEUNE DISEASE = autosomal recessive disorder

Incidence: 100 cases

Associated with: renal anomalies (hydroureter), PDA

• reduced thoracic mobility (abdominal breathing) + frequent pulmonary infections
• progressive renal failure + hypertension

@ Chest
√ markedly narrow + elongated bell-shaped chest
√ normal size of heart leaving little room for lungs
√ horizontal clavicles at level of 6th cervical vertebra
√ short horizontal ribs + irregular bulbous costochondral junction

@ Pelvis
√ trident pelvis (retardation of ossification of triradiate cartilage)
√ small iliac bone flared + shortened in cephalocaudal diameter ("wineglass" pelvis)
√ short ischial + pubic bones
√ reduced acetabular angle
√ premature ossification of capital femoral epiphysis

@ Extremities
√ rhizomelic brachymelia (humerus, femur) = long bones shorter + wider than normal
√ metaphyseal irregularity
√ postaxial hexadactyly
√ shortening of distal phalanges + cone-shaped epiphyses in hands + feet

@ Kidneys
√ enlarged kidneys with linear streaking on nephrogram

OB-US:
√ proportionate shortening of long bones
√ small thorax with decreased circumference
√ increased cardiothoracic ratio
√ occasionally polydactyly
√ polyhydramnios

Prognosis: neonatal death in 80% (respiratory failure + infections)

DDx: Ellis-van Creveld syndrome

AVASCULAR NECROSIS

= AVN = OSTEONECROSIS = ASEPTIC NECROSIS
= consequence of interrupted blood supply to bone with death of cellular elements

Histo:
(a) cellular ischemia leading to death of hematopoietic cells (in 6–12 hours), osteocytes (in 12–48 hours) and lipocytes (in 2–5 days)
(b) necrotic debris in intertrabecular spaces + proliferation and infiltration by mesenchymal cells + capillaries
(c) mesenchymal cells differentiate to osteoblasts on the surface of dead trabeculae synthesizing new bone layers + resulting in trabecular thickening

Pathogenesis:
(1) obstruction of extra- and intraosseous vessels by arterial embolism, venous thrombosis, traumatic disruption, external compression (increased marrow space pressure)
(2) cumulative stress from cytotoxic factors

Cause:
A. Traumatic interruption of arteries
@ femoral head:
1. Femoral neck fracture (60–75%)
2. Dislocation of hip joint (25%)
3. Slipped capital femoral epiphysis (15–40%)

@ carpal scaphoid:
4–6 months after fracture (in 10–15%), in 30–40% of nonunion of scaphoid fracture
Site: proximal fragment (most common)

@ humeral head (infrequent)

B. Embolization of arteries
   1. Hemoglobinopathy: sickle-cell disease
   2. Nitrogen bubbles: Caisson disease
C. Vasculitis
   1. Collagen-vascular disease: SLE
   2. Radiation exposure
D. Abnormal accumulation of cells
   1. Lipid-containing histiocytes: Gaucher disease
   2. Fat cells: steroid therapy
E. Idiopathic
   1. Spontaneous osteonecrosis of knee
   2. Legg-Calvé-Perthes disease
   3. Freiberg disease

mnemonic: "PLASTIC RAGS"
Pancreatitis, **P**regnancy
Legg-Perthes disease, **L**upus erythematosus
Alcoholism, **A**therosclerosis
Steroids
Trauma (femoral neck fracture, hip dislocation)
Idiopathic (Legg-Perthes disease), **I**nfection
Caisson disease, **C**ollagen disease (SLE)
Rheumatoid arthritis, **R**adiation treatment
Amyloid
Gaucher disease
Sickle cell disease

mnemonic: "GIVE INFARCTS"
Gaucher disease
Idiopathic (Legg-Calvé-Perthes, Köhler, Chandler)
Vasculitis (SLE, polyarteritis nodosa, rheumatoid arthritis)
Environmental (frostbite, thermal injury)
Irradiation
Neoplasia (-associated coagulopathy)
Fat (prolonged corticosteroid use increases marrow)
Alcoholism
Renal failure + dialysis
Caisson disease
Trauma (femoral neck fracture, hip dislocation)
Sickle cell disease

NO predisposing factors in 25%!
Location: femoral head (most common), humeral head, femoral condyles

Avascular Necrosis of Hip

◊ Involvement of one hip increases risk to contralateral hip to 70%!
Age: 20–50 years
• hip / groin / thigh / knee pain
• limited range of motion

Plain film (positive only several months after symptoms):
√ radiolucent crescent parallel to articular surface secondary to subchondral structural collapse of necrotic segment
  Site: anterosuperior portion of femoral head (best seen on frogleg view)
√ preservation of joint space (DDx: arthritis)
√ flattening of articular surface
√ increased density of femoral head (compression of bony trabeculae following microfracture of nonviable bone, calcification of dendritic marrow, creeping substitution = deposition of new bone)

Classification (Steinberg):
Stage O = normal
Stage I = normal / barely detectable trabecular mottling; abnormal bone scan / MRI
Stage IIA = focal <u>sclerosis</u> + osteopenia
Stage IIB = distinct sclerosis + osteoporosis + early crescent sign
Stage IIIA = subchondral undermining ("<u>crescent sign</u>") + cyst formation
Stage IIIB = mild alteration in femoral head contour / <u>subchondral fracture</u> + normal joint space
Stage IV = marked collapse of femoral head + significant <u>acetabular involvement</u>
Stage V = <u>joint space narrowing</u> + acetabular degenerative changes

NUC (80–85% sensitivity):
◊ Bone marrow imaging (with radiocolloid) more sensitive than bone imaging (with diphosphonates)
◊ More sensitive than plain films in early AVN (evidence of ischemia seen as much as 1 year earlier)
◊ Less sensitive than MR
Technique: imaging improved with double counts, pinhole collimation
√ <u>early</u>: cold = photopenic defect (interrupted blood supply)
√ <u>late</u>: "doughnut sign" = cold spot surrounded by increased uptake secondary to
  (a) capillary revascularization + new-bone synthesis
  (b) degenerative osteoarthritis

CT (utilized for staging of known disease):
√ staging upgrades in 30% compared with plain films

MR (90–100% sensitivity for symptomatic disease):
Prevalence of clinically occult disease: 6%
◊ MR imaging changes reflect the death of marrow fat cells (not death of osteocytes with empty lacunae)!
◊ Sagittal images particularly useful!

Classification (Mitchell):

Stage	*T1*	*T2*	*analogous to*
A	high	intermediate	fat
B	high	high	subacute blood
C	low	high	fluid / edema
D	low	low	fibrosis

EARLY AVN:
√ decreased Gd-enhancement on short-inversion-recovery (STIR) images (very early)

√ low-signal intensity band with sharp inner interface + blurred outer margin on T1WI within 12–48 hours (= mesenchymal + fibrous repair tissue, amorphous cellular debris, thickened trabecular bone) seen as
(a) band extending to subchondral bone plate
(b) complete ring (less frequent)
√ "double-line sign" on T2WI (in 80%) [MORE SPECIFIC] = juxtaposition of inner hyperintense band (granulation tissue) + outer hypointense band (chemical shift artifact / fibrosis + sclerosis)

ADVANCED AVN:
√ "pseudohomogeneous edema pattern" = inhomogeneous large areas of mostly decreased signal intensity on T1WI
√ hypo- to hyperintense lesion on T2WI
√ contrast-enhancement of interface + surrounding marrow + within lesion

SUBCHONDRAL FRACTURE:
√ predilection for anterosuperior portion of femoral head (sagittal images!)
√ cleft of low-signal intensity running parallel to the subchondral bone plate within areas of fatlike signal intensity on T1WI
√ hyperintense band (= fracture cleft filled with articular fluid / edema) within the intermediate- or low-signal-intensity necrotic marrow on T2WI
√ lack of enhancement within + around fracture cleft

EPIPHYSEAL COLLAPSE:
√ focal depression of subchondral bone

Cx: early osteoarthritis through collapse of femoral head + joint incongruity in 3–5 years if left untreated
Rx: (1) core decompression (for grade 0–II): most successful with <25% involvement of femoral head
(2) osteotomy (for grade 0–II)
(3) arthroplasty / arthrodesis / total hip replacement (for grade >III)
DDx: bone marrow edema (ill-delimited marrow changes, no reactive interface); epiphyseal fracture (speckled / linear hypointense areas, focal depression of epiphyseal contour)

Blount disease
= TIBIA VARA
= avascular necrosis of medial tibial condyle
Age: >6 years
• limping, lateral bowing of leg
√ medial tibial condyle enlarged + deformed (DDx: Turner syndrome)
√ irregularity of metaphysis (medially + posteriorly prolonged with beak)

Calvé-Kümmel-Verneuil disease
= VERTEBRAL OSTEOCHONDROSIS = VERTEBRA PLANA = avascular necrosis of vertebral body
Age: 2–15 years
√ uniform collapse of vertebral body into flat thin disk
√ increased density of vertebra
√ neural arches NOT affected
√ disks are normal with normal intervertebral disk space
√ intravertebral vacuum cleft sign (PATHOGNOMONIC)
DDx: Eosinophilic granuloma, metastatic disease

Freiberg disease
= osteochondrosis of head of 2nd (3rd / 4th) metatarsal
Age: 10–18 years; M:F = 1:3
• metatarsalgia, swelling, tenderness
Early:
√ flattening, increased density, cystic lesions of metatarsal head
√ widening of metatarsophalangeal joint
Late:
√ osteochondral fragment
√ sclerosis + flattening of metatarsal head
√ increased cortical thickening

Kienböck disease
= LUNATOMALACIA
= avascular necrosis of lunate bone
Predisposed: individuals engaged in manual labor with repeated / single episode of trauma
Age: 20–40 years
Associated with: ulna minus variant (short ulna) in 75%
• progressive pain + soft-tissue swelling of wrist
Location: uni- > bilateral (usually right hand)
√ initially normal radiograph
√ fracture / osteonecrosis of lunate
√ increased density + altered shape + collapse of lunate
Cx: scapholunate separation, ulnar deviation of triquetrum, degenerative joint disease in radiocarpal / midcarpal compartments
Rx: ulnar lengthening / radial shortening, lunate replacement

Köhler disease
= avascular necrosis of tarsal scaphoid
Age: 3–10 years; boys
√ irregular outline
√ fragmentation
√ disklike compression in AP direction
√ increased density
√ joint space maintained
√ decreased / increased uptake on radionuclide study

Legg-Calvé-Perthes disease
= COXA PLANA = idiopathic avascular necrosis of femoral head in children; one of the most common sites of AVN; 10% bilateral
Age: (a) 4–8 years: M:F = 5:1
(b) adulthood: **Chandler disease**

Cause: trauma in 30% (subcapital fracture, epiphyseolysis, esp. posterior dislocation), closed reduction of congenital hip dislocation, prolonged interval between injury and reduction

Pathophysiology:
femoral head blood supply insufficient (epiphyseal plate acts as a barrier in ages 4–10; ligamentum teres vessels become nonfunctional; blood supply is from medial circumflex artery + lateral epiphyseal artery only)

Stages:
- I = histologic + clinical diagnosis without radiographic findings
- II = sclerosis ± cystic changes with preservation of contour + surface of femoral head
- III = loss of structural integrity of femoral head
- IV = in addition loss of structural integrity of acetabulum

• 1 week–6 months (mean 2.7 months) duration of symptoms prior to initial presentation: limping, pain

NUC (may assist in early diagnosis):
√ decreased uptake (early) in femoral head = interruption of blood supply
√ increased uptake (late) in femoral head =
(a) revascularization + bone repair
(b) degenerative osteoarthritis
√ increased acetabular activity with associated degenerative joint disease

X-RAY:
Early signs:
√ femoral epiphysis smaller than on contralateral side (96%)
√ sclerosis of femoral head epiphysis (sequestration + compression) (82%)
√ slight widening of joint space due to thickening of cartilage, failure of epiphyseal growth, presence of joint fluid, joint laxity (60%)
√ ipsilateral bone demineralization (46%)
√ alteration of pericapsular soft-tissue outline due to atrophy of ipsilateral periarticular soft tissues (73%)
√ rarefaction of lateral + medial metaphyseal areas of neck
√ NEVER destruction of articular cortex as in bacterial arthritis

Late signs:
√ delayed osseous maturation of a mild degree
√ "radiolucent crescent line" of subchondral fracture = small archlike subcortical lucency (32%)
√ subcortical fracture on anterior articular surface (best seen on frogleg view)
√ femoral head fragmentation
√ femoral neck cysts (from intramedullary hemorrhage in response to stress fractures)
√ loose bodies (only found in males)
√ coxa plana = flattened collection of sclerotic fragments (over 18 months)
√ coxa magna = remodeling of femoral head to become wider + flatter in mushroom configuration to match widened metaphysis + epiphyseal plate

CT:
√ loss of "asterisk" sign (= starlike pattern of crossing trabeculae in center of femoral head) with distortion of asterisk and extension to surface of femoral head

MR:
√ normal signal intensity in marrow of femoral epiphysis replaced by low signal intensity on T1WI + high signal intensity on T2WI = "asterisk" sign
√ "double-line" sign (80%) = sclerotic nonsignal rim producing line between necrotic + viable bone edged by a hyperintense rim of granulation tissue
√ fluid within fracture plane
√ hip joint incongruity: lateral femoral head uncovering, labral inversion, femoral head deformity

Cx: severe degenerative joint disease in early adulthood

Panner disease
= osteonecrosis of capitellum

Preiser disease
= nontraumatic osteonecrosis of scaphoid

Spontaneous osteonecrosis of knee
= SONK

Cause: ? meniscal tear (78%), trauma with resultant microfractures, vascular insufficiency, degenerative joint disease, severe chondromalacia, gout, rheumatoid arthritis, joint bodies, intraarticular steroid injection (45–85%)

Age: 7th decade (range 13–83 years)

• acute onset of pain

Location: weight-bearing medial condyle more toward epicondylus (95%), lateral condyle (5%), may involve tibial plateau

√ radiographs usually normal (within 3 months after onset)
√ positive bone scan within 5 weeks (most sensitive)
√ flattening of weight-bearing segment of medial femoral epicondyle
√ radiolucent focus in subchondral bone + peripheral zone of osteosclerosis
√ horizontal subchondral fracture (within 6–9 months) + osteochondral fragment
√ periosteal reaction along medial side of femoral shaft (30–50%)

Cx: osteoarthritis

BASAL CELL NEVUS SYNDROME
= GORLIN SYNDROME = syndrome of autosomal dominant inheritance characterized by
(1) multiple cutaneous basal cell carcinomas
(2) jaw cysts
(3) ectopic calcifications
(4) skeletal anomalies

- multiple nevoid basal cell carcinomas (nose, mouth, chest, back) at mean age of 19 years; after puberty aggressive, may metastasize
- pitlike defects in palms + soles

Associated with: high incidence of medulloblastoma in children

√ multiple mandibular + maxillary cysts (dentigerous cysts + ectopic dentition)
√ anomalies of upper 5 ribs: bifid, fused, dysplastic
√ bifid spinous processes, spina bifida
√ scoliosis (cervical + upper thoracic)
√ hemivertebrae + block vertebrae
√ Sprengel deformity (scapula elevated, hypoplastic, bowed)
√ brachydactyly
√ extensive calcification of falx + tentorium
√ ectopic calcifications of subcutaneous tissue, ovaries, sacrotuberous ligaments, mesentery
√ bony bridging of sella turcica

BATTERED CHILD SYNDROME

= CAFFEY-KEMPE SYNDROME = CHILD ABUSE = PARENT / INFANT TRAUMATIC STRESS SYNDROME = NONACCIDENTAL TRAUMA

◊ Most common cause of serious intracranial injuries in children <1 year of age; 3rd most common cause of death in children after sudden infant death syndrome + true accidents

Prevalence: 1.7 million cases reported + 833,000 substantiated in United States in 1990 (45% neglected children, 25% physically abused, 16% sexually abused children); resulting in 2,500–5,000 deaths/year; 5–10% of children seen in emergency rooms

Age: usually <2 years

- skin burns, bruising, lacerations, hematomas (SNAT = suspected nonaccidental trauma)

@ Skeletal trauma (50–80%)

Site: multiple ribs, transverse fracture of sternum, costochondral / costovertebral separation, lateral end of clavicles, scapula, acromion, skull, anterior-superior wedging, vertebral compression, vertebral fracture dislocation, disk space narrowing, spinous processes, tibia, metacarpus

√ multiple asymmetric fractures in different stages of repair (HALLMARK = repeated injury)
√ separation of distal epiphysis
√ marked irregularity + fragmentation of metaphyses (DDx: osteochondritis stage of congenital syphilis; infractions of scurvy)
√ "corner" fracture (11%) = "bucket-handle" fracture = avulsion of an arcuate metaphyseal fragment overlying the lucent epiphyseal cartilage secondary to sudden twisting motion of extremity about knee, elbow, distal tibia, fibula, radius, ulna (periosteum easily pulled away from diaphysis but tightly attached to metaphysis)
√ isolated spiral fracture (15%) of diaphysis secondary to external rotatory force applied to femur / humerus
√ extensive periosteal reaction from large subperiosteal hematoma (DDx: scurvy, copper deficiency)
√ exuberant callus formation at fracture sites
√ cortical hyperostosis extending to epiphyseal plate (DDx: not in infantile cortical hyperostosis)
√ avulsion fracture of ligamentous insertion; frequently seen without periosteal reaction

@ Head trauma (13–25%)

Most common cause of death + physical disability

(1) Impact injury with translational force: skull fracture (flexible calvaria + meninges decrease likelihood of skull fractures), subdural hematoma, brain contusion, cerebral hemorrhage, infarction, generalized edema
(2) Whiplash injury with rotational force: shearing injuries + associated subarachnoid hemorrhage

- bulging fontanelles, convulsions

Skull film (associated fracture in 1%):

√ linear fracture > comminuted fracture > diastases (conspicuously absent)

CT:

√ subdural hemorrhage (most common): interhemispheric location most common
√ subarachnoid hemorrhage
√ epidural hemorrhage (uncommon)
√ cerebral edema (focal, multifocal, diffuse)
√ acute cerebral contusion as ovoid collection of intraparenchymal blood with surrounding edema

MR: more sensitive in identifying hematomas of differing ages

√ white matter shearing injuries as areas of prolonged T1 + T2 at corticomedullary junction, centrum semiovale, corpus callosum

@ Viscera (3%)

Second leading cause of death in child abuse

Cause: crushing blow to abdomen (punch, kick)

Age: often >2 years

√ small bowel / gastric rupture
√ hematoma of duodenum / jejunum
√ contusion / laceration of lung, pancreas, liver, spleen, kidney
√ traumatic pancreatic pseudocyst

Cx: (1) Brain atrophy (up to 100%)
(2) Infarction (50%)
(3) Subdural hygroma
(4) Encephalomalacia
(5) Porencephaly

DDx: normal periostitis of infancy, osteogenesis imperfecta, congenital insensitivity to pain, infantile cortical hyperostosis, Menke's kinky hair syndrome, Schmid-type chondrometaphyseal dysplasia, scurvy, congenital syphilitic metaphysitis

BENIGN CORTICAL DEFECT

= developmental intracortical bone defect

Age: usually 1st–2nd decade; uncommon in boys <2 years of age; uncommon in girls <4 years of age

• asymptomatic
Site: metaphysis of long bone
√ well-defined intracortical round / oval lucency
√ usually <2 cm long
√ sclerotic margins
Cx: pathologic / avulsion fracture following minor trauma (infrequent)
Prognosis: (1) Spontaneous healing resulting in sclerosis / disappearance
(2) Ballooning of endosteal surface of cortex = fibrous cortical defect
(3) Medullary extension resulting in nonossifying fibroma

BONE INFARCT

Etiology:
A. Occlusion of vessel:
(a) thrombus: thromboembolic disease, sickle cell anemia (SS + SC hemoglobin), polycythemia rubra vera
(b) fat: pancreatitis (intramedullary fat necrosis from circulating lipase), alcoholism
(c) gas: Caisson disease, astronauts
B. Vessel wall disease:
1. Arteritis: SLE, rheumatoid arthritis, polyarteritis nodosa, sarcoidosis
2. Arteriosclerosis
C. Vascular compression by deposition of:
(a) fat: corticosteroid therapy (eg, renal transplant, Cushing disease)
(b) blood: trauma (fractures + dislocations)
(c) inflammatory cells: osteomyelitis, infection, histiocytosis X
(d) edema: radiation therapy, hypothyroidism, frostbite
(e) substances: Gaucher disease (vascular compression by lipid-filled histiocytes), gout
D. Others: idiopathic, hypopituitarism, pheochromocytoma (microscopic thrombotic disease), osteochondroses

Medullary infarction

◊ Nutrient artery is the sole blood supply for diaphysis!
Location: distal femur, proximal tibia, iliac wings, ribs, humeri
(a) Acute phase:
√ NO radiographic changes without cortical involvement
√ area of rarefaction
√ bone marrow scan: diminished uptake in medullary RES for long period of time
√ bone scan: photon-deficient lesion within 24–48 hours; increased uptake after collateral circulation established
(b) Healing phase: (complete healing / fibrosis / calcification)
√ demarcation by zone of serpiginous / linear calcification + ossification parallel to cortex
√ dense bone indicating revascularization

Cortical infarction

◊ Requires compromise of (a) nutrient artery and (b) periosteal vessels!
Age: particularly in childhood where periosteum is easily elevated by edema
√ avascular necrosis = osteonecrosis
√ osteochondrosis dissecans
Cx: (1) Growth disturbances
√ cupped / triangular / coned epiphyses
√ "H-shaped" vertebral bodies
(2) Fibrosarcoma (most common), malignant fibrous histiocytoma, benign cysts
(3) Osteoarthritis

BONE ISLAND

= ENOSTOSIS = ENDOSTEOMA = COMPACT ISLAND = FOCAL SCLEROSIS = SCLEROTIC BONE ISLAND = CALCIFIED MEDULLARY DEFECT
= focal lesion of densely sclerotic (compact) bone nesting within spongiosa
Age: any age (mostly 20–80 years of age); grows more rapidly in children
Histo: nest of lamellar compacted bone with haversian system embedded within medullary canal
Pathogenesis:
? misplaced cortical hamartoma, ? developmental error of endochondral ossification as a coalescence of mature bone trabeculae with failure to undergo remodeling
• asymptomatic
Location: ilium + proximal femur (88–92%), ribs, spine (1–14%), humerus, phalanges (not in skull)
√ round / oval solitary osteoblastic lesion with abrupt transition to surrounding normal trabecular bone
√ long axis of bone island parallels long axis of bone
√ usually 2–10 mm in size; lesion >2 cm in longest axis = GIANT BONE ISLAND
√ "brush border" = "thorny radiations" = sharply demarcated margins with feathery peripheral radiations (HALLMARK)
√ may show activity on bone scan, esp. if large (33%)
√ may demonstrate slow growth / decrease in size (32%)
√ NO involvement of cortex / radiolucencies / periosteal reaction
Prognosis: may increase to 8–12 cm over years (40%); may decrease / disappear
DDx: (1) Osteoblastic metastasis (aggressive, break through cortex, periosteal reaction)
(2) Low-grade osteosarcoma (cortical thickening, extension beyond medullary cavity)
(3) Osteoid osteoma (pain relieved by aspirin, nidus)
(4) Benign osteoblastoma
(5) Involuted nonossifying fibroma replaced by dense bone scar
(6) Eccentric focus of monostotic fibrous dysplasia
(7) Osteoma (surface lesion)

BRUCELLOSIS

= multisystemic zoonosis of worldwide distribution; endemic in Saudi Arabia, Arabian Peninsula, South America, Spain, Italy (secondary to ingestion of raw milk / milk products)

Organism: small Gram-negative nonmotile, nonsporing, aflagellate, nonencapsulated coccobacilli: Brucella abortus, B. suis, B. canis, B. melitensis

Histo: small intracellular pathogens shed in excreta of infected animals (urine, stool, milk, products of conception) cause small noncaseating granuloma within RES

Location: commonest site of involvement is reticulo-endothelial system; musculoskeletal system

- 1–3 weeks between initial infection + symptoms
  ◊ Radiologic evidence of disease in 69% of symptomatic sites!

@ Brucellar spondylitis (53%)
  Age: 40 years is average age at onset
  - pain, localized tenderness, radiculopathy, myelopathy

  Location: lumbar (71%) > thoracolumbar (10%) > lumbosacral (8%) > cervical (7%) > thoracic (4%)

  (a) focal form
    √ bone destruction at diskovertebral junction (anterior aspect of superior endplate)
    √ associated with bone sclerosis + anterior osteophyte formation + small amount of gas

  (b) diffuse form: entire vertebral endplate / whole vertebral body affected with spread to adjacent disks + vertebral bodies
    √ bone destruction associated with sclerosis
    √ small amount of disk gas (25–30%)
    √ obliteration of paraspinal muscle-fat planes
    √ no / minimal epidural extension
    DDx: TB (paraspinal abscess, gibbus)

@ Extraspinal disease
  (a) Brucellar synovitis (81%)
    Location: knee > sacroiliac joint > shoulder > hip > sternoclavicular joint > ankle > elbow
    Site: organism localized in synovial membrane
    - serosanguinous sterile joint effusion

  (b) Brucellar destructive arthritis (9%)
    √ indistinguishable from tuberculous / pyogenic arthritis

  (c) Brucellar osteomyelitis (2%)
    - pain, tenderness, swelling

  (d) Brucellar myositis (2%)

Dx: serologic tests (enzyme-linked immunosorbent assay, counterimmunoelectrophoresis, rose bengal plate test

Rx: combination of aminoglycosides + tetracyclines

DDx: fibrous dysplasia, benign tumor, osteoid osteoma

CAISSON DISEASE

= DECOMPRESSION SICKNESS = THE BENDS

Etiology: during too rapid decompression = reduction of surrounding pressure (ascent from dive, exit from caisson / hyperbaric chamber, ascent to altitude) nitrogen bubbles form (nitrogen more soluble in fat of panniculus adiposus, spinal cord, brain, bones containing fatty marrow)

- "the bends" = local pain in knee, elbow, shoulder, hip
- neurologic symptoms (paresthesia, major cerebral / spinal involvement)
- "chokes" = substernal discomfort + coughing (embolization of pulmonary vessels)

Location: mostly in long tubular bones of lower extremity (distal end of shaft + epiphyseal portion); symmetrical lesions

√ early: area of rarefaction
√ healing phase: irregular new-bone formation with greater density
√ peripheral zone of calcification / ossification
√ ischemic necrosis of articular surface with secondary osteoarthritis

CALCIUM PYROPHOSPHATE DIHYDRATE CRYSTAL DEPOSITION DISEASE

= PSEUDOGOUT = FAMILIAL CHONDROCALCINOSIS
= most common crystalline arthropathy

Types:
1. Osteoarthritic form (35–60%)
2. Pseudogout = acute synovitis (10–20%)
3. Rheumatoid form (2–6%)
4. Pseudoneuropathic arthropathy (2%)
5. Asymptomatic with tophaceous pseudogout (common)

Associated with: hyperparathyroidism, hypothyroidism, hemochromatosis, hypomagnesemia

Prevalence: widespread in older population; M:F = 3:2

- calcium pyrophosphate crystals in synovial fluid + within leukocytes (characteristic weakly positive birefringent diffraction pattern)
- acute / subacute / chronic joint inflammation

Location:
  (a) knee (especially meniscus + cartilage of patellofemoral joint)
  (b) wrist (triangular fibrocartilage in distal radioulnar joint bilaterally)
  (c) pelvis (sacroiliac joint, symphysis)
  (d) spine (annulus fibrosis of lumbar intervertebral disk; NEVER in nucleus pulposus as in ochronosis)
  (e) shoulder (glenoid), hip (labrum), elbow, ankle, acromioclavicular joint

√ polyarticular chondrocalcinosis (in fibro- and hyaline cartilage)
√ disproportionate narrowing of patellofemoral joint
√ involvement of tendons, bursae, pinnae of the ear
√ pyrophosphate arthropathy resembles osteoarthritis: joint space narrowing, extensive subchondral sclerosis
√ large subchondral cyst (HALLMARK)
√ numerous intraarticular bodies (fragmentation of subchondral bone)

CAMPOMELIC DYSPLASIA

= sporadic / autosomal recessive dwarfism

Incidence: 0.05:10,000 births

Associated with:
1. Hydrocephalus (23%)
2. Congenital heart disease (30%): VSD, ASD, tetralogy, AS
3. Hydronephrosis (30%)

- pretibial dimple

√ macrocephaly, cleft palate, micrognathia (90–99%)
@ Chest & spine
√ hypoplastic scapulae (92%)
√ narrow bell-shaped chest
√ hypoplastic vertebral bodies + nonmineralized pedicles (especially lower cervical spine)
@ Pelvis
√ vertically narrowed iliac bones
√ vertical inclination of ischii
√ wide symphysis
√ narrow iliac bones with small wings
√ shallow acetabulum
@ Extremities (lower extremity more severely affected)
√ dislocation of hips + knees
√ anterior bowing (= campo) of long bones: marked in tibia + moderate in femur
√ hypoplastic fibula
√ small secondary ossification center of knee
√ small primary ossification center of talus
√ clubfoot
OB-US:
√ bowing of tibia + femur
√ decreased thoracic circumference
√ hypoplastic scapulae
√ ± cleft palate
Prognosis: death usually <5 months of age (within first year in 97%) due to respiratory insufficiency

CARPAL TUNNEL SYNDROME
= entrapment syndrome caused by chronic pressure on the median nerve within the carpal tunnel
Cause: repetitive wrist / finger flexion; carpal tunnel crowding by cyst / mass / flexor tendon tendinitis or tenosynovitis / anomalous origin of lumbrical muscles
Pathogenesis: probably ischemia with venous congestion (stage 1), nerve edema from anoxic damage to capillary endothelium (stage 2), impairment of venous + arterial blood supply (stage 3)
• nocturnal hand discomfort
• weakness, clumsiness, finger paresthesias
MR:
√ "pseudoneuroma" of median nerve = swelling of median nerve proximal to carpal tunnel
√ swelling of nerve within carpal tunnel
√ increased signal intensity of nerve on T2WI
√ volar bowing of flexor retinaculum
√ swelling of tendon sheath (due to tenosynovitis)
√ mass(es) within carpal tunnel
√ marked enhancement (nerve edema = breakdown of blood-nerve barrier)
√ no enhancement (ischemia) provoked by wrist held in an extended / flexed position

CARPENTER SYNDROME
= ACROCEPHALOPOLYSYNDACTYLY type 2
autosomal recessive
• retardation
• hypogonadism
√ patent ductus arteriosus
√ acro(oxy)cephaly
√ preaxial polysyndactyly + soft-tissue syndactyly

CHONDROBLASTOMA
= CODMAN TUMOR = BENIGN CHONDROBLASTOMA
= CARTILAGE-CONTAINING GIANT CELL TUMOR
Incidence: 1% of primary bone neoplasms (700 cases in world literature)
Age: peak in 2nd decade (range of 8–59 years); 10–26 years (90%); M:F = 2:1; occurs before cessation of enchondral bone growth
Path: derived from primitive cartilage cells
Histo: polyhedral chondroblasts + multinucleated giant cells + nodules of pink amorphous material (= chondroid) = epiphyseal chondromatous giant cell tumor (resembles chondromyxoid fibroma); "chicken wire" calcification = pericellular deposition of calcification is virtually PATHOGNOMONIC
• symptomatic for months to years prior to treatment
• mild joint pain, tenderness, swelling (joint effusion)
• limitation of motion
Location:
(a) long bones (80%): proximal femur + greater trochanter (23%), distal femur (20%), proximal tibia (17%), proximal humerus (17%)
◊ 2/3 in lower extremity, 50% about knee
◊ may occur in apophyses (minor + greater trochanter, patella, greater tuberosity of humerus)
(b) flat bones: near triradiate cartilage of innominate bone
(c) short tubular bones of hand + feet
Site: eccentric medullary, subarticular location with open growth plate (98% begin within epiphysis); tumor growth may continue to involve metaphysis (50%) + rarely diaphysis
√ oval / round eccentrically placed lytic lesion of epiphysis
√ 1–4 cm in diameter occupying < one-half of epiphysis
√ well-defined sclerotic margin, lobulated in 50%
√ punctate / irregular calcifications in 25–30–50% (cartilaginous clumps better visualized by CT)
√ intact cortical border
√ thick periosteal reaction in metaphysis (50%) / joint involvement
√ periostitis of adjacent metaphysis / diaphysis (30–50%)
√ open growth plate in majority of patients
MR:
◊ MR tends to overestimate extent + aggressiveness due to large area of reactive edema!
√ intermediate to low signal intensity on T2WI relative to fat
√ extensive intramedullary signal abnormalities consistent with bone marrow edema
√ peripheral rim of very low signal intensity
√ hypointense changes on T1WI + hyperintense on T2WI in adjacent soft tissues (muscle edema) in 50%
√ ± joint effusion
Prognosis: almost always benign; may become locally aggressive; rarely metastasizes

Dx: surgical biopsy
Rx: curettage + bone chip grafting (recurrence in 25%)
DDx: (1) Ischemic necrosis of femoral head (may be indistinguishable, more irregular configuration)
(2) Giant cell tumor (usually larger + less well demarcated, not calcified, older age group with closed growth plate)
(3) Chondromyxoid fibroma
(4) Enchondroma
(5) Osteomyelitis (less well-defined, variable margins)
(6) Aneurysmal bone cyst
(7) Intraosseous ganglion
(8) Langerhans cell histiocytosis (less well-defined, variable margins)
(9) Primary bone sarcoma

CHONDRODYSPLASIA PUNCTATA

= CONGENITAL STIPPLED EPIPHYSES
= DYSPLASIA EPIPHYSEALIS PUNCTATA
= CHONDRODYSTROPHIA CALCIFICANS CONGENITA
= proportional / mesomelic dwarfism
Etiology: peroxisomal disorder characterized by fibroblast plasmalogen deficiency
Incidence: 1:110,000 births

A. AUTOSOMAL RECESSIVE CHONDRODYSPLASIA PUNCTATA = RHIZOMELIC TYPE
Associated with: CHD (common)
• flat face
• congenital cataracts
• ichthyotic skin thickening
• mental retardation
• cleft palate
√ multiple small punctate calcifications of varying size in epiphyses (knee, hip, shoulder, wrist), in base of skull, in posterior elements of vertebrae, in respiratory cartilage and soft tissues (neck, rib ends) before appearance of ossification centers
√ prominent symmetrical shortening of femur + humerus (rarely all limbs symmetrically affected)
√ congenital dislocation of hip
√ flexion contractures of extremities
√ clubfeet
√ metaphyseal splaying of proximal tubular bones (in particular about knee)
√ thickening of diaphyses
√ prominent vertebral + paravertebral calcifications
√ coronal clefts in vertebral bodies
Prognosis: death usually <1 year of age
DDx: Zellweger syndrome

B. CONRADI-HÜNERMANN DISEASE
= NONRHIZOMELIC TYPE
more common milder nonlethal variety; autosomal dominant
• normal intelligence
√ more widespread but milder involvement as above
Prognosis: survival often into adulthood

Cx: respiratory failure (severe underdevelopment of ribs), tracheal stenosis, spinal cord compression

DDx: (1) Cretinism (may show epiphyseal fragmentation, much larger calcifications within epiphysis)
(2) Warfarin embryopathy
(3) Zellweger syndrome

CHONDROECTODERMAL DYSPLASIA

= ELLIS-VAN CREVELD SYNDROME = MESODERMAL DYSPLASIA
= autosomal recessive acromesomelic dwarfism
Incidence: 120 cases; in inbred Amish communities
Associated with: congenital heart disease in 50% (single atrium, ASD, VSD)
• ectodermal dysplasia:
 – absent / hypoplastic brittle spoon-shaped nails
 – irregular + pointed teeth, partial anodontia, teeth may be present at birth
 – scant / fine hair
• obliteration of maxillary mucobuccal space (thick frenula between alveolar mucosa + upper lip)
• strabismus
• genital malformations: epispadia, hypospadia, hypoplastic external genitalia, undescended testicles
√ hepatosplenomegaly
√ accelerated skeletal maturation
√ normal spine

@ Skull
 √ wormian bones
 √ cleft lip
@ Chest
 √ long narrow thorax in AP + transverse dimensions
 √ horizontal ribs + elevated clavicles
@ Pelvis
 √ small flattened ilium
 √ trident shape of acetabulum with indentation in roof + bony spur (almost pathognomonic)
 √ acetabular + tibial exostoses
@ Extremities
 √ thickening + shortening of all long bones, more severe in forearms + lower legs (radius + tibia > humerus + femur)
 √ excessive shortening of fibula
 √ widening of proximal tibial shaft + delayed development of tibial plateau
 √ dislocation of radial head (due to shortening of ulna)
 √ carpal / tarsal coalition = frequent fusion of two / more carpal (hamate + capitate) + tarsal bones
 √ supernumerary carpal bones
 √ hypoplasia / absence of terminal phalanges + cone-shaped epiphyses
 √ postaxial polydactyly common (usually finger, rarely toe) ± syndactyly of hands + feet
 √ carpal fusion (after complete ossification)

OB-US:
√ proportional shortening of long bones
√ small thorax with decreased circumference
√ increased cardiothoracic ratio
√ ASD
√ polydactyly

Prognosis: death within first month of life in 33% (due to respiratory / cardiac complications)
DDx: Asphyxiating thoracic dysplasia (difficult distinction); rhizomelic achondroplasia

CHONDROMALACIA PATELLAE

= pathologic softening of patellar cartilage
Cause: trauma, tracking abnormality of patella
- anterior knee pain
- asymptomatic (incidental arthroscopic diagnosis)

CHONDROMYXOID FIBROMA

Rare benign cartilaginous tumor; initially arising in cortex
Incidence: <1% of all bone tumors
Histo: chondroid + fibrous + myxoid tissue (related to chondroblastoma); may be mistaken for chondrosarcoma
Age: peak 2nd–3rd decade (range of 5–79 years); M:F = 1:1
- slowly progressive local pain, swelling, restriction of motion

Location: (a) long bones (60%): about knee (50%), proximal tibia (82% of tibial lesions), distal femur (71% of femoral lesions), fibula
(b) short tubular bones of hand + feet (20%)
(c) flat bones: pelvis, ribs (classic but uncommon)

Site: eccentric, metaphyseal (47–53%), metadiaphyseal (20–43%), metaepiphyseal (26%), diaphyseal (1–10%), epiphyseal (3%)

√ expansile ovoid lesion with radiolucent center + oval shape at each end of lesion
√ long axis parallel to long axis of host bone (1–10 cm in length and 4–7 cm in width)
√ geographic bone destruction (100%)
√ well-defined sclerotic margin (86%)
√ expanded shell = bulged + thinned overlying cortex (68%)
√ partial cortical erosion (68%)
√ scalloped margin (58%)
√ septations (57%) may mimic trabeculations
√ stippled calcifications within tumor in advanced lesions (7%)
√ NO periosteal reaction (unless fractured)

Prognosis: 25% recurrence rate following curettage
Cx: malignant degeneration distinctly unusual
DDx: (1) Aneurysmal bone cyst (2) Simple bone cyst (3) Nonossifying fibroma (4) Fibrous dysplasia (5) Enchondroma (6) Chondroblastoma (7) Eosinophilic granuloma (8) Fibrous cortical defect (9) Giant cell tumor

CHONDROSARCOMA

A. PRIMARY CHONDROSARCOMA
B. SECONDARY CHONDROSARCOMA
as a complication of a preexisting skeletal abnormality such as
1. Osteochondroma
2. Enchondroma
3. Parosteal chondroma

Metastases (uncommon) to: lung

CT:
√ chondroid matrix mineralization of "rings and arcs" (CHARACTERISTIC) in 70%
√ nonmineralized portion of tumor hypodense to muscle (high water content of hyaline cartilage)
√ extension into soft-tissues

MR:
√ low to intermediate signal intensity on T1WI
√ high signal intensity on T2WI + hypointense areas (due to mineralization)

Peripheral chondrosarcoma

= EXOSTOTIC CHONDROSARCOMA = malignant degeneration of hereditary multiple exostoses and rarely of a solitary exostosis (beginning in cartilaginous cap of osteochondroma)
Peak age: 5th–6th decade; M:F = 1.5:1
- asymptomatic / pain + swelling (45%)

Location: pelvis, scapula, sternum, ribs, ends of humerus / femur, skull, facial bones

Classification of Chondromalacia Patellae

Grade	Arthroscopic pathology	T1WI of MRI
1	softening + swelling of articular cartilage	focal hypointense areas not extending to cartilage surface / subcondral bone
2	blistering of articular cartilage producing deformity of surface	focal hypointense areas extending to cartilage surface with preservation of sharp cartilage margins
3	surface irregularity + cartilage fibrillation with minimal extension to subchondral bone ("brush-border sign")	focal hypointense areas extending to articular surface but not to osseous surface; loss of sharp dark margin between articular cartilage of patella + trochlea
4	ulceration with exposure of subchondral bone	focal hypointense areas extending from subchondral bone to cartilage surface; cartilage thinned to subchondral bone

√ unusually large soft-tissue mass attached to bone
√ flocculent / streaky chondroid calcification (CHARACTERISTIC)
√ dense radiopaque center with streaks radiating to periphery (not marginated)
√ thickening of cortex at site of attachment
√ late destruction of bone

DDx: (1) Osteochondroma (densely calcified with multiple punctate calcifications)
(2) Parosteal osteosarcoma (more homogeneous density of calcified osteoid)

Central chondrosarcoma

= ENDOSTEAL CHONDROSARCOMA

Incidence: 3rd most common primary bone tumor (1st multiple myeloma, 2nd osteosarcoma)

Histo: arises from chondroblasts (tumor osteoid is never formed)

Age: median 45 years; 50% >40 years; 10% in children (rapidly fatal); M:F = 2:1

• hyperglycemia as paraneoplastic syndrome (85%)

Location: neck of femur, pubic rami, proximal humerus, ribs, skull (sphenoid bone, cerebellopontine angle, mandible), sternum, spine (3–12%)

Site: central + meta- / diaphysis

√ expansile osteolytic lesion 1 to several cm in size
√ short transition zone ± sclerotic margin (well defined from host bone)
√ ± small irregular punctate / snowflake type of calcification; single / multiple
√ late: loss of definition + break through cortex
√ endosteal cortical thickening, sometimes at a distance from the tumor
√ presence of large soft-tissue mass

DDx: benign enchondroma, osteochondroma, osteosarcoma, fibrosarcoma

Clear cell chondrosarcoma

◊ Usually mistaken for chondroblastoma because of low grade malignancy (may be related)!

Histo: small lobules of tissue composed of cells with centrally filled vesicular nuclei surrounded by large clear cytoplasm

Age: 19–68 years, predominantly after epiphyseal fusion

Location: proximal femur, proximal humerus, proximal ulna, lamina vertebrae (5%); pubic ramus

Site: epiphysis

√ single lobulated oval / round sharply marginated lesion of 1–2 cm in size
√ surrounding increased bone density
√ aggressive rapid growth over 3 cm
√ may contain calcifications
√ bone often enlarged
√ indistinguishable from conventional chondrosarcoma / chondroblastoma (slow growth over years)

Extraskeletal chondrosarcoma

Incidence: 2% of all soft-tissue sarcomas

1. **Myxoid extraskeletal chondrosarcoma** (most common)

Histo: surrounded by fibrous capsule + divided into multiple lobules by fibrous septa; delicate strands of small elongated chondroblasts are suspended in an abundant myxoid matrix; foci of mature hyaline cartilage are rare

Mean age: 50 years (range 4–92 years); M > F

• slowly growing soft-tissue mass
• pain + tenderness (33%)

◊ Metastatic in 40–45% at time of presentation!

Location: extremities (thigh most common)

Site: deep soft tissues; subcutis (25%)

√ lobulated soft-tissue mass WITHOUT calcification / ossification
√ usually between 4 and 7 cm in diameter

MR:
√ approximately equal to muscle on T1WI + equal to fat on T2WI
√ may mimic a cyst / myxoma

Prognosis: 45% 10-year survival rate; 5–15 years survival after development of metastases

2. **Extraskeletal mesenchymal chondrosarcoma**

50% of all mesenchymal chondrosarcomas arise in soft tissues

Histo: proliferation of small primitive mesenchymal cells with scattered islands of cartilage; hemangiopericytoma-like vascular pattern

Bimodal age distribution: M = F
(a) tumors of head + neck in 3rd decade (common): meninges, periorbital region
(b) tumors of thigh + trunk in 5th decade

• frequently metastasized to lungs + lymph nodes

√ matrix mineralization (50–100%) characterized as rings + arcs / flocculent + stippled calcification / dense mineralization

MR:
√ approximately equal to muscle on T1WI + equal to fat on T2WI
√ signal voids from calcifications
√ homogeneous enhancement

Prognosis: 25% 10-year survival rate

CLEIDOCRANIAL DYSOSTOSIS

= CLEIDOCRANIAL DYSPLASIA = MUTATIONAL DYSOSTOSIS

= delayed ossification of midline structures (particularly of membranous bone)

Autosomal dominant disease

@ Skull
• large head
√ diminished / absent ossification of skull (in early infancy)
√ wormian bones
√ widened fontanelles + sutures with delayed closure
√ persistent metopic suture
√ brachycephaly + prominent bossing

√ large mandible
√ high narrow palate (± cleft)
√ hypoplastic paranasal sinuses
√ delayed / defective dentition

@ Chest
√ hypoplasia / absence (10%) of clavicles (defective development usually of lateral portion, R > L (DDx: congenital pseudarthrosis of clavicle)
√ thorax may be narrowed + bell-shaped
√ supernumerary ribs
√ incompletely ossified sternum
√ hemivertebrae, spondylosis (frequent)

@ Pelvis
√ delayed ossification of bones forming symphysis pubis (DDx: bladder exstrophy)
√ hypoplastic iliac bones

@ Extremities
√ radius short / absent
√ elongated second metacarpals
√ pseudoepiphyses of metacarpal bases
√ short hypoplastic distal phalanges of hand
√ pointed terminal tufts
√ coned epiphyses
√ coxa vara = deformed / absent femoral necks
√ accessory epiphyses in hands + feet (common)

OB-US:
√ cephalopelvic disproportion (large fetal head + narrow birth canal of affected maternal pelvis) necessitates cesarean section

COCCIDIOIDOMYCOSIS

Histo: chronic granulomatous process in bones, joints, periarticular structures

Location: (a) bones: most frequently in metaphyses of long bones + medial end of clavicle, spine, ribs, pelvis / bony prominences of patella, tibial tuberosity, calcaneus, olecranon, acromion
(b) weight-bearing joints (33%): knee, ankle, wrist, elbow
• "desert rheumatism"
(c) tenosynovitis of hand, bursitis

√ focal areas of destruction, formation of cavities (early) = bubbly bone lesion
√ bone sclerosis surrounding osteolysis (later, rare)
√ proliferation of overlying periosteum
√ destruction of vertebra with preservation of disk space
√ psoas abscess indistinguishable from tuberculosis, may calcify
√ joints rarely infected (usually monarticular from direct extension of osteomyelitic focus): synovial effusion, osteopenia, joint space narrowing, bone destruction, ankylosis
√ soft-tissue abscesses common

DDx: tuberculosis

CONGENITAL INSENSITIVITY TO PAIN WITH ANHYDROSIS

= rare autosomal recessive disorder presumably on the basis of abnormal neural crest development

Age: presenting at birth
Incidence: 15 reported cases
Path: absence of dorsal + sympathetic ganglia, deficiency of neural fibers <6 μm in diameter + disproportionate number of fibers of 6–10 μm in diameter

• history of painless injuries + burns (DDx: familial dysautonomia, congenital sensory neuropathy, hereditary sensory radicular neuropathy, acquired sensory neuropathy, syringomyelia)
• abnormal pain + temperature perception
• burns, bruises, infections are common
• biting injuries of fingers, lips, tongue
• absence of sweating
• mental retardation

CRITERIA: (1) defect must be present at birth
(2) general insensitivity to pain
(3) general mental / physical retardation

√ epiphyseal separation in infancy (epiphyseal injuries result in growth problems)
√ metaphyseal fractures in early childhood
√ diaphyseal fractures in late childhood
√ Charcot joints = neurotrophic joints (usually weight-bearing joints) with effusions + synovial thickening
√ ligamentous laxity
√ bizarre deformities + gross displacement + considerable hemorrhage (unnoticed fractures + dislocations)
√ osteomyelitis + septic arthritis may occur + progress extensively

DDx: (1) sensory neuropathies (eg, diabetes mellitus), (2) hysteria, (3) syphilis, (4) mental deficiency, (5) syringomyelia, (6) organic brain disease

CORNELIA DE LANGE SYNDROME

= Amsterdam dwarfism
• mental retardation (IQ <50)
• hirsutism; hypoplastic genitalia
• feeble growling cry
• high forehead; short neck
• arched palate
• bushy eyebrows meeting in midline + long curved eyelashes
• small nose with depressed bridge; upward tilted nostrils; excessive distance between nose + upper lip

√ small + brachycephalic skull
√ hypoplasia of long bones (upper extremity more involved)
√ forearm bones may be absent
√ short radius + elbow dislocation
√ thumbs placed proximally (hypoplastic 1st metacarpal)
√ short phalanges + clinodactyly of 5th finger

CORTICAL DESMOID

= AVULSIVE CORTICAL IRREGULARITY
= PERIOSTEAL / SUBPERIOSTEAL DESMOID
= SUBPERIOSTEAL / CORTICAL ABRASION
= SUBPERIOSTEAL CORTICAL DEFECT
= rare fibrous lesion of the periosteum

Age: peak 14–16 years (range of 3–17 years); M:F = 3:1

Histo: shallow defect filled with proliferating fibroblasts, multiple small fragments of resorbing bone (microavulsions) at tendinous insertions

- no localizing signs / symptoms

Location: posteromedial aspect of medial femoral epicondyle along medial ridge of linea aspera at attachment of adductor magnus aponeurosis; 1/3 bilateral

√ area of cortical thickening
√ 1–2 cm irregular, shallow, concave saucerlike crater with sharp margin
√ lamellated periosteal reaction
√ localized cortical hyperostosis proximally (healing phase)
◊ May be confused with a malignant tumor (eg, osteosarcoma) / osteomyelitis!

CRI-DU-CHAT SYNDROME

= deletion of short arm of 5th chromosome (5 p)

- generalized dwarfism due to marked growth retardation
- failure to thrive
- peculiar high-pitched cat cry (hypoplastic larynx)
- antimongoloid palpebral fissures
- strabismus
- profound mental retardation
- round facies
- low set ears

Associated with: congenital heart disease (obtain CXR!)

√ agenesis of corpus callosum
√ microcephaly
√ hypertelorism
√ small mandible
√ faulty long-bone development
√ short 3rd, 4th, 5th metacarpals
√ long 2nd, 3rd, 4th, 5th proximal phalanges
√ horseshoe kidney

Dx: made clinically

CROUZON DISEASE

= CRANIOFACIAL SYNOSTOSIS / DYSOSTOSIS
= Apert syndrome without syndactyly
= characterized by skull + cranial base deformities secondary to craniosynostosis, maxillary hypoplasia, shallow orbits, ocular proptosis

Prevalence: 1:25,000

Etiology: autosomal dominant inheritance (in 67%)

- parrot-beak nose
- strabismus
- deafness
- mental retardation
- dental abnormalities

√ acro(oxy)cephaly / brachycephaly / scaphocephaly / trigonocephaly / "cloverleaf" skull (premature craniosynostosis)
√ hypertelorism + exophthalmos
√ hypoplastic maxilla (relative prominence of mandible)

OB-US:

√ cloverleaf appearance (coronal view) + bilateral frontal indentations (axial view) of skull
√ increased interorbital distance + ocular proptosis
√ mild ventriculomegaly

CRUCIATE LIGAMENT INJURY

A. COMPLETE TEAR
√ failure to identify ligament
√ amorphous areas of high signal intensity on T1WI + T2WI with inability to define ligamentous fibers
√ focal discrete complete disruption of all visible fibers

B. PARTIAL / INTRASUBSTANCE TEAR
√ abnormal signal intensity within substance of ligament with some intact + some discontinuous fibers

Anterior cruciate ligament injury (ACL)

◊ If the ACL appears intact in one of the sagittal oblique sequences discordant findings in other sequences can be disregarded!

Site: intrasubstance tear near insertion of femoral condyle (frequently); bone avulsion (rarely)

√ hyperintense signal (= focal fluid collection / soft-tissue edema) replacing the tendon substance in acute tear
√ mass (hematoma + torn fibers) in intercondylar notch near femoral attachment
√ concavity of anterior margin of ligament

Indirect findings:

◊ The indirect signs of ACL injury have a low sensitivity but high specificity!
√ bone bruise in lateral compartment (posterolateral tibia + mid lateral femur) in >50%
√ deepening of lateral femoral sulcus >1.5 mm
√ posterior displacement of posterior horn of lateral meniscus >3.5 mm behind tibial plateau
√ anterior translation of tibia (= anterior drawer sign)
√ PCL bowing = angle between proximal + distal limbs of PCL <105°

False-positive Dx:

(1) slice thickness / interslice gap too great
(2) adjacent fluid / synovial proliferation
(3) cruciate ganglion / synovial cyst

Associated injuries:

meniscal tear (lateral > medial) in 65%

Chronic ACL tear

√ often complete absence of ligament
√ bridging fibrous scar within intercondylar notch (simulating an intact ligament)

Partial ACL tear (15%)

◊ Extremely difficult to diagnose! 40–50% of partial tears are missed on MR!

- positive Lachman test (in 12–30%)

√ MR primary signs positive for injury (in 33–43%)

Posterior cruciate ligament injury (PCL)

Prevalence: 2–23% of all knee injuries

√ midsubstance of PCL most frequently involved (best seen on sagittal images)
√ bone avulsion from posterior tibial insertion (<10%), best seen on lateral plain film

Mechanism:
(1) Direct blow to proximal anterior tibia with knee flexed (dashboard accident)
√ midsubstance PCL tear
√ injury to posterior joint capsule
√ bone contusion at anterior tibial plateau + femoral condyles farther posteriorly
(2) Hyperextension of knee
√ avulsion of tibial attachment of PCL (with preservation of PCL substance)
√ ± ACL rupture
√ bone contusion in anterior tibial plateau + anterior aspect of femoral condyles
(3) Severe ab-/adduction + rotational forces
√ + injury to collateral ligaments

Associated with: coexistent ligamentous injury in 70%

anterior cruciate ligament	27–38%
medial collateral ligament	20–23%
lateral collateral ligament	6–7%
medial meniscal tear	32–35%
lateral meniscal tear	28–30%
bone marrow injury	35–36%
effusion	64–65%

◊ In 30% of cases injury of PCL is isolated!
• posterior tibial laxity
• difficult to evaluate arthroscopically unless ACL torn

DERMATOMYOSITIS

= POLYMYOSITIS
= inflammatory myopathy of unknown etiology with diffuse nonsuppurative inflammation of striated muscle
Pathophysiology: damaged chondroitin sulfate no longer inhibits calcification
Path: atrophy of muscle bundles followed by edema and coagulation necrosis, fibrosis, calcification
Histo: mucoid degeneration with round cell infiltrates concentrated around blood vessels
Age: bimodal: 5–15 and 50–60 years; M:F = 1:2
• elevated muscle enzymes (creatinine kinase, aldolase)
• myositis-specific autoantibodies: anti-Jo-1
(a) anti-aminoacyl-tRNA synthetase
• arthritis, Raynaud phenomenon, fever, fatigue
• interstitial lung disease
Prognosis: requires prolonged treatment
(b) anti-Mi-2 antibodies:
• V-shaped chest rash (= shawl rash)
• cuticular overgrowth
Prognosis: good response to medication
(c) anti-signal recognition particle antibodies
• abrupt onset myositis ± heart involvement

@ Skeleton
√ linear + confluent calcifications in soft tissues of extremities (quadriceps, deltoid, calf muscles), elbows, knees, hands, abdominal wall, chest wall, axilla, inguinal region) in 75%
√ pointing + resorption of terminal tufts
√ rheumatoid-like arthritis (rare)
√ "floppy-thumb" sign
Cx: flexion contractures; soft-tissue ulceration

@ Chest
• respiratory muscle weakness
√ disseminated pulmonary infiltrates (reminiscent of scleroderma)

@ Myocardium
√ changes similar to skeletal muscle

@ GI tract
• dysphagia
√ atony + dilatation of esophagus
√ atony of small intestines + colon

ACUTE FORM
• fever, joint pain, lymphadenopathy, splenomegaly, subcutaneous edema
Prognosis: death within a few months

CHRONIC FORM
= insidious onset with periods of spontaneous remission and relapse
• low-grade fever, muscular aches + pains, edema
• muscle weakness (due to active inflammation, necrosis, muscle atrophy with fatty replacement, steroid-induced myopathy)
◊ first symptom in 50%
• skin erythema: heliotrope rash (= dusky erythema of eyelids) with periorbital edema, Gottron sign (= scaly erythematous papules of knuckles, major joints and upper body)
◊ first symptom in 25%

Cx: high incidence of malignant neoplasms in GI tract, lung, kidney, ovary, breast
Dx: muscle biopsy (normal in up to 15%)

DEVELOPMENTAL DYSPLASIA OF HIP (DDH)

= CONGENITAL DYSPLASIA OF HIP
= abnormal laxity of ligaments + joint capsule resulting in dislocation / subluxation / dysplasia irrespective of prenatal (congenital) or postnatal onset
Etiology:
(a) mechanical:
— oligohydramnios (restricted space in utero)
— firstborn (tight maternal musculature)
— breech position (hyperflexion of hip results in shortening of iliopsoas muscle; L > R)
(b) physiologic:
— maternal estrogen (not inactivated by immature fetal liver) blocking cross-linkage of collagen fibrils

Incidence: 0.15% of neonates
Increased risk:
(1) infants born in frank breech position (25%; risk of breech:vertex = 6:1)
(2) congenital torticollis (10%)
(3) skull-molding deformities, neuromuscular disorders (eg, myelodysplasia)
(4) family history of DDH (6%): 6% risk for subsequent sibling of normal parents, 36% risk for subsequent sibling of one affected parent; 12% risk for patient's own children
(5) foot deformities [metatarsus adductus, clubfoot](2%)

Increased prevalence: females, firstborns (60%), pregnancy with oligohydramnios

Age: most dislocations probably occur after birth; M:F = 1:4 – 1:8; Caucasians > Blacks

Classification:

Type 1 = DISLOCATABLE UNSTABLE HIP

Incidence: 0.25–0.85% of all newborn infants; 2/3 are firstborns

√ slight increase in femoral anteversion
√ mild marginal abnormalities in acetabular cartilage
√ early labral eversion

Prognosis: 60% will become stable after 1 week; 88% will become stable by age of 2 months

Type 2 = SUBLUXED HIP

√ loss of femoral head sphericity
√ increased femoral anteversion
√ early labral inversion
√ shallow acetabulum

Type 3 = DISLOCATED HIP

√ accentuated flattening of femoral head
√ shallow acetabulum
√ limbus formation (= inward growth + hypertrophy of labrum)

- positive Ortolani (reduction) test = reduction of proximal femur into the acetabulum by progressive abduction of flexed hips ± associated with audible "click"
- positive Barlow (dislocation) test = displacement of proximal femur by progressive adduction with downward pressure on flexed hips
- Alli sign = Galeazzi sign = affected knee is lower with knees bent in supine position
- asymmetric skin folds + shortening of thigh on dislocated side
- Trendelenburg test = visible drooping + shortening on dislocated side with child standing on both feet, then one foot

Location: left:right:bilateral = 11:1:4

Radiologic lines:

1. Line of Hilgenreiner
   = line connecting superolateral margins of triradiate cartilages
2. Acetabular angle / index
   = slope of acetabular roof = angle that lies between Hilgenreiner's line and a line drawn from most superolateral ossified edge of acetabulum to superolateral margin of triradiate cartilage
   √ >30° strongly suggests dysplasia
3. Perkin's line
   = vertical line to Hilgenreiner's line through the lateral rim of acetabulum
4. Shenton's curved line
   = arc formed by inferior surface of superior pubic ramus (= top of obturator foramen) + medial surface of proximal femoral metaphysis to level of lesser trochanter
   √ disruption of line (DDx: coxa valga)
5. Center-edge angle
   = angle subtended by one line drawn from the acetabular edge to center of femoral head + second line perpendicular to line connecting centers of femoral heads
   √ <25° suggests femoral head instability

Sonographic Hip Types

Type	Description	alpha- / beta angle	
1	mature hip	>60°	
1A	narrow cartilaginous roof		<55°
1B	wide cartilagenous roof		>55°
2	deficient bony acetabulum		
2A	physiologic <3 months	50 – 59°	
2B	delayed ossification >3 months		
2C	concentric but unstable; *critical range*	43 – 49°	70 – 77°
2D	decentered = subluxed		>77°
3	eccentric = dislocated	<43°	
4	severe dysplasia with inverted labrum		

(1) **alpha angle** = angle between straight lateral edge of ilium + bony acetabular margin (on coronal view); determines sonographic hip type

(2) **beta angle** = angle between straight lateral edge of ilium + fibrocartilaginous acetabulum; determines nuances of sonographic hip type

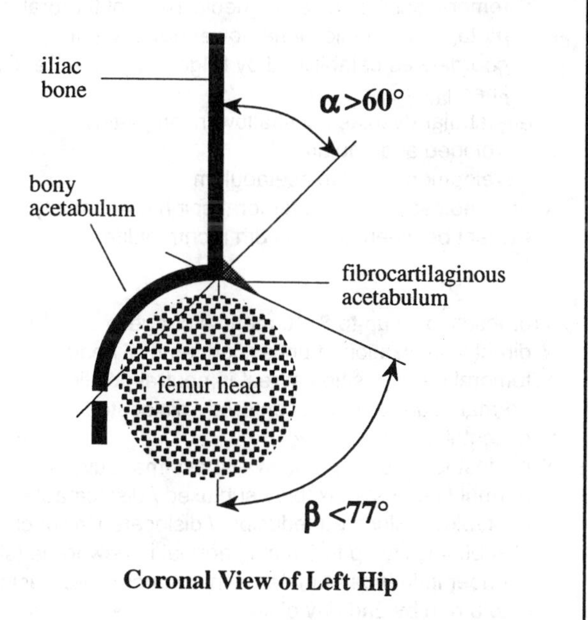

Coronal View of Left Hip

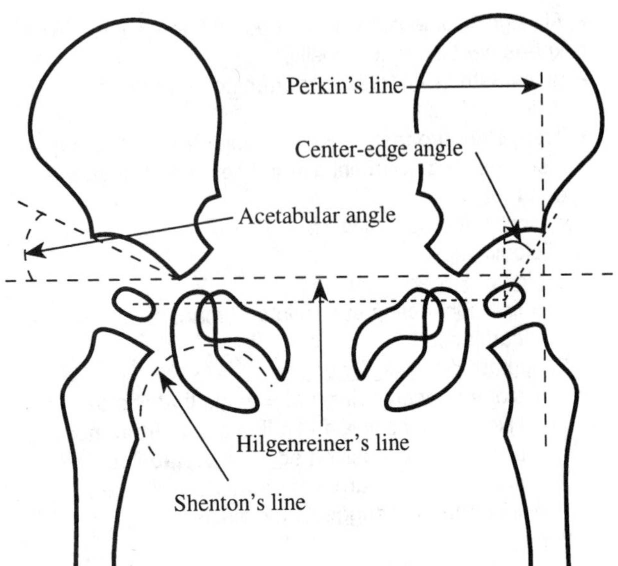

AP pelvic radiograph: >6–8 weeks of age (von Rosen view = legs abducted 45° + thighs internally rotated)
- √ proximal + lateral migration of femur
  - √ eccentric position of femoral epiphysis (position estimated by a circle drawn with a diameter equivalent to width of femoral neck)
  - √ interrupted discontinuous arc of Shenton's line
  - √ line drawn along axis of femoral shaft will not pass through upper edge of acetabulum but intersect the anterior-superior iliac spine (during Barlow maneuver)
  - √ apex of metaphysis lateral to edge of acetabulum
  - √ femoral shaft above horizontal line drawn through the Y-synchondroses
  - √ unilateral shortening of vertical distance from femoral ossific nucleus / femoral metaphysis to Hilgenreiner's line
  - √ femoral ossific nucleus / medial beak of femoral metaphysis outside inner lower quadrant of coordinates established by Hilgenreiner's + Perkin's lines
- √ acetabular dysplasia = shallow incompletely developed acetabulum
- √ development of false acetabulum
- √ delayed ossification of femoral epiphysis (usually evident between 2nd and 8th month of life)

US (practical only up to 8–10 months of age):
- √ direct visualization of unossified femoral head
- √ femoral head position at rest in neutral position: normal / subluxed = decentered / dislocated = eccentric
- √ hip instability under motion + stress maneuvers: normal / lax = subluxable / subluxed / dislocatable = unstable / dislocated reducible / dislocated irreducible
  - ◊ subluxability up to 6 mm is normal in newborns (still under influence of maternal hormones); decreasing to 3 mm by 2nd day of life
  - ◊ examination should be performed >2 weeks of age!
- √ dislocatable (= concentric but unstable) hip can be pushed out of hip joint (Barlow positive) by "piston" maneuver (= pushing / pulling in AP direction with hip flexed)
- √ posterior + superior dislocation of head against ilium
- √ dislocated (= eccentric) hip can be reduced (Ortolani positive)
- √ hypoechoic femoral head not centered over triradiate cartilage between pubis + ischium (on transverse view)
- √ increased amount of soft-tissue echoes ("pulvinar") between femoral head and acetabulum
- √ cartilaginous acetabular labrum interposed between head and acetabulum (inverted labrum)
- √ disparity in presence + size of ossific nucleus
- √ disparity in size of femoral head
- √ equator sign = <50% of femoral head lies medial to line drawn along iliac bone (on coronal view); 58% to 33% coverage is indeterminate, <33% coverage is abnormal
- √ delayed ossification of acetabular corner
- √ wavy contour of bony acetabulum with only slight curvature
- √ abnormally acute <u>alpha angle</u> (= angle between straight lateral edge of ilium + bony acetabular margin)
  - ◊ 4°–6° interobserver variation!

Prognosis: alpha-angle <50° at birth / 50° - 59° after 3 months indicates significant risk for dislocation without treatment; follow-up at 4-week intervals are recommended

CT:
<u>sector angle</u> = angle between line drawn from center of femoral head to acetabular rim + horizontal axis of pelvis (= reflection of acetabular support)
- √ anterior acetabular sector angle <50°
- √ posterior acetabular sector angle <90°

Cx:
(1) Avascular necrosis of femoral head
(2) Intra-articular obstacle to reduction
 (a) pulvinar = fibrofatty tissue at apex of acetabulum
 (b) hypertrophy of ligamentum teres
 (c) labral hypertrophy / inversion
(3) Extra-articular obstacle to reduction
 (a) iliopsoas tendon impingement on anterior joint capsule with infolding of joint capsule

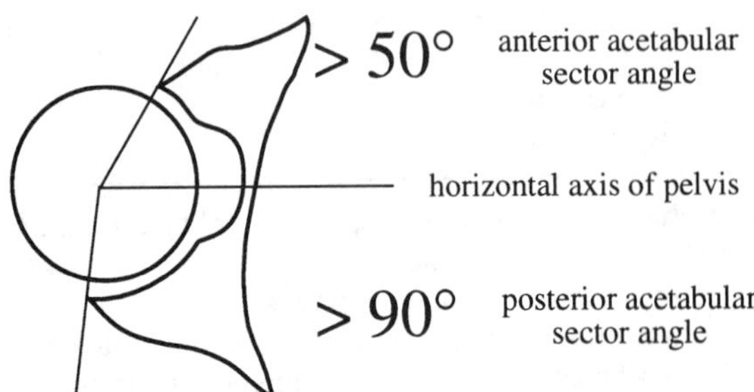

Acetabular sector angles (in normal right hip)

Rx: (1) Flexion-abduction-external rotation brace (Pavlik harness) / splint / spica cast
(2) Femoral varus osteotomy
(3) Pelvic (Salter) / acetabular rotation
(4) Increase in acetabular depth (Pemberton)
(5) Medialization of femoral head (Chiari)

DESMOPLASTIC FIBROMA

= INTRAOSSEOUS DESMOID TUMOR
= rare locally aggressive benign neoplasm of bone with borderline malignancy resembling soft-tissue desmoids / musculoaponeurotic fibromatosis

Incidence: 107 cases in world literature
Histo: intracellular collagenous material in fibroblasts with small nuclei
Age: mean of 21 years (range 15 months to 75 years); in 90% <30 years; M:F = 1:1

• slowly progressive pain + local tenderness
• palpable mass

Location: mandible (26%), ilium (14%), >50% in long bones (femur [14%], humerus [11%], radius [9%], tibia [7%], clavicle), scapula, vertebra, calcaneus
Site: central meta- / diaphyseal (if growth plate open); may extend into epiphysis with subarticular location (if growth plate closed)

√ geographic (96%) / moth-eaten (4%) bone destruction without matrix mineralization
√ narrow (96%) / poorly defined (4%) zone of transition
√ no marginal sclerosis (94%)
√ residual columns of bone with "pseudotrabeculae" are CLASSIC (91%)
√ bone expansion (89%); may grow to massive size (simulating aneurysmal bone cyst / metastatic renal cell carcinoma)
√ breach of cortex + soft-tissue mass (29%)

Cx: pathologic fracture (9%)
Prognosis: 52% rate of local recurrence
Rx: wide excision
DDx: (1) Giant cell tumor (round rather than oval, may extend into epiphysis + subchondral bone plate)
(2) Fibrous dysplasia (occupies longer bone, contains mineralized matrix, often with sclerotic rim)
(3) Aneurysmal bone cyst (eccentric blowout appearance rather than fusiform)
(4) Chondromyxoid fibroma (eccentric with delicate marginal sclerosis + scalloped border)

DIASTROPHIC DYSPLASIA

= DIASTROPHIC DWARFISM = EPIPHYSEAL DYSOSTOSIS
= autosomal recessive severe rhizomelic dwarfism secondary to generalized disorder of cartilage followed by fibrous scars + ossifications

• diastrophic = "twisted" habitus
• "cauliflower ear" = ear deformity from inflammation of pinna
• laryngomalacia
• lax + rigid joints with contractures
• normal intellectual development

@ Axial skeleton
√ cleft palate (25%)
√ cervical spina bifida occulta
√ hypoplasia of odontoid
√ severe progressive kyphoscoliosis of lumbar spine (not present at birth)
√ narrowed interpedicular space in lumbar spine
√ short + broad bony pelvis
√ posterior tilt of sacrum

@ Extremities
√ severe micromelia (predominantly rhizomelic = humerus + femur shorter than distal long bones
√ widened metaphysis
√ flattened epiphysis (retardation of epiphyseal ossification) with invagination of ossification centers into distal ends of femora
√ multiple joint flexion contractures (notably of major joints)
√ dislocation of one / more large joints (hip, elbow), lateral dislocation of patella
√ coxa vara (common)
√ medially bowed metatarsals
√ clubfoot = severe talipes equinovarus
√ ulnar deviation of hands
√ oval + hypoplastic 1st metacarpal bone + abducted proximally positioned thumb = "hitchhiker's thumb" (CHARACTERISTIC)
√ bizarre carpal bones with supernumerary centers
√ widely spaced fingers

OB-US:
√ proportionately shortened long bones
√ hitchhiker thumb
√ clubfeet
√ joint contractures
√ abnormal spinal curvature

Prognosis: death in infancy (due to abnormal softening of tracheal cartilage)

DIFFUSE IDIOPATHIC SKELETAL HYPEROSTOSIS

= DISH = FORESTIER DISEASE = ANKYLOSING HYPEROSTOSIS
= common ossifying diathesis characterized by bone proliferation at sites of tendinous + ligamentous attachment (enthesis)

Etiology:
(1) may be caused by altered vitamin A metabolism (elevated plasma levels of unbound retinol)
(2) long-term ingestion of retinoid derivatives for dermatologic disorders (eg, Accutane®);
? hypertrophic variant of spondylosis deformans

Age: >50 years; M:F = 3:1

• pain, tenderness in extraspinal locations
• restricted motion of vertebral column
• hyperglycemia
• positive HLA-B27 in 34%

Location: lower thoracic > lower cervical > entire lumbar spine

√ anterior + lateral right-sided osteophytes of vertebral column (not on left because of aorta)

√ disk spaces well preserved, no apophyseal ankylosis, no sacroiliitis
√ flowing ossification along anterior / anterolateral aspect of at least 4 contiguous vertebral bodies
√ "whiskering" at iliac crest, ischial tuberosity, trochanters
√ spurs of olecranon process of ulna + calcaneus (plantar + posterior surface) + anterior surface of patella
√ broad osteophytes at lateral acetabular edge, inferior portions of sacroiliac joints, superior aspect of symphysis pubis
√ ossification of iliolumbar + sacrotuberous + sacroiliac ligaments (high probability for presence of spinal DISH, DDx: fluorosis)
√ ossification of coracoclavicular ligament, patellar ligament, tibial tuberosity, interosseous membranes
√ increased incidence of hyperostosis frontalis interna

DDx: (1) Fluorosis (increased skeletal density)
(2) Acromegaly (posterior scalloping, skull features)
(3) Hypoparathyroidism
(4) X-linked hypophosphatemic vitamin D–resistant rickets
(5) Ankylosing spondylitis (squaring of vertebral bodies, coarser syndesmophytes, sacroiliitis, apophyseal alteration)
(6) Intervertebral osteochondrosis (vacuum phenomenon, vertebral body marginal sclerosis, decreased intervertebral disk height)

DISLOCATION

Hip dislocation

Incidence: 5% of all dislocations

A. POSTERIOR HIP DISLOCATION (80–85%)
Mechanism: classical dashboard injury (= flexed knee strikes dashboard)
Associated with: fractures of posterior rim of acetabulum, femoral head

B. ANTERIOR HIP DISLOCATION (5–10%)
1. anterior obturator dislocation
2. superoanterior / pubic hip dislocation
Associated with: fractures of acetabular rim, greater trochanter, femoral neck, femoral head (characteristic depression on posterosuperior and lateral portion)

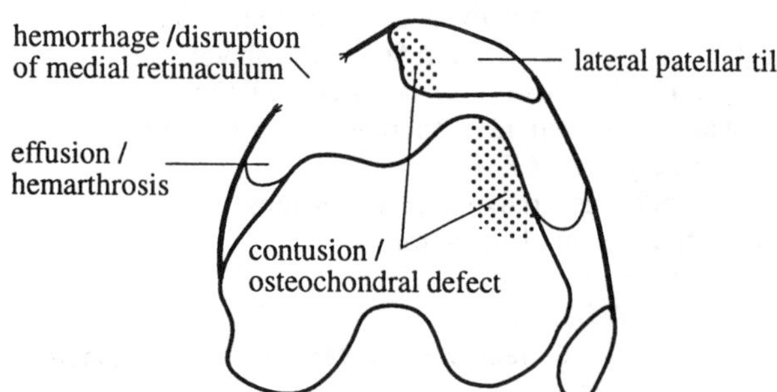

MR Imaging Signs of Patellar Dislocation

C. CENTRAL ACETABULAR FRACTURE-DISLOCATION
Mechanism: force applied to lateral side of trochanter

Patellar dislocation

= TRANSIENT LATERAL PATELLAR DISLOCATION

Incidence: 2–3% of all knee injuries
Mechanism: during attempt to slow forward motion while pivoting medially on a planted foot; internal rotation of femur and quadriceps contraction produces a net lateral force
Associated with: medial meniscal tear / major ligamentous injury in 31%
Age: young physically active people

• hemarthrosis (most common cause of hemarthrosis in young conscripts)
• swelling + tenderness of medial retinaculum

◊ >50% not clinically diagnosed initially!

√ increased signal intensity / thickening / disruption of medial patellar retinaculum
√ lateral patellar tilt
√ contusion / microfracture / osteochondral injury of nonarticular surface of lateral femoral condyle + medial articular surface of patella
√ hemarthrosis

Rx: (1) Temporary immobilization + rehabilitation: successful in 75%
(2) Surgery: fixation of osteochondral fragments, medial capsule repair, lateral retinacular release, vastus medialis et lateralis rearrangement, medial retinaculum reefing

Shoulder dislocation

Sternoclavicular dislocation (3%)
Acromioclavicular dislocation (12%)
Glenohumeral dislocation (85%)

◊ Glenohumeral joint dislocations make up >50% of all dislocations!

A. ANTERIOR / SUBCORACOID SHOULDER DISLOCATION (96%)
Types: subcoracoid, subglenoid, subclavicular, intrathoracic
Mechanism: external rotation + abduction; 40% recurrent
Age: in younger individuals
May be associated with:
√ fracture of greater tuberosity (15%)
√ Bankart lesion = fracture of anterior glenoid rim (originally only referring to injury of anterior band of glenohumeral ligament)
√ fracture of anterior rim of glenoid
√ Hill-Sachs defect (50%) = depression fracture of posterolateral surface of humeral head at / above level of coracoid process (impaction against glenoid rim in subglenoid type)

B. POSTERIOR SHOULDER DISLOCATION (2–4%)
Cause: (a) traumatic: convulsive disorders / electric shock therapy
(b) nontraumatic: voluntary, involuntary, congenital, developmental

Types: subacromial, subglenoid, subspinous
◊ In >50% unrecognized initially + subsequently misdiagnosed as frozen shoulder!
◊ Average interval between injury and diagnosis is 1 year!
√ rim sign (66%) = distance between medial border of humeral head + anterior glenoid rim <6 mm

May be associated with:
√ trough sign (75%) = "reverse Hill-Sachs" = compression fracture of anteromedial humeral head (tangential Grashey view of glenoid!)
√ fracture of posterior glenoid rim
√ avulsion fracture of lesser tuberosity

C. INFERIOR SHOULDER DISLOCATION (1–2%)
= LUXATIO ERECTA = extremity held over head in fixed position with elbow flexed
Mechanism: severe hyperabduction of arm resulting in impingement of humeral head against acromion
√ humeral articular surface faces inferiorly
Cx: rotator cuff tear; fracture of acromion ± inferior glenoid fossa ± greater tuberosity; neurovascular injury

D. SUPERIOR SHOULDER DISLOCATION (<1%)
= humeral head driven upward through rotator cuff
May be associated with: fracture of humerus, clavicle, acromion

DDx: drooping shoulder (transient phenomenon after fracture of surgical neck of humerus due to hemarthrosis / muscle imbalance)

Wrist dislocation

Mechanism: fall on outstretched hand
Incidence: 10% of all carpal injuries

A. LUNATE DISLOCATION

B. PERILUNATE DISLOCATION
2–3 times more common than lunate dislocation accompanied by fracture in 75% (= transscaphoid perilunate dislocation)
√ most commonly dorsal dislocation

C. ROTARY SUBLUXATION OF SCAPHOID
= tearing of interosseous ligaments of lunate, scaphoid, capitate
Mechanism: acute dorsiflexion of wrist; may be associated with rheumatoid arthritis
√ gap >4 mm between scaphoid + lunate (PA view)
√ foreshortening of scaphoid
√ ring sign of distal pole of scaphoid

D. MIDCARPAL DISLOCATION

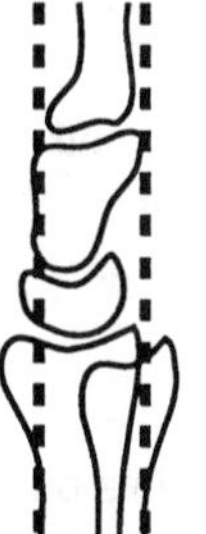
Normal

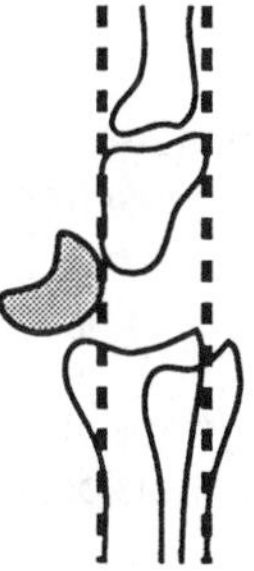
Lunate Dislocation

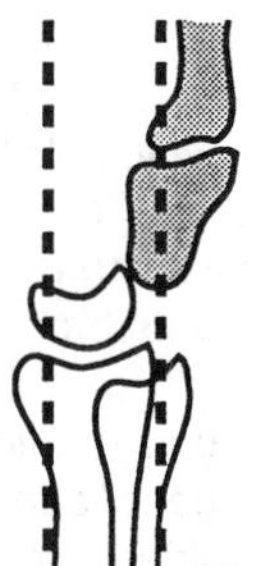
Perilunate Dislocation

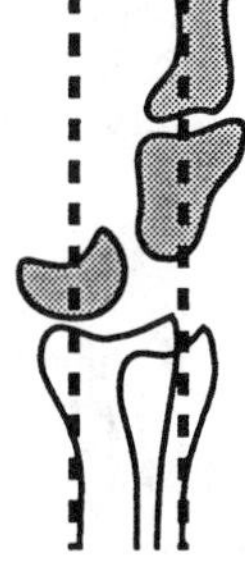
Midcarpal Dislocation

DOWN SYNDROME

= MONGOLISM = TRISOMY 21 (95% nondisjunction, 5% translocation)

Incidence: 1:870 liveborn infants, most common karyotype / chromosomal abnormality in U.S.

- mental retardation
- characteristic facies
- hypotonia in infancy
- Simian crease

@ Skull
√ hypotelorism
√ persistent metopic suture (40–79%) after age 10
√ hypoplasia of sinuses + facial bones
√ microcrania (brachycephaly)
√ delayed closure of sutures + fontanelles
√ dental abnormalities (underdeveloped tooth No. 2)
√ flat-bridged nose

@ Axial skeleton
√ atlantoaxial subluxation (25%)
√ anterior scalloping of vertebral bodies
√ "squared vertebral bodies" = centra high and narrow = positive lateral lumbar index (ratio of horizontal to vertical diameters of L2)

@ Chest
√ congenital heart disease (40%): endocardial cushion defect, VSD, tetralogy of Fallot
√ hypersegmentation of manubrium = 2–3 ossification centers (90%)
√ gracile ribs; 11 pairs of ribs (25%)

@ Pelvis
√ flaring of iliac wings (decreased iliac angle + index) = "Mickey Mouse ears" / "elephant ears"
√ flattening of acetabular roof (decreased acetabular angle)
√ tapering of ischial rami

@ Extremities
√ metaphyseal flaring
√ clinodactyly (50%); widened space between first two digits of hands + feet
√ hypoplastic and triangular middle + distal phalanges of 5th finger = acromicria (DDx: normal individuals, cretins, achondroplastic dwarfs)
√ pseudoepiphyses of 1st + 2nd metacarpals

@ Gastrointestinal
√ umbilical hernia
√ "double bubble" sign (8–10%) = duodenal atresia / stenosis / annular pancreas
√ tracheoesophageal fistula
√ anorectal anomalies
√ Hirschsprung disease

OB-US:
- triple-marker screening test:
  - low maternal alpha-fetoprotein (20–30%)
  - increased HCG (DDx: decreased in trisomy 18)
  - decreased unconjugated estriol (ue3)

- advanced maternal age
  - ◊ in 1:385 livebirths for women >35 years of age
  - ◊ HOWEVER: 80% of fetuses with Down syndrome are born to mothers <35 years of age
- √ occipital-nuchal skin thickening ≥6 mm during 19–24 weeks (in 45–80%) / ≥5 mm during 14–18 weeks on transcerebellar diameter view (69% positive predictive value, 0.5% false positives)
- √ ratio of measured-to-expected femur length ≤0.91 [expected femur length: -9.3105 + 0.9028 x BPD] (sensitivity 40%, specificity 95%, false-positive rate of 2–7%, 0.3% PPV for low-risk population [1:700], 1% PPV for high-risk population [1:250])
- √ elevated BPD / femur ratio (secondary to short femur)
- √ ratio of measured-to-expected humerus length ≤0.90 [expected humerus length: -7.9404 + 0.8492 x BPD] (1–2% PPV for low-risk population; 3% PPV for high-risk population)
- √ major structural malformations:
  - √ VSD / complete AV canal (50%)
  - √ cystic hygroma, resolved by 20th week MA
  - √ omphalocele
  - √ double bubble of duodenal atresia (8–10%), not apparent before 22 weeks GA
  - √ hydrothorax
  - √ mild cerebral ventricular dilatation
  - √ agenesis of corpus callosum
  - √ imperforate anus
- √ mild fetal pyelectasis (17–25%)
- √ hyperechoic bowel at <20 weeks GA (15%, in 0.6% of normals)
- √ intracardiac echogenic focus, usually in left ventricle = thickening of papillary muscle (18%, in 5% of normals)
- √ sandal-gap deformity = separation of great toe (45%)
- √ hypoplasia of middle phalanx of 5th digit resulting in clinodactyly (= inward curve) in 60%
- √ flared ilium = iliac wings rotated toward coronal plane at SIJ describing an angle of >70° with each other
- √ brachycephaly
- √ small cerebellum
- √ IUGR (in 30%)
- √ polyhydramnios

Cx: leukemia (increased frequency 3–20 x)

DYSCHONDROSTEOSIS

= LÉRI-LAYANI-WEILL SYNDROME = mesomelic long-bone shortening (forearm + leg); autosomal dominant

M:F = 1:4

- limited motion of elbow + wrist
- √ bilateral Madelung deformity
  - √ radial shortening in relation to ulna
  - √ bowing of radius laterally + dorsally
  - √ dorsal subluxation of distal end of ulna
  - √ carpal wedging between radius + ulna (due to triangular shape of distal radial epiphysis + underdevelopment of ulna)

DDx: Pseudo-Madelung deformity (from trauma / infection)

DYSPLASIA EPIPHYSEALIS HEMIMELICA

= TREVOR DISEASE = TARSOEPIPHYSEAL ACLASIS

= eccentric usually medial epiphyseal cartilaginous overgrowth of one / more epiphyses; spontaneous occurrence

Age: 2–4 years; M > F

May be associated with: hemihypertrophy

- limitation of joint mobility (due to localized painless mass)

Location: localized to tarsus, carpus, knee, ankle; occasionally generalized

- √ osteochondroma-like growth from one side of epiphysis

Cx: genu valgum

DDx: osteochondroma

ECHINOCOCCUS OF BONE

Occurs occasionally in the U.S.; usually in foreign-born individuals; bone involvement in 1%

Histo: no connective tissue barrier; daughter cysts extend directly into bone

@ Pelvis, sacrum, rarely long tubular bones
- √ round / irregular regions of rarefaction
- √ multiloculated lesion (bunch of grapes)
- √ no sharp demarcation (DDx: chondroma, giant cell tumor) with secondary infection
  - √ thickening of trabeculae with generalized perifocal condensation
  - √ cortical breakthrough with soft-tissue mass

@ Vertebra
- √ sclerosis without pathologic fracture
- √ intervertebral disks not affected
- √ vertebral lamina often involved
- √ frequently involvement of adjacent ribs

EHLERS-DANLOS SYNDROME

= group of autosomal dominant diseases of connective tissue characterized by abnormal collagen synthesis

Types: 10 types have been described that differ clinically, biochemically, and genetically

Age: present at birth; predominantly in males

- hyperelasticity of skin
- fragile brittle skin with gaping wounds and poor healing
- molluscoid pseudotumors over pressure points
- hyperextensibility of joints
- joint contractures with advanced age
- bleeding tendency (fragility of blood vessels)
- blue sclera, microcornea, myopia, keratoconus, ectopia lentis

@ Soft tissues
- √ multiple ovoid calcifications (2–10 mm) in subcutis / in fatty cysts ("spheroids"), most frequently in periarticular areas of legs
- √ ectopic bone formation

@ Skeleton
- √ hemarthrosis (particularly in knee)
- √ malalignment / subluxation / dislocation of joints on stress radiographs
- √ recurrent dislocations (hip, patella, shoulder, radius, clavicle)
- √ precocious osteoarthrosis (predominantly in knees)

√ ulnar synostosis
√ kyphoscoliosis
√ spondylolisthesis
√ spina bifida occulta

@ Chest
√ diaphragmatic hernia
√ panacinar emphysema + bulla formation
√ tracheobronchomegaly + bronchiectasis

@ Arteries
√ aneurysm of great vessels, aortic dissection, tortuosity of arch, ectasia of pulmonary arteries
◊ AORTOGRAPHY CONTRAINDICATED! (Cx following arteriography: aortic rupture, hematomas)

@ GI tract
√ ectasia of gastrointestinal tract

ELASTOFIBROMA

= benign tumorlike lesion forming as a reaction to mechanical friction

Incidence: in 24% of women + 11% of men >55 years (autopsy study)

Age: elderly; M:F = 1:2

Histo: enlarged irregular serrated elastic hypereosinophilic fibers, collagen, scattered fibroblasts, occasional lobules of adipose tissue

• asymptomatic
• may remain clinically inapparent

Location: between inferior margin of scapula + posterior chest wall; bilateral in 25%

√ inhomogeneous poorly defined lesion of soft-tissue attenuation similar to muscle
√ well-defined intermediate-signal intensity lesion with interlaced areas of fat-intensity signal on T1WI + T2WI

ENCHONDROMA

= benign cartilaginous growth in medullary cavity; bones preformed in cartilage are affected (NOT skull)

Age: 10–30 years; M:F = 1:1

Histo: lobules of hyaline cartilage

• usually asymptomatic, painless swelling

Location: (frequently multiple = enchondromatosis)
(a) in 40% small bones of wrists + hand (most frequent tumor here), distal + mid aspects of metacarpals, proximal / middle phalanges
(b) femur, tibia, humerus, radius, ulna, foot, rib

Site: central + diaphyseal, epiphysis only affected after closure of growth plate

√ oval / round lucency near epiphysis with fine marginal line
√ scalloped endosteum
√ ground-glass appearance
√ calcification: pinhead, stippled, flocculent, "rings and arcs" pattern
√ bulbous expansion of bone with thinning of cortex
√ Madelung deformity = bowing deformities of limb, discrepant length
√ NO cortical breakthrough / periosteal reaction

Cx: (1) pathologic fracture
(2) malignant degeneration in long-bone enchondromas in 15–20%

DDx: (1) Epidermoid inclusion cyst (phalangeal tuft, Hx of trauma, more lucent)
(2) Unicameral bone cyst (rare in hands, more radiolucent)
(3) Giant cell tumor of tendon sheath (commonly erodes bone, soft-tissue mass outside bone)
(4) Fibrous dysplasia (rare in hand, mostly polyostotic)
(5) Bone infarct
(6) Chondrosarcoma

ENCHONDROMATOSIS

= OLLIER DISEASE = DYSCHONDROPLASIA
= MULTIPLE ENCHONDROMATOSIS
= nonhereditary failure of cartilage ossification

Age: early childhood presentation

• growth disparity with leg / arm shortening
• hand + feet deformity

Location: predominantly unilateral monomelic distribution (a) localized (b) regional (c) generalized

√ rounded masses / columnar streaks of decreased density from epiphyseal plate into diaphysis of long bones = cartilaginous rests
√ bony spurs pointing toward the joint (DDx: exostosis points away from it)
√ cartilaginous areas show punctate calcifications with age
√ associated with dwarfing of the involved bone due to impairment of epiphyseal fusion
√ clublike deformity of metaphyseal region
√ cartilaginous metaphyseal expansion with cortical expansion + thinning + breakthrough
√ bowing deformities of limb bones
√ discrepancy in length = Madelung deformity (radius, ulna)
√ small bones of feet + hands: aggressive deforming tumors that may break through cortex secondary to tendency to continue to proliferate
√ fanlike radiation of cartilage from center to crest of ilium

Cx: sarcomatous transformation (in 25–50%): osteosarcoma (young adults); chondro- / fibrosarcoma (in older patients)

Maffucci syndrome

= nonhereditary mesodermal dysplasia characterized by enchondromatosis + multiple soft-tissue cavernous hemangiomas

Age: generally not before puberty; M > F

• multiple nodules particularly on digits + extremities (cavernous hemangiomas)
• normal intelligence

Location: unilateral involvement / marked asymmetry; distinct predilection for hands + feet

√ phleboliths may be present
√ striking tendency for enchondromata to be very large projecting into soft tissues
√ growth disturbance of long bones (common)

Cx: (1) malignant transformation of
(a) enchondroma to chondrosarcoma (15–20%)
(b) soft-tissue hemangioma to vascular sarcoma (in 3–5%)
(2) increased prevalence of ovarian carcinoma, pancreatic carcinoma, CNS glioma

ENGELMANN-CAMURATI DISEASE

= PROGRESSIVE DIAPHYSEAL DYSPLASIA
= ENGELMANN DISEASE = RIBBING DISEASE (as forme fruste)
Autosomal dominant
Age: 5–25 years, M > F
- neuromuscular dystrophy = delayed walking (18–24 months) with wide-based waddling gait; often misdiagnosed as muscular dystrophy / poliomyelitis
- weakness + easy fatigability
- bone pain + tenderness usually in midshaft of long bones
- underdevelopment of muscles secondary to malnutrition
- NORMAL laboratory values

Location: usually symmetrical; NO involvement of hands, feet, ribs, scapulae
@ Skull (initially affected)
√ amorphous increase in density at base of skull
@ Long bones (bilateral symmetrical distribution)
√ fusiform enlargement of diaphyses with cortical thickening (endosteal + periosteal accretion of mottled new bone) and progressive obliteration of medullary cavity; symmetrical involvement
√ progression of lesions along long axis of bone toward either end
√ abrupt demarcation of lesions (metaphyses + epiphyses spared)
√ relative elongation of extremities
√ NORMAL epiphyses + metaphyses

DDx: (1) Chronic osteomyelitis (single bone)
(2) Hyperphosphatasemia (high alkaline phosphatase levels)
(3) Paget disease (age, new-bone formation, increased alkaline phosphatase)
(4) Infantile cortical hyperostosis (fever; mandible, rib, clavicles; regresses, <1 year of age)
(5) Fibrous dysplasia (predominantly unilateral, subperiosteal new bone)
(6) Osteopetrosis (very little bony enlargement)
(7) Vitamin A poisoning

EPIDERMOID INCLUSION CYST

= INTRAOSSEOUS KERATIN CYST = IMPLANTATION CYST
Age: 2nd–4th decade;M > F
Histo: stratified squamous epithelium, keratin, cholesterol crystals (soft white cheesy contents)
- history of trauma (implantation of epithelium under skin with secondary bone erosion)
- asymptomatic

Location: superficially situated bones such as calvarium (typically in frontal / parietal bone), phalanx (usually terminal tuft of middle finger), L > R hand, occasionally in foot
√ well-defined round osteolysis with sclerotic margin
√ cortex frequently expanded + thinned
√ NO calcifications / periosteal reaction / soft-tissue swelling
√ pathologic fracture often without periosteal reaction

DDx: (a) in finger: glomus tumor, enchondroma (rare in terminal phalanx)
(b) in skull: infection, metastasis (poorly defined), eosinophilic granuloma (beveled margin)

EPIPHYSEOLYSIS OF FEMORAL HEAD

= SLIPPED CAPITAL FEMORAL EPIPHYSIS
= atraumatic fracture through hypertrophic zone of physeal plate
Frequency: 2:100,000 people
Etiology: growth spurt, renal osteodystrophy, rickets, childhood irradiation, growth hormone therapy, trauma (Salter-Harris type I epiphyseal injury)
Pathogenesis: widening of physeal plate during growth spurt + change in orientation of physis from horizontal to oblique increases shear forces
Age: overweight 8–17 year old boys (mean age for boys 13, for girls 11 years); M > F; black > white
Associated with:
(a) malnutrition, endocrine abnormality, developmental dysplasia of hip (during adolescence)
(b) delayed skeletal maturation (after adolescence)
- hip pain (50%) / knee pain (25%) for 2–3 weeks

Location: usually unilateral; bilateral in 20–37% (at initial presentation in 9–18%)
√ widening of epiphyseal plate (<u>preslip phase</u>)
√ irregularity + blurring of physeal physis
√ demineralization of neck metaphysis
√ posteromedial displacement of head (<u>acute slip</u>)
√ decrease in neck-shaft angle with alignment change in the growth plate to a more vertical orientation
√ line of Klein (= line drawn along superior edge of femoral neck) fails to intersect the femoral head
√ epiphysis appears smaller due to posterior slippage: early slips are best seen on cross-table LAT view
CAVE: positioning into a frogleg view may cause further displacement
√ sclerosis + irregularity of widened physis (<u>chronic slip</u>)
√ metaphyseal blanch sign = area of increased opacity in proximal part of metaphysis (healing response)

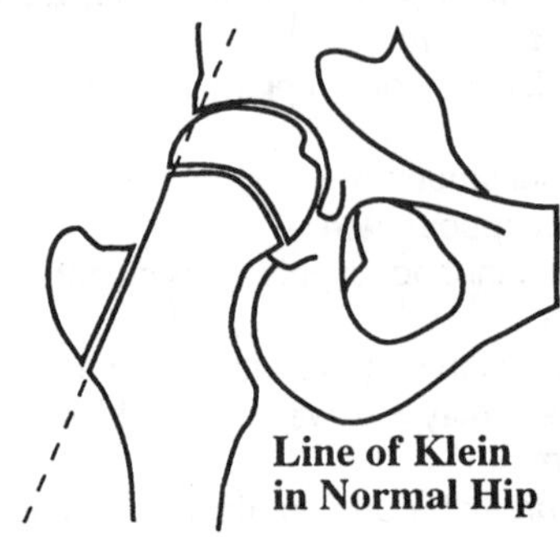
Line of Klein in Normal Hip

Grading (based on femoral head position):

mild	displaced by <1/3 of metaphyseal diameter
moderate	displaced by 1/3–2/3 of diameter
severe	displaced by >2/3 of metaphyseal diameter

Cx: (1) Chondrolysis = acute cartilage necrosis (7–10%) = rapid loss of >50% of thickness of cartilage
√ joint space <3 mm
(2) Avascular necrosis of femoral head (15%) risk increases with advanced degree of slip, delayed surgery for acute slip, anterior pin placement, large number of fixation pins, subcapital osteotomy
(3) Pistol-grip deformity = broadening + shortening of femoral neck in varus deformity
(4) Degenerative osteoarthritis (90%)
(5) Limb-length discrepancy due to premature physeal closure

Rx: (1) limitation of activity, (2) prophylactic pinning
Attempted reductions increase risk of AVN!

ESSENTIAL OSTEOLYSIS

Progressive slow bone-resorptive disease

Histo: proliferation + hyperplasia of smooth muscle cells of synovial arterioles

√ progressive osteolysis of carpal + tarsal bones
√ thinned pointed proximal ends of metacarpals + metatarsals
√ elbows show same type of destruction
√ bathyrocephalic depression of base of skull

DDx: (1) Massive osteolysis = Gorham disease (local destruction of contiguous bones, usually not affecting hands / feet) (2) Tabes dorsalis (3) Leprosy (4) Syringomyelia (5) Scleroderma (6) Raynaud disease (7) Regional posttraumatic osteolysis (8) Ulcero-mutilating acropathy (9) Mutilating forms of rheumatoid arthritis (10) Acrodynia mutilante (nonhereditary)

EWING SARCOMA

= EWING TUMOR

Incidence: 4–10% of all bone tumors (less common than osteo- / chondrosarcoma); most common malignant bone tumor in children

◊ Clinically, radiologically, and histologically very similar to PNET!

Histo:
small round cells, uniformly sized + solidly packed (DDx: lymphoma, osteosarcoma, myeloma, neuroblastoma, carcinoma, eosinophilic granuloma) invading medullary cavity and entering subperiosteum via Haversian canals producing periostitis, soft-tissue mass, osteolysis; glycogen granules present (DDx to reticulum cell sarcoma); absence of alkaline phosphatase (DDx to osteosarcoma)

Age: peak 15 years (range 5 months to 54 years); in 30% <10 years; in 39% 11–15 years; in 31% >15 years; in 50% <20 years; in 95% 4–25 years; M:F = 2:1; Caucasians in 96%

- severe localized pain
- soft-tissue mass
- fever, leukocytosis, anemia (in early metastases) simulating infection

Location:
femur (25%), pelvis-ilium (14%), tibia (11%), humerus (10%), fibula (8%), ribs (6%)
(a) long bones in 60%:
metadiaphysis (44%), middiaphysis (33%), metaphysis (15%), metaepiphyseal (6%), epiphyseal (2%); usually no involvement of epiphysis as tumor originates in medullary cavity with invasion of Haversian system
(b) flat bones in 40%: pelvis, scapula, skull, vertebrae (in 3–10%; sacrum > lumbar > thoracic > cervical spine); ribs (in 7% > age 10; in 30% < age 10)
◊ >20 years of age predominantly in flat bones
◊ <20 years of age predominantly in cylindrical bones (tumor derived from red marrow)

√ 8–10 cm long lytic lesion in shaft of long bone (62% lytic, 23% mixed density, 15% dense)
√ mottled "moth-eaten" destructive permeative lesion (72%) (late finding)
√ penetration into soft tissue (55%) with preservation of tissue planes (DDx: osteomyelitis with diffuse soft-tissue swelling)
√ early fusiform lamellated "onionskin" periosteal reaction (53%) / spiculated = "sunburst" / "hair-on-end" (23%), Codman triangle
√ cortical thickening (16%)
√ cortical destruction (18%)
√ ± cortical sequestration
√ reactive sclerotic new bone (30%)
√ bone expansion (12%)
√ Ewing sarcoma of rib: disproportionately large inhomogeneous soft-tissue mass with large intrathoracic + minimal extrathoracic component

Metastases to: lung, bones, regional lymph nodes in 11–30% at time of diagnosis, in 40–45% within 2 years of diagnosis

Cx: pathologic fracture (5–14%)

Prognosis: 60–75% 5-year survival

DDx: (1) Multiple myeloma (older age group)
(2) Osteomyelitis (duration of pain <2 weeks)
(3) Eosinophilic granuloma (solid periosteal reaction)
(4) Osteosarcoma (ossification in soft tissue, near age 20, no lamellar periosteal reaction)
(5) Reticulum cell sarcoma (clinically healthy, between 30 and 50 years, no glycogen)
(6) Neuroblastoma (< age 5)
(7) Anaplastic metastatic carcinoma (>30 years of age)
(8) Osteosarcoma
(9) Hodgkin disease

EXTRAMEDULLARY HEMATOPOIESIS

= compensatory response to deficient bone marrow blood cell production

Etiology: prolonged erythrocyte deficiency due to
(1) destruction of RBC:
acquired hemolytic anemia, sickle cell anemia, thalassemia, hereditary spherocytosis, idiopathic severe anemia, erythroblastosis fetalis
(2) inability of normal blood-forming organs to produce erythrocytes:
iron deficiency anemia, pernicious anemia, myelofibrosis, myelosclerosis, polycythemia, carcinomatous / lymphomatous replacement of bone marrow (leukemia, Hodgkin disease)
◊ NO hematologic disease in 25%
• absence of pain, bone erosion, calcification
• chronic anemia
Sites: in areas of fetal erythropoiesis
@ spleen, liver, lymph nodes
@ adrenal glands
@ mediastinum, heart, thymus
@ lung
@ renal pelvis
@ gastrointestinal lymphatics
@ dura mater (falx cerebri and over brain convexity)
@ cartilage, broad ligaments
@ thrombi, adipose tissue
√ frequently bilateral paraspinal masses with round + lobulated margins between T8 and T12
√ extramedullary hematopoiesis may compress cord
√ splenomegaly / absent spleen
√ lack of calcification / bone erosion

FAMILIAL IDIOPATHIC ACROOSTEOLYSIS
= HAJDU-CHENEY SYNDROME
= rare bizarre entity of unknown etiology
Location: may be unilateral
• fingernails remain intact
• sensory changes + plantar ulcers rare
√ pseudoclubbing of fingers + toes with osteolysis of terminal + more proximal phalanges
√ genu varum / valgum
√ hypoplasia of proximal end of radius
√ subluxation of radial head
√ scaphocephaly, basilar impression
√ wide sutures, persistent metopic suture, Wormian bones, poorly developed sinuses
√ kyphoscoliosis
√ severe osteoporosis + fractures at multiple sites (esp. of spine)
√ protrusio acetabuli

FANCONI ANEMIA
= autosomal recessive disease with severe hypoplastic anemia + skin pigmentation + skeletal and urogenital anomalies
• skin pigmentation (melanin deposits) in 74% (trunk, axilla, groin, neck)
• anemia onset between 17 months and 22 years of age
• bleeding tendency (pancytopenia)
• hypogonadism (40%)
• microphthalmia (20%)
√ anomalies of radial component of upper extremity (strongly suggestive):
√ absent / hypoplastic / supernumerary thumb
√ hypoplastic / absent radius
√ absent / hypoplastic navicular / greater multangular bone
√ slight / moderate dwarfism
√ minimal microcephaly
√ renal anomalies (30%): renal aplasia, ectopia, horseshoe kidney
Prognosis: fatal within 5 years after onset of anemia; patient's family shows high incidence of leukemia

FARBER DISEASE
= DISSEMINATED LIPOGRANULOMATOSIS
Histo: foam cell granulomas; lipid storage of neuronal tissue (accumulation of ceramide + gangliosides)
• hoarse weak cry
• swelling of extremities; generalized joint swelling
• subcutaneous + periarticular granulomas
• intermittent fever, dyspnea
• lymphadenopathy
√ capsular distension of multiple joints (hand, elbow, knee)
√ juxta-articular bone erosions from soft-tissue granulomas
√ subluxation / dislocation
√ disuse / steroid deossification
Prognosis: death from respiratory failure within 2 years

FIBROCHONDROGENESIS
= autosomal recessive lethal short-limb skeletal dysplasia
Incidence: 5 cases
√ severe micromelia + broad dumbbell-shaped metaphyses
√ flat + clefted pear-shaped vertebral bodies
√ short + cupped ribs
√ frontal bossing
√ low-set abnormally formed ears
Prognosis: stillbirth / death shortly after birth
DDx: (1) Thanatophoric dysplasia
(2) Metatropic dysplasia
(3) Spondyloepiphyseal dysplasia

FIBRODYSPLASIA OSSIFICANS PROGRESSIVA
= MYOSITIS OSSIFICANS PROGRESSIVA (misnomer since primarily connective tissues are affected)
= rare slowly progressive sporadic / autosomal dominant disease with variable penetrance characterized by remissions + exacerbations of fibroblastic proliferation, subsequent calcification + ossification of subcutaneous fat, skeletal muscle, tendons, aponeuroses, ligaments
Histo: edema with proliferating fibroblasts in a loose myxoid matrix; subsequent collagen deposition plus calcification + ossification of collagenized fibrous tissue in the center of nodules
Age: presenting by age 2 years (50%)
• initially subcutaneous painful masses on neck, shoulders, upper extremities

- progressive involvement of remaining musculature of back, chest, abdomen, lower extremities
- lesions may ulcerate and bleed
- muscles of back + proximal extremities become rigid followed by thoracic kyphosis
- inanition secondary to jaw trismus (masseter, temporal muscle)
- "wry neck" = torticollis (due restriction of sternocleidomastoid muscle)
- respiratory failure (thoracic muscles affected)
- conductive hearing loss (fusion of middle ear ossicles)

A. ECTOPIC OSSIFICATION
   √ rounded / linear calcification in neck / shoulders, paravertebral region, hips, proximal extremity, trunk, palmar + plantar fascia forming ossified bars + bony bridges
   √ ossification of voluntary muscles, complete by 20–25 years (sparing of sphincters + head)
B. SKELETAL ANOMALIES
   may appear before ectopic ossification
   - clinodactyly
   √ microdactyly of big toes (90%) and thumbs (50%) = usually only one large phalanx present / synostosis of metacarpal + proximal phalanx (first sign)
   √ phalangeal shortening of hand + foot (middle phalanx of 5th digit)
   √ shortened 1st metatarsal + hallux valgus (75%)
   √ shortened metacarpals + metatarsals
   √ shallow acetabulum
   √ short widened femoral neck
   √ thickening of medial cortex of tibia
   √ progressive fusion of posterior arches of cervical spine
   √ narrowed AP diameter of cervical + lumbar vertebral bodies
   √ ± bony ankylosis

CAVE: surgery is hazardous causing accelerated ossification at the surgical site

FIBROMA OF SOFT TISSUE

Histo: hypocellular highly collagenic tumor
Age: 3rd and 4th decades; M > F
Location: tendon sheath of distal upper extremity
√ slowly growing lesion 1–5 cm in size
MR:
   √ small hypointense nodule on all pulse sequences

FIBROMATOSIS

= DESMOID TUMOR
= benign aggressively growing lesion
Location: shoulder, pelvis, abdomen, thigh
Site: fascia in / around muscle
√ mostly <10 cm in diameter
MR:
   √ poorly defined (with invasion of fat / muscle) / lobulated well-defined lesion
   √ isointense with muscle on T1WI
   √ hyperintense (hypercellular) / hyperintense with areas of low intensity (intermixed with fibrous components) / hypointense (hypocellular) on T2WI

Cx: compresses / engulfs adjacent structures

FIBROSARCOMA

Incidence: 4% of all primary bone neoplasm
Etiology:
   A. PRIMARY FIBROSARCOMA (70%)
   B. SECONDARY FIBROSARCOMA (30%)
      1. following radiotherapy of giant cell tumor / lymphoma / breast cancer
      2. underlying benign lesion: Paget disease (common); giant cell tumor, bone infarct, osteomyelitis, desmoplastic fibroma, enchondroma, fibrous dysplasia (rare)
      3. dedifferentiation of low-grade chondrosarcoma

Histo: spectrum of well to poorly differentiated fibrous tissue proliferation; will not produce osteoid / chondroid / osseous matrix
Age: predominantly in 3rd–5th decade (range of 8–88 years); M:F = 1:1
Metastases to: lung, lymph nodes
- localized painful mass

Location: tubular bones in young, flat bones in older patients; femur (40%), tibia (16%) (about knee in 30–50%), jaw, pelvis (9%); rare in small bones of hand + feet or spinal column
Site: eccentric at diaphyseal-metaphyseal junction into metaphysis; intramedullary / periosteal

A. CENTRAL FIBROSARCOMA
   = intramedullary
   √ well-defined lucent bone lesion
   √ thin expanded cortex
   √ aggressive osteolysis with geographic / ragged / permeative bone destruction + wide zone of transition
   √ occasionally large osteolytic lesion with cortical destruction, periosteal reaction + soft-tissue invasion
   √ sequestration of bone may be present (DDx: eosinophilic granuloma, bacterial granuloma)
   √ sparse periosteal proliferation (uncommon)
   √ intramedullary discontinuous spread
   √ no calcification
   DDx: malignant fibrous histiocytoma, myeloma, telangiectatic osteosarcoma, lymphoma, desmoplastic fibroma, osteolytic metastasis
B. PERIOSTEAL FIBROSARCOMA
   = rare tumor arising from periosteal connective tissue
   Location: long bones of lower extremity, jaw
   √ contour irregularity of cortical border
   √ periosteal reaction with perpendicular bone formation may be present
   √ rarely extension into medullary cavity

Cx: pathologic fracture (uncommon)
Prognosis: 20% 10-year survival
DDx: (1) Osteolytic osteosarcoma (2nd–3rd decade)
   (2) Chondrosarcoma (usually contains characteristic calcifications)

(3) Aneurysmal bone cyst (eccentric blown-out appearance with rapid progression)
(4) Malignant giant cell tumor (begins in metaphysis extending toward joint)

FIBROUS CORTICAL DEFECT

Incidence: 30% of children; M:F = 2:1
Age: peak age of 7–8 years (range of 2–10 years); mostly before epiphyseal closure
Histo: fibrous tissue from periosteum invading underlying cortex

- asymptomatic

Location: metaphyseal cortex of long bone; posterior medial aspect of distal femur, proximal tibia, proximal femur, proximal humerus, ribs, ilium, fibula

√ round when small, average diameter of 1–2 cm
√ oval, extending parallel to long axis of host bone
√ cortical thinning + expansion may occur
√ smooth, well-defined / scalloped margins
√ larger lesions are multilocular
√ involution over 2–4 years

Prognosis:
(a) potential to grow and encroach on the medullary cavity leading to nonossifying fibroma
(b) bone islands in the adult may be residue of incompletely involuted cortical defect

FIBROUS DYSPLASIA

= LICHTENSTEIN-JAFFE DISEASE
= benign fibro-osseous developmental anomaly of the mesenchymal precursor of bone, manifested as a defect in osteoblastic differentiation and maturation

Cause: probable gene mutation during embryogenesis
Age: 1st–2nd decade (highest incidence between 3 and 15 years), 75% before age 30; progresses until growth ceases; M:F = 1:1
Histo: medullary cavity replaced by immature matrix of collagen with small irregularly shaped trabeculae of immature "woven" bone + inadequate mineralization; never replaced by mature lamellar bone

Types:

A. MONOSTOTIC FORM (70–80%)
- usually asymptomatic until 2nd–3rd decade

Location: ribs (28%), proximal femur (23%), craniofacial bones (10–25%)

B. POLYOSTOTIC FORM (20–30%)
Age: mean age of 8 years
- 2/3 symptomatic by age 10
- leg pain, limp, pathologic fracture (75%)
- abnormal vaginal bleeding (25%)

Location: unilateral + asymmetric; femur (91%), tibia (81%), pelvis (78%), foot (73%), ribs, skull + facial bones (50%), upper extremities, lumbar spine (14%), clavicle (10%), cervical spine (7%)
Site: metadiaphysis

√ leg length discrepancy (70%)
√ "shepherd's crook" deformity (35%)
√ facial asymmetry
√ tibial bowing
√ rib deformity

C. CRANIOFACIAL FORM = LEONTIASIS OSSEA
Incidence: in 10–25% of monostotic form / in 50% of polyostotic form / isolated
- cranial asymmetry
- facial deformity
- exophthalmos
- visual impairment

Location: sphenoid, frontal, maxillary, ethmoid bones > occipital, temporal bones
√ unilateral overgrowth of facial bones + calvarium (NO extracranial lesions)
√ outward expansion of outer table maintaining convexity (DDx: Paget disease with destruction of inner + outer table)
√ prominence of external occipital protuberance
Cx: neurologic deficit secondary to narrowed cranial foramina (eg, blindness)

D. CHERUBISM (special variant)
= autosomal dominant disorder of variable penetrance
Age: childhood; more severe in males
√ symmetric involvement of mandible + maxilla
Prognosis: regression after adolescence

May be associated with:
(a) endocrine disorders:
— precocious puberty in girls
— hyperthyroidism
— hyperparathyroidism: renal stones, calcinosis
— acromegaly
— diabetes mellitus
— Cushing syndrome: osteoporosis, acne
— growth retardation
(b) soft-tissue myxoma (rare): typically multiple intramuscular lesions

VARIANT: **McCune-Albright syndrome** (10%)
(1) polyostotic unilateral fibrous dysplasia
(2) "coast of Maine" café-au-lait spots (35%)
(3) endocrine dysfunction: menarche in infancy (20%), hyperthyroidism

- swelling + tenderness
- limp, pain (± pathologic fracture)
- increased alkaline phosphatase
- advanced skeletal + somatic maturation (early)
- coast of Maine café-au-lait spots = yellowish to brownish patches of cutaneous pigmentation with irregular / serrated border, predominantly on back of trunk (30–50%), buttocks, neck, shoulders; often ipsilateral to bone lesions (DDx: "coast of California" spots of neurofibromatosis)

Common location:
rib cage (30%), craniofacial bones [calvarium, mandible] (25%), femoral neck + tibia (25%), pelvis

Site: metaphysis is primary site with extension into diaphysis (rarely entire length)
√ normal bone architecture altered + remodeled
√ lesions in medullary cavity: radiolucent / "ground-glass" appearance / increased density
√ trabeculated appearance due to reinforced subperiosteal bone ridges in wall of lesion
√ expansion of bones (ribs, skull, long bones)
√ well-defined sclerotic margin of reactive bone = rind
√ endosteal scalloping with thinned / lost cortex (ribs, long bones) and intervening normal cortex is HALLMARK
√ lesion may undergo calcification + enchondral bone formation = fibrocartilaginous dysplasia
√ increased activity on bone scan during early perfusion + on delayed images

@ Skull
- skull deformity with cranial nerve compromise
- proptosis

Location: frontal bone > sphenoid bone; hemicranial involvement (DDx: Paget disease is bilateral)
√ sclerotic skull base, may narrow neural foramina (visual + hearing loss)
√ widened diploic space with displacement of outer table, inner table spared (DDx: Paget disease, inner table involved)
√ obliteration of sphenoid + frontal sinuses due to encroachment by fibrous dysplastic bone
√ inferolateral displacement of orbit
√ sclerosis of orbital plate + small orbit + hypoplasia of frontal sinuses (DDx: Paget disease, meningioma en plaque)
√ occipital thickening
√ cystic calvarial lesions, commonly crossing sutures
√ mandibular cystic lesion (very common) = osteocementoma, ossifying fibroma

@ Pelvis + ribs
√ cystic lesions (extremely common)
√ protrusio acetabuli

@ Extremities
- short stature as adult / dwarfism

√ premature fusion of ossification centers
√ epiphysis rarely affected before closure of growth plate
√ bowing deformities + discrepant limb length (tibia, femur) due to stress of normal weight bearing
√ "shepherd's crook" deformity of femoral neck = coxa vara
√ pseudarthrosis in infancy = osteofibrous dysplasia (DDx: neurofibromatosis)
√ premature onset of arthritis

Cx: (1) Transformation into osteo- / chondro- / fibrosarcoma or malignant fibrous histiocytoma (0.5–1%, more often in polyostotic form)
- increasing pain

√ enlarging soft-tissue mass
√ previously mineralized lesion turns lytic

(2) Pathologic fractures: transformation of woven into lamellar bone may be seen, subperiosteal healing without endosteal healing

DDx:
(1) HPT (chemical changes, generalized deossification, subperiosteal resorption)
(2) Neurofibromatosis (rarely osseous lesions, cystic intraosseous neurofibroma rare, café-au-lait spots smooth, familial disease)
(3) Paget disease (mosaic pattern histologically, radiographically identical to monostotic cranial lesion)
(4) Osteofibrous dysplasia (almost exclusively in tibia of infants, monostotic, lesion begins in cortex)
(5) Nonossifying fibroma
(6) Simple bone cyst
(7) Giant cell tumor (no sclerotic margin)
(8) Enchondromatosis
(9) Eosinophilic granuloma
(10) Osteoblastoma
(11) Hemangioma
(12) Meningioma

FIBROUS HISTIOCYTOMA

Benign fibrous histiocytoma

Incidence: 0.1% of all bone tumors
Histo: interlacing bundles of fibrous tissue in storiform pattern (whorled / woven) interspersed with mono- / multinucleated cells resembling histiocytes, benign giant cells, and lipid-laden macrophages; resembles nonossifying fibroma / fibroxanthoma
Age: 23–60 years
- localized intermittently painful soft-tissue swelling

Location: long bone, pelvis, vertebra (rare)
Site: typically in epiphysis / epiphyseal equivalent
√ well-defined radiolucent lesion with septa / soap-bubble appearance / no definable matrix
√ may have reactive sclerotic rim
√ narrow transition zone (= nonaggressive lesion)
√ no periosteal reaction
Rx: curettage
DDx: nonossifying fibroma (childhood / adolescence, asymptomatic, eccentric metaphyseal location)

Atypical benign fibrous histiocytoma

Histo: "atypical aggressive" features = mitotic figures present
√ lytic defect with irregular edges
Prognosis: may metastasize

Malignant fibrous histiocytoma

= MFH = MALIGNANT FIBROUS XANTHOMA
= XANTHOSARCOMA = MALIGNANT HISTIOCYTOMA = FIBROSARCOMA VARIANT
Histo: spindle-cell neoplasm of a mixture of fibroblasts + giant cells resembling histiocytes with nuclear atypia and pleomorphism in pinwheel arrangement; closely resembles high-grade fibrosarcoma (= fibroblastic cells arranged in uniform pattern separated by collagen fibers)

(a) pleomorphic-storiform subtype (50–60%)
(b) myxoid subtype (25%)
(c) giant cell subtype (5–10%)
(d) inflammatory subtype (5–10%)
(e) angiomatoid subtype (<5%)

Age: 10–90 (average 50) years; peak prevalence in 5th decade; more frequent in Caucasians; M:F = 3:2

Location: potential to arise in any organ (ubiquitous mesenchymal tissue); soft tissues >> bone

Soft-tissue MFH

Incidence: 20–30% of all soft-tissue sarcomas; most common primary malignant soft-tissue tumor of late adult life

◊ Any deep-seated invasive intramuscular mass in a patient >50 years of age is most likely MFH!

Location: extremities (75%), [lower extremity (50%), upper extremity (25%)], retroperitoneum (15%), head + neck (5%)

Site: within large muscle groups

- large painless soft-tissue mass with progressive enlargement over several months

√ mass usually 5–10 cm in size with increase over months / years
√ poorly defined curvilinear / punctate peripheral calcifications / ossifications (in 5–20%)
√ cortical erosion of adjacent bone (HIGHLY SUGGESTIVE FEATURE)

CT:
√ well-defined soft-tissue mass with central hypodense area = myxoid MFH (DDx: hemorrhage, necrosis, leiomyosarcoma with necrosis, myxoid lipo- / chondrosarcoma)
√ enhancement of solid components

MR:
√ inhomogeneous poorly defined lesion iso- / hyperintense to muscle on T1WI + hyperintense on T2WI

Prognosis for soft-tissue MFH:
larger + more deeply located tumors have a worse prognosis; 2-year survival rate of 60%; 5-year survival rate of 50%; local recurrence rate of 44%; metastatic rate of 42% (lung, lymph nodes, liver, bone)

DDx: (1) Liposarcoma (younger patient, presence of fat in >40%, calcifications rare)
(2) Rhabdomyosarcoma
(3) Synovial sarcoma (cortical erosion)

Osseous MFH

Prevalence: 5% of all primary malignant bone tumors

- painful, tender, rapidly enlarging mass
- pathologic fracture (20%)

Associated with:
prior radiation therapy, bone infarcts, Paget disease, fibrous dysplasia, osteonecrosis, fibroxanthoma (= nonossifying fibroma), enchondroma, chronic osteomyelitis

◊ 20% of all osseous MFH arise in areas of abnormal bone!

Location: femur (45%), tibia (20%), 50% about knee; humerus (10%); ilium (10%); spine; sternum; clavicle; rarely small bones of hand + feet

Site: central metaphysis of long bones (90%); eccentric in diaphysis of long bones (10%)

√ radiolucent defect with ill-defined margins (2.5–10 cm in diameter)
√ extensive mineralization / small areas of focal metaplastic calcification
√ permeation + cortical destruction
√ expansion in smaller bones (ribs, sternum, fibula, clavicle)
√ occasionally lamellated periosteal reaction (especially in presence of pathologic fracture)
√ soft-tissue extension

Cx: pathologic fracture (30–50%)

DDx: (1) metastasis (2) fibrosarcoma (often with sequestrum) (3) reticulum cell sarcoma (4) osteosarcoma (5) giant cell tumor (6) plasmacytoma

Pulmonary MFH (extremely rare)

√ solitary pulmonary nodule without calcification
√ diffuse infiltrate

NUC:
√ increased uptake of Tc-99m MDP (mechanism not understood)
√ increased uptake of Ga-67 citrate

US:
√ well-defined mass with hyperechoic + hypoechoic (necrotic) areas

CT:
√ mass of muscle density with hypodense areas (necrosis)
√ invasion of abdominal musculature, but not IVC / renal veins (DDx to renal cell carcinoma)

Angio:
√ hypervascularity + early venous return

FOCAL FIBROCARTILAGINOUS DYSPLASIA OF TIBIA

Associated with: tibia vara

Age: 9–28 months

Histo: dense hypocellular fibrous tissue resembling tendon with lacuna formation

- slight shortening of affected leg

Location: insertion of pes anserinus (= tendinous insertion of gracilis, sartorius, semitendinous muscles) distal to proximal tibial physis; unilateral involvement

√ unilateral tibia vara
√ well-defined elliptic obliquely oriented lucent defect in medial tibial metadiaphyseal cortex
√ sclerosis along lateral border of lesion
√ absence of bone margin superomedially

Prognosis: resolution in 1–4 years

DDx: (1) Unilateral Blount disease (typically bilateral in infants, varus angulation of upper tibia, decreased height of medial tibial metaphysis, irregular physis)
(2) Chondromyxoid fibroma, eosinophilic granuloma, osteoid osteoma, osteoma, fibroma, chondroma (not associated with tibia vara, soft-tissue mass)

FRACTURE

= soft-tissue injury in which there is a break in the continuity of bone or cartilage

General description:

(1) OPEN / [CLOSED]
open Fx = communication between fractured bone + skin

(2) [COMPLETE] / INCOMPLETE
complete Fx = all cortical surfaces disrupted
incomplete Fx = partial separation of bone
greenstick Fx = break of one cortical margin only due to tension
buckle / torus Fx = buckling of cortex due to compression
bowing Fx = plastic deformity of bone
lead-pipe Fx = combination of greenstick + torus Fx

(3) SIMPLE / COMMINUTED
simple Fx = noncomminuted
comminuted Fx = >2 fragments
segmental Fx = isolated segment of shaft
butterfly fragment = V-shaped fragment not completely circumscribed by cortex

(4) DIRECTION OF FRACTURE LINE in relation to long axis of bone:
transverse, oblique, oblique-transverse, spiral

Special terminology:
avulsion Fx = fragment pulled off by tendon / ligament from parent bone
transchondral Fx = cartilaginous surface involved
chondral Fx = cartilage alone involved
osteochondral Fx = cartilage + subjacent bone involved

Description of anatomic positional changes:
= change in position of distal fracture fragment in relation to proximal fracture fragment

LENGTH
= longitudinal change of fragments
distraction = increase from original anatomic length
shortening = decrease from original anatomic length
— impacted = fragments driven into each other
— overriding = also includes latitudinal changes
— overlapping = bayonet apposition

DISPLACEMENT
= latitudinal change of anatomic axis:
— undisplaced
— anterior, posterior, medial / ulnar, lateral / radial

ANGULATION / TILT
= long axes of fragments intersect at the fracture apex:
— medial / lateral, ventral / dorsal
— varus = angular deviation of distal fragment toward midline on frontal projection
— valgus = angular deviation of distal fragment away from midline on frontal projection
eg, "ventral angulation of fracture apex"
eg, "in anatomic / near anatomic alignment"

ROTATION
◊ Difficult to detect radiographically!
√ differences in diameters of apposing fragments
√ mismatch of fracture line geometry
— internal / external rotation

NUC:
Typical time course:
1. Acute phase (3–4 weeks)
abnormal in 80% <24 hours, in 95% <72 hours
◊ elderly patients show delayed appearance of positive scan
√ broad area of increased tracer uptake (wider than fracture line)
2. Subacute phase (2–3 months) = time of most intense tracer accumulation
√ more focal increased tracer uptake corresponding to fracture line
3. Chronic phase (1–2 years)
√ slow decline in tracer accumulation
√ in 65% normal after 1 year; >95% normal after 3 years

Return to normal:
◊ non–weight-bearing bone returns to normal more quickly than weight-bearing bone
◊ rib fractures return to normal most rapidly
◊ complicated fractures with orthopedic fixation devices take longest to return to normal
1. Simple fractures: 90% normal by 2 years
2. Open reduction / fixation: <50% normal by 3 years
3. Delayed union: slower than normal for type of fracture
4. Nonunion: persistent intense uptake in 80%
5. Complicated union (true pseudarthrosis, soft-tissue interposition, impaired blood supply, presence of infection)
√ intense uptake at fracture ends
√ decreased uptake at fracture site
6. Vertebral compression fractures: 60% normal by 1 year; 90% by 2 years; 97% by 3 years

Pathologic Fracture

= fracture at site of preexisting osseous abnormality
Cause: tumor, osteoporosis, infection, metabolic disorder

Stress Fracture

= fractures produced as a result of repetitive prolonged muscular action on bone that has not accommodated itself to such action

Insufficiency Fracture

= normal physiologic stress applied to bone with abnormal elastic resistance / deficient mineralization

Cause:

1. Osteoporosis
2. Rheumatoid arthritis
3. Paget disease
4. Fibrous dysplasia
5. Osteogenesis imperfecta
6. Osteopetrosis
7. Osteomalacia / rickets
8. Hyperparathyroidism
9. Renal osteodystrophy
10. Radiation therapy
11. Prolonged corticosteroid treatment

Location: lower extremity (calcaneus, tibia, fibula), thoracic vertebra, sacrum, ilium, pubic bone

Pelvic Insufficency Fracture

- severe pain in lower back, buttock, groin
- walking ability impaired

Incidence: 1.8–5% of women >55 years

Predisposed: postmenopausal women

Location: sacral ala, parasymphyseal region of os pubis, pubic rami, supra-acetabular region, iliac blades, superomedial portion of ilium

Types:

(a) occult fracture:

Site: sacrum > supra-acetabulum, ilium

√ sclerotic band, cortical disruption, fracture line

◊ Often obscured by overlying bowel gas!

(b) aggressive fracture:

Site: parasymphysis, pubic rami

√ exuberant callus formation, osteolysis + fragments (with prolonged or delayed healing / chronic nonunion)

CAVE: fracture may be misdiagnosed as neoplasm; interpretation also histologically difficult

NUC:

√ butterfly / H-shaped ("Honda sign") / asymmetric incomplete H-shaped pattern of sacral uptake

√ pelvic outlet view for parasymphyseal fx

CT (most accurate modality):

√ sclerotic band, linear fracture line, cortical disruption, fragmentation, displacement

◊ Excludes bone destruction + soft-tissue masses!

Prognosis: healing in 12–30 months

Fatigue Fracture

= normal bone subjected to repetitive stresses (none of which is singularly capable of producing a fracture) leading to mechanical failure over time

Risk factors: new / different / rigorous repetitive activity; female sex; increased age; Caucasian race; low bone mineral density; low calcium intake; fluoride treatment for osteoporosis; condition resulting in altered gait

- activity-related pain abating with rest
- constant pain with continued activity

1. **Clay shoveler's fracture**: spinous process of lower cervical / upper thoracic spine
2. **Clavicle**: postoperative (radical neck dissection)
3. **Coracoid process of scapula**: trap shooting
4. **Ribs**: carrying heavy pack, golf, coughing
5. **Distal shaft of humerus**: throwing ball
6. **Coronoid process of ulna**: pitching ball, throwing javelin, pitchfork work, propelling wheelchairs
7. **Hook of hamate**: swinging golf club / tennis racquet / baseball bat
8. **Spondylolysis** = pars interarticularis of lumbar vertebrae: ballet, lifting heavy objects, scrubbing floors
9. **Femoral neck**: ballet, long-distance running
10. **Femoral shaft**: ballet, marching, long-distance running, gymnastics
11. **Obturator ring of pelvis**: stooping, bowling, gymnastics
12. **Patella**: hurdling
13. **Tibial shaft**: ballet, jogging
14. **Fibula**: long-distance running, jumping, parachuting
15. **Calcaneus**: jumping, parachuting, prolonged standing, recent immobilization
16. **Navicular**: stomping on ground, marching, prolonged standing, ballet
17. **Metatarsal** (commonly 2nd MT): marching, stomping on ground, prolonged standing, ballet, postoperative bunionectomy
18. **Sesamoids of metatarsal**: prolonged standing

X-ray (15% sensitive in early fractures, increasing to 50% on follow-up):

– cancellous (trabecular) bone (notoriously difficult to detect)
  - √ subtle blurring of trabecular margins
  - √ faint sclerotic radiopaque area of peritrabecular callus (50% change in bone density needed)
  - √ sclerotic band (due to trabecular compression + callus formation) usually perpendicular to cortex

– compact (cortical) bone
  - √ "gray cortex sign" = subtle ill definition of cortex
  - √ intracortical radiolucent striations (early)
  - √ solid thick lamellar periosteal new bone formation
  - √ endosteal thickening (later)

√ follow-up radiography after 2–3 weeks of conservative therapy

NUC ("gold standard" = almost 100% sensitive):
- √ abnormal uptake within 6–72 hours of injury (prior to radiographic abnormality)
- √ "stress reaction" = focus of subtly increased uptake
- √ focal fusiform area of intense cortical uptake
- √ abnormal uptake persists for months

MR (very sensitive modality; fat saturation technique most sensitive to detect increase in water content of medullary edema / hemorrhage):
- √ diminished marrow signal intensity on T1WI
- √ increased marrow signal intensity on T2WI
- √ low-intensity band contiguous with cortex on T2WI = fracture line of more advanced lesion

CT (least sensitive modality):
helpful in: longitudinal stress fracture of tibia; in confusing pediatric stress fracture (to detect endosteal bone formation)

DDx:
(1) Shin splints (activity not increased in angiographic / blood-pool phase)
- √ long linear uptake on posteromedial (soleus muscle) / anterolateral (tibialis anterior muscle) tibial cortex on delayed images (from stress to periosteum at muscle insertion site)

(2) Osteoid osteoma (eccentric, nidus, solid periosteal reaction, night pain)
(3) Chronic sclerosing osteomyelitis (dense, sclerotic, involving entire circumference, little change on serial radiographs)
(4) Osteomalacia (bowed long bones, looser zones, gross fractures, demineralization)
(5) Osteogenic sarcoma (metaphyseal, aggressive periosteal reaction)
(6) Ewing tumor (lytic destructive appearance with soft-tissue component, little change on serial radiographs)

Epiphyseal plate injury

Prevalence: 6–18–30% of bone injuries in children <16 years of age
Peak age: 12 years
Location: distal radius (28%), phalanges of hand (26%), distal tibia (10%), distal phalanges of foot (7%), distal humerus (7%), distal ulna (4%), proximal radius (4%), metacarpals (4%), distal fibula (3%)
Mechanism: 80% shearing force; 20% compression
Resistance to trauma: ligament > bone > physis (hypertrophic zone most vulnerable)

Salter-Harris classification (considering probability of growth disturbance)
◊ Prognosis is worse in lower extremities (ankle + knee) irrespective of Salter-Harris type!

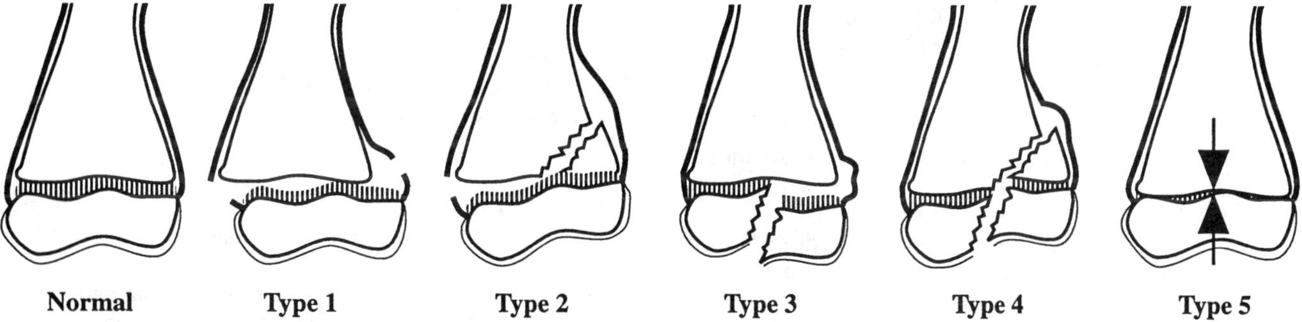

Salter -Harris Classifcation of Epiphyseal Plate Injuries

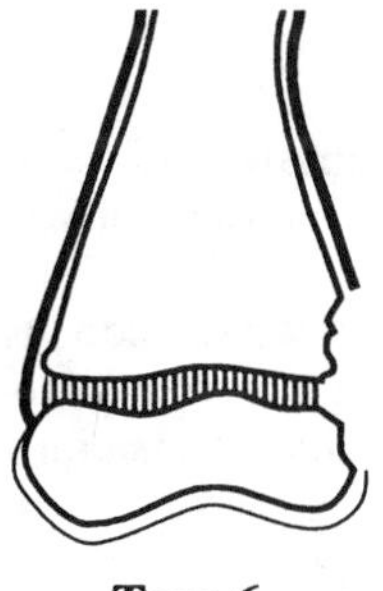

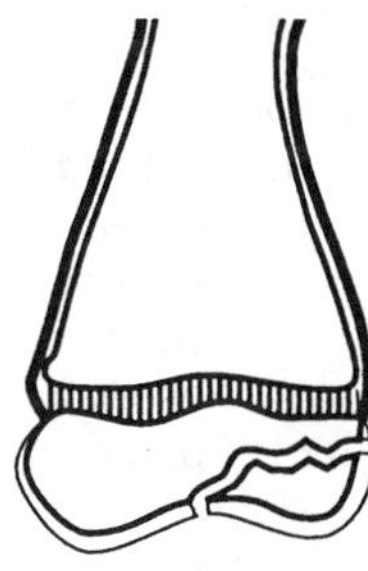

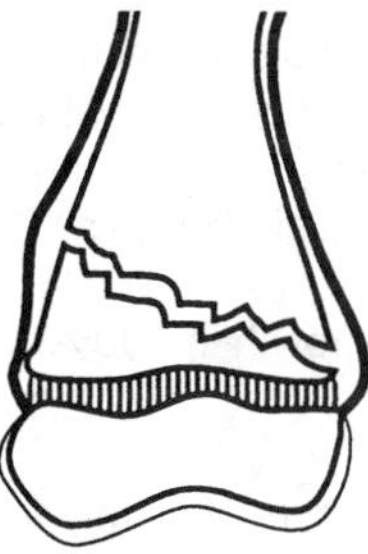

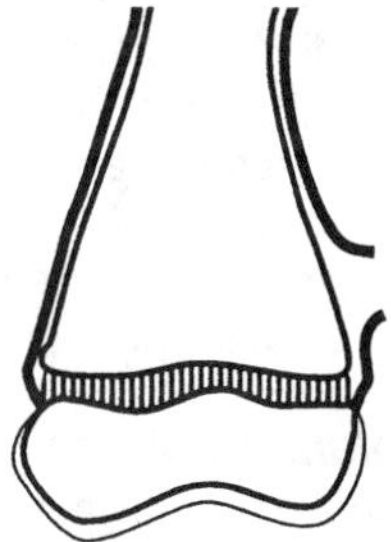

Rang and Ogden's Additions to Salter-Harris

mnemonic: "SALTR"

Slip of physis	= type 1
Above physis	= type 2
Lower than physis	= type 3
Through physis	= type 4
Rammed physis	= type 5

Salter Type 1 (*6–8.5%*)
= slip of epiphysis due to shearing force separating epiphysis from physis

Line of cleavage: confined to physis

Location: most commonly in phalanges, distal radius (includes: apophyseal avulsion, slipped capital femoral epiphysis)

√ displacement of epiphyseal ossification center

Prognosis: favorable irrespective of location

Salter Type 2 (*73–75%*)
= shearing force splits growth plate

Line of fracture: through physis + extending through margin of metaphysis separating a triangular metaphyseal fragment (= "corner sign")

Location: distal radius (33–50%), distal tibia + fibula, phalanges

Prognosis: good, may result in minimal shortening

Salter Type 3 (*6.5–8%*)
= intra-articular fracture, often occurring after partial closure of physis

Line of fracture: vertically / obliquely through epiphysis + extending horizontally to periphery of physis

Location: distal tibia, distal phalanx, rarely distal femur

√ epiphysis split vertically

Prognosis: fair (imprecise reduction leads to alteration in linearity of articular plane)

Salter Type 4 (*10–12%*)
Location: lateral condyle of humerus, distal tibia

√ fracture involves metaphysis + physis + epiphysis

Prognosis: guarded (may result in deformity + angulation)

Salter Type 5 (*<1%*)
= crush injury with injury to vascular supply

Location: distal femur, proximal tibia, distal tibia

Often associated with: fracture of adjacent shaft

√ no immediate radiographic finding

√ shortening of bone + cone epiphysis / angular deformity on follow-up

Prognosis: poor (impairment of growth in 100%)

Triplane Fracture (6%)
Location: distal tibia, lateral condyle of distal humerus

√ vertical fracture of epiphysis + horizontal cleavage plane within physis + oblique fracture of adjacent metaphysis

MR:

√ focal dark linear area (= line of cleavage) within bright physis on gradient echo images (GRE)

Cx:
(1) progressive angular deformity from segmental arrest of germinal zone growth with formation of a bone bridge across physis = "bone bar"
(2) limb length discrepancy from total cessation of growth
(3) articular incongruity from disruption of articular surface
(4) Bone infarction in metaphysis / epiphysis

Apophyseal Injury
Mechanism: avulsive force

◊ Physis under secondary ossification center is weakest part!

At risk: hurdlers, sprinters, cheerleaders (repetitive to and fro adduction / abduction + flexion / extension)

• pain, point tenderness, swelling

Location	*Muscle origin / insertion*
anterior superior iliac spine	sartorius muscle + tensor fasciae femoris m.
anterior inferior iliac spine	rectus femoris muscle
lesser trochanter	psoas muscle
ischial tuberosity	hamstring muscle
greater trochanter	gluteal muscle
iliac crest	abdominal muscle
symphysis pubis	adductor muscle

√ irregularity at site of avulsion

√ displaced pieces of bone of variable size

√ abnormal foci of ossification

Elbow Fracture
common among children 2–14 years of age

@ Soft-tissue

√ displacement of anterior + posterior fat pads (= elbow joint effusion with supracondylar / lateral condylar / proximal ulnar fractures)

√ supinator fat pad (= fracture of proximal radius)

√ focal edema medially (= medial epicondyle fx) / laterally (= lateral condyle fx)

@ Humerus (80%)

Supracondylar fracture (55%)

Mechanism: hyperextension with vertical stress

√ transverse fracture line

√ distal fragment posteriorly displaced / tilted

√ anterior humeral line intersecting anterior to posterior third of capitellum (on lateral x ray)

Lateral condylar fracture (20%)

Mechanism: hyperextension with varus stress

√ fracture line between lateral condyle + trochlea / through capitellum

Medial epicondylar fracture (5%)
Mechanism: hyperextension with valgus stress
√ avulsion of medial epicondyle (by flexor muscles of forearm)
√ may become trapped in joint space (after reduction of concomitant elbow dislocation)

@ Radius (10%)
Mechanism: hyperextension with valgus stress
√ Salter-Harris type II / IV fracture
√ transverse metaphyseal / radial neck fracture
Mechanism: hyperextension with varus stress
√ dislocation as part of Monteggia fracture (from rupture of annular ligament)

@ Ulna (10%)
√ longitudinal linear fracture through proximal shaft
Mechanism: hyperextension with vertical stress
√ transverse fracture through olecranon
Mechanism: hyperextension with valgus / varus stress; blow to posterior elbow in flexed position
√ coronoid process avulsion
Mechanism: hyperextension-rotation associated with forceful contraction of brachial m.

Forearm fracture

Barton fracture
Mechanism: fall on outstretched hand
√ intra-articular oblique fracture of dorsal lip of distal radius
√ carpus dislocates with distal fragment up and back on radius

Chauffeur fracture
= name derived from direct trauma to radial side of wrist sustained from recoil of crank used in era of hand-cranked automobiles
= HUTCHINSON FRACTURE
Mechanism: acute dorsiflexion + abduction of hand
√ triangular fracture of radial styloid process

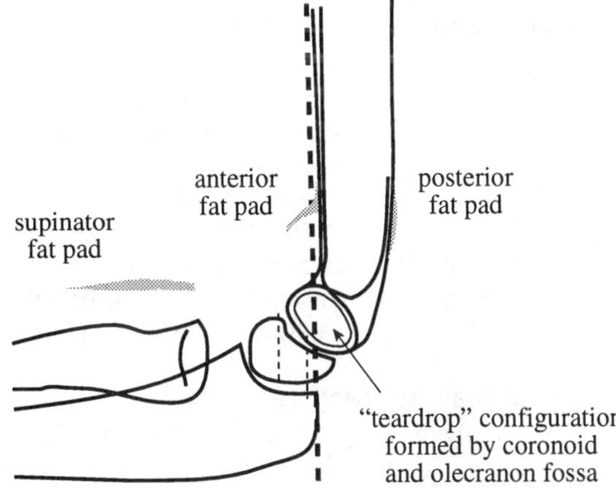

Anterior Humeral Line and Elbow Fat Pads

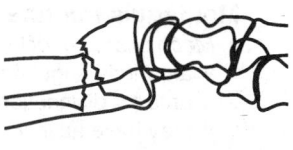

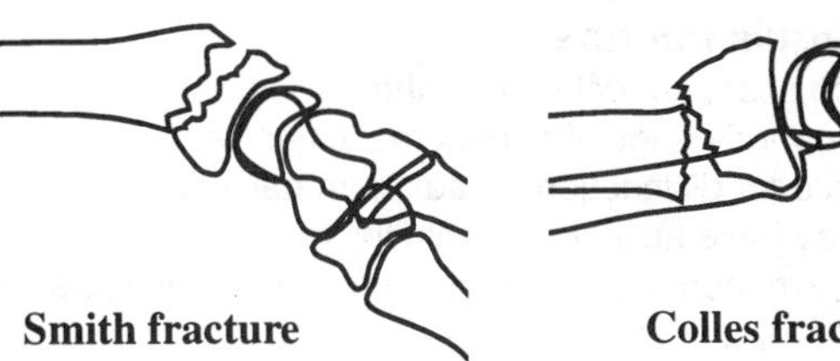

Smith fracture **Colles fracture**

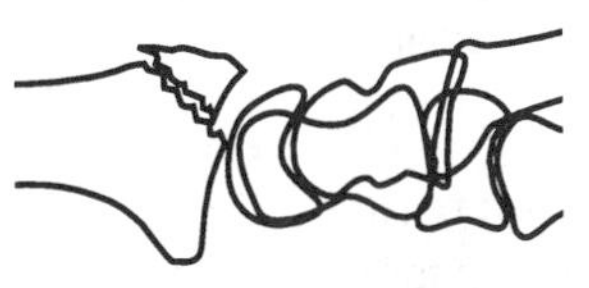

Barton fracture

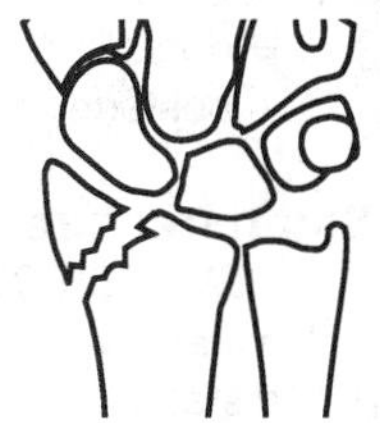

Chauffeur fracture

Colles fracture
Most common fracture of forearm
Mechanism: fall on outstretched hand
√ radial fracture in distal 2 cm ± ulnar styloid fracture
√ dorsal displacement of distal fragment
√ "silver-fork" deformity
Cx: posttraumatic arthritis
Rx: anatomic reduction important
Significant postreduction deformity:
1. Residual positive ulnar variance >5 mm indicates unsatisfactory outcome in 40%
2. Dorsal angulation of palmar tilt >15° decreases grip strength + endurance in >50%

Galeazzi fracture
Mechanism: fall on outstretched hand with elbow flexed
√ radial fracture in distal third + subluxation / dislocation of distal radioulnar joint
√ dorsal angulation
√ ulnar plus variance (= radial shortening) of >10 mm implies complete disruption of interosseous membrane = complete instability of radioulnar joint
Cx: (1) high incidence of nonunion, delayed union, malunion (unstable fracture)
(2) limitation of pronation / supination

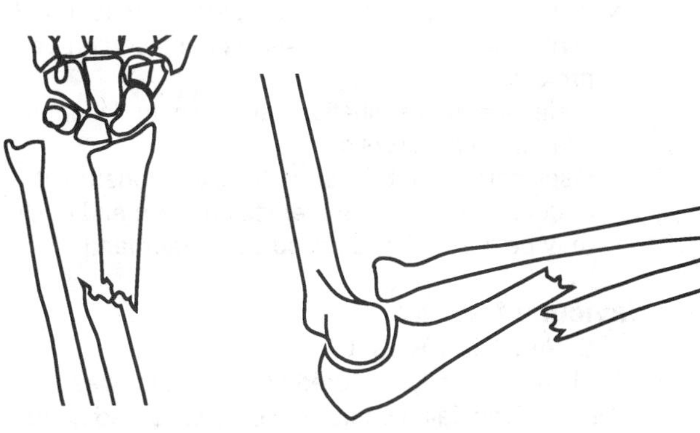

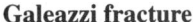

Galeazzi fracture **Monteggia fracture**

Monteggia fracture

Mechanism: direct blow to the forearm

√ anteriorly angulated proximal ulnar fracture + anterior dislocation of radiohumeral joint

√ may have associated wrist injury

Cx: nonunion, limitation of motion at elbow, nerve abnormalities

REVERSE MONTEGGIA FRACTURE

= dorsally angulated proximal ulnar fracture + posterior dislocation of radial head

Smith fracture

= REVERSE COLLES FRACTURE

Mechanism: hyperflexion with fall on back of hand

√ distal radial fracture

√ ventral displacement of fragment

√ radial deviation of hand

√ "garden spade" deformity

Cx: altered function of carpus

Hand fracture

Bennett fracture

Mechanism: forced abduction of thumb

√ intra-articular fracture / dislocation of base of 1st metacarpal

√ small fragment of 1st metacarpal continues to articulate with trapezium

√ lateral retraction of 1st metacarpal shaft by abductor pollicis longus

Rx: anatomic reduction important, difficult to keep in anatomic alignment

Cx: pseudarthrosis

Boxer's fracture

Mechanism: direct blow with clenched fist

√ transverse fracture of distal metacarpal (usually 5th)

Gamekeeper's thumb

= SKIER'S THUMB; originally described as chronic lesion in hunters strangling rabbits

Incidence: 6% of all skiing injuries; 50% of skiing injuries to the hand

Mechanism: violent abduction of thumb with injury to ulnar collateral ligament (UCL) in 1st MCP (faulty handling of ski pole)

√ disruption of ulnar collateral ligament of 1st MCP joint, usually occurring distally near insertion on proximal phalanx

√ radial stress examination necessary to document ligamentous disruption

√ displacement of UCL superficial to aponeurosis of adductor pollicis (= Stener lesion) [torn end of UCL may be marked by avulsed bone fragment]

Navicular fracture

= SCAPHOID FRACTURE

◊ Most frequently fractured of all carpal bones

Mechanism: fall on dorsiflexed outstretched hand

• pain + tenderness at anatomic snuff box

Radiographic misses: 25–33–65%

N.B.: If initial radiograph negative, reexamine in 2 + 6 weeks after treatment with short-arm spica cast!

MR: high sensitivity

Bone scan: up to 100% sensitive, 93% PPV after 2–3 days

Prognosis: dependent on

√ displaced fracture = >1 mm offset / angulation / rotation of fragments (less favorable)

√ location (blood supply derived from distal part):
- distal 1/3 (10%) = usually fragments reunite
- middle-third (70%) = failure to reunite in 30%
- proximal 1/3 (20%) = failure to reunite in 90%

√ orientation of fracture
- transverse / horizontal oblique = relatively stable
- vertical oblique (less common) = unstable

◊ Good prognosis with distal fracture + no displacement + no ligamentous injury!

◊ Less favorable prognosis with displaced / comminuted fracture + proximal pole fracture!

Cx: avascular necrosis of proximal fragment

Rolando fracture

√ comminuted intra-articular fracture through base of thumb

Prognosis: worse than Bennett's fracture (difficult to reduce)

Pelvic fracture

Malgaigne fracture

Mechanism: direct trauma

• shortening of involved extremity

√ vertical fractures through one side of pelvic ring
(1) superior to acetabulum
(2) inferior to acetabulum
(3) ± sacroiliac dislocation / fracture

Bucket handle fracture

√ double vertical fracture through superior and inferior pubic rami + sacroiliac joint dislocation on contralateral side

Knee fracture

Segond fracture

Mechanism: external rotation + varus stress causing excessive tension on the lateral capsular ligament

Associated with: lesion of anterior cruciate ligament (75–100%), meniscal tear (67%)

• anterolateral instability of the knee

√ small cortical avulsion fracture of proximal lateral tibial rim immediately distal to lateral plateau

Tibial plateau fracture (Schatzker classification)

Mechanism: valgus force ("bumper / fender fracture" from lateral force of automobile against a pedestrian's fixed knee) / compression force often in extension

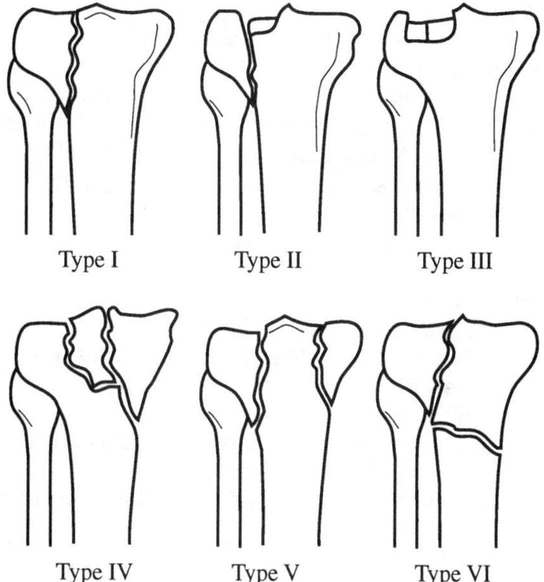

Type I	= wedge-shaped pure cleavage fracture	6%
Type II	= combined cleavage + median compression fracture	25%
Type III	= pure compression fracture	36%
Type IV	= medial plateau fracture with a split / depressed comminution	10%
Type V	= bicondylar fracture, often with inverted Y appearance	3%
Type VI	= transverse / oblique fracture with separation of metaphysis from diaphysis	20%

◊ Lateral plateau fractures (type I–III) are most common!

◊ Fractures of medial plateau are associated with greater violence and higher percentage of associated injuries!

Foot fracture

Ankle fracture

Incidence: ankle injuries account for 10% of all emergency room visits; 85% of all ankle sprains involve lateral ligaments

Ligamentous connections at ankle:

(a) binding tibia + fibula
   1. anterior inferior tibiofibular ligament (= tibiofibular syndesmosis)
   2. posterior inferior tibiofibular ligament
   3. transverse tibiofibular ligament
   4. interosseous membrane

(b) lateral malleolus
   85% of all ankle sprains involve these ligaments:
   1. anterior talofibular ligament
   2. posterior talofibular ligament
   3. calcaneofibular ligament

(c) medial malleolus = deltoid ligament with
   1. navicular portion
   2. sustentaculum portion
   3. talar portion

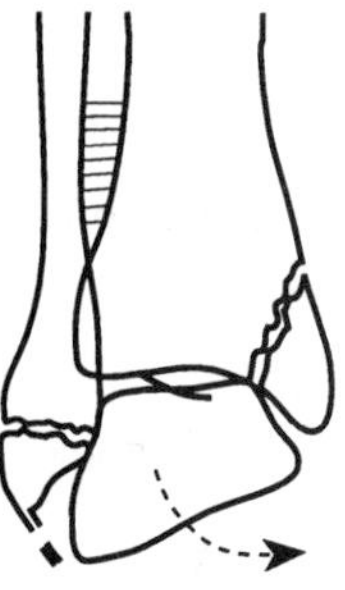
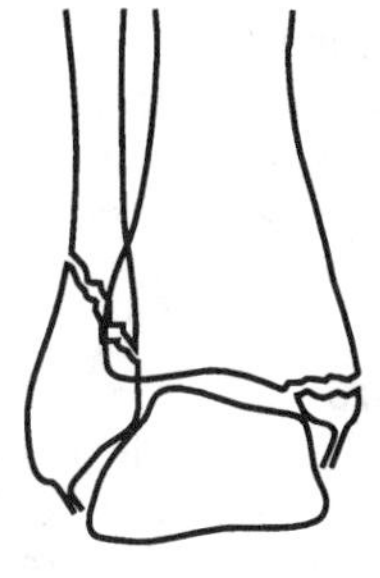
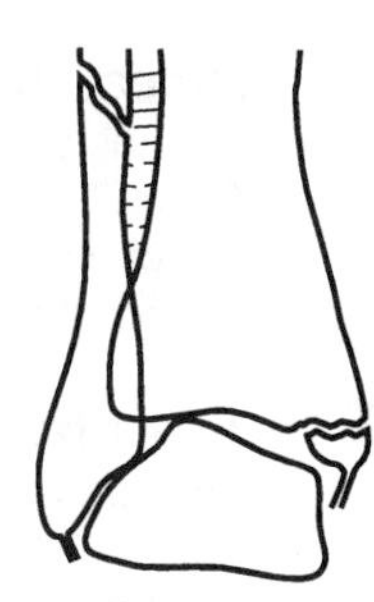

Supination-Adduction **Supination-Abduction** **Pronation-External Rotation**

A. SUPINATION-ADDUCTION
= INVERSION-ADDUCTION INJURY
Mechanism:
   (1) avulsive forces affect lateral ankle structures
   (2) impactive forces secondary to talar shift stress medial structures

√ sprain / rupture of lateral collateral ligament
   ◊ anterior tibiofibular ligament ruptures alone in 66%
   ◊ injury of all 3 lateral ligaments in 20%
   Prognosis: chronic lateral ankle instability in 10–20%

√ transverse avulsion of malleolus sparing tibiofibular ligaments

√ oblique fracture of medial malleolus ± posterior lip fracture

B. SUPINATION-ABDUCTION
= EVERSION / EXTERNAL ROTATION
Mechanism:
   (1) avulsive forces on medial structures
   (2) impacting forces on lateral structures (talar impact)

√ lateral subluxation of talus

√ oblique / spiral fracture of lateral malleolus

√ partial disruption of tibiofibular ligament

√ sprain / rupture / avulsion of deltoid ligament

√ transverse fracture of medial malleolus

(a) **Pott fracture**
   √ fracture of fibula above an intact tibiofibular ligament

(b) **Dupuytren fracture**
   √ fracture of fibula above a disrupted tibiofibular ligament

C. PRONATION-EXTERNAL ROTATION
= EVERSION + EXTERNAL ROTATION

√ tear of tibiofibular ligament / avulsion of anterior tubercle (Tillaux-Chaput) / avulsion of posterior tubercle (Volkmann)

√ tear of interosseous membrane = lateral instability

√ fibular fracture higher than ankle joint (Maisonneuve fracture if around knee)

Chopart fracture
√ fracture / dislocation through midtarsal joint (calcaneocuboid + talonavicular)
√ commonly associated with fractures of the bones abutting the joint

Jones fracture
Mechanism: plantar flexion + inversion (stepping off a curb)
√ transverse avulsion fracture of base of 5th metatarsal (insertion of peroneus brevis tendon)

Lisfranc fracture
Mechanism: metatarsal heads fixed and hindfoot forced plantarward and into rotation
√ fracture / dislocation of tarsometatarsal joints

Calcaneal fracture
Incidence: most commonly fractured tarsal bone; 60% of all tarsal fractures; 2% of all fractures in the body; commonly bilateral
Mechanism: fall from heights
May be associated with: lumbar vertebral fracture
Age: 95% in adults, 5% in children
— adulthood: intra-articular (75%), extra-articular (25%)
— childhood: extra-articular (63–92%)
Classification:
(a) Extra-articular fracture of calcaneal tuberosity: beak type, vertical, horizontal, medial avulsion
(b) Intra-articular fracture
— subtalar joint involvement: undisplaced, displaced, comminuted
— calcaneocuboid joint involvement
√ apex of lateral talar process does not point to "crucial angle" of Gissane
√ Boehler angle decreased below 28°–40°

FROSTBITE
Cause: (1) cellular injury + necrosis from freezing process
(2) cessation of circulation secondary to cellular aggregates + thrombi forming as a result of exposure to low temperatures below -13° Celsius (usually cold air)
• firm white numb areas in cutis (separation of epidermal-dermal interface)
Location: feet, hands (thumb commonly spared due to protection by clenched fist)

Early changes:
√ soft-tissue swelling + loss of tissue at tips of digits

CHILD
√ fragmentation / premature fusion / destruction of distal phalangeal epiphyses
√ secondary infection, articular cartilage injury, joint space narrowing, sclerosis, osteophytosis of DIP
√ shortening + deviation / deformity of fingers

ADULT
√ osteoporosis (4–10 weeks after injury)
√ periostitis
√ acromutilation (secondary to osteomyelitis + surgical removal) + tuftal resorption (result of soft-tissue loss)
√ small round punched-out areas near edge of joint
√ interphalangeal joint abnormalities (simulating osteoarthritis)
√ calcification / ossification of pinna

Angio:
√ vasospasm, stenosis, occlusion
√ proliferation of arterial + venous collaterals (in recovery phase)
Bone scintigraphy:
√ persistent absence of uptake (= lack of vascular perfusion) indicates nonviable tissue
Rx: selective angiography with intraarterial reserpine

GANGLION
Ganglion = mucin-containing cyst arising from tendon sheath / joint capsule / bursa / subchondral bone lined by flat spindle-shaped cells
Synovial cyst = cyst continuous with joint capsule lined by synovial cells (term is used by some synonymously with ganglion)

Soft-tissue ganglion
= cystic tumorlike lesion usually attached to a tendon sheath
Origin: synovial herniation / coalescence of smaller cysts formed by myxomatous degeneration of periarticular connective tissue
• uni- / multilocular swelling
Location: hand, wrist, foot
Site: arise from tendon, muscle, semilunar cartilage
√ soft-tissue mass with surface bone resorption
√ periosteal new-bone formation
√ arthrography may demonstrate communication with joint / tendon sheath
√ internal septations
Rx: steroid injection may improve symptomatology

Intraosseous ganglion
= benign subchondral radiolucent lesion WITHOUT degenerative arthritis
• mild localized pain (4% of patients with unexplained wrist pain)
Age: middle age
Origin: (1) mucoid degeneration of intraosseous connective tissue perhaps due to trauma / ischemia
(2) penetration of juxtaosseous soft-tissue ganglion into underlying bone (occasionally)
Path: uni- / multilocular cyst surrounded by fibrous lining, containing gelatinous material
Location: epiphysis of long bone (medial malleolus, femoral head, proximal tibia, carpal bones) / subarticular flat bone (acetabulum)

√ well-demarcated solitary 0.6–6 cm lytic lesion
√ sclerotic margin
√ NO communication with joint
√ increased radiotracer uptake on bone scintigraphy (in 10%)
DDx: posttraumatic / degenerative cyst

Periosteal ganglion
= cystic structure with viscid / mucinous contents
Incidence: 11 cases in literature
Age: 39–50 years; M > F
• swelling, mild tenderness
Location: long tubular bones of lower extremity
√ cortical erosion / scalloping / reactive bone formation
√ NO intraosseous component (endosteal surface intact)
CT:
√ well-defined soft-tissue mass adjacent to bone cortex with fluid contents
MR:
√ homogeneous isointense signal to muscle on T1WI
√ homogeneous hyperintense signal to fat on T2WI
√ NO internal septations (DDx to soft-tissue ganglion)
DDx: periosteal chondroma without matrix calcification, cortical desmoid, subperiosteal aneurysmal bone cyst, acute subperiosteal hematoma (history of trauma / blood dyscrasia), subperiosteal abscess (involvement of adjacent bone marrow)
Rx: surgical excision (local recurrence possible)

GARDNER SYNDROME
= autosomal dominant syndrome characterized by (1) osteomas (2) soft-tissue tumors (3) colonic polyps
Location of osteomas: paranasal sinuses; outer table of skull (frequent); mandible (at angle)
√ endosteal cortical thickening / osteomas in any bone
√ may have solid periosteal cortical thickening
√ osteomas / exostoses may protrude from periosteal surface
√ wavy cortical thickening of superior aspect of ribs
√ polyps: colon, stomach, duodenum, ampulla of Vater, small intestine
Cx: high incidence of carcinoma of duodenum / ampulla of Vater

GAUCHER DISEASE
= rare autosomal recessive disorder / dominant (in a few), common among Ashkenazi Jews; M < F
Etiology: deficiency of lysosomal hydrolase acid β-glycosidase (= glucocerebrosidase) leads to accumulation of glucosyl ceramide within cells of RES (liver, spleen, bone marrow, lung, lymph nodes)
Histo: bone-marrow aspirate shows Gaucher cells (kerasin-laden histiocytes)
Types:
(1) Rapidly fatal infantile form = type 2: 1–12 months
  • early onset of significant hepatosplenomegaly
  • severe progressive neurologic symptoms: seizures, mental retardation, spasticity
  Prognosis: fatal during first 2 years of life
(2) Juvenile form = type 3: 2–6 years
  • mild neurologic involvement
  Prognosis: survival into adolescence
(3) Adult form = type 1 (most common form in USA)
  Prognosis: longest time of survival; pulmonary involvement / hepatic failure may lead to early death
• hepatosplenomegaly, impairment of liver function, ascites
• elevated serum acid phosphatase
• pancytopenia, anemia, leukopenia, thrombocytopenia (hypersplenism)
• hemochromatosis (yellowish brown pigmentation of conjunctiva + skin)
• dull bone pain; bone involvement in 75%
Location: axial skeleton, distal femur, pelvis, predominantly proximal + other long bones
√ generalized osteopenia (decrease in trabecular bone density)
√ striking cortical thinning + bone widening
√ endosteal scalloping (due to marrow packing)
√ Erlenmeyer flask deformity of distal femur + proximal tibia
√ numerous sharply circumscribed lytic lesions resembling metastases / multiple myeloma (marrow replacement)
√ periosteal reaction = cloaking
√ weakening of subchondral bone + degenerative arthritis
√ bone infarction in long-bone metaphyses (common)
√ H-shaped / "step-off" / biconcave "fish-mouth" vertebra
@ Spleen
  √ multiple nodular lesions of low attenuation without enhancement on CT / hypoechoic or hyperechoic on US (= clusters of RES cells laden with glucosyl ceramide)
@ Lung
  √ diffuse reticulonodular infiltrates at lung bases (= infiltration with Gaucher cells)
Cx: ◊ >90% have orthopedic complications at some time
  (1) pathologic fractures + compression fractures of vertebrae
  (2) osteonecrosis of femoral head, humeral head, wrist, ankle (common)
  (3) osteomyelitis (increased incidence)
  (4) myelosclerosis in long-standing disease
  (5) repeated pulmonary infections
Prognosis: highly variable clinical course; strong relationship between splenic volume and disease severity

GIANT CELL REPARATIVE GRANULOMA
= GIANT CELL REACTION
Histo: numerous giant cells in exuberant fibrous matrix, osteoid formation, areas of hemorrhage
Peak age: 2nd + 3rd decade (range from childhood to 76 years); M:F = 1:1
Location: mandible, maxilla, small bones of hand + feet
• pain + mass in affected bone
√ expansile lytic defect with thinning of overlying cortex
√ periosteal reaction may be present
√ soft-tissue swelling / extension beyond cortex
√ no matrix calcification

Cx: pathologic fracture
Rx: curettage (50% recurrence rate) / local excision
DDx: (1) Enchondroma (same location, matrix calcification)
(2) Aneurysmal bone cyst (rare in small bones of hand + feet, typically prior to epiphyseal closure)
(3) Giant cell tumor (more aggressive appearance)
(4) Infection (clinical)
(5) Brown tumor of HPT (periosteal bone resorption, abnormal Ca + P levels)

GIANT CELL TUMOR

= OSTEOCLASTOMA = probably arise from zone of intense osteoclastic activity in skeletally immature patients
Incidence: 4.2% of all primary bone tumors; 21% of benign skeletal tumors
Histo: multinucleated osteoclastic giant cells intermixed throughout a spindle cell stroma (giant cells characteristic of all reactive bone disease, seen in pigmented villonodular synovitis, benign chondroblastoma, nonosteogenic fibroma, chondromyxoid fibroma, fibrous dysplasia)
Age: in 98.3% after (in 1.7% before) epiphyseal plate fusion; 14% < age 20; 70–80% between 20 and 40 years; M:F = 1:1
May be associated with: Paget disease (in 50–60% located in skull + facial bones)
- tenderness + pain at affected site
- weakness + sensory deficits (if in spine)

Location:
(a) 85% in long bones
— lower extremity (50–60% about knee): distal end of femur > proximal end of tibia
— upper extremity (away from elbow): distal end of radius > proximal end of humerus
(b) 15% in flat bones: pelvis, sacrum near SIJ (common, 2nd only to chordoma) > thoracic > cervical > lumbar spine (5–7%), rib (anterior / posterior end), skull

Site: eccentric in metaphysis of long bones, adjacent to / in ossified epiphyseal line, subarticular if epiphyseal plate is fused (MOST TYPICAL)
√ expansile solitary lytic bone lesion ("soap bubble"), large at diagnosis
√ conspicuous peripheral trabeculae without tumor matrix
√ no sclerosis / periosteal reaction (aggressive rapid growth) in absence of fracture
√ may break through bone cortex with cortical thinning, soft-tissue invasion (25%), pathologic fracture (5%)
√ destruction of vertebral body with secondary invasion of posterior elements (DDx: ABC, osteoblastoma)
√ frequently vertebral collapse
√ involves adjacent vertebral disks + vertebrae, crosses sacroiliac joint
√ may cross joint space in long bones (exceedingly rare)

NUC:
√ diffusely increased uptake ± "donut" sign of central photopenia

Angio:
√ hypervascular lesion

CT:
√ tumor of soft-tissue attenuation with foci of low attenuation (hemorrhage / necrosis)
√ well-defined margins ± thin rim of sclerosis

MR:
√ heterogeneous signal intensity with low to intermediate intensity on T1WI + T2WI (63–96%) due to collagen + hemosiderin content
√ focal cystic areas
√ low-signal-intensity pseudocapsule

Cx: 15% malignant within first 5 years (M:F = 3:1); metastases to lung
Prognosis: locally aggressive; 40–60% recurrence rate
Rx: complete resection; excision + radiation therapy
DDx: (1) Aneurysmal bone cyst (in posterior elements of spine with invasion of vertebral body)
(2) Brown tumor of HPT (lab values)
(3) Cartilage tumor: chondroblastoma, enchondroma (not epiphyseal), chondromyxoid fibroma, chondrosarcoma
(4) Bone abscess
(5) Hemangioma
(6) Fibrous dysplasia

GLOMUS TUMOR

= hamartoma composed of cells derived from neuromyo-arterial apparatus (regulating blood flow in skin)
Glomus body = encapsulated oval organ of 300 µm length; located in reticular dermis (= deepest layer of skin); concentrated in tips of digits (93–501/cm^2); composed of an afferent arteriole, an anastomotic vessel (= Sucquet-Hoyer canal lined by endothelium + surrounded by smooth muscle fibers), a primary collecting vein, the intraglomerular reticulum + capsule
Histo: (a) vascular (b) myxoid (c) solid form
Prevalence: 1–5% of soft-tissue tumors of hand
Age: mostly in 4–5th decade
- joint tenderness + pain (on average of 4–7 years duration prior to diagnosis)
- Love test = eliciting pain by applying precise pressure with a pencil tip
- Hildreth sign = disappearance of pain after application of a tourniquet proximally on arm (PATHOGNOMONIC)

@ SUBUNGUAL GLOMUS TUMOR
√ increased distance between dorsum of phalanx + underside of nail (25%)
√ extrinsic bone erosion (14–25–65%), often with sclerotic border
√ small hypoechoic tumor by US (>3 mm detectable)
√ homogeneously high-signal–intensity lesion on T2WI (detectable if >2 mm in diameter)

@ GLOMUS TUMOR OF BONE occasionally within bone
√ resembles enchondroma

DDx: (1) Mucoid cyst (painless, in proximal nail fold, communicating with DIP joint, associated with osteoarthritis)
(2) Angioma (more superficially located)

GOUT

= deposition of positively birefringent monosodium urate monohydrate crystals in poorly vascularized tissues (synovial membranes, articular cartilage, ligaments, bursae) leading to destruction of cartilage

Age: >40 years; males (in women gout may occur after menopause)

Cause:

A. Idiopathic Gout
Incidence: 0.3%; M:F = 20:1
(1) Overproduction of uric acid (phosphoribosyl transferase deficiency)
(2) Abnormality of renal urate excretion

B. Secondary Gout
rarely cause for radiographically apparent disease
(1) Myeloproliferative disorders + sequelae of their treatment: polycythemia vera, leukemia, lymphoma, multiple myeloma
(2) Blood dyscrasias
(3) Endocrinologic: myxedema, hyperparathyroidism
(4) Chronic renal failure
(5) Enzyme defects: glycogen storage disease
(6) Vascular: myocardial infarction, hypertension
(7) Lead poisoning

Stages:
(1) asymptomatic hyperuricemia
(2) acute monarticular gout
(3) polyarticular gout
(4) chronic tophaceous gout = multiple large urate deposits

Location: (a) joints: hands + feet (1st MTP joint most commonly affected = podagra), elbow, wrist (carpometacarpal compartment especially common), knee, shoulder, hip, sacroiliac joint (15%, unilateral)
(b) ear > bones, tendon, bursa
Involvement of hip + spine is rare

◊ Radiologic features usually not seen until 6–12 years after initial attack
◊ Radiologic features present in 50% of inflicted patients

@ Soft tissues
√ calcific deposits in gouty tophi in 50% (sodium urate crystals not radiopaque, only after calcium deposition)
√ eccentric juxta-articular lobulated soft-tissue masses (hand, foot, ankle, elbow, knee)
√ bilateral effusion of bursae olecrani (PATHOGNOMONIC)
√ aural calcification

@ Joint
√ preservation of joint space initially (important clue!)
√ absence of periarticular demineralization (DDx: rheumatoid arthritis)
√ erosion of joint margins (resembling rheumatoid arthritis) but with sclerosis
√ cartilage destruction (late in course of disease)
√ periarticular swelling (in acute monarticular gout)
√ chondrocalcinosis (menisci, articular cartilage of knee) resulting in secondary osteoarthritis
√ round / oval subarticular cysts up to 3 cm

@ Bone
√ "punched-out" lytic bone lesion ± sclerosis of margin = "mouse / rat bite" from erosion of long-standing soft-tissue tophus
√ "overhanging margin" (40%) = elevated osseous spicule in sites of tophus formation associated with erosion of adjacent bone (in intra- and extra-articular locations) (HALLMARK)
√ ischemic necrosis of femoral / humeral heads
√ bone infarction due to deposits at vascular basement membrane (DDx: bone island)

Coexisting disorders:
1. Psoriasis
2. Glycogen storage disease Type I
3. Hypo- and hyperparathyroidism
4. Down syndrome
5. Lesch-Nyhan syndrome (choreoathetosis, spasticity, mental retardation, self-mutilation of lips + fingertips)

◊ NOT associated with rheumatoid arthritis!

Rx: colchicine, allopurinol (effective treatment usually does not improve roentgenograms)

GRANULOCYTIC SARCOMA

= CHLOROMA = MYELOBLASTOMA
= solid tumor consisting of primitive precursors of the granulocytic series of WBCs (myeloblasts, promyelocytes, myelocytes)

Associated with: AML (3–8%), CML (1%), polycythemia rubra vera, myelofibrosis with myeloid metaplasia, hypereosinophilic syndrome

• 60% are of green color (chloroma) due to high levels of myeloperoxidase (30% are white / gray / brown depending on preponderance of cell type + oxidative state of myeloperoxidase)

Location: orbit, subcutaneous tissue, paranasal sinus, lymph node, bone, organs; often multiple

Site: propensity for bone marrow (arises from bone marrow traversing haversian canal + reaching the periosteum), perineural + epidural tissue

√ osteolysis with ill-defined margins
√ homogeneous enhancement on CT / MR (DDx to hematoma / abscess)

MR:
√ isointense to brain / bone marrow / muscle on T1WI + T2WI

Prognosis: resolution under chemotherapy ± radiation therapy; recurrence rate of 23%

DDx: osteomyelitis, histiocytosis X, neuroblastoma, lymphoma, multiple myeloma

HEMANGIOENDOTHELIAL SARCOMA

= HEMANGIOENDOTHELIOMA
= HEMANGIOEPITHELIOMA
= neoplasm of vascular endothelial cells of intermediate aggressiveness with either benign or malignant behavior

Histo: irregular anastomosing vascular channels lined by one / several layers of atypical anaplastic endothelial cells
Age: 4th–5th decade; M:F = 2:1
• history of trauma / irradiation

Soft-tissue hemangioendothelioma (common)
Location: deep tissues of extremities
Site: in 50% closely related to a vessel (often a vein)

Osseous hemangioendothelioma (rare)
Age: 2nd–3rd decade of life; M > F
Location: calvarium, spine, femur, tibia, humerus, pelvis; multicentric lesions in 30% often with regional distribution (less aggressive)
√ eccentric lesion in metaphysis of long bones
√ osteolytic aggressively destructive area with indistinct margins (high grade)
√ well-demarcated margins with scattered bony trabeculae (low grade)
√ osteoblastic area in vertebrae, contiguous through several vertebrae
Metastases to: lung (early)
Prognosis: 26% 5-year survival rate
DDx: aneurysmal bone cyst, poorly differentiated fibrosarcoma, highly vascular metastasis, alveolar rhabdomyosarcoma

HEMANGIOMA

A. CAPILLARY HEMANGIOMA (most common)
= small-caliber vessels lined by flattened epithelium
Site: skin, subcutaneous tissue; vertebral body
Age: first few years of life
(a) Juvenile capillary hemangioma = strawberry nevus
Prevalence: 1:200 births; in 20% multiple
Prognosis: involutes in 75–90% by age 7 years
(b) Verrucous capillary hemangioma
(c) Senile capillary hemangioma
√ enlarged arteries + arteriovenous shunting
√ pooling of contrast material

B. CAVERNOUS HEMANGIOMA
= dilated blood-filled spaces lined by flattened endothelium
Site: deeper soft tissues, frequently intramuscular; calvarium
Age: childhood
√ phleboliths = dystrophic calcification in organizing thrombus
√ large cystic spaces
√ enlarged arteries + arteriovenous shunting
√ pooling of contrast material
Prognosis: NO involution

C. ARTERIOVENOUS HEMANGIOMA
= persistence of fetal capillary bed with abnormal communications of an increased number of normal / abnormal arteries and veins
Etiology: (?) congenital arteriovenous malformation
Age: young patients
Site: soft tissues
(a) superficial lesion without arteriovenous shunting
(b) deep lesion with arteriovenous shunting
• limb enlargement, bruit
• distended veins, overlying skin warmth
• Branham sign = reflex bradycardia after compression
√ large tortuous serpentine feeding vessels
√ fast blood flow + dense staining
√ early draining veins

D. VENOUS HEMANGIOMA
= thick-walled vessels containing muscle
Site: deep soft tissues of retroperitoneum, mesentery, muscles of lower extremities
Age: adulthood
√ ± phleboliths
√ serpentine vessels with slow blood flow
√ vessels oriented along long axis of extremity (in 78%) + neurovascular bundle (in 64%)
√ multifocal involvement (in 37%)
√ muscle atrophy with increased subcutaneous fat
√ may be normal on arterial angiography

Osseous hemangioma
Incidence: 10%
Histo: mostly cavernous; capillary type is rare
Age: 4th–5th decade; M:F = 2:1
• usually asymptomatic

@ Vertebra (28% of all skeletal hemangiomas)
Incidence: in 5–11% of all autopsies; multiple in 1/3
Histo: capillary hemangioma interspersed in fatty matrix
◊ The larger the degree of fat overgrowth, the less likely the lesion will be symptomatic!
Age: >40 years; female
Location: in lower thoracic / upper lumbar spine
√ "accordion" / "corduroy" / "honeycomb" vertebra = coarse vertical trabeculae with osseous reinforcement adjacent to bone resorption caused by vascular channels (also in multiple myeloma, lymphoma, metastasis)
√ bulge of posterior cortex
√ extraosseous extension beyond bony lesion (with cord compression)
√ paravertebral soft-tissue extension
√ lesion enhancement
CT:
√ polka-dot appearance = small punctate areas of sclerosis (= thickened vertical trabeculae)
MR:
√ mottled pattern of low-to-high intensity on T1WI + very-high intensity on T2WI depending on degree of adipose tissue (CHARACTERISTIC)
Cx: vertebral collapse (unusual), spinal cord compression
@ Calvarium (20% of all hemangiomas)
Location: frontal / parietal region
Site: diploe

√ <4 cm round osteolytic lesion with sunburst / weblike / spoke-wheel appearance of trabecular thickening
√ expansion of outer table to a greater extent than inner table producing palpable lump

@ Flat bones & long bones (rare)
– ribs, clavicle, mandible, zygoma, nasal bones, metaphyseal ends of long bones (tibia, femur, humerus)
√ radiating trabecular thickening
√ bubbly bone lysis creating honeycomb / latticelike / "hole-within-hole" appearance

MR:
√ serpentine vascular channels with low signal intensity on T1WI + high signal intensity on T2WI (= slow blood flow) / low signal intensity on all sequences (= high blood flow)

NUC (bone / RBC-labeled scintigraphy):
√ photopenia / moderate increased activity

Soft-tissue hemangioma

Incidence: 7% of all benign tumors; most frequent tumor of infancy + childhood

Nonvascular elements: fat, smooth muscle, fibrous tissue, thrombus, bone

◊ Fat overgrowth may be so extensive that some areas of lesion may be misdiagnosed as lipoma!

Age: primarily in children; M < F

• intermittent change in size
• painful
• bluish discoloration of overlying skin (rare)
• may dramatically increase in size during pregnancy

Location: usually intramuscular; synovia (<1% of all hemangiomas); common in head and neck

√ nonspecific soft-tissue mass
√ may extend into bone
√ ± longitudinal / axial bone overgrowth (secondary to chronic hyperemia)
√ may contain phleboliths (30% of lesions, SPECIFIC)
√ nonspecific curvilinear / amorphous calcifications
√ may contain such large amounts of fat as to be indistinguishable from lipoma

CT:
√ poorly defined mass with attenuation similar to muscle
√ areas of decreased attenuation approximating subcutaneous fat (= fat overgrowth)

MR:
√ poorly marginated mass isointense to muscle on T1WI
√ areas with increased signal intensity on T1WI in periphery of lesion extending into septations (= fat)
√ well-marginated markedly hyperintense mass on T2WI (increased free water content in stagnant blood)
√ tubular structures with blood flow characteristics (flow void / inflow enhancement; contrast enhancement)
√ phleboliths as low-intensity areas inside lesion
√ high-signal-intensity areas on T1WI + T2WI (= hemorrhage)

US:
√ complex mass
√ low-resistance arterial signal (occasionally)

Synovial hemangioma

• repetitive bleeding into joint

Location: knee (60%), elbow (30%)

DDx: hemophilic arthropathy (polyarticular)

HEMANGIOPERICYTOMA

= borderline tumor with benign / locally aggressive / malignant behavior (counterpart of glomus tumor)

Age: 4th–5th decade; M:F = 1:1

Path: large vessels predominantly in tumor periphery

Histo: cells packed around vascular channels containing cystic + necrotic areas; arising from cells of Zimmerman that are located around vessels

@ Soft tissue
= deep-seated well-circumscribed lesion arising in muscle

Location: lower extremity in 35% (thigh), pelvic cavity, retroperitoneum

• painless slowly growing mass up to 20 cm

@ Bone (rare)

Location: lower extremity, vertebrae, pelvis, skull (dura similar to meningioma)

√ osteolytic lesions in metaphysis of long / flat bone
√ subperiosteal large blowout lesion (similar to aneurysmal bone cyst)

Angio:
√ displacement of main artery
√ pedicle of tumor feeder arteries
√ spider-shaped arrangement of vessels encircling tumor
√ small corkscrew arteries
√ dense tumor stain

DDx: hemangioendothelioma, angiosarcoma

HEMOCHROMATOSIS

1. PRIMARY HEMOCHROMATOSIS
   = autosomal recessive / indeterminate inheritance (abnormal iron-loading gene) in thalassemia, sideroblastic anemia
2. SECONDARY HEMOCHROMATOSIS
   = excessive iron absorption in anemias, myelofibrosis, portacaval shunt, exogenous administration of iron, porphyria cutanea tarda, beer brewed in iron vessels + deposition of excessive iron in liver, pancreas, spleen, GI tract, kidney, gonads, heart, endocrine glands (pituitary, hypothalamus)

Age: >40 years; M:F = 10:1 (females protected by menstruation)

• cirrhosis
• "bronzed diabetes"
• congestive heart failure
• skin pigmentation
• hypogonadism
• arthritic symptoms (30%)
• increase in serum iron

@ Skeleton
Site: most commonly in hands (metacarpal heads, particularly 2nd + 3rd MCP joints), carpal + proximal interphalangeal joints, knees, hips
√ generalized osteoporosis
√ small subchondral cystlike rarefactions with fine rim of sclerosis (metacarpal heads)
√ arthropathy in 50% with iron deposition in synovium
√ uniform joint space narrowing
√ enlargement of metacarpal heads
√ eventually osteophyte formation
√ chondrocalcinosis in >60%, knees most commonly affected
(a) calcium pyrophosphate deposition (inhibition of pyrophosphatase enzyme within cartilage which hydrolyzes pyrophosphate to soluble orthophosphate)
(b) calcification of triangular cartilage of wrist, menisci, annulus fibrosus, ligamentum flavum, symphysis pubis, Achilles tendon, plantar fascia
@ Brain MRI:
√ marked loss in signal intensity of anterior lobe of pituitary gland (iron deposition)
Cx: hepatoma (in 30%)
Prognosis: death from CHF (30%), death from hepatic failure (25%)
DDx: (1) Pseudogout (no arthropathy)
(2) Psoriatic arthritis (skin + nail changes)
(3) Osteoarthritis (predominantly distal joints in hands)
(4) Rheumatoid arthritis
(5) Gout (may also have chondrocalcinosis)

HEMOPHILIA

= X-linked deficiency / functional abnormality of coagulation factor VIII (= hemophilia A) in >80% / factor IX (= hemophilia B = Christmas disease)
Incidence: 1:10,000 males
@ Hemarthrosis (most common)
Histo: hypertrophic synovial membrane with pannus formation that erodes cartilage, loss of subchondral bone plate, formation of subarticular cysts
• tense red warm joint with decreased range of motion (muscle spasm)
• fever, elevated WBC (DDx: septic arthritis)
Location: in knee, ankle, elbow
√ soft-tissue swelling of joint
√ enlargement of epiphysis (secondary to synovial hyperemia)
√ thinning of joint cartilage (particularly patella) secondary to cartilage destruction
√ erosion of articular surface with multiple subchondral cysts
√ superimposed degenerative joint disease
√ "squared" patella
√ widening of intercondylar notch
√ medial "slanting" of tibiotalar joint
√ juxta-articular osteoporosis

@ Hemophilic pseudotumor (1–2%)
= posthemorrhagic cystic swelling within muscle + bone characterized by pressure necrosis + destruction
(a) juvenile form = usually multiple intramedullary expansile lesions without soft-tissue mass in small bones of hand / feet (before epiphyseal closure)
(b) adult form = usually single intramedullary expansile lesion with large soft-tissue mass in ilium / femur
(c) soft-tissue involvement of retroperitoneum (psoas muscle), bowel wall, renal collecting system
√ mixed cystic expansile lesion
√ bone erosion + pathologic fracture
CT:
√ sometimes encapsulated mass containing areas of low attenuation + calcifications
MR:
√ hemorrhage of varying age
N.B.: Needle aspiration / biopsy / excision may cause fistulae / infection / uncontrolled bleeding!
Rx: palliative radiation therapy (destroys vessels prone to bleed) + transfusion of procoagulation factor concentrate

HEREDITARY HYPERPHOSPHATASIA

= "JUVENILE PAGET DISEASE" = rare autosomal recessive disease with sustained elevation of serum alkaline phosphatase, especially in individuals of Puerto Rican descent
Histo: rapid turnover of lamellar bone without formation of cortical bone; immature woven bone is rapidly laid down, but simultaneous rapid destruction prevents normal maturation
Age: 1st–3rd year; usually stillborn
• rapid enlargement of calvarium + long bones
• dwarfism
• cranial nerve deficit (blind, deaf)
• hypertension
• frequent respiratory infections
• pseudoxanthoma elasticum
• elevated alkaline phosphatase
√ deossification = decreased density of long bones with coarse trabecular pattern
√ metaphyseal growth deficiency
√ wide irregular epiphyseal lines (resembling rickets in childhood), persistent metaphyseal defects (40% of adults)
√ bowing of long bones + fractures with irregular callus
√ widened medullary canal with cortical thinning (cortex modeled from trabecular bone)
√ skull greatly thickened with wide tables, cotton wool appearance
√ vertebra plana
OB-US:
√ diagnosis suspected in utero in 20%
Cx: pathologic fractures; vertebra plana universalis
DDx: (1) Osteogenesis imperfecta
(2) Polyostotic fibrous dysplasia
(3) Paget disease (> age 20, not generalized)
(4) Pyle disease (spares midshaft)

(5) van Buchem syndrome (only diaphyses > age 20, no long-bone bowing)
(6) Engelmann syndrome (lower limbs)

HEREDITARY MULTIPLE EXOSTOSES

= DIAPHYSEAL ACLASIS

Inheritance: autosomal dominant (unaffected female may be carrier)

Age: discovered between 2 and 10 years; M:F = 2:1

Path: ectopic cartilaginous rest in metaphysis + defect in periosteum; cap of hyaline cartilage; often bursa formation over cap

- usually painless mass near joints
- tendons, blood vessels, nerves may be impaired
- mechanical limitation of joint movement

Location: multiple + usually bilateral; common sites are knee, elbow, scapula, pelvis, ribs

Site: metaphyses of long bones near epiphyseal plate (distance to epiphyseal line increases with growth)

√ cortex + cancellous bone of exostosis contiguous to host bone
√ slope on epiphyseal side + right angle on diaphyseal side of stalk = points away from joint + toward center of shaft
√ occasionally small punctate calcifications in cartilaginous cap
√ shortening of 4th + 5th metacarpals
√ supernumerary fingers / toes
√ Madelung / reversed Madelung deformity = radius usually longer + bowed
√ occasionally results in disproportionate shortening of an extremity, radioulnar synostosis, dislocation of radial head

Prognosis: exostosis begins in childhood; stops growing when nearest epiphyseal center fuses

Cx: (1) Cord compression secondary to involvement of posterior spinal elements
(2) Malignant transformation to chondrosarcoma in <5%; iliac bone commonest site; growth with irregularity of outline + fuzziness; sudden painful growth spurt

HEREDITARY SPHEROCYTOSIS

= autosomal dominant congenital hemolytic anemia

Age: anemia begins in early infancy to late adulthood

- rarely severe anemia
- jaundice
- spherocytes in peripheral smear

√ bone changes rare (due to mild anemia); long bones rarely affected
√ widening of diploe with displacement + thinning of outer table
√ hair-on-end appearance

Rx: splenectomy corrects anemia even though spherocytemia persists
√ improvement in skeletal alterations following splenectomy

HERNIATION PIT

= SYNOVIAL HERNIATION PIT = CONVERSION DEFECT
= ingrowth of fibrous + cartilaginous elements from adjacent joint through perforation in cortex

Histo: fibroalveolar tissue

Age: usually in older individuals

- may be symptomatic
- no clinical significance

Location: anterior superolateral aspect of proximal femoral neck; uni- or bilateral

Site: subcortical

√ well-circumscribed round lucency
√ usually <1 cm in diameter
√ reactive thin sclerotic border
√ hyperintense area on T2WI
√ bone scan may be positive

HOLT-ORAM SYNDROME

Autosomal dominant; M < F

Associated with CHD: secundum type ASD (most common), VSD, persistent left SVC, tetralogy, coarctation

- intermittent cardiac arrhythmia
- bradycardia (50–60/min)

Location: upper extremity only involved; symmetry of lesions is the rule; left side may be more severely affected

√ aplasia / hypoplasia of radial structures: thumb, 1st metacarpal, carpal bones, radius
√ "fingerized" hypoplastic thumb / triphalangeal thumb
√ slender elongated hypoplastic carpals + metacarpals
√ hypoplastic radius; absent radial styloid
√ shallow glenoid fossa (voluntary dislocation of shoulder common)
√ hypoplastic clavicula
√ high arched palate
√ cervical scoliosis
√ pectus excavatum

HOMOCYSTINURIA

Autosomal recessive disorder

Etiology: cystathionine B synthetase deficiency results in defective methionine metabolism with accumulation of homocystine + homocysteine in blood and urine; causes defect in collagen / elastin structure

- thromboembolic phenomena due to stickiness of platelets
- ligamentous laxity
- downward + inward dislocation of lens (DDx: upward + outward dislocation in Marfan syndrome)
- mild / moderate mental retardation
- crowding of maxillary teeth and protrusion of incisors
- malar flush

√ arachnodactyly in 1/3 (DDx: Marfan syndrome)
√ microcephaly
√ enlarged paranasal sinuses
√ osteoporosis of vertebrae (biconcave / flattened / widened vertebrae)
√ scoliosis

	Marfan Syndrome	Homocystinuria
Inheritance:	autosomal dominant	autosomal recessive
Biochemical defect:	not known	cystathionine synthetase
Osteoporosis:	no	yes
Spine:	scoliosis	biconcave vertebrae
Lens dislocation:	upward	downward
Arachnodactyly:	100%	33%

√ pectus excavatum / carinatum (75%)
√ osteoporosis of long bones (75%) with bowing + fracture
√ children: metaphyseal cupping (50%); enlargement of ossification centers in 50% (knee, carpal bones); epiphyseal calcifications (esp. in wrist, resembling phenylketonuria); delayed ossification
√ Harris lines = multiple growth lines
√ genu valgum, coxa valga, coxa magna, pes cavus
√ premature vascular calcifications

Prognosis: death from occlusive vascular disease / minor vascular trauma

HYPERPARATHYROIDISM

= uncontrolled production of parathyroid hormone

Age: middle age; M:F = 1:3

Histo: decreased bone mass secondary to increased number of osteoclasts, increased osteoid volume (defect in mineralization), slightly increased number of osteoblasts

- increase in parathyroid hormone (100%)
- increase in serum alkaline phosphatase (50%)
- elevation of serum calcium (due to accelerated bone turnover and increased calcium absorption) + decrease in serum phosphate (30%)
- hypotonicity of muscles, weakness, constipation, difficulty in swallowing, duodenal / gastric peptic ulcer disease (secondary to hypercalcemia)
- polyuria, polydipsia (hypercalciuria + hyperphosphaturia)
- renal colic + renal insufficiency (nephrocalculosis + nephrocalcinosis)
- rheumatic bone pain + tenderness (particularly at site of brown tumor), pathologic fracture secondary to brown tumor

A. BONE RESORPTION

(a) subperiosteal (most constant + specific finding; virtually PATHOGNOMONIC of hyperparathyroidism):

√ lacelike irregularity of cortical margin; may progress to scalloping / spiculation (pseudoperiostitis)

Site: phalangeal tufts (earliest involvement), radial aspect of middle phalanx of 2nd + 3rd finger beginning in proximal metaphyseal region (early involvement), bandlike zone of resorption in middle / base of terminal tuft, distal end of clavicles, medial tibia plateau, medial humerus neck, medial femoral neck, distal ulna, superior + inferior margins of ribs in midclavicular line, lamina dura of skull and teeth

(b) subchondral

√ pseudowidening of joint space
√ collapse of cortical bone + overlying cartilage with development of erosion, cyst, joint narrowing (similar to rheumatoid arthritis)

Site: DIP joint (most commonly 4th + 5th digit), MCP joint, PIP joint, distal clavicle, acromioclavicular joint (clavicular side), "pseudowidening" of sacroiliac joint (iliac side), sternoclavicular joint, symphysis pubis, "scalloping" of posterior surface of patella, Schmorl nodes; typically polyarticular

(c) cortical (due to osteoclastic activity within haversian canal):

√ intracortical tunneling
√ scalloping along inner cortical surface (endosteal resorption)

(d) trabecular

√ spotty deossification with indistinct + coarse trabecular pattern
√ granular salt and pepper skull
√ loss of distinction between inner and outer table
√ ground-glass appearance

(e) subligamentous:

√ bone resorption with smooth scalloped / irregular ill-defined margins

Site: inferior surface of calcaneus (long plantar tendons + aponeurosis), inferior aspect of distal clavicle (coracoclavicular ligament), greater trochanter (hip abductors), lesser trochanter (iliopsoas), anterior inferior iliac spine (rectus femoris), humeral tuberosity (rotator cuff), ischial tuberosity (hamstrings), proximal extensor surface of ulna (anconeus), posterior olecranon (triceps)

B. BONE SOFTENING

√ basilar impression of skull
√ wedged vertebrae, kyphoscoliosis, biconcave vertebral deformities
√ bowing of long bones
√ slipped capital femoral epiphysis

C. BROWN TUMOR

= OSTEOCLASTOMA

Cause: PTH-stimulated osteoclastic activity (more frequent in 1° HPT; in 1.5% of 2° HPT)

Path: localized replacement of bone by vascularized fibrous tissue (osteitis fibrosa cystica) containing giant cells; lesions may become cystic following necrosis + liquefaction

Location: jaw, pelvis, rib, metaphyses of long bones (femur), facial bones, axial skeleton
Site: often eccentric / cortical; frequently solitary
√ expansile lytic well-marginated cystlike lesion (DDx: giant cell tumor)
√ endosteal scalloping
√ destruction of midportions of distal phalanges with telescoping

D. OSTEOSCLEROSIS
More frequent in 2° HPT
Cause: ? PTH-stimulated osteoblastic activity, ? role of calcitonin (poorly understood)
Site: strong predilection for axial skeleton, pelvis, ribs, clavicles, metaphysis + epiphysis of appendicular skeleton
√ "rugger jersey spine" (resembling the stripes on rugby jerseys) = sclerosis of vertebral endplates with intervening normal osseous density

E. SOFT-TISSUE CALCIFICATION
More frequent in 2° HPT; metastatic calcification when Ca x P product >70 mg/dL
(a) cornea, viscera (lung, stomach, kidney)
(b) periarticular in hip, knee, shoulder, wrist
(c) arterial tunica media (resembling diabetes mellitus)
(d) Chondrocalcinosis (15–18%) = calcification of hyaline / fibrous cartilage in menisci, wrist, shoulder, hip, elbow

F. EROSIVE ARTHROPATHY
• asymptomatic
√ simulates rheumatoid arthritis with preserved joint spaces

G. PERIOSTEAL NEW-BONE FORMATION
Cause: PTH-stimulation of osteoblasts
Site: pubic ramus along iliopectineal line (most frequent), humerus, femur, tibia, radius, ulna, metacarpals, metatarsals, phalanges
√ linear new bone paralleling cortical surface; may be laminated; often separated from cortex by radiolucent zone
√ increase in cortical thickness (if periosteal reaction becomes incorporated into adjacent bone)

Sequelae:
1. Renal stones / nephrocalcinosis (70%)
2. Increased osteoblastic activity (25%)
   • increased alkaline phosphatase
   (a) osteitis fibrosa cystica
      √ subperiosteal bone resorption + cortical tunneling
      √ brown tumors (primary HPT)
   (b) bone softening
      √ fractures
3. Peptic ulcer disease (increased gastric secretion from gastrinoma)
4. Calcific pancreatitis
5. Soft-tissue calcifications (2° HPT)
6. Marginal joint erosions + subarticular collapse (DIP, PIP, MCP)

Primary hyperparathyroidism

= pHPT = 1° HPT = hypercalcemia due to uncontrolled secretion of parathormone by one / more hyperfunctioning parathyroid glands featuring
(1) brown tumor
(2) chondrocalcinosis (20–30%)
◊ requires surgical Rx
Incidence: 25 / 100,000 per year; incidence of bone lesions in HPT is 25–40%
Etiology:
(a) Parathyroid adenoma (87%): single (80%); multiple (7%)
(b) Parathyroid hyperplasia (10%): chief cell (5%); clear cell (5%)
(c) Parathyroid carcinoma (3%)
Histo: increased number of osteoclasts, increased osteoid volume (defect in mineralization), slightly increased osteoblasts = decreased bone mass
Age: 3rd–5th decade; M:F = 1:3
Associated with:
(a) Wermer syndrome = MEA I (+ pituitary adenoma + pancreatic islet cell tumor)
(b) Sipple syndrome = MEA II (+ medullary thyroid carcinoma + pheochromocytoma)
X-ray (skeletal involvement in 20%):
√ thin cortices with lacy cortical pattern (subperiosteal bone resorption)
√ brown tumor (particularly in jaw + long bones)
√ osteitis cystica fibrosa (= intertrabecular fibrous connective tissue)
NUC:
√ normal bone scan in 80%
√ foci of abnormal uptake: calvarium (especially periphery), mandible, sternum, acromioclavicular joint, lateral humeral epicondyles, hands
√ increased uptake in brown tumors
√ extraskeletal uptake: cornea, cartilage, joint capsules, tendons, periarticular areas, lungs, stomach
√ normal renal excretion [except in stone disease / calcium nephropathy (10%)]
Rx: pathologic glands identified by experienced surgeons in 90–95% on initial neck exploration (ectopic + supernumerary glands often overlooked at operation; recurrent hypercalcemia in 3–10%)
Surgical risk for repeat surgery
6.6% recurrent laryngeal nerve injury
20.0% permanent hypoparathyroidism
<1.0% perioperative mortality

Secondary hyperparathyroidism

= sHPT = 2° HPT = diffuse / adenomatous hyperplasia of all four parathyroid glands as a compensatory mechanism in any state of hypocalcemia featuring (1) soft-tissue calcifications (2) osteosclerosis
◊ requires medical Rx

Etiology:
(a) renal osteodystrophy (renal insufficiency + osteomalacia / rickets)
(b) calcium deprivation, maternal hypoparathyroidism, pregnancy, hypovitaminosis D
(c) rise in serum phosphate leading to decrease in calcium by feedback mechanism

• low to normal calcium levels
• Ca^{2+} PO_4^{2-} solubility product often exceeded

NUC:
√ "superscan" in 2° HPT:
√ absent kidney sign
√ increased bone-to-soft tissue uptake ratio
√ increased uptake in calvarium, mandible, acromioclavicular region, sternum, vertebrae, distal third of long bones, ribs
√ diffuse Tc-99m MDP uptake in lungs (60%)

Tertiary hyperparathyroidism

= tHPT = 3° HPT = development of autonomous PTH adenoma in patients with chronically overstimulated hyperplastic parathyroid glands (renal insufficiency);
◊ requires surgical Rx

Clue: (a) intractable hypercalcemia
(b) inability to control osteomalacia by vitamin D administration

Ectopic parathormone production

= pseudohyperparathyroidism as paraneoplastic syndrome in bronchogenic carcinoma + renal cell carcinoma

HYPERTROPHIC OSTEOARTHROPATHY

= HYPERTROPHIC PULMONARY OSTEOARTHROPATHY

Etiology: (1) Release of vasodilators which are not metabolized by lung
(2) Increased flow through AV shunts
(3) Reflex peripheral vasodilation (vagal impulses)
(4) Hormones: estrogen, growth hormone, prostaglandin

A. THORACIC CAUSES
(a) malignant tumor (0.7–12%): bronchogenic carcinoma (88%), mesothelioma, lymphoma, pulmonary metastasis from osteogenic sarcoma, melanoma, renal cell carcinoma, breast cancer
(b) benign tumor: benign pleural fibroma, tumor of ribs, thymoma, esophageal leiomyoma, pulmonary hemangioma, pulmonary congenital cyst
(c) chronic infection / inflammation: pulmonary abscess, bronchiectasis, blastomycosis, TB (very rare); cystic fibrosis, interstitial fibrosis
(d) congenital heart disease with R-to-L shunt

B. EXTRATHORACIC CAUSES
(a) GI tract: ulcerative colitis, amebic + bacillary dysentery, intestinal TB, Whipple disease, Crohn disease, gastric ulcer, bowel lymphoma, gastric carcinoma
(b) liver disease: biliary + alcoholic cirrhosis, posthepatic cirrhosis, chronic active hepatitis, bile duct carcinoma, benign bile duct stricture, amyloidosis, liver abscess
(c) undifferentiated nasopharyngeal carcinoma, pancreatic carcinoma, chronic myelogenous leukemia

• burning pain, painful swelling of limbs, and stiffness of joints: ankles (88%), wrists (83%), knees (75%), elbows (17%), shoulders (10%), fingers (7%)
• peripheral neurovascular disorders: local cyanosis, areas of increased sweating, paresthesia, chronic erythema, flushing + blanching of skin
• hypocratic fingers + toes (clubbing)
• hypertrophy of extremities (soft-tissue swelling)

Location: tibia + fibula (75%), radius + ulna (80%), proximal phalanges (60%), femur (50%), metacarpus + metatarsus (40%), humerus + distal phalanges (25%), pelvis (5%); unilateral (rare)

Site: in diametaphyseal regions

√ periosteal proliferation of new bone, at first smooth then undulating + rough, most conspicuous on concavity of long bones (dorsal + medial aspects)
√ regression of periosteal reaction after thoracotomy
√ soft-tissue swelling ("clubbing") of distal phalanges

Bone scan (reveals changes early with greater sensitivity + clarity):
√ symmetric diffusely increased uptake along cortical margins of diaphysis + metaphysis of tubular bones of the extremities with irregularities
√ increased periarticular uptake (= synovitis)
√ scapular involvement in 2/3
√ mandible ± maxilla abnormal in 40%

HYPERVITAMINOSIS A

Age: usually infants + children

• anorexia, irritability
• loss of hair, dry skin, pruritus, fissures of lips
• jaundice, enlargement of liver

√ separation of cranial sutures secondary to hydrocephalus (coronal > lambdoid) in children <10 years of age, may appear within a few days
√ symmetrical solid periosteal new-bone formation along shafts of long + short bones (ulna, clavicle)
√ premature epiphyseal closure + thinning of epiphyseal plates
√ accelerated growth
√ tendinous, ligamentous, pericapsular calcifications
√ changes usually disappear after cessation of vitamin A ingestion

DDx: Infantile cortical hyperostosis (mandible involved)

HYPERVITAMINOSIS D

= excessive ingestion of vitamin D (large doses act like parathormone)

• loss of appetite, drowsiness, headaches
• polyuria, polydipsia, renal damage
• anemia
• diarrhea

- convulsions
- excessive phosphaturia (parathormone decreases tubular absorption)
- hypercalcemia + hypercalciuria

√ deossification
√ widening of provisional zone of calcification
√ cortical + trabecular thickening
√ alternating bands of increased + decreased density near / in epiphysis (zone of provisional calcification)
√ vertebra outlined by dense band of bone + adjacent radiolucent line within
√ dense calvarium
√ metastatic calcinosis in (a) arterial walls (between age 20 and 30) (b) kidneys = nephrocalcinosis (c) periarticular tissue (puttylike) (d) premature calcification of falx cerebri (most consistent sign!)

HYPOPARATHYROIDISM

Etiology:

A. Idiopathic Hypoparathyroidism
= rare condition of unknown cause
- round face, short dwarflike, obese
- mental retardation
- cataracts
- dry scaly skin, atrophy of nails
- dental hypoplasia (delayed tooth eruption, impaction of teeth, supernumerary teeth)

B. Secondary Hypoparathyroidism
= accidental removal / damage to parathyroid glands in thyroid surgery / radical neck dissection (5%); I-131 therapy (rare); external beam radiation; hemorrhage; infection; thyroid carcinoma; hemochromatosis (iron deposition)

- tetany = neuromuscular excitability (numbness, cramps, carpopedal spasm, laryngeal stridor, generalized convulsions)
- hypocalcemia + hyperphosphatemia
- normal / low serum alkaline phosphatase

√ premature closure of epiphyses
√ hypoplasia of tooth enamel + dentine; blunting of roots
√ generalized increase in bone density in 9%
  √ localized thickening of skull
  √ sacroiliac sclerosis
√ bandlike density in metaphysis of long bones (25%), iliac crest, vertebral bodies
√ thickened lamina dura (inner table) + widened diploe
√ deformed hips with thickening + sclerosis of femoral head + acetabulum

@ Soft tissue
  √ intracranial calcifications in basal ganglia, choroid plexus, occasionally in cerebellum
  √ calcification of spinal and other ligaments
  √ subcutaneous calcifications
  √ ossification of muscle insertions
  √ ectopic bone formation

HYPOPHOSPHATASIA

= autosomal recessive congenital disease with low activity of serum-, bone-, liver-alkaline phosphatase resulting in poor mineralization (deficient generation of bone crystals)

Incidence: 1:100,000
Histo: indistinguishable from rickets

- phosphoethanolamine in urine as precursor of alkaline phosphatase
- normal serum calcium + phosphorus

A. <u>GROUP I = neonatal = congenital lethal form</u>
  √ marked demineralization of calvarium ("caput membranaceum" = soft skull)
  √ lack of calcification of metaphyseal end of long bones
  √ streaky irregular spotty margins of calcification
  √ cupping of metaphysis
  √ angulated shaft fractures with abundant callus formation
  √ short poorly ossified ribs
  √ poorly ossified vertebrae (especially neural arches)
  √ small pelvic bones
  OB-US:
    √ high incidence of intrauterine fetal demise
    √ increased echogenicity of falx (enhanced sound transmission secondary to poorly mineralized calvarium)
    √ poorly mineralized short bowed tubular bones + multiple fractures
    √ poorly mineralized spine

	HypoPT	PseudoHypoPT	PseudopseudoHypoPT
Serum-Ca	down	down	norm
Serum-P	up	up	norm
AlkaPhos	down/norm	down/norm	norm

Response to PTH-Injection	Norm / HypoPT	PseudoHypoPT
Urine-AMP	up	norm
Urine-P	up	norm
Plasma-AMP	up	norm

√ short poorly ossified ribs
√ polyhydramnios
Prognosis: death within 6 months

B. GROUP II = juvenile severe form
onset of symptoms within weeks to months
• moderate / severe dwarfism
• delayed weight bearing
√ resembles rickets
√ separated cranial sutures; craniostenosis in 2nd year
Prognosis: 50% mortality

C. GROUP III = adult mild form
recognized later in childhood / adolescence / adulthood
• dwarfism
√ clubfoot, genu valgum
√ demineralization of ossification centers (at birth / 3–4 months of age)
Prognosis: excellent; after 1 year no further progression

D. GROUP IV = latent form
heterozygous state
• normal / borderline levels of alkaline phosphatase
• patients are small for age
• disturbance of primary dentition
√ bone fragility + healed fractures
√ enlarged chondral ends of ribs
√ metaphyseal notching of long bones
√ Erlenmeyer flask deformity of femur

HYPOTHYROIDISM

A. Childhood = CRETINISM:
Frequency: 1:4,000 live births have congenital hypothyroidism
Cause: sporadic hypoplasia / ectopia of thyroid
√ delayed skeletal maturation (appearance + growth of ossification centers, epiphyseal closure)
√ fragmented stippled epiphyses
√ wide sutures / fontanelles with delayed closure
√ delayed dentition
√ delayed / decreased pneumatization of sinuses + mastoids
√ hypertelorism
√ dense vertebral margins
√ demineralization
√ hypoplastic phalanges of 5th finger
MR:
√ reduced myelination of brain (usually beginning during midgestation)
OB-US:
√ fetal goiter (especially in hyperthyroid mothers treated with methimazole / propylthiouracil / I-131)

B. Adulthood:
√ calvarial thickening / sclerosis
√ wedging of dorsolumbar vertebral bodies
√ coxa vara with flattened femoral head
√ premature atherosclerosis
No skeletal changes with adult onset!

INFANTILE CORTICAL HYPEROSTOSIS

= CAFFEY DISEASE
= uncommon self-limiting proliferative bone disease of infancy; remission + exacerbations are common
Cause: ? infectious; ? autosomal dominant with variable expression + incomplete penetrance / sporadic occurrence (rare)
Age: <6 months, reported in utero; M:F = 1:1
Histo: inflammation of periosteal membrane, proliferation of osteoblasts + connective tissue cells, deposition of immature bony trabeculae
• sudden, hard, extremely tender soft-tissue swellings over bone
• irritability, fever
• ± elevated ESR, increased alkaline phosphatase
• leukocytosis, anemia
Location: mandible (80%) > clavicle > ulna + others (except phalanges + vertebrae + round bones of wrists and ankles)
Site: hyperostosis affects diaphysis of tubular bones asymmetrically, epiphyses spared
√ massive periosteal new-bone formation + perifocal soft-tissue swelling
√ "double-exposed" ribs
√ narrowing of medullary space (= proliferation of endosteum)
√ bone expansion with remodeling of old cortex
Prognosis: usually complete recovery by 30 months
Rx: mild analgesics, steroids

Chronic Infantile Hyperostosis

Disease may persist or recur intermittently for years
√ bowing deformities, osseous bridging, diaphyseal expansion
• delayed muscular development, crippling deformities

DDx: (1) Hypervitaminosis A (rarely <1 year of age) (2) Periostitis of prematurity (3) Healing rickets (4) Scurvy (uncommon <4 months of age) (5) Syphilis (focal destruction) (6) Child abuse (7) Prostaglandin administration (usually following 4–6 weeks of therapy) (8) Osteomyelitis (9) Leukemia (10) Neuroblastoma (11) Kinky hair syndrome (12) Hereditary hyperphosphatasia

INFANTILE MYOFIBROMATOSIS

= GENERALIZED HAMARTOMATOSIS = CONGENITAL MULTIPLE FIBROMATOSIS = MULTIPLE VASCULAR LEIOMYOMAS = DESMOFIBROMATOSIS
= rare disorder characterized by proliferation of fibroblasts
Cause: unknown
Frequency: most common fibromatosis in childhood
Age: at birth (in 60%), <2 years (in 89%)
Path: well-marginated soft-tissue lesion 0.5–3 cm in diameter with scarlike consistency ± infiltration of surrounding tissues
Histo: spindle-shaped cells in short bundles and fascicles in periphery of lesion; hemangiopericytoma-like pattern in center with necrosis, hyalinization, calcification

(1) Solitary lesion (50–75%)
dermis, subcutis, muscle (86%)
Location: head, neck, trunk, bone (9%), GI tract (4%)
Prognosis: spontaneous regression in 100%; recurrence after surgical excision in 7–10%

(2) Multicentric disease (25–50%)
Location: skin (98%), subcutis (98%), muscle (98%), bone (57%), viscera (25–37%): lung (28%), heart (16%), GI tract (14%), pancreas (9%), liver (8%)
Prognosis: related to extent + location of visceral lesions with cardiopulmonary + GI involvement as harbingers of poor prognosis (death in 75–80%); spontaneous regression (33%)

• firm nodules in skin, subcutis, muscle
• ± overlying scarring of skin with ulceration

@ Skeleton
Location: any bone may be involved; commonly in femur, tibia, rib, pelvis, vertebral bodies, calvarium; often symmetric
Site: metaphysis of long bones
√ eccentric lobulated lytic foci with smooth margins 0.5–1.0 cm in size
√ well-defined with narrow zone of transition
√ initially no sclerosis; sclerotic margin with healing
√ osseous foci may increase in size and number
√ healing leaves little residual abnormality
√ unusual osseous findings:
  √ periosteal reaction, pathologic fracture
  √ vertebra plana, kyphoscoliosis with posterior scalloping of vertebral bodies
NUC (bone scan):
  √ increased / little radiotracer uptake
DDx: (1) Langerhans cell histiocytosis (skin lesions)
(2) Neurofibromatosis (multiple masses)
(3) Osseous hemangiomas / lymphangiomatosis / lipomatosis
(4) Metastatic neuroblastoma
(5) Multiple nonossifying fibromas
(6) Enchondromatosis
(7) Unusual infection
(8) Fibrous dysplasia

@ Soft tissue
√ solid mass with central necrosis
√ central / peripheral solitary / multiple calcifications
  √ ± contrast enhancement
CT:
  √ attenuation similar to muscle
MR:
  √ hypo- to hyperintense mass on T1WI + T2WI
DDx: (1) Neurofibromatosis
(2) Infantile fibrosarcoma, leiomyosarcoma
(3) Angiomatosis

@ Lung
√ interstitial fibrosis, reticulonodular infiltrates
√ discrete mass
√ generalized bronchopneumonia

@ GI tract
√ diffuse narrowing with multiple small filling defects

IRON DEFICIENCY ANEMIA
Age: infants affected
Cause:
(1) inadequate iron stores at birth (2) deficient iron in diet (3) impaired gastrointestinal absorption of iron (4) excessive iron demands from blood loss (5) polycythemia vera (6) cyanotic CHD
√ widening of diploe + thinning of tables with sparing of occiput (no red marrow)
√ hair-on-end appearance of skull
√ osteoporosis in long bones (most prominent in hands)
√ absence of facial bone involvement

JACCOUD ARTHROPATHY
After subsidence of frequent severe attacks of rheumatic fever
Path: periarticular fascial + tendon fibrosis without synovitis
• rheumatic valve disease
Location: primarily involvement of hands; occasionally in great toe
√ muscular atrophy
√ periarticular swelling of small joints of hands + feet
√ ulnar deviation + flexion of MCP joints most marked in 4th + 5th finger
√ NO joint narrowing / erosion

JUVENILE APONEUROTIC FIBROMA
Rare benign fibrous tumor
Histo: cellular dense fibrous tissue with focal chondral elements infiltrating adjacent structures (= cartilaginous tumor)
Age: children + adolescents; male preponderance
Location: deep palmar fascia of hand + wrist
√ soft-tissue mass overlying inflamed bursa (often mistaken for calcified bursitis)
√ stippled calcifications
√ interosseous soft-tissue mass of forearm + wrist
√ bone erosion may occur
DDx: synovial sarcoma, chondroma, fibrosarcoma, osteosarcoma, myositis ossificans

KLINEFELTER SYNDROME
47,XXY (rarely XXYY) chromosomal abnormality
Incidence: 1:750 live births (probably commonest chromosomal aberration)
• testicular atrophy (hyalinization of seminiferous tubules) = small / absent testes, sterility (azoospermia)
• eunuchoid constitution: gynecomastia; paucity of hair on face + chest; female pubic escutcheon
• mild mental retardation
• high level of urinary gonadotropins + low level of 17-ketosteroids after puberty

◊ NO distinctive radiological findings!
√ may have delayed bone maturation

√ failure of frontal sinus to develop
√ small bridged sella turcica
√ ± scoliosis, kyphosis
√ ± coxa valga
√ ± metacarpal sign (short 4th metacarpal)
√ accessory epiphyses of 2nd metacarpal bilaterally

47,XXX = SUPERFEMALE SYNDROME
- usually over 6 feet tall; subnormal intelligence; frequently antisocial behavior

KLIPPEL-TRÉNAUNAY SYNDROME

= sporadic (nonhereditary) rare mesodermal abnormality that usually affects a single lower limb characterized by a triad of:
(1) port-wine nevus = unilateral large flat infiltrative cutaneous capillary hemangioma often in dermatomal distribution on affected limb; may fade in 2nd–3rd decade
(2) gigantism = overgrowth of distal digits / entire extremity (especially during adolescent growth spurt) involving soft-tissue + bone
(3) varicose veins on lateral aspect of affected limb; usually ipsilateral to hemangioma

Pathogenesis:
superficial lateral venous channel of large caliber thought to represent the fetal lateral limb bud vein that has failed to regress; tissue overgrowth is secondary to impaired venous return

Age: usually in children; M:F = 1:1

Associated with:
— polydactyly, syndactyly, clinodactyly, oligodactyly, ectrodactyly, congenital dislocation of hip
— hemangiomas of colon / bladder (3–10%)
— spinal hemangiomas + AVMs
— hemangiomas in liver / spleen
— lymphangiomas of limb

Location: lower extremity (10–15 x more common than upper extremity); bilateral in <5%

√ increased metatarsal / metacarpal + phalangeal size
√ cortical thickening
√ punctate calcifications (phleboliths) in pelvis (bowel wall, urinary bladder)
√ pulmonary vein varicosities
√ cystic lung lesions

Venogram:
√ aplasia / hypoplasia of lower extremity veins (18–40%): ? selective flow of contrast material up the lateral venous channel may fail to opacify the deep venous system
√ valveless collateral venous channels (? persistent lateral limb bud vein = Klippel-Trénaunay vein) draining into deep femoral vein / iliac veins

Color Doppler US:
√ normal deep veins

DDx: (1) **Parke-Weber syndrome**
= congenital persistence of multiple microscopic AV fistulas + spectrum of Klippel-Trénaunay-Weber syndrome
(2) Neurofibromatosis (café-au-lait spots, axillary freckling, cutaneous neurofibromas, macrodactyly secondary to plexiform neurofibromas, wavy cortical reaction, early fusion of growth plate, limb hypertrophy not as extensive / bilateral)
(3) Beckwith-Wiedemann syndrome (aniridia, macroglossia, cryptorchidism, Wilms tumor, broad metaphyses, thickened long-bone cortex, advanced bone age, periosteal new-bone formation, hemihypertrophy)
(4) Macrodystrophia lipomatosis (hyperlucency of fat, distal phalanges most commonly affected, overgrowth ceases with puberty, usually limited to digits)
(5) Maffucci syndrome (cavernous hemangiomas, soft tissue hypertrophy, phleboliths, multiple enchondromas)

LANGERHANS CELL HISTIOCYTOSIS

= HISTIOCYTOSIS X (former name)
= poorly understood group of disorders characterized by proliferation of Langerhans cells (normally responsible for first-line immunologic defense in the skin)

Cause: uncertain (? primary proliferative disorder possibly due to defect in immunoregulation; neoplasm)

Path: influx of eosinophilic leukocytes simulating inflammation; reticulum cells accumulate cholesterol + lipids (= foam cells); sheets or nodules of histiocytes may fuse to form giant cells, cytoplasm contains (? viral) Langerhans bodies

Histo: Langerhans cells are similar to mononuclear macrophages + dendritic cells as the two major types of nonlymphoid mononuclear cells involved in immune + nonimmune inflammatory response; derived from promonocytes (= bone marrow stem cell)

Age: any age, mostly presenting at 1–4 years; M:F = 1:1

Location: bone + bone marrow, lymph nodes, thymus, ear, liver and spleen, gallbladder, GI tract, endocrine system

DDx: osteomyelitis, Ewing sarcoma, leukemia, lymphoma, metastatic neuroblastoma

Letterer-Siwe disease

= acute disseminated, fulminant form of histiocytosis X characterized by wasting, pancytopenia (from bone marrow dysfunction), generalized lymphadenopathy, hepatosplenomegaly

Incidence: 1: 2,000,000; 10% of histiocytosis X

Age: several weeks after birth to 2 years

Path: generalized involvement of reticulum cells; may be confused with leukemia

- hemorrhage, purpura (secondary to coagulopathy)
- severe progressive anemia / pancytopenia
- intermittent fever
- failure to grow / malabsorption + hypoalbuminemia

- skin rash: scaly erythematous seborrhea-like brown to red papules
  Location: especially pronounced behind ears, in axillary, inguinal, and perineal areas

√ hepatosplenomegaly + lymphadenopathy (most often cervical)
√ obstructive jaundice
@ Bone involvement (50%):
√ widespread multiple lytic lesions; "raindrop" pattern in calvarium
Prognosis: 70% mortality rate

Hand-Schüller-Christian disease

= chronic disseminated form of histiocytosis X (15–40%) in 10% characterized by a triad of
(1) exophthalmos
(2) diabetes insipidus
(3) lytic skull lesions

Path: proliferation of histiocytes, may simulate Ewing sarcoma
Age at onset: 5–10 years (range from birth to 40 years); M:F = 1:1

- diabetes insipidus (30–50%) often with large lytic lesion in sphenoid bone / panhypopituitarism
- otitis media with mastoid + inner ear invasion
- exophthalmos (33%), sometimes with orbital wall destruction
- generalized eczematoid skin lesions (30%)
- ulcers of mucous membranes (gingiva, palate)

@ Bone
√ osteolytic skull lesions with overlying soft-tissue nodules
√ "geographic skull" = ovoid / serpiginous destruction of large area
√ "floating teeth" with mandibular involvement
√ destruction of petrous ridge + mastoids + sella turcica
@ Orbit
√ diffuse orbital disease with multiple osteolytic bone lesions
@ Soft tissue
√ hepatosplenomegaly (rare) with scattered granuloma
√ lymphadenopathy (may be massive)
√ gallbladder wall thickening (from infiltration)
@ Lung
√ cyst + bleb formation with spontaneous pneumothorax (25%)
√ ill-defined diffuse nodular infiltration often progressing to fibrosis + honeycomb lung
Prognosis: spontaneous remissions + exacerbations

Eosinophilic granuloma

= most benign variety of histiocytosis X (60–80%) localized to bone

Age: 5–10 years (highest frequency); range 2–30 years; <20 years (in 75%); M:F = 3:2
Path: bone lesions arise within medullary canal (RES)
Histo: proliferation of histiocytes + infiltrate by variable number of inflammatory cells (eosinophils, lymphocytes, neutrophils, plasma cells)

- eosinophilia in blood + CSF

Location: monostotic involvement in 50–75%; calvarium > mandible > large long bones of upper extremity > ribs > pelvis > vertebrae

@ Skull (50%)
Site: diploic space of parietal bone (most commonly involved) + temporal bone (petrous ridge, mastoid)
√ round / ovoid punched-out lesion with serrated + beveled edge
DDx: venous lake, arachnoid granulation, parietal foramen, epidermoid cyst, hemangioma
√ sharply marginated without sclerotic rim (DDx: epidermoid with bone sclerosis)
√ sclerotic margin during healing phase (50%)
√ "hole-within-hole" appearance = uneven involvement of inner + outer table
√ "button sequestrum" = central bone density within lytic lesion
√ soft-tissue mass overlying the lytic process in calvarium (often palpable)
√ isodense homogeneously enhancing mass in hypothalamus / pituitary gland
@ Orbit
√ benign focal mass ± infiltration of orbital bones
@ Mastoid process
- intractable otitis media with chronically draining ear (in temporal bone involvement)

√ destructive lesion near mastoid antrum
DDx: mastoiditis, cholesteatoma, metastasis
Cx: extension to middle ear may destroy ossicles leading to deafness
@ Jaw
- gingival + contiguous soft-tissue swelling

√ "floating" teeth, fracture
@ Axial skeleton (25%)
√ "vertebra plana" = "coin on edge" = Calvé disease (6%) = collapse of vertebra (most commonly thoracic); preserved disk space; rare involvement of posterior elements; no kyphosis; most common cause of vertebra plana in children
√ lytic lesion in supraacetabular region
@ Proximal long bones (15%)
- painful bone lesion + swelling

Site: mostly diaphyseal, epiphyseal lesions are uncommon
√ expansile lytic lesion with ill-defined / sclerotic edges
√ endosteal scalloping, widening of medullary cavity
√ cortical thinning, intracortical tunneling
√ erosion of cortex + soft-tissue mass
√ laminated periosteal reaction (frequent), may show interruptions
√ may appear rapidly within 3 weeks
√ lesions respect joint space + growth plate
@ Lung involvement (20%)
Incidence: 0.05 to 0.5 / 100,000 annually

Age: peak between 20 and 40 years
◊ Strong association between smoking + primary pulmonary Langerhans cell histiocytosis!
√ 3–10 mm nodules
√ reticulonodular pattern with predilection for apices
√ may develop into honeycomb lung
√ recurrent pneumothoraces (25%)
√ rib lesions with fractures (common)
√ pleural effusion, hilar adenopathy (unusual)

NUC:
√ negative bone scans in 35% (radiographs more sensitive)
√ bone lesions generally not Ga-67 avid
√ Ga-67 may be helpful for detecting nonosseous lesions

Prognosis: excellent with spontaneous resolution of bone lesions in 6–18 months

LAURENCE-MOON-BIEDL SYNDROME

• retardation
• obesity
• hypogonadism
√ craniosynostosis
√ polysyndactyly

LEAD POISONING

= PLUMBISM

Path: lead concentrates in metaphyses of growing bones (distal femur > both ends of tibia > distal radius) leading to failure of removal of calcified cartilaginous trabeculae in provisional zone

• loss of appetite, vomiting, constipation, abdominal cramps
• peripheral neuritis (adults), meningoencephalitis (children)
• anemia
• lead line at gums (adults)
√ bands of increased density at metaphyses of tubular bones (only in growing bone)
√ lead lines may persist
√ clubbing if poisoning severe (anemia)
√ bone-in-bone appearance

DDx: (1) Healed rickets
(2) Normal increased density in infants <3 years of age

LEPROSY

= HANSEN DISEASE

Organism: Mycobacterium leprae

Types:
(1) lepromatous: in cutis, mucous membranes, viscera
(2) neural: enlarged indurated nodular nerve trunks; anesthesia, muscular atrophy, neurotrophic changes
(3) mixed form

Osseous changes in 15–54% of patients:

SPECIFIC SIGNS

Location: center of distal end of phalanges / eccentric

√ ill-defined areas of decalcification, reticulated trabecular pattern, small rounded osteolytic lesions, cortical erosions
√ joint spaces preserved
√ healing phase: complete resolution / bone defect with sclerotic rim + endosteal thickening
√ nasal spine absorption + destruction of maxilla, nasal bone, alveolar ridge
√ enlarged nutrient foramina in clawlike hand
√ erosive changes of ungual tufts

NONSPECIFIC SIGNS
√ soft-tissue swelling; calcification of nerves
√ contractures / deep ulcerations
√ neurotrophic joints (distal phalanges in hands, MTP in feet, Charcot joints in tarsus)

LEUKEMIA OF BONE

A. CHILDHOOD

most common malignancy of children

Histo: acute lymphoblastic leukemia (in 75%)

• migratory paraarticular arthralgias (25–50%) due to adjacent metaphyseal lesions (may be confused with acute rheumatic fever / rheumatoid arthritis)
• fever, elevated erythrocyte sedimentation rate
• hepatosplenomegaly, occasionally lymphadenopathy
◊ Peripheral blood smears may be negative in aleukemic form!

Skeletal manifestations in 50–90%:

(a) Diffuse osteopenia (most common pattern)
√ diffuse demineralization of spine + long bones (= leukemic infiltration of bone marrow + catabolic protein / mineral metabolism)
√ coarse trabeculation of spongiosa (due to destruction of finer trabeculae)
√ multiple biconcave / partially collapsed vertebrae (14%)

(b) "Leukemic lines" (40–53% in acute lymphoblastic leukemia):
√ transverse radiolucent metaphyseal bands, uniform + regular across the width of metaphysis (= leukemic infiltration of bone marrow / osteoporosis at sites of rapid growth)
Location: large joints (proximal tibia, distal femur, proximal humerus, distal radius + ulna)
√ horizontal / curvilinear bands in vertebral bodies + edges of iliac crest
√ dense metaphyseal lines after treatment

(c) Focal destruction of flat / tubular bones:
√ multiple small clearly defined ovoid / spheroid osteolytic lesions (destruction of spongiosa, later cortex) in 30–60%
√ moth-eaten appearance, sutural widening, prominent convolutional markings of skull
◊ Lytic lesions distal to knee / elbow in children are suggestive of leukemia (rather than metastases)!

(d) Isolated periostitis of long bones (infrequent):
√ smooth / lamellated / sunburst pattern of periosteal reaction (cortical penetration by sheets of leukemic cells into subperiosteum) in 12–25%

(e) Metaphyseal osteosclerosis + focal osteoblastic lesion (very rare)
√ osteosclerotic lesions (late in disease due to reactive osteoblastic proliferation)
√ mixed lesions (lytic + bone-forming) in 18%

Dx: sternal marrow / peripheral blood smear
Cx: proliferation of leukemic cells in marrow leads to extraskeletal hematopoiesis
DDx: metastatic neuroblastoma, Langerhans cell histiocytosis

B. ADULTHOOD
Death usually occurs before skeletal abnormalities manifest
√ osteoporosis
√ solitary radiolucent foci (vertebral collapse)
√ permeating radiolucent mottling (proximal humerus)

LIPOBLASTOMA

= postnatal proliferation of mesenchymal cells with a spectrum of differentiation ranging from prelipoblasts (spindle cells) to mature adipocytes
Path: immature adipose tissue separated by septa into multiple lobules
Histo: uni- and multivacuolated lipoblasts interspersed between spindle / stellate mesenchymal cells; suspended in myxoid stroma
Age: <3 years of age; M:F = 2:1
Location: subcutaneous tissue of extremities, neck, trunk, perineum, retroperitoneum
√ fatty tumor with enhancing soft-tissue component
DDx: liposarcoma (extremely rare in children)

LIPOMA OF BONE

= INTRAOSSEOUS LIPOMA
Incidence: <1:1,000 primary bone tumors
Age: any (4–6th decade); M:F = 1:1
May be associated with: hyperlipoproteinemia
• asymptomatic / localized bone pain
Location: calcaneus, extremities (proximal femur > tibia, fibula, humerus), ilium, skull, mandible, maxilla, ribs, vertebrae, sacrum, coccyx, radius
Site: metaphysis
√ expansile nonaggressive radiolucent lesion
√ loculated / septated appearance (trabeculae)
√ thin well-defined sclerotic border
√ ± thinned cortex (NO cortical destruction)
√ NO periosteal reaction
√ may contain clump of calcification centrally (= dystrophic calcification from fat necrosis)
◊ VIRTUALLY DIAGNOSTIC:
@ Calcaneus
√ in triangular region between major trabecular groups (LAT projection)
√ calcified / ossified nidus
@ Proximal femur
√ on / above intertrochanteric line
√ marked ossification of margins of lesion
◊ Radiographic appearance similar to unicameral bone cyst (infarcted lipoma = unicameral bone cyst ?)
DDx: fibrous dysplasia, simple bone cyst, posttraumatic cyst, giant cell tumor, desmoplastic fibroma, chondromyxoid fibroma, osteoblastoma

LIPOMA OF SOFT TISSUE

Most common mesenchymal tumor composed of mature adipose tissue
Histo: mature fat cells (adipocytes) that are uniform in size + shape, occasionally have fibrous connective tissue as septations; fat unavailable for systemic metabolism
• stable size after initial period of discernible growth
Age: 5th–6th decade; M > F
Location:
(a) superficial = subcutaneous lipoma (more common) in posterior trunk, neck, proximal extremities
(b) deep lipoma in retroperitoneum, chest wall, deep soft tissue of hands + feet; multiple in 5–7% (up to several hundred tumors)
√ mass of fat opacity / density / intensity identical to subcutaneous fat
√ cortical thickening (with adjacent parosteal lipoma)
CT:
√ well-defined + homogeneous tumor with low attenuation coefficient (-65 to -120 HU)
√ no enhancement following IV contrast material
MR:
√ well-defined + homogeneous, often with septations
√ signal intensity characteristics similar to subcutaneous fat: hyperintense on T1WI + moderately intense on T2WI
√ differentiation from other lesions by fat suppression technique

Angiolipoma

= lesion composed of fat separated by small branching vessels
Age: 2nd + 3rd decade; 5% familial incidence
• tender
Location: upper extremity, trunk
√ signal characteristics of fat + mixed with varying numbers of large / small vessels
√ mostly encapsulated lesion, may infiltrate

Benign mesenchymoma

= long-standing lipoma with chondroid + osseous metaplasia

Infiltrating lipoma

= INTRAMUSCULAR LIPOMA = relatively common benign lipomatous tumor extending between muscle fibers that become variably atrophic
Peak age: 5–6th decade; M > F
Location: thigh (50%), shoulder, upper arm

Lipoma arborescens

= DIFFUSE SYNOVIAL LIPOMA = lipoma-like lesion composed of hypertrophic synovial villi distended with fat, probably reactive process to chronic synovitis

Location: knee; monarticular

Frequently associated with:
degenerative joint disease, chronic rheumatoid arthritis, prior trauma

Neural fibrolipoma

= FIBROLIPOMATOUS HAMARTOMA OF NERVE
= rare tumorlike condition characterized by sausage-shaped / fusiform enlargement of a nerve by fibrofatty tissue

Age: early adulthood before age 30 years / at birth
Histo: infiltration of epineurium + perineurium by fibrofatty tissue with separation of nerve bundles

- soft slowly enlarging mass
- pain, tenderness, decreased sensation, paresthesia

Location: volar aspect of hand, wrist, forearm
Site: median n. (most frequently), ulnar n., radial n., brachial plexus;

May be associated with:
macrodactyly (in 2/3) = **macrodystrophia lipomatosa**

√ may not be visible radiographically

MR:
√ longitudinally oriented, cylindrical, linear / serpiginous structures of signal void about 3 mm in diameter (= nerve fascicles with epi- and perineural fibrosis) separated by areas of fat signal intensity (= mature fat infiltrating the interfascicular connective tissue)

US:
√ "cablelike appearance" = alternating hyper- and hypoechoic bands on US

DDx: cyst, ganglion, lipoma, traumatic neuroma, plexiform neurofibroma, vascular malformation

LIPOSARCOMA

Malignant tumor of mesenchymal origin with bulk of tumor tissue differentiating into adipose tissue

Incidence: 12–18% of all malignant soft-tissue tumors; 2nd most common soft-tissue sarcoma in adults (after malignant fibrous histiocytoma)
Age: 5th–6th decade
Histo: (a) well-differentiated
(b) myxoid in 40–50% (most common): proliferating fibroblasts, plexiform capillary pattern, myxoid matrix, fat amount <10%
(c) round cell = poorly differentiated myxoid
(d) pleomorphic

- usually painless mass (may be painful in 10–15%)

Location: trunk (42%), lower extremity (41%), upper extremity (11%), head + neck (6%); particularly in thigh + retroperitoneum
Spread: hematogenous to lung, visceral organs; myxoid liposarcoma shows tendency for serosal + pleural surfaces, subcutaneous tissue, bone

√ nonspecific soft-tissue mass (frequently fat is radiologically not detectable)
√ inhomogeneous mass with soft-tissue + fatty components
√ enhancement after IV contrast material (contradistinction to lipoma)
√ concomitant mass in retroperitoneum / thigh (in up to 10% of myxoid liposarcomas) as multicentric lesion / metastasis
√ mass of near water density / hypoechoic / hypointense on T1WI + hyperintense on T2WI in myxoid liposarcoma (high content of myxoid cells)

LYME ARTHRITIS

Agent: spirochete Borrelia burgdorferi; transmitted by tick Ixodes dammini
Histo: inflammatory synovial fluid, hypertrophic synovia with vascular proliferation + cellular infiltration

- history of erythema chronicum migrans
- endemic areas: Lyme, Connecticut, first recognized location; now also throughout United States, Europe, Australia
- recurrent attacks of arthralgias within days to 2 years after tick bite (80%)

Location: mono- / oligoarthritis of large joints (especially knee)

√ erosion of cartilage / bone (4%)

Rx: antibiotics
DDx: (1) Rheumatic fever (2) Rheumatoid arthritis (3) Gonococcal arthritis (4) Reiter syndrome

LYMPHANGIOMA

= sequestered noncommunicating lymphoid tissue lined by lymphatic endothelium

Cause: congenital obstruction of lymphatic drainage

Subtypes:
(1) Capillary lymphangioma (rare)
Location: subcutaneous tissue
(2) Cavernous lymphangioma
Location: about the mouth + tongue
(3) Cystic lymphangioma (most common)
= cystic hygroma
Associated with: hydrops fetalis, Turner syndrome
Location: head, neck (75%), axilla (20%), extension into mediastinum (3–10%)

- soft fluctuant mass

◊ Lymphangiomas are frequently a mixture of subtypes!

Age: found at birth (50–65%); within first 2 years of life (90%)
Location: soft tissue; bone (rare)

√ multilocular cystic lesion with fibrous septations
√ occasionally serpentine vascular channels
√ opacification during lymphangiography / direct puncture
√ clear / milky fluid on aspiration

DDx: hemangioma (blood on aspiration)

LYMPHOMA OF BONE

= RETICULUM CELL SARCOMA = HISTIOCYTIC LYMPHOMA = PRIMARY LYMPHOMA OF BONE (the generalized form of reticulum cell sarcoma is lymphoma); 2–6% of all primary malignant bone tumors in children

Incidence of bone marrow involvement:
5–15% in Hodgkin disease;
25–40% in non-Hodgkin lymphoma
◊ bone marrow involvement indicates progression of disease
◊ bone marrow imaging-guidance for biopsy!
NUC: 40% sensitivity; 88% specificity
MR: 65% sensitivity; 90% specificity

Histo: sheets of reticulum cells, larger than those in Ewing sarcoma (DDx: myeloma, inflammation, osteosarcoma, eosinophilic granuloma)

Age: any age; peak age in 3rd–5th decade; 50% <40 years; 35% <30 years; M:F = 2:1

• striking contrast between size of lesion + patient's well-being

Location: lower femur, upper tibia (40% about knee), humerus, pelvis, scapula, ribs, vertebra

Site: dia- / metaphysis

√ cancellous bone erosion (earliest sign)
√ mottled permeative pattern of separate coalescent areas
√ late cortical destruction
√ lamellated / sunburst periosteal response (less than in Ewing sarcoma)
√ lytic / reactive new-bone formation
√ associated soft-tissue mass without calcification
√ synovitis of knee joint common

Cx: pathologic fracture (most common among malignant bone tumors)

Prognosis: 50% 5-year survival

DDx:
(1) Osteosarcoma (less medullary extension, younger patients)
(2) Ewing tumor (systemic symptoms, debility, younger patients)
(3) Metastatic malignancy (multiple bones involved, more destructive)

MACRODYSTROPHIA LIPOMATOSA

= rare nonhereditary congenital form of localized gigantism = neural fibrolipoma with macrodactyly

Path: striking increase in adipose tissue in a fine fibrous network involving periosteum, bone marrow, nerve sheath, muscle, subcutaneous tissue

May be associated with: syn-, clino-, polydactyly

• painless

Location: 2nd or 3rd digit of hand / foot; unilateral; one / few adjacent digits may be involved in the distribution of the median / plantar nerves

√ long + broad splayed phalanges with endosteal + periosteal bone deposition
√ overgrowth of soft tissue, greatest at volar + distal aspects
√ slanting of articular surfaces
√ lucent areas of fat (DIAGNOSTIC)

Prognosis: accelerated maturation possible; growth stops at puberty

DDx: fibrolipomatous hamartoma associated with macrodystrophia lipomatosa (indistinguishable), Klippel-Trénaunay-Weber syndrome, lymphangiomatosis, hemangiomatosis, neurofibromatosis, chronic vascular stimulation, Proteus syndrome

MARFAN SYNDROME

= ARACHNODACTYLY = autosomal dominant familial disorder of connective tissue with high penetrance but extremely variable expression, new mutations in 15%

Etiology: fibrillin gene defect on chromosome 15 resulting in abnormal cross-linking of collagen fibers

Prevalence: 5:100,000; M:F = 1:1

A. MUSCULOSKELETAL MANIFESTATIONS
- • tall thin stature with long limbs, arm span greater than height
- • muscular hypoplasia + hypotonicity
- • scarcity of subcutaneous fat (emaciated look)
- √ generalized osteopenia
- @ Skull
  - • elongated face
  - √ dolichocephaly
  - √ prominent jaw
  - √ high arched palate
- @ Hand
  - • Steinberg sign = protrusion of thumb beyond the confines of the clenched fist (found in 1.1% of normal population)
  - • metacarpal index (averaging the 4 ratios of length of 2nd through 5th metacarpals divided by their respective middiaphyseal width) >8.8 (male) or 9.4 (female)
  - √ arachnodactyly = elongation of phalanges + metacarpals
  - √ flexion deformity of 5th finger
- @ Foot
  - √ pes planus
  - √ clubfoot
  - √ hallux valgus
  - √ hammer toes
  - √ disproportionate elongation of 1st digit of foot
- @ Spine
  - • ratio of measurement between symphysis and floor + crown and floor >0.45
  - √ pectus carinatum / excavatum (common)
  - √ scoliosis / kyphoscoliosis (45–60%)
  - √ increased incidence of Scheuermann disease and spondylosis
  - √ dural ectasia
  - √ increased interpedicular distance
  - √ posterior scalloping
  - √ presacral + lateral sacral meningoceles
  - √ expansion of sacral spinal canal
  - √ enlargement of sacral foramina
  - √ winged scapulae

@ Joints
- ligamentous laxity + hypermobility + instability
√ premature osteoarthritis
√ patella alta
√ genu recurvatum
√ recurrent dislocations of patella, hip, clavicle, mandible
√ slipped capital femoral epiphysis
√ progressive protrusio acetabuli (50%), bilateral > unilateral, F > M

B. OCULAR MANIFESTATIONS
- bilateral ectopia lentis, usually upward + outward (secondary to poor zonular attachments)
- glaucoma, macrophthalmia
- hypoplasia of iris + ciliary body
- contracted pupils (absence of dilator muscle)
- myopia, retinal detachment
- strabismus, ptosis
- blue sclera
- megalocornea = flat enlarged thickened cornea

C. CARDIOVASCULAR MANIFESTATIONS (60–98%)
affecting mitral valve, ascending aorta, pulmonary artery, splenic + mesenteric arteries (occasionally)
◊ Cause of death in 93%!
- chest pain, palpitations, shortness of breath, fatigue
- mid-to-late systolic murmur + one / more clicks

Associated with congenital heart defect (33%): incomplete coarctation, ASD

@ Aorta (cause of death in 55%)
Histo: myxomatous degeneration of aortic annulus
√ "tulip bulb aorta" = symmetrical dilatation of aortic sinuses of Valsalva slightly extending into ascending aorta (58%)
√ annuloaortic ectasia = combination of aortic root dilatation + aortic regurgitation
√ fusiform aneurysm of ascending aorta, rarely beyond innominate artery (due to cystic medial necrosis)
√ aortic wall calcification rare
Cx: (1) Aortic regurgitation (in 81% if root diameter >5 cm; in 100% if root diameter >6 cm (2) Aortic dissection (3) Aortic rupture (secondary to progressive aortic root dilatation)

@ Mitral valve
Histo: myxomatous degeneration of valve leads to redundancy + laxness
- mid-to-late systolic murmur + one / more clicks
√ "floppy valve syndrome" (95%) = redundant chordae tendineae with mitral valve prolapse + regurgitation
Cx: (1) Mitral regurgitation (2) Rupture of chordae tendineae (rare)

@ Coarctation (mostly not severe)
@ Pulmonary artery aneurysm + dilatation of pulmonary arterial root (43%)
@ Cor pulmonale (secondary to chest deformity)

D. PULMONARY MANIFESTATIONS
√ cystic lung disease
√ recurrent spontaneous pneumothoraces

E. ABDOMINAL MANIFESTATION
√ recurrent biliary obstruction

DDx: (1) Homocystinuria (osteoporosis)
(2) Ehlers-Danlos syndrome
(3) Congenital contractural arachnodactyly (ear deformities, NO ocular / cardiac abnormalities)
(4) Type III MEN (medullary thyroid carcinoma, mucosal neuromas, pheochromocytoma, marfanoid habitus)

MASSIVE OSTEOLYSIS

= GORHAM DISEASE = "VANISHING BONE" SYNDROME = PHANTOM BONE = HEMANGIOMA OF BONE
= infrequent disorder of unknown etiology with unpredictable course + progression

Incidence: >100 cases described
Histo: massive proliferation of hemangiomatous / lymphangiomatous tissue with large sinusoid spaces + fibrosis
Age: children + adults <40 years
Associated with: soft-tissue hemangiomas without calcifications
- frequently history of severe trauma (50%)
- little / no pain

Location: any bone; most commonly major long bones (humerus, shoulder, mandible), innominate bone, spine, thorax, short tubular bones of hand + feet (unusual)
√ progressive relentless destruction of bone
√ lack of reaction (no periosteal reaction, no repair)
√ advancing edge of destruction not sharply delineated
√ tapering margins of bone ends at sites of osteolysis with conelike spicule of bone (early changes)
√ no respect for joints
√ may destroy all bones in a particular area

MASTOCYTOSIS

= URTICARIA PIGMENTOSA
= mast cell accumulation in multiple organs

Age: <6 months (50%)
Associated with: myeloproliferative disorders, acute non-lymphatic leukemia, malignant lymphoma, mast cell leukemia
- hyperpigmented skin lesions exhibiting "wheal and flare" phenomenon when disturbed
- pruritus, flushing
- pancytopenia (chronic neutropenia)

@ Skeletal involvement (70%)
- bone and joint pain
√ osteoporosis (due to release of heparin + prostaglandin by mast cells activating osteoclasts)

√ scattered well-defined sclerotic foci with focal / diffuse involvement (due to release of histamine by mast cells promoting osteblastic activity); often alternating with areas of bone rarefaction
Predilected sites: skull, spine, ribs, pelvis, humerus, femur

@ Abdomen
- √ hepatosplenomegaly
- √ lymphadenopathy: retroperitoneal, periportal, mesenteric
- √ thickening of omentum, + mesentery
- √ ascites

@ GI tract
- • nausea, vomiting, diarrhea
- √ thickened nodular irregular folds in small bowel (due to infiltration by mast cells, lymphocytes, plasma cells)
- √ duodenal ulcers (due to release of histamine increasing gastric acid secretion)

MELORHEOSTOSIS

Nonhereditary disease of unknown etiology; often incidental finding

Age: slow chronic course in adults; rapid progression in children

Associated with: osteopoikilosis, osteopathia striata, tumors / malformations of blood vessels (hemangioma, vascular nevi, glomus tumor, AVM, aneurysm, lymphedema, lymphangiectasia)

- • severe pain + limited joint motion (bone may encroach on nerves, blood vessels, or joints)
- • thickening + fibrosis of overlying skin (resembling scleroderma)
- • muscle atrophy (frequent)

Location: diaphysis, usually monomelic with at least two bones involved in dermatomal distribution (follows spinal sensory nerve sclerotomes); entire cortex / limited to one side of cortex; more common in lower limb; skull, spine, ribs rarely involved

- √ "candle wax dripping" = continuous / interrupted streaks / blotches of sclerosis along tubular bone beginning at proximal end extending distally with slow progression
- √ may cross joint with joint fusion
- √ small opacities in scapula + hemipelvis (similar to osteopoikilosis)
- √ discrepant limb length
- √ flexion contractures of hip + knee
- √ genu valgum / varus
- √ dislocated patella
- √ ossified soft-tissue masses (27%)

DDx:
(1) Osteopoikilosis (generalized)
(2) Fibrous dysplasia (normal bone structure not lost, not as dense)
(3) Engelmann disease
(4) Hyperostosis of neurofibromatosis, tuberous sclerosis, hemangiomas
(5) Osteoarthropathy

MENISCAL TEAR

Type of tear:

A. LONGITUDINAL TEAR
1. Horizontal cleavage tear
   Cause: usually degenerative
   Associated with: meniscal cyst
   Site: primarily involving the central horizontal plane of meniscus beginning at inner margin
2. Bucket handle tear
   Cause: traumatic
   Site: usually in medial rarely in lateral meniscus
   √ longitudinal vertical tear with unstable displaced inner fragment
3. Peripheral tear
   Cause: traumatic
   √ vertical tear in peripheral third of meniscus

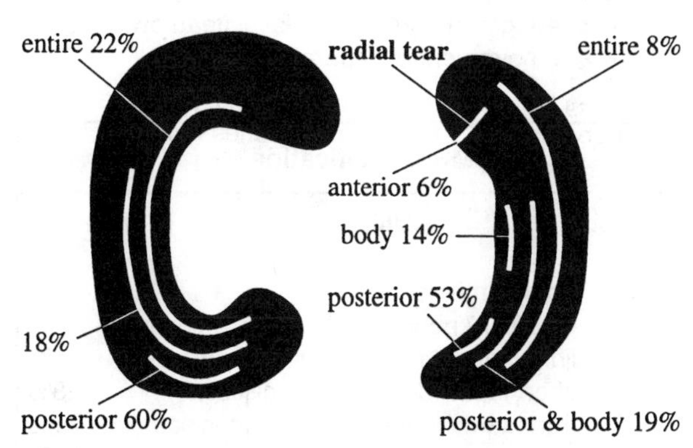

Medial Meniscus Tears **Lateral Meniscus Tears**

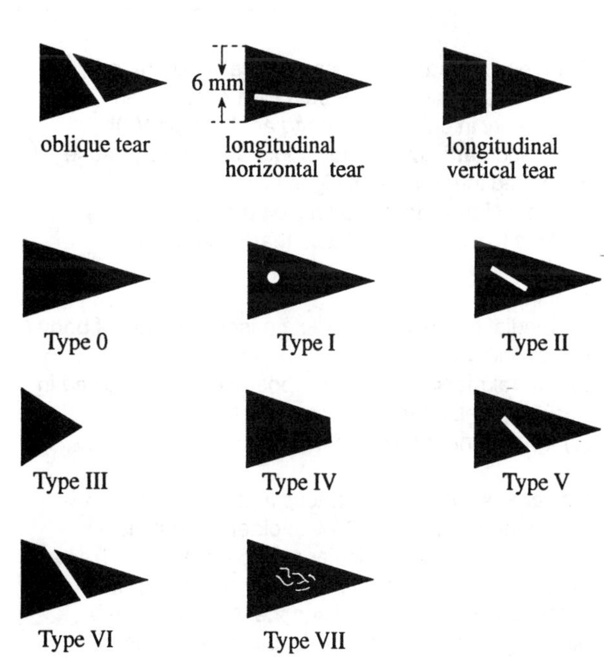

B. OBLIQUE TEAR
Site: common in midportion of medial meniscus
√ both horizontal and vertical components
√ commonly extending to inferior surface of meniscus
1. Parrot beak tear
Cause: usually degenerative
Site: in body of lateral meniscus near the junction of body + posterior horn
√ fraying of free edge
2. Flap tear = oblique + incomplete tear
Cause: traumatic, at times degenerative

C. TRANSVERSE TEAR = RADIAL TEAR
Site: posterior + midportion of lateral meniscus
√ peripheral displacement of meniscus
√ "absent" / gray meniscus posteriorly
Cx: lack of resistance to hoop stresses

D. MENISCOCAPSULAR SEPARATION
= tearing of peripheral attachments of meniscus
√ linear regions of fluid separating meniscus from capsule
√ uncovering of a portion of tibial plateau owing to inward movement of separated meniscus

MR Classification

Grade	Type	MR finding	PPV for tear
0	0	normal meniscus	1%
1	I	globular / punctate intrameniscal signal	2%
2	II	linear signal not extending to surface	5%
	III	short tapered apex of meniscus	23%
	IV	truncated / blunted apex of meniscus	71%
3	V	signal extending to only one surface	85%
3	VI	signal extending to both surfaces	95%
3	VII	comminuted reticulated signal pattern	82%

◊ Diagnosis of tear hinges on surface involvement!
◊ Intrameniscal signal may be a sign of persistent vascularity in children + young adults (type VII)!
◊ Truncation artifact + magic angle artifact may cause increased intrameniscal signal!
◊ Grade 3 signal identified only on a single image is unlikely to be confirmed as a tear at surgery!

Site of injury:
(a) medial meniscus in 45%: no isolated tears of body / anterior horn
(b) lateral meniscus in 22%: posterior horn involved in 80% of all lateral meniscal tears
(c) both menisci involved in 33%

Associated with: ligamentous injury
• asymptomatic in up to 20% of older individuals
√ signal extending to articular surface (type V + VI)
√ notch sign = linear signal intensity becoming wider as it extends toward meniscal surface indicates type V finding (tapering toward surface = type II finding)

√ meniscal cyst = implies presence of meniscal tear
DDx: synovial cyst, tendon sheath fluid, fluid within normal synovial recess, fluid collection remote from meniscus

MR sensitivity, specificity, and accuracy:

Tear of	Sensitivity	Specificity	Accuracy
medial meniscus	95%	88%	59–92%
lateral meniscus	81%	96%	87–92%
anterior cruciate lig.			91–96%
posterior cruciate lig.			up to 99%

◊ MR has a high negative predictive value!
◊ 60–97% accuracy for arthrography
◊ 84–99% accuracy for arthroscopy (poor at posterior horn of medial meniscus)

Interpretative errors (12% for experienced radiologist):
Lateral meniscus: 5.0% FN (middle + posterior horn)
1.5% FP (posterior horn)
Medial meniscus: 2.5% FN (posterior horn)
2.5% FP (posterior horn)

PITFALLS:
A. Normal variants simulating tears:
1. Superior recess on posterior horn of medial meniscus
2. Popliteal hiatus
√ hiatus of popliteal tendon separates lateral meniscus from joint capsule
◊ Seen above posterior aspect of lateral meniscus on most superficial sagittal slice!
◊ Tendon moves behind + inferior to meniscus on adjacent deeper sections!
3. Transverse ligament
Course: connects anterior horns of both menisci
√ overrides superior aspect of menisci before completely fusing to menisci
◊ Trace the cross section of the transverse ligament through the infrapatellar fat pad on more central images!
4. Meniscofemoral ligaments
Origin: superior + medial aspect of posterior horn of lateral meniscus
Attachment: medial femoral condyle
√ demonstrated in 1/3 of cases on SAG images
(a) Wrisberg ligament
√ posterior to posterior cruciate ligament
(b) Humphry ligament
√ anterior to posterior cruciate ligament
◊ Finding usually limited to single most medial image!
5. Soft tissue between capsule + medial meniscus

B. Healed meniscus
√ persistent grade 3 signal at least up to 6 months
√ S/P meniscectomy (false-positive type IV finding)

C. Degenerative changes
√ grade 1 signal = globular increase in intensity
√ grade 2 signal = linear signal not extending to articular surface

D. Discoid meniscus
= abnormally shaped enlarged discus-like meniscus
Prevalence: in 1.5–15.5%
Age: children, adolescents
Side: lateral >> medial meniscus
√ centrally displaced fragment with meniscus apparently of normal size (coronal images)

MESOMELIC DWARFISM
= heritable bone dysplasia with shortening of intermediate segments (radius + ulna or tibia + fibula)

A. **Langer type** autosomal recessive
• mental impairment
√ mesomelic shortening of limbs
√ hypoplasia of ulna + fibula
√ hypoplasia of mandible with short condyles

B. **Nievergelt type** autosomal dominant
√ severe mesomelic shortening of lower limbs
√ marked thickening of tibia + fibula in central portion
√ clubfoot (frequent)

C. Reinhardt type: autosomal dominant
D. Robinow type: autosomal dominant
E. Werner type: autosomal dominant
F. **Lamy-Bienenfeld type** autosomal dominant
• ligamentous laxity
√ shortening of radius + ulna + tibia
√ absent fibula
√ normal femur + humerus

√ shortening of all long bones at birth, most marked in tibia + radius
√ modeling deformity with widening of diaphysis
√ mild to moderate bowing
√ hypoplasia of fibula with absent lateral malleolus
√ short + thick ulna with hypoplastic distal end
√ Madelung deformity of wrist
√ hypoplasia of a vertebral body may be present

METAPHYSEAL CHONDRODYSPLASIA
= severe short-limbed dwarfism
√ metaphyseal flaring (Erlenmeyer flask deformity) extending into diaphysis

A. **Schmid type** (most common)
autosomal dominant
• waddling gate
Distribution: more marked in lower limbs; mild involvement of hands + wrists
√ shortened bowed long bones
√ widened epiphyseal growth plates
√ irregular widened cupped metaphyses
√ coxa vara
√ genu varum
DDx: vitamin D–refractory rickets

B. **McKusick type**
autosomal recessive (eg, in Amish)
• sparse brittle hair, deficient pigmentation
• normal intelligence
√ shortening of long bones with normal width
√ cupped + widened metaphyses with lucent defects
√ short middle phalanges + narrow distal phalanges becoming triangular and bullet-shaped (more frequent in hands than feet)
√ widened costochondral junctions + cystic lucencies

C. **Jansen type** (less common)
sporadic occurrence with wide spectrum
• intelligence normal / retarded
• serum calcium levels often elevated
Distribution: symmetrical involvement of all long + short tubular bones
√ widened epiphyseal plates
√ expanded irregular + fragmented metaphyses (unossified cartilage extending into diaphyses)
DDx: rickets

D. **Pyle disease** = Metaphyseal dysplasia
• often tall
• often asymptomatic
Distribution: major long bones, tubular bones of hands, medial end of clavicle, sternal end of ribs, innominate bone
√ splaying of proximal + distal ends of long bones with thinned cortex
√ relative constriction of central portion of shafts
√ craniofacial hyperostosis
√ genu valgum

METASTASES TO BONE
◊ 15–100 times more common than primary skeletal neoplasms!

Frequency:

if primary known		if primary unknown	
breast	35%	prostate	25%
prostate	30%	lymphoma	15%
lung	10%	breast	10%
kidney	5%	lung	10%
uterus	2%	thyroid	2%
stomach	2%	colon	1%
others	13%		

METASTASES OF PRIMARY BONE TUMORS
1. Osteosarcoma: 2% with distant metastases, adjuvant therapy has changed the natural history of the disease in that bone metastases occur in 10% of osteosarcomas without metastases to the lung
2. Ewing sarcoma: 13% with distant metastases

SOLITARY BONE LESION
◊ of all causes only 7% due to metastasis
◊ in patients with known malignancy due to metastasis (55%), due to trauma (25%), due to infection (10%)
Location: axial skeleton (64–68%), ribs (45%), extremities (24%), skull (12%)

mnemonic: "**S**everal **K**inds **O**f **H**orribly **N**asty **T**umors **L**eap **P**romptly **T**o **B**one"
Sarcoma, **S**quamous cell carcinoma
Kidney tumor
Ovarian cancer
Hodgkin disease
Neuroblastoma
Testicular cancer
Lung cancer
Prostate cancer
Thyroid cancer
Breast cancer

Breast cancer: extensive osteolytic lesions; involvement of entire skeleton; pathologic fractures common
Thyroid / kidney: often solitary; rapid progression with bone expansion (bubbly); frequently associated with soft-tissue mass (distinctive)
Rectum / colon: may resemble osteosarcoma with sunburst pattern + osteoblastic reaction
Hodgkin tumor: upper lumbar + lower thoracic spine, pelvis, ribs; osteolytic / occasionally osteoblastic lesions
Neuroblastoma: extensive destruction, resembles leukemia (metaphyseal band of rarefaction), mottled skull destruction + increased intracranial pressure, perpendicular spicules of bone
Ewing tumor: extensive osteolytic / osteoblastic reaction

Mode of spread: through bloodstream / lymphatics / direct extension
Location: predilection for marrow-containing skeleton (skull, spine, ribs, pelvis, humeri, femora)
√ single / multiple lesions of variable size
√ usually nonexpansile
√ joint spaces + intervertebral spaces preserved (cartilage resistant to invasion)

Osteolytic Bone Metastases

Most common cause: neuroblastoma (in childhood); lung cancer (in adult male); breast cancer (in adult female), thyroid cancer; kidney; colon
√ may begin in spongy bone (associated with soft tissue mass in ribs)
√ vertebral pedicles often involved (not in multiple myeloma)

Osteoblastic Bone Metastases

= evidence of slow-growing neoplasm
Primary: prostate, breast, lymphoma, malignant carcinoid, medulloblastoma, mucinous adenocarcinoma of GI tract, TCC of bladder, pancreas, neuroblastoma
Most common cause: prostate cancer (in adult male); breast cancer (in adult female)

mnemonic: "5 **B**ees **L**ick **P**ollen"
Brain (medulloblastoma)
Bronchus
Breast
Bowel (especially carcinoid)
Bladder
Lymphoma
Prostate
√ frequent in vertebrae + pelvis
√ may be indistinguishable from Paget disease

Mixed Bone Metastases

breast, prostate, lymphoma

Expansile / Bubbly Bone Metastases

kidney, thyroid

Permeative Bone Metastases

Burkitt lymphoma, Mycosis fungoides

Bone Metastases With "Sunburst" Periosteal Reaction (infrequent)

prostatic carcinoma, retinoblastoma, neuroblastoma (skull), GI tract

Bone Metastases With Soft-tissue Mass

thyroid, kidney

Calcifying Metastases

mnemonic: "BOTTOM"
Breast
Osteosarcoma
Testicular
Thyroid
Ovary
Mucinous adenocarcinoma of GI tract

Skeletal Metastases In Children

1. Neuroblastoma (most often)
2. Retinoblastoma
3. Embryonal rhabdomyosarcoma
4. Hepatoma
5. Ewing tumor

Skeletal Metastases In Adult

mnemonic: "**C**ommon **B**one **L**esions **C**an **K**ill **T**he **P**atient"
Colon
Breast
Lung
Carcinoid
Kidney
Thyroid
Prostate

Role Of Bone Scintigraphy In Bone Metastases

Pathophysiology: accumulation of tracer at sites of reactive bone formation
False-negative scan: very aggressive metastases

False-positive scan: degeneration, healing fractures, metabolic disorders

Baseline bone scan:

(a) high sensitivity for many metastatic tumors to bone (particularly carcinoma of breast, lung, prostate); 5% of metastases have normal scan; 5–40% occur in appendicular skeleton

(b) substantially less sensitive than radiographs in infiltrative marrow lesions (multiple myeloma, neuroblastoma, histiocytosis)

(c) screening of asymptomatic patients
- — useful in: prostate cancer, breast cancer
- — not useful in: non–small-cell bronchogenic carcinoma, gynecologic malignancy, head and neck cancer

√ multiple asymmetric areas of increased uptake
√ axial > appendicular skeleton (dependent on distribution of bone marrow); vertebrae, ribs, pelvis involved in 80%
√ superscan in diffuse bony metastases

Follow-up bone scan:

√ stable scan = suggestive of relatively good prognosis
√ increased activity in:
(a) enlargement of bone lesions / appearance of new lesions indicate progression of the disease
(b) "healing flare" phenomenon (in 20–61%) = transient increase in lesion activity secondary to healing under antineoplastic treatment concomitant with increased sclerosis, detected at 3.2 ± 1.4 months after initiation of hormonal / chemotherapy, of no additional favorable prognostic value
(c) avascular necrosis particularly in hips, knees, shoulders caused by steroid therapy
(d) osteoradionecrosis / radiation-induced osteosarcoma

√ decreased activity in:
(a) predominately osteolytic destruction
(b) metastases under radiotherapy; as early as 2–4 months with minimum of 2000 rads

ROLE OF BONE SCAN IN BREAST CANCER

Routine preoperative bone scan not justified:

Stage I : unsuspected metastases in 2%, mostly single lesion
Stage II : unsuspected metastases in 6%
Stage III : unsuspected metastases in 14%

Follow-up bone scan:

At 12 months no new cases; at 28 months in 5% new metastases; at 30 months in 29% new metastases

Conversion from normal: Stage I : in 7%
Stage II : in 25%
Stage III : in 58%

◊ With axillary lymph node involvement conversion rate 2.5 x that of those without!
◊ Serial follow-up examinations are important to assess therapeutic efficacy + prognosis!

ROLE OF BONE SCAN IN PROSTATE CANCER

Stage B : 5% with skeletal metastases
Stage C : 10% with skeletal metastases
Stage D : 20% with skeletal metastases

Test sensitivities for detection of osseous metastases:
(a) Scintigraphy 1.0
(b) Radiographic survey 0.68
(c) Alkaline phosphatase 0.5
(d) Acid phosphatase 0.5

DDx: pulmonary metastasis (SPECT helpful in distinguishing nonosseous lung from overlying rib uptake)

Role Of Magnetic Resonance Imaging

ideal for bone marrow imaging due to high contrast between bone marrow fat + water-containing metastatic deposits

(1) Focal lytic lesion:
√ hypointense on T1WI + hyperintense on T2WI
(2) Focal sclerotic lesion:
√ hypointense on T1WI + T2WI
(3) Diffuse inhomogeneous lesions:
√ inhomogeneously hypointense on T1WI + hyperintense on T2WI
(4) Diffuse homogeneous lesions:
√ homogeneously hypointense on T1WI + hyperintense on T2WI

METATROPHIC DYSPLASIA

= HYPERPLASTIC ACHONDROPLASIA
= METATROPHIC DWARFISM

metatrophic = "changeable" (change in proportions of trunk to limbs over time secondary to developing kyphoscoliosis in childhood)

• longitudinal double skin fold overlying coccyx
√ long bones short with dumbbell-like / trumpet-shaped configuration (exaggerated metaphyseal flaring)
√ "hourglass" phalanges (short with widened ends)
√ wide separation of major joint spaces (thick articular cartilage)
√ delayed ossification of flat irregular epiphyses

@ Chest
√ cylindrical narrowed elongated thorax
√ short + wide ribs
√ pectus carinatum

@ Vertebrae
√ odontoid hypoplasia with atlantoaxial instability
√ progressive kyphoscoliosis
√ platyspondyly + very wide intervertebral spaces
√ wedge- / keel-shaped vertebral bodies

@ Pelvis
√ coccygeal appendage similar to a tail (rare but CHARACTERISTIC)
√ short squared iliac bones + irregular acetabula
√ narrowed greater sciatic notch

Prognosis: compatible with life, increased disability from kyphoscoliosis

DDx: achondroplasia, mucopolysaccharidoses

MUCOPOLYSACCHARIDOSES

= lysosomal storage disorder from deficiency of specific lysosomal enzymes involved in degradation of mucopolysaccharides

Type I = Hurler
Type II = Hunter
Type III = Sanfilippo
Type IV = Morquio
Type V = Scheie
Type VI = Maroteaux-Lamy
Type VII = Sly

◊ All autosomal recessive except for Hunter (X-linked)!

Associated with: valvular heart disease

- corneal clouding
- retardation (prominent in types I, II, III, VII)
- skeletal involvement dominates in types IV and VI

√ scaphocephaly, macrocephaly; thick calvarium; hypertelorism
√ platyspondyly with kyphosis + dwarfism
√ irregularity at anterior aspect of vertebral bodies
√ atlantoaxial subluxation (laxity of transverse ligament / hypoplasia or absence of odontoid)
√ limb contractures
√ broad hands
√ hepatosplenomegaly

@ Brain
- √ brain atrophy
- √ varying degree of hydrocephalus
- √ multiple white matter changes within cerebral hemispheres (diffuse hypodense areas, prolongation of T1 + T2)

Cx: cord compression at atlantoaxial joint (types IV + VI)

Dx: combination of clinical features, radiographic abnormalities correlated with genetic + biochemical studies

Prenatal Dx: occasionally successful analysis of fibroblasts cultured from amniotic fluid

Hurler Syndrome

= GARGOYLISM = PFAUNDLER-HURLER DISEASE
= MPS I-H; autosomal recessive disease

Cause: homozygous for MPS III gene with excess chondroitin sulfate B due to deficient X-L iduronidase (= Hurler corrective factor)

Incidence: 1:10,000 births

Age: usually appears >1st year

- dwarfism
- progressive mental deterioration after 1–3 years
- large head; sunken bridge of nose; hypertelorism
- early corneal clouding progressing to blindness
- "gargoyle" features = everted lips + protruding tongue
- teeth widely separated + poorly formed
- progressive narrowing of nasopharyngeal airway
- protuberant abdomen (secondary to dorsolumbar kyphosis + hepatosplenomegaly)
- urinary excretion of chondroitin sulfate B (dermatan sulfate) + heparan sulfate
- Reilly bodies (metachromic granules) in white blood cells or bone marrow cells

@ Skull (earliest changes >6 months of age)
- √ frontal bossing
- √ calvarial thickening
- √ premature fusion of sagittal + lambdoid sutures
- √ deepening of optic chiasm
- √ enlarged J-shaped sella (undermining of anterior clinoid process)
- √ small facial bones

Mucopolysaccharidoses

Type	Eponym	Inheritance	Enzyme Deficiency	Urinary Glycosaminoglycan	Neurologic Signs
I-H	Hurler	autosomal recessive	alpha-L-iduronidase	dermatan sulfate	marked
II	Hunter	X-linked recessive	iduronate sulfatase	dermatan / heparan sulfate	mild to moderate
III	Sanfilippo	autosomal recessive		heparan sulfate	mental deterioration
	A		heparan sulfate sulfatase		
	B		N-acetyl-alpha-D-glucosaminidase		
	C		alpha-glucosamine-N-acetyl-transferase		
	D		N-acetylglucosamine-6-sulfate sulfatase		
IV	Morquio A–D	autosomal recessive	N-acetylgalactosamine-6-sulfate sulfatase beta-galactosidase	keratan sulfate	none
I-S(V)	Scheie	autosomal recessive	alpha-L-iduronidase	heparan sulfate	none
VI	Maroteaux-Lamy	autosomal recessive	arylsulfatase B	dermatan sulfate	none
VII	Sly	autosomal recessive	beta-glucuronidase	dermatan sulfate heparan sulfate	variable

√ wide mandibular angle + underdevelopment of condyles
√ communicating hydrocephalus

@ Extremities
√ thick periosteal cloaking of long-bone diaphyses (early changes)
√ swelling of diaphyses + tapering of either end: distal humerus, radius, ulna, proximal ends of metacarpals, ribs
√ enlargement of shaft due to dilatation of medullary canal with cortical thinning
√ deossification
√ flexion deformities of knees + hips
√ trident hands; clawing (occasionally)
√ delayed maturation of irregular carpal bones

@ Spine
√ thoracolumbar kyphosis with lumbar gibbus
√ oval centra with normal / increased height + anterior beak at T12/L1/L2
√ long slender pedicles
√ spatulate rib configuration

@ Pelvis
√ widely flared iliac wings
√ constriction of iliac bones
√ coxa valga

Prognosis: death by age 10–15 years

Morquio Syndrome

= KERATOSULFATURIA = MPS IV;
autosomal recessive; excess keratosulfate

Incidence: 1:40,000 births

Etiology: N-acetylgalactosamine-6-sulfatase deficiency resulting in defective degradation of keratin sulfate (mainly in cartilage, nucleus pulposus, cornea)

Age: normal at birth; skeletal changes manifest within first 18 months

• excessive urinary excretion of keratan sulfate
• normal intelligence
• weakness + hypotonia
• dwarfism with short trunk (<4 feet tall)
• head thrust forward + sunken between high shoulders
• normal intelligence
• corneal opacities evident around age 10
• progressive deafness
• short nose, wide mouth, spacing between teeth
• semicrouching stance + knock knees from flexion deformities of knees + hips

@ Skull
√ mild dolichocephaly
√ hypertelorism
√ poor mastoid air cell development
√ short nose + depression of bridge of nose
√ prominent maxilla

@ Chest
√ increased AP diameter + marked pectus carinatum
√ slight lordosis with wide short ribs
√ bulbous costochondral junctions
√ failure of fusion of sternal segments

@ Spine
√ hypoplasia / absence of odontoid process of C2
√ C1-C2 instability with anterior subluxation
√ thick C2-body with narrowing of vertebral canal
√ atlas close to occiput / posterior arch of C1 within foramen magnum
√ platyspondyly = universal vertebra plana esp. affecting lumbar spine (DDx: normal height in Hurler syndrome)
√ ovoid vertebral bodies with central anterior beak / tongue at lower thoracic / upper lumbar vertebrae
√ mild gibbus at thoracolumbar transition = low dorsal kyphosis
√ exaggerated lumbar lordosis
√ widened intervertebral disk spaces

@ Pelvis
√ "goblet-shaped" / "wineglass" pelvis = constricted iliac bodies + elongated pelvic inlet + flared iliac wings
√ oblique hypoplastic acetabular roofs

@ Femur
√ initially well-formed femoral head epiphysis, involution + fragmentation by age 3–6 years
√ lateral subluxation of femoral heads; later hip dislocation
√ wide femoral neck + coxa valga deformity

@ Tibia
√ delayed ossification of lateral proximal tibial epiphysis
√ sloping of superior margin of tibia plateau laterally + severe genu valgum

@ Hand & foot
√ short bones of forearm with widening of proximal ends
√ delayed appearance + irregularity of carpal centers
√ small irregular carpal bones
√ proximally pointed short metacarpals 2–5
√ enlarged joints; hand + foot deformities (flat feet)
√ ulnar deviation of hand

Cx: cervical myelopathy (traumatic quadriplegia / leg pains / subtle neurologic abnormality) most common cause of death secondary to C2 abnormality; frequent respiratory infections (from respiratory paralysis)

Rx: early fusion of C1–C2

Prognosis: may live to adulthood

DDx: (1) Hurler syndrome (normal / increased vertebral height; vertebral beak inferior)
(2) Spondyloepiphyseal dysplasia (autosomal dominant, present at birth, absent flared ilia / deficient acetabular ossification, small acetabular angle, deficient ossification of pubic bones, varus deformity of femoral neck, minimal involvement of hand + foot, myopia)

MULTIPLE EPIPHYSEAL DYSPLASIA

= FAIRBANK DISEASE = ? tarda form of chondrodystrophia calcificans congenita
√ mild limb shortening

√ irregular mottled calcifications of epiphyses (in childhood + adolescence)
√ epiphyseal irregularities + premature degenerative joint disease, especially of hips (in adulthood)
√ short phalanges
DDx: Legg-Perthes disease, hypothyroidism

MULTIPLE MYELOMA

Most common primary malignant neoplasm in adults
Histo: normal / pleomorphic plasma cells (not pathognomonic), may be mistaken for lymphocytes (lymphosarcoma, reticulum cell sarcoma, Ewing tumor, neuroblastoma)
(a) diffuse infiltration: myeloma cells intimately admixed with hematopoietic cells
(b) tumor nodules: displacement of hematopoietic cells by masses entirely composed of myeloma cells
Age: usually 5th– 8th decade; 98% >40 years; rare < age 30; M:F = 2:1
(a) DISSEMINATED FORM: >40 years of age (98%); M:F = 3:2
(b) SOLITARY FORM: mean age 50 years
- bone pain (68%)
- normochromic normocytic anemia (62%)
- RBC rouleau formation
- renal insufficiency (55%)
- hypercalcemia (30–50%)
- proteinuria (88%)
- Bence-Jones proteinuria (50%)
- increased globulin production (monoclonal gammopathy)

Location:
A. DISSEMINATED FORM:
scattered; axial skeleton predominant site; vertebrae (50%) > ribs > skull > pelvis > long bones (distribution correlates with normal sites of red marrow)
B. SOLITARY FORM:
vertebrae > pelvis > skull > sternum > ribs
C. SPINAL PLASMA CELL MYELOMA
√ sparing of posterior elements (no red marrow) (DDx: metastatic disease)
√ paraspinal soft-tissue mass with extradural extension
√ scalloping of anterior margin of vertebral bodies (osseous pressure from adjacent enlarged lymph nodes)

√ generalized osteoporosis with accentuation of trabecular pattern, especially in spine (early)
√ punched out appearance of widespread osteolytic areas (skull, long bones) with endosteal scalloping and uniform size
√ diffuse osteolysis (pelvis, sacrum)
√ expansile osteolytic lesions (ballooning) in ribs, pelvis, long bones
√ soft-tissue mass adjacent to bone destruction (= extrapleural + paraspinal mass adjacent to ribs / vertebral column)
√ periosteal new-bone formation exceedingly rare
√ involvement of mandible (rarely affected by metastatic disease)
√ sclerosis may occur after chemotherapy, radiotherapy, fluoride administration
√ sclerotic form of multiple myeloma (1–3%)
(a) solitary sclerotic lesion: frequently in spine
(b) diffuse sclerosis
associated with **POEMS syndrome**:
Polyneuropathy
Organomegaly
Endocrine abnormalities
M-protein
Skin changes

MR (recognition dependent on knowledge of normal range of bone marrow appearance for age):
√ hypointense focal areas on T1WI (25%)
√ hyperintense focal areas on T2WI (53%)
√ absence of fatty infiltration (nonspecific)

SENSITIVITY OF BONE SCANS VS. RADIOGRAPHS
Radiographs : in 90% of patients and 80% of sites
Bone scan : in 75% of patients and 24–54% of sites
Gallium scan : in 55% of patients and 40% of sites
◊ 30% of lesions only detected on radiographs
◊ 10% of lesions only detected on bone scans

Cx: (1) renal involvement frequent
(2) predilection for recurrent pneumonias (leukopenia)
(3) secondary amyloidosis in 6–15%
(4) pathologic fractures occur often

Prognosis: 20% 5-year survival; death from renal insufficiency, bacterial infection, thromboembolism

DDx:
— with osteopenia: (1) Postmenopausal osteoporosis (2) Hyperparathyroidism
— with lytic lesion: (1) Metastatic disease (2) Amyloidosis (3) Myeloid metaplasia
— with sclerotic lesion: (1) Osteopoikilosis (2) Lymphoma (3) Osteoblastic metastasis (4) Mastocytosis (5) Myelosclerosis (6) Fluorosis (7) Lymphoma (8) Renal osteodystrophy

Myelomatosis

√ generalized deossification without discrete tumors
√ vertebral flattening

MYELOPROLIFERATIVE DISORDERS

= autonomous clonal disorder initiated by an acquired pluripotential hematopoietic stem cell
Types:
1. Polycythemia vera
2. Chronic granulomatous leukemia = chronic myelogenous leukemia

3. Essential idiopathic thrombocytopenia
4. Agnogenic myeloid metaplasia (= primary myelofibrosis + extramedullary hematopoiesis in liver + spleen)

Pathophysiology:
— self-perpetuating intra- and extramedullary hematopoietic cell proliferation without stimulus
— trilinear panmyelosis (RBCs, WBCs, platelets)
— myelofibrosis with progression to myelosclerosis
— myeloid metaplasia = extramedullary hematopoiesis (normocytic anemia, leukoerythroblastic anemia, reticulocytosis, low platelet count, normal / reduced WBC count)

MYELOSCLEROSIS

= AGNOGENIC MYELOID METAPLASIA
= MYELOPROLIFERATIVE SYNDROME
= PSEUDOLEUKEMIA
= hematologic disorder of unknown etiology with gradual replacement of bone marrow elements by fibrosis

Characterized by
(1) extramedullary hematopoiesis
(2) progressive splenomegaly
(3) anemia
(4) variable changes in number of granulocytes + platelets; often predated by polycythemia vera

Age: usually >50 years
Path: fibrous / bony replacement of bone marrow; extramedullary hematopoiesis
Associated with: metastatic carcinoma, chemical poisoning, chronic infection (TB), acute myelogenous leukemia, polycythemia vera, McCune-Albright syndrome, histiocytosis

• dyspnea, weakness, fatigue, weight loss, hemorrhage
• normochromic normocytic anemia; polycythemia may precede myelosclerosis in 59%
• dry marrow aspirate

Location: red marrow–containing bones in 40% (thoracic cage, pelvis, femora, humeral shafts, lumbar spine, skull, peripheral bones)

√ splenomegaly
√ widespread diffuse increase in density (ground glass)
√ "jail-bar" ribs
√ sandwich / rugger jersey spine
√ generalized increase in bone density in skull + obliteration of diploic space; scattered small rounded radiolucent lesions; or combination of both

NUC:
√ diffuse increased uptake of bone tracer in affected skeleton, possibly "superscan"
√ increased uptake at ends of long bones

DDx: (a) with splenomegaly: chronic leukemia, lymphoma, mastocytosis
(b) without splenomegaly: osteoblastic metastases, fluorine poisoning, osteopetrosis, chronic renal disease

MYOSITIS OSSIFICANS

= PSEUDOMALIGNANT OSSEOUS TUMOR OF SOFT TISSUE = EXTRAOSSEOUS LOCALIZED NONNEOPLASTIC BONE AND CARTILAGE FORMATION = MYOSITIS OSSIFICANS CIRCUMSCRIPTA = HETEROTOPIC OSSIFICATION
= benign solitary self-limiting ossifying soft-tissue mass typically occurring within skeletal muscle

Age: adolescents, young athletic adults; M > F
Path: lesion rimmed by compressed fibrous connective tissue + surrounded by atrophic skeletal muscle (myositis = misnomer since no primary inflammation of muscle present)

Histo:
(a) early: focal hemorrhage + degeneration + necrosis of damaged muscle; histiocytic invasion; central nonossified core of proliferating benign fibroblasts + myofibroblasts; mesenchymal cells enclosed in ground substance assume characteristics of osteoblasts with subsequent mineralization + peripheral bone formation
(b) intermediate age (3–6 weeks): "zone phenomenon" with central area of cellular variation and atypical mitotic figures (impossible to differentiate from soft-tissue sarcoma); middle zone of immature osteoid; outer zone of well-formed mature trabeculated dense bone

• history of direct trauma (75%)
• pain, tenderness, soft-tissue mass

Location: large muscles of extremities (80%)
(a) within muscle: anterolateral aspect of thigh + arm; temporal muscle; small muscles of hands; gluteal muscle; **"rider's bone"** (adductor longus); **"fencer's bone"** (brachialis); **"dancer's bone"** (soleus); breast, elbow, knee
(b) periosteal at tendon insertion: **Pellegrini-Stieda disease** (medial collateral ligament of knee)

√ faint calcifications develop in 2–6 weeks after onset of symptoms
√ well-defined partially ossified soft-tissue mass apparent by 6–8 weeks, becoming smaller + mature by 5–6 months
√ radiolucent zone separating lesion from bone (DDx: periosteal sarcoma on stalk)
√ ± periosteal reaction

CT:
√ well-defined mineralization at periphery of lesion after 4–6 weeks + less distinct lucent center (DDx: sarcoma with ill-defined periphery + calcified ossific center)
√ diffuse ossification in mature lesion

MR:
Early phase:
√ mass with poorly defined margins
√ inhomogeneously hyperintense to fat on T2WI
√ isointense to muscle on T1WI
√ contrast enhancement

Intermediate phase:
√ isointense / slightly hyperintense core on T1WI, increasing in intensity on T2WI

√ rim of curvilinear areas of decreased signal intensity surrounding the lesion (= peripheral mineralization / ossification)
√ increased peritumoral signal intensity on T2WI (= edema of diffuse myositis)
√ focal signal abnormality within bone marrow (= marrow edema)

Mature phase:
√ well-defined inhomogeneous mass with signal intensity approximating fat
√ decreased signal intensity surrounding lesion + within (dense ossification + fibrosis, hemosiderin from previous hemorrhage)

NUC:
√ intense tracer accumulation on bone scan (directly related to deposition of calcium in damaged muscle)
√ in phase of mature ossification activity becomes reduced + surgery may be performed with little risk of recurrence

Angio:
√ diffuse tumor blush + fine neovascularity in early active phase
√ avascular mass in mature healing phase

Prognosis: ? resorption in 1 year
DDx:
◊ In early stages difficult to differentiate histologically + radiologically from soft-tissue sarcomas!
(1) Osteosarcoma
(2) Synovial sarcoma
(3) Fibrosarcoma
(4) Chondrosarcoma
(5) Rhabdomyosarcoma
(6) Parosteal sarcoma (usually metaphyseal with thick densely mineralized attachment to bone)
(7) Posttraumatic periostitis (ossification of subperiosteal hematoma with broad-based attachment to bone)
(8) Acute osteomyelitis (substantial soft-tissue edema + early periosteal reaction)
(9) Tumoral calcinosis (periarticular calcific masses of lobular pattern with interspersed lucent soft-tissue septa)
(10) Osteochondroma (stalk contiguous with normal adjacent cortex + medullary space)

MYOSITIS OSSIFICANS VARIANTS
1. **Panniculitis ossificans**
Location: subcutis of mostly upper extremities
√ less prominent zoning phenomenon
2. **Fasciitis ossificans**
Location: fascia
3. **Fibro-osseous pseudotumor of digits**
= FLORID REACTIVE PERIOSTITIS
Age: mean age of 32 years (range 4–64 years); M:F = 1:2
• fusiform swelling / mass
Location: predominantly fingers (2nd > 3rd > 5th), occasionally toes
Site: proximal > distal > middle phalanx
√ radiopaque soft-tissue mass with radiolucent band between mass + cortex
√ visible calcifications (50%)
√ focal periosteal thickening (50%)
√ cortical erosion (occasionally)

NAIL-PATELLA SYNDROME

= FONG DISEASE = ILIAC HORNS = FAMILIAL / HEREDITARY OSTEO-ONYCHODYSPLASIA
= OSTEO-ONYCHODYSOSTOSIS = HOOD SYNDROME
= ELBOW-PATELLA SYNDROME
= rare autosomal dominant disorder characterized by symmetrical meso- and ectodermal anomalies

Etiology: ? enzymatic defect in collagen metabolism
Age: evident in 2nd + 3rd decades
• aplasia / hypoplasia of thumb + index fingernails
• bilateral spooning / splitting / ridging of fingernails
• abnormal gait
• abnormal pigmentation of iris
• renal dysfunction (secondary to abnormal glomerular basement membrane): proteinuria, hematuria, failure later in life

√ bilateral posterior iliac horns in 80% (occasionally capped by an epiphysis) DIAGNOSTIC
√ flared iliac crest with protuberant anterior iliac spines
√ genu valgum due to asymmetrical development of femoral condyles
√ prominent tibial tubercles
√ fragmentation / hypoplasia / absence of patella; frequently with recurrent lateral dislocations
√ radial head / capitellum hypoplasia with subluxation / dislocation of radial head dorsally and increased carrying angle of elbow (DDx: congenital dislocation of radial head)
√ clinodactyly of 5th finger
√ short 5th metacarpal
√ flexion contractures of hip, knee, elbow, fingers, foot
√ deltoid, triceps, quadriceps hypoplasia
√ mandibular cysts (occasionally)
√ scoliosis
√ renal osteodystrophy

DDx: (1) Seckel syndrome
(2) "Bird-headed dwarfism" (absence of patella, radial head dislocation)
(3) Popliteal pterygium syndrome (absence of patella, toenail dysplasia)

NECROTIZING FASCIITIS

Incidence: 500 cases (in literature)
Age: 58 ± 14 years; M>F
Cause: deep internal infection / malignancy (perforated duodenal ulcer / retroperitoneal appendix, retroperitoneal / perirectal infection, infiltrating rectal / sigmoid carcinoma
Predisposed: patients with diabetes, cancer, alcohol / drug abuse, poor nutrition
Organism: Staphylococcus, E. coli, Bacteroides, Streptococcus, Peptostreptococcus, Klebsiella, Proteus, C. perfringens (5–15%) (multiple organisms in 75%)

Histo: necrotic superficial fascia, leukocytic infiltration of deep fascial layers; fibrinoid thrombosis of arterioles + venules with vessel wall necrosis; microbial infiltration of destroyed fascia
- indolent (1–21 days delay before diagnosis)
- nonspecific symptoms: severe pain, fever, leukocytosis, shock, altered mental status
- crepitus (50%), overlying skin may be completely intact

Location: lower extremity, arm, neck, back, male perineum / scrotum (= **Fournier gangrene**)
√ asymmetric fascial thickening with fat stranding (80%) from fluid
√ gas in soft-tissues dissecting along fascial planes from gas-forming organisms (in 55%)
√ associated deep abscess (35%)
√ ± secondary muscle involvement

Prognosis: poor with delay in diagnosis
Rx: extensive surgical débridement
DDx: (1) myonecrosis (infection originating in muscle)
(2) fasciitis-panniculitis syndromes (chronic swelling of skin + underlying soft-tissues + fascial planes in arm + calf)
(3) soft-tissue edema of CHF / cirrhosis (symmetrical diffuse fat stranding)

NEUROPATHIC OSTEOARTHROPATHY

= NEUROTROPHIC JOINT = CHARCOT JOINT
= traumatic arthritis due associated with loss of sensation + proprioception of affected limb

Pathogenesis: (1) decreased pain sensation produces repetitive trauma
(2) sympathetic dysfunction results in local hyperemia + bone resorption

Cause:
A. Congenital
1. Myelomeningocele
2. Congenital indifference to pain = asymbolia

B. Acquired
(a) central neuropathy
1. Injury to brain / spinal cord
2. Syringomyelia (in 1/3 of patients): shoulder, elbow
3. Neurosyphilis = tabes dorsalis (in 15–20% of patients): hip, knee, ankle, tarsals
4. Spinal cord tumors / infection

(b) peripheral neuropathy
1. Diabetes mellitus (most common cause, although incidence low): ankle, foot, hand
2. Leprosy
3. Peripheral nerve injury

(c) others
1. Scleroderma, Raynaud disease, Ehlers-Danlos syndrome
2. Rheumatoid arthritis, psoriasis
3. Amyloid infiltration of nerves, adrenal hypercorticism

C. Iatrogenic
prolonged use of pain-relieving drugs

mnemonic: "DS6"
Diabetes
Syphilis | **S**pina bifida
Steroids | **S**yringomyelia
Spinal cord injury | **S**cleroderma

Pathology:
(a) atrophic resorptive / hyperemic phase: osteoclasts + macrophages remove bone + cartilage debris making bone susceptible to fractures + joint destruction
(b) hypertrophic reparative sclerotic phase
- no history of trauma
- swollen + warm joint with normal WBC count + ESR (infection may coexist)
- usually painless joint; pain at presentation (in 1/3) with decreased response to deep pain + proprioception
- joint changes frequently precede neurologic deficit
- synovial fluid: frequently xanthochromic / bloody, lipid crystals (from bone marrow)

√ persistent joint effusion (first sign)
√ narrowing of joint space
√ speckled calcification in soft tissue (= calcification of synovial membrane)
√ fragmentation of eburnated subchondral bone
√ NO juxtaarticular osteoporosis (unless infected)
√ "bag-of-bones" appearance in late stage (= marked deformities around joint)
mnemonic: "6 Ds"
√ **D**ense subchondral bone (= sclerosis)
√ **D**egeneration (= attempted repair by osteophytes)
√ **D**estruction of articular cortex (with sharp margins resembling those of surgical amputation)
√ **D**eformity ("pencil point" deformity of metatarsal heads)
√ **D**ebris (loose bodies)
√ **D**islocation (nontraumatic)
√ subluxation of joints (laxity of periarticular soft tissues)
√ talonavicular displacement with midfoot arthropathy (common in diabetic neuropathy)
√ progressive rapid bone resorption
√ joint distension (by fluid, hypertrophic synovitis, osteophytes, subluxation)

MR:
√ decreased signal intensity in bone marrow on T1WI + T2WI (due to osteosclerotic changes)

@ Spine (involved in 6–21%):
√ lysis / sclerosis of intervertebral + facet joints
√ scoliosis
√ large osteophytes with beaking

NODULAR SYNOVITIS

= GIANT CELL TUMOR OF TENDON SHEATH

Histo: very cellular tumor with a capsule that separates the tumor into lobules

Location: soft tissue of hand, occasionally lower extremity
√ lobulated lesion with well-defined nodules up to 4 cm in size
√ located along tendon sheath (CHARACTERISTIC)

MR:
√ low signal intensity on T1WI + T2WI (hemosiderin deposition)

NONOSSIFYING FIBROMA

= FIBROXANTHOMA = NONOSTEOGENIC FIBROMA
= XANTHOMA = XANTHOGRANULOMA OF BONE
= FIBROUS METAPHYSEAL-DIAPHYSEAL DEFECT
= FIBROUS MEDULLARY DEFECT

Incidence: up to 40% of all children >2 years of age

Etiology: lesion resulting from proliferative activity of a fibrous cortical defect that has expanded into medullary cavity

Histo: whorled bundles of spindle-shaped fibroblasts + scattered multinucleated giant cells + foamy xanthomatous cells

Age: 8–20 years; 75% in 2nd decade of life

• usually asymptomatic

Location: shaft of long bone; mostly in bones of lower extremity, especially about knee (distal femur + proximal tibia); distal tibia; fibula

Site: eccentric metaphyseal, several cm shaftward from epiphysis, mostly intramedullary, rarely purely diaphyseal

Multiple fibroxanthomas (in 8–10%)

Associated with: neurofibromatosis, fibrous dysplasia, Jaffe-Campanacci syndrome

√ multilocular ovoid bubbly osteolytic area
√ alignment along long axis of bone, about 2 cm in length
√ dense sclerotic border toward medulla; V- or U-shaped at one end
√ endosteal scalloping + thinning ± overlying bulge
√ migrates toward center of diaphysis
√ resolves with age
√ minimal / mild uptake on bone scan

Prognosis: spontaneous healing in most cases

Cx: (1) Pathologic fracture (not uncommon)
(2) Hypophosphatemic vitamin D–resistant rickets + osteomalacia (tumor may secrete substance that increases renal tubular resorption of phosphorus)

DDx: (1) Adamantinoma (midshaft of tibia)
(2) Chondromyxoid fibroma (bulging of cortex more striking)

JAFFE-CAMPANACCI SYNDROME

= nonossifying fibroma with extraskeletal manifestations in children

• mental retardation
• hypogonadism
• ocular defect
• cardiovascular congenital defect
• café-au-lait spots

NOONAN SYNDROME

= PSEUDO–TURNER = MALE TURNER SYNDROME
= phenotype similar to Turner syndrome but with normal karyotype (occurs in both males + females)

Striking familial incidence

• short / may have normal height
• webbed neck
• agonadism / normal gonads
• delayed puberty
• mental retardation

√ osteoporosis
√ retarded bone age
√ cubitus valgus

@ Skull
√ mandibular hypoplasia with dental malocclusion
√ hypertelorism
√ biparietal foramina
√ dolichocephaly, microcephaly / cranial enlargement
√ webbed neck

@ Chest
√ sternal deformity: pectus excavatum / carinatum
√ right-sided congenital heart disease (valvar pulmonic stenosis, ASD, eccentric hypertrophy of left ventricle, PDA, VSD)
√ coronal clefts of spine
√ may have pulmonary lymphangiectasis

@ Gastrointestinal tract
√ intestinal lymphangiectasia
√ eventration of diaphragm
√ renal malrotation, renal duplication, hydronephrosis, large redundant extrarenal pelvis

DDx: Turner syndrome (mental retardation rare, renal anomalies frequent)

OCHRONOSIS

= ALKAPTONURIA = inherited absence of homogentisic acid oxidase with excessive homogentisic acid production + deposition in connective tissue including cartilage, synovium, and bone

Histo: abnormally pigmented cartilage subject to deterioration resulting in calcification + denudation of cartilaginous tissue

M:F = 2:1

• black pigment in soft tissues (in 2nd decade): yellowish skin; gray pigmentation of sclera; bluish tinge of ears + nose cartilage
• alkaptonuria with black staining of diapers
• heart failure, renal failure (pigment deposition)

@ Spine
Age: middle age
Site: lumbar region with progressive ascension
√ laminated calcification of multiple intervertebral disks
√ disk space drastically narrowed
√ multiple "vacuum" phenomena (common)
√ osteoporosis of adjoining vertebrae
√ massive osteophytosis + ankylosis of spine (in older patient)
√ spotty calcifications in tissue anterior to vertebral bodies

@ Joints
√ hypertrophic changes in humeral head
√ severe premature progressive osteoarthritic changes in shoulder, knee, hip, spine of young patients
√ intraarticular osseous bodies

√ small calcifications in paraarticular soft tissues + tendon insertions

OROD IGITOFACIAL SYNDROME

= OROFACIODIGITAL SYNDROME
= group of heterogeneous defects, probably representing varying expressivity, involving face, oral cavity, and limbs

Etiology: autosomal trisomy of chromosome No. 1 with 47 chromosomes; X-linked dominant
Sex: nuclear chromatin pattern female (lethal in male)
Associated with: renal polycystic disease

- mental retardation
- hypertelorism
- cleft lip + tongue, lingual hamartoma
- bifid nasal tip

√ cleft in palate + jaw bone
√ hypoplasia of mandible (micrognathia) + occiput of skull
√ hypodontia
√ clinodactyly, syndactyly, brachydactyly (metacarpals may be elongated), polysyndactyly, duplication of hallux

OSGOOD-SCHLATTER DISEASE

= traumatically induced disruption of the attachment of the patellar ligament to the tibial tuberosity (NOT osteonecrosis); bilateral in 25%

Age: 10–15 years; M > F
Cause: trauma (common in sports that involve jumping, kicking, squatting) = ? cartilaginous avulsion fracture, ? tendinitis

- local pain + tenderness on pressure
- swelling of overlying soft tissue

√ soft-tissue swelling in front of tuberosity (= edema of skin + subcutaneous tissue)
√ thickening of distal portion of patellar tendon
√ indistinct margin of patellar tendon
√ increased radiodensity of infrapatellar fat pad
√ avulsion with separation of small ossicles from the developing ossification center of tibial tuberosity
√ single / multiple ossifications in avulsed fragment
√ comparison with other side (irregular development normal)

MR:
√ increased signal intensity at tibial insertion site of patellar tendon on T1WI + T2WI
√ distension of deep infrapatellar bursa
√ bone marrow signal changes in tibial tuberosity + tibial apophysis (rare)

Cx: nonunion of bone fragment, patellar subluxation, chondromalacia, avulsion of patellar tendon, genu recurvatum
Rx: immobilization / steroid injection
DDx: (1) normal ossification pattern of tibial tuberosity between ages 8–14 (no symptoms)
(2) Osteitis: tuberculous / syphilitic
(3) Soft-tissue sarcoma with calcifications

OSLER-WEBER-RENDU SYNDROME

= HEREDITARY HEMORRHAGIC TELANGIECTASIA
= autosomal dominant systemic fibrovascular dysplasia of all vessels resulting in
(1) telangiectasias
(2) arteriovenous malformations (AV hemangiomas)
(3) aneurysms

- frequent bleeding into mucous membranes, skin, lungs, genitourinary system, gastrointestinal system (due to vascular weakness)
- congestive heart failure (due to AV shunting)

OSSIFYING FIBROMA

Closely related to fibrous dysplasia + adamantinoma

Age: 2nd–4th decade; M < F
Histo: maturing cellular fibrous spindle cells with osteoblastic activity producing many calcific cartilaginous + bone densities

Location: frequently in face

@ Mandible, maxilla
- painless expansion of tooth-bearing portion of jaw

√ 1–5 cm well-circumscribed round / oval tumor
√ moderate expansion of intact cortex
√ homogeneous tumor matrix
√ dislodgment of teeth

@ Tibia
√ eccentric ground-glass lesion (resembling fibrous dysplasia)

Cx: frequent recurrences

OSTEITIS CONDENSANS ILII

Incidence: 2% of population
Cause: chronic stress secondary to instability of pubic symphysis
Age: young multiparous women

- associated with low back pain when instability of pubic symphysis present

√ triangular area of sclerosis along inferior anterior aspect of ileum adjacent to SI joint (joint space uninvolved)
√ similar triangle of reparative bone on sacral side
√ usually bilateral + symmetric; occasionally unilateral
√ sclerosis dissolves in 3–20 years following stabilization of pubic symphysis

DDx: (1) Ankylosing spondylitis (affects ilium + sacrum, joint space narrowing, involvement of other bones)
(2) Rheumatoid arthritis (asymmetric, joint destruction)
(3) Paget disease (thickened trabecular pattern)

OSTEOARTHRITIS

= DEGENERATIVE JOINT DISEASE = decreased chondroitin sulfate with age creates unsupported collagen fibrils followed by cartilage degeneration

√ joint space narrowing
√ sclerosis / eburnation of subchondral bone in areas of stress
√ subchondral cyst formation (geodes)
√ osteophytosis at articular margin / nonstressed area

@ Hand + foot
Target area: 1st MCP; trapezioscaphoid; DIP > PIP; 1st MTP

√ radial subluxation of 1st metacarpal base
√ Bouchard nodes = osteophytosis at PIP joint
√ Heberden nodes = osteophytosis at DIP joint: M:F = 1:10

@ Hip
√ superior migration of femoral head (less frequently medial / axial)
√ femoral + acetabular osteophytes, sclerosis, cyst formation
√ thickening / buttressing of medial femoral cortex

@ Knee
√ medial femorotibial compartment usually first to be involved
√ varus deformity

@ Spine
√ sclerosis + narrowing of intervertebral apophyseal joints
√ osteophytosis usually associated with discogenic disease

Erosive Osteoarthritis

= inflammatory form of osteoarthrosis

Predisposed: postmenopausal females

Site: DIP + PIP joints of hands; bilateral + symmetric

√ "bird-wing" / "sea-gull" joint configuration = central erosions
√ may lead to bony ankylosis

DDx: Rheumatoid arthritis, Wilson disease, chronic liver disease, hemochromatosis

Early Osteoarthritis

mnemonic: "**E**arly **O**steo**A**rthritis"
Epiphyseal dysplasia, multiple
Ochronosis
Acromegaly

OSTEOBLASTOMA

= GIANT OSTEOID OSTEOMA = OSTEOGENIC FIBROMA OF BONE = OSSIFYING FIBROMA
= rare benign tumor with unlimited growth potential + capability of malignant transformation

Incidence: <1% of all primary bone tumors; 3% of all benign bone tumors

Age: mean age of 16–19 years; 6–30 years (90%); 2nd decade (55%); 3rd decade (20%); M:F = 2:1

Path: lesion >1.5 cm; smaller lesions are classified as osteoid osteoma

Histo: numerous multinucleated giant cells (osteoclasts), irregularly arranged osteoid + bone; very vascular connective tissue stroma with interconnecting trabecular bone; trabeculae broader + longer than in osteoid osteoma

- asymptomatic in <2%
- dull localized pain of insidious onset (84%), worse at night in 7–13%
- response to salicylates in 7%
- localized swelling, tenderness, decreased range of motion (29%)
- painful scoliosis in 50% (with spinal / rib location) secondary to muscle spasm, may be convex toward side of tumor
- paresthesias, mild muscle weakness, paraparesis, paraplegia (due to cord compression)
- occasional systemic toxicity (high WBC, fever)

Location: (rarely multifocal)
(a) spine (33–37%): 62–94% in posterior elements, secondary extension into vertebral body (28–42%); cervical spine (31%), thoracic spine (34%), lumbar spine (31%), sacrum (3%)
(b) long bones (26–32%): femur (50%), tibia (19%), humerus (19%), radius (8%), fibula (4%); unusual in neck of femur
(c) small bones of hand + feet (15–26%): dorsal talus neck (62%), calcaneus (4%), scaphoid (8%), metacarpals (8%), metatarsals (8%)
(d) calvarium + mandible (= cementoblastoma)

Site: diaphyseal (58%), metaphyseal (42%); eccentric (46%), intracortical (42%), centric (12%), may be periosteal

√ similar to osteoid osteoma:
 √ radiolucent nidus >2 cm (range of 2–12 cm) in size
 √ well demarcated (83%)
 √ ± stippled / ringlike small flecks of matrix calcification
 √ reactive sclerosis (22–91%) / no sclerosis (9–56%)
√ progressive expansile lesion that may rapidly increase in size (25%):
 √ cortical expansion (75–94%) / destruction (20–22%)
 √ tumor matrix radiolucent (25–64%) / ossified (36–72%)
 √ sharply defined soft-tissue component
 √ thin shell of periosteal new bone (58–77%) / no periosteal reaction
√ scoliosis (35%)
√ osteoporosis due to disuse + hyperemia in talar location
√ rapid calcification after radiotherapy

CT:
 √ multifocal matrix mineralization, sclerosis
 √ expansile bone remodeling, thin osseous shell

NUC:
 √ intense focal accumulation of bone agent (100%)

Angio:
 √ tumor blush in capillary phase (50%)

MR:
 √ low to intermediate signal intensity on T1WI
 √ mixed intermediate to high intensity on T2WI
 √ surrounding edema

Prognosis: 10% recurrence after excision; incomplete curettage can effect cure due to cartilage production + trapping of host lamellar bone

DDx:
(1) Osteo- / chondrosarcoma (periosteal new bone)
(2) Osteoid osteoma (dense calcification + halo of bone sclerosis, stable lesion size <2 cm due to limited growth potential)
(3) Cartilaginous tumors (lumpy matrix calcification

(4) Giant cell tumor (no calcification, epiphyseal involvement)
(5) Aneurysmal bone cyst
(6) Osteomyelitis
(7) Hemangioma
(8) Lipoma
(9) Epidermoid
(10) Fibrous dysplasia
(11) Metastasis
(12) Ewing sarcoma

OSTEOCHONDROSIS DISSECANS

= OSTEOCHONDRITIS DISSECANS
= OSTEOCHONDRAL FRACTURE
= fragmentation + possible separation of a portion of the articular surface

Etiology:
(1) subchondral fatigue fracture as a result of shearing, rotatory / tangentially aligned impaction forces
(2) ? autosomal dominant trait associated with short stature, endocrine dysfunction, Scheuermann disease, Osgood-Schlatter disease, tibia vara, carpal tunnel syndrome

Age: adolescence; M > F

• asymptomatic / vague complaints
• clicking, locking, limitation of motion
• swelling, pain aggravated by movement

Location: (a) knee: medial (in 10% lateral) femoral condyle close to fossa intercondylaris; bilateral in 20–30%
(b) humeral head
(c) capitellum of elbow
(d) talus

√ purely cartilaginous fragment unrecognized on plain film
√ fracture line parallels joint surface
√ mouse = osteochondrotic fragment
Location: posterior region of knee joint, olecranon fossa, axillary / subscapular recess of glenohumeral joint
√ mouse bed = sclerosed pit in articular surface
√ soft-tissue swelling, joint effusion

DDx: spontaneous osteonecrosis, neuroarthropathy, degenerative joint disease, synovial osteochondromatosis

OSTEOFIBROUS DYSPLASIA

= entity previously mistaken for fibrous dysplasia

Age: newborn up to 5 years
Histo: fibrous tissue surrounding trabeculae in a whorled storiform pattern
Location: normally confined to tibia (middiaphysis in 50%), lesion begins in anterior cortex; ipsilateral fibula affected in 20%

√ enlargement of tibia with anterior bowing
√ cortex thin / invisible
√ periosteal expansion
√ sclerotic margin (DDx: nonosteogenic fibroma, chondromyxoid fibroma)
√ spontaneous regression in 1/3

Cx: pathologic fracture in 25%, fractures will heal with immobilization; infrequently complicated by pseudarthrosis
DDx: fibrous dysplasia, Paget disease

OSTEOGENESIS IMPERFECTA

= PSATHYROSIS = FRAGILITAS OSSIUM = LOBSTEIN DISEASE
= heterogeneous group of a generalized connective tissue disorder leading to micromelic dwarfism characterized by bone fragility, blue sclerae, and dentinogenesis imperfecta

Incidence: overall in 1:28,500 (20,000–60,000) live births; M:F = 1:1
Histo: immature collagen matrix
Clinical types:
1. OSTEOGENESIS IMPERFECTA CONGENITA
= disease manifest at birth (occurring in utero); autosomal dominant; corresponds to type II; lethal variety
2. OSTEOGENESIS IMPERFECTA TARDA
= usually not manifest at birth; recessive / sporadic corresponds to type I + IV; nonlethal variety

• soft skull (caput membranaceum)
• hyperlaxity of joints
• blue sclerae
• poor dentition
• otosclerosis
• thin loose skin

√ diffuse demineralization, deficient trabecular structure, cortical thinning
√ defective cortical bone: increase in diameter of proximal ends of humeri + femora; slender fragile bone; multiple cystlike areas
√ multiple fractures + pseudarthrosis with bowing (vertebral bodies, long bones)
√ normal / exuberant callus formation
√ rib thinning / notching
√ thin calvarium
√ sinus + mastoid cell enlargement
√ thickened undermineralized otic capsule (= otosclerosis)
√ wormian bones persisting into adulthood
√ basilar impression (= platybasia)
√ biconcave vertebral bodies + Schmorl nodes, increased height of intervertebral disk space
√ bowing deformities after child begins to walk

Cx: (1) impaired hearing / deafness from otosclerosis (20–60%)
(2) death from intracranial hemorrhage (abnormal platelet function)
Dx: choricnic villous sampling

Osteogenesis imperfecta type I

Autosomal dominant; compatible with life

Age at presentation: 2–6 years

• blue sclerae
• presenile deafness
• normal / abnormal dentinogenesis

√ infants of normal weight + length
√ osteoporosis

√ fractures in neonate (occurring during delivery)
OB-US:
- √ marked bowing of long bones
- √ NO IUGR

Osteogenesis imperfecta type II

= CONGENITAL LETHAL OI

Autosomal recessive / sporadic; perinatal lethal form

Incidence: 1:54,000 births; most frequent variety

- • blue sclerae
- • ligamentous laxity + loose skin
- √ shortened broad crumpled long bones
- √ bone angulations, bowing, demineralization
- √ localized bone thickening from callus formation
- √ thin beaded ribs ± fractures resulting in bell-shaped / narrow chest
- √ thin poorly ossified skull
- √ spinal osteopenia
- √ platyspondyly

OB-US:

A normal sonogram after 17 weeks MA excludes the diagnosis!
- √ increased through-transmission of skull (extremely poor mineralization)
  - √ unusually good visualization of brain surface
  - √ unusually good visualization of orbits
  - √ increased visualization of intracranial arterial pulsations
- √ abnormal compressibility of skull vault with transducer
- √ decreased visualization of skeleton
- √ multiple fetal fractures + deformities of long bones + ribs
  - √ wrinkled appearance of bone (= more than one fracture in single bone)
  - √ beaded ribs (callus formation around fractures)
- √ abnormally short limbs
- √ small thorax (collapse of thoracic cage)
- √ decreased fetal movement
- √ infants small for gestational age (frequent)
- √ polyhydramnios

Prognosis: stillborn / death shortly after birth due to pulmonary hypoplasia

DDx: congenital hypophosphatasia, achondrogenesis type I

Osteogenesis imperfecta type III

= SEVERE PROGRESSIVELY DEFORMING OI

Autosomal recessive / dominant; progressively deforming disorder compatible with life

- • bluish sclerae during infancy which turn pale with time
- • joint hyperlaxity (50%)
- √ decreased ossification of skull
- √ normal vertebrae + pelvis
- √ progressive deformities of limbs + spine into adulthood
- √ shortened + bowed long bones
- √ ± rib fractures
- √ multiple fractures present at birth in 2/3 of cases
- √ fractures heal well

OB-US:
- √ short + bowed long bones
- √ fractures
- √ humerus almost normal in shape
- √ normal thoracic circumference

Prognosis: progressive limb + spine deformities during childhood / adolescence

Osteogenesis imperfecta type IV

Autosomal dominant; mildest form with best prognosis

- • normal scleral color
- • little tendency to develop hearing loss
- √ tubular bones of normal length; mild femoral bowing may occur
- √ osteoporosis

OB-US:
- √ bowing of long bones

OSTEOID OSTEOMA

= benign skeletal neoplasm composed of osteoid + woven bone less than 1.5 cm in diameter per definition

Incidence: 12% of benign skeletal neoplasms

Etiology: ? inflammatory response

Histo: small nidus of osteoid-laden interconnected trabeculae with a background of highly vascularized fibrous connective tissue surrounded by zone of reactive bone sclerosis; osteoblastic rimming; indistinguishable from osteoblastoma

Age: 10–20 years (51%); 2nd + 3rd decade (73%); 5–25 years (90%); range of 19 months–56 years; uncommon <5 and >40 years of age; M:F = 2:1; uncommon in Blacks

- • tender to touch + pressure
- • local pain (95–98%), weeks to years in duration, worse at night, decreased by activity
- • salicylates give relief in 20–30 minutes in 75–90%
- • prostaglandin E2 elevated 100–1000 x normal within nidus (probable cause of pain and vasodilatation)

Location:
- (a) meta- / diaphysis of long bones (73%): upper end of femur (43%), hands (8%), feet (4%); frequent in proximal tibia + femoral neck, fibula, humerus; no bone exempt
- (b) spine (10–14%): predominantly in posterior elements (50% in pedicle + lamina + spinous process; 20% in articular process) of lumbar (59%), cervical (27%), thoracic (12%), sacral (2%) segments
  - •painful scoliosis, focal / radicular pain
  - •gait disturbance, muscle atrophy
- (c) skull, rib, ischium, mandible, patella

Classification:

Cortical osteoid osteoma (most common)

= nidus within cortex
- √ solid / laminated periosteal reaction
- √ fusiform sclerotic cortical thickening in shaft of long bone
- √ radiolucent area within center of osteosclerosis

Cancellous osteoid osteoma (intermediate frequency)
= intramedullary
◊ Intra-articular lesion difficult to identify with delay in diagnosis of 4 months–5 years!
Site: juxta- / intra-articular at femoral neck, vertebral posterior elements, small bones of hands + feet
√ little osteosclerosis / sclerotic cortex distant to nidus (functional difference of intra-articular periosteum)
√ joint space widened (effusion, synovitis)

Subperiosteal osteoid osteoma (rare)
= round soft-tissue mass adjacent to bone
Site: juxta- / intra-articular at medial aspect of femoral neck, hands, feet (neck of talus)
√ juxtacortical mass excavating the cortex (bony pressure atrophy) with almost no reactive sclerosis

√ round / oval radiolucent nidus (75%) of <1.5 cm in size
√ variable surrounding sclerosis ± central calcification
√ painful scoliosis concave toward lesion / kyphoscoliosis / hyperlordosis / torticollis with spinal location (due to spasm)
√ may show extensive synovitis + effusion + premature loss of cartilage with intra-articular site (lymphofollicular synovitis)
√ osteoarthritis (50%) with intra-articular site 1.5–22 years after onset of symptomatology
√ regional osteoporosis (probably due to disuse)
◊ Radiographically difficult areas: vertebral column, femoral neck, small bones of hand + feet
NUC:
√ intensely increased radiotracer uptake (increased blood flow + new-bone formation)
√ double density sign = small area of focal activity (nidus) superimposed on larger area of increased tracer uptake
CT (for detection + precise localization of nidus):
√ small well-defined round / oval nidus surrounded by variable amount of sclerosis
√ nidus enhances on dynamic scan
√ nidus with variable amount of mineralization (50%): punctate / amorphous / ringlike / dense
MR (diminished conspicuity of lesion compared with CT):
√ nidus isointense to muscle on T1WI
√ signal intensity increases to between that of muscle + fat / remains low on T2WI
√ perinidal inflammation of bone marrow (63%)
√ perinidal soft-tissue inflammation / edema (47%)
√ synovitis + joint effusion with intra-articular site
Angio:
√ highly vascularized nidus with intense circumscribed blush appearing in early arterial phase + persisting late into venous phase
Prognosis: no growth progression, infrequent regression
Rx: (1) complete surgical excision of nidus (reactive bone regresses subsequently)
(2) percutaneous CT-guided removal
(3) percutaneous ablation with radio-frequency electrode / laser / alcohol

DDx:
(1) Cortical osteoid osteoma: Brodie abscess, sclerosing osteomyelitis, syphilis, bone island, stress fracture, osteosarcoma, Ewing sarcoma, osteoblastic metastasis, lymphoma, subperiosteal aneurysmal bone cyst, osteoblastoma (progressive growth)
(2) Intra-articular osteoid osteoma: inflammatory / septic / tuberculous / rheumatoid arthritis, nonspecific synovitis / Legg-Calvé-Perthes disease

OSTEOMA
= benign tumor of membranous bone (hamartoma)
Age: adult life
Associated with: Gardner syndrome (multiple osteomas + colonic polyposis)
Location: inner / outer table of calvarium (usually from external table), paranasal sinuses (frontal / ethmoid sinuses), mandible, nasal bones
√ well-circumscribed round extremely dense structureless lesion usually <2 cm in size

FIBROUS OSTEOMA
Probably a form of fibrous dysplasia
Age: childhood
√ less dense than osteoma / radiolucent
√ expanding external table without affecting internal table
DDx: endostoma, bone island, bone infarct (located in medulla)

OSTEOMYELITIS
Acute osteomyelitis
Age: most commonly affects children
Organisms:
(a) newborns: S. aureus, Group B streptococcus, Escherichia coli
(b) children: S. aureus (blood cultures in 50% positive)
(c) adults: S. aureus (60%), enteric species (29%), Streptococcus (8%)
(d) drug addicts: Pseudomonas (86%), Klebsiella, Enterobacteriae; (57 days average delay in diagnosis)
(e) sickle cell disease: Salmonella
Cause:
(1) Genitourinary tract infection (72%)
(2) Lung infection (14%)
(3) Dermal infection (14%): direct contamination from a soft-tissue lesion in diabetic patient
Pathogenesis:
(a) hematogenous spread
(b) direct implantation from a traumatic / iatrogenic source
(c) extension from adjacent soft-tissue infection
Location:
@ Lower extremity (75%): over pressure points in diabetic foot
@ Vertebrae (53%): lumbar (75%) > thoracic > cervical

@ Radial styloid (24%)
@ Sacroiliac joint (18%)
• leukocytosis + fever (66%)

A. ACUTE NEONATAL OSTEOMYELITIS
Age: onset <30 days of age
• little / no systemic disturbance
√ multicentric involvement more common; often joint involvement
√ bone scan falsely negative / equivocal in 70%

B. ACUTE OSTEOMYELITIS IN INFANCY
Age: <18 months of age
Pathomechanism: spread to epiphysis because transphyseal vessels cross growth plate into epiphysis
√ striking soft-tissue component
√ subperiosteal abscess with extensive periosteal new bone
Cx: frequent joint involvement
Prognosis: rapid healing

C. ACUTE OSTEOMYELITIS IN CHILDHOOD
Age: 2–16 years of age
Pathomechanism:
transphyseal vessels closed; metaphyseal vessels adjacent to growth plate loop back toward metaphysis locating the primary focus of infection into metaphysis; abscess formation in medulla with cortical spread
√ sequestration frequent
√ periosteal elevation (with disruption of periosteal blood supply)
√ small single / multiple osteolytic areas in metaphysis
√ extensive periosteal reaction parallel to shaft (after 3–6 weeks); may be "lamellar nodular" (DDx: osteoblastoma, eosinophilic granuloma)
√ shortening of bone with destruction of epiphyseal cartilage
√ growth stimulation by hyperemia + premature maturation of adjacent epiphysis
√ midshaft osteomyelitis less frequent site
√ serpiginous tract with small sclerotic rim (PATHOGNOMONIC)

D. ACUTE OSTEOMYELITIS IN ADULTHOOD
√ delicate periosteal new bone
√ joint involvement common

Radiographs:
√ initial radiographs often normal (notoriously poor in early phase of infection for as long as 10 days)
√ localized soft-tissue swelling adjacent to metaphysis with obliteration of usual fat planes (after 3–10 days)
√ area of bone destruction (lags 7–14 days behind pathologic changes)
√ involucrum = cloak of laminated / spiculated periosteal reaction (develops after 20 days)
√ sequestrum = detached necrotic cortical bone (develops after 30 days)
√ cloaca formation = space in which dead bone resides

MR:
√ bone marrow hypointense on T1WI + hyperintense on T2WI (= water-rich inflammatory tissue)
DDx: neuropathic osteoarthropathy, aseptic arthritis, acute fracture, recent surgery
√ focal / linear cortical involvement hyperintense on T2WI
√ hyperintense halo surrounding cortex on T2WI = subperiosteal infection
√ hyperintense line on T2WI extending from bone to skin surface + enhancement of borders (= sinus tract)

Abscess characteristics:
√ hyperintense enhancing rim (= hyperemic zone) around a central focus of low intensity (= necrotic / devitalized tissue) on contrast-enhanced T1WI
√ hyperintense fluid collection surrounded by hypointense pseudocapsule on T2WI + contrast-enhancement of granulation tissue
√ hyperintense adjacent soft tissues on T2WI
√ fat-suppressed contrast-enhanced imaging (88% sensitive + 93% specific compared with 79% + 53% for nonenhanced MR imaging)

NUC (accuracy approx. 90%):
(1) Ga-67 scans: 100% sensitivity; increased uptake 1 day earlier than for Tc-99m MDP
◊ Gallium helpful for chronic osteomyelitis!
(2) Static Tc-99m diphosphonate: 83% sensitivity 5–60% false-negative rate in neonates + children because of (a) masking effect of epiphyseal plates (b) early diminished blood flow with infection (c) spectrum of uptake pattern from hot to cold
(3) Three-phase skeletal scintigraphy: 92% sensitivity, 87% specificity
Phase 1: Radionuclide angiography = perfusion phase of regional blood flow
Phase 2: "blood pool" images
Phase 3: "bone uptake"
Limitations: diagnostic difficulties in children, in posttraumatic / postoperative state, diabetic neuropathy (poor blood supply), neoplasia, septic arthritis, Paget disease, healed osteomyelitis, noninfectious inflammatory process
DDx: cellulitis (decrease in activity over time)
(4) WBC-scan:
(a) In-111–labeled leukocytes: best agent for acute infections
(b) Tc-99m labeled leukocytes: preferred over In-111–leukocyte imaging especially in extremities
◊ WBC scans have largely replaced gallium imaging for acute osteomyelitis due to improved photon flux + improved dosimetry (higher dose allowed relative to In-111) allowing faster imaging + greater resolution

√ "cold" area in early osteomyelitis subsequently becoming "hot" if localized to long bones / pelvis (not seen in vertebral bodies)

√ local increase in radiopharmaceutical uptake (positive within 24–72 hours)

Cx: (1) Soft-tissue abscess (2) Fistula formation (3) Pathologic fracture (4) Extension into joint (5) Growth disturbance due to epiphyseal involvement (6) Neoplasm (7) Amyloidosis (8) Severe deformity with delayed treatment

Chronic osteomyelitis

√ thick irregular sclerotic bone with radiolucencies, elevated periosteum, chronic draining sinus

Sclerosing osteomyelitis of Garré

= low-grade infection, no purulent exudate

Location: mandible (most commonly)

√ focal bulge of thickened cortex (sclerosing periosteal reaction)

DDx: osteoid osteoma, stress fracture

Chronic recurrent multifocal osteomyelitis

= benign self-limited disease of unknown etiology

Age: children + adolescents; M:F = 1:2

Histo: nonspecific subacute / chronic osteomyelitis

• pain, soft-tissue swelling, limited motion

Location: tibia > femur > clavicle > fibula

Site: metaphyses of long bones; often symmetric

√ small areas of bone lysis, often confluent

Brodie abscess

= subacute pyogenic osteomyelitis (smoldering indolent infection)

Organism: S. aureus (most common)

Histo: granulation tissue + eburnation

Age: more common in children; M > F

Location: predilection for ends of tubular bones (proximal / distal tibial metaphysis most common); carpal + tarsal bones

Site: metaphysis, rarely traversing the open growth plate; epiphysis (children + infants)

√ central area of lucency surrounded by dense rim of reactive sclerosis

√ lucent channel-like / tortuous configuration extending toward growth plate (PATHOGNOMONIC)

√ periosteal new-bone formation

√ ± adjacent soft-tissue swelling

√ may persist for many months

MR:

√ "double line" effect = high signal intensity of granulation tissue surrounded by low signal intensity of bone sclerosis on T2WI

√ well-defined low- to intermediate-signal lesion outlined by low-signal rim on T1WI

DDx: Osteoid osteoma

Epidermoid carcinoma

Etiology: complication of chronic osteomyelitis (0.2–1.7%)

Histo: squamous cell carcinoma (90%); occasionally: basal cell carcinoma, adenocarcinoma, fibrosarcoma, angiosarcoma, reticulum cell sarcoma, spindle cell sarcoma, rhabdomyosarcoma, parosteal osteosarcoma, plasmacytoma

Age: 30–80 (mean 55) years; M >> F

Latent period: 20–30 (range of 1.5–72) years

• history of childhood osteomyelitis

• exacerbation of symptoms with increasing pain, enlarging mass

• change in character / amount of sinus drainage

Location: at site of chronically / intermittently draining sinus; tibia (50%), femur (21%)

√ lytic lesion superimposed on changes of chronic osteomyelitis

√ soft-tissue mass

√ pathologic fracture

Prognosis:

(1) early metastases in 14–20–40% (within 18 months)

(2) no recurrence in 80%

OSTEOPATHIA STRIATA

= VOORHOEVE DISEASE

• usually asymptomatic (similar to osteopoikilosis)

Location: all long bones affected; the only bone sclerosis primarily involving metaphysis (with extension into epi- and diaphysis)

√ longitudinal striations of dense bone in metaphysis

√ radiating densities of "sunburst" appearance from acetabulum into ileum

OSTEOPETROSIS

= ALBERS-SCHÖNBERG DISEASE = MARBLE BONE DISEASE = rare hereditary disorder

Path: defective osteoclast function with failure of proper reabsorption + remodeling of primary spongiosum; bone sclerotic + thick but structurally weak + brittle

A. INFANTILE AUTOSOMAL RECESSIVE TYPE
 • failure to thrive
 • premature senile appearance of facies
 • severe dental caries
 • anemia, leukocytopenia, thrombocytopenia (severe marrow depression)
 • cranial nerve compression (optic atrophy, deafness)
 • hepatosplenomegaly (extramedullary hematopoiesis)
 • lymphadenopathy
 • subarachnoid hemorrhage (due to thrombocytopenia)

 May be associated with:
 renal tubular acidosis + cerebral calcification

 Prognosis: survival beyond middle life uncommon (death due to recurrent infection, massive hemorrhage, terminal leukemia)

B. BENIGN ADULT AUTOSOMAL DOMINANT TYPE
 • 50% asymptomatic
 • recurrent fractures, mild anemia
 • occasionally cranial nerve palsy

 Prognosis: normal life expectancy

√ diffuse osteosclerosis = generalized dense amorphous structureless bones with obliteration of normal trabecular pattern; mandible least commonly involved
√ cortical thickening with medullary encroachment
√ Erlenmeyer flask deformity = clublike long bones due to lack of tubulization + flaring of ends
√ bone-within-bone appearance
√ "sandwich" vertebrae
√ alternating sclerotic + radiolucent transverse metaphyseal lines (phalanges, iliac bones) as indicators of fluctuating course of disease
√ longitudinal metaphyseal striations
√ obliteration of mastoid cells, paranasal sinuses, basal foramina by osteosclerosis
√ sclerosis predominantly involving base of skull; calvaria often spared

Cx: (1) usually transverse fractures (common because of brittle bones) with abundant callus + normal healing
(2) crowding of marrow (myelophthisic anemia + extramedullary hematopoiesis)
(3) frequently terminates in acute leukemia

Rx: bone marrow transplant

DDx: (1) Heavy metal poisoning
(2) Melorheostosis (limited to one extremity)
(3) Hypervitaminosis D
(4) Pyknodysostosis
(5) Fibrous dysplasia of skull / face

OSTEOPOIKILOSIS

= OSTEOPATHIA CONDENSANS DISSEMINATA
Often autosomal dominant; M > F
• asymptomatic
Histo: compact bone islands
Location: in most metaphyses + epiphyses (rarely extending into midshaft); concentrated at glenoid + acetabulum, wrist, ankle, pelvis; rare in skull, ribs, vertebral centra, mandible
√ small foci of ovoid / lenticular opacification (2–10 mm) in cancellous bone
√ long axis of lesions parallel to long axis of bone
Prognosis: not progressive, no change after cessation of growth
DDx: (1) Epiphyseal dysplasia (metaphyses normal)
(2) Melorheostosis (diaphyseal involvement)

OSTEORADIONECROSIS

Cause: deleterious effect of radiation on osteoblasts, osteoclasts, vascular damage, increased susceptibility of irradiated bone to infection
Time of onset: 1–3 years following radiation therapy
Dose: >6,000 cGy in adults; >2,000 cGy in children
√ focal lytic area with abnormal bone matrix
√ ± cortical thinning from chronic infection
√ ± pathologic fracture
DDx: neoplastic involvement (soft-tissue mass)

OSTEOSARCOMA

Most common malignant primary bone tumor in young adults + children; 2nd most common primary malignant bone tumor after multiple myeloma
Prevalence: 4–5:1,000,000; 15% of all primary bone tumors confirmed at biopsy

Types & Frequency:

A. Conventional osteosarcoma:		
– high-grade intramedullary		75%
– telangiectatic		4.5–11%
– low-grade intraosseous		4–5%
– small cell		1–4%
– osteosarcomatosis		3–4%
– gnathic		6–9%
B. Surface / juxtacortical osteosarcoma:		4–10%
– intracortical	rare	
– parosteal	65%	
– periosteal	25%	
– high-grade surface	10%	
C. Extraskeletal		4%
D. Secondary osteosarcoma		5–7%

Prognosis: dependent on age, sex, tumor size, site, classification; best predictor is degree of tissue necrosis in postresection specimen following chemotherapy (91% survival with tumor necrosis >90%, 14% survival with <90% tumor necrosis)

Extraskeletal osteosarcoma

= located within soft tissue without attachment to bone / periosteum
Incidence: 1% of soft-tissue sarcomas
Histo: variable amounts of neoplastic osteoid + bone + cartilage; frequently associated with fibrosarcoma, malignant fibrous histiocytoma, malignant peripheral nerve sheath tumor
Mean age: 50 years; 94% >30 years of age; M > F
Location: lower extremity (thigh in 42–47%), upper extremity (12–23%), retroperitoneum (8–17%), buttock, back, orbit, submental, axilla, abdomen, neck, kidney, breast
• slowly growing soft-tissue mass
• painful + tender (25–50%)
• history of trauma (12–31%): in preexisting myositis ossificans / site of intramuscular injection
√ often deep-seated + fixed soft-tissue tumor (average diameter of 9 cm)
√ focal / massive area of mineralization (>50%)
√ increased radionuclide uptake on bone scan
Prognosis:
(1) multiple local recurrences (in 80–90%) after interval of 2 months to 10 years
(2) metastases after interval of 1 month to 4 years: lungs (81–100%), lymph nodes (25%), bone, subcutis, liver
(3) death within 2–3 years (>50%) with tumor size as major predictor

High-grade intramedullary osteosarcoma

= CENTRAL OSTEOSARCOMA = CONVENTIONAL OSTEOSARCOMA

Histo: arising from undifferentiated mesenchymal tissue; forming fibrous / cartilaginous / osseous matrix (mostly mixed) that produces osteoid / immature bone
(a) osteoblastic (50–80%)
(b) chondroblastic (5–25%)
(c) fibroblastic-fibrohistiocytic (7–25%)

Age: bimodal distribution 10– 25 years and >60 years; 21% <10 years; 68% <15 years; 70% between 10 and 30 years; M:F = 3:2 to 2:1; >35 years: related to preexisting condition

• painful swelling (1–2 months' duration)
• fever (frequent)
• slight elevation of alkaline phosphatase
• diabetes mellitus (paraneoplastic syndrome) in 25%

Location: long bones (70–80%), femur (40–45%), tibia (16–20%); 50–55% about knee; proximal humerus (10–15%); cylindrical bone <30 years; flat bone (ilium) >50 years
Site: origin in metaphysis (90–95%) / diaphysis (2–11%) /epiphysis (<1%); growth through open physis with extension into epiphysis (75–88%)
Doubling time: 20–30 day

√ usually large bone lesion >5–6 cm when first detected
√ cloudlike density (90%) / almost normal density / osteolytic (fibroblastic type)
√ aggressive periosteal reaction: sunburst / hair-on-end / onion-peel = laminated / Codman triangle
√ moth-eaten bone destruction + cortical disruption
√ soft-tissue mass with tumor new bone (osseous / cartilaginous type)
√ transepiphyseal spread before plate closure (75–88%); physis does NOT act as a barrier to tumor spread
√ spontaneous pneumothorax (due to subpleural metastases)

NUC (bone scintigraphy):
√ intensely increased activity on blood flow, blood pool, delayed images (hypervascularity, new-bone formation)
√ soft-tissue extension demonstrated, especially with SPECT
√ bone scan establishes local extent (extent of involvement easily overestimated due to intensity of uptake), skip lesions, metastases to bone + soft tissues

CT:
√ soft-tissue attenuation (nonmineralized portion) replacing fatty bone marrow
√ low attenuation (higher water content of chondroblastic component / hemorrhage / necrosis)
√ very high attenuation (mineralized matrix)

MR (preferred modality):
√ tumor of intermediate signal intensity on T1WI + high signal intensity on T2WI
√ clearly defines marrow extent (best on T1WI), vascular involvement, soft-tissue component (best on T2WI)

Evaluate for:
(1) extent of marrow + soft-tissue involvement
(2) invasion of epiphysis
(3) joint (19–24%) + neurovascular involvement
(4) viable tumor + mineralized matrix for biopsy

Metastases (in 2% at presentation):
(a) hematogenous lung metastases (15%): calcifying; spontaneous pneumothorax secondary to subpleural cavitating nodules rupturing into pleural space
(b) lymph nodes, liver, brain (may be calcified)
(c) skeletal metastases uncommon (unlike Ewing sarcoma); skip lesions = discontinuous tumor foci in marrow cavity in 1–25%

Cx: (1) pathologic fracture (15–20%)
(2) radiation-induced osteosarcoma (30 years delay)

Rx: chemotherapy followed by wide-surgical resection

Prognosis: 60–80% 5-year survival
(1) amputation: 20% 5-year survival; 15% develop skeletal metastases; 75% dead within <2 years
(2) multidrug chemotherapy: 55% 4-year survival more proximal lesions carry higher mortality (0% 2-year survival for axial primary)

Predictors of poor outcome:
metastasis at presentation, soft-tissue mass >20 cm, pathologic fracture, skip lesions in marrow

Predictors of poor response to chemotherapy:
no change / increase in size of soft-tissue mass, increase in bone destruction

DDx: Osteoid osteoma, sclerosing osteomyelitis, Charcot joint

High-grade surface osteosarcoma

Location: femur, humerus, fibula
Site: diaphysis
√ similar to periosteal osteosarcoma
√ often involve entire circumference of bone
√ frequent invasion of medullary canal

Prognosis: identical to conventional intramedullary osteosarcoma

Intracortical osteosarcoma

Rarest form of osteosarcoma

Histo: sclerosing variant of osteosarcoma which may contain small foci of chondro- or fibrosarcoma

Location: femur, tibia
√ tumor <4 cm in diameter
√ intracortical geographic bone lysis
√ tumor margin may be well defined with thickening of surrounding cortex
√ metastases in 29%

Low-grade intraosseous osteosarcoma

= WELL-DIFFERENTIATED / SCLEROSING OSTEOSARCOMA

Age: most frequently 3rd decade; M:F = 1:1

- protracted clinical course with nonspecific symptoms

Location: about the knee
Site: metaphysis; often with extension into epiphysis
√ may have well-defined margins + sclerotic rim
√ diffuse sclerosis
√ expansile remodeling of bone
√ subtle signs of aggressiveness: bone lysis, focally indistinct margin, cortical destruction, soft-tissue mass, periosteal reaction
Cx: transformation into high-grade osteosarcoma
DDx: fibrous dysplasia, nonossifying fibroma, chondrosarcoma, chondromyxoid fibroma

Osteosarcoma of jaw

= GNATHIC OSTEOSARCOMA
Average age: 34 years (10–15 years older than in conventional osteosarcoma)
Histo: chondroblastic predominance (~50%), osteoblastic predominance (~25%); better differentiated (grade 2 or 3) than conventional osteosarcoma (grade 3 or 4)

- simulating periodontal disease: rapidly enlarging mass, lump, swelling
- paresthesia (if inferior alveolar nerve involved)
- painful / loose teeth, bleeding gum

Location: body of mandible (lytic), alveolar ridge of maxilla (sclerotic), maxillary antrum
√ osteolytic / osteoblastic / mixed pattern
√ osteoid matrix (60–80%)
√ aggressive periosteal reaction for mandibular lesion
√ soft-tissue mass (100%)
√ opacification of maxillary sinus (frequent in maxillary lesions)
Prognosis: 40% 5-year survival rate (lower probability of metastases, lower grade)
DDx: metastatic disease (lung, breast, kidney), multiple myeloma, direct invasion by contiguous tumor from oral cavity, Ewing sarcoma, primary lymphoma of bone, chondrosarcoma, fibrosarcoma, acute osteomyelitis, ameloblastoma, Langerhans cell histiocytosis, giant cell reparative granuloma, "brown tumor" of HPT

Osteosarcomatosis

= MULTIFOCAL OSTEOSARCOMA
= MULTIPLE SCLEROTIC OSTEOSARCOMA
Etiology: (a) multicentric type of osteosarcoma
(b) multiple metastatic bone lesions
Classification (Amstutz):
Type I multiple synchronous bone lesions occurring within 5 months + patient ≤18 years of age
Type II multiple synchronous bone lesions occurring within 5 months + patient >18 years of age
Type IIIa early metachronous metastatic osteosarcoma occurring 5 to 24 months after diagnosis
Type IIIb late metachronous metastatic osteosarcoma occurring >24 months after diagnosis
Age: Amstutz type I = 4–18 (mean 11) years
Amstutz type II = 19–63 (mean 30) years
Site: metaphysis of long bones; may extend into epiphyseal plate / begin in epiphysis
√ multicentric simultaneously appearing lesions with a radiologically dominant tumor (97%)
√ smaller lesions are densely opaque (osteoblastic)
√ lesions bilateral + symmetrical
√ early: bone islands
√ late: entire metaphysis fills with sclerotic lesions breaking through cortex
√ lesions are of same size
√ lung metastases (62%)
Prognosis: uniformly poor with mean survival of 12 (range, 6–37) months
DDx: heavy metal poisoning, sclerosing osteitis, progressive diaphyseal dysplasia, melorheostosis, osteopoikilosis, bone infarction, osteopetrosis

Parosteal osteosarcoma

Frequency: 4% of all osteosarcomas; 65% of all juxtacortical osteosarcomas
Origin: outer layer of periosteum slowly growing lesion with fulminating course if tumor reaches medullary canal
Histo: low-grade lesion with higher-grade regions (22–64%), invasion of medullary canal (8–59%); fibrous stroma + extensive osteoid with small foci of cartilage
Age: peak age 38 years (range of 12–58 years); 50% > age 30 (for central osteosarcoma 75% < age 30); M:F = 2:3
Location: posterior aspect of distal femur (50–65%), either end of tibia, proximal humerus, fibula, rare in other long bones
Site: metaphysis (80–90%)

- palpable mass

√ large lobulated "cauliflower-like" homogeneous ossific mass extending away from cortex
√ "string sign" = initially fine radiolucent line separating tumor mass from cortex (30–40%)
√ tumor stalk (= attachment to cortex) grows with tumor obliterating the radiolucent cleavage plane
√ cortical thickening without aggressive periosteal reaction
√ tumor periphery less dense than center (DDx: myositis ossificans with periphery more dense than center + without attachment to cortex)
√ large soft-tissue component with osseous + cartilaginous elements
Prognosis: 80–90% 5- and 10-year survival rates (best prognosis of all osteosarcomas)
DDx: osteochondroma, myositis ossificans, juxtacortical hematoma, extraosseous osteosarcoma

Periosteal Osteosarcoma

Origin: deep layer of periosteum
Histo: intermediate-grade lesion; highly chondroblastic lesion with smaller areas of osteoid formation
Age: peak 10–20 years (range of 13–70 years)
Location: femur and tibia (85–95%), ulna and humerus (5–10%)
Site: diaphysis / metadiaphysis of long bone; limited to periphery of cortex with normal endosteal margin + medullary canal (resembles parosteal sarcoma)
√ tumor 7–12 cm in length, 2–4 cm in width, involving 50% of osseous circumference
√ tumor base closely attached to cortex over entire extent of tumor
√ tumor lies in apparent depression on bone surface causing scalloped surface of thickened diaphyseal cortex
√ short spicules of new bone perpendicular to shaft extending into broad-based elliptical soft-tissue mass
√ solid (cortical thickening) / aggressive periosteal reaction (Codman triangle) at upper and lower margins of lesion
√ NO cortical destruction / medullary cavity invasion
√ chondroblastic areas of low attenuation on CT, hypointense on T1WI, very hyperintense on T2WI
Prognosis: 80–90% cure rate (better prognosis than central osteosarcoma with 50% 5-year survival but worse than parosteal osteosarcoma)
DDx: juxtacortical chondrosarcoma

Secondary Osteosarcoma

Cause: malignant transformation within benign process
(1) Paget disease (67–90%)
◊ 0.2–7.5% of patients with Paget disease develop osteosarcoma dependent on extent of disease
(2) sequela of irradiation (6–22%) 2–40 years ago (malignant fibrous histiocytoma most common; fibrosarcoma 3rd most common)
◊ 0.02–4% of patients with radiation therapy develop osteosarcoma related to exposure dose (usually >1,000 cGy)
(3) osteonecrosis, fibrous dysplasia, metallic implants, osteogenesis imperfecta, chronic osteomyelitis, retinoblastoma (familial bilateral type)
Path: high-grade anaplastic tissue with little / no mineralization
Age: middle-aged / late adulthood
√ aggressive bone destruction in area of preexisting condition associated with large soft-tissue mass
Prognosis: <5% 5-year survival rate

Small-cell Osteosarcoma

Age: similar to conventional osteosarcoma; M:F = 1:1
Histo: small round blue cells (similar to Ewing sarcoma) lacking cellular uniformity and consistently producing fine reticular osteoid
Location: distal femur
Site: metaphysis with frequent extension into epiphysis; diaphysis (in 15%)
√ predominantly permeative lytic medullary lesion
√ cortical breakthrough
√ aggressive periosteal reaction
√ associated soft-tissue mass
Prognosis: extremely poor

Telangiectatic Osteosarcoma

= MALIGNANT BONE ANEURYSM
Frequency: 4–11% of all osteosarcomas
Age: 3–67 (mean 20) years; M:F = 3:2
Path: malignant osteoid-forming sarcoma of bone with large blood-filled vascular channels
Histo: hemorrhagic + cystic + necrotic spaces occupying >90% of the lesion before therapy; blood-filled cavernous vessels lined with osteoclastic giant cells
Location: about knee (62%); distal femur (48%), proximal tibia (14%), proximal humerus (16%)
Site: metaphysis (90%); extension into epiphysis (87%)
√ geographic bone destruction with a wide zone of transition
√ marked aneurysmal expansion of bone (19%)
√ fluid-fluid levels (90%)
√ nodular calcific foci of osteoid (61–81%)
√ "doughnut sign" = peripherally increased uptake with central photopenia on bone scan
DDx: aneurysmal bone cyst (no enhancing rim of viable tumor along lesion periphery)

OXALOSIS

Rare inborn error of metabolism
Etiology: excessive amounts of oxalic acid combine with calcium and deposit throughout body (kidneys, soft tissue, bone)
• hyperoxaluria = urinary excretion of oxalic acid >50 mg/day
• progressive renal failure
√ osteoporosis = cystic rarefaction + sclerotic margins in tubular bones on metaphyseal side, may extend throughout diaphysis
√ erosions on concave side of metaphysis near epiphysis (DDx: hyperparathyroidism)
√ bone-within-bone appearance of spine
√ nephrocalcinosis (2° HPT: subperiosteal resorption, rugger jersey spine, sclerotic metaphyseal bands)
Cx: pathologic fractures

PACHYDERMOPERIOSTOSIS

= OSTEODERMOPATHIA HYPERTROPHICANS (TOURAINE-SOLENTE-GOLE) = PRIMARY HYPERTROPHIC OSTEOARTHROPATHY
Autosomal dominant
Age: 3–38 years with progression into late 20s / 30s; M >> F
• large skin folds of face + scalp
Location: epiphyses + diametaphyseal region of tubular bones; distal third of bones of legs + forearms (early); distal phalanges rarely involved
√ enlargement of paranasal sinuses

√ irregular periosteal proliferation of phalanges + distal long bones (hand + feet) beginning in epiphyseal region at tendon / ligament insertions
√ thick cortex, BUT NO narrowing of medulla
√ clubbing
√ may have acroosteolysis

Prognosis: progression ceases after several years
DDx: pulmonary osteoarthropathy, thyroid acropachy

PAGET DISEASE

= OSTEITIS DEFORMANS = multifocal chronic skeletal disease due to chronic paramyxoviral infection

Prevalence: 3% of individuals >40 years; 10% of persons >80 years; higher prevalence in northern latitudes
Age: >55 years (in 3%); >85 years (in 10%); unusual <40 years; M:F = 2:1
Histo: increased resorption + increased bone formation; newly formed bone is abnormally soft with disorganized trabecular pattern ("mosaic pattern") causing deformity

(a) ACTIVE PHASE = OSTEOLYTIC PHASE
= aggressive bone resorption with lytic lesions, replacement of hematopoietic bone marrow by fibrous connective tissue with numerous large vascular channels

(b) INACTIVE PHASE = QUIESCENT PHASE
= decreased bone turnover with skeletal sclerosis + cortical accretion + loss of excessive vascularity

(c) MIXED PATTERN (common)
= lytic + sclerotic phases usually coexist

- asymptomatic (1/5)
- fatigue
- enlarged hat size
- peripheral nerve compression
- neurologic disorders from compression of brainstem (basilar invagination)
- hearing loss, blindness, facial palsy (narrowing of neural foramina) — rare
- pain from (a) primary disease process — rare
  (b) pathologic fracture
  (c) malignant transformation
  (d) degenerative joint disease / rheumatic disorder aggravated by skeletal deformity
- local hyperthermia of overlying skin
- high-output congestive heart failure from markedly increased perfusion (rare)
- increased alkaline phosphatase (increased bone formation)
- hydroxyproline increased (increased bone resorption)
- normal serum calcium + phosphorus

Sites: usually polyostotic + asymmetric; pelvis (75%) > lumbar spine > thoracic spine > proximal femur > calvarium > scapula > distal femur > proximal tibia > proximal humerus

Sensitivity: scintigraphy + radiography (60%)
scintigraphy only (27%)
radiography only (13%)

√ thick coarse trabeculae + cortical thickening
√ cystlike areas (fat-filled marrow cavity / blood-filled sinusoids / liquefactive degeneration + necrosis of proliferating fibrous tissue)

@ Skull (involvement in 29–65%)
√ inner + outer table involved
√ diploic widening
√ osteoporosis circumscripta = well-defined lysis, most commonly in calvarium anteriorly, occasionally in long bones (destructive active stage)
√ "cotton wool" appearance = mixed lytic + blastic pattern of thickened calvarium (late stage)
√ basilar invagination with encroachment on foramen magnum
√ deossification + sclerosis in maxilla
√ sclerosis of base of skull

@ Long bones (almost invariable at end of bone; rarely in diaphysis)
√ "candle flame" / "blade of grass" lysis = advancing tip of V-shaped lytic defect in diaphysis of long bone originating in subarticular site (CHARACTERISTIC)
√ lateral curvature of femur, anterior curvature of tibia (commonly resulting in fracture)

@ Small / flat bones
√ bubbly destruction + periosteal successive layering

@ Pelvis
√ thickened trabeculae in sacrum, ilium; rarefaction in central portion of ilium
√ thickening of ileopectineal line
√ acetabular protrusion (DDx: metastatic disease not deforming) + secondary degenerative joint disease

@ Spine (upper cervical, low dorsal, midlumbar)
√ lytic / coarse trabeculations at periphery of bone
√ "picture-frame vertebra" = bone-within-bone appearance = enlarged square vertebral body with reinforced peripheral trabeculae + radiolucent inner aspect, typically in lumbar spine
√ "ivory vertebra" = blastic vertebra with increased density
√ ossification of spinal ligaments, paravertebral soft tissue, disk spaces

Bone scan:
√ usually markedly increased uptake (symptomatic lesions strikingly positive)
√ normal scan in some sclerotic burned-out lesions
√ marginal uptake in lytic lesions
√ enlargement + deformity of bones

Bone marrow scan:
√ sulfur colloid bone marrow uptake is decreased (marrow replacement by cellular fibrovascular tissue)

MR:
√ hypointense area / area of signal void on T1WI + T2WI (cortical thickening, coarse trabeculation)
√ widening of bone
√ reduction in size + signal intensity of medullary cavity (replacement of high-signal-intensity fatty marrow by increased medullary bone formation)
√ focal areas of higher signal intensity than fatty marrow (= cystlike fat-filled marrow spaces)

√ areas of decreased signal intensity within marrow on T1WI + increased intensity on T2WI (= fibrovascular tissue resembling granulation tissue)

Cx: (1) Associated neoplasia (0.7–20%)
(a) sarcomatous transformation into osteosarcoma (22–90%), fibrosarcoma / malignant fibrous histiocytoma (29–51%), chondrosarcoma (1–15%)
√ osteolysis in pelvis, femur, humerus
(b) giant cell tumor (3–10%)
√ lytic expansile lesion in skull, facial bones
(c) lymphoma, plasma cell myeloma
(2) Fracture
(a) "banana fracture" = tiny horizontal cortical infractions on convex surfaces of lower extremity long bones (lateral bowing of femur, anterior bowing of tibia);
(b) compression fractures of vertebrae (soft bone despite increased density)
(3) Extradural spinal block (bone-forming phase / compression fractures) with neurologic deficits
(4) Early-onset osteoarthritis

Rx: calcitonin, diphosphonate, mithramycin

Detection of recurrence:
(a) in 1/3 detected by bone scan
(b) in 1/3 detected by biomarkers (alkaline phosphatase, urine hydroxyproline)
(c) in 1/3 by scan + biomarkers simultaneously
√ diffuse (most common) / focal increase in tracer uptake
√ extension of uptake beyond boundaries of initial lesion

DDx: Osteosclerotic metastases, Hodgkin disease, vertebral hemangioma

PARAOSTEOARTHROPATHY

= HETEROTOPIC BONE FORMATION = ECTOPIC OSSIFICATION = MYOSITIS OSSIFICANS

Common complication following surgical manipulation, total hip replacement (62%) and chronic immobilization (spinal cord injury / neuromuscular disorders)

Mechanism: pluripotent mesenchymal cell lays down matrix for formation of heterotopic bone similar to endosteal bone

Causes: para- / quadriplegia (40–50%), myelomeningocele, poliomyelitis, severe head injury, cerebrovascular disease, CNS infections (tetanus, rabies), surgery (commonly following total hip replacement)

Evolution: calcifications seen 4–10 weeks following insult; progression for 6–14 months; trabeculations by 2–3 months; stable lamellar bone ankylosis in 5% by 12–18 months

√ largest quantity of calcifications around joints, especially hip, along fascial planes
√ disuse osteoporosis of lower extremities
√ renal calculi (elevation of serum calcium levels)

Radiographic grading system (Brooker):
0 no soft-tissue ossification
I separate small foci of ossification
II >1 cm gap between opposing bone surfaces of heterotopic ossifications
III <1 cm gap between opposing bone surfaces
IV bridging ossification

Bone scan:
√ tracer accumulation in ectopic bone
√ assessment of maturity for optimal time of surgical resection (indicated by same amount of uptake as normal bone)

Cx: Ankylosis in 5%

Rx: 1000–2000 rad within 4 days following surgical removal

PHENYLKETONURIA

High incidence of x-ray changes in phenylalanine-restricted infants:
√ metaphyseal cupping of long bones (30–50%), especially wrist
√ calcific spicules extending vertically from metaphysis into epiphyseal cartilage (DDx to rickets)
√ sclerotic metaphyseal margins
√ osteoporosis
√ delayed skeletal maturation

DDx: Homocystinuria

PHOSPHORUS POISONING

Etiology: (1) ingestion of metallic phosphorus (yellow phosphorus)
(2) treatment of rachitis or TB with phosphorized cod liver oil

Location: long tubular bones, ilium
√ multiple transverse lines (intermittent treatment with phosphorus)
√ lines disappear after some years

PIERRE ROBIN SYNDROME

May be associated with: CHD, defects of eye and ear, hydrocephalus, microcephaly
• glossoptosis
√ micrognathia = hypoplastic receding mandible
√ arched ± cleft palate
√ rib pseudarthrosis

Cx: airway obstruction (relatively large tongue), aspiration

PIGMENTED VILLONODULAR SYNOVITIS

= PVNS = benign highly vascular synovial proliferation

Cause: frequent history of antecedent trauma

Histo: (1) hyperplasia of undifferentiated connective tissue with multinucleated large cells ingesting hemosiderin / lipoid (foam / giant cells)
(2) villonodular appearance of synovial membrane ± fibrosis
(3) pressure erosion / invasion of adjoining bone

Age: mainly 2nd–4th decade (range 12–68 years); 50% <40 years; M < F

- hemorrhagic "chocolate" effusion without trauma
- insidious onset of swelling, pain of long duration
- decreased range of motion, joint locking

Location: knee, ankle, hip, elbow, shoulder, tarsal + carpal joints; predominantly monarticular (DDx: degenerative arthritis)

√ soft-tissue swelling around joint (effusion + synovial proliferation)
√ dense soft-tissues (hemosiderin deposits)
√ subchondral pressure erosion at margins of joint
√ multiple sites of deossification appearing as cysts
√ NO calcifications, osteoporosis, joint space narrowing (until late)

MR:
√ masses of synovial tissue in a joint with effusion
√ scalloping / truncation of prefemoral fat pad
√ predominantly low signal intensity on all sequences (due to presence of iron) is CHARACTERISTIC
√ often heterogeneous low + high signal intensity on T2WI (hemosiderin deposits in masses + para-articular fat)
DDx: hemosiderin deposits in other diseases (eg, rheumatoid arthritis)

Rx: synovectomy, arthrodesis, arthroplasty, radiation
DDx: Synovial sarcoma (solitary calcified mass outside joint); synovial hemangioma

INTRA-ARTICULAR LOCALIZED NODULAR SYNOVITIS
= synovial lining without hemosiderin

POLAND SYNDROME

May be associated with: aplasia of mamilla / breast
Autosomal recessive
√ unilateral absence of the sternocostal head of the pectoralis major muscle
√ ipsilateral syndactyly + brachydactyly
√ rib anomalies

POLIOMYELITIS

√ osteoporosis
√ soft-tissue calcification / ossification
√ intervertebral disk calcification
√ rib erosion commonly on superior margin of 3rd + 4th rib (secondary to pressure from scapula)
√ "bamboo" spine (resembling ankylosing spondylitis)
√ sacroiliac joint narrowing

POPLITEAL CYST

= BAKER CYST = synovial cyst in the posterior aspect of knee joint communicating with posterior joint capsule

Prevalence: 19% in general orthopedic patients, 61% in patients with rheumatoid arthritis

Pathophysiology:
formed by escape of synovial effusion into one of the bursae; fluid trapped by one-way valvular mechanism
(a) Bunsen-type valve = expanding cyst compresses the communicating channel
(b) ball-type valve = ball composed of fibrin + cellular debris plugs the communication channel

Etiology: (1) arthritis (rheumatoid arthritis most common)
(2) internal derangement (meniscal / anterior cruciate ligament tears)
(3) pigmented villonodular synovitis

- pseudothrombophlebitis syndrome (= pain + swelling in calf)
- cellulitis (after leakage / rupture)

Location: (a) gastrocnemio-semimembranous bursa = posterior to gastrocnemius muscle at level of medial condyle
(b) supralateral bursa = between lateral head of gastrocnemius muscle + distal end of biceps muscle superior to lateral condyle (uncommon)
(c) popliteal bursa = beneath lateral meniscus + anterior to popliteal muscle (uncommon)

√ communication with bursa (documented on arthrogram)
√ hypointense collection on T1WI + hyperintense on T2WI

Types:
1. Intact cyst
√ smooth contour
2. Dissected cyst
√ smooth contour extending along fascial planes (usually between gastrocnemius + soleus)
3. Ruptured cyst
√ leakage into calf tissues

DDx of other synovial cysts about the knee:
(1) Meniscal cyst (at lateral / medial side of joint line; associated with horizontal cleavage tears)
(2) Tibiofibular cyst (at proximal tibiofibular joint which communicates with knee joint in 10%)
(3) Cruciate cyst (surrounding anterior / posterior cruciate ligaments following ligamentous injury)

PROGERIA

= HUTCHINSON-GILFORD SYNDROME
= autosomal recessive inheritance; most commonly in populations with consanguineous marriages (Japanese, Jewish)

Age: shortly after adolescence; M:F = 1:1

Characteristic habitus + stature:
- symmetric retardation of growth
- absent adolescent growth spurt
- dwarf with short stature + light body weight
- spindly extremities with stocky trunk
- beak-shaped nose + shallow orbits

Premature senescence:
- birdlike appearance
- graying of hair + premature baldness
- hyperpigmentation
- voice alteration
- diffuse arteriosclerosis
- bilateral cataracts
- osteoporosis

Scleroderma-like skin changes:
- atrophic skin + muscles
- circumscribed hyperkeratosis
- telangiectasia
- tight skin
- cutaneous ulcerations

- localized soft-tissue calcifications

Endocrine abnormalities:
- diabetes
- hypogonadism

√ generalized osteoporosis

@ Skull
- √ thin cranial vault
- √ delayed sutural closure + wormian bones
- √ hypoplastic facial bones (maxilla + mandible)

@ Chest
- √ narrow thorax + slender ribs
- √ progressive resorption with fibrous replacement of outer portions of thinned clavicles (HALLMARK)
- √ coronary artery + heart valve calcifications with cardiac enlargement

@ Extremities & joints
- √ short + slender long bones
- √ coxa valga
- √ valgus of humeral head
- √ acroosteolysis of terminal phalanges (occasionally)
- √ flexion + extension deformities of toes (hallux valgus, pes planus)
- √ excessive degenerative joint disease of major + peripheral joints
- √ neurotrophic joint lesions (feet)
- √ widespread osteomyelitis + septic arthritis (hands, feet, limbs)

@ Soft tissue
- √ soft-tissue atrophy of extremities
- √ soft-tissue calcifications around bony prominences (ankle, wrist, elbow, knee)
- √ peripheral vascular calcifications = premature atherosclerosis

Prognosis: most patients die in their 30s / 40s from complications of arteriosclerosis (myocardial infarction, stroke) or neoplasm (sarcoma, meningioma, thyroid carcinoma)

DDx: Cockayne syndrome (mental retardation, retinal atrophy, deafness, family history)

PSEUDOACHONDROPLASIA

- normal face + head

√ limb shortening
√ irregular epiphyses
√ scoliosis
√ coxa vara
√ marked shortening of bones in hands + feet

PSEUDOFRACTURES

= LOOSER LINES = LOOSER ZONES = OSTEOID SEAMS = MILKMAN SYNDROME = insufficiency stress fractures + nonunion (incomplete healing due to mineral deficiency)

Path: area of unmineralized woven bone occurring at sites of mechanical stress / nutrient vessel entry

Associated with:
(1) Osteomalacia / rickets (2) Paget disease ("banana fracture") (3) Osteogenesis imperfecta tarda (4) Fibrous dysplasia (5) Organic renal disease in 1% (6) Renal tubular dysfunction (7) Congenital hypophosphatasia (8) Congenital hyperphosphatasia ("juvenile Paget disease") (9) Vitamin D malabsorption / deficiency (10) Neurofibromatosis

mnemonic: "POOF"
Paget disease
Osteomalacia
Osteogenesis imperfecta
Fibrous dysplasia

Common locations:
scapulae (axillary margin, lateral + superior margin), medial femoral neck + shaft, pubic + ischial rami, ribs, lesser trochanter, ischial tuberosity, proximal 1/3 of ulna, distal 1/3 of radius, phalanges, metatarsals, metacarpals, clavicle

√ typically bilateral + symmetric at right angles to bone margin
√ paralleled by marginal sclerosis in later stages
√ healing fracture with little or no callus response
√ 2–3 mm stripe of lucency at right angle to cortex (= osteoid seams formed within stress-induced infractions (PATHOGNOMONIC) + nonunion (= incomplete healing due to mineral deficiency)

PSEUDOHYPOPARATHYROIDISM

= PHypoPT = congenital X-linked dominant abnormality with renal + skeletal resistance to PTH due to (1) end organ resistance (2) presence of antienzymes (3) defective hormone

May be associated with: hyperparathyroidism due to hypocalcemia; F > M

- short obese stature
- mental retardation
- corneal + lenticular opacity
- abnormal dentition (hypoplasia, delayed eruption, excessive caries)
- hypocalcemia + hyperphosphatemia (resistant to PTH injection)

	PHypoPT	PPHypoPT
√ calcification of basal ganglia	44%	8%
√ soft-tissue calcifications	55%	40%
√ metacarpal shortening (4 + 5 always involved)	75%	90%
√ metatarsal shortening (3 + 4 involved)	70%	99%

• normal levels of PTH
√ brachydactyly in bones in which epiphysis appears latest (metacarpal, metatarsal bones I, IV, V) (75%)
√ accelerated epiphyseal maturation resulting in dwarfism + coxa vara / valga
√ multiple diaphyseal exostoses (occasionally)
√ calcification of basal ganglia + dentate nucleus
√ calcification / ossification of skin + subcutaneous tissue

PSEUDOPSEUDOHYPOPARATHYROIDISM

= PPHypoPT = different expression of same familial disturbance with identical clinical + radiographic features as pseudohypoparathyroidism
• short stature, round facies
• NO blood chemical changes (normal calcium + phosphorus)
• normal response to injection of PTH
√ brachydactyly

PSORIATIC ARTHRITIS

Uncommon disease involving synovium + ligamentous attachments with propensity for sacroiliitis / spondylitis classified as seronegative spondyloarthropathy 6/c

Incidence: <5% of patients with psoriasis (peripheral arthritis in 5%, sacroiliitis in 29%, peripheral arthritis + sacroiliitis in 10%)

Path: synovial inflammation (less prominent than in rheumatoid arthritis) with early fibrosis of proliferative synovium; bony proliferation at joint margins / tendon insertions / subperiosteum

Types:
(1) true psoriatic arthritis (31%)
(2) psoriatic arthritis resembling rheumatoid arthritis (38%)
(3) concomitant rheumatoid + psoriatic arthritis (31%)

• skin rash precedes / develops simultaneously with onset of arthritis in 85%
◊ Arthritis antedates dermatological changes by an interval of up to 20 years!
• pitting, discoloration, hyperkeratosis, subungual separation, ridging of nails (in 80%)
• positive HLA-B27 in 80%
• negative rheumatoid factor

Location: widely variable distribution + asymmetry with involvement of lower + upper extremities
distinctive pattern: terminal interphalangeal joints, ray distribution, unilateral polyarticular asymmetrical distribution

√ NO / minimal juxtaarticular osteoporosis (early stage); frequent osteoporosis (later stages)
√ periosteal reaction frequent

@ Hand + foot
Target area: DIP, PIP, MCP
√ "sausage digit" = soft-tissue swelling of entire digit
√ asymmetrical destruction of distal interphalangeal joints (erosive polyarthritis) + osseous resorption
√ bony ankylosis (10%)
√ "pencil-in-cup" deformity = erosions with ill-defined margins + adjacent proliferation at periosteal new bone (CHARACTERISTIC)
√ ivory phalanx = sclerosis of terminal phalanx (28%)
√ destruction of interphalangeal joint of 1st toe with exuberant periosteal reaction + bony proliferation at distal phalangeal base (PATHOGNOMONIC)
√ poorly defined diffuse new bone formation at attachment of Achilles tendon + plantar aponeurosis
√ erosions at superior / posterior margin of calcaneus (20%)
√ acroosteolysis (occasionally)

@ Axial skeleton
√ "floating" osteophyte = large bulky vertically oriented asymmetrical paravertebral soft-tissue calcification involving the disk annulus (not endplates), separate from edges of vertebrae
Location: lower cervical, thoracic, upper lumbar spine
√ squaring of vertebrae in lumbar region
√ sacroiliitis (40%) = asymmetrical / unilateral sacroiliac joint widening, increased density, fusion
√ apophyseal joint narrowing + sclerosis
√ atlantoaxial subluxation + odontoid abnormalities

DDx: (1) Reiter syndrome (affects only lower extremity)
(2) Rheumatoid arthritis (bilaterally symmetric well-defined erosions, juxtaarticular osteoporosis)

PYKNODYSOSTOSIS

= autosomal recessive disease; probably variant of cleidocranial dysostosis

Age: children; M:F = 2:1
• dwarfism (resembling osteopetrosis)
• mental retardation (10%)
• widened hands + feet
• dystrophic nails
• yellowish discoloration of teeth
• characteristic facies (beaked nose, receding jaw)
√ brachycephaly + platybasia
√ wide cranial sutures, wormian bones
√ thick skull base
√ hypoplasia of mandible + obtuse mandibular angle
√ hypoplasia + nonpneumatization of paranasal sinuses
√ nonsegmentation of C1/2 and L5/S1
√ generalized increased density of long bones with thickened cortices
√ clavicular dysplasia
√ hypoplastic tapered terminal tufts
√ multiple spontaneous fractures

DDx: (1) Osteopetrosis (no mandibular / skull abnormality, no phalangeal hypoplasia, no transverse metaphyseal bands, anemia, Erlenmeyer flask deformity; "bone-within-bone" appearance)
(2) Cleidocranial dysostosis (no dense bones / terminal phalangeal hypoplasia, short stature)

RADIATION INJURY TO BONE

Pathogenesis: vascular compromise with obliterative endarteritis + periarteritis followed by damage to osteoblasts with decreased matrix production (growing bone + periosteal new bone most sensitive)

Dose effects:
- >300 rad: microscopic changes
- >400 rad: growth retardation
- <600–1200 rad: histological recovery retained
- >1200 rad: pronounced cellular damage to chondrocytes; bone marrow atrophy + cartilage degeneration after >6 months; vascular fibrosis

A. BONE GROWTH DISTURBANCE
- √ growth plate widening in 1–2 months, often returning to normal by 6 months
- √ joint space widening after 8–10 months
- √ metaphyseal bowing
- √ ricketlike irregularity + fraying of metaphysis
- √ abnormal tubulation + premature fusion of physis

B. RADIATION OSTEITIS
= bone mottling due to osteopenia + coarse trabeculation + focally increased bone density
- √ osteopenia about 1 year after radiation
- √ periostitis
- √ increased fragility with sclerosis (= insufficiency fx)
- √ avascular necrosis
- √ osteoradionecrosis

MR:
- √ increased intensity of spinal bone marrow on T1WI + T2WI corresponding to radiation port (fatty infiltration)

DDx: recurrent malignancy, radiation-induced sarcoma, infection

C. BENIGN NEOPLASM
Most likely in patients <2 years of age at treatment; with doses of 1600–6425 rads
Latent period: 1.5–14 years
1. Exostosis = Osteochondroma
2. Osteoblastoma

D. MALIGNANT NEOPLASM
= RADIATION-INDUCED SARCOMA
Latency period: 3–55 (average of 11–14) years
Minimum dose: 1,660–3,000 rad
Criteria: (a) malignancy occurring within irradiated field
(b) latency period of >5 years
(c) histologic proof of sarcoma
(d) microscopic evidence of altered histology of the original lesion

Histo: 1. Osteosarcoma (90%) = 4–11% of all osteogenic sarcomas
2. Fibrosarcoma > chondrosarcoma > malignant fibrous histiocytoma
- • pain, soft-tissue mass, rapid progression of lesion

REFLEX SYMPATHETIC DYSTROPHY

= CAUSALGIA = SHOULDER-HAND SYNDROME = POSTTRAUMATIC OSTEOPOROSIS = SUDECK DYSTROPHY
= serious + potentially disabling condition with poorly understood origin + cause

Etiology:
(1) Trauma in >50% (fracture, frostbite; may be trivial)
◊ affects 0.01% of all trauma patients
(2) Idiopathic in 27% (immobilization, infection)
(3) Myocardial ischemia in 6%
(4) CNS disorders in 6%
◊ affects 12–21% of patients with hemiplegia
(5) Discogenic disease in 5%

- • burning pain, tenderness, allodynia, hyperpathia
- • soft-tissue swelling ± pitting edema out of proportion to degree of injury
- • dystrophic skin + nail changes
- • sudomotor changes: hyperhidrosis + hypertrichosis
- • vasomotor instability (Raynaud phenomenon, local vasoconstriction / -dilatation)
- • end-stage (after 6–12 months): contractures, atrophy of skin + soft tissues

Location: hands and feet distal to injury
- √ periarticular soft-tissue swelling
- √ patchy osteopenia (50%) as early as 2–3 weeks after onsets of symptoms (DDx: disuse osteopenia)
- √ generalized osteopenia = ground-glass appearance (endosteal + intracortical excavation; subperiosteal bone resorption; lysis of juxta-articular + subchondral bone)

NUC (3-phase bone scan):
- √ increased flow + increased blood pool + increase in periarticular uptake on delayed images in affected part (60%)
- √ diminished flow / delayed uptake (15–20%)

Rx: sympathetic block, a-/b-adrenergic blocking agents, nonsteroidal anti-inflammatory drugs, radiation therapy, hypnosis, acupuncture, acupressure, transcutaneous nerve stimulation, physiotherapy, calcitonin, corticosteroids, early mobilization

REITER SYNDROME

= triad of (1) arthritis (2) uveitis (3) urethritis; 98% male

Types:
(1) endemic (venereal)
(2) epidemic (postdysenteric)

- • Hx of sexual exposure / diarrhea 3–11 days before onset of urethritis
- • mucocutaneous lesions (keratosis blennorrhagia, balanitis circinata sicca)
- • uveitis, conjunctivitis
- • positive HLA-B27 in 76%

Location: asymmetric mono- / pauciarticular
- √ polyarthritis
- √ articular soft-tissue swelling + joint space narrowing in 50% (particularly knees, ankles, feet)
- √ widening + inflammation of Achilles + patella tendons
- √ "fluffy" periosteal reaction (DISTINCTIVE) at metatarsal necks, proximal phalanges, calcaneal spur, tibia + fibula at ankle and knee
- √ juxta-articular osteoporosis (rare in acute stage)

CHRONIC CHANGES
- recurrent joint attacks in a few cases
- √ calcaneal spur at insertion of plantar fascia + Achilles tendon
- √ periarticular deossification
- √ marginal erosions, loss of joint space
- √ bilateral sacroiliac changes indistinguishable from ankylosing / psoriatic spondylitis
- √ isolated osteophyte usually in thoracolumbar area, separated from vertebral body

Cx: gastric ulcer + hemorrhage; aortic incompetence; heart block; amyloidosis

RELAPSING POLYCHONDRITIS

= generalized recurring inflammation + destruction of cartilage in joints, ears, nose, larynx, airways

Etiology: acquired metabolic disorder (? abnormal acid mucopolysaccharide metabolism / hypersensitivity / altered immunity

Histo: loss of cytoplasm in chondrocytes; plasma cell + lymphocyte infiltration

- saddle-nose deformity
- swollen + tender ears, cauliflower ears
- hearing loss (obstruction of external auditory meatus)
- cough, hoarseness, dyspnea (collapse of trachea)
- arthralgia

@ Head
- √ calcification of pinna of ear

@ Chest
- √ ectasia + collapsibility with narrowing of trachea and mainstem bronchi
- √ generalized + localized emphysema
- √ aortic aneurysm (10%), mostly in ascending aorta, may be multiple / dissecting
- √ costochondritis

@ Bone
- √ periarticular osteoporosis
- √ erosive changes in carpal bones resembling rheumatoid arthritis
- √ soft-tissue swelling around joints + styloid process of ulna
- √ erosive irregularities in sacroiliac joints
- √ disk space erosion + increased density of articular plates

Rx: corticosteroids

RENAL OSTEODYSTROPHY

= constellation of musculoskeletal abnormalities that occur with chronic renal failure as a combination of
(a) osteomalacia (adults) / rickets (children)
(b) 2° HPT with osteitis cystica fibrosa + soft-tissue calcifications
(c) osteosclerosis (d) soft-tissue + vascular calcifications

Classification:
(1) Glomerular form = acquired renal disease: chronic glomerulonephritis (common)
(2) Tubular form = congenital renal osteodystrophy:
1. Vitamin D–resistant rickets = hypophosphatemic rickets
2. Fanconi syndrome = impaired resorption of glucose, phosphate, amino acids, bicarbonate, uric acid, sodium, water
3. Renal tubular acidosis

Pathogenesis:
(a) Renal insufficiency causes a decrease in vitamin D conversion into the active $1,25(OH)_2D_3$ (done by 25-OH-D-1-a hydroxylase, which is exclusive to renal tissue mitochondria); vitamin D deficiency slows intestinal calcium absorption; *vitamin D resistance predominates* and calcium levels stay low (Ca x P product remains almost normal secondary to hyperphosphatemia); low calcium levels lead to OSTEOMALACIA; additional factors responsible for osteomalacia are inhibitors to calcification produced in the uremic state, aluminium toxicity, dysfunction of hepatic enzyme system
(b) Renal insufficiency with diminished filtration results in phosphate retention; maintenance of Ca x P product lowers serum calcium directly, which in turn increases PTH production (2° HPT); *2° HPT predominates* associated with mild vitamin D resistance and leads to an increase in Ca x P product with SOFT-TISSUE CALCIFICATION in kidney, lung, joints, bursae, blood vessels, heart as well as OSTEITIS FIBROSA
(c) Mixture of (a) and (b): increased serum phosphate inhibits vitamin D activation via feedback regulation

- phosphate retention
- hypocalcemia

A. OSTEOPENIA (in 0–25–83%)
= diminution in number of trabeculae + thickening of stressed trabeculae = increased trabecular pattern

Cause: combined effect of
(1) Osteomalacia (reduced bone mineralization due to acquired insensitivity to vitamin D / antivitamin D factor)
(2) Osteitis fibrosa cystica (bone resorption)
(3) Osteoporosis (decrease in bone quantity)
Contributing factors:
chronic metabolic acidosis, poor nutritional status, pre- and posttransplantation azotemia, use of steroids, hyperparathyroidism, low vitamin D levels

Cx: fracture predisposition (lessened structural strength) with minor trauma / spontaneously; fracture prevalence increases with duration of hemodialysis + remains unchanged after renal transplantation

Site: vertebral body (3–25%), pubic ramus, rib (5–25%)
- √ Milkman fracture / Looser zones (in 1%)
- √ metaphyseal fractures

Prognosis: osteopenia may remain unchanged / worsen after renal transplantation + during hemodialysis

B. RICKETS (children)

Cause: in CRF normal vessels fail to develop orderly along cartilage columns in zone of provisional calcification; this results in disorganized proliferation of the zone of maturing + hypertrophying cartilage and disturbed endochondral calcification

Location: most apparent in areas of rapid growth such as knee joints

√ diffuse bone demineralization
√ widening of growth plate
√ irregular zone of provisional calcification
√ metaphyseal cupping + fraying
√ bowing of long bones, scoliosis
√ diffuse concave impression at multiple vertebral endplates, basilar invagination
√ slipped epiphysis (10%): capital femoral, proximal humerus, distal femur, distal radius, heads of metacarpals + metatarsals
√ general delay in bone age

C. SECONDARY HPT (in 6–66%)

Cause: inability of kidneys to adequately excrete phosphate leads to hyperplasia of parathyroid chief cells (2° HPT); excess PTH affects the development of osteoclasts, osteoblasts, osteocytes

• hyperphosphatemia
• hypocalcemia
• increased PTH levels

√ subperiosteal, cortical, subchondral, trabecular, endosteal, subligamentous bone resorption
√ osteoclastoma = brown tumor = osteitis fibrosa cystica in 1.5–1.7% (due to PTH-stimulated osteoclastic activity; more common in 1° HPT)
√ periosteal new-bone formation (8–25%)
√ chondrocalcinosis (more common in 1° HPT)

D. OSTEOSCLEROSIS (9–34%)

One of the most common radiologic manifestations; most commonly with chronic glomerulonephritis; may be the sole manifestation of renal osteodystrophy

√ diffuse chalky density: thoracolumbar spine in 60% (rugger jersey spine); also in pelvis, ribs, long bones, facial bones, base of skull (children)

Prognosis: may increase / regress after renal transplantation

E. SOFT-TISSUE CALCIFICATIONS

(a) metastatic secondary to hyperphosphatemia (solubility product for calcium + phosphate [Ca^{2+} x PO_4^{-2}] exceeds 60–75 mg/dL in extracellular fluid), hypercalcemia, alkalosis with precipitation of calcium salts

(b) dystrophic secondary to local tissue injury

Location:

(a) arterial (27–83%): in medial + intimal elastic tissue

Location: dorsal pedis a., forearm, hand, wrist, leg

√ pipestem appearance without prominent luminal involvement

(b) periarticular (0–52%): multifocal, frequently symmetric, may extend into adjacent joint

• chalky fluid / pastelike material
• inflammatory response in surrounding tenosynovial tissue

√ discrete cloudlike dense areas
√ fluid-fluid level in tumoral calcinosis

Prognosis: often regresses with treatment

(c) visceral (79%): heart, lung, stomach, kidney

√ fluffy amorphous "tumoral" calcification

Rx:
1. Decrease of phosphorus absorption in bowel (in hyperphosphatemia)
2. Vitamin D_3 administration (if vitamin D resistance predominates)
3. Parathyroidectomy for 3° HPT (= autonomous HPT)

Congenital Renal Osteodystrophy

Vitamin D–resistant rickets

= PHOSPHATE DIABETES = PRIMARY HYPOPHOSPHATEMIA = FAMILIAL HYPOPHOSPHATEMIC RICKETS

= rare X-linked dominant disorder of renal tubular reabsorption characterized by

(1) impaired resorption of phosphate in proximal renal tubule (due to defect in renal brush-border membrane)

(2) inappropriately low synthesis of 1,25 dihydroxyvitamin D_3 [$1,25(OH)_2D_3$] in renal tubules resulting in decreased intestinal resorption of calcium + phosphate

Age: <1 year

• hypophosphatemia + hyperphosphaturia
• elevated serum alkaline phosphatase
• normal plasma + urine calcium
• normal / low serum $1,25(OH)_2D_3$

√ classic rachitic changes
√ skeletal deformity, particularly bowed legs
√ retarded bone age; dwarfism if untreated
√ osteosclerosis / bone thickening (from overabundance of incompletely calcified matrix)

Rx: phosphate infusion + large doses of vitamin D

DDx: vitamin-D–deficient and –dependent rickets (absence of muscle weakness + seizures + tetany)

Fanconi syndrome

Triad of

(1) hyperphosphaturia
(2) amino aciduria
(3) renal glucosuria (normal blood glucose)

Etiology: renal tubular defect

√ rickets, osteomalacia, osteitis fibrosa, osteosclerosis

Prognosis: functional renal impairment likely when bone changes occur

Rx: large doses of vitamin D + alkalinization

Renal Tubular Acidosis

- systemic acidosis, bone lesions

√ rickets, osteomalacia, pseudofractures, nephrocalcinosis, osteitis fibrosa (rare)

(a) Lightwood syndrome = salt-losing nephritis (self-limited form)
- NO nephrocalcinosis

(b) Butler-Albright syndrome (severe form)
- nephrocalcinosis

RHEUMATOID ARTHRITIS

= generalized connective tissue disease
= Type III hypersensitivity = delayed hypersensitivity
= immune complex disease (= formation of antigen-antibody complexes with complement fixation)

Cause: genetic predisposition; ? reaction to antigen from Epstein-Barr virus / certain strains of E. coli
Age: highest incidence 40–50 years; M:F = 1:3 if <40 years; M:F = 1:1 if >40 years
Pathogenesis: injury to synovial endothelial cells; synovitis with synovial hypertrophy leads to impaired nutrition with chondronecrosis, joint narrowing, subluxation, and ankylosis

Diagnostic criteria of American Rheumatism Association (at least 4 criteria should be present):
(1) morning stiffness for ≥1 hour
(2) swelling of ≥3 joints, particularly of wrist, metatarsophalangeal or proximal interphalangeal joints for >6 weeks
(3) symmetric swelling
(4) typical radiographic changes
(5) rheumatoid nodules
(6) positive rheumatoid factor

- morning stiffness
- fatigue, weight loss, anemia
- carpal tunnel syndrome
- rheumatoid factor (positive in 85–94%) = IgM-antibody = agglutination of sensitized sheep RBCs closely correlating with disease severity;
  false positive: normal (5%), asbestos workers with fibrosing alveolitis (25%), viral / bacterial / parasitic infection, other inflammatory diseases
- antinuclear antibodies (positive in many)
- LE cells (positive in some)
- positive latex flocculation test
- hormonal influence:
  (a) decrease in activity during pregnancy
  (b) men with RA have low testosterone levels

Location: symmetric involvement of diarthrodial joints
Target areas:
all five MCP, PIP, interphalangeal joint of thumb, all wrist compartments (especially radiocarpal, inferior radioulnar, pisiform-triquetral joints); medial aspect of MTP + interphalangeal joints of foot (esp. great toe); earliest changes seen in 2nd + 3rd MCP, 3rd PIP

EARLY SIGNS:
√ fusiform periarticular soft-tissue swelling (result of effusion)
√ regional osteoporosis (disuse + local hyperthermia)
√ widened joint space
√ marginal + central bone erosions (less common in large joints); site of first erosion is classically base of proximal phalanx of 4th finger
√ changes in the ulnar styloid + distal radioulnar joint
√ atlantoaxial subluxation >2.5 mm (in >6%)
√ giant synovial cyst

LATE SIGNS:
√ diffuse loss of interosseous space
√ flexion + extension contractures with ulnar subluxation + dislocation
√ marked destruction + fractures of joint space
√ extensive destruction of bone ends
√ bony fusion
√ elevation of humeral heads (tear / atrophy of rotator cuff)
√ resorption of distal clavicle
√ erosion of superior margins of posterior portions of ribs 3–5
√ destruction + narrowing of disk spaces + irregular vertebral body outlines + absence of osteophytosis
√ destruction of zygapophyseal joints without osteophyte formation
√ resorption of spinous processes
√ "stepladder appearance" of cervical spine due to subaxial subluxations
√ protrusio acetabuli (from osteoporosis)
√ synovial herniation + cysts (eg, popliteal cyst)
√ calcaneal plantar spur

DDx: SLE, psoriatic arthritis, seronegative spondylarthropathies

EXTRA-ARTICULAR MANIFESTATIONS (76%)
(a) **Felty syndrome** (<1%)
= rheumatoid arthritis (present for >10 years) + splenomegaly + neutropenia
Age: 40–70 years; F > M; rare in Blacks
- rapid weight loss
- therapy refractory leg ulcers
- brown pigmentation over exposed surfaces of extremities

(b) Sjögren syndrome (15%)
= keratoconjunctivitis + xerostomia + rheumatoid arthritis

(c) Pulmonary manifestations
√ pleural effusion, mostly unilateral, without change for months, usually not associated with parenchymal disease
√ interstitial fibrosis with lower lobe predominance
√ rheumatoid nodules (30%): well-circumscribed, peripheral, with frequent cavitation
√ Caplan syndrome (= hyperimmune reactivity to silica inhalation with rapidly developing multiple pulmonary nodules)
√ pulmonary hypertension secondary to arteritis

(d) Subcutaneous nodules
(in 5–35% with active arthritis) over extensor surfaces of forearm + other pressure points (eg, olecranon) without calcifications (DDx to gout)

(e) Cardiovascular involvement
1. Pericarditis (20–50%)
2. Myocarditis (arrhythmia, heart block)
3. Aortitis (5%) of ascending aorta ± aortic valve insufficiency

(f) Rheumatoid vasculitis
Mimics periarteritis nodosa
• polyneuropathy, cutaneous ulceration, gangrene, polymyopathy, myocardial / visceral infarction

(g) Neurologic sequelae
1. Distal neuropathy (related to vasculitis)
2. Nerve entrapment (atlantoaxial subluxation, carpal tunnel syndrome, Baker cyst)

(h) Lymphadenopathy (up to 25%)
√ splenomegaly (1–5%)

Cystic Rheumatoid Arthritis

= intraosseous cystic lesions as dominant feature

Pathogenesis: increased pressure in synovial space from joint effusion decompresses through microfractures of weakened marginal cortex into subarticular bone

◊ increase in size + extent of cysts correlates with increased level of activity + absence of synovial cysts

Age: as above; M:F = 1:1

• seronegative in 50%

√ juxta-articular subcortical lytic lesions with well-defined sclerotic margins

√ relative lack of cartilage loss, osteoporosis, joint disruption

DDx: gout (presence of urate crystals), pigmented villonodular synovitis (monarticular)

Juvenile Rheumatoid Arthritis

= rheumatoid arthritis in patients <16 years of age; M < F

Classification:

(1) <u>Juvenile-onset adult type</u> (10%)
• IgM RA factor positive; age 8–9; poor prognosis
√ erosive changes; perfuse periosteal reaction; hip disease with protrusio

(2) <u>Polyarthritis of the ankylosing spondylitic type</u>
• iridocyclitis; boys age 9–11 years
√ peripheral arthritis; fusion of greater trochanter; complete fusion of both hips; heel spur

(3) **Still disease**
(a) systemic
(b) polyarticular
(c) pauciarticular + iridocyclitis (30%)
• fever, rash, lymphadenopathy, hepatosplenomegaly; pericarditis, dwarfism
• fatal kidney disease in 20%

Age: 2–4 and 8–11 years of age; M < F

Location: involvement of carpometacarpal joints ("squashed carpi" in adulthood), hind foot, hip (40–50%)

√ periosteal reaction of phalanges; broadening of bones; accelerated bone maturation + early fusion (stunting of growth)

• morning stiffness, arthralgia
• subcutaneous nodules (10%)
• skin rash (50%)
• fever, lymphadenopathy

Location: early involvement of large joints (hips, knees, ankles, wrists, elbows); later of hands + feet

√ radiologic signs similar to rheumatoid arthritis (except for involvement of large joints first, late onset of bony changes, more ankylosis, wide metaphyses)
√ periarticular soft-tissue swelling
√ thinning of joint cartilage
√ large cystlike lesions removed from articular surface (invasion of bone by inflammatory pannus); rare in children
√ articular erosions at ligamentous + tendinous insertion sites
√ joint destruction may resemble neuropathic joints
√ juxta-articular osteoporosis
√ "balloon epiphyses" + "gracile bones" (epiphyseal overgrowth + early fusion with bone shortening secondary to hyperemia)

@ Hand / foot
√ "rectangular" phalanges (periostitis + cortical thickening)
√ ankylosis in carpal joints

@ Axial skeleton
√ ankylosis of cervical spine (apophyseal joints), sacroiliac joints
√ subluxation of atlantoaxial joint (66%)
√ thoracic spinal compression fractures

@ Chest
√ ribbon ribs
√ pleural + pericardial effusions
√ interstitial pulmonary lesions (simulating scleroderma, dermatomyositis)
√ solitary pulmonary nodules, may cavitate

Prognosis: complete recovery (30%); secondary amyloidosis

RICKETS

= osteomalacia during enchondral bone growth

Age: 4–18 months

Histo: zone of preparatory calcification does not form, heap up of maturing cartilage cells; failure of osteoid mineralization also in shafts so that osteoid production elevates periosteum

• irritability, bone pain, tenderness
• craniotabes
• rachitic rosary
• bowed legs
• delayed dentition
• swelling of wrists + ankles

Location: metaphyses of long bones subjected to stress are particularly involved (wrists, ankles, knees)

√ poorly mineralized epiphyseal centers with delayed appearance
√ irregular widened epiphyseal plates (increased osteoid)
√ increase in distance between end of shaft and epiphyseal center
√ cupping + fraying of metaphysis with threadlike shadows into epiphyseal cartilage (weight-bearing bones)
√ cortical spurs projecting at right angles to metaphysis
√ coarse trabeculation (NO ground-glass pattern as in scurvy)
√ periosteal reaction may be present
√ deformities common (bowing of soft diaphysis, molding of epiphysis, fractures)
√ bowing of long bones
√ frontal bossing

mnemonic: "RICKETS"
Reaction of periosteum may occur
Indistinct cortex
Coarse trabeculation
Knees + wrists + ankles mainly affected
Epiphyseal plates widened + irregular
Tremendous metaphysis (fraying, splaying, cupping)
Spur (metaphyseal)

Causes Of Rickets

I. *ABNORMALITY IN VITAMIN D METABOLISM*
Associated with reactive hyperparathyroidism
- A. VITAMIN D DEFICIENCY
  - (a) Dietary lack of vitamin D = famine osteomalacia
  - (b) Lack of sunshine exposure
  - (c) Malabsorption of vitamin D = gastroenterogenous rickets
    1. pancreatitis + biliary tract disease
    2. steatorrhea, celiac disease, postgastrectomy
    3. inflammatory bowel disease
- B. DEFECTIVE CONVERSION OF VITAMIN D TO 25-OH-CHOLECALCIFEROL IN LIVER
  1. Liver disease
  2. Anticonvulsant drug therapy (= induction of hepatic enzymes that accelerate degradation of biologically active vitamin D metabolites)
- C. DEFECTIVE CONVERSION OF 25-OH-D3 TO 1,25-OH-D3 IN KIDNEY
  1. Chronic renal failure = renal osteodystrophy
  2. Vitamin D–dependent rickets = autosomal recessive enzyme defect of 1-OHase

II. *ABNORMALITY IN PHOSPHATE METABOLISM*
not associated with hyperparathyroidism secondary to normal serum calcium
- A. PHOSPHATE DEFICIENCY
  1. Intestinal malabsorption of phosphates
  2. Ingestion of aluminum salts [$Al(OH)_2$] forming insoluble complexes with phosphate
  3. Low phosphate feeding in prematurely born infants
  4. Severe malabsorption state
  5. Parenteral hyperalimentation
- B. DISORDERS OF RENAL TUBULAR REABSORPTION OF PHOSPHATE
  1. Renal tubular acidosis (renal loss of alkali)
  2. deToni-Debré-Fanconi syndrome = hypophosphatemia, glucosuria, aminoaciduria
  3. Vitamin D–resistant rickets
  4. Cystinosis
  5. Tyrosinosis
  6. Lowe syndrome
- C. HYPOPHOSPHATEMIA WITH NONENDOCRINE TUMORS
  = Oncogenic rickets = elaboration of humeral substance which inhibits tubular reabsorption of phosphates
  1. Sclerosing hemangioma
  2. Hemangiopericytoma
  3. Ossifying mesenchymal tumor
  4. Nonossifying fibroma
- D. HYPOPHOSPHATASIA

III. *CALCIUM DEFICIENCY*
1. Dietary rickets = milk-free diet (extremely rare)
2. Malabsorption
3. Consumption of substances forming chelates with calcium

Classification Of Rickets

I. Primary vitamin D–deficiency rickets
II. Gastrointestinal malabsorption
- A. Partial gastrectomy
- B. Small intestinal disease: gluten-sensitive enteropathy / regional enteritis
- C. Hepatobiliary disease: chronic biliary obstruction / biliary cirrhosis
- D. Pancreatic disease: chronic pancreatitis

III. Primary hypophosphatemia; vitamin D–deficiency rickets
IV. Renal disease
- A. Chronic renal failure
- B. Renal tubular disorders: renal tubular acidosis
- C. Multiple renal defects

V. Hypophosphatasia + pseudohypophosphatasia
VI. Fibrogenesis imperfecta osseum
VII. Axial osteomalacia
VIII. Miscellaneous
Hypoparathyroidism, hyperparathyroidism, thyrotoxicosis, osteoporosis, Paget disease, fluoride ingestion, ureterosigmoidostomy, neurofibromatosis, osteopetrosis, macroglobulinemia, malignancy

ROTATOR CUFF LESIONS

SUBACROMIAL PAIN SYNDROME
(1) Impingement syndrome
(2) Rotator cuff tendinitis
(3) Degeneration without impingement
(4) Shoulder instability with secondary impingement
(5) Instability without impingement

Impingement syndrome

= lateral shoulder pain with abduction; common cause of rotator cuff tears; NOT radiographic diagnosis

Age: lifelong process; 1st stage <25 years; 2nd stage 25–40 years; complete rotator cuff tear >40 years

Pathophysiology:
movement of humerus impinges rotator cuff tendons against coracoacromial arch resulting in microtrauma, which causes inflammation of subacromial bursa (= fibrous thickening of subacromial bursa) / rotator cuff (critical zone of rotator cuff = supraspinatus tendon 2 cm from its attachment to humerus)
◊ Impingement pathophysiology may be secondary to primary instability!

Impingement anatomy:
narrowing of subacromial space secondary to
(1) acquired degenerative subacromial osteophyte / enthesophyte from
  (a) bony outgrowth along coracoacromial ligament
  (b) acromioclavicular joint osteoarthritis
(2) congenital subacromial hook of anterior acromion (= subacromial spur)
◊ Impingement syndrome may exist without impingement anatomy!

• painful arc of motion
√ subacromial enthesophyte
√ alteration in acromial shape + orientation
√ thickening of coracoacromial ligament

Cx: (1) partial / complete tear (may be precipitated by acute traumatic event on preexisting degenerative changes)
(2) cuff tendinitis / degenerative tendinosis

Dx: Lidocaine impingement test (= subacromial lidocaine injection relieves pain)

Rx: acromioplasty (= removal of a portion of the acromion), removal of subacromial osteophytes, removal / lysis / débridement of coracoacromial ligament, resection of distal clavicle, removal of acromioclavicular joint osteophtyes

Glenohumeral instability

Glenohumeral stability is dependent on a functional anatomic unit (= anterior capsular mechanism) formed by: glenoid labrum, joint capsule, superior + middle + anteroinferior + posteroinferior glenohumeral ligaments, coracohumeral ligament, subscapularis tendon, rotator cuff

Age: <35 years

Frequency: acute, recurrent, fixed

Cause: traumatic, microtraumatic, atraumatic

Direction: anterior > multidirectional > inferior > posterior

Type of lesions:
labral abnormalities (compression, avulsion, shearing), capsular / ligamentous tear / avulsion

Associated lesions:
Hill-Sachs fracture, trough line fracture, glenoid fracture, labral cyst
◊ Normal clefts may exist within labrum!

False positive for labral separation:
(1) Articular cartilage deep to labrum
(2) Glenohumeral ligaments passing adjacent to labrum

Rotator cuff tear

Etiology: (1) Attritional change + tendon degeneration due to aging, repeated microtrauma as a result of impingement between humeral head + coracoacromial arch, overuse of shoulder from professional / athletic activities
(2) Acute trauma (rare)

Age: most commonly >50 years

Location: "critical zone" of supraspinatus tendon 1 cm medial to tendon attachment (area of relative hypovascularity)

Classification:
EXTENT OF TEAR
(a) incomplete rupture = **partial tear** involves either bursal or synovial surface or remains intratendinous
(b) complete rupture = **full-thickness** tear bridging subacromial bursa and glenohumeral joint
  — pure transverse tear
  — pure vertical / longitudinal tear
  — tear with retraction of tendon edges
  — global tear = **massive tear** / avulsion of cuff involving more than one of the tendons

TOPOGRAPHY OF TEAR
(a) extent in frontal plane: nondisplaced, minimally displaced, dramatically displaced
(b) extent in anterior direction: supraspinatus tendon + coracohumeral ligament + subscapularis tendon
(c) extent in posterior direction: supraspinatus tendon + infraspinatus + teres minor tendon

Arthrography (71–100% sensitive, 71–100% specific for combined full + partial thickness tears)
√ opacification of subacromial-subdeltoid bursa

MR (41–100% sensitive and 79–100% specific for combined full + partial thickness tears):
√ discontinuity of cuff with retraction of musculotendinous junction
√ focal / generalized intense / markedly increased signal intensity on T2WI (= fluid within cuff defect) in <50%
√ fluid within subacromial-subdeltoid bursa (MOST SENSITIVE)
√ low / moderate signal intensity on T2WI (= severely degenerated tendon, intact bursal / synovial surface, granulation / scar tissue filling the region of torn tendinous fibers)
√ cuff defect with contour irregularity
√ abrupt change in the signal character at boundary of the lesion
√ supraspinatus muscle atrophy (MOST SPECIFIC)

PITFALLS:
- √ hyperintense focus in distal supraspinatus tendon
- √ gray signal isointense to muscle on all pulse sequences
  - (a) partial volume averaging with superior + lateral infraspinatus tendon
  - (b) vascular "watershed" area
  - (c) magic angle effect = orientation of collagen fibers at 55° relative to main magnetic field
- √ hyperintense focus within rotator cuff on T2WI
  - (a) partial volume averaging with fluid in biceps tendon sheath / subscapularis bursa
  - (b) partial volume averaging with fat of peribursal fat
  - (c) motion artifacts: respiration, vascular pulsation, patient movement
- √ fatty atrophy of muscle
  - (a) impingement of axillary / suprascapular nn. = quadrilateral space syndrome

US (scans in hyperextended position, 75–100% sensitive, 43–97% specific, 65–95% negative predictive value, 55–75% positive predictive value):
- √ nonvisualization of rotator cuff (large tear), most reliable sign
  - √ deltoid muscle directly on top of humeral head
  - √ defect filled with hypoechoic thickened bursa + fat (with hypervascularity on color Doppler) between deltoid and humeral head
- √ focal nonvisualization of rotator cuff, reliable sign
  - √ "naked tuberosity sign" = retracted tendon leaves a bare area of bone
  - √ folding of bursal + peribursal fat tissue into focal defect
- √ discontinuity of rotator cuff filled with joint fluid / hypoechoic reactive tissue
- √ abrupt + sharply demarcated focal thinning
- √ small comma-shaped area of hyperechogenicity (small tear filled with granulation tissue / hypertrophied synovium)

False negative: longitudinal tear, partial tear
False positive: intraarticular biceps tendon, soft-tissue calcification, small scar / fibrous tissue

Subacromial-subdeltoid bursitis

common finding in rotator cuff tears
- √ peribursal fat totally / partially obliterated + replaced by low-signal-intensity tissue on all pulse sequences
- √ fluid accumulation within bursa

Supraspinatus tendinopathy / tendinosis

Cause: impingement, acute / chronic stress
Histo: mucinous + myxoid degeneration
- √ increase in signal intensity in tendon on proton-density images without disruption of tendon
- √ tendinous enlargement + inhomogeneous signal pattern

RUBELLA

= GERMAN MEASLES
Incidence: endemic rate of 0.1%
Age: infants (in utero transmission)
- • neonatal dwarfism (intrauterine growth retardation)
- • failure to thrive
- • retinopathy, cataracts, deafness
- • mental deficiency with encephalitis + microcephaly
- • thrombocytopenic purpura, petechiae, anemia
- √ "celery-stalk" sign (50%) = metaphyseal irregular margins + coarsened trabeculae extending longitudinally from epiphysis; distal end of femur > proximal end of tibia, humerus
- √ no periosteal reaction
- √ hepatosplenomegaly + adenopathy
- √ pneumonitis

@ Cardiovascular:
- √ congenital heart disease (PDA)
- √ peripheral pulmonary artery stenosis
- √ necrosis of myocardium

@ CNS
- √ punctate / nodular calcifications
- √ porencephalic cysts
- √ occasionally microcephaly

Prognosis: osseous manifestations disappear in 1–3 months
DDx: (1) CMV
(2) Congenital syphilis (diaphysitis + epiphysitis)
(3) Toxoplasmosis

RUBINSTEIN-TAYBI SYNDROME

= BROAD THUMB SYNDROME
= rare sporadic syndrome without known chromosomal / biochemical markers; M:F = 1:1
- • small stature
- • mental, motor, language retardation

@ Characteristic facies
- • beaked / straight nose ± low nasal septum
- • antimongoloid slant of palpebral fissures
- • epicanthic folds
- • broad fleshy nasal bridge
- • high-arched palate
- • dental abnormalities

@ Ophthalmologic findings
- • strabismus, ptosis, refractive errors

@ Cutaneous findings
- • keloids, hirsutism, simian crease
- • flat capillary hemangioma on forehead / neck

@ Musculoskeletal findings
- √ short broad "spatulate" terminal phalanges of thumb and great toe ± angulation deformity (MOST CONSISTENT + CHARACTERISTIC FINDING)
- √ radial angulation of distal phalanx (50%) caused by trapezoid / delta shape of proximal phalanx
- √ tufted "mushroom-shaped" fingers + webbing
- √ thin tubular bones of hand + feet
- √ club feet
- √ skeletal maturation retardation
- √ dysplastic ribs

√ spina bifida occulta
√ scoliosis
√ flat acetabular angle + flaring of ilia
@ Genitourinary tract anomalies
√ bilateral renal duplication
√ renal agenesis
√ bifid ureter
√ incomplete / delayed descent of testes
@ Cardiovascular abnormalities
√ atrial septal defect
√ patent ductus arteriosus
√ coarctation of aorta
√ valvular aortic stenosis
√ pulmonic stenosis
OB-US:
√ decreased head circumference
√ small for gestational age
Cx in infancy: obstipation, feeding problems, recurrent upper respiratory infection

SAPHO SYNDROME

= **S**ynovitis, **A**cne, **P**almoplantar pustulosis, **H**yperostosis, **O**steitis
= PUSTULOTIC ARTHROOSTEITIS
= STERNOCLAVICULAR HYPEROSTOSIS
= association between rheumatologic and cutaneous lesions (= seronegative spondyloarthropathy)
◊ Delay of several years can separate osseous from cutaneous lesions!
Etiology: ? variant of psoriasis
Age: young to middle-aged adults; M:F = 1:1
• palmoplantar pustulosis (52%) = chronic eruption of yellowish intradermal sterile pustules on palms + soles
• severe acne (15%) = acne fulminans, acne conglobata
• pain, soft-tissue swelling, limitation of motion at skeletal site of involvement
@ Sternoclavicular joint (70–90%)
Site: insertion of costoclavicular ligament, clavicles, manubrium sterni
√ osteolysis at beginning of disease
√ hyperostosis + osteosclerosis
√ arthritis + ankylosis of sternoclavicular joint
@ Axial skeleton (33%)
√ osteosclerosis of one / more vertebral bodies
√ disk space narrowing + endplate erosion
√ paravertebral ossifications (mimicking marginal / nonmarginal syndesmophytes / massive bridging)
√ unilateral sacroiliitis + associated osteosclerosis of adjacent iliac bone
@ Appendicular skeleton (30%)
Location: distal femur, proximal tibia, fibula, humerus, radius, ulna
Site: metaphysis
√ osteosclerosis / osteolysis + periosteal new bone formation with aggressive appearance
@ Joints
Location: knee, hip, ankle, DIP of hand
√ synovial inflammation with juxta-articular osteoporosis (early)
√ joint narrowing, marginal erosion, hyperostosis, enthesopathy (later)
Prognosis: chronic course with unpredictable exacerbations + remissions
Rx: nonsteroidal anti-inflammatory drugs, corticosteroids, analgesics, cyclosporine
DDx: infectious osteomyelitis / spondylitis, osteosarcoma, Ewing sarcoma, metastasis, Paget disease, aseptic necrosis of clavicle

SARCOIDOSIS

Osseous involvement in 6–15–20%
• unimpaired joint function, joints are rarely involved
Location: small bones of hands + feet (middle + distal phalanges)
√ reticulated "lacelike" trabecular pattern in metaphyseal ends of middle + distal phalanges, metacarpals, metatarsals
√ well-defined cystlike lesions of varying size
√ neuropathy-like destruction of terminal phalanges (DDx: scleroderma)
√ phalangeal endosteal sclerosis + periosteal new bone (infrequent)
√ vertebral involvement unusual: destructive lesions with sclerotic margin
√ diffuse sclerosis of multiple vertebral bodies
√ paravertebral soft-tissue mass (DDx: indistinguishable from tuberculosis)
√ osteolytic changes in skull

SCURVY

= BARLOW DISEASE = vitamin C deficiency with defective osteogenesis from abnormal osteoblast function
Age: 6–9 months (maternal vitamin C protects for first 6 months)
• irritability
• tenderness + weakness of lower limbs
• scorbutic rosary of ribs
• bleeding of gums (teething)
• legs drawn up + widely spread = pseudoparalysis
Location: distal femur (esp. medial side), proximal and distal tibia + fibula, distal radius + ulna, proximal humerus, sternal end of ribs
√ Wimberger ring = sclerotic ring around epiphysis indicating loss of epiphyseal density
√ white line of Fränkel = metaphyseal zone of preparatory calcification (DDx: lead / phosphorus poisoning, bismuth treatment, healing rickets)
√ Trümmerfeld zone = radiolucent zone on shaft side of Fränkel's white line (site of subepiphyseal infraction)
√ Parke corner sign = subepiphyseal infraction / comminution resulting in mushrooming / cupping of epiphysis (DDx: syphilis, rickets)
√ Pelkan spurs = metaphyseal spurs projecting at right angles to shaft axis
√ "ground-glass" osteoporosis (CHARACTERISTIC)
√ cortical thinning

√ subperiosteal hematoma with calcification of elevated periosteum (sure radiographic sign of healing)
√ soft-tissue edema (rare)

SEPTIC ARTHRITIS

Organism:
most often due to S. aureus; Gonorrhea (indistinguishable from tuberculous arthritis, but more rapid); Brucellar arthritis (indistinguishable from tuberculosis, slow infection); Salmonella (commonly associated with sickle cell disease / Gaucher disease)
(a) <4 years of age: Streptococcus pyogenes, S. aureus, Haemophilus influenzae
(b) >4 years of age: S. aureus
(c) >10 years of age: S. aureus, Neisseria gonorrhoeae

Location: lower extremity (75%) with hip + knee in 90%

- pain, limp, pseudoparalysis
- warmth, swelling
- septic clinical picture
- bacteremia, leukocytosis

ACUTE SIGNS:
√ initial radiographs frequently normal
√ soft-tissue swelling (first sign secondary to local hyperemia + edema)
√ joint distension (effusion) ± subluxation of hip and humerus in children
√ joint space narrowing = rapid development of destruction of articular cartilage (not in tuberculous arthritis)

SUBACUTE SIGNS after 8–10 days:
√ small erosions in articular cortex / loss of entire cortical outline (marginal erosions in tuberculosis)
√ reactive bone sclerosis in underlying bone
√ subchondral bone destruction (by synovial proliferation)
√ defective reparation / ankylosis (if entire cartilage is destroyed)
√ local bone atrophy (immobility)
√ metaphyseal bone destruction (if osteomyelitis is source of septic joint)

Dx: prompt arthrocentesis + blood culture
Cx: (1) bone growth disturbance (lengthening, shortening, angulation)
(2) chronic degenerative arthritis
(3) ankylosis
(4) osteonecrosis

SHIN SPLINTS

= SHIN SORENESS = MEDIAL TIBIAL STRESS SYNDROME = SOLEUS SYNDROME
= nonspecific term describing exertional lower leg pain

Incidence: 75% of exertional leg pain
Cause: ? atypical stress fracture, traction periostitis, compartment syndrome

- diffuse tenderness along posteromedial tibia in its middle to distal aspect

Location: posterior / posteromedial tibial cortex

Plain radiographs:
√ normal / longitudinal periosteal new bone

Bone scintigraphy:
√ normal radionuclide angiogram + blood-pool phase (DDx to stress fracture)
√ linear longitudinal uptake on delayed images

MR:
√ marrow edema / hemorrhage
√ periosteal fluid

SHORT–RIB POLYDACTYLY SYNDROME

= group of autosomal recessive disorders characterized by short limb dysplasia, constricted thorax, postaxial polydactyly (on ulnar / fibular side)

TYPE I = SALDINO-NOONAN SYNDROME
TYPE II = MAJEWSKI TYPE
TYPE III = NAUMOFF TYPE
TYPE BEEMER

√ severe micromelia
√ pointed femurs at both ends (type I); widened metaphyses (type III)
√ narrow thorax
√ extremely short horizontally oriented ribs
√ distorted underossified vertebral bodies + incomplete coronal clefts
√ polydactyly
√ cleft lip / palate

Prognosis: uniformly lethal

SICKLE CELL DISEASE

Abnormal hemoglobins:
HbS = DNA mutation substituting glutamic acid in position 6 on β-chain with valine
HbC = DNA mutation substituting glutamic acid in position 6 on β-chain with lysine
(a) homozygous = HbSS = sickle cell anemia
(b) heterozygous = HbSA = sickling trait but no anemia
(c) heterozygous variants:
— HbSC (less severe form)
— HbS β-thalassemia anemia (seen occasionally)

Incidence: 8–13% of American Blacks carry sickling factor (HbS); 1:40 with sickle cell trait will manifest sickle cell anemia (HbSS); 1:120 with sickle cell trait will manifest HbSC disease

Pathogenesis:
altered shape + plasticity of RBCs under lowered oxygen tension lead to increased blood viscosity, stasis, "log jam" occlusion of small blood vessels, infarction, necrosis, superinfection; damage of intima occurs most frequently in vessels with high flow rates (terminal ICA); sickling occurs in areas of
(a) slow flow (spleen, liver, renal medulla)
(b) rapid metabolism (brain, muscle, fetal placenta)

- chronic hemolytic anemia (increased sequestration of sickled RBCs in spleen), jaundice
- chronic leg ulcers, priapism
- abdominal crisis
- rheumatism-like joint pain
- skeletal pain (osteomyelitis, cellulitis, bone marrow infarction)

• splenomegaly (in children + infants), later organ atrophy
Cx: high incidence of infections (lung, bone, brain)
Prognosis: death <40 years

(1) DEOSSIFICATION DUE TO MARROW HYPERPLASIA
√ porous decrease in bone density of skull (25%)
√ widening of diploe with decrease in width of outer table (22%)
√ vertical hair-on-end striations (5%)
√ osteoporosis with thinning of trabeculae
√ biconcave "fish" vertebrae (bone softening) in 70%
√ widening of medullary space + thinning of cortices
√ coarsening of trabecular pattern in long + flat bones
√ rib notching
√ pathologic fractures

(2) THROMBOSIS AND INFARCTION
Location: in diaphysis of small tubular bones (children); in metaphysis + subchondrium of long bones (adults)
√ osteolysis (in ACUTE infarction)
√ dystrophic medullary calcification
√ periosteal reaction (bone-within-bone appearance)
√ juxtacortical sclerosis
√ Lincoln log = Reynold sign = H-vertebrae = steplike endplate depression
√ articular disintegration
√ collapse of femoral head (DDx: Perthes with involvement of metaphysis)
MR:
√ diffusely decreased signal of marrow on short + long TR/TE images (= hematopoietic marrow replacing fatty marrow)
√ focal areas of decreased signal intensity on short TR/TE + increased intensity on long TR/TE (= acute marrow infarction)
√ focal areas of decreased signal intensity on short TR/TE + long TR/TE images (= old infarction / fibrosis)

(3) SECONDARY OSTEOMYELITIS
Organism: Salmonella in unusual frequency, also Staphylococcus
√ periostitis (DDx: indistinguishable from bone infarction)
√ dactylitis = hand-foot syndrome

(4) GROWTH EFFECTS (secondary to diminished blood supply)
Location: particularly in metacarpal / phalanx
√ bone shortening = premature epiphyseal fusion
√ epiphyseal deformity with cupped metaphysis
√ cup / peg-in-hole defect of distal femur
√ diminution in vertebral height (shortening of stature + kyphoscoliosis)

@ Chest
√ cardiomegaly + CHF
@ Gallbladder
√ cholelithiasis

@ Brain
Pathophysiology:
chronic anemia produces cerebral hyperemia, hypervolemia, impaired autoregulation
(a) cerebral blood flow cannot be increased leading to infarction in time of crisis
(b) increased cerebral blood flow produces epithelial hyperplasia of large intracranial vessels (terminal ICA / proximal MCA) resulting in thrombus formation
• stroke (5–17%): ischemic infarction (70%), ischemia of deep white matter (25%), hemorrhage (20%), embolic infarction
Angio (in 87% abnormal):
√ arterial stenosis / occlusion of supraclinoid portion of ICA + proximal segments of ACA and MCA
√ moyamoya syndrome (35%)
√ distal branch occlusion (secondary to thrombosis / embolism)
√ aneurysm (rare)
CT:
√ cerebral infarction (mean age of 7.7 years)
√ subarachnoid hemorrhage (mean age of 27 years)
@ Kidney
• hematuria
• hyposthenuria
• nephrotic syndrome
• renal tubular acidosis (distal)
• hyperuricemia
• progressive renal insufficiency
√ normal urogram (70%)
√ papillary necrosis (20%)
√ focal renal scarring (20%)
√ smooth large kidney (4%)
MR:
√ decreased cortical signal on T2-weighted images (renal cortical iron deposition)

@ Spleen
√ splenomegaly < age 10 (in patients with heterozygous sickle cell disease)
Cx: splenic rupture
√ splenic infarction
√ hemosiderosis

Functional asplenia
= anatomically present nonfunctional spleen
• Howell-Jolly bodies, siderocytes, anisocytosis, irreversibly sickled cells
√ normal-sized / enlarged spleen on CT
√ absence of tracer uptake on sulfur colloid scan

Autosplenectomy
= autoinfarction of spleen in homozygous sickle cell disease (function lost by age 5)
Histo: extensive perivascular fibrosis with deposition of hemosiderin + calcium
√ small (as small as 5–10 mm) densely calcified spleen

Acute splenic sequestration crisis
= sudden trapping of large amount of blood in spleen
Cause: obstruction of small intrasplenic veins / sinusoids
Age: (a) homozygous: infancy / childhood
(b) heterozygous: any age
• sudden splenic enlargement
• rapid fall in hematocrit + rise in reticulocytes
√ enlarged spleen
√ multiple lesions at periphery of spleen: hypoechoic by US, of low attenuation by CT, hyperintense on T1WI + T2WI (due to hemorrhage)
Prognosis: in 50% death <2 years of age (due to hypovolemic shock)

Bone marrow scintigraphy:
√ usually symmetric marked expansion of hematopoietic marrow beyond age 20 involving entire femur, calvarium, small bones of hand + feet (normally only in axial skeleton + proximal femur and humerus)
√ bone marrow defects indicative of acute / old infarction

Tc-99m diphosphonate scan:
√ increased overall skeletal uptake (high bone-to-soft tissue ratio)
√ prominent activities at knees, ankles, proximal humerus (delayed epiphyseal closure / increased blood flow to bone marrow)
√ bone marrow expansion (calvarial thickening with relative decrease in activity along falx insertion)
√ decreased / normal uptake on bone scan within 24 hours in acute infarction / posthealing phase following infarction (cyst formation)
√ increased uptake on bone scan after 2–10 days persistent for several weeks in healing infarction
√ increased uptake on bone scan within 24–48 hours in osteomyelitis
√ increased blood-pool activity + normal delayed image on bone scan in cellulitis
√ renal enlargement with marked retention of tracer in renal parenchyma (medullary ischemia + failure of countercurrent system) in 50%
√ persistent splenic uptake (secondary to degeneration, atrophy, fibrosis, calcifications)

SICKLE CELL TRAIT
Hb SA carrier; mild disease with few episodes of crisis + infection; sickling provoked only under extreme stress (unpressurized aircraft, anoxia with CHD, prolonged anesthesia, marathon running)
Incidence: in 8–10% of American Blacks
• may have normal blood count
• recurrent gross hematuria
√ splenic infarction

SC DISEASE
Hb SC carrier
Incidence: 3% of American Blacks
• retinal hemorrhages
• hematuria due to multiple infarctions
√ aseptic necrosis of hip

SICKLE-THAL DISEASE
Resembling clinically Hb SS patients
• anemia (no normal adult hemoglobin)
√ persistent splenomegaly

SINDING-LARSEN-JOHANSSON DISEASE

= osteochondrosis of inferior pole of patella, often bilateral (NOT osteonecrosis / epiphysitis / osteochondritis)
Cause: traction with contusion + subsequent tendinitis / traumatic avulsion of bone; repeated subluxation ± dislocation of patella
Age: adolescents (often 10–14 years)
Predisposed: cerebrospastic children
• tenderness + soft-tissue swelling over lower pole of patella
√ peripatellar soft-tissue swelling
√ calcification / ossification of patellar tendon
√ small bone fragments at lower pole of patella (LAT view)
MR:
√ hypointense area on T1WI + hyperintense on T2WI in inferior pole of patella + surrounding soft tissues

SMALLPOX

5% of infants
Location: elbow bilateral; metaphysis of long bones
√ rapid bone destruction spreading along shaft
√ periosteal reaction
√ endosteal + cortical sclerosis frequent
√ premature epiphyseal fusion with severe deformity
√ ankylosis is frequent

SOFT-TISSUE CHONDROMA

= EXTRASKELETAL CHONDROMA = CHONDROMA OF SOFT PARTS
Incidence: 1.5% of all benign soft-tissue tumors
Age: 30–60 years (range 1–85 years); M:F = 1.2:1
Histo: adult-type hyaline cartilage with areas of calcification + ossification; myxoid change; regions of increased cellularity + cytologic atypia
• slow-growing soft-tissue mass
• occasionally pain + tenderness
Location: hand (54–64%) + foot (20–28%)
√ lobulated well-defined extraskeletal mass <2 cm in size
√ may contain calcifications (33–70%) with ringlike appearance / ossifications
√ scalloping of adjacent bone with sclerotic reaction
MR:
√ high signal intensity on T2WI
√ intermediate signal intensity on T1WI
Rx: local excision
Prognosis: 15–25% recurrence rate
DDx: (1) Extraskeletal myxoid chondrosarcoma (deep-seated in large muscles of upper + lower extremities, pelvic + shoulder girdles)
(2) Periosteal chondroma

SOFT-TISSUE OSTEOMA

= OSTEOMA OF SOFT PARTS (extremely rare)

Histo: mature lamellar bone with well-defined haversian system; bone marrow, myxoid, vascular, fibrous connective tissue between bone trabeculae; collagenous capsule blending into benign hyaline cartilage

Location: head (usually posterior part of tongue), thigh

√ ossified mass

NUC:

√ intense tracer accumulation, greater than adjacent bone

SOLITARY BONE CYST

= UNICAMERAL / SIMPLE BONE CYST

Incidence: up to 5% of primary bone lesions

Etiology: ? trauma (synovial entrapment at capsular reflection), ? vascular anomaly (blockage of interstitial drainage)

Histo: cyst filled with clear yellowish fluid often under pressure, wall lined with fibrous tissue + hemosiderin, giant cells may be present

Age: 3–19 years (80%); occurs during active phase of bone growth; M:F = 3:1

• asymptomatic, unless fractured

Location: proximal femur + proximal humerus (60–75%), fibula, at base of calcaneal neck (4%, >12 years of age), talus; rare in ribs, ilium, small bones of hand + feet (rare), NOT in spine / calvarium; solitary lesion

Site: intramedullary centric metaphyseal, adjacent to epiphyseal cartilage (during active phase) / migrating into diaphysis with growth (during latent phase), does not cross epiphyseal plate

√ 2–3 cm oval radiolucency with long axis parallel to long axis of host bone

√ fine sclerotic boundary

√ scalloping + erosion of internal aspect of underlying cortex

√ photopenic area on bone scan (if not fractured)

√ "fallen fragment" sign if fractured (20%) = centrally dislodged fragment falls into a dependent position

Prognosis: mostly spontaneous regression

Cx: pathologic fracture (65%)

DDx: (1) Enchondroma (calcific stipplings) (2) Fibrous dysplasia (more irregular lucency) (3) Eosinophilic granuloma (4) Chondroblastoma (epiphyseal) (5) Chondromyxoid fibroma (more eccentric + expansile) (6) Giant cell tumor (7) Aneurysmal bone cyst (eccentric) (8) Hemorrhagic cyst (9) Brown tumor

SOLITARY OSTEOCHONDROMA

= OSTEOCARTILAGINOUS EXOSTOSIS

= hyperplastic / dysplastic bone disturbance; growth ends when nearest epiphyseal plate fuses

◊ Most common benign growth of the skeleton!

Etiology: displaced or aberrant physeal cartilage (? microtrauma); radiation induced with latency period of 17 months to 9 years in patient younger than 2 years receiving >2,500 cGy

Age: 1st–3rd decade; M>F

Path: continuity of lesion with marrow + cortex of host bone (HALLMARK)

Histo: cartilage cap containing a basal surface with enchondral ossification (cortex + marrow space)

• usually painless mass; painful with impingement of nerves / blood vessels

Location: long-bone metaphysis of femur, humerus, proximal radius, tibia (50% about knee); scapula; rib; pelvis; spine (1–5%, commonly cervical, esp. C2); in any bone that develops by enchondromal calcification

Type: (a) pedunculated form (b) broad-based sessile form (c) calcific form

√ cortical bone with cartilaginous cap

√ grows at right angles + toward diaphysis (tendon pull)

√ continuity of bone cortex to host bone

√ continuity of medullary marrow space to host bone

√ metaphyseal widening

Cx: (1) Impingement on nerves / blood vessels
(2) Malignant transformation into chondro- / osteosarcoma (<1%)

<u>Signs of malignant degeneration</u>

mnemonic: "GLAD PAST"

Growth after epiphyseal fusion
Lucency (new radiolucency)
Additional scintigraphic activity
Destruction (cortical)
Pain after puberty
And
Soft-tissue mass
Thickened cartilaginous cap

Rx: surgical excision (recurrence unusual)

SOLITARY PLASMACYTOMA

= represents early stage of multiple myeloma, precedes multiple myeloma by 1–20 years

Age: 5th–7th decade

• negative marrow aspiration; no IgG spike in serum / urine

A. SOLITARY MYELOMA OF BONE

Site: thoracic / lumbar spine (most common) > pelvis > ribs > sternum, femora, humeri (common)

√ solitary "bubbly" osteolytic grossly expansile lesion

√ poorly defined margins, Swiss-cheese pattern

√ frequently pathologic fracture (collapse of vertebra)

DDx: giant cell tumor, aneurysmal bone cyst, osteoblastoma, solitary metastasis from renal cell / thyroid carcinoma

B. EXTRAMEDULLARY PLASMACYTOMA

Location: majority in head + neck; 80% in nasal cavity, paranasal sinuses, upper airways of trachea, lung parenchyma

SPONDYLOEPIPHYSEAL DYSPLASIA

Spondyloepiphyseal dysplasia congenita

Autosomal dominant / sporadic (most)
- disproportionate dwarfism with spine + hips more involved than extremities
- waddling gait + muscular weakness
- flat facies
- short neck
- deafness

√ cleft palate

@ Axial skeleton
- √ ovoid vertebral bodies + severe platyspondyly (incomplete fusion of ossification centers + flattening of vertebral bodies)
- √ hypoplasia of odontoid process (Cx: cervical myelopathy)
- √ progressive kyphoscoliosis (short trunk) involving thoracic + lumbar spine
- √ narrowing of disk spaces (resulting in short trunk)
- √ broad iliac bases + deficient ossification of pubis
- √ flat acetabular roof

@ Chest
- √ bell-shaped thorax
- √ pectus carinatum

@ Extremities
- √ normal / slightly shortened limbs
- √ severe coxa vara + genu valgum
- √ multiple accessory epiphyses in hands + feet
- √ talipes equinovarus

Cx: (1) Retinal detachment, myopia (50%)
(2) Secondary arthritis in weight-bearing joints

Spondyloepiphyseal dysplasia tarda

Sex-linked recessive form with milder manifestation + later clinical onset

Age: apparent by 10 years; exclusive to males

√ hyperostotic new bone along posterior 2/3 of vertebral endplate (PATHOGNOMONIC)
√ platyspondyly with depression of anterior 1/3 of vertebral body
√ narrowing with calcification of disk spaces + spondylitic bridging
√ short trunk
√ dysplastic joints (eg, flattened femoral heads)
√ premature osteoarthritis

DDx: Ochronosis

SPRENGEL DEFORMITY

= failure of descent of scapula secondary to fibrous / osseous omovertebral connection

Associated with: Klippel-Feil syndrome, renal anomalies
- webbed neck
- shoulder immobility

√ elevation of scapula

SYNOVIAL OSTEOCHONDROMATOSIS

= SYNOVIAL CHONDROMATOSIS = JOINT CHONDROMA

= benign self-limiting proliferative + metaplastic changes in the synovium with formation of intrasynovial cartilaginous / osteocartilaginous nodules

Cause: hyperplastic synovium with cartilage metaplasia (foci <2–3 cm); loose body may remain free floating / conglomerate with other loose bodies into large mass / reattach to synovium with either reabsorption or continued growth

Histo: foci of hyaline cartilage with mineralized chondroid matrix beneath synovial surface + within subsynovial connective tissue; hypercellularity + nuclear atypia may be confused with malignancy

Age: presents in 3rd–5th decade; M:F = 2–4:1
- slow-growing soft-tissue mass in joint
- progressive joint pain for several years with limitation of motion / locking
- ± hemorrhagic joint effusion

Location: knee (most common with >50%, in 10% bilateral) elbow > hip > shoulder > ankle > wrist; usually monarticular, occasionally bilateral

Sites: within joint / tendon sheath / ganglion / bursa

√ multiple calcified / ossified loose bodies in a single joint (bony shell of remodeled lamellar bone is rare)
√ size of nodules varies between a few mm to several cm
√ varying degrees of bone mineralization (1/3 of chondromas show no radiopacity)
√ pressure erosion of adjacent bone in joints with tight capsule (eg, hip)
√ widening of joint space (from accumulation of loose bodies)
√ NO osteoporosis

CT:
- √ intra-articular soft-tissue mass of near water attenuation containing multiple small calcifications

MR:
- √ lobulated intra-articular mass isointense to muscle on T1WI + hyperintense to muscle on T2WI containing multiple foci of low signal intensity

Cx: (1) long-standing disease may lead to degenerative arthritis (from chronic mechanical irritation + destruction of articular cartilage by loose bodies)
(2) malignant dedifferentiation to chondrosarcoma

Rx: removal of loose bodies (recurrence is common)

DDx: (1) Synovial sarcoma, chondrosarcoma
(2) Osteochondral fracture (Hx of trauma), osteochondritis dissecans, osteonecrosis
(3) Secondary chondromatosis = joint surface disintegration (rheumatoid arthritis, neuropathic arthropathy, tuberculous arthritis, degenerative joint disease)
(4) Pigmented villonodular synovitis, synovial hemangioma, lipoma arborescens

SYNOVIOMA

= SYNOVIAL SARCOMA

= slow-growing expansile malignant tumor originating in the synovial lining / bursa / tendon sheath; uncommonly intra-articular

Incidence: 10% of soft-tissue sarcomas

Histo: fibrosarcomatous + synovial component
Age: 3rd–5th decade; M:F = 2:3
• painful soft-tissue mass
Location: knee (most common), hip, ankle, elbow, wrist, hands, feet; usually solitary
√ large spheroid well-defined soft-tissue mass
√ lesion about 1 cm removed from joint cartilage
√ amorphous calcifications (1/3), often at periphery
√ involvement of adjacent bone (11–20%):
  √ periosteal reaction
  √ bone remodeling (pressure from tumor)
  √ invasion of cortex with wide zone of transition
√ juxta-articular osteoporosis
MR:
  √ low signal intensity on T1WI
  √ inhomogeneously increased signal intensity on T2WI
  √ multilocular appearance with internal septation
  √ fluid-fluid levels (previous hemorrhage)
Rx: local excision / amputation + radiation / chemotherapy

SYPHILIS OF BONE

Congenital syphilis

Transplacental transmission cannot occur <16 weeks gestational age
• positive rapid plasma reagin (measures quantity of antibodies to assess new infection / efficacy of Rx)
• positive microhemagglutination test for Treponema pallidum (remains reactive for life)
√ pneumonia alba
√ hepatomegaly
Location: symmetrical bilateral osteomyelitis involving multiple bones (HALLMARK)

A. Early phase
  ◊ Skeletal radiography abnormal in 19% of infected newborns without overt disease!
  1. Metaphysitis
    √ lucent metaphyseal band adjacent to thin / widened zone of provisional calcification (disturbance in enchondral bone growth)
    √ frayed edge of metaphyseal-physeal junction (osteochondritis) = erosions + lytic defects
  2. Diaphyseal periostitis = "luetic diaphysitis"
    √ solid / lamellated periosteal new-bone growth = bone-within-bone appearance
  3. Spontaneous epiphyseal fractures causing Parrot pseudopalsy (DDx: battered child syndrome)
  4. Bone destruction
    √ marginal destruction of spongiosa + cortex along side of shaft with widening of medullary canal (in short tubular bones)
    √ patchy rarefaction in diaphysis
  5. Wimberger sign
    √ symmetrical focal bone destruction of medial portion of proximal tibial metaphysis (ALMOST PATHOGNOMONIC)

B. Late phase
  • Hutchinson triad = dental abnormality, interstitial keratitis, 8th nerve deafness
  √ frontal bossing of Parrot = diffuse thickening of outer table
  √ saddle nose + high palate (syphilitic chondritis + rhinitis)
  √ short maxilla (maxillary osteitis)
  √ thickening at sternal end of clavicle
  √ "saber-shin" deformity = anteriorly convex bowing in upper 2/3 of tibia with bone thickening

Acquired syphilis

= TERTIARY SYPHILIS resembles chronic osteomyelitis
√ dense bone sclerosis of long bones
√ irregular periosteal proliferation + endosteal thickening with narrow medulla
√ extensive calvarial bone proliferation with mottled pattern (anterior half + lateral skull) in outer table (DDx: fibrous dysplasia, Paget disease)
√ ill-defined lytic destruction in skull, spine, long bones (gumma formation)
√ enlargement of clavicle (cortical + endosteal new bone)
√ Charcot arthropathy = neuropathic joints (lower extremities + spine)

TARSAL COALITION

= abnormal fibrous / cartilaginous / bony fusion of two or more tarsal ossification centers
Most important congenital problem of calcaneus clinically
• asymptomatic / painful pes planus with peroneal spasm
Age: fibrous coalition at birth, ossification during 2nd decade of life
√ bone bars on lateral radiographs between calcaneus, talus, navicular (CT superior to other imaging)
√ both feet affected in 20%
Types:
  (1) calcaneonavicular coalition (30%)
    M:F = 1:1
    • rigid flat foot ± pain in 2nd decade of life
    √ hypoplastic talar head
    √ narrowed calcaneonavicular joint with indistinct articular margins
  (2) talocalcaneal coalition (60%)
    • painful peroneal spastic flat foot, relieved by rest
    Site: middle facet (most frequently)
    √ prominent talar beak (66%) arising from dorsal aspect of head / neck of talus
    √ "ball-and-socket" ankle mortise
    √ asymmetric anterior talocalcaneal joint
DDx: acquired intertarsal ankylosis (infection, trauma, arthritis, surgery)

THALASSEMIA SYNDROMES

PHYSIOLOGIC HEMOGLOBINS
  (a) in adulthood:
    Hb A (98% = 2 α- and 2 β-chains);
    Hb A_2 (2% = 2 α- and 2 δ-chains)
  (b) in fetal life, rapidly decreasing up to 3 months of newborn period:
    Hb F (= 2 α- and 2 γ-chains)

A. ALPHA-THALASSEMIA
   = decreased synthesis of a-chains leading to excess of β-chains + γ-chains (Hb H = 4 β-chains; Hb Bart = 4 γ-chains)
   • disease begins in intrauterine life as no fetal hemoglobin is produced
   • homozygosity is lethal (lack of oxygen transport)

B. BETA-THALASSEMIA
   = decreased synthesis of β-chains leading to excess of α-chains + γ-chains (= fetal hemoglobin)
   • disease manifest in early infancy
   (a) homozygous defect = thalassemia major = Cooley anemia
   (b) heterozygous defect = thalassemia minor

Thalassemia major

= COOLEY ANEMIA = MEDITERRANEAN ANEMIA
= HEREDITARY LEPTOCYTOSIS = beta-thalassemia trait inherited from both parents (= homozygous)

Incidence: 1% for American Blacks; 7.4% for Greek population; 10% for certain Italian populations

Age: develops after newborn period

• retarded growth
• elevated serum bilirubin
• hyperpigmentation of skin
• hyperuricemia
• secondary sexual characteristics retarded, normal menstruation rare (primary gonadotropin insufficiency from iron overload in pituitary gland)
• hypochromic microcytic anemia (Hb 2–3 g/dL), nucleated RBC, target cells, reticulocytosis, decrease in RBC survival, leukocytosis
• susceptible to infection (leukopenia secondary to splenomegaly)
• bleeding diathesis (secondary to thrombocytopenia)

@ Skull:
   √ widening of diploic space with coarsened trabeculations and displacement + thinning of outer table (from marrow hyperplasia)
   √ severe hair-on-end appearance (frontal bone, NOT inferior to internal occipital protuberance)
   √ impediment of pneumatization of maxillary antra + mastoid sinuses
   √ lateral displacement of orbits
   √ rodent facies = ventral displacement of incisors (marrow overgrowth in maxillary bone) with dental malocclusion

@ Peripheral skeleton:
   √ earliest changes in small bones of hands + feet (>6 months of age)
   √ widened medullary spaces with thinning of cortices
   √ osteoporosis = atrophy + coarsening of trabeculae (marrow hyperplasia)
   √ Erlenmeyer flask deformity = bulging of normally concave outline of metaphyses
   √ premature fusion of epiphyses (10%), usually at proximal humerus + distal femur
   √ arthropathy (secondary to hemochromatosis + CPPD + acute gouty arthritis)
   √ regression of peripheral skeletal changes (as red marrow becomes yellow)

@ Chest:
   √ cardiac enlargement + congestive heart failure (secondary to anemia)
   √ paravertebral masses (= extramedullary hematopoiesis)
   √ costal osteomas = expanded posterior aspect of ribs with thinned cortices

@ Abdomen:
   √ hepatosplenomegaly
   √ gallstones

Cx: (1) Pathologic fractures
   (2) Sequelae of iron overload from transfusion therapy (absent puberty, diabetes mellitus, adrenal insufficiency, myocardial insufficiency)

Prognosis: usually death within 1st decade

Thalassemia minor

= beta-thalassemia trait inherited from one parent (= heterozygous)
• usually asymptomatic except for periods of stress (pregnancy, infection)
• microcytic hypochromic anemia (Hb 9–11 g/dL)
• occasionally jaundice + splenomegaly

THANATOPHORIC DYSPLASIA

= sporadic lethal skeletal dysplasia characterized by severe rhizomelia (micromelic dwarfism)

Incidence: 6.9:100,000 births; 1:6,400–16,700 births; most common lethal bone dysplasia

• hypotonic infants
• protuberant abdomen
• extended arms + abducted externally rotated thighs

@ Head
   √ large head with short base of skull + prominent frontal bone
   √ occasionally trilobed cloverleaf skull = "Kleeblattschädel"

@ Chest
   √ narrow chest
   √ short horizontal ribs with cupped anterior ends
   √ small scapula + normal clavicles

@ Spine
   √ normal length of trunk
   √ reduction of interpediculate space of last few lumbar vertebrae
   √ extreme generalized platyspondyly = severe H-shaped vertebra plana
   √ excessive intervertebral space height

@ Pelvis
   √ iliac wings small + square (vertical shortening but wide horizontally)
   √ flat acetabulum
   √ narrow sacrosciatic notch
   √ short pubic bones

@ Extremities
   √ severe micromelia + bowing of extremities

√ metaphyseal flaring = "telephone handle" appearance of long bones
√ thornlike projections in metaphyseal area

OB-US (findings may be seen very early in pregnancy):
√ polyhydramnios (71%)
√ short-limbed dwarfism with extremely short + bowed "telephone receiver"-like femurs
√ extremely small hypoplastic thorax with short ribs + narrowed in anteroposterior dimension
√ protuberant abdomen
√ macrocrania with frontal bossing ± hydrocephalus (increased HC:AC ratio)
√ "cloverleaf skull" (in 14%) (DDx: encephalocele)
√ diffuse platyspondyly
√ redundant soft tissues

Prognosis: often stillborn; uniformly fatal within a few hours / days after birth (respiratory failure)

DDx: (1) Ellis-van Creveld syndrome (extra digit, acromesomelic short limbs)
(2) Asphyxiating thoracic dysplasia (less marked bone shortening, vertebrae spared)
(3) Short-rib polydactyly syndrome
(4) Homozygous achondroplasia (both parents affected)

THROMBOCYTOPENIA-ABSENT RADIUS SYNDROME

= TAR SYNDROME = rare autosomal recessive disorder

Age: presentation at birth

May be associated with: CHD (33%): ASD, tetralogy

- platelet count <100,000/mm^3 (decreased production by bone marrow)

√ usually bilateral radial aplasia / hypoplasia
√ uni- / bilaterally hypoplastic / absent ulna / humerus
√ defects of hands, feet, legs

Prognosis: death in 50% in early infancy (hemorrhage)

THYROID ACROPACHY

Onset: after 18 months following thyroidectomy for hyperthyroidism (does not occur with antithyroid medication)

Incidence: 1–10%

- clubbing, soft-tissue swelling
- eu- / hypo- / hyperthyroid state

Location: diaphyses of phalanges + metacarpals of hand; less commonly feet, lower legs, forearms

√ thick spiculated lacy periosteal reaction

DDx: (1) Pulmonary osteoarthropathy (painful)
(2) Pachydermoperiostosis
(3) Fluorosis (ligamentous calcifications)

TRANSIENT REGIONAL OSTEOPOROSIS

Cause: unknown; ? overactivity of sympathetic nervous system + local hyperemia similar to reflex sympathetic dystrophy syndrome, trauma, synovitis, transient ischemia

Regional migratory osteoporosis

= rapid onset of self-limiting episodes of severe localized osteoporosis and pain but repetitive occurrence of same symptoms in other regions of the same or opposite lower extremity

- rapid onset of local pain
- diffuse erythema, swelling, increased heat
- significant disability due to severe pain on weight-bearing

Age: middle-aged males

Location: usually lower extremity (ie, ankle, knee, hip, foot)

√ rapid localized osteoporosis within 4–8 weeks after onset migrating from one joint to another; may affect trabecular / cortical bone
√ linear / wavy periosteal reaction
√ preservation of subchondral cortical bone
√ no joint space narrowing, bone erosion

MR:
√ affected area has low signal intensity on T1WI, high signal intensity on T2WI (= bone marrow edema)

NUC:
√ increased activity

Prognosis: persists for 6–9 months in one area; cycle of symptoms may last for several years

Rx: variable response to analgesics / corticosteroids

PARTIAL TRANSIENT OSTEOPOROSIS
= variant of regional migratory osteoporosis with more focal pattern of osteoporosis, which may eventually become more generalized
(a) Zonal form = portion of bone involved, ie, one femoral condyle / one quadrant of femoral head
(b) Radial form = only one / two rays of hand / foot involved

Transient osteoporosis of hip

= self-limiting disease of unknown etiology

Age: typically in middle-aged males / in 3rd trimester of pregnancy in females involving left hip; M > F

- spontaneous onset of hip and groin pain, usually progressive over several weeks
- painful swelling of joint followed by progressive demineralization
- rapid development of disability, limp, decreased range of motion

Site: hip most commonly affected; generally only one joint at a time

√ progressive marked osteoporosis of femoral head, neck, acetabulum (3–8 weeks after onset of illness)
√ virtually PATHOGNOMONIC striking loss of subchondral cortex of femoral head + neck region
√ NO joint space narrowing / subchondral bone collapse

NUC:
√ markedly increased uptake on bone scan without cold spots / inhomogeneities (positive before radiograph)

MR:
√ diffuse bone marrow edema involving femoral head + neck + sometimes intertrochanteric region

√ small joint effusion

Cx: pathologic fracture common

Prognosis: spontaneous recovery within 2–6 months; recurrence in another joint within 2 years possible

DDx: (1) AVN (cystic + sclerotic changes, early subchondral undermining)
(2) Septic / tuberculous arthritis (joint aspiration)
(3) Monarticular rheumatoid arthritis
(4) Metastasis
(5) Reflex sympathetic dystrophy
(6) Disuse atrophy
(7) Synovial chondromatosis
(8) Villonodular synovitis

TRANSIENT SYNOVITIS OF HIP

= OBSERVATION HIP = TRANSITORY SYNOVITIS = TOXIC SYNOVITIS = COXITIS FUGAX

= nonspecific inflammatory reaction; most common nontraumatic cause of acute limp in a child

Etiology: unknown

Age: 5–10 (average 6) years; M:F = 2:1

• developing limp over 1–2 days
• pain in hip, thigh, knee
• Hx of recent viral illness (65%)
• mild fever (25%)

√ radiographs usually normal
√ joint effusion
  √ displacement of femur from acetabulum
  √ displacement of psoas line
  √ lateral displacement of gluteal line (least sensitive + least reliable)
√ regional osteoporosis (? hyperemia, disuse)

Prognosis: complete recovery within a few weeks

Dx: per exclusion

Rx: non–weight-bearing treatment

DDx: trauma, Legg-Perthes disease, acute rheumatoid arthritis, acute rheumatic fever, septic arthritis, tuberculosis, malignancy

TREACHER COLLINS SYNDROME

= MANDIBULOFACIAL DYSOSTOSIS

= autosomal dominant disease (with new mutations in 60%) characterized by bilateral malformations of eyes, malar bones, mandible, and ears resulting in birdlike face

Cause: defect in growth of 1st + 2nd branchial arches before the 7th to 8th week of gestation

• antimongoloid eye slant (drooping lateral lower eyelids due to hypoplasia of lateral canthal tendon of orbicular muscle)
• sparse / absent lashes in lower eye lids, coloboma
• dysplastic low-set auricles
• preauricular skin tags / fistulas
• conductive hearing loss (common)
• extension of scalp hair growth onto cheek

√ craniosynostosis
√ egg-shaped orbits = drooping of outer inferior orbital rim
√ sunken cheek due to marked hypoplasia of zygomatic arches (= malar hypoplasia)
√ hypoplasia of lateral wall of orbits + shallow / incomplete orbital floor
√ hypoplasia of maxilla + maxillary sinus
√ pronounced micrognathia = mandibular hypoplasia with broad concave curve on lower border of body
√ microtia with small middle ear cavity
√ deformed / fused / absent auditory ossicles
√ atresia / stenosis of external auditory canal
√ high-arched / cleft palate

OB-US:
  √ polyhydramnios (from swallowing difficulty)

Prognosis: early respiratory problems (tongue relatively too large for hypoplastic mandible)

DDx: (1) Goldenhar-Gorlin syndrome (unilateral microtia + midface anomalies, hemivertebrae, block vertebrae, vertebral hypoplasia, microphthalmia, coloboma of upper lid)
(2) Acrofacial dysplasia (limb malformations)
(3) Crouzon disease (maxillary hypoplasia with protrusion of mandible, hypertelorism, exophthalmos, craniosynostosis)

TRISOMY D SYNDROME

= Trisomy 13–15 group syndrome

Etiology: additional chromosome in D group; high maternal age

• severe mental retardation
• hypertonic infant
• cleft lip + palate

Associated with: capillary hemangioma of face + upper trunk

• hypotelorism
• coloboma, cataract, microphthalmia
• malformed ear with hypoplastic external auditory canal
• hyperconvex nails

√ postaxial polydactyly

@ Skull
  √ deficient ossification of skull
  √ cleft / absent midline structures of facial bones
  √ poorly formed orbits
  √ slanting of frontal bones
  √ microcephaly
  √ arhinencephaly
  √ holoprosencephaly

@ Chest
  √ thin malformed ribs
  √ diaphragmatic hernia (frequent)
  √ congenital heart disease

Prognosis: death within 6 months of age

TRISOMY E SYNDROME

= Trisomy 16–18 group syndrome

Etiology: additional chromosome at 18 or E group location

Sex: usually female

• hypertonic infants

- mental + psychomotor retardation
- typical facies: micrognathia, high narrow palate with small buccal cavity, low-set deformed ears
- flexed ulnar-deviated fingers + short adducted thumb
- 2nd finger overlapping of 3rd (CHARACTERISTIC)

Associated with: congenital heart disease in 100% (PDA, VSD); hernias; renal anomalies; eventration of diaphragm

√ stippled epiphyses

@ Skull
- √ thin calvarium
- √ persistent metopic suture
- √ prominent occiput
- √ hypoplastic mandible (most constant feature) + maxilla

@ Chest
- √ increase in AP diameter of thorax
- √ hypoplastic sternum
- √ hypoplastic clavicles (DDx: cleidocranial dysostosis)
- √ slender + tapered ribs
- √ diaphragmatic eventration (common)

@ Pelvis
- √ small pelvis with forward rotation of iliac wings
- √ increased obliquity of acetabulum

@ Hand & foot
- √ adducted thumb = short 1st metacarpal + phalanges (DIAGNOSTIC)
- √ overlap of 2nd on 3rd finger (DIAGNOSTIC)
- √ flexed ulnar-deviated fingers
- √ short 1st toe
- √ varus deformities of forefoot + dorsiflexion of toes
- √ rocker bottom foot / extreme pes planus (frequent)

OB-US:
- √ hydrocephalus
- √ cystic hygroma
- √ diaphragmatic hernia
- √ clubfoot
- √ overlapping index finger
- √ choroid plexus cyst (30%)

Prognosis: child rarely survives beyond 6 months of age

TUBERCULOSIS OF BONE

Incidence: 3–5% of tuberculous patients, 30% in patients with extrapulmonary tuberculosis

Age: any, rare in 1st year of life, M:F = 1:1

- negative skin test excludes diagnosis
- history of active pulmonary disease (in 50%)

Location: vertebral column, hip, knee, wrist, elbow

Pathogenesis:
1. Hematogenous spread from
   (a) primary infection of lung (particularly in children)
   (b) quiescent primary pulmonary site / extraosseous focus
2. Reactivation: especially in hip

Tuberculous arthritis

= joint involvement usually secondary to adjacent osteomyelitis

Incidence: 84% of skeletal tuberculosis

Pathophysiology: synovitis with pannus formation leads to chondronecrosis

Age: middle-aged / elderly

- chronic pain, weakness, muscle wasting
- soft-tissue swelling, draining sinus
- joint fluid: high WBC count, low glucose level, poor mucin clot formation (similar to rheumatoid arthritis)

Location: hip, knee > elbow, wrist, sacroiliac joint, glenohumeral, articulation of hand + foot

√ Phemister triad:
1. gradual narrowing of joint space due to slow cartilage destruction (DDx: cartilage destruction in pyogenic arthritis is much quicker)
2. peripherally located (= marginal) bone erosions
3. juxtaarticular osteoporosis

Early radiographs:
- √ joint effusion (hip in 0%, knee in 60%, ankle in 80%)
- √ extensive osteopenia (deossification) adjacent to primarily weight-bearing joints
- √ soft tissues normal

Late radiographs:
- √ small cystlike erosions along joint margins in non–weight-bearing line opposing one another (DDx: pyogenic arthritis erodes articular cartilage)
- √ no joint space narrowing for months
- √ articular cortical bone destruction earlier in joints with little unopposed surfaces (hip, shoulder)
- √ infection of subchondral bone forming "kissing sequestra"
- √ increased density with extensive soft-tissue calcifications in healing phase

Cx: fibrous ankylosis, leg shortening

Dx: synovial biopsy (in 90% positive), culture of synovial fluid (in 80% positive)

Tuberculous osteomyelitis

Incidence: 16% of skeletal tuberculosis

Age: children <5 years (0.5–14%), rare in adults

- painless swelling of hand / foot

Location: any bone

Site: (a) epiphysis with spread to joint / spread from adjacent affected joint (most common)
(b) metaphysis with transphyseal spread (in child) (DDx: pyogenic infections usually do not extend across physis)
(c) diaphysis (<1%)

- √ initially round / oval poorly defined lytic lesion with minimal / no surrounding sclerosis
- √ varying amounts of eburnation + periostitis
- √ advanced epiphyseal maturity / overgrowth (due to hyperemia) ± limb shortening from premature physeal fusion
- √ cystic tuberculosis = well-marginated osseous lesions
  (a) in children (frequent): in peripheral skeleton, ± symmetric distribution, no sclerosis
  (b) in adults: in skull / shoulder / pelvis / spine, with sclerosis

√ spina ventosa = tuberculous dactylitis = digit with exuberant periosteal new-bone formation of fusiform appearance secondary to erosion of endosteal cortex with lamellated / solid periosteal thickening in hands + feet

Tuberculous spondylitis

= POTT DISEASE
= destruction of vertebral body + intervertebral disk by tuberculous mycobacterium

Incidence: <1% of patients with tuberculosis; 25–60% of all skeletal tuberculosis

Age: children / adults; M > F

- insidious onset of back pain, stiffness
- local tenderness
- NO pulmonary lesions in 50%

Location: thoracolumbar area (L1 most common), frequent involvement of multiple contiguous segments

Site: vertebral body (82%) > posterior elements (18%)

Spread:
(a) hematogenous spread via paravertebral venous plexus of Batson: separate foci in 1–4%
(b) contiguous into disk by penetrating subchondral bone plate + cartilaginous endplate
(c) subligamentous spread beneath paraspinal ligaments to adjacent vertebral bodies

√ erosion and collapse of vertebral endplates leads to narrowing of vertebral interspaces (first change)
N.B.: vertebral disk space maintained longer than in pyogenic arthritis (disk itself preserved but fragmented)
√ destruction of centra
√ vertebra plana in children
√ angular kyphotic deformity (= gibbus) in adults
√ vertebra within a vertebra (= growth recovery lines)
√ ivory vertebra (= reossification as healing response to osteonecrosis)
√ large cold fusiform abscess in paravertebral gutters / psoas, commonly bilateral, ± anterolateral scalloping of vertebral bodies
√ amorphous / teardrop-shaped calcification in paraspinal area between L1 + L5 (DDx: nontuberculous abscess rarely calcifies)
√ "gouge defect" = mild contour irregularity of anterior and lateral aspect of vertebral body (= erosion from subligamentous extension of tuberculous abscess)

Cx: angular kyphosis (= gibbus deformity), scoliosis, ankylosis, osteonecrosis, paralysis (spinal cord compression from abscess, granulation tissue, bone fragments, arachnoiditis)

Prognosis: 26–30% mortality rate

DDx:
1. Pyogenic spondylitis (rapid destruction, multiple abscess cavities, no thickening / calcification of abscess rim, little new-bone formation, posterior elements not involved)
2. Neoplasia (multiple noncontiguous lesions, no disk destruction, little soft-tissue involvement)

TUMORAL CALCINOSIS

= LIPOCALCINOGRANULOMATOSIS
= rare disease with progressive large nodular juxtaarticular calcified soft-tissue masses in patients with normal serum calcium + phosphorus and no evidence of renal, metabolic, or collagen-vascular disease

Etiology: autosomal dominant (1/3) with variable clinical expressivity; unknown biochemical defect of phosphorus metabolism responsible for abnormal phosphate reabsorption + 1,25-dihydroxy-vitamin D formation

Path: multilocular cystic lesions with creamy white fluid (hydroxyapatite) + many giant cells (granulomatous foreign body reaction) surrounded by fibrous capsule

Age: onset mostly within 1st / 2nd decade (range of 1–79 years); M:F = 1:1; predominantly in Blacks

- progressive painful / painless soft-tissue mass with overlying skin ulceration + sinus tract draining chalky milklike fluid
- swelling
- limitation of motion
- hyperphosphatemia + hypervitaminosis D
- normal serum calcium, alkaline phosphatase, renal function, parathyroid hormone

@ Soft tissue
Location: paraarticular in hips > elbows > shoulders > feet, ribs, ischial spines; single / multiple joints; ALMOST NEVER knees; usually along extensor surface of joints (? initially a calcific bursitis)
√ dense loculated multiglobular homogeneously calcified soft-tissue mass of 1–20 cm in size
√ radiolucent septa (= connective tissue)
√ ± fluid-fluid levels with milk-of-calcium consistency
√ underlying bones NORMAL
√ increased tracer uptake of soft-tissue masses on bone scan

@ Bone
√ diaphyseal periosteal reaction (diaphysitis)
√ patchy areas of calcification in medullary cavity (calcific myelitis)

@ Teeth
√ bulbous root enlargement
√ pulp stones = intrapulp calcifications

@ Pseudoxanthoma elasticum-like features
√ calcinosis cutis = skin calcifications
√ vascular calcifications
√ angioid streaks of retina

Prognosis: tendency for recurrence after incomplete excision

Rx: phosphate depletion

DDx: Chronic renal failure on hemodialysis, CPPD, paraosteoarthropathy, hyperparathyroidism

TURNER SYNDROME

= due to nondisjunction of sex chromosomes as
(1) complete monosomy (45,XO)
(2) partial monosomy (structurally altered second X chromosome)
(3) mosaicism (XO + another sex karyotype)

Incidence: 1:3,000–5,000 livebirths

Associated with: coarctation, aortic stenosis, horseshoe kidney (most common)

- sexual infantilism: primary amenorrhea, absent secondary sex characteristics
- short stature; absence of prepubertal growth spurt
- webbed neck; low irregular nuchal hair line
- shield-shaped chest + widely spaced nipples
- mental deficiency (occasionally)
- high palate; thyromegaly
- multiple pigmented nevi; keloid formation
- idiopathic hypertension; elevated urinary gonadotropins

@ General
√ normal skeletal maturation with growth arrest at skeletal age of 15 years
√ delayed fusion of epiphyses > age 20 years
√ osteoporosis during / after 2nd decade (gonadal hormone deficiency)
√ coarctation of aorta (10%); aortic stenosis
√ renal ectopia / horseshoe kidney
√ lymphedema

@ Skull
√ basilar impression; basal angle >140°
√ parietal thinning
√ small bridged sella
√ hypertelorism

@ Axial skeleton
√ hypoplasia of odontoid process + C1
√ osteochondrosis of vertebral plates
√ squared lumbar vertebrae; kyphoscoliosis
√ deossification of vertebrae
√ small iliac wings; late fusion of iliac crests
√ android pelvic inlet with narrowed pubic arch + small sacrosciatic notches

@ Chest
√ thinning of lateral aspects of clavicles
√ thinned + narrowed ribs with pseudonotching

@ Hand + arm
√ positive metacarpal sign = relative shortening of 4th metacarpal = tangential line along heads of 5th + 4th metacarpals intersects 3rd metacarpal
√ positive carpal sign = narrowing of scaphoid-lunate-triquetrum angle <117°
√ phalangeal preponderance = length of proximal + distal phalanx exceeds length of 4th metacarpal by >3 mm
√ shortening of 2nd + 5th middle phalanx (also in Down syndrome)
√ "drumstick" distal phalanges = slender shaft + large distal head
√ "insetting" of epiphyses into bases of adjacent metaphyses (phalanges + metacarpals)
√ Madelung deformity = shortening of ulna / absence of ulnar styloid process
√ cubitus valgus = bilateral radial tilt of articular surface of trochlea
√ deossification of carpal bones

@ Knee
√ tibia vara = enlarged medial femoral condyle + depression of medial tibial plateau (DDx: Blount disease)
√ small exostosis-like projection from medial border of proximal tibial metaphysis

@ Foot
√ deossification of tarsal bones
√ shortening of 1st, 4th, and 5th metatarsals
√ pes cavus

OB-US:
√ large nuchal cystic hygroma
√ lymphangiectasia with generalized hydrops
√ symmetrical edema of dorsum of feet
√ CHD (20%): coarctation of aorta (70%), left heart lesions
√ horseshoe kidney

BONNEVIE-ULLRICH SYNDROME

= infantile form of Turner syndrome
(1) congenital webbed neck
(2) widely separated nipples
(3) lymphedema of hands + feet

VAN BUCHEM DISEASE

= GENERALIZED CORTICAL HYPEROSTOSIS
may be related to hyperphosphatasemia

- paralysis of facial nerve
- auditory + ocular disturbances (in late teens secondary to foraminal encroachment)
- increased alkaline phosphatase

Location: skull, mandible, clavicles, ribs, long-bone diaphyses

√ symmetrical generalized sclerosis + thickening of endosteal cortex
√ obliteration of diploe
√ spinous processes thickened + sclerotic

DDx: (1) Osteopetrosis (sclerosis of all bones, not confined to diaphyses)
(2) Generalized hyperostosis with pachydermia (involves entire long bones, considerable pain, skin changes)
(3) Hyperphosphatasia (infancy, widened bones but decreased cortical density)
(4) Engelmann disease (rarely generalized, involves lower limbs)
(5) Pyle disease (does not involve middiaphyses)
(6) Polyostotic fibrous dysplasia (rarely symmetrically generalized, paranasal sinuses abnormal, skull involvement)

WILLIAMS SYNDROME

= IDIOPATHIC HYPERCALCEMIA OF INFANCY

- elfin facies, dysplastic dentition
- neonatal hypercalcemia
- mental retardation

@ Skeletal manifestations
√ osteosclerosis (secondary to trabecular thickening)
√ dense broad zone of provisional calcification
√ radiolucent metaphyseal bands
√ dense vertebral endplates + acetabular roofs
√ bone islands in spongiosa
√ metastatic calcification
√ craniostenosis

@ Cardiovascular manifestations
√ supravalvular aortic stenosis, aortic hypoplasia
√ pulmonic stenosis
√ stenoses of major vessels (innominate, carotids, renal arteries)

@ GI and GU tract:
√ colonic diverticula
√ bladder diverticula

Prognosis: spontaneous resolution after 1 year in most
Rx: withhold vitamin D + calcium
DDx: Hypervitaminosis D

WILSON DISEASE

= HEPATOLENTICULAR DEGENERATION
= autosomal recessive disease with excessive copper retention (= copper toxicosis)

Prevalence: 1:33,000–200,000; 1:90 persons is a heterozygous carrier

Cause: alteration of chromosome 13 resulting in inability of liver to excrete copper into bile hypothetically due to either
(a) lysosomal defect in hepatocytes, or
(b) deficiency of biliary copper-binding proteins, or
(c) persistence of fetal mode of copper metabolism, or
(d) hepatic synthesis of high-affinity copper-binding proteins)

Age of onset: 7–50 years; hepatic manifestations predominate in children; neuropsychiatric manifestations predominate in adolescents + adults

Histo: macrovesicular fat deposition in hepatocytes, glycogen degeneration of hepatocyte nuclei, Kupffer cell hypertrophy

Stage 1 asymptomatic copper accumulation in hepatocytic cytosol
Stage 2 redistribution of copper into hepatic lysosomes + circulation from saturated hepatocytic cytosol
(a) gradual redistribution is asymptomatic
(b) rapid redistribution causes fulminant hepatic failure / acute intravascular hemolysis
Stage 3 cirrhosis, neurologic, ophthalmologic, renal dysfunction may be reversible with therapy

• tremor, rigidity, dysarthria, dysphagia (excessive copper deposition in lenticular region of brain)
• intellectual impairment, emotional disturbance
• Kayser-Fleischer ring (= green pigmentation surrounding limbus corneae) is DIAGNOSTIC
• jaundice / portal hypertension (liver cirrhosis)
• elevated copper concentration in serum ceruloplasmin (BEST SCREENING TEST)
• decreased incorporation of orally administered radiolabeled copper into newly synthesized ceruloplasmin

Skeletal manifestations (in 2/3):
√ generalized deossification may produce pathologic fractures

@ Joints: shoulder (frequent), knee, hip, wrist, 2nd–4th MCP joints
• articular symptoms in 75%: pain, stiffness, gelling of joints
√ subarticular cysts
√ premature osteoarthritis (narrowing of joint space + osteophyte formation)
√ osteochondritis dissecans
√ chondrocalcinosis
√ premature osteoarthrosis of spine, prominent Schmorl nodes, wedging of vertebrae, irregularities of vertebral plates

@ Brain
Location: basal ganglia, rarely thalamus
√ cerebral white matter atrophy
√ hypodensities, prolongation of T1 + T2

Cx: rickets + osteomalacia (secondary to renal tubular dysfunction) in minority of patients
Rx: life long pharmacologic therapy with chelation agents (penicillamine / trientine / zinc); liver transplantation

DIFFERENTIAL DIAGNOSIS OF SKULL AND SPINE DISORDERS

Lumbosacral postsurgical syndrome
= signs of dysfunction and disability + pain and paresthesia following surgery

Cause:

A. Biomechanical failure
  1. Primary disk herniation
  2. Recurrent disk herniation (onset 1 week – 1 month)

B. Failure of surgical treatment
  1. Residual disk herniation (onset <1 week)
  2. Perioperative intraspinal hemorrhage (onset <1 week)
  3. Spinal / meningeal / neural inflammation (onset 1 week – 1 month)
  4. Intraspinal scar formation (onset >1 month)
     (a) Epidural fibrosis
        √ enhancing epidural plaque / mass
     (b) Fibrosing arachnoiditis
        √ clumping of nerve roots
        √ adhesion of roots to wall of thecal sac
        √ abnormal enhancement of thickened meninges + matted nerve roots
  5. Remote phenomena unrelated to spine

Failed back surgery syndrome
= failure of improvement following back surgery in 5–15%

◊ Interpretation in immediate postoperative period difficult, stabilization of findings occurs in 2–6 months

A. OSSEOUS CAUSES
  1. Spondylolisthesis
  2. Central stenosis
  3. Foraminal stenosis
  4. Pseudarthrosis

B. SOFT-TISSUE CAUSES
  1. Adhesive arachnoiditis
     √ thickened irregular clumped nerve roots
  2. Infection
  3. Hemorrhage
  4. Epidural fibrosis (scarring)
     √ heterogeneous enhancement on early T1WI (maximum at about 5 minutes post injection)
  5. Recurrent disk herniation
     √ no enhancement on early T1WI (appears enhanced ≥30 minutes post injection)

C. SURGICAL ERRORS
  1. Wrong level / side of surgery
  2. Direct nerve injury

mnemonic: "ABCDEF"

Arachnoiditis
Bleeding
Contamination (infection)
Disk (residual / recurrent / new level)
Error (wrong disk excised)
Fibrosis (scar)

Cauda equina syndrome
= constellation of signs + symptoms resulting from compressive lesion in lower lumbar spinal canal

Cause:

(1) Displaced disk fragment
(2) Intra- / extramedullary tumor
(3) Osseous: Paget disease, osteomyelitis, osteoarthrosis of facet joints, complication of ankylosing spondylitis

- diminished sensation in lower lumbar + sacral dermatomes
- wasting + weakness of muscles
- decreased ankle reflexes
- impotence
- disturbed sphincter function + overflow incontinence
- decreased sphincter tone

MANDIBLE & MAXILLA

Mandibular hypoplasia = micrognathia

A. WITH ABNORMAL EARS
  1. Treacher-Collins syndrome
  2. Goldenhar syndrome = facio-auriculo-vertebral spectrum (x-rays of vertebrae!)
  3. Langer-Giedion syndrome (IUGR, protruding ears)

B. ABNORMALITIES OF EARS + OTHER ORGANS
  1. Miller syndrome (severe postaxial hand anomalies)
  2. Velo-cardio-facial syndrome (hand + cardiac lesions)
  3. Otopalatodigital syndrome - type II (hand abnormalities)
  4. Stickler syndrome (ear anomalies not severe)
  5. Pierre-Robin syndrome (large fleshy ears)

C. NO EAR ANOMALIES
  1. Pyknodysostosis

Destruction of temporomandibular joint
mnemonic: "HIRT"

Hyperparathyroidism
Infection
Rheumatoid arthritis
Trauma

Radiolucent lesion of mandible

A. SHARPLY MARGINATED LESION
  (a) around apex of tooth
    1. Radicular cyst
    2. Cementinoma
  (b) around unerupted tooth
    1. Dentigerous cyst
    2. Ameloblastoma

(c) unrelated to tooth
1. Simple bone cyst
2. Fong disease
3. Basal cell nevus syndrome

B. POORLY MARGINATED LESIONS
√ "floating teeth": suggestive of primary / secondary malignancy
√ resorption of tooth root: hallmark of benign process
(a) Infection
1. Osteomyelitis: actinomycosis
(b) Radiotherapy
1. Osteoradionecrosis
(c) Malignant neoplasm
1. Osteosarcoma (1/3 lytic, 1/3 sclerotic, 1/3 mixed)
2. Local invasion from gingival / buccal neoplasms (more common)
3. Metastasis from breast, lung, kidney in 1% (in 70% adenocarcinoma)
(d) Other
1. Eosinophilic granuloma: "floating tooth"
2. Fibrous dysplasia
3. Osteocementoma
4. Ossifying fibroma (very common)

Tooth mass

A. CYSTIC LESION
1. **Radicular cyst** (commonest)
Cause: deep carious lesion / deep filling / trauma
Site: intimately associated with apex of nonvital tooth
√ apical lucency
2. **Ameloblastoma = adamantinoma of jaw**
locally aggressive lesion from enamel-type epithelial tissue elements around tooth; 1/3 arise from dentigerous cyst
Age: 4 – 5th decade; M:F = 1:1
Location: mandible (75%), maxilla (25%), in region of bicuspids + molars (angle of mandible commonly affected)
√ uni- / multilocular lytic lesion with scalloped margin + cortical expansion
√ may be associated with impacted tooth / resorption of the root of a tooth
Prognosis: frequently local recurrence even more aggressive after excision
3. **Primordial cyst**
arising from follicle of tooth that never developed
√ absent tooth
4. **Giant cell reparative granuloma**
unrelated to tooth (nonodontogenic)
√ lucent smooth multiloculated lesion
5. **Traumatic bone cyst**
in association with vital tooth
√ sharply marginated lucent lesion with fingerlike projections between roots
6. **Dentigerous cyst**
= epithelial-lined cyst from odontogenic epithelium developing around unerupted tooth
Location: maxilla (may expand into maxillary sinus), posterior mandible
√ cystic expansile lesion containing tooth
Cx: may degenerate into ameloblastoma (rare)

B. SCLEROTIC LESION
1. **Cementinoma** = fibro-osteoma = periapical cemental dysplasia
Histo: spindle-cell fibroblastic proliferation + cementum
Age: 30–40 years of age; most common in women
Location: in anterior portion of mandible, at apex of vital tooth
√ often multicentric
√ mixed lucent + sclerotic lesion with little expansion, calcifies with time
DDx: ossifying fibroma, fibrous dysplasia, Paget disease
2. True cementoma = benign cementoblastoma
3. Gigantiform cementoma
4. **Hypercementosis**
= bulbous enlargement of a root
(a) idiopathic
(b) associated with Paget disease
5. Benign fibro-osseous lesions
(a) ossifying fibroma: young adults; mandible > maxilla
(b) monostotic fibrous dysplasia: M < F, younger patients
(c) condensing osteitis = focal chronic sclerosing osteitis
√ near apex of nonvital tooth
6. Paget disease
involvement of jaw in 20%; maxilla > mandible
Location: bilateral, symmetric involvement
√ widened alveolar ridges
√ flat palate
√ loosening of teeth
√ hypercementosis
√ may cause destruction of lamina dura
7. **Torus mandibularis** = exostosis
Site: midline of hard palate; lingual surface of mandible in region of bicuspids

SKULL

Sutural abnormalities

Wide sutures

= >10 mm at birth, >3 mm at 2 years, >2 mm at 3 years of age; (sutures are splittable up to age 12–15; complete closure by age 30)
A. NORMAL VARIANT
in neonate + prematurity; growth spurt occurs at 2–3 years and 5–7 years

B. CONGENITAL UNDEROSSIFICATION
osteogenesis imperfecta, hypophosphatasia, rickets, hypothyroidism, pyknodysostosis, cleidocranial dysplasia

C. METABOLIC DISEASE
hypoparathyroidism; lead intoxication; hypo- / hypervitaminosis A

D. RAISED INTRACRANIAL PRESSURE
Cause: (1) intracerebral tumor (2) subdural hematoma (3) hydrocephalus
Age: seen only if <10 years of age
Location: coronal > sagittal > lambdoid > squamosal suture

E. INFILTRATION OF SUTURES
Cause: metastases to meninges from (1) neuroblastoma (2) leukemia (3) lymphoma
√ poorly defined margins

F. RECOVERY
from (1) deprivational dwarfism (2) chronic illness (3) prematurity (4) hypothyroidism

Craniosynostosis

= CRANIOSTENOSIS = premature closure of sutures (normally at about 30 years of age)

Age: often present at birth; M:F = 4:1

Etiology:

A. Primary craniosynostosis
B. Secondary craniosynostosis
(a) hematologic: sickle cell anemia, thalassemia
(b) metabolic: rickets, hypercalcemia, hyperthyroidism, hypervitaminosis D
(c) bone dysplasia: hypophosphatasia, achondroplasia, metaphyseal dysplasia, mongolism, Hurler disease, skull hyperostosis, Rubinstein-Taybi syndrome
(d) syndromes: Crouzon, Apert, Carpenter, Treacher-Collins, cloverleaf skull, craniotelencephalic dysplasia, arrhinencephaly
(e) microcephaly: brain atrophy / dysgenesis
(f) after shunting procedures

Types:

Sagittal suture most commonly affected followed by coronal suture

1. **Scaphocephaly = Dolichocephaly** (55%)
premature closure of sagittal suture (long skull)
2. **Brachycephaly = Turricephaly** (10%)
premature closure of coronal / lambdoid sutures (short tall skull)
3. **Plagiocephaly** (7%)
unilateral early fusion of coronal + lambdoidal suture (lopsided skull)
4. **Trigonocephaly**: premature closure of metopic suture (forward pointing skull)
5. **Oxycephaly**: premature closure of coronal, sagittal, lambdoid sutures
6. **Cloverleaf skull** = Kleeblattschädel:
intrauterine premature closure of sagittal, coronal, lambdoid sutures;
May be associated with: thanatophoric dwarfism
√ sharply defined thickened sclerotic suture margins
√ delayed growth of BPD in early pregnancy

Wormian bones

= intrasutural ossicles in lambdoid, posterior sagittal, temporosquamosal sutures; normal up to 6 months of age (most frequently)

mnemonic: "PORK CHOPS I"

Pyknodysostosis
Osteogenesis imperfecta
Rickets in healing phase
Kinky hair syndrome
Cleidocranial dysostosis
Hypothyroidism / **H**ypophosphatasia
Otopalatodigital syndrome
Primary acroosteolysis (Hajdu-Cheney) / **P**achydermoperiostosis / **P**rogeria
Syndrome of Down
Idiopathic

Increased skull thickness

A. GENERALIZED
1. Chronic severe anemia (eg, thalassemia, sickle cell disease)
2. Cerebral atrophy following shunting of hydrocephalus
3. Engelmann disease: mainly skull base
4. Hyperparathyroidism
5. Acromegaly
6. Osteopetrosis

B. FOCAL
1. Meningioma
2. Fibrous dysplasia
3. Paget disease
4. Dyke-Davidoff-Mason syndrome
5. Hyperostosis frontalis interna
= dense hyperostosis of inner table of frontal bone; M < F

mnemonic: "HIPFAM"

Hyperostosis frontalis interna
Idiopathic
Paget disease
Fibrous dysplasia
Anemia (sickle cell, iron deficiency, thalassemia, spherocytosis)
Metastases

Hair-on-end skull

mnemonic: "HI NEST"

Hereditary spherocytosis
Iron deficiency anemia
Neuroblastoma
Enzyme deficiency (glucose-6-phosphate dehydrogenase deficiency causes hemolytic anemia)
Sickle cell disease
Thalassemia major

Leontiasis ossea
= overgrowth of facial bones causing leonine (lionlike) facies
1. Fibrous dysplasia
2. Paget disease
3. Craniometaphyseal dysplasia
4. Hyperphosphatasia

Abnormally thin skull
A. GENERALIZED
1. Obstructive hydrocephalus
2. Cleidocranial dysostosis
3. Progeria
4. Rickets
5. Osteogenesis imperfecta
6. Craniolacunia

B. FOCAL
1. Neurofibromatosis
2. Chronic subdural hematoma
3. Arachnoid cyst

Inadequate calvarial calcification
1. Achondroplasia
2. Osteogenesis imperfecta
3. Hypophosphatasia

Osteolytic lesion of skull
A. NORMAL VARIANT
1. Emissary vein
connecting venous systems inside + outside skull
√ bony channel <2 mm in width
2. Venous lake
= outpouching of diploic vein
√ extremely variable in size, shape, and number
√ irregular well-demarcated contour
3. Pacchionian granulations
√ usually multiple lesions with irregular contour in parasagittal location (within 3 cm of superior sagittal sinus) primarily involving the inner table
Associated with: impressions by arachnoid granulations
4. Parietal foramina
nonossification of embryonal rests in parietal fissure; bilateral at superior posterior angles of parietal bone; hereditary transmission

B. TRAUMA
1. Surgical burr hole
2. Leptomeningeal cyst

C. INFECTION
1. Osteomyelitis
2. Hydatid disease
3. Syphilis
4. Tuberculosis

D. CONGENITAL
1. Epidermoid / dermoid
2. Neurofibromatosis (asterion defect)
3. Meningoencephalocele
4. Fibrous dysplasia
5. Osteoporosis circumscripta of Paget disease

E. BENIGN TUMOR
1. Hemangioma
2. Brown tumor
3. Eosinophilic granuloma

F. MALIGNANT TUMOR
1. Solitary / multiple metastases
2. Multiple myeloma
3. Leukemia
4. Neuroblastoma

Solitary lytic lesion ion skull
mnemonic: "HELP MFT HOLE"
Hemangioma
Epidermoid / dermoid
Leptomeningeal cyst
Postop, **P**aget disease
Metastasis, **M**yeloma
Fibrous dysplasia
Tuberculosis
Hyperparathyroidism
Osteomyelitis
Lambdoid defect (neurofibromatosis)
Eosinophilic granuloma

Multiple lytic lesions in skull
mnemonic: "BAMMAH"
Brown tumor
AVM
Myeloma
Metastases
Amyloidosis
Histiocytosis

Lytic area in bone flap
mnemonic: "RATI"
Radiation necrosis
Avascular necrosis
Tumor
Infection

Button sequestrum
mnemonic: "TORE ME"
Tuberculosis
Osteomyelitis
Radiation
Eosinophilic granuloma
Metastasis
Epidermoid

Absent greater sphenoid wing
mnemonic: "M FOR MARINE"
Meningioma
Fibrous dysplasia
Optic glioma
Relapsing hematoma
Metastasis
Aneurysm

Retinoblastoma
Idiopathic
Neurofibromatosis
Eosinophilic granuloma

Absence of innominate line

= OBLIQUE CAROTID LINE
= vertical line projecting into orbit (on PA skull film) produced by orbital process of sphenoid

A. CONGENITAL
   1. Fibrous dysplasia
   2. Neurofibromatosis
B. INFECTION
C. TUMOR

Widened superior orbital fissure

mnemonic: "A FAN"
Aneurysm (internal carotid artery)
Fistula (cavernous sinus)
Adenoma (pituitary)
Neurofibroma

Tumors of the central skull base

A. DEVELOPMENTAL
   1. Encephalocele
B. INFECTION / INFLAMMATION
   1. Extension from paranasal sinus / mastoid infection
   2. Complication of trauma
   3. Fungal disease: mucormycosis in diabetics, aspergillosis in immunosuppressed patients
   4. Sinus + nasopharyngeal sarcoidosis
   5. Radiation necrosis
C. BENIGN
   1. Juvenile angiofibroma
   2. Meningioma
   3. Chordoma
   4. Pituitary tumor
   5. Paget disease
   6. Fibrous dysplasia
D. MALIGNANT
   1. Metastasis: prostate, lung, breast
   2. Chondrosarcoma
   3. Nasopharyngeal carcinoma
   4. Rhabdomyosarcoma
   5. Perineural tumor spread: head + neck neoplasm

CRANIOVERTEBRAL JUNCTION

Craniovertebral junction anomaly

Basilar invagination

= primary developmental anomaly with abnormally high position of vertebral column prolapsing into skull base

Associated with: Chiari malformation, syringohydromyelia in 25–35%

Cause:

1. Condylus tertius = ossicle at distal end of clivus
   √ pseudojoint with odontoid process / anterior arch of C1
2. Condylar hypoplasia
   √ lateral masses of atlas may be fused to condyles
   √ violation of Chamberlain line
   √ widening of atlantooccipital joint axis angle
   √ tip of odontoid >10 mm above bimastoid line
3. Basiocciput hypoplasia
   √ shortening of clivus
   √ violation of Chamberlain line
   √ clivus-canal angle typically decreased
4. Atlantooccipital assimilation
   = complete / partial failure of segmentation between skull + 1st cervical vertebra
   √ violation of Chamberlain line
   √ clivus-canal angle decreased
   May be associated with: fusion of C2 + C3
   Cx: atlantoaxial subluxation (50%); sudden death

• limitation in range of motion of CVJ
√ abnormal craniometry
√ C-spine + foramen magnum bulge into cranial cavity
√ elevation of posterior arch of C1

Basilar impression

= acquired form of basilar invagination with bulging of C-spine and foramen magnum into cranial cavity

Cause: Paget disease, Osteomalacia, rickets, fibrous dysplasia, hyperparathyroidism, Hurler syndrome, osteogenesis imperfecta, skull base infection

mnemonic: "PF ROACH"
Paget disease
Fibrous dysplasia
Rickets
Osteogenesis imperfecta, **O**steomalacia
Achondroplasia
Cleidocranial dysplasia
Hyperparathyroidism, **H**urler syndrome

Platybasia

= anthropometric term referring to flattening of skull base

May be associated with: basilar invagination

• cord symptoms
√ craniovertebral = clivus-canal angle becomes acute (<150°)
√ Welcher basal angle = sphenoid angle >140°
√ bowstring deformity of cervicomedullary junction

ATLAS AND AXIS

Atlas anomalies

A. POSTERIOR ARCH ANOMALIES
   1. Posterior atlas arch rachischisis (4%)
      Location: midline (97%), lateral through sulcus of vertebral artery (3%)
      √ absence of arch-canal line (LAT view)
      √ superimposed on odontoid process / axis body simulating a fracture (open-mouth odontoid view)

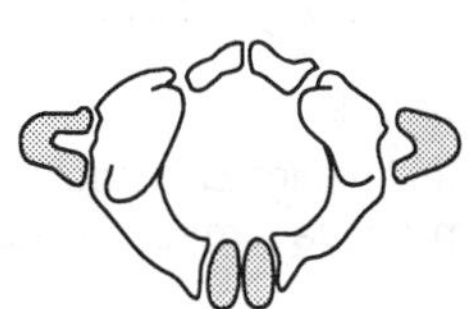
Atlas Ossification Center
secondary centers

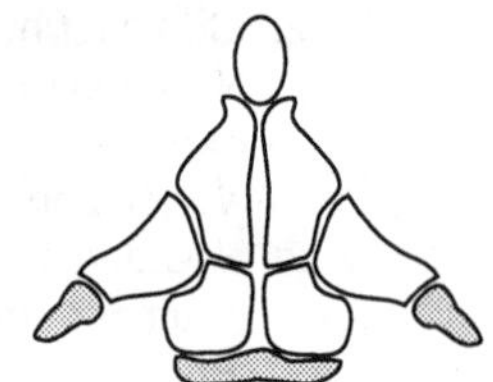
Axis Ossification Center
secondary centers

2. Total aplasia of posterior atlas arch
3. Keller-type aplasia with persistence of posterior tubercle
4. Aplasia with uni- / bilateral remnant + midline rachischisis
5. Partial / total hemiaplasia of posterior arch

B. ANTERIOR ARCH ANOMALIES
1. Isolated anterior arch rachischisis (0.1%)
2. Split atlas = anterior + posterior arch rachischisis
   √ plump rounded anterior arch overlapping the odontoid process making identification of predental space impossible (LAT view)
   √ duplicated anterior margins (LAT view)

Axis anomalies
1. Persistent ossiculum terminale = Bergman ossicle
   √ unfused odontoid process >12 years of age
   DDx: type 1 odontoid fracture
2. Odontoid aplasia (extremely rare)
3. Os odontoideum
   = independent os cephalad to axis body in location of odontoid process
   √ absence of odontoid process
   √ anterior arch of atlas hypertrophic + situated too far posterior in relation to axis body
   Cx: atlantoaxial instability
   DDx: type 2 odontoid fracture (uncorticated margin)

Odontoid erosion
mnemonic: "P LARD"
Psoriasis
Lupus erythematosus
Ankylosing spondylitis
Rheumatoid arthritis
Down syndrome

Atlantoaxial subluxation
= displacement of atlas with respect to axis
(1) Posterior atlantoaxial subluxation (rare)
(2) Anterior atlantoaxial subluxation (common)
   = distance between dens + anterior arch of C1 (measurement along midplane of atlas on lateral view):
   (a) predental space: >2.5 mm; >4.5 mm (in children)
   (b) retrodental space: <18 mm

Causes of subluxation:
(a) Congenital
   1. Occipitalization of atlas
      0.75% of population; fusion of basion + anterior arch of atlas
   2. Congenital insufficiency of transverse ligament
   3. Os odontoideum / aplasia of dens
   4. Down syndrome (20%)
   5. Morquio syndrome
   6. Bone dysplasia
(b) Arthritis
   due to laxity of transverse ligament or erosion of dens
   1. Rheumatoid arthritis
   2. Psoriatic arthritis
   3. Reiter syndrome
   4. Ankylosing spondylitis
   5. SLE
   rare: in gout + CPPD
(c) Inflammatory process
   Pharyngeal infection in childhood, retropharyngeal abscess, coryza, otitis media, mastoiditis, cervical adenitis, parotitis, alveolar abscess
   √ dislocation 8–10 days after onset of symptoms
(d) Trauma (very rare without odontoid fracture)
(e) Marfan disease

mnemonic: "JAP LARD"
Juvenile rheumatoid arthritis
Ankylosing spondylitis
Psoriatic arthritis
Lupus erythematosus
Accident (trauma)
Retropharyngeal abscess, **R**heumatoid arthritis
Down syndrome

PSEUDOSUBLUXATION
= ligamentous laxity in infants allows for movement of the vertebral bodies on each other, esp. C2 on C3

SPINAL DYSRAPHISM
= abnormal / incomplete fusion of midline embryologic mesenchymal, neurologic, bony structures

External signs (in 50%)
- subcutaneous lipoma
- hypertrichosis
- pigmented nevi
- skin dimple
- bladder + bowel dysfunction
- pathologic plantar response
- spastic gait disturbance
- foot deformities
- absent tendon reflexes
- sinus tract

Spina bifida
= incomplete closure of bony elements of the spine (lamina + spinous processes) posteriorly

Spina bifida occulta
= OCCULT SPINAL DYSRAPHISM
= skin covered defect; 15% of spinal dysraphism
- rarely leads to neurologic deficit in itself

Associated with:
vertebral defect (85 – 90%), lumbosacral dermal lesion (80%), ie, hairy tuft, dimple, sinus, nevus, hyperpigmentation, hemangioma, subcutaneous mass

1. Diastematomyelia
2. Lipomeningocele
3. Tethered cord syndrome
4. Filum terminale lipoma
5. Intraspinal dermoid
6. Epidermoid cyst
7. Myelocystocele
8. Split notochord syndrome
9. Meningocele
10. Dorsal dermal sinus
11. Tight filum terminale syndrome

Spina bifida aperta

= SPINA BIFIDA CYSTICA
= posterior protrusion of all / parts of the contents of the spinal canal through a bony spina bifida; 85% of spinal dysraphism

• associated with neurologic deficit in >90%

1. Simple meningocele
   = herniation of CSF-filled sac without neural elements
2. Myelocele
   = midline plaque of neural tissue lying exposed at the skin surface
3. Myelomeningocele
   = a myelocele elevated above skin surface by expansion of subarachnoid space ventral to neural plaque
4. Myeloschisis
   = surface presentation of neural elements completely uncovered by meninges

Segmentation anomalies of vertebral bodies

during 9 – 12th week of gestation two ossification centers form for the ventral + dorsal half of vertebral body

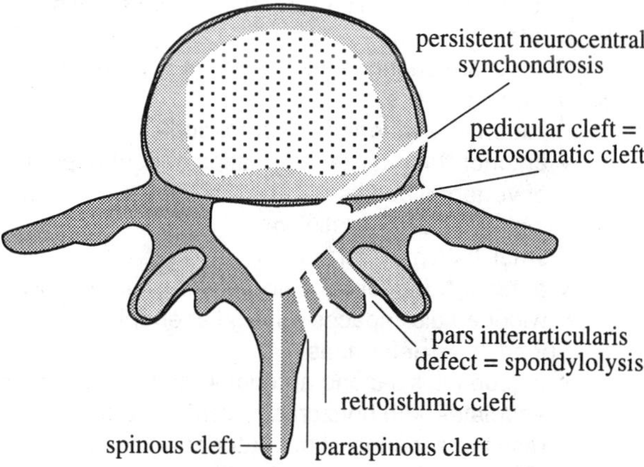

Clefts in Neural Arch

1. **Asomia** = agenesis of vertebral body
   √ complete absence of vertebral body
   √ hypoplastic posterior elements may be present
2. **Hemivertebra**
   (a) Unilateral wedge vertebra
      √ right / left hemivertebra
      √ scoliosis at birth
   (b) Dorsal hemivertebra
      √ rapidly progressive kyphoscoliosis
   (c) Ventral hemivertebra (extremely rare)
3. **Coronal cleft**
   = failure of fusion of anterior + posterior ossification centers
   May be associated with: premature male infant, Chondrodystrophia calcificans congenita
   Location: usually in lower thoracic + lumbar spine
   √ vertical radiolucent band just behind midportion of vertebral body; disappears mostly by 6 months of life
4. **Butterfly vertebra**
   = failure of fusion of lateral halves secondary to persistence of notochordal tissue
   May be associated with: anterior spina bifida ± anterior meningocele
   √ widened vertebral body with butterfly configuration (AP view)
   √ adaptation of vertebral endplates of adjacent vertebral bodies
5. **Block vertebra**
   = congenital vertebral fusion
   Location: lumbar / cervical
   √ height of fused vertebral bodies equals the sum of heights of involved bodies + intervertebral disk
   √ "waist" at level of intervertebral disk space
6. Hypoplastic vertebra
7. Klippel-Feil syndrome

VERTEBRAL BODY

Small vertebral body

1. Radiation therapy
   during early childhood in excess of 1000 rads
2. Juvenile rheumatoid arthritis
   Location: cervical spine
   √ atlantoaxial subluxation may be present
   √ vertebral fusion may occur
3. Eosinophilic granuloma
   Location: lumbar / lower thoracic spine
   √ compression deformity / vertebra plana
4. Gaucher disease
   = deposits of glucocerebrosides within RES
   √ compression deformity
5. Platyspondyly generalisata
   = flattened vertebral bodies associated with many hereditary systemic disorders (achondroplasia, spondyloepiphyseal dysplasia tarda, mucopolysaccharidosis, osteopetrosis, neurofibromatosis, osteogenesis imperfecta, thanatophoric dwarfism)
   √ disk spaces of normal height

VERTEBRA PLANA
mnemonic: " FETISH"
Fracture (trauma, osteogenesis imperfecta)
Eosinophilic granuloma
Tumor (metastasis, myeloma, leukemia)
Infection
Steroids (avascular necrosis)
Hemangioma

Signs of acute vertebral collapse on MRI

1. OSTEOPOROSIS
   √ retropulsion of posterior bone fragment
2. MALIGNANCY
   √ epidural soft-tissue mass
   √ no residual normal marrow signal intensity
   √ abnormal enhancement

Enlarged vertebral body

1. Paget disease
   √ "picture framing"; bone sclerosis
2. Gigantism
   √ increase in height of body + disk
3. Myositis ossificans progressiva
   √ bodies greater in height than width
   √ osteoporosis
   √ ossification of ligamentum nuchae

Enlarged vertebral foramen

1. Neurofibroma
2. Congenital absence / hypoplasia of pedicle
3. Dural ectasia (Marfan syndrome, Ehlers-Danlos syndrome)
4. Intraspinal neoplasm
5. Metastatic destruction of pedicle

Cervical spine fusion

mnemonic: "SPAR BIT"
Senile hypertrophic ankylosis (DISH)
Psoriasis, **P**rogressive myositis ossificans
Ankylosing spondylitis
Reiter disease, **R**heumatoid arthritis (juvenile)
Block vertebra (Klippel-Feil)
Infection (TB)
Trauma

Vertebral border abnormality

Straightening of anterior border

1. Ankylosing spondylitis
2. Paget disease
3. Psoriatic arthritis
4. Reiter disease
5. Rheumatoid arthritis
6. Normal variant

Anterior scalloping of vertebrae

1. Aortic aneurysm
2. Lymphadenopathy
3. Tuberculosis
4. Multiple myeloma (paravertebral soft-tissue mass)

Posterior scalloping of vertebrae

in conditions associated with dural ectasia

A. INCREASED INTRASPINAL PRESSURE
   1. Communicating hydrocephalus
   2. Ependymoma
B. MESENCHYMAL TISSUE LAXITY
   1. Neurofibromatosis (secondary to dural ectasia / spinal tumor)
   2. Marfan syndrome
   3. Ehlers-Danlos syndrome
   4. Posterior meningocele
C. BONE SOFTENING
   1. Mucopolysaccharidoses: Hurler, Morquio, Sanfilippo
   2. Acromegaly (lumbar vertebrae)
   3. Ankylosing spondylitis (lax dura acting on osteoporotic vertebrae)
   4. Achondroplasia

mnemonic: "DAMN MALE SHAME"
Dermoid
Ankylosing spondylitis
Meningioma
Neurofibromatosis

Marfan syndrome
Acromegaly
Lipoma
Ependymoma

Syringohydromyelia
Hydrocephalus
Achondroplasia
Mucopolysaccharidoses
Ehlers-Danlos syndrome

Bony projections from vertebra

1. Hurler syndrome = gargoylism
   √ rounded appearance of vertebral bodies
   √ mild kyphotic curve with smaller vertebral body at apex of kyphosis displaying tonguelike beak at anterior half (usually at T12 / L1)
   √ "step-off" deformities along anterior margins
2. Hunter syndrome
   less severe changes than in Hurler syndrome
3. Morquio disease
   √ flattened + widened vertebral bodies
   √ anterior "tonguelike" elongation of central portion of vertebral bodies
4. Hypothyroidism = cretinism
   √ small flat vertebral bodies
   √ anterior "tonguelike" deformity (in children only)
   √ widened disk spaces + irregular endplates
5. Spondylosis deformans
   √ osteophytosis along anterior + lateral aspects of endplates with horizontal + vertical course as a result of shearing of the outer annular fibers (Sharpey fibers connecting the annulus fibrosus to adjacent vertebral body)

6. Diffuse idiopathic skeletal hyperostosis (DISH)
   = Forestier disease
   √ flowing calcifications + ossifications along anterolateral aspect of >4 contiguous thoracic vertebral bodies ± osteophytosis
7. Ankylosing spondylitis
   √ bilateral symmetric syndesmophytes (ossification of annulus fibrosus)
   √ "bamboo spine"
   √ "discal ballooning" = biconvex intervertebral disks secondary to osteoporotic deformity of endplates
   √ straightening of anterior margins of vertebral bodies (erosion)
   √ ossification of paraspinal ligaments
8. Fluorosis
   √ vertebral osteophytosis + hyperostosis
   √ sclerotic vertebral bodies + kyphoscoliosis
   √ calcification of paraspinal ligaments

Spine ossification

1. Syndesmophyte = ossification of annulus fibrosus
   Associated with: ankylosing spondylitis, ochronosis
2. Osteophyte
   = ossification of anterior longitudinal ligament
   Associated with: osteoarthritis
3. Flowing anterior ossification
   = ossification of disk, anterior longitudinal ligament, paravertebral soft tissues
   Associated with: diffuse idiopathic skeletal hyperostosis
4. Paravertebral ossification
   Associated with: psoriatic arthritis, Reiter syndrome

Vertebral endplate abnormality

1. Osteoporosis (senile / steroid-induced)
   √ "fish-mouth vertebrae" (DDx: osteomalacia, Paget disease, hyperparathyroidism)
   √ bone sclerosis along endplates
2. Sickle cell disease
   √ "H-vertebrae" = compression of central portions from subchondral infarcts (DDx: other anemias, Gaucher disease)
3. Schmorl node
   = intraosseous herniation of nucleus pulposus at center of weakened endplate in disk herniation / Scheuermann disease
4. Limbus vertebrae
   = intraosseous herniation of disk material at junction of vertebral bony rim of centra + endplate (anterosuperior corner)
5. "Ring" epiphysis
   = normal aspect of developing vertebra (between 6 and 12 years of age)
   √ small steplike recess at corner of anterior edge of vertebral body
6. Renal osteodystrophy
   √ "rugger-jersey spine" = horizontal bands of increased opacity subjacent to vertebral endplates
7. Myelofibrosis
   √ "rugger-jersey spine"
8. Osteopetrosis
   √ "sandwich" / "hamburger" vertebrae = sclerotic endplates alternate with radiolucent midportions of vertebral bodies

Bullet-shaped vertebral body

mnemonic: "HAM"
- **H**ypothyroidism
- **A**chondroplasia
- **M**orquio syndrome

Bone-within-bone vertebra

= "ghost vertebra" following stressful event during vertebral growth phase in childhood

1. Stress line of unknown cause
2. Leukemia
3. Heavy metal poisoning
4. Thorotrast injection, TB
5. Rickets
6. Scurvy
7. Hypothyroidism
8. Hypoparathyroidism

Ivory vertebra

mnemonic: "LOST FROM CHOMP"
- **L**ymphoma
- **O**steopetrosis
- **S**ickle cell disease
- **T**rauma
- **F**luorosis
- **R**enal osteodystrophy
- **O**steoblastic metastasis
- **M**yelosclerosis
- **C**hronic sclerosing osteomyelitis
- **H**emangioma
- **O**steosarcoma
- **M**yeloma
- **P**aget disease

TUMORS OF VERTEBRA

Expansile lesion of vertebrae

A. INVOLVEMENT OF MULTIPLE VERTEBRAE
   Metastases, multiple myeloma / plasmacytoma, lymphoma, hemangioma, Paget disease, angiosarcoma, eosinophilic granuloma
B. INVOLVEMENT OF TWO / MORE CONTIGUOUS VERTEBRAE
   Osteochondroma, chordoma, aneurysmal bone cyst, myeloma
C. BENIGN LESION
   1. Osteochondroma (1–5% with solitary osteochondromas, 7–9% with hereditary multiple exostoses) commonly cervical, esp. C2; commonly rising from posterior elements

2. Osteoblastoma (30–40% in spine)
   M:F = 2:1; equal distribution in spine; posterior elements (lamina, pedicle), may involve body if large; expansile lesion with sclerotic / shell-like rim, foci of calcified tumor matrix in 50%
3. Giant cell tumor (5–7% in spine)
   commonly sacrum, expansile lytic lesion of vertebral body with well-defined borders; secondary invasion of posterior elements; malignant degeneration in 5–20% after radiation therapy
4. Osteoid osteoma (10–25% in spine)
   commonly lower thoracic / upper lumbar spine, posterior elements (pedicle, lamina, spinous process), painful scoliosis with concavity toward lesion
5. Aneurysmal bone cyst (12–30% in spine)
   thoracic > lumbar > cervical spine, posterior elements with frequent extension into vertebral bodies, well-defined margins, may arise from primary bone lesion (giant cell tumor, fibrous dysplasia) in 50%, may involve two contiguous vertebrae
6. Hemangioma (30% in spine)
   10% incidence in general population; commonly lower thoracic / upper lumbar spine, vertebral body, "accordion" / "corduroy" appearance
7. Hydatid cyst (1% in spine)
   slow-growing destructive lesion, well-defined sclerotic borders, endemic areas
8. Paget disease
   vertebral body ± posterior elements, enlargement of bone, "picture framing"; bone sclerosis
9. Eosinophilic granuloma (6% in spine)
   most often cervical / lumbar spine, vertebral body, "vertebra plana"; multiple involvement common
10. Fibrous dysplasia (1% in spine)
    vertebral body, nonhomogeneous trabecular "ground glass" appearance
11. Enostosis (1–14% in spine)
    Location: T1–T7 > L2–L3

D. MALIGNANT
1. Chordoma (15% in spine)
   most common nonlymphoproliferative primary malignant tumor of the spine in adults; particularly C2, within vertebral body; violates disk space
2. Metastases (especially from lung, breast)
   Age: >50 years of age;
   Clue: pedicles often destroyed
3. Multiple myeloma / plasmacytoma
   Clue: vertebral pedicles usually spared
4. Angiosarcoma
   10% involve spine, most commonly lumbar
5. Chondrosarcoma (3–12% in spine)
   2nd most common nonlymphoproliferative primary malignant tumor of the spine in adults
   Site: vertebral body (15%), posterior elements (40%), both (45%)
   √ involvement of adjacent vertebra by extension through disk (35%)
6. Ewing sarcoma and PNET
   most common nonlymphoproliferative primary malignant tumor of the spine in children; metastases more common than primary
   Site: vertebral body with extension to posterior elements
   √ diffuse sclerosis + osteonecrosis (69%)
7. Osteosarcoma (0.6–3.2% in spine)
   Average age: 4th decade
   Location: lumbosacral segments
   Site: vertebral body, posterior elements (10–17%)
   √ may present as "ivory vertebra"
8. Lymphoma

Blowout lesion of posterior elements
mnemonic: "GO APE"
Giant cell tumor
Osteoblastoma
Aneurysmal bone cyst
Plasmacytoma
Eosinophilic granuloma

Bone tumors favoring vertebral bodies
mnemonic: "CALL HOME"
Chordoma
Aneurysmal bone cyst
Leukemia
Lymphoma
Hemangioma
Osteoid osteoma, **O**steoblastoma
Myeloma, **M**etastasis
Eosinophilic granuloma

Primary vertebral tumors in children
in order of frequency:
1. Osteoid osteoma
2. Benign osteoblastoma
3. Aneurysmal bone cyst
4. Ewing sarcoma

Primary tumor of posterior elements
mnemonic: "A HOG"
Aneurysmal bone cyst
Hydatid cyst, **H**emangioma
Osteoblastoma, **O**steoid osteoma
Giant cell tumor

INTERVERTEBRAL DISK

Vacuum phenomenon in intervertebral disk space
= liberation of nitrogen gas from surrounding tissues into clefts with an abnormal nucleus or annulus attachment
Incidence: in up to 20% of plain radiographs / in up to 50% of spinal CT in patients > age 40

Cause:
1. Primary / secondary degeneration of nucleus pulposus
2. Intraosseous herniation of disk (= Schmorl node)
3. Spondylosis deformans
4. Adjacent vertebral metastatic disease with vertebral collapse
5. Infection (extremely rare)

Intervertebral disk calcification

mnemonic: " A DISC SO WHITE"

Amyloidosis, **A**cromegaly
Degenerative
Infection
Spinal fusion
CPPD
Spondylitis ankylosing
Ochronosis
Wilson disease
Hemochromatosis, **H**omocystinuria, **H**yperparathyroidism
Idiopathic skeletal hyperostosis
Traumatic
Etceteras: Gout and other causes of chondrocalcinosis

Intervertebral disk ossification

Associated with: fusion of vertebral bodies
1. Ankylosing spondylitis
2. Ochronosis
3. Sequela of trauma
4. Sequela of disk-space infection
5. Degenerative disease

Schmorl node

= chondrification defects where periosteal vessels penetrate cartilage plates of disk
√ concave defects at upper and lower vertebral endplates with sharp margins produced by superior / inferior herniation of disk material

MR:
- √ node of similar signal intensity as disk
- √ low signal intensity of rim
- √ associated with narrowed disk space

DDx: mnemonic: "SHOOT"
Scheuermann disease
Hyperparathyroidism
Osteoporosis
Osteomalacia
Trauma

SPINAL CORD

Intramedullary lesion

15% of spinal canal tumors in adults; 6% of spinal cord tumors in children (1/3 of spinal neoplasms in childhood)

A. TUMOR
  (a) primary:
    1. Ependymoma (60% of all spinal cord tumors)
    2. Astrocytoma (25%)
    3. Oligodendroglioma (3%)
    4. Epidermoid, dermoid, teratoma (1–2%)
    5. Lipoma (1%)

    Location: — cervical region: astrocytoma
    — thoracic region: teratoma-dermoid, astrocytoma
    — lumbar region: ependymoma, dermoid
  (b) metastatic: eg, malignant melanoma, breast, lung

B. CYSTIC LESION
  may show delayed filling of cystic space on CT-myelography
  1. Syringomyelia
  2. Hydromyelia
  3. Reactive cyst
  4. Hemangioblastoma (2 – 4%)

C. VASCULAR
  1. Cord concussion = reversible local edema
  2. Hemorrhagic contusion
  3. Cord transection
  4. AVM

D. CHRONIC INFECTION
  1. Sarcoid
  2. Transverse myelitis
  3. Multiple sclerosis

mnemonic: "I'M ASHAMED"
Inflammation (multiple sclerosis, sarcoidosis, myelitis)
Medulloblastoma
Astrocytoma
Syringomyelia / hydromyelia
Hematoma, **H**emangioblastoma
Arteriovenous malformation
Metastasis
Ependymoma
Dermoid

Intradural extramedullary mass

1. Neurofibroma (25–35%)
2. Meningioma (25–45% of all spinal tumors)
3. Lipoma
4. Dermoid
   commonly conus / cauda equina; associated with spinal dysraphism (1/3)
5. Ependymoma
   commonly filum terminale; NO spinal dysraphism
6. "Drop metastases" from CNS tumors
7. Metastases from outside CNS
8. Arachnoid cyst
9. Neurenteric cyst
10. Hemangioblastoma

mnemonic: "MAMA N"
Metastasis
Arachnoiditis
Meningioma
AVM, **A**rachnoid cyst
Neurofibroma

Epidural extramedullary lesion

Epidural space = space between dura mater + bone containing epidural venous plexus, lymphatic channels, connective tissue, fat

Incidence: 30% of all spinal tumors

A. TUMOR
  (a) benign
    1. Dermoid, epidermoid
    2. Lipoma: over several segments
    3. Fibroma
    4. Neurinoma (with intradural component)
    5. Meningioma (with intradural component)
    6. Ganglioneuroblastoma, ganglioneuroma
  (b) malignant
    1. Hodgkin disease
    2. Lymphoma: most commonly in dorsal space
    3. Metastasis: breast, lung — most commonly from involved vertebrae without extension through dura
    4. Paravertebral neuroblastoma
B. DISK DISEASE
  1. Bulging disk
  2. Herniated nucleus pulposus
  3. Sequestered nucleus pulposus
C. OSSEOUS: spinal stenosis, spondylosis
D. INFLAMMATION: epidural abscess
E. HEMATOMA
F. SYNOVIAL CYST

mnemonic: "MANDELIN"
Metastasis (drop mets from CNS tumor), **M**eningioma
Arachnoiditis, **A**rachnoid cyst
Neurofibroma
Dermoid / epidermoid
Ependymoma
Lipoma
Infection (TB, Cysticercosis)
Normal but tortuous roots

Tumors of nerve roots and nerve sheaths

= NEURINOMA

A. ARISING FROM NERVE SHEATH
  1. **Schwannoma**
     = encapsulated benign slowly growing neoplasm arising from Schwann cells
     Schwann cell = cell that surrounds cranial, spinal, and peripheral nerves producing myelin sheath around axons thus providing mechanical protection, serving as a tract for nerve regeneration
     ◊ NOTE that myelin sheaths within brain substance are made by oligodendrocytes!
     ◊ Usually sporadic tumor, but 5 – 20% of patients with solitary intracranial schwannomas have type 2 neurofibromatosis!
     Histo: cellular component (Antoni type A tissue) + myxoid component (Antoni type B tissue)
     Location:
       (a) extracranial: (most commonly) cervical spine roots, vagus nerve, sympathetic plexus
       (b) intracranial: mostly from sensory nerves, vestibulocochlear (VIII) cranial nerve (most common), trigeminal (V) cranial nerve (2nd most common)
     √ solitary fusiform well-encapsulated lesion
     MR:
       √ dark line surrounding the lesion (= capsule) frequently seen
  2. **Neurofibroma**
     = tumor of nerve sheath composed of Schwann cells + fibroblasts with involvement of nerve, nerve fibers run through mass
     Histo: swirls of neuronal elements
     Associated with: neurofibromatosis type 1;
     M:F = 1:1
     ◊ Potential for malignant transformation!
     ◊ The spinal neurofibroma is rarely sporadic and usually a sign of type 1 neurofibromatosis!
     ◊ Only 10% of patients with neurofibromas have von Recklinghausen disease!
     Location: any level, but particularly cervical
     (a) peripheral nerves
       √ nonencapsulated well-circumscribed fusiform mass of peripheral nerves
     (b) intradural extramedullary mass
       √ well-defined mass with dumbbell configuration (= extradural component extends through neural foramen)
       √ widening of intervertebral foramen + erosion of pedicles
       √ scalloping of vertebral bodies
       √ hypodense (CHARACTERISTIC) approaching characteristics of water / isodense to skeletal muscle
       √ usually NO contrast enhancement
       MR:
         √ homogeneous mass isointense to cord on T1WI
         √ hyperintense tumor on T2WI compared with surrounding fat
         √ "target sign" = low signal-intensity center on T2WI (due to collagen + condensed Schwann cells)
     DDx: conjoined nerve root sleeve
B. ORIGINATING FROM NERVE
  1. **Neuroma**
     = posttraumatic lesion forming at end of severed nerve
  2. **Neurilemmoma**
     = nerve fibers diverge and course over the surface of the tumor mass

Cord lesions

A. INFLAMMATION
  1. Multiple sclerosis
  2. Acute disseminated encephalomyelitis

3. Acute transverse myelitis
   √ involves half the cross-sectional area of cord
4. Lyme disease
5. Devic syndrome

B. INFECTION
1. Cytomegalovirus
2. Progressive multifocal leukoencephalopathy
3. HIV

C. VASCULAR
1. Anterior spinal artery infarct
   √ affects central gray matter first
   √ extends to anterior two-thirds of cord
2. Venous infarct / ischemia
   √ starts centrally progressing centripetally

D. NEOPLASM

Cord atrophy
1. Multiple sclerosis
2. Amyotrophic lateral sclerosis
3. Cervical spondylosis
4. Sequelae of trauma
5. Ischemia
6. Radiation therapy
7. AVM of cord

Delayed uptake of water-soluble contrast in cord lesion
1. Syringohydromyelia
2. Cystic tumor of cord
3. Osteomalacia

exceedingly rare:
4. Demyelinating disease
5. Infection
6. Infarction

Extra-arachnoid myelography
A. SUBDURAL INJECTION
√ spinal cord, nerve roots, blood vessels not outlined
√ irregular filling defects
√ slow flow of contrast material
√ CSF pulsations diminished
√ contrast material pools at injection site within anterior / posterior compartments

B. EPIDURAL INJECTION
√ contrast extravasation along nerve roots
√ contrast material lies near periphery of spinal canal
√ intraspinal structures are not well outlined

SACRUM

Destructive sacral lesion
mnemonic: "SPACEMON"

Sarcoma
Plasmacytoma
Aneurysmal bone cyst
Chordoma
Ependymoma
Metastasis
Osteomyelitis
Neuroblastoma

Sacral neoplasms
1. Metastases from breast, prostate, kidney, cervix, colon
2. Multiple myeloma
3. Chordoma (most common primary)
4. Giant cell tumor (most common benign tumor)
5. Sacrococcygeal teratoma

SPINAL FIXATION DEVICES

Function:
(1) to restore anatomic alignment in fractures (fracture reduction)
(2) to stabilize degenerative disease
(3) to correct congenital deformities (scoliosis)
(4) to replace diseased / abnormal vertebrae (infection, tumor)

Posterior fixation devices
using paired / unpaired rods attached with

1. Sublaminar wiring
   = passing a wire around lamina + rod
2. Interspinous wiring
   = passing a wire through a hole in the spinous process; a Drummond button prevents the wire from pulling through the bone
3. Subpars wiring
   = passing a wire around the pars interarticularis
4. Laminar / sublaminar hooks
   used on rods for compression / distraction forces to be applied to pedicles / laminae
   (a) upgoing hook curves under lamina
   (b) downgoing hook curves over lamina
5. Pedicle / transpedical screws
6. Rods
   (a) Luque rod = straight / L-shaped smooth rod 6–8 mm in diameter
   (b) O-ring fixator, rhomboid-shaped bar, Luque rectangle, segmental rectangle = preshaped loop to form a flat rectangle
   (c) Harrington distraction rod
   (d) Harrington compression rod
   (e) Knodt rod = threaded distraction rod with a central fixed nut (turnbuckle) and opposing thread pattern
   (f) Cotrel-Dubousset rods = a pair of rods with a serrated surface connected by a cross-link with ≥4 laminar hooks / pedicle screws
7. Plates
   (a) Roy-Camille plates
   = simple straight plates with round holes
   (b) Luque plates
   = long oval holes with clips encircling the plate
   (c) Steffee plates = straight plates with long slots
8. Translaminar screw
   = cancellous screws for single level fusion
9. Percutaneous pinning
   = (hollow) interference screws placed across disk level

Anterior fixation devices

1. Dwyer device
   = screws threaded into vertebral body over staples embedded into vertebral body connected by braided titanium wire; placed on convex side of spine
2. Zielke device
   = modified Dwyer system replacing cable with solid rod
3. Kaneda device
   = 2 curved vertebral plates with staples attached to vertebral bodies with screws, plates connected by 2 threaded rods attached to screw heads
4. Dunn device
   (similar to Kaneda device, discontinued)

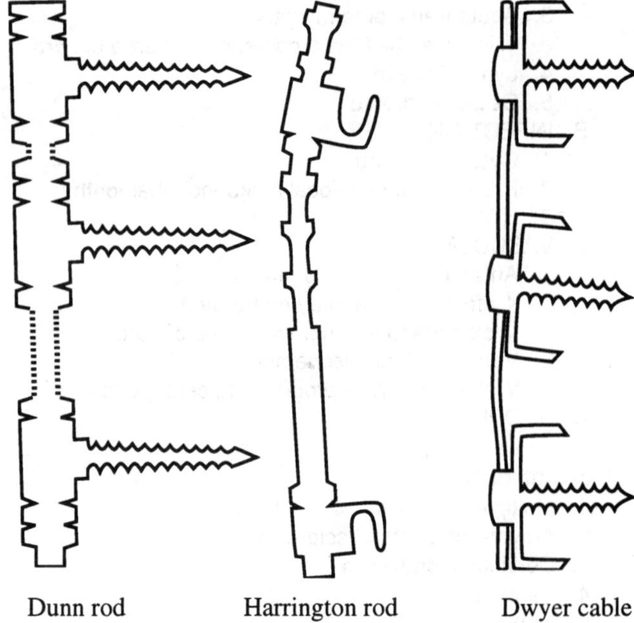

Dunn rod Harrington rod Dwyer cable

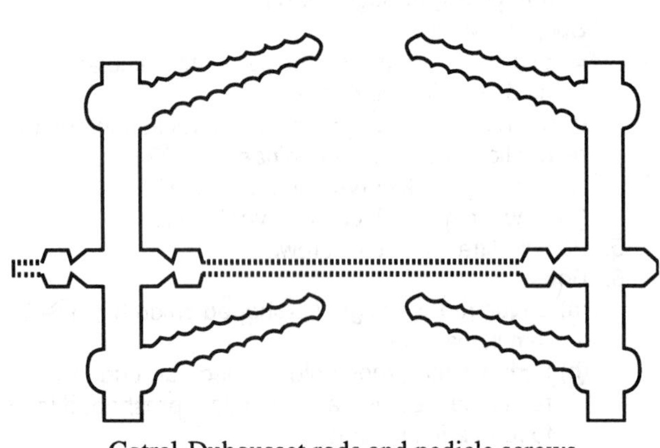

Cotrel-Dubousset rods and pedicle screws

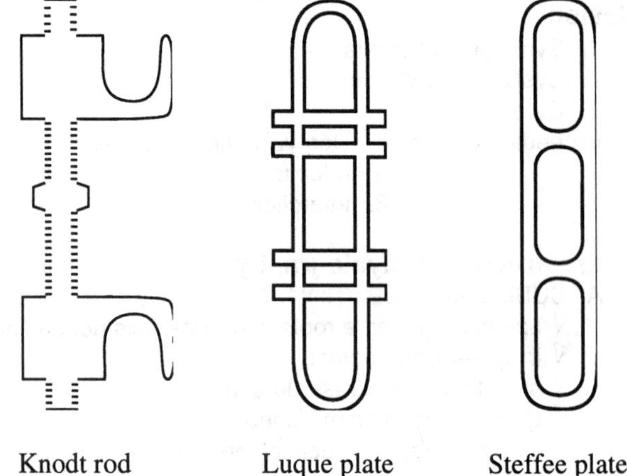

Knodt rod Luque plate Steffee plate

ANATOMY OF SKULL AND SPINE

FORAMINA OF BASE OF SKULL

on inner aspect of middle cranial fossa 3 foramina are oriented along an oblique line in the greater sphenoidal wing from anteromedial behind the superior orbital fissure to posterolateral

mnemonic: "rotos"

foramen **rot**undum
foramen **o**vale
foramen **s**pinosum

Foramen rotundum

= canal within greater sphenoid wing connecting middle cranial fossa + pterygopalatine fossa

Location: inferior and lateral to superior orbital fissure

Course: extends obliquely forward + slightly inferiorly in a sagittal direction parallel to superior orbital fissure

Contents:

(a) nerves: V_2 (maxillary nerve)
(b) vessels: (1) artery of foramen rotundum
(2) emissary vv.

√ best visualized by coronal CT

Foramen ovale

= canal connecting middle cranial fossa + infratemporal fossa

Location: medial aspect of sphenoid body, situated posterolateral to foramen rotundum (endocranial aspect) + at base of lateral pterygoid plate (exocranial aspect)

Contents:

(a) nerves: (1) V_3 (mandibular nerve)
(2) lesser petrosal nerve (occasionally)
(b) vessels: (1) accessory meningeal artery
(2) emissary vv.

Foramen spinosum

Location: on greater sphenoid wing posterolateral to foramen ovale (endocranial aspect) + lateral to eustachian tube (exocranial aspect)

Contents:

(a) nerves: (1) recurrent meningeal branch of mandibular nerve
(2) lesser superficial petrosal nerve
(b) vessels: (1) middle meningeal a.
(2) middle meningeal v.

Foramen lacerum

Fibrocartilage cover (occasionally), carotid artery rests on endocranial aspect of fibrocartilage

Location: at base of medial pterygoid plate

Contents: (inconstant)

(a) nerve: nerve of pterygoid canal (actually pierces cartilage)
(b) vessel: meningeal branch of ascending pharyngeal a.

Foramen magnum

Contents:

(a) nerves: (1) medulla oblongata
(2) cranial nerve XI (spinal accessory n.)
(b) vessels: (1) vertebral a.
(2) anterior spinal a.
(3) posterior spinal a.

Pterygoid canal

= VIDIAN CANAL
= within sphenoid body connecting pterygopalatine fossa anteriorly to foramen lacerum posteriorly

Location: at base of pterygoid plate below foramen rotundum

Contents:

(a) nerves: Vidian nerve = nerve of pterygoid canal
= continuation of greater superficial petrosal nerve (from cranial nerve VII) after its union with deep petrosal nerve
(b) vessel: Vidian artery = artery of pterygoid canal
= branch of terminal portion of internal maxillary a. arises in pterygopalatine fossa + passes through foramen lacerum posterior to Vidian n.

Hypoglossal canal

= ANTERIOR CONDYLAR CANAL

Location: in posterior cranial fossa anteriorly above condyle starting above anterolateral part of foramen magnum, continuing in an anterolateral direction + exiting medial to jugular foramen

Contents:

(a) nerves: cranial nerve XII (hypoglossal nerve)
(b) vessels: (1) pharyngeal artery
(2) branches of meningeal artery

Jugular foramen

Location: at the posterior end of petro-occipital suture directly posterior to carotid orifice

(a) anterior part:
(1) inferior petrosal sinus
(2) meningeal branches of pharyngeal artery + occipital artery
(b) intermediate part:
(1) cranial nerve IX (glossopharyngeal nerve)
(2) cranial nerve X (vagus nerve)
(3) cranial nerve XI (spinal accessory nerve)
(c) posterior part: internal jugular vein

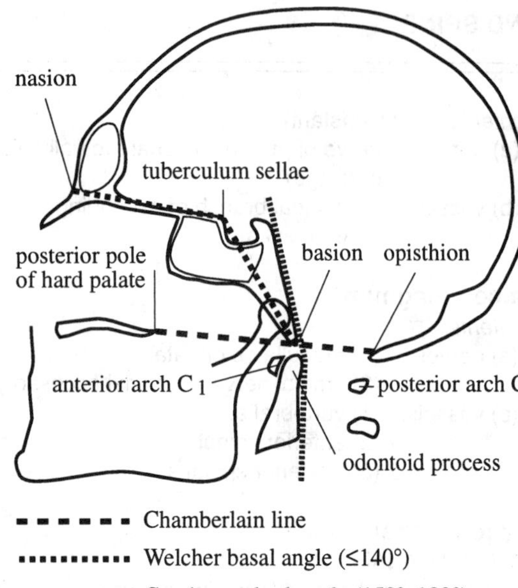

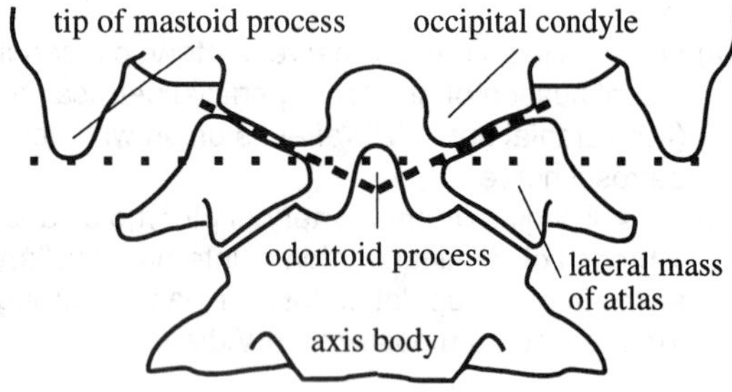

CRANIOVERTEBRAL JUNCTION

Craniometry:

— LATERAL VIEW

1. **Chamberlain line** = line between posterior pole of hard palate + opisthion (= posterior margin of foramen magnum)
   √ tip of odontoid process usually lies below / tangent to Chamberlain line
   √ tip of odontoid process may lie up to 1 ± 6.6 mm above the Chamberlain line
2. **McGregor line** = line between posterior pole of hard palate + most caudal portion of occipital squamosal surface
   ◊ substitute to Chamberlain line if opisthion not visible
   √ tip of odontoid <5 mm above this line
3. **Wackenheim clivus baseline**
   = BASILAR LINE = line along clivus
   √ usually falls tangent to posterior aspect of tip of odontoid process
4. **Craniovertebral angle** = clivus-canal angle
   = angle formed by line along posterior surface of axis body and odontoid process + basilar line
   √ ranges from 150° in flexion to 180° in extension
   √ ventral spinal cord compression may occur at <150°
5. **Welcher basal angle**
   = formed by nasion-tuberculum line and tuberculum-basion line
   √ angle averages 132° (should be <140°)
6. **McRae line** = line between anterior lip (= basion) to posterior lip (= opisthion) of foramen magnum
   √ tip of odontoid below this line

— ANTEROPOSTERIOR VIEW

7. **Atlanto-occipital joint axis angle**
   = formed by lines drawn parallel to both atlanto-occipital joints
   √ lines intersect at center of odontoid process
   √ average angle of 125° (range of 124° to 127°)
8. **Digastric line** = line between incisurae mastoideae (origin of digastric muscles)
   √ tip of odontoid below this line
9. **Bimastoid line** = line connecting the tips of both mastoid processes
   √ tip of odontoid <10 mm above this line

MENINGES OF SPINAL CORD

A. PERIOSTEUM
   = continuation of outer layer of cerebral dura mater

B. EPIDURAL SPACE
   consists of loose areolar tissue + rich plexus of veins
   (a) cervical + thoracic spine: spacious posteriorly, potential space anteriorly
   (b) lower lumbar + sacral spine: may occupy more than half of cross-sectional area

C. DURA
   = continuation of meningeal / inner layer of cerebral dura mater; ends at 2nd sacral vertebra + forms coccygeal ligament around filum terminale; sends tubular extensions around spinal nerves; is continuous with epineurium of peripheral nerves
   Attachment: at circumference of foramen magnum, bodies of 2nd + 3rd cervical vertebrae, posterior longitudinal ligament (by connective tissue strands)

D. SUBARACHNOID SPACE
   = space between arachnoid and pia mater containing CSF, reaching as far lateral as spinal ganglia
   dentate ligament partially divides CSF space into an anterior + posterior compartment extending from foramen magnum to 1st lumbar vertebra, is continuous with pia mater of cord medially + dura mater laterally (between exiting nerves)
   dorsal subarachnoid septum connects the arachnoid to the pia mater (cribriform septum)

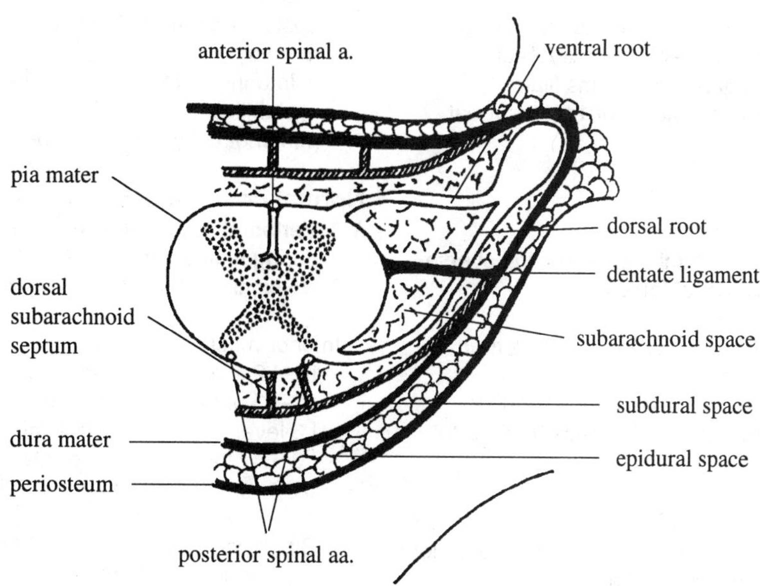

Meninges of Spinal Cord

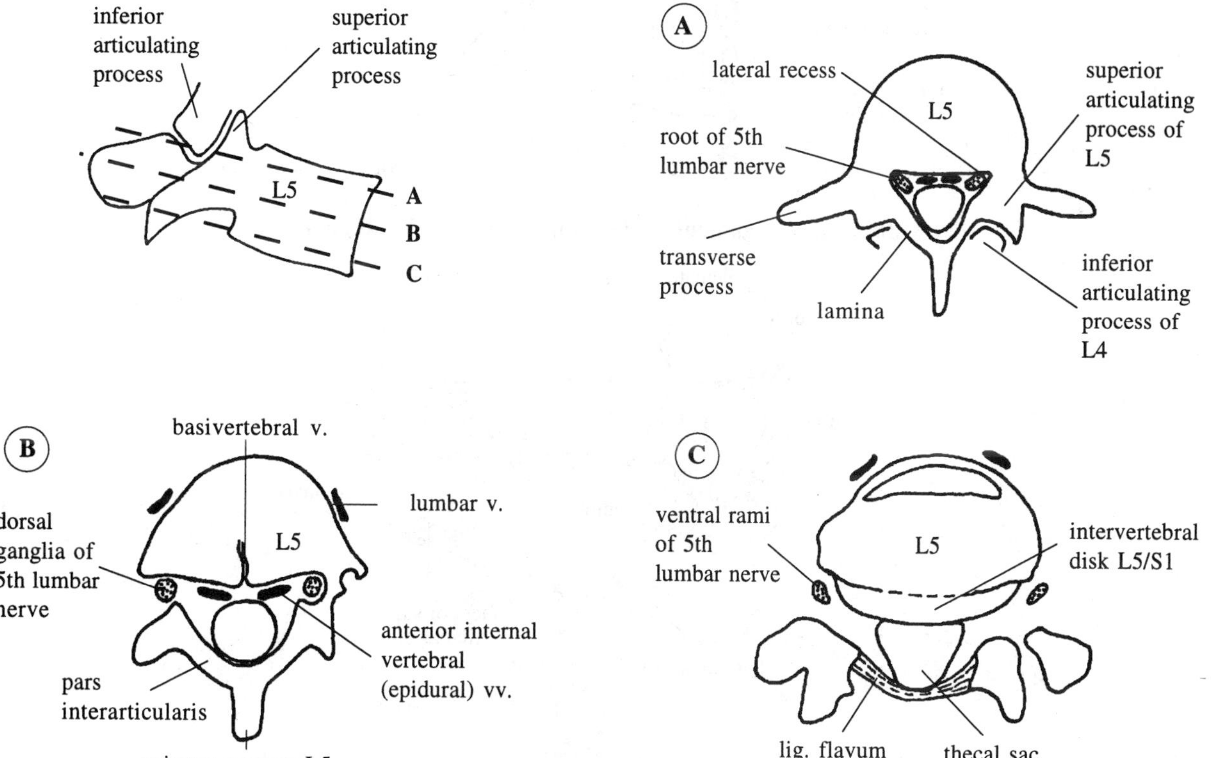

Cross-Sections Through 5th Lumbar Vertebra

E. PIA MATER
= firm vascular membrane intimately adherent to spinal cord, blends with dura mater in intervertebral foramina around spinal ganglia, forms filum terminale, fuses with periosteum of 1st coccygeal segment

Thoracic spine
- 12 load-bearing vertebrae
- posterior arch (= pedicles, laminae, facets, transverse processes) handles tensional forces
- vertebral bodies:
  (a) height of vertebrae anteriorly 2–3 mm less than posteriorly = mild kyphotic curvature
  (b) AP diameter: gradual increase from T1 to T12
  (c) transverse diameter: gradual increase from T3 to T12

Thoracolumbar spine (T11–L2)
- anterior column = anterior longitudinal ligament, anterior annulus fibrosus, anterior vertebral body
- middle column = posterior longitudinal ligament, posterior annulus fibrosus, posterior vertebral body margin
  ◊ Integrity of the middle column is synonymous with stability!
- posterior column = posterior elements + ligaments

Normal position of conus medullaris
◊ Vertebral bodies grow more quickly than spinal cord during fetal period of <19 weeks MA!
◊ No significant difference regardless of age!

Inferior-most aspect of conus:

L1–L2 level:	normal (range T12 to L3)
L2–L3 or higher:	in 97.8%
L3 level:	indeterminate (in 1.8%)
L3–L4 / lower:	abnormal
by 3 month:	above inferior endplate of L2 (in 98%)

N.B.: If conus is at / below L3 level, a search should be made for tethering mass, bony spur, thick filum!

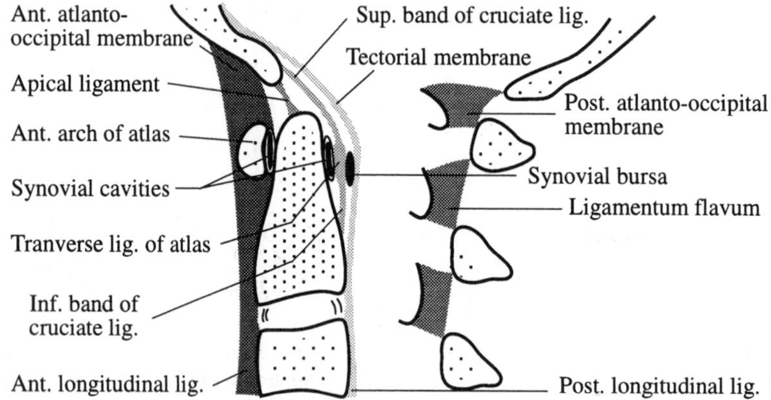

Joints and Ligaments of Occipito-atlanto-axial Region

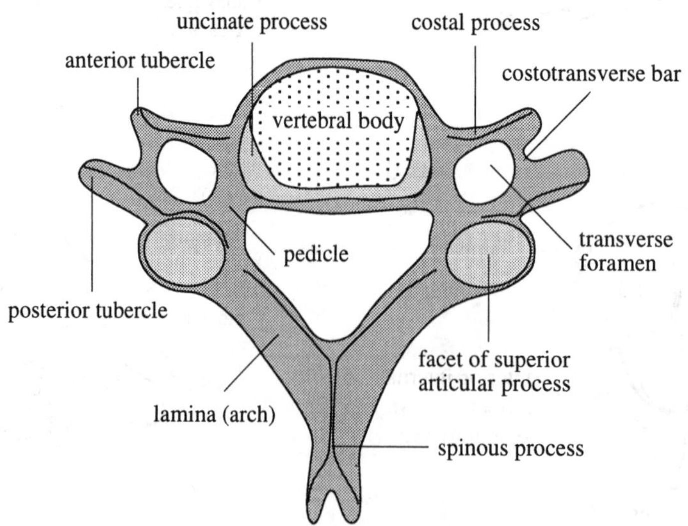

Typical Cervical Vertebra
(cranial aspect)

SKULL AND SPINE DISORDERS

ARACHNOIDITIS

Etiology: back surgery, hemorrhage, trauma, Pantopaque (inflammatory effect potentiated by blood), idiopathic

Associated with: syrinx

Myelo:
- √ blunting of nerve root sleeves
- √ blocked nerve roots without cord displacement (2/3)
- √ streaking + clumping of contrast

CT:
- √ fusion / clumping of nerve roots
- √ featureless empty-looking sac with roots adherent to wall (final stage)

ARACHNOID CYST OF SPINE

Location: dorsal to cord in thoracic region

Site:
- (a) extradural cyst secondary to congenital / acquired dural defect
- (b) intradural secondary to congenital deficiency within arachnoid (= true arachnoid cyst) / adhesion from prior infection or trauma (= arachnoid loculation)

- √ oval sharply demarcated extramedullary mass
- √ immediate / delayed contrast filling depending upon size of opening between cyst + subarachnoid space
- √ local displacement + compression of spinal cord
- √ higher signal intensity than CSF (from relative lack of CSF pulsations)

ARACHNOID DIVERTICULUM

= widening of root sheath with arachnoid space occupying >50% of total transverse diameter of root + sheath together

Cause: ? congenital / traumatic, arachnoiditis, infection

Pathogenesis: hydrostatic pressure of CSF

- √ scalloping of posterior margins of vertebral bodies
- √ myelographic contrast material fills diverticula

ARTERIOVENOUS MALFORMATION OF SPINAL CORD

Classification:

1. True intramedullary AVM
   = nidus of abnormal intermediary arteriovenous structure with multiple shunts
   Age: 2nd–3rd decade
   Cx: subarachnoid hemorrhage, paraplegia
   Prognosis: poor (especially in midthoracic location)
2. Intradural arteriovenous fistula
   = single shunt between one / several medullary arteries + single perimedullary vein
3. Dural arteriovenous fistula
   = single shunt between meningeal arteries + intradural vein
4. Metameric angiomatosis

ATLANTOAXIAL ROTARY FIXATION

- • history of insignificant cervical spine trauma / upper respiratory tract infection
- • limited painful neck motion
- • head held in "cock-robin" position + inability to turn head
- √ atlanto-odontoid asymmetry (open mouth odontoid view):
  - √ decrease in atlanto-odontoid space + widening of lateral mass on side ipsilateral to rotation
  - √ increase in atlanto-odontoid space + narrowing of lateral mass on side contralateral to rotation
- √ atlantoaxial asymmetry remains constant with head turned into neutral position

Types:
- I <3 mm anterior displacement of atlas on axis
- II 3–5 mm anterior displacement
- III >5 mm anterior displacement
- IV posterior displacement of atlas on axis

DDx: torticollis (atlantoaxial symmetry reverts to normal with head turned into neutral position)

BRACHIAL PLEXUS INJURY

1. Erb-Duchenne: adduction injury affecting C5/6 (downward displacement of shoulder)
2. Klumpke: abduction injury at C7, C8, T1 (arm stretched over head)

- √ pouchlike root sleeve at site of avulsion
- √ asymmetrical nerve roots
- √ contrast extravasation collecting in axilla
- √ metrizamide in neural foramina (CT myelography)

CAUDAL REGRESSION SYNDROME

= midline closure defect of neural tube with a spectrum of anomalies

Etiology: disturbance of caudal mesoderm <4th week of gestation from toxic / infectious / ischemic insult

Incidence: 1:7,500 births; 0.005–0.01%

Predisposed: infants of diabetic mothers (16–22%)

◊ NOT associated with VATER syndrome!

A. Musculoskeletal anomalies
   - @ Lower extremity
     - • symptoms from minor muscle weakness to complete sensorimotor paralysis of both lower extremities
     - √ hip dislocation
     - √ foot deformities
     - √ hypoplasia of extremities
   - @ Lumbosacral spine
     - √ spina bifida (myelomeningocele often not in combination with hydrocephalus)
     - √ total / partial sacral agenesis
     - √ total / partial agenesis of lumbosacral spine
     - √ fusion of caudal-most 2 or 3 vertebrae
     - √ narrowing of spinal canal rostral to last intact vertebra

√ characteristic wedge-shaped cord terminus (hypoplasia of distal spinal cord)
√ spinal cord may be tethered ± associated lipoma
√ ± dural sac stenosis with high termination
√ ± spinal cord lipoma, teratoma, cauda equina cyst

B. Genitourinary anomalies
- neurogenic bladder (if >2 segments are missing)
- malformed external genitalia
- lack of bowel control

√ ± bilateral renal aplasia with pulmonary hypoplasia + Potter facies
√ anal atresia

OB-US:
- normal / imperforate anus

√ normal / mildly dilated urinary system
√ normal / increased amniotic fluid
√ 2 umbilical arteries
√ 2 hypoplastic nonfused lower extremities
√ sacral agenesis, absent vertebrae from lower thoracic / upper lumbar spine caudally

Sirenomelia

= recently considered a distinct separate entity from caudal regression syndrome
◊ NOT associated with maternal diabetes mellitus!
- Potter facies
- absence of anus
- absent genitalia

√ bilateral renal agenesis / dysgenesis (lethal)
√ marked oligohydramnios
√ single aberrant umbilical artery
√ single / fused lower extremity
√ sacral agenesis, absent pelvis, lumbosacral "tail", lumbar rachischisis

Prognosis: incompatible with life

CHORDOMA

◊ Chordoma is the most common primary malignant tumor of the spine in adults excluding lymphoproliferative neoplasms!

Prevalence: 1:2,000,000; 1–2–4% of all primary malignant neoplasms of bone; 1% of all intracranial tumors

Etiology: originates from embryonic remnants of notochord / ectopic cordal foci (notochord appears between 4th and 7th week of embryonic development, extends from Rathke pouch to coccyx and forms nucleus pulposus)

Age: 30–70 years (peak age in 6th decade); M:F = 2:1; highly malignant in children

Path: lobulated tumor contained within pseudocapsule

Histo:
(1) typical chordoma: cords + clusters of large bubblelike vacuolated (physaliferous) cells containing intracytoplasmic mucous droplets; abundant extracellular mucus deposition + areas of hemorrhage
(2) chondroid chordoma: cartilage instead of mucinous extracellular matrix

Location: (a) 50% in sacrum (b) 35% in skull base (c) 15% spinal axis (d) other sites (5%) in mandible, maxilla, scapula

√ enhancement after contrast administration

CT:
√ low-attenuation within soft-tissue mass (due to myxoid-type tissue)
√ higher attenuation fibrous pseudocapsule

MR (modality of choice):
√ heterogeneous low to intermediate intensity on T1WI, occasionally hyperintense (due to high protein content)
√ very high signal intensity on T2WI (similar to nucleus pulposus with high water content)

NUC:
√ cold lesion on bone scan
√ no uptake on gallium scan

Metastases (in 5–43%) to: liver, lung, regional lymph nodes, peritoneum, skin (late), heart

Prognosis: almost 100% recurrence rate despite radical surgery

Sacrococcygeal Chordoma (50–70%)

40% of all sacral tumors
Peak age: 40–60 years; M:F = 2:1
- low back pain (70%)
- constipation / fecal incontinence
- rectal bleeding (42%)
- sciatica
- frequency, urgency, straining on micturition
- sacral mass (17%)

Location: esp. in 4th + 5th sacral segment
√ presacral mass with average size of 10 cm extending superiorly + inferiorly; rarely posterior location
√ displacement of rectum + bladder
√ solid tumor with cystic areas (in 50%)
√ osteolytic midline mass in sacrum + coccyx
√ amorphous peripheral calcifications (15–89%)
√ secondary bone sclerosis in tumor periphery (50%)
√ honeycomb pattern with trabeculations (10–15%)
√ may cross sacroiliac joint

Prognosis: 8–10 years average survival; 66% 5-year survival rate (adulthood)

DDx: Giant cell tumor, plasmacytoma, lymphoma, metastatic adenocarcinoma, aneurysmal bone cyst, atypical hemangioma, chondrosarcoma, osteomyelitis, ependymoma

Spheno-occipital Chordoma (15–35%)

Age: younger patient (peak age of 20–40 years); M:F - 1:1
- orbitofrontal headache
- visual disturbances, ptosis
- 6th nerve palsy / paraplegia

Location: clivus, spheno-occipital synchondrosis
√ bone destruction (in 90%): clivus > sella > petrous bone > orbit > floor of middle cranial fossa > jugular fossa > atlas > foramen magnum

√ reactive bone sclerosis (rare)
√ calcifications / bone fragments (20–70%)
√ soft-tissue extension into nasopharynx (common), into sphenoid + ethmoid sinuses (occasionally), may reach nasal cavity + maxillary antrum
√ variable degree of enhancement

MR:
- √ large intraosseous mass extending into prepontine cistern, sphenoid sinus, middle cranial fossa, nasopharynx
- √ posterior displacement of brainstem
- √ usually isointense to brain / occasionally inhomogeneously hyperintense on T1WI
- √ hyperintense on T2WI

Prognosis: 4–5 years average survival
DDx: meningioma, metastasis, plasmacytoma, giant cell tumor, sphenoid sinus cyst, nasopharyngeal carcinoma, chondrosarcoma

Vertebral / Spinal Chordoma (15–20%)

more aggressive than sacral / cranial chordomas
Age: younger patient; M:F = 2:1
- low back pain + radiculopathy

Location: cervical (8% – particularly C2), thoracic spine (4%), lumbar spine (3%)
√ solitary midline spinal mass
√ tumor calcification in 30%
√ sclerosis / "ivory vertebra" in 43–62%
√ total destruction of vertebra, initially unaccompanied by collapse
√ variable extension into spinal canal
√ violates disk space to involve adjacent bodies (10–14%) simulating infection
√ anterior soft-tissue mass

Cx: complete spinal block
Prognosis: 4–5 years average survival
DDx: Metastasis, primary bone tumor, primary soft-tissue tumor, neuroma, meningioma

CSF FISTULA

Cause:
(1) Trauma to skull base (most commonly)
◊ 2% of all head injuries develop CSF fistula
(2) Tumor: especially those arising from pituitary gland
(3) Congenital anomalies: encephalocele

- traumatic leak: usually unilateral; onset within 48 hours after trauma, usually scanty; resolve in 1 week
- nontraumatic leak: profuse flow; may persist for years
- anosmia (in 78% of trauma cases)

Location: fractures through frontoethmoidal complex + middle cranial fossa (most commonly)
√ high-resolution thin-section CT in coronal plane followed by rescanning after low-dose intrathecal contrast material instilled into lumbar subarachnoid space

Cx: infection (in 25–50% of untreated cases)

DEGENERATIVE DISK DISEASE

◊ Therapeutic decision-making should be based on clinical assessment alone!
◊ There are no prognostic indicators on images in patients with acute lumbar radiculopathy!
35% of individuals without back trouble have abnormal findings (HNP, disk bulging, facet degeneration, spinal stenosis)
◊ Imaging tests are only justified in patients for whom surgery is considered!

Pathophysiology:
loss of disk height leads to malalignment (= rostrocaudal subluxation) of facet joints causing spine instability with arthritis, capsular hypertrophy, hypertrophy of posterior ligaments, facet fracture

Plain film:
- √ narrowing of disk space
- √ disk calcification
- √ vacuum disk phenomenon = radiolucent interspace accumulation of nitrogen gas at sites of negative pressure
- √ intervertebral osteochondrosis = loss of disk space height + bone sclerosis of adjacent vertebral bodies
- √ cartilaginous nodes = intraosseous disk herniation
- √ spondylosis deformans = endplate osteophytosis secondary to anterolateral disk displacement resulting in traction osteophytes at sites of osseous attachment of annulus fibrosus fibers of Sharpey

Myelography:
- √ delineation of thecal sac, spinal cord, exiting nerve roots

CT (accuracy >90%):
- √ facet joint disease (marginal sclerosis, joint narrowing, cyst formation, bony overgrowth)

MR:
- √ endplate changes (Modic & DeRoos):
  - (a) Type I (4%) with decreased signal on T1WI + increased signal on T2WI (= vascularized fibrous tissue), contrast-enhancement of marrow
  - (b) Type II (16%) with increased signal on T1WI + isointensity on T2WI (= local fatty replacement of marrow)
  - (c) Type III with decreased signal on T1WI + T2WI (= advanced sclerosis)

NUC:
SPECT imaging of vertebrae can aid in localizing increased uptake to vertebral bodies, posterior elements, etc.
- √ eccentrically placed increased uptake on either side of an intervertebral space (osteophytes, discogenic sclerosis)

Sequelae: (1) disk bulging (2) disk herniation (3) spinal stenosis (4) facet joint disease

TERMINOLOGY:
1. Disk bulge
   = concentric smooth circumferential expansion of softened disk material beyond the confines of endplates

2. Disk protrusion
   = focal protrusion of disk material maintaining broad base with parent disk due to focally weakened / ruptured annulus but intact posterior longitudinal ligament
3. Disk extrusion
   = prominent focal extrusion of disk material with only an isthmus of connection to parent disk due to
   (a) ruptured annulus + intact posterior longitudinal ligament
   (b) ruptured annulus + ruptured posterior longitudinal ligament
4. Free fragment
   = frank separation of disk material from parent disk
5. Free fragment migration
   = separated disk material travels above / below intervertebral disk space

Bulging disk

= broad-based disk extension outward in all directions with intact but weakened annulus fibrosus + posterior longitudinal ligament

Age: common finding in individuals >40 years of age

Location: lumbar, cervical spine

√ rounded symmetric defect localized to disk space level

√ concave anterior margin of thecal sac

MR:

√ nucleus pulposus hypointense on T1WI + hyperintense on T2WI (water loss through degeneration)

Herniation of nucleus pulposus

= HNP = focal protrusion of disk material beyond margins of adjacent vertebral endplates secondary to rupture of annulus fibrosus confined within posterior longitudinal ligament

◊ 21% of asymptomatic population has disk herniation!

- local somatic spinal pain = sharp / aching, deep, localized
- centrifugal radiating pain = sharp, well-circumscribed, superficial, "electric," confined to dermatome
- centrifugal referred pain = dull, ill-defined, deep or superficial, aching or boring, confined to somatome (= dermatome + myotome + sclerotome)

Location: L4/5 (35%) > L5/S1 (27%) > L3/4 (19%) > L2/3 (14%) > L1/2 (5%); thoracic spine affected in 3:1,000 disk operations
   (a) posterolateral (49%) = weakest point along posterolateral margin of disk at lateral recess of spinal canal (posterior longitudinal ligament tightly adherent to posterior margins of disk)
   (b) posterocentral (8%)
   (c) bilateral (on both sides of posterior ligament)
   (d) lateral / foraminal (<10%)
   (e) intraosseous / vertical = Schmorl node (14%)
   (f) extraforaminal = anterior (commonly overlooked) (29%)

Myelography:

√ sharply angular indentation on lateral aspect of thecal sac with extension above or below level of disk space (ipsilateral oblique projection best view)

√ asymmetry of posterior disk margin

√ double contour secondary to superimposed normal + abnormal side (horizontal beam lateral view)

√ narrowing of intervertebral disk space (most commonly a sign of disk degeneration)

√ deviation of nerve root / root sleeve

√ enlargement of nerve root secondary to edema ("trumpet sign")

√ amputated / truncated nerve root (nonfilling of root sleeve)

MR:

√ herniated disk material of low signal intensity displaces the posterior longitudinal ligament and epidural fat of relative high signal intensity on T1WI

Cx: spinal stenosis

Prognosis:

conservative therapy reduces size of herniation by
   0–50% in 11% of patients,
   50–75% in 36% of patients,
   75–100% in 46% of patients
(secondary to growth of granulation tissue)

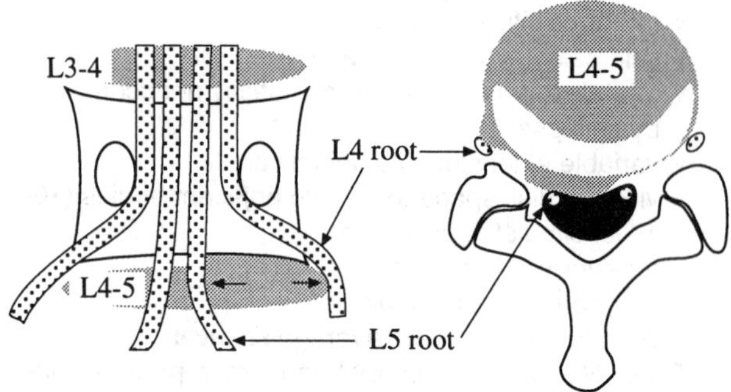

Lateral Disk Herniation

Nerve compression usually occurs posterolaterally (here at L4-5); therefore an atypical lateral compression (here of L4 root) directs surgery to the wrong more cephalad level (L3-4 disk)

Free fragment herniation

= DISK SEQUESTRATION

= complete separation of disk material with rupture through posterior longitudinal ligament into epidural space

◊ Missed free fragments are a common cause of failed back surgery!

√ migration superiorly / inferiorly away from disk space with compression of nerve root above / below level of disk herniation

√ disk material noted >9 mm away from intervertebral disk space

√ soft-tissue density with higher value than thecal sac

DDx: (1) Postoperative scarring (retraction of thecal sac to side of surgery)
   (2) Epidural abscess
   (3) Epidural tumor

(4) Conjoined nerve root (2 nerve roots arising from thecal sac simultaneously representing mass in ventrolateral aspect of spinal canal; normal variant in 1–3% of population)
(5) Tarlov cyst (dilated nerve root sleeve)

Cervical Disk Herniation

Peak age: 3rd–4th decade
- neck stiffness, muscle splinting
- dermatomic sensory loss
- weakness + muscle atrophy
- reflex loss

Sites: C6-7 (69%); C5-6 (19%); C7-T1 (10%); C4-5 (2%)

Sequelae: (1) compression of exiting nerve roots
(2) cord compression (spinal stenosis + massive disk rupture)

DERMOID OF SPINE

= uni- / multilocular cystic tumor lined by squamous epithelium containing skin appendages (hair follicles, sweat glands, sebaceous glands)

Cause:
(a) congenital dermal rest / focal expansion of dermal sinus
(b) acquired from implantation of viable dermal tissue (by spinal needle without trocar)

Incidence: 1% of spinal cord tumors
Age at presentation: <20 years; M:F = 1:1
May be associated with: dermal sinus (in 20%)
- slowly progressive myelopathy
- acute onset of chemical meningitis (secondary to rupture of inflammatory cholesterol crystals from cyst into CSF)

Location: lumbosacral (60%), cauda equina (20%)
Site: extramedullary (60%), intramedullary (40%)
√ almost always complete spinal block on myelography
√ intensity of fat
√ occasionally hypointense on T1WI + hypodense on CT (secretions from sweat glands within tumor)
√ NO contrast enhancement
√ CT myelography facilitates detection

DIASTEMATOMYELIA

= SPLIT CORD = MYELOSCHISIS
= sagittal division of spinal cord into two hemicords, each of which contains a central canal, one dorsal horn + one ventral horn

Etiology: congenital malformation as a result of split notochord; M:F = 1:3

Path:
(a) 2 hemicords each covered by layer of pia within single subarachnoid space + dural sac (60%); not accompanied by bony spur / fibrous band
(b) 2 hemicords each with its own pial, subarachnoidal + dural sheath (40%); accompanied by fibrous band (in 25%), cartilaginous / bony spurs (in 75%)

Associated with: myelomeningocele
- hypertrichosis, nevus, lipoma, dimple, hemangioma overlying the spine (26–81%)
- clubfoot (50%)
- muscle wasting, ankle weakness in one leg

Location: lower thoracic / upper lumbar > upper thoracic > cervical spine
√ congenital scoliosis (50–75%)
◊ 5% of patients with congenital scoliosis have diastematomyelia
√ spina bifida over multiple levels
√ anteroposterior narrowing of vertebral bodies
√ widening of interpediculate distance
√ narrowed disk space with hemivertebra, butterfly vertebra, block vertebra
√ fusion + thickening of adjacent laminae (90%)
(a) fusion to ipsilateral lamina at adjacent levels
(b) diagonal fusion to contralateral adjacent lamina = intersegmental laminar fusion
√ bony spur through center of spinal canal arising from posterior aspect of centra (<50%)
√ thickened filum terminale >2 mm (>50%)
√ tethered cord (>50%)
√ low conus medullaris below L2 level (>75%)
√ the 2 hemicords usually reunite caudal to cleft
√ defect in thecal sac on myelogram

Cx: progressive spinal cord dysfunction

DISCITIS

most common pediatric spine problem

Etiology:
(1) Bloodborne bacterial invasion of vertebrae infecting disk via communicating vessels through endplate
(2) invasive procedure: surgery, discography, myelography, chemonucleolysis

Agents:
(a) pyogenic: Staphylococcus aureus (by far most frequent), Gram-negative rods (in IV drug abusers / immunocompromised patients)
(b) nonpyogenic: tuberculosis, coccidioidomycosis

Pathogenesis: infection starts in disk (still vascularized in children) / in anterior inferior corner of vertebral body (in adults) with spread across disk to adjacent vertebral endplate

Age peak: 6 months to 4 years and 10–14 years; average age of 6 years at presentation
- over 2–4 weeks gradually progressing irritability, malaise, fever
- back / referred hip pain, limp
- refusal to bear weight

Location: L3/4, L4/5, unusual above T9; usually involvement of one disk space (occasionally 2)

Plain film (positive 2–4 weeks after onset of symptoms):
√ decrease in disk space height (earliest sign) = intraosseous herniation of nucleus pulposus into vertebral body through weakened endplate
√ indistinctness of adjacent endplates with destruction
√ endplate sclerosis (during healing phase beginning anywhere from 8 weeks to 8 months after onset)
√ bone fusion (after 6 months to 2 years)

CT:
- √ paravertebral inflammatory mass
- √ epidural soft-tissue extension with deformity of thecal sac

MR (preferred modality; 93% sensitive, 97% specific, 95% accurate):
- √ decreased marrow intensity on T1WI in two contiguous vertebrae
- √ in early stage preserved disk height with variable intensity on T2WI (often increased)
- √ in later stages loss of disk height with increased intensity on T2WI

NUC (41% sensitive, 93% specific, 68% accurate on Tc-99m MDP + Tc-99m WBC scans):
- √ positive before radiographs
- √ increased uptake in disk space + contiguous vertebra
- √ bone scan usually positive in adjacent vertebrae (until age 20) secondary to vascular supply via endplates; may be negative after age 20

Cx: kyphosis
Rx: immobilization in body cast for ~4 weeks
DDx: osteomyelitis of vertebra

Postoperative Discitis

Frequency: 0.75–2.8%
Organism: Staphylococcus aureus; many times no organism recovered

- severe recurrent back pain 7–28 days after surgery accompanied by decreased back motion, muscle spasm, positive straight leg raising test
- fever (33%)
- wound infection (8%)
- persistently elevated / increasing ESR

MR:
- √ decreased signal intensity within disk + adjacent vertebral body marrow on T1WI
- √ increased signal intensity in disk + adjacent marrow on T2WI often with obliteration of intranuclear cleft
- √ contrast-enhancement of vertebral bone marrow ± disk space

DDx: degenerative disk disease type I (no gadolinium-enhancement of disk)

DISLOCATION

Atlanto-occipital Dislocation

= ATLANTO-OCCIPITAL DISTRACTION INJURY
= disruption of tectorial membrane + paired alar ligaments

Cause: rapid deceleration with either hyperextension or hyperflexion
Age: childhood (due to larger size of head relative to body, increased laxity of ligaments, horizontally oriented occipito-atlanto-axial joint, hypoplastic occipital condyles)

- neurologic symptoms: range from respiratory arrest with quadriplegia to normal neurologic exam
- discomfort, stiffness

√ retropharyngeal swelling (80%)
√ dens-basion distance (BD) >12.5 mm without traction placed on head / neck
√ BC/OA ratio >1 = ratio of distance between basion + posterior arch of C1 divided by distance between opisthion + anterior arch of C1

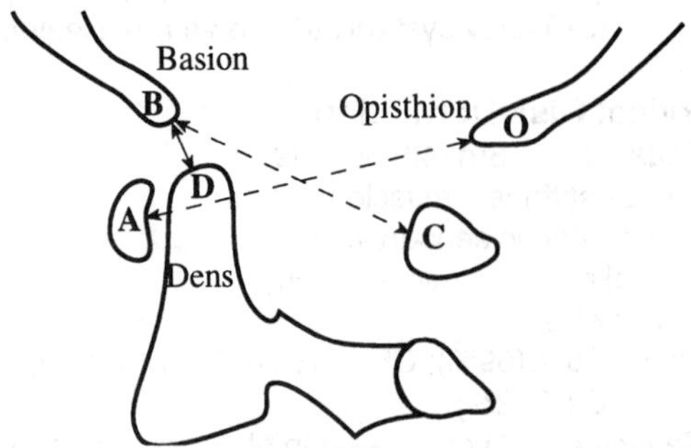

CT:
- √ blood in region of tectorial membrane + alar ligaments

Cx: injury to caudal cranial nerves, upper 3 cervical nerves, brainstem, upper part of spinal cord

DORSAL DERMAL SINUS

= epithelium-lined dural tube extending from skin surface to intracanalicular space + frequently communicating with CNS / its coverings

Cause: focal area of incomplete separation of cutaneous ectoderm from neural ectoderm during neurulation
Age: encountered in early childhood–3rd decade; M:F = 1:1

- midline dimple / pinpoint ostium
- hyperpigmented patch / hairy nevus / capillary angioma

Location: lumbosacral (60%), occipital (25%), thoracic (10%), cervical (2%), sacrococcygeal (1%), ventral (8%)

CT myelography (best modality to define intraspinal anatomy):
- √ groove in upper surface of spinous process + lamina of vertebra
- √ hypoplastic spinous process
- √ single bifid spinous process
- √ focal multilevel spina bifida
- √ laminar defect
- √ dorsal tenting of dura + arachnoid
- √ sinus may terminate in conus medullaris / filum terminale / nerve root / fibrous nodule on dorsal aspect of cord / dermoid / epidermoid
- √ nerve roots bound down to capsule of dermoid / epidermoid cyst
- √ displacement / compression of cord by extramedullary dermoids / epidermoids
- √ expansion of cord by intramedullary dermoids / epidermoids
- √ clumping of nerve roots from adhesive arachnoiditis

◊ 50% of dorsal dermal sinuses end in dermoid / epidermoid cysts!
◊ 20–30% of dermoid cysts / dermoid tumors are associated with dermal sinus tracts!

Cx: (1) Meningitis (bacterial / chemical)
(2) Subcutaneous / epidural / subdural / subarachnoid / subpial abscess (bacterial ascent)
◊ Dermal sinus accounts for up to 3% of spinal cord abscesses!
(3) Compression of neural structures

EPIDERMOID OF SPINE

= cystic tumor lined by a membrane composed of epidermal elements of skin

Cause:
(a) congenital dermal rest / focal expansion of dermal sinus
(b) acquired from implantation of viable epidermal tissue (by spinal needle without trocar)

Incidence: 1% of spinal cord tumors
Age at presentation: 3rd–5th decade; M > F
May be associated with: dermal sinus

- slowly progressive myelopathy
- acute onset of chemical meningitis (secondary to rupture of inflammatory cholesterol crystals from cyst into CSF)

Location: upper thoracic (17%), lower thoracic (26%), lumbosacral (22%), cauda equina (35%)
Site: extramedullary (60%), intramedullary (40%)

√ almost always complete spinal block on myelography
√ displacement of spinal cord / nerve roots
√ small tumors isointense to CSF
√ NO contrast enhancement
√ CT myelography facilitates detection

EPIDURAL HEMATOMA OF SPINE

Etiology: (1) vertebral fracture / dislocation (2) traumatic lumbar puncture (3) hypertension (4) AVM (5) vertebral hemangioma (6) bleeding diathesis / anticoagulation / hemophilia (7) idiopathic (45%)
Peak age: 40–50 years

- acute radicular pain
- paraplegia

Location: thoracic spine (most common)

√ compression of posterior aspect of cord
√ high attenuation lesion on CT
√ iso- / slightly hypointense lesion on T1WI with marked increase in intensity on T2WI

FRACTURES OF SKULL

1. Linear fracture (most common type)
   √ deeply black sharply defined line
   DDx: (1) vascular groove, esp. temporal artery (gray line, slightly sclerotic margin, branching like a tree, typical location (temporal artery projects behind dorsum sellae)
   (2) suture
2. Depressed fracture
   - often palpable

   √ bone-on-bone density
   Rx: surgery indicated if depression >3–5 mm (due to arachnoid tear / brain injury)
   N.B.: CT / MR mandatory to assess extent of underlying brain injury
3. Skull-base fracture

LeFort Fracture

= all LeFort fractures involve pterygoid process

A. LeFort I = Transverse maxillary fracture caused by blow to premaxilla
   Fracture line: (a) alveolar ridge
   (b) lateral aperture of nose
   (c) inferior wall of maxillary sinus
   √ detachment of alveolar process of maxilla
B. LeFort II = "Pyramidal fracture"
   Fracture line: arch through
   (a) posterior alveolar ridge
   (b) medial orbital rim
   (c) across nasal bones
   √ separation of midportion of face
C. LeFort III = "craniofacial disjunction"
   Fracture line: horizontal course through
   (a) nasofrontal suture
   (b) maxillo-frontal suture
   (c) orbital wall
   (d) zygomatic arch
   √ separation of entire face from base of skull

Sphenoid Bone Fracture

Incidence: involved in 15% of skull-base fractures

- CSF rhinorrhea / otorrhea
- hematotympanum
- battle sign = mastoid region ecchymosis
- raccoon eyes = periorbital ecchymosis
- 7th / 8th nerve palsy
- muscular dysfunction: problems with ocular motility, mastication, speech, swallowing, eustachian tube function

√ air-fluid level in sinuses + mastoid
√ axial thin-slice high-resolution CT for best delineation of fractures
√ water-soluble intrathecal contrast material for CSF fistula

Zygomaticomaxillary Fracture

= "TRIPOD" FRACTURE = MALAR / ZYGOMATIC COMPLEX FRACTURE

Cause: direct blow to malar eminence

- loss of sensibility of face below orbit
- deficient mastication
- double vision / ophthalmoplegia
- facial deformity

Fracture line:
(a) lateral wall of maxillary sinus
(b) orbital rim close to infraorbital foramen
(c) floor of orbit (d) zygomatico-frontal suture / zygomatic arch

Blowout Fracture

= isolated fracture of orbital floor

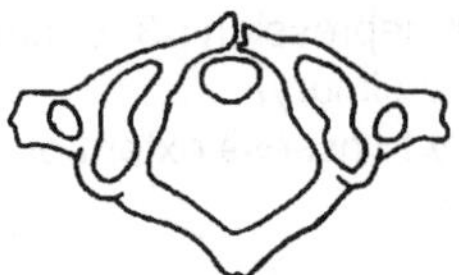
Anterior arch fracture

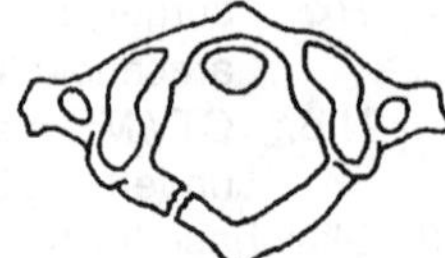
Posterior arch fracture

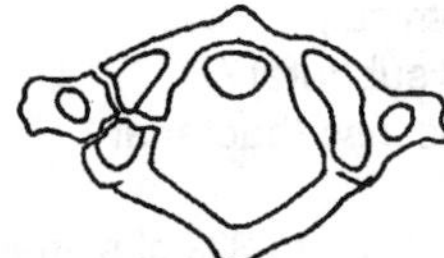
Lateral mass fracture

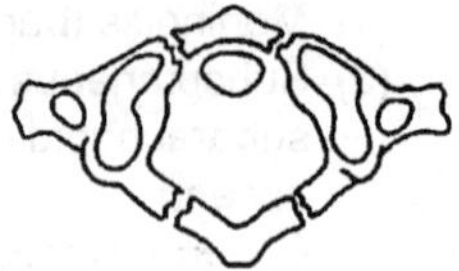
Jefferson fracture

Atlas Fractures

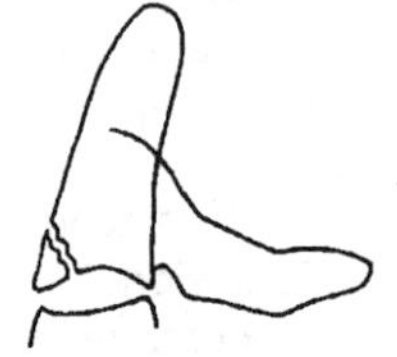
Teardrop fracture

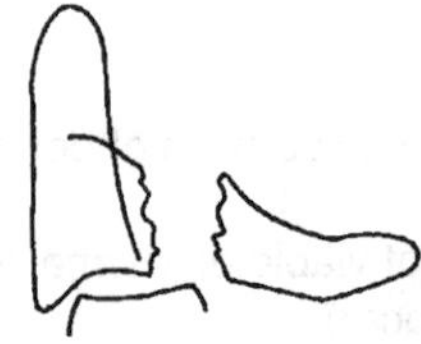
Hangman's fracture

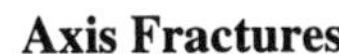
Axis Fractures

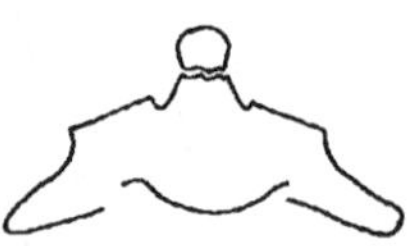
Type I

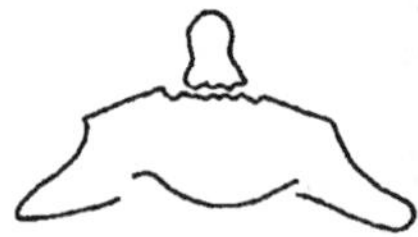
Type II

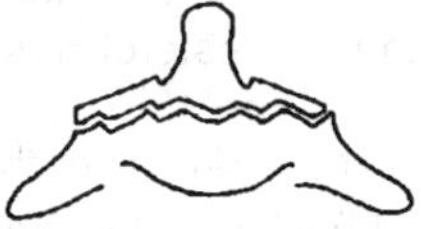
Type III

Dens Fractures

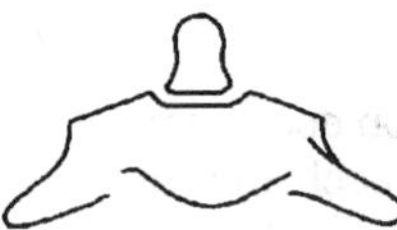
Os odontoideum

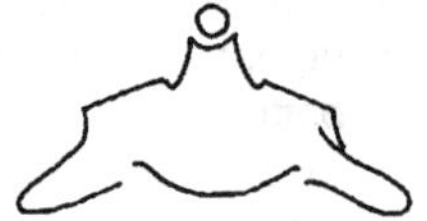
Ossiculum terminale

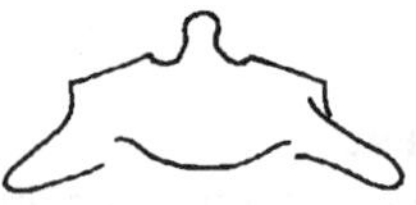
Hypoplasia of dens

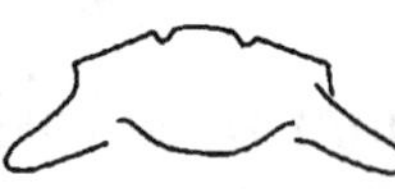
Aplasia of dens

Cause: sudden direct blow to globe with increase in intraorbital pressure transmitted to the weak orbital floor, often associated with fracture of the thin lamina papyracea

- diplopia on upward gaze (entrapment of inferior rectus + inferior oblique muscles)
- enophthalmos
- facial anesthesia

√ soft-tissue mass extending into maxillary sinus
√ complete opacification of maxillary sinus (edema + hemorrhage)
√ depression of orbital floor
√ posttraumatic atrophy of orbital fat leads to enophthalmos

FRACTURES OF CERVICAL SPINE

Frequency: C2, C6 > C5, C7 > C3, C4 > C1
Location:
(a) upper cervical spine = C1/2 (19–25%): atlas (4%), odontoid (6%)
(b) lower cervical spine = C3–7 (75–81%)
(c) multiple noncontiguous spine fractures (15–20%)

Site: vertebral arch (50%), vertebral body (30%), intervertebral disk (25%), posterior ligaments (16%), dens (14%), locked facets (12%), anterior ligament (2%)

Associated with: thoracic / lumbar spine fracture in 5–15%

N.B.: Plain radiography misses 20–30% of cervical spine injuries!

◊ Most missed fractures involve C1 (8%), C2 (34%), C4 (12%), C6-7 (14%), occipital condyles !

A. HYPERFLEXION INJURY (46–79%)
1. Odontoid fracture
2. Simple wedge fracture (stable)
3. Teardrop fracture: most severe + unstable injury of C-spine
4. Anterior subluxation
5. Bilateral locked facets (unstable)

6. Anterior disk space narrowing
7. Widened interspinous distance
8. Spinous process fracture = clay shoveler's fracture = sudden load on flexed spine with avulsion fracture of C6 / C7 / T1 (stable)

B. HYPEREXTENSION INJURY (20–38%)
1. Anteriorly widened disk space
2. Prevertebral swelling
3. **Teardrop fracture** = avulsion of anteroinferior corner by anterior ligament (unstable) typically at C2
4. Neural arch fracture of C1 (stable = anterior ring + transverse ligament intact)
5. Subluxation (anterior / posterior)
6. **Hangman's fracture** = bilateral neural arch fracture of C2 (unstable)
   √ prevertebral soft-tissue swelling
   √ anterior subluxation of C2 on C3
   √ avulsion of anteroinferior corner of C2 (rupture of anterior longitudinal ligament)

C. FLEXION-ROTATION INJURY (12%)
1. Unilateral locked facets (oblique views!, stable)

D. VERTICAL COMPRESSION (4%)
1. **Jefferson fracture** = comminuted fracture of ring of C1 (unstable)
   √ lateral displacement of lateral massa (self-decompressing)
   (*DDx:* Pseudo-Jefferson fracture = lateral offset of lateral masses of atlas without fracture in fusion anomalies of anterior / posterior arches of C1, in children as lateral masses of atlas ossify earlier than C2)
2. Burst fracture = intervertebral disk driven into vertebral body below (stable)
   √ several fragments, fragment from posterior superior margin often in spinal canal

E. LATERAL FLEXION / SHEARING (4–6%)
1. Uncinate fracture
2. Isolated pillar fracture
3. Transverse process fracture
4. Lateral vertebral compression

Significant signs of cervical vertebral trauma

(a) most reliable + specific
   √ widening of interspinous space (43%)
   √ widening of facet joint (39%)
   √ displacement of prevertebral fat stripe (18%)
(b) reliable but nonspecific
   √ wide retropharyngeal space >7 mm (31%)
   (DDx: mediastinal hemorrhage of other cause, crying in children, S/P difficult intubation)
(c) nonspecific
   √ loss of lordosis (63%)
   √ anterolisthesis / retrolisthesis (36%)
   √ kyphotic angulation (21%)
   √ tracheal deviation (13%)
   √ disk space: narrow (24%), wide (8%)

Atlas Fracture

Incidence: 4% of cervical spine injuries
Site: posterior arch, anterior arch, massa lateralis, Jefferson fracture
Associated with: fractures of C7 (25%), C2 pedicle (15%), extraspinal fractures (58%)

Axis Fracture

Incidence: 6% of cervical spine injuries
Associated with: fractures of C1 in 8%
Type I = avulsion of tip of odontoid (5–8%)
   √ difficult to detect
Type II = fracture through base of dens (54–67%)
   Cx: nonunion
Type III = subdental fracture (30–33%)
   Prognosis: good
DDx: os odontoideum, ossiculum terminale, hypoplasia of dens, aplasia of dens

FRACTURES OF THORACOLUMBAR SPINE

40% of all vertebral fractures that cause neurologic deficit, mostly complex (body + posterior elements involved)
Location: 2/3 at thoracolumbar junction
√ diastasis of apophyseal joints
√ disruption of interspinal ligament
√ retropulsion of body fragments into spinal canal
√ "burst" fragments at superior surface of body

Fracture of Upper Thoracic Spine (T1 to T10)

Types:
1. compression / axial loading fracture (most common)
   √ wedging of vertebral body
   √ retropulsion of bone fragments
   √ posttraumatic disk herniation
2. burst fracture
   √ associated fracture of posterior neural arch
   √ comminuted retropulsed bone fragments
3. sagittal slice fracture
   √ vertebra above telescopes into vertebra below, displacing it laterally
4. anterior / posterior dislocation
   √ torn anterior / posterior longitudinal ligament
   √ facet dislocation

◊ Relatively stable fractures due to rib cage + strong costovertebral ligaments + more horizontal orientation of facet joints!

Signs of spinal instability:
= inability to maintain normal associations between vertebral segments while under physiologic load
√ displaced vertebra
√ widening of interspinous / interlaminar distance
√ facet dislocation
√ disruption of posterior vertebral body line

Fracture of Thoracolumbar Junction (T11 to L2)

= area of transition between a stiff + mobile segment of the spine
• neurologic deficit (in up to 40%)

Classification based on injury to the middle column:
(1) Hyperflexion injury (most common)
= compression of anterior column + distraction of posterior spinal elements
(a) hyperflexion-compression fracture
√ loss of height of vertebral body anteriorly + laterally
√ focal kyphosis / scoliosis
√ fracture of anterosuperior end plate
(b) flexion-rotation injury (unusual)
◊ Very unstable!
• catastrophic neurologic sequela: paraplegia
√ subluxation / dislocation
√ widening of interspinous distance
√ fractures of lamina, transverse process, facets, adjacent ribs
(c) shearing fracture-dislocation
= damage of all 3 columns secondary to horizontally impacting force
(d) flexion-distraction injury: Chance fracture
2. Hyperextension injury (extremely uncommon)
√ widened disc space anteriorly
√ posterior subluxation
√ vertebral anterior superior corner avulsion
√ posterior arch fracture
3. Axial compression fracture
◊ Unstable!
√ burst fracture with herniation of intervertebral disc through end plates + comminution of vertebral body
√ marked anterior vertebral body wedging
√ retropulsed bone fragment
√ increase in interpediculate distance
√ ± vertical fracture through vertebral body, pedicle, lamina

Chance Fracture
= SEATBELT FRACTURE
Mechanism: shearing flexion-distraction injury (lap-type seatbelt injury in back-seat passengers)
• neurologic deficit infrequent (20%)
Location: L2 or L3
√ horizontal splitting of spinous process, pedicles, laminae + superior portion of vertebral body
√ disruption of ligaments
√ distraction of intervertebral disc + facet joints
◊ Fracture often unstable!
Often associated with:
(1) bone injury
rib fractures along the course of diagonal strap; sternal fractures; clavicular fractures
(2) soft-tissue injury
transverse tear of rectus abdominis muscle; anterior peritoneal tear; diaphragmatic rupture
(3) vascular injury
mesenteric vascular tear; transection of common carotid artery; injury to internal carotid artery, subclavian artery, superior vena cava; thoracic aortic tear; abdominal aortic transection
(4) visceral injury
perforation of jejunum + ileum > large intestine > duodenum (free intraperitoneal fluid in 100%, mesenteric infiltration in 88%, thickened bowel wall in 75%, extraluminal air in 56%); laceration / rupture of liver, spleen, kidneys, pancreas, distended urinary bladder; uterine injury

Chance Equivalent
= purely ligamentous disruption leading to lumbar subluxation / dislocation
√ mild widening of posterior aspect of affected disk space
√ widened facet joints
√ splaying of spinous processes = "empty hole sign" on AP view

GLIOMA OF SPINAL CORD
Often associated with: syrinx
1. Ependymoma (60–70%)
Location: lower spinal cord, conus medullaris, filum terminale; extends over several vertebral segments
√ well-demarcated / diffusely infiltrating tumor
√ occupies whole width of spinal cord
√ focal mass with areas of extensive cystic degeneration, hemorrhage, and calcification
√ erosion of vertebral body (uncommon)
MR:
√ intense homogeneous sharply marginated focal enhancement on Gd-enhanced MR
√ hypointense tumor margin on T1WI + T2WI
2. Astrocytoma (30%)
Histo: low-grade astrocytoma I and II (75%), high-grade astrocytoma III and IV (8%)
Location: cervical + thoracic spine; often extending into lower brainstem
√ usually homogeneous extensive cord tumor with widening of spinal cord
√ eccentric location within spinal cord
√ dilated veins on surface of cord
√ mass may be cystic with water-soluble myelographic contrast entering cystic space on delayed CT images
√ patchy irregular Gd enhancement on MR

HEMANGIOBLASTOMA OF SPINE
= ANGIOBLASTOMA = ANGIORETICULOMA
Incidence: 2% of all spinal cord tumors; mostly sporadic
Associated with: von Hippel-Lindau disease (in 1/3)
Age: middle age; M:F = 1:1
Location: intramedullary (75%), radicular (20%), intradural extramedullary (5%); solitary in >90%; mostly in cervicothoracic spine
√ increased interpediculate distance (mass effect)
√ expanded cord
√ intratumoral cystic component (50–60%)
√ large draining veins form sinuous mass along posterior aspect of cord
√ densely staining tumor nodule
√ frequently accompanies syrinx

MR:
- √ well-demarcated Gd-enhancing mass
- √ curvilinear area of signal void

Cx: intramedullary hemorrhage

KLIPPEL-FEIL SYNDROME

= BREVICOLLIS
= synostosis of two / more cervical segments
May be associated with:
platybasia, syringomyelia, encephalocele, facial + cranial asymmetry, Sprengel deformity (25–40%), syndactyly, clubbed foot, hypoplastic lumbar vertebrae; renal anomalies in 50% (agenesis, dysgenesis, malrotation, duplication, renal ectopia); congenital heart disease in 5% (atrial septal defect, coarctation)

- clinical triad of
  (1) short neck
  (2) restriction of cervical motion
  (3) low posterior hairline
- deafness (30%)
- webbed neck

Location: cervical spine
- √ fusion of vertebral bodies and posterior elements
- √ ± hemivertebrae
- √ may have cervicothoracic / cervical / atlanto-occipital fusion
- √ torticollis
- √ scoliosis
- √ rib fusion
- √ Sprengel deformity (25–40%) = elevation + medial rotation of scapula (may be related to presence of anomalous omovertebral bone)
- √ ear anomalies: absent auditory canal, microtia, deformed ossicles, underdevelopment of bony labyrinth

KÜMMELL DISEASE

= intravertebral vacuum phenomenon
Cause: 1. Osteonecrosis
2. Weeks to months following acute fracture
Pathophysiology: likely to represent gaseous release into bony clefts within a nonhealed fracture underneath endplate
Age: >50 years
Location: most commonly at thoracolumbar junction
- √ gas collection increasing with extension + traction, decreasing with flexion

LEPTOMENINGEAL CYST

= "Growing" fracture
Incidence: 1% of all pediatric skull fractures
Pathogenesis: skull fracture with dural tear leads to arachnoid herniation into dural defect; CSF pulsations produce fracture diastasis + erosion of bone margins (apparent 2–3 months after injury)
Age: usually <3 years
- √ skull defect with indistinct scalloped margins
- √ CSF-density cyst adjacent to / in skull, may contain cerebral tissue

MR:
- √ cyst isointense with CSF + communicating with subarachnoid space
- √ area of encephalomalacia underlying fracture (frequent)
- √ intracranial tissue extending between edges of bone

LIPOMA OF SPINE

= partially encapsulated mass of fat + connective tissue with connection to leptomeninges / spinal cord
Types:
(a) intradural lipoma (4%)
(b) lipomyelomeningocele (84%)
(c) fibrolipoma of filum terminale (12%)
◊ Intradural lipomas + lipomyelomeningoceles represent 35% of skin-covered lumbosacral masses + 20–50% of occult spinal dysraphism!

Intradural Lipoma

= subpial juxtamedullary mass totally enclosed in intact dural sac
Incidence: <1% of primary intraspinal tumors
Age peaks: first 5 years of life (24%), 2nd + 3rd decade (55%), 5th decade (16%)
- slow ascending mono- / paraparesis, spasticity, cutaneous sensory loss, defective deep sensation (with cervical + thoracic intradural lipoma)
- flaccid paralysis of legs, sphincter dysfunction (with lumbosacral intradural lipoma)
- overlying skin most often normal
- elevation of protein in CSF (30%)

Location: cervical (12%) / cervicothoracic (24%) / thoracic (30%); dorsal aspect of cord (75%), lateral / anterolateral (25%)
- √ spinal cord open in midline dorsally
- √ lipoma in opening between lips of placode
- √ exophytic component at upper / lower pole of lipoma
- √ syringohydromyelia (2%)
- √ focal enlargement of spinal canal ± adjacent neural foramina
- √ narrow localized spina bifida

Lipomyelomeningocele

= lipoma tightly attached to exposed dorsal surface of neural placode blending with subcutaneous fat
Incidence: 20% of skin-covered lumbosacral masses; up to 50% of occult spinal dysraphism
Age: typically <6 months of age; M < F
- semifluctuant lumbosacral mass with overlying skin intact
- sensory loss in sacral dermatomes, motor loss, bladder dysfunction
- foot deformities, leg pain

Location: lumbosacral; longitudinal extension over entire length of spinal canal (in 7%)
- √ lipoma may enter central canal and extend rostrally (= "intradural intramedullary lipoma")
- √ lipoma may extend upward within spinal canal external to dura (= "epidural lipoma")
- √ tethered cord

√ large spinal canal
√ erosion of vertebral body + pedicles
√ posterior scalloping (50%)
√ focal spina bifida
√ segmental anomalies / butterfly vertebra (up to 43%)
√ confluent sacral foramina / partial sacral agenesis (up to 50%)

Fibrolipoma of Filum Terminale

Incidence: 6% of autopsies
• asymptomatic
Location: intradural filum, extradural filum, involvement of both portions
Prognosis: potential for development of symptoms of tethered cord

LÜCKENSCHÄDEL

= CRANIOLACUNIA = LACUNAR SKULL = mesenchymal dysplasia of calvarial ossification (developmental disturbance)
Age: present at birth
Associated with: (1) meningocele / myelomeningocele (2) encephalocele (3) spina bifida (4) cleft palate (5) Arnold-Chiari II malformation
• normal intracranial pressure
Location: particularly upper parietal area
√ honeycombed appearance about 2 cm in diameter (thinning of diploic space)
√ premature closure of sutures (turricephaly / scaphocephaly)
Prognosis: spontaneous regression within first 6 months of life
DDx: (1) Convolutional impressions = "digital" markings (visible at 2 years, maximally apparent at 4 years, disappear by 8 years of age)
(2) "Beaten brass" = "hammered silver" appearance of increased intracranial pressure

MENINGIOMA OF SPINE

Incidence: 25–45% of all spine tumors; 2–3% of pediatric spinal tumors; 12% of all meningiomas
Age: >40 years + female (80%)
Location: thoracic region (82%); cervical spine on anterior cord surface near foramen magnum (2nd most common location); 90% on lateral aspect
Site: intradural extramedullary (50%); entirely epidural; intradural + epidural
• spinal cord / nerve root compression
√ bone erosion in <10%
√ scalloping of posterior aspect of vertebral body
√ widening of interpedicular distance
√ enlargement of intervertebral foramen
√ may calcify (not as readily as intracranial meningioma)
CT:
√ solid smoothly marginated mass isodense to skeletal muscle
√ marked enhancement
MR:
√ isointense to grey matter on T1WI + T2WI
√ rapid + dense enhancement after Gd-DTPA

METASTASES TO SPINE

Source:
(a) Metastatic tumors: breast, prostate, lung, kidney, lymphoma, malignant melanoma
(b) Primary tumor: multiple myeloma
Pathogenesis: hematogenous spread to vertebral bodies (bones with greatest vascularity)
MR:
√ patchy multifocal relatively well defined lesions
√ diminished signal on T1WI + increased signal on T2WI (except for blastic metastases with diminished T1 + T2 signals)
DDx: (1) Infection (centered around disk space)
(2) Primary vertebral tumor (rare in older patients, almost always benign in patients <21 years of age)

METASTASES TO SPINAL CORD

Metastases from Outside CNS

(a) with subarachnoid hemorrhage: malignant melanoma, choriocarcinoma, hypernephroma, bronchogenic carcinoma
(b) others: breast, lymphoma
√ predominantly dorsal location
√ single / multiple nodules
√ thickening of meninges
√ matted nerve roots

CSF Seeding of Intracranial Neoplasms

Age: occurs more frequently in pediatric age group than in adults
CNS-tumors causing drop metastases:
1. Medulloblastoma: up to 33%
2. Ependymoma: after local recurrence, more common in infra- than supratentorial ependymomas
3. Anaplastic glioma
4. Germinoma
5. Pineoblastoma, pineocytoma

Less common: malignant choroid plexus papilloma, angioblastic meningioma

mnemonic: "MEGO TP"
Medulloblastoma
Ependymoma
Glioblastoma multiforme
Oligodendroglioma
Teratoma
Pineoblastoma

Location: lumbosacral + dorsal thoracic spine
√ thickened + nodular nerve roots
√ nodular + irregularly narrowed thecal sac
√ enlarged cord (from coating of outer wall of spinal cord)
√ Gd-DTPA enhancement

MYELOCYSTOCELE

= SYRINGOCELE

= hydromyelic spinal cord + arachnoid herniated through posterior spina bifida; least common form of spinal dysraphism

May be associated with: GI tract anomalies, GU tract anomalies

- cystic skin-covered mass over spine
- cloacal exstrophy (frequent)

Location: lower spine > cervical > thoracic spine

√ direct continuity of meningocele with subarachnoid space

√ cyst communicating with widened central canal of spinal cord typically posteriorly + inferiorly to meningocele

√ lordosis, scoliosis, partial sacral agenesis (common)

MYELOMENINGOCELE

= sac covered by leptomeninges containing CSF + variable amount of neural tissue; herniated through a defect in the posterior / anterior elements of spine

Incidence: 1:1,000–2,000 births (in Great Britain 1:200 births); twice as common in infants of mothers >35 years of age; Caucasians > Blacks > Orientals; most common congenital anomaly of CNS

Etiology: localized defect of closure of caudal neuropore (usually closed by 28 days)

- positive family history in 10%
- neural placode = reddish neural tissue in the middle of back made up of open spinal cord
- normal skin / cutaneous abnormality: pigmented nevus, abnormal distribution of hair, skin dimple, angioma, lipoma
- MS-AFP (≥ 2.5 S.D. over mean) permits detection in 80% (positive predictive value of 2–5%) if defect not covered by full skin thickness

Recurrence rate: 3–7% chance of NTD with previously affected sibling / in fetus of affected parent

Associated with:

(1) Hydrocephalus (70–90%): requiring ventriculoperitoneal shunt in 90%
◊ 25% of patients with hydrocephalus have spina bifida!

(2) Chiari II malformation (100%)

(3) Congenital / acquired kyphoscoliosis (90%)

(4) Vertebral anomalies (vertebral body fusion, hemivertebrae, cleft vertebrae, butterfly vertebrae)

(5) Diastematomyelia (31–46%): spinal cord split above (31%), below (25%), at the same level (22%) as the myelomeningocele

(6) Duplication of central canal (5%) cephalic to + at level of placode

(7) **Hemimyelocele** (10%) = two hemicords in separate dural tubes separated by fibrous / bony spur: one hemicord with myelomeningocele on one side of midline, one hemicord normal / with smaller myelomeningocele at a lower level
- impaired neurological function on side of hemimyelocele

(8) Hydromyelia (29–77%) depending on efficacy of hydrocephalus treatment

(9) Chromosomal anomalies (10–17%): trisomy 18, trisomy 13, triploidy, unbalanced translocation
◊ In 20% no detectable associated anomalies!

Location:

(a) **dorsal meningocele**: lumbosacral (70% below L2), suboccipital

(b) **anterior sacral meningocele** = prolapse through anterior sacral bony defect; occasionally associated with neurofibromatosis type 1, Marfan syndrome, partial sacral agenesis, imperforate anus, anal stenosis, tethered spinal cord, GU tract / colonic anomalies; M:F = 1:4

(c) **lateral thoracic meningocele** through enlarged intervertebral foramen into extrapleural aspect of thorax; right > left side, in 10% bilateral; often associated with neurofibromatosis (85%) + sharply angled scoliosis convex to meningocele
√ expanded spinal canal
√ erosion of posterior surface of vertebral body
√ thinning of neural arch
√ enlarged neural foramen

(d) **lateral lumbar meningocele** through enlarged neural foramina into subcutaneous tissue / retroperitoneum; often associated with neurofibromatosis / Marfan syndrome
√ expanded spinal canal
√ erosion of posterior surface of vertebral body
√ thinning of neural arch
√ enlarged neural foramen

(e) **traumatic meningocele** = avulsion of spinal nerve roots secondary to tear in meningeal root sheath; in C-spine after brachial plexus injury (most commonly)
√ small irregular arachnoid diverticulum with extension outside the spinal canal

(f) **cranial meningocele** = encephalocele

OB-US:

detection rate of 85–90%; sensitivity dependent on GA (fetal spine may be adequately visualized after 16–20 weeks GA); false-negative rate of 24%

√ spinal level estimated by counting up from last sacral ossification center = S4 in 2nd trimester + S5 in 3rd trimester (79% accuracy for ± spinal level)

√ may have clubfoot / rocker-bottom foot

√ polyhydramnios

@ Spine:

√ loss of dorsal epidermal integrity

√ soft-tissue mass protruding posteriorly + visualization of sac

√ widening of lumbar spine with fusiform enlargement of spinal canal
- √ splaying (= divergent position) of ossification centers of laminae with cup- / wedge-shaped pattern (in transverse plane = most important section for diagnosis)
- √ absence of posterior line = posterior vertebral elements (in sagittal plane)

√ gross irregularity in parallelism of lines representing laminae of vertebrae (in coronal plane)
√ anomalies of segmentation / hemivertebrae (33%) with short-radius kyphoscoliosis
√ tethered cord (with lumbar / lumbosacral myelomeningocele)

@ Head:
√ "lemon sign" = concave / linear frontal contour abnormality located at coronal suture associated with nonskin covered myelomeningocele (in 98% of fetuses ≤24 weeks + 13% of fetuses >24 weeks; positive predictive value 81–84%, in 0.7–1.3% of normal fetuses)
√ "banana sign" = obliteration of cisterna magna with cerebellum wrapped around posterior brainstem secondary to downward traction of spinal cord in Arnold-Chiari malformation type II (in 96% of fetuses ≤24 weeks + in 91% of fetuses >24 weeks)

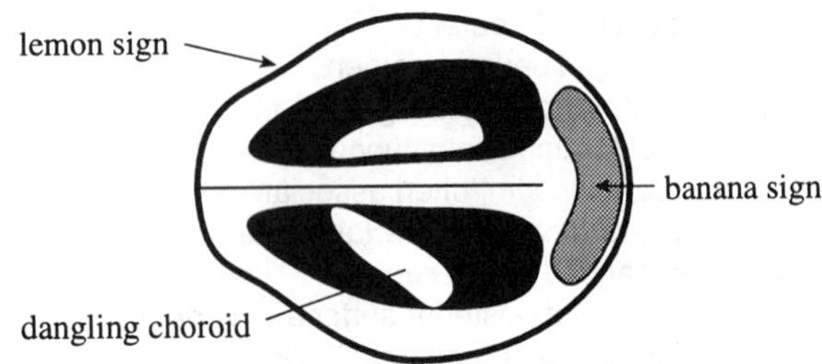

√ nonvisualization of cerebellum
√ effaced cisterna magna (100% sensitivity)
◊ the normal cisterna magna is 3–10 mm deep and usually visualized in 97% at 15–25 weeks GA
√ BPD <5th percentile during 2nd trimester (65–79% sensitivity)
√ HC <5th percentile (35% sensitivity)
√ ventriculomegaly (40–90%) with choroid plexus incompletely filling the ventricles (54–63% sensitivity) = "dangling" choroid on dependent side; in 44% of myelomeningoceles <24 weeks GA; in 94% of myelomeningoceles during 3rd trimester

Plain films:
√ bony defect in neural arch
√ deformity + failure of fusion of lamina
√ absent spinous process
√ widened interpedicular distance
√ widened spinal canal

Rx: (1) Possibly elective cesarean section at 36–38 weeks GA (may decrease risk of contaminating / rupturing the meningomyelocele sac)
(2) Repair within 48 hours

Postoperative complications:
(1) Postoperative tethering of spinal cord by placode / scar
(2) Constricting dural ring
(3) Cord compression by lipoma / dermoid / epidermoid cyst
(4) Ischemia from vascular compromise
(5) Syringohydromyelia

Prognosis:
(1) Mortality 15% by age 10 years
(2) Intelligence: IQ <80 (27%); IQ >100 (27%); learning disability (50%)
(3) Urinary incontinence: 85% achieve social continence (scheduled intermittent catheterization)
(4) Motor function: some deficit (100%); improvement after repair (37%)
(5) Hindbrain dysfunction associated with Chiari II malformation (32%)
(6) Ventriculitis: 7% in initial repair within 48 hours, more common in delayed repair >48 hours

NEURENTERIC CYST

= incomplete separation of foregut and notochord with persistence of canal of Kovalevski between yolk sac + notochord; cyst connected to meninges through midline defect

Incidence: rarest of bronchopulmonary foregut malformations (pulmonary sequestration, bronchogenic cyst, enteric cyst)

Associated with: neurofibromatosis; meningocele; spinal malformation (stalk connects cyst and neural canal; usually no stalk between cyst and esophagus)

Location: anterior to spinal canal on mesenteric side of gut

√ posterior mediastinal mass
√ air-fluid level (if communicating with GI-tract through diaphragmatic defect)
√ spinal dysraphism at the same level:
√ midline cleft in centra (accommodates stalk)
√ anterior / posterior spina bifida
√ vertebral body anomalies: absent vertebra, butterfly vertebra, hemivertebra, scoliosis
√ diastematomyelia
√ thoracic myelomeningocele

OSSIFYING FIBROMA

Peak incidence: first 2 decades of life

Histo: areas of osseous tissue intermixed with a highly cellular fibrous tissue

Sites: maxilla > frontal > ethmoid bone > mandible (rarely seen elsewhere)

√ areas of increased + decreased attenuation
√ intact inner + outer table
√ slow-growing expansile lesion
√ usually unilateral + monostotic

DDx: may be impossible to differentiate from fibrous dysplasia

OSTEOMYELITIS OF VERTEBRA

Incidence: 2–10% of all cases of osteomyelitis

Causes:
(1) direct penetrating trauma (most common); following surgical removal of nucleus pulposus

(2) hematogenous: associated with urinary tract infections / following GU surgery / instrumentation; diabetes mellitus; drug abuse

Pathophysiology: infection begins in low-flow end-vascular arcades adjacent to subchondral plate

Organism: Staphylococcus aureus, Salmonella

Peak age: 5th–7th decade

- pain in back, neck, chest, abdomen, flank, hip
- neurologic deficit
- fever (most common presenting symptom), leukocytosis
- increased erythrocyte sedimentation rate
- positive blood / urine culture

√ disk space narrowing (earliest radiographic sign)
√ demineralization of adjacent vertebral endplates
√ bulging of paraspinal lines
√ tracer uptake in adjacent portions of two vertebral bodies
√ decreased marrow signal on T1WI
√ iso- / hyperintense marrow signal on T2WI

Cx: secondary infection of intervertebral disk is frequent

Rx: >4 weeks course of IV antibiotics

DDx: discitis

PERINEURAL SACRAL CYST

= TARLOV CYST = cyst arising from posterior rootlets (S2 + S3 most common) = dilated nerve-root sleeve as normal variant

√ sacral erosion
√ may communicate with thecal sac

SACRAL AGENESIS

= CAUDAL REGRESSION SYNDROME = midline closure defect of neural tube

Incidence: 0.005–0.01%

Predisposed: infants of diabetic mothers (16%)

Associated with:

(1) musculoskeletal anomalies: hip dislocation, foot deformities, hypoplasia of extremities
(2) lack of bladder / bowel control
(3) spina bifida (myelomeningocele often not in combination with hydrocephalus) NOT associated with VATER syndrome

√ sacral agenesis
√ ± dural sac stenosis with high termination
√ ± tethered cord with associated lipoma, teratoma, cauda equina cyst

Cx: neurogenic bladder (if >2 segments are missing)

SACROCOCCYGEAL TERATOMA

Incidence: 1:40,000 livebirths; Type I + II (80%); most common congenital solid tumor in the newborn; M:F = 1:4

Pathogenesis:

(1) growth of residual primitive pluripotential cells derived from the primitive streak + knot (Hensen node) of very early embryonic development
(2) attempt at twinning
   - increased prevalence of twins in family

Histo:

(1) Mature teratoma (55–75%) with elements from glia, bowel, pancreas, bronchial mucosa, skin appendages, striated + smooth muscle, bowel loops, bone components (metacarpal bones + digits), well-formed teeth, choroid plexus structures (production of CSF)
   ◊ MATURE TERATOMA = benign tumor composed of tissues foreign to the anatomic site in which they arise, usually containing tissues from at least 2 germ cell layers
(2) Immature teratoma (11–28%): admixed with primitive neuroepithelial / renal tissue
   ◊ IMMATURE TERATOMA = benign teratoma with embryonic elements
(3) Malignant germ cell tumor
   (a) mixed malignant teratoma (7–17%): elements of endodermal sinus tumor (= yolk sac tumor) + either form of teratoma
   (b) pure endodermal sinus tumor (rare)
   (c) seminoma (dysgerminoma), embryonal carcinoma, choriocarcinoma (extremely rare)
   Metastases to: lung, bone, lymph nodes (inguinal, retroperitoneal), liver, brain

Age: 50–70% during first few days of life; 80% by 6 months of age; <10% >2 years of age; M:F = 1:4

Classification (Altman):

Type I	predominantly external lesion covered by skin with only minimal presacral component (47%)
Type II	predominantly external tumor with significant presacral component (35%)
Type III	predominantly sacral component + external extension (8%)
Type IV	presacral tumor with no external component (10%)

Associated with: other congenital anomalies (in 18%):

(1) musculoskeletal (5–16%): spinal dysraphism, sacral agenesis, dislocation of hip
(2) renal anomalies: hydronephrosis, renal cystic dysplasia, Potter syndrome
(3) GI tract: imperforate anus, gastroschisis, constipation
(4) fetal hydrops (due to high-output cardiac failure)
(5) placentomegaly (due to fetal hydrops)
(6) curvilinear sacrococcygeal defect (rare autosomal dominant inheritance with equal sex incidence, low malignant potential, absence of calcifications) + anorectal stenosis / atresia, vesicoureteral reflux

- AFP elevated with mixed malignant teratoma + endodermal sinus tumor (CAVE: fetal + newborn serum contains AFP which reaches adult levels not until about 8 months of age)
- premature labor (due to polyhydramnios + large mass)
- uterus large for dates
- radicular pain, constipation, urinary frequency / incontinence

Plain film:
√ amorphous, punctate, spiculated calcifications, possibly resembling bone (36–50%); suggestive of benign tumor
√ soft-tissue mass in pelvis protruding anteriorly + inferiorly
BE:
√ anterosuperior displacement of rectum
√ luminal constriction
IVP:
√ displacement of bladder anterosuperiorly
√ development of bladder neck obstruction
Myelography:
√ intraspinal component may be present
Angio:
√ neovascularity (arterial supply by middle + lateral sacral + gluteal branches of internal iliac artery, branches of profunda femoris artery)
√ enlargement of feeding vessels
√ arterial encasement
√ arteriovenous shunting
√ early venous filling with serpiginous dilated tumor veins
US / CT:
√ solid (25%) / mixed (60%) / cystic (15%) sacral mass
√ 1–30 cm (average size of 8 cm) in diameter
√ polyhydramnios (2/3)
√ oligohydramnios, fetal hydronephrosis, fetal hydrops with ascites, pleural effusions, skin edema, placentomegaly are poor prognostic factors
MR:
√ lobulated + sharply demarcated tumor extremely heterogeneous on T1WI as a result of high signal from fat, intermediate signal from soft tissue, low signal from calcium
√ best modality to detect spinal canal invasion

Prognosis: prevalence of malignant germ cell tumors increases with patient's age
◊ predominantly fatty tissue tumors are usually benign
◊ hemorrhage / necrosis is suggestive of malignancy
◊ cystic lesions are less likely malignant
◊ sacral destruction indicates malignancy
◊ patients >2 months of age have a malignant tumor with a 50–90% probability
Cx: (1) dystocia in 6–13%
(2) massive intratumoral hemorrhage
(3) fetal death in utero / stillbirth
Rx: 1. Complete tumor resection + coccygectomy + reconstruction of pelvic floor: up to 37% recurrence rate, esp. without coccygectomy
2. Multiagent chemotherapy (in malignancy) with long-term survival rate of 50%
DDx: 1. Myelomeningocele (superior to sacrococcygeal region, not septated, axial bone changes)
2. Rectal duplication, anterior meningocele (purely cystic)
3. Hemangioma, lymphangioma, lipomeningocele, lipoma, epidermal cyst, chordoma, sarcoma, ependymoma, neuroblastoma

SCHEUERMANN DISEASE

= SPINAL OSTEOCHONDROSIS = KYPHOSIS DORSALIS JUVENILIS = VERTEBRAL EPIPHYSITIS
= disorder consisting of vertebral wedging + endplate irregularity + narrowing of intervertebral disk space
Incidence: in 31% of male + 21% of female patients with back pain
Age: onset at puberty
Location: lower thoracic / upper lumbar vertebrae; in mild cases limited to 3–4 vertebral bodies
√ anterior wedging of vertebral body of >5°
√ increased anteroposterior diameter of vertebral body
√ slight narrowing of disk space
√ kyphosis of >40°/ loss of lordosis; scoliosis
√ Schmorl nodes (intravertebral herniation of nucleus pulposus into vertebral body) = depression in contour of endplate in posterior half of vertebral body; found in up to 30% of adolescents + young adults
√ flattened area in superior surface of epiphyseal ring anteriorly = avulsion fracture of ring apophysis due to migration of nucleus pulposus through weak point between ring apophysis + vertebral endplate (fusion of ring apophysis usually occurs at about 18 years of age)
√ detached epiphyseal ring anteriorly
DDx: (1) Developmental notching of anterior vertebrae (NO wedging or Schmorl nodes)
(2) Osteochondrodystrophy (earlier in life, extremities show same changes)

SPINAL STENOSIS

= encroachment on central spinal canal, lateral recess, or neuroforamen by bone / soft tissue
Cause:
A. Congenitally short pedicles
(a) idiopathic
(b) developmental: Down syndrome, achondroplasia, hypochondroplasia, Morquio disease
B. Acquired:
1. Hypertrophy of ligamentum flavum = buckling of ligament secondary to joint slippage in facet joint osteoarthritis (most common)
2. Facet joint hypertrophy
3. Degenerated bulging disk
4. Spondylosis, spondylolisthesis
5. Surgical fusion
6. Fracture
7. Ossification of posterior longitudinal ligament
8. Paget disease
9. Epidural lipomatosis
Age: middle-aged for congenital cause / elderly during 6th–8th decade for acquired cause; M > F
Location: generally involves lumbar spinal canal; cervical spinal canal may be similarly affected
√ distorted shape of thecal sac
√ obliteration of epidural fat
√ narrowing of cervical canal <13 mm, of lumbar canal <16 mm (AP diameter)
√ interpedicular distance <25 mm
◊ Measurements are not a valid indicator of disease!

Lumbar Spinal Stenosis

Cause:

1. Achondroplasia:
   √ narrowed interpediculate distance progressive toward lumbar spine
2. Paget disease: bony overgrowth
3. Spondylolisthesis
4. Operative posterior spinal fusion
5. Herniated disk
6. Metastasis to vertebrae
7. Developmental / congenital

Age: presentation between 30–50 years of age

- low back pain
- "neurogenic claudication" = bilateral lower extremity pain, numbness, weakness worse during walking / standing + relieved in supine position and flexion
- cauda equina syndrome: paraparesis, incontinence, sensory findings in saddlelike pattern, areflexia

√ sagittal diameter of spinal canal <12 mm (normal range in adults: 15–23 mm)
√ dural sac area <100 mm^2
√ diminished amount of CSF + crowding of nerve roots
√ unusual small quantity of contrast material to fill thecal sac
√ anteroposterior + interpediculate diameter spinal canal constricted
√ hourglass configuration of thecal sac (SAG view)
√ triangular / trefoil shape of thecal sac (AXIAL view)
√ redundant serpiginous nerve roots above + below stenosis
√ may appear as spinal block in hyperextended neck on AP views
√ thickened articular process, pedicles, laminae, ligaments
√ bulging disks

SPLIT NOTOCHORD SYNDROME

= spectrum of anomalies with persistent connection between gut + dorsal ectoderm

Etiology: failure of complete separation of ectoderm from endoderm with subsequent splitting of notochord and mesoderm around the adhesion about 3rd week of gestation

√ fistula / isolated diverticula / duplication / cyst / fibrous cord / sinus along the tract

Types:

1. **Dorsal enteric fistula**
   = fistula between intestinal cavity + dorsal midline skin traversing prevertebral soft tissue, vertebral body, spinal canal, posterior elements of spine
   - bowel ostium / exposed pad of mucous membrane in dorsal midline in newborn
   - opening passes meconium + feces

   √ dorsal bowel hernia into a skin- / membrane-covered dorsal sac after passing through a combined anterior + posterior spina bifida
2. **Dorsal enteric sinus**
   = blind remnant of posterior part of tract with midline opening to dorsal external skin surface
3. **Dorsal enteric enterogenous cyst**
   = prevertebral / postvertebral / intraspinal enteric-lined cyst derived from intermediate part of tract

   Intraspinal enteric cyst

   Age at presentation: 20–40 years
   - intermittent local / radicular pain worsened by elevation of intraspinal pressure

   Location: intraspinal in lower cervical / upper thoracic region

   √ enlarged spinal canal at site of cyst
   √ hemivertebrae, segmentation defect, partial fusion, scoliosis in region of cyst
4. **Dorsal enteric diverticulum**
   = tubular / spherical diverticulum arising from dorsal mesenteric border of bowel as a persistent portion of tract between gut + vertebral column
5. **Dorsal enteric cyst**
   = involution of portion of diverticulum near gut
   - mass in abdomen / mediastinum (due to bowel rotation)

SPONDYLOLISTHESIS

= forward displacement of one vertebra over another

Incidence: 4% of general population

Location: L5/S1 or L4/L5

Grades I–IV (Meyerding method): each grade equals 1/4 anterior subluxation of superior on inferior vertebral body

Isthmic Spondylolisthesis = open-arch type

Cause: usually bilateral spondylolysis

= separation of anterior part (vertebral body, pedicles, transverse processes, superior articular facet) from posterior part (inferior facet, laminae, dorsal spinous process)

Age: often <45 years

- symptomatic if intervertebral disk + posterosuperior aspect of vertebral body encroaches on superior portion of neuroforamen

√ elongation of spinal canal in anteroposterior diameter
√ bilobed configuration of neuroforamen
√ ratio of maximum anteroposterior diameter of spinal canal at any level divided by diameter at L1 >1.25

Degenerative Spondylolisthesis = closed-arch type

= PSEUDOSPONDYLOLISTHESIS

Cause: degenerative / inflammatory joint disease (eg, rheumatoid arthritis)

Pathophysiology: excess motion of facet joints

Age: usually >60 years

- commonly symptomatic

√ narrowing of spinal canal
√ hypertrophy of facet joints
√ ratio of maximum anteroposterior diameter of spinal canal at any level divided by diameter at L1 <1.25

SPONDYLOLYSIS

= pars interarticularis defect between superior + inferior articulating processes as the weakest portion of spinal unit

Incidence: 3–7% of population; in 30–70% other family members afflicted
Age: early childhood; M:F = 3:1; Whites:Blacks = 3:1
Cause:
(a) pseudarthrosis following stress (fatigue) fracture of pars (in most) from repetitive minor trauma; common in gymnastics (30%), diving, contact sports (football, soccer, hockey, lacrosse)
(b) hereditary hypoplasia of pars leads to insufficiency fracture; eg, pars defect in 34% of Eskimos
(c) secondary spondylolysis: neoplasm, osteomyelitis, Paget disease, osteomalacia, osteogenesis imperfecta
(d) congenital malformation: frequently associated with spina bifida occulta of S1, dorsally wedge-shaped body of L5, hypoplasia of L5; HOWEVER: no pars defects have been identified in fetal cadavers

- symptomatic in 50% (if associated with degenerative disk disease / spondylolisthesis)

Location: L5 (67–95%); L4 (15–30%); L3 (1–2%); in 75% bilateral
Plain film:
√ radiolucent band ± sclerotic margin resembling the collar of the "Scottie dog" (on oblique view)
√ may be associated with spondylolisthesis
√ subluxation of involved vertebra (if pars defect bilateral)
√ Wilkinson syndrome = reactive sclerosis + bony hypertrophy of contralateral pedicle + lamina (produced by stress changes related to weakening of neural arch in unilateral pars defect)
◊ Planar / SPECT bone scintigraphy may be useful!
CT:
√ pars defect located 10–15 mm above disk space
√ inner contour of spinal canal interrupted

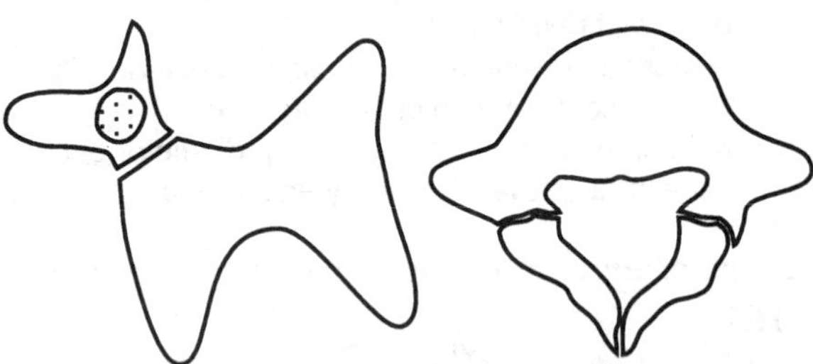

Spondylolysis
oblique radiograph of L5 — CT scan through mid-vertebral body

Spondylolysis of Cervical Spine
= progressive degeneration of intervertebral disks leading to proliferative changes of bone + meninges; more common than disk herniation as a cause for cervical radiculopathy
Incidence: 5–10% at age 20–30; >50% at age 45; >90% by age 60

- spastic gait disorder
- neck pain

Location: C4-5, C5-6, C6-7 (greater normal cervical motion at these levels)
Sequelae: (a) direct compression of spinal cord
(b) neural foraminal stenosis
(c) ischemia due to vascular compromise
(d) repeated trauma from normal flexion / extension
DDx of myelopathy:
rheumatoid arthritis, congenital anomalies of craniocervical junction, intradural extramedullary tumor, spine metastases, cervical spinal cord tumor, arteriovenous malformation, amyotrophic lateral sclerosis, multiple sclerosis, neurosyphilis

SYRINGOHYDROMYELIA
= SYRINGOMYELIA = SYRINX (used in a general manner reflecting difficulty in classification)
= longitudinally oriented CSF-filled cavities + gliosis within spinal cord frequently involving both parenchyma + central canal
Age: primarily childhood / early adult life

- loss of sensation to pain + temperature (interruption of spinothalamic tracts)
- trophic changes [skin lesions; Charcot joints in 25% (shoulder, elbow, wrist)]
- muscle weakness (anterior horn cell involvement)
- spasticity, hyperreflexia (upper motor neuron involvement)
- abnormal plantar reflexes (pyramidal tract involvement)

Location: predominantly lower end of cervical cord; extension into brainstem (= syringobulbia)
CT:
√ distinct area of decreased attenuation within spinal cord (100%)
√ swollen / normal-sized / atrophic cord
√ no contrast enhancement
√ flattened vertebral border (rare) with increased transverse diameter of cord
√ change in shape + size of cord with change in position (rare)
√ filling of syringohydromyelia with intrathecal contrast
(a) early filling via direct communication with subarachnoid space
(b) late filling after 4–8 hours (80–90%) secondary to permeation of contrast material
Myelography:
√ enlarged cord (DDx: intramedullary tumor)
√ "collapsing cord sign" = collapsing of cord with gas myelography as fluid content moves caudad in the erect position (rare)
MR:
√ cystic area of low signal intensity on T1WI, increased intensity on T2WI
√ presence of CSF flow-void (= low signal on T2WI) within cavity from pulsations
√ beaded cavity from multiple incomplete septations
√ cord enlargement

Hydromyelia
= PRIMARY SYRINGOHYDROMYELIA
= CONGENITAL SYRINGOHYDROMYELIA

= dilatation of persistent central canal of spinal cord (in 70–80% obliterated) which communicates with 4th ventricle (= communicating syringomyelia)

Histo: lined by ependymal tissue

Associated with:
(1) Chiari malformation in 20–70%
√ metameric haustrations within syrinx on sagittal T1WI
(2) Spinal dysraphism
(3) Myelocele
(4) Dandy-Walker syndrome
(5) Diastematomyelia
(6) Scoliosis in 48–87%
(7) Klippel-Feil syndrome
(8) Spinal segmentation defects
(9) Tethered cord (in up to 25%)

Syringomyelia

= ACQUIRED / SECONDARY SYRINGOHYDROMYELIA
= any cavity within substance of spinal cord which may communicate with the central canal, usually extending over several vertebral segments

Histo: not lined by ependymal tissue

Pathophysiology: interrupted flow of CSF through the perivascular spaces of cord between subarachnoid space + central canal

Cause:
1. Posttraumatic syringomyelia
Incidence: in 3.2% after spinal cord injury
Location: 68% in thoracic cord
√ 0.5–40 cm (average 6 cm) in length
√ syrinx may be septated (parallel areas of cavitation) on transverse T1WI
√ loss of sharp cord-CSF interface (obliteration of arachnoid space by adhesions)
√ in 44% associated with arachnoid loculations (extramedullary arachnoid cysts) at upper aspect of syrinx
2. Postinflammatory syringomyelia
subarachnoid hemorrhage, arachnoid adhesions, S/P surgery, infection (tuberculosis, syphilis)
3. Tumor-associated syringomyelia
spinal cord tumors, herniated disk; secondary to circulatory disturbance + thoracic spinal cord atrophy
4. Vascular insufficiency

Reactive Cyst

= POSTTRAUMATIC SPINAL CORD CYST
= CSF-filled cyst adjacent to level of trauma; usually single (75%)
• late deterioration in patients with spinal cord injury (not related to severity of original injury)

Rx: shunting leads to clinical improvement

TETHERED CORD

= TIGHT FILUM TERMINALE SYNDROME = LOW CONUS MEDULLARIS
= abnormally short + thickened filum terminale with low position of conus medullaris

Etiology: failure of ascent of conus (normal location of tip of conus medullaris: L 4/5 at 16 weeks of gestation, L 2/3 at birth, L1/2 >3 months of age)

Pathophysiology: mechanical + metabolic + vascular insults with stretching of cord

Age at presentation: 5–15 years (in years of growth spurt); M:F = 2:3

Associated with: lipoma in 29–78%, diastematomyelia, imperforate anus

• dorsal nevus, dermal sinus tract, hair patch (50%)
• bowel + bladder dysfunction in childhood
• spastic gait with muscle stiffness
• lower extremity weakness + muscle atrophy
• asymmetric hyporeflexia + fasciculations
• orthopedic anomalies: scoliosis, pes cavus, tight Achilles tendon
• hypalgesia, dysesthesia
• paraplegia, paraparesis
• radiculopathy (adults)
• hyperactive deep tendon reflexes
• extensor plantar responses
• anal / perineal pain (in adults)
• back pain (particularly with exertion)

√ lumbar spina bifida occulta with interpedicular widening
√ scoliosis (20%)
√ diameter of filum terminale >2 mm at L5-S1 level (55%), small fibrolipoma within thickened filum (23%), small filar cyst (3%), spinal cord ending in a small lipoma (13%)
√ posteriorly located tethered conus medullaris + filum terminale (supine views)
√ conus medullaris below level of L2 by age 12 (86%)
√ abnormal lateral course of nerve roots (>15° angle relative to spinal cord)
√ widened triangular thecal sac tented posteriorly (thecal sac pulled posteriorly by filum)

MR:
√ prolonged T1 relaxation in center of spinal cord on T1WI in 25% (? myelomalacia / mild hydromyelia)

Rx: decompressive laminectomy / partial removal of lipoma ± freeing of cord

TERATOMA OF SPINE

= neoplasm containing tissue belonging to all 3 germinal layers at sites where these tissues do not normally occur

Incidence: 0.15% (excluding sacrococcygeal teratoma)

Age: all ages; M:F = 1:1

Path: solid, thin- / thick-walled partially / wholly cystic with clear / milky / dark cyst fluid, uni- / multilocular, presence of bone / cartilage

Location: intra- / extramedullary

√ complete block at myelography
√ syringomyelia above level of tumor
√ spinal canal may be focally widened

DIFFERENTIAL DIAGNOSIS OF BRAIN DISORDERS

Birth trauma

1. **Caput succedaneum**
   = localized edema in presenting portion of scalp, frequently associated with microscopic hemorrhage + subcutaneous hyperemia
   Cause: common after vaginal delivery
   • soft superficial pitting edema
   √ crosses suture lines
2. **Subgaleal hemorrhage**
   = hemorrhage subjacent to aponeurosis covering scalp beneath the occipito-frontalis muscle
   • may become symptomatic secondary to blood loss
   • firm fluctuant mass increasing in size after birth
   • may dissect into subcutaneous tissue of neck
   • usually resolves over 2–3 weeks
3. **Cephalohematoma**
   = hematoma beneath outer layer of periosteum
   Cause: incorrect application of obstetric forceps / skull fracture during birth
   Incidence: 1–2% of all deliveries
   Location: most commonly parietal
   • firm tense mass
   • usually increase in size after birth
   • resolution in few weeks to months
   √ crescent-shaped lesion adjacent to outer table of skull
   √ will not cross cranial suture line
   √ may calcify / ossify causing thickening of diploe
4. Skull fracture
   Incidence: 1% of all deliveries
   √ CT shows associated intracranial hemorrhage
5. Subdural hemorrhage
   (a) convexity hematoma (b) interhemispheric hematoma (c) posterior fossa hematoma
6. **Benign subdural effusion**
   = benign condition that resolves spontaneously
   • clear / xanthochromic fluid with elevated protein level
   √ extracerebral fluid collection accompanied by ventricular dilatation (= communicating hydrocephalus caused by impaired CSF absorption of these subdural fluid collections)

Increased intracranial pressure

1. Intracranial mass
2. Hydrocephalus
3. Malignant hypertension
4. Diffuse cerebral edema
5. Increased venous pressure
6. Elevated CSF protein
7. Pseudotumor cerebri

• papilledema
√ enlargement of perioptic nerve subarachnoid space

Prolactin elevation

Normal level: up to 25 ng/mL

Cause:
1. Interference with hypothalamic-pituitary axis:
   (a) hypothalamic tumor
   (b) parasellar tumor
   (c) pituitary adenoma
   (d) sarcoidosis
   (e) histiocytosis
   (f) traumatic infundibular transection
2. Pharmacologic agents
   alpha-methyldopa, reserpine, phenothiazine, butyrophenone, tricyclic antidepressants, oral contraceptives
3. Hypothyroidism (TRH also stimulates prolactin)
4. Renal failure
5. Cirrhosis
6. Stress / recent surgery
7. Breast examination
8. Pregnancy
9. Lactation

Stroke

= generic term designating a heterogeneous group of cerebrovascular disorders
Incidence:
3rd leading cause of death in United States (after heart disease + cancer); 2nd leading cause of death due to cardiovascular disease in U.S.; 2nd leading cause of death in patients >75 years of age; 450,000 new cases per year; 160 new strokes per 100,000 population per year; leading cause of death in Orient
Age: >55 years; M:F = 2:1
Risk factors: heredity, hypertension (50%), smoking, diabetes (15%), obesity, familial hypercholesterolemia, myocardial infarction, atrial fibrillation, congestive heart failure, alcoholic excess, oral contraceptives, high anxiety + stress
Etiology:
A. NONVASCULAR (5%): eg, tumor, hypoxia
B. VASCULAR (95%)
   1. Brain infarction = ischemic stroke (80%)
      (a) Occlusive atheromatous disease of extracranial (35%) / intracranial (10%) arteries
      = large vessel disease between aorta + penetrating arterioles
      — critical stenosis, thrombosis,
      — plaque hemorrhage / ulceration / embolism
      (b) Small vessel disease of penetrating arteries (25%) = lacunar infarct
      (c) Cardiogenic emboli (6–15–23%)
      Ischemic heart disease with mural thrombus
      — acute myocardial infarction (3% risk/year)
      — cardiac arrhythmia
      Valvular heart disease
      — postinflammatory (rheumatic) valvulitis
      — infective endocarditis (20% risk/year)

— nonbacterial thrombotic endocarditis (30% risk/year)
— mitral valve prolapse (low risk)
— mitral stenosis (20% risk/year)
— prosthetic valves (1–4% risk/year)
Nonvalvular atrial fibrillation (6% risk/year)
Left atrial myxoma (27–55% risk/year)
(d) Nonatheromatous disease (5%)
— elongation, coil, kinks (up to 20%)
— fibromuscular dysplasia (typically spares origin + proximal segment of ICA)
— aneurysm (rare) may occur in cervical / petrous portion / intracranially
— dissection: traumatic / spontaneous (2%)
— cerebral arteritis (Takayasu, collagen disease, lymphoid granulomatosis, temporal arteritis, Behçet disease, chronic meningitis, syphilis)
— postendarterectomy thrombosis / embolism / restenosis
(e) Overactive coagulation (5%)
2. Hemorrhagic stroke (20%)
(a) Primary intracerebral hemorrhage (15%)
— Hypertensive hemorrhage (40–60%)
— Amyloid angiopathy (15–25%)
— Vascular malformation (10–15%)
— Drugs: eg, anticoagulants (1–2%)
— Bleeding diathesis (<1%): eg, hemophilia
(b) Vasospasm due to nontraumatic SAH (4%)
— Ruptured aneurysm (75–80%)
— Vascular malformation (10–15%)
— "Nonaneurysmal" SAH (5–15%)
(c) Veno-occlusive disease (1%): sinus thrombosis

May be preceded by TIA
◊ 10–14% of all strokes are preceded by TIA!
◊ 60% of all strokes ascribed to carotid disease are preceded by TIA!

Prognosis:
(1) death during hospitalization (25%): alteration in consciousness, gaze preference, dense hemiplegia have a 40% mortality rate
(2) survival with varying degrees of neurologic deficit (75%)
(3) good functional recovery (40%)
◊ Hypodensity involving >50% of MCA territory has a fatal outcome in 85%!

◊ Clinical diagnosis inaccurate in 13%!

Role of imaging:
1. Confirm clinical diagnosis
2. Identify primary intracerebral hemorrhage
3. Detect structural lesions mimicking stroke: tumor, vascular malformation, subdural hematoma
4. Detect early complications of stroke: cerebral herniation, hemorrhagic transformation

Indications for cerebrovascular testing:
1. TIA = transient ischemic attack
2. Progression of carotid disease to 95–98% stenosis
3. Cardiogenic cerebral emboli

Temporal classification:
1. **TIA** = transient ischemic attack
2. **RIND** = reversible ischemic neurologic deficit
= fully reversible prolonged ischemic event resulting in minor neurologic dysfunction for >24 hours
Incidence: 16 per 100,000 population per year
3. **Progressing stroke** = stepwise / gradually progressing accumulative neurologic deficit evolving over hours / days
4. **Slow stroke** = rare clinical syndrome presenting as developing neuronal fatigue with weakness in lower / proximal upper extremity after exercise; occurs in patients with occluded internal carotid artery
5. **Completed stroke** = severe + persistent stable neurologic deficit = cerebral infarction (death of neuronal tissue) as end stage of prolonged ischemia
• level of consciousness correlates well with size of infarction
Prognosis: 6–11% recurrent stroke rate

Transient ischemic attack

= brief episode of transient focal neurological deficit owing to ischemia of <24 hours duration with return to pre-attack status

Incidence: 31 per 100,000 population per year; increasing with age up to 300; 105,000 new cases per year in United States; M > F

Cause: (1) embolic: usually from ulcerative plaque at carotid bifurcation
(2) hemodynamic: fall in perfusion pressure distal to a high-grade stenosis / occlusion

Risk factors:
(1) Hypertension (linear increase in probability of stroke with increase in diastolic blood pressure)
(2) Cardiac disorders (prior myocardial infarction, angina pectoris, valvular heart disease, dysrhythmia, congestive heart failure)
(3) Diabetes mellitus
(4) Cigarette smoking (weak)

Prognosis: 5.3% stroke rate per year for 5 years after first TIA; per year 12% increase of stroke / myocardial infarction / death; complete stroke in 33% within 5 years; complete stroke in 5% in 1 month

A. CAROTID TIA (2/3)
• carotid attacks <6 hours in 90%
• transient weakness / sensory dysfunction CLASSICALLY in
(a) hand / face with embolic event
(b) proximal arm + lower extremity with hemodynamic event (watershed area)
— motor dysfunction = weakness, paralysis, clumsiness of one / both limbs on same side
— sensory alteration = numbness, loss of sensation, paresthesia of one / both limbs on same side
— speech / language disturbance = difficulty in speaking (dys- / aphasia) / writing, in comprehension of language / reading / performing calculations

— visual disturbance = loss of vision in one eye, homonymous hemianopia, amaurosis fugax
- paresis (mono-, hemiparesis) in 61%
- paresthesia (mono-, hemiparesthesia) in 57%
- amaurosis fugax (= transient premonitory attack of impaired vision due to retinal ischemia) in 12% caused by transient hypotension or emboli of platelets / cholesterol crystals which may be revealed by funduscopy
- facial paresthesia in 30%

B. VERTEBROBASILAR TIA (1/3)
- vertebrobasilar events <2 hours in 90%

— motor dysfunction = as with carotid TIA but sometimes changing from side to side including quadriplegia, diplopia, dysarthria, dysphagia

— sensory alteration = as with carotid TIA usually involving one / both sides of face / mouth / tongue

— visual loss = as with carotid TIA including uni- / bilateral homonymous hemianopia

— disequilibrium of gait / postural disturbance, ataxia, imbalance / unsteadiness

— drop attack = sudden fall to the ground without loss of consciousness
- binocular visual disturbance in 57%
- vertigo in 50%
- paresthesia in 40%
- diplopia in 38%
- ataxia in 33%
- paresis in 33%
- headaches in 25%
- seizures in 1.5%

Accelerating / crescendo TIA

= repeated periodic events of neurologic dysfunction with complete recovery to normal in interphase

Rx: 1. Carotid endarterectomy (1% mortality, 5% stroke)
2. Anticoagulation
3. Antiplatelet agent: aspirin, ticlopidine

— in patients with recently symptomatic TIA / minor stroke + >70% carotid artery stenosis: prophylactic carotid endarterectomy + chronic low-dose aspirin therapy

Infection in immunocompromised patients

Cause: underlying malignancy, collagen disease, cancer therapy, AIDS, immunosuppressive therapy in organ transplants

Organism: Toxoplasma, Nocardia, Aspergillus, Candida, Cryptococcus

√ poorly defined hypodense zones with rapid enlargement in size + number, particularly affecting basal ganglia + centrum semiovale (poorly localized + encapsulated infection with poor prognosis)

√ ring / nodular enhancement (sufficient immune defenses): Toxoplasma, Nocardia

√ enhancement may be blunted by steroid Rx

AIDS may be associated with:
thrombocytopenia, lymphoma, plasmacytoma, Kaposi sarcoma, progressive multifocal leukoencephalopathy

Trigeminal neuropathy

- facial pain, numbness, weakness of masticatory muscles, trismus
- diminished / absent corneal reflex
- abnormal jaw reflex
- decreased pain / touch / temperature sensation
- atrophy of masticatory muscles
- **tic douloureux** = paroxysmal facial pain (usually confined to V_2 and V_3) mainly caused by neurovascular compression (tortuous elongated superior cerebellar artery / anterior inferior cerebellar artery / vertebrobasilar dolichoectasia / venous compression)

A. BRAIN STEM LESION
1. Vascular: infarct, AVM
2. Neoplastic: glioma, metastasis
3. Inflammatory: multiple sclerosis (1–8%), herpes rhombencephalitis
4. Other: syringobulbia

B. CISTERNAL CAUSES
1. Vascular: aneurysm, AVM, vascular compression
2. Neoplastic: acoustic schwannoma, meningioma, trigeminal schwannoma, epidermoid cyst, lipoma, metastasis
3. Inflammatory: neuritis

C. MECKEL CAVE + CAVERNOUS SINUS
1. Vascular: carotid aneurysm
2. Neoplastic: meningioma, trigeminal schwannoma, epidermoid cyst, lipoma, pituitary adenoma, base of skull neoplasm, metastasis, perineural tumor spread
3. Inflammatory: Tolosa-Hunt syndrome

D. EXTRACRANIAL
1. Neoplastic: neurogenous tumor, squamous cell carcinoma, adenocarcinoma, lymphoma, adenoid cystic carcinoma, mucoepidermoid carcinoma, melanoma, metastasis, perineural tumor spread
2. Inflammatory: sinusitis
3. Other: masticator space abscess, trauma

Dementia

1. Alzheimer disease
2. Pick disease
3. Normal pressure hydrocephalus
4. Subdural hematoma
5. Brain mass

CLASSIFICATION OF CNS ANOMALIES

A. DORSAL INDUCTION ANOMALY
= defects of neural tube closure
1. Chiari malformation: at 4 weeks
2. Encephalocele: at 4 weeks
3. Anencephaly
4. Spinal dysraphism
5. Hydromyelia

B. VENTRAL INDUCTION ANOMALY
1. Holoprosencephaly: 5 – 6 weeks
2. Septo-optic dysplasia: 6 – 7 weeks
3. Dandy-Walker malformation: 7 – 10 weeks
4. Agenesis of septum pellucidum

C. NEURONAL PROLIFERATION & HISTOGENESIS
1. Neurofibromatosis: 5 weeks – 6 months
2. Tuberous sclerosis: 5 weeks – 6 months
3. Primary hydranencephaly: >3 months
4. Neoplasia
5. Vascular malformation (vein of Galen, AVM, hemangioma)

D. NEURONAL MIGRATION ANOMALY
due to infection, ischemia, metabolic disorders
1. Schizencephaly: 2 months
2. Agyria + pachygyria: 3 months
3. Gray matter heterotopia: 5 months
4. Dysgenesis of corpus callosum: 2 – 5 months
5. Lissencephaly
6. Polymicrogyria
7. Unilateral megalencephaly

E. DESTRUCTIVE LESIONS
1. Hydranencephaly
2. Porencephaly
3. Hypoxia
4. Toxicosis
5. Inflammatory disease (TORCH)
   (a) **To**xoplasmosis
   (b) **R**ubella
      √ punctate / nodular calcifications
      √ porencephalic cysts
      √ occasionally microcephaly
   (c) **C**ytomegalic inclusion disease
      √ typically punctate / stippled / curvilinear periventricular calcifications
      √ often hydrocephalus
   (d) **H**erpes simplex

Absence of septum pellucidum

1. Holoprosencephaly
2. Callosal agenesis
3. Septo-optic dysplasia
4. Schizencephaly
5. Severe chronic hydrocephalus
6. Destructive porencephaly

Phakomatoses

= NEUROCUTANEOUS SYNDROMES
= NEUROECTODERMAL DYSPLASIAS
= development of benign tumors / malformations especially in organs of ectodermal origin
1. Neurofibromatosis
2. Tuberous sclerosis
3. von Hippel-Lindau disease
4. Sturge-Weber-Dimitri syndrome
5. Ataxia-telangiectasia

DEGENERATIVE DISEASES OF CEREBRAL HEMISPHERES

= progressive fatal disease characterized by destruction / alteration of gray and white matter

Etiology: genetic; viral infection; nutritional disorders (eg, anorexia nervosa, Cushing syndrome); immune system disorders (eg, AIDS); exposure to toxins (eg, CO); exposure to drugs (eg, alcohol, methotrexate + radiation)

Leukodystrophy
= degenerative diffuse sclerosis with symmetrical bilateral white matter lesions

Leukoencephalopathy
= disease of white matter

A. DEMYELINATING DISEASE
= normal myelin destroyed by disease process
1. Multiple sclerosis (most frequent primary demyelinating disease)
2. Alzheimer disease (most common of diffuse gray matter degenerative diseases)
3. Parkinson disease (most common subcortical degenerative disease)
4. Creutzfeldt-Jakob disease
5. Menkes disease (sex-linked recessive disorder of copper metabolism)
6. Progressive multifocal leukoencephalopathy
7. Disseminated necrotizing leukoencephalopathy
8. Globoid cell leukodystrophy
9. Spongiform degeneration
10. Cockayne syndrome
11. Spongiform leukoencephalopathy
12. Myelinoclastic diffuse sclerosis (Schilder disease)

B. DYSMYELINATING DISEASE
= metabolic disorder (= enzyme deficiency) resulting in deficient / absent myelin sheaths
(a) macrencephalic:
   1. Alexander disease (frontal areas affected first)
   2. Canavan disease (white matter diffusely affected)
(b) hyperdense thalami, caudate nuclei, corona radiata
   1. Krabbe disease
(c) family history (X-linked recessive)
   1. X-linked adrenoleukodystrophy
   2. Pelizaeus-Merzbacher disease
(d) others
   1. Metachromatic leukodystrophy (most common hereditary leukodystrophy)
   2. Binswanger disease (SAE)
   3. Multi-infarct dementia (MID)
   4. Pick disease
   5. Huntington disease
   6. Wilson disease
   7. Reye syndrome
   8. Mineralizing microangiopathy
   9. Diffuse sclerosis

BRAIN ATROPHY

Cerebral atrophy

= irreversible loss of brain substance + subsequent enlargement of intra- and extracerebral CSF-containing spaces (hydrocephalus ex vacuo = ventriculomegaly)

A. DIFFUSE BRAIN ATROPHY

Cause:

(a) Trauma, radiation therapy
(b) Drugs (dilantin, steroids, methotrexate, marijuana, hard drugs, chemotherapy), alcoholism, hypoxia
(c) Demyelinating disease (multiple sclerosis, encephalitis)
(d) Degenerative disease
eg, Alzheimer disease, Pick disease, Jakob-Creutzfeldt disease
(e) Cerebrovascular disease + multiple infarcts
(f) Advancing age, anorexia, renal failure
√ enlarged ventricles + sulci

B. FOCAL BRAIN ATROPHY

Cause: vascular / chemical / metabolic / traumatic / idiopathic (Dyke-Davidoff-Mason syndrome)

C. REVERSIBLE PROCESS SIMULATING ATROPHY (in younger people)

Cause: anorexia nervosa, alcoholism, catabolic steroid treatment, pediatric malignancy

√ prominent sulci
√ ipsilateral dilatation of basal cisterns + ventricles
√ ex vacuo dilatation of ventricles
√ thinning of gyri

Cerebellar atrophy

A. WITH CEREBRAL ATROPHY
= generalized senile brain atrophy

B. WITHOUT CEREBRAL ATROPHY

1. Olivopontocerebellar degeneration / Marie ataxia / Friedreich ataxia
   • onset of ataxia in young adulthood
2. Ataxia-telangiectasia
3. Ethanol-toxicity: predominantly affecting midline (vermis)
4. Phenytoin-toxicity: predominantly affecting cerebellar hemispheres
5. Idiopathic degeneration secondary to carcinoma (= paraneoplastic), usually oat cell carcinoma of lung
6. Radiotherapy
7. Focal cerebellar atrophy:
   (a) infarction (b) traumatic injury

EXTRA-AXIAL LESIONS

Extra-axial tumor

mnemonic: "MABEL"

Meningioma
Arachnoid cyst
Bony lesion
Epidermoid
Leukemic / lymphomatous infiltration

Leptomeningeal disease

A. INFLAMMATION

1. Langerhans cell histiocytosis
2. Sarcoidosis
3. Wegener granulomatosis
4. Chemical meningitis: rupture of epidermoid

B. INFECTION

1. Bacterial meningitis
2. Tuberculous meningitis
3. Fungal meningitis
4. Neurosyphilis

C. TUMOR

(a) Primary meningeal tumor:
1. Meningioma
2. Glioma: primary leptomeningeal glioblastomatosis / gliosarcomatosis
3. Melanoma / melanocytoma
4. Sarcoma
5. Lymphoma

(b) CSF-spread from primary CNS tumor
1. Medulloblastoma
2. Germinoma
3. Pineoblastoma

(c) Metastasis
1. Breast carcinoma
2. Lymphoma / leukemia
3. Lung carcinoma
4. Malignant melanoma
5. Gastrointestinal carcinoma
6. Genitourinary carcinoma

D. TRAUMA

1. Old subarachnoid hemorrhage
2. Surgical scarring from craniotomy
3. Lumbar puncture

Intra- versus extra-axial mass

	intra-axial	extra-axial
Relationship to dura / bone	no attachment until advanced	contiguous
Local bony changes	uncommon	common
Displacement of cortex	toward dura / bone	away from bone
Subarachnoid cistern	effaced	widened
Feeding arteries	pial feeding arteries	dural feeding arteries

Pericerebral Fluid Collection In Childhood

A. ENLARGED SUBARACHNOID SPACE
  (a) due to macrocephaly
  (b) due to brain atrophy
  √ superficial cortical veins cross subarachnoid space to reach superior sagittal sinus
  √ wide sulci, normal configuration of gyri
  √ normal / prominent size of ventricles

B. SUBDURAL FLUID COLLECTION
  (1) Subdural hygroma
  (2) Subdural empyema / abscess (due to meningitis)
  (3) Subdural hematoma
  √ superficial cortical veins are prevented to cross subarachnoid by presence of arachnoid / neomembrane
  √ wide interhemispheric fissure

VENTRICLES

Ventriculomegaly

A. MACROCEPHALY
  • increased intraventricular pressure
  (a) Obstruction to CSF flow
    1. Communicating hydrocephalus
    2. Noncommunicating hydrocephalus
  (b) Overproduction of CSF = nonobstructive hydrocephalus
  (c) Neoplasm

B. MICROCEPHALY
  • normal intraventricular pressure
  (a) Primary failure of brain growth
    — dysgenesis
      1. Holoprosencephaly
      2. Aneuploidy syndromes (trisomies)
      3. Migrational (<6 layers)
    — environment: alcohol, drugs, toxins
    — infection: TORCH
  (b) Loss of brain mantle
    — Infection: TORCH
    — Vascular accident:
      1. Hydranencephaly
      2. Schizencephaly
      3. Porencephaly
    — Hemorrhage:
      1. Porencephaly
      2. Leukomalacia

C. NORMOCEPHALY

Colpocephaly

= dilatation of trigones + occipital horns + posterior temporal horns of lateral ventricles

1. Agenesis of corpus callosum
2. Arnold-Chiari malformation
3. Holoprosencephaly

Intraventricular tumor

Prevalence: 10% of all intracranial neoplasms

1. Ependymoma	20%
2. Astrocytoma	18%
3. Colloid cyst	12%
4. Meningioma	11%
5. Choroid plexus papilloma	7%
6. Epidermoid / dermoid	6%
7. Craniopharyngioma	6%
8. Medulloblastoma	5%
9. Cysticercosis	5%
10. Arachnoid cyst	4%
11. Subependymoma	2%
12. AVM	2%
13. Teratoma	1%
14. Metastasis	
15. Intraventricular neurocytoma	
16. Oligodendroglioma	

Tumor In 4th Ventricle

1. Choroid plexus papilloma
2. Ependymoma / glioma
3. Hemangioblastoma
4. Vermian metastasis
5. AVM
6. Epidermoid tumor (rare)
7. Inflammatory mass
8. Cyst

Tumor In 3rd Ventricle

1. Colloid cyst
2. Glioma
3. Aneurysm
4. Craniopharyngioma
5. Ependymoma
6. Meningioma
7. Choroid plexus papilloma
8. Intraventricular neurocytoma

PERIVENTRICULAR REGION

Periventricular Hypodensity

1. Encephalomalacia
   √ slightly denser than CSF
2. Porencephaly
   = cavity communicating with ventricle / cistern from intracerebral hemorrhage
   Associated with: dilated ventricle, sulci, and fissures
   √ CSF density
3. Resolving hematoma
   • Hx of previously demonstrated hematoma
   √ may show ring enhancement + compression of adjacent structures
4. Cystic tumor
   √ mass effect + contrast enhancement

Enhancing Ventricular Margins

(a) Subependymal spread of metastatic tumor
  1. Bronchogenic carcinoma (especially small cell carcinoma)
  2. Melanoma
  3. Breast carcinoma
(b) Subependymal seeding of CNS primary
  1. Glioma
  2. Ependymoma

(c) Ependymal seeding of CNS primary
1. Medulloblastoma
2. Germinoma
(d) Primary CNS lymphoma / systemic lymphoma
(e) Inflammatory ventriculitis

Periventricular calcifications in a child

1. Tuberous sclerosis
2. Congenital infection: CMV, toxoplasmosis

Periventricular T2WI-hyperintense lesions

A. YOUNG PATIENTS
1. Multiple sclerosis
2. Migraine: in 41% with classic migraine, in 57% with complicated migraine; presumed to represent vasculitis-induced small infarcts
3. Vasculitic disorder: SLE, Behçet disease, sickle cell disease
√ triad of deep white matter lesions + cortical infarcts + hemorrhage
4. Acute disseminated encephalomyelitis (ADE)
= postviral leukoencephalopathy
5. Virchow-Robin space
= small invaginations of subarachnoid space following pia mater along perforating nutrient end vessels into brain substance
Location: inferior third of putamen; usually bilateral
√ 1–2 mm round lesions isointense to CSF (well seen on coronal sections through centrum semiovale + on low-axial sections at level of anterior commissure)
6. Leukodystrophy: in children
√ symmetric diffuse confluent involvement
7. Ependymitis granularis
= symmetrically focal areas of hyperintensity on T2WI anterior + lateral to frontal horns in normal individuals
Histo: patchy loss of ependyma with paucity of hydrophobic myelin, which allows migration of fluid out of the ventricle into interstitium

B. ELDERLY
1. **État criblé** (sievelike) / gliosis
= deep white matter ischemia
= extensive number of perivascular fluid spaces predominantly at arteriolar level as part of subacute arteriosclerotic encephalopathy
Cause: chronic ischemia due to arteriosclerosis of long penetrating arteries arising from circle of Willis (lenticulostriate + thalamo-perforators) = small vessel disease
Predisposed: cigarette smoker, hypertensive patient
Histo: lipohyalin deposits within vessel walls followed by partial demyelination, gliosis, interstitial edema
Incidence: in 10% without risk factors, in 84% with risk factors and symptoms
Age: >60 years (in 30–60%)
Location: periventricular white matter > optic radiation > basal ganglia > centrum semiovale > brainstem (usually spares corpus callosum + subcortical U-fibers)
√ multiple focal lesions <2 mm
2. Lacunar infarction

C. PATIENTS WITH AIDS
1. HIV encephalitis:
√ well-defined "patchy" / ill-defined "dirty white matter"
√ central atrophy
2. Toxoplasmosis
3. Lymphoma
4. Progressive multifocal leukoencephalopathy (PML)

D. PATIENTS WITH TRAUMA
1. Diffuse axonal / shearing injury
2. Diffuse white matter injury
= radiation-induced demyelination of periventricular white matter
Cause: whole-brain irradiation
• subclinical
3. Diffuse necrotizing leukoencephalopathy
Cause: intrathecal methotrexate ± whole brain irradiation
• rapidly deteriorating clinical course
√ confluent pattern with scalloped margins within periventricular white matter extending out to subcortical U-fibers

E. PATIENTS WITH HYDROCEPHALUS
1. Transependymal CSF flow
√ smooth halo of even thickness

HYPODENSE BRAIN LESIONS

Diffusely swollen hemispheres

A. METABOLIC
1. Metabolic encephalopathy: eg, uremia, Reye syndrome, ketoacidosis
2. Anoxia: cardiopulmonary arrest, near-drowning, smoke inhalation, ARDS

B. NEUROVASCULAR
1. Hypertensive encephalopathy
2. Superior sagittal sinus thrombosis
3. Head trauma
4. Pseudotumor cerebri

C. INFLAMMATION
eg, herpes encephalitis, CMV, toxoplasmosis

Edema of brain

= increase in brain volume due to increased tissue-water content (80% for gray matter + 68% for white matter is normal)
Etiology:
(a) Cytotoxic edema
reversible increase in intracellular water content secondary to ischemia / anoxia (axonal pallor)

(b) Vasogenic edema (most common form)
increase in pinocytotic activity with passage of protein across vessel wall into intercellular space (lack of contrast enhancement means breakdown of blood-brain barrier is not the cause); associated with primary brain neoplasm, metastases, hemorrhage, infarction, inflammation

Types:

1. Hydrostatic edema
   rapid increase / decrease in intracranial pressure
2. Interstitial edema
   increase in periventricular interstitial spaces secondary to transependymal flow of CSF with elevated intraventricular pressure
3. Hypoosmotic edema
   produced by overhydration from IV fluid / inappropriate secretion of antidiuretic hormone
4. Congestive brain swelling
   rapid accumulation of extravascular water as a result of head trauma; may become irreversible (brain death) if intracranial pressure equals systolic blood pressure

√ decreased distinction between gray + white matter
√ compressed slitlike lateral ventricles
√ compression of cerebral sulci + perimesencephalic cisterns

CT:
- √ areas of hypodensity
- ◊ Edema is always greatest in white matter!
- √ mass effect: flattening of gyri, displacement + deformation of ventricles, midline shift
- √ return to normal from nonhemorrhagic edema / brain atrophy from white matter shearing injury

MR:
- √ decreased intensity on T1WI, increased intensity on T2WI
- √ enhancement with gadolinium

US:
- √ generalized / focal increase of parenchymal echogenicity with featureless appearance
- √ decreased resistive indices

Brain herniation

1. Subfalcine
   contralateral shift of midline structures under falx cerebri
2. Transtentorial
   (a) upward: displacement of cerebellum through tentorial incisura
   (b) downward
   - anterior: uncal herniation (most common) caused by lesions in anterior half of brain
   - posterior: herniation of parahippocampal gyrus
   - total: herniation of entire hippocampus
3. Retroalar
   herniation of frontal lobe posteriorly across edge of sphenoid ridge
4. Transforaminal
   herniation of inferior mesial portions of cerebellum downward through foramen magnum

Cholesterol-containing CNS lesions

1. Epidermoid inclusion cyst
2. Cholesterol granuloma
3. Acquired epidermoid of middle ear
4. Congenital cholesteatoma of middle ear
5. Craniopharyngioma

Cyst with a mural nodule

1. Pilocytic astrocytoma (childhood)
2. Ganglioglioma
3. Pleomorphic xanthoastrocytoma
4. Glioblastoma multiforme
5. Hemangioblastoma (posterior fossa, spinal cord)

Midline cyst

1. **Cavum septi pellucidi** = "5th ventricle"
   = thin triangular membrane consisting of two glial layers covered laterally with ependyma separating the frontal horns of lateral ventricles
   Incidence: in 80% of term infants; in 15% of adults
   Location: posterior to genu of corpus callosum, inferior to body of corpus callosum, anterosuperior to anterior pillar of fornix
   √ extends to foramen of Monro
   √ may dilate + cause obstructive hydrocephalus (rare)
2. **Cavum vergae** = "6th ventricle"
   = cavity posterior to columns of fornix; contracts after about 6th gestational month
   Incidence: in 30% of term infants; in 15% of adults
   Location: posterior to fornix, anterior to splenium of corpus callosum, inferior to body of corpus callosum, superior to transverse fornix
   √ posterior midline continuation of cavum septi pellucidi beyond foramen of Monro
3. **Cavum veli interpositi**
   = extension of quadrigeminal plate cistern above 3rd ventricle to foramen of Monro, laterally bounded by columns of fornix + thalamus
4. Colloid cyst: anterior + superior to cavum septi pellucidi
5. Arachnoid cyst: in region of quadrigeminal plate cistern
   √ curvilinear margins

Posterior fossa cystic malformation

1. Dandy-Walker malformation
2. Dandy-Walker variant
3. Megacisterna magna
4. Arachnoid pouch

Suprasellar low-density lesion with hydrocephalus

A. CYST
   1. Arachnoid cyst
   2. Ependymal cyst of 3rd ventricle

3. Parasitic cyst of 3rd ventricle (cysticercosis)
4. Dilated 3rd ventricle (in aqueductal stenosis)

B. CYSTIC MASS
1. Epidermoid
2. Hypothalamic pilocytic astrocytoma
3. Cystic craniopharyngioma

Nota bene: Cystic lesion may be inapparent within surrounding CSF; metrizamide cisternography is helpful in detection + to exclude aqueduct stenosis

Mesencephalic low-density lesion

1. Normal: decussation of superior cerebellar peduncles at level of inferior colliculi
2. Syringobulbia
   found in conjunction with syringomyelia, Arnold-Chiari malformation, trauma
   √ CSF density centrally
   √ intrathecal contrast enters central cavity
3. Brainstem infarction
   √ abnormal contrast enhancement after 1 week
   √ well-defined low-attenuation region without enhancement after 2–4 weeks
4. Central pontine myelinolysis
   comatose patient receiving rapid correction / overcorrection of severe hyponatremia (following prolonged IV fluid administration / alcoholism)
   Pathophysiology:
   rapid correction of sodium releases myelinotoxic compounds by gray matter components resulting in loss of myelin (osmotic myelinolysis) with preservation of neurons + axons
   • spastic quadriparesis + pseudobulbar palsy
   • progression to pseudocoma (locked-in syndrome) in 3–5 days
   √ diminished attenuation in central region of pons
   √ ± extrapontine lesions in basal ganglia, thalami
   Prognosis: 10% survival rate beyond 6 months
5. Brainstem glioma
   √ mass with indistinct margins + vague enhancement
6. Metastasis
   √ well-defined contrast enhancement
7. Granuloma in TB / sarcoidosis (rare)

Intracranial pneumocephalus

Cause:

A. TRAUMA (74%):
(a) fracture
in 3% of all skull fractures; in 8% of fractures involving paranasal sinuses (frontal > ethmoid > sphenoid > mastoid) or base of skull
(b) penetrating injury

B. NEOPLASM INVADING SINUS (13%):
1. Osteoma of frontal / ethmoid sinus
2. Pituitary adenoma
3. Mucocele, epidermoid
4. Malignancy of paranasal sinuses

C. INFECTION WITH GAS-FORMING ORGANISM (9%):
in mastoiditis, sinusitis

D. SURGERY (4%):
hypophysectomy, paranasal sinus surgery

Mechanism (dural laceration):
(1) ball-valve mechanism during straining, coughing, sneezing
(2) vacuum phenomenon secondary to loss of CSF

Time of onset: on initial presentation (25%), usually seen within 4–5 days, delay up to 6 months (33%)

Mortality: 15%

Cx:
1. CSF rhinorrhea (50%)
2. Meningitis / epidural / brain abscess (25%)
3. Extracranial pneumocephalus = air collection in subaponeurotic space

HYPERDENSE INTRACRANIAL LESIONS

Intracranial calcifications

mnemonic: "PINEEAL"
Physiologic
Infection
Neoplasm
Endocrine
Embryologic
Arteriovenous
Leftover Ls

A. PHYSIOLOGIC INTRACRANIAL CALCIFICATIONS

B. INFECTION
TORCH (toxoplasmosis, CMV, rubella, herpes), healed abscess, hydatid cyst, granuloma (tuberculoma, actinomycosis, coccidioidomycosis, cryptococcosis, mucormycosis), cysticercosis, trichinosis, paragonimiasis
mnemonic:
CMV calcifications are circumventricular
Toxoplasma calcifications are intraparenchymal

C. NEOPLASM
Craniopharyngioma (40–80%), oligodendroglioma (50–70%), chordoma (25–40%), choroid plexus papilloma (10%), meningioma (20%), pituitary adenoma (3–5%), pinealoma (10–20%), dermoid (20%), lipoma of corpus callosum, ependymoma (50%), astrocytoma (15%), after radiotherapy, metastases (1–2%, lung > breast > GI tract)
N.B.: astrocytomas calcify less frequently but are the most common tumor
mnemonic: "Ca^{2+} COME"
Craniopharyngioma
Astrocytoma, **A**neurysm,
Choroid plexus papilloma
Oligodendroglioma
Meningioma, **M**edulloblastoma
Ependymoma

D. ENDOCRINE
Hyperparathyroidism, hypervitaminosis D, hypoparathyroidism, pseudohypoparathyroidism, CO poisoning, lead poisoning

E. EMBRYOLOGIC
Neurocutaneous syndromes (tuberous sclerosis, Sturge-Weber, neurofibromatosis), Fahr disease, Cockayne syndrome, basal cell nevus syndrome

F. ARTERIOVENOUS
Atherosclerosis, aneurysm, AVM, occult vascular malformation, hemangioma, subdural + epidural hematomas, intracerebral hemorrhage

G. LEFTOVER Ls
Lipoma, lipoid proteinosis, lissencephaly

Physiologic intracranial calcification

1. Pineal calcification
   Age: no calcification <5 years of age, in 8–10% at 8–14 years of age, in 40% by 20 years of age, 2/3 of adult population
   √ amorphous / ringlike calcification <3 mm from midline usually <10 mm in diameter
   √ approximately 30 mm above highest posterior elevation of pyramids
   CAVE: pineal calcification >14 mm suggests pineal neoplasm (teratoma / pinealoma)
2. Habenula
   Incidence: approximately in 1/3 of population
   Age: >10 years of age
   √ posteriorly open C-shaped calcification 4–6 mm anterior to pineal gland
3. Choroid plexus
   may calcify in all ventricles: most commonly in glomus within atrium of lateral ventricles, near foramen of Monro, tela choroidea of 3rd ventricle, roof of 4th ventricle, along foramina of Luschka
   Age: >3 years of age
   √ 20–30 mm behind + slightly below pineal on lateral projection, symmetrical on AP projection
   DDx: neurofibromatosis
4. Dura, falx cerebri, falx cerebelli, tentorium
   Incidence: 10% of population
   Age: >3 years of age
   DDx: basal cell nevus syndrome (Gorlin syndrome), pseudoxanthoma elasticum, congenital myotonic dystrophy
5. Petroclinoid ligament (= reflection of tentorium) between tip of dorsum sellae and apex of petrous bone
   Age: >5 years of age
6. Interclinoid ligament
   = interclinoid bridging
7. Arteriosclerosis: particularly intracavernous segment of ICA, basilar a., vertebral a.
8. Basal ganglia

Increased density of falx

1. Subarachnoid hemorrhage
2. Interhemispheric subdural hematoma
3. Diffuse cerebral edema (= increased density relative to low-density brain)
4. Dural calcifications (hypercalcemia from chronic renal failure, basal cell nevus syndrome, hyperparathyroidism)
5. Normal falx (can be normal in pediatric population)

Intraparenchymal hemorrhage

mnemonic: "ITHACANS"
- **I**nfarction (hemorrhagic)
- **T**rauma
- **H**ypertensive hemorrhage
- **A**rteriovenous malformation
- **C**oagulopathy
- **A**neurysm, **A**myloid angiopathy
- **N**eoplasm: metastasis / primary neoplasm
- **S**inus thrombosis

Dense cerebral mass

Substrate: calcification / hemorrhage / dense protein

A. VESSEL
   1. Aneurysm
   2. Arteriovenous malformation
   3. Hematoma (acute / subacute)

B. TUMOR
   1. Lymphoma
   2. Medulloblastoma
   3. Meningioma
   4. Metastasis
      (a) from mucinous-producing adenocarcinoma
      (b) hemorrhagic metastases: melanoma, choriocarcinoma, hypernephroma, bronchogenic carcinoma, breast carcinoma (rarely)

Dense lesion near foramen of Monro

A. INTRAVENTRICULAR LESION
   1. Colloid cyst
   2. Meningioma
   3. Choroid plexus tumor / granuloma
   4. AVM of septal, thalamostriate, internal cerebral veins

B. PERIVENTRICULAR MASS
   1. Primary CNS lymphoma
   2. Tuberous sclerosis
      (a) subependymal tuber
      (b) giant cell astrocytoma
   3. Metastasis from mucin-producing adenocarcinoma / hemorrhagic metastasis (melanoma, choriocarcinoma, hypernephroma, bronchogenic carcinoma, breast carcinoma)
   4. Glioblastoma of septum pellucidum

C. MASSES PROJECTING SUPERIORLY FROM SKULL BASE
   1. Pituitary adenoma
   2. Craniopharyngioma
   3. Aneurysm
   4. Dolichoectatic basilar artery

BRAIN MASSES

Classification of primary CNS tumors

A. TUMORS OF BRAIN AND MENINGES
   (a) Gliomas
      Astrocytoma (50%)
         1. Astrocytoma (astrocytoma grades I – II)
         2. Glioblastoma (astrocytoma grades III – IV)
      Oligodendroglioma

Paraglioma
1. Ependymoma
2. Choroid plexus papilloma
Ganglioglioma
Medulloblastoma
(b) Pineal tumor
1. Germinoma
2. Teratoma
3. Pineocytoma
4. Pineoblastoma
(c) Pituitary tumor
1. Pituitary adenoma
2. Pituitary carcinoma
(d) Meningioma
(e) Nerve sheath tumor
1. Schwannoma
2. Neurofibroma
(f) Miscellaneous
1. Sarcoma
2. Lipoma
3. Hemangioblastoma

B. TUMORS OF EMBRYONAL REMNANTS
(a) Craniopharyngioma
(b) Colloid cyst
(c) Teratoid tumor
1. Epidermoid
2. Dermoid
3. Teratoma

Incidence Of Brain Tumors

= 9% of all primary neoplasms (5th most common primary neoplasm); 5–10 cases per 100,000 population per year; account for 1.2% of autopsied deaths

IN ALL AGE GROUPS:	
Glioma	34%
Meningioma	17%
Metastasis	12%
Pituitary adenoma	6%
Neurinoma	4%
Sarcoma	3%
Granuloma	3%
Craniopharyngioma	2%
Hemangioblastoma	2%

IN PEDIATRIC AGE GROUP:	
Astrocytoma	50%
Medulloblastoma	15%
Ependymoma	10%
Craniopharyngioma	6%
Choroid plexus papilloma	2%

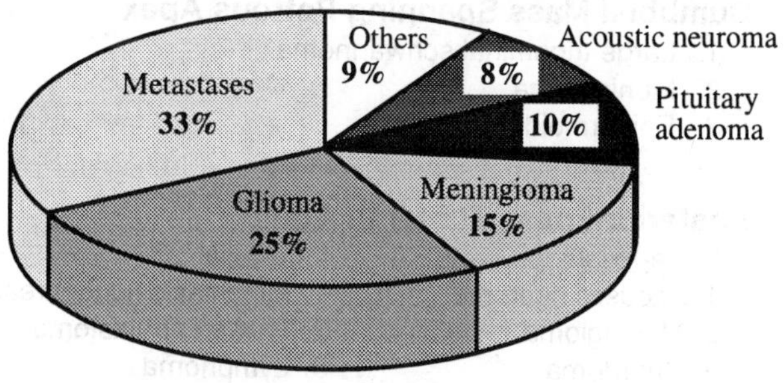

Intracranial Tumors in Adult Population

CNS Tumors Presenting At Birth

1. Hypothalamic astrocytoma
2. Choroid plexus papilloma / carcinoma
3. Teratoma
4. Primitive neuroectodermal tumor
5. Medulloblastoma
6. Ependymoma
7. Craniopharyngioma

CNS Tumors In Pediatric Age Group

Incidence:
2.4:100,000 (<15 years of age); 2nd most common pediatric tumor (after leukemia); 15% of all pediatric neoplasms; 15–20% of all primary brain tumors; M > F

- increased intracranial pressure
- increasing head size

A. SUPRATENTORIAL (50%)
Age: first 2–3 years of life

Covering of brain	dural sarcoma, schwannoma, meningioma (3%)
Cerebral hemisphere	astrocytoma (37%), oligodendroglioma
Corpus callosum	astrocytoma
3rd ventricle	colloid cyst, ependymoma
Lateral ventricle	ependymoma (5%), choroid plexus papilloma (12%)
Optic chiasm	craniopharyngioma (12%), optic nerve glioma (13%), teratoma, pituitary adenoma
Hypothalamus	glioma (8%), hamartoma
Pineal region	germinoma, pinealoma, teratoma (8%)

B. INFRATENTORIAL (50%)
Age: 4–11 years

Cerebellum	astrocytoma (31–33%), medulloblastoma (26–31%)
Brainstem	glioma (16–21%)
4th ventricle	ependymoma (6–14%), choroid plexus papilloma

mnemonic: "BE MACHO"
Brainstem glioma
Ependymoma
Medulloblastoma
AVM
Cystic astrocytoma
Hemangioblastoma
Other

Supratentorial MidlineTumors

1. Optic + hypothalamic glioma (39%)
2. Craniopharyngioma (20%)
3. Astrocytoma (9%)
4. Pineoblastoma (9%)
5. Germinoma (6%)
6. Lipoma (6%)
7. Teratoma (3.5%)
8. Pituitary adenoma (3.5%)
9. Meningioma (2%)
10. Choroid plexus papilloma (2%)

Supratentorial IntraventricularTumors

(a) Lateral ventricle (3/4)
1. Choroid plexus tumor (44%)
2. Giant cell astrocytoma in tuberous sclerosis (19%)
3. Hemangioma in Sturge-Weber syndrome (12%)

(b) Third ventricle (1/4)
1. Astrocytoma (13%)
2. Choroid plexus tumor (6%)
3. Meningioma (6%)

CLASSIFICATION BY HISTOLOGY
1. Astrocytic tumors (33.5%)
2. "Primitive" neuroectodermal tumor = PNET (21%) highly malignant neoplasms originating from germinal matrix + containing glial + neural elements
   — Medulloblastoma (16%)
   — Ependymoblastoma (2.5%)
   — PNET of cerebral hemisphere (2.5%)
3. Mixed gliomas (16%)
4. Malformative tumors (11.5%)
   — Craniopharyngioma (5.5%)
   — Lipoma (4.5%)
   — Dermoid cyst (1%)
   — Epidermal cyst (0.5%)
5. Choroid plexus tumors (4%)
6. Ependymal tumors (4%)
7. Tumors of meningeal tissues (3.5%)
   — Meningioma (3%)
   — Meningeal sarcoma (0.5%)
8. Germ cell tumors (2.5%)
   — Germinoma (1.5%)
   — Teratomatous tumor (1%)
9. Neuronal tumors
   — Gangliocytoma (1.5%)
10. Tumors of neuroendocrine origin
   — Pituitary adenoma (1%)
11. Oligodendroglial tumors (0.5%)
12. Tumors of blood vessel
   — Hemangioma (1%)

Multifocal CNS Tumors

A. METASTASES FROM PRIMARY CNS TUMOR
   (a) via commissural pathways: corpus callosum, internal capsule, massa intermedia
   (b) via CSF: ventricles / subarachnoid cisterns
   (c) satellite metastases

B. MULTICENTRIC CNS TUMOR
   (a) true multicentric gliomas (4%)
   (b) concurrent tumors of different histology (coincidental)

C. MULTICENTRIC MENINGIOMAS (3%) without neurofibromatosis

D. MULTICENTRIC PRIMARY CNS LYMPHOMA

E. PHAKOMATOSES
1. Generalized neurofibromatosis:
   meningiomatosis, bilateral acoustic neuromas, bilateral optic nerve gliomas, cerebral gliomas, choroid plexus papillomas, multiple spine tumors, AVMs
2. Tuberous sclerosis:
   subependymal tubers, intraventricular gliomas (giant cell astrocytoma), ependymomas
3. von Hippel-Lindau disease:
   retinal angiomatosis, hemangioblastomas, congenital cysts of pancreas + liver, benign renal tumors, cardiac rhabdomyomas

CNS Tumors Metastasizing Outside CNS

mnemonic: "MEGO"
Medulloblastoma
Ependymoma
Glioblastoma multiforme
Oligodendroglioma

Calcified Intracranial Mass

mnemonic: "Ca^{2+} COME"
Craniopharyngioma
Astrocytoma, **A**neurysm
Choroid plexus papilloma
Oligodendroglioma
Meningioma
Ependymoma

Avascular Mass Of Brain

mnemonic: "TEACH"
Tumor: astrocytoma, metastasis, oligodendroglioma
Edema
Abscess
Cyst, **C**ontusion
Hematoma, **H**erpes

Jugular Foramen Mass

1. Glomus tumor
2. Meningioma
3. Neuroma
4. Metastasis

Dumbbell Mass Spanning Petrous Apex

1. Large trigeminal schwannoma
2. Meningioma
3. Epidermoid cyst

Posterior Fossa Tumor In Adult

Extra-axial	Intra-axial
1. Acoustic neuroma	1. Metastasis (lung, breast)
2. Meningioma	2. Hemangioblastoma
3. Chordoma	3. Lymphoma
4. Choroid plexus papilloma	4. Lipoma
5. Epidermoid	

Cystic mass in cerebellar hemisphere

1. Hemangioblastoma
2. Cerebellar astrocytoma
3. Metastasis
4. Lateral medulloblastoma (= "cerebellar sarcoma")
5. Choroid plexus papilloma with lateral extension

Cerebellopontine angle tumor

= extra-axial tumor arising in CSF-filled space bound by pons + cerebellar hemisphere + petrous bone

Incidence: 5–10% of all intracranial tumors

- cranial neuropathy: high frequency hearing loss (n. VIII), tinnitus + facial motor dysfunction (n. V II), facial sensory dysfunction (n. V), taste disturbance (chorda tympani)
- signs of posterior fossa mass effect: headache, nausea, vomiting, disequilibrium, ataxia
- hemifacial spasm, trigeminal neuralgia (tic douloureux)

√ may widen CSF space (cistern) in 25%
√ bone erosion / hyperostosis
√ sharp margination with brain

Types:

1. Acoustic neuroma = schwannoma (80–90%): from intracanalicular portion of 8th cranial nerve
2. Meningioma (10–18%)
   2nd most common extra-axial mass in posterior fossa; <5% of all intracranial meningiomas; larger + more hemispheric in shape + more homogeneously enhancing than acoustic neuroma
3. Epidermoid inclusion cyst (5–9%)
4. Arachnoid cyst (<1%)
5. Aneurysm of basilar / vertebral / posterior inferior cerebellar artery:
   congenital berry aneurysm / saccular aneurysm / atherosclerotic dolichoectasia
6. Choroid plexus papilloma
7. Ependymoma
8. Trigeminal neuroma
   from gasserian ganglion within Meckel cave in the most anteromedial portion of petrous pyramid / trigeminal nerve root
9. Glomus jugulare tumor
   within adventitia of bulb of jugular vein at base of petrous bone with invasion of posterior fossa
10. Chordoma
11. Exophytic brainstem glioma
    Histo: usually diffuse fibrillary astrocytoma
12. Metastasis (0.2–2%)
13. Lipoma (<1%)

mnemonic: "**E**ver **G**rave **C**erebello**P**ontine **A**ngle **M**asses"

Epidermoid
Glomus jugulare tumor
Chondroma, **C**hordoma, **C**holesteatoma
Pituitary tumor, **P**ontine glioma (exophytic)
Acoustic + trigeminal neuroma, **A**neurysm of basilar / vertebral artery, **A**rachnoid cyst
Meningioma, **M**etastasis

LOW-ATTENUATION EXTRA-AXIAL LESION:

1. Acoustic schwannoma (occasionally low-density mass)
2. Epidermoid tumor
3. Arachnoid cyst

Lesion expanding cavernous sinus

A. TUMOR
   1. Trigeminal schwannoma
   2. Pituitary adenoma
   3. Parasellar meningioma
   4. Parasellar metastasis
   5. Invasion by tumor of skull base
B. VESSEL
   1. Internal carotid artery aneurysm
   2. Carotid-cavernous fistula
   3. Cavernous sinus thrombosis
C. TOLOSA-HUNT SYNDROME
   = granulomatous invasion of cavernous sinus

ENHANCING BRAIN LESIONS

Gyral enhancement

A. MENINGEAL TUMOR
   (a) Meningeal carcinomatosis from systemic tumor: eg, breast carcinoma, small cell carcinoma of lung, malignant melanoma, lymphoma / leukemia
   (b) Seeding primary CNS tumor:
      1. Medulloblastoma
      2. Pineoblastoma
      3. Ependymoma
B. MENINGITIS
   pyogenic, tuberculous, fungal, cysticercosis, sarcoidosis
C. SEQUELAE OF SUBARACHNOID HEMORRHAGE (from fibroblastic proliferation)
D. SUBACUTE BRAIN INFARCT

mnemonic: "CAL MICE"

Cerebritis
Arteriovenous malformation
Lymphoma
Meningitis
Infarct
Carcinomatosis
Encephalitis

Ring-enhancing lesion of brain

Cause:

A. NEOPLASM
   1. Primary neoplasm: high-grade glioma, meningioma, lymphoma, leukemia, pituitary macroadenoma, acoustic neuroma, craniopharyngioma
   2. Metastatic carcinoma + sarcoma
B. ABSCESS
   1. Abscess: bacterial, fungal, parasitic
   2. Empyema of epidural / subdural / intraventricular spaces

C. HEMORRHAGIC-ISCHEMIC LESION
  1. Resolving infarction
  2. Aging hematoma
  3. Operative bed following resection
  4. Thrombosed aneurysm

D. DEMYELINATING DISORDER
  1. Radiation necrosis
  2. Tumefactive demyelinating lesion ("singular sclerosis")
  3. Necrotizing leukoencephalopathy after methotrexate

Pathogenesis:
(1) hypervascular margin of lesion = granulation tissue / peripheral vascular channels / hypervascular tumor capsule
(2) breakdown of blood-brain barrier = leakage of contrast out of abnormally permeable vessels into extracellular fluid space
(3) hypodense center = avascular / hypovascular (requires time to fill) / cystic degeneration

Incidence of ring blush:
abscess (in 73%); glioblastoma (in 48%); metastasis (in 33%); grade II astrocytoma (in 26%) [NOT in grade I astrocytoma]

mnemonic: "MAGIC DR"
Metastasis
Abscess / cerebritis
Glioma, **G**lioblastoma multiforme
Impact, **I**nfarct (resolving)
Contusion
Demyelinating disease
Resolving hematoma

Ring-enhancing lesion crossing corpus callosum

mnemonic: "GAL"
Glioblastoma multiforme (butterfly glioma)
Astrocytoma
Lymphoma

Dense and enhancing lesions

1. Aneurysm
2. Meningioma
3. CNS lymphoma
4. Medulloblastoma
5. Metastasis

Multifocal enhancing lesions

1. Multiple infarctions
2. Arteriovenous malformations
3. Multifocal primary / secondary neoplasms
4. Multifocal infectious processes
5. Demyelinating diseases: eg, multiple sclerosis

Innumerable small enhancing cerebral nodules

A. METASTASES
B. PRIMARY CNS LYMPHOMA
C. DISSEMINATED INFECTION
  1. Cysticercosis
  2. Histoplasmosis
  3. Tuberculosis
D. INFLAMMATION
  1. Sarcoidosis
  2. Multiple sclerosis
E. SUBACUTE MULTIFOCAL INFARCTION
  from hypoperfusion, multiple emboli, cerebral vasculitis (SLE), meningitis, cortical vein thrombosis

Enhancing lesion in internal auditory canal

A. NEOPLASTIC
  1. Acoustic schwannoma
  2. Ossifying hemangioma
B. NONNEOPLASTIC
  1. Sarcoidosis
  2. Meningitis
  3. Postmeningitic / postcraniotomy fibrosis
  4. Vascular loop of anterior inferior cerebellar a.

VASCULAR DISEASE

Classification of vascular CNS anomalies

A. VASCULAR MALFORMATION
  (a) arterial = arteriovenous malformation (AVM)
    1. Facial / brain arteriovenous malformation
    2. Vein of Galen malformation
  (b) capillary = telangiectasia
    1. Facial port wine stain
    • commonly asymptomatic
  (c) venous = venous malformation
    = tangle of abnormal varices of a "caput-medusae" / "spoked-wheel" configuration draining into a dilated cortical vein
    • soft + compressible without thrills / pulsations
    • distension with Valsalva maneuver
    • commonly asymptomatic
    Location: white matter with normal intervening brain parenchyma
    Cx (uncommon): hemorrhage, ischemia
    1. Venous angioma
    2. Sinus pericranii
  (d) lymphatic
    1. Cystic hygroma
  (e) combinations
    1. Sturge-Weber disease
    2. Rendu-Osler-Weber disease
B. VASCULAR TUMOR
  1. Hemangioma
    (a) capillary hemangioma: seen in children, involution by 7 years of age in 95%
    (b) cavernous hemangioma: seen in adults, no involution
      √ thrombosed blood + hemosiderin
      √ normal angiogram
  2. Hemangiopericytoma
  3. Hemangioendothelioma
  4. Angiosarcoma

<u>Occult / cryptic vascular malformation</u>
1. Cavernous hemangioma
2. Capillary telangiectasia

Occlusive vascular disease

(a) Embolic state:
√ single vascular territory
(b) Hypoperfusive state:
√ multiple vascular territories

Cause:

1. <u>Vasospasm</u> from subarachnoid hemorrhage
2. <u>Embolic infarction</u> (50%)
   (a) thrombus (atrial fibrillation, valvular disease, Atheromatous plaques of extracerebral arteries, fibromuscular dysplasia, intracranial aneurysm, surgery, paradoxic emboli, sickle cell disease, atherosclerosis, thrombotic thrombocytopenic purpura)
   - fluctuating blood pressures
   - hypercoagulability
   √ cerebral petechial hemorrhage within cortical / basal gray matter during 2nd week (from fragments of embolus) in up to 40%; initial ischemia is followed by reperfusion (= HALLMARK of embolic infarction)
   √ "supernormal artery" on NECT = high-density material lodged in cerebral vessel near major bifurcations
   √ atheromatous narrowing of vessels
   (b) fat
   (c) nitrogen
3. <u>Watershed infarct</u>
   involving deep white matter between two adjacent vascular beds in global hypoperfusion secondary to poor cardiac output / cervical carotid artery occlusion
   ◊ 6% of cerebral infarcts have hemorrhage (red infarct)
   - stroke (3rd most common cause of death in USA, 5% of stroke syndromes are caused by underlying tumor)
   - TIA = transitory ischemic attack: clears within 24 hours
   - RIND = reversible ischemic neurologic deficit: still evident >24 hours with eventual total recovery
   - amaurosis fugax = transient monocular blindness
   - weakness / numbness in an extremity
   - aphasia
   - dizziness, diplopia, dysarthria (Vertebrobasilar ischemia)
4. <u>Hypertension</u>
   (a) Hypertensive encephalopathy
   √ diffuse white matter hypodensity (edema secondary to arterial spasm)
   (b) Hypertensive hemorrhage
   Location: basal ganglia (putamen, external capsule), thalamus, pons, cerebellum

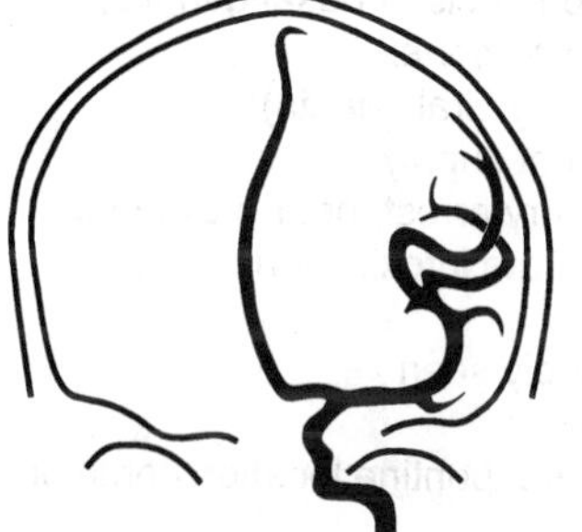
Round shift

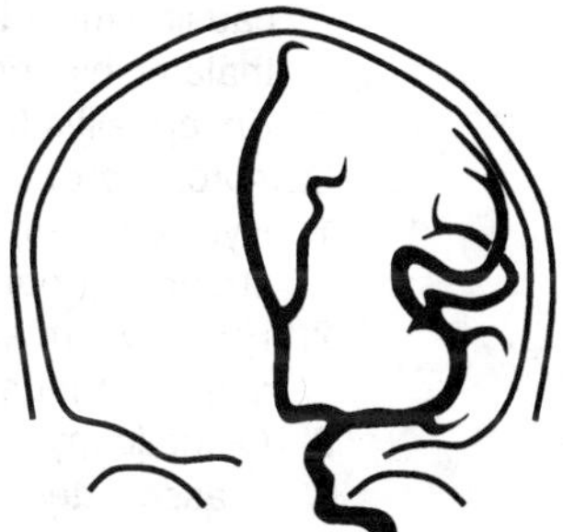
Distal shift

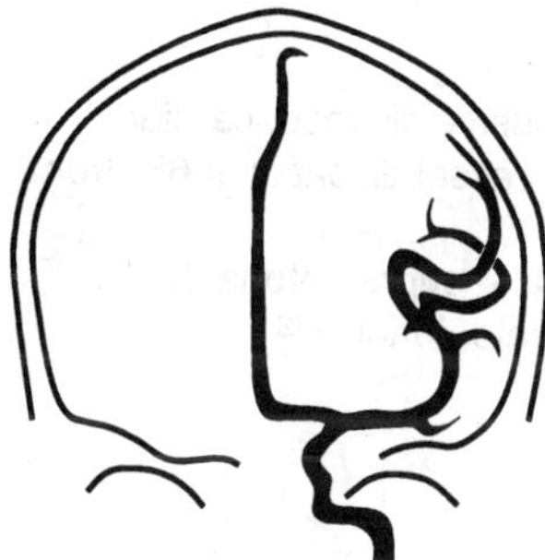
Square shift

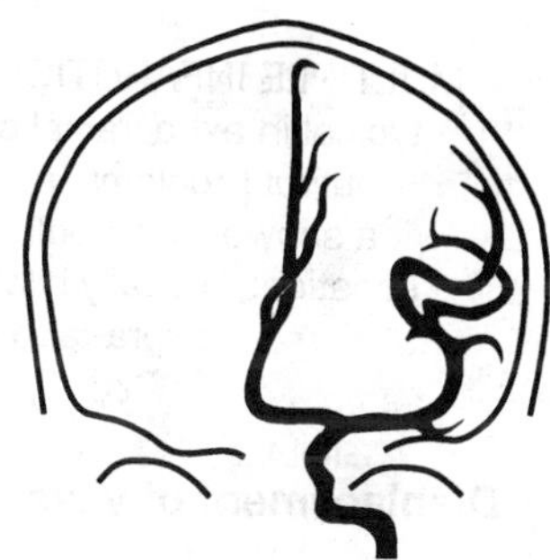
Proximal shift

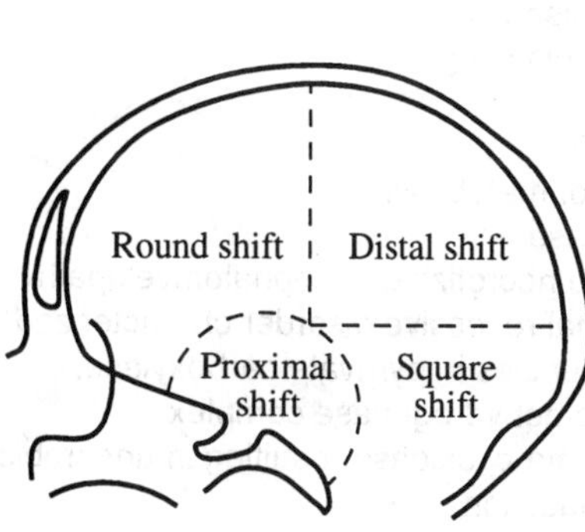

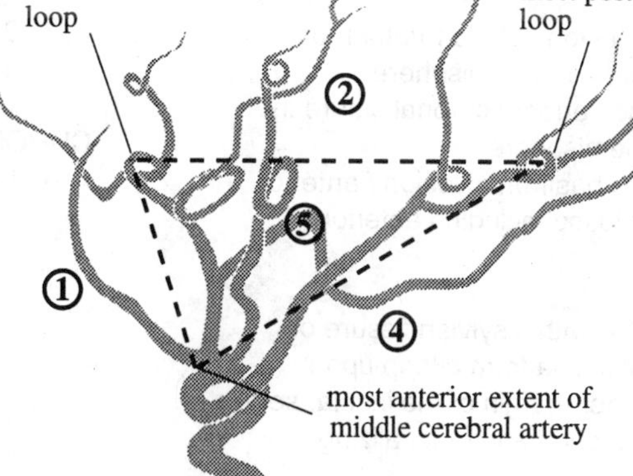

Sylvian Triangle

(c) Lacunar infarction
(d) Subcortical arteriosclerotic encephalopathy

5. Amyloidosis
involvement of small- + medium-sized arteries of meninges + cortex
• normotensive patient >65 years of age
√ multiple simultaneous / recurrent cortical hemorrhages
6. Vasculitis
(a) Bacterial meningitis, TB, syphilis, fungus, virus, rickettsia
(b) Collagen-vascular disease: Wegener granulomatosis, polyarteritis nodosa, SLE, scleroderma, dermatomyositis
(c) Granulomatous angitis: giant cell arteritis, sarcoidosis, Takayasu disease, temporal arteritis
(d) Inflammatory arteritis: rheumatoid arteritis, hypersensitivity arteritis, Behçet disease, lymphomatoid granulomatosis
(e) Drug-induced: IV amphetamine, ergot preparations, oral contraceptives
(f) Radiation arteritis = mineralizing microangiopathy
(g) Moyamoya disease
7. Anoxic encephalopathy
cardiorespiratory arrest, near-drowning, drug overdose, CO poisoning
8. Venous thrombosis

MULTIPLE INFARCTIONS
typical in extracranial occlusive disease, cardiac output problems, small vessel disease; in 6% from a shower of emboli
Location: usually bilateral + supratentorial (3/4); supra- and infratentorial (1/4)

Displacement of vessels

A. ARTERIAL SHIFT
(a) Pericallosal arteries
1. Round shift = frontal lesion anterior to coronal suture
2. Square shift = lesion behind foramen of Monro in lower half of hemisphere
3. Distal shift = posterior to coronal suture in upper half of hemisphere
4. Proximal shift = basifrontal lesion / anterior middle cranial fossa including anterior temporal lobe

(b) Sylvian triangle
= branches of MCA within sylvian fissure on outer surface of insula form a loop upon reaching the upper margin of the insula; serves as angiographic landmark for localizing supratentorial masses
Location of lesion:
- anterior sylvian — frontal region
- suprasylvian — posterior frontal + parietal
- retrosylvian — occipital, parieto-occipital
- infrasylvian — temporal lobe + extracerebral region
- intrasylvian — usually due to meningioma
- lateral sylvian — frontal, frontotemporal, parietotemporal
- central sylvian — deep posterior frontal, basal ganglia

B. CEREBRAL VEINS
= indicate the midline of the posterior part of the forebrain showing the exact location of the roof of the 3rd ventricle

BASAL GANGLIA

Bilateral basal ganglia lesions in childhood

Basal ganglia are susceptible to damage during childhood because of high energy requirements (ATP) mandating a rich blood supply + high concentration of trace metals (iron, copper, manganese)
• increased irritability, lethargy, dystonia
• seizure, behavioral changes
√ bilateral necrosis of basal ganglia

ACUTE CAUSES
A. Compromise of vascular supply
1. Hemolytic-uremic syndrome
causing microthrombosis of basal ganglia, thalami, hippocampi, cortex
2. Encephalitis (usually viral agents)
B. Compromise of nutrient supply
1. Hypoxia: respiratory arrest, near drowning, strangling, barbiturate intoxication
2. Hypoglycemia
√ hemorrhage rarely seen
3. Osmotic myelinolysis
√ associated central pontine location common
C. Acute poisoning
1. Carbon monoxide
√ preferentially affects globus pallidus
rare in children:
2. Hydrogen sulfide
3. Cyanide poisoning
4. Methanol poisoning

CHRONIC CAUSES
A. Inborn errors of metabolism
1. Leigh disease
= subacute necrotizing encephalomyelopathy
= autosomal recessive disorder characterized by deficiencies in pyruvate carboxylase, pyruvate dehydrogenase complex, cytochrome *c* oxidase resulting in anaerobic ATP production
• lactic acidosis (elevated ratio of lactate to pyruvate in CSF + serum)
√ propensity to involve putamen

2. Wilson disease
   = hepatolenticular degeneration
   = increased deposition of copper in brain + liver
   • decreased levels of serum copper + ceruloplasmin
   • increased urinary copper excretion
   √ cell damage of lenticular nucleus (= lenslike configuration of putamen + globus pallidus)
3. Mitochondrial encephalomyelopathies
   = subset of lactic acidemias with structurally abnormal mitochondria
   • "ragged red" fibers in muscle biopsy
4. Maple syrup urine disease
   = inability to catabolize branched-chain amino acids (leucine, isoleucine, valine)
   • urine smells of maple syrup
5. Methylmalonic acidemia
   = group of genetically distinct autosomal recessive disorders of organic acid metabolism affecting conversion of methylmalonyl-CoA to succinyl-CoA
   • accumulation of methylmalonic acid in blood + urine

B. Degenerative disease
   1. Huntington disease
   2. Dystrophic calcifications

C. Dysmyelinating disease
   basal ganglia are a mixture of gray + white matter
   1. Canavan disease
   2. Metachromatic leukodystrophy

D. Others
   1. Neurofibromatosis type 1

Low-attenuation lesion in basal ganglia

1. Poisoning: carbon monoxide, barbiturate intoxication, hydrogen sulfide poisoning, cyanide poisoning, methanol intoxication
2. Hypoxia
3. Hypoglycemia
4. Hypotension (lacunar infarcts)
5. Wilson disease

Basal ganglia calcification

Prevalence in children: 1.1 – 1.6%

A. PHYSIOLOGIC WITH AGING

B. ENDOCRINE
   1. Hypoparathyroidism, pseudo~, pseudopseudo~ (60%)
   2. Hyperparathyroidism
   3. Hypothyroidism

C. METABOLIC
   1. Leigh disease
   2. Mitochondrial cytopathy
      (a) Kearns-Sayre syndrome = ophthalmoplegia, retinal pigmentary degeneration, complete heart block, short stature, mental deterioration
      (b) MELAS = **M**itochondrial myopathy, **E**ncephalopathy, **L**actic acidosis, **A**nd **S**troke
      (c) MERRF = **M**yoclonic **E**pilepsy with **R**agged **R**ed **F**ibers
   3. Fahr disease = familial cerebrovascular ferrocalcinosis

D. CONGENITAL / DEVELOPMENTAL
   1. Familial idiopathic symmetric basal ganglia calcification
   2. Hastings-James syndrome
   3. Cockayne syndrome
   4. Lipoid proteinosis = hyalinosis cutis
   5. Neurofibromatosis
   6. Tuberous sclerosis
   7. Oculocraniosomatic disease
   8. Methemoglobinopathy
   9. Down syndrome

E. INFLAMMATION / INFECTION
   1. Toxoplasmosis, congenital rubella, CMV
   2. Measles, chicken pox
   3. Pertussis, Coxsackie B virus
   4. Cysticercosis
   5. Systemic lupus erythematosus
   6. AIDS

F. TRAUMA
   1. Childhood leukemia following methotrexate therapy
   2. S/P radiation therapy
   3. Birth anoxia, hypoxia
   4. Cardiovascular event

G. TOXIC
   1. Carbon monoxide poisoning
   2. Lead intoxication
   3. Nephrotic syndrome

mnemonic: "BIRTH"
Birth anoxia
Idiopathic (most common), **I**nfarct
Radiation therapy
Toxoplasmosis / CMV
Hypoparathyroidism / pseudoHPT

Linear echogenic foci in thalamus + basal ganglia

A. IN UTERO INFECTION
   = destruction of wall of lenticulostriate arteries + replacement by deposits of amorphous granular material
   1. TORCH agents: Toxoplasma, rubella virus, cytomegalovirus, herpes virus
   2. Syphilis
   3. Human immunodeficiency virus

B. CHROMOSOMAL ABNORMALITY
   1. Down syndrome
   2. Trisomy 13

C. OTHERS (anoxic injury?)
   1. Perinatal asphyxia, respiratory distress syndrome, cyanotic congenital heart disease, necrotizing enterocolitis
   2. Fetal alcohol syndrome
   3. Nonimmune hydrops

SELLA

Destruction of sella

1. Pituitary adenoma
2. Suprasellar tumor
3. Carcinoma of sphenoid + posterior ethmoid sinus
   √ opacification of sinus + destruction of walls
   √ associated with nasopharyngeal mass (common)
4. Nasopharyngeal carcinoma
   (a) squamous cell carcinoma
   (b) lymphoepithelioma = Schmincke tumor = non-keratinizing form of squamous cell carcinoma
   √ sclerosis of adjacent bone
5. Metastasis to sphenoid
   from breast, kidney, thyroid, colon, prostate, lung, esophagus
6. Primary tumor of sphenoid bone (rare)
   osteogenic sarcoma, giant cell tumor, plasmacytoma
7. Chordoma
8. Mucocele of sphenoid sinus (uncommon)
9. Enlarged 3rd ventricle
   aqueductal stenosis from infratentorial mass, maldevelopment

J-shaped sella

mnemonic: "CONMAN"

Chronic hydrocephalus
Optic glioma, **O**steogenesis imperfecta
Neurofibromatosis
Mucopolysaccharidosis
Achondroplasia
Normal variant

Enlarged sella

A. PRIMARY TUMOR
   1. Pituitary adenoma
   2. Craniopharyngioma
   3. Meningioma: hyperostosis
   4. Optic glioma: J-shaped sella
B. PITUITARY HYPERPLASIA
   1. Hypothyroidism
   2. Hypogonadism
   3. Nelson syndrome (occurring in 7% of patients subsequent to adrenalectomy)
C. CSF-SPACE
   1. Enlarged 3rd ventricle
   2. Hydrocephalus
   3. Empty sella
D. VESSEL
   1. Arterial aneurysm
   2. Ectatic internal carotid artery

mnemonic: "CHAMPS"

Craniopharyngioma
Hydrocephalus (empty sella)
AVM, **A**neurysm
Meningioma
Pituitary adenoma
Sarcoidosis, TB

Pituitary gland enlargement

1. Neoplasm: eg, pituitary gland adenoma
2. Hypertrophy: primary precocious puberty, primary hypothyroidism
3. Lymphocytic hypophysitis
4. Infection
5. Severe dural AV fistula

Intrasellar mass

1. Pituitary adenoma / carcinoma (most common cause)
2. Craniopharyngioma (2nd most common cause)
3. Meningioma: from surface of diaphragm / tuberculum sellae
4. Chordoma
5. Metastasis: lung, breast, prostate, kidney, GI tract, spread from nasopharynx
6. Intracavernous ICA aneurysm: bilateral in 25%
7. Pituitary abscess: rapidly expanding mass associated with meningitis
8. Empty sella
9. Rathke cleft cyst: commonly at junction of anterior + posterior pituitary gland
10. Granular cell tumor = myeloblastoma: benign neoplasm of posterior pituitary gland
11. Granuloma: sarcoidosis, giant cell granuloma, TB, syphilis, eosinophilic granuloma
12. Lymphoid adenohypophysitis
13. Pituitary hyperplasia, eg, in Nelson syndrome

Hypointense lesion of sella

1. Empty sella
2. Pituitary stone (= pituilith)
   = sequela of autonecrosis of pituitary adenoma
3. Intrasellar aneurysm
4. Persistent trigeminal artery
5. Calcified meningioma
6. Pituitary hemochromatosis (anterior pituitary lobe only)

Parasellar mass

1. Meningioma: tentorium cerebelli
2. Neurinoma (III, IV, V_1, V_2, VI)
3. Metastasis: lung, breast, kidney, GI tract, spread from nasopharynx
4. Epidermoid
5. Aneurysm
6. Carotid-cavernous fistula

mnemonic: "SATCHMO"

Sella neoplasm with superior extension, **S**arcoidosis
Aneurysm, ectatic carotid, carotid-cavernous sinus fistula, **A**rachnoid cyst
Teratoma: dysgerminoma (usually), dermoid, epidermoid
Craniopharyngioma, **C**hordoma
Hypothalamic glioma, **H**istiocytoma, **H**amartoma
Metastatic disease, **M**eningioma, **M**ucocele
Optic nerve glioma, neuroma

Suprasellar mass

1. Meningioma
2. Craniopharyngioma: in 80% suprasellar
3. Chiasmal + optic nerve glioma
   in 38% of neurofibromatosis; adolescent girls;
   DDx: chiasmal neuritis
4. Hypothalamic glioma
5. Hamartoma of tuber cinereum
6. Infundibular tumor
   metastasis (esp. breast); glioma; lymphoma / leukemia; histiocytosis X; sarcoidosis, tuberculosis
   √ diameter of infundibulum >4.5 mm immediately above level of dorsum; cone-shaped (on coronal scan)
7. Germinoma
   malignant tumor similar to seminoma (= "ectopic pinealoma")
   √ frequently calcified (teratoma)
   √ CSF spread (germinoma + teratocarcinoma)
   √ enhancement on CECT (common)
8. Epidermoid / dermoid
   √ cystic lesion containing calcifications + fat
   √ minimal / no contrast enhancement
9. Arachnoid cyst
   - hydrocephalus (common), visual impairment
   - endocrine dysfunction

   Age: most common in infancy
10. Enlarged 3rd ventricle extending into pituitary fossa
11. Suprasellar aneurysm
    √ rim calcification + eccentric position

Suprasellar mass with low attenuation

1. Craniopharyngioma
2. Dermoid / epidermoid
3. Arachnoid cyst
4. Lipoma
5. Simple pituitary cyst
6. Glioma of hypothalamus

Suprasellar mass with mixed attenuation

A. IN CHILDREN
   1. Hypothalamic-chiasmatic glioma
   2. Craniopharyngioma
   3. Hamartoma of tuber cinereum
   4. Histiocytosis

B. IN ADULTS
   1. Suprasellar extension of pituitary adenoma
   2. Craniopharyngioma
   3. Epidermoid cyst
   4. Thrombosed aneurysm
   5. Low-grade hypothalamic / optic glioma
   6. Inflammatory lesion: sarcoidosis, TB, sphenoid mucocele

Suprasellar mass with calcification

A. CURVILINEAR
   1. Giant carotid aneurysm
   2. Craniopharyngioma

B. GRANULAR
   1. Craniopharyngioma
   2. Meningioma
   3. Granuloma
   4. Dermoid cyst / teratoma
   5. Optic / hypothalamic glioma (rare)

Enhancing supra- and intrasellar mass

1. Pituitary adenoma
2. Meningioma
3. Germinoma
4. Hypothalamic glioma
5. Craniopharyngioma

Perisellar vascular lesion

1. ICA aneurysm
   Giant aneurysms are >2.5 cm in diameter
   √ destruction of bony sella / superior orbital fissure
   √ calcified wall / thrombus
   √ CECT enhancement, nonuniform with thrombosis
2. Ectatic carotid artery
   √ curvilinear calcifications
   √ encroachment upon sella turcica
3. Carotid-cavernous sinus fistula

PINEAL GLAND

Classification of pineal gland tumors

Incidence of pineal mass:
<1% of all intracranial tumors, 4% of all childhood intracranial masses, 9% of all intracranial masses in Asia

A. PRIMARY TUMOR
   (a) Germ cell origin (2/3)
      — forming embryonic tissue
         1. Germinoma (40 – 50%)
         2. Embryonal cell carcinoma
         3. Teratoma (15%): benign mature teratoma, benign immature teratoma, malignant teratoma

      — forming extraembryonic tissue
         4. Choriocarcinoma (<5%)
         5. Endodermal sinus tumor = yolk sac tumor

   (b) Pineal parenchymal cell origin (<15%)
      1. Pineocytoma
      2. Pineoblastoma

   (c) Other cell origin
      1. Retinoblastoma (trilateral retinoblastoma = left eye + right eye + pineal gland
      2. Astrocytoma
      3. Ependymoma
      4. Meningioma
      5. Hemangiopericytoma

   (d) Cysts
      1. Pineal cyst
      2. Malignant teratoma
      3. AVM, vein of Galen aneurysm
      4. Arachnoid cyst
      5. Inclusion cyst (dermoid / epidermoid)

B. SECONDARY TUMOR
Metastasis: eg, lung carcinoma

DDx considerations:

— female:	likely NOT germ cell tumor
— hypodense matrix:	likely NOT pineal cell tumor
— distinct tumor margins:	probably pineocytoma / teratoma / germinoma
— calcification:	likely NOT teratocarcinoma, metastasis, germinoma
— CSF seeding:	NOT teratoma
— intense enhancement:	likely NOT teratoma

Intensely enhancing mass in pineal region

1. Germinoma
2. Pineocytoma / -blastoma
3. Pineal teratocarcinoma
4. Glioma of brainstem / thalamus
5. Subsplenial meningioma
6. Vein of Galen aneurysm

ANATOMY OF BRAIN

Embryology

NEURULATION

neural plate = CNS originates as a plate of thickened ectoderm on the dorsal aspect of the embryo

neural crest = elevation of the lateral margins of the neural plate; forms the peripheral nervous system

neural tube = invagination between the two neural crests; its wall forms the brain + spinal cord; its lumen forms the ventricles + spinal canal

4.6 weeks MA: formation of neural tube

5.6 weeks MA: rostral neuropore closes

5.9 weeks MA: caudal neuropore closes

6.0 weeks MA: 3 primary brain vesicles develop (prosencephalon, mesencephalon, rhombencephalon) development of cervical flexure

7.0 weeks MA: 2 additional primary brain vesicles form out of rhombencephalon (pontine flexure divides into myelencephalon, metencephalon)

15 weeks MA: dorsal portion of alar plates bulging into 4th ventricle have fused in midline to form cerebellar vermis

BRAIN GROWTH

= increase in thickness of brain mantle with relative constant ventricular width

◊ Most rapid brain growth from 12 to 24 weeks MA!

NEURONAL MIGRATION

7th week subependymal neuronal proliferation = germinal matrix

8th week radial migration to cortex along radial glial fibers

Classification of brain anatomy

A. PROSENCEPHALON = forebrain
  √ cerebrum, lateral ventricles, choroid, thalami, cerebellum sonographically visible at 12 weeks MA
  1. **Telencephalon** = cerebrum
     = cerebral hemispheres, putamen, caudate nucleus
  2. **Diencephalon**
     = thalamus, hypothalamus, epithalamus (= pineal gland + habenula), globus pallidus

B. MESENCEPHALON = midbrain
  = short segment of brainstem above pons; traverses the hiatus in tentorium cerebelli; contains cerebral peduncles, tectum, colliculi (corpora quadrigemina)

C. RHOMBENCEPHALON = hindbrain
  √ posterior cystic space of 4th ventricle sonographically detectable between 8 and 10 weeks MA
  1. **Metencephalon** = cerebellar hemispheres, vermis
  2. **Myelencephalon** = medulla oblongata, pons

D. BRAINSTEM = mesencephalon + myelencephalon
  contains
  (a) cranial nerve nuclei
  (b) sensory and motor tracts between thalamus, cerebral cortex, and spinal cord
  (c) reticular formation controlling respiration, blood pressure, gastrointestinal function, centers for arousal and wakefulness

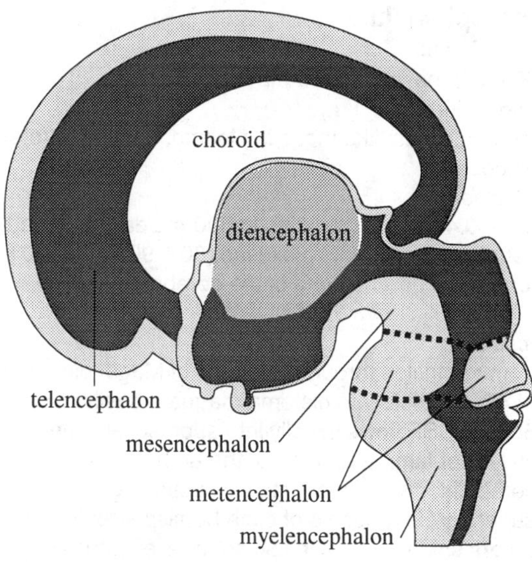

Sagittal Section Through Brain at 10–11 Weeks GA

Meninges of brain

A. CALVARIA

B. EPIDURAL SPACE
  = created when dura becomes detached from calvaria

C. PACHYMENINGES = DURA
  (a) outer dural layer
     = highly vascularized periosteum of calvaria
  (b) space for venous sinuses
  (c) inner dural layer
     = meningeal layer derived from meninx

D. SUBDURAL SPACE
  = cleft formed in pathologic states within inner layer of dura

E. LEPTOMENINGES
  1. Arachnoid
     = closely applied to inner surface of dura
  2. Subarachnoid space
     Histo: fine connective tissue + cellular septa link pia and arachnoid
     - contains CSF that drains through the valves of arachnoid granulations into venous sinuses
     - forms basal cisterns
  3. Pia mater

F. SUBPIAL SPACE
  = perivascular (Virchow-Robin) space

CNS

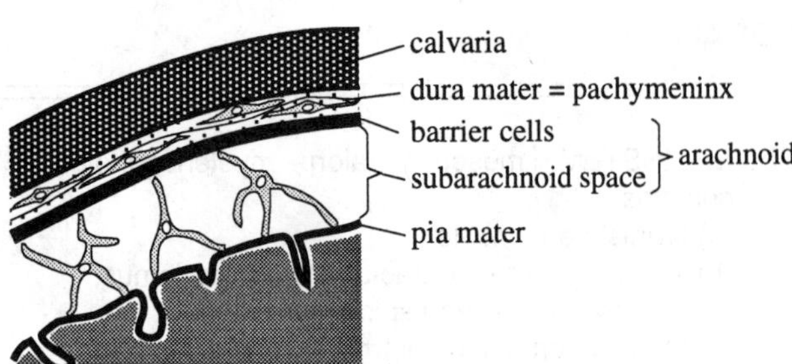

Meninges of Brain

Cerebrospinal fluid

Total volume:
50 mL in newborn, 150 mL in adult

Composition:
inorganic salts like those in plasma, traces of protein + glucose

Production:
0.3 – 0.4 mL/min resulting in 500 mL/day; secreted into ventricles by choroid plexuses (80 – 90%), 10–20% formed by parenchyma of the cerebrum + spinal cord

Circulation:
from ventricles through foramina of Magendie + Luschka of 4th ventricle into cisterna magna + basilar cisterns; 80% of CSF flows initially into suprasellar cistern + cistern of lamina terminalis, the ambient / superior cerebellar cisterns, eventually ascending over superolateral aspects of each hemisphere; 20% initially enters spinal subarachnoid space + eventually recirculates into cerebral subarachnoid space

Cerebral aqueduct:
pulsatile flow (due to brain motion during cardiac cycle) + net outflow into 4th ventricle; diameter of 2.6–4.2 mm; peak outflow velocity of 6–51 mm/sec; inflow velocity of 3–28 mm/sec

Absorption:
into venous system by
(a) arachnoid villi of superior sagittal sinus (villi behave as one-way valves with an opening pressure between 20 – 50 mm of CSF)
(b) cranial + spinal nerves with eventual absorption by lymphatics (50%)

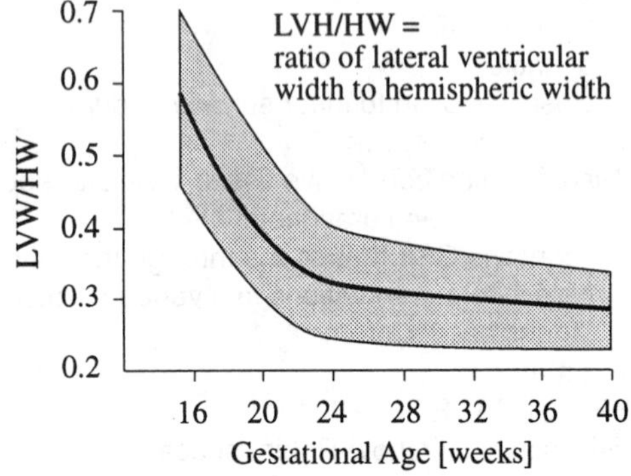

(c) prelymphatic channels of capillaries within brain parenchyma
(d) vertebral venous plexuses, intervertebral veins, posterior intercostal + upper lumbar veins into azygos + hemiazygos veins

Pituitary gland

= HYPOPHYSIS CEREBRI within hypophysial fossa of sphenoid, covered superiorly by sellar diaphragm (= dura mater) which has an aperture for the infundibulum centrally

Size:
adult size is achieved at puberty
Height in adult females = 7 (range 4–10) mm
Height in adult males = 5 (range 3– 7) mm

Shape:
√ flat / downwardly convex superior border
√ upwardly convex during puberty, pregnancy, in hypothyroidism (due to hyperplasia)

A. ANTERIOR LOBE
= larger anterior portion of adenohypophysis comprising 80% of pituitary gland volume
Origin: ectodermal derivative of stomodeum
Function:
(a) chromophil cells
1. acidophil cells = α cells
growth hormone = somatotropin (STH), prolactin = lactogenic hormone (LTH)
2. basophil cells = β cells
adrenocorticotropin = adrenocorticotropic hormone (ACTH), thyrotropin = thyroid-stimulating hormone (TSH), follicle-stimulating hormone (FSH), interstitial-cell-stimulating hormone (ICSH), luteinizing hormone (LH), melanocyte-stimulating hormone (MSH)
(b) chromophobe cells = 50% of epithelial cell population, of unknown significance

MRI:
√ larger homogeneous component isointense to white matter on T1WI + T2WI
√ prominent contrast enhancement (during first 3 minutes) due to lack of blood-brain barrier
√ hyperintense in the newborn fading to normal adult signal by 2nd month of life

B. PARS INTERMEDIA
= posterior portion of adenohypophysis; separated from anterior lobe by hypophysial cleft in fetal life
Origin: pouch of Rathke
Function: termination point of short hypothalamic axons elaborating tropic hormones (= releasing factors + prolactin inhibiting factor), which are carried to anterior lobe via the portal system
√ not visible with imaging techniques

C. POSTERIOR LOBE
= major portion of neurohypophysis
Origin: diencephalic outgrowth (termination point of axons from supraoptic + paraventricular nuclei of hypothalamus)

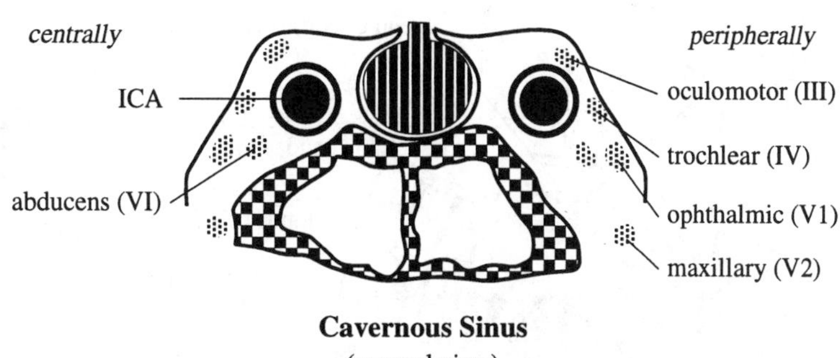

Cavernous Sinus
(coronal view)

Function: storage site for vasopressin (= antidiuretic hormone [ADH]) + oxytocin transported from paraventricular + supraoptic nuclei of hypothalamus along neurosecretory hypothalamohypophysial tract

MRI:
- √ hyperintense on T1WI + isointense on T2WI in comparison with anterior lobe (? due to relaxing agent of phospholipid / neurosecretory granules / vasopressin)
- √ isointense in 10% of normal individuals

D. PITUITARY STALK = INFUNDIBULUM

arises from anterior aspect of floor of 3rd ventricle (infundibular recess)

Histo: formed from axons of cells lying in supraoptic + paraventricular nuclei of hypothalamus

- √ joins posterior lobe at junction of anterior + posterior lobes
- √ up to 3 mm thick superiorly, up to 2 mm thick inferiorly
- √ usually in midline, may be slightly tilted to one side

MRI:
- √ prominent contrast enhancement

Basal nuclei

= BASAL GANGLIA (earlier incorrect designation)

A. Amygdaloid body
B. Claustrum
C. Corpus striatum
  (1) Caudate
  (2) Lentiform nucleus
    (a) pallidum = globus pallidus
    (b) putamen

Pineal gland

Development:

from area of ependymal thickening at the most caudal portion of roof of 3rd ventricle that evaginates into a pinecone-shaped mass during 7th week of gestation; initially contains ependyma lining in central cavity that connects with 3rd ventricle

Function:

1. regulation of long-term biologic rhythm (eg, onset of puberty)
2. regulation of short-term biologic rhythm (eg, diurnal / circadian) due to photoperiodic clues via accessory optic pathway

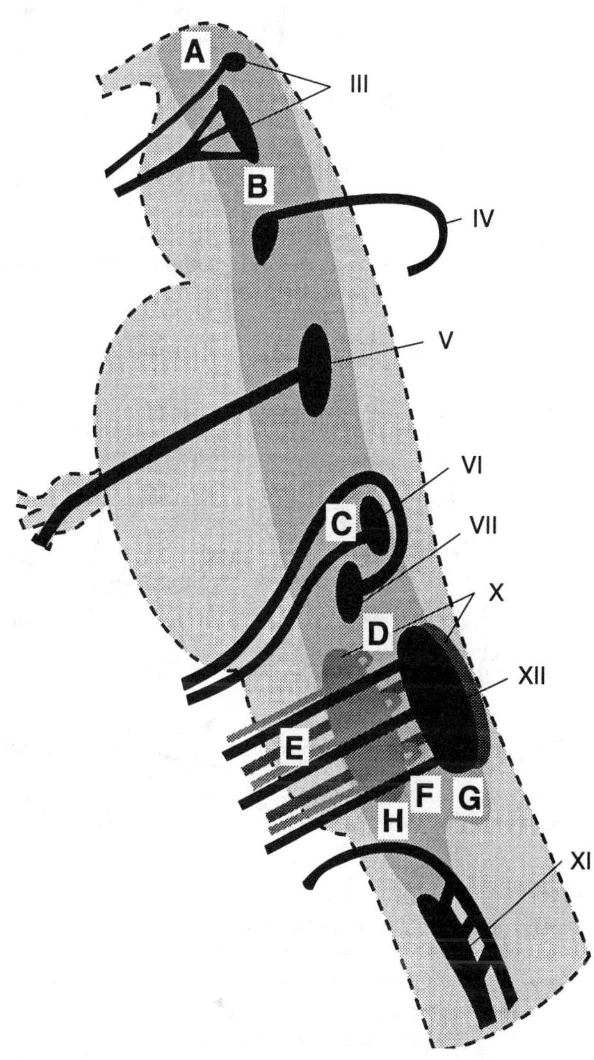

Cranial Nuclei of Brainstem and Reticular Formation

A = sleep, wakefulness, consciousness
B = visual spatial orientation, higher autonomic coordination of food intake
C = pneumotaxic center, coordination of breathing and circulation
D = swallowing
E = blood pressure, cardiac activity, vascular tone
F = expiration
G = area postrema = trigger zone for vomiting
H = inspiration

CNS

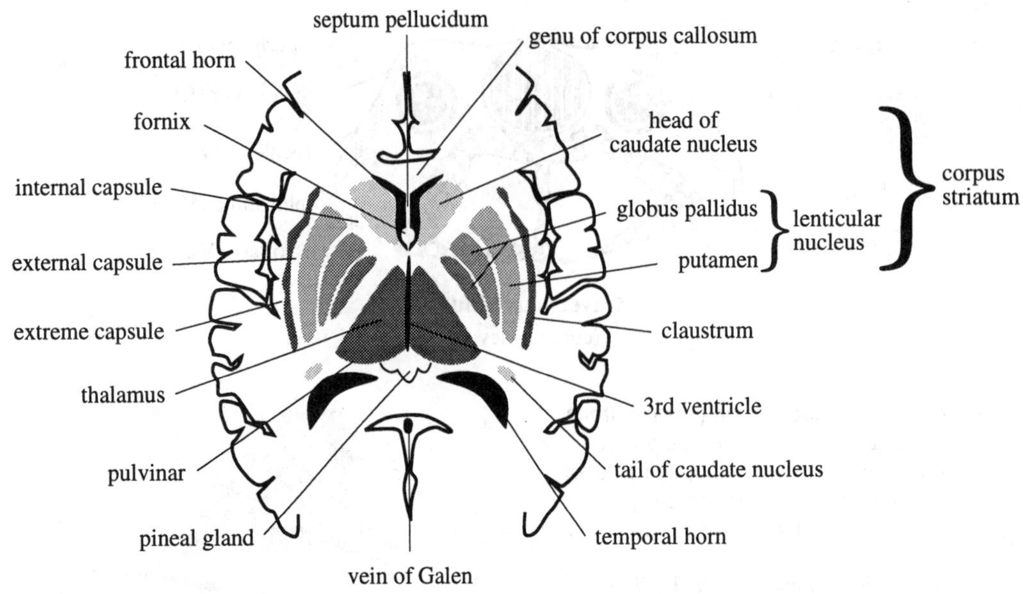

Axial Section Through Level of 3rd Ventricle

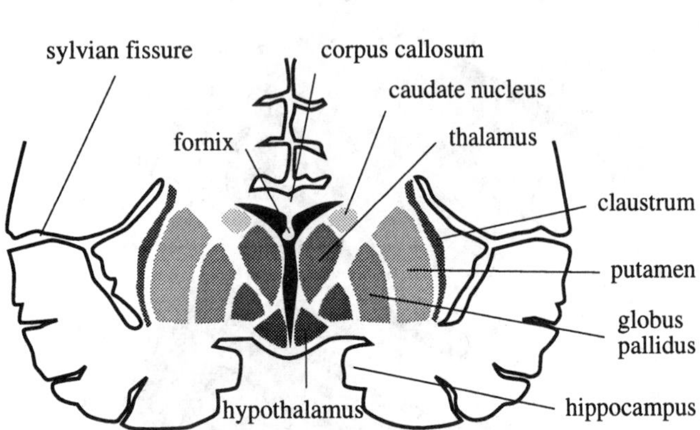

Coronal Section Through Level of Basal Ganglia

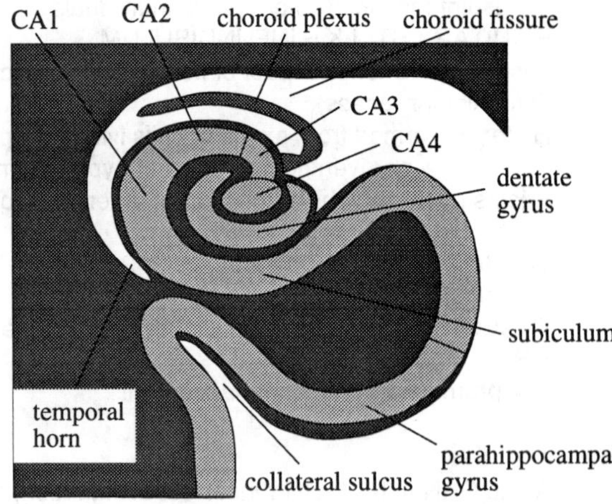

Right Medial Temporal Lobe

Histo:
(a) pinealocytes with dendritic processes (= neuronal cells) make up 95% of population
(b) neuroglial supporting cells make up 5% of population

Location: attached to upper aspect of posterior border of 3rd ventricle, lies within CSF of quadrigeminal cistern, anterior to pineal gland is cistern of velum interpositum (= cistern of transverse fissure)

Size: 8 mm long, 4 mm wide

Trigeminal nerve (V)

Nuclei:
(1) mesencephalic nucleus: proprioception extends to level of inferior colliculus
(2) main sensory nucleus: tactile sensation
(3) motor nucleus: motor innervation
(4) spinal nucleus: pain + temperature sensation extends to level of 2nd cervical vertebra
Location: in tegmentum of lateral pons, along anterolateral aspect of 4th ventricle

Course:
— through prepontine cistern
— exits through porus trigeminus (= opening in dura)
— enters Meckel cave with dura mater + leptomeninges forming trigeminal cistern (= CSF-filled subarachnoid space)
— forms gasserian ganglion (= trigeminal ganglion) which contains cell bodies of sensory fibers except those for proprioception

Trifurcation into 3 principal branches:
(1) **ophthalmic nerve** (V_1)
Course: in lateral wall of cavernous sinus
Exit: superior orbital fissure

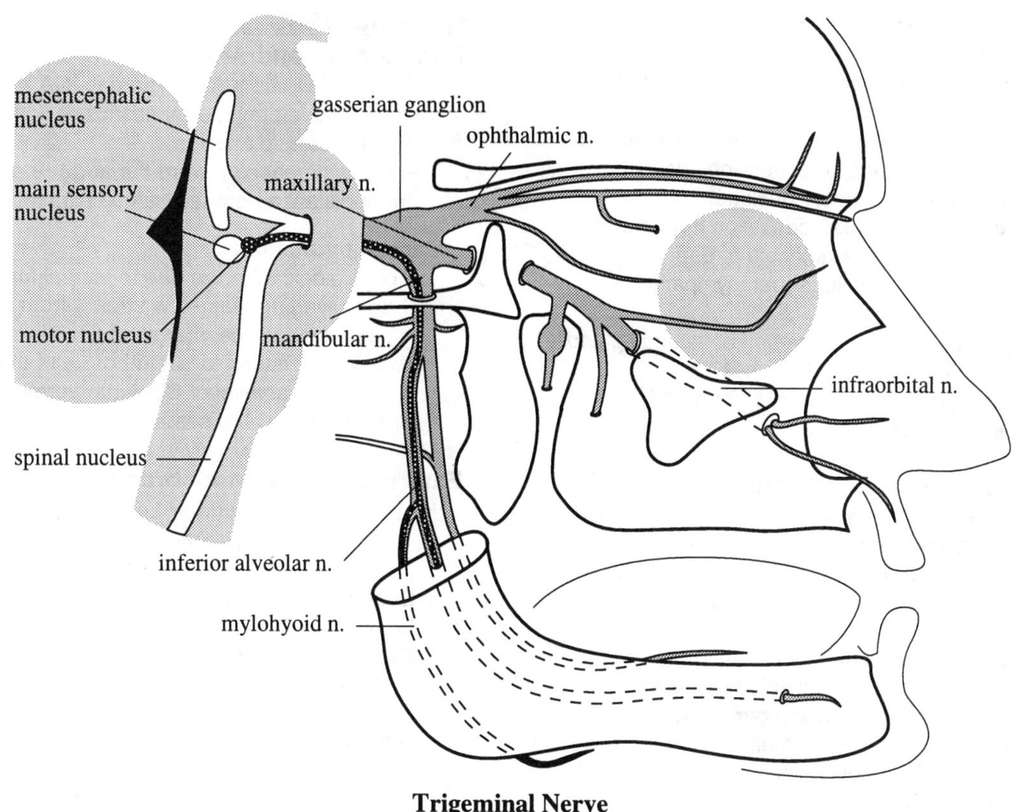

Trigeminal Nerve

Supply: sensory innervation of scalp, forehead, nose, globe
- mediates afferent aspect of corneal reflex

(2) **maxillary nerve** (V_2)
Course: between lateral dural wall of cavernous sinus + skull base
Exit: through foramen rotundum into pterygopalatine fossa
Supply: sensory innervation of middle third of face, upper teeth
Main trunk: infraorbital nerve

(3) **mandibular nerve** (V_3)
Course: NOT through cavernous sinus
Exit: through foramen ovale into masticator space
Supply: (a) sensory innervation of lower third of face, tongue, floor of mouth, jaw
(b) motor innervation of muscles of mastication (masseter, temporalis, medial + lateral pterygoid), mylohyoid m., anterior belly of digastric m., tensor tympani m., tensor veli palatini m.

Facial nerve (VII)

Nuclei:

(1) Motor nucleus: ventrolateral deep in reticular formation of the caudal part of the pons
Intrapontine course:
— dorsomedially towards 4th ventricle
— curving anterolaterally around upper pole of abducent nucleus (= **geniculum**)

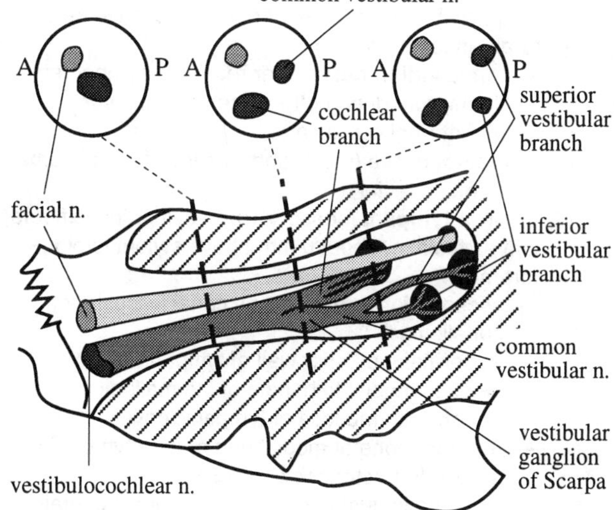

Internal Auditory Canal

Posterior wall of IAC is removed; cross sections through IAC are displayed above; A = anterior, P = posterior

— descending anterolaterally through reticular formation

Innervation to: stapedius m., stylohyoid m., posterior belly of digastric m., occipitalis m., buccinator, muscles of facial expression, platysma

(2) Nucleus solitarius (sensory nucleus):
— **nervus intermedius**: sensation from anterior 2/3 of tongue, skin on + adjacent to ear

(3) Superior salivatory nucleus (parasympathetic secretomotor innervation)
- greater petrosal n.: secretion of lacrimal glands, nasal cavity, paranasal sinuses
— chorda tympani: submandibular gland, sublingual glands

Course:
— from lateral aspect of pontomedullary junction
— coursing anterolaterally in cerebellopontine angle cistern to internal auditory canal (IAC)
— motor root of facial n. in anterosuperior groove of vestibulocochlear n. with nervus intermedius between them
mnemonic: "seven up"
— labyrinthine segment (in fallopian canal) travels anteromedially to **geniculate ganglion**
— turns posteriorly and horizontally along medial wall of mesotympanum (= anterior tympanic segment) below lateral semicircular canal just above the oval window
— turns inferiorly at second genu in pyramidal eminence + descends through anterior mastoid (= medial wall of aditus ad antrum)

Exit: from skull base through stylomastoid foramen

Branches:

(1) **Greater superficial petrosal nerve** (parasympathetic + motor fibers) arises from geniculate ganglion, runs anteromedially, and exits at the facial hiatus on the anterior surface of the temporal bone + passes under Meckel cave near foramen lacerum
— forms **vidian nerve** after receiving sympathetic fibers from deep petrosal nerve which surrounds the internal carotid artery

(2) **Stapedial nerve** (motor fibers) arises from proximal descending facial n.

(3) **Chorda tympani** (sensory + parasympathetic fibers) leaves facial n. about 6 mm above stylomastoid foramen
— ascends forward in a bony canal (= posterior canaliculus)
— perforates posterior wall of tympanic cavity
— crosses medial to handle of the malleolus underneath mucosa of tympanic cavity
— reenters bone at medial end of petrotympanic fissure (= posterior canaliculus)
— joins the lingual nerve (= branch of V_3) containing sensory fibers from anterior 2/3 of tongue + secretomotor fibers for submandibular and sublingual glands

CEREBRAL VESSELS

Common Carotid Artery

• 70% of blood flow is delivered to ICA
√ shares waveform characteristics of both internal + external carotid arteries
√ velocity increases toward the aorta (9 cm/sec for each cm of distance from the carotid bifurcation)

Carotid bifurcation

= physiologic stenosis due to inertial forces of blood flow diverting main-flow stream from midvessel to a path along vessel margin at flow divider

Location: lateral to upper border of thyroid cartilage; at level of C3-4 intervertebral disc

Branches: ECA arises anterior + medial to ICA (95%)

External carotid artery branches

mnemonic: "**A**ll **S**ummer **L**ong **E**mily **O**gled **P**eter's **S**porty **I**suzu"

Ascending pharyngeal artery
Superior thyroid artery
Lingual artery
External maxillary = facial artery
Occipital artery
Posterior auricular artery
Superficial temporal artery
Internal maxillary artery

Internal carotid artery

A. CERVICAL SEGMENT
ascends posterior and medial to ECA; enters carotid canal of petrous bone; NO branches

B. PETROUS SEGMENT
ascends briefly, in carotid canal bends anteromedially in a horizontal course (anterior to tympanic cavity + cochlea); exits near petrous apex through posterior portion of foramen lacerum; ascends to juxtasellar location where it pierces dural layer of cavernous sinus
Branches:
1. **Caroticotympanic a.**: to tympanic cavity, anastomoses with anterior tympanic branch of maxillary a. + stylomastoid a.
2. **Pterygoid (vidian) a.**: through pterygoid canal; anastomoses with recurrent branch of greater palatine a.

C. CAVERNOUS SEGMENT
ascends to posterior clinoid process, then turns anteriorly + superomedially through cavernous sinus; exits medial to anterior clinoid process piercing dura
Branches:
1. **Meningohypophyseal trunk**
(a) tentorial branch
(b) dorsal meningeal branch
(c) inferior hypophysial branch
2. **Anterior meningeal a.**: supplies dura of anterior fossa; anastomoses with meningeal branch of posterior ethmoidal a.
3. Cavernous rami supply trigeminal ganglion, walls of cavernous + inferior petrosal sinuses

D. SUPRACLINOID SEGMENT
ascends posterior + lateral between oculomotor + optic nerve
Branches:
mnemonic: "OPA"
Ophthalmic a.
Posterior communicating a.
Anterior choroidal a.

1. **Ophthalmic a.** exits from ICA medial to anterior clinoid process, travels through optic canal inferolateral to optic nerve
   (a) recurrent meningeal branch: dura of anterior middle cranial fossa
   (b) posterior ethmoidal a.: supplies dura of planum sphenoidale
   (c) anterior ethmoidal a.
2. **Superior hypophysial a.**: optic chiasm, anterior lobe of pituitary
3. **Posterior communicating a.** (pCom)
4. **Anterior choroidal a.**
5. **Middle + anterior cerebral arteries** (MCA, ACA)

CAROTID SIPHON
flow direction: C4 — C1

(a) C4 segment = before origin of ophthalmic a.
(b) C3 segment = genu of ICA
(c) C2 segment = supraclinoid segment after origin of ophthalmic a.
(d) C1 segment = terminal segment of ICA between pCom + ACA

Anterior cerebral artery (ACA)
A. HORIZONTAL PORTION = A 1 SEGMENT
= segment between origin and anterior communicating a. (aCom)
(a) Inferior branches
supply superior surface of optic nerve + chiasm
(b) superior branches
penetrate brain to supply anterior hypothalamus, septum pellucidum, anterior commissure, fornix columns, anterior inferior portion of corpus striatum (largest striatal artery = medial lenticulostriate artery = recurrent **artery of Heubner** for anteroinferior portion of head of caudate, putamen, anterior limb of internal capsule)

B. INTERHEMISPHERIC PORTION = A 2 SEGMENT
= segment after origin of anterior communicating a. (aCom); ascends in cistern of lamina terminalis
Branches:

1. **Medial orbitofrontal a.**: along gyrus rectus
2. **Frontopolar a.**
3. **Callosomarginal a.**: within cingulus gyrus
4. **Pericallosal a.**: over corpus callosum within callosal cistern
   (a) Superior internal parietal a.: anterior portion of precuneus + convexity of superior parietal lobule
   (b) Inferior internal parietal a.
   (c) Posterior pericallosal a.
   from callosomarginal / pericallosal artery:
   — Anterior + middle + posterior internal frontal aa.
   — Paracentral a.: supplies precentral + postcentral gyri

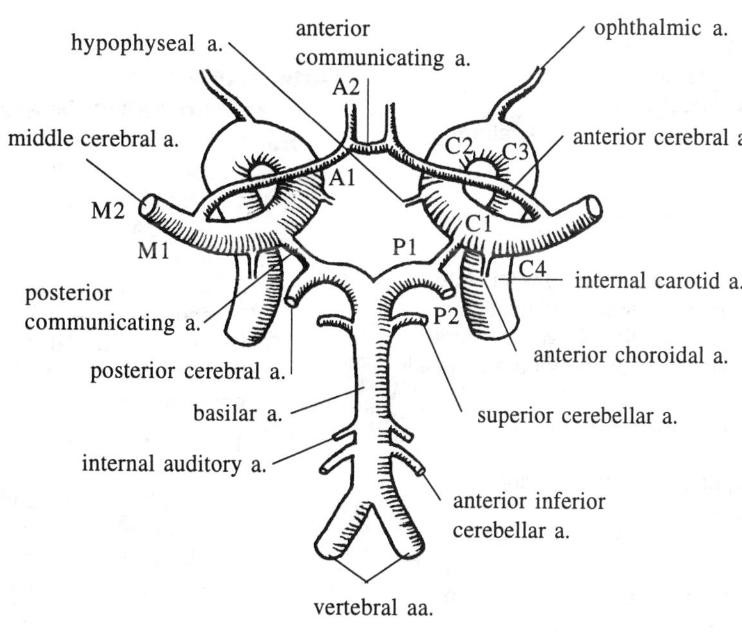

Circle of Willis

CNS

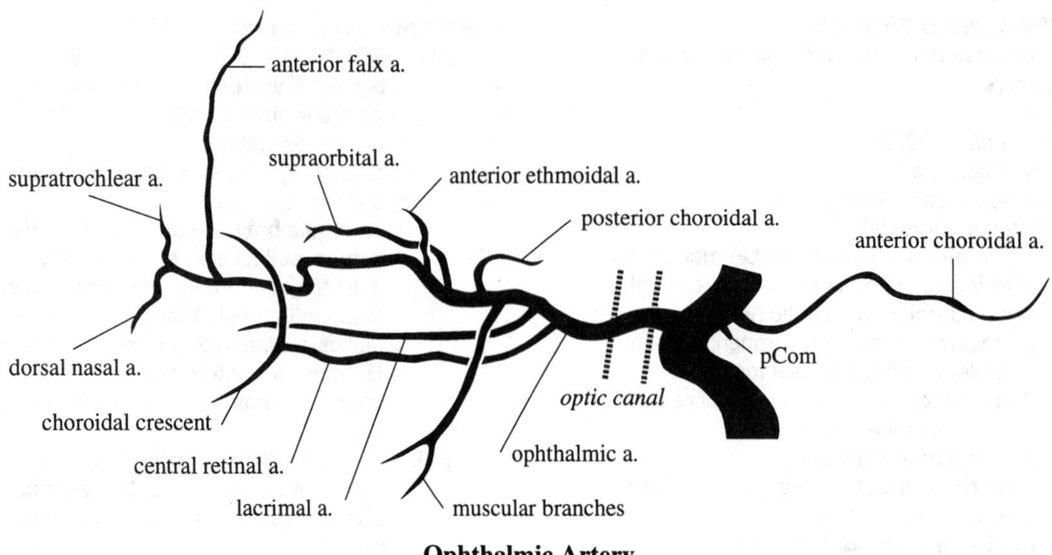

Ophthalmic Artery

Supply: anterior 2/3 of medial cerebral surface + 1 cm of superomedial brain over convexity

Middle cerebral artery

= largest branch of ICA arising lateral to optic chiasm; passes horizontal in lateral direction just ventral to anterior perforated substance to enter sylvian fissure where it divides into 2 / 3 / 4 branches

Branches:
1. **Anterior temporal a.**
2. **Ascending frontal a.** (candelabra) / prefrontal a.
3. **Precentral a.** = Pre-Rolandic a.
4. **Central a.** = Rolandic a.
5. **Anterior parietal a.** = Post-Rolandic a.
6. **Posterior parietal a.**
7. **Angular a.**
8. **Middle temporal a.**
9. **Posterior temporal a.**
10. **Temporo-occipital a.**

Supply: lateral cerebrum, insula, anterior + lateral temporal lobe

Posterior cerebral artery

originates from bifurcation of basilar artery within interpeduncular cistern (in 15% as a direct continuation of posterior communicating artery); lies above oculomotor nerve and circles midbrain above the tentorium cerebelli

Branches:
1. Mesencephalic perforating branches: tectum + cerebral peduncles
2. Posterior thalamoperforating aa.: midline of thalamus + hypothalamus
3. Thalamogeniculate aa.: geniculate bodies + pulvinar
4. Posterior medial choroidal a.: circles midbrain parallel to PCA; enters lateral aspect of quadrigeminal cistern; passes lateral and above pineal gland and enters roof of 3rd ventricle; supplies quadrigeminal plate + pineal gland
5. Posterior lateral choroidal a.: courses lateral and enters choroidal fissure; anterior branch to temporal horn + posterior branch to choroid plexus of trigone and lateral ventricle + lateral geniculate body
6. Cortical branches: (a) Anterior inferior temporal a.
   (b) Posterior inferior temporal a.
   (c) Parieto-occipital a.
   (d) Calcarine a.
   (e) Posterior pericallosal a.

Supply: medial + posterior temporal lobe, medial parietal lobe, occipital lobe

Arterial anastomoses of the brain

Anastomoses via the arteries at the base of the brain

A. CIRCLE OF WILLIS
   1. right ICA — right ACA — aCom — left ACA — left ICA
   2. ICA — pCom — basilar a.
   3. ICA — anterior choroidal a. — posterior choroidal a. — PCA — basilar a.

B. DEVELOPMENTAL ANOMALY
   three transient embryonal carotid-basilar anastomoses appearing consecutively in fetal life:
   1. **Primitive hypoglossal artery**
      = arterial connection between the intrapetrosal portion of ICA and proximal portion of basilar artery
   2. **Primitive acoustic (otic) artery**
      = arterial connection between cervical portion of ICA + vertebral artery in region of 12th nerve

3. **Persistent primitive trigeminal artery**
   Incidence: 1–2 / 1000 angiograms
   √ short wide connection between the cavernous portion of ICA and upper third of basilar artery (beneath posterior communicating artery)
   √ enlargement of ipsilateral ICA
   √ ectopic vessel crossing the pontine cistern to anastomose with basilar artery

Anastomoses via surface vessels

A. Leptomeningeal anastomoses of the cerebrum: ACA — MCA — PCA
B. Leptomeningeal anastomoses of the cerebellum: Superior cerebellar a. — AICA — PICA

Rete mirabile

ECA — middle meningeal a. / superficial temporal a. — leptomeningeal aa. — ACA / MCA

Cerebral veins

Important vascular markers:

1. Pontomesencephalic v. = anterior border of brainstem
2. Precentral cerebellar v. = position of tectum
   ◊ colliculocentral point = midpoint of Twining's line at knee of precentral cerebellar vein
3. Venous angle = acute angle at junction of thalamostriate with internal cerebral v. = posterior aspect of foramen of Monro
4. Internal cerebral vv. = demarcate caudad border of splenium of corpus callosum superiorly + pineal gland inferiorly
5. Copular point = junction of inferior + superior retrotonsillar tributaries draining cerebellar tonsils in region of copular pyramids of vermis

CEREBELLAR VESSELS

Vertebral artery

originates from subclavian a. proximal to thyrocervical trunk; left vertebral a. usually greater than right cerebral a.; left vertebral a. may originate directly from aorta (5%)

A. PREVERTEBRAL SEGMENT
   ascends posterosuperiorly between longus colli + anterior scalene muscle; enters transverse foramina at C6
   Branches: muscular branches
B. CERVICAL SEGMENT
   ascends through transverse foramina in close proximity to uncinate processes
   Branches: 1. **Anterior meningeal a.**
C. ATLANTIC SEGMENT
   exits transverse foramen of atlas; passes posteriorly in a groove on superior surface of posterior arch of atlas; pierces atlanto-occipital membrane + dura mater to enter cranial cavity
   Branches: 1. **Posterior meningeal branch** to posterior falx + tentorium
D. INTRACRANIAL SEGMENT
   ascends anteriorly + laterally around medulla to reach midline at pontomedullary junction; anastomoses with contralateral side to form basilar artery at clivus

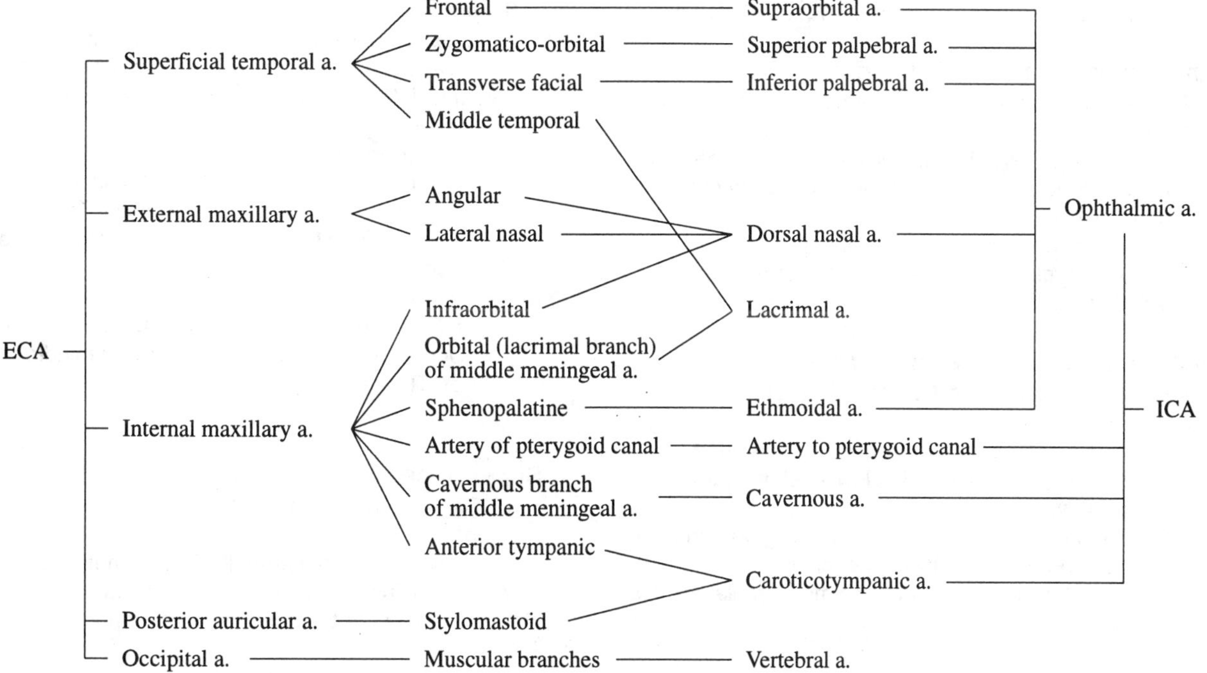

Anastomoses Between ICA and ECA and Vertebral Artery

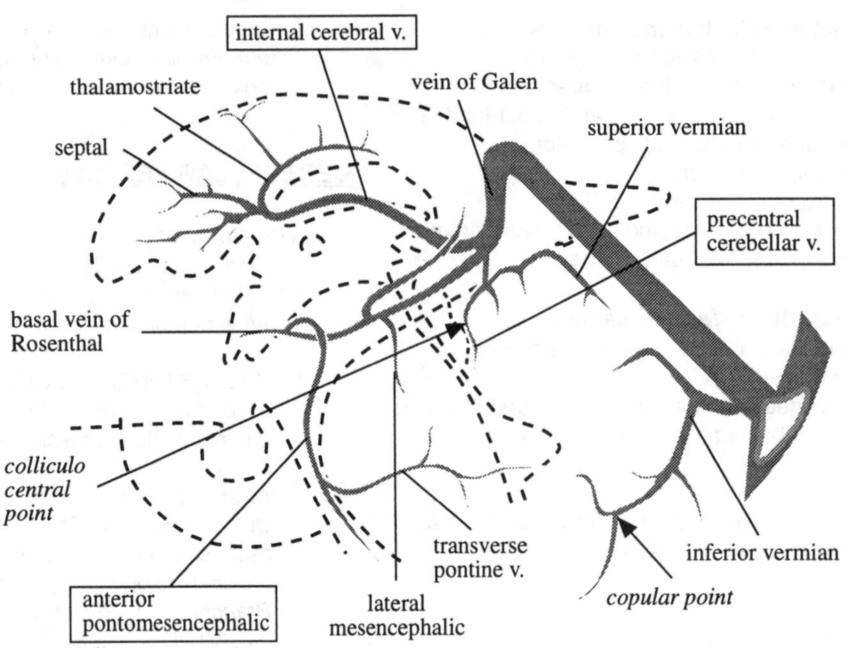

Cerebral Veins

Branches:

1. **Anterior + posterior spinal a.**
2. **Posterior inferior cerebellar a.** (PICA)
3. **Anterior inferior cerebellar a.** (AICA)
4. **Internal auditory a.**
5. **Superior cerebellar a.**
6. **Posterior cerebral a.** (PCA)
7. Medullary + pontine perforating branches

◊ may terminate in common AICA-PICA trunk

Anterior inferior cerebellar artery

= AICA = first branch of basilar artery

Supply:
lateroinferior part of pons, middle cerebellar peduncle, floccular region, anterior petrosal surface of cerebellar hemisphere

◊ Quite variable course + vascular supply with reciprocal relation between vascular territories of AICA + PICA!

Posterior inferior cerebellar artery

= PICA = last and largest branch of vertebral artery

Parts:

1. Premedullar segment = caudal loop around medulla, may descend below level of foramen magnum
2. Retromedullar segment = ascending portion up to the level of 4th ventricle and tonsils
3. Supratonsillar segment = the most cranial point is the choroidal point

P1 segment = horizontal segment between origin of PICA + pCom

P2 segment = segment downstream from pCom take-off

Variations: commonly asymmetric; hypoplastic / absent in 20% [vascular supply then provided by anterior inferior cerebellar artery (AICA)]

Supply:
inferoposterior surface of cerebellar hemisphere adjacent to occipital bone, ipsilateral part of inferior vermis, inferior portion of deep white matter only

Orthotopic **choroid point** established by:

1. perpendicular line from choroid point onto Twining's line = TTT-line (Twining's Tuberculum-Torcular line) bisects TTT-line (length of anterior portion 52 – 60%)
2. perpendicular line from choroid point cuts CT-line (Clivus-Torcular line) <1 mm anterior / <3 mm posterior to junction of anterior and middle thirds of CT-line

Superior cerebellar artery

= SCA = last but one branch of basilar artery

Supply:
superior aspect of cerebellar hemisphere (tentorial surface), ipsilateral superior vermis, largest part of deep white matter including dentate nucleus, pons

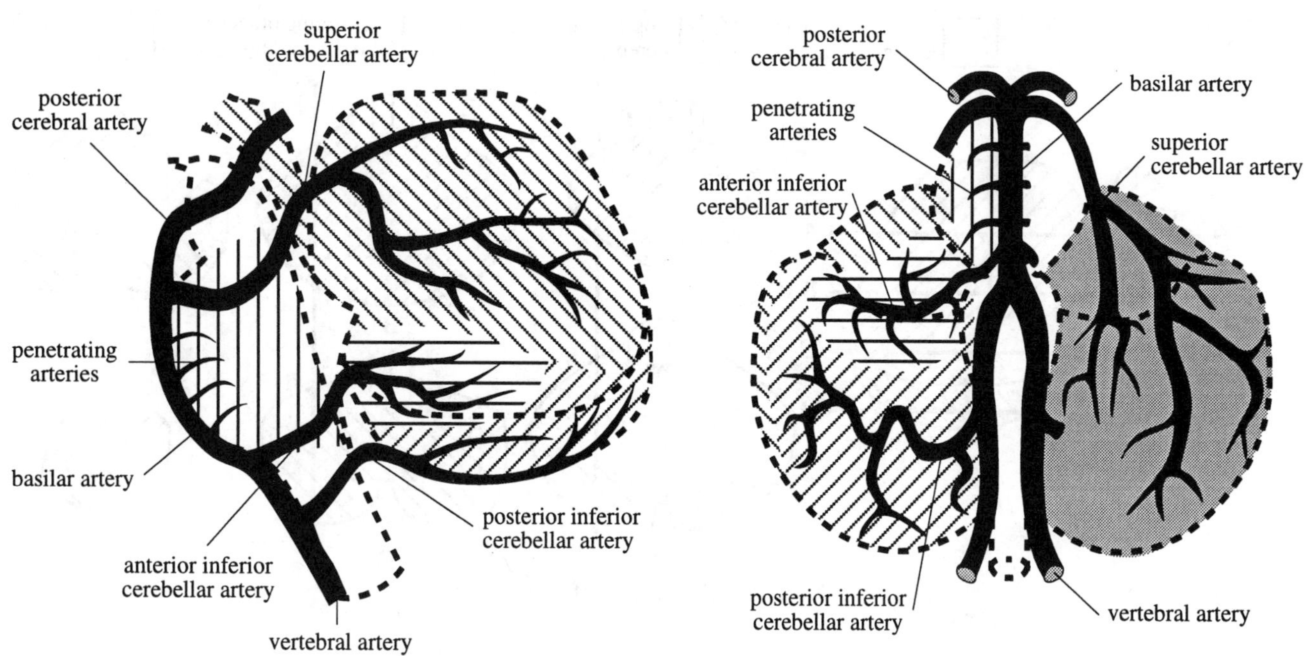

Blood Supply to the Cerebellum

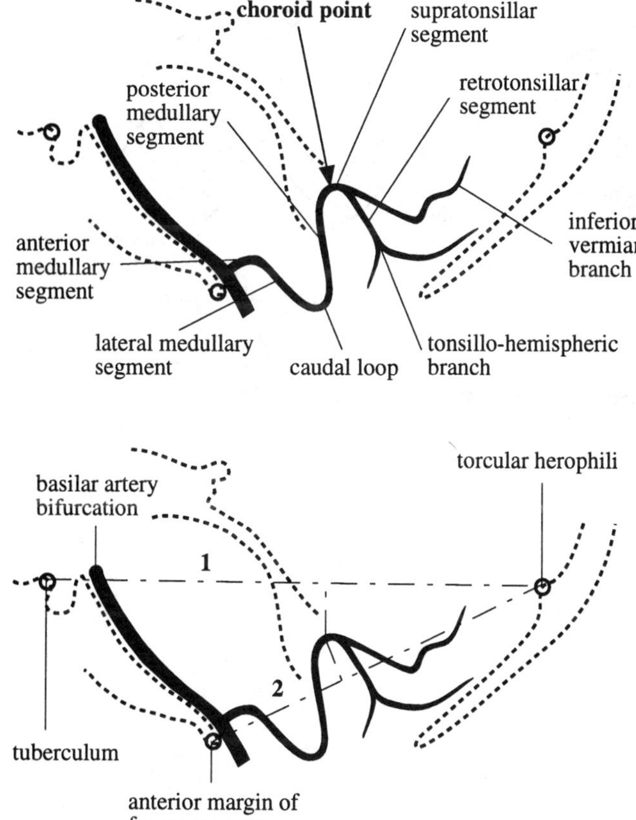

Posterior Inferior Cerebellar Artery

1, 2 = lines to establish orthotopic choroid point (see text)

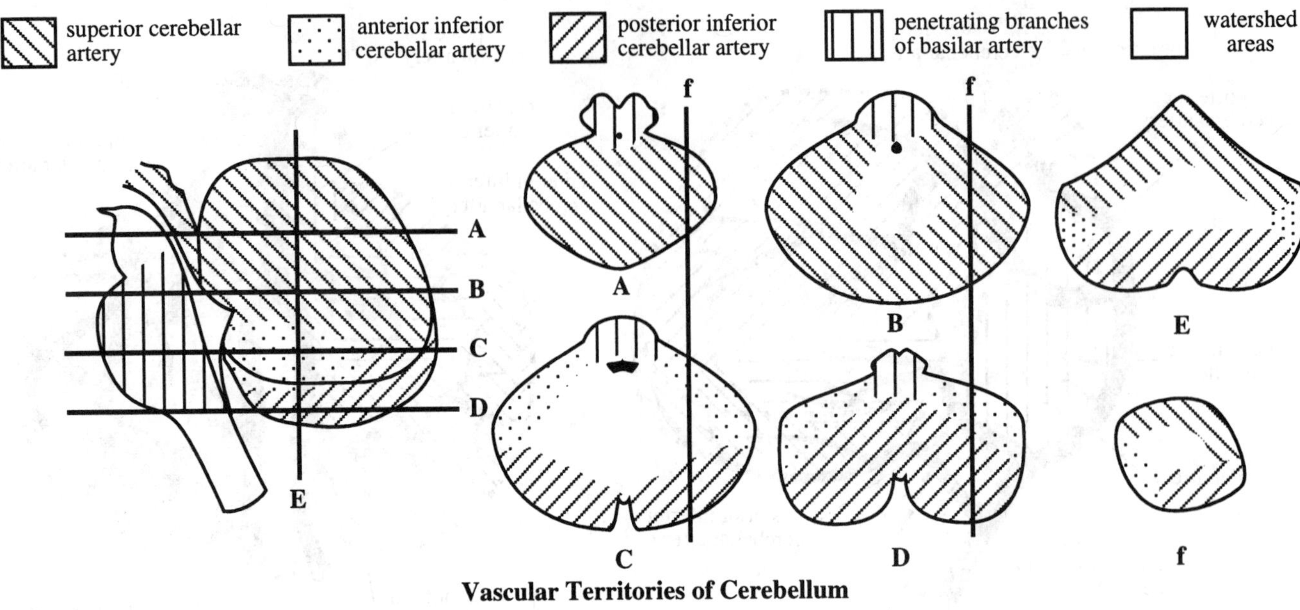
superior cerebellar artery
anterior inferior cerebellar artery
posterior inferior cerebellar artery
penetrating branches of basilar artery
watershed areas
A
B
C
D
E
f
A
B
C
D
E
f
f
f

Vascular Territories of Cerebellum

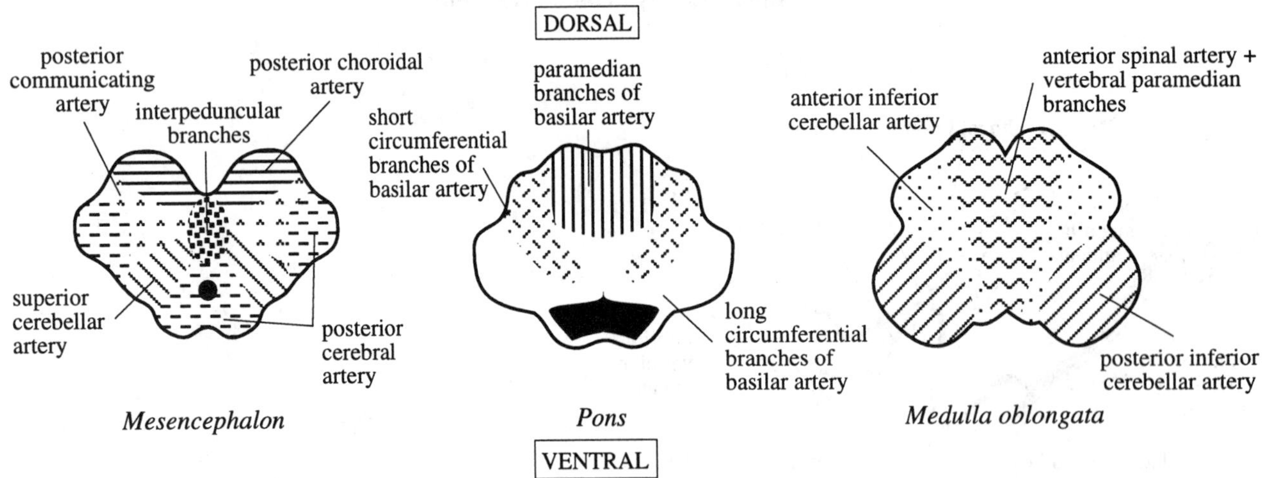
DORSAL
posterior communicating artery
posterior choroidal artery
interpeduncular branches
superior cerebellar artery
posterior cerebral artery
Mesencephalon
short circumferential branches of basilar artery
paramedian branches of basilar artery
long circumferential branches of basilar artery
Pons
anterior inferior cerebellar artery
anterior spinal artery + vertebral paramedian branches
posterior inferior cerebellar artery
Medulla oblongata
VENTRAL

Vascular Territories of Brainstem

BRAIN DISORDERS

ABSCESS OF BRAIN

Pyogenic Abscess

= focal area of necrosis beginning in area of cerebritis with formation of surrounding membrane

Cause:

1. Extension from paranasal sinus infection (41%) / mastoiditis / otitis media (5%) / facial soft-tissue infection / dental abscess
2. Generalized septicemia (32%):
   (a) lung (most common): bronchiectasis, empyema, lung abscess, bronchopleural fistula, pneumonia
   (b) heart (less common): CHD with R-L shunt, AVM, bacterial endocarditis
   (c) osteomyelitis
3. Penetrating trauma or surgery
4. Cryptogenic (25%)

Predisposed: diabetes mellitus, patients on steroids / immunosuppressive drugs, congenital / acquired immunologic deficiency

Organism: Anaerobic streptococcus (most common), Bacteroides, Staphylococcus; in 20% multiple organisms; in 25% sterile contents

Pathophysiology:

Stage I: vascular congestion, petechial hemorrhage, edema

Stage II: cerebral softening + necrosis

Stage III: (after 2–3 weeks) liquefaction, cavitation + capsule consisting of inner layer of granulation tissue, a middle collagenous layer and an outer astroglial layer; edema outside abscess capsule

Location: typically at corticomedullary junction; frontal + temporal lobes; supratentorial : infratentorial = 2:1

NCCT:

√ zone of low density with mass effect (92%)
√ slightly increased rim density (4%), development of collagen layer takes 10–14 days
√ gas within lesion (4%) is diagnostic of gas-forming organism

CECT:

√ ring enhancement (90%) with peripheral zone of edema
√ homogeneous enhancement in lesions <0.5 cm
√ edema + contrast enhancement suppressed by steroids
√ smooth regular 1–3 mm thick wall with relative thinning of medial wall (secondary to poorer blood supply of white matter)
√ multiloculation + subjacent daughter abscess in white matter

MR: (most sensitive modality)

√ centrally increased / variable intensity with hypointense rim on T2WI
√ outside border of increased signal intensity on T2WI (edema)

Cx: (1) Development of daughter abscesses toward white matter
(2) Rupture into ventricular system / subarachnoid space (thinner abscess capsule formation on medial wall of abscess related to fewer blood vessels) producing ventriculitis ± meningitis

Dx helpful features:

- multiple lesions at gray-white matter border
- clinical history of altered immune status
- R-to-L shunt: eg, pulmonary AV fistula
- foreign travel
- high-risk behavior: eg, IV drug abuse

DDx: primary / metastatic neoplasm, subacute infarction, resolving hematoma

Granulomatous Abscess

1. Tuberculoma
2. Sarcoid abscess
3. Fungal abscess: eg, Cryptococcus

Predisposed: immunocompromised patients

√ enhancement of leptomeningeal surface
√ nodular / ring-enhancing parenchymal lesion

Cx: Communicating hydrocephalus (secondary to thick exudate blocking basal cisterns)

ACRANIA

= EXENCEPHALY

= developmental anomaly characterized by partial / complete absence of membranous neurocranium + complete but abnormal development of brain tissue

Incidence: 25 cases reported

Cause: impaired migration of mesenchyme to its normal location under the calvarial ectoderm resulting in failure for development of dura mater + skull + musculature

Time: develops after closure of anterior neuropore during 4th week

May be associated with:

cleft lip, bilateral absence of orbital floors, metatarsus varus, talipes, cervicothoracic spina bifida

• ± elevation of maternal serum AFP

√ absence of calvarium
√ normal ossification of chondrocranium (face, skull base)
√ hemispheres surrounded by thin membrane

Prognosis: uniformly lethal; progression to anencephaly (brain destruction secondary to exposure to amniotic fluid + mechanical trauma)

DDx: encephalocele, anencephaly, osteogenesis imperfecta, hypophosphatasia

ADRENOLEUKODYSTROPHY

= BRONZED SCLEROSING ENCEPHALOMYELITIS

= inherited metabolic disorder characterized by progressive demyelination of cerebral white matter + adrenal insufficiency

Etiology: defective peroxisomal fatty acid oxidation due to impaired function of lignoceryl-coenzyme A ligase with accumulation of saturated very long chain fatty acids (cholesterol esters) in white matter + adrenal cortex + testes

Dx: assay of plasma, red cells, cultured skin fibroblasts for the presence of increased amounts of very long chain fatty acids

Mode of inheritance:
(a) X-linked recessive in boys (common)
(b) autosomal recessive in neonates (uncommon)

Histo: PAS cytoplasmic inclusions in brain, adrenals, other tissues

Age: 3–10 years (X-linked recessive)

- deteriorating vision (27%), loss of hearing (50%)
- ataxia
- optic disk pallor
- adrenal gland insufficiency (abnormal increased pigmentation, elevated ACTH levels)
- altered behavior, attention disorder, mental deterioration, death

Location: disease process usually starts in central occipital white matter, advances anteriorly through internal + external capsules + centrum semiovale, centripetal progression to involve subcortical white matter, interhemispheric spread via corpus callosum particularly splenium, involvement of optic radiation ± auditory system ± pyramidal tract

CT:
√ large symmetric low-density lesions in occipitoparietotemporal white matter (80%) advancing toward frontal lobes + cerebellum
√ thin curvilinear / serrated enhancing rims near edges of lesion
√ initial frontal lobe involvement (12%)
√ calcifications within hypodense areas (7%)
√ cerebral atrophy in late stage (progressive loss of cortical neurons)

MR:
√ hypointensity on T1WI in affected areas (hypointense atrophic splenium of corpus callosum)
√ hyperintense bilateral confluent areas on T2WI

Prognosis: usually fatal within several years after onset of symptoms

Adrenomyeloneuropathy

= clinically milder form with later age of onset
- symptoms of spinal cord demyelination + peripheral neuropathy

AGENESIS OF CORPUS CALLOSUM

= COMPLETE DYSGENESIS OF CORPUS CALLOSUM
= failure of formation of corpus callosum originating from the lamina terminalis at 7–13 weeks from where a phalanx of callosal tissue extends backward arching over the diencephalon; usually developed by 20 weeks

Incidence: 0.7–5.3%

Cause: congenital, acquired (infarction of ACA)

Histo: axons from cerebral hemispheres that would normally cross continue along medial walls of lateral ventricles as longitudinal callosal bundles of Probst that terminate randomly in occipital + temporal lobes

Associated with:
(a) CNS anomalies (85%):
1. Dandy-Walker cyst (11%)
2. Interhemispheric arachnoid cyst may be continuous with 3rd and lateral ventricles
3. Hydrocephalus (30%)
4. Midline intracerebral lipoma of corpus callosum often surrounded with ring of calcium (10%)
5. Arnold-Chiari II malformation (7%)
6. Midline encephalocele
7. Porencephaly
8. Holoprosencephaly
9. Hypertelorism median cleft syndrome
10. Polymicrogyria, gray-matter heterotopia

(b) Cardiovascular, gastrointestinal, genitourinary anomalies (62%)
(c) Abnormal karyotype (trisomy 13, 15, 18)

- normal brain function in isolated agenesis
- intellectual impairment; seizures

√ absence of septum pellucidum + corpus callosum + cavum septi pellucidi
√ longitudinal bundles of Probst create crescentic lateral ventricles
  √ colpocephaly (= dilatation of trigones + occipital horns + posterior temporal horns in the absence of splenium
  √ "bat-wing" appearance of lateral ventricles (= wide separation of lateral ventricles with straight parallel parasagittal orientation with absent callosal body)
  √ laterally convex frontal horns in case of absent genu of corpus callosum
√ "high-riding third ventricle" = upward displacement of widened 3rd ventricle often to level of bodies of lateral ventricle
√ anterior interhemispheric fissure adjoins elevated 3rd ventricle ± communication (PATHOGNOMONIC)
√ "interhemispheric cyst" = interhemispheric CSF collection as an upward extension of 3rd ventricle
√ enlarged foramina of Monro
√ "sunburst gyral pattern" = dysgenesis of cingulate gyrus with characteristic radial orientation of cerebral sulci from the roof of the 3rd ventricle (on sagittal images)
√ failure of normal convergence of calcarine + parieto-occipital sulci
√ persistent eversion of cingulate gyrus (rotated inferiorly + laterally) with absence on midsagittal images
√ incomplete formation of Ammon's horn in the hippocampus

OB-US (>22 weeks GA):
√ absence of septum pellucidum
√ "teardrop" ventriculomegaly = disproportionate enlargement of occipital horns = colpocephaly
√ dilated + elevated 3rd ventricle
√ radial array pattern of medial cerebral sulci

Angio:
- √ wandering straight posterior course of pericallosal arteries (lateral view)
- √ wide separation of pericallosal arteries secondary to intervening 3rd ventricle (anterior view)
- √ separation of internal cerebral veins
- √ loss of U-shape in vein of Galen

DDx: (1) Prominent cavum septi pellucidi + cavum vergae (should not be mistaken for 3rd ventricle)
(2) Arachnoid cyst in midline (suprasellar, collicular plate) raising and deforming the 3rd ventricle and causing hydrocephalus

Partial Agenesis of Corpus Callosum

= milder form of callosal dysgenesis (best seen on MR) depending on time of arrested growth (anteroposterior development of genu + body + splenium, however, rostrum forming last)
- (a) genu only
- (b) genu + part of the body
- (c) genu + entire body
- (d) genu + body + splenium (without rostrum)

AIDS

= DNA retrovirus infection attacking monocytes + macrophages which leads to deficient cell-mediated immunity

Incidence: 1% of population in United States is HIV-seropositive; 187,000 new cases in 1991

Histo: formation of microglial nodules instead of granulomas in 75–80% of autopsied brains

- • neurologic symptoms as initial complaint in 10%, ultimately afflict up to 40–60%: headache, memory loss, confusion, dementia, focal deficit from mass lesion
- ◊ Any male with neurologic symptoms between age 20 and 50 has AIDS until proven otherwise
- ◊ Unusual presentations are clues to HIV infection: pan-sinusitis, mastoiditis, parotid cysts, cervical adenopathy, hypointense spine

DIFFUSE CHANGES:
(1) HIV / CMV encephalopathy (most common complication)
both viruses occur always in combination
- • dementia in up to 60% during course of disease
- • cognitive dysfunction in up to 90%
- √ patchy white matter lesions (= subacute leukoencephalitis) in 31%

FOCAL CHANGES:
(1) Toxoplasmosis (50–70%)
(2) Primary CNS lymphoma (20–30%)
Prevalence: in 75% at autopsy
- ◊ Initial manifestation in 0.6% of AIDS patients
- ◊ 2% of AIDS patients develop primary CNS lymphoma at some point during their illness

(3) Progressive multifocal leukoencephalopathy (10–20%)
(4) Fungal, granulomatous, viral, bacterial infection
(a) Cryptococcosis
Location: extension along Virchow-Robin spaces
- √ hydrocephalus + cortical / central atrophy (with inadequate immune response)
- √ enhancing granulomatous meningitis (with sufficient immune response)
- √ bilateral nonenhancing hyperintense abnormalities in lenticulostriate region (= gelatinous pseudocyst) on T2WI

(b) Other opportunistic CNS infections: tuberculosis, neurosyphilis
- ◊ With multiple CNS lesions toxoplasmic encephalitis is the more likely diagnosis!
- ◊ With a single CNS lesion the probability of lymphoma is at least equal to toxoplasmosis!

Rx: azidothymidine (AZT)

ALEXANDER DISEASE

= FIBRINOID LEUKODYSTROPHY

Age: as early as first few weeks of life
- • macrocephaly
- • failure to attain developmental milestones
- • progressive spastic quadriparesis
- • intellectual failure

Location: frontal white matter gradually extending posteriorly into parietal region + internal capsule

CT:
- √ low-density white matter lesion
- √ contrast enhancement near tip of frontal horn

MR:
- √ prolonged T1 + T2 relaxation times

Prognosis: death in infancy / early childhood

ALZHEIMER DISEASE

most common of diffuse gray matter diseases with large loss of cells from cerebral cortex + other areas
- • slowly progressing memory loss, dementia
- √ "cracked walnut" appearance = symmetrically enlarged sulci in high-convexity area
- √ focal atrophic change in medial temporal lobe
- √ smooth periventricular halo of hyperintensity (50%)

ANENCEPHALY

= lethal anomaly with failure of closure of the rostral end of the neural tube by 5.6 weeks MA
- ◊ Associated with highest AF-AFP and MS-AFP values; >90% will be detected with MS-AFP ≥2.5 MoM

Incidence: 1:1,000 births (3.5:1,000 in South Wales); M:F = 1:4; most common congenital defect of CNS; 50% of all neural tube defects

Recurrence rate: 3–4%

Etiology: multifactorial (genetic + environmental)

Path: absence of cerebral hemispheres + cranial vault; partial / complete absence of diencephalic + mesencephalic structures; hypophysis + rhombencephalic structures usually preserved

Risk factors: family history of neural tube defect; twin pregnancy
Associated anomalies:
spinal dysraphism (17–50%), cleft lip / palate (2%), clubfoot (2%), umbilical hernia, amniotic band syndrome
√ absence of bony calvarium cephalad to orbits
√ ± cranial soft-tissue mass (= angiomatous stroma)
√ bulging froglike eyes
√ short neck
√ polyhydramnios (40–50%) after 26 weeks GA (due to failure of normal fetal swallowing) / oligohydramnios
Dx: in 100% >14 weeks GA
Prognosis: uniformly fatal within hours to days of life; in 53% premature birth; in 68% stillbirth
DDx: acrania, encephalocele, amniotic band syndrome

ANEURYSM OF CNS

Etiology:
(a) congenital (97%) = "berry aneurysm" in 2% of population (in 20% multiple); associated with aortic coarctation + adult polycystic kidney disease
(b) infectious (3%) = mycotic aneurysm
(c) arteriosclerotic: fusiform shape
(d) traumatic
(e) neoplastic
(f) fibromuscular disease
(g) collagen vascular disease

Risk factors:
(1) family history for aneurysms in 1st- / 2nd-degree relatives
(2) female gender
(3) age >50 years
(4) cigarette smoking
(5) oral contraceptives / pregnancy
(6) Marfan syndrome, pseudoxanthoma elasticum, Ehlers-Danlos syndrome
(7) polycystic kidney disease
(8) asymmetry of circle of Willis
(9) cerebral arteriovenous malformation

Pathogenesis: arterial wall deficient in tunica media + external elastic lamina (natural occurrence with advancing age)

Location of aneurysm:
A. by autopsy:
(a) circle of Willis (85%):
MCA bifurcation (25%), aCom (25%), pCom (18%), distal ACA (5%), ICA at bifurcation (4%), ophthalmic a. (4%), anterior choroidal a. (4%)
(b) posterior fossa (15%)
basilar bifurcation (7%), basilar trunk (3%), vertebral-PICA (3%), PCA (2%)
B. by angiography (= symptomatic aneurysms):
pCom (38%) > aCom (36%) > MCA bifurcation (21%) > ICA bifurcation > tip of basilar artery (2.8%)
C. by risk of bleeding: 1–2% per year
aCom (70% bleed), pCom (2nd highest risk)
◊ Aneurysms at bifurcations / branching points are at greatest risk for rupture!

MULTIPLE ANEURYSMS
Cause: congenital in 20–30%, mycotic in 22%
mnemonic: "FECAL P"
Fibromuscular dysplasia
Ehlers-Danlos syndrome
Coarctation
Arteriovenous malformation
Lupus erythematosus
Polycystic kidney disease (adult)
◊ 35% of patients with one MCA aneurysm have one on the contralateral side (= mirror image aneurysms)!
◊ simultaneous aneurysm + AVM in 4–15%

CECT: detection rate of aneurysms at pCom (40%), aCom / MCA, basilar artery (80%)
Angio (all 4 cerebral vessels):
√ contrast outpouching
√ <2 mm infundibuli typically occur at pCom / anterior choroidal a. origin
√ mass effect in thrombosed aneurysm
◊ 2nd arteriogram within 1–2 weeks detects aneurysm in 10–20% following negative 1st angiogram!

Prognosis:
(1) Death in 10% within 24 hours from concomitant intracerebral hemorrhage, extensive brain herniation, massive infarcts + hemorrhage within brainstem; 45% mortality within 30 days (25% prior to admission)
(2) Complete recovery in 58% of survivors
(3) Cerebral ischemia + infarction
(4) Rebleeding rate: 12–20% within 2 weeks, 11–22% within 30 days, up to 50% within 6 months (increased mortality); thereafter 4% risk/year

Surgical mortality rate: 50% for ruptured, 1–3% for unruptured aneurysms
Cx: subdural hematoma

Ruptured Berry Aneurysm

Incidence: 28,000 cases/year = 10 cases/10,000 people/year
Age: 50–60 years of age; M:F = 1:2
Rupture size: 5–15 mm
• "worst headache of one's life"
• neck stiffness, nausea, vomiting
• sudden loss of consciousness (in up to 45%)
• history of warning leak / sentinel hemorrhage hours to days earlier

Clues for which aneurysm is bleeding:
(a) the largest aneurysm (87%)
(b) anterior communicating artery (70%)
(c) contralateral side of all visualized aneurysms (60%), nonvisualization due to spasm
mnemonic: "BISH"
Biggest
Irregular contour
Spasm (adjacent)
Hematoma location

Location of blood suggesting accurately in 70% the site of the ruptured aneurysm:

(a) according to location of subarachnoid hemorrhage:

1. Anterior chiasmatic cistern : aCom
2. Septum pellucidum : aCom
3. Intraventricular : aCom, ICA, MCA
4. Sylvian fissure : MCA, ICA, pCom
5. Anterior pericallosal cistern : ACA, aCom
6. Symmetric distribution in subarachnoid space : ACA + basilar a.

(b) according to location of cerebral hematoma:

1. inferomedial frontal lobe : aCom
2. temporal lobe : MCA
3. corpus callosum artery : pericallosal

(c) intraventricular hemorrhage
from aneurysms at aCom, MCA, pericallosal artery (CAVE: blood may have entered in retrograde manner from subarachnoid location)

Giant Aneurysm

= aneurysm larger than 2.5 cm in diameter, usually presenting with intracranial mass effect

Incidence: 25% of all aneurysms

Age: no age predilection; M:F = 2:1

Location: (arise from arteries at the base of the brain)

(a) middle fossa: cavernous segment of ICA (43%), supraclinoid segment of ICA, terminal bifurcation of ICA, middle cerebral artery

(b) posterior fossa: at tip of basilar artery, AICA, vertebral artery

Skull film:

√ predominantly peripheral curvilinear calcification (22%)

√ bone erosion (44%)

√ pressure changes on sella turcica (18%)

CECT:

√ "target sign" = centrally opacified vessel lumen + ring of thrombus + enhanced fibrous outer wall

√ simple ring-blush (75%) of fibrous outer wall with total thrombosis

√ little / no surrounding edema

MR:

√ mixed signal intensity (combination of subacute + chronic hemorrhage, calcification)

Cx: subarachnoid hemorrhage in <30%

Mycotic Aneurysm

= 3% of all intracranial aneurysms, multiple in 20%

Source: subacute bacterial endocarditis (65%), acute bacterial endocarditis (9%), meningitis (9%), septic thrombophlebitis (9%), myxoma

Location: peripheral to first bifurcation of major vessel (64%); often located near surface of brain especially over convexities

(a) suprasellar cistern = circle of Willis

(b) inferolateral sylvian fissure = middle cerebral artery trifurcation

(c) genu of corpus callosum = origin of callosomarginal artery

(d) bottom of 3rd ventricle = pericallosal a.

NCCT:

√ aneurysm rarely visualized; indirect evidence from focal hematoma secondary to rupture

√ zone of increased density / calcification

√ increased density in subarachnoid, intraventricular, intracerebral spaces (extravasated blood)

√ focal / diffuse lucency of brain (edema / infarction / vasospasm)

CECT:

√ intense homogeneous enhancement within round / oval mass contiguous to vessels

√ incomplete opacification with mural thrombus

Cx: develop recurrent bleeding more frequently than congenital aneurysms

Supraclinoid Carotid Aneurysm

= 38% of intracranial aneurysms

Site: (a) at origin of pCom (65%)

(b) at bifurcation of internal carotid artery (23%)

(c) at origin of ophthalmic artery (12%) medial to anterior clinoid process; most likely to become giant aneurysm

Presentation: bitemporal hemianopia (extrinsic compression on chiasm)

√ calcification is rare (frequent in atherosclerotic cavernous sinus aneurysm)

Cavernous Sinus Aneurysm

Age: 20–70 years, peak 5th–6th decade; F >> M

Cause: sinus thrombophlebitis

- progressive visual impairment
- cavernous sinus syndrome: trigeminal nerve pain, oculomotor nerve paralysis

Site: extradural portion of cavernous sinus ICA

√ undercutting of anterior clinoid process

√ erosion of lateral half of sella

√ erosion of posterior clinoid process

√ invasion of middle cranial fossa

√ enlargement of superior orbital fissure

√ erosion of tip of petrous pyramid

√ rimlike calcification (33%)

√ displacement of thin bony margins without sclerosis

Rx: often inoperable; balloon embolization ± parent artery occlusion

AQUEDUCTAL STENOSIS

= focal reduction in size of aqueduct at level of superior colliculi / intercollicular sulcus (normal range of 0.2–1.8 mm^2)

Embryology:

aqueduct develops about the 6th week of gestation + decreases in size until birth due to growth pressure from adjacent mesencephalic structures

Incidence: 0.5–1:1,000 births; most frequent cause of congenital hydrocephalus (20–43%); recurrence rate in siblings of 1–4.5%; M:F = 2:1

Etiology:
(a) postinflammatory (50%): secondary to perinatal infection (toxoplasmosis, CMV, syphilis, mumps, influenza virus) or intracranial hemorrhage
= destruction of ependymal lining of aqueduct with adjacent marked fibrillary gliosis
(b) developmental: aqueductal forking (= marked branching of aqueduct into channels) / narrowing / transverse septum (X-linked recessive inheritance in 25% of males)
(c) neoplastic (extremely rare): pinealoma, meningioma, tectal astrocytoma (may be missed on routine CT scans, easily differentiated by MR)

May be associated with: other congenital anomalies (16%): thumb deformities

√ enlargement of lateral + 3rd ventricles with normal-sized 4th ventricle (4th ventricle may be normal with communicating hydrocephalus)

Prognosis: 11–30% mortality

ARACHNOID CYST

= CSF-containing intra-arachnoid cyst without ventricular communication / brain maldevelopment

Incidence: 1% of all intracranial masses

Origin:
(1) congenital: arising from clefts / duplication / "splitting" of arachnoid membrane with expansion by CSF due to secretory activity of arachnoid cells
= **true arachnoid cyst**
(2) acquired: following surgery / trauma / subarachnoid hemorrhage / infection in neonatal period / associated with extra-axial neoplasm = loculation of CSF surrounded by arachnoidal scarring with expansion by osmotic filtration / ball-valve mechanism = **leptomeningeal cyst = secondary arachnoid cyst = acquired arachnoid cyst**

Histo: cyst filled with clear fluid, thin wall composed of cleaved arachnoid membrane lined by ependymal / meningothelial cells

Age: presentation at any time during life

- often asymptomatic
- symptomatic due to mass effect, hydrocephalus, seizures, headaches, hemiparesis, intracranial hypertension, craniomegaly, developmental delay, visual loss, precocious puberty, bobble-head doll syndrome

Location: (arise in CSF cisterns between brain + dura)
(a) floor of middle fossa near tip of temporal lobe (sylvian fissure) in 50%
(b) suprasellar / chiasmatic cistern (may produce endocrinopathy) in 10%
(c) posterior fossa (1/3): cerebellopontine angle (11%), quadrigeminal plate cistern (10%), in relationship to vermis (9%), prepontine / interpeduncular cistern (3%)
(d) interhemispheric fissure, cerebral convexity, anterior infratentorial midline

√ forward bowing of anterior wall of cranial fossa + elevation of sphenoid ridge
√ extra-axial unilocular thin-walled CSF-density cyst with well-defined smooth angular margins
√ compression of subarachnoid space + subjacent brain (minimal mass effect)
√ may erode inner table of calvarium
√ NO enhancement (intrathecal contrast penetrates into cyst on delayed scans)
√ NO calcifications

MR (best modality):
√ well-circumscribed lesion with same uniform signal intensity as CSF ± mass effect

Cx: (1) hydrocephalus (30–60%)
(2) concurrent subdural / intracystic hemorrhage

Prognosis: favorable if removed before onset of irreversible brain damage

Rx: fenestration / cyst-peritoneal shunting

CT-DDx:
epidermoid cyst, dermoid, subdural hygroma, infarction, porencephaly

US-DDx:
choroid plexus cyst, porencephalic cyst (communicates with ventricle), cystic tumor (solid components), midline cyst associated with agenesis of corpus callosum, dorsal cyst associated with holoprosencephaly, Dandy-Walker cyst (extension of 4th ventricle, developmental delay), vein of Galen aneurysm

ARTERIOVENOUS FISTULA

= abnormal communication between artery + vein resulting in tremendous amount of flow due to high pressure gradient; leading to enlargement + elongation of draining veins

Cause:
(1) Vessel laceration (delay between trauma + clinical manifestation due to delayed lysis of hematoma surrounding arterial laceration)
(2) Angiodysplasia: fibromuscular disease, neurofibromatosis, Ehlers-Danlos syndrome
(3) Congenital fistula

- pulsatile mass + thrill / bruit
- ± neurologic symptoms / deficit (due to arterial steal)

Location:
(a) carotid-cavernous sinus fistula (most common)
(b) vertebral artery fistula
(c) external carotid fistula (rare)

ARTERIOVENOUS MALFORMATION

= congenital abnormality consisting of a nidus of abnormal dilated tortuous arteries + veins with racemose tangle of closely packed pathologic vessels resulting in shunting of blood from arterial to venous side without intermediary capillary bed

Prevalence: most common vascular lesion

Histo: affected arteries have thin walls (no elastica, small amount of muscularis); intervening gliotic brain parenchyma between vessels

Age: 80% by end of 4th decade; 20% <20 years of age

- headaches, seizures (nonfocal in 40%), mental deterioration
- progressive hemispheric neurologic deficit (50%)
- ictus from acute intracranial hemorrhage (50%)

Location:
(a) supratentorial (90%): parietal > frontal > temporal lobe > paraventricular > intraventricular region > occipital lobe
(b) infratentorial (10%)

Vascular supply:
(a) pial branches of ICA in 73% of supratentorial location, in 50% of posterior fossa location
(b) dural branches of ECA in 27% with infratentorial lesions

√ NO mass effect

Skull film:
√ speckled / ringlike calcifications (15–30%)
√ thinning / thickening of skull at contact area with AVM
√ prominent vascular grooves on inner table of skull (dilated feeding arteries + draining veins) in 27%

NCCT:
√ irregular lesion with large feeding arteries + draining veins
√ mixed density (60%): dense large vessels + hemorrhage + calcifications
√ isodense lesion (15%): may be recognizable by mass effect
√ low density (15%): brain atrophy due to ischemia
√ not visualized (10%)

CECT:
√ serpiginous dense enhancement in 80% (tortuous dilated vessels)
√ No enhancement in thrombosed AVM
√ No avascular spaces within AVM
√ lack of mass effect / edema (unless thrombosed / bleeding)
√ rapid shunting
√ thickened arachnoid covering
√ adjacent atrophic brain

MR:
√ flow void (imaging with GRASS gradient echo + long TR sequences)

Angio:
√ grossly dilated efferent + afferent vessels with a racemose tangle ("bag of worms")
√ arteriovenous shunting into at least one early draining vein
√ negative angiogram (compression by hematoma / thrombosis)

Cx: (1) Hemorrhage (common): bleeding on venous side due to increased pressure / ruptured aneurysm (5%)
(2) Infarction

Prognosis: 10% mortality; 30% morbidity; 2–3% yearly chance of bleeding increasing to 6% in year following 1st bleed + 25% in year following 2nd bleed

Wyburn-Mason Syndrome

= telangiectasias of skin + retinal cirsoid aneurysm + AVM involving entire optic tract (optic nerve, thalamus, geniculate bodies, calcarine cortex);

May be associated with: AVMs of posterior fossa, neck, mandible / maxilla presenting in childhood

ASTROCYTOMA

Incidence: 70–75% of all primary intracranial tumors; most common brain tumor in children (40–50% of all primary pediatric intracranial neoplasms)

Location:
cerebral hemisphere (lobar), thalamus, pons, midbrain, may spread across corpus callosum (incidence of occurrence proportional to amount of white matter); no particular lobar distribution;
(a) in adults: central white matter of cerebrum (15–30% of all gliomas)
(b) in children: cerebellum (40%) + brainstem (20%), supratentorial (30%)

Well-differentiated = Low-grade Astrocytoma

Incidence: 9% of all primary intracranial tumors
Age: 20– 40 years; M > F

WHO Classification of Astrocytomas

Grade	Type	Features
Grade I	Circumscribed astrocytoma	generally benign well-circumscribed tumor, specific unique histologic features for each tumor, **pilocytic astrocytoma** (most common), subependymal **giant cell astrocytoma**; no tendency to progress to higher grade; low rate of recurrence
Grade II	Astrocytoma	diffusely infiltrating; well-differentiated; minimal pleomorphism or nuclear atypia; no vascular proliferation / necrosis
Grade III	Anaplastic astrocytoma	pleomorphism and nuclear atypia; increased cellularity; mitotic activity; vascular proliferation + necrosis absent
Grade IV	Glioblastoma multiforme	marked vascular proliferation and necrosis; increased cellularity; anaplasia + pleomorphism; variable mitotic activity; cell type may be poorly differentiated, fusiform, round or multinucleated

Path: benign nonmetastasizing; poorly defined borders with infiltration of white matter + basal ganglia + cortex; NO significant tumor vascularity / necrosis / hemorrhage; blood-brain barrier may remain intact
Histo: homogeneous relatively uniform appearance with proliferation of well-differentiated multipolar fibrillary / protoplasmic astrocytes; mild nuclear pleomorphism + mild hypercellularity; mitoses rare
Location: posterior fossa in children, supratentorial in adults (typically lobar); distribution proportional to amount of white matter
√ may develop a cyst with high-protein content (rare)
CT:
√ usually hypodense lesion with minimal mass effect + NO peritumoral edema
√ well-defined tumor margins
√ central calcifications (frequent)
√ minimal / no contrast enhancement (normal capillary endothelial cells)
MR:
√ well-defined hypointense lesion with little mass effect / vasogenic edema / heterogeneity on T1WI
√ hyperintense on T2WI
√ little / no enhancement on Gd-DTPA
√ cyst with content hyperintense to CSF (protein content)
√ hyperintense area within tumor mass (paramagnetic effect of methemoglobin)
√ inhomogeneous gadolinium-DTPA enhancement of tumor nodule
Angio:
√ majority avascular
Prognosis: 3–10 years postoperative survival; occasionally converting into more malignant form several years after presentation

Anaplastic Astrocytoma

Incidence: 11% of all primary intracranial neoplasms
Path: frequently vasogenic edema; NO necrosis / hemorrhage
Histo: less well differentiated with greater degree of hypercellularity + pleomorphism, multipolar fibrillary / protoplasmic astrocytes; mitoses + vascular endothelial proliferation common
Location: typically lobar
Distribution: proportional to amount of white matter
MR:
√ well-defined slightly heterogeneous hypointense lesion on T1WI with prevalent vasogenic edema
√ hyperintense on T2WI
√ ± enhancement on Gd-DTPA
Prognosis: 2 years postoperative survival

Pilocytic Astrocytoma

= JUVENILE PILOCYTIC ASTROCYTOMA
= most benign histologic subtype of astrocytoma without progression to high-grade glioma
Histo: alternating pattern of compact bipolar pilocytic (hairlike) astrocytes arranged mostly around vessels + loosely aggregated protoplasmic astrocytes undergoing microcystic degeneration
Age: predominantly in children + young adults; peak age between birth and 9 years of age; M:F = 1:1
Associated with: neurofibromatosis
Location: cerebellum, hypothalamus (around 3rd ventricle), optic nerve / chiasm
√ mural tumor nodule located in wall of cerebellar cyst
√ multilobulated / dumbbell appearance along optic pathway
√ rarely calcifies
√ micro- / macrocysts in cerebellar location
√ increased heterogeneous signal intensity on early Gd-DTPA enhanced T1WI; homogeneous enhancement on delayed images
Prognosis: relatively benign clinical course, almost never recurs after surgical excision; NO malignant transformation to anaplastic form
DDx: metastasis, hemangioblastoma, atypical medulloblastoma

ATAXIA-TELANGIECTASIA

= autosomal recessive disorder characterized by telangiectasias of skin + eye, cerebellar ataxia, sinus + pulmonary infections, immunodeficiencies, propensity to develop malignancies
Incidence: 1:40,000 livebirths
Path: neuronal degradation + atrophy of cerebellar cortex (? from vascular anomalies)
• cerebellar ataxia at beginning of walking age
• progressive neurologic deterioration
• oculomotor abnormalities, dysarthric speech, choreaathetosis, myoclonic jerks
• mucocutaneous telangiectasias: bulbar conjunctiva, ears, face, neck, palate, dorsum of hands, antecubital + popliteal fossa
• recurrent bacterial + viral sinopulmonary infections
√ cerebellar cortical atrophy: diminished cerebellar size, dilatation of 4th ventricle, increased cerebellar sulcal prominence
√ cerebral hemorrhage (rupture of telangiectatic vessels)
√ cerebral infarct (emboli shunted through vascular malformations in lung)
Cx:
1. Bronchiectasis + pulmonary failure (most common cause of death)
2. Malignancies (10–15%): lymphoma, leukemia, epithelial malignancies

BINSWANGER DISEASE

= ENCEPHALOPATHIA SUBCORTICALIS PROGRESSIVA
= LEUKOARIAOSIS = SUBCORTICAL ARTERIOSCLEROTIC ENCEPHALOPATHY (SAE)
Cause: arteriosclerosis affecting the poorly collateralized distal penetrating arteries (perforating medullary arteries, thalamoperforators, lenticulostriates, pontine perforators); positive correlation with hypertension + aging

Path: ischemic demyelination / infarction
Age: >60 years
• psychiatric changes, intellectual impairment, slowly progressive dementia, transient neurologic deficits, seizures, spasticity, syncope
Location: periventricular white matter, centrum semiovale, basal ganglia; subcortical white matter "U" fibers + corpus callosum are spared
√ multifocal hypodense lesions (periventricular, centrum semiovale) with sparing of U fibers
√ lacunar infarcts in basal ganglia
√ sulcal enlargement + dilated lateral ventricles (brain atrophy)
MR:
√ focal areas of increased signal intensity on T2WI (= "unidentified bright objects")
DDx: leukodystrophy, progressive multifocal leukoencephalopathy, multiple sclerosis

CANAVAN DISEASE

= SPONGIFORM LEUKODYSTROPHY
= rare form of leukodystrophy as an autosomal recessive disorder, most common in Ashkenazi Jews
Incidence: <100 reported cases
Cause: deficiency of aspartoacyclase leading to accumulation of *N*-acetylaspartic acid in brain, plasma, urine, CSF
Histo: spongy degeneration of white matter with astrocytic swelling + mitochondrial elongation
Age: 3–6 months
• marked hypotonia
• progressive megalencephaly
• seizures
• failure to attain motor milestones
• spasticity
• intellectual failure
• optic atrophy with blindness
• swallowing impairment
√ diffuse symmetric white matter abnormality
√ may involve basal ganglia
√ cortical atrophy
CT:
√ low-density white matter
MR:
√ white matter hypointense on T1WI + hyperintense on T2WI
Prognosis: death in 2nd–5th year of life
Dx: (1) elevation of *N*-acetylaspartic acid in urine
(2) deficiency of aspartoacyclase in cultured skin fibroblasts

CAPILLARY TELANGIECTASIA

= CAPILLARY ANGIOMA
= abnormal dilated capillaries separated by normal neural tissue; commonly "cryptic"
May be associated with:
hereditary Rendu-Osler-Weber syndrome, ataxia-telangiectasia syndrome, irradiation (latency period of 5 months to 22 years)
Age: typically in elderly
• usually asymptomatic (incidental finding at necropsy)
Location: mostly in pons / midbrain; usually multiple / may be solitary
√ poorly defined area of dilated vessels (resembling petechiae)
√ best delineated with MR (due to hemorrhage)
Cx: punctate hemorrhage (uncommon), gliosis + calcifications (rare)
Prognosis: bleeding in pons usually fatal
DDx: cavernous angioma (identical on images)

CAVERNOUS HEMANGIOMA OF BRAIN

= CAVERNOUS ANGIOMA = CAVERNOMA
Path: well-circumscribed nodule of honeycomblike large sinusoidal vascular spaces separated by fibrous collagenous bands <u>without</u> intervening neural tissue; slow blood flow in vascular channels
Age: 3rd–6th decade; M > F
• seizures (commonly presenting symptom)
Location: cerebrum (mainly subcortical) > pons > cerebellum; solitary > multiple
√ NO obvious mass effect / edema
NCCT:
√ extensive calcifications = hemangioma calcificans (20%)
√ small round hyperdense region (CLUE)
√ minimal surrounding edema
CECT:
√ minimal / intense enhancement
√ low-attenuation areas due to thrombosed portions
MR:
√ well-defined area of mixed signal intensity centrally (= "mulberry"-shaped lesion) with a mixture of
√ increased signal intensity (= extracellular methemoglobin / slow blood flow / thrombosis)
√ decreased intensity (= deoxyhemoglobin / intracellular methemoglobin / hemosiderin / calcification)
√ surrounded by hypointense rim (= hemosiderin) on T2WI
Angio:
√ negative = "cryptic / occult vascular malformation"
Cx: hemorrhage of varying ages
DDx: (1) Hemorrhagic neoplasm (edema, mass effect)
(2) Small AVM (thrombosed / small feeding vessels, associated hemorrhage)
(3) Capillary angioma (no difference)

CEPHALOCELE

= mesodermal defect in skull + dura with extracranial extension of intracranial structures
ENCEPHALOCELE = herniation of brain tissue + meninges + CSF
CRANIAL MENINGOCELE = herniation of meninges + CSF only
Prevalence:
1–4 per 10,000 livebirths; 5–6–20% of all craniospinal malformations; predominant neural axis anomaly in fetuses spontaneously aborted <20 weeks GA

Cause:
failure of surface ectoderm to separate from neuroectoderm early in embryonic development
@ Skull base
(1) faulty closure of neural tube (without mesenchyme membranous cranial bone cannot develop)
(2) failure of basilar ossification centers to unite
@ Calvarium
(1) defective induction of bone
(2) pressure erosion of bone by intracranial mass / cyst

In 60% associated with:
(1) Spina bifida (7–30%)
(2) Corpus callosum dysgenesis
(3) Chiari malformation
(4) Dandy-Walker malformation
(5) Meckel-Gruber syndrome (= occipital encephalocele + microcephaly + cystic dysplastic kidneys + polydactyly)
(6) Amniotic band syndrome: multiple irregular asymmetric off-midline encephaloceles
(7) Migrational abnormalities
(8) Chromosomal anomalies in 44% (trisomy 18)

- MS-AFP elevated in 3% (skin-covered in 60%)
- CSF rhinorrhea
- meningitis

Prognosis: dependent on associated malformations + size and content of lesion; 21% liveborn; 50% survival in liveborns, 74% retarded
Risk of recurrence: 3% (25% with Meckel syndrome)
DDx: teratoma, cystic hygroma, iniencephaly, scalp edema, hemangioma, branchial cleft cyst, cloverleaf skull

Occipital Encephalocele (75%)

Most common encephalocele in Western Hemisphere
Associated with: Dandy-Walker malformation, Chiari malformation

- external occipital mass

Location: supra- and infratentorial structures involved with equal frequency
√ skull defect (visualized in 80%)
√ flattening of basiocciput
√ ventriculomegaly
√ lemon sign = inward depression of frontal bones (33%)
√ cyst-within-a-cyst (ventriculocele = herniation of 4th ventricle into cephalocele)
√ acute angle between mass + skin line of neck and occiput
DDx: cystic hygroma

Frontoethmoidal Encephalocele (13–15%)

= sincipital cephalocele
Most common variety in Southeast Asia
Cause: failure of anterior neuropore located near optic recess to close normally at 4th week GA
Types: nasoethmoidal, nasofrontal, naso-orbital, interfrontal
Associated with: midline craniofacial dysraphism (dysgenesis of corpus callosum, interhemispheric lipoma, anomalies of neural migration)
√ external mass near dorsum of nose, orbits, forehead
√ hypertelorism = increase in interorbital distance

Sphenoidal Encephalocele (10%)

= basal encephalocele
Age: present at end of first decade of life

- clinically occult
- mass in nasal cavity, nasopharynx, mouth, posterior portion of orbit
- mouth breathing due to nasopharyngeal obstruction
- nasopharyngeal mass increasing with Valsalva
- diminished visual acuity with hypoplasia of optic discs
- hypothalamic-pituitary dysfunction

Associated with: agenesis of corpus callosum (80%)
Types:
(a) sphenopharyngeal = through sphenoid body
(b) spheno-orbital = through superior orbital fissure
(c) sphenoethmoidal = through sphenoid + ethmoid
(d) transethmoidal = through cribriform plate
(e) sphenomaxillary = through maxillary sinus

Parietal Encephalocele (10–12%)

Associated with: dysgenesis of corpus callosum, large interhemispheric cyst
√ hole in sphenoid bone (seen on submentovertex film)
√ cranium bifidum = cranioschisis = “split cranium” (= skull defect) = smooth opening with well-defined sclerotic rim of cortical bone
√ hydrocephalus in 15–80% (from associated aqueductal stenosis, Arnold-Chiari malformation, Dandy-Walker cyst)
√ nonenhancing expansile homogeneous paracranial mass
√ mantle of cerebral tissue often difficult to image in encephalocele (except with MR)
√ intracranial communication often not visualized
√ metrizamide / radionuclide ventriculography diagnostic
√ microcephaly (20%)
√ polyhydramnios
DDx: (1) sonographic refraction artifact at skull edge
(2) clover leaf skull (temporal bone may be partially absent)

CEREBELLAR ASTROCYTOMA

2nd most frequent tumor of posterior fossa in children
Incidence: 10–20% of pediatric brain tumors
Histo: mostly grade I
Age: children > adults; no specific age peak; M:F = 1:1
Path:
(1) cystic lesion with tumor nodule (“mural nodule”) in cyst wall (50%); (midline astrocytomas cystic in 50%, hemispheric astrocytomas cystic in 80%)
(2) solid mass with cystic (= necrotic) center (40–45%)
(3) solid tumor without necrosis (<10%)

- cerebellar signs: truncal ataxia, dysdiadochokinesia

Location: originating in midline with extension into cerebellar hemisphere (30%) > vermis > tonsils > brainstem
√ calcifications (20%): dense / faint / reticular / punctate / globular; mostly in solid variety
√ may develop extreme hydrocephalus (quite large when finally symptomatic)
CT:
√ round / oval cyst with density of cyst fluid > CSF
√ round / oval / plaquelike mural nodule with intense homogeneous enhancement
√ cyst wall slightly hyperdense + nonenhancing (= compressed cerebellar tissue)
√ uni- / multilocular cyst (= necrosis) with irregular enhancement of solid tumor portions
√ round / oval lobulated fairly well-defined iso- / hypodense solid tumor with hetero- / homogeneous enhancement
MR:
√ hypointense on T1WI + hyperintense on T2WI
√ enhancement of solid tumor portion
Angio: √ avascular
Prognosis:
malignant transformation exceedingly rare
— 40% 25-year survival rate for solid cerebellar astrocytoma
— 90% 25-year survival rate for cystic juvenile pilocytic astrocytoma
DDx of solid astrocytoma:
(1) medulloblastoma (hyperdense mass, noncalcified)
(2) ependymoma (fourth ventricle, 50% calcify)
DDx of cystic astrocytoma:
(1) Hemangioblastoma (lesion <5 cm)
(2) Arachnoid cyst
(3) Trapped 4th ventricle
(4) Megacisterna magna
(5) Dandy-Walker cyst

CEREBRITIS

= focal area of inflammation within brain substance
CT:
√ area of decreased density ± mass effect
√ no contrast enhancement (initially) / central or patchy enhancement (later)
MR:
√ focal area of increased intensity on T2WI
Cx: brain abscess

CHIARI MALFORMATION

Chiari I Malformation (adulthood)

= "cerebellar tonsillar ectopia" = herniation of cerebellar tonsils below a line connecting basion with opisthion (= foramen magnum)
◊ Frequently isolated hindbrain abnormality of little consequence without supratentorial anomalies!
Proposed causes:
(a) small posterior fossa
(b) disproportionate CSF absorption from subarachnoid spinal space
(c) cerebellar overgrowth
Associated with:
(1) syringohydromyelia (20–30%)
(2) hydrocephalus (25–44%)
(3) malformation of skull base + cervical spine:
(a) basilar impression (25%)
(b) craniovertebral fusion, eg, occipitalization of C1 (10%), incomplete ossification of C1-ring (5%)
(c) Klippel-Feil anomaly (10%)
(d) platybasia
◊ NOT associated with myelomeningocele!
• benign cerebellar ectopia <3 mm of no clinical consequence; 3–5 mm of uncertain significance; >5 mm clinical symptoms likely
• no symptoms in childhood (unless associated with hydrocephalus / syringomyelia)
• may have cranial nerve dysfunction / dissociated anesthesia of lower extremities in adulthood
√ downward displacement of cerebellar tonsils + medial part of the inferior lobes of the cerebellum 5 mm below the level of the foramen magnum
√ inferior pointing peglike / triangular tonsils
√ obliteration of cisterna magna
√ elongation of 4th ventricle which remains in normal position
√ slight anterior angulation of lower brainstem

Chiari II Malformation (childhood)

= ARNOLD-CHIARI MALFORMATION
= most common and serious complex of anomalies secondary to a too small posterior fossa involving hindbrain, spine, mesoderm
HALLMARK is dysgenesis of hindbrain with
(1) caudally displaced 4th ventricle
(2) caudally displaced brainstem
(3) tonsillar + vermian herniation through foramen magnum
Associated with:
(a) spinal anomalies
(1) lumbar myelomeningocele (>95%)
(2) syringohydromyelia
(b) supratentorial anomalies
(1) dysgenesis of corpus callosum (80–85%)
(2) obstructive hydrocephalus (50–98%) following closure of myelomeningocele
(3) absence of septum pellucidum (40%)
(4) excessive cortical gyration (stenogyria = histologically normal cortex; polymicrogyria = histologically abnormal cortex)
NOT associated with basilar impression / C1-assimilation / Klippel-Feil deformity!
• newborn: respiratory distress, apneic spells, bradycardia, impaired swallowing, poor gag reflex, retrocollis, spasticity of upper extremities
• teenager: gradual loss of function + spasticity of lower extremities
Skull film:
√ Lückenschädel (most prominent near torcular herophili / vertex) in 85% = dysplasia of membranous skull disappearing by 6 months of age

√ scalloping of clivus + posterior aspect of petrous pyramids (from pressure of cerebellum) in 70–90% leading to shortening of IAC
√ small posterior fossa
√ enlarged foramen magnum + enlarged upper spinal canal secondary to molding in 75%
√ absent / hypoplastic posterior arch of C1 (70%)

@ Supratentorial
√ hydrocephalus (duct of Sylvius dysfunctional but probe patent); may not become evident until after repair of myelomeningocele (90%)
√ colpocephaly (= enlargement of occipital horns + atria) due to maldeveloped occipital lobes
√ hypoplasia / absence of splenium + rostrum of corpus callosum (80–90%)
√ "bat-wing" configuration of frontal horns on coronal views = frontal horns pointing inferiorly with blunt superolateral angle secondary to prominent impressions by enlarged caudate nucleus
√ "hourglass ventricle" = small biconcave 3rd ventricle secondary to large massa intermedia
√ interdigitation of medial cortical gyri (hypoplasia + fenestration of falx in up to 100%)
√ wide prepontine + supracerebellar cisterns
√ nonvisualization of aqueduct (in up to 70%)
√ stenogyria = multiple small closely spaced gyri at medial aspect of occipital lobe secondary to dysplasia (in up to 50%)

@ Cerebellum
√ "cerebellar peg" = protrusion of vermis + hemispheres through foramen magnum (90%) resulting in craniocaudal elongation of cerebellum
√ hypoplastic poorly differentiated cerebellum (poor visualization of folia on sagittal images) secondary to severe degeneration
√ elongated / obliterated vertically oriented thin-tubed 4th ventricle with narrowed AP diameter exiting below foramen magnum (40%)
√ obliteration of CPA cistern + cisterna magna by cerebellum growing around brainstem
√ dysplastic tentorium with wide U-shaped incisura inserting close to foramen magnum (95%)
√ "tectal beaking" = fusion of midbrain colliculi into a single beak pointing posteriorly and invaginating into cerebellum
√ V-shaped widened quadrigeminal plate cistern (due to hypoplasia of cingulate gyri)
√ "towering cerebellum" = "pseudomass" = cerebellar extension above incisura of tentorium
√ triple peak configuration = corners of cerebellum wrapped around brainstem pointing anteriorly + laterally (on axial images)
√ flattened superior portion of cerebellum secondary to temporoparietal herniation
√ vertical orientation of shortened straight sinus

@ Spinal cord
√ medulla + pons displaced into cervical canal
√ "cervicomedullary kink" = herniation of medulla posterior to spinal cord (up to 70%) at level of dentate ligaments
√ widened anterior subarachnoid space at level of brainstem + upper cervical spine (40%)
√ AP diameter of pons narrowed
√ upper cervical nerve roots ascend toward their exit foramina
√ syringohydromyelia
√ low-lying often tethered conus medullaris below L2

OB-US:
√ "banana sign" = cerebellum wrapped around posterior brainstem + obliteration of cisterna magna due to small posterior fossa
√ hydrocephalus

Chiari III Malformation

most severe rare abnormality; probably unrelated to type I and II Chiari malformation
√ low occipital / high cervical meningomyelo-encephalocele

Prognosis: survival usually not beyond infancy

Chiari IV Malformation

extremely rare anomaly probably erroneously included as type of Chiari malformation
√ agenesis of cerebellum
√ hypoplasia of pons
√ small + funnel-shaped posterior fossa

CHOROID PLEXUS CYST

= cyst arising from folding of neuroepithelium with trapping of secretory products + desquamated cells

Incidence: 0.9–3.6% in sonographic population; 50% of autopsied brains

Histo: no epithelial lining, filled with clear fluid ± debris

May be associated with:
aneuploidy (76% with trisomy 18, 17% with trisomy 21, 7% with triploidy / Klinefelter syndrome)
◊ In absence of other anomalies 1% of fetuses with choroid plexus cysts will have trisomy 18!
◊ In presence of other anomalies 4% of fetuses with choroid plexus cysts will have trisomy 18!
◊ 40–71% of autopsied fetuses with trisomy 18 have choroid plexus cysts bilaterally >10 mm in diameter
◊ Risk of chromosomal abnormality not linked to size, bilaterality, gestational age at appearance / disappearance

• usually asymptomatic

Location: frequently at level of atrium; uni- / bilateral
√ single / multiple round anechoic cysts
√ ≥3 mm in size (average 4.5 mm, up to 25 mm)

Cx: hydrocephalus (if cyst large)

Prognosis: 90% disappear by 28th week; may persist; in 95% of no significance

OB-management:
a choroid plexus cyst should stimulate a thorough sonographic examination at >19 weeks; if no other sonographic abnormalities are identified, the yield of abnormal karyotype is low so that the risk of trisomy 18 (1:450–500) is lower than risk of fetal loss due to amniocentesis (approximately 1:200–300)

Risk of karyotype abnormality:
10 x with 1 additional defect
600 x with ≥2 additional defects
DDx: Choroid plexus pseudocyst in the inferolateral aspect of atrium (? corpus striatum) on oblique coronal plane which elongates by turning transducer

CHOROID PLEXUS PAPILLOMA

Incidence: 0.5–0.6% of all intracranial tumors; 2–5% of brain tumors in childhood
Age: 20–40% <1 year of age; 86% <5 years of age; middle age; in 75% <2 years of age; M >> F
Path: large aggregation of choroidal fronds producing great quantities of CSF; occasionally found incidentally on postmortem examination
Pathophysiology: abnormal rate of CSF production of 1.0 mL/min (normal rate = 0.2 mL/min)
• signs of increased intracranial pressure
Location:
(a) glomus of choroid plexus in trigone of lateral ventricles, L > R (in children)
(b) 4th ventricle + cerebellopontine angle (in adults)
(c) 3rd ventricle (unusual)
(d) multiple in 7%
√ large mass with smooth lobulated border
√ small foci of calcifications (common)
√ engulfment of glomus of choroid plexus (distinctive feature)
√ asymmetric diffuse ventricular dilatation (CSF overproduction / decreased absorption secondary to obstruction of arachnoid granulations from repeated occult hemorrhage)
√ dilatation of temporal horn in atrial location (obstruction)
√ growth into surrounding white matter (occasionally, more common a feature of choroid plexus carcinoma)
CT:
√ iso- / mildly hyperdense with intense homogeneous enhancement on CECT
MR:
√ isointense / slightly hyperintense lesion on T1WI + slightly hypointense on T2WI relative to white matter
√ surrounded by hypointense signal on T1WI + hyperintense signal on T2WI (CSF)
√ intraventricular enhancing island of tumor on Gd-DTPA
US:
√ echogenic mass adjacent to normal choroid plexus
Angio:
√ supplied by anterior + posterior choroidal arteries
Cx: (1) transformation into malignant choroid plexus papilloma = choroid plexus carcinoma
(2) hydrocephalus (in children) secondary to increased intracranial pressure from CSF-overproduction
Rx: surgical removal (24% operative mortality) cures hydrocephalus
DDx: intraventricular meningioma, ependymoma, metastasis, cavernous angioma, xanthogranuloma, astrocytoma

COCKAYNE SYNDROME

= autosomal recessive diffuse demyelinating disease
Age: beginning at age 1
• dwarfism
• progressive physical + mental deterioration
• retinal atrophy + deafness
√ brain atrophy / microcephaly
√ calcifications in basal ganglia + cerebellum
√ skeletal changes superficially similar to progeria
DDx: Progeria

COLLOID CYST

Incidence: 2% of glial tumors of ependymal origin; 0.5–1% of CNS tumors
Histo: ciliated + columnar epithelium; mucin-secreting; squamous cells of ependymal origin; tough fibrous capsule
Age: young adults; M > F
• positional headaches (transient obstruction secondary to ball-valve mechanism at foramen of Monro)
• gait apraxia
• change in mental status ± dementia (related to increased intracranial pressure)
• papilledema (may become medical emergency with acute herniation)
Location: exclusively arising from inferior aspect of septum pellucidum protruding into anterior portion of 3rd ventricle between columns of fornix

√ ± sellar erosion
√ spherical iso- / hyperdense lesion on NCCT with smooth surface
√ fluid contents:
(a) in 20% similar to CSF (= isodense)
(b) in 80% mucinous fluid, proteinaceous debris, hemosiderin, desquamated cells (= hyperdense)
√ may show enhancement of border (draped choroid plexus / capsule)
√ 3rd ventricular enlargement (to accommodate cyst anteriorly)
√ asymmetric lateral ventricular enlargement (invariably)
√ occasionally widens septum pellucidum
MR:
√ lesion hyperintense on T1WI + hyperintense on T2WI in 60% (related to large protein molecules / paramagnetic effect of magnesium, copper, iron in cyst)
DDx: meningioma, ependymoma of 3rd ventricle (rare) with enhancement

CORTICAL CONTUSION

= traumatic injury to cortical surface of brain
Incidence: most common type of primary intra-axial lesion; in 21% of head trauma patients; children:adults = 2:1
Path: tissue necrosis, capillary disruption, petechial hemorrhage followed by liquefaction + edema after 4–7 days

Mechanism: linear acceleration-deceleration forces / penetrating trauma
1. **Coup** = direct impact on stationary brain
2. **Contrecoup** = impact of moving brain on stationary calvarium opposite to the site of the coup

Location: multiple bilateral lesions;
— common: along anterior + lateral + inferior surfaces of frontal lobe (in orbitofrontal, inferior frontal, and rectal gyri above cribriform plate, planum sphenoidale, lesser sphenoid wing) and temporal lobe (just above petrous bone / posterior to greater sphenoid wing)
— less frequent: in parietal + occipital lobes, cerebellar hemispheres, vermis, cerebellar tonsils
— often bilateral / beneath an acute subdural hematoma

• confusion (mild initial impairment)
• focal cerebral dysfunction
• seizures, personality changes
• focal neurologic deficits (late changes)

CT (sensitive only to hemorrhage in acute phase):
◊ Look for scalp swelling to focus your attention on the location of the coup!
√ focal / multiple (29%) poorly defined areas of low attenuation with irregular contour (edema) intermixed with a few tiny areas of increased density (petechial hemorrhage)
√ diffuse cerebral swelling without hemorrhage in immediate posttraumatic period (common in children) due to hyperemia / ischemic edema
√ some degree of contrast enhancement (leaking new capillaries)
√ isodense hemorrhage after 2–3 weeks
√ true extent of lesions becomes more evident with progression of edema + cell necrosis + mass effect over ensuing weeks

MR (best modality for initial detection of contusional edema + accurate portrayal of extent of lesions):
√ hemorrhagic lesions (detected in 50% of all contusions):
  √ initially decreased intensity (deoxyhemoglobin of acute hemorrhage) surrounded by hyperintense edema on T2WI
  √ hyperintense on T1WI + T2WI in subacute phase (secondary to Met-Hb)
  √ hyperintense gliosis + hypointense hemosiderin on T2WI in chronic phase
√ nonhemorrhagic lesions hypointense on T1WI + hyperintense on T2WI

Cx: (1) Encephalomalacia (= scarred brain)
(2) Porencephaly (= formation of cystic cavity lined with gliotic brain and communicating with ventricles / subarachnoid space)
(3) Hydrocephalus as a result from adhesions caused by subarachnoid blood

CRANIOPHARYNGIOMA

Incidence: 3–4% of all intracranial neoplasms; 15% of supratentorial + 50% of suprasellar tumors in children; most common suprasellar mass

Origin: from epithelial rests along vestigial craniopharyngeal duct (Rathke cleft / pouch within intermediate lobe of pituitary gland)

Path: benign tumor originating from neuroepithelium in craniopharyngeal duct + primitive buccal epithelium

Histo: cystic (rich in liquid cholesterol) / complex / solid

Age: from birth–7th decade; bimodal age distribution: age peaks in 1st–2nd decade (75%) + in 5th decade (25%); M > F

• diabetes insipidus (compression of pituitary gland)
• growth retardation (compression of hypothalamus)
• bitemporal hemianopia (compression of optic nerve chiasm)
• headaches from hydrocephalus (compression of foramen of Monro / aqueduct of Sylvius)

Location:
(a) pituitary stalk / tuber cinereum
(b) suprasellar (20%)
(c) intrasellar (10%)
(d) intra- and suprasellar (70%)

Ectopic craniopharyngioma:
(e) floor of anterior 3rd ventricle (more common in adults)
(f) sphenoid bone

Skull films:
√ normal sella (25%)
√ enlarged J-shaped sella with truncated dorsum
√ thickening + increased density of lamina dura in floor of sella (10%)
√ extensive sellar destruction (75%)
√ curvilinear / flocculent / stippled calcifications / lamellar ossification; calcifications seen in youth in 70–90%, in adults in 30–40%

CT:
√ multilobulated inhomogeneous suprasellar mass
√ solid (15%) / mixed (30%) / cystic lesion (54–75%) [cystic appearance secondary to cholesterol, keratin, necrotic debris with higher density than CSF]
√ enhancement of solid lesion, peripheral enhancement of cystic lesion
√ marginal hyperdense lesion (calcification / ossification) in 70–90% in childhood tumors + 30–50% of adult tumors
√ ± obstructive hydrocephalus
√ extension into middle > anterior > posterior cranial fossa (25%)

MR (relatively ineffective in demonstrating calcifications):
√ mostly hyperintense, but also iso- / hypointense on T1WI (variable secondary to hemorrhage / cholesterol-containing proteinaceous fluid)
√ markedly hyperintense on T2WI
√ marginal enhancement of solid components with gadopentetate dimeglumine

Angio:
√ usually avascular
√ lateral displacement, elevation, narrowing of supraclinoid segment of ICA
√ posterior displacement of basilar artery

DDx: (1) Epidermoid (no contrast enhancement)
(2) Rathke cleft cyst (small intrasellar lesion)

CYSTICERCOSIS OF BRAIN

larva of pork tapeworm (Taenia solium) frequently involving CNS, muscles, heart, fat tissue

Infection:

(1) Ingestion of ova by fecal-oral route; embryophore is dissolved by gastric acid and enzymes + oncosphere is liberated

(2) Ingestion of uncooked contaminated pork containing cysticerci; tapeworm develops in intestinal lumen + releases eggs

Organism:

embryos invade intestinal wall + enter circulation + disseminate in varies parts of body; embryo develops into a cysticercus (= complex wall surrounding a cavity containing vesicular fluid + scolex); following ingestion of cysticercus by definitive host a tapeworm develops within the intestinal tract

Incidence: CNS involvement in up to 90%

Location: meninges (39%) esp. in basal cisterns, parenchyma (20%), intraventricular (17%), mixed (23%), intraspinal (1%)

A. ACUTE PAHSE (= focal meningoencephalitis)
- focal seizures
- √ single / multiple small focal enhancing lesions; transitory with resolution in a few months
- √ diffusely edematous white matter
- √ homogeneously enhancing small nodules often with extensive edema (DDx: metastases without edema)

B. CHRONIC PHASE (= involution with subsequent calcification + cyst formation)
- √ small focal calcifications (= probably dead larvae); may appear within 8 months to 10 years after acute infection along gray-white matter junction
- √ well-defined cystic areas of CSF density without associated edema (= living larvae)
- √ "ricelike" muscle calcifications rarely visible
- ◊ Cysts incite edema upon death of larvae!

RADIOGRAPHIC TYPES

1. Parenchymal type
   - √ multiple / solitary cystic lesions up to 6 cm in size; many terminate as calcified granulomata (larvae not dead unless completely calcified)
   - √ encephalitic form may occur in children
2. Meningeal / racemose type
   - √ ventricular dilatation indicating diffuse meningeal inflammatory process
   - √ lucent cystic lesions in basal cisterns (= racemose cysts) with variable enhancement, usually located in cerebellopontine angle / suprasellar cistern
3. Intraventricular type
   - √ obstructive hydrocephalus caused by blockage within various portions of ventricular system from solitary / multiple cysts
4. Mixed type (frequent)

CYTOMEGALOVIRUS INFECTION

Most common intrauterine infection

Incidence: 0.4–2.3% of liveborn infants

- asymptomatic (90%)
- sensorineural hearing loss, chorioretinitis, mental retardation, neurologic deficits
- √ intrauterine growth retardation
- √ ascites
- √ hydrops

@ CNS
- √ periventricular calcifications
- √ ventricular dilatation
- √ microcephaly

DANDY-WALKER MALFORMATION

= characterized by (1) enlarged posterior fossa with high position of tentorium (2) dys- / agenesis of cerebellar vermis (3) cystic dilatation of 4th ventricle filling nearly entire posterior fossa

Cause: dysmorphogenesis of roof of 4th ventricle with failure to incorporate the area membranacea into developing choroid plexus; proposed originally as congenital atresia of foramina of **L**uschka (**l**ateral) + **M**agendie (**m**edian) not likely since foramina are not patent until 4th month

Incidence: 12% of all congenital hydrocephaly

Path: defect in vermis connecting an ependyma-lined retrocerebellar cyst with 4th ventricle (PATHOGNOMONIC)

Associated anomalies :

— midline CNS anomalies (in >60%)

(1) dysgenesis of corpus callosum (20–25%), lipoma of corpus callosum
(2) holoprosencephaly (25%)
(3) malformation of cerebral gyri (dysplasia of cingulate gyrus) (25%)
(4) cerebellar heterotopia + malformation of cerebellar folia (25%)
(5) malformation of inferior olivary nucleus
(6) hamartoma of tuber cinereum
(7) syringomyelia
(8) cleft palate
(9) occipital encephalocele (<5%)

— other CNS anomalies:

(1) polymicrogyria / gray matter heterotopia (5–10%)
(2) schizencephaly
(3) lumbosacral meningocele

— non-CNS anomalies (25%)

(1) polydactyly, syndactyly
(2) Klippel-Feil syndrome
(3) Cornelia de Lange syndrome
(4) cleft palate
(5) facial angioma
(6) cardiac anomalies

Skull film:
- √ large skull secondary to hydrocephalus + dolichocephaly
- √ diastatic lambdoid suture
- √ disproportionately large expanded posterior fossa
- √ torcular herophili and lateral sinuses high above lambdoid angle = torcular-lambdoid inversion

CT / US / MR:
- √ absence / hypoplasia of cerebellar vermis: total (25%), partial (75%)
- √ superiorly displaced superior vermis cerebelli
- √ small + widely separated cerebellar hemispheres
- √ anterior + lateral displacement of ± hypoplastic cerebellar hemispheres
- √ large posterior fossa cyst with extension through foramen magnum = diverticulum of roofless 4th ventricle
- √ elevated insertion of tentorium cerebelli
- √ cerebellar hemispheres in apposition without intervening vermis following shunt procedure
- √ absence of falx cerebelli
- √ scalloping of petrous pyramids
- √ ventriculomegaly (in 72% open communication with 3rd ventricle; in 39% patent 4th ventricle; in 28% aqueductal stenosis; in 11% incisural obstruction); present prenatally in 30%, by 3 months of age in 75%
- √ anterior displacement of pons

Angio:
- √ high position of transverse sinus
- √ elevated great vein of Galen
- √ elevated posterior cerebral vessels
- √ anterosuperiorly displaced superior cerebellar arteries above the posterior cerebral arteries
- √ small / absent PICA with high tonsillar loop

Cx: trapping of cyst above tentorium = "keyhole configuration"

Prognosis: fetal demise in 66%; 22–50% mortality during 1st year of life

DDx:
(1) Posterior fossa extra-axial cyst
(2) Arachnoid cyst (normal 4th ventricle, patent foramina, intact vermis)
(3) Isolated 4th ventricle
(4) Megacisterna magna = giant cisterna magna (enlarged posterior fossa, enlarged cisterna magna, intact vermis, normal 4th ventricle)
(5) Porencephaly

Dandy-Walker Variant

characterized by
(1) variable hypoplasia of posteroinferior portion of vermis leading to communication between 4th ventricle and cisterna magna
(2) cerebellar dysgenesis
(3) cystic dilatation of 4th ventricle
(4) NO enlargement of posterior fossa

◊ More common than Dandy-Walker malformation; accounts for 1/3 of all posterior fossa malformations

Cause: focal insult to developing cerebellum

Associated CNS anomalies:
agenesis of corpus callosum (21%), cerebral gyral malformation (21%), heterotopia, holoprosencephaly (10%), diencephalic cyst (10%), posterior fossa meningoencephalocele (10%)

Other associated anomalies:
polydactyly; cardiac, renal, facial anomalies; abnormal karyotype (29%)

- √ 4th ventricle smaller + better formed
- √ retrocerebellar cyst smaller
- √ communication between retrocerebellar cyst and subarachnoid space through a patent foramen of Magendie may be present
- √ posterior fossa smaller than in usual Dandy-Walker syndrome

OB-US:
- √ incomplete closure of vermis is normal until 18 weeks GA!

Dandy-Walker Complex

= continuum of anomalies, including Dandy-Walker malformation + Dandy-Walker variant + megacisterna magna, characterized by partial / complete dysgenesis of vermis cerebelli

Cause: broad insult to alar plate from a variety of abnormalities

Associated with:

A. Inherited genetic syndromes
- — autosomal recessive:
  1. Meckel-Gruber syndrome
  2. Ellis-van Creveld syndrome
  3. Walker-Warburg syndrome
- — autosomal dominant:
  1. X-linked cerebellar hypoplasia
  2. Aicardi syndrome

B. Abnormal karyotype (33%)
  1. Duplications of chromosomes 5p, 8p, 8q
  2. Trisomies 9, 13, 18

C. Infection
  1. Virus: CMV, rubella
  2. Protozoan: toxoplasmosis

D. Teratogen: alcohol, sodium warfarin

E. Multifactorial

Pseudo-Dandy-Walker Malformation

= developing rhombencephalon during 1st trimester
- √ fluid-filled space in posterior aspect of fetal head

DERMOID OF CNS

= pilosebaceous mass lined with skin appendages originating from inclusion of epithelial cells + skin appendages during closure of neural tube

Incidence: 1% of all intracranial tumors

Path: ectodermal + mesodermal lesion = squamous epithelium, mesodermal cells (hair follicles, sweat + sebaceous glands)

Age: <30 years (appears in adulthood secondary to slow growth); M < F

Location:
(a) spinal canal (most common): extra- / intramedullary in lumbosacral region
(b) posterior fossa within vermis / 4th ventricle (predilection for midline)
(c) posterior to superior orbital fissure, may be associated with bone defect

- • bouts of chemical / bacterial meningitis possible
- √ thick-walled inhomogeneous mass with focal areas of fat
- √ mural / central calcifications / bone (possible)

√ may have sinus tract to skin surface (dermal sinus) if located in midline at occipital / nasofrontal region
√ fat-fluid level if cyst ruptures into ventricles, fat droplets in subarachnoid space
√ NO contrast enhancement
MR:
√ variointense on T1WI (hyperintense with contents of liquefied cholesterol products)
√ shortened T1 + T2 relaxation times (= fat)

DIFFUSE AXONAL INJURY

= WHITE MATTER SHEARING INJURY
Incidence: most common type of primary traumatic injury in patients with severe head trauma (48%)
Cause: indirect injury due to rotational acceleration / deceleration forces (not necessarily with direct impact to head)
Pathogenesis:
cortex and deep structures move at different speed resulting in shearing stress along the course of white matter tracts especially at gray-white matter junction with axonal tears followed by wallerian degeneration
Path: much of the injury is only microscopic
Histo: multiple axonal retraction balls (HALLMARK), numerous perivascular hemorrhages
• severe impairment of consciousness

Location (according to severity of trauma):
(a) lobar white matter at corticomedullary junction (67%): parasagittal region of frontal lobe + periventricular region of temporal lobe; occasionally in parietal + occipital lobes
(b) internal + external capsule, corona radiata, cerebellar peduncles
(c) corpus callosum (21%): 3/4 of lesions in posterior body + splenium
√ often associated with intraventricular hemorrhage
(d) brainstem: posterolateral quadrants of midbrain + upper pons; superior cerebellar peduncles especially vulnerable

√ sparing of cortex
√ 20% of lesions with small central areas of petechial hemorrhage
CT:
√ foci of decreased density (usually seen when >1.5 cm in size)
MR (most sensitive modality):
√ multiple small oval / round foci of decreased signal intensity on T1WI + increased signal on T2WI
Prognosis: poor due to sequelae (may go on to die without signs of high intracranial pressure)

DIFFUSE SCLEROSIS

sporadic, young adults, fulminant course
• dementia, deafness
√ low-attenuation regions in both hemispheres without symmetry

DYKE-DAVIDOFF-MASON SYNDROME

= CEREBRAL HEMIATROPHY = INFANTILE / CONGENITAL HEMIPLEGIA = SYNDROME OF HEMICONVULSIONS, HEMIPLEGIA, AND EPILEPSY
= unilateral cerebral atrophy with ipsilateral small skull
Cause: insult to immature brain resulting in neuronal loss + impaired brain growth:
(a) prenatal: congenital malformation, infection, vascular insult
(b) perinatal: birth trauma, anoxia, hypoxia, intracranial hemorrhage
(c) postnatal: trauma, tumor, infection, prolonged febrile seizures
• seizures
• hemiparesis (typically spastic hemiplegia)
• mental retardation
Age: presents in adolescence
√ unilateral thickening of skull
√ unilateral decrease in size of cranial fossa
√ unilateral overdevelopment of sinuses
√ contraction of a hemisphere / lobe
√ compensatory enlargement of adjacent ventricle + sulci with midline shift

EMPTY SELLA SYNDROME

= extension of subarachnoid space into sella turcica, which becomes exposed to CSF pulsations secondary to defect in diaphragma sellae; characterized by normal / molded pituitary gland + normal or enlarged sella (empty sella = misnomer)
Incidence: 24% in autopsy study

A. PRIMARY EMPTY SELLA (anatomic spectrum)
Incidence: 10% of adult population; M:F = 1:4
Probable causes:
(1) pituitary enlargement followed by regression during pregnancy
(2) involution of a pituitary tumor
(3) congenital weakness of diaphragma sellae
◊ occurs more frequently in patients with increased intracranial pressure
• usually asymptomatic
• increased risk for CSF rhinorrhea
• NO endocrine abnormalities
B. SECONDARY EMPTY SELLA
= postsurgical when diaphragma sellae has been disrupted
• visual disturbance
• headaches

√ slowly progressive symmetrical / asymmetrical (double floor) enlargement of sella
√ remodeled lamina dura remains mineralized
√ small rim of pituitary tissue displaced posteriorly + inferiorly
√ infundibulum sign = infundibulum extends to floor of sella
DDx: cystic tumor, large herniated 3rd ventricle (displaced infundibulum)

EMPYEMA OF BRAIN

Subdural Empyema

20% of all intracranial bacterial infections

Cause: paranasal sinusitis, otitis media, calvarial osteomyelitis, infection after craniotomy or ventricular shunt placement, penetrating wound, contamination of meningitis-induced subdural effusion

Location: frontal + inferior cranial space in close proximity to paranasal sinuses; 80% over convexity extending into interhemispheric fissure or posterior fossa

√ hypo- / isodense crescentic / lentiform zone adjacent to inner table

√ may show mass effect (sulcal effacement, ventricular compression, shift)

√ thin curvilinear rim of enhancement (7–10 days later) adjacent to brain

√ severe sinusitis / mastoiditis (may be most significant indicator)

Mortality: 30% (neurosurgical emergency)

Cx: venous thrombosis, infarction, seizures, hemiparesis, hemianopia, aphasia, brain abscess

DDx: subacute / chronic subdural hematoma

Epidural Empyema

Cause: same as above

- no neurologic deficits (dura minimizes pressure exerted on brain)

√ thick enhancing rim

ENCEPHALITIS

= term generally reserved for diffuse inflammatory process of viral etiology (herpes simplex, California encephalitis, Eastern equine encephalitis, St. Louis encephalitis, Western equine encephalitis)

√ diffuse mild cerebral edema

√ small infarctions / hemorrhage (less frequent)

Acute Hemorrhagic Leukoencephalitis

= fulminant myelinoclastic disease of CNS

= hyperacute form of acute disseminated encephalomyelitis

Cause: immunoreactive disease following prodromal illness (minor upper respiratory viral infection, ulcerative colitis)

Path: marked edema, brain softening

Histo: necrotizing angiitis of venules + capillaries within white matter with extravasation of PMNs + lymphocytes; fibrinoid necrosis of affected capillaries + surrounding tissues; confluent hemorrhages with ball-and-ring configuration due to diapedesis of RBCs

- progressive coma, motor disturbance, speech difficulty, seizures
- pyrexia, leukocytosis
- pleocytosis, elevated protein in spinal fluid

Location: unilateral disease; parietal + posterior frontal white matter at level of centrum semiovale (sparing subcortical U-fibers + cortex) > basal ganglia, cerebellum, brainstem, spinal cord

√ rapid development of profound mass effect resembling infarction

√ multiple punctate white matter hemorrhages

√ extensive hypoattenuation virtually confined to hemispheric white matter

Prognosis: usually results in death

DDx: (1) Herpes simplex encephalitis (cortical lesions in temporal + inferior frontal lobes + insular region, no imaging findings until 3–5 days after onset of significant symptoms)
(2) Tumefactive multiple sclerosis
(3) Osmotic demyelination
(4) Toxic encephalopathy: lipophilic solvent, methanol
(5) Hypertensive encephalopathy: eclampsia, thrombotic thrombocytopenic purpura

Herpes Simplex Encephalitis (HSE)

= most common cause of nonepidemic necrotizing meningoencephalitis in USA

Organism: HSV type I (in adults); HSV type II (in neonates from transplacental infection)

- confusion, disorientation
- preceding viral syndrome, fever, headache, seizures

Location: temporal > frontal > parietal lobes; propensity for limbic system (olfactory tract, temporal lobes, cingulate gyrus, insular cortex); predominantly unilateral

CT (principal role is to identify biopsy site):

√ may be negative in first 3 days

√ poorly defined bilateral areas of decreased attenuation

√ spared putamen forms sharply defined concave / straight border (DDx: infarction, glioma)

√ compression of lateral ventricles, sylvian fissure (brain edema)

√ patchy peripheral / gyral / cisternal enhancement (50%), may persist for several months

√ tendency for hemorrhage + rapid dissemination in brain

MR:

√ increased signal intensity on T2WI

NUC:

Agents: standard brain imaging (eg, Tc-99m DTPA), newer brain agents (eg, I-123 iodoamphetamine / Tc-99m HMPAO)

SPECT imaging improves sensitivity

√ characteristic focal increase in activity in temporal lobes on brain scintigraphy (blood-brain barrier breakdown)

Dx: fluorescein antibody staining / viral culture from brain biopsy

Mortality: 70%

Rx: adenine arabinoside

DDx: low-grade glioma, infarct, abscess

Human Immunodeficiency Virus Encephalitis

often in combination with CMV encephalitis

Histo: microglial nodules + perivascular multinucleated giant cells accompanying gliosis of deep white + gray matter

√ predominantly central CNS atrophy

√ symmetric periventricular / diffuse white matter disease without mass effect (hypodense on CT, high intensity on T2WI)

Postinfectious Encephalitis

following exanthematous viral illness / vaccination

Acute disseminated encephalomyelitis (ADEM)

= autoimmune reaction against patient's white matter following measles, mumps, varicella, pertussis, rubella infection / vaccination

• seizures + focal neurologic signs 7–14 days after clinical onset of viral infection

Histo: diffuse perivenous inflammatory process resulting in areas of demyelination

Location: subcortical white matter of both hemispheres asymmetrically

CT:

√ hypodense white matter

MR:

√ focal areas of hyperintensity on T2WI

√ may demonstrate contrast enhancement

Rx: corticosteroids result in dramatic improvement

Prognosis: complete recovery / some permanent neurologic damage (10–20%)

DDx: simulating multiple sclerosis (rarely recurrent episodes as in multiple sclerosis)

EPENDYMOMA

= in majority benign slow-growing neoplasm of mature well-differentiated ependymal cells lining the ventricles

Incidence: most commonly in children; 5–9% of all primary CNS neoplasms; 15% of posterior fossa tumors in children; 63% of spinal intramedullary gliomas

Histo: benign aggregates of ependymocytes in form of perivascular pseudorosettes; may have papillary pattern (difficult DDx from choroid plexus papilloma)

Age: (a) supratentorial: at any age (atrium / foramen of Monro)

(b) posterior fossa: <10 years; age peaks at 5 and 34 years; M:F = 0.8:1

Associated with: neurofibromatosis

• increased intracranial pressure (90%)

Location:

(a) infratentorial: floor of 4th ventricle (70% of all intracranial ependymomas)

(b) supratentorial: frontal > parietal > temporoparietal juxtaventricular region (uncommonly intraventricular), lateral ventricle, 3rd ventricle

(c) conus (40–65% of all spinal intramedullary gliomas)

<u>in children</u>: infratentorial in 70%, supratentorial in 30%

√ small cystic areas in 15–50% (central necrosis)

√ fine punctate multifocal calcifications (25–50%)

√ intratumoral hemorrhage (10%)

√ frequently grows into brain parenchyma extending to cortical surface (particularly in frontal + parietal lobes)

√ may invaginate into ventricles

√ expansion frequently through foramen of Luschka into cerebellopontine angle (15%) or through foramen of Magendie caudad into cisterna magna (up to 60%) (CHARACTERISTIC)

√ direct invasion of brainstem / cerebellum (30–40%)

√ insinuation around blood vessels + cranial nerves

√ communicating hydrocephalus (100%) secondary to protein exudate elaborated by tumor clogging resorption pathways

CT:

√ sharply marginated multilobulated iso- / slightly hyperdense 4th ventricular mass

√ thin well-defined low-attenuation halo (distended effaced 4th ventricle)

√ heterogeneous / moderately uniform enhancement of solid portions (80%)

MR:

√ low to intermediate heterogeneous signal intensity on T1WI

√ hypointense tumor margins on T1WI + T2WI in 64% (hemosiderin deposits)

√ foci of high-signal intensity on T2WI (= necrotic areas / cysts) + low signal intensity (= calcification / hemorrhage)

√ fluid-fluid level within cysts

√ homogeneous Gd-DTPA enhancement of tumor

Cx: subarachnoid dissemination via CSF (rare) (DDx: malignant ependymoma, ependymoblastoma)

Rx: surgery (difficult to resect due to adherence to surrounding brain) + radiation (partially radiosensitive) + chemotherapy

DDx of cerebellar ependymoma:

(1) Astrocytoma (hypodense, displaces 4th ventricle from midline, cystic lucency, intramedullary)

(2) Medulloblastoma (hyperdense, calcifications in only 10%)

(3) Trapped 4th ventricle (no contrast enhancement)

EPIDERMOID OF CNS

= EPIDERMOID [INCLUSION] CYST

= benign tumor with extremely slow linear growth resulting from desquamation of epithelial cells from tumor wall

Incidence: 0.2–1.8% of all primary intracranial neoplasms; most common congenital intracranial tumor

Etiology: inclusion of ectodermal epithelial tissue from pharyngeal pouch of Rathke / pluripotential cells during closure of neural tube in 5th week of fetal life (early inclusion results in midline lesion, later inclusion results in more lateral location)

Path: "pearly tumor" = well-defined solid lesion with glistening irregular nodular surface; soft flaky desquamated keratinaceous debris rich in cholesterol + triglycerides = PRIMARY / CONGENITAL CHOLESTEATOMA

Histo: tumor lined by simple stratified cuboidal squamous epithelium; surrounded by thin band of collagenous connective tissue; tumor center of lamellar appearance due to desquamation

Age: 10–60 years, peak age in 4th–5th decade; tumor slowly expands over decades by continued desquamation of the lining thus becoming symptomatic in adulthood; M:F = 1:1

- facial pain
- cranial nerve palsies from CP angle epidermoids (50%)
- hydrocephalus in suprasellar epidermoids
- chemical meningitis (secondary to leakage of tumor contents into subarachnoid space) in middle cranial fossa epidermoids

Site: midline / paramidline; intradural (90%) / extradural; transspatial growth (= extension from one into another intracranial space)

Location: (a) cerebellopontine angle (40%, account for 5% of CP angle tumors)
(b) suprasellar region, perimesencephalic cisterns (14%)
(c) within ventricles, brainstem, brain parenchyma
(d) skull vault

√ soft lesion conforming to + molding itself around brain surfaces
√ may intimately surround vessels + cranial nerves rather than displacing them (limited resectability)
√ little mass effect, no edema / hydrocephalus
√ NO contrast enhancement
√ may be associated with dermal sinus tract at occipital / nasofrontal region if midline in location

CT:
√ typically lobulated round homogeneous mass with density similar to CSF (between water and -20 HU)
√ occasionally hyperdense due to high protein content, saponification of keratinaceous debris, prior hemorrhage into cyst, ferrocalcium / iron-containing pigment, abundance of PMNs
√ bony erosion with sharply defined well-corticated margins
√ calcification (25%)
√ peripheral enhancement (perilesional inflammation)

MR:
√ lamellated onionskin appearance with septations (layer-on-layer accretion of desquamated material)
√ "black epidermoid" = signal intensity similar to CSF: heterogeneously hypointense lesion on T1WI + hyperintense on T2WI (due to cholesterol in solid crystalline state + keratin within tumor + CSF within tumor interstices)
√ "white epidermoid" (rare) = hyperintense on T1WI + isointense on T2WI due to presence of triglycerides + polyunsaturated fatty acids
√ hypointense on T2WI (very rare) due to calcification, low hydration, viscous secretion, paramagnetic iron-containing pigment

Angio:
√ avascular

Cisternography:
√ papillary / frondlike surface with contrast material extending into tumor interstices

Rx: surgical resection (complicated by adherence to surrounding brain + cranial nerves, spillage of cyst contents with chemical meningitis, CSF seeding + implantation)

DDx: arachnoid cyst (smooth surface, earlier diffusion), cystic schwannoma, adenomatoid tumor, atypical meningioma, chondroma, chondrosarcoma, chordoma, calcified neurogenic tumor, teratoma, calcified astrocytoma, ganglioglioma

EPIDURAL HEMATOMA OF BRAIN

= EXTRADURAL HEMATOMA = within potential space between naked inner table + calvarial periosteum (dura layer), which is bound down at suture margins

Incidence: 2% of all serious head injuries; in <1% of all children with cranial trauma; uncommon in infants

Age: more common in younger patients (dura more easily stripped away from skull)

Associated with:
(1) skull fracture in 75–85 –95% (best demonstrated on skull radiographs)
◊ Skull fractures frequently not visible in children!
(2) subdural hemorrhage
(3) contusion

Mechanism of injury:
(a) laceration of (middle) meningeal artery / vein adjacent to inner table from fracture of calvarium (91%)
(b) avulsion of venous vessels from points of calvarial perforations
(c) disruption of dural venous sinuses (transverse / superior sagittal sinus) due to diastatic fracture of lambdoid / coronal suture [major cause in younger children]

Time of presentation: within first few days of injury (80%), 4–21 days (20%)

- transient loss of consciousness (= brief period of unconsciousness from concussion of brainstem)
- lucent interval (in <33%)
- somnolence (24–96 hours after accident) due to accumulation of epidural hematoma:
  ◊ DANGEROUS because of focal mass effect + rapid onset (neurosurgical emergency unless small)!
- progressive deterioration of consciousness to coma
- focal neurologic signs: 3rd nerve palsy (sign of cerebral herniation), hemiparesis

◊ Most commonly clinically significant if located in temporoparietal region!

◊ Only a minority of skull fractures across the middle meningeal artery groove result in epidural hematomas!

Types:

I	acute epidural hematoma	(58%) from arterial bleeding
II	subacute hematoma	(31%)
III	chronic hematoma	(11%) from venous bleeding

Location:
(a) in 66% temporoparietal (most often from laceration of middle meningeal artery)
(b) in 29% at frontal pole, parieto-occipital region, between occipital lobes, posterior fossa (most often from laceration of dural sinuses by fracture)
◊ NO crossing of sutures unless diastatic fracture of suture present!

CT:
√ fracture line in area of epidural hematoma
√ expanding biconvex (lenticular = elliptical) extra-axial fluid collection (most frequent) = under high pressure
√ usually does not cross suture lines
√ fresh extravasating blood (30–50 HU) / coagulated blood (50–80 HU) in acute stage
√ hematoma usually homogeneous / rarely inhomogeneously "swirled" (due to mixture of clotted + unclotted blood indicating active bleeding)
√ mass effect ("compression cone effect") with effacement of gyri + sulci from:
— epidural hematoma (57%)
— hemorrhagic contusion (29%)
— cerebral edematous swelling (14%)
√ separation of venous sinuses / falx from inner table of skull
◊ The ONLY hemorrhage displacing falx / venous sinuses away from inner table!
√ marked stretching of vessels
√ signs of arterial injury (rare): contrast extravasation, arteriovenous fistula, middle meningeal artery occlusion, formation of false aneurysm

MR:
√ low intensity of fibrous dura mater allows differentiation of epidural from subdural blood in the late subacute phase (extracellular methemoglobin) with hyperintensity on T1WI + T2WI

Angio:
√ meningeal arteries displaced away from inner table of skull

Rx: after surgical evacuation return of ventricular system to midline
◊ Epidural hematoma at another site may be unmasked following surgical decompression!

DDx: Chronic subdural hematoma (may have similar biconvex shape, crosses suture lines, stops at falx, no associated skull fracture, no displaced dura on MRI)

FIBROMUSCULAR DYSPLASIA

= nonatherosclerotic angiopathy of unknown pathogenesis

Incidence: <1% of cerebral angiographies

Age: 2/3 >50 years; M:F = 1:9

Associated with: brain ischemia (up to 50%), intracranial aneurysms (up to 30%), intracranial tumors (30%), bruits, trauma

Location: cervical + intracranial ICA (85%), vertebral artery (7%); both anterior + posterior circulation (8%); bilateral (60–65%)
◊ simultaneous involvement of renal / muscular arteries in 3%

Angio:
√ length of affected vessel from 0.5 cm to several cm

Types:
1. Medial fibroplasia = fibromuscular hyperplasia (80%)
   √ string of beads = alternating zones of widening + narrowing
   √ tubular narrowing
2. Intimal fibroplasia
   √ smooth concentric tubular narrowing (DDx: Takayasu arteritis, sclerosing arteritis, vessel spasm, arterial hypoplasia)
3. Subadventitial hyperplasia
4. Atypical fibromuscular dysplasia (= ? variant of intimal fibroplasia)
   √ web = smooth / corrugated mass involving only one wall of vessel + projecting into lumen (DDx: atherosclerotic disease, posttraumatic aneurysm)

Cx: dissection (in 3%), macroaneurysm

Prognosis: tends to remain stable / minimal progression

Rx: only when symptoms progress

GLIOBLASTOMA MULTIFORME

Most malignant form of all gliomas / astrocytomas; end stage of progressive severe anaplasia of preexisting Grade I / II astrocytoma (not from embryologic glioblasts)

Incidence: most common primary brain tumor; 50% of all intracranial tumors; 1–2% of all malignancies; 20,000 cases per year

Age: all ages; peak incidence at 65–75 years; M:F = 3:2; more frequently in whites

Genetics: Turcot syndrome, neurofibromatosis type 1, Li-Fraumeni syndrome (familial neoplasms in various organs based on abnormal p53 tumor-suppressor gene)

Path: multilobulated appearance; quite extensive vasogenic edema (transudation through structurally abnormal tumor vascular channels); deeply infiltrating neoplasm; hemorrhage; necrosis is essential for pathologic diagnosis (HALLMARK)

Histo: highly cellular, often bizarrely pleomorphic / undifferentiated multipolar astrocytes; common mitoses + prominent vascular endothelial proliferation; no capsule; pseudopalisading (= viable neoplastic cells forming an irregular border around necrotic debris as the tumor outgrows its blood supply)

Subtypes:
(a) giant cell GBM = monstrocellular sarcoma
(b) small cell GBM = gliosarcoma = Feigin tumor

Location:
(a) hemispheric: white matter of centrum semiovale: frontal > temporal lobes; common in pons, thalamus, quadrigeminal region; relative sparing of basal ganglia + gray matter
DDx: solitary metastasis, tumefactive demyelinating lesion ("singular sclerosis"), atypical abscess
(b) callosal: "butterfly glioma" may grow exophytically into ventricle
(c) posterior fossa: pilocytic astrocytoma, brainstem astrocytoma

(d) extra-axial: primary leptomeningeal glioblastomatosis
(e) multifocal: in 2–5%

Spread:
(a) direct extension following white matter tracts into corpus callosum (36%); readily crosses midline = "butterfly" glioma (clue: invasion of septum pellucidum); frontal + temporal gliomas tend to invade basal ganglia; may invade pia, arachnoid and dura (mimicking meningioma)
(b) subependymal carpet after reaching the surface of the ventricles
(c) via CSF (<2%)
(d) hematogenous (extremely rare)
√ osteoblastic bone lesion

NECT:
√ inhomogeneous low-density mass with irregular shape + poorly defined margins (hypodense solid tumor / cavitary necrosis / tumor cyst / peritumoral "fingers of edema")
√ considerable mass effect: compression + displacement of ventricles, cisterns, brain parenchyma
√ iso- / hyperdense portions (hemorrhage) in 5%
√ rarely calcifies (if coexistent with lower-grade glioma / after radio- or chemotherapy)

CECT:
Enhancement pattern: contrast enhancement due to breakdown of blood-brain barrier / neovascularity / areas of necrosis
(a) diffuse homogeneous enhancement
(b) nonhomogeneous enhancement
(c) ring pattern (occasionally enhancing mass within the ring)
(d) low-density lesion with contrast fluid level (leakage of contrast)
√ almost always ring blush of variable thickness: multiscalloped ("garland"), round / ovoid; may be seen surrounding ventricles (subependymal spread); tumor usually extends beyond margins of enhancement
√ sedimentation level secondary to cellular debris / hemorrhage / accumulated contrast material in tumoral cyst

MR:
√ poorly defined lesion with some mass effect / vasogenic edema / heterogeneity
√ hemosiderin deposits (gradient echo images)
√ hemorrhage (hypointensity on T2WI and T2*-WI)
√ T1WI + gadolinium-DTPA enhancement separate tumor nodules from surrounding edema, central necrosis and cyst formation

Angio:
√ wildly irregular neovascularity + early draining veins
√ avascular lesion

PET:
√ increase in glucose utilization rate

Rx: surgery + radiation therapy + chemotherapy
Prognosis: 16–18 months postoperative survival (frequent tumor recurrence due to uncertainty during surgery about tumor margins)

Multifocal GBM
(1) Spread of primary GBM
(2) Multiple areas of malignant degeneration in diffuse low-grade astrocytoma ("gliomatosis cerebri")
(3) Inherited / acquired genetic abnormality

GANGLION CELL TUMOR

Gangliocytoma
rare benign tumor
Incidence: 0.1%
Histo: purely neuronal tumor (no glial components); ganglion cells without stain for glial fibrillary acetic protein

Ganglioglioma
glial component that may show neoplastic differentiation
√ cyst formation + calcifications
√ contrast enhancement

GLIOMA
= malignant tumors of glial cells growing along white matter tracts, tendency to increase in grade with time; may be multifocal
Incidence: 30–40% of all primary intracranial tumors
√ contrast enhancement:
◊ increases in proportion to degree of anaplasia
◊ diminished intensity of enhancement with steroid therapy

CELL OF ORIGIN
1. Astrocyte .... Astrocytoma
2. Oligodendrocyte .... Oligodendroglioma
3. Ependyma .... Ependymoma
4. Medulloblast .... Medulloblastoma; (PNET = primitive neuroectodermal tumor)
5. Choroid plexus .... Choroid plexus papilloma

FREQUENCY OF INTRACRANIAL GLIOMAS

Glioblastoma multiforme	51%
Astrocytoma	25%
Ependymoma	6%
Oligodendroglioma	6%
Spongioblastoma polare	3%
Mixed gliomas	3%
Astroblastoma	2%

Age peak: middle adult life
Location: cerebral hemispheres; spinal cord; brainstem + cerebellum (in children)

Brainstem Glioma
Incidence: 1%; 12–15% of all pediatric brain tumors; 20–30% of infratentorial brain tumors
Histo: usually anaplastic astrocytoma / glioblastoma multiforme with infiltration along fiber tracts
Age: in children + young adults; peak age 3–13 years; M:F = 1:1

• become clinically apparent early before ventricular obstruction occurs
• ipsilateral progressive multiple cranial nerve palsies
• contralateral hemiparesis
• cerebellar dysfunction: ataxia, nystagmus
• eventually respiratory insufficiency

Location: pons > midbrain > medulla; often unilateral at medullopontine junction
◊ Medullary + mesencephalic gliomas are more benign than pontine gliomas!

Growth pattern:
(a) diffuse infiltration of brainstem with symmetric expansion + rostrocaudal spread into medulla / thalamus + spread to cerebellum
(b) focally exophytic growth into adjacent cisterns (cerebellopontine, prepontine, cisterna magna)

√ asymmetrically expanded brainstem
√ flattening + posterior displacement of 4th ventricle + aqueduct of Sylvius
√ compression of prepontine + interpeduncular cistern (in upward transtentorial herniation)
√ paradoxical widening of CP angle cistern with tumor extension into CP angle
√ paradoxical anterior displacement of 4th ventricle with tumor extension into cisterna magna

CT:
√ isodense / hypodense mass with indistinct margins
√ hyperdense foci (= hemorrhage) uncommon
√ absent / minimal / patchy contrast enhancement (50%)
√ ring enhancement in necrotic / cystic tumors (most aggressive)
√ prominent enhancement in exophytic lesion
√ hydrocephalus uncommon (because of early symptomatology)

MR: (better evaluation in subtle cases)
√ hypointense on T1WI + hyperintense on T2WI
√ ± engulfment of basilar artery

Angio:
√ anterior displacement of basilar artery + anterior pontomesencephalic vein
√ posterior displacement of precentral cerebellar vein
√ posterior displacement of posterior medullary + supratonsillar segments of PICA
√ lateral displacement of lateral medullary segment of PICA

Prognosis: 10–30% 5-year survival rate
Rx: radiation therapy
DDx: focal encephalitis, resolving hematoma, vascular malformation, tuberculoma, infarct, multiple sclerosis, metastasis, lymphoma

Hypothalamic / Chiasmatic Glioma

Point of origin often undeterminable: hypothalamic gliomas invade chiasm, chiasmatic gliomas invade hypothalamus

Incidence: 10–15% of supratentorial tumors in children
Age: 2–4 years; M:F = 1:1
Associated with: von Recklinghausen disease (20–50%)

• diminished visual acuity (50%) with optic atrophy
• diencephalic syndrome (in up to 20%): marked emaciation, pallor, unusual alertness, hyperactivity, euphoria
• obese child
• sexual precocity
• diabetes insipidus

√ obstructive hydrocephalus
√ suprasellar hypodense lobulated mass with dense inhomogeneous enhancement
√ hypointense on T1WI + hyperintense on T2WI
√ cyst formation, necrosis, calcifications render lesion inhomogeneous

DDx: hypothalamic hamartoma

GLOBOID CELL LEUKODYSTROPHY

= KRABBE DISEASE

Cause: deficiency of galactosylceramide beta-galactosidase resulting in cerebroside accumulation + destruction of oligodendrocytes
Dx: biochemical assay from white blood cells / skin fibroblasts
Age: 3–6 months

• restlessness + irritability
• marked spasticity
• optic atrophy
• hyperacusis

√ symmetric hyperdense lesions in thalami, caudate nuclei, corona radiata
√ decreased attenuation of white matter
√ brain atrophy with enlargement of ventricles

Prognosis: death within first few years of life

HALLERVORDEN-SPATZ DISEASE

rare metabolic disorder with abnormal iron retention in basal ganglia

Age: 2nd decade of life
Histo: hyperpigmentation + symmetrical destruction of globus pallidus + substantia nigra

• progressive gait impairment + rigidity of limbs
• slowing of voluntary movements, dysarthria
• choreoathetotic movement disorder
• mental deterioration

CT:
√ low- (= tissue destruction) / high-density (= dystrophic calcification) foci in globus pallidus

MR:
√ initially hypointense globus pallidus on T2WI (= iron deposition)
√ later hyperintense foci on T2WI (= tissue destruction + gliosis)

HAMARTOMA OF CNS

rare tumor
(a) sporadic
(b) associated with tuberous sclerosis; may degenerate into giant cell astrocytoma

Age: 0–30 years
Location: temporal lobe, hamartoma of tuber cinereum, subependymal in tuberous sclerosis
√ cyst with little mass effect, possibly with focal calcifications
√ usually no enhancement

HEAD TRAUMA

Incidence: 0.2–0.3% annually in United States; peak at 550/100,000 people aged 15–24 years; second peak >50 years of age

Classification:

A. Primary traumatic lesion
 (a) primary neuronal injury
  1. Cortical contusion
  2. Diffuse axonal injury
  3. Subcortical gray matter injury
   = injury to thalamus ± basal ganglia
  4. Primary brainstem injury
 (b) primary hemorrhages (from injury to a cerebral artery / vein / capillary)
  1. Subdural hematoma
  2. Epidural hematoma
  3. Intracerebral hematoma
  4. Diffuse hemorrhage (intraventricular, subarachnoid)
 (c) primary vascular injuries
  1. Carotid-cavernous fistula
  2. Arterial pseudoaneurysm
   Location: branches of ACA + MCA, intracavernous portion of ICA, pCom
  3. Arterial dissection / laceration / occlusion
  4. Dural sinus laceration / occlusion
 (d) traumatic pia-arachnoid injury
  1. Posttraumatic arachnoid cyst
  2. Subdural hygroma
 (e) cranial nerve injury

B. Secondary traumatic lesion
 • deterioration of consciousness / new neurologic signs some time after initial injury
  1. Major territorial arterial infarction
   Cause: prolonged transtentorial / subfalcine herniation pinching the artery against a rigid dural margin
   Location: PCA, ACA territory
  2. Boundary + terminal zone infarction
  3. Diffuse hypoxic injury
  4. Diffuse brain swelling / edema
  5. Pressure necrosis from brain herniation
   Cause: increased intracranial pressure
   Location: cingulate, uncal, parahippocampal gyri, cerebellar tonsils
  6. Secondary "delayed" hemorrhage
  7. Secondary brainstem injury (mechanical compression, secondary (Duret) hemorrhage in tegmentum of rostral pons + midbrain, infarction of median / paramedian perforating arteries, necrosis)
  8. Other (eg, fatty embolism, infection)
 • **Duret hemorrhage** = hemorrhage in lateral brainstem due to massive temporal lobe herniation
 • **Kernahorn notch** = contusion of contralateral brainstem caused by pressure of free edge of tentorium

Pathomechanism:

A. Direct impact on brain due to fracture / skull distortion
 √ superficial neural damage localized to immediate vicinity of calvarial injury
 1. Cortical laceration due to depressed fracture fragment
 2. Epidural hematoma

B. Indirect injury irrespective of skull deformation
 (a) compression-rarefaction strain = change in cell volume without change in shape (rare)
 (b) shear strain = change in shape without change in volume by
  — rotational acceleration forces (more common)
   √ bilateral multiple superficial / deep lesions possibly remote from the site of impact
   1. Cortical contusion (brain surface)
   2. Diffuse axonal injury (white matter)
   3. Brainstem + deep gray matter nuclei
  — linear acceleration forces (less common)
   1. Subdural hematoma
   2. Small superficial contusion

Intracerebral Hemorrhage

1. Hematoma
 = blood separating relatively normal neurons
  (a) shear-strain injury (most common)
  (b) blunt / penetrating trauma (bullet, ice pick, skull fracture fragment)
 Incidence: 2–16% of trauma victims
 Location: low frontal + anterior temporal white matter / basal ganglia (80–90%)
 • frequently no loss of consciousness
 • development may be delayed in 8% of head injuries
 √ well-defined homogeneously increased density
2. Cortical contusion
 = blood mixed with edematous brain
 √ poorly defined area of mixed high and low densities, may increase with time
3. Intraventricular hemorrhage
 = potential complication of any intracranial hemorrhage
 ◊ For earliest detection focus on occipital horns!

Extracerebral Hemorrhage

1. Subdural hematoma
 in adults: dura inseparable from skull
2. Epidural hematoma
 in children: dura easily stripped away from skull
3. Subarachnoid hemorrhage
 common accompaniment to severe cerebral trauma

Other posttraumatic lesions

1. Pneumocephalus
2. Penetrating foreign body

Indications for radiographic skull series:
Only in conjunction with positive CT scan findings!
1. Evaluation of depressed skull fracture / fracture of base of the skull

Indications for CT:
1. Loss of consciousness (more than transient)
2. Altered mental status during observation
3. Focal neurologic signs
4. Clinically suspected basilar fracture
5. Depressed skull fracture (= outer table of fragment below level of inner table of calvarium)
6. Penetrating wound (eg, bullet)
7. Suspected acute subarachnoid hemorrhage, epidural / subdural / parenchymal hematoma

CT report addresses:
√ midline shift
√ localized mass effect
√ distortion / effacement of basal, perimesencephalic, suprasellar, quadrigeminal cisterns
√ pressure on brainstem, brainstem abnormality
√ hemorrhage / contusion: extra-axial, intra-axial, subarachnoid, intraventricular
√ edema: generalized / localized
√ hydrocephalus
√ presence of foreign bodies, bullet, bone fragments, air
√ base of skull, face, orbit
√ scalp swelling

Indications for MR:
1. Postconcussive symptomatology
2. Diagnosis of small sub- / epidural hematoma
3. Suspected diffuse axonal (shearing) injury, cortical contusion, primary brainstem injury
4. Vascular damage (eg, pseudoaneurysm formation due to basilar skull fracture)

Sequelae of head injury:
1. Posttraumatic hydrocephalus (1/3)
   = obstruction of CSF pathways secondary to intracranial hemorrhage; develops within 3 months
2. Generalized cerebral atrophy (1/3)
   = result of ischemia + hypoxia
3. Encephalomalacia
   √ focal areas of decreased density, but usually higher density than CSF
4. Pseudoporencephaly
   = CSF-filled space communicating with ventricle / subarachnoid space from cystic degeneration
5. Subdural hygroma
   = localized collection of CSF in subdural space secondary to (a) result of chronic subdural hematoma (b) arachnoidal tear acting as a ball valve
   Age: most often in elderly + young children
   √ may resolve spontaneously
6. Leptomeningeal cyst
   = progressive protrusion of leptomeninges through traumatic calvarial defect
7. Cerebrospinal fluid leak
   • rhinorrhea, otorrhea (indicating basilar fracture with meningeal tear)
8. Posttraumatic abscess
   secondary to (a) penetrating injury (b) basilar skull fracture (c) infection of traumatic hematoma
9. Parenchymal injury
   brain atrophy, residual hemoglobin degradation products, wallerian-type axonal degeneration, demyelination, cavitation, microglial scarring

Prognosis: up to 10% fatal; 5–10% with some degree of neurologic deficit
Mortality: 25/100,000 per year (traffic-related in 20–50%, gunshot 20–40%; falls)

HEMANGIOBLASTOMA OF CNS

= benign autosomal dominant tumor of vascular origin
Incidence: 1–2.5% of all intracranial neoplasms
Age: (a) adulthood (>80%): 20–50 years, average age of 33 years; M > F
(b) childhood (<20%): in von Hippel-Lindau disease (10–20%); girls

Associated with:
(a) von Hippel-Lindau disease, may have multiple hemangioblastomas (only 20% of patients show other stigmata)
(b) pheochromocytoma (often familial)
(c) syringomyelia
(d) spinal cord hemangioblastomas

• erythrocythemia in 20% (tumor elaborates stimulant)

Location: paravermian cerebellar hemisphere > spinal cord > cerebral hemisphere / brainstem; multiple lesions in 10%

√ solid (1/3) / cystic / cystic + mural nodule
√ solid portion often intensely hemorrhagic
√ almost never calcifies

CT:
√ cystic sharply marginated mass of CSF-density (2/3)
√ peripheral mural nodule with homogeneous enhancement (50%
√ occasionally solid with intense homogeneous enhancement

MR:
√ well-demarcated tumor mass moderately hypointense on T1WI + T2WI
√ hyperintense areas on T1WI (= hemorrhage)
√ hypointense areas on T1WI + hyperintense areas on T2WI (= cyst formation)
√ intralesional vermiform areas of signal dropout (= high-velocity blood flow)
√ heterogeneous enhancement on Gd-DTPA with nonenhancing foci of cyst formation + calcification + rapidly flowing blood
√ perilesional Gd-DTPA enhancing areas of slow-flowing blood vessels feeding + draining the tumor
√ peripheral hyperintense rim on T2WI (= edema)

Angio:
- √ densely stained tumor nidus within cyst ("contrast loading")
- √ staining of entire rim of cyst
- √ draining vein

DDx: (1) Cystic astrocytoma (>5 cm, calcifications, larger nodule, thick-walled lesion, no angiographic contrast blush of mural nodule, no erythrocythemia)
(2) Arachnoid cyst (if mural nodule not visualized)
(3) Metastasis (more surrounding edema)

HEMATOMA OF BRAIN

= INTRACEREBRAL HEMATOMA

Etiology:

A. Very common
1. Chronic hypertension
   Age: >60 years
   Location: external capsule and basal ganglia (putamen in 50%) / thalamus (25%), pons + brainstem (10%), cerebellum (10%), cerebral hemisphere (5%)
2. Trauma
3. Aneurysm
4. AVM

B. Common
1. Hemorrhagic infarction = hemorrhagic transformation of stroke
2. Amyloid angiopathy: elderly patients
3. Coagulopathy
4. Drug abuse: methamphetamines, cocaine
5. Bleeding into tumor (eg, metastasis, glioma)

C. Uncommon
1. Venous infarction
2. Eclampsia
3. Septic emboli
4. Vasculitis (especially fungal)
5. Encephalitis

Stages of Cerebral Hematomas

Progression: hematoma gradually "snowballs" in size, dissects along white matter tracts; may decompress into ventricular system / subarachnoid space

Resolution: resorption from outside toward the center; rate depends on size of hematoma (usually 1–6 weeks)

FALSE-NEGATIVE CT:
1. impaired clotting
2. anemia
- √ iso- / hypodense stage

Hyperacute Hemorrhage

Time period: <24 hours

Substrate: fresh oxygenated arterial blood contains 95% diamagnetic (= no unpaired electrons) intracellular oxyhemoglobin (Fe^{2+}) with higher water contents than white matter; oxyhemoglobin persists for 6–12 hours)

NCCT:
- √ homogeneous consolidated high-density lesion (50–70 HU) with irregular well-defined margins increasing in density during day 1–3 (hematoma attenuation dependent on hemoglobin concentration + rate of clot retraction)
- √ usually surrounded by low attenuation (edema, contusion) appearing within 24–48 hours
  (a) irregular shape in trauma
  (b) spherical + solitary in spontaneous hemorrhage
- √ less mass effect compared with neoplasms

MR (less sensitive than CT during first hours):
- √ little difference to normal brain parenchyma = center of hematoma iso- to hypointense on T1WI + minimally hyperintense on T2WI
- √ peripheral rim of hypointensity (= degraded blood products as clue for presence of hemorrhage)

Acute Hematoma

Time period: 1–3 days

Substrate: paramagnetic (= 4 unpaired electrons) intracellular deoxyhemoglobin (Fe^{2+}); deoxyhemoglobin persists for 3 days

MR:
- √ slightly hypo- / isointense on T1WI (= paramagnetic deoxyhemoglobin within clotted intact hypoxic RBCs does not cause T1 shortening)
- √ very hypointense on T2WI (progressive concentration of RBCs, blood clot retraction, and fibrin production shorten T2)
- √ surrounding tissue isointense on T1WI / hyperintense on T2WI (edema)

Early Subacute Hematoma

Time period: 3–7 days

Substrate: intracellular strongly paramagnetic (= 5 unpaired electrons) methemoglobin (Fe^{3+}); (inhomogeneously distributed within cells)

NCCT:
- √ increase in size of hemorrhagic area over days / weeks
- √ high-density lesion within 1st week; often with layering

MR:
- √ very hyperintense on T1WI (= oxidation of deoxyhemoglobin to methemoglobin results in marked shortening of T1)
  (a) beginning peripherally in parenchymal hematomas
  (b) beginning centrally in partially thrombosed aneurysm (oxygen tension higher in lumen)
  DDx: melanin, high-protein concentration, flow-related enhancement, gadolinium-based contrast agent
- √ very hypointense on T2WI (= intracellular methemoglobin causes T2 shortening)

Late Subacute Hematoma

Time period: 7–14 days

Substrate: extracellular strongly paramagnetic methemoglobin (homogeneously distributed)

NCCT:
- √ gradual decrease in density from periphery inward (1–2 HU per day) during 2nd + 3rd week

CECT:
- √ peripheral rim enhancement at inner border of perilesional lucency (1–6 weeks after injury) in 80% (secondary to blood-brain barrier breakdown / luxury perfusion / formation of hypervascular granulation tissue)
- √ ring blush may be diminished by administration of corticosteroids

MR:
- √ hyperintense on T1WI (= RBC lysis allows free passage of water molecules across cell membrane)
- √ hyperintense on T2WI (= compartmentalization of methemoglobin is lost due to RBC lysis)
- √ surrounding edema isointense on T1WI + hyperintense on T2WI

Chronic Hematoma

Time period: >14 days

Substrate: superparamagnetic **ferritin** (= soluble + stored in intracellular compartment) and **hemosiderin** (= insoluble + stored in lysosomes) cause marked field inhomogeneities

NCCT:
- √ isodense hematoma from 3rd–10th week with perilesional ring of lucency

CT:
- √ hypodense phase (4–6 weeks) secondary to fluid uptake by osmosis
- √ decreased density (3–6 months) / invisible
- √ after 10 weeks lucent hematoma (encephalomalacia due to proteolysis and phagocytosis + surrounding atrophy) with ring blush (DDx: tumor)

MR:
- √ rim slightly hypointense on T1WI + very hypointense on T2WI (= superparamagnetic hemosiderin + ferritin within macrophages); rim gradually increases over weeks in thickness, eventually fills in entire hematoma = HALLMARK
- √ center hyperintense on T1WI + T2WI (= extracellular methemoglobin of lysed RBCs just inside the darker hemosiderin ring); present for months to 1 year
- √ surrounding hyperintensity on T2WI (= edema + serum extruded from clot) with associated mass effect should resorb within 4–6 weeks (DDx: malignant hemorrhage)

Prognosis: (1) herniation (if 3–4 cm in size)
(2) death (if >5 cm in size)

Basal Ganglia Hematoma

= rupture of small distal microaneurysms in the lenticulostriate arteries in patients with poorly controlled systemic arterial hypertension

Cx: (1) Dissection into adjacent ventricles (2/3)
(2) Porencephaly
(3) Atrophy with ipsilateral ventricular dilatation

HETEROTOPIC GRAY MATTER

= collection of cortical neurons in an abnormal location secondary to arrest of migrating neuroblasts from ventricular walls to brain surface between 7–24 weeks of GA

MR Appearance of Intracerebral Hematoma

Phase	Age	Compartment	Hemoglobin	T1	T2	Comments
hyperacute	<24 hr	intracellular	oxyhemoglobin	iso	hyper	hyperacute bleed in <1 hr
						deoxygenation
acute	1 – 3 d	intracellular	deoxyhemoglobin	**hypo**	**hypo**	within clotted intact hypoxic RBCs
		extracellular	deoxyhemoglobin	iso	iso	after lysis of RBCs
subacute						oxidation
early	>3 d	intracellular	methemoglobin	**hyper**	**hypo**	within intact RBCs inside retracting clot
late	>7 d	extracellular	methemoglobin	**hyper**	**hyper**	after lysis of RBCs
chronic	>14 d					
center		extracellular	hemichromes	iso	hyper	non–iron-containing heme pigments
rim		intracellular	hemosiderin	**hypo**	**hypo**	within macrophages, present for years
		fibrous tissue		hypo	hypo	
		edema		iso	hyper	

mnemonic: "DD-BD-BB-DD on T1/T2"

Dark-**D**ark	acute	0–2 days	deoxyhemoglobin
Bright-**D**ark	early subacute	3 – 7 days	intracellular methemoglobin
Bright-**B**right	late subacute	8 – 14 days	extracellular methemoglobin
Dark-**D**ark	chronic	>14 days	hemosiderin

Frequency: 3% of healthy population
May be associated with: agenesis of corpus callosum, aqueductal stenosis, microcephaly, schizencephaly

• seizures

Location:
(1) nodular form: usually symmetric bilaterally in subependymal region / periventricular white matter with predilection for posterior + anterior horns
(2) laminar form: deep / subcortical regions within white matter (less common)

√ single / multiple bilateral subependymal nodules along lateral ventricles
√ NO surrounding edema, isointense with gray matter on all sequences, no contrast enhancement

DDx: subependymal spread of neoplasm, subependymal hemorrhage, vascular malformation, tuberous sclerosis, intraventricular meningioma, neurofibromatosis

HOLOPROSENCEPHALY

= lack of cleavage / diverticulation of the forebrain (= prosencephalon) laterally (cerebral hemispheres), transversely (telencephalon, diencephalon), horizontally (optic + olfactory structures) as a consequence of arrested lateral ventricular growth in 6-week embryo; cortical brain tissue develops to cover the monoventricle and fuses in the midline; posterior part of the monoventricle becomes enlarged and saclike

◊ Septum pellucidum always absent!

Incidence: 1:16,000; M:F = 1:1

A. ALOBAR = no hemispheric development
B. SEMILOBAR = some hemispheric development
C. LOBAR = frontal and temporal lobation + small monoventricle

Associated with: polyhydramnios (60%), renal + cardiac anomalies; chromosomal anomalies (predominantly trisomy 13 + 18)

Associated borderline syndromes secondary to diencephalic malformation:
1. Anophthalmia
2. Microphthalmia
3. Aplasia of pituitary gland
4. Olfactogenital dysplasia
5. Septo-optic dysplasia

DDx:
1. Severe hydrocephalus (roughly symmetrically thinned cortex)
2. Dandy-Walker cyst (normal supratentorial ventricular system)
3. Hydranencephaly (frontal + parietal cortex most severely affected)
4. Agenesis of corpus callosum with midline cyst (lateral ventricles widely separated with pointed superolateral margin)

Alobar Holoprosencephaly

= extreme form in which the prosencephalon does not divide

• minimal motor activity, little sensory response (ineffective brain function); seizures
• severe facial anomalies ("the face predicts the brain"):
  1. Normal face in 17%
  2. Cyclopia (= midline single orbit); may have proboscis (= fleshy supraorbital prominence) + absent nose
  3. Ethmocephaly = 2 hypoteloric orbits + proboscis between eyes and absence of nasal structures
  4. Cebocephaly = 2 hypoteloric orbits + single nostril with small flattened nose + absent nasal septum
  5. Median cleft lip + cleft palate + hypotelorism
  6. Others: micrognathia, trigonocephaly (early closure of metopic suture), microphthalmia, microcephaly

√ thalami fused
  √ protrusion of anteriorly placed fused thalami + basal ganglia into monoventricle
√ absence of: septum pellucidum, 3rd ventricle, falx cerebri, interhemispheric fissure, corpus callosum, fornix, optic tracts, olfactory bulb (= arrhinencephaly), internal cerebral veins, superior + inferior straight sagittal sinus, vein of Galen, tentorium, sylvian fissure, opercular cortex
√ crescent-shaped holoventricle = single large ventricle without occipital or temporal horns
√ large dorsal cyst occupying most of calvarium + widely communicating with single ventricle
√ "horseshoe" / "boomerang" configuration of brain = peripheral rim of cerebral cortex displaced rostrally (coronal plane)
  (a) pancake configuration = cortex covers monoventricle to edge of dorsal cyst
  (b) cup configuration = more cortex visible posteriorly
  (c) ball configuration = complete covering of monoventricle without dorsal cyst

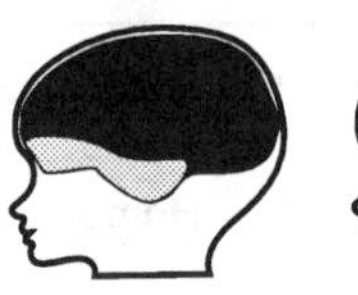
pancake

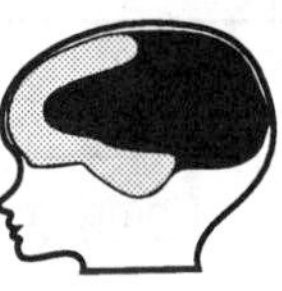
cup

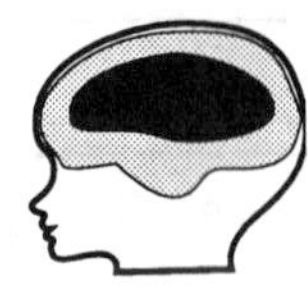
ball

√ midbrain, brainstem, cerebellum structurally normal
√ pancakelike cerebrum in posterior cranium
√ cerebral mantle pachygyric
√ midline clefts in maxilla + palate

Prognosis: death within 1st year of life / stillborn
DDx: massive hydrocephalus, hydranencephaly

Semilobar Holoprosencephaly

= intermediate form with incomplete cleavage of prosencephalon (more midline differentiation + beginning of sagittal separation)

• mild facial anomalies: midline cleft lip + palate
• hypotelorism
• mental retardation

√ single ventricular chamber with partially formed occipital horns + rudimentary temporal horns

√ peripheral rim of brain tissue is several cm thick
√ partially fused thalami anteriorly situated + abnormally rotated resulting in small 3rd ventricle
√ absence of septum pellucidum + corpus callosum + olfactory bulb
√ rudimentary falx cerebri + interhemispheric fissure form caudally with partial separation of occipital lobes
√ incomplete hippocampal formation

Prognosis: infants survive frequently into adulthood

Lobar Holoprosencephaly

= mildest form with two cerebral hemispheres + two distinct lateral ventricles

◊ May be part of septo-optic dysplasia!

• usually not associated with facial anomalies except for hypotelorism
• mild to severe mental retardation, spasticity, athetoid movements

√ closely apposed bodies of lateral ventricles with distinct occipital + frontal horns
√ mild dilatation of lateral ventricles
√ colpocephaly
√ unseparated frontal horns of angular squared shape + flatroof (on coronal images) due to dysplastic frontal lobes
√ dysplastic anterior falx + interhemispheric fissure
√ absence of septum pellucidum + sylvian fissures
√ corpus callosum usually present
√ hippocampal formation nearly normal
√ basal ganglia + thalami may be fused / separated
√ pachygyria (= abnormally wide + plump gyri), lissencephaly (= o gyri)

Prognosis: survival into adulthood

HYDATID DISEASE OF BRAIN

= canine tapeworm (Echinococcus granulosus) in sheep- and cattle-grazing areas

Location: liver (60%), lung (25%), CNS (2%) subcortical

√ usually single, large round, sharply marginated smooth-walled hypodense cyst
√ no significant surrounding edema; no rim enhancement
√ development of daughter cysts (after rupture / following diagnostic puncture)

HYDRANENCEPHALY

= liquefaction necrosis of cerebral hemispheres replaced by a thin membranous sac of leptomeninges in outer layer + remnants of cortex and white matter in inner layer, filled with CSF + necrotic debris

Incidence: 0.2% of infant autopsies

Etiology: absence of supraclinoid ICA system (? vascular occlusion / infection with toxoplasmosis or CMV) = ultimate form of porencephaly

• seizures; respiratory failure; generalized flaccidity
• decerebrate state with vegetative existence

√ normal skull size / macrocrania / microcrania
√ complete filling of hemicranium with membranous sac
√ absence of cortical mantle (inferomedial aspect of temporal lobe, inferior aspect of frontal lobe, occipital lobe may be identified in some patients)
√ brainstem usually atrophic
√ cerebellum almost always intact
√ thalamic, hypothalamic, mesencephalic structures usually preserved + project into cystic cavity
√ central brain tissue can be asymmetric
√ choroid plexus present
√ falx cerebri + tentorium cerebelli usually intact, may be deviated in asymmetric involvement, may be incomplete / absent

Prognosis: not compatible with prolonged extrauterine life (no intellectual improvement from shunting)

DDx: (1) Severe hydrocephalus (some identifiable cortex present)
(2) Alobar holoprosencephaly (facial midline anomalies)
(3) Schizencephaly (some spared cortical mantle)

HYDROCEPHALUS

= excess of CSF due to imbalance of CSF formation + absorption resulting in increased intraventricular pressure

Pathophysiology:

A. Overproduction (rare)
B. Impaired absorption
 1. Blockage of CSF flow within ventricular system, cisterna magna, basilar cisterns, cerebral convexities
 2. Blockage of arachnoid villi / lymphatic channels of cranial nerves, spinal nerves, adventitia of cerebral vessels

Compensated hydrocephalus = new equilibrium established at higher intracranial pressure due to opening of alternate pathways (arachnoid membrane / stroma of choroid plexus / extracellular space of cortical mantle = transependymal flow of CSF)

Skull film: signs of raised intracranial pressure

A. YOUNG INFANT / NEWBORN
 √ increase in craniofacial ratio
 √ bulging of anterior fontanelle
 √ sutural diastasis
 √ macrocephaly + frontal bossing
 √ "hammered silver" appearance = prominent digital impressions (wide range of normals in 4–10 years of age)
B. ADOLESCENT / ADULT (changes in sella turcica)
 √ atrophy of anterior wall of dorsum sellae
 √ shortening of the dorsum sellae producing pointed appearance
 √ erosion / thinning / discontinuity of floor of sella
 √ depression of floor of sella with bulging into sphenoid sinus
 √ enlargement of sella turcica
 DDx: osteoporotic sella (aging, excessive steroid hormone)

Signs favoring hydrocephalus over white matter atrophy:

√ commensurate dilatation of temporal horn with lateral ventricles (most reliable sign)

√ narrowing of ventricular angle (= angle between anterior / superior margins of frontal horns at level of foramen of Monro) due to concentric enlargement
√ Mickey Mouse ears on axial scans
√ enlargement of frontal horn radius (= widest diameter of frontal horns taken at 90° angle to long axis of frontal horn)
√ rounding of frontal horn shape
√ enlargement of ventricular system disproportionate to enlargement of cortical sulci (due to compression of brain tissue against skull + consequent sulcal narrowing)
√ interstitial edema from transependymal flow of CSF
√ periventricular hypodensity
√ rim of prolonged T1 + T2 relaxation times surrounding lateral ventricles

Hydrocephalic distortion of ventricles + brain:
√ atrial diverticulum = herniation of ventricular wall through choroidal fissure of ventricular trigone into supracerebellar + quadrigeminal cisterns
√ dilatation of suprapineal recess expanding into posterior incisural space resulting in inferior displacement of pineal gland / shortening of tectum in rostral-caudal direction / elevation of vein of Galen
√ enlargement of anterior recess of 3rd ventricle extending into suprasellar cistern

Obstructive Hydrocephalus

= obstruction to normal CSF flow + absorption

Communicating Hydrocephalus

= EXTRAVENTRICULAR HYDROCEPHALUS
= elevated intraventricular pressure secondary to blockade beyond the outlet of 4th ventricle within the subarachnoid pathways

Incidence: 38% of congenital hydrocephaly

Pathophysiology:
unimpeded CSF flow through ventricles, impeded CSF flow over convexities / impeded reabsorption by arachnoid villi

Cause:
subarachnoid hemorrhage (most common cause), meningeal carcinomatosis (medulloblastoma, germinoma, leukemia, lymphoma, adenocarcinoma), purulent / tuberculous meningitis, subdural hematoma, craniosynostosis, achondroplasia, Hurler syndrome, venous obstruction (obliteration of superior sagittal sinus), absence of Pacchioni granulations

√ symmetric enlargement of lateral, 3rd, and often 4th ventricles
√ dilatation of subarachnoid cisterns
√ normal / effaced cerebral sulci
√ symmetric low attenuation of periventricular white matter (transependymal CSF flow)
√ delayed ascent of radionuclide tracer over convexities
√ persistence of radionuclide tracer in lateral ventricles for up to 48 hours

Changes after successful shunting:
√ diminished size of ventricles + increased prominence of sulci
√ cranial vault may thicken

Cx: subdural hematoma (result from precipitous decompression)

Noncommunicating Hydrocephalus

= INTRAVENTRICULAR HYDROCEPHALUS
= blockade of CNS flow within the ventricular system with dilatation of ventricles proximal to obstruction

Pathogenesis: increased CSF pressure causes ependymal flattening with breakdown of CSF-brain barrier leading to myelin destruction + compression of cerebral mantle (brain damage)

Location:
(a) Lateral ventricular obstruction
Cause: ependymoma, intraventricular glioma, meningioma
(b) Foramen of Monro obstruction
Cause: 3rd ventricular colloid cyst, tuber, papilloma, meningioma, septum pellucidum cyst / glioma, fibrous membrane (post infection), giant cell astrocytoma
(c) Third ventricular obstruction
Cause: large pituitary adenoma, teratoma, craniopharyngioma, glioma of 3rd ventricle, hypothalamic glioma
(d) Aqueductal obstruction
Cause: Congenital web / atresia (often associated with Chiari malformation), fenestrated aqueduct, tumor of mesencephalon / pineal gland, tentorial meningioma, S/P intraventricular hemorrhage or infection
(e) Fourth ventricular obstruction
Cause: Congenital obstruction, Dandy-Walker syndrome, inflammation (TB), tumor within 4th ventricle (ependymoma), extrinsic compression of 4th ventricle (astrocytoma, medulloblastoma, large CPA tumors, posterior fossa mass), isolated / trapped 4th ventricle

√ enlarged lateral ventricles (enlargement of occipital horns precedes enlargement of frontal horns)
√ effaced cerebral sulci
√ periventricular edema with indistinct margins (especially frontal horns)
√ radioisotope cisternography: no obstruction if tracer reaches ventricle
√ change in RI indicates increased intracranial pressure (ΔRI 47–132% versus 3–29% in normals)

Nonobstructive Hydrocephalus

= secondary to rapid CSF production

Cause: Choroid plexus papilloma

√ ventricle near papilloma enlarges
√ intense radionuclide uptake in papilloma
√ enlarged anterior / posterior choroidal artery and blush

Congenital hydrocephalus

= multifactorial CNS malformation during the 3rd / 4th week after conception

Etiology:
(1) aqueductal stenosis (43%)
(2) communicating hydrocephalus (38%)
(3) Dandy-Walker syndrome (13%)
(4) other anatomic lesions (6%)
(a) Genetic factors: spina bifida, aqueductal stenosis (X-linked recessive trait with a 50% recurrence rate for male fetuses), congenital atresia of foramina of Luschka and Magendie (Dandy-Walker syndrome; autosomal recessive trait with 25% recurrence rate), cerebellar agenesis, cloverleaf skull, trisomy 13–18
(b) Nongenetic etiology: tumor compressing 3rd / 4th ventricle, obliteration of subarachnoid pathway due to infection (syphilis, CMV, rubella, toxoplasmosis), proliferation of fibrous tissue (Hurler syndrome), Chiari malformations, vein of Galen aneurysm, choroid plexus papilloma, vitamin A intoxication

Incidence: 0.3–1.8:1,000 pregnancies

Associated with:
(a) Intracranial anomalies (37%): hypoplasia of corpus callosum, encephalocele, arachnoid cyst, arteriovenous malformation
(b) extracranial anomalies (63%): spina bifida in 25 – 30% (with spina bifida hydrocephalus is present in 80%), renal agenesis, multicystic dysplastic kidney, VSD, tetralogy of Fallot, anal agenesis, malrotation of bowel, cleft lip / palate, Meckel syndrome, gonadal dysgenesis, arthrogryposis, sirenomelia
(c) chromosomal anomalies (11%): trisomy 18 + 21, mosaicism, balanced translocation

• elevated amniotic alpha-fetoprotein level

OB-US: (assessment difficult prior to 20 weeks GA as ventricles ordinarily constitute a large portion of cranial vault)
√ "dangling choroid plexus sign" = choroid plexus not touching medial + lateral walls of lateral ventricles with downside choroid falling away from medial wall + upside choroid falling away from lateral wall
√ lateral width of ventricular atrium ≥10 mm (size usually constant between 16 weeks MA and term)
◊ 88% of fetuses with sonographically detected neural axis anomalies have atrial width >10 mm
√ BPD >95th percentile (usually not before third trimester)
√ polyhydramnios (in 30%)

Recurrence rate: <4%

Mortality: (1) fetal death in 24%
(2) neonatal death in 17%

Prognosis: poor with
(1) associated anomalies
(2) shift of midline (porencephaly)
(3) head circumference >50 cm
(4) absence of cortex (hydranencephaly)
(5) cortical thickness <10 mm

Infantile hydrocephalus

• ocular disturbances: paralysis of upward gaze, abducens nerve paresis, nystagmus, ptosis, diminished pupillary light response
• spasticity of lower extremities (from disproportionate stretching of paracentral corticospinal fibers)

Etiology:
mnemonic: "**A** **VP**-**S**hunt **C**an **D**ecompress **T**he **H**ydrocephalic **C**hild"
Aqueductal stenosis
Vein of Galen aneurysm
Postinfectious
Superior vena cava obstruction
Chiari II malformation
Dandy-Walker syndrome
Tumor
Hemorrhage
Choroid plexus papilloma

Normal pressure hydrocephalus

= NPH = ADAM SYNDROME
= pressure gradient between ventricle + brain parenchyma in spite of normal CSF pressure

Cause: communicating hydrocephalus with incomplete arachnoidal obstruction from neonatal intraventricular hemorrhage, spontaneous subarachnoid hemorrhage, intracranial trauma, infection, surgery, carcinomatosis
mnemonic: "PAM the HAM"
Paget disease
Aneurysm
Meningitis
Hemorrhage (from trauma)
Achondroplasia
Mucopolysaccharidosis

Pathophysiology of CSF:
(?) brain pushed toward cranium from ventricular enlargement; brain unable to expand during systole thus compressing lateral + 3rd ventricles + expressing large CSF volume through aqueduct; reverse dynamic during diastole; "water-hammer" force of recurrent ventricular expansion damages periventricular tissues

Age: 50–70 years

• normal opening pressure at lumbar puncture
• dementia, gait apraxia, incontinence
mnemonic: wacky, wobbly and wet

√ communicating hydrocephalus with prominent temporal horns
√ ventricles dilated out of proportion to any sulcal enlargement
√ upward bowing of corpus callosum

√ flattening of cortical gyri against inner table of calvarium (DDx: rounded gyri in generalized atrophy)

MR:

- √ pronounced aqueductal flow void (due to diminished compliance of normal pressure hydrocephalus)
- √ periventricular hyperintensity (due to transependymal CSF flow)

Rx: CSF shunting (only 50% improved)

HYPOTHALAMIC HAMARTOMA

= HAMARTOMA OF TUBER CINEREUM

= rare congenital malformation composed of normal neuronal tissue arising from posterior hypothalamus in region of tuber cinereum

Age: <2 years of age; M > F

Histo: heterotopic collection of neurons, astrocytes, oligodendroglial cells (closely resembling histologic pattern of tuber cinereum)

- isosexual precocious puberty (due to LRH secretion)
- gelastic seizures, hyperactivity
- neurodevelopmental delay

Location: mamillary bodies / tuber cinereum of thalamus, rarely within hypothalamus itself

√ well-defined round / oval mass projecting from base of brain into suprasellar / interpeduncular cistern

√ attached to tuber cinereum / mamillary bodies by thin stalk (pedunculated)

√ remain stable in size over time; up to 4 cm in diameter

CT:

- √ round homogeneous mass isodense with brain tissue
- √ NO enhancement

MR:

- √ well-defined round pedunculated mass suspended from tuber cinereum / mamillary bodies
- √ isointense on T1WI + iso- / slightly hyperintense on T2WI (imaging characteristics of gray matter)
- √ no gadolinium-enhancement

IDIOPATHIC INTRACRANIAL HYPERTENSION

= PSEUDOTUMOR CEREBRI = BENIGN INTRACRANIAL HYPERTENSION (BIH)

secondary to

(a) elevation in blood volume (85%)

(b) decrease in regional cerebral blood flow with delayed CSF absorption (10%)

Etiology:

1. Sinovenous occlusive disease, SVC occlusion, obstruction of dural sinus, obstruction of both internal jugular veins
2. Dural AVM
3. S/P brain biopsy with edema
4. Endocrinopathies
5. Hypervitaminosis A
6. Hypocalcemia
7. Menstrual dysfunction, pregnancy, menarche, birth control pills
8. Drug therapy

Predilection for: obese young to middle-aged women

- headache
- papilledema
- elevated opening pressures on lumbar puncture

√ normal ventricular size / pinched ventricles

√ increased volume of subarachnoid space

INFARCTION OF BRAIN

= brain cell death leading to coagulation necrosis

Pathophysiology:

distal microstasis occurs within 2 minutes after occlusion of cerebral artery; regional cerebral blood flow is acutely decreased in area of infarction + remains depressed for several days at center of infarct; arterial circulation time may be prolonged in entire hemisphere; rapid development of vasodilatation due to hypoxia, hypercapnia, tissue acidosis; delayed filling + emptying of arterial channels in area of infarction (= arteriolar-capillary block) well into venous phase; by end of 1st week regional blood flow commonly increases to rates even above those required for metabolic needs (= hyperemic phase = luxury perfusion)

Detection rate by CT:

80% for cortex + mantle, 55% for basal ganglia, 54% for posterior fossa

◊ positive correlation between degree of clinical deficit and CT sensitivity

CT sensitivity:

on day of ictus: 48%
1–2 days later: 59%
7–10 days later: 66%
10–11 days later: 74%

Location: cerebrum:cerebellum = 19:1;

(a) supratentorial

— cerebral mantle (70%) in territory of MCA (50%), PCA (10%), watershed between MCA + ACA (7%), ACA (4%)

— basal ganglia + internal capsule (20%)

(b) infratentorial (10%)

upper cerebellum (5%), lower cerebellum (3%), pons + medulla (2%)

Hyperacute Ischemic Infarction

Time period: <12 hours

CT:

- √ normal (in 10–60%)
- √ "hyperdense artery sign" = acute intraluminal thrombus (25–50% of acute MCA occlusions)
- √ obscuration of lentiform nucleus (50–80% of MCA occlusions)
- √ calcified intraluminal embolus (rare)

MR (more sensitive than CT):

- √ parenchymal swelling due to cytotoxic edema (= increased intracellular water) can be seen by 2 hours post ictus (best on T1WI)

NUC:

◊ Newer imaging agents (eg, Tc-99m HM-PAO) may be positive within minutes of the event, while CT and MR are normal

√ hemispheric hypoperfusion throughout all phases

√ defect corresponding to nonperfused vascular territory
√ "flip-flop sign" in radionuclide angiogram (15%) = decreased uptake during arterial + capillary phase followed by increased uptake during venous phase
√ "luxury perfusion syndrome" (14%) = increased perfusion

Angio:
- √ narrowed / occluded vessels supplying the area of infarction
- √ delayed filling + emptying of involved vessels
- √ early draining vein
- √ luxury perfusion of infarcted area (rare) = loss of small vessel autoregulation due to local increase in pH

Acute Ischemic Infarction

Histo: cortical cytotoxic edema (from loss of vascular autoregulation) followed by white matter vasogenic edema

(a) Substage I (12–24 hours)

NCCT:
- √ low-density basal ganglia
- √ effacement of gray-white matter junction, eg, "insular ribbon sign" = hypodense extreme capsule no longer distinguishable from insular cortex)
- √ subtle sulcal effacement (8%)

CECT:
- √ no iodine accumulation in affected cortical region

MR (routinely positive by 4–6 hours post ictus):
- √ subtle narrowing of sulci
- √ increase in thickness of cortex (= gyral swelling)
- √ blurring of gray-white matter junction on T2- and proton-density images
- √ contrast-enhanced cortical arterial vessels in area of brain injury (due to slow arterial blood flow provided by collateral circulation via leptomeningeal anastomoses)
- √ subtle low-signal intensity on T1WI, high-signal intensity on T2WI (masking of gyral infarcts on heavily T2WI due to sulcal CSF intensity)

MRA:
- √ absence of flow for infarcts >2 cm in diameter

(b) Substage II (1–7 days)

NCCT:
- √ hypodense wedge-shaped lesion with base at cortex in a vascular distribution (in 70%) due to vasogenic + cytotoxic edema
- √ mass effect (23–75%): sulcal effacement, transtentorial herniation, displaced subarachnoid cisterns + ventricles
- √ "bland infarct" may be transformed into hemorrhagic infarct after 2–4 days (due to leakage of blood from ischemically damaged capillary endothelium following lysis of intraluminal clot + arterial reperfusion)

CECT:
- √ gyral enhancement along cortex

MR:
- √ intravascular enhancement sign (77%) = Gd-pentetate enhancement of vessels supplying infarct after 1–3 days
- √ meningeal enhancement sign = Gd-pentetate enhancement of meninges adjacent to infarct after 2–6 days

Subacute Ischemic Infarction

Time period: 7–30 days = paradoxical phase with resolution of edema + onset of coagulation necrosis

NCCT:
- √ "fogging phenomenon" = low-density area less apparent
- √ decrease of mass effect + ex vacuo dilatation of ventricles (in 57%)
- √ ± transient calcification (especially in children)

CECT:
- √ gyral blush + ring enhancement (breakdown of blood-brain barrier + luxury perfusion) for 2–8 weeks (in 65–80% within first 4 weeks)
- √ no enhancement in 1/5 of patients

MR:

Histo: vasogenic edema (= increased extracellular water) due to disruption of blood-brain barrier

- √ hypointense on T1WI, hyperintense on T2WI
- √ gyriform parenchymal Gd-pentetate enhancement
  - ◊ Gyriform parenchymal enhancement permits differentiation of subacute from chronic infarction!

Chronic Ischemic Infarction

Time period: >30 days

Histo: demyelination + gliosis complete (focal brain atrophy after 8 weeks)

√ cerebral atrophy + encephalomalacia + gliosis (HALLMARKS)

NCCT:
- √ cystic foci of CSF-density (= encephalomalacia) in vascular distribution

MR:
- √ patchy region with increased intensity on T2WI
- √ gliosis (hyperintense on T2WI) often surrounding encephalomalacic region
- √ wallerian degeneration (= anterograde degeneration of axons secondary to neuronal injury) of corticospinal tracts in the wake of old large infarcts that involve the motor cortex

Hemorrhagic Infarction

Etiology: lysis of embolus / opening of collaterals / restoration of normal blood pressure following hypotension / hypertension / anticoagulation causes extravasation in reperfused ischemic brain

Incidence: 6% of clinically diagnosed brain infarcts, 20% of autopsied brain infarcts

Path: petechial hemorrhages in various degrees of coalescence
Location: corticomedullary junction
CT:
√ hyperdensity appearing within a previously imaged hypodense acute ischemic infarct = hemorrhagic transformation (in 50–72%)
MR:
√ hypointense area on T2WI within edema marking gyri = deoxyhemoglobin of acute hemorrhage
√ hyperintense area on T1WI = methemoglobin of subacute hematoma

Basal Ganglia Infarct

= occlusion of small penetrating arteries at base of brain (lenticulostriate / thalamoperforating arteries)
= lacunar infarct (infarcts <1 cm in size)
Cause:
(1) Embolism (2) Hypoperfusion (3) Carbon monoxide poisoning (4) Drowning (5) Vasculopathy (hypertension, microvasculopathy, aging)
√ dense homogeneous enhancement outlining caudate nucleus, putamen, globus pallidus, thalamus
√ dense round nodular enhancement / peripheral ring enhancement

Laminar Necrosis

= ischemic changes affecting deep layers of the cortex (layers 3, 5, 6 very sensitive to oxygen deprivation)
MR:
(a) acute stage
√ linear cortical hyperintensity on T1WI
√ contrast enhancement
√ white matter edema on T2WI
(b) chronic stage
√ thin hypointense cortex
√ hyperintense white matter
√ enlargement of CSF spaces

Lacunar Infarction

= small deep infarcts in the distal distribution of penetrating vessels (lenticulostriate, thalamoperforating, pontine perforating arteries, recurrent artery of Heubner)
Cause: occlusion of small penetrating end arteries at base of brain due to fibrinoid degeneration
Predisposed: hypertensive / diabetic patients
Incidence: 20% of cerebral infarctions
Path: lacune = cavitated infarct resulting in small hole traversed by cobweblike fibrous strands
Histo: "microatheroma" = hyalinization + arteriolar sclerosis resulting in thickening of vessel wall + luminal narrowing
• pure motor / pure sensory stroke
• ataxic hemiparesis
Location: upper two-thirds of putamen > caudate > thalamus > pons > internal capsule
√ small discrete foci of hypodensity between 3 mm and 15 mm in size (most <1 cm in diameter)
√ higher in signal intensity than CSF (due to marginal gliosis)
√ unilateral pontine infarcts are sharply marginated at midline

TIA and RIND

√ hypodense small lesions located peripherally near / within cortex without enhancement
√ lesions detected in only 14%, contralateral lesion present in 14% (CT of marginal value)

INIENCEPHALY

= complex developmental anomaly characterized by (1) exaggerated lordosis (2) rachischisis (3) imperfect formation of skull base at foramen magnum
M:F = 1:4
Associated with other anomalies in 84%:
anencephaly, encephalocele, hydrocephalus, cyclopia, absence of mandible, cleft lip / palate, diaphragmatic hernia, omphalocele, gastroschisis, single umbilical artery, CHD, polycystic kidney disease, arthrogryposis, clubfoot
√ dorsal flexion of head
√ abnormally short + deformed spine
Prognosis: almost uniformly fatal
DDx: (1) Anencephaly
(2) Klippel-Feil syndrome
(3) Cervical myelomeningocele

INTRAVENTRICULAR NEUROCYTOMA

= INTRAVENTRICULAR NEUROBLASTOMA
= benign primary neoplasm of lateral + 3rd ventricles
Incidence: unknown; tumor frequently mistaken for intraventricular oligodendroglioma
Age: 20–40 years
Histo: uniform round cells with central round nucleus + fine chromatin stippling ± perivascular pseudorosettes, focal microcalcifications (closely resembling oligodendroglioma but with neuronal differentiation into synapselike junctions)
Location: body ± frontal horn of lateral ventricle, may extend into 3rd ventricle
√ entirely intraventricular well-circumscribed tumor, coarsely calcified (69%), containing cystic spaces (85%)
√ mild to moderate contrast enhancement
√ attachment to septum pellucidum CHARACTERISTIC
√ ± hemorrhage into tumor / ventricle
√ hydrocephalus
√ peritumoral edema extremely uncommon
MR:
√ isointense relative to cortical gray matter on T1WI + T2WI with heterogeneous areas due to calcifications, cystic spaces, vascular flow voids (62%)
Rx: complete surgical resection
DDx:
(1) Intraventricular oligodendroglioma (no hemorrhage)
(2) Astrocytoma (peritumoral edema in 20%)
(3) Meningioma (almost exclusively in trigone, >30 years of age)

(4) Ependymoma (in + around 4th ventricle / trigone, in childhood)
(5) Subependymoma (in + around 4th ventricle, young adults)
(6) Choroid plexus papilloma (body + posterior horn of lateral ventricle, intense enhancement, younger patient)
(7) Colloid cyst (anterior 3rd ventricle / foramen of Monroe, calcifications uncommon)
(8) Craniopharyngioma (extraventricular origin)
(9) Teratoma + dermoid cyst (fat attenuation)

JAKOB-CREUTZFELDT DISEASE

= rare transmissible disease developing over weeks

Cause: "prion" = protein devoid of functional nucleic acid; ? slow-virus infection

Age: older adults

Histo: classified as "spongiform encephalopathy"

• rapidly progressive dementia, ataxia, myoclonus

√ hyperintense lesions in head of caudate nucleus + putamen, bilaterally on T2WI

√ NO gadolinium-enhancement of lesions

√ NO white matter involvement

Prognosis: usually fatal within 1 year of onset

JOUBERT SYNDROME

• episodic hyperpnea
• abnormal eye movement
• ataxia, mental retardation

Path: (1) nearly total aplasia of cerebellar vermis
(2) dysplasia + heterotopia of cerebellar nuclei
(3) near total absence of pyramidal decussation
(4) anomalies in structure of inferior olivary nuclei, descending trigeminal tract, solitary fascicle, dorsal column nuclei

√ 4th ventricle triangle-shaped at mid-level + bat-wing–shaped superiorly

√ cerebellar hemispheres appose one another in midline

√ superior cerebellar peduncles surrounded by CSF

LIPOMA

= congenital tumor developing within subarachnoid space as a result of abnormal differentiation of the meninx primitiva (which differentiates into pia mater, arachnoid, inner meningeal layer of dura mater)

Incidence: <1% of brain tumors

Age: presentation in childhood / adulthood

Associated with congenital anomalies:
(a) in anterior location: various degrees of agenesis of corpus callosum (in 50–80%)
(b) in posterior location (in <33%)

• asymptomatic in 50%

Location:
(usually in subarachnoid space) callosal cistern (25–50%), sylvian fissure, quadrigeminal cistern, chiasmatic cistern, interpeduncular cistern, CP angle cistern, cerebellomedullary cistern, tuber cinereum, choroid plexus of lateral ventricle

CT:
√ well-circumscribed mass with CT density of -100 HU
√ occasionally calcified rim (esp. in corpus callosum)
√ no enhancement

MR:
√ hyperintense mass on T1WI + less hyperintense on T2WI (CHARACTERISTIC)

Lipoma of Corpus Callosum

= congenital pericallosal tumor not actually involving the corpus callosum as a result of faulty disjunction of neuroectoderm from cutaneous ectoderm during process of neurulation

Incidence: approx. 30% of intracranial lipomas

Associated with:
(1) anomalies of corpus callosum (30% with small posterior lipoma, 90% with large anterior lipoma)
(2) frontal bone defect (frequent) = encephalocele
(3) cutaneous frontal lipoma

• in 50% symptomatic:
  • seizure disorders, mental retardation, dementia
  • emotional lability, headaches
  • hemiplegia

Plain film:
√ midline calcification with associated lucency of fat density

CT:
√ area of marked hypodensity immediately superior to lateral ventricles with possible extension inferiorly between ventricles / anteriorly into interhemispheric fissure
√ curvilinear peripheral / nodular central calcification within fibrous capsule (more common in anterior compared with posterior lipomas)

MR:
√ hyperintense midline mass superior + posterior to corpus callosum on T1WI
√ no callosal fibers dorsal to lipoma
√ branches of pericallosal artery frequently course through lipoma

DDx: dermoid (denser, extra-axial), teratoma

LISSENCEPHALY

= "smooth brain" = AGYRIA-PACHYGYRIA COMPLEX

= most severe of neuronal migration anomalies; autosomal recessive disease with abnormal cortical stratification

agyria = absence of gyri on brain surface

pachygyria = focal / diffuse area of few broad flat gyri

A. COMPLETE LISSENCEPHALY = AGYRIA
most frequently parieto-occipital in location

B. INCOMPLETE LISSENCEPHALY
= areas of both agyria + pachygyria, pachygyric areas most frequently in frontal + temporal regions

Histo: thick gray + thin white matter with only four cortical layers I, III, V, VI (instead of six layers)

Often associated with:
(1) CNS anomalies: microcephaly, hydrocephalus, agenesis of corpus callosum, hypoplastic thalami
(2) micromelia, clubfoot, polydactyly, camptodactyly, syndactyly, duodenal atresia, micrognathia, omphalocele, hepatosplenomegaly, cardiac + renal anomalies
- micrencephaly
- severe mental retardation
- hypotonia + occasional myoclonic spasm
- early seizures refractory to medication

√ smooth thickened cortex with diminished white matter
√ figure-eight appearance of cerebrum on axial images due to shallow widened vertically oriented sylvian fissures
√ absent / shallow sulci and gyri (brain looks similar to that in fetuses <23 weeks GA)
√ middle cerebral arteries close to inner table of calvarium (absence of sulci)
√ small splenium + absent rostrum of corpus callosum
√ hypoplastic brainstem (lack of formation of corticospinal + corticobulbar tracts)
√ ventriculomegaly (atrium + occipital horns)
√ midline round calcification in area of septum pellucidum (CHARACTERISTIC)
√ polyhydramnios (50%)
Prognosis: death by age 2
DDx: Polymicrogyria (= formation of multiple small gyri mimicking pachygyria on CT + MR, most common around sylvian fissures, broad thickened gyri with frequent gliosis subjacent to polymicrogyric cortex as the most important differentiating feature)

LYMPHOID HYPOPHYSITIS

= rare inflammatory autoimmune disorder with lymphocytic infiltration of pituitary gland
Associated with: thyrotoxicosis + hypopituitarism
Age: almost exclusively in early postpartum women
- headaches, vision loss, inability to lactate / to resume normal menses

√ enlarged homogeneously enhancing pituitary gland
Prognosis: spontaneous regression
Rx: steroids (reduction in pituitary size on follow-up)

LYMPHOMA

A. PRIMARY LYMPHOMA (93%) = RETICULUM CELL SARCOMA = HISTIOCYTIC LYMPHOMA = MICROGLIOMA
increased incidence (350-fold) in immunocompromised patients: AIDS, renal transplant, Wiskott-Aldrich syndrome, immunoglobulin deficiency A, rheumatoid arthritis, progressive multifocal leukoencephalopathy
Associated with: intraocular lymphoma
B. SECONDARY (7%) = SYSTEMIC LYMPHOMA
Location: tendency for dura mater + leptomeninges
- palsies of cranial nerves III, VI, VII

◊ Primary lymphoma is indistinguishable from secondary!
Clues: (1) multicentric involvement of deep hemispheres
(2) association with immunosuppression
(3) rapid regression with corticosteroids / radiation therapy = "ghost tumor"

Prevalence: 0.3–2% of all intracranial tumors; 7–15% of all primary brain tumors (equivalent to meningioma + low-grade astrocytoma); M > F
◊ Only 0.8% of lymphomas are primary CNS lesions
Peak age: 30–50 years; M:F = 2:1
Histo: atypical pleomorphic B-cells mixed with reactive T-cells infiltrate blood vessel walls + cluster within perivascular (Virchow-Robin) spaces simulating vasculitis
- symptoms of rapidly enlarging mass (60%)
- symptoms of encephalitis (<25%)
- stroke (7%)
- cranial nerve palsy, demyelinating disease
- personality changes, headaches, seizures
- cerebellar signs, motor dysfunction
- CSF cytology positive in 4–25–43%: elevated protein, mononuclear / blast / other lymphoma cells

Location: suapratentorial:posterior fossa = 3–9:1; paramedian structures preferentially affected; white matter + corpus callosum (55%), deep central gray matter of basal ganglia + thalamus + hypothalamus (17%), posterior fossa + cerebellum (11%), spinal cord (1%); multicentricity in 11–47%
Site: tendency to abut ependyma + meninges (12–30%); "butterfly pattern" of frontal lobe lymphoma; dural involvement may mimic meningioma (rare)
Spread: typically infiltrating; may cross anatomic boundaries + midline, diffuse leptomeningeal spread; subependymal spread + ventricular encasement

√ commonly large discrete solitary lesion (57%)
◊ Large lesion suggests lymphoma!
√ small + symmetric multiple nodular lesions (43–81%)
√ diffusely infiltrating lesion with blurred margins
√ usually mildly hyperdense (33%) / occasionally isodense / low-density area (least common)
√ little mass effect with significant peritumoral edema
√ homogeneously dense + well-defined / irregular + patchy periventricular contrast enhancement
√ commonly thick-walled ring enhancement
√ spontaneous regression (unique feature)
MR (superior to CT):
√ well-demarcated round / oval / gyral-shaped (rare) mass
√ relatively little mass effect for size
√ isointense / slightly hypointense relative to gray matter on T1WI
√ hypo- to isointense / hyperintense (less common) relative to gray matter on T2WI
√ ring pattern (= central necrosis with densely cellular rim in hyperintense "sea of edema") typical in immunocompromised patients
√ intense ring-shaped contrast enhancement on T1WI
√ irregular sinuous / gyral-like contrast enhancement or homogeneous enhancement
√ solid homogeneous enhancement in immunocompetent patient

√ irregular heterogeneous ringlike mass in immunocompromised patient
√ periventricular enhancement is highly SPECIFIC (DDx: CMV ependymitis)

Angio:
√ avascular mass / tumor neovascularity
√ focal blush in late arterial-to-capillary phase persisting well into venous phase
√ arterial encasement
√ dilated deep medullary veins

NUC:
√ increased uptake of C-11 methionine on PET
√ increased uptake of thallium-201 on SPECT

Prognosis: median survival of 45 days for AIDS patients; median survival of 3.3 months for immuno-competent patients; improved with radiation therapy (4.5–20 months) + chemotherapy

DDx:
A. Neoplastic disorders
(1) Glioma (may be bilateral with involvement of basal ganglia + corpus callosum, may show dense homogeneous enhancement with vascularity)
(2) Metastases (known primary, at gray-white matter junction)
(3) Primitive neuroectodermal tumor
(4) Meningioma
B. Infectious disease (multicentricity)
(1) Abscess, especially toxoplasmosis (large edema)
(2) Sarcoidosis
(3) Tuberculosis
C. Demyelinating disease
(1) Multiple sclerosis
(2) Progressive multifocal leukoencephalopathy

Spinal Epidural Lymphoma

(a) invasion of epidural space through intervertebral foramen from paravertebral lymph nodes
(b) destruction of bone with vertebral collapse (less common)
(c) direct involvement of CNS (rare)

Leukemia

CNS affected in 10% of patients with acute leukemia
√ enlargement of ventricles + sulci due to atrophy (31%)
√ sulcal / fissural / cisternal enhancement (meningeal infiltration) in 5%

Prognosis: 3–5 months survival if untreated

MESIAL TEMPORAL SCLEROSIS

Cause: long-standing temporal lobe epilepsy

Histo: marked neuronal loss throughout hippocampal subfields with relative sparing of the CA2 subfield

Mechanism for excitotoxicity-induced neuronal death: seizures cause excessive neuronal depolarization which cause overproduction of excitory amino acid neurotransmitters which cause excessive activation of N-methyl-D-aspartate receptors which cause unregulated entry of Ca^{2+} which causes neuronal swelling with cytotoxic edema

√ increased signal intensity + decreased volume of hippocampus compared to contralateral side on T2WI

Associated limbic system findings:
√ ipsilateral atrophy of fornix (55%)
√ ipsilateral atrophy of mamillary body (26%)

Associated extrahippocampal abnormalities:
√ increased signal intensity of anterior temporal lobe cortex (38%)
√ cerebral hemiatrophy (1%)

MEDULLOBLASTOMA

most malignant infratentorial neoplasm; most common neoplasm of posterior fossa in childhood (followed by cerebellar astrocytoma)

Incidence: 15–20% of all pediatric intracranial tumors; 30–40% of all posterior fossa neoplasms in children; 2–10% of all intracranial gliomas

Origin: from external granular layer of inferior medullary velum (= roof of 4th ventricle)

Histo: completely undifferentiated cells (50%), desmoplastic variety (25%), glial / neuronal differentiation (25%)

Age: 40% within first 5 years of life; 75% in first decade; between ages 5–14 (2/3); between ages 15–35 (1/3); M:F = 2–4:1

• duration of symptoms <1 month prior to diagnosis: nausea, vomiting, headache, increasing head size, ataxia

Site: (a) vermis cerebelli + roof of 4th ventricle (younger age group) in 91%
(b) cerebellar hemisphere (older age group)

Size: usually >2 cm in diameter

√ well-defined vermian mass with widening of space between cerebellar tonsils
√ encroachment on 4th ventricle / aqueduct with hydrocephalus (85–95%)
√ shift / invagination of 4th ventricle
√ rapid growth with extension into cerebellar hemisphere / brainstem (more often in adults)
√ extension into cisterna magna + upper cervical cord, occasionally through foramina of Luschka into cerebellopontine angle cistern
√ mild / moderate surrounding edema (90%)

CT:
<u>Classic features</u> in 53%:
√ slightly hyperdense (70%) / isodense (20%) / mixed (10%) lesion
√ rapid intense homogeneous enhancement (97%) due to usually solid tumor

<u>Atypical features</u>:
√ cystic / necrotic areas (10–16%) with lack of enhancement
√ calcifications in 13%
√ hemorrhage in 3%
√ supratentorial extension

MR:
√ mixed / hypointense on T1WI
√ hypo- / iso- / hyperintense on T2WI
√ usually homogeneous Gd-DTPA enhancement with hypointense rim
√ cerebellar folia blurred

Cx: (1) Subarachnoid metastatic spread (30–100%) via CSF pathway to spinal cord + cauda equina ("drop metastases" in 40%), cerebral convexities, sylvian fissure, suprasellar cistern, retrograde into lateral + 3rd ventricle
√ continuous "frosting" of tumor on pia
(2) Metastases outside CNS (axial skeleton, lymph nodes, lung) after surgery

Rx: surgery + radiation therapy (extremely radiosensitive)

DDx of midline medulloblastoma:
ependymoma, astrocytoma (hypodense)

DDx of eccentric medulloblastoma:
astrocytoma, meningioma, acoustic neuroma

MENINGIOMA

Incidence: most common extra-axial tumor; 15–18% of intracranial tumors in adults; 1–2% of primary brain tumors in children; 33% of all incidental intracranial neoplasms

Origin: derived from meningothelial cells concentrated in arachnoid villi (= "arachnoid cap cells") which penetrate the dura (villi are numerous in large dural sinuses, in smaller veins, along root sleeves of exiting cranial + spinal nerves, choroid plexus)

Histologic classification:
— benign behavior pattern
(a) fibroblastic type = fibrous type
interwoven bands of spindle cells + collagen + reticulin fibers
(b) transitional type = mixed type
features of meningothelial + fibroblastic forms
— aggressive imaging appearance
(c) meningothelial = syncytial type
forming a syncytium of closely packed cells with indistinct borders
(d) angioblastic / malignant type
probably hemangiopericytoma / hemangioblastoma arising from vascular pericytes

Age: peak incidence 45 years (range 35–70 years); rare <20 years (in children >50% malignant, M > F); M:F = 1:2 to 1:4

Associated with: type 2 neurofibromatosis (multiple meningiomas, occurrence in childhood)
◊ 10% of patients with multiple meningiomas have type 2 neurofibromatosis!
◊ Most common radiation-induced CNS tumor with latency period of 19–35 years varying with dosage!

Types:
(1) Globular meningioma (most common):
compact rounded mass with invagination of brain; flat at base; contact to falx / tentorium / basal dura / convexity dura
(2) Meningioma en plaque:
pronounced hyperostosis of adjacent bone particularly along base of skull; difficult to distinguish hyperostosis from tumor cloaking the inner table (DDx: Paget disease, chronic osteomyelitis, fibrous dysplasia, metastasis)
(3) Multicentric meningioma (2–9%):
16% in autopsy series; tendency to localize to a single hemicranium; present clinically at earlier age; global / mixed; CSF seeding is exceptional; in 50% associated with neurofibromatosis type 2

Location:
(a) convexity = lateral hemisphere (20–34%)
(b) parasagittal = medial hemisphere (18–22%)
— falcine meningioma (5%) below superior sagittal sinus, usually extending to both sides
(c) sphenoid ridge + middle cranial fossa (17–25%)
(d) frontobasal (10%)
(e) posterior fossa (9–15%)
— cerebellar convexity (5%)
— tentorium cerebelli (2–4%)
— cerebellopontine angle (2–4%)
— clivus (<1%)
(f) spine (12%)

Atypical location:
(a) cerebellopontine angle (<5%)
(b) optic nerve sheath (<2%)
(c) intraventricular (2–5%): 80% in lateral (L > R), 15% in 3rd, 5% in 4th ventricle; from infolding of meningeal tissue during formation of choroid plexus
◊ Most common trigonal intraventricular mass in adulthood!
(d) ectopic = extradural (<1%): intradiploic space, outer table of skull, scalp, paranasal sinus, parotid gland, parapharyngeal space, mediastinum, lung, adrenal gland

Plain film:
√ hyperostosis at site close to / within bone (exostosis, enostosis, sclerosis)
◊ Hyperostosis does NOT indicate tumor infiltration!
√ blistering at paranasal sinuses (ethmoid, sphenoid) ± sclerosis (= pneumosinus dilatans)
√ enlarged meningeal grooves (if location in vault), enlarged foramen spinosum
√ calcification (= psammoma bodies)

CT:
√ sharply demarcated well-circumscribed slowly growing mass
√ wide attachment to adjacent dura mater
√ "cortical buckling" of underlying brain
√ isodense / hyperdense lesion (psammomatous calcifications) on NECT
√ calcifications in circular / radial pattern (20%) (DDx: osteoma)
√ "intraosseous meningioma" = permeation of bone with intra- and extracerebral soft-tissue component (DDx: fibrous dysplasia)
√ hyperostosis of adjacent bone (18%)
√ intense uniform enhancement on CECT (absence of blood-brain barrier)
√ minimal peritumoral edema (in up to 75%): NO correlation between tumor size + amount of edema (DDx: intra-axial lesion)
√ cystic component: major in 2%, minor in 15%

MR (100% detection rate with gadolinium DTPA):
- √ hypo- to isointense on T1WI + iso- to hyperintense on T2WI (intensity depends on amount of cellularity versus collagen elements)
- √ homogeneous / heterogeneous texture (tumor vascularity, cystic changes, calcifications)
- √ arcuate bowing of white matter + cortical effacement
- √ tumor-brain interface of low-intensity vessels + high-intensity cerebrospinal cleft on T2WI
- √ contrast enhancement for 3–60 minutes on T1WI as high as 148% over brain parenchyma
- √ "dural tail" sign = curvilinear area of enhancement tapering off from the margin of tumor along dural surface in 60% (= dural tumor infiltration / reactive hypervascularity / reactive hyperplastic changes)

Angio:
- √ "mother-in-law" phenomenon (contrast material shows up early and stays late into venous phase)
- √ "sunburst" / "spoke-wheel" pattern of tumor vascularity with hypervascular cloudlike stain
- √ early draining vein (rare: perhaps in angioblastic meningioma)
- √ en plaque meningioma is poorly vascularized

Vascular supply:
- A. External carotid artery (almost always):
  1. vault: middle meningeal artery
  2. sphenoid plane + tuberculum: recurrent meningeal branch of ophthalmic a.
  3. tentorium: meningeal branch of meningohypophyseal trunk of ICA
  4. clivus + posterior fossa: vertebral artery / ascending pharyngeal artery
  5. falx: partly middle meningeal artery + others
- B. Internal carotid artery (rare):
  1. intraventricular: choroidal vessels

Cx: local invasion of venous sinuses

ATYPICAL MENINGIOMA (15%)
1. Low attenuation area of necrosis, old hemorrhage, cyst formation, fat (DDx: malignant glioma, metastasis)
   - (a) **Cystic meningioma** (2–4%)
     Frequency: 55–65% in 1st year of life; 10% in children
     type I = intratumoral central / eccentric cyst (ischemic necrosis, microcystic degeneration, breakdown of hemorrhagic products); often associated with meningothelial / microcystic / atypical / malignant histologic subtypes
     type II = extratumoral intraparenchymal cyst (arachnoid cyst / reactive gliosis / liquefactive necrosis of adjacent brain)
     type III = trapped CSF (DDx: cystic / necrotic glioma)
   - (b) **Lipoblastic meningioma** (5%)
     metaplastic change of meningothelial cells into adipocytes
2. Heterogeneous / ring enhancement (secondary to bland tumor infarction / necrosis in aggressive histologic variants / true cyst formation from benign fluid accumulation)
3. "En plaque" morphology
4. "Comma shape" = combination of semilunar component bounded by dural interface + spherical component growing beyond dural margin
5. Sarcomatous transformation with spread over hemisphere + invasion of cerebral parenchyma (leptomeningeal supply)
6. **Meningeal hemangiopericytoma**
   - √ multilobulated contour
   - √ narrow dural base / "mushroom" shape
   - √ large intratumoral vascular signals
   - √ bone erosion
   - √ prominent peritumoral edema
   - √ multiple irregular feeding vessels on angiogram

Sphenoid Wing Meningioma

1. Hyperostotic meningioma en plaque
   - slowly progressive unilateral painless exophthalmos
   - numbness in distribution of cranial nerve $V_1 + V_2$
   - headaches, seizures
2. Meningioma arising from middle third of sphenoid ridge
   - headaches, seizures
   - √ compression of regional frontal + temporal lobes
3. Meningioma arising from clinoid process
   - √ encasement of carotid + middle cerebral arteries
   - √ compression of optic nerve + chiasm
4. Meningioma of planum sphenoidale
   - √ subfrontal growth + posterior growth into sella turcica and clivus
   - √ hyperostotic blistering of planum sphenoidale

Suprasellar Meningioma

Incidence: 10% of all intracranial meningiomas
Origin: from arachnoid + dura along tuberculum sellae / clinoids / diaphragma sellae / cavernous sinus with secondary extension into sella; NOT from within pituitary fossa

- • hypothalamic / pituitary dysfunction (rare)
- √ irregular hyperostosis = blistering adjacent to sinus (HALLMARK of meningiomas at planum sphenoidale / tuberculum sellae)
- √ pneumatosis sphenoidale = increased pneumatization of sphenoid in area of anterior clinoids + dorsum sellae (DDx: normal variant)
- √ broad base of attachment
- √ intense homogeneous enhancement (may be impossible to differentiate from supraclinoid carotid aneurysm on CT)
- √ blood supply: posterior ethmoidal branches of ophthalmic artery, branches of meningohypophyseal trunk

MR:
- √ large mass isointense to gray matter on T1WI + T2WI

√ hyperintense flattened pituitary gland within floor of sella
√ marked homogeneous enhancement on T1WI
DDx: metastasis, glioma, lymphoma

MENINGITIS

1. Pachymeningitis: affecting dura mater
2. Leptomeningitis: affecting pia matter / arachnoid (most common)

• headaches, stiff neck
• confusion, disorientation
• positive CSF lab analysis

ROLE of CT and MR:
(1) to exclude parenchymal abscess, ventriculitis, localized empyema
(2) to evaluate paranasal sinuses / temporal bone as source of infection
(3) to monitor complications: hydrocephalus, subdural effusion, infarction

Purulent Meningitis

Cause: otitis media / sinusitis
Organism:
(a) adults: Meningococcus, Streptococcus pneumoniae, Haemophilus influenzae, Neisseria meningitidis, Staphylococcus aureus
(b) children: Escherichia coli, Citrobacter, b-hemolytic Streptococcus

NECT:
√ often normal
√ increased density in subarachnoid space (increased vascularity), esp. in children
√ small ventricles secondary to diffuse cerebral edema

CECT:
√ marked curvilinear meningeal enhancement over cerebrum (frontal + parietal lobes) and interhemispheric + sylvian fissures
√ obliteration of basal cisterns with enhancement (common)

MR (most sensitive modality):
√ hyperintense plaques on T2WI
√ leptomeningeal enhancement with Gd-DTPA

Cx:
(1) Cerebritis
(2) Ventriculitis = ependymitis (secondary to retrograde spread)
(3) Brain atrophy
(4) Brain infarction (arteritis, venous thrombosis)
(5) Subdural effusion [sterile subdural effusion secondary to H. influenzae meningitis (in children) may turn into empyema]
(6) Hydrocephalus (cellular debris blocking foramen of Monro, aqueduct, 4th ventricular outlet / intraventricular septa / arachnoid adhesions)
(7) Cranial nerve dysfunction

Prognosis:
◊ Cerebral infarction + edema are predictive of poor outcome
◊ Enlargement of ventricles + subarachnoid spaces + subdural effusions have no predictive value

Mortality: 10% (5th common cause of death in children between 1 and 4 years of age)
DDx: meningeal carcinomatosis

Granulomatous Meningitis

Histo: thick exudate, perivascular inflammation, granulation tissue + reactive fibrosis
(1) Tuberculous meningitis = basilar meningitis: part of generalized miliary tuberculosis / primary tuberculous infection; in infants + small children
(2) Sarcoidosis
may be associated with single / multiple intracerebral masses
(3) Fungal meningitis: cryptococcosis, candidiasis, coccidioidomycosis (endemic), blastomycosis, mucormycosis (diabetics), nocardiosis, actinomycosis, aspergillosis (under chronic corticosteroid therapy)

• acute life-threatening process / chronic indolent disease

May be associated with: cerebritis, abscess formation
√ hydrocephalus

CT:
√ obliteration of basal cisterns, sylvian fissure, suprasellar cistern (isodense cisterns secondary to filling with debris)
√ intense contrast enhancement of gyri + involved subarachnoid spaces
√ calcification of meninges
√ decreased attenuation of white matter

MR:
√ high-signal intensity of basilar cisterns on T2WI
√ enhancement with gadopentetate dimeglumine

Cx: (1) hydrocephalus (obliteration of basal cisterns; blocking of CSF flow + CSF absorption)
(2) infarction (due to arteritis)

METACHROMATIC LEUKODYSTROPHY

= MLD = most common hereditary (autosomal recessive) leukodystrophy (dysmyelinating disorder)

Cause: deficiency of arylsulfatase A resulting in severe deficiency of myelin lipid sulfatide within macrophages + Schwann cells
Age of presentation: before age 3 (2/3), in adolescence (1/3)

A. LATE INFANTILE FORM
Age: 2nd year of life
• gait disorder + strabismus
• impairment of speech
• spasticity + tremor
• intellectual deterioration

Prognosis: death within 4 years of onset

B. JUVENILE FORM
Age: 5–7 years

C. ADULT FORM
• organic mental syndrome

- progressive corticospinal, corticobulbar, cerebellar, extrapyramidal signs

√ progressive loss of hemispheric brain tissue
CT:
√ symmetric low density of white matter adjacent to ventricles (esp. centrum ovale and frontal horns)
√ progressive atrophy
√ no contrast enhancement
MR:
√ progressive symmetrical areas of hypointensity on T1WI
√ hyperintensity on T2WI (increased water)
Prognosis: death within several years

METASTASES TO BRAIN

Incidence: 14–37% of all intracranial tumors
Metastatic primary:
Six tumors account for 95% of all brain metastases:
1. Bronchial carcinoma (47%): RARELY squamous cell carcinoma
2. Breast carcinoma (17%)
3. GI-tract tumors (15%): colon, rectum
4. Hypernephroma (10%)
5. Melanoma (8%)
6. Choriocarcinoma

In childhood:
1. Leukemia / lymphoma
2. Neuroblastoma

◊ Brain metastases from sarcomas are exceptionally rare!
Location:
(a) corticomedullary junction of brain (most characteristic)
(b) subarachnoid space = carcinomatous meningitis (15%)
(c) subependymal spread (frequent in breast carcinoma)
(d) skull (5%)

HEMORRHAGIC METASTASES (in 3–4%):
1. Malignant melanoma
2. Choriocarcinoma
3. Oat cell carcinoma of lung
4. Renal cell carcinoma
5. Thyroid carcinoma

√ hyperdense without contrast
√ hypervascular with contrast
mnemonic: "MATCH"
Melanoma
Anaplastic lung carcinoma
Thyroid carcinoma
Choriocarcinoma
Hypernephroma

CYSTIC METASTASES:
1. Squamous cell carcinoma of lung
2. Adenocarcinoma of lung

CALCIFIED METASTASES:
1. Mucin-producing neoplasm
2. Cartilage- / bone-forming sarcoma
3. Effective radiochemotherapy

Presentation:
— multiple lesions (2/3), single lesion (1/3)
— cerebral hemispheres (57%), cerebellum (29%), brainstem (32%)
— nodular deposits to dura are common

√ multiple lesions of different sizes + locations
√ surrounding edema usually exceeds tumor volume
CT:
√ solid enhancement in small tumors / ringlike enhancement in large tumors
MR: (a combination of T2WI + contrast-enhanced T1WI offer greatest sensitivity)
√ hypointense mass relative to edema on T2WI
√ hypointensity more pronounced in melanoma + mucinous adenocarcinoma (paramagnetic effect)
√ homogeneous / ring / nodular mixed enhancement after Gd-DTPA; often more than one metastatic focus identified in region of colliding edema
√ asymmetric enhancement of dura with dural spread
√ leptomeningeal enhancement (eg, in metastatic ependymoma)

MICROCEPHALY

= clinical syndrome characterized by a head circumference below the normal range
Incidence: 1.6:1,000 or 1:6,200–1:8,500 births
Etiology:
(1) Undiagnosed intrauterine infection (toxoplasmosis, rubella, CMV, herpes, syphilis), toxic agents, drugs hypoxia, radiation, maternal phenylketonuria
(2) Premature craniosynostosis
(3) Chromosomal abnormalities (trisomies 13, 18, 21)
(4) Meckel-Gruber syndrome

Often associated with:
micrencephaly, macrogyria, pachygyria, atrophy of basal ganglia, decrease in dendritic arborization, holoprosencephaly
√ AC:HC discrepancy
√ head circumference <3 S.D. below the mean
√ apelike sloping of forehead
√ dilatation of lateral ventricles
√ poor growth of fetal cranium
√ intracranial contents may not be visible (rare)
Prognosis: normal to severe mental retardation (depending on degree of microcephaly)

MINERALIZING MICROANGIOPATHY

= RADIATION-INDUCED LEUKOENCEPHALOPATHY
= sequelae of radiotherapy combined with methotrexate therapy for leukemia
Incidence: in 25–30% after >9 months after treatment
Age: childhood
Cause: deposition of calcium within small vessels of previously irradiated brain parenchyma
- 85% without neurologic deficits

CT:
√ thin reticular / serrated linear / punctate calcifications near corticomedullary junction, especially in basal ganglia + frontal and posterior parietal lobes

√ symmetric low-attenuation process in white matter near corticomedullary area

MR:

√ confluent diffuse periventricular distribution spreading peripherally with an irregular scalloped edge

MOYAMOYA DISEASE

= progressive obstructive / occlusive cerebral arteritis affecting distal ICA at bifurcation into its branches (anterior 2/3 of circle of Willis), usually involving both hemispheres

Etiology: unknown

Age: predominantly in children + young adults

Path: endothelial hyperplasia + fibrosis without associated inflammatory reaction

- headaches
- behavioral disturbances
- recurrent hemiparetic attacks

√ bilateral stenosis / occlusion of supraclinoid portion of internal carotid extending to proximal portions of middle + anterior cerebral arteries

√ large network of vessels in basal ganglia ("puff of smoke") + upper brainstem fed by basilar artery, anterior + middle cerebral arteries (dilatation of lenticulostriate + thalamoperforating arteries)

√ anastomoses between dural meningeal + leptomeningeal arteries

Cx: subarachnoid hemorrhage (occasionally)

Moyamoya Syndrome

Etiology: neurocutaneous syndromes (neurofibromatosis), bacterial meningitis, periarteritis nodosa, head trauma, tuberculosis, oral contraceptives, atherosclerosis, sickle cell anemia

MULTIPE SCLEROSIS

= most frequent form of chronic inflammatory demyelinating disease of unknown etiology, which reduces the lipid content and brain volume; characterized by a relapsing + remitting course

Prevalence: 6:10,000 (higher frequency in cooler climates; increased incidence with positive family history)

Cause: ? viral / autoimmune mechanism

Peak age: 25–30 (range of 20–50) years; M:F = 2:3

Histo:

(a) acute stage: perivenular inflammation (at junctions of pial veins) with
  — hypercellularity (= infiltration of lipid-laden macrophages + lymphocytes)
  — well-demarcated demyelination (destruction of oligodendroglia with loss of myelin sheath)
  — reactive astrocytosis (= gliosis), initially with preservation of axons (= denuded axons) resulting in scar (= white matter plaque)

(b) chronic stage: plaques advance to fibrillary gliosis with reduction in inflammatory component

Clinical forms: (a) relapsing remitting
(b) relapsing progressive
(c) chronic progressive

- waxing and waning course with
  - numbness, dysesthesia, burning sensations
  - signs of brain neoplasm: headaches, seizures, dizziness, nausea, weakness, altered mental status
  - ataxia, diplopia
  - optic neuritis = retrobulbar pain, central loss of vision, afferent pupillary defect (Marcus Gunn pupil)
  - trigeminal neuralgia (1–2%)
- Schumacher criteria:
  (1) CNS dysfunction (2) involvement of two / more parts of CNS (3) predominant white matter involvement (4) two / more episodes lasting >24 hours less than 1 month apart (5) slow stepwise progression of signs + symptoms (6) at onset 10–50 years of age
- Rudick red flags (suggests diagnosis other than MS):
  (1) no eye findings (2) no clinical remission (3) totally local disease (4) no sensory findings (5) no bladder involvement (6) no CSF abnormality

@ Brain

◊ number + extent of plaques correlate with duration of disease + degree of cognitive impairment

Location:
subependymal periventricular location (along lateral aspects of atria + occipital horns), corpus callosum, internal capsule, centrum semiovale, corona radiata, optic nerves, chiasm, optic tract, brainstem (ventrolateral aspect of pons at 5th nerve root entry), cerebellar peduncles, cerebellum; rather symmetric involvement of cerebral hemispheres; subcortical U fibers NOT spared

√ lesion size: 1–25 (majority between 5 and 10) mm
  √ large lesions may masquerade as brain tumors

√ lesions usually without mass effect / edema unless acute

√ ovoid lesions (86%) oriented with their long axis perpendicular to ventricular walls (due to perivenous demyelination; pathologically described as "Dawson fingers")

√ chronic plaques do not enhance (due to intact blood-brain barrier)

CT:

√ normal CT scan (18%)

√ nonspecific atrophy of brain (45%): enlarged ventricles, prominent sulci

√ periventricular (near atria) multifocal nonconfluent lesions with distinct margins (location not always correlating well with symptoms)
  (a) NECT: isodense / lucent
  (b) CECT: transient enhancement during acute stage (active demyelination) for about 2 weeks; may require double dose of contrast; ultimately disappearance / permanent scar

MR (modality of choice; 95% specific):

√ well-marginated discrete foci of varying size with high-signal intensity on T2WI + proton density images (= loss of hydrophobic myelin produces increase in water content); hypointense on T1WI

√ Gd-DTPA enhancement of lesions on T1WI (up to 8 weeks following acute demyelination with breakdown of blood-brain barrier)
√ lesions on undersurface of corpus callosum (CHARACTERISTIC sagittal images)

@ Spinal cord
◊ Most common demyelinating process of spinal cord!
◊ In 12% without coexistent intracranial plaques!
• number + extent of plaques correlate with degree of disability
Location: predilection for cervical region
Site: eccentric involvement of dorsal + lateral elements abutting subarachnoid space
√ atrophic plaques oriented along spinal cord axis
√ length of plaque usually less than 2 vertebral body segments + width less than half of cross section
√ acute tumefactive MS = cord swelling + enhancement
DDx: (1) Cord tumor (follow-up after 6 weeks without decrease in size of lesion)
(2) Infection
(3) Acute transverse myelitis (after viral illness / vaccination)

Rx: steroids (inciting rapid decrease in size of lesions + loss of enhancement)
DDx:
(1) White matter ischemic disease (patients >50 years of age, lesions <5 mm, not infratentorial)
(2) Acute disseminated encephalomyelitis, subacute sclerosing panencephalitis (lesions of similar age)
(3) AIDS, CNS vasculitis, migraine, radiation injury, lymphoma, sarcoidosis, tuberculosis, systemic lupus erythematosus, cysticercosis, metastases, multifocal glioma, neurofibromatosis, contusions

MYELINOCLASTIC DIFFUSE SCLEROSIS
= SCHILDER DISEASE
= rare demyelinating disorder with episodic recurrence and remission
Age: children > adults; M:F = 1:1
Histo: selective confluent demyelination with relative axonal sparing, perivascular inflammatory infiltrate, reactive astrocytosis (indistinguishable from multiple sclerosis)
• hemiplegia, aphasia, ataxia, blindness
• swallowing difficulties, progressive dementia
• increased intracranial pressure
Location: centrum semiovale
√ large bilateral white matter lesions with mass effect
√ enhancement with IV contrast material
Rx: usually responsive to corticosteroids
DDx: (1) Acute disseminated encephalomyelitis (history of recent viral illness, monophasic course, lesions less confluent, no mass effect / enhancement)
(2) Adrenoleukodystrophy (bilaterally symmetric, confluent lesions, parietal location)
(3) Tumor, abscess, infarct

NEONATAL INTRACRANIAL HEMORRHAGE
Germinal Matrix Bleed
= GERMINAL MATRIX–RELATED HEMORRHAGE

Germinal matrix
= highly vascular gelatinous subependymal tissue adjacent to lateral ventricles in which the cells that compose the brain are generated; has its largest volume around 26 weeks GA; decreases in size with increasing fetal maturity; usually involutes by 32–34 weeks of gestation
Location: greatest portion of germinal matrix above caudate nucleus in floor of lateral ventricle, tapering as it sweeps from frontal horn posteriorly into temporal horn, roof of 3rd + 4th ventricle
Arterial supply: via Heubner artery from ACA, striate branches of MCA, anterior choroidal a., perforating branches from meningeal aa.
Capillary network: persisting immature vascular rete = large irregular endothelial-lined channels devoid of connective tissue support (collagen and muscle)
Venous drainage: terminal vv., choroidal v., thalamostriate v. course anteriorly + feed into internal cerebral v. which has a posterior course

Risk factors:
(1) prematurity (2) low birth weight (3) sex (M:F = 2:1)
(4) multiple gestations (5) trauma at delivery
(6) prolonged labor (7) hyperosmolarity
(8) hypocoagulation (9) pneumothorax (10) patent ductus arteriosus
Etiology: hypoxia with loss of autoregulation
Pathogenesis: rupture of friable vascular bed due to
(1) fluctuating cerebral blood flow in preterm infants with respiratory distress
(2) increase in cerebral blood flow with
(a) systemic hypertension (pneumothorax, REM sleep, handling, tracheal suctioning, ligation of PDA, seizures, instillation of mydriatics)
(b) Rapid volume expansion (blood, colloid, hyperosmolar glucose / sodium bicarbonate)
(c) Hypercarbia (RDS, asphyxia)
(3) increase in cerebral venous pressure with labor and delivery, asphyxia (= impairment in exchange of oxygen and carbon dioxide), respiratory disturbances
(4) decrease in cerebral blood flow with systemic hypotension followed by reperfusion
(5) platelet and coagulation disturbance

Incidence: in premature neonates <32 weeks of age; in 43% of infants <1,500 g (in 65% of 500–700 g infants, in 25% of 701–1,500 g infants) ; in up to 50% without prenatal care, in 5–10% with prenatal care

Location: region of the caudate nucleus and thalamostriate groove (= caudothalamic notch) remains metabolically active the longest; in 80–90% in infants <28 weeks of MA age

Time of onset: 36% on first day, 32% on second day, 18% on first 3 day of life; by 6th day 91% of all intracranial bleeds have occurred

GRADES (Papile classification)

- I : subependymal hemorrhage confined to germinal matrix (GMH) on one / both sides
- II : subependymal hemorrhage ruptured into nondilated ventricle (IVH)
- III : intraventricular hemorrhage (IVH) with ventricular enlargement: (a) mild, (b) moderate, (c) severe
- IV : extension of germinal matrix hemorrhage into brain parenchyma (IPH)

Serial scans: 5–10-day intervals

US (100% sensitivity + 91% specificity for lesions >5 mm; 27% sensitivity + 88% specificity for lesions ≤5 mm):

Germinal matrix hemorrhage (grade I)

√ well-defined ovoid area of increased echogenicity (= fibrin mesh within clot) inferolateral to floor of frontal horn ± body of lateral ventricle
√ bulbous enlargement of caudothalamic groove anterior to termination of choroid plexus
DDx: choroid plexus (attached to inferomedial aspect of ventricular floor, tapers toward caudothalamic groove, never anterior to foramen of Monro)
√ resolving bleed develops central sonolucency
√ outcome: (1) complete involution (2) thin echogenic scar (3) subependymal cyst

Mild intraventricular hemorrhage (grade II)

√ echogenic material filling a portion of lateral ventricles (acute phase) becoming sonolucent in a few weeks
√ clot may gravitate into occipital horns
√ vertical band of echogenicity between thalami on coronal scans (blood in 3rd ventricle)
√ irregular bulky choroid plexus (clot layered on surface of choroid plexus)
√ temporarily increased echogenicity of ventricular wall (= subependymal white halo between 7 days and 6 weeks after hemorrhagic event)

Extensive intraventricular hemorrhage (grade III)

√ intraventricular cast of blood distending the lateral ventricles
√ ± extension of hemorrhage into basal cisterns, cavum septi pellucidi
√ hemorrhage becomes progressively less echogenic
√ temporarily thickened echogenic walls of ventricles ("ventriculitis")

Intraparenchymal hemorrhage (grade IV)

Cause: (a) extension of hemorrhage originating from germinal matrix (unusual)
(b) separate hemorrhage within infarcted periventricular tissue (frequent)

Location: on side of largest amount of IVH, commonly lateral to frontal horns / in parietal lobe, rare in occipital lobe + thalamus

√ homogeneous highly echogenic intraparenchymal mass with irregular margins
√ central hypoechogenicity (liquefying hematoma after 10–14 days)
√ retracted clot settles to dependent position (3–4 weeks)
√ complete resolution by 8–10 weeks results in anechoic area (= porencephalic cyst)

CT:

Most sensitive + definite means to define site + extent of hemorrhage, especially in subdural hemorrhage, cerebral parenchymal hemorrhage, posterior fossa lesion

√ hyperdense bleed only visible up to 7 days before it becomes isodense

Cx:

(1) Posthemorrhagic hydrocephalus (30–70%)
◊ Severity of hydrocephalus directly proportional to size of original hemorrhage!
Cause:
(a) temporary blockage of arachnoid villi by particulate blood clot (within days), often transient with partial / total resolution
(b) obliterative fibrosing arachnoiditis often in cisterna magna (within weeks); frequently leads to permanent progressive ventricular dilatation (50%)
√ thickened echogenic ventricular walls
Time of onset: by 14 days (in 80%)
• delayed clinical signs because of compressible premature brain parenchyma
√ ventricular dilatation, particularly affecting the occipital horns (amount of compressible immature white matter is larger posteriorly)
DDx: ventriculomegaly secondary to periventricular cerebral atrophy (occurring slowly over several weeks)
(2) Cyst formation
(a) cavitation of hemorrhage
(b) unilocular subependymal cyst
(c) unilocular porencephalic cyst
(3) Mental retardation, cerebral palsy
(4) Death in 25% (IVH most common cause of neonatal death)

Prognosis:

(1) Grade I + II: good with normal developmental scores (12–18% risk of handicap)
(2) Grade III + IV: 54% mortality; 30–40% risk of handicap (spastic diplegia, spastic quadriparesis, intellectual retardation)

Choroid Plexus Hemorrhage

affects primarily full-term infants

Cause: birth trauma, asphyxia, apnea, seizures

√ echogenicity of choroid plexus same as hemorrhage
√ nodularity of choroid plexus
√ enlargement of choroid plexus >12 mm in AP diameter
√ left-right asymmetry >5 mm
√ intraventricular hemorrhage without subependymal hemorrhage

Cx: intraventricular hemorrhage (25%)

Intracerebellar Hemorrhage

Cause:
(a) full-term infant: traumatic delivery, intermittent positive pressure ventilation, coagulopathy
(b) premature infant: subependymal germinal matrix hemorrhage up to 30 weeks gestation

Incidence: 16–21% of autopsies

√ echogenicity of vermis same as hemorrhage
√ echogenic mass in less echogenic cerebellar hemisphere (coronal scan most useful)
√ nonvisualization / deformity of 4th ventricle
√ asymmetry in thickness of paratentorial echogenicity is a sign of subarachnoid hemorrhage

Prognosis: poor + frequently fatal

Intraventricular Hemorrhage

Etiology:
(a) germinal matrix hemorrhage ruptures through ependymal lining at multiple sites
(b) bleeding from choroid plexus

Route of hemorrhage: blood dissipates throughout ventricular system + aqueduct of Sylvius, passes through foramina of 4th ventricle, collects in basilar cistern of posterior fossa

- seizures, dystonia, obtundation, intractable acidosis
- bulging anterior fontanelle, drop in hematocrit, bloody / proteinaceous CSF

√ IVH usually cleared within 7–14 days

Cx: (1) Intracerebral hemorrhage
(2) Hydrocephalus

Periventricular Leukoencephalopathy

Periventricular Leukomalacia

= PVL = perinatal hypoxic-ischemic encephalopathy
= principal ischemic lesion of the premature infant characterized by focal coagulation necrosis of deep white matter as a result of ischemic infarction involving the watershed (= arterial border) zones between central and peripheral vascularity

Vascular supply:
(a) ventriculopedal branches penetrating cerebrum from pial surface are derived from MCA ± PCA ± ACA
(b) ventriculofugal branches extending from ventricular surface are derived from choroidal arteries ± striate arteries

Incidence:
7–22% at autopsy (88% of infants between 900 and 2,200 g surviving beyond 6 days); in 34% of infants <1,500 g; in 59% of infants surviving longer than 1 week on assisted ventilation; only 28% detected by cranial sonography

Histo: edema, white matter necrosis, evolution of cysts + cavities / diminished myelin; nonhemorrhagic : hemorrhagic PVL = 3:1

Pathogenesis:
immature autoregulation of periventricular vessels secondary to deficient muscularis of arterioles limits vasodilation in response to hypoxemia + hypercapnia + hypotension of perinatal asphyxia (hypoxic-ischemic encephalopathy)

- "cerebral palsy" (in 6.5% of infants <1,800 g)
  - spastic diplegia (81%) > quadriparesis (necrosis of descending fibers from motor cortex)
  - choreaathetosis, ataxia
  - ± mental retardation
- severe visual / hearing impairment
- convulsive disorders

Location:
bilateral white matter subjacent to external angle of lateral ventricular trigones, involving particularly the centrum semiovale (frontal horn + body), optic (occipital horn), and acoustic (temporal horn) radiations

US (50% sensitivity + 87% specificity):

Early changes (2 days to 2 weeks after insult)
√ increased periventricular echogenicity (PVE) (DDx: echogenic periventricular halo / blush of fiber tracts in normal neonates, white matter gliosis, cortical infarction extending into deep white matter)
√ bilateral often asymmetric zones, occasionally extending to cortex
√ infrequently accompanied by IVH

Late changes (1–3–6 weeks after development of echodensities):
√ periventricular cystic PVL = cystic degeneration of ischemic areas (= multiple small never septated periventricular cysts in relationship to lateral ventricles; the larger the echodensities, the sooner the cyst formation)
√ brain atrophy secondary to thinning of periventricular white matter always at trigones, occasionally involving centrum semiovale
√ ventriculomegaly (after disappearance of cysts) with irregular outline of body + trigone of lateral ventricles
√ deep prominent sulci abutting the ventricles with little / no interposed white matter (DDx: schizencephaly)
√ enlarged interhemispheric fissure

CT (not sensitive in early phase):
√ periventricular hypodensity (DDx: immature brain with increased water + incomplete myelination)

MR (not sensitive in early phase):
√ hypointense areas on T1WI
√ hyperintense periventricular signals on T2WI in peritrigonal region
√ thinning of posterior body + splenium of corpus callosum (= degeneration of transcallosal fibers)

Prognosis:
major neurologic problem / death in up to 62%; PVL localized to frontal lobes show relative normal development; generalized PVL results in neurologic deficits in close to 100%

DDx: tissue damage from ventriculitis (sequelae of meningitis), metabolic disorders, in utero ischemia (eg, maternal cocaine abuse)

Periventricular Hemorrhagic Infarction

= hemorrhagic necrosis of periventricular white matter, usually large + asymmetric

Incidence: in 15–25% of infants with IVH

Pathogenesis:
(a) germinal matrix hemorrhage with intraventricular blood clot (in 80%)
(b) ischemic periventricular leukomalacia
lead to obstruction of terminal veins with sequence of venous congestion + thrombosis + infarction

Histo: perivascular hemorrhage of medullary veins near ventricular angle

Associated with: the most severe cases of intraventricular hemorrhage

Age: peak occurrence on 4th postnatal day

• spastic hemiparesis (affecting lower + upper extremities equally) / asymmetric quadriparesis (in 86% of survivors)

Location: lateral to external angle of lateral ventricle on side of more marked IVH: 67% unilateral; 33% bilateral but asymmetric

Early changes (hours to days after major IVH):
√ unilateral / asymmetric bilateral triangular "fan-shaped" echodensities
√ extension from frontal to parietooccipital regions / localized (particularly in anterior portion of lesion)

Late changes:
√ single large cyst = porencephaly
√ bumpy ventricle / false accessory ventricle

Prognosis: 59% overall mortality with echodensities >1 cm; in 64% major intellectual deficits

Encephalomalacia

= more extensive brain damage than PVL; may include all of white matter in subcortex + cortex

Associated with:
(1) Neonatal asphyxia
(2) Vasospasm
(3) Inflammation of CNS

√ small ventricles (edema) with diffuse damage
√ increased parenchymal echogenicity making it difficult to define normal structures
√ decreased vascular pulsations
√ transcranial Doppler:
(a) group I (good prognosis)
√ normal flow profile, normal velocities, normal resistive index
(b) group II (guarded prognosis)
√ increase in peak-systolic + end-diastolic flow velocities + decreased resistive index
(c) group III (unfavorable prognosis)
√ reduced diastolic flow + decreased peak systolic and diastolic velocities + increased resistive index
√ ventricular enlargement + atrophy
√ extensive multicystic encephalomalacia with cysts often not communicating

NEUROBLASTOMA

Age at presentation: <2 years (50%); <4 years (75%); <8 years (90%); peak age <3 years

• abdominal mass (45%)
• neurologic signs (20%)
• bone pain / limp (20%)
• orbital ecchymosis / proptosis (12%)
• catecholamine production (95%) with paroxysmal episodes of flushing, tachycardia, hypertension, headaches, sweating, intractable diarrhea, acute cerebellar encephalopathy
• positive bone marrow aspiration (70%)

Location: adrenal gland (67%), chest (13%), neck (5%), intracranial (2%); commonly involvement of multiple skeletal sites

NUC (overall sensitivity of detection better than radiography):
CAVE: symmetric lytic neuroblastoma metastases occur frequently in metaphyseal areas where normal epiphyseal activity obscures lesions
√ purely lytic lesions may present as photopenic areas
√ soft-tissue uptake of Tc-99m phosphate in 60%
√ frequently Ga-67 uptake in primary site of neuroblastoma

Prognosis: 2-year survival (a) in 60% for age <1 year (b) in 20% for ages 1–2 years (c) in 10% for ages >2 years

A. PRIMARY CEREBRAL NEUROBLASTOMA (rare)
Age: childhood / early adolescence
√ large hypodense / mixed-density mass with well-defined margins
√ intratumoral coarse dense calcifications
√ central cystic / necrotic zones with hemorrhage
Cx: metastasizes via subarachnoid space to dura + calvarium

B. SECONDARY NEUROBLASTOMA (common)
metastatic to:
@ liver
@ skeleton
√ osteolysis with periosteal new-bone formation
√ sutural diastasis
√ hair-on-end appearance of skull

@ orbit:
√ unilateral proptosis
◊ Neuroblastoma usually not metastatic to brain!

Olfactory Neuroblastoma

= very malignant tumor arising from olfactory mucosa
Types: 1. Esthesioneuroepithelioma
2. Esthesioneurocytoma
3. Esthesioneuroblastoma
√ mass in superior nasal cavity with extension into ethmoid + maxillary sinuses
Cx: distant metastases in 20%

NEUROFIBROMATOSIS

= autosomal dominant inherited disorder, probably of neural crest origin affecting all 3 germ cell layers, capable of involving any organ system
Path:
pure neurofibromas (= tumor of nerve sheath with involvement of nerve, nerve fibers run through mass) + neurilemomas (nerve fibers diverge and course over the surface of the tumor mass); frequently combined
(1) discrete round mass
(2) plexiform = tortuous tangles / fusiform enlargement of peripheral nerves (PATHOGNOMONIC of neurofibromatosis type 1)
Histo: proliferation of fibroblasts + Schwann cells

Peripheral Neurofibromatosis (90%)

= NEUROFIBROMATOSIS TYPE 1 = NF-1
= VON RECKLINGHAUSEN DISEASE
= dysplasia of mesodermal + neuroectodermal tissue with potential for diffuse systemic involvement; autosomal dominant with abnormalities of long arm of chromosome **17**: *von Recklinghausen* has **17** letters; 50% spontaneous mutants; variable expressivity
Incidence: 1:2,000–4,000; M:F = 1:1; most common of phakomatoses

Diagnostic criteria (at least two must be present):
(1) >6 café-au-lait spots >5 mm in greatest diameter (>15 mm in postpubertal individuals)
(2) ≥2 neurofibromas of any type / one plexiform neurofibroma
(3) freckling in axilla / inguinal region
(4) optic glioma
(5) ≥2 Lisch nodules (= pigmented hamartomas of iris)
(6) distinctive osseous lesion (eg, sphenoid dysplasia / thinning of long bone cortex) ± pseudarthrosis
(7) first-degree relative (parent, sibling, child) with peripheral neurofibromatosis

May be associated with:
(1) MEA IIb (pheochromocytoma + medullary carcinoma of thyroid + multiple neuromas)
(2) CHD (10 fold increase): pulmonary valve stenosis, ASD, VSD, IHSS

A. CNS MANIFESTATIONS
@ Intracranial
1. Optic pathway glioma
isolated to single optic nerve ± extension to other optic nerve, chiasm, optic tracts
Histo: pilocytic astrocytoma with perineural / subarachnoid spread (optic nerve is embryologically part of hypothalamus and develops gliomas instead of schwannomas)
◊ in up to 30% of all neurofibromatosis patients
◊ 10% of all optic nerve gliomas are associated with neurofibromatosis
2. Cerebral gliomas
astrocytomas of tectum, brainstem, gliomatosis cerebri (= unusual confluence of astrocytomas)
3. Hydrocephalus
obstruction usually at aqueduct of Sylvius
Cause: benign aqueductal stenosis, glioma of tectum / tegmentum of mesencephalon
4. Vascular dysplasia
= occlusion / stenosis of distal internal carotid artery, proximal middle / anterior cerebral artery
√ moyamoya phenomenon (60–70%)
5. Schwannomas of cranial nerves 3–12 (most commonly 5 + 8)
6. Craniofacial plexiform neurofibromas
= locally aggressive congenital lesion composed of tortuous cords of Schwann cells, neurons + collagen with progression along nerve of origin (usually small unidentified nerves)
Location: commonly orbital apex, superior orbital fissure
7. CNS hamartomas (up to 75–90%)
= probably dysmyelinating lesions (may resolve)
Location: pons, basal ganglia (most commonly in globus pallidus), thalamus, cerebellar white matter
√ multiple foci of isointensity on T1WI + hyperintensity on T2WI without mass effect (= "unidentified bright objects")
8. Vacuolar / spongiotic myelinopathy (in 66%)
Location: basal ganglia (esp. in globus pallidus), cerebellum, internal capsule, brainstem
√ nonenhancing hyperintense foci on T2WI

@ Spine
1. Paraspinal neurofibromas
√ tumors of varying sizes at nearly every level throughout the spinal canal
√ enlargement of neural foramina due to "dumbbell" neurofibroma of spinal nerves
√ fusiform / spherical low-attenuation mass (20–30 HU)

√ slightly hyperintense to muscle on T1WI, hyperintense periphery + hypointense core on T2WI
√ hypoechoic well-circumscribed cylindrical lesion
√ spinal cord displaced to contralateral side

2. Lateral / intrathoracic meningocele
= diverticula of thecal sac extending through widened neural foramina
Cause: dysplasia of meninges focally stretched by CSF pulsations
Location: thoracic level (most common)
√ erosion of bony elements with marked posterior scalloping
√ widening of neural foramina (due to protrusion of spinal meninges)

B. SKELETAL MANIFESTATIONS (in 30–40–80%)
• dwarfism caused by scoliosis

@ Orbit
√ Harlequin appearance to orbit = partial absence of greater and lesser wing of sphenoid bone + orbital plate of frontal bone (failure of development of membranous bone)
√ hypoplasia + elevation of lesser wing of sphenoid
√ defect in sphenoid bone ± extension of middle cranial fossa structures into orbit
√ concentric enlargement of optic foramen (optic glioma)
√ enlargement of orbital margins + superior orbital fissure (plexiform neurofibroma of peripheral and sympathetic nerves within orbit / optic nerve glioma)
√ sclerosis in the vicinity of optic foramen (optic nerve sheath meningioma)
√ deformity + decreased size of ipsilateral ethmoid + maxillary sinus

@ Skull
√ macrocranium + macroencephaly
√ calvarial defect adjacent to left lambdoid suture = parietal mastoid (rare)

@ Spine
√ sharply angled kyphoscoliosis (50%) in lower thoracic + lumbar spine; kyphosis predominates over scoliosis; incidence increases with age
Cause: abnormal development of vertebral bodies
√ hypoplasia of pedicles, transverse + spinous processes
√ posterior scalloping of vertebral bodies with dural ectasia (secondary to weakened meninges allowing transmission of normal CSF pulsations)

@ Chest
√ twisted "ribbonlike" ribs in upper thoracic segments accompanying kyphoscoliosis
√ localized cortical notches / depression of inferior margins of ribs (DDx: aortic coarctation)
√ intrathoracic meningoceles
√ lung + mediastinal neurofibromas
√ progressive pulmonary interstitial fibrosis

@ Appendicular skeleton
√ anterolateral bowing of lower half of tibia (most common) / fibula (frequent) / upper extremity (uncommon) ± pseudarthrosis secondary to deossification with bowing-fracture in 1st year of life
√ atrophic thinned / absent fibulas
√ periosteal dysplasia = traumatic subperiosteal hemorrhage with abnormal easy detachment of periosteum from bone
√ subendosteal sclerosis
√ bone erosion from periosteal / soft-tissue neurofibromas
√ intramedullary longitudinal streaks of increased density
√ single / multiple cystic lesions within bone (? deossification / nonossifying fibroma)
√ focal gigantism = unilateral overgrowth of a limb bone; marked enlargement of a digit in a hand / foot (overgrowth of ossification center)

C. NEURAL CREST TUMORS
1. Pheochromocytoma: • hypertension in adults
2. Parathyroid adenomas: • hyperparathyroidism

D. VASCULAR LESIONS
Schwann cell proliferation within vessel wall
1. Cranial artery stenosis
2. Renal artery stenosis: very proximal, funnel-shaped (one of the most common causes of hypertension in childhood)
3. Renal artery aneurysm
4. Thoracic / abdominal aortic coarctation

E. GI TRACT MANIFESTATIONS (10–25%)
• pain, intestinal bleeding
• obstruction (simulating Hirschsprung disease (with plexiform neurofibromas of colon)
Location: jejunum > stomach > ileum > duodenum; retroperitoneal / paraspinal
Associated with: increased prevalence of carcinoid tumors + GI stromal tumors
(a) solitary pattern = single neurofibroma, neuroma, ganglioneuroma, schwannoma
√ subserosal / submucosal filling defect ("mucosal ganglioneurofibromatosis")
(b) plexiform pattern = regional enlargement of nerve root trunks
√ mass effect on adjacent barium-filled loops
√ multiple eccentric polypoid filling defects involving mesenteric side of small bowel
√ mesenteric fat trapped within entangled network (15–30 HU) CHARACTERISTIC
√ multiple leiomyomas ± ulcer
Cx: intussusception

F. OCULAR MANIFESTATIONS (6%)
- pulsatile exophthalmos / unilateral proptosis (herniation of subarachnoid space + temporal lobe into orbit)
- buphthalmos = congenital glaucoma (aberrant mesodermal tissue obstructing canal of Schlemm)

1. Plexiform neurofibroma (most common)
2. Pigmented iris hamartomas <2 mm (Lisch nodules) in >90%, mostly bilateral; appear in childhood
3. Optic glioma: in 12% of patients, in 4% bilateral; 75% in 1st decade
   √ extension into optic chiasm (up to 25%), optic tracts + optic radiation
   √ increased intensity on T2WI if chiasm + visual pathways involved
4. Perioptic meningioma
5. Choroidal hamartoma: in 50% of patients

G. SKIN MANIFESTATIONS
1. Café-au-lait spots
   of "coast of California" type (= smooth outline):
   ≥6 in number >5 mm in greatest diameter
   usually develop within 1st year of life / >15 mm in size in postpubertal individuals
2. Axillary freckling (in 66%)
3. Cutaneous neurofibroma
   begin to appear around puberty
   (a) localized = fibroma molluscum = string of pearls along peripheral nerve
   (b) plexiform neurofibroma = elephantiasis neuromatosa

Cx: malignant transformation to malignant neurofibromas + malignant schwannomas (3–15%), glioma, xanthomatous leukemia

Neurofibromatosis with Bilateral Acoustic Neuromas

= NEUROFIBROMATOSIS TYPE 2 = NF-2
= CENTRAL NEUROFIBROMATOSIS
= rare autosomal dominant syndrome characterized by propensity for developing multiple schwannomas, meningiomas, and gliomas of ependymal derivation

mnemonic: "MISME"
Multiple **I**nherited **S**chwannomas
Meningiomas
Ependymomas

Incidence: 1:50,000 births
Etiology: deletion on the long arm of chromosome 22; in 50% new spontaneous mutation
◊ Neurofibromatosis **2** is located on chromosome **22**!
Symptomatic age: during 2nd / 3rd decade of life
Diagnostic criteria:
(1) Bilateral 8th cranial nerve masses
(2) First-degree relative with unilateral 8th nerve mass, neurofibroma, meningioma, glioma (spinal ependymoma), schwannoma, juvenile posterior subcapsular lenticular opacity

- NO Lisch nodules, skeletal dysplasia, optic pathway glioma, vascular dysplasia, learning disability
- café-au-lait spots (<50%): pale, <5 in number
- cutaneous neurofibroma: minimal in size + number / absent

@ Intracranial
1. Bilateral acoustic schwannomas (*sine qua non*)
   Site: superior / inferior division of vestibular n.
   √ usually asymmetric in size
2. Schwannoma of other cranial nerves
   Frequency: trigeminal n. > facial n.
   ◊ Nerves without Schwann cells are excluded: olfactory nerve, optic nerve
3. Multiple meningiomas: intraventricular in choroid plexus of trigone, parasagittal, sphenoid ridge, olfactory groove, along intracranial nerves
4. Meningiomatosis = dura studded with innumerable small meningiomas
5. Glioma of ependymal derivation

@ Spinal
- symptoms of cord compression

A. Extramedullary
   1. Multiple paraspinal neurofibromas
   2. Meningioma of spinal cord (thoracic region)
B. Intramedullary
   1. Spinal cord ependymomas

NEUROMA

Prevalence: 8% of all intracranial tumors
Age: 20–50 years
- slow growth; not painful

Acoustic Neuroma

= VESTIBULAR SCHWANNOMA = ACOUSTIC SCHWANNOMA = NEURILEMMOMA
◊ Most common neoplasm of internal auditory canal / cerebellopontine angle!
Prevalence: 5–10% of all intracranial tumors; 85% of all intracranial neuromas; 80–90% of all cerebellopontine angle tumors
Age: (a) sporadic tumor: 35–60 years; M:F = 1:2
(b) type 2 neurofibromatosis: 2nd decade
Histo:
encapsulated neoplasm composed of proliferating fusiform Schwann cells with
(a) highly cellular dense regions (Antoni A) with reticulin + collagen, and
(b) loose areas with widely separated cells (Antoni B) in a reticulated myxoid matrix; common degenerative changes with cyst formation, vascular features, lipid-laden foam cells
May be associated with: central neurofibromatosis
◊ Solitary intracranial schwannoma is associated with type 2 neurofibromatosis in 5–25%!
◊ Bilateral acoustic schwannomas allow a presumptive diagnosis of type 2 neurofibromatosis!

- long history of slowly progressive unilateral sensorineural hearing loss affecting high-frequency sounds more severely (in 95%)

- tinnitus
- diminished corneal reflex
- unsteadiness, vertigo, ataxia, dizziness (<10%)
- pain

Doubling time: 2 years

Location:
(a) arises from within internal auditory canal (IAC)
(b) may arise in cerebellopontine angle cistern at opening of IAC (= porus acusticus) with intracanalicular extension in 5%

Site: (a) in 85% from the vestibular portion of 8th nerve (around vestibular ganglion of Scarpa / at the glial-Schwann cell junction)
(b) in 15% from the cochlear portion

√ round mass centered on long axis of IAC forming acute angles with petrous bone
√ funnel-shaped component extending into IAC
√ IAC enlargement / erosion (70–90%)
√ widening / obliteration of ipsilateral cerebellopontine angle cistern
√ shift / asymmetry of 4th ventricle with hydrocephalus
√ degenerative changes (cystic areas ± hemorrhage) with tumors >2–3 cm

Plain film:
√ erosion of IAC: a difference in canal height of >2 mm is abnormal + indicates a schwannoma in 93%

CT:
√ isodense small / hypodense large solid tumor
√ cyst formation in tumor (= central necrosis) / adjacent to tumor (= extramural arachnoid cyst) in 15% of large tumors
√ usually uniformly dense tumor enhancement with small tumors (50% may be missed without CECT) / ring enhancement with large tumors
√ NO calcification
√ intrathecal contrast / carbon dioxide insufflation (for tumors <5 mm)

MR (most sensitive test with Gd-DTPA enhancement):
√ iso- / slightly hypointense on T1WI relative to brain
√ intensely enhancing homogeneous mass / ringlike enhancement (if cystic) after Gd-DTPA
√ hyperintense on T2WI (DDx: meningioma remains hypo- / isointense)

Angio:
√ elevation + posterior displacement of anterior inferior cerebellar artery (AICA) on basal view
√ elevation of the superior cerebellar artery (large tumors)
√ displacement of basilar artery anteriorly / posteriorly + contralateral side
√ compression / posterior + lateral displacement of petrosal vein
√ posterior displacement of choroid point of PICA
√ vascular supply frequently from external carotid artery branches
√ rarely hypervascular tumor with tumor blush

DDx: ossifying hemangioma (bony spiculations)

Trigeminal Neuroma

= TRIGEMINAL SCHWANNOMA

Incidence: 2–5% of intracranial neuromas, 0.26% of all brain tumors

Origin: arising from gasserian ganglion within Meckel cave at the most anteromedial portion of the petrous pyramid / trigeminal nerve root

Age: 35–60 years; M:F = 1:2

Symptoms of location in middle cranial fossa:
- facial paresthesia / hypesthesia
- exophthalmos, ophthalmoplegia

Symptoms of location in posterior cranial fossa:
- facial nerve palsy
- hearing impairment, tinnitus
- ataxia, nystagmus

Location: (in any segment of trigeminal nerve)
(a) middle cranial fossa (46%) = gasserian ganglion
(b) posterior cranial fossa (29%)
(c) in both fossae (25%)
(d) pterygoid fossa / paranasal sinuses (10%)

√ erosion of petrous tip
√ enlargement of contiguous fissures, foramina, canals
√ dumbbell / saddle-shaped mass (extension into middle cranial fossa + through tentorial incisura into posterior fossa)
√ isodense mass with dense inhomogeneous enhancement (tumor necrosis + cyst formation)
√ distortion of ipsilateral quadrigeminal cistern
√ displacement + cutoff of posterior 3rd ventricle
√ anterior displacement of temporal horn
√ angiographically avascular / hypervascular mass

OLIGODENDROGLIOMA

= uncommon form of slowly growing glioma; presenting with large size at time of diagnosis

Incidence: 2–10% of intracranial gliomas; 5–7% of all primary intracranial neoplasms

Histo: mixed glial cells (50%), astrocytic components (30%); hemorrhage + cyst formation infrequent

Age: 30–50 years

- seizures

Location: most commonly in cerebral hemispheres (propensity for periphery of frontal lobes) involving cortex + white matter, thalamus, corpus callosum; occasionally around / in ventricles ("subependymal oligodendroglioma") rare in cerebellum + spinal cord

√ large nodular clumps of calcifications (in 45% on plain film; in 90% on CT)

CT:
√ round / oval hypodense lesion with mass effect (75%)
√ commonly no / minimal tumor enhancement (75%), pronounced in high-grade tumors
√ may be adherent to dura (mimicking meningiomas)
√ ± erosion of inner table of skull
√ cystic changes (uncommon)
√ edema (in 50% of low-grade, in 80% of high-grade tumors)

MR:
√ well-circumscribed heterogeneous hypointense lesion on T1WI + hyperintense on T2WI
√ little edema / mass effect
√ solid / peripheral / mixed enhancement
√ calcification may not be detected

Cx: malignant metaplasia + CSF seeding

DDx: (1) Astrocytoma (no large calcifications)
(2) Ganglioglioma (in temporal lobes + deep cerebral tissues
(3) Ependymoma (enhancing tumor, often with internal bleeding producing fluid levels)
(4) Glioblastoma (infiltrating, enhancing, edema, no calcifications)

PARAGONIMIASIS OF BRAIN

Oriental lung fluke (Paragonimus westermani) producing arachnoiditis, parenchymal granulomas, encapsulated abscesses
√ isodense / inhomogeneous masses surrounded by edema
√ ring enhancement

PELIZAEUS-MERZBACHER DISEASE

= rare X-linked sudanophilic leukodystrophy (5 types with different times of onset, rate of progression, genetic transmission)

Age: neonatal period

- bizarre pendular nystagmus + head shaking
- cerebellar ataxia
- slow psychomotor development

CT:
√ hypodense white matter
√ progressive white matter atrophy

MR:
√ lack of myelination (appearance of newborn retained)
√ hyperintense internal capsule, optic radiations, proximal corona radiata on T1WI
√ near complete absence of hypointensity in supratentorial region on T2WI
√ mild / moderate prominence of cortical sulci

Prognosis: death in adolescence / early adulthood

PICK DISEASE

= rare form of presenile dementia similar to Alzheimer disease; may be inherited with autosomal dominant mode; M < F
√ focal cortical atrophy of anterior frontal + anterior temporal lobes
√ dilatation of frontal + temporal horns of lateral ventricle

PINEAL CYST

= small nonneoplastic cyst of pineal gland

Incidence: 25–40% on autopsy, 4% on MRI

Types:
(a) developmental = persistence of ependymal-lined pineal diverticulum
(b) degenerative = glial-lined secondary cavitation within area of gliosis

- never associated with Parinaud syndrome
- never cause of hydrocephalus
- may be symptomatic when large

CT:
√ normal-sized gland (80%), slightly >1 cm in 20%
√ isodense to CSF in surrounding cistern (infrequently noted)

MR:
√ sharply marginated ovoid mass in pineal region
√ slight impression on superior colliculi (sagittal image)
√ isointense to CSF on T1WI + slightly hyperintense to CSF on T2WI (due to phase coherence in cysts but not in moving CSF)
√ may have higher signal intensity than CSF due to high protein content
√ contrast may diffuse from enhanced rim of residual pineal tissue into fluid center (no blood-brain barrier) on delayed sequence images

PINEAL GERMINOMA

= DYSGERMINOMA = PINEALOMA = ATYPICAL TERATOMA (former inaccurate names)
◊ "pinealoma" = misnomer referring to any pineal mass
= malignant primitive germ cell neoplasm

Incidence: most common pineal tumor (>50% of all pineal tumors)

Histo: identical to testicular seminoma + ovarian dysgerminoma, NO capsule facilitates invasion

Age: 10–25 years; M:F = 10:1

May be associated with: ectopic pinealoma = secondary focus in inferior portion of 3rd ventricle

- precocious puberty frequent in children <10 years of age
- Parinaud syndrome = paralysis of upward gaze (compression of mesencephalic tectum)

Location of germinomas: pineal gland (80%), suprasellar region (20%), basal ganglia, thalamus

√ displacement of calcified pineal gland
√ hydrocephalus (compression of aqueduct of Sylvius)
√ well-defined lesion restricted to pineal gland
√ may infiltrate quadrigeminal plate / thalamus

CT:
√ infiltrating variodense homogeneous mass (attenuation usually similar to gray matter)
√ rarely psammomatous calcifications within tumor, but pineal calcifications in 100% (40% in normal population)
√ moderate / marked uniform contrast enhancement

MR:
√ round / lobular well-circumscribed relatively homogeneous mass isointense to gray matter
√ hypointense mass on T2WI (occasionally)
√ strong Gd-DTPA enhancement

Cx: metastatic spread via CSF (frequent)

Rx: combination of irradiation (very radiosensitive) + chemotherapy (adriamycin, cisplatin, cyclophosphamide)

Prognosis: 75% survival after radiation therapy alone

PINEAL TERATOCARCINOMA

= highly malignant variant of germ cell tumors

Types: 1. Choriocarcinoma
2. Embryonal cell carcinoma
3. Endodermal sinus tumor

Histo: arising from primitive germ cells, frequently containing more than one cell type

Age: <20 years; males

• Parinaud syndrome
• tumor markers elevated in serum + CSF
√ intratumoral hemorrhage (esp. choriocarcinoma)
√ invasion of adjacent structures
√ intense homogeneous contrast enhancement

Cx: seeding via CSF

PINEAL TERATOMA

= benign tumor containing one / all three germ cell layers (pineal region most common site of teratomas)

Incidence: 15% of all pineal masses (2nd most common tumor in pineal region)

Age: <20 years; M:F = 2–8:1

• Parinaud syndrome = paralysis of upward gaze (compression / infiltration of superior colliculi)
• hypothalamic symptoms
• headache
• somnolence (related to hydrocephalus)

Location: pineal, parapineal, suprasellar, 3rd ventricle

√ well-defined rounded / irregular lobulated extremely heterogenous mass of fat, cartilage, hair, linear / nodular calcifications + cysts
◊ Fat is absent in all other pineal tumors!
√ may show heterogeneous / rimlike contrast enhancement (limited to solid-tissue areas)

Angio:
√ elevation of internal cerebral vein
√ posterior displacement of precentral vein

CT:
√ heterogeneous mass with fat, calcification, cystic + solid areas

MR:
√ variegated appearance on all pulse sequences with hyperintense areas of fat on T1WI

Cx: chemical meningitis with spontaneous rupture

PINEOBLASTOMA

= highly malignant tumor derived from primitive pineal parenchymal cells

Histo: unencapsulated highly cellular primitive small round cell tumor (similar to medulloblastoma, neuroblastoma, retinoblastoma)

Age: any age, more common in children; M < F

CT:
√ poorly marginated iso- / slightly hyperdense mass
√ may contain dense tumor calcifications
√ peripherally displaced preexisting normal pineal calcification (= "exploded pineal pattern")
√ intense homogeneous contrast enhancement

MR:
√ iso- / moderately hypointense on T1WI + iso- / hyperintense on T2WI
√ dense homogeneous Gd-DTPA enhancement

Spread:
(1) direct extension posteriorly with invasion of cerebellar vermis + anteriorly into 3rd ventricle
(2) throughout CSF (frequent) along meninges / via ventricles

PINEOCYTOMA

= rare slow-growing unencapsulated tumor composed of mature pineal parenchymal cells

Age: any age; M:F = 1:1

√ well-marginated slightly hyperdense / isodense mass
√ dense focal tumor calcifications possible
√ peripherally displaced preexisting normal pineal calcification (= "exploded pineal pattern")
√ well-defined homogeneous enhancement

MR:
√ intermediate intensity on T1WI + T2WI
√ may be isointense to CSF but containing trabeculations (DDx to pineal cyst)
√ mild to moderate Gd-DTPA enhancement

Cx: some metastasize via CSF

PITUITARY ADENOMA

= benign slow-growing neoplasm arising from adenohypophysis (= anterior lobe); most common tumor of adenohypophysis

Prevalence: 5–10–18% of all intracranial neoplasms

• pituitary hyperfunction / hypofunction / visual field defect

FORMER CLASSIFICATION:
(a) Chromophobe adenoma (80%)
associated with hypopituitarism;
elevation of prolactin, TSH, GH serum levels
√ greatest sella enlargement; calcified in 5%
however: functioning microadenomas are part of chromophobe adenomas
(b) Acidophilic / eosinophilic adenoma (15%)
increased GH secretion (acromegaly), prolactin, TSH
√ tumor of intermediate size
(c) Basophilic adenoma (5%)
associated with ACTH secretion (Cushing syndrome), LH, FSH
√ small tumor

Plain film: (UNRELIABLE !)
√ enlargement of sella + sloping of sella floor
√ erosion of anterior + posterior clinoid processes
√ erosion of dorsum sellae
√ calcification in <10%
√ may present with mass in nasopharynx

Functioning Pituitary Adenoma

Adenoma may secrete multiple hormones!

1. PROLACTINOMA (30%)
most common of pituitary adenomas; approximately 50% of all cranial tumors at autopsy; M << F
• prolactin levels do not closely correlate with tumor size

◊ Any mass compressing the hypothalamus / pituitary stalk diminishes the tonic inhibitory effect of dopaminergic factors, which originate there, resulting in hyperprolactinemia!

Female:
Age: 15–44 years (during childbearing age)
- infertility
- amenorrhea
- galactorrhea
- elevated prolactin levels (normal <20 ng/mL)

◊ >75% of patients with serum prolactin levels >200 ng/mL will show a pituitary tumor!

Male:
- headache
- impotence + decreased libido
- visual disturbance

√ characteristic lateral location, anteriorly / inferiorly; variable in size

Rx: bromocriptine

2. CORTICOTROPHIC ADENOMA (14%)
Function: ACTH-secreting tumor
Age: 30–40 years; M:F = 1:3
√ central location; posterior lobe; usually <5 mm in size
√ sampling of inferior petrosal sinuses (95% diagnostic accuracy compared with 65% for MRI)
- **Cushing disease**
= truncal obesity, abdominal striae, glycosuria, osteoporosis, proximal muscle weakness, hirsutism, amenorrhea, hypertension, elevated cortisol levels in plasma and urine

Rx: (1) suppression by high doses of dexamethasone of 8 mg/day
(2) surgical resection difficult because ACTH adenomas usually require resection of an apparently normal gland (tumor small + usually not on surface)

3. SOMATOTROPHIC ADENOMA (14%)
- gigantism, acromegaly, elevated GH >10 ng/mL, no rise in GH after administration of glucose / TRH

Histo: (a) densely granulated type
(b) sparsely granulated type: clinically more aggressive
√ hypodense region, may be less well-defined, variable size

4. GONADOTROPH CELL ADENOMA (7%)
secrets follicle-stimulating hormone (FSH) / luteinizing hormone (LH)
√ slow-growing often extending beyond sella

5. THYROTROPH CELL ADENOMA (<1%)
secrets thyroid-stimulating hormone (TSH)
√ often large + invasive pituitary adenoma

6. PLURIHORMONAL PITUITARY ADENOMA (>5%)

CECT (dynamic bolus injection):
√ upward convexity of gland
√ increased height >10 mm
√ deviation of pituitary stalk
√ floor erosion of sella
√ gland asymmetry
√ focal hypodensity (most specific for adenoma)
√ shift of pituitary tuft / density change in region of adenoma

MR:
Highest sensitivity on coronal nonenhanced T1WI (70%) + 3 D FLASH sequence (69%) + combination of both (90%)
◊ 1/3 of lesions are missed with enhancement
◊ 1/3 of lesions are missed without enhancement
√ focus of low signal intensity on T1WI
√ focus of high-signal intensity on T2WI
√ focal hypointensity within normally enhancing gland

DDx: simple pituitary cyst (= Rathke cleft cyst)

Nonfunctioning Pituitary Adenoma

1. NULL CELL ADENOMA
= hormonally inactive pituitary tumor with no histologic / immunologic / ultrastructural markers to indicate its cellular derivation
Prevalence: 17% of all pituitary tumors
Age: older patient
√ slow-growing
2. ONCOCYTOMA
Prevalence: 10% of all pituitary tumors
- clinically + morphologically similar to null cell adenoma

Pituitary Macroadenoma

= tumor >10 mm in size, usually endocrinologically inactive (70–80% of pituitary adenomas)
Incidence: 10%; M:F = 1:1
Age: 2560 years
- symptoms of mass effect: hypopituitarism, bitemporal hemianopia (with superior extension), pituitary apoplexy, hydrocephalus, cranial nerve involvement (III, IV, VI)

Extension into: suprasellar cistern / cavernous sinus / sphenoid sinus + nasopharynx (up to 67% are invasive)
√ occasionally tumor hemorrhage
√ lucent areas correspond to cysts / focal necrosis
√ invasion of cavernous sinus: encasement of carotid artery (surest sign)

CT:
√ tumor isodense to brain tissue
√ erosion of bone (eg, floor of sella)
√ calcifications infrequent

MR: (allows differentiation from aneurysm)
√ homogeneous enhancement

Cx:
(1) Obstructive hydrocephalus (at foramen of Monro)
(2) Encasement of carotid artery
(3) Pituitary apoplexy (rare)

DDx:
(1) Metastasis (more bone destruction, rapid growth)
(2) Pituitary abscess

Pituitary Microadenoma
= very small adenomas <10 mm
• usually become clinically apparent by hormone production (20–30% of all pituitary adenomas)
◊ prolactin elevation (>25 ng/mL in females)
4–8 x normal: adenoma demonstrated in 71%
>8 x normal: adenoma demonstrated in 100%
• **incidentaloma** = nonfunctioning microadenoma / pituitary cyst
√ NO imaging features to distinguish between different types o adenomas
MRI:
√ small mass of hypointensity on pre- and postcontrast T1WI (nonenhancing)
√ occasionally isointense on precontrast images + hyperintense on postcontrast images
√ enhancement on delayed images
√ focal bulge on surface of gland
√ focal depression of sellar floor
√ deviation of pituitary stalk

PITUITARY APOPLEXY
Cause: massive hemorrhage into pituitary adenoma (especially in patients on bromocriptine for pituitary adenoma) / dramatic necrosis / sudden infarction of pituitary gland
◊ 25% of patients with pituitary hemorrhage will present with apoplexy!
Sheehan syndrome = postpartum infarction of anterior pituitary gland
• severe headache, nausea, vomiting
• hypertension
• stiff neck
• sudden visual-field defect, ophthalmoplegia
• obtundation (frequent)
• hypopituitarism (eg, secondary hypothyroidism)
◊ Area of destruction must be >70% to produce pituitary insufficiency!
√ enlargement of pituitary gland
NCCT:
√ increased density ± fluid level
MR:
√ bright signal from presence of hemoglobin on T1WI with persistence over hyperintensity on T2WI
√ intermediate signal intensity from deoxyhemoglobin on T1WI + T2WI

PORENCEPHALY
= focal cavity as a result of localized brain destruction
A. AGENETIC PORENCEPHALY
= Schizencephaly (= true porencephaly)
B. ENCEPHALOCLASTIC PORENCEPHALY
Time of injury: during first half of gestation
Histo: necrotic tissue completely reabsorbed without surrounding glial reaction (= liquefaction necrosis)
MR:
√ smooth-walled cavity filled with CSF on all pulse sequences (= porencephalic cyst)
√ lined by white matter
C. ENCEPHALOMALACIA
= Pseudoporencephaly = Acquired porencephaly
Cause: infectious, vascular
Time f injury: after end of 2nd trimester (brain has developed capacity for glial response)
Location: parasagittal watershed areas with sparing of periventricular region + ventricular wall
CT:
√ hypodense regions
MR:
√ hypointense on T1WI + hyperintense on T2WI
√ surrounding hyperintense rim on T2WI = gliosis)
√ glial septa coursing through cavity identified on T1WI + proton density images
US:
√ septations in cavity well visualized

POSTVIRAL LEUKOENCEPHALOPATHY
= ACUTE DISSEMINATED ENCEPHALOMYELITIS
= autoimmune process
• several weeks following an exanthematous viral infection / vaccination (measles, rubella, chickenpox, Epstein-Barr virus, mumps, pertussis)
• seizures, focal neurologic deficits
√ multifocal white matter abnormalities, occasionally deep gray matter involvement
√ sparing of cortical gray matter
√ no additional lesions on follow-up exam
Prognosis: resolution of neurologic deficits within 1 month (80–90%)

PRIMITIVE NEUROECTODERMAL TUMOR
= PNET = group of very undifferentiated tumors arising from germinal matrix cells of primitive neural tube
Incidence: <5% of supratentorial neoplasms in children
Age: mainly in children <5 years of age; M:F = 1:1
Histo: highly cellular tumors composed of >90–95% of undifferentiated cells (histologically similar to medulloblastoma, pineoblastoma, peripheral neuroblastoma)
• signs of increased intracranial pressure / seizures
Location:
(a) supratentorial: deep cerebral white matter (most commonly in frontal lobe), pineal gland, in thalamic + suprasellar territories (least frequently)
(b) posterior fossa (= medulloblastoma)

√ large cellular lesion with tendency for necrosis (65%), cyst formation, calcifications (71%), hemorrhage (10%)
√ thin rim of edema
√ contrast enhancement of solid tumor portion
CT:
√ solid tumor portions hyperdense (due to high nuclear to cytoplasmic ratio)
MR:
√ mildly hypointense on T1WI + hyperintense on T2WI

√ remarkably inhomogeneous due to cyst formation + necrosis
√ areas of signal dropout due to calcifications
√ hyperintense areas on T1WI + variable intensity on T2WI due to hemorrhage
√ inhomogeneously enhancing mass with tumor nodules + ringlike areas surrounding central necrosis after Gd-DTPA

PROGRESSIVE MULTIFOCAL LEUKOENCEPHALOPATHY

= PML = rapidly progressive fatal demyelinating disease in patients with impaired immune system (chronic lymphocytic leukemia, lymphoma, Hodgkin disease, carcinomatosis, AIDS, tuberculosis, sarcoidosis, organ transplant)

Etiology: virus infection (probably latent papovavirus = JC virus)

Pathophysiology: destruction of oligodendrogliocytes leading to areas of demyelination + edema

Histo: intranuclear inclusion bodies within swollen oligodendrocytes (viral particles in nuclei), absence of significant perivenous inflammation

• progressive neurologic deficits, visual disturbances, dementia, ataxia, spasticity
• normal CSF fluid

Location: predilection for parietooccipital region

Site: subcortical white matter spreading centrally

√ NO contrast enhancement

CT:
√ multicentric confluent white matter lesions of low attenuation with scalloped borders along cortex
√ NO mass effect

MR:
√ patchy high-intensity lesions of white matter away from ependyma in asymmetric distribution on T2WI
√ sparing of cortical gray matter

Prognosis: death usually within 6 months

DDx in early stages: primary CNS lymphoma

REYE SYNDROME

= hepatitis + encephalitis following viral upper respiratory tract infection with Hx of large doses of aspirin ingestion

Age: in children + young adults

• obtundation rapidly progressing to coma
√ initially (within 2–3 days) small ventricles
√ later progressive enlargement of lateral ventricles + sulci
√ markedly diminished attenuation of white matter

Mortality: 15–85% (from white matter edema + demyelination)

Dx: liver biopsy

SARCOIDOSIS OF CNS

= inflammatory disorder characterized by presence of noncaseating granulomas; mostly in Blacks

Incidence: CNS involvement in 1–8% (in up to 15% of autopsies)

• cranial neuropathy (facial > acoustic > optic > trigeminal nerves) secondary to granulomatous infiltration + leptomeningeal fibrosis (50–75%)
• peripheral neuropathy + myopathy
• aseptic meningitis (20%)
• diffuse encephalopathy, dementia
• pituitary + hypothalamic dysfunction (eg, diabetes insipidus in 5–10%)
• generalized / focal seizures (herald poorer prognosis)
• multiple sclerosislike symptoms (from multifocal parenchymal involvement)
• prompt improvement following therapy with steroids

Location: dura mater, leptomeninges, subarachnoid space, peripheral nerves, brain parenchyma, ventricular system

◊ Affects meninges + cranial nerves more often than the brain!

√ diffuse meningeal enhancement (most common) / meningeal nodules (less common) from leptomeningeal invasion
  Site: particularly in basal cisterns (suprasellar, sellar, subfrontal regions) with extension to optic chiasm, hypothalamus, pituitary gland, cranial nerves where exiting brainstem
√ focal / widespread infarcts of peripheral gray matter / at gray-white matter junction (periarteritis)
√ dense enhancement of falx + tentorium (granulomatous invasion of dura)
√ isodense / hyperdense homogeneously enhancing small single / multiple nodules (invasion of brain parenchyma via perivascular spaces of Virchow-Robin)
  Site: periphery of parenchyma, intraspinal
√ communicating / obstructive hydrocephalus is the most common finding (from arachnoiditis / adhesions)

SCHIZENCEPHALY

= AGENETIC PORENCEPHALY = TRUE PORENCEPHALY = "split brain"

= full-thickness CSF-filled parenchymal cleft lined by gray matter extending from subarachnoid space to subependyma of lateral ventricles

Frequency: 1:1,650

Cause: segmental developmental failure of cell migration to form cerebral cortex / vascular ischemia of portion of germinal matrix

Time of injury: 30–60 days of gestation

Often associated with: polymicrogyria, microcephaly, gray matter heterotopia

Types:
(a) clefts with fused lips
  (may be missed in imaging planes parallel to the plane of cleft)
  √ walls appose one another obliterating CSF space
(b) clefts with separated / open lips
  √ CSF fills cleft from lateral ventricle to subarachnoid space

• seizure disorder
• mild / moderate developmental delay
• range of normal mentation to severe mental retardation
• blindness possible (optic nerve hypoplasia in 33%)

Location: most commonly near pre- and postcentral gyri (sylvian fissure); uni- / (mostly) bilateral; in middle cerebral artery distribution
√ polymicrogyria / pachygyria of cortex adjacent to cleft
√ full-thickness cleft through hemisphere with irregular margins
√ gray-matter lining of cleft (PATHOGNOMONIC) extending through entire hemisphere
√ bilateral often symmetric intracranial cysts, usually around sylvian fissure
√ asymmetrical dilatation of lateral ventricles with midline shift
√ wide separation of lateral ventricles + squaring of frontal lobes
√ absence of cavum septi pellucidi (80 - 90%) + corpus callosum

Prognosis: severe intellectual impairment, spastic tetraplegia, blindness

DDx: (1) Pseudoporencephaly = Acquired porencephaly = local parenchymal destruction secondary to vascular / infectious / traumatic insult (almost always unilateral)
(2) Arachnoid cyst
(3) Cystic tumor

SEPTO-OPTIC DYSPLASIA

= DeMORSIER SYNDROME
= rare anterior midline anomaly with (1) hypoplasia of optic nerves (2) hypoplasia / absence of septum pellucidum; often considered a mild form of lobar holoprosencephaly

M:F = 1:3

Cause: insult between 5–7th week of GA

Associated with: schizencephaly (50%)

• hypothalamic hypopituitarism (66%): diabetes insipidus (in 50%), growth retardation (deficient secretion of growth hormone + thyroid stimulating hormone)
• diminished visual acuity (hypoplasia of optic discs), nystagmus, occasionally hypotelorism
• seizures, hypotonia
√ small optic canals
√ hypoplasia of optic nerves + chiasm + infundibulum
√ dilatation of chiasmatic + suprasellar cisterns
√ fused dilated boxlike frontal horns squared off dorsally + pointing inferiorly
√ bulbous dilatation of anterior recess of 3rd ventricle
√ hypoplastic / absent septum pellucidum
√ thin corpus callosum

SINUS PERICRANII

= subperiosteal venous angiomas adherent to skull and connected by anomalous diploic veins to a sinus / cortical vein
• soft painless scalp mass that reduces under compression

Location: frontal bone
√ calvarial thinning + defect

CT:
√ sessile sharply marginated homogeneous densely enhancing mass adjacent to outer table of skull, perforating it and connecting it with another similar structure beneath the inner table

Angio:
√ extracalvarial sinus may not opacify secondary to slow flow

SPONGIFORM LEUKOENCEPHALOPATHY

rare, hereditary, > age 40
• deteriorating mental function
√ confluent areas of diminished attenuation

STURGE-WEBER-DIMITRI SYNDROME

= ENCEPHALOTRIGEMINAL ANGIOMATOSIS
= MENINGOFACIAL ANGIOMATOSIS
= vascular malformation with capillary venous angiomas involving face, choroid of eye, leptomeninges

Cause: persistence of transitory primordial sinusoidal plexus stage of vessel development; usually sporadic

• seizures (80%) in 1st year of life: usually focal involving the side of the body contralateral to nevus flammeus
• mental deficiency (>50%)
• increasing crossed hemiparesis (35–65%)
• hemiatrophy of body contralateral to facial nevus (secondary to hemiparesis)
• homonymous hemianopia

@ FACIAL MANIFESTATION
  • congenital facial port-wine stain (nevus flammeus)
  = telangiectasia of trigeminal region; usually 1st ± 2nd division of 5th nerve; usually unilateral
  — V_1 associated with occipital lobe angiomatosis
  — V_2 associated with parietal lobe angiomatosis
  — V_3 associated with frontal lobe angiomatosis

@ CNS MANIFESTATION
  √ leptomeningeal venous angiomas confined to pia mater
  Location: parietal > occipital > frontal lobes
  Angio:
    √ capillary blush
    √ abnormally large veins in subependymal + periventricular regions
    √ abnormal deep medullary veins draining into internal cerebral vein (= venous shunt)
    √ failure to opacify superficial cortical veins in calcified region (markedly slow blood flow / thrombosis of dysgenetic superficial veins)
  √ cortical hemiatrophy beneath meningeal angioma due to anoxia (steal)
  √ "tram track" gyriform cortical calcifications >2 years of age; in layers 2-3(-4-5) of opposing gyri underlying pial angiomatosis; bilateral in up to 20%
    Location: temporo-parieto-occipital area, occasionally frontal, rare in posterior fossa
  √ subjacent white matter hypodense on CT with slight prolongation of T1 + T2 relaxation times (gliosis)

√ choroid plexus enlargement ipsilateral to angiomatosis
√ ipsilateral thickening of skull + orbit (bone apposition as result of subdural hematoma secondary to brain atrophy)
√ elevation of sphenoid wing + petrous ridge
√ enlarged ipsilateral paranasal sinuses + mastoid air cells
√ thickened calvarium (= widening of diploic space)

@ ORBITAL MANIFESTATION (30%)
ipsilateral to nevus flammeus:
- congenital glaucoma (30%)

√ choroidal hemangioma (71%)
√ dilatation + tortuosity of conjunctival + episcleral + iris + retinal vessels
√ buphthalmos = enlarged + elongated globe as result of increased intraocular pressure

Cx: retinal detachment

@ VISCERAL MANIFESTATION
localized / diffuse angiomatous malformation located in intestine, kidneys, spleen, ovaries, thyroid, pancreas, lungs

DDx: Klippel-Trenaunay syndrome, Wyburn-Mason syndrome

SUBARACHNOID HEMORRHAGE

Cause:

A. Spontaneous
(1) ruptured aneurysm (72%) (2) AV malformation (10%) (3) hypertensive hemorrhage (4) hemorrhage from tumor (5) embolic hemorrhagic infarction (6) blood dyscrasia, anticoagulation therapy (7) eclampsia (8) intracranial infection (9) spinal vascular malformation (10) cryptogenic in 6% (negative 4-vessel angiography; seldom recurrent)

B. Trauma (common)
concomitant to cerebral contusion
(a) injury to leptomeningeal vessels at vertex
(b) rupture of major intracerebral vessels (less common)

Location: (a) focal, overlying site of contusion
(b) interhemispheric fissure, paralleling falx cerebri
(c) spread diffusely throughout subarachnoid space (rare in trauma)

Pathophysiology: irritation of meninges by blood + extra fluid volume increases intracranial pressure

- acute severe headache ("worst in life"), vomiting
- altered state of consciousness: drowsiness, sleepiness, stupor, restlessness, agitation, coma
- spectrophotometric analysis of CSF obtained by lumbar puncture

NCCT (60–90% accuracy of detection depending on time of scan; sensitivity depends on amount of blood; accuracy high within 4–5 days of onset):
◊ May occur in only two locations if subtle!
√ increased density in basal cisterns, superior cerebellar cistern, sylvian fissure, cortical sulci, intraventricular, intracerebral
√ along interhemispheric fissure = on lateral aspect irregular dentate pattern due to extension into paramedian sulci with rapid clearing after several days

MR (relatively insensitive within first 48 hours):
√ deoxyhemoglobin effects not appreciable in acute phase (secondary to higher oxygen tension in CSF, counterbalancing effects of very long T2 of CSF, pulsatile flow effects of CSF)
√ low-signal intensity on brain surfaces in recurrent subarachnoid hemorrhages (hemosiderin deposition)

Prognosis: clinical course depends on amount of subarachnoid blood

Cx:
(1) Acute obstructive hydrocephalus (in <1 week) secondary to intraventricular hemorrhage / ependymitis obstructing aqueduct of Sylvius or outlet of 4th ventricle
(2) Delayed communicating hydrocephalus (after 1 week) secondary to fibroblastic proliferation in subarachnoid space and arachnoid villi interfering with CSF resorption
(3) Cerebral vasospasm + infarction (develops after 72 hours, at maximum between 5–17 days, amount of blood is prognostic parameter)
(4) Transtentorial herniation (cerebral hematoma, hydrocephalus, infarction, brain edema)

SUBDURAL HEMATOMA OF BRAIN

Incidence: in 5% of head trauma patients; in 15% of closed head injuries; in 65% of head injuries with prolonged interruption of consciousness

Age: predominantly in infants + elderly (large subarachnoid space with freedom to move in cerebral atrophy)

Cause: direct trauma, sudden de-/acceleration; forceful coughing / sneezing / vomiting in elderly; occasionally in blood clotting disorder / during anticoagulation therapy
◊ No consistent relationship to skull fractures!

Pathogenesis:
differential movement of brain + adherent cortical veins with respect to skull + attached dural sinuses tears the "bridging veins" (= subdural veins), which connect cerebral cortex to dural sinuses and travel through the subarachnoid and subdural space

Location: subdural space = potential space between pia-arachnoid membrane (leptomeninges) + dura mater; freely extending across suture lines, limited only by interhemispheric fissure and tentorium

DDx: (1) Arachnoid cyst (extension into sylvian fissure)
(2) Subarachnoid hemorrhage (extension into sulci)

Acute Subdural Hematoma

Usually follows severe trauma, manifest within hours after injury

Time frame: <3–4 days old

Associated with: underlying brain injury (50%) with worse long-term prognosis than epidural hematoma, skull fracture (1%)

Location:

(a) over cerebral convexity, frequent extension into interhemispheric fissure, along tentorial margins, beneath temporal + occipital lobes; NO crossing of midline

(b) bilateral in 15–25% of adults (common in elderly) and in 80–85% in infants

√ extra-axial peripheral crescentic fluid collection between skull and cerebral hemisphere usually with
- √ concave inner margin (hematoma minimally pressing into brain substance)
- √ convex outer margin following normal contour of cranial vault
- √ occasionally with blood-fluid level
- √ after surgical evacuation: underlying parenchymal injury becomes more obvious
- √ after healing: ventricular + sulcal enlargement

CT:
- √ hyperdense (<1 week) / isodense (1–2 weeks) / hypodense (3–4 weeks)

False-negative CT scan:

high-convexity location, beam-hardening artifact, volume averaging with high density of calvarium obscuring flat "en plaque" hematoma, too narrow window setting, isodense hematoma due to delay in imaging 10–20 days post injury / due to low hemoglobin content of blood / lack of clotting, CSF-dilution from associated arachnoid tear

◊ 38% of small subdural hematomas are missed!

Aids in detection of acute subdural hematoma:
- √ thickening of ipsilateral portion of skull (hematoma of similar pixel brightness as bone)
- √ "subdural window" setting = window level of 40 HU + window width of 400 HU
- √ effacement of adjacent sulci
- √ sulci not traceable to brain surface
- √ ipsilateral ventricular compression / distortion
- √ displacement of gray-white matter interface away from ipsilateral inner table
- √ midline shift (often greater than width of subdural hematoma due to underlying brain contusion)
- √ contrast enhancement of cortex but not of subdural hematoma

Aids in detection of bilateral subdural hematomas:
- √ "parentheses" ventricles
- √ ventricles too small for patient's age

MR: refer to HEMATOMA OF BRAIN

US (neonate):

Limitations:

(a) convexity hematoma may be obscured by pie-shaped display + loss of near-field resolution

◊ Use contralateral transtemporal approach!

(b) small loculations may be missed

- √ linear / elliptical space between cranial vault + brain
- √ flattened gyri + prominent sulci
- √ ± distortion of ventricles, extension into interhemispheric space

Cx: Arteriovenous fistula (meningeal artery + vein caught in fracture line)

Prognosis: may progress to subacute + chronic stage / may disappear spontaneously

Mortality: 35–50% (higher number due to associated brain injury, mass effect, old age, bilateral lesions, rapid rate of hematoma accumulation, surgical evacuation >4 hours)

Interhemispheric Subdural Hematoma

Most common acute finding in child abuse (whiplash forces on large head with weak neck muscles)
- √ predominance for posterior portion of interhemispheric fissure
- √ crescentic shape with flat medial border
- √ unilateral increased attenuation with extension along course of tentorium
- √ anterior extension to level of genu of corpus callosum

Subdural Hemorrhage in Newborn

Cause: mechanical trauma during delivery (excessive vertical molding of head)

1. Posterior fossa hemorrhage
   (a) tentorial laceration with rupture of vein of Galen / straight sinus / transverse sinus
   (b) occipital osteodiastasis = separation of squamous portion from exoccipital portion of occipital bone
   - √ high-density thickening of affected tentorial leaf extending down posterior to cerebellar hemisphere (better seen on coronal views)
   - √ mildly echogenic subtentorial collection

   Cx: death from compression of brainstem, acute hydrocephalus
2. Supratentorial hemorrhage
   (a) laceration of falx near junction with tentorium with rupture of inferior sagittal sinus (less common than tentorial laceration)
   - √ hematoma over corpus callosum in inferior aspect of interhemispheric fissure

   (b) convexity hematoma from rupture of superficial cortical veins
   - √ usually unilateral subdural convexity hematoma accompanied by subarachnoid blood
   - √ underlying cerebral contusion
   - √ sonographic visualization of convexities difficult

Subacute Subdural Hematoma

Time frame: 4–20 days

CT:
- √ isodense hematoma (1–3 weeks) may be recognizable by mass effect with effacement of cortical sulci, deviation of lateral ventricle, midline shift, white matter buckling, displacement of gray-white matter junction

√ contrast enhancement of inner membrane
AID in Dx: contrast enhancement defines cortical-subdural interface

MR:
√ modality of choice in subacute stage because of high sensitivity for Met-Hb on T1WI (esp. superior to CT during isodense phase, for small subdural hematoma, for hematomas oriented in the CT scan plane, eg, tentorial subdural hematoma)

Chronic Subdural Hematoma

= result of (a) resolving phase of medically managed acute subdural hematoma
(b) repeated episodes of subclinical hemorrhage until becoming symptomatic

Time frame: >20 days old = 3 weeks and older

Histo: hematoma enclosed by thick + vascular membrane which forms after 3–6 weeks

Pathogenesis: vessel fragility accounts for repeated episodes of rebleeding following minor injuries that tear fragile capillary bed within neomembrane surrounding subdural hematoma

Predisposing factors:
alcoholism, increased age, epilepsy, coagulopathy, prior placement of ventricular shunt
◊ >75% occur in patients >50 years of age!

- history of antecedent trauma often absent (25–48%)
- ill-defined neurologic signs + symptoms: cognitive deficit, behavioral abnormality, nonspecific headache

√ crescent-shaped configuration (early) conforming to contour of brain
√ often biconvex lenticular = medially concave configuration (late), esp. after compartmentalization secondary to formation of fibrous septa
√ different attenuations within compartments
√ low-density lesion of intermediate attenuation between CSF + brain, sometimes as low as CSF
√ high-density components of collection (after common rebleeding)
√ fluid-sedimentation levels (sedimented fresh blood with proteinaceous fluid layered above)
√ displacement / absence of sulci, displacement of ventricles + parenchyma
√ No midline shift if bilateral (25%)
√ CECT demonstrates medially displaced cortical vein or membrane around hematoma (1–4 weeks after injury)

DDx: Acute epidural hematoma (similar biconvex shape)

SUBDURAL HYGROMA

= CSF-fluid collection within subdural space; common in children

Cause: traumatic tear in arachnoid with secondary ball valve mechanism

Time of onset: 6–30 days following trauma

√ radiolucent crescent-shaped collection (as in acute subdural hematoma)
√ no evidence of blood products (DDx to subdural hematoma)

MR:
√ isointense to CSF / hyperintense to CSF on T1WI (increased protein content)

Prognosis: often spontaneous resorption

DDx: (1) Enlarged subarachnoid space
(2) Subdural empyema
(3) Subdural hematoma

TERATOMA OF CNS

Incidence: 0.5% of primary intracranial neoplasms; 2% of intracranial tumors before age 15

Histo: mostly benign, occasionally containing primitive elements + highly malignant

Location: pineal + parapineal region > floor of 3rd ventricle > posterior fossa > spine (associated with spina bifida)

√ heterogeneous midline lesion, occasionally homogeneous soft-tissue mass (DDx: astrocytoma)
√ contains fat + calcium
√ hydrocephalus (common)

TOXOPLASMOSIS OF BRAIN

Organism: obligate intracellular protozoan parasite Toxoplasma gondii, can live in any cell except for nonnucleated RBCs; felines are definite host

Infection: ingestion of undercooked meat containing cysts or sporulated oocysts / transplacental transmission of trophozoites; acquired through blood transfusion + organ transplantation

Prevalence of seropositivity:
11–16% of urban adults in United States;
up to 90% of European adults

Histo: inflammatory solid / cystic granulomas as a result of glial mesenchymal reaction surrounded by edema + microinfarcts due to vasculitis

Affected tissue:
@ Gray + white matter of brain
◊ Most common cause of focal CNS infection in patients with AIDS!
@ Retina: most common retinal infection in AIDS
@ Alveolar lining cells (4%):
mimics Pneumocystis carinii pneumonia
@ Heart (rare):
cardiac tamponade / biventricular failure
@ Skeletal muscle

- asymptomatic
- lymphadenopathy
- malaise, fever

A. AIDS INFECTION = toxoplasmic encephalitis
= reactivation of a chronic latent infection in >95%
Path: well-localized indolent granulomatous process / diffuse necrotizing encephalitis
- focal neurologic deficit of subacute onset (50–89%)
- seizures (15–25%)
- pseudotumor cerebri syndrome

Location: basal ganglia (75%), scattered throughout brain parenchyma at gray-white matter junction
√ multiple / solitary (up to 39%) lesions with nodular / thin-walled (common) ring enhancement
√ surrounding white matter edema
√ double-dose delayed CT scans with higher detection rate for multiple lesions (64–72%)
√ ± hemorrhage and calcifications after therapy
Dx: improvement on therapy with pyrimethamine + sulfadiazine within 1–2 weeks / biopsy
DDx: CNS lymphoma (particularly with single lesion)
◊ Multiple lesions suggest toxoplasmosis!

B. INTRAUTERINE INFECTION
Time of fetal infection: chances of transplacental transmission greater in late pregnancy
Screening: impractical due to high false-positive rate
• Toxoplasma gondii found in ventricular fluid
• chorioretinitis
• mental retardation
√ multiple irregular, nodular / cystlike / curvilinear calcifications in periventricular area + choroid plexus (= necrotic foci); bilateral; 1–20 mm in size; increasing in number + size (usually not developed at time of birth)
√ hydrocephalus with return to normal / persistence of large head size
√ thickened vault, sutures apposed / overlapping
OB-US (as early as 20 weeks MA):
√ sonographic findings in only 36%
√ evolving symmetric ventriculomegaly
√ intracranial periventricular + hepatic densities
√ increased thickness of placenta
√ ascites
◊ Microcephaly is NOT a feature of toxoplasmosis!
Dx: elevated toxospecific IgM levels in fetal blood
Dx: demonstration of elongated teardrop-shaped trophozoites in histologic sections of tissue

TUBERCULOMA OF BRAIN

= result of granuloma formation within cerebral substance
Incidence: 0.15% of intracranial masses in Western countries, 30% in underdeveloped countries
Age: infant, small child, young adult
Associated with: tuberculous meningitis in 50%
• history of previous extracranial TB (in 60%)
Location: more common in posterior fossa (62%), cerebellar hemispheres; may be associated with tuberculous meningitis
√ solitary (70%) / multiple (30–60%) lesions; may be multiloculated
NCCT:
√ isodense (72%) / hyperdense lesion of 0.5–4 cm in diameter with mass effect (93%)
√ surrounding edema (72%) less marked than in pyogenic abscess
√ central calcification (29%)
CECT:
√ homogeneous enhancement
√ ring blush (nearly all) with smooth / slightly shaggy margins + thick wall around an isodense center (DDx: in pyogenic abscess less thick + more regular)
√ "target sign" = central calcification in isodense lesion + ring-blush (DDx: giant aneurysm)
√ homogeneous blush in tuberculoma en plaque along dural plane (6%) (DDx: meningioma en plaque)
MR:
√ isointense lesion on T1WI
√ hypointense lesion ± hyperintense core on T2WI
DDx: other CNS infection (esp. toxoplasmosis), lymphoma, atypical meningioma, radiation necrosis

TUBEROUS SCLEROSIS

= BOURNEVILLE DISEASE = EPIPLOIA
= neuroectodermal disorder characterized by TRIAD consisting of
(1) Adenoma sebaceum (30%)
(2) Seizures (80%)
(3) Mental retardation (70%)
mnemonic: zits, fits, nitwits
Frequency: 1:150,000 livebirths
Cause: autosomal dominant with low penetrance (frequent skips in generations); gene loci 9q34 and 16p13; spontaneous mutations in 50–80%
Prognosis: 30% dead by age 5; 75% dead by age 20

@ CNS INVOLVEMENT
• myoclonic seizures (80–90%): often first + most common sign of tuberous sclerosis with onset at 1st–2nd year, decreasing in frequency with age
• mental retardation (50–82%): mild to moderate (1/3) moderate to severe (2/3); progressive; observed in adulthood; common if onset of seizures before age 5 years

1. **Subependymal hamartomas**
Location: along ventricular surface of caudate nucleus, on lamina of sulcus thalamostriatus immediately posterior to foramen of Monro (most often), along frontal + temporal horns or 3rd + 4th ventricle (less commonly)
√ multiple subependymal nodules with "candle drippings" appearance at lining of lateral ventricles
√ calcification with increasing age (in up to 88%)
M:
√ subependymal nodules protruding into adjacent ventricle isointense with white matter
√ minimal / no contrast enhancement

2. **Giant cell astrocytoma**
= large subependymal nodule located near foramen of Monro with tendency for enlargement + growth into ventricle
Incidence: 5–15%; M:F = 1:1
√ hydrocephalus (obstruction at foramen of Monro)
√ hypo- / isodense well-demarcated rounded lesion in the region of foramen of Monro

√ hypo- / isointense on T1WI + hyperintense on T2WI
√ uniformly enhancing mass
√ frequent extension into frontal horn / body of lateral ventricle
Cx: degeneration into higher grade astrocytoma

3. **Tubers** (in 56%)
= CORTICAL / SUBCORTICAL HAMARTOMAS
Histo: clusters of atypical glial cells surrounded by giant cells with frequent calcifications (if >2 years of age) = hamartomas
Frequency: multiple (75%); bilateral (30%)
√ noncalcified hypodense brain lesions of abnormal myelination within broadened cortical gyri
√ cortical tubers calcified (in 15% <1 year of age, in 50% by age 10)
MR:
√ relaxation time similar to white matter (if uncalcified)
√ multiple nodules of high-signal intensity on T2WI, iso- / hypointense on T1WI (fibrillary gliosis / demyelination)

4. **Heterotopic gray matter islands in white matter**
Histo: grouping of bizarre and gigantic neuronal cells associated with gliosis + areas of demyelination
CT:
√ hypodense well-defined regions within cerebral white matter without contrast enhancement
√ calcification of all / part of nodule
MR:
√ subtle hypointense region on T1WI + well-defined hyperintense area on T2WI

DDx of CNS lesions:
(1) Intrauterine CMV / Toxoplasma infection (smaller lesions, brain atrophy, microcephaly)
(2) Basal ganglia calcification in hypoparathyroidism / Fahr disease (location)
(3) Sturge-Weber, calcified AVM (diffuse atrophy, not focal)
(4) Heterotopic gray matter (along medial ventricular wall, isodense, associated with agenesis of corpus callosum, Chiari malformation)

@ SKIN INVOLVEMENT
• Adenoma sebaceum (80–90%) = wartlike nodules of brownish red color averaging 4 mm in size with bimalar distribution ("butterfly rash")
Age: first discovered at age 1–5 years; family history in 30%
Path: small hamartomas from neural elements with blood vessel hyperplasia = angiofibromas
Location: nasolabial folds, eventually covers nose + middle of cheeks
• Shagreen rough skin patches (80%) = "pigskin" = "peau d'orange" = patches of fibrous hyperplasia; in intertriginous + lumbar location
• Ash leaf patches = hypopigmented macules shaped like ash / spearmint leaf on trunk + extremities (earliest manifestation in infancy); may be visible only under ultraviolet light
• Ungual fibromas (15–50%): sub- / periungual with erosion of distal tuft
• Café-au-lait spots: incidence similar to that in general population

@ OCULAR INVOLVEMENT
• Phakoma (>50%) = whitish disk-shaped retinal hamartoma = astrocytic proliferation in / near optic disc, often multiple + usually in both eyes
√ small calcifications in region of optic nerve head
√ optic nerve glioma

@ RENAL INVOLVEMENT
• renal failure in severe cases (5%); hypertension
1. Angiomyolipoma (38%): usually multiple + bilateral; risk of spontaneous hemorrhage (subcapsular / perinephric)
2. Multiple cysts of varying size in cortex + medulla mimicking adult polycystic kidney disease (15%)
Path: cysts lined by columnar epithelium with foci of hyperplasia projecting into cyst lumen
3. Renal cell carcinoma (3%), bilateral in 40%

@ LUNG INVOLVEMENT (1%)
√ interstitial fibrosis in lower lung fields + miliary nodular pattern may progress to honeycomb lung (lymphangioleiomyomatosis = smooth muscle proliferation around blood vessels)
√ cystic changes of lung parenchyma
√ spontaneous pneumothorax (50%)
√ chylothorax
√ cor pulmonale

@ HEART INVOLVEMENT
• congenital cardiomyopathy
√ circumscribed / diffuse subendocardial rhabdomyoma (in 5%)
√ aortic aneurysm

@ BONE INVOLVEMENT
√ sclerotic calvarial patches (45%) = "bone islands" involving diploe + internal table; frontal + parietal location
√ thickening of diploe (long-term phenytoin therapy)
√ bone islands in pelvic brim, vertebrae, long bones
√ periosteal thickening of long bones
√ bone cysts with undulating periosteal reaction in distal phalanges (most common), metacarpals, metatarsals (DDx: sarcoid, neurofibromatosis)

@ OTHER VISCERAL INVOLVEMENT
1. Adenomas + lipomyomas of liver
2. Adenomas of pancreas
3. Tumors of spleen

@ VASCULAR INVOLVEMENT (rare)
√ thoracic + abdominal arterial aneurysms
Path: vascular dysplasia with intimal + medial abnormalities of large muscular + musculoelastic arteries

UNILATERAL MEGALENCEPHALY

= hamartomatous overgrowth of all / part of a cerebral hemisphere with neuronal migration defects
• intractable seizure disorder at early age, hemiplegia
• developmental delay
√ moderately / marked enlargement of hemisphere
√ ipsilateral ventriculomegaly proportionate to enlargement of affected hemisphere
straightened frontal horn of ipsilateral ventricle pointing anterolaterally
√ neuronal migration defects
√ polymicrogyria
√ pachygyria
√ heterotopia of gray matter
√ white matter gliosis (low density in white matter on CT, prolonged T1 + T2 relaxation times on MR)
Rx: partial / complete hemispheric resection

VEIN OF GALEN ANEURYSM

= central AVM directly draining into secondarily enlarged vein of Galen (aneurysm is a misnomer)
Anatomical types:
type 1 = AV fistula fed by enlarged arterial branches leading to dilatation of vein Galen + straight sinus + torcular herophili
type 2 = angiomatous malformation involving basal ganglia + thalami ± midbrain draining into vein of Galen
type 3 = transitional AVM with both features
Feeding vessels:
(a) posterior cerebral artery, posterior choroidal artery (90%)
(b) anterior cerebral artery + anterior choroidal artery
(c) middle cerebral artery + lenticulostriate + thalamic perforating arteries (least common)
Age at presentation: detectable in utero >30 weeks GA; M:F = 2:1
(a) neonatal pattern (0–1 month)
• high-output cardiac failure (36%) due to massive shunting
(b) infant pattern (1–12 months)
• macrocrania from obstructive hydrocephalus
• seizures
(c) adult pattern (>1 year)
• headaches ± intracranial hemorrhage
• ± hydrocephalus
• focal neurologic deficits (5%) due to steal of blood from surrounding structures
• cranial bruit
May be associated with: porencephaly, nonimmune hydrops
√ smoothly marginated midline mass posterior to indented 3rd ventricle
√ prominent serpiginous network in basal ganglia, thalami, midbrain
√ dilated straight + transverse sinus + torcular herophili
√ dilatation of lateral + 3rd ventricle (37%)
NCCT:
√ round well-circumscribed homogeneous slightly hyperdense mass in region of 3rd ventricular outlet
√ hyperdense intracerebral hematoma (ruptured AVM)
√ focal hypodense zones (ischemic changes)
√ rim calcification (14%)
CECT:
√ marked homogeneous enhancement of serpentine structures + vein of Galen + straight sinus
OB-US:
√ median tubular cystic space with high-velocity turbulent flow demonstrated by pulsed / color Doppler
√ brain infarction / leukomalacia (steal phenomenon with hypoperfusion)
√ cardiac enlargement (high-output heart failure)
√ dilated veins of head + neck
√ hydrocephalus (aqueductal obstruction / posthemorrhagic impairment of CSF absorption)
MR:
√ areas of signal void
Angio:
necessary to define vascular anatomy for surgical / endovascular intervention

Cx: subarachnoid hemorrhage
Rx: ligation, excision, embolization of vessels from transtorcular / transarterial approach
Prognosis: 56% overall mortality; 91% neonatal mortality
DDx: pineal tumor, arachnoid / colloid / porencephalic cyst

VENOUS ANGIOMA

= cluster of dilated medullary veins, which drain into an enlarged vein; bleed rarely
◊ Can be considered a normal variant!
Histo: venous channels without internal elastic lamina, separated by gliotic neural tissue that may calcify; probably representing persistent fetal venous system
√ no arterial vessels
√ "umbrella" configuration = multiple small radially oriented veins at periphery of lesion converging to a single larger vein
◊ Associated with increased incidence of cavernous angiomas which can bleed!
DDx: Sturge-Weber disease (diffuse pial angiomatosis with venous-type capillaries)

VENOUS SINUS THROMBOSIS

Septic causes (esp. in childhood):
mastoiditis, sub- / epidural empyema, meningitis, encephalitis, brain abscess, face + scalp cellulitis, septicemia
Aseptic causes:
(a) Tumor compressing sinuses: meningioma, leukemia
(b) Trauma: fracture through sinus wall, cranial surgery
(c) Low-flow state: CHF, CHD, dehydration, shock

(d) Hypercoagulability: polycythemia vera, idiopathic thrombocytosis, thrombocytopenia, sickle cell disease, cryofibrinogenemia, pregnancy, contraceptive steroids, disseminated intravascular coagulopathy
(e) Chemotherapy: eg, ARA-C

- headaches, drowsiness, fever, nausea, vomiting
- stroke symptomatology, seizures

NCCT:
√ high-attenuation material (clotted blood) in sagittal sinus / straight sinus / cerebral cortical vein = "cord sign" (rare)
√ compression of lateral ventricles in 32% (infarction / edema)
√ unilateral (2/3) / bilateral (1/3) parenchymal hemorrhage involving gray + white matter (20%)

CECT:
√ "delta sign" / "empty triangle" = filling defect in straight sinus / superior sagittal sinus (in 70%)
√ gyral enhancement in periphery of infarction (30–40%)
√ intense tentorial enhancement secondary to collaterals (rare)
√ dense transcortical medullary vein

Angio:
√ nonfilling of thrombosed sinus
√ filling of cortical veins, deep venous system, cavernous sinus
√ parasagittal hemorrhages (highly specific for superior sagittal sinus thrombosis) secondary to cortical venous infarction

MR:
√ high signal within sinus on T1WI + T2WI

Prognosis: high mortality

VENTRICULITIS

= EPENDYMITIS = inflammation of ependymal lining of one / more ventricles

Cause: (1) rupture of periventricular abscess (thinner capsule wall medially)
(2) retrograde spread of infection from basal cisterns

CECT (necessary for diagnosis):
√ thin uniform enhancement of involved ependymal lining
√ often associated with intraventricular inflammatory exudate + septations

Cx: obstructive hydrocephalus (occlusion at foramen of Monro / aqueduct)

DDx: ependymal metastases, lymphoma, infiltrating glioma

VENTRICULOPERITONEAL SHUNT

A. SHUNT MALFUNCTION

Cause: occlusion of catheter by choroid plexus / glial tissue, disconnection of tubes

- symptoms of increased intracranial pressure
- persistent bulging of anterior fontanelle
- excessive rate of head growth

√ increasing ventricular size
√ shuntogram (by scintigram / contrast radiography) determines site of obstruction
√ brain edema tracking along shunt + within interstices of centrum semiovale (with partial obstruction)
√ formation of white matter cyst surrounding ventricular catheter

B. SHUNT INFECTION

Incidence: 1–5%

- intermittent low-grade fever
- anemia, dehydration, hepatosplenomegaly
- stiff neck
- swelling + redness over shunting tract
- peritonitis

√ ventriculitis (= enlarged ventricles with irregular enhancing ventricular wall ± septations)

C. ABDOMINAL COMPLICATIONS

1. Ascites
2. Pseudocyst formation
3. Perforation of viscus / abdominal wall
4. Intestinal obstruction

D. SUBDURAL HEMATOMA

Cause: precipitous drainage of markedly enlarged ventricles

Age: usually seen in children >3 years of age

Prognosis: small hematomas are insignificant

E. GRANULOMATOUS LESION

= rare granulomatous reaction adjacent to shunt tube within / near ventricle
√ irregular contrast-enhancing mass along course of shunt tube

F. SLIT VENTRICLE SYNDROME

= symptoms from shunt failure in absence of ventricular enlargement (poorly defined syndrome)
√ normal imaging studies

VISCERAL LARVA MIGRANS OF BRAIN

roundworm nematode (Toxocara canis)
√ small calcific nodules, especially in basal ganglia + periventricular

DDx: tuberous sclerosis

VON HIPPEL-LINDAU DISEASE

= vHL = RETINOCEREBELLAR ANGIOMATOSIS
= inherited neurocutaneous dysplasia complex; autosomal dominant (gene located on chromosome 3p25-p26) with 80–100% penetrance + variable delayed expressivity; grouped under hereditary phakomatosis; in 20% familial

Age at onset: 2nd–3rd decade; M:F = 1:1

Diagnostic criteria:
(a) >1 hemangioblastoma of CNS
(b) 1 hemangioblastoma + visceral manifestation
(c) 1 manifestation + known family history

@ CNS MANIFESTATION
Age at presentation: 25–35 years
- cerebellar symptoms: vertigo, dysdiadochokinesia, dysmetria, Romberg sign
- signs of increased intracranial pressure: headache, vomiting
- vision changes: reactive retinal inflammation with exudate + hemorrhage, retinal detachment, glaucoma, cataract, uveitis, decreasing visual acuity, eye pain
- spinal cord symptoms (uncommon): loss of sensation, impaired proprioception

1. Retinal angiomatosis = **von Hippel tumor** (>45%)
   earliest manifestation of disease; multiple in up to 66%, bilateral in up to 50%
   Dx: indirect ophthalmoscopy + fluorescein angiography
   √ small tumors rarely detected by imaging studies
   √ globe distortion
   √ thick calcified retinal density (calcified angioma-induced hematoma)
   US:
   √ small hyperechoic solid masses, most in temporal retina
   Cx: (1) repeated vitreous hemorrhage (frequent)
   (2) exudative retinal detachment posteriorly

2. Hemangioblastomas of CNS = **Lindau tumor** (40%)
   = most commonly recognized manifestation of vHL disease
   Age: 15–40 years
   Site: cerebellum (65%), brainstem (20%), spinal cord (15%); multiple lesions in 10–15%
   ◊ 4–20% of single hemangioblastomas occur in von Hippel-Lindau disease!
   CT:
   √ large cystic lesion with 3–15 mm mural nodule (75%)
   √ solid enhancing lesion (10%)
   √ enhancing lesion with multiple cystic areas (15%)
   √ intense tumor blush / blushing mural nodule
   √ NO calcifications (DDx: cystic astrocytoma calcifies in 25%)
   MR (modality of choice):
   √ hypointense cystic component on T1WI (slightly hyperintense to CSF due to protein content); hyperintense on T2WI
   √ small tubular areas of flow void within mural nodule (= enlarged feeding + draining vessels); intense contrast enhancement of mural nodule
   √ slightly hypointense solid lesion on T1WI; hyperintense on T2WI; intense contrast enhancement
   Angio:
   √ intense staining of mural nodule ("mother-in-law phenomenon" = tumor blush comes early, stays late, very dense)
   √ presence of feeding vessels
   Prognosis: most frequent cause of morbidity and mortality; frequent recurrence after resection

@ LABYRINTH
1. Endolymphatic sac neoplasm
   = aggressive adenomatous tumor with mixed histologic features
   - sensorineural hearing loss
   Location: retrolabyrinthine temporal bone
   Site: endolymphatic sac
   √ aggressive lytic lesion containing intratumoral osseous spicules + areas of hemorrhage
   √ heterogeneous enhancement with hyperintense areas on T1WI + T2WI (due to hemorrhage)

@ HEART
1. Rhabdomyoma

@ KIDNEYS
- polycythemia due to elevated erythropoietin level (in 15% with hemangioblastoma, in 10% with renal cell carcinoma)
1. Cortical renal cysts (75%)
   multiple + bilateral (may be confused with adult polycystic kidney disease)
2. Renal cell carcinoma (20–45%)
   Age: 20–50 years
   √ multicentric in 87%, bilateral in 10–75%, may arise from cyst wall
   √ sensitivity: 35% for angiography, 37% for US, 45% for CT (due to inability to reliably distinguish between cystic RCC, cancer within cyst, atypical cyst)
   √ 50% metastatic at time of discovery
   Prognosis: RCC is cause of death in 30–50% as the second most frequent cause of mortality!
3. Renal adenoma
4. Renal hemangioma

@ ADRENAL pheochromocytoma (in up to 10–17%), bilateral in up to 40%; confined to certain families

@ EPIDIDYMIS
1. Cystadenoma of epididymis

@ PANCREAS
1. Pancreatic cystadenoma / cystadenocarcinoma
2. Pancreatic islet cell tumor
3. Pancreatic hemangioblastoma
4. Pancreatic cysts (in 30%); incidence in autopsies up to 72%

√ usually multiple and multilocular cysts

@ LIVER
1. Liver hemangioma
2. Adenoma

@ OTHERS
1. Paraganglioma
2. Cysts in virtually any organ: liver, spleen, adrenal, epididymis, omentum, mesentery, lung, bone

MULTIPLE ORGAN NEOPLASMS

@ Kidney : renal cell carcinoma (up to 40%), renal angioma (up to 45%)

@ Liver : adenoma, angioma

@ Pancreas : cystadenoma / adenocarcinoma

@ Epididymis : adenoma

@ Adrenal gland: pheochromocytoma

MULTIPLE ORGAN CYSTS

(1) Kidney (usually multiple cortical cysts in 75–100% at early age, most common abdominal manifestation)

(2) Pancreas (in 9–72% often numerous cysts; second most common affected abdominal organ)

(3) Others: liver, spleen, omentum, mesentery, epididymis, adrenals, lung, bone

DIFFERENTIAL DIAGNOSIS OF OCULAR AND ORBITAL DISORDERS

OPHTHALMOPLEGIA

Lesions of

1. Oculomotor nerve (III)
   innervates medial rectus, superior rectus, inferior rectus, inferior oblique muscle, pupilloconstrictor, levator palpebrae
2. Trochlear nerve (IV)
   innervates superior oblique muscle
3. Abducens nerve (VI)
   innervates lateral rectus muscle

ANOPIA

[numbers are referring to drawing]

A. MONOCULAR DEFECTS
  1 = monocular blindness (optic nerve lesion in fracture of optic canal, amaurosis fugax)

B. BILATERAL HETERONYMOUS DEFECTS
  2 = bitemporal hemianopia (chiasmatic lesion)

C. BILATERAL HOMONYMOUS DEFECTS
  3 = homonymous hemianopia
  4 = upper right-sided quadrantanopia
  5 = central hemianoptic scotoma
  3,4,5 = most common type of hemianopia (CVA, brain tumor)

OCULAR TRAUMA

Types: (a) Simple / complicated contusion with rupture of ocular wall
(b) Simple / perforating injury to the globe
(c) Foreign body

Evaluate for:

(1) vitreous hemorrhage

(2) retinal detachment

(3) choroidal detachment

(4) alteration in position / texture of lens

(5) thickening / rupture of ocular wall

(6) Hematoma in retro-ocular space

(7) Vascular complications: central renal artery occlusion, carotid-cavernous fistula, fistula of angular vein

(8) Foreign body in globe (95% sensitivity for US) / orbit (50% sensitivity for US)

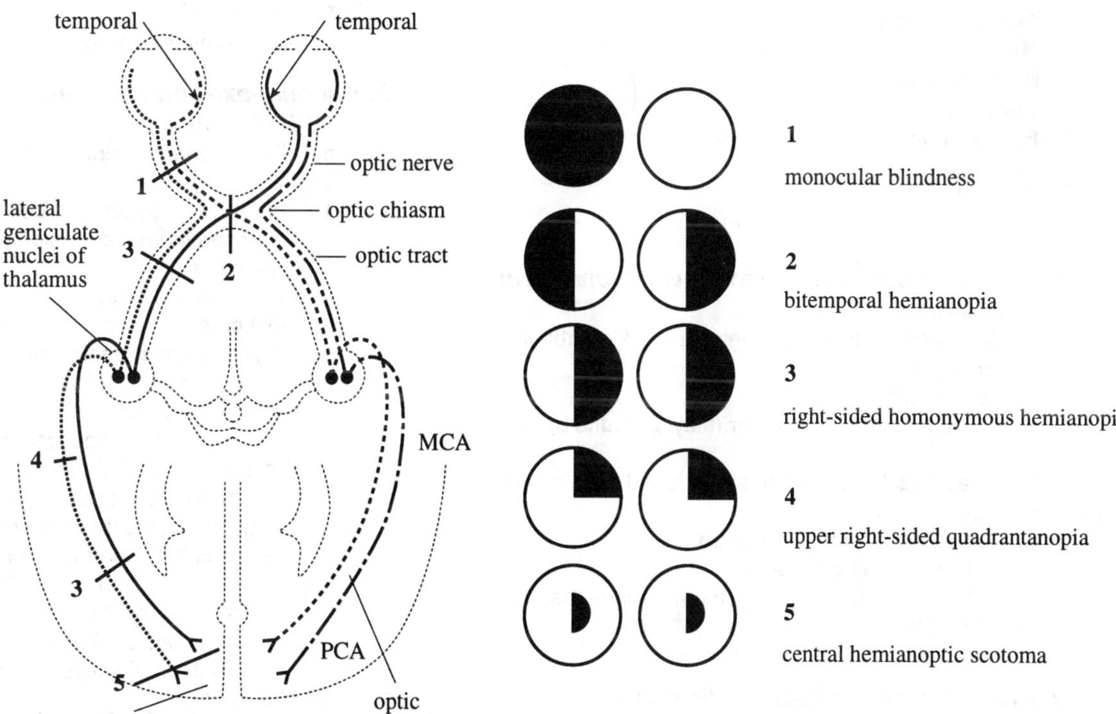

Types of Anopia

EYE

ORBIT

Spectrum of orbital disorders

A. INFLAMMATORY DISEASE
  1. Tissue-specific inflammation:
     orbital cellulitis, optic neuritis, scleritis, myositis
  2. Panophthalmitis
  3. Pseudotumor of orbit

B. CYSTIC DISEASE
  1. Dermoid cyst
  2. Mucocele
  3. Retro-ocular cyst (developmental)

C. VASCULAR DISEASE
  1. Cavernous angioma
  2. Capillary angioma
  3. Lymphangioma
  4. Varix
  5. Carotid-cavernous fistula

D. TUMORS
  1. Rhabdomyosarcoma
  2. Optic nerve glioma
  3. Meningioma
  4. Lymphoma
  5. Metastasis

Intraconal lesion

mnemonic: "**M**el **M**et **R**ita **M**ending **H**ems **O**n **P**oor **C**harlie's **G**rave"

Melanoma
Metastasis
Retinoblastoma
Meningioma
Hemangioma
Optic glioma
Pseudotumor
Cellulitis
Grave disease

Intraconal lesion with optic nerve involvement

1. Optic nerve glioma
2. Optic nerve sheath meningioma (10% of orbital neoplasm)
3. Optic neuritis
4. Inflammatory pseudotumor (may surround optic nerve)
5. Intraorbital lymphoma (may surround optic nerve, older patient)
6. Elevated intracranial pressure
   = distension of optic sheath
   √ bilateral tortuous enlarged optic nerve-sheath complex

Intraconal lesion without optic nerve involvement

1. Cavernous hemangioma
2. Orbital varix
3. Carotid-cavernous fistula
4. Arteriovenous malformation
   least common of orbital vascular malformations (congenital, idiopathic, traumatic)
   √ irregularly shaped intensely enhancing mass of enlarged vessels
   √ associated with dilated superior / inferior ophthalmic vein
5. Hematoma
6. Lymphangioma
7. Neurilemoma
   √ commonly adjacent to superior orbital fissure, inferior to optic nerve
   √ local bone erosion

Extraconal lesion

Extraconal-intraorbital lesion

A. BENIGN TUMOR
  1. Dermoid cyst
  2. **Teratoma**
     <1% of all pediatric orbital tumors
     √ ± areas of fat, cartilage, bone
     √ expansion of bony orbit ± bone defect
  3. Capillary hemangioma
  4. Lymphangioma
  5. Plexiform neurofibroma
  6. Inflammatory orbital pseudotumor
  7. Histiocytosis X
     lesion usually arises from bone

B. MALIGNANT TUMOR
  1. Lymphoma / Leukemia
  2. Metastasis
  3. Rhabdomyosarcoma

Extraconal-extraorbital lesion

A. FROM SINUS
  maxillary / sphenoid sinuses are rare locations of origin
  1. Tumor: squamous cell carcinoma (80%), adenocarcinoma, adenoid cystic carcinoma, lymphoma
  2. Paranasal sinusitis:
     most common cause of orbital infection;
     Origin: from ethmoid sinuses (in children), from frontal sinus (in adolescence)
     Organism: Staphylococcus, Streptococcus, Pneumococcus
     √ preseptal / orbital edema / cellulitis
     √ subperiosteal / orbital abscess
     √ mucormycosis (in diabetics) destroys bone + extends into cavernous sinus
     Cx: (1) epidural abscess (2) subdural empyema (3) cavernous sinus thrombosis (4) meningitis (5) cerebritis (6) brain abscess
  3. Mucocele

B. FROM SKIN
  1. Orbital cellulitis

C. FROM LACRIMAL GLAND
  √ mass arising from superolateral aspect of orbit

mnemonic: "MOLD"
Metastasis
Others (rhabdomyosarcoma, lymphangioma, sinus lesion)
Lymphoma, **L**acrimal gland tumor
Dermoid

Orbital Mass In Childhood

1.	Dermoid cyst	46%
2.	Inflammatory lesion	16%
3.	Dermolipoma	7%
4.	Capillary hemangioma	4%
5.	Rhabdomyosarcoma	4%
6.	Leukemia / lymphoma	2%
7.	Optic nerve glioma	2%
8.	Lymphangioma	2%
9.	Cavernous hemangioma	1%

mnemonic: "LO VISHON"
Leukemia, **L**ymphoma
Optic nerve glioma
Vascular malformation: hemangioma, lymphangioma
Inflammation
Sarcoma: ie, rhabdomyosarcoma
Histiocytosis
Orbital pseudotumor, **O**steoma
Neuroblastoma

Primary Malignant Orbital Tumors

1.	Retinoblastoma	86.0%
2.	Rhabdomyosarcoma	8.1%
3.	Uveal melanoma	2.3%
4.	Sarcoma	1.7%

Secondary Malignant Orbital Tumors

1.	Leukemia	36.7%
2.	Sarcoma	14.3%
3.	Hodgkin lymphoma	11.0%
4.	Neuroblastoma	9.2%
5.	Wilms tumor	6.7%
6.	Non-Hodgkin lymphoma	5.6%
7.	Histiocytosis	3.9%
8.	Medulloblastoma	3.5%

Orbital Cystic Lesion

1. Abscess
2. Intraorbital hematoma
3. Dermoid cyst
4. Lacrimal cyst
5. Lymphangioma
6. Hydatid cyst

Orbital Vascular Tumors

1. Orbital varix
2. Arteriovenous malformation
3. Carotid-cavernous fistula
4. Hemangioma: capillary / cavernous
5. Blood cyst
6. Arterial malformation
7. Glomus tumor
8. Hemangiopericytoma

Mass In Superolateral Quadrant Of Orbit

1. Lacrimal gland tumor
2. Dermoid cyst
3. Metastasis (breast, prostate, lung)
4. Lymphoma
5. Leukemic infiltration of lacrimal gland
6. Sarcoidosis
7. Wegener granulomatosis
8. Pseudotumor
9. Frontal sinus mucocele

Extraocular Muscle Enlargement

A. ENDOCRINE
   1. Grave disease (50%)
   2. Acromegaly

B. INFLAMMATION
   1. **Myositis**
      - rapid onset of proptosis, erythema of lids, conjunctival injection

      Location: single muscle (in adults); multiple muscles (in children)
      √ enlarged extraocular muscle
      √ positive response to steroids
   2. Orbital cellulitis
   3. Sjögren disease, Wegener granulomatosis, lethal midline granuloma, SLE
   4. Sarcoidosis
   5. Foreign-body reaction

C. TUMOR
   1. Pseudotumor
   2. Rhabdomyosarcoma
   3. Metastasis, lymphoma, leukemia

D. VASCULAR
   1. Spontaneous / traumatic hematoma
   2. Arteriovenous malformation
   3. Carotid-cavernous sinus fistula

GLOBE

Spectrum Of Ocular Disorders

A. CONGENITAL
   1. Persistent hyperplastic primary vitreous
   2. Coats disease
   3. Coloboma
   4. Congenital cataract

B. VITREORETINAL
   1. Vitreous hemorrhage
   2. Retinal detachment
   3. Choroidal detachment
   4. Endophthalmitis
   5. Retinoschisis
   6. Retrolental fibroplasia

C. TUMOR
   1. Retinoblastoma
   2. Choroidal hemangioma
   3. Retinal angiomatosis
   4. Melanocytoma
   5. Choroidal osteoma

D. TRAUMA

Microphthalmia

= congenital underdevelopment / acquired diminution of globe

A. BILATERAL with cataract
   1. Congenital rubella
   2. Persistent hyperplastic vitreous
   3. Retinopathy of prematurity
   4. Retinal folds
   5. Lowe syndrome
      √ small globe + small orbit

B. UNILATERAL
   1. Trauma / surgery / radiation therapy
   2. Inflammation with disorganization of eye (phthisis bulbi)
      √ shrunken calcified globe + normal orbit

Macrophthalmia

= enlargement of globe

A. WITHOUT INTRAOCULAR MASS
   (a) generalized enlargement
      1. Axial myopia (most common cause)
         √ enlargement of globe in AP direction
         √ ± thinning of sclera
      2. Buphthalmos
      3. Juvenile glaucoma
      4. Connective tissue disorder: Marfan syndrome, Ehlers-Danlos syndrome, Weill-Marchesani syndrome (congenital mesodermal dysmorphodystrophy), homocystinuria
         √ "wavy" contour of sclera
   (b) focal enlargement
      1. **Staphyloma**
         = sacculation of posterior pole of globe (or berrylike protrusion of cornea)
         Prevalence: increasing with size of globe
         Cause: axial myopia (temporal side of optic disc / anteriorly / along equator), trauma, scleritis, necrotizing infection
         √ focal bulge + thinning of sclera
         Cx: advanced chorioretinal degeneration (77%), choroid retraction from optic disc, posterior vitreous detachment, choroidal hemorrhage, retinal detachment, cataract, glaucoma
      2. Apparent enlargement due to contralateral microphthalmia

B. WITH INTRAOCULAR MASS
   (rare cause for enlargement)
   (a) with calcifications:
      1. Retinoblastoma
   (b) without calcifications:
      1. Melanoma
      2. Metastasis

Ocular Lesion

Intraocular Calcifications

1. Retinoblastoma (>50% of all cases)
2. Astrocytic hamartoma
3. **Choroidal osteoma**
   = rare juxtapapillary tumor of mature bone
   Age: young woman; may be bilateral
   √ small flat very dense curvilinear mass aligned with choroidal margin of globe
   DDx: calcified choroidal angioma
4. **Optic drusen**
   = accretions of hyaline material on / near surface of optic disc; often familial
   • headache, visual field defects
   • pseudopapilledema
   √ small flat / round calcification at junction of retina + optic nerve
   √ bilateral in 75%
5. Scleral calcifications
   (a) in systemic hypercalcemic states (HPT, hypervitaminosis D, sarcoidosis, secondary to chronic renal disease)
   (b) in elderly: at insertion of extraocular muscles
6. Retrolental fibroplasia
7. **Phthisis bulbi**
   secondary to trauma or infection
   √ small contracted calcified disorganized nonfunctioning globe

mnemonic: "NMR CT"
Neurofibromatosis
Melanoma (hyperdense melanin)
Retinoblastoma
Choroidal osteoma
Tuberous sclerosis

Noncalcified Ocular Process

1. Uveal melanoma
2. Metastasis
   86% of ocular lesions within globe; usually in vascular choroid
   Origin: breast, lung, GI tract, GU tract, cutaneous melanoma, neuroblastoma
   √ bilateral in 30%
3. Choroidal hemangioma
4. **Vitreous lymphoma**
   √ diffuse ill-defined soft-tissue density
5. Developmental anomalies
   (a) **Primary glaucoma** = enlargement of eye secondary to narrowing of Schlemm canal
   (b) Coloboma
   (c) Staphyloma

Vitreous Hemorrhage

Cause: trauma, surgical intervention, arterial hypertension, retinal detachment, ocular tumor, Coats disease

US:
√ numerous irregular, poorly defined, mobile low-intensity echoes
√ voluminous hyperechoic fibrin clots not fixed to optic nerve (DDx to retinal detachment)

Prognosis: complete absorption / development of vitreous membranes (repetitive episodes)

Dense vitreous in pediatric age group
1. Retinoblastoma
2. Persistent hyperplastic primary vitreous
3. Coats disease
4. Norrie disease
5. Retrolental fibroplasia
6. Sclerosing endophthalmitis

Retinal detachment
Cause: trauma, tumor, exudative / inflammatory process, scar

US:
- √ curvilinear area of high echogenicity fixed at optic disk (= papilla) + extending to ora serrata
- √ V-shaped (with total detachment)
- √ in one quadrant only (partial detachment)
- √ thick folded retina with loss of mobility (long-standing detachment)
- √ subretinal space normal / occupied by blood, inflammation / tumor (depending on cause)

DDx: vitreous membranes, choroidal detachment (point of fixation not at papilla)

Choroidal detachment
Cause: trauma, surgical intervention, spontaneous

US:
- √ two convex lines emerging from both walls of the vitreous + advancing to ciliary body with posterior fixation outside the macula
- √ minimal / no choroidal membrane mobility

Leukokoria
= abnormal white / pinkish / yellowish pupillary light reflex [from Greek *leuko* = white and *koria* = pupil]

A. TUMOR
1. Retinoblastoma (most common cause – 58%)
2. Retinal astrocytic hamartoma (3%): associated with tuberous sclerosis + von Recklinghausen disease
2. Medulloepithelioma (rare)

B. DEVELOPMENTAL
1. Persistent hyperplastic primary vitreous (2nd most common cause – 28%)
2. Coats disease (16%)
3. Retrolental fibroplasia (3–5%)
4. Coloboma of choroid / optic disc

C. INFECTION
1. Uveitis
2. Larval granulomatosis (16%)

D. DEGENERATIVE
1. Posterior cataract

E. TRAUMA
1. Retinopathy of prematurity (5%)
2. Organized vitreous hemorrhage
3. Long-standing retinal detachment

Leukokoria in normal-sized eye
A. CALCIFIED MASS
1. Retinoblastoma
2. Retinal astrocytoma

B. NONCALCIFIED MASS
1. Toxocaral endophthalmitis
2. Coats disease

Leukokoria with microphthalmia
A. UNILATERAL
1. Persistent hyperplastic primary vitreous (PHPV)

B. BILATERAL
1. Retinopathy of prematurity
2. Bilateral PHPV

OPTIC NERVE

Optic nerve enlargement
A. TUMOR:
1. Optic nerve glioma
2. Optic nerve sheath meningioma
3. Infiltration by leukemia / lymphoma

B. FLUID:
1. Perineural hematoma
2. Papilledema of intracranial hypertension
3. Patulous subarachnoid space

C. INFLAMMATION:
1. Optic neuritis
2. Sarcoidosis

- √ fusiform thickening
  = lens-shaped thickening of nerve-sheath complex
  (a) with central lucency: meningioma
  (b) without central lucency: optic nerve glioma
- √ excrescentic thickening
  = single / multiple nodules along nerve-sheath complex usually due to tumor
- √ tubular enlargement
  = uniform enlargement of nerve-sheath complex
  (a) with central lucency: subarachnoid process (metastases, perineuritis, meningioma, perineural hemorrhage)
  (b) without central lucency: papilledema, leukemia, lymphoma, sarcoid, optic nerve glioma

LACRIMAL GLAND

Lacrimal gland lesion
A. INFLAMMATION
1. Dacryoadenitis
2. **Mikulicz syndrome**
   = nonspecific enlargement of lacrimal + salivary glands
   Associated with: sarcoidosis, lymphoma, leukemia
3. **Sjögren syndrome**
   = lymphocytic infiltration of lacrimal + salivary glands
   • decreased lacrimation, xerostomia
   Often associated with:
   rheumatoid arthritis, systemic lupus erythematosus, scleroderma, polymyositis
4. Sarcoidosis

EYE

B. TUMOR
- (a) benign: granuloma, cyst, benign mixed tumor (= pleomorphic adenoma)
- (b) malignant: malignant mixed tumor (= pleomorphic adenocarcinoma), adenoid cystic carcinoma, lymphoma, metastasis (rare)

Lacrimal gland enlargement

mnemonic: "MELD"

Metastasis
Epithelial tumor
Lymphoid tumor
Dermoid

BILATERAL LACRIMAL GLAND MASSES

mnemonic: "LACS"

Lymphoma
And
Collagen-vascular disease
Sarcoidosis

ANATOMY OF ORBIT

Orbital connections

Superior orbital fissure

Boundaries (Gray's Anatomy):
- — medial : sphenoid body
- — above : lesser wing of sphenoid = optic strut
- — below : greater wing of sphenoid
- — lateral : small segment of frontal bone

Contents:

(a) nerves:
- III oculomotor n.
- IV trochlear n.
- V_1 ophthalmic branch of trigeminal n.:
  - (a) lacrimal nerve
  - (b) frontal nerve
- VI abducens n.
- sympathetic filaments of internal carotid plexus

(b) veins: superior + inferior ophthalmic vein

(c) arteries:
1. meningeal branch of lacrimal artery
2. orbital branch of middle meningeal artery

Inferior orbital fissure

Location: between floor + lateral wall of orbit; connects with pterygopalatine + infratemporal fossa

Contents:

(a) nerves: infraorbital + zygomatic nn.
branches from pterygopalatine ganglion

(b) veins: connection between inferior orbital v. + pterygoid plexus

superior rectus m..
superior ophthalmic v.
levator palpebrae superioris m.
ophthalmic a.
superior oblique m.
lateral rectus m.
medial rectus m.
inferior rectus m.
optic n.
infraorbital n.

Coronal Orbital Tomogram Through Midorbit

Optic canal

completely formed by lesser wing of sphenoid

Contents:
- (a) nerve: optic nerve (I)
- (b) vessel: ophthalmic a.

Normal orbit measurements

Muscles
- medial rectus muscle .... 4.1 ± 0.5 mm
- inferior rectus muscle .... 4.9 ± 0.8 mm
- superior rectus muscle .... 3.8 ± 0.7 mm
- lateral rectus muscle .... 2.9 ± 0.6 mm
- superior oblique muscle .... 2.4 ± 0.4 mm

Superior ophthalmic vein
- axial CT .... 1.8 ± 0.5 mm
- coronal CT .... 2.7 ± 1.0 mm

Optic nerve sheath
- retrobulbar............................... 5.5 ± 0.8 mm
- waist....................................... 4.2 ± 0.6 mm

Globe position
- behind interzygomatic line .... 9.9 ± 1.7 mm

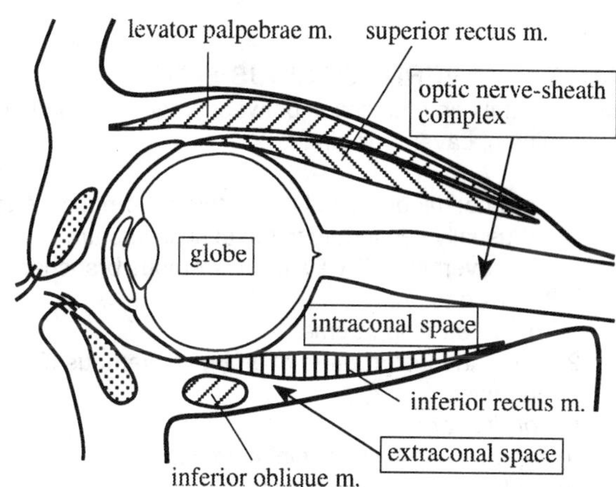

Orbital Spaces

globe:	subdivided into anterior + posterior segments by lens
optic nerve-sheath complex:	optic nerve surrounded by meningeal sheath as extension from cerebral meninges
intraconal space:	orbital fat, ophthalmic a., superior ophthalmic v., nerves I, III, IV, V_1, VI
conus:	incomplete fenestrated musculofascial system extending from bony orbit to anterior third of globe, consists of extraocular muscles + interconnecting fascia
extraconal space:	between muscle cone + bony orbit containing fat, lacrimal gland, lacrimal sac, portion of superior ophthalmic v.

EYE

EYE

ORBITAL DISORDERS

BUPHTHALMOS
= HYDROPHTHALMOS = MEGOPHTHALMOS
= diffuse enlargement of eye in children secondary to increased intraocular pressure
Cause:
1. Congenital / infantile glaucoma
2. Neurofibromatosis type 1: obstruction of canal of Schlemm by membranes / masses composed of aberrant mesodermal tissue
3. Sturge-Weber syndrome
4. Lowe (cerebrohepatorenal) syndrome
5. Ocular mesodermal dysplasia (eg, Axenfeld or Rieger anomalies)
6. Homocystinuria
7. Aniridia
8. Acquired glaucoma (rare)

Pathophysiology:
obstruction of canal of Schlemm located between cornea + iris leads to decreased resorption of aqueous humor (= anterior chamber fluid) with scleral distension
√ uniformly enlarged globe without mass of round / oval / bizarre shape

Rx: goniotomy (increases the angle of anterior chamber); trabeculotomy (lyses adhesions)

CAROTID-CAVERNOUS SINUS FISTULA
= abnormal communication between internal carotid artery + veins of cavernous sinus
Etiology:
(1) Trauma: laceration of ICA within cavernous sinus
  (a) usually secondary to basal skull fracture (cavernous ICA + small cavernous branches fixed to dura)
  (b) penetrating trauma
(2) Spontaneous: rupture of an intracavernous ICA aneurysm

Route of drainage:
(a) superior ophthalmic vein (common)
(b) contralateral cavernous sinus
(c) petrosal sinus
(d) cortical veins (rare)

• pulsating exophthalmos, chemosis, conjunctival edema
• persistent orbital bruit
• restricted extraocular movement
• decrease in vision due to increase in intraocular pressure (50%) = indication for emergent treatment

√ enlarged edematous extraocular muscles
√ dilatation of superior ophthalmic vein / facial veins / internal jugular vein
√ focal / diffuse enlargement of cavernous sinus
√ occasionally sellar erosion / enlargement
√ enlargement of superior orbital fissure (in chronic phase)

US + MR:
√ arterial flow in cavernous sinus + superior ophthalmic vein

Angio:
√ ipsilateral ICA contrast injection shows wall of ICA to be incomplete
√ contralateral ICA contrast injection + compression of involved ICA
√ early opacification of veins of cavernous sinus
√ retrograde flow through dilated superior ophthalmic v.

Rx: latex / silicone balloon detached inside cavernous sinus to plug laceration (ocular signs resolve within 7–10 days)

CHOROIDAL HEMANGIOMA
= vascular hamartoma
Age: 10–20 years (most common benign tumor in adults)
May be associated with: Sturge-Weber syndrome
Location: posterior pole temporal to optic disk (70%)
√ 0.5–3-mm small tumor
√ focal thickening of posterior wall of globe
√ enhancement similar to choroid
√ retinal detachment (frequent)

US:
√ hyperechoic homogeneous mass

DDx: melanoma (choroidal excavitation)

COATS DISEASE
= RETINAL TELANGIECTASIA
= Pseudoglioma = congenital idiopathic primary vascular malformation of the retina characterized by
(1) multiple abnormal telangiectatic retinal vessels
(2) lack of blood-retina barrier causing leakage of a lipoproteinaceous exudate into retina + subretinal space with secondary detachment of retina

Age: 6–8 years (but present at birth); M:F = 2:1
• strabismus
• may present with leukokoria (if retina massively detached) [16% of leukokoria cases]
• loss of vision, secondary glaucoma
• cholesterol crystals at funduscopy

Location: unilateral in 90%
Associated with:
√ retinal detachment
√ slight microphthalmia

√ NO focal mass / calcification (HALLMARK)

US:
√ clumpy particulate echoes in subretinal space (due to cholesterol crystals suspended in fluid)
√ vitreous + subretinal hemorrhage (frequent)
DDx: unilateral noncalcifying retinoblastoma (before 3 years of age, no microphthalmia)

CT:
√ unilateral dense vitreous in normal-sized globe

MR:
√ hyperintense subretinal exudate on T1WI + T2WI (due to mixture of protein + lipid) / hypointense on T2WI (cholesterol crystals + membranous lipids)
√ abnormal enhancement of retina at ora serrata + of detached retinal leaves

DDx: (1) Persistent hyperplastic primary vitreous (thick tubular retrolental mass)
(2) Retinopathy of prematurity
Rx: photocoagulation / cryotherapy to obliterate telangiectasias (in early stages)

COLOBOMA

[Greek koloboun, to mutilate]
= incomplete closure of embryonic choroidal fissure affecting eyelid / lens / iris / choroid / retina / macula; autosomal dominant trait with variable penetrance (30%) and expression; bilateral in 60%
Time of insult: 6th week of GA
May be associated with: encephalocele, agenesis of corpus callosum
Location: in 50% bilateral
√ cystic outpouching (= herniation) of vitreous at site of optic nerve attachment
√ small globe
DDx: microphthalmos with cyst = duplication cyst, axial (high) myopia

CONGENITAL CATARACT

= opacification of lens
Etiology: infection, hereditary
Location: frequently bilateral
US:
√ increase in thickness + echogenicity of posterior wall of lens ± intralenticular echoes

DACRYOADENITIS

= infection of lacrimal gland
Organism: staphylococci (most common), mumps, infectious mononucleosis, influenza
√ homogeneous enlargement of lacrimal gland
√ ± compression of globe

DERMOID CYST OF ORBIT

Most common benign orbital tumor in childhood (45% of all masses)
Age: 1st decade
Histo: contains keratin, hair, stratified epithelium + dermal appendages within thick capsule; usually arises in fetal cleavage planes (sutures)
Location: in anterior extraconal orbit, upper temporal quadrant (60%), upper nasal quadrant (25%)
√ well-defined cystic mass ± negative HU numbers
√ thick surrounding capsule
√ ± expansion / erosion of bony orbit
US:
√ encapsulated heterogeneous mass with variable cystic component
MR:
√ high signal intensity on T1WI + T2WI

ENDOPHTHALMITIS

Infectious endophthalmitis

Organism: bacteria (rare in childhood, trauma, idiopathic), fungi, parasites
Cause:
(a) exogenous endophthalmitis: most commonly related to eye injury / surgery
(b) endogenous endophthalmitis: hematogenous spread from distant source of infection
US:
√ medium- to high-intensity echoes dispersed throughout vitreous (DDx: echoes in vitreous hemorrhage are more mobile)
CT:
√ increased attenuation of vitreous
√ uveal-scleral thickening
√ decreased attenuation of lens

Sclerosing endophthalmitis

= TOXOCARA CANIS ENDOPHTHALMITIS
= granulomatous uveitis resulting in subretinal exudate, retinal detachment, organized vitreous
Age: 2–6–12 years
Mode of infection:
playing in soil contaminated by viable infective eggs from dog excrement (common in playgrounds)
Organism: helminthic nematode Toxocara canis causing visceral / ocular larva migrans (0.5 mm long, 20 μm wide); endemic throughout world; especially common in southeastern United States
Life cycle:
egg hatches into larva within intestines of definite host (dog) + develops into adult worm; alternatively dog may eat infective-stage larvae from intestines / viscera of other animals; in noncanine host larvae will not develop into adult worm, but burrow through intestinal wall and migrate to liver, lung, and other tissue including brain + eye
Pathophysiology:
migration through human tissue produces a severe eosinophilic reaction that becomes granulomatous; spreads hematogenously to temporal choroid
Path: retina elevated + distorted + partially replaced by an inflammatory mass containing abundant dense scar tissue; subjacent choroid infiltrated with chronic inflammatory cells including eosinophils; proteinaceous subretinal exudate
• red "hot" eye, photophobia, pain
• anterior chamber flare cells, keratic precipitates
• vitreous synechia
• vitreitis = accumulation of cellular debris in vitreous
• leukokoria (16% of cases of childhood leukokoria)
• fever, hepatomegaly, pneumonitis, convulsions
• peripheral blood eosinophilia
Location: usually unilateral
√ eye of normal size without calcifications
√ secondary retinal detachment
US:
√ hypoechoic mass in peripheral fundus
√ ± calcifications
CT:
√ intravitreal mass

√ focal uveoscleral thickening (granulomatous reaction around larva) with contrast enhancement
√ increased density of vitreous cavity

MR:
√ enhancing granuloma isointense to vitreous on T1WI
√ mass usually hyperintense relative to vitreous on T2WI, occasionally hypointense (due to dense fibroconnective tissue)

Cx: retinal detachment (due to subretinal fluid / vitreoretinal traction), cataract
Dx: (1) Enzyme-linked immunosorbent assay (ELISA) on blood serum / vitreous aspirate
(2) Histologic identification of organism
DDx: retinoblastoma

GRAVES DISEASE OF ORBIT

= THYROID OPHTHALMOPATHY
= ENDOCRINE EXOPHTHALMOS
= increase in orbital pressure produces ischemia, edema, fibrosis of muscles

Etiology: produced by long-acting thyroid-stimulating factor (LATS); probably immunologic cross-reactivity against antigens shared by thyroid + orbital tissue
Age: adulthood; 5% younger than 15 years; M:F = 1:4
Histo: deposition of hygroscopic mucopolysaccharides + glycoprotein (early) + collagen (late); infiltration by mast cells and lymphocytes, edema, muscle fiber necrosis, lipomatosis, fatty degeneration
Time of onset: signs + symptoms usually develop within one year of the onset of hyperthyroidism

• proptosis
◊ Most common cause of uni- / bilateral proptosis in adult!
• lid lag = upper eyelid retraction
• periorbital swelling
• conjunctival injection
• restricted ocular motility (correlates with increase in mean muscle diameters)
• progressive optic neuropathy (5%)
• hyperthyroidism; euthyroidism (in 10–15%); severity of orbital involvement unrelated to degree of thyroid dysfunction

STAGING (Werner's modified classification):
Stage I : eyelid retraction without symptoms
Stage II : eyelid retraction with symptoms
Stage III : proptosis >22 mm without diplopia
Stage IV : proptosis >22 mm with diplopia
Stage V : corneal ulceration
Stage VI : loss of sight

Location:
bilateral in 70–85%; single muscle in 10%; asymmetrical involvement in 10–30%; all muscles equally affected with similar proportional enlargements; superior muscle group most commonly when only single muscle involved [former notion: inferior > medial > superior rectus muscle + levator palpebrae > lateral rectus muscle

mnemonic: "I'M SLow"
Inferior
Medial
Superior
Lateral]

√ proptosis = globe protrusion >21 mm anterior to interzygomatic line on axial scans at level of lens
√ swelling of muscles maximally in midportion (relative sparing of tendinous insertion at globe) = "Coke-bottle" sign
√ slight uveal-scleral thickening
√ apical crowding = orbital apex involved late (pressure on optic nerve)
√ dilatation of superior ophthalmic vein (compromised orbital venous drainage at orbital apex due to enlarged extraocular muscles)
√ increase in diameter of retrobulbar optic nerve sheath (dural distension due to accumulation of CSF in subarachnoid space with optic neuropathy)
√ increased density of orbital fat (late)
√ anterior displacement of lacrimal gland
√ intracranial fat herniation through superior ophthalmic fissure (best correlation with compressive neuropathy

MR:
√ high signal intensity in enlarged eye muscles on T2WI (edema in acute inflammation)

Prognosis: in 90% spontaneous resolution within 3–36 months; in 10% decrease in visual acuity (corneal ulceration / optic neuropathy)
Rx: short- and long-term steroid therapy, cyclosporine, radiation, surgical decompression, correction of eyelid position
DDx: pseudotumor (usually includes tendon of eye muscles)

HEMANGIOMA OF ORBIT

Most common benign orbital tumor
Location: 83–94% retrobulbar (intraconal)
√ sharply demarcated oval mass in superior-temporal portion of conus (2/3) often sparing orbital apex
√ displacement (not involvement) of optic nerve
√ expansion of bony orbit
√ uniform / inhomogeneous (when thrombosed) enhancement
√ small calcifications (phleboliths)
√ puddling of contrast material on angiography

US:
√ well-defined encapsulated mass of intermediate echogenicity
√ absent / poor predominantly venous flow

Capillary Hemangioma Of Orbit

most common vascular tumor of orbit in children; 5–15% of all pediatric orbital masses
Age: first 2 weeks of life; 95% in <6 months of age; M < F
Histo: proliferation of endothelial cells with multiple capillaries
• proptosis, chemosis (= edema) of eyelid + conjunctiva exaggerated by crying

• associated with skin angioma (90%)

Location: anterior part of orbit, occasionally posterior

√ mass with enhancement equal to / greater than orbital muscle

√ poorly marginated (suggesting malignant cause)

√ activity in radionuclide flow studies

US:

√ poorly defined heterogeneous mass of intermediate echogenicity

√ abundant internal flow decreasing with age

Prognosis: often increase in size for 6–10 months followed by spontaneous involution within 1–2 years

Cavernous Hemangioma Of Orbit

Frequency: usually tumor of adulthood; 12–15% of all orbital masses; 1–2% of childhood orbital masses

Age: 20–40 years; F > M

Histo: large dilated venous channels with flattened endothelial cells surrounded by fibrous pseudocapsule

• slowly progressive unilateral proptosis, diplopia, diminished visual acuity (optic nerve compression)

INFECTION OF ORBIT

Cause: bacterial infection extending from paranasal sinuses (especially ethmoid + frontal sinuses), face, eyelid, nose, teeth, lacrimal sac through thin lamina papyracea + valveless facial veins into orbit

Organism: staphylococci, streptococci, pneumococci

• lid edema, ocular pain, ophthalmoplegia

• fever, elevated WBC

Location: preseptal = periorbital soft tissue; subperiosteal; peripheral = extraconal fat; extraocular muscles; central = intraconal fat; optic nerve complex; globe; lacrimal gland

Cx: epidural abscess, subdural empyema, cavernous sinus thrombosis, cerebral abscess, osteomyelitis

Abscess Of Orbit

Location: most commonly in subperiosteal space on medial wall

√ subperiosteal fluid collection

√ displacement of thickened periosteal membrane + increased enhancement

√ displacement of adjacent fat + extraocular muscles

MR:

√ hyperintensity on T1WI + T2WI

Cellulitis Of Orbit

• limitation of ocular movements

• fever

√ thickening of eyelids + septum

√ proptosis

√ scleral thickening

√ enlargement + displacement of extraocular muscles (frequently medial rectus muscle)

√ increased attenuation of retro-orbital fat + obliteration of fat planes

√ opacification of ethmoid + maxillary sinuses

US:

√ diffuse hypoechoic area invading retrobulbar fat

Rx: antibiotics + corticosteroids

DDx: cannot be differentiated from edema, chloroma, leukemic infiltrate

Edema Of Orbit

Location: usually confined to preseptal structures (eyelid, face); involvement of orbital structures (rare)

√ swelling of eyelids / face

√ increased attenuation of orbital fat + obliteration of fat planes

√ displacement + enlargement of extraocular muscles

MR:

√ hyperintensity on T2WI

LYMPHANGIOMA OF ORBIT

Incidence: 3.5:100,000; 1–2% of orbital childhood masses; 8% of expanding orbital lesions

Histo: dilated lymphatics, dysplastic venous vessels, smooth muscle, areas of hemorrhage

(a) simple / capillary lymphangioma
= lymphatic channels of capillary size

(b) cavernous lymphangioma
= dilated microscopic channels

(c) cystic hygroma
= macroscopic multilocular cystic mass

Age: 1st decade or later (mean age of 6 years)

• proptosis (sudden proptosis from spontaneous intratumoral hemorrhage = CARDINAL FEATURE; exacerbated during upper respiratory infections [rare])

• associated with lesions on lid, conjunctiva, cheek

• coincident lymphangiomatous cysts in oral mucosa

Location: usually medial to optic nerve with intra- and extraconal component, crossing anatomic boundaries (conal fascia / orbital septum); may involve conjunctiva + lid

√ poorly defined multilobulated inhomogeneous lesion

√ single / multiple cystlike areas with rim enhancement (after hemorrhage) = blood cyst = "chocolate cyst"

√ areas of enhancement (= venous channels) / ring enhancement (after hemorrhage)

√ rarely contains phleboliths (DDx: hemangioma, orbital varix)

√ mild to moderate enlargement of orbit

US:

√ area of predominantly cystic heterogeneous texture with infiltrative borders

MR:

√ may show hematoma of various duration within lesion

Prognosis: no involution, progression slows with termination of body growth

DDx: orbital varix

LYMPHOMA OF ORBIT

Usually presents without evidence of systemic disease; subsequent development of systemic disease frequent

Incidence: 3rd most common cause of proptosis after orbital pseudotumor + cavernous hemangioma; in 8% of leukemia; in 3–4% of lymphoma

Age: 50 years on average

Type: usually non-Hodgkin B-cell lymphoma; Burkitt lymphoma with orbit as primary manifestation; Hodgkin disease rare

- painless swelling of eyelid
- exophthalmos (late in course of disease)

Location: extraconal (especially lacrimal gland, anterior extraconal space, retrobulbar) > intraconal > optic nerve-sheath complex; may be bilateral

◊ Lacrimal gland is a common site for leukemic infiltration!

Growth types:

(a) well-defined high-density mass (most commonly about lacrimal gland)

(b) diffuse infiltration (tends to involve entire intraconal region)

√ slight to moderate enhancement

US:

√ solitary / multiple hypoechoic homogeneous masses with infiltrative borders

METASTASIS TO ORBIT

Origin: only in 50% known; carcinoma of breast + lung (adults); neuroblastoma > Ewing sarcoma, leukemia, Wilms tumor (children)

Location: 12% intraorbital, 86% intraocular especially in posterior temporal portion of uvea (vascular layer between retina + sclera) near macula; may be bilateral

CT:

√ small areas of thickening + increased density

√ subretinal fluid

NORRIE DISEASE

= RETINAL DYSPLASIA

= X-linked recessive disease with; ? inherited form of persistent hyperplastic primary vitreous

- seizures, mental retardation (50%)
- hearing loss, deafness by age 4 (30%)
- bilateral leukokoria + microphthalmia
- cataract, blindness (absence of retinal ganglion cells)

√ microphthalmia

√ dense vitreous with blood-fluid level

√ cone-shaped central retinal detachment

√ calcifications

OCULAR TRAUMA

- clinical evaluation: testing of visual acuity, slit-lamp evaluation of cornea + anterior segment, intraocular pressure measurement, funduscopy

US (used if ocular media opaque due to vitreous hemorrhage / hyphema / traumatic cataract)

1. Vitreous hemorrhage (53%)
   - visual loss frequent

   √ echogenic material moving freely within vitreous chamber during eye movement

   Cx: retinal detachment (vitreous traction secondary to fibrovascular ingrowth following hemorrhage)

   Rx: vitrectomy
2. Total retinal detachment (18%)

   √ slightly thick line of "V" shape with apex at optic disk

   √ retina remains bound down at ora serrata
3. Vitreous detachment (11%)

   √ thin undulate mobile line moving away from posterior aspect of globe during eye motion
4. Intraocular foreign body (7%)

   Cx: siderosis (if metallic); endophthalmitis
5. Choroidal detachment (5%)

   √ convex lines projecting into the eye from periphery of globe, with most posterior aspect at some distance anterior to + separate from optic disk

   √ immobile during eye movement
6. Lens dislocation (3%)
7. Retrohyaloid hemorrhage (2%)

   √ echogenic material remaining behind detached vitreous capsule during eye movement
8. Focal retinal detachment (2%)

   √ elevated immobile line close to sclera at periphery of globe

OPTIC NERVE GLIOMA

= JUVENILE PILOCYTIC ASTROCYTOMA

= most common cause of optic nerve enlargement

Incidence: 1% of all intracranial tumors, 2% of childhood orbital masses; 80% of primary tumors of optic nerve

Histo: proliferation of well-differentiated astrocytes = low-grade glial neoplasm; most commonly pilocytic astrocytoma (in children) + glioblastoma (in adults)

Age: 1st decade (80%); peak age around 5 years; M < F

Associated with: neurofibromatosis in 10–50% (± bilateral optic gliomas)

◊ 15% of patients with neurofibromatosis have optic nerve gliomas!

- decreased visual acuity, minimal axial proptosis

√ tubular / fusiform / excrescentic well-circumscribed enlargement of optic nerve

√ posterior extension along optic tracts in 60–70% (indicates nonresectability)

√ calcifications (rare)

√ same attenuation as normal optic nerve; slight contrast enhancement

√ ipsilateral optic canal enlargement (90%) >3 mm / 1 mm difference compared with contralateral side

US:

√ well-defined homogeneous mass of medium echogenicity inseparable from optic nerve

MR: more sensitive than CT in detecting intracanalicular + intracranial extent

√ isointense to muscle on T1WI

√ hyperintense on T2WI

DDx: optic nerve sheath meningioma (no intracranial extension along optic pathway)

OPTIC NERVE SHEATH MENINGIOMA

= PERIOPTIC MENINGIOMA

Incidence: 10% of all intraorbital neoplasms; <2% of intracranial meningiomas

Age: middle-aged + elderly females; slightly more aggressive in children

Occasionally associated with:
neurofibromatosis (usually in teenagers)

Primary origin: arising from arachnoid rests in the meningeal investiture of optic nerves in orbit / middle fossa

• progressive loss of visual acuity over months (optic atrophy), proptosis

√ ± enlargement of optic canal
√ tubular (most commonly) / fusiform / excrescentic thickening of optic nerve
√ sphenoid bone hyperostosis
√ frequently calcified (HIGHLY SUGGESTIVE)

US:
√ hypoechoic tumor with irregular border

CECT: enhancement is the rule
√ dense linear bands (axial view) as "tram tracks" / ringlike (coronal view) due to tumor enhancement around nonenhancing optic nerve
√ minimal extension into optic canal (not uncommon)

MR:
√ extrinsic soft-tissue mass surrounding optic nerve
√ hypointense to fat on T1WI

OPTIC NEURITIS

= nerve involvement by inflammation, degeneration, demyelination

Etiology: (1) multiple sclerosis (involves optic nerve in 1/3)
(2) inflammation secondary to ocular infection
(3) degeneration (toxic, metabolic, nutritional)
(4) ischemia (5) meningitis / encephalitis

◊ 45–80% of patients develop multiple sclerosis within 15 years of their first episode of optic neuritis!

• ipsilateral orbital pain on eye movement
• sudden onset of unilateral loss of vision over several hours to several days

CT:
√ normal / mildly enlarged optic nerve + chiasm
√ may show enhancement

MR:
√ mild enlargement + enhancement of optic nerve well demonstrated on axial T1WI

Prognosis: spontaneous improvement of visual acuity within 1–2 weeks

PERSISTENT HYPERPLASTIC PRIMARY VITREOUS

= rare condition with persistence + proliferation of embryonic hyaloid vascular system of primary vitreous due to arrest of normal regression

May be associated with:
any severe ocular malformation / optic dysplasia / trisomy 13

◊ Bilaterality is a feature of a congenital syndrome (Norrie disease, Warburg disease)!

— Primary vitreous
= fibrillar ectodermal meshwork + mesodermal tissue consisting of embryonic hyaloid vascular system; appears during 1st month of life; extends between lens + retina; involutes by 6th month of gestation

— Hyaloid artery
= important source of intraocular nutrition until 8th month of gestation; arises from dorsal ophthalmic artery at 3rd week of gestation; grows anteriorly with branches supplying vitreous + posterior aspect of lens

— Secondary / adult vitreous
begins to form during 3rd gestational month; a watery mass of loose collagen fibers + hyaluronic acid gradually replaces primary vitreous, which is reduced to a small S-shaped remnant (hyaloid canal = Cloquet canal) and serves as lymph channel

• unilateral leukokoria (2nd most common cause) [2–3% of leukokoria cases]
• seizures, mental deficiency, hearing loss
• ± cataract
• ophthalmoscopy: S-shaped tubular mass extending between posterior surface of lens + region of optic nerve head; lens opacity may preclude diagnosis

√ microphthalmia = small hypoplastic globe
√ retinal detachment (due to vitreoretinal traction in 30%)

US:
√ hyperechoic band extending from posterior pole of globe to posterior surface of lens (= embryonic rest of primary vitreous)
√ central anechoic line (= persistent hyaloid artery) visible in cases of echogenic vitreous hemorrhage
√ hyperechoic band extending from papilla to ora serrata (= retinal detachment)

CT:
√ enhancing cone-shaped central retrolental density extending from lens through vitreous body to back of orbit, just lateral to optic nerve
√ small optic nerve
√ deformity of globe + lens
√ hyperdense vitreous (from previous hemorrhage)
√ fluid-fluid levels from breakdown of recurrent hemorrhage in subhyaloid (between vitreous + retina) / subretinal space (between sensory + pigment epithelium)
√ NO calcifications

MR:
√ hyperintense vitreous body on T1WI + T2WI from chronic blood degradation products (methemoglobin) / proteinaceous fluid
√ hypo- to isointense thin triangular band with base near optic disc and apex at posterior surface of lens
√ marked enhancement of fibrovascular mass within vitreous

Cx: (1) Glaucoma, cataract from recurrent spontaneous intravitreal hemorrhage (due to friable vessels)
(2) Proliferation of embryonic tissue
(3) Retinal detachment from organizing hemorrhage / traction
(4) Hydrops / atrophy of globe + resorption of lens
(5) Phthisis bulbi (scarred shrunken eye)

PSEUDOTUMOR OF ORBIT

= IDIOPATHIC INFLAMMATORY PSEUDOTUMOR
= nongranulomatous inflammatory process affecting all intraorbital soft tissues

Etiology:
(a) cause not apparent at time of study: bacterial, viral, foreign body
(b) systemic disease presently not apparent: sarcoidosis, collagen, endocrine
(c) idiopathic: probably abnormal immune response

Incidence: 25% of all cases of unilateral exophthalmos; most common cause of an intraorbital mass lesion in adult
Age: young female
Histo: lymphocytic infiltrate
May be associated with:
Wegener granulomatosis, sarcoidosis, fibrosing mediastinitis, retroperitoneal fibrosis, thyroiditis, cholangitis, vasculitis, lymphoma

• unilateral painful ophthalmoplegia
• proptosis, chemosis, lid injection
• limitation of ocular movement

Location: retrobulbar fat (76%), extraocular muscle (57%), optic nerve (38%), uveal-scleral area (33%), lacrimal gland (5%)
(a) tumefactive type (common)
√ discrete / poorly defined intra- / extraconal mass = "pseudotumor" close to surface margin of globe
(b) myositic type (unusual)
√ enlargement of one / more extraocular muscles close to insertion in globe with ill-defined margins
√ typically involves muscles + tendon insertions (DDx to Graves disease with muscle involvement only)

√ increased density of retro-orbital fat (may involve anterior compartment)
√ thickening and enhancement of sclera near Tenon capsule
√ enlarged lacrimal gland
√ proptosis

MR:
√ lesion isointense to fat on T2WI

Prognosis:
(1) remitting / chronic + progressive course
(2) rapid dramatic + lasting response to steroid therapy

DDx: (1) lymphoma (may be confused with lymphoma clinically, radiographically, pathologically)
(2) thyroid ophthalmopathy (tapering of distal muscles, painless proptosis)
(3) radiation therapy

RETINAL ASTROCYTOMA

= low-grade neoplasm / hamartoma arising from the nerve fiber layer of retina / optic nerve, usually associated with tuberous sclerosis

Etiology: tuberous sclerosis (53%); neurofibromatosis type 1 (14%); sporadic (33%)
Path: usually multiple + bilateral in tuberous sclerosis;
(1) small flat noncalcified semitranslucent lesion in posterior / peripheral retina
(2) "mulberry" lesion = raised white tumor in posterior retina with fine nodularity containing calcifications + cystic fluid accumulations

Histo: spindle-shaped fibrous astrocytes

• leukokoria (3% of all childhood cases of leukokoria)
• asymptomatic, progressive loss of vision

Location: retina near optic disc
√ retinal mass ± enhancement
√ typically unilateral (DDx to drusen)

Cx: (1) Central retinal vein occlusion + secondary hemorrhage
(2) Neovascular glaucoma
(3) Extensive tumor necrosis

RETINOBLASTOMA

= rare malignant congenital intraocular tumor arising from primitive photoreceptor cells of retina (included in primitive neuroectodermal tumor group)

Types:
(A) Nonheritable form (66%)
(1) Sporadic postzygotic somatic mutation (subsequent generations unaffected)
Mean age at presentation: 23 months
√ unilateral disease
(2) Chromosomal anomaly
= monosomy 13 / deletions of 13q
Associated with: microcephaly, ear changes, facial dysmorphism, mental retardation, finger + toe abnormalities, malformation of genitalia

(B) Heritable form
(1) Heritable sporadic form (20–25%)
= sporadic germinal mutation (50% chance to occur in subsequent generations)
Mean age at presentation: 12 months
√ bilateral retinoblastomas in 66%
(2) Familial retinoblastoma (5–10%)
= autosomal dominant with abnormality of band 14 in chromosome 13 (95% penetrance)
Mean age at presentation: 8 months
√ usually 3 to 5 ocular tumors per eye
√ bilateral tumors in 66%
Risk of secondary nonocular malignancy:
osteo~, chondro~, fibrosarcoma, malignant fibrous histiocytoma (20% risk within 10 years, >90% by 30 years of age)

Trilateral retinoblastoma (rare variant)
= bilateral retinoblastomas + neuroectodermal pineal tumor (pineoblastoma)

Quadrilateral retinoblastoma
= trilateral retinoblastoma + 4th focus in suprasellar cistern

Incidence: 1:15,000–34,000 livebirths; most common intraocular neoplasm in childhood; 1% of all pediatric malignancies
Age: mean age at presentation is 18 months; 98% in children <5 years of age; M:F = 1:1
Path: (1) Exophytic form = proliferation into subretinal space with detachment of retina + invasion of vascular choroid (hematogenous spread)
(2) Endophytic form = centripetal tumor invasion causing floating islands of tumor within semiliquid vitreous ± anterior chamber
(3) Diffuse form = thin en-plaque lesion extending along retina
Histo: (a) Flexner-Wintersteiner rosettes (in 50%)
= neuronal cells line up around an empty central zone filled with polysaccharides
◊ Very specific for retinoblastomas!
(b) Homer-Wright rosettes = neuronal cells line up around a central area containing a cobweb of filaments (also found in other primitive neuroectodermal tumors)
(c) "fleurettes" = flowerlike groupings of tumor cells that form photoreceptor elements (specific for retinal differentiation)
- "cat's eye" = leukokoria (whitish mass behind lens) in 60%
  ◊ About 50% of all childhood leukokoria are caused by retinoblastoma!
- decreased visual acuity, heterochromia iridis
- strabismus (crossed eyes), proptosis (less common)
- hyphema
- iris neovascularization, phthisis bulbi
- ocular pain from secondary angle-closure glaucoma

Location: posterolateral wall of globe (most commonly); 60% unilateral; 40% bilateral + frequently synchronous (90% bilateral in inherited forms)
√ normal ocular size
US:
√ heterogeneous hyperechoic solid intraocular mass
√ cystic appearance upon tumor necrosis
√ secondary retinal detachment in all cases
√ acoustic shadowing (in 75%)
√ vitreous hemorrhage frequent
CT:
√ solid smoothly marginated lobulated retrolental hyperdense mass in endophytic type (rarer exophytic type grows subretinally causing retinal detachment)
√ partial punctate / nodular calcification (50–75–95%)
◊ Retinoblastoma is the most common cause of orbital calcifications!
√ dense vitreous (common)
√ extraocular extension (in 25%): optic nerve enlargement, abnormal soft tissue in orbit, intracranial extension
√ contrast enhancement usual
√ ± macrophthalmia
MR:
√ iso- to mildly hyperintense tumor on T1WI relative to vitreous + moderate to marked enhancement
√ distinctly hypointense on T2WI (similar to uveal melanoma)
√ subretinal exudate usually hyperintense on T1WI + T2WI (proteinaceous fluid)
Cx: (1) Metastases to: meninges (via subarachnoid space), bone marrow, lung, liver, lymph nodes
(2) Radiation-induced sarcomas develop in 15–20%
Prognosis: spontaneous regression in 1%;
√ calcifications = favorable prognostic sign
√ contrast enhancement = poor prognostic sign
Mortality:
(a) choroidal invasion: 65% if significant, 24% if slight
(b) optic nerve invasion:
<10% if not invaded
15% if through lamina cribrosa
44% if significantly posterior to lamina cribrosa
(c) margin of resection not free of tumor: >65%
DDx: (1) Retinoma = retinocytoma (benign variant)
(2) Toxocara canis infection (no calcification)
(3) Retrolental fibroplasia (microphthalmia)
(4) Coats disease (subretinal exudation, no calcification)
(5) Norrie disease (retinal dysplasia)
(6) Persistent hyperplastic primary vitreous (hypoplastic globe, no calcification)

RETROLENTAL FIBROPLASIA
= RETINOPATHY OF PREMATURITY
= bilateral often asymmetric postnatal fibrovascular organization of vitreous humor which usually leads to retinal detachment
Pathophysiology:
retinal vascularization occurs in 4th–9th months of fetal life progressing from the papilla to the periphery; vascularization is incomplete in premature neonates especially in temporal sectors
Predisposed: premature infants with respiratory distress syndrome requiring prolonged oxygen therapy
Severity directly related to:
(1) degree of prematurity
(2) birth weight
(3) amount of oxygen used in therapy
- leukokoria in severe cases (traction retinal detachment, usually bilateral + temporal) [3–5% of all childhood leukokoria cases]
- Ophthalmoscopic stages:
  1st stage = arteriolar narrowing of most immature vessels at the border of the vascular-avascular retina (from spasm as a reaction to hyperoxygenation)
  2nd stage = dilatation + elongation + tortuosity of retinal vessels (after oxygen withdrawal)
  3rd stage = retinal neovascularization with growth into vitreous leads to vitreous hemorrhage
  4th stage = fibrosis with retraction of fibrovascular tissue + retinal detachment

EYE

√ bilateral microphthalmia ± retinal detachment

US:

√ hyperechoic tracts extending from temporal side of periphery of retina to vitreous behind the lens

CT:

√ dense vitreous bilaterally (neovascular ingrowth)

√ ± dystrophic calcifications in choroid + lens (late stage)

MR:

√ hyperintense vitreous on T1WI + T2WI (from chronic subretinal hemorrhage)

√ hypointense retrolental mass (apposition of detached leaves of retina displaced from retinal pigment layer)

Prognosis:
(1) spontaneous regression of vitreous neovascularization (85–95%) ± retinal detachment
(2) progression to cicatricial stage characterized by formation of dense membrane of gray-white vascularized tissue in retrolental vitreous + retinal detachment + microphthalmia

DDx: (1) Retinoblastoma (calcifications in eye of normal size)

RHABDOMYOSARCOMA

Most common primary malignant orbital tumor in childhood

◊ 10% occur primarily in orbit

◊ 10% metastasize to / invade orbit

Incidence: 3–4% of all pediatric orbital masses

Histo: arising from undifferentiated mesenchyma of orbital soft tissues (not from striated muscle)
(1) embryonal type (75%)
(2) alveolar type (15%)
(3) pleomorphic type (10%)

Age at presentation: average 7 years; 90% by 16 years of age; M > F

Rarely associated with: neurofibromatosis

• rapidly progressive exophthalmos + proptosis of upper lid

Location: superior orbit / retrobulbar (71%), lid (22%), conjunctiva (7%)

√ large soft-tissue density mass with ill-defined margins (extraocular muscles not involved)

√ ± extension into preseptal space, adjacent sinus, nasal cavity, intracranial cavity with bony erosion

√ may show significant enhancement

US:

√ heterogeneous well-defined irregular mass of low to medium echogenicity

Metastases: lung, bone marrow, cervical lymph nodes (rare)

Prognosis: (1) 40% survival after exenteration
(2) 80–90% survival after radiation therapy (4,000–5,000 rad) + chemotherapy (vincristine, cyclophosphamide, adriamycin)

DDx: pseudotumor, lymphoma

UVEAL MELANOMA

Most common primary intraocular neoplasm in adult Caucasian

Age: 50–70 years

Location: choroid (85–93%) > ciliary body (4–9%) > iris (3–6%); almost always unilateral

• retinal detachment, vitreous hemorrhage

• astigmatism, glaucoma

US:

√ small flat hyperechoic solid mass

CT:

√ ill-defined hyperdense thickening of wall of globe with inward bulge

MR:

√ sharply circumscribed hyperintense lesion on T1WI (paramagnetic properties of melanin)

Metastases to: globe, optic nerve; liver, lung, subcutis

VARIX OF ORBIT

Etiology: (a) Congenital: venous malformation / venous wall weakness
(b) Acquired: intraorbital / intracranial AVM

• intermittent exophthalmos associated with straining

• frequent blindness

√ involvement of superior / inferior orbital vein; phleboliths rare

√ may produce bony erosion without sclerotic reaction

√ enlargement of mass during Valsalva maneuver / jugular vein compression

√ well-defined markedly enhancing mass

√ spontaneous thrombosis (common)

US:

√ anechoic tubular / oval structure ± thrombus

√ venous flow increasing with Valsalva

MR:

√ flow void (rapid flow) / flow-related enhancement (slow flow)

WARBURG DISEASE

= autosomal recessive syndrome characterized by
(1) bilateral persistent hyperplastic primary vitreous
(2) hydrocephalus, lissencephaly
(3) mental retardation

• bilateral leukokoria + microphthalmia

EAR, NOSE, AND THROAT

DIFFERENTIAL DIAGNOSIS OF EAR, NOSE, AND THROAT DISORDERS

Facial nerve paralysis

A. INTRACRANIAL SEGMENT
   (a) intra-axial
      brainstem glioma, metastasis, multiple sclerosis, cerebrovascular accident, hemorrhage
      • cranial nerve VI also involved
   (b) extra-axial
      CPA tumor (acoustic neuroma, meningioma, epidermoid), CPA inflammation (sarcoidosis, basilar meningitis), vertebrobasilar dolichoectasia, AVM, aneurysm
      • cranial nerve VIII also involved

B. INTRATEMPORAL SEGMENT
   fracture, cholesteatoma, paraganglioma, hemangioma, facial nerve schwannoma, metastasis, Bell palsy, otitis media
   • loss of lacrimation, hyperacusis, loss of taste

C. EXTRACRANIAL PAROTID SEGMENT
   forceps delivery, penetrating facial trauma, parotid surgery, parotid malignancy, malignant otitis externa
   • preservation of lacrimation, stapedius reflex, taste

EAR

Hearing deficit

A. CONDUCTIVE HEARING LOSS
   • decrease in air conduction via EAC, tympanic membrane, ossicular chain, oval window (sound via headphones)
   • normal bone conduction (sound via bone oscillator)
      (a) destruction of ossicular chain: otitis media
      (b) restriction of ossicular chain: fenestral otosclerosis
   ◊ CT is the modality of choice!

B. SENSORINEURAL HEARING LOSS (most common)
   • elevated conduction thresholds for bone + air
   (a) sensory / cochlear SNHL = damage to cochlea / organ of Corti (less common)
      – bony labyrinth
         (1) demineralization: otosclerosis (otospongiosis), osteogenesis imperfecta, Paget disease, syphilis
         (2) congenital deformity: cochlear dys- / aplasia, Michel anomaly, Mondini dysplasia, enlarged vestibular aqueduct syndrome, X-linked sensorineural hearing loss
         (3) traumatic lesion: transverse fracture, perilymphatic fistula, cochlear concussion
         (4) destructive lesion: inflammatory lesion, neoplastic lesion
         ◊ CT is the modality of choice!
      – membranous labyrinth
         (1) enhancement: labyrinthitis, Cogan syndrome (early phase of autoimmune interstitial keratitis), intralabyrinthine schwannoma, site of postinflammatory perilymphatic fistula
         (2) obliteration: labyrinthitis ossificans, Cogan syndrome (late phase)
         (3) hemorrhage: trauma, labyrinthitis, coagulopathy, tumor fistulization
         (4) Meniere disease (vertigo + fluctuating sensory sensorineural hearing loss)
         ◊ MRI is the modality of choice!
   (b) neural / retrocochlear SNHL (more common)
      = abnormalities of neurons of spiral ganglion + central auditory pathways
      – IAC / cerebellopontine angle
         (1) Neoplastic lesions: vestibular / trigeminal schwannoma (acoustic neuroma in 1%), meningioma, arachnoid cyst, epidermoid cyst, leptomeningeal carcinomatosis, lymphoma, lipoma, hemangioma
         (2) nonneoplastic lesion: sarcoidosis, meningitis, vascular loop, siderosis
      – intra-axial auditory pathway
         (brain stem, thalamus, temporal lobe)
         (1) ischemic lesion
         (2) neoplastic lesion
         (3) traumatic lesion
         (4) demyelinating lesion
      ◊ MRI is the modality of choice!

Pulsatile tinnitus ± vascular tympanic membrane

= perception of a rhythmic cardiac synchronous sound

A. No abnormality (20%)
B. Congenital vascular variants (21%)
   1. Aberrant ICA
      = result of anastomosis of enlarged inferior tympanic artery with enlarged caroticotympanic artery when cervical ICA is underdeveloped
   2. Dehiscent jugular bulb
      √ absence of bony plate separating jugular bulb from middle ear cavity
      √ jugular bulb bulges into middle ear cavity
   3. High-riding nondehiscent jugular bulb (= jugular megabulb)
      √ high jugular bulb with diverticulum projecting cephalad into petrous temporal bone
C. Acquired vascular lesions (25%)
   1. Dural AVM
   2. Extracranial arteriovenous fistula
   3. High-grade stenotic vascular lesion: carotid artery atherosclerosis, fibromuscular dysplasia, carotid artery dissection

4. Aneurysm involving horizontal segment of petrous ICA

D. Temporal bone tumors (31%)
1. Paraganglioma (27%): glomus tympanicum, glomus jugulare
2. Meningioma
3. Hemangioma

E. Miscellaneous
1. Cholesterol granuloma

Temporal bone sclerosis

1. Otosclerosis = otospongiosis
2. **Paget disease** = osteoporosis circumscripta
   - sensorineural / mixed hearing loss (cochlear involvement / stapes fixation in oval window)
   - √ usually lytic changes beginning in petrous pyramid + progressing laterally; otic capsule last to be affected
   - √ calvarial changes ± basilar impression
3. **Fibrous dysplasia**
   monostotic with temporal bone involvement
   - painless mastoid swelling
   - conductive hearing loss (from narrowing of EAC / middle ear)
   - √ homogeneously dense thickened bone (fibro-osseous tissue less dense than calvarial bone)
   - √ expanded bone with preserved cortex
   - √ lytic lesions (less frequent)
   - √ sparing of membranous labyrinth, facial nerve canal, IAC is the rule
4. Osteogenesis imperfecta
   - √ changes similar to otosclerosis

   van der Hoeve syndrome = osteogenesis imperfecta + otosclerosis + blue sclera
5. Meningioma
6. Otosyphilis: labyrinthitis + osteitis
7. Metastasis
8. Ossifying fibroma
9. Osteosarcoma
10. Osteopetrosis

External ear masses

A. CONGENITAL
1. Atresia

B. INFLAMMATORY
1. Malignant external otitis
2. **Keratosis obturans**
   bilateral process in association with chronic sinusitis + bronchiectasis
   Age: <40 years
3. Cholesteatoma

C. BENIGN TUMOR
1. **Exostosis** = surfer's ear
   Cause: irritation by cold water
   - √ bony mass projecting into EAC; often multiple + bilateral
2. **Osteoma**
   - √ may invade adjacent bone; single in EAC / mastoid
3. **Ceruminoma**
   from apocrine + sebaceous glands; bone erosion mimics malignancy

D. MALIGNANT TUMOR
1. Squamous cell carcinoma
   - often long history of chronic suppurative otitis media = "malignant otitis"
2. Basal cell carcinoma
3. Melanoma, adenocarcinoma, adenoid cystic carcinoma
4. Metastases
   (a) hematogenous: breast, prostate, lung, kidney, thyroid
   (b) direct spread: skin, parotid, nasopharynx, brain, meninges
   (c) systemic: leukemia, lymphoma, myeloma
5. Histiocytosis X: in 15% of patients

Middle ear masses

A. CONGENITAL
1. **Aberrant internal carotid artery**
   - vascular tympanic membrane
   - pulsatile tinnitus
   - √ tubular soft-tissue density entering middle ear cavity posterolateral to cochlea, crossing mesotympanum along cochlear promontory, exiting anteromedial to become horizontal portion of carotid canal
   - √ protrusion into middle ear without bony margin
2. **Dehiscent jugular bulb**
   - pulsatile tinnitus
   - vascular tympanic membrane
   - √ middle ear soft-tissue mass contiguous with jugular foramen
   - √ absence of bony plate separating jugular bulb from posteroinferior middle ear

   DDx: Jugular megabulb (rises above floor of EAC but with preservation of bony plate)

B. INFLAMMATORY
1. Cholesteatoma
2. Cholesterol granuloma
3. Granulation tissue
   - √ linear strands partially opacifying middle ear cavity without bony erosion

C. BENIGN TUMOR
1. Glomus tumor (multiple in 10%; 8% malignant)
   (a) Glomus tympanicum: at cochlear promontory
   - √ seldom erodes bone

   (b) Glomus jugulare: at jugular foramen
   - √ invasion of middle ear from below
   - √ destruction of bony roof of jugular fossa + bony spur separating vein from carotid artery
2. Facial neuroma
   - persistent Bell palsy (in 5% caused by neurinoma)

   Location: intracanalicular > IAC
   - √ tubular mass in enlarged / scalloped facial canal

3. Ossifying hemangioma
4. Choristoma = ectopic mature salivary tissue
5. Meningioma

D. MALIGNANT TUMOR
1. Squamous cell carcinoma
2. Metastasis
3. Rhabdomyosarcoma
Location: orbit > nasopharynx > ear
4. Adenocarcinoma (rare), adenoid cystic carcinoma

Mass on the promontory

[promontory = bone over basal turn of cochlea]
1. Glomus tympanicum
2. Congenital cholesteatoma
3. Aberrant carotid artery
4. Persistent stapedial artery

Inner ear masses

A. CONGENITAL
1. Congenital / primary cholesteatoma = epidermoid tumor (3rd most common CPA tumor)

B. INFLAMMATION
1. Cholesterol granuloma
2. Petrous apex mucocele

C. TUMOR
1. Glomus jugulare tumor
2. Hemangioma, fibro-osseous lesion
3. Metastasis
4. Facial nerve neurinoma
5. Large CPA tumors: acoustic neuroma, meningioma (2nd most common CPA tumor)

SINUSES

Opacification of maxillary sinus

A. WITHOUT BONE DESTRUCTION
1. Sinus aplasia / hypoplasia
Age: NOT routinely visualized at birth, by age 6 antral floor at level of middle turbinate, by age 15 of adult size
Location: uni- / bilateral
√ depression of orbital floor with enlargement of orbit
√ lateral displacement of lateral wall of nasal fossa with large turbinate
2. Maxillary dentigerous cyst
usually containing a tooth / crown; without tooth = primordial dentigerous cyst
3. Ameloblastoma
4. Acute sinusitis
√ air-fluid level

B. WITH BONE DESTRUCTION
1. Maxillary sinus tumor
2. Infection: aspergillosis, mucormycosis, TB, syphilis
3. Wegener granulomatosis; lethal midline granuloma
4. Blowout fracture

Paranasal sinus masses

1. Mucocele
2. Mucous retention cyst
= smoothly marginated soft-tissue mass from obstruction of small seromucinous gland (commonly in floor of maxilla)
3. Sinonasal polyp
4. Antrochoanal polyp
5. Inverting papilloma
6. Sinusitis
7. Carcinoma

Granulomatous lesions of sinuses

A. Chronic irritants
1. Beryllium
2. Chromate salts

B. Infection
1. Tuberculosis
2. Actinomycosis
3. Rhinoscleroma
4. Yaws
5. Blastomycosis
6. Leprosy
7. Rhinosporidiosis
8. Syphilis
9. Leishmaniosis
10. Glanders

C. Autoimmune disease
1. Wegener granulomatosis

D. Lymphoma-like lesions
1. Midline granuloma

E. Unclassified
1. Sarcoidosis

Hyperdense sinus secretions

1. Inspissated secretions
2. Fungal sinusitis
3. Hemorrhage into sinus
4. Chronic sinusitis infected with bacteria (in particular in very long-standing disease / cystic fibrosis)

Opacified sinus + expansion / destruction

mnemonic: "PLUMP FACIES"
Plasmacytoma
Lymphoma
Unknown etiology: Wegener granulomatosis
Mucocele
Polyp
Fibrous dysplasia, **F**ibroma (ossifying)
Aneurysmal bone cyst, **A**ngiofibroma
Cancer
Inverting papilloma
Esthesioneuroblastoma
Sarcoma: ie, rhabdomyosarcoma

ENT

NOSE

Nasal Vault Masses

A. BENIGN
1. Sinonasal polyp
2. Inverted papilloma
3. Hemangioma
   • history of epistaxis
4. Pyogenic granuloma
   √ pedunculated lobular mass
5. Granuloma gravidarum
   = nasal hemangioma of pregnancy
6. Hemangiopericytoma
7. Juvenile nasopharyngeal angiofibroma
   √ arises in superior nasopharynx with extension into nose via posterior choana

B. MALIGNANT
1. Lymphoma
2. Melanoma
3. Vascular metastasis

Mass In Nasopharynx

mnemonic: "NASAL PIPE"
Nasopharyngeal carcinoma
Angiofibroma (juvenile)
Spine / skull fracture
Adenoids
Lymphoma
Polyp
Infection
Plasmacytoma
Extension of neoplasm (sphenoid / ethmoid sinus ca.)

PHARYNX

Parapharyngeal Space Mass

1. Asymmetric pterygoid venous plexus
   √ racemose, enhancing area along medial border of lateral pterygoid muscle
2. Abscess
   Origin: pharyngitis (most common), dental infection, parotid calculus disease, penetrating trauma
3. Atypical second branchial cleft cyst
   Age: child / young adult
   • protruding parotid gland
   • bulging posterolateral pharyngeal wall
   √ cystic mass projecting from deep margin of faucial tonsil toward skull base
4. Pleomorphic adenoma of ectopic salivary tissue

Pharyngeal Mucosal Space Mass

1. Asymmetric fossa of Rosenmüller
   = lateral pharyngeal recess = asymmetry in amount of lymphoid tissue
2. Tonsillar abscess
   • sore throat, fever, painful swallowing
3. Postinflammatory retention cyst
   √ 1–2-cm well-circumscribed cystic mass
4. Postinflammatory calcification
   • remote history of severe pharyngitis
   √ multiple clumps of calcification
5. Benign mixed tumor
   • pedunculated mass arising from minor salivary glands
   √ oval / round well-circumscribed mass protruding into airway
6. Squamous cell carcinoma
   √ infiltrating mass with epicenter medial to + invading parapharyngeal space
   √ middle-ear fluid (eustachian tube malfunction)
   √ cervical adenopathy
7. Non-Hodgkin lymphoma
8. Minor salivary gland malignancy
9. Thornwaldt cyst

Masticator Space Mass

1. Asymmetric accessory parotid gland
   Incidence: 21% of general population
   Location: usually on surface of masseter muscle
   √ prominent salivary gland tissue
2. Benign masseteric hypertrophy
   Cause: bruxism (= nocturnal gnashing of teeth)
   √ homogeneous enlargement of one / both masseters
3. Odontogenic abscess
   • bad dentition + trismus
4. Sarcoma (chondro-, osteo-, soft-tissue sarcoma)
   √ infiltrating mass with mandibular destruction
5. Malignant schwannoma
   √ tubular mass along cranial nerve V_3
6. Non-Hodgkin lymphoma
7. Infiltrating squamous cell carcinoma

Carotid Space Mass

A. VASCULAR LESION
1. Ectatic common / internal carotid artery
2. Carotid artery aneurysm / pseudoaneurysm
3. Asymmetric internal jugular vein
4. Jugular vein thrombosis

B. BENIGN TUMOR
1. Paraganglioma (carotid body tumor + glomus vagale)
2. Schwannoma
3. Neurofibroma of cranial nerves IX, X, XI

C. MALIGNANT TUMOR
1. Nodal metastasis from squamous cell carcinoma
2. Non-Hodgkin lymphoma

Retropharyngeal Space Mass

A. INFECTION
1. Reactive lymph adenopathy
   √ nodes >10 mm in diameter
2. Abscess
   √ bow-tie shape

B. BENIGN TUMOR
1. Hemangioma
2. Lipoma

C. MALIGNANT TUMOR
1. Metastasis from squamous cell carcinoma, melanoma, thyroid carcinoma

2. Non-Hodgkin lymphoma
3. Direct invasion by squamous cell carcinoma

Prevertebral Space Mass

A. PSEUDOTUMOR
  1. Anterior disk herniation
  2. Vertebral body osteophyte

B. INFLAMMATION
  1. Vertebral body osteomyelitis
  2. Abscess

C. TUMOR
  1. Chordoma
  2. Vertebral body metastasis: lung, breast, prostate, non-Hodgkin lymphoma

AIRWAYS

Inspiratory Stridor In Children

1. Croup
2. Congenital subglottic stenosis
3. Subglottic hemangioma
4. Airway foreign body
5. Esophageal foreign body
6. Epiglottitis

Airway Obstruction In Children

Nasopharyngeal Narrowing

(a) Congenital: Choanal atresia, choanal stenosis, encephalocele
(b) Inflammatory: Adenoidal enlargement, polyps
(c) Neoplastic: Juvenile angiofibroma, rhabdomyosarcoma, teratoma, neuroblastoma, lymphoepithelioma
(d) Traumatic: Foreign body, hematoma, rhinolith

Oropharyngeal Narrowing

(a) Congenital: Glossoptosis + micrognathia (Pierre Robin, Goldenhar, Treacher Collins syndrome), macroglossia (cretinism, Beckwith-Wiedemann syndrome)
(b) Inflammatory: Abscess, tonsillar hypertrophy
(c) Neoplastic: Lingular tumor / cyst
(d) Traumatic: Hematoma, foreign body

Retropharyngeal Narrowing

= potential space (normally <3/4 of AP diameter of adjacent cervical spine in infants / <3 mm in older children)
(a) Congenital: Branchial cleft cyst, ectopic thyroid
(b) Inflammatory: Retropharyngeal abscess
(c) Neoplastic: Cystic hygroma (originating in posterior cervical triangle with extension toward midline + into mediastinum), neuroblastoma, neurofibromatosis, hemangioma
(d) Traumatic: Hematoma, foreign body
(e) Metabolic: Hypothyroidism

Vallecular Narrowing

= valleys on each side of glossoepiglottic folds between base of tongue + epiglottis
(a) Congenital: Congenital cyst, ectopic thyroid, thyroglossal cyst
(b) Inflammatory: Abscess
(c) Neoplastic: Teratoma
(d) Traumatic: Foreign body, hematoma

Supraglottic Narrowing

= area between epiglottis and true vocal cords
(a) Congenital: Aryepiglottic fold cyst
(b) Inflammatory: Acute bacterial epiglottitis, angioneurotic edema
(c) Neoplastic: Retention cyst, cystic hygroma, neurofibroma
(d) Traumatic: Foreign body, hematoma, radiation, caustic ingestion
(e) Idiopathic: Laryngomalacia

Glottic Narrowing

= area of true vocal cords
(a) Congenital: Laryngeal atresia, laryngeal stenosis, laryngeal web (anterior commissure)
(b) Neoplastic: Laryngeal papillomatosis
(c) Neurogenic: Vocal cord paralysis (most common)
(d) Traumatic: Foreign body, hematoma

Subglottic Narrowing

= short segment between undersurface of true vocal cords + inferior margin of cricoid cartilage is the narrowest portion of child's airway
(a) Congenital: Congenital subglottic stenosis
(b) Inflammatory: Croup
(c) Neoplastic: Hemangioma, papillomatosis
(d) Traumatic: Acquired stenosis (result of prolonged endotracheal intubation in 5%), granuloma
(e) Idiopathic: Mucocele = mucous retention cyst (rare complication of prolonged endotracheal intubation)

Tracheal Narrowing

A. ANTERIOR COMPRESSION
  (a) Congenital
    1. Congenital goiter
    2. Innominate artery syndrome
       Cause: crowding of thoracic inlet by cervical herniation of an enlarged thymus with development of focal tracheomalacia
       • ablation of right radial pulse by rigid endoscopic pressure
       √ posterior tracheal displacement
       √ focal collapse of trachea at fluoroscopy
       √ pulsatile indentation of anterior tracheal wall by innominate artery on MRI
       Rx: surgical attachment of innominate artery to manubrium

ENT

(b) Inflammatory
1. Cervical / mediastinal abscess
(c) Neoplastic
1. Cervical / intrathoracic teratoma
√ amorphous calcifications + ossifications
2. Thymoma
3. Thyroid tumors
4. Lymphoma
(d) Traumatic: Hematoma
B. POSTERIOR TRACHEAL COMPRESSION
(a) Congenital
1. Vascular ring
— complete: double aortic arch, right aortic arch
— incomplete: anomalous right subclavian artery
√ posterior indentation of esophagus + trachea
2. Pulmonary sling
= anomalous left pulmonary artery arising from right pulmonary artery, passing between trachea + esophagus en route to left lung
3. Bronchogenic cyst
most common between esophagus + trachea at level of carina
(b) inflammatory: abscess
(c) neoplastic: neurofibroma
(d) traumatic: esophageal foreign body, esophageal stricture, hematoma
C. INTRINSIC TRACHEAL CAUSES
(a) Congenital:
1. Congenital tracheal stenosis: generalized / segmental
= complete cartilaginous ring (instead of horseshoe shape)
2. Congenital tracheomalacia = immaturity of tracheal cartilage
• expiratory stridor
√ tracheal collapse on expiration
(b) Neoplastic: papilloma, fibroma, hemangioma
(c) Traumatic: acquired stenosis (endotracheal + tracheostomy tubes), granuloma, acquired tracheomalacia (cartilage degeneration after inflammation, extrinsic pressure, bronchial neoplasia, TE fistula, foreign body)

Tracheal Tumor
1. Adenomatoid cystic carcinoma
2. Squamous cell carcinoma
3. Carcinoid
4. Squamous cell papilloma
5. Mucoepidermoid carcinoma

LARYNX
Vocal Cord Paralysis
1. Birth injury
2. Arnold-Chiari malformation
3. Intracranial tumor
4. Mediastinal mass / cyst
5. Vascular ring
6. Thyroidectomy
7. Malignancy
√ fixed vocal cords (fluoroscopy)

Epiglottic Enlargement
A. NORMAL VARIANT
1. Prominent normal epiglottis
2. Omega epiglottis
B. INFLAMMATION
1. Acute / chronic epiglottitis
2. Angioneurotic edema
3. Stevens-Johnson syndrome
4. Caustic ingestion
5. Radiation therapy
C. MASSES
1. Epiglottic cyst
2. Aryepiglottic cyst
3. Foreign body

Aryepiglottic Cyst
1. Retention cyst
2. Lymphangioma
3. Cystic hygroma
4. Thyroglossal cyst
• may be symptomatic at birth
√ well-defined mass in aryepiglottic fold

NECK
Solid Neck Masses In Childhood
1. Lymphadenopathy
2. Fibromatosis colli
3. Malignancy: neuroblastoma (most common), lymphoma
4. Teratoma
5. Hemangioma
6. Lipoma
7. Thyroid mass
8. Ectopic thymus

Lymph Node Enlargement Of Neck
A. NORMAL LYMPH NODES
√ few small oval hypoechoic
√ ± central linear echogenicity (= invaginating hilar fat)
√ larger in transverse than anteroposterior dimension
B. MALIGNANT LYMPH NODES
√ increased anteroposterior diameter
√ prominent calcifications suggestive of medullary thyroid cancer
√ minimal axial diameter of 11 mm (in squamous cell carcinoma)
CT:
√ marginal enhancement

Congenital Cystic Lesions Of Neck
◊ 95% of all branchial cleft anomalies arise from 2nd branchial apparatus!

ENT

1. **Second branchial cleft cyst**
   = incomplete obliteration of 2nd branchial cleft tract (cervical sinus) resulting in sinus tract / fistula / cyst
   Age: young to middle-aged adult
   Location: parotid space near mandibular angle, parapharyngeal space
   • history of multiple parotid abscesses unresponsive to drainage + antibiotics
   • otorrhea (if connected to external auditory canal)
   √ cystic oval / round mass near mandibular angle
   √ displacement of sternocleidomastoid muscle posteriorly, carotid artery + jugular vein posteromedially, submandibular gland anteriorly
   √ may insinuate between internal + external carotid artery (PATHOGNOMONIC)
   √ cyst may enlarge after upper respiratory tract infection / injury
   DDx: necrotic neural tumor, cervical abscess, submandibular gland cyst, cystic lymphangioma, necrotic metastatic / inflammatory lymphadenopathy

2. **First branchial cleft cyst**
   Residual embryonic tract begins near submandibular triangle + ascends through the parotid gland, terminates at junction of cartilaginous + bony external auditory canal
   Incidence: 8% of all branchial cleft anomalies
   Age: middle-aged women
   • enlarging mass near lower pole of parotid gland
   DDx: inflammatory parotid cyst, benign cystic parotid tumor, necrotic metastatic lymphadenopathy

3. **Cervical thymic cyst**
   forms along migratory tract of thymic tissue into mediastinum
   Age: <5 years of age; M > F
   No association with myasthenia gravis!
   Location: from angle of mandible to anterior mid-neck
   √ uni- / multilocular mostly unilateral cyst

4. **Parathyroid cyst**
   Age: 30–50 years
   • hormonally inactive
   √ noncolloidal cyst near lower pole of thyroid gland

5. Thyroglossal duct cyst
6. Lymphangioma / cystic hygroma

7. **Dermoid cyst**
   (1) Cystic teratoma
      (a) epidermoid cyst = lined by simple squamous epithelium without adnexal structures
      (b) dermal cyst = epithelial-lined cyst containing hair + sebaceous glands
      (c) teratoid cyst = lined with squamous / respiratory epithelium containing derivatives of skin appendages + endoderm + mesoderm
   (2) Nonteratomatous epithelial-lined cyst
      Location:
      — dorsum of nose in infants (most common)
      — midline anterior floor of mouth:
      (a) sublingual between mylohyoid muscle + tongue (DDx: inclusion cyst, ranula)
      (b) submental between platysma + mylohyoid muscle

8. Ectopic bronchogenic cyst
   • stridor
   √ indentation of trachea

Branchial Fistula

1. Third branchial fistula
   Internal opening: piriform fossa anterior to fold formed by internal laryngeal nerve
   Course: through thyrohyoid membrane, over hypoglossal nerve, between internal + external carotid arteries, caudolateral / posterolateral to proximal internal + common carotid arteries
   External opening: at base of neck anterior to sternocleidomastoid muscle
2. Fourth branchial fistula
   Internal opening: apex of piriform sinus
   Course: between cricoid + thyroid cartilage, below cricothyroid muscle, caudal course between trachea + carotid vessels, deep to clavicle into mediastinum, looping forward below aorta (left side) / right subclavian artery (right side), ascending posterior to common carotid artery, passing over hypoglossal nerve
   External opening: at base of neck anterior to sternocleidomastoid muscle

Air-containing Masses Of Neck

1. Laryngocele
2. Tracheal diverticulum
   arising from anterior wall of trachea close to thyroid
3. Zenker diverticulum
4. Lateral pharyngeal diverticulum
   located in tonsillar fossa / vallecula / pyriform fossa

PAROTID GLAND

Parotid Gland Enlargement

A. LOCALIZED INFLAMMATORY DISEASE
   1. Chronic recurrent sialadenitis
   2. Sialosis
   3. Sarcoidosis
   4. Tuberculosis
   5. Cat-scratch fever
   6. Syphilis
   7. Abscess
   8. Reactive adenopathy

ENT

B. SYSTEMIC AUTOIMMUNE RELATED DISEASE
   1. Sjögren disease (= myoepithelial sialadenitis)
   2. Mikulicz disease
C. NEOPLASM
   (a) benign tumor
      1. Pleomorphic / monomorphic adenoma
      2. Cystadenolymphoma (= Warthin tumor)
      3. Benign lymphoepithelial cysts (AIDS)
      4. Lipoma
      5. Facial neuroma
      6. Oncocytoma
   (b) primary malignant tumor
      1. Mucoepidermoid carcinoma
      2. Adenoid cystic carcinoma (= cylindroma)
      3. Malignant mixed tumor
      4. Adenocarcinoma
      5. Acinus cell carcinoma
   (c) metastatic tumor
      ◊ Parotid gland undergoes late encapsulation, which leads to incorporation of lymph nodes!
      1. Squamous cell carcinoma
      2. Melanoma
      3. Non-Hodgkin lymphoma
D. LYMPHOPROLIFERATIVE DISORDER
   1. Lymphoma
   2. Primary Non-Hodgkin lymphoma
E. CONGENITAL
   1. First branchial cleft cyst

Multiple Lesions Of Parotid Gland

1. Warthin tumor
2. Metastases to lymph nodes: squamous cell carcinoma of skin, malignant melanoma, Non-Hodgkin lymphoma
3. Benign lymphoepithelial cysts (AIDS)

THYROID

Congenital Dyshormonogenesis

1. Trapping defect
   = defective cellular uptake of iodine into thyroid, salivary glands, gastric mucosa;
   ◊ high doses of inorganic iodine facilitate diffusion into thyroid permitting a normal rate of thyroid hormone synthesis
   ◊ normal ratio of iodine concentrations for gastric juice:plasma = 20:1
   √ nearly entire dose of administered radioiodine is excreted within 24 hours
2. Organification defect
   = deficient peroxidase activity, which catalyzes the oxidation of iodide by H_2O_2 to form monoiodotyrosine (MIT) / diiodotyrosine (DIT)
   • high serum TSH
   • low serum T_4
   • diffuse symmetric thyromegaly
   √ high thyroidal uptake of radioiodine / pertechnetate
   √ rapid I-131 turnover
   √ positive perchlorate washout test

   Pendred syndrome = autosomal recessive trait of deficient peroxidase regeneration characterized by hypothyroidism + goiter + nerve deafness
3. Deiodinase (dehalogenase) defect
   = deficient deiodination of MIT / DIT to release iodide which is reutilized to synthesize thyroid hormone production
   • hypothyroidism
   • identification of MIT + DIT in serum + urine following administration of I-131
   • "intrinsic" iodine deficiency goiter
   √ high thyroidal I-131 uptake
   √ rapid intrathyroidal turnover of I-131
4. Thyroxin-binding globulin (TBG) deficiency
   • abnormal T_4 transport
   • low bound serum T_4 concentration
   • euthyroid
5. End-organ resistance to thyroid hormone
   • high serum T_4
   • euthyroid / hypothyroid
   • growth retardation
   √ goiter
   √ stippled epiphyses

Hyperthyroidism

1. Graves disease (most common)
2. Toxic nodular goiter
3. Iodine-induced hyperthyroidism = Jod-Basedow
4. Thyroiditis
   (a) Hashimoto thyroiditis = chronic lymphocytic thyroiditis
   (b) Subacute thyroiditis = de Quervain thyroiditis
   (c) Painless thyroiditis
   US:
      √ decrease in overall echogenicity
      √ discrete nodules (50%)
5. Thyrotoxicosis medicamentosa / factitia surreptitious self-administration of thyroid hormones
6. Struma ovarii
   = ovarian teratoma containing thyroid tissue
7. Hydatidiform mole / choriocarcinoma / testicular trophoblastic carcinoma
   = stimulation of thyroid by HCG
8. Pituitary hyperthyroidism = pituitary neoplasm
   • ± acromegaly
   • ± hyperprolactinemia
9. Thyroid carcinoma / hyperfunctioning metastases very rare (25 cases)

Hypothyroidism

A. PRIMARY HYPOTHYROIDISM (most common)
   = thyroid's inability to produce sufficient thyroid hormone
   1. Agenesis of thyroid
   2. Congenital dyshormonogenesis
   3. Chronic thyroiditis
   4. Previous radioiodine therapy
   5. Ectopic thyroid (1:4,000)

ENT

B. SECONDARY HYPOTHYROIDISM
   = failure of anterior pituitary to release sufficient quantities of TSH
   1. Sheehan syndrome
   2. Head trauma
   3. Pituitary tumor (primary / secondary)
   4. Aneurysm
   5. Surgery

C. TERTIARY / HYPOTHALAMIC HYPOTHYROIDISM
   = failure of hypothalamus to produce sufficient amounts of TRH

Decreased / No Uptake Of Radiotracer

A. BLOCKED TRAPPING FUNCTION
   1. Iodine load (most common)
      = dilution of tracer within flooded iodine pool (from administration of radiographic contrast / iodine-containing medication)
      ◊ Suppression usually lasts for 4 weeks!
   2. Exogenous thyroid hormone (replacement therapy)
      suppresses TSH release

B. BLOCKED ORGANIFICATION
   1. Antithyroid medication (propylthiouracil (PTU) / methimazole) / goitrogenic substances
   √ Tc-99m uptake not inhibited

C. DIFFUSE PARENCHYMAL DESTRUCTION
   1. Subacute / chronic thyroiditis

D. HYPOTHYROIDISM
   1. Congenital hypothyroidism
   2. Surgical / radioiodine ablation
   3. Thyroid ectopia (struma ovarii, intrathoracic goiter)

mnemonic: "H MITTE"
- **H**ypothyroidism (congenital)
- **M**edications: PTU, perchlorate, Cytomel, Synthroid, Lugol solution
- **I**odine overload (eg, after IVP)
- **T**hyroid ablation (surgery, radioiodine)
- **T**hyroiditis (subacute / chronic)
- **E**ctopic thyroid hormone production

Increased Uptake Of Radiotracer

mnemonic: "THRILLEr"
- **T**hyroiditis (early Hashimoto)
- **H**yperthyroidism (diffuse / nodular)
- **R**ebound after withdrawal of antithyroid medication
- **I**odine starvation
- **L**ow serum albumin
- **L**ithium therapy
- **E**nzyme defect

Prominent Pyramidal Lobe

= distal remnant of thyroid descent tract
1. Normal variant: present in 10%
2. Hyperthyroidism
3. Thyroiditis
4. S/P thyroid surgery
   DDx: esophageal activity from salivary excretion (disappears after glass of water)

Thyroid Calcifications

= benign calcifications = stromal calcifications in adenoma
√ coarse calcifications with rough outline
√ alignment along periphery of lesion
√ irregular distribution

Psammoma Bodies

= microcalcifications (<1 mm) occur in 54% of thyroid neoplasms
√ seen on xeroradiography in 94%
1. Papillary carcinoma 61%
2. Follicular carcinoma 26%
3. Undifferentiated carcinoma 13%

Cystic Areas In Thyroid

15–25% of all thyroid nodules!

A. Anechoic fluid + smooth regular wall:
   1. Colloid accumulation in goiter = colloid-filled dilated macrofollicle
   2. Simple cyst (extremely uncommon)

B. Solid particles + irregular outline:
   1. Hemorrhagic colloid nodule
   2. Hemorrhagic adenoma (30%)
   3. Necrotic papillary cancer (15%)
   4. Liquefaction necrosis in adenoma / goiter
   5. Abscess
   6. Cystic parathyroid tumor

- bloody fluid = benign / malignant lesion
- clear amber fluid = benign lesion

◊ Cystic lesions often yield insufficient numbers of cells!

Thyroid Nodule

Incidence: (increasing with age)
   (a) 4–8% by palpation (>2 cm in 2%, 1–2 cm in 5%, <1 cm in 1%); M:F = 1:4
   (b) 50% by autopsy / thyroid US if clinically normal: multiple in 38%, solitary in 12% (occult small cancers found in 4%)

A. THYROID ADENOMA
   1. Colloid / adenomatous nodule = adenomatous hyperplasia / degenerative involuted nodule (42–77%)
   2. Follicular adenoma (15–40%)
   3. Ectopic parathyroid adenoma

B. INFLAMMATION / HEMORRHAGE
   1. Inflammatory lymph node in subacute + chronic thyroiditis
   2. Hemorrhage / hematoma: frequently associated with adenomas
   3. Abscess

C. CARCINOMA (8–17%)
   1. Thyroid carcinoma
      (a) papillary carcinoma (70%)
      (b) follicular (15%)
      (c) medullary carcinoma (5–10%)
      (d) anaplastic carcinoma (5%)
      (e) thyroid lymphoma (5%)

2. Nonthyroidal neoplasm
   metastasis from breast, lung, kidney, malignant melanoma, Hodgkin disease
3. Hürthle cell carcinoma
   √ very thin hypoechoic halo
4. Carcinoma in situ
   √ echogenic area inside a goiter nodule

Role of fine-needle aspiration biopsy (FNAB):
(large-needle biopsy has more complications with no increase in diagnostic yield)
◊ FNAB as initial test leads to a better selection of patients for surgery than any other test!
Diagnostic accuracy of 70–97%:
(a) 70–80% negative
(b) 10% positive specimens (3–6% false-positive rate often due to Hashimoto thyroiditis)
(c) 10–20% indeterminate
Up to 20% nondiagnostic (too few cells) material

Role of imaging:
◊ Imaging cannot reliably distinguish malignant + benign nodules!
(a) radionuclide scanning
   — useful in indeterminate cytology
   ◊ Hyperfunctioning nodule is almost always benign!
(b) ultrasound
   — best method to determine volume of nodule
   — useful during follow-up to distinguish nodular growth from intranodular hemorrhage

Discordant Thyroid Nodule

= nodule hyperfunctioning on Tc-99m pertechnetate scan + hypofunctioning on I-131 scan, which indicates reduced organification capacity

Cause:
1. Malignancy : follicular / papillary carcinoma
2. Benign lesion : follicular adenoma / adenomatous hyperplasia
   (autonomous nontoxic nodules have accelerated iodine turnover and discharge radioiodine as hormone within 24 hours)

Hot Thyroid Nodule

Incidence: 8% of Tc-99m pertechnetate scans
1. Adenoma
   (a) Autonomous adenoma = TSH-independent
      • euthyroid (80%), thyrotoxicosis (20%)
      √ partial / total suppression of remainder of gland
   (b) Adenomatous hyperplasia = TSH-dependent secondary to defective thyroid hormone production
2. Thyroid carcinoma (extremely rare)
   √ discordant uptake

N.B.: any hot nodule on Tc-99m scan must be imaged with I-123 to differentiate between autonomous or cancerous lesion

Cold Thyroid Nodule

A. BENIGN TUMOR
   1. Nonfunctioning adenoma
   2. Cyst (11–20%)
   3. Involutional nodule
   4. Parathyroid tumor
B. INFLAMMATORY MASS
   1. Focal thyroiditis
   2. Granuloma
   3. Abscess
C. MALIGNANT TUMOR
   1. Carcinoma
   2. Lymphoma
   3. Metastasis

US features of cold nodule:
√ hypoechoic (71%)
√ isoechoic (22%)
√ mixed echogenicity (4%)
√ hyperechoic (3%)
√ cystic (rarely malignant)

◊ A palpable hypofunctioning nodule in a patient with Graves' disease is likely malignant!

mnemonic: "CATCH LAMP"
Colloid cyst
Adenoma (most common)
Thyroiditis
Carcinoma
Hematoma
Lymphoma, **L**ymph node
Abscess
Metastasis (kidney, breast)
Parathyroid

PROBABILITY OF A COLD NODULE TO REPRESENT THYROID CANCER:
◊ Solitary cold nodules by scintigraphy are multinodular by US in 20–25%!
(a) 15–25% for solitary cold nodule
(b) 1–6% for multiple nodules (DDx: multinodular goiter)
(c) with history of neck irradiation in childhood
   — solitary nodule found in 70% (cancerous in 31%)
   — multiple nodules found in 25% (cancerous in 37%)
   — normal thyroid scan found in 5% (cancer detected in 20%)

ANATOMY AND FUNCTION OF NECK ORGANS

PARANASAL SINUSES

Mucus production of 1 L/day; mucus blanket turns over every 20–30 minutes; irritants are propelled toward nasopharynx at a rate of 1 cm/minute

Maxillary Sinus

Size: 6–8 cm at birth
Walls: roof = floor of orbit; posterior wall abuts pterygopalatine fossa
Extension: 4–5 mm below level of nasal cavity by age 12
Ostium: maxillary ostium + infundibulum enter middle meatus within posterior aspect of hiatus semilunaris; additional ostia may be present
Plain film: present at birth; visible at 4–5 months; completely developed by 15 years of age
Variations: sinus hypoplasia in 9%; aplasia in 0.4%

Ethmoid Sinuses

Size: adult size by age 12; 3–18 air cells per side
Walls: roof = floor of anterior cranial fossa; lateral wall = lamina papyracea
Plain film: very small at birth; visible at 1 year of age; completely developed by puberty

(a) **anteromedial ethmoid air cells**

2–8 cells with a total area of 24 x 23 x 11 mm
Ostia: opening into anterior aspect of hiatus semilunaris of middle meatus (anterior group), opening into ethmoid bulla (middle group)

Agger nasi cells
= anteriormost ethmoid air cells in front of the attachment of middle turbinate to cribriform plate near the lacrimal duct
= anterior, lateral + inferior to frontoethmoidal recess = anteromedial margin of orbit
Prevalence: present in >90%

Ethmoidal bulla
= ethmoidal air cell above + posterior to infundibulum + hiatus semilunaris, located outside the lamina papyracea at the lateral wall of the middle meatus

Haller cells
= anterior ethmoid air cells inferolateral to ethmoidal bulla, on lateral wall of infundibulum, along inferior margin of orbit / roof of maxillary sinus, protruding into maxillary sinus
Prevalence: 10–45%

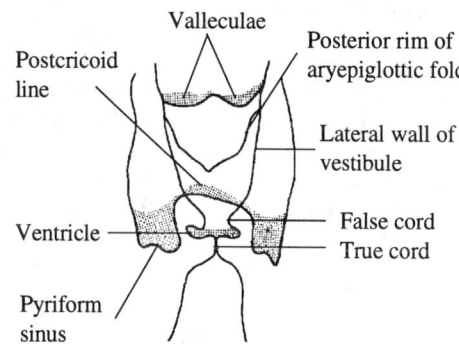

Frontal Laryngopharyngogram During Phonation

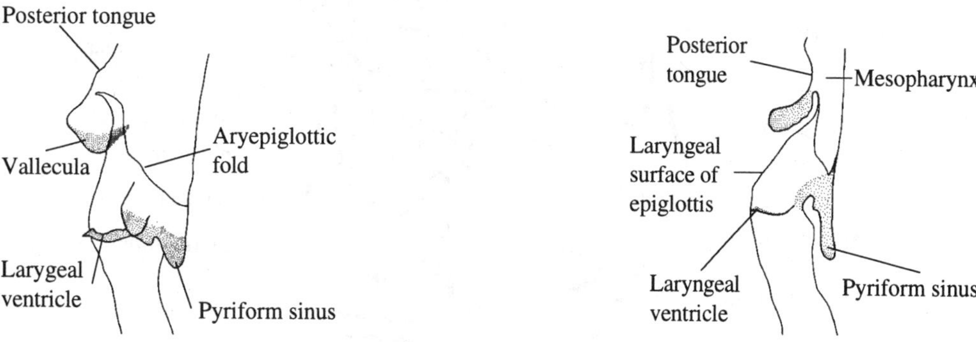

Lateral Laryngogram

during phonation

during quiet breathing

(b) **posterior ethmoid air cells**
1–8 cells, larger cells, total area smaller than that of anteromedial group
Location: behind the basal (= ground) lamella of the middle turbinate
Ostium: into superior meatus / supreme meatus, ultimately draining into sphenoethmoidal recess of nasal cavity

Onodi cell
= most posterior ethmoid air cell pneumatized into sphenoid bone ± surrounding the optic canal
Location: superolateral to sphenoid sinus

Frontal Sinus
Size: 28 x 24 x 20 mm in adults, rapid growth until the late teens
Walls: posterior wall = anterior cranial fossa; inferior wall = anterior portion of roof of orbit
Ostium: into frontal recess of middle meatus via frontoethmoidal recess (= nasofrontal duct)
Plain film: visible at age 6 years
Variations: sinus aplasia in up to 4% (in 90% with Down syndrome)

Sphenoid Sinus
Size: 20 x 23 x 17 mm in adults, small evagination of sphenoethmoidal recess at birth, invasion of sphenoid bone begins at age 5 years; aerated extensions into pterygoid plates (44%) + into clinoid processes (13%)
Walls: roof = floor of sella turcica; anterior wall shared with ethmoid sinuses; posterior wall = clivus; inferior wall = roof of nasopharynx
Ostium: 10 mm above sinus floor into sphenoethmoidal recess posterior to superior meatus at level of sphenopalatine foramen
Plain film: appears by 3 years of age; continues to grow posteriorly + inferiorly into the sella until adulthood

OSTIOMEATAL UNIT
= area of superomedial maxillary sinus + middle meatus as the common mucociliary drainage pathway of frontal maxillary, and anterior + middle ethmoid air cells into the nose
Coronal CT: visualized on two or three 3-mm-thick sections

Components:
1. Infundibulum
   = flattened conelike passage between inferomedial border of orbit / ethmoid bulla (laterally) + uncinate process (medially) + maxillary sinus (inferiorly) + hiatus semilunaris (superiorly)
2. Uncinate process
   = key bony structure in lateral nasal wall below hiatus semilunaris in middle meatus defines hiatus semilunaris together with adjacent ethmoid bulla
   √ pneumatized in <2.5% of patients
3. Ethmoid bulla
   √ located in cephalad recess of middle meatus
4. Hiatus semilunaris
   final segment for drainage of maxillary sinus; located just inferior to ethmoid bulla in middle meatus
   Ostia:
   (1) multiple ostia from anterior ethmoid air cells (at its anterior aspect)
   (2) maxillary ostium infundibulum (at its posterior aspect)

<u>Anatomic variations predisposing to ostiomeatal narrowing</u>:
1. Concha bullosa (4–15%) = aerated / pneumatized middle turbinate
2. Intralamellar cell = air cell within vertical portion of middle turbinate
3. Oversized ethmoid bulla
4. Haller cells
5. Uncinate process bulla
6. Bowed nasal septum

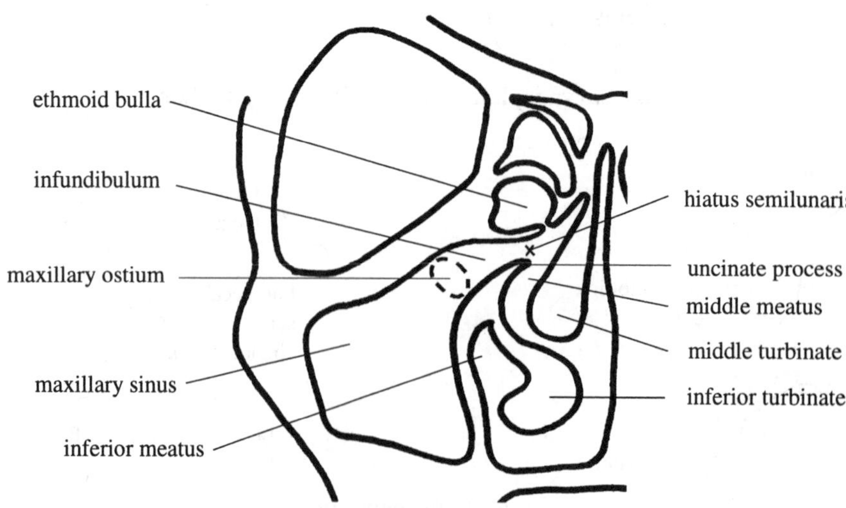

Coronal Scan of Ostiomeatal Unit

7. Paradoxical middle turbinate = convexity of turbinate directed toward lateral nasal wall (10–26%)
8. Deviation of uncinate process

◊ These conditions are not disease states per se!

BRANCHIAL CLEFT DEVELOPMENT

— 6 paired branchial arches are responsible for formation of lower face + neck
— each branchial cleft arch contains a central core of cartilage + muscle, a blood vessel and a nerve
— arches form 5 ectodermal "clefts" / grooves on outer aspect of neck + 5 endodermal pharyngeal pouches separated by a membrane

Formation: during 4th–6th week of embryonic development

1st Branchial Arch = maxillomandibular arch

(a) large ventral / mandibular prominence
forms: mandible, incus, malleus, muscles of mastication
(b) small dorsal / maxillary prominence
forms: maxilla, zygoma, squamous portion of temporal bone, cheek, portions of external ear

nerve: mandibular division of trigeminal nerve
pouch forms: mastoid air cells + eustachian tube
cleft forms: external auditory canal + tympanic cavity

2nd Branchial Arch = Hyoid Arch

nerve: facial nerve
arch forms: thyroid gland, stapes, portions of external ear, muscles of facial expression
pouch forms: palatine tonsil + tonsillar fossa
cleft involutes completely by 9th fetal week; 2nd arch overgrows 2nd + 3rd + 4th clefts to form *cervical sinus* which creates a tract that runs from supraclavicular area just lateral to carotid sheath, turns medially at mandibular angle between external + internal carotid artery, terminates in tonsillar fossa

3rd Branchial Arch

sunk into retrohyoid depression
nerve: glossopharyngeal nerve
arch forms: glossoepiglottic fold, superior constrictor m., internal carotid a., parts of hyoid bone
pouch forms:
(a) thymus gland, which descends into mediastinum by 9th fetal week
(b) inferior parathyroid glands passing down with the thymus

4th Branchial Arch

sunk into retrohyoid depression
nerve: superior laryngeal branch of vagus nerve
arch forms: epiglottis + aryepiglottic folds, thyroid cartilage, cricothyroid m., left component of aortic arch, right component of right proximal subclavian a.

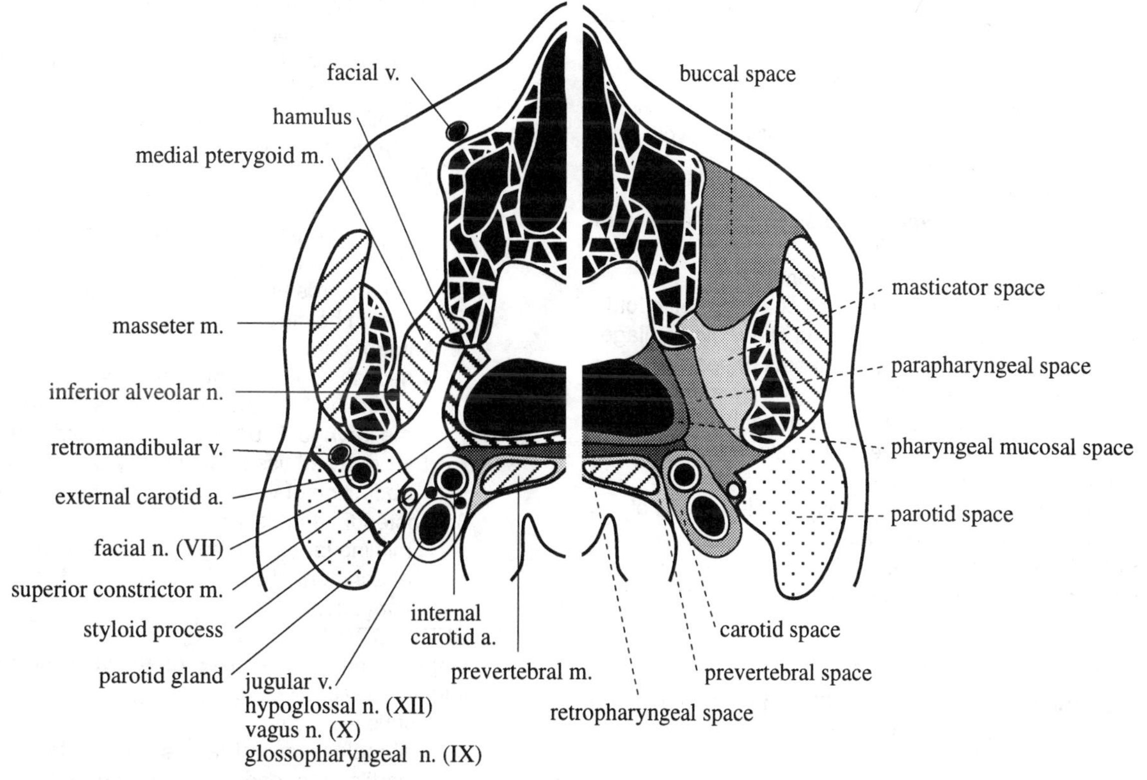

Transaxial Scan Through Level of Lower Nasopharynx

pouch forms: superior parathyroid glands, apex of piriform fossa
cleft forms: ultimobranchial body, which provides parafollicular = "C" cells of thyroid

5th + 6th Branchial Arches
cannot be recognized externally
nerve: recurrent laryngeal branch of vagus nerve

ORAL CAVITY
comprises lip, upper + lower gingiva, buccal mucosa, hard palate, floor of mouth, anterior 2/3 of tongue

OROPHARYNX
consists of
(a) pharyngeal wall between nasopharynx + pharyngoepiglottic fold
(b) soft palate
(c) tonsillar region
(d) tongue base

Borders:
(a) superior: soft palate and Passavant ridge (= ridge of pharyngeal muscle that opposes the soft palate when soft palate is elevated)
(b) anterior: plane that joins the posterior border of soft palate, anterior tonsillar pillars, circumvallate papillae
(c) posterior: posterior pharyngeal wall
(d) inferior: vallecula
(e) lateral: tonsillar region consisting of anterior tonsillar pillar (= palatoglossus muscle) + palatine / faucial tonsil + posterior tonsillar pillar (= palatopharyngeus muscle)

HYPOPHARYNX
= compartment of aerodigestive tract between hyoid bone + inferior aspect of cricoid cartilage
1. Pyriform sinuses
   = two symmetric lateral stalactites of air hanging from hypopharynx behind larynx
   — inferior wall: level of cricoarytenoid joint
   — anteromedial wall: lateral wall of aryepiglottic fold
   — lateral wall: abuts posterior ala of thyroid cartilage
   — posterior wall: most lateral aspect of posterior hypopharyngeal wall
2. Postcricoid area = pharyngoesophageal junction extends from level of arytenoid cartilages to inferior border of cricoid cartilage
   — anterior wall of hypopharynx = posterior wall of lower larynx = "party wall"
3. Posterior hypopharyngeal wall extends from level of valleculae to cricoarytenoid joints

LARYNX
Vertical length: 44 mm (males), 36 mm (females), at 4th–6th cervical vertebrae

A. SUPRAGLOTTIS
extends from tongue base + valleculae to laryngeal ventricle
1. Vestibule
   = airspace within supraglottic larynx
2. Epiglottis
   = leaf-shaped cartilage that functions as a lid to endolarynx
   (a) petiole = stem of epiglottis
   (b) thyroepiglottic ligament = connects petiole to thyroid cartilage inferiorly
   (c) hyoepiglottic ligament = connects epiglottis to hyoid bone anteriorly, covered by a mucosal fold between the valleculae (glossoepiglottic fold)
   (d) "free margin" = superior portion of epiglottis
3. False vocal cords
   = ventricular folds = inferior continuation of aryepiglottic folds = mucosal surface of ventricular ligaments; forming superior border of laryngeal ventricle
4. Arytenoid cartilages
5. Aryepiglottic folds
   = mucosal reflections between cephalad portion (= arytenoid processes) of arytenoid cartilage + inferolateral margin of epiglottis
   √ soft-tissue folds forming border between lateral pyriform sinuses + central laryngeal lumen
6. Laryngeal ventricle
   = fusiform fossa bounded by crescentic edge of false cords superiorly + straight margin of true cords inferiorly
   √ generally not visible on axial scans
7. Preepiglottic space
   √ low-density tissue between anterior margin of epiglottis + thyroid cartilage
8. Paralaryngeal space
   √ low-density tissue between true + false cords and thyroid cartilage
   √ continuous with preepiglottic space anteriorly + aryepiglottic folds superiorly

B. GLOTTIS
1. True vocal cords
   = extend from vocal process of arytenoid cartilage to anterior commissure
   √ vocal cords adduct during phonation of "E" / breath holding
2. Anterior commissure
   = midline laryngeal mucosa covering anterior portions of the true vocal cords where they abut the laryngeal surface of the thyroid cartilage
   √ <1 mm soft tissue behind thyroid cartilage (during abduction of vocal cords with quiet breathing)
3. Posterior commissure
   = midline laryngeal mucosal surface between attachment of true vocal cords to the arytenoid cartilages

C. SUBGLOTTIS
extends from undersurface of true vocal cords to inferior surface of cricoid cartilage
1. Conus elasticus
   = fibroelastic membrane extending from cricoid cartilage to medial margin of true vocal cords + forming lateral wall of subglottis

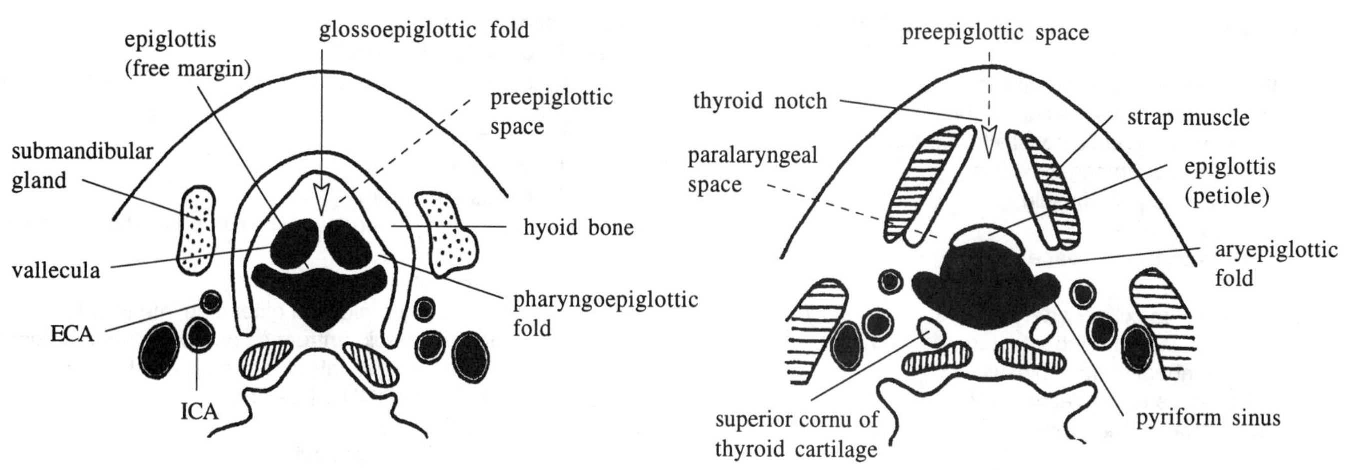

epiglottis
(free margin)
glossoepiglottic fold
preepiglottic
space
submandibular
gland
hyoid bone
vallecula
pharyngoepiglottic
fold
ECA
ICA

Hyoid Bone Level

preepiglottic space
thyroid notch
strap muscle
paralaryngeal
space
epiglottis
(petiole)
aryepiglottic
fold
superior cornu of
thyroid cartilage
pyriform sinus

High Supraglottic Level

thyroid notch
sternohyoid m.
thyroid lamina
omohyoid &
thyrohoid m.
hyoepiglottic
ligament
aryepiglottic
fold
paralaryngeal
space
pyriform sinus
posterior
pharyngeal wall

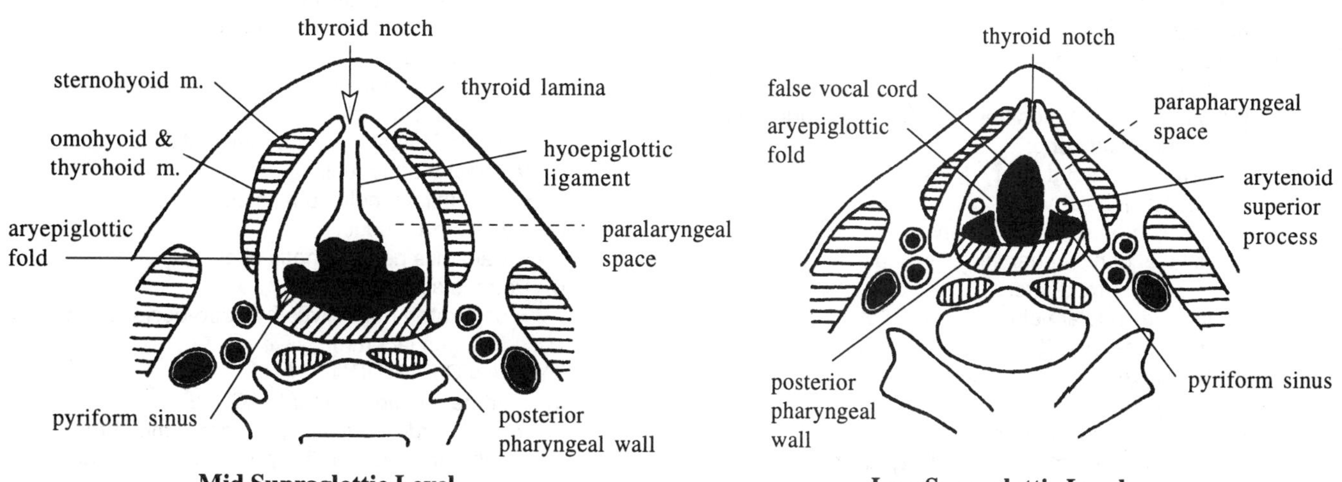

Mid Supraglottic Level

thyroid notch
false vocal cord
parapharyngeal
space
aryepiglottic
fold
arytenoid
superior
process
posterior
pharyngeal
wall
pyriform sinus

Low Supraglottic Level

anterior commissure
thyroid lamina
thyroid m.
true vocal
cord
CCA
IJV
arytenoid
cartilage
cricoarytenoid
joint
cricoid
cartilage
longus capitis & colli m.

Glottic Level

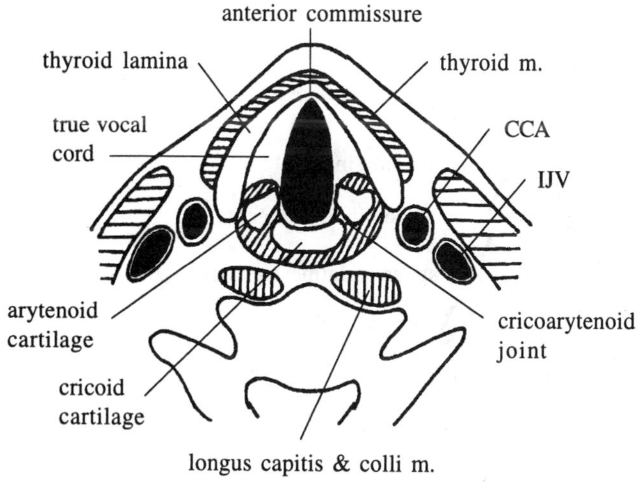

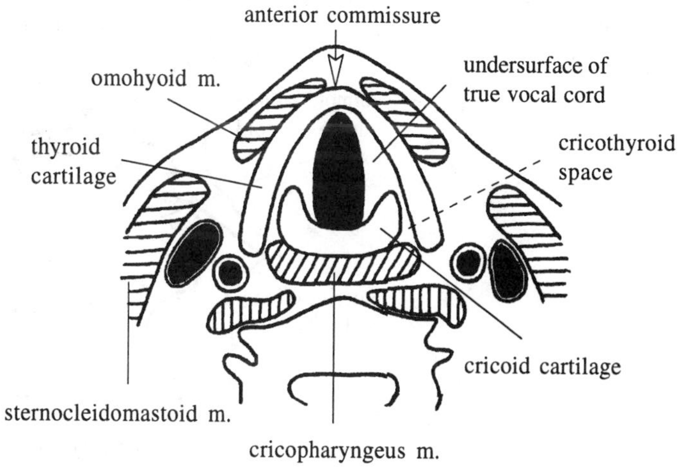

anterior commissure
omohyoid m.
undersurface of
true vocal cord
thyroid
cartilage
cricothyroid
space
cricoid cartilage
sternocleidomastoid m.
cricopharyngeus m.

Undersurface of True Cord

ENT

ENT

Deep spaces of suprahyoid head & neck

Pharyngeal mucosal space
adenoids, faucial + lingual tonsils
superior + middle constrictor muscles
salpingopharyngeal muscle
levator palatini muscle
torus tubarius

Parapharyngeal space
fat
internal maxillary artery
ascending pharyngeal artery
pharyngeal venous plexus
branches of cranial nerve V_3

Retropharyngeal space
fat
medial + lateral retropharyngeal nodes

Prevertebral space
prevertebral muscles
scalene muscles
vertebral artery + vein
brachial plexus
phrenic nerve

Carotid space
Carotid fascia extends from skull base to aortic arch
(a) below hyoid bone:
common carotid artery
internal jugular vein
cranial nerve X (vagus nerve)
(b) at level of nasopharynx:
internal carotid artery
internal jugular vein
cranial nerves IX — XII

Parotid space
parotid gland
intraparotid lymph nodes
external carotid + internal maxillary arteries
retromandibular vein
facial nerve

Temporal bone

A. SQUAMOUS PORTION
= lateral wall of middle cranial fossa + floor of temporal fossa

B. MASTOID PORTION
1. Mastoid antrum
2. Aditus ad antrum
connects epitympanum (= attic) of middle ear cavity to mastoid antrum
3. Körner septum
= small bony projection extending inferiorly from roof of mastoid antrum as part of petrosquamosal suture between lateral + medial mastoid air cells

C. PETROUS PORTION = inner ear
1. Tegmen tympani
= roof of tympanic cavity
2. Arcuate eminence
= prominence of bone over superior semicircular canal
3. Internal auditory canal (IAC)
(a) Porus acusticus internus
= opening of internal auditory canal
(b) Modiolus
= entrance to cochlea
(c) Crista falciformis
= horizontal bony septum in IAC
4. Vestibular aqueduct
= transmits endolymphatic duct
5. Cochlear aqueduct
= transmits perilymphatic duct
6. Petrous apex
= separated from clivus by petro-occipital fissure + foramen lacerum

D. TYMPANIC PORTION
1. External auditory canal (EAC)
medial border formed by tympanic membrane, which attaches superiorly at scutum + inferiorly at tympanic annulus

E. STYLOID PORTION

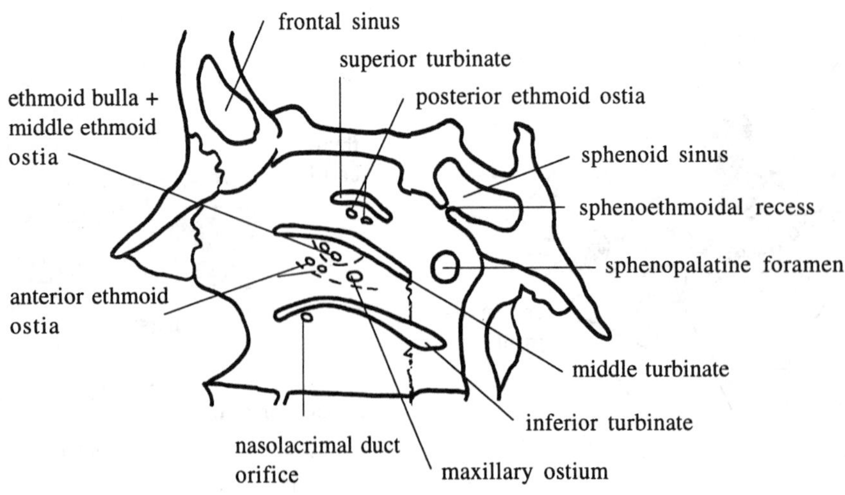

View of Lateral Nasal Wall (turbinates removed)

MIDDLE EAR

Borders:
- — anterior wall = carotid wall
- — posterior wall = mastoid wall including
  - (a) facial nerve recess for descending facial nerve
  - (b) pyramidal eminence for stapedius muscle
  - (c) sinus tympani (clinically blind spot)
- — superior wall = tegmen tympani
- — inferior wall = jugular wall
- — lateral wall = tympanic membrane
- — medial wall = labyrinthine wall

A. EPITYMPANUM
= tympanic cavity above the line drawn between the inferior tip of scutum + tympanic portion of facial nerve
Contents: malleus head, body + short process of incus, Prussak space (= area between incus + lateral wall of epitympanum)

B. MESOTYMPANUM
= tympanic cavity between inferior tip of scutum + line drawn parallel to inferior aspect of bony EAC
Contents: manubrium of malleus, long process of incus, stapes, tensor tympani muscle (innervated by V_3), stapedius muscle (innervated by VII)

C. HYPOTYMPANUM
= shallow trough in floor of middle ear

INNER EAR

1. Cochlea
2 1/2 turns, basal first turn opens into round window posteriorly, encircles central bony axis of modiolus
2. Vestibule
= largest part of membranous labyrinth with subunits of utricle + saccule (not separately visualized); separated from middle ear by oval window
3. Semicircular canals
   - — superior semicircular canal forms convexity of arcuate eminence
   - — posterior semicircular canal points posteriorly along line of petrous ridge
   - — lateral / horizontal semicircular canal juts into epitympanum
4. Cochlear aqueduct
contains 8 mm long perilymphatic duct, extends from basal turn of cochlea to lateral border of jugular foramen paralleling IAC
Function: regulates CSF + perilymphatic fluid pressure
5. Vestibular aqueduct
encompasses endolymphatic duct, extends from vestibule to endolymphatic sac
Function: equilibration of endolymphatic fluid pressure

FACIAL NERVE

Segments:
- (a) intracranial segment
  = from brainstem to porus acusticus internus
- (b) internal auditory canal
  = in anterosuperior portion of IAC
- (c) labyrinthine segment
  = short segment curling anteriorly over top of cochlea; terminates in anterior genu (geniculate ganglion)
- (d) tympanic segment
  = segment from anterior to posterior genu just underneath lateral semicircular canal
- (e) mastoid segment
  = from posterior genu to stylomastoid foramen
- (f) parotid segment
  = extracranial segment between superficial + deep lobes of parotid gland

Function:
1. Lacrimation (via greater superficial petrosal nerve)
2. Stapedius reflex: sound damping
3. Taste of anterior 2/3 of tongue (via chorda tympani nerve to lingual nerve)
4. Facial expression (platysma)
5. Secretion of lacrimal + submandibular + sublingual glands (via nervus intermedius)

THYROID HORMONES

free hormone	: T_4	(0.03%)
	T_3	(0.4%)
Thyroxin-binding globulin (TBG)	: binds T_4	(70%)
	and T_3	(38%)
Thyroxin-binding prealbumin (TBPA)	: binds T_4	(10%)
	and T_3	(27%)
Albumin	: binds T_4	(20%)
	and T_3	(35%)

A. ELEVATION OF TBG
1. Pregnancy
2. Estrogen administration
3. Genetic trait

B. REDUCTION IN TBG
1. Androgens
2. Anabolic steroids
3. Glucocorticoids
4. Nephrotic syndrome
5. Chronic hepatic disease

C. INHIBITION OF T_4 BINDING TO TBG: salicylates

PARATHYROID GLANDS

A. SUPERIOR PARATHYROID GLANDS
Embryology: derived from 4th pharyngeal pouches, descending together with thyroid gland in close relationship to its posterolateral lobes
Location: superior dorsal surface of thyroid gland / intrathyroidal

B. INFERIOR PARATHYROID GLANDS
Embryology: derived from 3rd pharyngeal pouches migrating caudally with thymus
Location: anywhere near / in thyroid, carotid bifurcation, lower neck, mediastinum

ENT

C. SUPERNUMERARY PARATHYROID GLANDS
5th / 6th gland may occupy an ectopic site
◊ Up to 12 parathyroids may be present!

Embryology: parathyroid glands develop by 6 weeks GA + migrate into neck at 8 weeks

Size: 6 x 4 x 1 mm = 25–40 mg

Surgical success rates for finding parathyroid glands:
— 95% for initial cervical exploration
— 60% for repeat surgical exploration
Cause for failure: overlooking an adenoma, multiple abnormal glands, diffuse hyperplasia

Localization technique:
US (75% sensitivity), thallium-technetium subtraction scintigraphy, MR (88% sensitivity)

Duplex Identification

Criteria	**External Carotid Artery**	**Internal Carotid Artery**
SIZE	usually smaller than ICA	usually larger than ECA
LOCATION	oriented medially + anteriorly toward face	oriented laterally + posteriorly toward mastoid process
BRANCHES	gives off arterial branches (superior thyroidal a. as 1st branch)	NO arterial branches
WAVE FORM	high-resistance flow pattern supplying capillary beds in skin + muscle √ forward systolic component √ early diastolic flow reversal occasionally followed by another forward component √ little / no flow in late diastole	low-resistance flow pattern supplying capillary bed in brain √ high-velocity forward systolic component √ sustained strong forward flow in diastole √ stagnant eddy with flow reversal opposite to flow divider in carotid bulb
MANEUVER	oscillations on temporal tap maneuver	

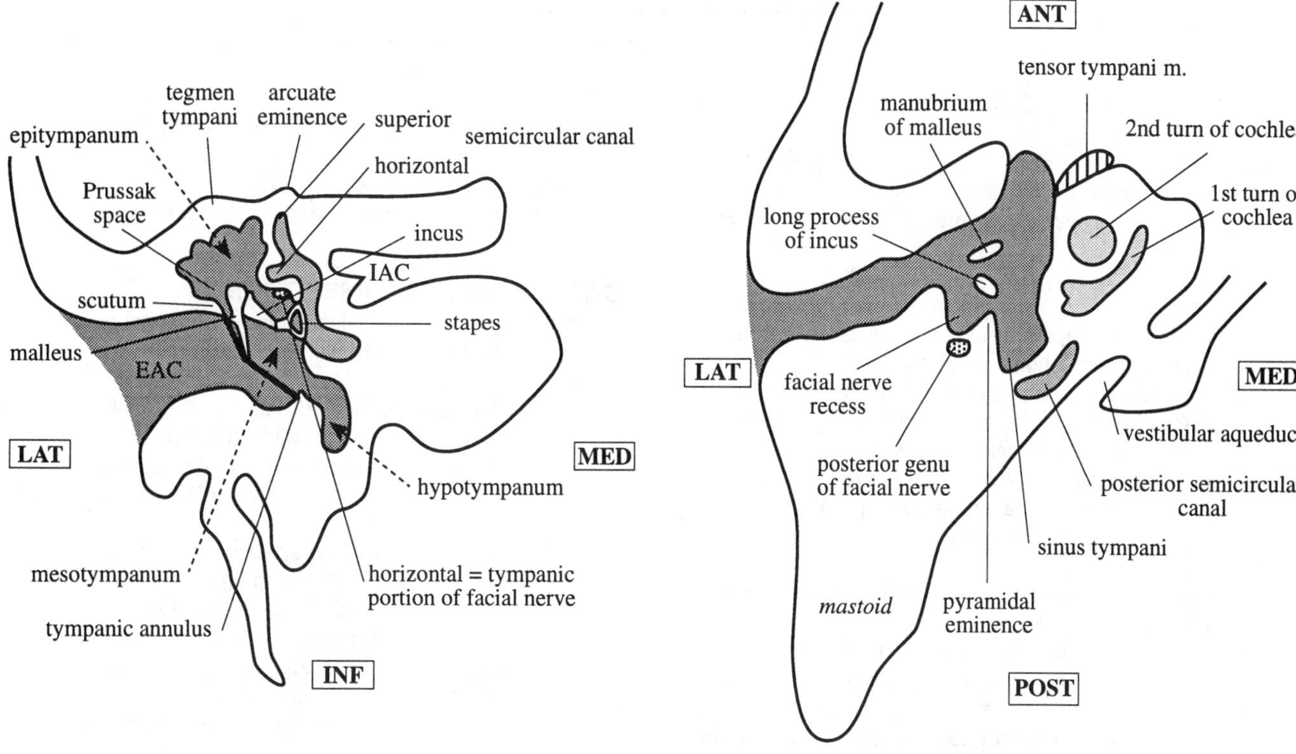

Coronal Tomogram of Temporal Bone **Axial Tomogram of Temporal Bone**

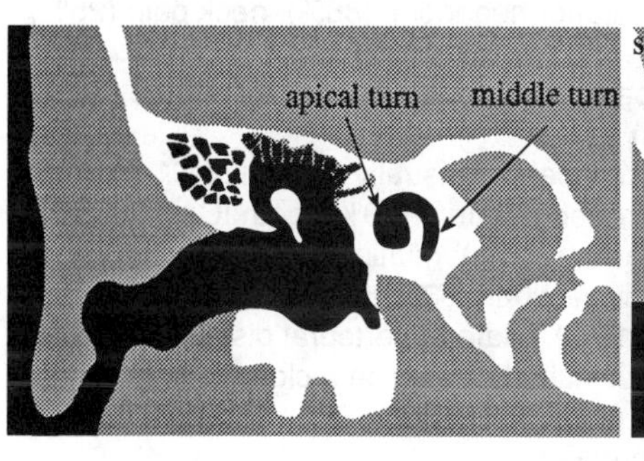

Most anterior scan through the cochlea

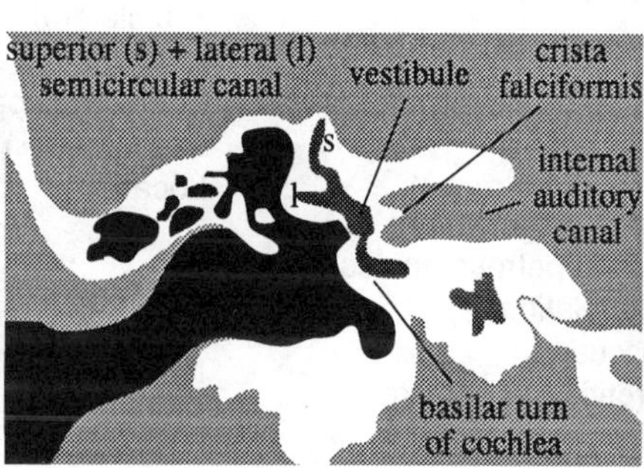

Scan at vestibular level

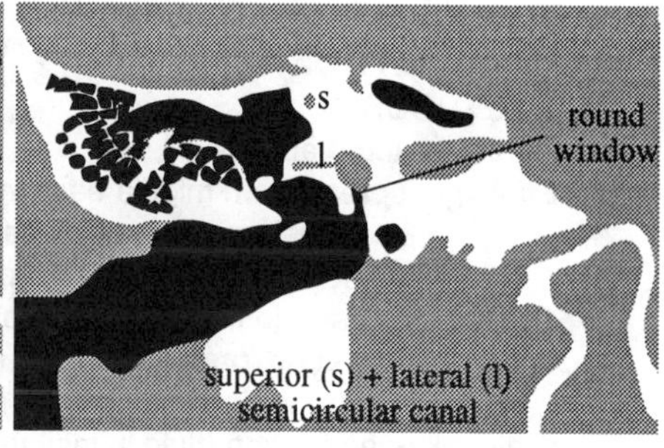

Most posterior scan through round window

Coronal Scan of Normal Rigth Ear

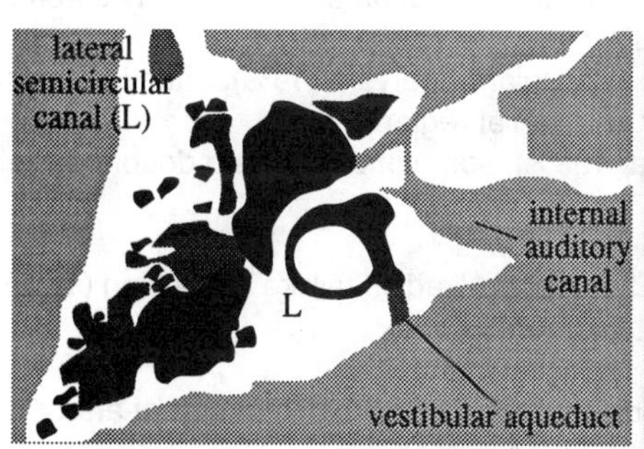

Most superior scan through lateral semicircular canal

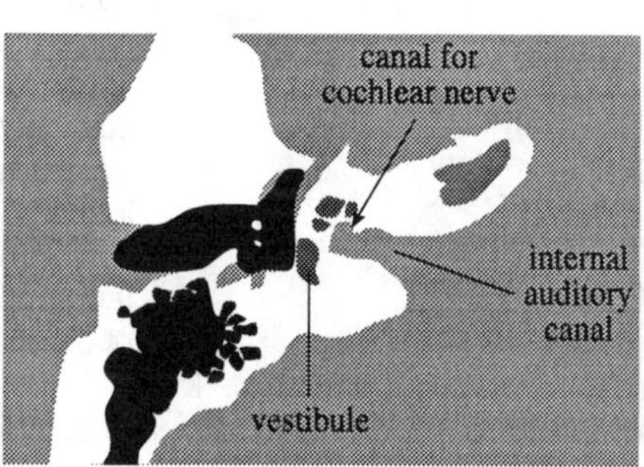

Scan through the vestibular level

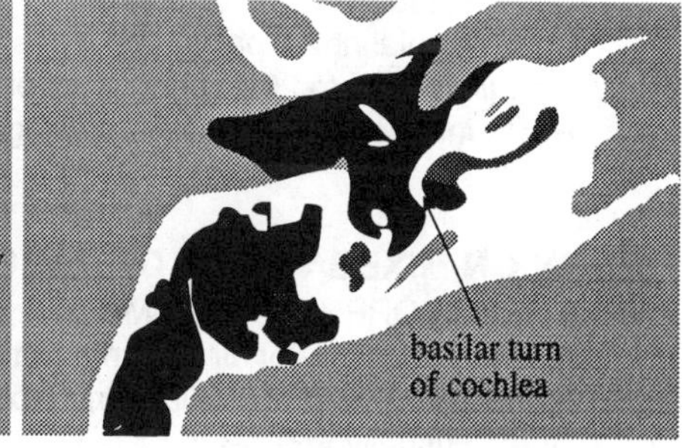

Most inferior scan through the basilar turn of cochlea

Axial Scan of Normal Rigth Ear

ENT

EAR, NOSE, AND THROAT DISORDERS

ADENOID CYSTIC CARCINOMA

= CYLINDROMA

Incidence: 4–15% of all salivary gland tumors

Histo: (a) tubular (b) cribriform (c) solid

Age: 3rd–9th decade; maximum between 40 and 70 years

Location:

@ Minor salivary glands (most common; 25–31% of malignant neoplasms in minor salivary glands)
- nasal obstruction + swelling

@ Submandibular gland (15% of tumors in this gland)

@ Parotid gland (2–6% of tumors in this gland; arises from peripheral parotid ducts with propensity for perineural spread along facial nerve)
- hard mass + facial nerve pain / paralysis

√ infiltrating parotid mass

MR:

√ hypo- to hyperintense (high signal corresponds to low cellularity) on T2WI

Metastases to: lung, cervical lymph nodes, bone, liver

Prognosis: slow relentless malignant course with repeat recurrences; the greater the cellularity, the worse the prognosis (requires entire tumor); 60–69% 5-year survival rate; 40% 10-year survival rate

Rx: repeat surgical excision + radiation therapy

APICAL PETROSITIS

= PETROUS APICITIS

chronic > acute apicitis

Etiology: spread from middle ear + mastoid infection; requires presence of air cells in petrous apices (which is found in 30% of population)

Organism: Pseudomonas, enterococcus

- **Gradenigo syndrome** = otorrhea (otitis media) + retro-orbital pain (trigeminal pain) + 6th nerve palsy

√ air cell opacification (fluid in ipsilateral middle ear + mastoid)

√ bone destruction (osteomyelitis)

MR:

√ enhancing mass about petrous tip

Cx: epidural abscess;
cranial nerve palsy (abducens, trigeminal, vagus)

Mortality: up to 20% (prior to antibiotic era)

Rx: intravenous antibiotics, myringotomy, surgery

BENIGN MIXED TUMOR OF PAROTIS

= PLEOMORPHIC ADENOMA

Incidence: 80% of all benign parotid tumors

Histo: mixture of epithelial + myoepithelial cells

Age: usually >50 years

- slow-growing lump in cheek

√ round / oval / lobulated sharply marginated mass

√ rarely dystrophic calcifications

√ variable contrast enhancement

CT:

√ low-density center if large (mucoid matrix)

MR:

√ hyperintense mass on T2WI

√ hyperintense areas in center (mucoid matrix)

CAROTID ARTERY DISSECTION

= hematoma within media splitting off the vessel wall and causing a false lumen within media

Etiology:

A. SPONTANEOUS CAROTID DISSECTION
(1) nonrecalled minor / trivial trauma
(2) primary arterial disease: Marfan syndrome (fibromuscular dysplasia in 15%), cystic medial necrosis
Associated with: hypertension (36%), smoking (47%), migraine (11%)

B. TRAUMATIC CAROTID DISSECTION
blunt / penetrating trauma (automobile accident, boxing, accidental hanging, diagnostic carotid compression, manipulative therapy)
Associated with: fracture through carotid canal

Incidence: 2% of strokes in persons aged 40–60 years

Age: 18–76 years (66% between 35 and 50 years)

- unilateral anterior headache (86%), neck pain (25%)
- TIA / stroke (58%), amaurosis fugax (12%)
- oculosympathetic paresis = Horner syndrome (52%)
- bruit (48%)

Location: cervical ICA usually at level of C1-2 (60%), vertebral artery (20%), both ICA + vertebral artery (10%); multiple simultaneous dissections (33%); bilateral carotid dissections (15%), bilateral vertebral dissections (5%)

Site: (a) Subintimal dissection = close to intima
(b) Subadventitial dissection = close to adventitia

US (50% accuracy)

Angiography:

√ string sign = elongated tapered irregular luminal stenosis extending to base of skull (76%)

√ abrupt luminal reconstitution at level of bony carotid canal (42%)

√ fingerlike / saccular aneurysm (40%), often in upper cervical / subcranial region

√ intimal flap (29%), sometimes creating double-barrel lumen

√ slow ICA-MCA flow

√ tapered "flamelike" / "radish taillike" occlusion (17%), often distal to carotid bulb

MR:

√ pseudoenlargement of external diameter of artery (= intramural hematoma)

Cx: (1) Thromboemboli due to stenosis
(2) Subarachnoid hemorrhage (with intracranial location)
(3) Secondary aneurysm

Prognosis: complete / excellent recovery (8%)
Rx: best therapy not clear; anticoagulants

CAROTID ARTERY STENOSIS

High-grade ICA stenosis is associated with increased risk for TIA, stroke, carotid occlusion, embolism arising from thrombi forming at site of narrowing

Increased risk for stroke:

(a) significant ICA stenosis (compromised blood flow)
Reduction of blood flow occurs at 50–60% diameter stenosis / 75% area stenosis
◊ 2% risk of stroke with nonsignificant stenosis
◊ 16% incidence of stroke with significant stenosis
◊ 2% incidence of subsequent stroke following endarterectomy

(b) intraplaque hemorrhage (embolic stroke)

Histo:

arteriosclerosis = generic term for all structural changes resulting in hardening of the arterial wall

1. Diffuse intimal thickening
= growth of intima through migration of medial smooth muscle cells into subendothelial space through fenestrations in internal elastic lamella associated with increasing amounts of collagen, elastic fibers, glycosaminoglycans
Age: beginning at birth slowly progressing to adult life
2. Atherosclerosis
= intimal pool of necrotic, proteinaceous + fatty substances within hardened arterial wall
Location: large + medium-sized elastic and muscular arteries
(a) fatty streak = superficial yellow-gray flat intimal lesion characterized by focal accumulation of subendothelial smooth muscle cells + lipid deposits
(b) fibrous plaque = whitish protruding lesion consisting of central core of lipid + cell debris surrounded by smooth muscle cells, collagen, elastic fibers, proteoglycans; a fibrous cap separates the lipid core (= atheroma) from the vessel lumen
(c) complicated lesion = fibrous plaque with degenerative changes such as calcification, plaque hemorrhage, intimal ulceration / rupture, mural thrombosis
Plaque hemorrhage from thin-walled blood vessels in vascularized plaque may cause ulceration, thrombosis + embolism, and luminal narrowing
◊ in 93% of symptomatic patients
◊ in 27% of asymptomatic patients
Plaque ulceration exposes thrombogenic subendothelial collagen + lipid-rich material
◊ frequent in plaques occupying >85% of lumen
◊ 12.5% stroke incidence per year
3. Mönckeberg sclerosis = medial calcification
4. Hypertensive arteriosclerosis

Predilection sites of arterial stenosis:

	Incidence of lesions	
	Stenosis	Occlusion
Right ICA origin	33.8%	8.6%
Left ICA origin	34.1%	8.7%
Right vertebral artery origin	18.4%	4.8%
Left vertebral artery origin	22.3%	2.2%
Right carotid siphon	6.7%	9.0%
Left carotid siphon	6.6%	9.2%
Basilar artery	7.7%	0.8%
Right MCA	3.5%	2.2%
Left MCA	4.1%	2.1%

COURSE OF CAROTID ARTERY STENOSIS
1. Stable stenosis (68%)
2. Progressive stenosis to >50% diameter reduction (25%)

Angiography:
@ Extracranial
√ smooth asymmetrical excrescence encroaching upon vessel lumen
√ crater / niche = ulceration
√ mound within base of crater = mural thrombus

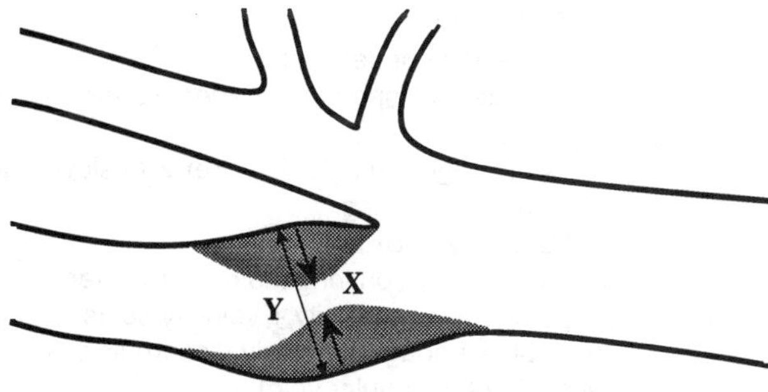

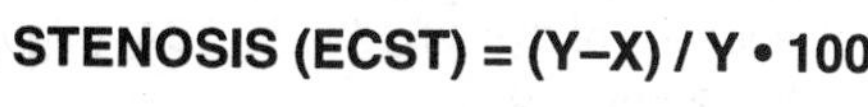
% STENOSIS (ECST) = (Y–X) / Y • 100

ECST = European Carotid Surgery Trial

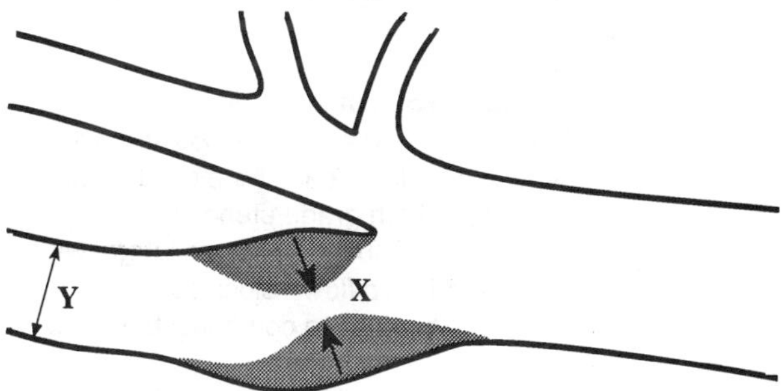

% STENOSIS (NASCET) = (Y–X) / Y • 100

NASCET = North American Symptomatic Carotid Endarterectomy Trial

√ Holman carotid slim sign = diffuse narrowing of entire ICA distal to high-grade stenosis due to decrease in perfusion pressure
√ occlusion of ICA

@ Intracranial
√ carotid siphon stenosis
√ retrograde flow in ophthalmic artery filled from ECA
√ small vessel occlusion
√ focal areas of slow flow
√ early draining vein = reactive hyperemia = "luxury perfusion" due to shunting between arterioles + venules surrounding an area of ischemia
√ ICA-MCA slow flow = delayed arrival + washout of ICA-MCA distribution in comparison to ECA

Carotid endarterectomy:
Benefit: 17% reduction of ipsilateral stroke at 2 years in patients with >70% carotid stenosis (NASCET = North American Symptomatic Carotid Endarterectomy Trial)
Risk: 1% mortality; 2% risk of intraoperative neurologic deficit

Carotid Duplex Ultrasound

Indications for carotid duplex US:
(1) Screening for suspected extracranial carotid disease
(a) high-grade flow-limiting stenosis
(b) low-grade stenosis with hemorrhage
(2) Nonhemispheric neurologic symptomatology
(3) History of transient ischemic attack / stroke
(4) Asymptomatic carotid bruit
(5) Retinal cholesterol embolus
(6) Preoperative evaluation before major cardiovascular surgery
(7) Intraoperative monitoring of vascular patency during endarterectomy
(8) Sequential evaluation after endarterectomy
(9) Monitoring of known plaque during medical treatment

Grading Of Carotid Stenosis

= severity of stenosis is primarily graded as a ratio of lumen diameter narrowing NOT reduction in cross sectional area

Limitations:
1. Calcifications >1 cm in length
◊ A jet associated with an >70% stenosis usually travels at least 1 cm downstream!
2. Contralateral high grade stenosis
= ipsilateral ICA functions as collateral with increased blood flow velocities
◊ Use velocity ratios to compensate for this effect!

Accuracy of duplex scans: (in comparison to arteriography for ICA lesions)
91–94% sensitivity, 85–99% specificity for >50% ICA diameter stenosis

Incorporating B-mode and Doppler spectrum analysis
A. NO LESION
√ peak systolic velocity (PSV) < 125 cm/sec
√ clear window under systole
√ no spectral broadening
√ no evidence of plaque
B. MINIMAL DISEASE
= 0–15% diameter reduction
√ PSV < 125 cm/sec
√ clear window under systole
√ minimal spectral broadening in deceleration phase of systole
√ minimal plaque
C. MODERATE DISEASE
= 16–49% diameter reduction
√ peak systole <125 cm/sec
√ no window under systole
√ poststenotic spectral broadening throughout systole
◊ End-diastolic velocity (EDV) remains normal in <50% diameter reduction!
√ moderate plaque
D. SEVERE DISEASE = HEMODYNAMICALLY SIGNIFICANT LESION
(a) 50–59% stenosis
√ PSV 120–130 cm/sec
√ EDV 30–40 cm/sec
(b) 60–79% stenosis
√ PSV of 131–250 cm/sec
√ EDV of 40–100 cm/sec
(c) ≥60 % stenosis
√ end diastolic velocity of >80 cm/sec
(d) 50–79% diameter reduction
√ peak velocity ratio of ICA/CCA >1.5
√ peak systole >125 cm/s
√ marked poststenotic spectral broadening throughout cardiac cycle
(e) **>70% stenosis** (benefit of endarterectomy documented in NASCET study)
√ peak systole >230 cm/s
√ end diastole >100 cm/sec
√ peak velocity ratio of ICA/CCA >4.0
√ peak systolic velocity ICA Π end diastolic velocity CCA >15
(f) 80–99% diameter reduction
√ PSV of >250 cm/sec
√ EDV of >100 cm/sec
√ no window under systole
√ poststenotic spectral broadening throughout systole
√ "string sign" on color Doppler with slow-flow sensitivity setting
E. OCCLUDED VESSEL
√ no signal in ICA on longitudinal / transverse images (color sensitivity + velocity scale must be set low enough to clearly discern flow signals within internal jugular vein)
√ absence of diastolic flow in CCA (high impedance flow)
√ diastolic flow reversal in CCA

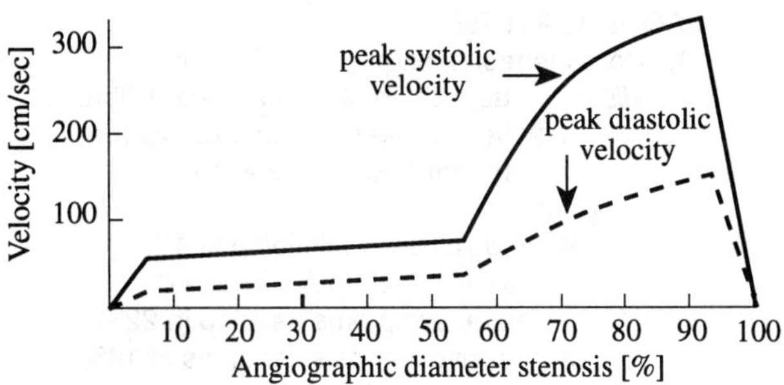

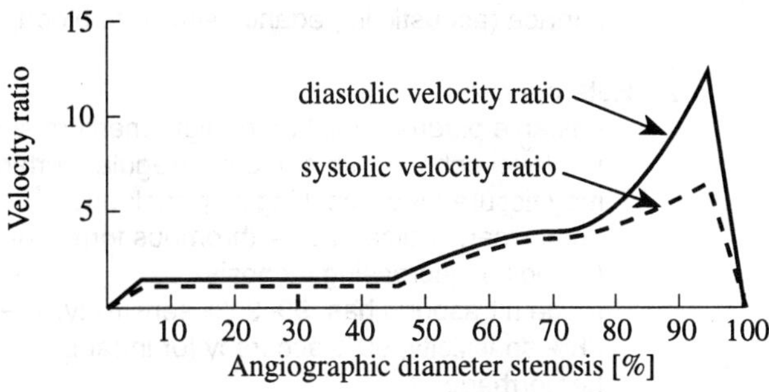

Doppler Parameters in Internal Carotid Artery Stenosis

√ increased diastolic flow in ECA (if ECA assumes the role of primary supplier of blood to brain)
√ increase in peak systolic velocities in contralateral ICA (due to collateral flow)

Limitations:
poor visualization due to calcification, tortuosity, increased depth of artery, "high" bifurcation

Common carotid waveform analysis

A. DISTAL OBSTRUCTION
   √ high-pulsatility waveform (pulsatility changes occur only with >80% stenosis)
   √ reduced amplitude
B. PROXIMAL OBSTRUCTION
   √ low-amplitude damped waveform

Hemodynamic variations of carotid artery stenosis

A. MORPHOLOGY OF STENOSIS
   1. Degree of stenosis: velocities increase up to a luminal diameter of 1.0–1.5 mm
   2. Length of stenosis: peak velocities decrease with length of stenosis
   √ use the same angle + steering direction when following a patient for disease progression

Doppler Spectrum Analysis

Diameter stenosis classification	(%)	ICA/CCA peak systolic ratio	ICA/CCA peak diastolic ratio	Peak systolic velocity (cm/sec)	kHz[†]	Peak diastolic velocity (cm/sec)	kHz[†]
normal – mild	0 – 40	<1.5	<2.6	<110 > 25	<3.5	<40	<1.5
moderate	41 – 59	<1.8	<2.6	>120	>3.5	<40	<1.5
severe	60 – 79	>1.8	>2.6	>130	>5.0	>40	>1.5
critical	80 – 99	>3.7	>5.5	>250	>8.0	>80 – 135	>4.5

† = based on 5MHz pulsed Doppler carrier frequency at 60° flow angle (Blackshear)

	(%)	ICA/CCA peak systolic ratio	ICA/CCA peak diastolic ratio	Peak systolic velocity (cm/sec)	kHz	Peak diastolic velocity (cm/sec)	kHz
	0 – 39	<1.8	<2.4	<110		<40	
	40 – 59	<1.8	<2.4	<130		<40	
	60 – 79	>1.8	>2.4	>130		>40	
	80 – 99	>3.7	>5.5	>250		>100	
(Bluth)							

	(%)	ICA/CCA peak systolic ratio	ICA/CCA peak diastolic ratio	Peak systolic velocity (cm/sec)	kHz	Peak diastolic velocity (cm/sec)	kHz
	0 – 50	<2:1		<125		<40	
	50 – 75	>2:1		125 – 225		40 – 100	
	75 – 90	>3:1	>5:1	225 – 325		>100	
	>90	>4:1	>9:1	>325		>100	
	>95	resistive CCA	distortion	may be decreased		may be decreased	
(Gosink)							

	(%)	ICA/CCA peak systolic ratio	ICA/CCA peak diastolic ratio	Peak systolic velocity (cm/sec)	kHz[†]	Peak diastolic velocity (cm/sec)	kHz[†]
	1 – 15						
	16 – 49			(<125)	<4.0		
	50 – 79			(≥125)	≥4.0	(<140)	<4.5
(Fell)	80 – 99					(≥140)	≥4.5
(Strandness)	occlusion			no flow detected			

† = based on 5MHz pulsed Doppler carrier frequency at 60° flow angle (University of Washington)

ENT

B. PHYSIOLOGIC VARIABILITY

◊ A range of velocities may be encountered with a given degree of stenosis!

◊ ICA/CCA ratio obviates effects of physiologic variability!

◊ Compare left with right waveforms to avoid errors!

◊ Measure volume flow (more sensitive because of contralateral compensatory flow increase)

Cause:

1. Cardiac output
2. Pulse rate
3. Flow velocity: increased with obstruction in collateral vessels, decreased with proximal obstruction in same vessel
4. Normal helical nature of blood flow with many different velocity vectors + nonaxial blood flow not detectable by color Duplex imaging
5. Peripheral resistance
6. Arterial compliance
7. Hypertension
8. Blood viscosity

Carotid Plaque

FORMATION THEORY

1. Stagnant eddy that rotates at outer vessel margin (opposite to the flow divider in area of flow separation + low shear stress) leads to net influx of fluid into subendothelial tissue with progressive deposition of lipids + smooth muscle cell proliferation
2. Increased likelihood of intraplaque hemorrhage (vascularization of plaque with fragile vessels derived from vasa vasorum / from lumen) + fissuring from a critical size on
   ◊ As the degree of stenosis increases, it is more likely that plaques become denser + more heterogeneous demonstrating an irregular surface!

PLAQUE DENSITY

1. Hypoechoic = low-echogenicity plaque
   = fibrofatty plaque / hemorrhage
   √ echogenicity less than sternocleidomastoid muscle
   √ flow void / flow disturbance on color Duplex
2. Isoechoic plaque
   = smooth muscle cell proliferation / laminar thrombus
   √ echogenicity equal to sternocleidomastoid muscle + lower than adventitia
3. Hyperechoic = moderately echogenic plaque
   = fibrous plaque
   √ echogenicity higher than sternocleidomastoid muscle + similar to adventitia
4. Calcification = strongly echogenic plaque
   √ acoustic shadow impairs visualization of intima

PLAQUE TEXTURE

1. Homogeneous plaque = stable plaque
   Histo: deposition of fatty streaks + fibrous tissue; rarely shows intraplaque hemorrhage / ulcerations
   Prognosis:
   ◊ neurologic deficits develop in 4%
   ◊ ipsilateral infarction on CT in 12%
   ◊ ipsilateral symptoms develop in 22%
   ◊ progressive stenosis develops in 18%
   √ homogeneous uniform echo pattern with smooth surface (acoustic impedance similar to blood)
2. Heterogeneous plaque
   = unstable plaque = mixture of high, medium and low level echoes with smooth / irregular surface; may fissure / tear resulting in intraplaque hemorrhage / ulceration + thrombus formation (embolus / increasing stenosis)
   B-mode ultrasound has 90–94% sensitivity, 75–88% specificity, 90% accuracy for intraplaque hemorrhage
   Histo: lipid-laden macrophages, monocytes, leukocytes, necrotic debris, cholesterol crystals, calcifications
   Prognosis:
   ◊ neurologic deficits develop in 27%
   ◊ ipsilateral infarction on CT in 24%
   ◊ ipsilateral symptoms develop in 50%
   ◊ progressive stenosis develops in 77%
   √ anechoic areas within plaque (= hemorrhage / lipid deposition / focal plaque degeneration)
   √ heterogeneous complex echo pattern

PLAQUE SURFACE CHARACTERISTICS

= US unreliable due to poor visualization of intima

Categories:
— smooth
— mildly irregular
— markedly irregular
— ulcerated

1. Intimal thickening
   Histo: fatty streaks
   √ wavy / irregular line paralleling vessel wall extending >1 mm into vessel lumen
2. Ulcerated plaque
   Accuracy: 60% sensitive, 60–70% specific
   ◊ The presence of intraplaque hemorrhage is much more common than normally appreciated
   ◊ Neither arteriography nor US has proved reliable!
   √ isolated crater of >2 mm within surface of plaque demonstrated on transverse + longitudinal images
   √ reversed flow vortices extending into plaque crater demonstrated by color Doppler
   √ proximal + distal undercutting of plaque
   √ anechoic area within plaque extending to surface

Errors in duplex ultrasound

1. Error in proper localization of stenosis (6%)
   Cause: ECA stenosis placed into ICA / carotid bifurcation or vice versa
2. Mistaking patent ECA branches for carotid bifurcation (4%)
   Cause: complete occlusion of ICA not recognized
   √ disparity in position of bifurcation
   √ no difference in pulsatility waveform
   √ high-resistance waveform in CCA
3. Interpreter error in estimating severity of stenosis (2.5%)
   usually overestimation, rarely underestimation
   √ absence of one / more components for diagnosis which are
   (a) significant elevation of peak velocity
   (b) poststenotic turbulence
   (c) extension of high velocity into diastole
4. Superimposition of ECA + ICA (2%)
   Cause: strict coronal orientation of ECA + ICA
   √ superimposition can be avoided by rotation of head to opposite side
5. Severe stenosis mistaken for occlusion
   minimal flow not detectable; angiogram necessary with delayed images
6. Weak signals misinterpreted as occlusion
7. Normal / weak signals in severe stenosis
   Cause: severe stenosis causes a decrease in blood flow + peak velocity with return to normal velocity levels
   √ high resistivity in CCA
8. Point of maximum frequency shift not identified
   Cause: extremely small lumen / short segment of stenosis
   √ unexplained (poststenotic) coarse turbulence
   √ ipsilateral ECA collateral flow
   √ abnormal CCA resistivity
9. Stenosis obscured by plaque / strong Doppler shift in overlying vessel
10. Inaccessible stenosis
    √ abnormal CCA resistivity
    √ abnormal oculoplethysmography
11. Unreliable velocity measurements
    (a) higher velocities: hypertension, severe bradycardia, obstructive contralateral carotid disease
    (b) lower velocities: arrhythmia, aortic valvular lesion, severe cardiomyopathy, proximal obstructive carotid lesion ("tandem lesion"), >95% ICA stenosis
    (c) aliasing = high velocities are displayed in reversed direction below zero baseline due to Doppler frequency exceeding half the pulse repetition frequency
    Remedy: shift zero baseline, increase pulse repetition frequency, increase Doppler angle, decrease transducer frequency, use continuous-wave Doppler probe

INDIRECT METHODS OF EVALUATION
1. Oculoplethysmography (OPG)
   = measurement of ophthalmic artery pressure + pulse arrival time by air calibrated system
   Contraindications: glaucoma, retinal detachment, recent eye surgery / trauma, lens implants
2. Periorbital bidirectional Doppler
   = insonation of frontal + supraorbital arteries to assess flow direction around orbit and to detect crossover flow through the circle of Willis (through contra- and ipsilateral compression)
3. Transcranial Doppler
   = insonation to establish flow direction in basal cerebral arteries through temporal bone (MCA, ACA, PCA, terminal portion of ICA), foramen magnum (both vertebral arteries, basilar artery), orbit (carotid siphon)
   ◊ Nondiagnostic in up to 35%!

CHOANAL ATRESIA

Etiology: failure of perforation of oronasal membrane which normally perforates by 7th week EGA
◊ Associated with other anomalies in 50%!
A. BONY SEPTATION (85%)
B. MEMBRANOUS SEPTATION (15%)

CHOLESTEATOMA

= KERATOMA = epithelium-lined sac filled with keratin debris leading to bone destruction by pressure + demineralizing enzymes

Primary cholesteatoma

= CONGENITAL CHOLESTEATOMA = EPIDERMOID CYST (2%)
= derived from aberrant embryonic ectodermal rests in temporal bone (commonly petrous apex) / epidural space / meninges
- conductive hearing loss in child with NO history of middle ear inflammatory disease
- cholesteatoma seen through intact tympanic membrane

Associated with: EAC dysplasia
Location:
(a) epitympanum
(b) petrous pyramid: internal auditory canal first involved
(c) meninges: scooped out appearance of petrous ridge
(d) cerebellopontine angle: erosion of porus, shortening of posterior canal wall
(e) jugular fossa: erosion of posteroinferior aspect of petrous pyramid

ENT

ENT

Secondary cholesteatoma

= INFLAMMATORY CHOLESTEATOMA
= ACQUIRED EPIDERMOID (98%)

Cause:
ingrowth of squamous cell epithelium of EAC through tympanic membrane (= eardrum) secondary to
(a) repeated episodes of ear inflammation with invagination of posterosuperior retraction pocket
(b) marginal perforation of eardrum

Age: usually >40 years

- whitish pearly mass behind intact tympanic membrane (invasion of middle ear cavity and mastoid) diagnosed otoscopically in 95%
- facial paralysis (compression of nerve VII at geniculate ganglion)
- conductive hearing loss (compromise of nerve VIII in internal auditory canal / involvement of cochlea or labyrinth)
- severe vertigo (labyrinthine fistula)

Types:

1. **Pars flaccida cholesteatoma** = Primary acquired cholesteatoma = Attic cholesteatoma (most common)
   √ increasing width of attic
   √ initially destruction of lateral wall of attic, particularly the drum spur (scutum) with invasion of Prussak space
   √ extension posteriorly through aditus ad antrum into mastoid antrum
   √ destruction of Körner septum
2. **Pars tensa cholesteatoma** = Secondary acquired cholesteatoma (less frequent)
   √ displacement of auditory ossicles
   √ erosion of ossicular chain: first affecting long process of incus

√ nondependent homogeneous mass
√ perforation of tympanic membrane posterosuperiorly (pars flaccida = Shrapnell membrane)
√ poorly pneumatized mastoid (frequent association)
√ erosion of tegmen tympani (with more extensive cholesteatoma) producing an extradural mass
√ destruction of labyrinthine capsule (less common) involving the lateral semicircular canal first
√ erosion of facial canal

MRI:
√ iso- / hypointense relative to cortex on T1WI
√ no enhancement with Gd-DTPA (enhancement is related to granulation tissue)

Cx: (1) Intratemporal: ossicular destruction, facial nerve paralysis (1%), labyrinthine fistula, automastoidectomy, complete hearing loss
(2) Intracranial: meningitis, sigmoid sinus thrombosis, temporal lobe abscess, CSF rhinorrhea

DDx: chronic otitis media, granulation tissue = cholesterol granuloma, brain herniation through tegmen defect, neoplasm (rhabdomyosarcoma, squamous cell carcinoma)

CHOLESTEROL GRANULOMA

= CHOLESTEROL CYST
= acquired inflammatory lesion of petrous bone

Histo: cholesterol crystals surrounded by foreign-body giant cells; embedded in fibrous connective tissue with varying proportions of hemosiderin-laden macrophages, chronic inflammatory cells and blood vessels; brownish fluid contains cholesterol crystals + blood (= "chocolate cyst")

- blue (vascular) tympanic membrane without pulsatile tinnitus

√ ossicles remain intact

CT: √ nonenhancing middle ear mass

MRI:
√ hyperintense signal on T1WI + T2WI secondary to methemoglobin (DDx to cholesteatoma, which is isointense to brain on T1WI)

CHRONIC RECURRENT SIALADENITIS

- painful periodic unilateral enlargement of parotid gland
- milky discharge may be expressed

Sialography:
√ Stensen duct irregularly enlarged / sausage-shaped
√ pruning of distal parotid ducts
√ ± calculi

CT:
√ diffusely enlarged dense gland
√ dilated Stensen duct ± calculi

Cx: Mucocele

COGAN SYNDROME

= AUTOIMMUNE INTERSTITIAL KERATITIS

MR: √ membranous labyrinthine enhancement

CROUP

= ACUTE LARYNGOTRACHEOBRONCHITIS
= ACUTE VIRAL SPASMODIC LARYNGITIS
= lower respiratory tract infection

Organism: parainfluenza, respiratory syncytial virus
Age: >6 months of age, peak incidence 2–3 years

- history of viral lower respiratory infection
- hoarse cry + "brassy" cough
- inspiratory difficulty with stridor
- fever

√ thickening of vocal cords
√ NORMAL epiglottis + aryepiglottic folds
√ "steeple sign" = subglottic "inverted V" = symmetrical funnel-shaped narrowing 1–1.5 cm below lower margins of pyriform sinuses on AP radiograph (loss of normal "shouldering" of air column caused by mucosal edema + external restriction by cricoid), accentuated on expiration, paradoxical inspiratory collapse, less pronounced during expiration
√ narrow + indistinct subglottic trachea on lateral radiograph
√ inspiratory ballooning of hypopharynx (nonspecific sign of any acute upper airway obstruction)
√ distension of cervical trachea on expiration

Prognosis: usually self-limiting

CYSTIC HYGROMA

= CYSTIC LYMPHANGIOMA = most common form of lymphangioma
= single / multiloculated fluid-filled cavities on either side of fetal neck + head (localized form) ± trunk (generalized form)

Cause: congenital blockage of lymphatic drainage (= noncommunication of jugular lymphatic sac with jugular vein)
Incidence: 1:6,000 pregnancies
Age: 50–65% present at birth; up to 90% evident by age 2
Histo: hugely dilated cystic lymphatic spaces

Associated with:
- (a) chromosomal abnormalities in 60–80% (in particular when detected in 2nd trimester)
  - (1) Turner syndrome (45 XO, mosaic) in 40–80%
  - (2) Trisomies 13, 18, 21, 13q, 18p, 22
  - (3) Noonan syndrome
  - (4) Distichiasis-lymphedema syndrome
  - (5) Familial pterygium colli
  - (6) Roberts, Cumming, Cowchock syndrome
  - (7) Achondrogenesis type II
  - (8) Lethal pterygium syndrome
- (b) exposure to teratogens
  - (1) Fetal alcohol syndrome
  - (2) aminopterin
  - (3) trimethadione

Types:
- (1) Cystic hygroma with abnormal peripheral lymphatic system
  - √ lymphangioma in posterior compartment of neck
  - √ septations (indicate high probability for aneuploidy, development of hydrops, and perinatal death)
- (2) Diffuse lymphangiectasia
  - √ lymphangioma of chest + extremities
  - √ peripheral lymphedema + nonimmune hydrops
- (3) Isolated cystic hygroma
  - (a) axillary lymph sac malformation
    - √ lymphangioma restricted to axilla
  - (b) jugular lymph sac malformation
    - √ lymphangioma restricted to lateral neck
  - (c) internal thoracic + paratracheal lymph sac malformation
    - √ lymphangioma within mediastinum
  - (d) combined lymph sac malformation
  - (e) thoracic duct malformation
    - √ thoracic duct cyst

- • AF- / MS-AFP may be elevated
- • ± dyspnea / dysphagia with encroachment upon trachea, pharynx, esophagus
- • rapid increase in size (from infection / hemorrhage)

Location: posterior neck (75%), mediastinum (3–10%, in 1/2 extension from neck), axilla (20%), chest wall (14%), face (10%), retroperitoneum, abdominal viscera, groin, scrotum, bones

√ thin-walled fluid-filled structure with multiple septa + solid cyst wall components
√ isolated nuchal cysts
√ webbed neck (= pterygium colli) following later communication with jugular veins
√ nonimmune hydrops (43%)
√ progressive peripheral edema
√ fetal ascites
√ oligo- / polyhydramnios / normal amount of fluid
√ bradycardia

MR:
- √ hyperintense on T2WI
- √ low to high signal intensity on T1WI (depending on protein content of fluid)
- √ ± fluid-fluid level (if hemorrhage present)

Cx: (1) Compression of airways / esophagus
(2) Slow growth / sudden enlargement (hemorrhage, inflammation)

Prognosis:
(1) Intrauterine demise (33%)
(2) Mortality of 100% with hydrops
(3) Spontaneous regression (10–15%)
Favorable for localized lesions of anterior neck + axilla
◊ Only 2–3% of fetuses with posterior cystic hygroma become healthy living children!

Rx: surgical excision (difficult since mass does not follow tissue planes)
DDx: twin sac of blighted ovum, cervical meningocele, encephalocele, cystic teratoma, nuchal edema, branchial cleft cyst, vascular malformation, lipoma, abscess

PSEUDOCYSTIC HYGROMA = PSEUDOMEMBRANE
= anechoic space bordered by specular reflection on posterior aspect of fetal neck during 1st trimester
Cause: ? developing integument
√ NO prominent posterior bulge / internal septations

EPIGLOTTITIS

= ACUTE BACTERIAL EPIGLOTTITIS = life-threatening infection with edema of epiglottis + aryepiglottic folds

Organism: Haemophilus influenzae type B, Pneumococcus, Streptococcus group A
Age: >3 years, peak incidence 6 years

- • abrupt onset of respiratory distress with inspiratory stridor
- • severe dysphagia

Location: purely supraglottic lesion; associated subglottic edema in 25%

Lateral radiograph should be taken in erect position only! (frontal view irrelevant)
- √ enlargement of epiglottis + thickening of aryepiglottic folds
- √ circumferential narrowing of subglottic portion of trachea during inspiration
- √ ballooning of hypopharynx + pyriform sinuses
- √ cervical kyphosis

Cx: Mortal danger of suffocation secondary to hazard of complete airway closure; patient needs to be accompanied by physician experienced in endotracheal intubation

ENT

EXTERNAL AUDITORY CANAL DYSPLASIA

Incidence: 1:10,000 births; family history in 14%

Etiology: (a) isolated (b) Trisomy 13, 18, 21 (c) Turner syndrome (d) Maternal rubella (e) Craniofacial dysostosis (f) Mandibulofacial dysostosis

SPECTRUM

1. Stenosis of EAC
2. Fibrous atresia of EAC
3. Bony atresia (in position of tympanic membrane)
4. Decreased pneumatization of mastoid (mastoid cells begin to form in 7th fetal month)
5. Decreased size / absence of tympanic cavity
6. Ossicular changes (rotation, fusion, absence)
7. Ectopic facial nerve = anteriorly displaced vertical (mastoid) portion of facial nerve canal
8. Decrease in number of cochlear turns / absence of cochlea
9. Dilatation of lateral semicircular canal

- bilateral in 29%; M:F = 6:4
- pinna deformity
- stenotic / absent auditory canal

Cx: congenital cholesteatoma (infrequent)

FIBROMATOSIS COLLI

Cause: pressure necrosis with secondary fibrosis of sternocleidomastoid muscle from birth trauma

- history of difficult delivery (forceps)
- anterior neck mass during first 2 weeks of life, which may grow over 2–4 additional weeks
- torticollis (14–20%)

Location: lower 2/3 of sternocleidomastoid muscle

US:
- √ well-defined mass within sternocleidomastoid muscle
- √ hypo- over iso- to hyperechoic mass depending on duration of disorder

CT:
- √ isoattenuating muscle enlargement

Prognosis: gradual spontaneous resolution over 4–8 months with / without treatment

Rx: (1) muscle stretching exercise (2) surgery in 10%

DDx:
(1) Neuroblastoma (heterogeneous solid mass with calcifications)
(2) Rhabdomyosarcoma
(3) Lymphoma (well-defined round /oval masses along cervical lymph node chain)
(4) Cystic hygroma (anechoic region with septations)
(5) Branchial cleft cyst
(6) Hematoma

FRACTURE OF TEMPORAL BONE

Longitudinal fracture of temporal bone (75%)

= fracture parallel to the axis of petrous pyramid arising in squamosa of temporal bone through tegmen tympani, EAC (external auditory canal), middle ear, terminating in foramen lacerum

- bleeding from EAC (disruption of tympanic membrane)
- NO neurosensory hearing loss
- otorrhea (CSF leak with ruptured tympanic membrane; rare)
- conductive hearing loss (dislocation of auditory ossicles — most commonly incus as the least anchored ossicle)
- facial nerve palsy (10–20%) due to edema / fracture of facial canal near geniculate ganglion; frequent spontaneous recovery

√ pneumocephalus
√ herniation of temporal lobe
√ incudostapedial joint dislocation (weakest joint)
  √ "ice cream" (malleus) has fallen off the "cone" (incus) on direct coronal CT scan
  √ fracture of "molar tooth" on direct sagittal CT scan
√ mastoid air cells opaque / with air-fluid level

Plain film views: Stenvers / Owens projection

Transverse fracture of temporal bone (25%)

= fracture perpendicular to axis of petrous pyramid originating in occipital bone extending anteriorly across the base of skull + across the petrous pyramid

- irreversible neurosensory hearing loss (fracture line across apex of IAC / labyrinthine capsule)
- persistent vertigo
- facial nerve palsy in 50% (injury in IAC); less frequent spontaneous recovery because of disruption of nerve fibers
- rhinorrhea (CSF leak with intact tympanic membrane)
- bleeding into middle ear

Plain film views: posteroanterior (transorbital) + Towne projection

GLOMUS TUMOR

= CHEMODECTOMA = NONCHROMAFFIN PARAGANGLIOMA = GLOMERULOCYTOMA
= slow-growing vascular lesion arising from glomus body

Origin: tumor arising from nonchromaffin paraganglion cells of neuroectodermal origin; differs from adrenal medulla only in its nonchromaffin feature

Histo: acidophil-epitheloid cells in contact with endothelial cells of a vessel; storage of catecholamines (usually nonfunctioning); histologically similar to pheochromocytoma

Age: range of 6 months to 80 years; peak age in 5–6th decade; F:M = 4:1

Associated with: pheochromocytoma

Location: anywhere in paraganglionic tissue between glomus jugulotympanicum and base of bladder: carotid body, skull base, temporal region, trachea, periaortic region, mandible, ciliary ganglion of the eye, retroperitoneal region, cervical vagus nerve, laryngeal branches of vagus nerve

Synchronous multicentricity in 3–26%:
(a) autosomal dominant in 25–35%
(b) nonhereditary in <5%

Glomus tympanicum tumor

Most common tumor in middle ear

- hearing loss, pulsatile tinnitus

- reddish purple mass behind tympanic membrane

Location: tympanic plexus on cochlear promontory of middle ear

CT (bone algorithm preferred):
- √ globular soft-tissue mass abutting promontory
- √ intense enhancement
- √ usually small at presentation (early involvement of ossicles)
- √ erosion + displacement of ossicles
- √ inferior wall of middle ear cavity intact

Angio:
- √ difficult to visualize because of small size

Glomus jugulare tumor

Most common tumor in jugular fossa with intracranial extension

Glomus jugulotympanicum tumor = large glomus jugulare tumor growing into the middle ear

Origin: adventitia of jugular vein
- tinnitus, hearing loss
- vascular tympanic membrane

Location: at dome of jugular bulb
- √ soft-tissue mass in jugular bulb region / hypotympanum / middle ear space
- √ intense enhancement
- √ destruction of posteroinferior petrous pyramid + corticojugular spine of jugular foramen
- √ destruction of ossicles (usually incus), otic capsule, posteromedial surface of petrous bone

MR:
- √ "salt and pepper" appearance due to multiple small tumor vessels

Angio: (film entire neck for concurrent glomus tumors!)
- √ hypervascular mass with persistent homogeneous reticular stain
- √ invasion / occlusion of jugular bulb by thrombus / tumor
- √ supplied by tympanic branch of ascending pharyngeal artery, meningeal branch of occipital artery, posterior auricular artery via stylomastoid branch, internal carotid artery, internal maxillary artery
- √ arteriovenous shunting

Cx: malignant transformation with metastases to regional lymph nodes (in 2–4%)

Glomus vagale tumor

Origin: near ganglion nodosum of vagus nerve at base of skull close to jugular foramen

Extension: (a) downward into parapharyngeal space (2/3)
(b) intracranially (dumbbell shape)
- slow growing + asymptomatic
- √ spherical / ovoid mass with sharp interfacing margins and homogeneous enhancement
- √ highly vascular mass + neovascularity + intense tumor blush

Cx: malignant transformation with metastases in 15% to regional lymph nodes + lung (other paragangliomas in 10%)

Carotid body tumor

Embryology:
derived from mesoderm of 3rd branchial arch + neural crest ectoderm cells, which differentiate into sympathogonia (= forerunner of paraganglionic cells)
- ◊ Chemodectoma is misnomer (not derived from chemoreceptor cells)!

Histo: nests of epithelioid cells ("Zellballen") with granular eosinophilic cytoplasm separated by trabeculated vascularized connective tissue
- ◊ chromaffin-positive granules (= catecholamines) may be present

Function of carotid body:
5 x 3 x 2 mm carotid body regulates pulmonary ventilation through afferent input by way of glossopharyngeal nerve to the medullary reticular formation

Stimulus: hypoxia > hypercapnia > acidosis

Effect: increase in respiratory rate + tidal volume; increase in sympathetic tone (heart rate, blood pressure, vasoconstriction, elevated catecholamines)
- painless pulsatile firm neck mass below the angle of the jaw, laterally mobile but vertically fixed

Location: adventitia of carotid bifurcation; bilateral in 5% with sporadic occurrence, in 32% with autosomal dominant transmission
- √ enhancing oval mass with splaying of ICA + ECA

Cx: malignant transformation in 6% with metastases to regional lymph nodes, brachial plexus, cerebellum, lung, bone, pancreas, thyroid, kidney, breast

GOITER

Adenomatous goiter

= MULTINODULAR GOITER

US: (89% sensitivity, 84% specificity, 73% positive predictive value, 94% negative predictive value)
- √ increased size + asymmetry of gland
- √ multiple 1–4 cm solid nodules
- √ areas of hemorrhage + necrosis
- √ coarse calcifications may occur within adenoma (secondary to hemorrhage + necrosis)

Diffuse goiter

US:
- √ increase in glandular size, R lobe > L lobe
- √ NO focal textural changes
- √ calcifications not associated with nodules

Iodine-deficiency goiter

Not a significant problem in United States because of supplemental iodine in food

Etiology: chronic TSH stimulation
- low serum T_4
- √ high I-131 uptake

ENT

JOD-BASEDOW PHENOMENON (2%)
= development of thyrotoxicosis (= excessive amounts of T_4 synthesized + released) if normal dietary intake is resumed / iodinated contrast medium administered
Incidence: most common in individuals with long-standing multinodular goiter
Age: >50 years
√ multinodular goiter with in- / decreased uptake (depending on iodine pool)

Toxic nodular goiter
= PLUMMER DISEASE
= autonomous function of one / more thyroid adenomas
Peak age: 4–5th decade; M:F = 1:3
• elevated T_4
• suppressed TSH
√ nodular thyroid with hot nodule + suppression of remainder of gland
√ stimulation scan will disclose normal uptake in remainder of gland
√ increased radioiodine uptake by 24 hours of approximately 80%
Rx:
(1) I-131 treatment with empirical dose of 25–29 mCi (hypothyroidism in 5–30%)
(2) Surgery (hypothyroidism in 11%)
(3) Percutaneous ethanol injection (hypothyroidism in <1%, transient damage of recurrent laryngeal nerve in 4%)

Intrathoracic goiter
= extension of cervical thyroid tissue / ectopic thyroid tissue (rare) into mediastinum
Incidence: 5% of resected mediastinal masses; most common cause of mediastinal masses
Location: usually anterior, 25% posterior exclusively on right side
• mostly asymptomatic
• symptoms of tracheal + esophageal + recurrent laryngeal nerve compression
√ continuity with cervical thyroid / lack of continuity (with narrow fibrous / vascular pedicle)
√ mass of high HU + well-defined borders
√ frequent focal calcifications
√ inhomogeneous texture with low-density areas (= degenerative cystic areas)
√ marked + prolonged enhancement

GRAVES DISEASE
= DIFFUSE TOXIC GOITER
= autoimmune disorder with thyroid stimulating antibodies (LATS) producing hyperplasia + hypertrophy of thyroid gland
Peak age: 3rd–4th decade; M:F = 1:7
• elevated $T_3 + T_4$
• depressed TSH production
• dermopathy = pretibial myxedema (5%)
• ophthalmopathy = periorbital edema, lid retraction, ophthalmoplegia, proptosis, malignant exophthalmos
√ diffuse thyroid enlargement
√ uniformly increased uptake
√ incidental nodules superimposed on preexisting adenomatous goiter (5%)
US: (identical to diffuse goiter)
√ global enlargement of 2–3 x the normal size
√ normal / diffusely hypoechoic pattern
√ hyperemia on color Doppler
Rx: I-131 treatments (for adults):
Dose: 80–120 µCi/g of gland with 100% uptake (taking into account estimated weight of gland + measured radioactive iodine uptake for 24 hours)
Cx: 10–30% develop hypothyroidism within 1st year + 3%/year rate thereafter

HYPOPHARYNGEAL CARCINOMA
Histo: squamous cell carcinoma
May be associated with: Plummer-Vinson syndrome (= atrophic mucosa, achlorhydria, sideropenic anemia) affecting women in 90%
• sore throat, intolerance to hot / cold liquids (early signs)
• dysphagia, weight loss (late signs)
• cervical adenopathy (in 50% at presentation)
Stage:
T1 tumor limited to one subsite
T2 tumor involves >1 subsite / adjacent site without fixation of hemilarynx
T3 same as T2 with fixation of hemilarynx
T4 invasion of thyroid / cricoid cartilage / soft tissue of neck

Pyriform sinus carcinoma
Incidence: 60% of hypopharyngeal carcinomas
• may escape clinical detection if located at inferior tip; often origin of "cervical adenopathy with unknown primary" (next to primaries in lingual + faucial tonsils and nasopharynx)
√ invasion of posterior ala of thyroid cartilage, cricothyroid space, soft tissue of neck in T4 lesion
Prognosis: poor due to early soft-tissue invasion

Postcricoid carcinoma
Incidence: 25% of hypopharyngeal carcinomas
√ difficult assessment due to varying thickness of inferior constrictor + prevertebral muscles
Prognosis: 25% 5-year survival (worst prognosis)

Posterior pharyngeal wall carcinoma
Incidence: 15% of hypopharyngeal carcinomas
√ invasion of retropharyngeal space with extension into oro- and nasopharynx
√ retropharyngeal adenopathy

INVERTED PAPILLOMA
= INVERTING PAPILLOMA = ENDOPHYTIC PAPILLOMA = SQUAMOUS CELL PAPILLOMA = TRANSITIONAL CELL PAPILLOMA = CYLINDRICAL EPITHELIOMA = SCHNEIDERIAN PAPILLOMA

Incidence: 4% of all nasal neoplasms; most common of epithelial papillomas; commonly occurring after nasal surgery
Cause: unknown; association with human papillomavirus-11
Age: 40–60 years; M:F = 3–5:1
Path: vascular mass with prominent mucous cyst inclusions interspersed throughout epithelium
Histo: hyperplastic epithelium inverts into underlying stroma rather than in an exophytic direction; high intracellular glycogen content
◊ Squamous cell carcinoma coexistent in 5.5–27%!
Location: uniquely unilateral (bilateral in <5%)
(a) most often arising from the lateral nasal wall with extension into ethmoid / maxillary sinuses, at junction of antrum + ethmoid sinuses
(b) paranasal sinus (most frequently maxillary antrum)
(c) nasal septum (5.5–18%)
• unilateral nasal obstruction, epistaxis, postnasal drip, recurrent sinusitis, sinus headache
• distinctive absence of allergic history
√ commonly involves antrum + ethmoid sinus
√ widening of infundibulum / outflow tract of antrum
√ destruction of medial antral wall / lamina papyracea of orbit, anterior cranial fossa (pressure necrosis) in up to 30%
√ septum may be bowed to opposite side (NO invasion)
√ homogeneous enhancement
MR:
√ may have intermediate to low intensity on T2WI (DDx: squamous cell carcinoma, olfactory neuroblastoma, melanoma, small cell carcinoma)
Cx: (1) cellular atypia / squamous cell carcinoma (10%)
(2) recurrence rate of 15–78%
Rx: complete surgical extirpation (lateral rhinotomy with en bloc excision of lateral nasal wall)

JUVENILE ANGIOFIBROMA

= most common benign nasopharyngeal tumor, can grow to enormous size and locally invade vital structures
Incidence: 0.5% of all head and neck neoplasms
Age: teenagers (mean age of 15 years); almost exclusively in males
• recurrent + severe epistaxis (59%)
• nasal speech due to nasal obstruction (91%)
• facial deformity (less common)

Location: nasopharynx / posterior nares
Extension: posterolateral wall of nasal cavity; via pterygopalatine fossa into retroantral region / orbit / middle cranial fossa; laterally into infratemporal fossa
√ widening of pterygopalatine fossa (90%) with anterior bowing of posterior antral wall
√ invasion of sphenoid sinus (2/3) from tumor erosion through floor of sinus
√ widening of inferior + superior orbital fissures (spread into orbit via inferior orbital fissure + into middle cranial fossa via superior orbital fissure)
√ highly vascular nasopharyngeal mass (only enhances on CT scan immediately after bolus injection); supplied primarily by internal maxillary artery
MR:
√ intermediate signal intensity on T1WI with discrete punctate areas of hypointensity (secondary to highly vascular stroma)
NOTE: Biopsy contraindicated!

LABYRINTHITIS

Cause: viral infection (mumps, measles) > bacterial infection > syphilis, autoimmune, toxins
• sudden hearing loss, vertigo, tinnitus
MR: √ faint diffuse enhancement of labyrinth on T1WI (HALLMARK)

Ramsay Hunt syndrome = herpes zoster oticus
• mucosal vesicles of external auditory canal
√ intracanalicular 8th nerve enhancement

Tympanogenic labyrinthitis

Cause: agent enters through oval / round window in middle ear infection

Meningogenic labyrinthitis

Cause: agent propagates along IAC / cochlear aqueduct in meningitis
Location: often bilateral

Labyrinthitis ossificans

= LABYRINTHITIS OBLITERANS = SCLEROSING LABYRINTHITIS = CALCIFIC / OSSIFYING COCHLEITIS
Cause: suppurative infection (tympanogenic, meningogenic, hematogenic) in 90%, trauma, surgery, tumor, severe otosclerosis
Pathophysiology: progressive fibrosis + ossification of granulation tissue within labyrinth
• bi - / unilateral profound deafness
√ loss of normal fluid signal within labyrinth on T2WI (early in course of disease)
√ inner ear structures filled with bone

LARYNGEAL CARCINOMA

98% of all malignant laryngeal tumors; in 2% sarcomas
Risk factors: smoking, alcohol abuse, airborne irritants
Histo: squamous cell carcinoma
Suggestive of lymph node metastasis:
√ lymph node >1.5 cm in cross section
√ proximity to laryngeal mass
√ cluster of >3 lymph nodes 6–15 mm in size

Supraglottic carcinoma

Incidence: 20–30% of all laryngeal cancers
Metastases: early to lymph nodes of deep cervical chain, in 25–55% at time of presentation
• symptomatic late in course of disease (often T3 / T4)

ENT

Stage:
- T1 tumor confined to site of origin
- T2 involvement of adjacent supraglottic site / glottis without cord fixation
- T3 tumor limited to larynx with cord fixation or extension to postcricoid area / medial wall of pyriform sinus / preepiglottic space
- T4 extension beyond larynx with involvement of oropharynx (base of tongue) / soft tissue of neck / thyroid cartilage

A. ANTERIOR COMPARTMENT
1. **Epiglottic carcinoma**
   √ circumferential relatively symmetric growth
   √ extension into preepiglottic space ± base of tongue ± paraglottic space
   Prognosis: better than for tumors of posterolateral compartment

B. POSTEROLATERAL COMPARTMENT
1. **Aryepiglottic fold (marginal supraglottic) carcinoma**
   √ exophytic growth from medial surface of aryepiglottic fold
   √ growth into fixed portion of epiglottis + paraglottic (= paralaryngeal) space
2. **False vocal cord / laryngeal ventricle carcinoma**
   √ submucosal spread into paraglottic space
   √ ± destruction of thyroid cartilage
   √ ± involvement of true vocal cords
   Prognosis: poorer than for cancer of the anterior compartment

Glottic carcinoma

Incidence: 50–60% of all laryngeal cancers
- early detection due to hoarseness

Stage:
- T1 tumor confined to vocal cord with normal mobility
- T2 supra- / subglottic extension ± impaired mobility
- T3 fixation of true vocal cord
- T4 destruction of thyroid cartilage / extension outside larynx

Patterns of tumor invasion:
(1) anterior extension into anterior commissure
   √ >1 mm thickness of anterior commissure
   √ invasion of contralateral vocal cord via anterior commissure
(2) posterior extension to arytenoid cartilage, posterior commissure, cricoarytenoid joint
(3) subglottic extension
   √ tumor >5 mm inferior to level of vocal cords
(4) deep lateral extension into paralaryngeal space

Prognosis: T1 carcinoma rarely metastasizes (0–2%) due to absence of lymphatics within true vocal cords

Subglottic carcinoma

Incidence: 5% of all laryngeal cancers
- late detection due to minimal symptomatology

Stage:
- T1 confined to subglottic area
- T2 extension to vocal cords ± mobility
- T3 tumor confined to larynx + cord fixation
- T4 cartilage destruction / extension beyond larynx

Prognosis: poor due to early metastases to cervical lymph nodes (in 25% at presentation)

LARYNGEAL PAPILLOMATOSIS

= RECURRENT RESPIRATORY PAPILLOMATOSIS

◊ Squamous papilloma is the most common benign tumor of the larynx!

Etiology: human papilloma virus types 6 + 11 (Papova virus causing genital condyloma acuminatum)

Histo: core of vascular connective tissue covered by stratified squamous epithelium

Age of onset: 1–54 years; M:F = 1:1; bimodal distribution
(a) <10 years (diffuse involvement) = juvenile onset papillomatosis; probably caused by transmission from mother to child during vaginal delivery
(b) 21–50 years (usually single papilloma)

- progressive hoarseness / aphonia
- repeated episodes of respiratory distress
- inspiratory stridor, asthmalike symptoms
- cough
- recurrent pneumonia
- hemoptysis

Location: (a) uvula, palate (b) vocal cord (c) subglottic extension (50–70%) (d) pulmonary involvement (1–6%)

√ thickened lumpy cords
√ bronchiectasis

Cx:
(1) Tracheobronchial papillomatosis (2–5%)
   Location: lower lobe + posterior predilection
   √ solid pulmonary nodules in mid + posterior lung fields
   √ 2–3 cm large thin-walled cavity with 2–4 mm thick nodular wall (foci of squamous papillomas enlarge centrifugally, undergo central necrosis, cavitate)
   √ peripheral atelectasis + obstructive pneumonitis
(2) Pulmonary papillomatosis
   from aerial dissemination (bronchoscopy, laryngoscopy, tracheal intubation) 10 years after initial diagnosis
   √ irregularities of tracheal / bronchial walls
   √ noncalcified granulomata progressing to cavitation
(3) Malignant transformation into invasive squamous cell carcinoma

Rx: CO_2 laser resection / surgical excision

LARYNGOCELE

= abnormally dilated appendix / sacculus of laryngeal ventricle (= anteriorly located blind pouch within laryngeal ventricle between false + true vocal cords; normal appendix relatively large in infancy, visible in 10% of adults during phonation)

Pathogenesis: chronic increase in intraglottic pressure

Cause: excessive coughing, playing wind instrument, blowing glass, obstruction of appendicular ostium (= secondary laryngocele) by chronic granulomatous disease, laryngeal neoplasm

Types:

(a) internal = in parapharyngeal space confined within thyrohyoid membrane + supraglottis

(b) external = protrusion above thyroid cartilage + through thyrohyoid membrane presenting as lateral neck mass near hyoid bone

(c) mixed (44%) = internal + external component joined through connection at thyrohyoid membrane

- hoarseness / stridor (internal laryngocele)
- anterior neck mass just below angle of mandible (external laryngocele)

Site: unilateral (80%), bilateral (20%)

√ cystic mass that can be followed to level of ventricle
√ increase in size during Valsalva maneuver
√ decrease in size during compression
√ may be filled with fluid

Cx: infection (pyolaryngocele), formation of mucocele

LARYNGOMALACIA

= immaturity of cartilage; most common cause of stridor in neonate + young infant

- only cause of stridor to get worse at rest

√ hypercollapsible larynx during inspiration (supraglottic portion only)
√ backward bent of epiglottis + anterior kink of aryepiglottic folds during inspiration

Prognosis: transient (disappears by age 1 year)

LINGUAL THYROID

= solid embryonic rest of thyroid tissue, which remains ectopic along the tract of thyroglossal duct

Incidence: in 10% of autopsies (within tongue <3 mm); M << F

- may be only functioning thyroid tissue (70–80%)
- asymptomatic (usually)
- may enlarge causing dysphagia / dyspnea

Location: midline dorsum of tongue near foramen cecum (majority), thyroglossal duct, trachea

CT: √ small focus of intrinsic high attenuation

Cx: malignancy in 3% (papillary carcinoma)

LYMPHANGIOMA

= congenital lymphatic malformation

Incidence: 5.6% of all benign lesions of infancy + childhood

Age: present at birth in 50–65%, clinically apparent by end of 2nd year in 80–90%

Lymphatic development:
endothelial buds from veins in jugular region form confluent plexuses, which develop into rapidly enlarging bilateral juguloaxillary lymph sacs (7.5 weeks GA); these fused lymph sacs extend craniad and dorsolateral with extensive outgrowth of lymph vessels in all directions; connection with internal jugular vein at level of confluence with external jugular vein persists on the left side

Pathogenesis:
failure of drainage from primordial lymph sacs into veins / sequestration of lymphatic tissue with failure to join central lymphatic channels / abnormal budding of lymph vessels with loss of connection with lymphatic primordia

Classification (on basis of size of lymphatic spaces):

(1) Cystic lymphangioma = cystic hygroma
= multilocular mass with enormously dilated lymphatic channels of varying size
Location: neck, axilla, mediastinum
√ low signal intensity on T1WI
√ high signal intensity on T2WI

(2) Cavernous lymphangioma
= mildly dilated cavernous lymphatic spaces with cysts of intermediate size
Location: tongue, floor of mouth, salivary glands
√ penetration of contiguous structures
√ same signal intensities as cystic lymphangioma + fibrous stromal component of low intensity on T1WI + T2WI

(3) Capillary / simple lymphangioma (least common)
= capillary-sized lymphatic channels
Location: epidermis + dermis of proximal limbs

(4) Vasculolymphatic malformation
composed of lymphatic + vascular elements, eg, lymphangiohemangioma

Histo: endothelial-lined lymphatic channels containing serous / milky fluid + separated by connective tissue stroma

- asymptomatic soft / semifirm mass
- may cause dyspnea / dysphagia

Location: anywhere in developing lymphatic system

(a) posterior triangle of neck (most common), with extension into mediastinum in 3–10%
- visible at birth in 65%
- clinically apparent by end of 2nd decade in 90%

(b) anterior mediastinum (<1%)

(c) axilla, chest wall, groin

Cx: infection, airway compromise, chylothorax, chylopericardium

Prognosis: spontaneous regression (10–15%)

Rx: surgical excision (treatment of choice) with recurrence rate of up to 15%

MALIGNANT EXTERNAL OTITIS

= severe bacterial infection of the soft tissues + bones of base of skull

Organism: almost always Pseudomonas aeruginosa

Age: elderly

Predisposed: diabetes mellitus / immunocompromised

- unrelenting otalgia, headache
- purulent otorrhea unresponsive to topical antibiotics
- may cause malfunction of nerves VII, IX, X, XI

Location: at bone-cartilage junction of EAC

Spread of infection:

(a) inferiorly into soft tissues inferior to temporal bone, parotid space, nasopharyngeal masticator space

(b) posteriorly into mastoid

ENT

(c) anteriorly into temporomandibular joint
(d) medially into petrous apex

CT:
- √ soft-tissue density in external auditory canal (100%)
- √ fluid in mastoid / middle ear (89%)
- √ disease around eustachian tube (64%)
- √ obliteration of fat planes beneath temporal bone (64%)
- √ involvement of parapharyngeal space (54%)
- √ masticator space disease (27%)
- √ mass effect in nasopharynx (54%)
- √ bone erosion of clivus (9%)
- √ intracranial extension (9%)

Cx: bone destruction, osteomyelitis, abscess
Prognosis: 20% recurrence rate
DDx: malignant neoplasm

MUCOCELE

= end stage of a chronically obstructed sinus

Incidence: most common lesion to cause expansion of paranasal sinus; increased incidence in cystic fibrosis
Etiology: obstructed paranasal sinus ostium
Path: expanded sinus cyst lined by mucosa with accumulated secretions and desquamations
Age: usually adulthood

- history of chronic nasal polyposis + pansinusitis
- commonly present with unilateral proptosis
- decreased visual acuity, visual field defect
- palpable mass in superomedial aspect of orbit (frontal mucocele)
- intractable headaches

Location:
mnemonic: "fems"
frontal (60%) > **e**thmoid (30%) > **m**axillary (10%) > **s**phenoid (rare)

- √ soft-tissue density mass
- √ sinus cavity expansion (DDx: never in sinusitis)
- √ bone demineralization + remodeling at late stage but NO bone destruction (impossible DDx from neoplasm)
- √ surrounding zone of bone sclerosis / calcification of edges of mucocele (from chronic infection)
- √ macroscopic calcification in 5% (especially with superimposed fungal infection)
- √ uniform enhancement of thin rim

US:
- √ homogeneous hypoechoic mass

MR:
- √ signal intensity varies with state of hydration, protein content, hemorrhage, air content, calcification, fibrosis
- √ hypointense on T1WI + signal void on T2WI due to inspissated debris + fungus
- √ peripheral enhancement pattern (DDx from solid enhancement pattern of neoplasms)

Cx: (1) protrusion into orbit displacing medial rectus muscle laterally
(2) expansion into subarachnoid space resulting in CSF leak
(3) mucopyocele = superimposed infection (rare)

DDx: paranasal sinus carcinoma, Aspergillus infection (enlargement of medial rectus muscle + optic nerve, focal / diffuse areas of increased attenuation), chronic infection, inverting papilloma

MUCOEPIDERMOID CARCINOMA

= most common malignant lesion of parotid gland
Path: arises from glandular ductal epithelium

- rock-hard mass
- pain / itching over course of facial nerve
- facial nerve paralysis
- √ well-circumscribed parotid mass (low-grade lesion) / infiltrating poorly marginated lesion (high-grade lesion)

OTIC CAPSULE DYSPLASIA

Cochlear aplasia

= **Michel aplasia** = Michel anomaly = agenesis of osseous + membranous labyrinth (rare)
Cause: arrested development at 4 weeks GA

- total sensorineural hearing loss
- √ region of otic capsule normally occupied by cochlea is replaced by dense labyrinthine + pneumatized bone
- √ flat medial wall of middle ear (= undeveloped horizontal semicircular canal)
- √ hypoplasia of internal auditory canal
- √ dysplasia of vestibule = marked enlargement into region of lateral + superior semicircular canals

DDx: labyrinthitis obliterans (no loss of lateral convexity of medial wall of middle ear)

Single-cavity cochlea

= saccular defect / cavity in otic capsule in the position normally occupied by cochlea without recognizable modiolus, osseous spiral lamina, interscalar septum

- profound hearing loss discovered in early childhood

May be associated with: recurrent bacterial meningitis, perilymphatic fistula of oval window

- √ cystic cochlea (= developed basal turn, middle + apical turn occupy common nondeveloped space)

Insufficient cochlear turns

= normal basilar turn + varying degrees of hypoplasia of middle and apical turns

Mondini malformation

= absence of anterior 1 1/2 turns of cochlea often with preservation of the basilar turn
Cause: in utero insult at 7 weeks GA
Frequency: 2nd most common imaging finding in children with sensorineural hearing loss

- some high-frequency hearing preserved
- vertigo
- otorrhea, rhinorrhea, recurrent meningitis (perilymphatic fistula caused by absence / defect of stapes footplate)
- √ absence of cochlear apex

May be associated with: deformity of vestibule + semicircular canals + vestibular aqueduct

Anomalies of membranous labyrinth

Scheibe dysplasia = abnormal cochlea + saccule
Alexander dysplasia = dysplasia of basal turn
√ normal CT findings

Small internal auditory canal

= decrease in the diameter of IAC due to hypoplasia / aplasia of cochlear nerve (portion of cranial nerve VIII)
- total sensorineural hearing loss

√ hypoplastic anteroinferior quadrant of IAC

Large vestibule

Associated with: underdeveloped lateral semicircular canal
- sensorineural hearing deficit (most common cause)

√ lateral semicircular canal smaller
√ vestibule extends further into lateral + superior aspects of otic capsule

Large vestibular aqueduct

= Enlarged vestibular aqueduct syndrome
Age: manifests around 3 years
Frequency: most common imaging abnormality detected in children with sensorineural hearing loss
- unilateral congenital deafness (commonly missed)
- vertigo, tinnitus (in 50%)

Location: bilateral in 50–66%
√ vestibular aqueduct >1.4–2 mm in diameter measured halfway between posterior petrous bone and common crus at level of vestibule
√ vestibular aqueduct larger than superior and posterior semicircular canals

OTOSCLEROSIS

= OTOSPONGIOSIS
= replacement of dense otic capsule by highly vascular spongy bone in active phase (misnomer) with restoration of density during reparative sclerotic phase
Etiology: unknown; frequently hereditary
Age: adolescent / young adult Caucasian; M:F = 1:2

A. STAPEDIAL = FENESTRAL OTOSCLEROSIS (80–90%)
Location: anterior oval window margin (= fissula ante fenestram); bilateral in 85%
- tinnitus early in course (2/3)
- progressive conductive hearing loss (stapes fixation in oval window)

√ oval window too wide (lytic phase)
√ new bone formation on anterior oval window margin ± posterior oval window margin ± round window
√ complete plugging of oval window = obliterative otosclerosis (in 2%)

B. COCHLEAR = RETROFENESTRAL OTOSCLEROSIS (10–20%)
Invariably associated with: fenestral otosclerosis
- progressive sensorineural hearing loss (involvement of otic capsule / cytotoxic enzyme diffusion into fluid of membranous labyrinth)
- Schwartze sign = reddish hue behind tympanic membrane when promontory involved

√ "double ring / double lucent" = lucent halo around cochlea (may appear as 3rd turn to cochlea) in early phase
√ bony proliferation in reparative sclerotic phase difficult to diagnose because of same density as cochlea

DDx: Paget disease, osteogenesis imperfecta, syphilis

PARANASAL SINUS CARCINOMA

Location: maxillary sinus (80%), nasal cavity (10%), ethmoid sinus (5–6%), frontal + sphenoid sinus (rare)

Maxillary sinus carcinoma

Incidence: 80% of all paranasal sinus carcinomas
Histo: squamous cell carcinoma (80%)
Age: >40 years in 95%; M:F = 2:1
- asymmetry of face, tumor in oral / nasal cavity

√ bone destruction (in 90%) predominates over expansion
√ nodal metastases in 10–18%

Nasopharyngeal carcinoma

Incidence: 10% of paranasal sinus carcinomas; 0.25–0.5% of all malignant tumors in whites; M>F
Predisposed: Chinese population
Histo: squamous cell carcinoma (>85%), nonkeratinizing ~, undifferentiated carcinoma
Mean age: 40 years
- asymptomatic for a long time
- history of chronic sinusitis / nasal polyps (15%)
- unilateral nasal obstruction

Location: turbinates (50%) > septum > vestibule > posterior choanae > floor
Extension:
(a) lateral + superior: through sinus of Morgagni (= natural defect in superior portion of lateral nasopharyngeal wall) into cartilaginous portion of eustachian tube + levator veli palatini muscle
± masticator space and pre- and poststyloid parapharyngeal spaces
± involvement of levator + tensor veli palatini muscle, 3rd division of nerve V, petroclinoid fissure
± foramen lacerum of skull base encasing internal carotid artery
± cavernous sinus (along ICA / mandibular nerve / direct skull base invasion)
(b) anterior: posterior nasal cavity + pterygopalatine fossa
(c) inferior (1/3): submucosal spread along lateral pharyngeal wall + anterior and posterior tonsillar pillars

ENT

√ polypoid or papillary (2/3)
√ bone invasion (1/3)
MR:
√ signal intensity similar to that of adjacent mucosa

Ethmoid sinus carcinoma

Incidence: 5–6% of paranasal sinus carcinomas
Histo: squamous cell carcinoma (>90%), sarcoma, adenocarcinoma, adenoid cystic carcinoma; frequently secondarily involved from maxillary sinus carcinoma
- nasal obstruction, bloody discharge
- anosmia, broadening of nose

PHARYNGEAL ABSCESS

Etiology: spread of infection from tonsils / pharynx
Age: children > adults
- trismus (most common presenting symptom) from involvement of pterygoid muscle
- sore throat
- low-grade fever

√ isodense / low-density mass with unsharp margins
√ rim enhancement
Cx: Mycotic aneurysm of carotid artery (within 10 days)

RAMSAY-HUNT SYNDROME

= HERPES ZOSTER OTICUS
- vesicles in mucosa of external auditory canal

√ intracanalicular 8th nerve enhancement

RETROPHARYNGEAL ABSCESS / HEMORRHAGE

Etiology: upper respiratory tract infection, perforating injury of pharynx / esophagus, suppuration of infected lymph node
Organism: Staphylococcus, mixed flora
Age: usually <1 year
- fever, neck stiffness, dysphagia

√ thickness of retropharyngeal space >3/4 of AP diameter of vertebral body
√ reversal of cervical lordosis
√ anterior displacement of airway
√ may contain gas and gas-fluid level

RHABDOMYOSARCOMA

= most common soft-tissue tumor in children;
Frequency:
5–10% of all malignant solid tumors in children <15 years of age (ranking 4th after CNS neoplasm, neuroblastoma, Wilms tumor); 3rd most common primary childhood malignancy of head + neck (following brain tumors + retinoblastomas); 10–25% of all sarcomas; annual incidence of 4.5:1,000,000 white + 1.3:1,000,000 black children
Age: 2–5 years (peak prevalence); <10 years (70%); M:F = 2:1
Histo:
(a) embryonal rhabdomyosarcoma (>50%)
subtype: polyploidal form = sarcoma botryoides = grapelike
(b) alveolar rhabdomyosarcoma (worst prognosis)
(c) pleomorphic rhabdomyosarcoma (mostly in adults)

- cranial nerve palsy

Location: head + neck (28–36%), trigone + bladder neck (18–21%), orbit (10%), extremities (18–23%), trunk (7–8%), retroperitoneum (6–7%), perineum + anus (2%), other sites (7%)
Site: paranasal sinus, middle ear, nasopharyngeal musculature (1/3); most common primary extracranial tumor invading the cranial vault in childhood
Metastases: lymph nodes (50%), lung, bone

√ bulky nasopharyngeal mass
√ extension into cranial vault through fissures + foramina (up to 35%) usually involving cavernous sinus
√ bone destruction
√ uniform enhancement
CT:
√ isodense with brain
√ expanded foramen / fissure
MR (imaging modality of choice):
√ signal intensity intermediate between muscle and fat on T1WI + hyperintense on T2WI

Prognosis: 12.5% 5-year survival

RHINOCEREBRAL MUCORMYCOSIS

= paranasal sinus infection caused by nonseptated fungi Rhizopus arrhizus and Rhizopus oryzae
Spread: fungus first involves nasal cavity, then extends into maxillary / ethmoid sinuses / orbits / intracranially along ophthalmic artery / cribriform plate (frontal sinuses are spared)
Predisposed:
(1) poorly controlled diabetes mellitus (2) chronic renal failure (3) cirrhosis (4) malnutrition (5) cancer (6) prolonged antibiotic therapy (7) steroid therapy (8) cytotoxic drug therapy (9) AIDS (10) extensive burns
- black crusting of nasal mucosa (in diabetics)
- small ischemic areas (invasion of arterioles + small arteries)

√ nodular thickening involving nasal septum + turbinates
√ mucoperiosteal thickening + clouding of ethmoids
√ focal areas of bone destruction
Cx: (1) blindness (2) cranial nerve palsy (3) hemiparesis
Prognosis: high mortality rate

SARCOIDOSIS

Blacks:Whites = 10:1
Location: eye, lacrimal glands, salivary glands (40%), larynx (5%), involvement of intra- and extraparotid lymph nodes (rare)
√ granulomas may enhance
√ enlargement of optic canal (optic neuritis)
√ thickening of larynx with enhancement of granulomas
√ multiple small granulomas of septum + turbinates

Heerfordt syndrome

(1) Parotid enlargement
- diffuse bilateral painless enlargement (10–30%)
- xerostomia

CT:
√ diffusely dense multinodular gland / enlargement of lymph nodes within gland

(2) Uveitis
(3) Facial nerve paralysis

SIALOSIS

= nontender noninflammatory recurrent enlargement of parotid gland

Cause: cirrhosis, alcoholism, diabetes, malnutrition, hormonal insufficiency (ovarian / pancreatic / thyroid), drugs (sulfisoxazole, phenylbutazone), radiation therapy

Histo: serous acinar hypertrophy + fatty replacement of gland

Sialography:
√ sparse peripheral ducts

CT:
√ enlarged / normal-sized gland
√ diffusely dense gland in end stage

SINONASAL POLYPOSIS

= benign sinonasal mucosal lesion

Incidence: in 25% of patients with allergic rhinitis; in 15% of patients with asthma

Cause: allergic rhinitis (atopic hypersensitivity), asthma, cystic fibrosis (child), Kartagener syndrome, nickel exposure, nonneoplastic hyperplasia of inflamed mucous membranes

Location: commonly maxillary antrum

√ rounded masses within nasal cavity enlarging sinus ostium
√ expansion of sinus
√ thinning of bony trabeculae ± erosive changes at anterior skull base
√ usually peripheral / occasionally solid heterogeneous enhancement

DDx: cancer, fungal infection

Antrochoanal polyp

= benign antral polyp, which widens the sinus ostium and extends into nasal cavity; 5% of all nasal polyps

Age: teenagers + young adults

√ antral clouding
√ ipsilateral nasal mass
√ smooth mass enlarging the sinus ostium
√ NO sinus expansion

Angiomatous polyp

= derivative of choanal polyp (following ischemia of polyp with secondary neovascularity along its surface)

DDx: juvenile angiofibroma (involvement of pterygopalatine fossa)

SINUSITIS

Incidence:
most common paranasal sinus problem; most common chronic disease diagnosed in United States (31,000,000 people affected each year); complicating common colds in 0.5% (3–4 colds/year in adults, 6–8 colds/year in children)

Pathogenesis:
mucosal congestion as a result of viral infection leads to apposition of mucosal surfaces resulting in retention of secretions with bacterial superinfection

(1) Obstruction of major ostia
  (a) middle meatus draining frontal, maxillary, anterior ethmoid sinus
  (b) sphenoethmoidal recess draining posterior ethmoid sphenoid sinus
(2) Ineffective mucociliary clearing secondary to contact of two mucosal surfaces

Predisposing anatomic variants:
(1) greater degree of nasal septal deviation
(2) horizontally oriented uncinate process
NOT concha bullosa, paradoxical turbinate, Haller cells, uncinate pneumatization

Location:
(1) Infundibular pattern (26%)
  = isolated obstruction of inferior infundibulum just above the maxillary sinus ostium
  √ limited maxillary sinus disease
(2) Ostiomeatal unit pattern (25%)
  √ middle meatus opacification
(3) Sphenoethmoidal recess obstruction (6%)
  √ sphenoid / posterior ethmoid sinus inflammation
(4) Sinonasal polyposis pattern
  √ enlargement of ostia, thinning of adjacent bone
  √ air-fluid levels

Plain films (Waters, Caldwell, lateral, submental vertex views):

1. **Acute sinusitis**
   √ air-fluid level [from retention of secretions secondary to mucosal swelling leading to ostial dysfunction] (54% sensitive, 92% specific in maxillary sinus)
   √ hyperintense secretions on T2WI (95% water content + 5% proteinaceous macromolecules)
2. **Chronic sinusitis**
   √ mucosal swelling >5 mm thick on Waters view (99% sensitive, 46% specific in maxillary sinus)
   √ bone remodeling + sclerosis (from osteitis)
   √ polyposis
   √ hyperattenuating lesion on NCCT (due to inspissated secretions / fungal disease)
   √ hypointense secretions on T1WI + T2WI due to inspissated material with chronic obstruction (DDx: air)

CT: to map bony anatomy for surgical planning

MR:
√ sinus thickening with high signal intensity on T2WI + low intensity on T1WI
√ near solid secretions with >28% protein concentration are hypointense on both T1WI + T2WI simulating air

ENT

√ rim gadolinium enhancement (DDx to neoplasms which enhance centrally)

A. ALLERGIC SINUSITIS
   √ involves multiple sinuses
   √ bilaterally symmetric
   √ uniform enhancement
   √ sinonasal polyposis
B. BACTERIAL SINUSITIS
   Organism:
   (a) acute phase: Streptococcus pneumoniae + Haemophilus influenzae (>50%), beta-hemolytic streptococcus, Moraxella catarrhalis
   (b) chronic phase: staphylococcus, streptococcus, corynebacteria, Bacteroides, fusobacteria
   √ solitary antral disease (obstruction of sinus ostium)
   √ uniform enhancement
C. MYCOTIC / FUNGAL SINUSITIS
   Organism: Aspergillus fumigatus, mucormycosis, bipolaris, Drechslera, Curvularia, Candida
   √ polypoid lesion / fungus ball (= extramucosal infection due to saprophytic growth on retained secretions, usually caused by Aspergillus)
   √ infiltrating fungal sinusitis (in immune-competent host)
   √ fulminant fungal sinusitis (aggressive infection in immune-compromised individual / diabetics)
   CT:
      √ punctate calcifications (= calcium phosphate / calcium sulfonate deposition near mycelium)
   MR:
      √ dark on T2WI secondary to high fungal mycelial iron, magnesium, manganese content from aminoacid metabolism
      (DDx: inspissated secretions / polypoid disease)
   Dx: failure to respond to antibiotic therapy

Cx:
   (1) Mucous retention cyst (10%)
   (2) Mucocele
   (3) Orbital extension through neurovascular foramina, dehiscences, or thin bones: orbital cellulitis,
   (4) Septic thrombophlebitis
   (5) Intracranial extension: meningitis, epidural abscess, subdural empyema, venous sinus thrombosis, cerebral abscess
Rx: functional endoscopic sinus surgery (amputation of uncinate process, enlargement of infundibulum + maxillary ostium, creation of common channel for anterior ethmoid air cells, complete / partial ethmoidectomy)

SUBGLOTTIC HEMANGIOMA

Most common subglottic soft-tissue mass causing upper respiratory tract obstruction in neonates
• crouplike symptoms in neonatal period
• hemangiomas elsewhere (skin, mucosal membranes) in 50%
√ eccentric thickening of subglottic portion of trachea (AP view)
√ arises from posterior wall below true cords (lateral view)

SUBGLOTTIC STENOSIS

A. CONGENITAL SUBGLOTTIC STENOSIS
   • crouplike symptoms, often self-limiting disease
   Location: 1–2 cm below vocal cords
   √ circumferential symmetrical narrowing of subglottic portion of trachea during inspiration
   √ NO change in degree of narrowing with expiration
B. ACQUIRED SUBGLOTTIC STENOSIS
   following prolonged endotracheal intubation (in 5%)

THORNWALDT CYST

= midline congenital pouch / cyst lined by ectoderm within nasopharyngeal mucosal space
Origin: persistent focal adhesion between notochord + ectoderm extending to the pharyngeal tubercle of the occipital bone
Incidence: 4% of autopsies
Peak age: 15–30 years
• asymptomatic incidental finding
• persistent nasopharyngeal drainage
• halitosis
• foul taste in mouth
Location: posterior roof of nasopharynx
√ smoothly marginated cystic mass of few mm to 3 cm in size
√ low density, not enhancing
√ NO bone erosion
Cx: infection of cyst
DDx: Rathke pouch (occurs in craniopharyngeal canal located anteriorly + cephalad to Thornwaldt cyst)

THYROGLOSSAL DUCT CYST

Embryogenesis:
   thyroglossal duct = duct along which thyroid gland descends to its final position from foramen cecum at base of tongue passing anteriorly / posteriorly / through precursor of hyoid bone; duct usually involutes by 8th week of fetal life; thyroid elements remain in thyroglossal duct in 5%
Histo: cyst lined by squamous cell mucosa
Age: <10 years in 50%; 2nd peak at 20–30 years
• midline neck mass
• ± history of previous incision and drainage of an "abscess" in area of cyst
Location: suprahyoid (20%), hyoid (15%), infrahyoid (65%)
√ midline / paramedian cystic mass of 2–4 cm
√ infrahyoid strap muscles beak over edge of cyst
Cx: infection; thyroglossal duct carcinoma (<1%)
Rx: complete surgical removal

THYROID ADENOMA

Adenomatous nodule (42–77%)

= COLLOID NODULE = ADENOMATOUS HYPERPLASIA = DEGENERATIVE INVOLUTED NODULE

Cytology: abundant colloid + benign follicular cells with uniform slightly large nuclei, arranged in a honeycomb pattern (difficult DDx from follicular tumors)

√ often multiple nodules by US / scintigraphy / surgery
√ mostly hypofunctioning, rarely hyperfunctioning
√ solid form = incompletely encapsulated, poorly demarcated nodules merging with surrounding tissue
√ cystic form (= colloid cyst) = anechoic areas in nodule (hemorrhage / colloid degeneration
√ calcific deposits

Follicular Adenoma (15–40%)

= monoclonal tumor arising from follicular epithelium

Path: single lesion with well-developed fibrous capsule

Histo subtypes:

(a) Simple colloid (macrofollicular) adenoma: most common form
(b) Microfollicular (fetal) adenoma
(c) Embryonal (trabecular) adenoma
(d) Hürthle-cell (oxyphil / oncocytic) adenoma: large single polygonal cells with abundant granular cytoplasm + uniform eccentric nuclei + no colloid
(e) Atypical adenoma
(f) Adenoma with papillae
(g) Signet-ring adenoma

◊ 5% of microfollicular adenomas, 5% of Hürthle-cell adenomas, 25% of embryonal adenomas prove to be follicular cancers with careful study!

Functional status:

(1) Toxic adenoma
(2) Toxic multinodular goiter = hyperfunctioning adenoma within multinodular goiter; usually occurs in nodule >2.5 cm in size
(3) Nonfunctioning adenoma

√ mass with increased / decreased echogenicity
√ "halo sign" = complete hypoechoic ring with regular border surrounding isoechoic solid mass

THYROID CARCINOMA

Incidence: 12,000 new cancers/year in United States; clinically silent cancers in up to 35% at autopsy / surgery (usually papillary carcinomas of <1.0 cm in size)

Age: <30 years; M > F

• history of neck irradiation
• rapid growth
• stone-hard nodule

√ hypoechoic mass
√ irregular ill-defined border without halo
√ NO hemorrhage / liquefaction necrosis

RADIATION-INDUCED THYROID CANCER

Incidence increases with doses of thyroidal irradiation from 6.5–1,500 rad (higher doses are associated with hypothyroidism)

Peak occurrence: 5–30 (up to 50) years post irradiation

Thyroid abnormalities in 20%:

(a) in 14% adenomatous hyperplasia, follicular adenoma, colloid nodules, thyroiditis
(b) in 6% thyroid cancer

◊ Nondetectable microscopic foci of cancer in 25% of patients operated on for benign disease!
◊ In patients with multiple cold nodules frequency of cancer is 40%

WHOLE-BODY SCAN in metastatic thyroid carcinoma

Indication: to detect metastases of thyroid carcinoma after total thyroidectomy; preferred over bone scan (only detects 40%) for skeletal metastases

◊ Metastases not detectable in presence of normal functioning thyroid tissue because uptake is much less in metastases
◊ Tc-99m pertechnetate is useless because of high background activity + lack of organification
◊ False-negative I-131 scan in 24% secondary to nonfunctioning metastases

Technique:

(1) T_4 replacement therapy discontinued
(2) short-acting T_3 is administered for 4–6 weeks
(3) T_3 replacement therapy discontinued 10–14 days prior to whole-body scan
(4) measurement of TSH level to confirm adequate elevation (TSH >50 mIU/mL; administration of exogenous TSH not desirable because of uneven stimulation)
(5) oral administration of 5–10 mCi I-131
(6) whole-body scan after 24, 48, 72 hours (low background activity)

N.B.: posttherapy scan (1 week after therapeutic dose) identifies more lesions than diagnostic scan

Normal sites of accumulation: nasopharynx, salivary glands, stomach, colon, bladder, liver (I-131-labeled thyroxine produced by carcinoma is metabolized in liver), breasts in lactating women (breast feeding must be terminated after administration of I-131)

CONTRAINDICATED during pregnancy!

TREATMENT for follicular / papillary cancer:

(1) Surgery: total thyroidectomy + modified radical neck dissection
(2) Postoperative radioiodine treatment with I-131 (multiple treatments are usually necessary)

◊ Radioiodine therapy only appropriate for papillary / mixed / follicular thyroid carcinomas (NOT for medullary or anaplastic carcinomas)

(a) ablative dose to destroy remaining thyroid tissue 6 weeks following surgery; no thyroid hormone replacement 3–4 weeks prior to therapy

Dose = [(weight (g) x 80–120 μCi/g) ÷ % uptake of I-123 by 24 hours] x 100
approx. 100 mCi I-131 orally

ENT

(b) treatment of metastases
Dose: 100–200 mCi (dose increase with regional lymph node / lung / bone metastases to 150, 175, 200 mCi)
Administration of 150 mCi of I-131 with an uptake of 0.5% per gram of tumor tissue and a biologic half-life of 4 days will produce 25,000 rads to tumor)
◊ Rapid turnover rates may exist in some metastases (lower dose advisable)
◊ Treatment of large tumors incomplete (range of beta radiation is a few mm)
Cx: radiation thyroiditis, radiation parotitis, GI-symptoms (nausea, diarrhea), minimal bone marrow depression, leukemia (2%), anaplastic transformation (uncommon), lung fibrosis (with extensive pulmonary metastases and dose >200 mCi)
(3) Thyroid replacement therapy
exogenous thyroid hormone to suppress TSH stimulation of metastases
(4) External radiation therapy for anaplastic carcinoma + metastases without iodine uptake

FOLLOW-UP: thyroglobulin >50 ng/mL indicates functioning metastases following complete ablation of thyroid tissue

Papillary carcinoma of thyroid

60% of all thyroid carcinomas
Peak age: 5th decade; F > M
Histo: unencapsulated well-differentiated tumor
(a) purely papillary
(b) mixed with follicular elements (more common, especially under age 40)
Metastases:
(1) Lymphogenic spread to regional lymph nodes (40%, in children almost 90%)
(2) Hematogenous spread to lung (4%), bone (rare)
• carcinoma elaborates thyroglobulin
NUC:
√ tumor usually concentrates radioiodine (even some purely papillary tumors)
US:
√ tumor of decreased echogenicity
√ purely solid / complex mass with areas of necrosis, hemorrhage, cystic degeneration
X-ray:
√ punctate / linear psammomatous calcifications at tumor periphery
Rx: lobectomy + isthmectomy for papillary cancer <1.5 to 2.0 cm in size isolated to one lobe
Prognosis: 90% 10-year survival for occult + intrathyroidal cancer; 60% 10-year survival for extrathyroidal cancer; worse prognosis with increasing age

Follicular carcinoma of thyroid

20% of all thyroid cancers; slow growing
Peak age: 5th decade; F > M
Histo: encapsulated well-differentiated tumor without papillary elements; in 25% multifocal; cytologically impossible to distinguish between well-differentiated follicular carcinoma + follicular adenoma (vascular invasion is only criteria)
Early hematogenous spread to:
(a) lung
(b) bone (30%): almost always osteolytic (more frequent than in papillary carcinoma)
• carcinoma elaborates thyroglobulin
√ psammoma bodies + stromal calcium deposits
NUC:
√ usually concentrates pertechnetate, but fails to accumulate I-123
US:
√ indistinguishable from benign follicular adenoma
Prognosis: 90% 10-year survival with slight / equivocal angioinvasion; 35% 10-year survival with moderate / marked angioinvasion

Anaplastic carcinoma of thyroid

4–15% of all thyroid cancers
Age: 6–7th decade; M:F = 1:1
√ intrathoracic extension in up to 50%
√ ± invasion of carotid a., internal jugular v., larynx
NUC:
√ NO radioiodine uptake
CT:
√ mass with inhomogeneous attenuation
√ areas of necrosis (74%)
√ calcifications (58%)
√ regional lymphadenopathy (74%)
Prognosis: 5% 5-year survival; average survival time of 6–12 months

Medullary carcinoma of thyroid

1–5% of all thyroid cancers; sporadic / familial
Histo: arises from parafollicular C-cells, associated with amyloid deposition in primary + metastatic sites
Mean age: 60 years for sporadic variety; in adolescence with MEN
May be associated with:
(1) MEN IIa = pheochromocytoma + parathyroid hyperplasia (Sipple syndrome)
(2) MEN IIb = without parathyroid component
Metastases: early spread to lymph nodes (50%), lung, liver, bone
• elevated calcitonin (from tumor production) stimulated by pentagastrin + calcium infusion
√ mass of 2 to 26 mm
√ granular calcifications within fibrous stroma / amyloid masses (50%)
NUC:
√ NO uptake by radioiodine / pertechnetate
√ frequently shows increased uptake of Tl-201
CT:
√ mass of low attenuation (no iodine concentration)

Prognosis:
90% 10-year survival without nodal metastases
42% 10-year survival with nodal metastases
Rx: total thyroidectomy + modified radical neck dissection

THYROIDITIS

Hashimoto thyroiditis

= CHRONIC LYMPHOCYTIC THYROIDITIS

Most frequent cause of goitrous hypothyroidism in adults in the USA (iodine-deficiency is the more common cause worldwide)

Etiology: autoimmune process with marked familial predisposition; antibodies are typically present; functional organification defect

Peak age: 4–5th decade; M > F

- firm rubbery lobular goiter
- gradual painless enlargement
- thyrotoxicosis in early stage (4%)
- decreased thyroid reserve
- hypothyroidism at presentation (20%)

√ moderate enlargement of both lobes (18%)

NUC:
- √ low tracer uptake (occasionally increased) with poor visualization (4%)
- √ prominent pyramidal lobe
- √ positive perchlorate washout test
- √ patchy tracer distribution
- √ multiple (40%) / single cold defects (28%) / normal thyroid (8%)

US:
- √ initially heterogeneous diffusely decreased echogenicity + slight lobulation of contour
- √ marked hyperemia on color Doppler
- √ later densely echogenic (fibrosis) + acoustical shadows

Cx: hypothyroidism

De Quervain thyroiditis

= SUBACUTE THYROIDITIS

Etiology: probably viral

Histo: lymphocytic infiltration + granulomas + foreign body giant cells

Peak age: 2–5th decade; M:F = 1:5

- upper respiratory tract infection precedes onset of symptoms by 2–3 weeks
- painful tender gland + fever; only mild enlargement
- hyperthyroidism (50%) secondary to severe destruction
- short-lived hypothyroidism (25%) secondary to hormone depletion of gland

NUC:
- √ abnormally low radioiodine uptake with clinical and laboratory evidence of hyperthyroidism
- √ poor visualization of thyroid (initially)
- √ single / multiple hypofunctional areas (occasionally)
- √ increased uptake during phase of hypothyroidism (late event)

Cx: permanent hypothyroidism (rare)

Prognosis: usually full recovery

Painless thyroiditis

Histo: resembles chronic lymphocytic thyroiditis

- clinical presentation similar to subacute thyroiditis
- NOT painful / tender

Acute suppurative thyroiditis

US:
- √ focal / diffuse enlargement; possibly abscess
- √ decreased echogenicity

WARTHIN TUMOR

= PAPILLARY CYSTADENOMA LYMPHOMATOSUM

Incidence: 2nd most common benign tumor of parotid gland; bilateral in 10%

Age: about 50 years; M > F

Origin: from heterotopic salivary gland tissue within parotid lymph nodes

- slow-growing mass

√ well-circumscribed single / multiple tumors in parotid region usually 3–4 cm in size

MR:
- √ hypointense compared with fat / surrounding parotid tissue on T2WI

DIFFERENTIAL DIAGNOSIS OF CHEST DISORDERS

HEMOPTYSIS

Source: bronchial a. (most common), pulmonary a.

A. TUMOR
   1. Carcinoma (35%)
   2. Bronchial adenoma
B. BRONCHIAL WALL INJURY
   1. Foreign body erosion
   2. Bronchoscopy / biopsy
C. VASCULAR
   1. COPD
   2. Pulmonary embolus with infarction
   3. Venous hypertension (most common)
   4. Arteriovenous malformation
   5. Rupture of pulmonary artery aneurysm: TB, vasculitis, trauma, neoplasm, abscess, septic embolus, indwelling catheter
D. INFECTION
   1. Chronic bronchitis
   2. Bronchiectasis, mouthful (15%)
   3. Tuberculosis (Rasmussen aneurysm)
   4. Aspergillosis
   5. Abscess

◊ In the majority of patients no cause is found!
◊ The two most common identifiable causes are bronchial carcinoma + bronchiectasis!

PULMONARY DISEASE ASSOCIATED WITH CIGARETTE SMOKING

1. Bronchogenic carcinoma
2. Chronic bronchitis
3. Centrilobular emphysema
4. Panacinar emphysema with α-1-antitrypsin deficiency
5. Respiratory bronchiolitis-associated interstitial lung disease
6. Pulmonary Langerhans cell histiocytosis

ABNORMAL LUNG PATTERNS

1. Mass
   = any localized density not completely bordered by fissures / pleura
2. Consolidative (alveolar) pattern
   = commonly produced by filling of air spaces with fluid (transudate / exudate) / cells / other material, ALSO by alveolar collapse, airway obstruction, confluent interstitial thickening
   ground glass = hazy area of increased attenuation not obscuring bronchovascular structures
   consolidation = marked increase in attenuation with obliteration of underlying anatomic features
3. Interstitial pattern
4. Vascular pattern
   (a) increased vessel size: CHF, pulmonary arterial hypertension, shunt vascularity, lymphangitic carcinomatosis
   (b) decreased vessel size: emphysema, thromboembolism
5. Bronchial pattern
   √ wall thickening: bronchitis, asthma, bronchiectasis
   √ density without air bronchogram (= complete airway obstruction)
   √ lucency of air trapping (= partial airway obstruction with ball-valve mechanism)

ALVEOLAR (CONSOLIDATIVE) PATTERN

Classic appearance of airspace consolidation:
mnemonic: "A^{2}BC^3"
√ **A**cinar rosettes: rounded poorly defined nodules in size of acini (6–10 mm), best seen at periphery of densities
√ **A**ir alveologram / bronchogram
√ **B**utterfly / bat-wing distribution: perihilar / bibasilar
√ **C**oalescent / confluent cloudlike ill-defined opacities
√ **C**onsolidation in diffuse, perihilar / bibasilar, segmental / lobar, multifocal / lobular distribution
√ **C**hanges occur rapidly (labile / fleeting)

HRCT:
√ poorly marginated densities within primary lobule (up to 1 cm in size)
√ rapid coalescence with neighboring lesions in segmental distribution
√ predominantly central location with sparing of subpleural zones
√ air bronchograms

Diffuse Airspace Disease

A. INFLAMMATORY EXUDATE = "PUS"
   1. Lobar pneumonia
   2. Bronchopneumonia: especially Gram-negative organisms
   3. Unusual pneumonias
      (a) viral: extensive hemorrhagic edema especially in immunocompromised patients with hematologic malignancies + transplants
      (b) Pneumocystis
      (c) fungal: Aspergillus, Candida, Cryptococcus, Phycomycetes
      (d) tuberculosis
   4. Aspiration
B. HEMORRHAGE = "BLOOD"
   1. Trauma: contusion
   2. Pulmonary embolism, thromboembolism
   3. Bleeding diathesis: leukemia, hemophilia, anticoagulants, DIC

4. Vasculitis: Wegener granulomatosis, Goodpasture syndrome, SLE, mucormycosis, aspergillosis, Rocky Mountain spotted fever, infectious mononucleosis
5. Idiopathic pulmonary hemosiderosis
6. Bleeding metastases: choriocarcinoma

C. TRANSUDATE = "WATER"
1. Cardiac edema
2. Neurogenic edema
3. Hypoproteinemia
4. Fluid overload
5. Renal failure
6. Radiotherapy
7. Shock
8. Toxic inhalation
9. Drug reaction
10. Adult respiratory distress syndrome

D. SECRETIONS = "PROTEIN"
1. Alveolar proteinosis
2. Mucus plugging

E. MALIGNANCY = "CELLS"
1. Bronchioloalveolar cell carcinoma
2. Lymphoma

F. INTERSTITIAL DISEASE simulating airspace disease, eg, "alveolar sarcoid"

mnemonics:

"**P**lease **P**ut **A** **H**ot-**L**ight **At** **T**he **S**ithouse **F**irst"
- **P**ulmonary edema
- **P**neumonia
- **A**lveolar proteinosis, carcinoma, microlithiasis
- **H**yaline membrane disease, **H**emorrhage, **H**eroin
- **L**ymphoma
- **A**spiration
- **Tu**berculosis
- **S**arcoidosis
- **F**ungus

"AIRSPACED"
- **A**spiration
- **I**nhalation, **I**nflammatory
- **R**enal (uremia)
- **S**arcoidosis
- **P**roteinosis (alveolar)
- **A**lveolar cell carcinoma
- **C**ardiovascular (CHF)
- **E**mboli
- **D**rug reaction, **D**rowning

Localized Airspace Disease

mnemonic: "4P'S & TAIL"
- **P**neumonia
- **P**ulmonary edema
- **P**ulmonary contusion
- **P**ulmonary interstitial edema
- **T**uberculosis
- **A**lveolar cell carcinoma
- **I**nfant
- **L**ymphoma

Acute Alveolar Infiltrate

mnemonic: "I 2 CHANGE FAST"
- **I**nfarct
- **I**nfection
- **C**ontusion
- **H**emorrhage
- **A**spiration
- **N**ear drowning
- **G**oodpasture syndrome
- **E**dema
- **F**ungus
- **A**llergic sensitivity
- **S**hock lung
- **T**uberculosis

Chronic Alveolar Infiltrate

mnemonics:

"PALS GET MOD"
- **P**roteinosis
- **A**lveolar cell carcinoma
- **L**ymphoma
- **S**arcoidosis
- **G**ranulomatosis
- **E**osinophilic granuloma
- **T**uberculosis
- **M**icrolithiasis
- **O**il aspiration
- **D**IP (not consolidative)

"STALLAG"
- **S**arcoidosis
- **T**uberculosis
- **A**lveolar cell ca.
- **L**ymphoma
- **L**ipoid pneumonia
- **A**lveolar proteinosis
- **G**oodpasture syndr.

CT Angiogram Sign

= homogeneous low attenuation of lung consolidation which allows vessels to be clearly seen
1. Lobar bronchioloalveolar cell carcinoma
2. Lobar pneumonia
3. Pulmonary lymphoma
4. Extrinsic lipid pneumonia
5. Pulmonary infarction
6. Pulmonary edema

HRCT Of Small Airway Disease

Cause:
1. Bronchiolitis obliterans
2. Bronchiolitis obliterans with organizing pneumonia
3. Small airway disease of smokers
4. Asthma
5. Infection: TB, aspiration pneumonia, viral pneumonia
6. Diffuse panbronchiolitis
7. Extrinsic allergic alveolitis

A. DIRECT SIGNS
- √ ringlike tubular structures in lung periphery (= wall thickening + dilatation of bronchioles)
- √ nodules / branching linear structures in lung periphery (= obliterated airways through wall thickening / filling with mucus or debris)

B. INDIRECT SIGNS
- √ air trapping = area of decreased attenuation from collateral air drift / ball-valve effect distal to occluded / stenotic airway more prominent on expiration
- √ mosaic perfusion = scattered areas of air trapping
- √ subsegmental atelectasis = wedge-shaped area of ground-glass attenuation
- √ centrilobular emphysema = destruction of small airways + surrounding parenchyma in the center of the pulmonary lobule

√ centrilobular airspace nodule = acinar nodule = <1 cm ill-defined nodule of ground-glass attenuation (from inflammation within alveolar space) less prominent on expiration

DDx: 1. Cystic lung disease (thin septum surrounds area of air attenuation, central vessel not present)
2. Panlobular emphysema (distortion of vascular + septal architecture, bullae)

Inhomogeneous Lung Attenuation On HRCT

A. GROUND-GLASS OPACITY DUE TO INFILTRATIVE LUNG DISEASE
√ areas of higher attenuation with nodular / centrilobular distribution
√ pulmonary vessels uniform in size in areas of differing attenuation
√ increase in lung attenuation in low- and high-attenuation areas on expiratory HRCT

B. MOSAIC PERFUSION = patchwork of normal and air-attenuated segments
√ vessels in areas of low attenuation are smaller in 94% (due to differential blood flow)
√ normal / dilated arteries in areas of hyperattenuation in 77%
1. Mosaic perfusion due to air trapping
√ attenuation differences are accentuated on expiratory HRCT
2. Mosaic perfusion due to vascular obstruction
√ increase in lung attenuation in low- and high-attenuation areas on expiratory HRCT

EOSINOPHILIC LUNG DISEASE

= PULMONARY INFILTRATION WITH BLOOD / TISSUE EOSINOPHILIA (PIE)

Classification:

1. IDIOPATHIC EOSINOPHILIC LUNG DISEASE
(a) Transient pulmonary eosinophilia = Löffler syndrome
• peripheral eosinophilia
(b) Acute / chronic eosinophilic pneumonia
• no peripheral eosinophilia
2. EOSINOPHILIC LUNG DISEASE OF SPECIFIC ETIOLOGY
(a) drug induced: nitrofurantoin, penicillin, sulfonamides, ASA, tricyclic antidepressants, hydrochlorothiazide, cromolyn sodium, mephenesin
(b) parasite induced: tropical eosinophilia (ascariasis, schistosomiasis), strongyloidiasis, ancylostomiasis (hookworm), filariasis, Toxocara canis (visceral larva migrans), Dirofilaria immitis, amebiasis (occasionally — in right lower + middle lobe)
(c) fungus induced: allergic bronchopulmonary aspergillosis, bronchocentric granulomatosis
(d) Pulmonary eosinophilia with asthma
3. EOSINOPHILIC LUNG DISEASE ASSOCIATED WITH ANGIITIS ± GRANULOMATOSIS
(a) Wegener granulomatosis
(b) Polyarteritis nodosa
(c) Churg-Strauss syndrome
(d) Lymphomatoid granulomatosis
may lead to lymphoma
√ CXR similar to Wegener granulomatosis
(e) Bronchocentric granulomatosis
= granulomas forming around bronchi + vasculitis
• often associated with long history of asthma
√ bronchial obstruction
(f) Necrotizing "sarcoidal" angiitis
(g) Rheumatoid disease
(h) Scleroderma
(i) Dermatomyositis
(j) Sjögren syndrome
(k) CREST

INTERSTITIAL LUNG DISEASE

= thickening of lung interstices (= interlobular septa)

◊ Over 200 diseases affect the interstitium of the lung!

A. MAJOR LYMPHATIC TRUNKS
1. Lymphangitic carcinomatosis
2. Congenital pulmonary lymphangiectasia

B. PULMONARY VEINS (increased pulmonary venous pressure)
1. Left ventricular failure
2. Venous obstructive disease

C. SUPPORTING CONNECTIVE TISSUE NETWORK
1. Interstitial edema
2. Chronic interstitial pneumonia
3. Pneumoconioses
4. Collagen-vascular disease
5. Interstitial fibrosis
6. Amyloid
7. Tumor infiltration within connective tissue
8. Desmoplastic reaction to tumor

Path: stereotypical inflammatory response of alveolar wall to injury
(a) acute phase: fluid + inflammatory cells exude into alveolar space, mononuclear cells accumulate in edematous alveolar wall
(b) organizing phase: hyperplasia of type II pneumocytes attempt to regenerate alveolar epithelium, fibroblasts deposit collagen
(c) chronic stage: dense collagenous fibrous tissue remodels normal pulmonary architecture

Characterizing criteria:
(a) zonal distribution:
– upper / lower lung zones
– axial (core) / parenchymal (middle) / peripheral
(b) volume loss
(c) time course
(d) interstitial lung pattern

Interstitial Lung Pattern On CXR

1. LINEAR FORM
(a) reticulations
= network of interlacing lines in all directions

CHEST

(b) Kerley lines = septal lines
= thickened connective septa
√ Kerley A lines = relatively long fine linear shadows in upper lungs, deep within lung parenchyma
√ Kerley B lines = short horizontally oriented lines extending to pleura, perpendicular to pleura in costophrenic angles + retrosternal clear space
√ Kerley C lines = "spider web" appearance covering entire lung

2. NODULAR FORM
= small sharp numerous uniform nodules with even distribution
3. DESTRUCTIVE FORM = honeycomb lung

Signs Of Acute Interstitial Disease

√ peribronchial cuffing = thickened bronchial wall + peribronchial sheath (when viewed end on)
√ thickening of interlobular fissures
√ Kerley-lines
√ perihilar haze = blurring of hilar shadows
√ blurring of pulmonary vascular markings
√ increased density at lung bases
√ small pleural effusions

Signs Of Chronic Interstitial Disease

√ irregular visceral pleural surface
√ **reticulations** = innumerable interlacing line shadows suggesting a mesh
(a) fine reticulations = early potentially reversible / minimal irreversible alveolar septal abnormality
(b) coarse reticulations
in 75% related to environmental disease, sarcoidosis, collagen-vascular disorders, chronic interstitial pneumonia
√ **nodularity**
in 90% related to infectious / noninfectious granulomatous process, metastatic malignancy, pneumoconioses, amyloidosis
√ **linearity**
cardiogenic / noncardiogenic interstitial pulmonary edema, lymphangitic malignancy, diffuse bronchial wall disorders (cystic fibrosis, bronchiectasis, hypersensitivity asthma)
√ **honeycombing** = usually subpleural clustered cystic air spaces <1 cm in diameter with thick well-defined walls set off against a background of increased lung density (end-stage lung)
◊ HRCT approximately 60% more sensitive than CXR

Distribution Of Interstitial Disease

A. MIDLUNG / PERIHILAR DISEASE
(a) Acute rapidly changing
1. Pulmonary edema
2. Pneumocystis pneumonitis
3. Early extrinsic allergic alveolitis
(b) Chronic slowly progressive
1. Lymphangitic carcinomatosis
often unilateral, associated with adenopathy, pleural effusion

B. PERIPHERAL LUNG DISEASE
(a) Acute rapidly changing
1. Interstitial pulmonary edema with Kerley B lines (most common)
2. Active fibrosing alveolitis
(b) Chronic slowly progressive
1. Secondary pulmonary hemosiderosis

C. UPPER LUNG DISEASE
(a) Chronic slowly progressive ± volume loss
1. Postprimary TB (common)
2. Silicosis (common)
(b) Chronic slowly progressive with volume loss
1. Sarcoidosis (common)
2. Ankylosing spondylitis (rare)
3. Sulfa drugs (rare)
(c) Chronic slowly progressive without volume loss
1. Extrinsic allergic alveolitis
2. Eosinophilic granuloma
3. Aspiration pneumonia
4. Postradiation pneumonitis
5. Recurrent Pneumocystis carinii pneumonia (PCP) in a patient receiving aerosolized pentamidine prophylaxis

mnemonic: "SHIRT CAP"
Sarcoidosis
Histoplasmosis
Idiopathic
Radiation therapy
Tuberculosis (postprimary)
Chronic extrinsic alveolitis
Ankylosing spondylitis
Progressive massive fibrosis

D. LOWER LUNG DISEASE
Usually chronic slowly progressive + with volume loss
1. Usual interstitial pneumonia (common)
2. Rheumatoid lung disease (common)
3. Scleroderma (common)
4. Chronic aspiration pneumonia with fibrosis more regional / unilateral
5. Asbestosis (posterior aspect of lung base)

mnemonics:

Basilar distribution
"BAD LASS RIF"
Bronchiectasis
Aspiration
Dermatomyositis
Lymphangitic spread
Asbestosis
Sarcoidosis
Scleroderma
Rheumatoid arthritis
Idiopathic pulmonary fibrosis
Furadantin

Apical distribution
"CASSET"
Cystic fibrosis
Ankylosing spondylitis
Silicosis
Sarcoidosis
Eosinophilic granuloma
Tuberculosis, fungus

CHEST

Chronic diffuse infiltrative lung disease on HRCT

maximum resolution = 300 μm

1. Interlobular septal thickening
   = interstitial fluid / fibrosis / cellular infiltrates
   (a) smooth septal thickening: pulmonary edema, lymphangitic carcinomatosis
   (b) beaded septa / septal nodules: lymphangitic carcinomatosis
   (c) irregular septa imply fibrosis
   — distorted lobules: fibrosis
   — no architectural distortion of lobules: edema / infiltration
2. Reticular densities
   (a) predominantly subpleural small reticular elements of 6–10 mm in diameter with small cystic changes ("honeycombing")
   Associated with: interstitial fibrosis, lymphangioleiomyomatosis, amyloidosis
   (b) fine diffusely distributed network of 2–3 mm basic elements
   Associated with: miliary TB, reactions to methotrexate
   — lower lung zones in subpleural areas: idiopathic pulmonary fibrosis, collagen vascular disease, asbestosis
   — mid lung zone / all lung zones: chronic extrinsic allergic alveolitis
   – mid + upper lung zones: sarcoidosis
3. Nodules
   (a) interstitial nodules
   sarcoidosis, histiocytosis X, silicosis, coal worker pneumoconiosis, tuberculosis, hypersensitivity pneumonitis, metastatic tumor, amyloidosis
   √ perihilar peribronchovascular, centrilobular, interlobular septa, subpleural
   (b) airspace nodules
   lobular pneumonia, transbronchial spread of TB, bronchiolitis obliterans organizing pneumonia (BOOP), pulmonary edema
   √ ill-defined nodules, a few mm to 1 cm in size
   √ peribronchiolar + centrilobular
   — along bronchoarterial bundles + interlobular septa + subpleural: sarcoidosis
   — upper zone: silicosis, coal-worker's pneumoconiosis
   — centrilobular: extrinsic allergic alveolitis
4. Ground-glass attenuation
   = hazy increase in lung opacity without obscuration of underlying vessels
   ◊ Often indicative of an acute, active, and potentially treatable process!
   (a) minimal alveolar wall thickening = early interstitial lung disease
   (b) minimal airspace filling = alveolitis
   (c) partial collapse of alveoli
   (d) increased capillary blood volume = edema
   (e) normal expiration
   — peripheral in lower lung zones: DIP, UIP
   — mid + upper lung zones: sarcoidosis
   — "crazy paving" appearance: alveolar proteinosis
   — mosaic perfusion: chronic thromboembolism, bronchiolitis obliterans
5. Consolidation
   = increase in lung opacity with obscuration of underlying vessels ± air bronchograms
   — subpleural in mid + upper lung zones: chronic eosinophilic pneumonia
   — subpleural + peribronchial: BOOP
   — focal: bronchioloalveolar cell carcinoma, lymphoma
6. Cystic airspaces
   = circumscribed air-containing lesions with well-defined walls
   Associated with: lymphangioleiomyomatosis, pulmonary Langerhans-cell granulomatosis, honeycomb lung

Generalized interstitial disease

mnemonic: "HIDE FACTS"

Hamman-Rich, **H**emosiderosis
Infection, **I**rradiation, **I**diopathic
Dust, **D**rugs
Eosinophilic granuloma, **E**dema
Fungal, **F**armer's lung
Aspiration (oil), **A**rthritis (rheumatoid, ankylosing spondylitis)
Collagen disease
Tumor, **T**B, **T**uberous sclerosis
Sarcoidosis, **S**cleroderma

Interstitial lung disease with increased lung volume

mnemonic: "ELECTS"

Emphysema with interstitial lung disease
Lymphangiomyomatosis
Eosinophilic granuloma
Cystic fibrosis
Tuberous sclerosis
Sarcoidosis

Diffuse fine reticulations

Acute diffuse fine reticulations

A. ACUTE INTERSTITIAL EDEMA
   1. Congestive heart failure
   2. Fluid overload
   3. Uremia
   4. Hypersensitivity
B. ACUTE INTERSTITIAL PNEUMONIA
   1. Viral pneumonia
   2. Mycoplasma pneumonia
   3. Pneumocystis carinii pneumonia

mnemonic: "HELP"

Hypersensitivity
Edema
Lymphoproliferative
Pneumonitis (viral)

Chronic diffuse fine reticulations

A. VENOUS OBSTRUCTION
1. Atherosclerotic heart disease
2. Mitral stenosis
3. Left atrial myxoma
4. Pulmonary veno-occlusive disease
5. Sclerosing mediastinitis

B. LYMPHATIC OBSTRUCTION
1. Lymphangiectasia (pediatric patient)
2. Mediastinal mass (lymphoma)
3. Lymphoma / leukemia
4. Lymphangitic carcinomatosis: predominantly basilar distribution
   (a) bilateral (breast, stomach, colon, pancreas)
   (b) unilateral (lung tumor)
5. Lymphocytic interstitial pneumonitis

C. INHALATIONAL DISEASE
1. Silicosis: small nodules + reticulations
2. Asbestosis: basilar distribution, pleural thickening + calcifications
3. Hard metals
4. Allergic alveolitis

D. GRANULOMATOUS DISEASE
from a nodular to a reticular pattern if
   (a) nodules line up along bronchovascular bundles
   (b) interlobular septa show fibrotic changes
1. Sarcoidosis: hilar + mediastinal adenopathy (may have disappeared)
2. Eosinophilic granuloma: upper lobe distribution

E. CONNECTIVE-TISSUE DISEASE
reticulations in late stages
1. Rheumatoid lung
2. Scleroderma
3. Systemic lupus erythematosus

F. DRUG REACTIONS

G. IDIOPATHIC
1. Usual interstitial pneumonitis (UIP)
2. Desquamative interstitial pneumonitis (DIP)
3. Tuberous sclerosis: smooth muscle proliferation
4. Lymphangiomyomatosis
5. Idiopathic pulmonary hemosiderosis
6. Alveolar proteinosis (late complication)
7. Amyloidosis
8. Interstitial calcification (chronic renal failure)

mnemonic: "LIFE lines"
Lymphangitic spread
Inflammation / infection
Fibrosis
Edema

Coarse reticulations

= architectural destruction of interstitium = end-stage scarring of lung = interstitial pulmonary fibrosis = **honeycomb lung**

√ coarse reticular interstitial densities with intervening cystic spaces
√ rounded radiolucencies <1 cm in areas of increased lung density
√ small lung volume (decreased compliance)

Cx: (1) intercurrent pneumothoraces
(2) bronchogenic carcinoma = scar carcinoma

Cause:

A. INHALATIONAL DISEASE
(a) Pneumoconioses
   1. Asbestosis: basilar distribution, shaggy heart, pleural thickening + calcifications
   2. Silicosis: upper lobe predominance, ± pleural thickening, ± hilar and mediastinal lymphadenopathy
   3. Berylliosis
(b) Chemical inhalation (late)
   1. Silo-filler's disease (nitrogen dioxide)
   2. Sulfur dioxide, chlorine, phosgene, cadmium
(c) Extrinsic allergic alveolitis (= hypersensitivity to organic dusts)
(d) Oxygen toxicity
   sequelae of RDS therapy with oxygen
(e) Chronic aspiration
   eg, mineral oil: localized process in medial basal segments / middle lobe

B. GRANULOMATOUS DISEASE
1. Sarcoidosis
2. Eosinophilic granuloma

C. COLLAGEN-VASCULAR DISEASE
1. Rheumatoid lung
2. Scleroderma
3. Ankylosing spondylitis: upper lobes
4. SLE: rarely produces honeycombing

D. IATROGENIC
1. Drug hypersensitivity
2. Radiotherapy

E. IDIOPATHIC
1. Usual interstitial pneumonitis (UIP)
   honeycombing in 50%, severe volume loss in 45%
2. Desquamative interstitial pneumonitis (DIP)
   honeycombing in 12.5%, severe volume loss in 23%
3. Lymphangiomyomatosis
4. Tuberous sclerosis (rare)
5. Neurofibromatosis (rare)
6. Pulmonary capillary hemangiomatosis (rare)

DDx: bronchiectasis, cavitary metastases (rare)

Reticulations + pleural effusion

A. ACUTE
1. Edema
2. Infection: viral, Mycoplasma (very rare)

B. CHRONIC
1. Congestive heart failure
2. Lymphangitic carcinomatosis
3. Lymphoma / leukemia
4. SLE
5. Rheumatoid disease
6. Lymphangiectasia
7. Lymphangiomyomatosis
8. Asbestosis

Reticulations & Hilar Adenopathy

1. Sarcoidosis
2. Silicosis
3. Lymphoma / leukemia
4. Lung primary: particularly oat cell carcinoma
5. Metastases: lymphatic obstruction / spread
6. Fungal disease
7. Tuberculosis
8. Viral pneumonia (rare combination)

Reticulonodular Disease

mnemonic: "**P**lease **D**on't **E**at **S**tale **T**una **F**ish **S**andwiches **E**very **M**orning"

Pneumoconiosis
Drugs
Eosinophilic granuloma
Sarcoidosis
Tuberculosis
Fungal disease
Schistosomiasis
Exanthem (measles, chickenpox)
Metastases (thyroid)

Reticulonodular Pattern & Lower Lobe Predominance

mnemonic: "CIA"

Collagen vascular disease
Idiopathic
Asbestosis

Nodular Disease

= round moderately well marginated opacity <3 cm in maximum diameter

A. GRANULOMATOUS LUNG DISEASE
   (a) Infections: eg, tuberculosis
   (b) Fungal disease: eg, histoplasmosis
   (c) Silicosis
   (d) Vasculitis: eg, Wegener granulomatosis
B. NEOPLASM
   (a) metastatic lung diseases: eg, thyroid cancer
   (b) lymphoma
   (c) bronchioloalveolar cell carcinoma
C. OTHER DISEASE
   (a) drug-induced: methotrexate
   (b) nongranulomatous vasculitis
   (c) sarcoidosis

Macronodular Disease

√ nodules >5 mm in diameter

mnemonic: "GAMMA WARPS"

Granuloma (EG, fungus)
Abscess
Metastases
Multiple myeloma
AVM
Wegener granulomatosis
Amyloidosis
Rheumatoid lung
Parasites (Echinococcus, Paragonimiasis)
Sarcoidosis

Micronodular Disease

= discrete 3–5–7 mm small round focal opacity of at least soft-tissue attenuation

1. Granulomatous disease (miliary tuberculosis, histoplasmosis)
2. Hypersensitivity (organic dust)
3. Pneumoconiosis (inorganic dust, thesaurosis = prolonged hair spray exposure)
4. Sarcoidosis
5. Metastases (thyroid, melanoma)
6. Histiocytosis X
7. Chickenpox

Diffuse Fine Nodular Disease & Miliary Nodules

√ very small 1–4 mm sharply defined nodules of interstitial disease

(a) Inhalational disease
   1. Silicosis + coal worker's pneumoconiosis
   2. Beryllios
   3. Siderosis
   4. Extrinsic allergic alveolitis (chronic phase)
(b) Granulomatous disease
   1. Eosinophilic granuloma
   2. Sarcoidosis (with current / previous adenopathy)
(c) Infectious disease
   1. Tuberculosis
   2. Fungus: histoplasmosis, coccidioidomycosis, blastomycosis, aspergillosis (rare), cryptococcosis (rare)
   3. Bacteria: salmonella, nocardiosis
   4. Virus: varicella (more common in adults), Mycoplasma pneumonia
(d) Metastases
   Thyroid carcinoma, melanoma, adenocarcinoma of breast, stomach, colon, pancreas
(e) Alveolar microlithiasis (rare)
(f) Bronchiolitis obliterans
(g) Gaucher disease

mnemonic: "TEMPEST"

Tuberculosis + fungal disease
Eosinophilic granuloma
Metastases (thyroid, lymphangitic carcinomatosis)
Pneumoconiosis, Parasites
Embolism of oily contrast
Sarcoidosis
Tuberous sclerosis

Fine Nodular Disease In Afebrile Patient

1. Inhalational disease
2. Eosinophilic granuloma
3. Sarcoidosis
4. Metastases
5. Fungal infection (late stage)
6. Miliary tuberculosis (rare)

FINE NODULAR DISEASE IN FEBRILE PATIENT
1. Tuberculosis
2. Fungal infection (early stage)
3. Pneumocystis
4. Viral pneumonia

Chronic Interstitial Disease Simulating Airspace Disease

A. REPLACEMENT OF LUNG ARCHITECTURE BY AN INTERSTITIAL PROCESS
(a) Neoplastic
Hodgkin disease, histiocytic lymphoma
(b) Benign cellular infiltrate
lymphocytic interstitial pneumonia, pseudolymphoma
(c) Granulomatous disease
alveolar sarcoidosis
(d) Fibrosis

B. EXUDATIVE PHASE OF INTERSTITIAL PNEUMONIA
1. UIP
2. Adult respiratory distress syndrome
3. Radiation pneumonitis
4. Drug reaction
5. Reaction to noxious gases

C. CELLULAR FILLING OF AIR SPACE
1. Desquamative interstitial pneumonia
2. Pneumocystis carinii pneumonia

End-stage Lung Disease

A. DISTRIBUTION
1. Usual interstitial pneumonia
√ subpleural distribution + lower lobe predominance
2. Asbestosis
√ subpleural distribution + lower lobe predominance + pleural thickening
3. Sarcoidosis
√ peribronchovascular distribution + upper lobe predominance
4. Extrinsic allergic alveolitis
√ diffuse random distribution + patchy areas of ground-glass attenuation

B. CYSTIC SPACES WITH WELL-DEFINED WALLS
1. Langerhans cell histiocytosis
√ upper lobe predominance
2. Lymphangioleiomyomatosis
√ no zonal predominance

C. CONGLOMERATE FIBROTIC MASSES
1. Sarcoidosis
√ peribronchovascular distribution
2. Silicosis
√ bronchi splayed around masses
3. Talcosis
√ areas of high attenuation (= talc deposits)

Honeycomb Lung

mnemonic:

"HIPS RDS"
Histiocytosis X
Interstitial pneumonia
Pneumoconiosis
Sarcoidosis

Rheumatoid lung
Dermatomyositis
Scleroderma

"SHIPS BOATS"
Sarcoidosis
Histiocytosis
Idiopathic (UIP)
Pneumoconiosis
Scleroderma
Bleomycin, **B**usulfan
Oxygen toxicity
Arthritis (rheumatoid), **A**myloidosis, **A**llergic alveolitis
Tuberous sclerosis, **T**B
Storage disease (Gaucher)

DENSE LUNG LESION

Ground-glass Attenuation

1. Desquamative interstitial pneumonia
2. Extrinsic allergic alveolitis
3. Sarcoidosis
4. Usual interstitial pneumonia
5. Alveolar proteinosis
6. Cryptogenic organizing pneumonia

Opacification Of Hemithorax

mnemonic: "FAT CHANCE"
Fibrothorax
Adenomatoid malformation
Trauma (ie, hematoma)
Collapse, **C**ardiomegaly
Hernia
Agenesis of lung
Neoplasm (ie, mesothelioma)
Consolidation
Effusion

Atelectasis

Cause:

A. TUMOR
1. Bronchogenic carcinoma (2/3 of squamous cell carcinoma occur as endobronchial mass with persistent / recurrent atelectasis or recurrent pneumonia)
2. Bronchial carcinoid
3. Metastases: primary tumor of kidney, colon, rectum, breast, melanoma
4. Lymphoma (usually as a late presentation)
5. Lipoma, granular cell myoblastoma, amyloid tumor, fibroepithelial polyp

B. INFLAMMATION
1. Tuberculosis (endobronchial granuloma, broncholith, bronchial stenosis)
2. Right middle lobe syndrome (chronic right middle lobe atelectasis)
3. Sarcoidosis (endobronchial granuloma — rare)

C. MUCUS PLUG
1. Severe chest / abdominal pain (postoperative patient)

2. Respiratory depressant drug (morphine; CNS illness)
3. Chronic bronchitis / bronchiolitis obliterans
4. Asthma
5. Cystic fibrosis
6. Bronchopneumonia (peribronchial inflammation)

D. OTHER
1. Large left atrium (mitral stenosis + left lower lobe atelectasis)
2. Foreign body (aspiration of food, endotracheal intubation)
3. Broncholithiasis
4. Amyloidosis
5. Wegener granulomatosis
6. Bronchial transection

√ local increase in lung density
√ crowding of pulmonary vessels
√ bronchial rearrangement
√ displacement of fissures
√ displacement of hilus
√ mediastinal shift
√ elevation of hemidiaphragm
√ cardiac rotation
√ approximation of ribs
√ compensatory overinflation of normal lung

Types:

A. OBSTRUCTIVE ATELECTASIS

Resorptive atelectasis

Pathophysiology:

sum of partial gas pressures in venous blood perfusing atelectatic region is less than atmospheric pressure, which is responsible for gradual resorption of air trapped distal to site of obstruction; continuing secretion into small airways leads to consolidation (postobstructive pneumonitis / bacterial infection)

Cause: bronchiolar obstruction by
1. Tumor
2. Stricture
3. Foreign body
4. Mucus plug
5. Bronchial rupture

• airless collapse within minutes to hours

MR:
√ high signal intensity on T2WI in atelectatic area

B. NONOBSTRUCTIVE ATELECTASIS

Pathophysiology:

pathway between bronchial system + alveoli is maintained because bronchi are less compliant than lung parenchyma + remain patent; secretions can be eliminated + convective airflow to distal bronchioles remains

• collapsed lung not completely airless (up to 40% residual air)

MR:
√ low-signal intensity on T2WI in atelectatic area

Passive atelectasis

= pleural space-occupying process
1. Pneumothorax
2. Hydrothorax / hemothorax
3. Diaphragmatic hernia
4. Pleural masses: metastases, mesothelioma

Adhesive atelectasis

= decrease in surfactant production
1. Respiratory distress syndrome of the newborn (hyaline membrane disease)
2. Pulmonary embolism: edema, hemorrhage, atelectasis
3. Intravenous injection of hydrocarbon

Cicatrizing atelectasis

= parenchymal fibrosis causing decreased lung volume
1. Tuberculosis / histoplasmosis (upper lobes)
2. Silicosis (upper lobes)
3. Scleroderma (lower lobes)
4. Radiation pneumonitis (nonanatomical distribution)
5. Idiopathic pulmonary fibrosis

Discoid atelectasis

mnemonic: "EPIC"
Embolus
Pneumonia
Inadequate inspiration
Carcinoma, obstructing

Multifocal ill-defined densities

= densities 5–30 mm resulting in airspace filling

A. INFECTION
1. Bacterial bronchopneumonia
2. Fungal pneumonia:
histoplasmosis, blastomycosis, actinomycosis, coccidioidomycosis, aspergillosis, cryptococcosis, mucormycosis, sporotrichosis
3. Viral pneumonia
initially may have interstitial appearance
= tracheitis, bronchitis, bronchiolitis, peribronchial infiltrate, interstitial septa infiltrates, injury to alveolar cells, hyaline membranes, necrosis of alveolar walls with blood, edema, fibrin, macrophages in alveoli
(a) Influenza: cavitary lesion confirms superimposed infection
(b) Varicella / herpes zoster: 10% of adults; 2–5 days after rash
(c) Rubeola (measles) = before / with onset of rash; following overt measles = giant cell pneumonia
(d) Cytomegalic inclusion virus: features suggestive of bronchopneumonia
(e) Coxsackie, parainfluenza, adenovirus, respiratory syncytial virus

CHEST

4. Tuberculosis (primary infection)
5. Rocky Mountain spotted fever
6. Pneumocystis carinii

B. GRANULOMATOUS DISEASE
1. Sarcoidosis (alveolar form secondary to peribronchial granulomas)
2. Eosinophilic granuloma

C. VASCULAR
1. Thromboembolic disease
2. Septic emboli
3. Vasculitis
(a) Wegener granulomatosis
(b) Wegener variants: limited Wegener, lymphomatoid granulomatosis
(c) Infectious vasculitis = invasion of pulmonary arteries: mucormycosis, invasive form of aspergillosis, Rocky Mountain spotted fever
(d) Goodpasture syndrome
(e) Scleroderma

D. NEOPLASTIC
1. Bronchioloalveolar cell carcinoma
= only primary lung tumor to produce multifocal ill-defined densities with air bronchograms
2. Alveolar type of lymphoma
= massive accumulation of tumor cells in interstitium with compression atelectasis + obstructive pneumonia
3. Metastases
(a) Choriocarcinoma: hemorrhage (however rare)
(b) Vascular tumors: malignant hemangiomas
4. Waldenström macroglobulinemia
5. Angioblastic lymphadenopathy
6. Mycosis fungoides
7. Amyloid tumor

E. IDIOPATHIC INTERSTITIAL DISEASE
1. Lymphocytic Interstitial Pneumonitis (LIP)
2. Desquamative Interstitial Pneumonitis (DIP)
3. Pseudolymphoma = localized form of LIP
4. Usual Interstitial Pneumonitis (UIP)

F. INHALATIONAL DISEASE
1. Allergic alveolitis: acute stage (eg, farmer's lung)
2. Silicosis
3. Eosinophilic pneumonia

G. DRUG REACTIONS

Diffuse infiltrates in immunocompromised cancer patient

mnemonic: "FOLD"
Failure (CHF)
Opportunistic infection
Lymphangitic tumor spread
Drug reaction

Segmental + lobar densities

A. PNEUMONIA
1. Lobar pneumonia
2. Lobular pneumonia
3. Acute interstitial pneumonia
4. Aspiration pneumonia
5. Primary tuberculosis

B. PULMONARY EMBOLISM
(rarely multiple / larger than subsegmental)

C. NEOPLASM
1. Obstructive pneumonia
2. Bronchioloalveolar cell carcinoma

D. ATELECTASIS

Chronic infiltrates

Chronic infiltrates in childhood

mnemonic: "ABC'S"
Asthma, **A**gammaglobulinemia, **A**spiration
Bronchiectasis
Cystic fibrosis
Sequestration, intralobar

Chronic multifocal ill-defined opacities

1. Organizing pneumonia
2. Granulomatous disease
3. Allergic alveolitis
4. Bronchioloalveolar cell carcinoma
5. Lymphoma

Chronic diffuse confluent opacities

1. Alveolar proteinosis
2. Hemosiderosis
3. Sarcoidosis

Ill-defined densities with holes

A. INFECTION
1. Necrotizing pneumonias:
Staphylococcus aureus, ß-hemolytic streptococcus, Klebsiella pneumoniae, E. coli, Proteus, Pseudomonas, anaerobes
2. Aspiration pneumonia:
mixed Gram-negative organisms
3. Septic emboli
4. Fungus:
histoplasmosis, blastomycosis, coccidioidomycosis, cryptococcosis
5. Tuberculosis

B. NEOPLASM
1. Primary lung carcinoma
2. Lymphoma (cavitates very rarely)

C. VASCULAR + COLLAGEN-VASCULAR DISEASE
1. Emboli with infarction
2. Wegener granulomatosis
3. Necrobiotic rheumatoid nodules

D. TRAUMA
1. Contusion with pneumatoceles

Perihilar "bat-wing" infiltrates

mnemonic: "**P**lease, **P**lease, **P**lease, **S**tudy **L**ight, **D**on't **G**et **A**ll **U**ptight"
Pulmonary edema
Proteinosis
Periarteritis
Sarcoidosis
Lymphoma

Drugs
Goodpasture syndrome
Alveolar cell carcinoma
Uremia

Peripheral "Reverse Bat-wing" Infiltrates

mnemonic: "REDS"
Resolving pulmonary edema
Eosinophilic pneumonia
Desquamative interstitial pneumonia
Sarcoidosis

Recurrent Fleeting Infiltrates

1. Löffler disease
2. Bronchopulmonary aspergillosis / bronchocentric granulomatosis
3. Asthma
4. Subacute bacterial endocarditis with pulmonary emboli

Tubular Density

A. Mucoid impaction
B. Vascular malformation
  1. Arteriovenous malformation
  2. Pulmonary varix

PULMONARY EDEMA

Transcapillary flow dependent on (1) hydrostatic pressure (2) colloid osmotic pressure (3) capillary permeability

A. INCREASED HYDROSTATIC PRESSURE
  (a) cardiogenic (most common)
    = pulmonary venous hypertension
    1. Heart disease: left ventricular failure, mitral valve disease, left atrial myxoma
    2. Pulmonary venous disease: primary veno-occlusive disease, mediastinal fibrosis
    3. Pericardial disease: pericardial effusion, constrictive pericarditis (extremely rare)
    4. Drugs: antiarrhythmic drugs; drugs depressing myocardial contractility (beta-blocker)
  (b) noncardiogenic
    1. Renal failure
    2. IV fluid overload
    3. Hyperosmolar fluid (eg, contrast medium)
  (c) neurogenic
    ? sympathetic venoconstriction in cerebrovascular accident, head injury, CNS tumor, postictal state
B. DECREASED COLLOID OSMOTIC PRESSURE
  1. Hypoproteinemia
  2. Transfusion of crystalloid fluid
  3. Rapid reexpansion of lung
C. INCREASED CAPILLARY PERMEABILITY
  Endothelial injury from
  (a) physical trauma: parenchymal contusion, radiation therapy
  (b) aspiration injury:
    1. Mendelson syndrome (gastric contents)
    2. Near drowning in sea water / fresh water
    3. Aspiration of hypertonic contrast media
  (c) inhalation injury:
    1. Nitrogen dioxide = silo-filler's disease
    2. Smoke (pulmonary edema may be delayed by 24–48 hours)
    3. Sulfur dioxide, hydrocarbons, carbon monoxide, beryllium, cadmium, silica, dinitrogen tetroxide, oxygen, chlorine, phosgene, ammonia, organophosphates
  (d) injury via bloodstream
    1. Vessel occlusion: shock (trauma, sepsis, ARDS) or emboli (fat, amniotic fluid, thrombus)
    2. Circulating toxins: snake venom, paraquat
    3. Drugs: heroin, morphine, methadone, aspirin, phenylbutazone, nitrofurantoin, chlorothiazide
    4. Anaphylaxis: transfusion reaction, contrast medium reaction, penicillin
    5. Hypoxia: high altitude, acute large airway obstruction

mnemonic: "ABCDEFGHI - PRN"
Aspiration
Burns
Chemicals
Drugs (heroin, nitrofurantoin, salicylates)
Exudative skin disorders
Fluid overload
Gram-negative shock
Heart failure
Intracranial condition
Polyarteritis nodosa
Renal disease
Near drowning

Interstitial Pulmonary Edema

◊ often marked dissociation between clinical signs + symptoms + roentgenographic evidence
◊ nothing differentiates it from other interstitial lesions
◊ does not necessarily develop before alveolar pulmonary edema
◊ NOT typical for bacterial pneumonia

Pulmonary Edema With Cardiomegaly

1. Cardiogenic
2. Uremic (with cardiomegaly from pericardial effusion / hypertension)

Pulmonary Edema Without Cardiomegaly

mnemonic: "U DOPA"
Uremia
Drugs
Overhydration
Pulmonary hemorrhage
Acute myocardial infarction, **A**rrhythmia

Noncardiogenic Pulmonary Edema

mnemonic: "The alphabet"

ARDS, **A**lveolar proteinosis, **A**spiration, **A**naphylaxis
Bleeding diathesis, **B**lood transfusion reaction
CNS (increased pressure, trauma, surgery, CVA, cancer)
Drowning (near), **D**rug reaction
Embolus (fat, thrombus)
Fluid overload, **F**oreign-body inhalation
Glomerulonephritis, **G**oodpasture syndrome, **G**astrografin aspiration
High altitude, **H**eroin, **H**ypoproteinemia
Inhalation (SO_2, smoke, CO, cadmium, silica)
-
Narcotics, **N**itrofurantoin
Oxygen toxicity
Pancreatitis
-
Rapid reexpansion of pneumothorax / removal of pleural effusion
-
Transfusion
Uremia

Unilateral Pulmonary Edema

A. IPSILATERAL = on side of preexisting abnormality
- (a) filling of airways
  1. Unilateral aspiration / pulmonary lavage
  2. Bronchial obstruction (drowned lung)
  3. Pulmonary contusion
- (b) increased pulmonary venous pressure
  1. Unilateral venous obstruction
  2. Prolonged lateral decubitus position
- (c) pulmonary arterial overload
  1. Systemic artery-to-pulmonary artery shunt (Waterston, Blalock-Taussig, Pott procedure)
  2. Rapid thoracentesis (rapid reexpansion)

B. CONTRALATERAL = opposite to side of abnormality
- (a) pulmonary arterial obstruction
  1. Congenital absence / hypoplasia of pulmonary artery
  2. Unilateral arterial obstruction
  3. Pulmonary thromboembolism
- (b) loss of lung parenchyma
  1. Swyer-James syndrome
  2. Unilateral emphysema
  3. Lobectomy
  4. Pleural disease

PNEUMONIA

"Classic" pneumonia pattern:

1. Lobar distribution : Streptococcus pneumoniae
2. Bulging fissure : Klebsiella
3. Pulmonary edema: Viral pneumonia, Pneumocystis pneumonia
4. Pneumatocele : Staphylococcus
5. Alveolar nodules : Varicella, bronchogenic spread of TB

Distribution:

A. SEGMENTAL / LOBAR
- — Normal host: S. pneumoniae, Mycoplasma, virus
- — Compromised host: S. pneumoniae

B. BRONCHOPNEUMONIA
- — Normal host: Mycoplasma, virus, Streptococcus, Staphylococcus, S. pneumoniae
- — Compromised host: Gram-negative, Streptococcus, Staphylococcus
- — Nosocomial: Gram-negative, Pseudomonas, Klebsiella, Staphylococcus
- — Immunosuppressed: Gram-negative, Staphylococcus, Nocardia, Legionella, Aspergillus, Phycomycetes

C. EXTENSIVE BILATERAL
- — Normal host: virus (eg, influenza), Legionella
- — Compromised host: candidiasis, Pneumocystis, tuberculosis

D. BILATERAL LOWER LOBE
- — Normal host: anaerobic (aspiration)
- — Compromised host: anaerobic (aspiration)

E. PERIPHERAL
- — Noninfectious eosinophilic pneumonia

Transmission:

A. COMMUNITY-ACQUIRED PNEUMONIA
Organism: viruses, S. pneumoniae, Mycoplasma
Mortality: 10%

B. NOSOCOMIAL PNEUMONIA
- (a) Gram-negative organism (>50%): Klebsiella pneumoniae, P. aeruginosa, E. coli, Enterobacter
- (b) Gram-positive organism (10%): S. aureus, S. pneumoniae, H. influenzae

Lobar Pneumonia

= ALVEOLAR PNEUMONIA
= pathogens reach peripheral air space, incite exudation of watery edema into alveolar space, centrifugal spread via small airways, pores of Kohn + Lambert into adjacent lobules + segments

√ nonsegmental sublobar consolidation
√ round pneumonia (= uniform involvement of contiguous alveoli)
- (a) Streptococcus pneumoniae
- (b) Klebsiella pneumoniae (more aggressive); in immunocompromised + alcoholics
- (c) any pneumonia in children
- (d) atypical measles

√ expansion of lobe with bulging of fissures
√ lung necrosis with cavitation

DDx: Aspiration, pulmonary embolus

Lobular Pneumonia

= BRONCHOPNEUMONIA
= combination of interstitial + alveolar disease (injury starts in airways involves bronchovascular bundle, spills into alveoli, which may contain edema fluid, blood, leukocytes, hyaline membranes, organisms)

Organisms:
(a) Staphylococcus aureus, Pseudomonas pneumoniae: thrombosis of lobular artery branches with necrosis + cavitation
(b) Streptococcus, Klebsiella, Legionnaires' bacillus, Bacillus proteus, E. coli, anaerobes (Bacteroides + Clostridia), Nocardia, actinomycosis
(c) Mycoplasma

√ small fluffy ill-defined acinar nodules, which enlarge with time
√ lobar + segmental densities with volume loss from airway obstruction secondary to bronchial narrowing + mucus plugging

Interstitial Pneumonia

Acute Interstitial Pneumonia

= NONBACTERIAL PNEUMONIA
initially predominantly affecting interstitial tissues
Organisms: viruses, Mycoplasma, Pneumocystis
• often subacute atypical pneumonia
√ diffuse interstitial process with peribronchial thickening
√ segmental / lobar densities (mucus plugging + damage of surfactant-producing type 2 alveolar cells)

Chronic Interstitial Pneumonia

= diverse group of inflammatory disorders that can progress to pulmonary fibrosis
Modified Liebow classification:
1. Usual interstitial pneumonia (UIP)
2. Desquamative interstitial pneumonia (DIP)
3. Bronchiolitis obliterans with organizing pneumonia (BOOP)

added:
4. Acute interstitial pneumonia = Hamman-Rich syndrome
5. Nonspecific interstitial pneumonitis
6. Respiratory bronchiolitis-associated interstitial lung disease

no longer included:
1. Lymphoid interstitial pneumonia (LIP)
   = potentially malignant lymphoproliferative disorder
2. Giant cell interstitial pneumonia (GIP)
   = manifestation of hard-metal pneumoconiosis

Cavitating Pneumonia

1. Staphylococcus aureus
2. Haemophilus influenzae
3. S. pneumoniae

other Gram-negative organisms (eg, Klebsiella)

Cavitating Opportunistic Infections

A. FUNGAL INFECTIONS
   1. Aspergillosis
   2. Nocardiosis
   3. Mucormycosis (= phycomycosis)
B. SEPTIC EMBOLI
   1. Anaerobic organisms
C. STAPHYLOCOCCAL ABSCESS
D. TUBERCULOSIS
   nummular form

◊ Repeated infections in same patient are not necessarily due to same organism!
DDx: Metastatic disease in carcinoma / Hodgkin lymphoma

Pulmonary Infiltrates In Neonate

mnemonic: "I HEAR"
Infection (pneumonia)
Hemorrhage
Edema
Aspiration
Respiratory distress syndrome

Recurrent Pneumonia In Childhood

A. IMMUNE PROBLEM
   1. Immune deficiency
   2. Chronic granulomatous disease of childhood (males)
   3. Alpha 1-antitrypsin deficiency
B. ASPIRATION
   1. Gastroesophageal reflux
   2. H-type tracheoesophageal fistula
   3. Disorder of swallowing mechanism
   4. Esophageal obstruction, impacted esophageal foreign body
C. UNDERLYING LUNG DISEASE
   1. Sequestration
   2. Bronchopulmonary dysplasia
   3. Cystic fibrosis
   4. Atopic asthma
   5. Bronchiolitis obliterans
   6. Sinusitis
   7. Bronchiectasis
   8. Ciliary dysmotility syndromes
   9. Pulmonary foreign body

Gram-negative Pneumonia

In 50% cause of nosocomial necrotizing pneumonias (including staphylococcal pneumonia)
Predisposed: elderly, debilitated, diabetes, alcoholism, COPD, malignancy, bronchitis, Gram-positive pneumonia, treatment with antibiotics, respirator therapy
Organisms:
1. Klebsiella
2. Pseudomonas
3. E. coli
4. Proteus
5. Haemophilus
6. Legionella

√ airspace consolidation (Klebsiella)
√ spongy appearance (Pseudomonas)
√ affecting dependent lobes (poor cough reflex without clearing of bronchial tree)
√ bilateral
√ cavitation common
Cx: (1) exudate / empyema (2) bronchopleural fistula

CHEST

Mycotic Infections Of Lung

A. IN HEALTHY SUBJECTS
1. Histoplasmosis
2. Coccidioidomycosis
3. Blastomycosis

B. OPPORTUNISTIC INFECTION
1. Aspergillosis
2. Candidiasis
3. Mucormycosis (phycomycosis)

Growth: (a) mycelial form
(b) yeast form (depending on environment)

Source of contamination:
(a) soil
(b) growth in moist areas (apart from Coccidioides immitis)
(c) contaminated bird / bat excreta

Hypersensitivity To Organic Dusts

A. TRACHEOBRONCHIAL HYPERSENSITIVITY
large particles reaching the tracheobronchial mucosa (pollens, certain fungi, some animal / insect epithelial emanations)
1. Extrinsic asthma
2. Hypersensitivity aspergillosis
3. Bronchocentric granulomatosis
4. Byssinosis in cotton-wool workers

B. ALVEOLAR HYPERSENSITIVITY
= HYPERSENSITIVITY PNEUMONITIS
= EXTRINSIC ALLERGIC ALVEOLITIS
small particles of <5 μ reaching alveoli

Drug-induced Pulmonary Damage

A. CHEMOTHERAPEUTIC AGENTS
1. BUSULFAN = Myleran® (for CML)
Dose-dependent toxicity after 3–4 years on the drug in 1–10%
√ diffuse linear pattern (occasionally reticulonodular / nodular pattern)
√ partial / complete clearing after withdrawal of drug
DDx: Pneumocystis pneumonia, interstitial leukemic infiltrate
2. BLEOMYCIN (for squamous cell carcinoma, lymphoma, testicular tumor)
Toxicity at doses >300 mg (in 3–6%); increased toxicity with age + radiation therapy + high oxygen concentrations
√ subpleural linear / nodular opacities in lower lung zones occurring after 1–3 months following beginning of therapy
3. NITROSOUREAS = BCNU, CCNU (for glioma, lymphoma, myeloma)
Incidence of 50% after doses >1500 mg/m^2
√ linear / finely nodular opacities (following treatment of 2–3 years)
√ high incidence of pneumothorax
4. METHOTREXATE, PROCARBAZINE (for AML, psoriasis, pemphigus)
Not dose-related, usually self-limited despite continuation of therapy
• blood eosinophilia (common)
√ linear / reticulonodular process (time delay of 12 days to 5 years, usually early)
√ acinar filling pattern (later)
√ transient hilar adenopathy + pleural effusion (on occasion)
DDx: Pneumocystis pneumonia

B. NITROFURANTOIN (Macrodantin®)
(a) acute disorder with fever + eosinophilia (common)
(b) chronic reaction with interstitial fibrosis (less common), may not be associated with peripheral eosinophilia
• positive for ANA + LE cells
√ bilateral basilar interstitial opacities
√ prompt resolution after withdrawal from drug

C. HEROIN, PROPOXYPHENE, METHADONE
Overdose followed by pulmonary edema in 30–40%
√ bilateral widespread airspace consolidation
√ aspiration pneumonia in 50–75%

D. SALICYLATES
• asthma
√ pulmonary edema (with chronic ingestion)

E. INTRAVENOUS CONTRAST AGENT
√ pulmonary edema

F. AMIODARONE (for refractory ventricular arrhythmia)
• pulmonary insufficiency after 1–12 months in 14–18% on long-term therapy
√ alveolar + interstitial infiltrates
√ peripheral consolidation
√ pleural thickening adjacent to consolidation
√ consolidated lung parenchyma has attenuation values of iodine

PULMONARY MASS

Differential-diagnostic Features Of Lung Masses

DDx Of Lung Masses On CXR

√ corona radiata = spiculations strongly suggestive of primary malignancy
◊ 89% of irregular / spiculated lesions are malignant!
√ lucencies / air bronchogram
(a) cavitation
◊ A thin-walled cavity of ≤4 mm is benign in 94%!
(b) infiltrative spread with air bronchogram: bronchioloalveolar cell carcinoma, lymphoma, resolving pneumonia
√ calcifications
(a) central / complete: granuloma
(b) peripheral: granuloma, tumor
√ decrease in size with time: benign lesion
◊ Bronchogenic carcinoma may show temporary decrease in size due to infarction - necrosis - fibrosis - retraction sequence!
√ absence of growth over 2 years: benign lesion
√ increase in size with time:
masses with "doubling times" (refers to volume not diameter) of <1 month / >16 months are unlikely to be malignant

(a) very rapid growth:
osteosarcoma, choriocarcinoma, testicular neoplasm, organizing infectious process, infarct (thromboembolism, Wegener granulomatosis)
(b) very slow growth:
hamartoma, bronchial carcinoid, inflammatory pseudotumor, granuloma, low-grade adenocarcinoma, metastases from renal cell carcinoma

√ nodule >3 cm is suspect for malignancy
√ satellite nodules (in association with larger peripheral nodule):
— in 99% due to inflammatory disease (often TB)
— in 1% due to primary lung cancer
√ lobulation
(a) organizing mass
(b) tumor with multiple cell types growing at different rates (eg, hamartoma)
◊ 79% of sharply defined marginated lesions are benign!
√ bubblelike areas of low attenuation: bronchioloalveolar cell carcinoma (in 50%)
√ focal collection of fat within smoothly marginated lung nodule: hamartoma
√ vessel leading to mass: pulmonary varix, AVM

DDx Of Lung Masses On Thin-section CT

√ air bronchogram in nodules <2 cm in diameter: in 65% malignant, in 5% benign
√ spiculation: in 87% malignant, in 55% benign
√ pleural tag: in 25% malignant, in 9% benign
√ presence of calcification, fat, smooth edge are suggestive of benignancy
√ in 31% calcifications (usually >164 HU) were not detected on CXR
√ CECT (2–5 minutes after administration):
benign neoplasms + granulomas enhance <15 HU; malignant neoplasms enhance >25 HU

Benign Lung Tumor

A. CENTRAL LOCATION
1. Bronchial polyp
2. Bronchial papilloma
3. **Granular cell myoblastoma**
= cell of origin from neural crest
Age: middle-aged, esp. Black women
√ endobronchial lesion in major bronchi

B. PERIPHERAL LOCATION
1. Hamartoma
2. Leiomyoma
benign metastasizing leiomyoma, history of hysterectomy
3. Amyloid tumor
not associated with amyloid of other organs / rheumatoid arthritis / myeloma
4. Intrapulmonary lymph node
5. Arteriovenous malformation
6. Endometrioma, fibroma, neural tumor, chemodectoma

C. CENTRAL / PERIPHERAL
1. Lipoma: (a) subpleural (b) endobronchial

D. PSEUDOTUMOR
1. Fibroxanthoma / xanthogranuloma
2. Plasma cell granuloma
3. Sclerosing hemangioma
middle-aged woman, RML / RLL (most commonly), may be multiple
4. Pseudolymphoma
5. Round atelectasis
6. Pleural pseudotumor = accumulation of pleural fluid within interlobar fissure

Solitary Nodule / Mass

Incidence:
(a) roentgenographic survey of low-risk population: <5% of masses are cancerous
(b) on surgical resection: 40% malignant tumors, 40% granulomas

A. INFLAMMATION / INFECTION
1. Granuloma (most common lung mass): Sarcoidosis (1/3), tuberculosis, histoplasmosis, coccidioidomycosis, nocardiosis, cryptococcosis, talc, Dirofilaria immitis (dog heartworm), gumma, atypical measles infection
2. Fluid-filled cavity: abscess, hydatid cyst, bronchiectatic cyst, bronchocele
3. Mass in preformed cavity: fungus ball, mucoid impaction
4. Rounded atelectasis
5. Inflammatory pseudotumor: fibroxanthoma, histiocytoma, plasma cell granuloma, sclerosing hemangioma
6. Paraffinoma = lipoid granuloma
7. Focal organizing pneumonia

B. MALIGNANT TUMORS
(a) Malignant primaries of lung
1. Bronchogenic carcinoma (66%, 2nd most common mass)
2. Lymphoma
3. Primary sarcoma of lung
4. Plasmacytoma (primary / secondary)
5. Clear cell carcinoma, carcinoid, giant cell ca.

(b) Metastases (4th most common cause)
<u>in adults:</u> kidney, colon, ovary, testes
<u>in children:</u> Wilms tumor, osteogenic sarcoma, Ewing sarcoma, rhabdomyosarcoma

C. BENIGN TUMORS
(a) lung tissue : hamartoma (6%, 3rd most common lung mass)
(b) fat tissue : lipoma (usually pleural lesion)
(c) fibrous tissue : fibroma
(d) muscle tissue : leiomyoma
(e) neural tissue : schwannoma, neurofibroma, paraganglioma
(f) lymph tissue : intrapulmonary lymph node
(g) deposits : amyloid, splenosis, endometrioma, extramedullary hematopoiesis

D. VASCULAR
   1. Arteriovenous malformation
   2. Hemangioma
   3. Hematoma
   4. Organizing infarct
   5. Pulmonary venous varix
   6. Pseudoaneurysm of pulmonary artery
   7. Rheumatoid / vasculitic nodule

E. DEVELOPMENTAL
   1. Bronchogenic cyst (fluid-filled)
   2. Pulmonary sequestration

F. INHALATIONAL
   1. Silicosis (conglomerate mass)
   2. Mucoid impaction (allergic aspergillosis)

G. MIMICKING DENSITIES
   1. Fluid in interlobar fissure
   2. Mediastinal mass
   3. Pleural mass (mesothelioma)
   4. Chest wall density: nipple, rib lesion, skin tumor (mole, neurofibroma, lipoma)
   5. Artifacts: buttons, snaps

mnemonic: "**B**ig **S**olitary **P**ulmonary **M**asses **C**ommonly **A**ppear **H**opeless **A**nd **L**onely"

Bronchogenic carcinoma
Solitary metastasis, **S**equestration
Pseudotumor
Mesothelioma
Cyst (bronchogenic, neurenteric, echinococcal)
Adenoma, **A**rteriovenous malformation
Hamartoma, **H**istoplasmosis
Abscess, **A**ctinomycosis
Lymphoma

Large Pulmonary Mass

mnemonic: "CAT PIES"

Carcinoma (large cell, squamous cell, cannon ball metastasis
Abscess
Toruloma (Cryptococcus)
Pseudotumor, **P**lasmacytoma
Inflammatory
Echinococcal disease
Sarcoma, **S**equestration

Cavitating Lung Nodule

A. NEOPLASM
   (a) Lung primary:
      1. Squamous cell carcinoma
      2. Adenocarcinoma
      3. Bronchioloalveolar carcinoma (rare)
      4. Hodgkin disease (rare)
   (b) Metastases (4% cavitate):
      1. Squamous cell carcinoma (2/3) nasopharynx (males), cervix (females), esophagus
      2. Adenocarcinoma (colorectal)
      3. Sarcoma: Ewing sarcoma, osteo-, myxo-, angiosarcoma
      4. Melanoma
      5. Seminoma, teratocarcinoma
      6. Wilms tumor

B. COLLAGEN-VASCULAR DISEASE
   1. Wegener granulomatosis + Wegener variant
   2. Rheumatoid nodules + Caplan syndrome
   3. SLE
   4. Periarteritis nodosa (rare)

C. GRANULOMATOUS DISEASE
   1. Histiocytosis X
   2. Sarcoidosis (rare)

D. VASCULAR DISEASE
   1. Pulmonary embolus with infarction
   2. Septic emboli (Staphylococcus aureus)

E. INFECTION
   1. Bacterial: pneumatoceles from staphylococcal / Gram-negative pneumonia
   2. Mycobacterial: TB
   3. Fungal: nocardiosis, cryptococcosis, coccidioidomycosis (in 10%), aspergillosis
   4. Parasitic: echinococcosis (multiple in 20–30%), paragonimiasis

F. TRAUMA
   1. Traumatic lung cyst (after hemorrhage)
   2. Hydrocarbon ingestion (lower lobes)

G. BRONCHOPULMONARY DISEASE
   1. Infected bulla
   2. Cystic bronchiectasis
   3. Communicating bronchogenic cyst

mnemonic: "CAVITY"

Carcinoma (squamous cell), **C**ystic bronchiectasis
Autoimmune disease (Wegener granulomatosis, rheumatoid lung)
Vascular (bland / septic emboli)
Infection (abscess, fungal disease, TB, Echinococcus)
Trauma
Young = congenital (sequestration, diaphragmatic hernia, bronchogenic cyst)

Pulmonary Mass With Air Bronchogram

1. Bronchioloalveolar carcinoma
2. Lymphoma
3. Pseudolymphoma
4. Kaposi sarcoma
5. Blastomycosis

Air-crescent Sign

= air in a crescentic shape separating the outer wall of a nodule / mass from an inner sequestrum

1. Invasive pulmonary aspergillosis
2. Noninvasive mycetoma
3. Septic emboli
4. Cavitating benign + malignant neoplasms
5. Echinococcal cyst
6. TB with Rasmussen aneurysms (most are too small to be identified on CXR)

Shaggy Pulmonary Nodule

mnemonic: "**S**haggy **S**ue **M**ade **L**oving **A** **R**eally **W**ild **F**antasy **T**oday"

Sarcoidosis, alveolar type
Septic emboli
Metastasis
Lymphoma, **L**ung primary, **L**ymphomatoid granulomatosis
Alveolar cell carcinoma
Rheumatoid lung
Wegener granulomatosis
Fungus
Tuberculosis

Hemorrhagic Pulmonary Nodule

√ CT halo sign = central area of soft-tissue attenuation surrounded by a halo of ground-glass attenuation

Causes:

A. HEMORRHAGIC INFARCTION
1. Early invasive aspergillosis
2. Hematogenous candidiasis
3. Herpes simplex, CMV, varicella-zoster virus

B. VASCULITIS
1. Wegener granulomatosis

C. FRAGILITY OF NEOVASCULAR TISSUE
1. Kaposi sarcoma
2. Metastatic angiosarcoma

D. BRONCHOARTERIAL FISTULA
1. Coccidioidomycosis

E. TRAUMA
1. Following lung biopsy

Multiple Nodules And Masses

√ homogeneous masses with sharp border
√ no air alveolo- / bronchogram

A. TUMORS
(a) malignant
1. Metastases:
from breast, kidney, GI tract, uterus, ovary, testes, malignant melanoma, sarcoma, Wilms tumor
2. Lymphoma (rare)
3. Multiple primary bronchogenic carcinomas (synchronous in 1% of all lung cancers)

(b) benign
1. Hamartoma (rarely multiple)
2. AV malformations
3. Amyloidosis

B. VASCULAR LESIONS
1. Thromboemboli with organizing infarcts
2. Septic emboli with organized infarcts

C. COLLAGEN-VASCULAR DISEASE
1. Wegener granulomatosis: vasculitis with organizing infarcts
2. Wegener variants
3. Rheumatoid nodules: tendency for periphery, occasionally cavitating

D. INFLAMMATORY GRANULOMAS
1. Fungal: coccidioidomycosis, histoplasmosis, cryptococcosis
2. Bacterial: nocardiosis, tuberculosis
3. Viral: atypical measles
4. Parasites: hydatid cysts, paragonimiasis
5. Sarcoidosis: large accumulation of interstitial granulomas
6. Inflammatory pseudotumors: fibrous histiocytoma, plasma cell granuloma, hyalinizing pulmonary nodules, pseudolymphoma

mnemonic: "SLAM DA PIG"

Sarcoidosis
Lymphoma
Alveolar proteinosis
Metastases
Drugs
Alveolar cell carcinoma
Pneumonias
Infarcts
Goodpasture syndrome

Small Pulmonary Nodules

mnemonic: "MALTS"

Metastases (esp. thyroid)
Alveolar cell carcinoma
Lymphoma, **L**eukemia
TB
Sarcoid

Pulmonary Nodules & Pneumothorax

1. Osteosarcoma
2. Wilms tumor
3. Histiocytosis

Pneumoconiosis Classification

according to ILO (International Labour Office)

A. TYPE OF OPACITIES
1. Silicosis, coal worker's pneumoconiosis
<u>nodular opacities</u>:
p = <1.5 mm
q = 1.5–3 mm
r = 3–10 mm
2.. Asbestosis
<u>linear opacities</u>:
s = fine
t = medium
u = coarse / blotchy

B. PROFUSION / SEVERITY
0 = normal
1 = slight
2 = moderate
3 = advanced

intermediate grading:
2/2 = definitely moderate profusion
2/3 = moderate, possibly advanced profusion

CHEST

Pneumoconiosis With Mass

Anthracosilicosis with:
1. Granuloma (histoplasmosis, TB, sarcoidosis)
2. Bronchogenic carcinoma (incidence same as in general population)
3. Metastasis
4. Progressive massive fibrosis
5. Caplan syndrome (rheumatoid nodules)

Pleura-based Lung Nodule

√ ill-defined / sharply defined lesion mimicking a true pleural mass
√ associated linear densities in lung parenchyma

Cause:
1. Granuloma (fungus, tuberculosis)
2. Inflammatory pseudotumor
3. Metastasis
4. Rheumatoid nodule
5. Pancoast tumor
6. Lymphoma
7. Infarct: Hampton hump
8. Atelectatic pseudotumor

Focal Area Of Ground-glass Attenuation

1. Bronchioloalveolar cell carcinoma
2. Pulmonary infiltrate with eosinophilia syndrome
   (a) simple pulmonary eosinophilia
   (b) idiopathic hypereosinophilic syndrome
   (c) parasitic infection
3. Lymphoma
4. Hemorrhagic nodule

Intrathoracic Mass Of Low Attenuation

A. CYSTS
   1. Bronchogenic / neurenteric / pericardial cyst
   2. Hydatid disease
B. FATTY SUBSTRATE
   1. Hamartoma
   2. Lipoma
   3. Tuberculous lymph node
   4. Lymphadenopathy in Whipple disease
C. NECROTIC MASSES
   1. Resolving hematoma
   2. Treated lymphoma
   3. Metastases from ovary, stomach, testes

PULMONARY CALCIFICATIONS

Multiple Pulmonary Calcifications

A. INFECTION
   1. Histoplasmosis
   2. Tuberculosis
   3. Chickenpox pneumonia
B. INHALATIONAL DISEASE
   1. Silicosis
C. MISCELLANEOUS
   1. Hypercalcemia
   2. Mitral stenosis
   3. Alveolar microlithiasis

Calcified Pulmonary Nodules

mnemonic: "**HAM TV S**tation"

Histoplasmosis, **H**amartoma
Amyloid, **A**lveolar microlithiasis
Mitral stenosis, **M**etastasis (thyroid, osteosarcoma, mucinous carcinoma)
Tuberculosis
Varicella
Silicosis

◊ Central / laminated / popcorn / diffuse calcifications are characteristic of benign solitary lung nodules!

LUCENT LUNG LESIONS

Hyperlucent Lung

Bilateral Hyperlucent Lung

A. FAULTY RADIOLOGIC TECHNIQUE
   1. Overpenetrated film
B. DECREASED SOFT TISSUES
   1. Thin body habitus
   2. Bilateral mastectomy
C. CARDIAC CAUSE of decreased pulmonary blood flow
   1. Right-to-left shunt:
      Tetralogy of Fallot (small proximal pulmonary vessels), pseudotruncus, truncus type IV, Ebstein malformation, tricuspid atresia
   2. Eisenmenger physiology of left-to-right shunt:
      ASD, VSD, PDA (dilated proximal pulmonary vessels)
D. PULMONARY CAUSE of decreased pulmonary blood flow
   (a) Decrease of vascular bed:
      1. Pulmonary embolism
         bilaterality is rare; localized areas of hyperlucency (Westermark sign)
   (b) Increase in air space:
      1. Air trapping (reversible changes):
         acute asthmatic attack, acute bronchiolitis (pediatric patient)
      2. Emphysema
      3. Bulla
      4. Bleb
      5. Interstitial emphysema

Unilateral Hyperlucent Lung

A. FAULTY RADIOLOGIC TECHNIQUE
   1. Rotation of patient
B. CHEST WALL DEFECT
   1. Mastectomy
   2. Absent pectoralis muscle (Poland syndrome)
C. INCREASED PULMONARY AIR SPACE with decreased pulmonary blood flow
   (a) Large airway obstruction with air trapping
      @ Bronchial compression:
         hilar mass (rare), cardiomegaly compressing LLL bronchus

@ Endobronchial obstruction with air trapping (collateral air drift):
foreign body, broncholith, bronchogenic carcinoma, carcinoid, bronchial mucocele

(b) Small airway obstruction
1. Bronchiolitis obliterans
2. Swyer-James / Macleod syndrome
3. Emphysema (particularly bullous emphysema)
4. Emphysema + unilateral lung transplant

(c) Pneumothorax (in supine patient)

D. PULMONARY VASCULAR CAUSE of decreased pulmonary blood flow
1. Pulmonary artery hypoplasia
2. Pulmonary embolism
3. Congenital lobar emphysema
4. Compensatory overaeration

Localized Lucent Lung Defect

A. CAVITY = tissue necrosis with bronchial drainage

(a) Infection

BACTERIAL PNEUMONIA
1. Pyogenic infection = abscess = necrotizing pneumonia:
Staphylococcus, Klebsiella, Pseudomonas, anaerobes, b-hemolytic streptococcus, E. coli, mixed Gram-negative organisms
2. Aspiration pneumonia = gravitational pneumonia:
mixed Gram-negative organisms, anaerobes

GRANULOMATOUS INFECTION
1. Tuberculosis
cavitation indicates active infectious disease with risk for hematogenous / bronchogenic dissemination
2. Fungal infection:
nocardiosis (in immunocompromised), coccidioidomycosis (any lobe, desert Southwest), histoplasmosis, blastomycosis, mucormycosis, sporotrichosis, aspergillosis, cryptococcosis
√ very thin-walled cavities less likely to follow apical distribution of TB / histoplasmosis
3. Sarcoidosis (stage IV, upper lobe predominance)
4. Angioinvasive organism (septic lung infarction followed by cavity formation):
Aspergillus, Mucorales, Candida, Torulopsis, P. aeruginosa

PARASITIC INFESTATION: hydatid disease

(b) Neoplasm

PRIMARY LUNG TUMOR: 16% of peripheral lung cancers (in particular in squamous cell carcinoma (30%); also in bronchioloalveolar cell carcinoma

METASTASIS (usually multiple)
1. Squamous cell carcinoma (nasopharynx, esophagus, cervix) in 2/3
2. Adenocarcinoma (lung, breast, GI)
3. Osteosarcoma (rare)
4. Melanoma
5. Lymphoma (rare): with adenopathy; cavities often secondary to opportunistic infection with nocardiosis + cryptococcosis

(c) Vascular occlusion
1. Infarct (thromboembolic, septic)
2. Wegener granulomatosis
3. Rheumatoid arthritis

(d) Inhalational
1. Silicosis with coal worker's pneumoconiosis
— complicating tuberculosis
— ischemic necrosis of center of conglomerate mass (rare)

B. CYST

(a) Cystic bronchiectasis
1. Cystic fibrosis (more obvious in upper lobes)
2. Agammaglobulinemia (predisposed to recurrent bacterial infections)
3. Recurrent bacterial pneumonias
√ multiple thin-walled lucencies with air-fluid levels in lower lobes
4. Childhood infection: tuberculosis, pertussis
5. Allergic bronchopulmonary aspergillosis (in asthmatic patients)
√ involvement of proximal perihilar bronchi
6. Kartagener syndrome (ciliary dysmotility)

(b) Pneumatocele
1. Postinfectious pneumatocele
2. Traumatic pneumatocele: lung hematoma / hydrocarbon inhalation

(c) Congenital lesion (rare)
1. Multiple bronchogenic cysts
2. Intralobar sequestration: multicystic structure in lower lobes
3. Congenital cystic adenomatoid malformation (CCAM) Type I
4. Diaphragmatic hernia (congenital / traumatic)

(d) Centrilobular / bullous emphysema

(e) Honeycomb lung

Multiple Lucent Lung Lesions

for details see causes of localized lucent lung defect

A. CAVITIES

(a) Infection
1. Bacterial pneumonia: cavitating pneumonia, lung abscess
2. Granulomatous infection: TB, sarcoidosis
3. Fungal infection: coccidioidomycosis
4. Parasitic infection: echinococcosis
5. Protozoan infection: pneumocystosis

(b) Neoplasm

(c) Vascular
1. Thromboembolic + septic infarcts
2. Wegener granulomatosis

CHEST

3. Rheumatoid arthritis
4. Angioinvasive organism (septic lung infarction followed by cavity formation): Aspergillus, Mucorales, Candida, Torulosis, P. aeruginosa

B. CYSTS
(a) Cystic bronchiectasis
1. Cystic fibrosis (more obvious in upper lobes)
2. Agammaglobulinemia (predisposed to recurrent bacterial infections)
3. Recurrent bacterial pneumonias
4. Tuberculosis
5. Allergic bronchopulmonary aspergillosis (in asthmatic patients)

(b) Pneumatoceles
(c) Congenital lesions (rare)
1. Multiple bronchogenic cysts
2. Intralobar sequestration: multicystic structure in lower lobes
3. Congenital cystic adenomatoid malformation (CCAM) Type I
4. Diaphragmatic hernia (congenital / traumatic)

(d) Centrilobular / bullous emphysema: blebs, bullae
(e) Tuberous sclerosis + lymphangiomyomatosis
(f) Honeycomb lung
(g) Juvenile pulmonary polyposis

Pulmonary Cyst

= round circumscribed space surrounded by an epithelial / fibrous wall of uniform / varied thickness containing air / liquid / semisolid / solid material

A. CONGENITAL CYST
1. Cystic adenomatoid malformation
2. Congenital lobar emphysema
3. Bronchial atresia
4. Bronchogenic cyst
5. Sequestration

B. ACQUIRED CYST
1. Pneumatocele (traumatic / infectious)
2. Pseudocyst (from interstitial emphysema)
3. Hydatid disease
4. **Bleb** = cystic air collection within visceral pleura; mostly apical with narrow neck; associated with spontaneous pneumothorax
5. **Bulla** = sharply demarcated dilated air space within lung parenchyma >1 cm in diameter with epithelialized wall <1 mm thick due to destruction of alveoli (= air cyst in localized / centrilobular / panlobular emphysema)
   • usually asymptomatic
   √ typically at lung apex
   √ slow progressive enlargement
   Cx: 1. Spontaneous pneumothorax
   2. "Vanishing lung" = large area of localized emphysema causing atelectasis + dyspnea
   Rx: surgical resection if bulla >33% of hemithorax

Multiple Pulmonary Cysts

A. INFECTION
1. Tuberculosis
2. Pneumocystis carinii pneumonia in AIDS

B. VASCULAR-EMBOLIC
1. Cavitating septic emboli
   √ often seen at end of feeding vessel
2. Angioinvasive infection (invasive pulmonary aspergillosis, candida, P. aeruginosa)
3. Pulmonary vasculitis (Wegener granulomatosis)

C. DILATATION OF BRONCHI = bronchiectasis
√ bronchial wall thickening

D. DISRUPTION OF ELASTIC FIBER NETWORK
1. Centrilobular emphysema
2. Panlobular emphysema
   √ lobular architecture preserved with bronchovascular bundle in central position, areas of lung destruction without arcuate contour
3. Lymphangiomyomatosis
   √ randomly scattered cysts in otherwise normal lung
4. Tuberous sclerosis
   √ associated skin abnormalities, mental retardation, epilepsy
5. Air-block disease (adult respiratory distress syndrome, asthma, bronchiolitis, viral / bacterial pneumonia)

E. REMODELING OF LUNG ARCHITECTURE
= honeycombing of idiopathic pulmonary fibrosis (= fibrosing alveolitis)
√ 3–10 mm small irregular thick-walled cystic air spaces usually of comparable diameter surrounded by abnormal lung parenchyma
√ predominantly peripheral + basilar distribution

F. MULTIFACTORIAL / UNKNOWN
1. Langerhans cell histiocytosis
   √ cysts with walls of variable thickness
   √ combination of nodules ± cavitation
   √ septal thickening
   √ predominant distribution in upper lung zones
2. Klippel-Trenaunay syndrome
3. Juvenile tracheolaryngeal papillomatosis
4. Neurofibromatosis
   √ cystic air spaces predominantly apical

Cystlike Pulmonary Lesions

mnemonic: "C.C., I BAN WHIPS"
Coccidioidomycosis
Cystic adenomatoid malformation
Infection
Bronchogenic cyst, **B**ronchiectasis, **B**owel
Abscess
Neoplasm
Wegener granulomatosis
Hydatid cyst, **H**istiocytosis X
Infarction
Pneumatocele
Sequestration

Multiple Thin-walled Cavities

mnemonic: "BITCH"

Bullae + pneumatoceles
Infection (TB, cocci, staph)
Tumor (squamous cell carcinoma)
Cysts (traumatic, bronchogenic)
Hydrocarbon ingestion

Mass Within Cavity

1. Mycetoma = aspergilloma
2. Tissue fragment within carcinoma
3. Necrotic lung within abscess
4. Disintegrating hydatid cyst
5. Intracavitary blood clot

MEDIASTINUM

Mediastinal Shift

= displacement of heart, trachea, aorta, hilar vessels
◊ expiration film, lateral decubitus film (expanded lung down), fluoroscopy help to determine side of abnormality

A. DECREASED LUNG VOLUME
  1. Atelectasis
  2. Postoperative (lobectomy, pneumothorax)
  3. Hypoplastic lung / lobe
     √ small pulmonary artery + small hilum
     √ decreased peripheral pulmonary vasculature
     √ irregular reticular vascular pattern (bronchial origin) without converging on the hilum
  4. Bronchiolitis obliterans = Swyer-James syndrome

B. INCREASED LUNG VOLUME
  = **air trapping** = retention of excess gas in all / part of the lung, especially during expiration, as a result of (a) complete / partial airway obstruction, or (b) local abnormalities in pulmonary compliance
  @ Major bronchus
    1. Foreign body obstructing main-stem bronchus (common in children) with ball-valve mechanism + collateral air drift
       √ contralateral mediastinal shift increasing with expiration
  @ Emphysema
    1. Bullous emphysema (localized form)
       √ large avascular areas with thin lines
    2. Congenital lobar emphysema: only in infants
    3. Interstitial emphysema
       √ pattern of diffuse coarse lines;
       Cx of positive pressure ventilation therapy
  @ Cysts / masses
    1. Bronchogenic cyst: with bronchial connection + check-valve mechanism
    2. Cystic adenomatoid malformation
    3. Large mass (pulmonary, mediastinal)

C. PLEURAL SPACE ABNORMALITY
  1. Large unilateral pleural effusion:
     opaque hemithorax through empyema, congestive failure, metastases
  2. Tension pneumothorax:
     not always complete collapse of lung
  3. Large diaphragmatic hernia:
     usually detected in neonatal period
  4. Large mass

D. Partial absence of pericardium / pectus excavatum
  √ shift of heart without shift of trachea, aorta, or mediastinal border

Pneumomediastinum

Pathophysiology:
alveolar rupture with air tracking along bronchovascular sheath into mediastinum + facial planes of the neck producing subcutaneous emphysema

Frequency: in 1% of patients with pneumothorax

√ streaky lucencies of air in mediastinum (look at thoracic inlet on PA + retrosternal space on LAT film)
√ "continuous diaphragm" sign = lucency connecting both domes of hemidiaphragms
√ "V-sign of Naclerio" = air between lower thoracic aorta + diaphragm
√ "spinnaker-sail" sign in children = air outlining the thymus

A. SPONTANEOUS PNEUMOMEDIASTINUM
  Age: neonates (0.05-1%), 2nd–3rd decade
  Causes:
  (a) rupture of marginally situated alveoli from sudden rise in intraalveolar pressure (acute asthma, aspiration pneumonia, hyaline membrane disease, measles, giant cell pneumonia, coughing, vomiting, strenuous exercise, parturition, diabetic acidosis)
  (b) tumor erosion of trachea / esophagus
  (c) pneumoperitoneum / retropneumoperitoneum = extension from peritoneal / retroperitoneal / deep fascial planes of the neck
  Cx: **air block** = buildup of pressure impeding blood flow in low-pressure veins; particularly common in neonatal period

B. TRAUMATIC PNEUMOMEDIASTINUM (rare)
  1. Pulmonary interstitial emphysema
     = disruption of marginal alveoli with gas traveling toward mediastinum due to positive pressure ventilation
  2. Bronchial / tracheal rupture
     √ commonly associated with pneumothorax
  3. Esophageal rupture (diabetic acidosis, alcoholic, Boerhaave syndrome)
  4. Iatrogenic - accidental
     neck / chest / abdominal surgery, subclavian vein catheterization, mediastinoscopy, bronchoscopy, gastroscopy, recto-sigmoido-colonoscopy, electrosurgery with intestinal gas explosion, positive pressure ventilation, intubation, barium enema

Mediastinal Fat

A. MEDIASTINAL LIPOMATOSIS
B. FAT HERNIATION
  = omental fat herniating into chest
  1. Foramen of Morgagni
     = cardiophrenic-angle mass, R >> L side

2. Foramen of Bochdalek
   = costophrenic-angle mass, almost always on left
3. Paraesophageal hernia = perigastric fat through phrenicoesophageal membrane

CT:
√ fat with fine linear densities (= omental vessels)

C. LIPOMA
un- / encapsulated with variable amount of fibrous septa
√ smooth + sharply defined boundaries
DDx: Liposarcoma, lipoblastoma (infancy), fat-containing teratoma, thymolipoma (inhomogeneous, higher CT numbers, poor demarcation, ± invasion of surrounding structures)

D. MULTIPLE SYMMETRIC LIPOMATOSIS
rare entity without involvement of anterior mediastinal / cardiophrenic / paraspinal areas
√ compression of trachea
√ periscapular lipomatous masses

Acute Mediastinal Widening

1. Rupture of aorta / brachiocephalic arteries
2. Venous hemorrhage: traumatic / iatrogenic (malpositioning of central venous line)
3. Congestive heart failure (venous dilatation)
4. Rupture of esophagus
5. Rupture of thoracic duct
6. Magnification on supine radiograph

Mediastinal Mass

(excluding hyperplastic thymus glands, granulomas, lymphoma, metastases)

1. Neurogenic tumors (28%) : malignant in 16%
2. Teratoid lesions (19%) : malignant in 15%
3. Enterogenous cysts (16%)
4. Thymomas (13%) : malignant in 46%
5. Pericardial cysts (7%)

◊ 75% of all mediastinal tumors are benign (in all age groups)
◊ 1/3 diagnosed on routine chest x-ray
◊ 2/3 found in association with symptoms (pain, cough, shortness of breath)
◊ 80% of malignant tumors are symptomatic

Thoracic Inlet Lesions

1. Thyroid mass
   1–3% of all thyroidectomies have a mediastinal component; 1/3 of goiters are intrathoracic
   Location: anterior (80%) / posterior (20%) mediastinum
   √ displacement of trachea posteriorly + laterally (anterior goiter)
   √ displacement of trachea anteriorly + esophagus posteriorly + laterally (posterior goiter)
   √ inhomogeneous density (cystic spaces, high-density iodine contents of >100 HU)
   √ focal calcifications (common)
   √ marked + prolonged contrast enhancement
   √ connection to thyroid gland
   √ vascular displacement + compression
   NUC (rarely helpful as thyroid tissue may be nonfunctioning):
   √ ± uptake on I-123 / I-131 scan (pertechnetate sufficient with modern gamma cameras, SPECT imaging may be helpful)
2. Cystic hygroma
   3–10% involve mediastinum; childhood
3. Lymphoma
4. Other tumors: adenoma, carcinoma, ectopic thymoma

Anterior Mediastinal Mass

mnemonic: "4 T's"
Thymoma
Teratoma
Thyroid tumor / goiter
Terrible lymphoma

A. SOLID THYMIC LESIONS
   1. Thymoma (benign, malignant): most common
   2. Normal thymus (neonate)
   3. Thymic hyperplasia (child)
   4. Thymolipoma
   5. Lymphoma
B. SOLID TERATOID LESIONS
   1. Teratoma
   2. Embryonal cell carcinoma
   3. Choriocarcinoma
   4. Seminoma
C. THYROID / PARATHYROID
   1. Substernal thyroid / intrathoracic goiter (10% of all mediastinal masses)
   2. Thyroid adenoma / carcinoma
   3. **Ectopic parathyroid adenoma**: ectopia in 10–22% (62–81% in anterior mediastinum / thymus, 30% within thyroid tissue, 8% in posterior superior mediastinum)
D. LYMPH NODES
   1. Lymphoma (Hodgkin, NHL): may arise in thymus, more common in young adults
   2. Metastases
   3. Benign lymph node hyperplasia
   4. Angioblastic lymphadenopathy
   5. Mediastinal lymphadenitis: sarcoidosis / granulomatous infection
E. CARDIOVASCULAR
   1. Tortuous brachiocephalic artery
   2. Aneurysm of ascending aorta
   3. Aneurysm of sinus of Valsalva
   4. Dilated SVC
   5. Cardiac tumor
   6. Epicardial fat-pad
F. CYSTS
   1. Cystic hygroma
   2. Bronchogenic cyst
   3. Extralobar sequestration
   4. Thymic cysts / dermoid cysts

5. Pericardial cyst: (a) true cyst
   (b) pericardial diverticulum
6. Pancreatic pseudocyst

G. OTHERS
1. Neural tumor (vagus, phrenic nerve)
2. Paraganglioma
3. Hemangioma / lymphangioma
4. Mesenchymal tumor (fibroma, lipoma)
5. Sternal tumors
   (a) metastases from breast, bronchus, kidney, thyroid
   (b) malignant primary (chondrosarcoma, myeloma, lymphoma)
   (c) benign primary (chondroma, aneurysmal bone cyst, giant cell tumor)
6. Primary lung / pleural tumor (invading mediastinum)
7. Mediastinal lipomatosis:
   (a) Cushing disease
   (b) Corticosteroid therapy
8. Morgagni hernia / localized eventration
9. Abscess

Middle Mediastinal Mass

mnemonic: "HABIT[5]"

Hernia, **H**ematoma
Aneurysm
Bronchogenic cyst / duplication cyst
Inflammation (sarcoidosis, histoplasmosis, coccidioidomycosis, primary TB in children)
Tumors - remember the 5 L's:
- **L**ung, especially oat cell carcinoma
- **L**ymphoma
- **L**eukemia
- **L**eiomyoma
- **L**ymph node hyperplasia

A. LYMPH NODES

◊ 90% of masses in the middle mediastinum are malignant

(a) Neoplastic adenopathy
1. Lymphoma (Hodgkin: NHL = 2 : 1)
2. Leukemia (in 25%): lymphocytic > granulocytic
3. Metastasis (bronchus, lung, upper GI, prostate, kidney)
4. Angioimmunoblastic lymphadenopathy

(b) Inflammatory adenopathy
1. Tuberculosis / histoplasmosis (may lead to fibrosing mediastinitis)
2. Blastomycosis (rare) / coccidioidomycosis
3. Sarcoidosis (predominant involvement of paratracheal nodes)
4. Viral pneumonia (particularly measles + cat-scratch fever)
5. Infectious mononucleosis / pertussis pneumonia
6. Amyloidosis
7. Plague / tularemia
8. Drug reaction
9. Giant lymph node hyperplasia = Castleman disease
10. Connective tissue disease (rheumatoid, SLE)
11. Bacterial lung abscess

(c) Inhalational disease adenopathy
1. Silicosis (eggshell calcification also in sarcoidosis + tuberculosis)
2. Coal worker's pneumoconiosis
3. Berylliosis

B. FOREGUT CYST
1. Bronchogenic / respiratory cyst: cartilage, respiratory epithelium
2. Enteric cyst = esophageal duplication cyst
3. Extralobar sequestration (anomalous feeding vessel)
4. Hiatal hernia
5. Esophageal diverticula: Zenker, traction, epiphrenic

C. PRIMARY TUMORS (infrequent)
1. Carcinoma of trachea
2. Bronchogenic carcinoma
3. Esophageal tumor: leiomyoma, carcinoma, leiomyosarcoma
4. Mesothelioma
5. Granular cell myoblastoma of trachea (rare)

D. VASCULAR LESIONS
1. Aneurysm of transverse aorta
2. Distended veins (SVC, azygos vein)
3. Hematoma

Posterior Mediastinal Mass

A. NEOPLASM

NEUROGENIC TUMOR (largest group): 30% malignant

(a) Tumor of peripheral nerve origin
- more common in adulthood
- √ 80% appear as round masses with sulcus
- √ lower attenuation than muscle (in 73%)

1. Schwannoma = neurilemoma (32%): derived from sheath of Schwann without nerve cells
2. Neurofibroma (10%): contains Schwann cells + nerve cells, 3rd + 4th decade
3. Malignant schwannoma

(b) Tumor of sympathetic ganglia origin
- more common in childhood
- √ 80% are elongated with tapered borders

1. Ganglioneuroma (23–38%): second most common tumor of posterior mediastinum after neurofibroma
2. Neuroblastoma (15%): highly malignant undifferentiated small round cell tumor originating in sympathetic ganglia, <10 years of age
3. Ganglioneuroblastoma (14%): both features, spontaneous maturation possible

(c) Tumors of paraganglia origin (rare)
1. Chemodectoma = paraganglioma (4%)

2. Pheochromocytoma
√ rib spreading, erosion, destruction
√ enlargement of neural foramina (dumbbell lesion)
√ scalloping of posterior aspect of vertebral body
√ scoliosis
CT: √ low-density soft-tissue mass (lipid contents)

SPINE TUMOR: metastases (eg, bronchogenic carcinoma, multiple myeloma), ABC, chordoma, chondrosarcoma, Ewing sarcoma
LYMPHOMA
INVASIVE THYMOMA
MESENCHYMAL TUMOR (fibroma, lipoma, leiomyoma)
HEMANGIOMA
LYMPHANGIOMA
THYROID TUMOR

B. INFLAMMATION / INFECTION
1. Infectious spondylitis: pyogenic, tuberculous, fungal
√ destruction of endplates + disk space
√ paravertebral soft-tissue mass
2. Mediastinitis
3. Lymphoid hyperplasia
4. Sarcoidosis (in 2%, typically asymptomatic patient)
5. Pancreatic pseudocyst

C. VASCULAR MASS
1. Aneurysm of descending aorta (curvilinear calcification; elderly)
2. Enlarged azygos + accessory hemiazygos vein
3. Esophageal varices
4. Congenital vascular anomalies: aberrant subclavian artery, double aortic arch, pulmonary sling, interruption of IVC with azygos / hemiazygos continuation

D. TRAUMA
1. Aortic aneurysm / pseudoaneurysm
2. Hematoma
3. Loculated hemothorax
4. Traumatic pseudomeningocele

E. FOREGUT CYST
√ cysts may demonstrate peripheral rimlike calcifications
1. Bronchogenic cyst
2. Enteric cyst
3. Neurenteric cyst
4. Extralobar sequestration

F. FATTY MASS
1. Bochdalek hernia
2. Mediastinal lipomatosis
3. Fat-containing tumors: lipoma, liposarcoma, teratoma (rare)

G. OTHER
1. Loculated pleural effusion
2. Pancreatic pseudocyst
3. Lateral meningocele (neurofibromatosis; enlarged neural foramen)
4. Extramedullary hematopoiesis: in chronic bone marrow deficiency; paraspinal area rich in RES-elements
√ splenomegaly; widening of ribs
5. "Pseudomass" of the newborn

mnemonic: "BELLMAN"
Bochdalek hernia
Extramedullary hematopoiesis
Lymphadenopathy
Lymphangioma
Meningocele (lateral)
Aneurysm
Neurogenic tumor

Aorticopulmonary Window Mass

1. Adenopathy
2. Traumatic aortic pseudoaneurysm
3. Pulmonary artery aneurysm
4. Bronchogenic cyst
5. Tumor of tracheobronchial tree
6. Esophageal tumor
7. Neurogenic tumor
8. Mediastinal abscess

Hypervascular Mediastinal Mass

1. Paraganglioma
2. Metastasis: typically renal cell carcinoma
3. Castleman disease
4. Hemangioma
5. Sarcoma
6. Tuberculosis
7. Sarcoidosis

Cardiophrenic-angle Mass

A. Lesion of pericardium
1. Pericardial cyst
2. Intrapericardiac bronchogenic cyst
3. Benign intrapericardiac neoplasm: teratoma, leiomyoma, hemangioma, lipoma
4. Malignant neoplasm: mesothelioma, metastasis (lung, breast, lymphoma, melanoma)

B. Cardiac lesion: aneurysm

C. Others: masses arising from lung, pleura, diaphragm, abdomen

RIGHT CARDIOPHRENIC-ANGLE MASS

A. Heart
1. Aneurysm (cardiac ventricle, sinus of Valsalva)
2. Dilated right atrium

B. Peri- / epicardium
1. Epicardial fat-pad / lipoma (most common cause)
√ triangular opacity in cardiophrenic angle less dense than heart
√ increase in size under corticosteroid treatment
2. Pericardial cyst

CHEST

C. Diaphragm
  1. Diaphragmatic hernia (Morgagni)
  2. Diaphragmatic lymph node (esp. in Hodgkin disease + breast cancer)
D. Anterior mediastinal mass
E. Primary lung mass
F. Paracardiac varices

Low-attenuation mediastinal mass

A. FLUID
  1. Foregut cyst
  2. Lymphocele
  3. Seroma
  4. Hematoma
  5. Abscess
  6. Hydatid disease
B. LYMPH NODE
  1. Tuberculous lymph nodes
  2. Metastasis from thyroid / testicular tumor
  3. Lymphoma: treated / untreated
C. PRIMARY NEOPLASM
  1. Neurogenic tumor
  2. Fat-containing neoplasm

Mediastinal cysts

= 21% of all primary mediastinal tumors, mostly developmental
1. Pericardial cyst
2. Thymic cyst
3. FOREGUT CYST
   (a) Bronchogenic cyst (54–63%)
   (b) Esophageal duplication cyst
   (c) Neurenteric cyst (least common)
4. **Lateral meningocele**
   = outpouching of leptomeninges through intervertebral foramen
   Etiology: in 75% neurofibromatosis
   √ spinal abnormalities (kyphoscoliosis, scalloping of dorsal vertebrae, enlargement of intervertebral foramen, pedicle erosion, thinning of ribs)
5. **Hydatid cyst**
   Location: paravertebral gutter
   √ erosion of ribs + vertebrae
6. **Thoracic duct cyst**
   rare, filled with chyle
   Etiology: degenerative / lymphangiomatous
7. Posttraumatic lymphocele
   = contained pleural / mediastinal lymph collection
   • history of prolonged chylous chest tube drainage
   Time of onset: several months after injury
8. Cystic hygroma
9. Parathyroid cyst
   uncommon as mediastinal mass

Hilar mass

A. LARGE PULMONARY ARTERIES
   √ enlargement of main pulmonary artery
   √ abrupt change in vessel caliber
   √ enlarged pulmonary artery compared with bronchus (in same bronchovascular bundle)
   √ cephalization
   √ enlargement of right ventricle (RAO 45°, LAO 60°)
   Cause:
   1. Chronic obstructive disease (emphysema)
   2. Chronic restrictive interstitial lung disease (idiopathic fibrosis, cystic fibrosis, rheumatoid arthritis, sarcoidosis)
   3. Pulmonary embolic disease (acute massive / chronic)
   4. Idiopathic pulmonary hypertension
   5. Left-sided heart failure + mitral stenosis
   6. Congenital heart disease with left-to-right shunt
      (a) acyanotic: ASD, VSD, PDA
      (b) cyanotic (admixture lesions): transposition of great vessels, truncus arteriosus
B. DUPLICATION CYST
C. UNILATERAL HILAR ADENOPATHY
   (a) NEOPLASTIC
      1. Bronchogenic carcinoma (most common)
      2. Metastases (lack of mediastinal involvement exceptional)
      3. Lymphoma
   (b) INFLAMMATORY
      1. Tuberculosis (primary) in 80%
      2. Fungal infection: histoplasmosis, coccidioidomycosis, blastomycosis
      3. Viral infections: atypical measles
      4. Infectious mononucleosis
      5. Drug reaction
      6. Sarcoidosis (in 1–3%)
      7. Bilateral lung abscess
   mnemonic: "**F**at **H**ila **S**uck"
      Fungus
      Hodgkin disease
      Squamous / oat cell carcinoma

D. BILATERAL HILAR ADENOPATHY
   (a) NEOPLASTIC
      1. Lymphoma (50% in Hodgkin disease)
      2. Metastases
      3. Leukemia
      4. Primary bronchogenic carcinoma
      5. Plasmacytoma
   (b) INFLAMMATORY
      1. Sarcoidosis (in 70–90%)
      2. Silicosis
      3. Histiocytosis X
      4. Idiopathic pulmonary hemosiderosis
      5. Chronic berylliosis
   (c) INFECTIOUS
      1. Rubella, ECHO virus, varicella, mononucleosis

   mnemonic: "**P**lease **H**elen **L**ick **M**y **P**opsicle **S**tick"
      Primary TB
      Histoplasmosis
      Lymphoma
      Metastases
      Pneumoconiosis
      Sarcoidosis

CHEST

Eggshell Calcification Of Nodes

A. PNEUMOCONIOSIS
  1. Silicosis (5%)
  2. Coal worker's pneumoconiosis (1.3–6%)
     not seen in: asbestosis, berylliosis, talcosis, baritosis
B. SARCOIDOSIS (5%)
C. FUNGAL + BACTERILA INFECTION (rare):
  1. Tuberculosis
  2. Histoplasmosis
  3. Coccidioidomycosis
D. FIBROSING MEDIASTINITIS
E. LYMPHOMA FOLLOWING RADIATION THERAPY

Enlargement Of Azygos Vein

Normal azygos vein (on upright CXR): ≤7 mm

A. COLLATERAL CIRCULATION
  1. Portal hypertension
  2. SVC obstruction / compression below azygos vein
  3. IVC obstruction / compression
  4. Interrupted IVC with azygos continuation
  5. Partial anomalous venous return (rare)
  6. Pregnancy
  7. Hepatic vein occlusion
B. RIGHT ATRIAL HYPERTENSION
  1. Right-sided heart failure
  2. Constrictive pericarditis
  3. Large pericardial effusion

THYMUS

Thymic Mass

1. Thymoma
2. Thymolipoma
3. Thymic cyst
4. Thymic carcinoid

Diffuse Thymic Enlargement

1. Thymic hyperplasia
2. Thymic infiltration
   by leukemia, Hodgkin lymphoma, non-Hodgkin lymphoma, histiocytosis
   • presence of adenopathy elsewhere
   √ no pleural implants
3. Thymic hemorrhage

TRACHEA & BRONCHI

Tracheal Tumor

• asthma symptomatology
• hoarseness, cough
• wheeze (inspiratory with extrathoracic lesion, expiratory with intrathoracic lesion)
• hemoptysis

A. BENIGN
  1. Cartilaginous tumor (hamartoma)
  2. Squamous cell papilloma
  3. Fibroma / lipoma
  4. Hemangioma
  5. Granular cell myoblastoma
  6. Granuloma (inflammatory, TB, fungus)
  7. Amyloid tumor
B. MALIGNANT
  1. Squamous-cell carcinoma (commonest primary)
  2. Adenoid cystic carcinoma = cylindroma
  3. Metastasis from renal cell carcinoma, colon cancer, malignant melanoma
  4. Lymphoma
  5. Plasmacytoma

Endobronchial Tumor

1. Neuroendocrine tumor (typical / atypical carcinoid)
2. Mucoepidermoid carcinoma
3. Adenoid cystic carcinoma
4. Hamartoma
5. Leiomyoma
6. Myoblastoma
7. Mucous gland adenoma
8. Squamous cell carcinoma

Bronchial Obstruction

1. Foreign body: most commonly in young children
2. Granulomatous disease: due to granuloma formation in bronchial wall / extrinsic compression by adenopathy
3. Broncholiths = erosion of calcified nodes into bronchial lumen
4. Stenosis / atresia
5. Neoplasm
   (a) Bronchogenic carcinoma
   (b) Adenoid cystic carcinoma
   (c) Mucoepidermoid tumor
   (d) Hamartoma

mnemonic: "MEATFACE"
Mucus plug
Endobronchial granulomatous disease
Adenoma
Tuberculosis
Foreign body
Amyloid, **A**tresia (bronchial)
Cancer (primary)
Endobronchial metastasis

Mucoid Impaction

= BRONCHIAL MUCOCELE = BRONCHOCELE
= accumulation of inspissated secretions (mucus / pus / inflammatory products) within bronchial lumen; usually associated with bronchial dilatation

A. WITH BRONCHIAL OBSTRUCTION in the presence of collateral air drift
  1. Bronchial obstruction by neoplasm: bronchogenic carcinoma / adenoma
  2. Bronchial atresia
B. WITHOUT BRONCHIAL OBSTRUCTION
  1. Asthma (most frequent cause): esp. during acute attack or convalescent phase
  2. Fluid-filled bronchiectasis: history of childhood pneumonia; peripheral distribution

3. Bronchopulmonary aspergillosis: central perihilar bronchiectasis
4. Cystic fibrosis
5. Chronic bronchitis

Signet-ring sign

= ring of opacity in association with smaller round soft-tissue opacity (usually thick-walled bronchus + adjacent pulmonary artery / dilated bronchial artery)

1. Bronchiectasis
2. Multifocal bronchioloalveolar carcinoma
3. Metastatic adenocarcinoma

HRCT classification of bronchiolar disease

[CT findings are nonspecific and must be interpreted in the appropriate clinical context]

√ nodules and branching lines
1. Acute infectious bronchiolitis in infants and young children (RSV, adenovirus, Mycoplasma)
2. Diffuse panbronchiolitis in Orientals
3. Chronic inflammation: asthma, chronic bronchitis, bronchiectasis

√ ground-glass attenuation and consolidation
1. BOOP
2. Respiratory bronchiolitis = smokers' bronchiolitis

√ low attenuation and mosaic perfusion
1. Constrictive bronchiolitis
2. Swyer-James syndrome

√ bronchiolocentric infiltrates
1. Extrinsic allergic alveolitis
2. Sarcoidosis (perivenular nodules)
3. Pneumoconiosis: asbestosis, silicosis

Bronchial wall thickening

◊ Apparent thickness of bronchial wall varies with lung window chosen on CT: a mean window that is too low can make bronchial wall appear abnormal!

A. PERIBRONCHOVASCULAR
   1. Sarcoidosis
   2. Lymphangitic carcinomatosis
   3. Kaposi sarcoma
   4. Lymphoma
   5. Pulmonary edema
B. BRONCHIAL WALL
   1. Airway disease
C. MUCOSA

Broncholithiasis

1. Histoplasmosis
2. Tuberculosis
3. Cryptococcosis
4. Actinomycosis
5. Coccidioidomycosis

√ calcified lymph node within / adjacent to affected bronchus
√ bronchial obstruction: atelectasis, airspace disease, bronchiectasis, air trapping
√ absence of associated soft-tissue mass

PLEURA

Pneumothorax

= accumulation of air in the pleural space

Pathophysiology: disruption of visceral pleura / trauma to parietal pleura

• pleuritic back / shoulder pain, dyspnea (in 80–90%)

Etiology:
1. Penetrating trauma
2. Blunt trauma
   (a) rib fracture
   (b) increased intrathoracic pressure against closed glottis: lung contusion / laceration
   (c) bronchial rupture
      √ fallen lung sign = hilum of lung below expected level within chest cavity
      √ persistent pneumothorax with functioning chest tube
      √ mediastinal pneumothorax
3. Iatrogenic
   tracheostomy, central venous catheter, PEEP ventilator (3–16%), thoracic irradiation
4. **Primary / idiopathic spontaneous pneumothorax**
   Cause: rupture of subpleural blebs in apical region of lung
   Age: 20–40 years; M:F = 8:1; esp. in patients with tall asthenic stature; mostly in smokers
   • chest pain (69%)
   • dyspnea
   Prognosis: recurrence in 30% on same side, in 10% on contralateral side
   Rx: simple aspiration (in >50% success) / tube thoracostomy (in 90% effective)
5. Other causes:
   (a) Neonatal disease: meconium aspiration, respirator therapy for hyaline membrane disease
   (b) Malignancy: primary lung cancer, lung metastases (esp. osteosarcoma, pancreas, adrenal, Wilms tumor)
   (c) Pulmonary infections: tuberculosis, necrotizing pneumonia, coccidioidomycosis, hydatid disease, pertussis, acute bacterial pneumonia, staphylococcal septicemia, AIDS (Pneumocystis carinii, Mycobacterium tuberculosis, atypical mycobacteria)
   (d) Cx of honeycomb lung: pulmonary fibrosis, cystic fibrosis, sarcoidosis, scleroderma, eosinophilic granuloma, interstitial pneumonitis, histiocytosis X, rheumatoid lung, idiopathic pulmonary hemosiderosis, pulmonary alveolar proteinosis, biliary cirrhosis
   (e) Spasmodic asthma, diffuse emphysema
      ◊ Chronic obstructive pulmonary disease is the most common predisposing disorder of secondary spontaneous pneumothorax
   (f) **Catamenial pneumothorax** = recurrent spontaneous pneumothorax during menstruation associated with endometriosis of the diaphragm; R >> L
   (g) Marfan syndrome, Ehlers-Danlos syndrome

(h) Pulmonary infarction
(i) Lymphangiomyomatosis + tuberous sclerosis

mnemonic: "THE CHEST SET"

Trauma
Honeycomb lung, **H**amman-Rich syndrome
Emphysema, **E**sophageal rupture
Chronic obstructive pulmonary disease
Hyaline membrane disease
Endometriosis
Spontaneous, **S**cleroderma
Tuberous sclerosis
Sarcoma (osteo-), **S**arcoidosis
Eosinophilic granuloma
Tuberculosis + fungus

Types:

1. Closed pneumothorax = intact thoracic cage
2. Open pneumothorax = "sucking" chest wound
3. **Tension pneumothorax**
   = accumulation of air within pleural space due to free ingress + limited egress of air
   Pathophysiology:
   intrapleural pressure exceeds atmospheric pressure in lung during expiration (check-valve mechanism)
   Frequency: in 3–5% of patients with spontaneous pneumothorax, higher in barotrauma
   √ displacement of mediastinum / anterior junction line
   √ deep sulcus sign = on frontal view larger lateral costodiaphragmatic recess than on opposite side
   √ diaphragmatic inversion
   √ total / subtotal lung collapse
   √ collapse of SVC / IVC / right heart border (decreased systemic venous return + decreased cardiac output)
   N.B.: Medical emergency!
4. **Tension hydropneumothorax**
   √ sharp delineation of visceral pleural by dense pleural space
   √ mediastinal shift to opposite side
   √ air-fluid level in pleural space on erect CXR

PNEUMOTHORAX SIZE

Average Interpleural Distance (AID) = (A + B + C) ÷ 3 [in cm] converts to percentage of pneumothorax

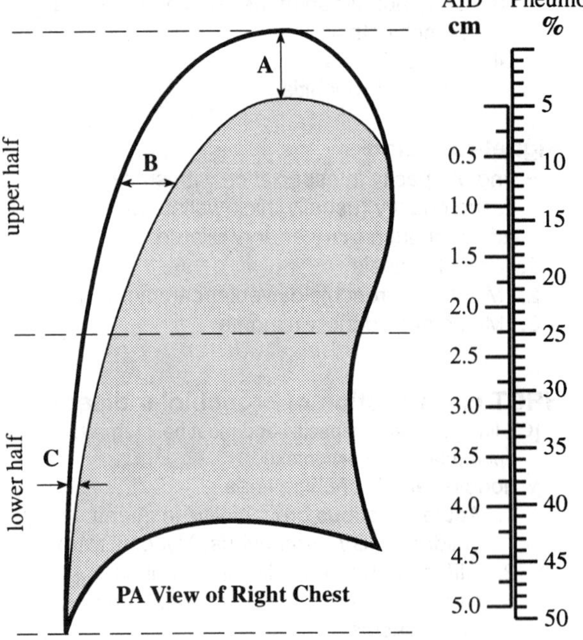

A = maximum apical interpleural distance
B = interpleural distance at midpoint of upper half of lung
C = interpleural distance at midpoint of lower half of lung

Radiographic signs in upright position:

√ white margin of visceral pleura separated from parietal pleura
DDx: skin fold, air trapped between chest wall soft tissues, hair braid)
√ absence of vascular markings beyond visceral pleural margin

Radiographic signs in supine position:

1. Anteromedial pneumothorax (earliest location)
   √ outline of medial diaphragm under cardiac silhouette
   √ sharp delineation of mediastinal contours (SVC, azygos vein, left subclavian artery, anterior junction line, superior pulmonary vein, heart border, IVC, deep anterior cardiophrenic sulcus, pericardial fat-pad)
2. Subpulmonic pneumothorax (second most common location)
   √ hyperlucent upper abdominal quadrant
   √ deep lateral costophrenic sulcus
   √ sharply outlined diaphragm in spite of parenchymal disease
   √ visualization of anterior costophrenic sulcus
   √ visualization of inferior surface of lung
3. Apicolateral pneumothorax (least common location)
   √ visualization of visceral pleural line
4. Posteromedial pneumothorax (in presence of lower lobe collapse)
   √ lucent triangle with vertex at hilum
   √ V-shaped base delineating costovertebral sulcus
5. Pneumothorax outlines pulmonary ligament

Prognosis: resorption of pneumothorax occurs at a rate of 1.25% per day (accelerated by increasing inspired oxygen concentrations)

Pleural Effusion

A. TRANSUDATE (protein level of 1.5–2.5 g/dL)
   Pathophysiology: result of systemic abnormalities causing an outpouring of low-protein fluid

(a) Increased hydrostatic pressure
1. Congestive heart failure (in 65%)
bilateral (88%); right-sided (8%); left-sided (4%); least amount on left side due to cardiac movement, which stimulates lymphatic resorption
2. Constrictive pericarditis (in 60%)

(b) Decreased colloid-oncotic pressure
— decreased protein production
1. Cirrhosis with ascites (in 6%): right-sided (67%)

— protein loss / hypervolemia
1. Nephrotic syndrome (21%), overhydration, glomerulonephritis (55%), peritoneal dialysis
2. Hypothyroidism

(c) Chylous effusion
◊ Most frequent cause of isolated pleural effusion in newborn with 15–25% mortality!
• chylomicrons + lymphocytes in fluid

B. EXUDATE
Pathophysiology: increased permeability of abnormal pleural capillaries with release of high-protein fluid into pleural space
Criteria:
• pleural fluid total protein / serum total protein ratio of >0.5
• pleural fluid LDH / serum LDH ratio of >0.6
• pleural fluid LDH >2/3 of upper limit of normal for serum LDH (upper limit for LDH ~200 IU)
• pleural fluid specific gravity >1.016
• protein level >3 g/dL

√ effusion with septation / low-level echoes
√ "split pleura" sign on CECT = thickened enhancing visceral + parietal pleura separated by fluid
√ extrapleural fat thickening of >2 mm + increased attenuation (edema / inflammation)

(a) Infection
1. **Empyema**
= parapneumonic effusion characterized by presence of pus ± positive culture
— *exudative phase* = inflammation of visceral pleura results in increased capillary permeability with weeping of high-protein fluid into pleural space
— *fibrinopurulent phase* = inflammatory cells + neutrophils pour into pleural space + fibrin deposition on pleural surfaces
— *organizing phase* = recruitment of fibroblasts + capillaries results in deposition of collagen + granulation tissue on pleural surfaces = pleural fibrosis
Rx: decortication if active infection persists
Organism: S. aureus, gram-negative + anaerobic bacteria
• positive Gram stain
• positive culture (anaerobic bacteria most frequent)
• gross pus (WBC >15, 000/cm³)
• pH <7.0
• LDH >1000 IU/L
• glucose <40 mg/dL
2. Parapneumonic effusion (in 40%)
= any effusion associated with pneumonia / lung abscess / bronchiectasis without criteria for an empyema
3. Tuberculosis (in 1%):
high protein content (75 g/dL), lymphocytes >70%, positive culture (only in 20–25%)
4. Fungi: Actinomyces, Nocardia
5. Parasites: amebiasis (secondary to liver abscess in 15–20%), Echinococcus
6. Mycoplasma, rickettsia (in 20%)

empyema necessitatis = chronic empyema attempting to decompress through chest wall (in TB, actinomycosis, aspergillosis, blastomycosis, nocardiosis)

(b) Malignant disease (in 60%)
• positive cytologic results
Cause: lung cancer (26–49%), breast cancer (8–24%), lymphoma (10–28%, in 2/3 chylothorax), ovarian cancer (10%), malignant mesothelioma containing hyaluronic acid (5%)
Pathogenesis:
— pleural metastases (increase pleural permeability)
— lymphatic obstruction (pleural vessels, mediastinal nodes, thoracic duct disruption)
— bronchial obstruction (loss of volume + resorptive surface)
— hypoproteinemia (secondary to tumor cachexia)
Rx: sclerosing agents: doxycycline, bleomycin, talc

(c) Vascular
Pulmonary emboli (in 15–30% of all embolic events): often serosanguinous

(d) Abdominal disease
1. Pancreatitis / pancreatic pseudocyst / pancreaticopleural fistula (in 2/3):
√ usually left-sided pleural effusion
• high amylase levels
2. Boerhaave syndrome:
left-sided esophageal perforation
3. Subphrenic abscess
√ pleural effusion (79%)
√ elevation + restriction of diaphragmatic motion (95%)
√ basilar platelike atelectasis / pneumonitis (79%)
4. Abdominal tumor with ascites

5. **Meigs-Salmon syndrome**
   = primary pelvic neoplasms (ovarian fibroma, thecoma, granulosa cell tumor, Brenner tumor, cystadenoma, adenocarcinoma, fibromyoma of uterus) cause pleural effusion in 2–3%; ascites + hydrothorax resolve with tumor removal
6. Endometriosis
7. Bile fistula

(e) Collagen-vascular disease
1. Rheumatoid arthritis (in 3%):
   unilateral; R > L (in 75%), recurrent alternating sides; pleural effusion relatively unchanged in size for months; predominantly in men; LOW GLUCOSE content of 20–50 mg/dL (in 70–80%) without increase following IV infusion of glucose (DDx: TB, metastatic disease, parapneumonic effusion)
2. SLE (in 15–74%)
   most common collagenosis to give pleural effusion, bilateral in 50%; L > R
   √ enlargement of cardiovascular silhouette (in 35–50%)
3. Wegener granulomatosis (in 50%)
4. Sjögren syndrome
5. Mixed connective tissue disease
6. Periarteritis nodosa
7. Postmyocardial infarct syndrome

(f) Traumatic
hemorrhagic, chylous, esophageal rupture, thoracic / abdominal surgery, intrapleural infusion = "infusothorax" (0.5%), radiation pneumonitis

(g) Miscellaneous
1. Sarcoidosis
2. Uremic pleuritis (in 20% of uremic patients)
3. Drug-induced effusion

CHEST

CXR:
√ first 300 ml not visualized on PA view (collect in subpulmonic region first, then spill into posterior costophrenic sinus)
√ lateral decubitus views may detect as little as 25 ml
√ hemidiaphragm + costophrenic sinuses obscured
√ extension upward around posterior > lateral > anterior thoracic wall (mediastinal portion fixed by pulmonary ligament + hilum)
√ meniscus-shaped semicircular upper surface with lowest point in midaxillary line
√ associated collapse of ipsilateral lung

Massive pleural effusion:
√ enlargement of ipsilateral hemithorax
√ displacement of mediastinum to contralateral side
√ severe depression / flattening / inversion of ipsilateral hemidiaphragm
√ visible air bronchogram

Subpulmonic / subdiaphragmatic / infrapulmonary pleural effusion:
√ peak of dome of pseudodiaphragm laterally positioned
√ acutely angulated costophrenic angle
√ increased distance between stomach bubble and lung
√ blunted posterior costophrenic sulcus
√ thin triangular paramediastinal opacity (mediastinal extension of pleural effusion)
√ flattened pseudodiaphragmatic contour anterior to major fissure (on lateral CXR)

CT:
√ fluid outside diaphragm
√ fluid elevating crus of diaphragm
√ indistinct fluid-liver interface
√ fluid posteromedial to liver (= bare area of liver)
CAVE: "central oval" sign of ascites may be seen in subpulmonic effusion with inverted diaphragm

Unilateral pleural effusion
◊ The majority of massive unilateral pleural effusions are malignant (lymphoma, metastatic disease, primary lung cancer)!
1. Neoplasm
2. Infection: TB
3. Collagen vascular disease
4. Subdiaphragmatic disease
5. Pulmonary emboli
6. Trauma: fractured rib
7. Chylothorax

Left-sided pleural effusion
1. Spontaneous rupture of the esophagus
2. Dissecting aneurysm of the aorta
3. Traumatic rupture of aorta distal to left subclavian artery
4. Transection of distal thoracic duct
5. Pancreatitis: left-sided (68%), right-sided (10%), bilateral (22%)
6. Pancreatic + gastric neoplasm

Right-sided pleural effusion
1. Congestive heart failure
2. Transection of proximal thoracic duct
3. Pancreatitis

Pleural effusion + large cardiac silhouette
1. Congestive heart failure (most common)
   √ cardiomegaly
   √ prominence of upper lobe vessels + constriction of lower lobe vessels
   √ prominent hilar vessels
   √ interstitial edema (fine reticular pattern, Kerley lines, perihilar haze, peribronchial thickening)
   √ alveolar edema (perihilar confluent ill-defined densities, air bronchogram)
   √ "phantom tumor" = fluid localized to interlobar pleural fissure (in 78% in right horizontal fissure)

2. Pulmonary embolus with right-sided heart enlargement
3. Myocarditis / pericarditis with pleuritis
   (a) viral infection
   (b) tuberculosis
   (c) rheumatic fever (poststreptococcal infection)
4. Tumor: metastatic, mesothelioma
5. Collagen-vascular disease
   (a) SLE (pleural + pericardial effusion)
   (b) rheumatoid arthritis

Pleural effusion + subsegmental atelectasis
1. Postoperative (thoracotomy, splenectomy, renal surgery) secondary to thoracic splinting + small airway mucous plugging
2. Pulmonary embolus
3. Abdominal mass
4. Ascites
5. Rib fractures

Pleural effusion + lobar densities
1. Pneumonia with empyema
2. Pulmonary embolism
3. Neoplasm
   (a) bronchogenic carcinoma (common)
   (b) lymphoma
4. Tuberculosis

Pleural effusion + hilar enlargement
1. Pulmonary embolus
2. Tumor
   (a) bronchogenic carcinoma
   (b) lymphoma
   (c) metastasis
3. Tuberculosis
4. Fungal infection (rare)
5. Sarcoidosis (very rare)

Hemothorax
A. TRAUMA
   1. Closed / penetrating injury
   2. Surgery
   3. Interventional procedures: thoracentesis, pleural biopsy, catheter placement

B. BLEEDING DIATHESIS
   1. Anticoagulant therapy
   2. Thrombocytopenia
   3. Factor deficiency

C. VASCULAR
   1. Pulmonary infarct
   2. Arteriovenous malformation
   3. Aortic dissection
   4. Leaking atherosclerotic aneurysm

D. MALIGNANCY
   1. Mesothelioma
   2. Lung cancer
   3. Metastasis
   4. Leukemia

E. OTHER
   1. Catamenial hemorrhage
   2. Extramedullary hematopoiesis

√ rapidly enlarging high-attenuation pleural effusion on CT
√ heterogeneous attenuation
√ hyperattenuating areas of debris
√ fluid-hematocrit level

Solitary pleural mass
= density with incomplete border and tapered superior + inferior borders, difficult to distinguish from chest wall mass (rib destruction reliable sign of chest wall mass)

1. Loculated pleural effusion ("vanishing tumor")
2. Organized empyema
3. Metastasis
4. Local benign mesothelioma
5. Subpleural lipoma: may erode adjacent rib
6. Hematoma
7. Mesothelial cyst
8. Neural tumor: schwannoma, neurofibroma
9. **Localized fibrous tumor of pleura**
10. **Fibrin bodies**
    = 3–4 cm large tumorlike concentrations of fibrin forming in serofibrinous pleural effusions; usually near lung base

Multiple pleural densities
√ diffuse pleural thickening with lobulated borders

1. Loculated pleural effusion:
   infectious, hemorrhagic, neoplastic
2. Pleural plaques
3. Metastasis (most common cause)
   Origin: lung (40%), breast (20%), lymphoma (10%), melanoma, ovary, uterus, GI tract, pancreas, sarcoma
   ◊ Metastatic adenocarcinoma histologically similar to malignant mesothelioma!
4. Diffuse malignant mesothelioma
   almost always unilateral, associated with asbestos exposure
5. Invasive thymoma (rare)
   √ contiguous spread, invasion of pleura, spreads around lung
   √ NO pleural effusion
6. **Thoracic splenosis**
   = autotransplantation of splenic tissue to pleural space following thoracoabdominal trauma; discovered 10–30 years later
   • asymptomatic / recurrent hemoptysis
   √ one or several nodules in left pleura / fissures measuring several mm to 6 cm
   √ positive Tc-99m–sulfur colloid scan, indium-111–labeled platelets, Tc-99m–labeled heat-damaged RBCs

CHEST

mnemonic: "**M**ary **T**yler **M**oore **L**ikes **L**emon"
Metastases (especially adenocarcinoma)
Thymoma (malignant)
Malignant mesothelioma
Loculated pleural effusion
Lymphoma

Pleural Thickening

A. TRAUMA
  1. **Fibrothorax** (most common cause)
     = organizing effusion / hemothorax / pyothorax
     √ dense fibrous layer of approx. 2 cm thickness; almost always on visceral pleura
     √ frequent calcification on inner aspect of pleural peel
B. INFECTION
  1. Chronic empyema: over bases; history of pneumonia; parenchymal scars
  2. Tuberculosis / histoplasmosis: lung apex; associated with apical cavity
  3. Aspergilloma: in preexisting cavity concomitant with pleural thickening
C. COLLAGEN-VASCULAR DISEASE
  1. Rheumatoid arthritis: pleural effusion fails to resolve
D. INHALATIONAL DISORDER
  1. Asbestos exposure: lower lateral chest wall; basilar interstitial disease (<25%); thickening of parietal pleura with sparing of visceral pleura
  2. Talcosis
E. NEOPLASM
  (a) Metastases: often nodular appearance; may be obscured by effusion
  (b) Diffuse malignant mesothelioma
  (c) Pancoast tumor
F. OTHER
  1. **Pleural hyaloserositis**
     Path: hyaline sclerotic tissue = cartilagelike whitish sugar icing appearance (Zuckerguss) with occasional calcification
  2. Mimicked by extrathoracic musculature, 1st + 2nd rib companion shadow, subpleural fat, focal scarring around old rib fractures

mnemonic: "TRINI"
Trauma (healed hemothorax)
Rheumatoid arthritis (collagen vascular disease)
Inhalation disease (asbestosis, talcosis)
Neoplasm
Infection

Apical Cap

1. Inflammatory process: TB, healed empyema
2. Postradiation fibrosis
3. Neoplasm
4. Vascular abnormality
5. Mediastinal hemorrhage
6. Mediastinal lipomatosis
7. Peripheral upper lobe collapse

Pleural Calcification

A. INFECTION
  1. Healed empyema
  2. Tuberculosis (and Rx for TB: pneumothorax / oleothorax), histoplasmosis
B. TRAUMA
  1. Healed hemothorax = fibrothorax:
     • Hx of significant chest trauma
     √ irregular plaques of calcium usually in visceral pleura
     √ healed rib fracture
  2. Radiation therapy
C. PNEUMOCONIOSIS
  1. Asbestos-related pleural disease (most common):
     √ combination of basilar reticular interstitial disease (<1/3) + pleural thickening
     √ calcifications of parietal pleura frequently diagnostic (diaphragmatic surface of pleura, bilateral but asymmetric)
  2. Talcosis: similar to asbestos-related disease
  3. Bakelite
  4. Muscovite mica
D. HYPERCALCEMIA
  1. Pancreatitis
  2. Secondary hyperparathyroidism in chronic renal failure / scleroderma
E. MISCELLANEOUS
  1. Mineral oil aspiration
  2. Pulmonary infarction

mnemonic: "TAFT"
Tuberculosis
Asbestosis
Fluid (effusion, empyema, hematoma)
Talc

DIAPHRAGM

Bilateral Diaphragmatic Elevation

A. Shallow inspiration (most frequent)
B. Abdominal causes
   Obesity, pregnancy, ascites, large abdominal mass
C. Pulmonary causes
   (1) Bilateral atelectasis
   (2) Restrictive pulmonary disease (SLE)
D. Neuromuscular disease
   (1) Myasthenia gravis
   (2) Amyotrophic lateral sclerosis

Unilateral Diaphragmatic Elevation

1. Subpulmonic pleural effusion
   √ dome of pseudodiaphragm migrates toward the costophrenic angle and flattens
2. Altered pulmonary volume
   (a) Atelectasis
       √ associated pulmonary density
   (b) Postoperative lobectomy / pneumonectomy
       √ rib defects, metallic sutures

CHEST

(c) Hypoplastic lung
√ small hemithorax (more often on the right), crowding of ribs, mediastinal shift, absent / small pulmonary artery, frequently associated with dextrocardia + anomalous pulmonary venous return
3. Phrenic nerve paralysis
(a) Primary lung tumor
(b) Malignant mediastinal tumor
(c) Iatrogenic
(d) Idiopathic
√ paradoxic motion on fluoroscopy (patient in lateral position sniffing)
4. Abdominal disease
(a) Subphrenic abscess: history of surgery, accompanied by pleural effusion
(b) Distended stomach / colon
(c) Interposition of colon
(d) Liver mass (tumor, echinococcal cyst, abscess)
5. Diaphragmatic hernia
6. Eventration of diaphragm
7. Traumatic rupture of diaphragm
Associated with rib fractures, pulmonary contusion, hemothorax
8. Diaphragmatic tumor
Mesothelioma, fibroma, lipoma, lymphoma, metastases

CHEST WALL

Chest Wall Lesions

A. EXTERNAL
1. Cutaneous lesion: moles, neurofibroma
2. Nipples
3. Artifact

B. NEOPLASTIC
1. Mesenchymal tumor
(a) Lipoma (common): growing between ribs presenting as intrathoracic + subcutaneous mass; CT diagnostic)
(b) Muscle tumor, fibroma
2. Neural tumor
Schwannoma, neurofibroma (may erode ribs inferiorly with sclerotic bone reaction), neuroma, neuroblastoma
3. Vascular tumor
Hemangioma, lymphangioma, hemangiopericytoma, aneurysm, false aneurysm
4. Bone tumor *(see also Rib lesion)*

C. TRAUMATIC
1. Hematoma
2. Rib fracture

D. INFECTIOUS
cellulitis, pyomyositis, abscess, necrotizing fasciitis
1. Actinomycosis (parenchymal infiltrate, pleural effusion, chest wall mass, rib destruction, cutaneous fistulas)
2. Aspergillosis, nocardiosis, blastomycosis, tuberculosis (rare)
3. Pyogenic: Staphylococcus, Klebsiella

E. CHEST WALL INVASION
1. Peripheral lung cancer (eg, Pancoast tumor)
2. Recurrent breast cancer
3. Lymphomatous nodes

√ incomplete border sign (due to obtuse angle)
√ smooth tapering borders (tangential views)
√ tumor pedicle suggests a benign tumor

Lung Disease With Chest Wall Extension

A. Infectious
1. Actinomycosis
2. Nocardia
3. Blastomycosis
4. Tuberculosis

B. Malignant tumor
1. Bronchogenic carcinoma
2. Lymphoma
3. Metastases
4. Mesothelioma
5. Breast carcinoma
6. Internal mammary node

C. Benign tumor
1. Capillary hemangioma of infancy
2. Cavernous hemangioma
3. Extrapleural lipoma
4. Abscess
5. Hematoma

Malignant Tumors Of Chest Wall In Children

1. Ewing sarcoma of rib (most common)
(a) older child: rib involvement in 7%, predominant involvement of pelvis + lower extremity
(b) child <10 years: rib involvement in 30%
2. Rhabdomyosarcoma
relatively common in children + adolescents
√ sclerosis / destruction / scalloping of cortex (local extension to contiguous bone)
√ may calcify
Metastases to: lung, occasionally lymph nodes
Prognosis: infiltrative growth with high risk of local recurrence
3. Neuroblastoma
10% present as chest wall mass
√ may calcify
4. **Askin tumor**
= uncommon tumor probably arising from intercostal nerves in young Caucasian females
Path: neuroectodermal small cell tumor containing neuron-specific enolase (may also be found in neuroblastoma)
√ rib destruction
√ pleural effusion
Metastases to: bone, CNS, liver, adrenal

DDx: Chest wall hamartoma in infancy

Pancoast Syndrome

= superior sulcus tumor invading brachial plexus + sympathetic stellate ganglion

CHEST

CLINICAL TRIAD:
1. Ipsilateral arm pain
2. Muscle wasting of hand
3. Horner syndrome = enophthalmos, ptosis, miosis, anhidrosis

Cause: lung cancer (most common), breast cancer, multiple myeloma, metastases, lymphoma, mesothelioma

PULMONARY MALFORMATION
= SEQUESTRATION SPECTRUM
1. Congenital lobar emphysema
2. Bronchogenic cyst
3. Congenital cystic adenomatoid malformation
4. Bronchopulmonary sequestration
5. Hypogenetic lung syndrome
6. Pulmonary arteriovenous malformation

NEONATAL LUNG DISEASE

Mediastinal Shift & Abnormal Aeration
A. SHIFT TOWARD LUCENT LUNG
   1. Diaphragmatic hernia
   2. Chylothorax
   3. Cystic adenomatoid malformation

B. SHIFT AWAY FROM LUCENT LUNG
   1. Congenital lobar emphysema
   2. Persistent localized pulmonary interstitial emphysema
   3. Obstruction of main-stem bronchus (by anomalous or dilated vessel / cardiac chamber)

Reticulogranular Densities In Neonate
1. Respiratory distress syndrome (90%): premature infant, inadequate surfactant
2. Immature lung: premature infant, normal surfactant
3. Transient tachypnea of the newborn
4. Neonatal group-B streptococcal pneumonia
5. Idiopathic hypoglycemia
6. Congestive heart failure
7. Early pulmonary hemorrhage
8. Infant of diabetic mother

Hyperinflation In Newborn
1. Fetal aspiration syndrome
2. Neonatal pneumonia
3. Pulmonary hemorrhage
4. Congenital heart disease
5. Transient tachypnea (mild)

Hyperinflation In Child
mnemonic: "BUMP FAD"

Bronchiectasis
Upper airway obstruction
Mucoviscidosis
Pneumonia (esp. staph)
Foreign body (ball-valve mechanism)
Asthma
Dehydration (diarrhea, acidosis)

PULMONARY HEMORRHAGE
A. WITHOUT RENAL DISEASE
   1. Bleeding diathesis: leukemia
   2. Anticoagulation therapy
   3. Disseminated intravascular coagulation
   4. Blunt trauma
   5. Idiopathic pulmonary hemosiderosis
   6. Limited Wegener granulomatosis
   7. Infectious diseases
   8. Exogenous agents: D-penicillamine, lymphangiography

B. WITH RENAL DISEASE
   1. Goodpasture syndrome = anti-basement membrane antibody disease
   2. Collagen vascular disease + systemic vasculitides: SLE, Wegener granulomatosis, polyarteritis nodosa, Henoch-Schönlein purpura, Behçet disease
   3. Rapidly progressive glomerulonephritis ± immune complexes

C. HEMORRHAGIC PNEUMONIA
   1. Bacteria: Legionnaires' disease
   2. Viruses: CMV, herpes
   3. Fungi: Aspergillosis, mucormycosis

BEDSIDE CHEST RADIOGRAPHY
Unexpected findings: in 37–43%
Change in diagnostic approach / therapy: in 27%
Indications:

A. Apparatus position + complications
   1. Malposition of tracheal tube (12%)
   2. Malposition of central venous line (9%)

B. Cardiopulmonary disease
   1. Congestive heart failure
   2. Pleural effusion
   3. Atelectasis
   4. Alveolar disease
   5. Air leak
   6. Lung trauma
   7. Thoracic bleeding
   8. Mediastinal disease

FUNCTION AND ANATOMY OF LUNG

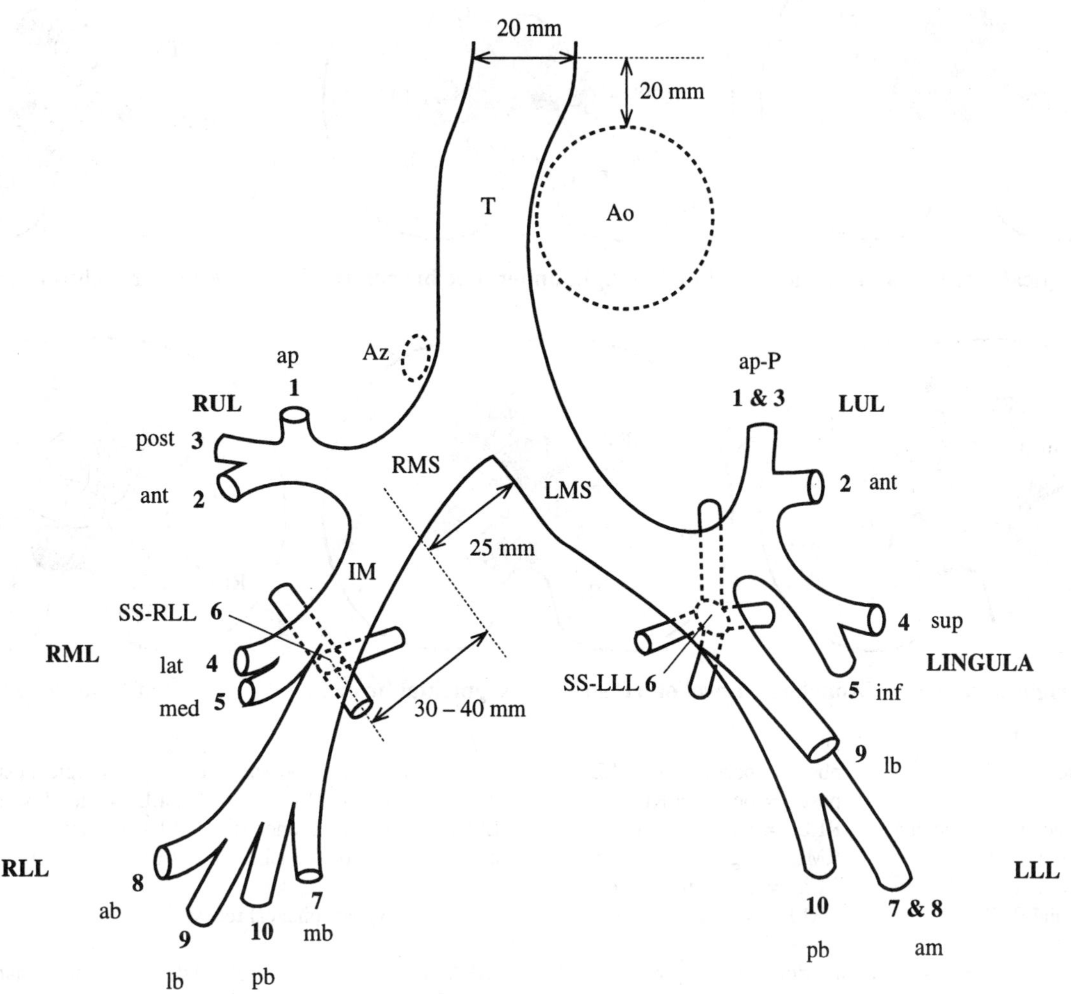

Bronchopulmonary Anatomy

Ao	=	aortic arch	RMS	=	right mainstem bronchus (2nd order bronchus)
Az	=	azygos vein	LMS	=	left mainstem bronchus
T	=	trachea (1st order bronchus)	IM	=	intermediate bronchus
SS-RLL	=	superior segment right lower lobe	SS-LLL	=	superior segment left lower lobe

RUL = right upper lobe
- 1 = apical
- 2 = anterior
- 3 = posterior

RML = right middle lobe
- 4 = lateral
- 5 = medial

RLL = right lower lobe
- 6 = superior
- 7 = mediobasal
- 8 = anterobasal
- 9 = laterobasal
- 10 = posterobasal

LUL = left upper lobe (3rd order bronchus)
- 1&3 = apicoposterior segment
- 2 = anterior (4th order bronchus)
- 4 = superior lingula
- 5 = inferior lingula

LLL = left lower lobe
- 6 = superior
- 7&8 = anteromedial
- 9 = laterobasal
- 10 = posterobasal

Order of lower lobe bronchi in frontal projection from lateral to medial:
mnemonic "ALPm" = **A**nterior-**L**ateral-**P**osterior-medial

CHEST

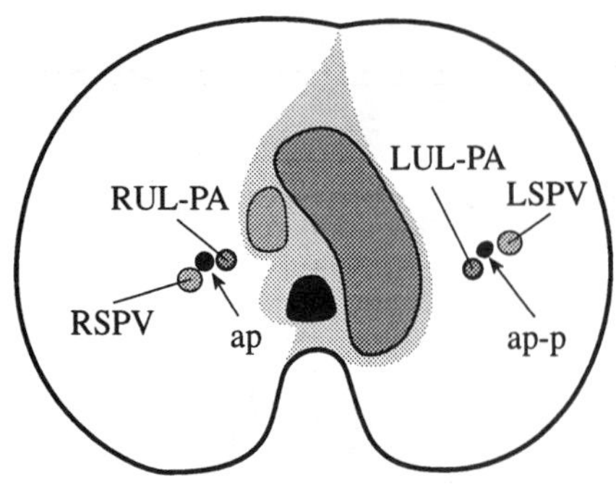

Level of apical segmental bronchus

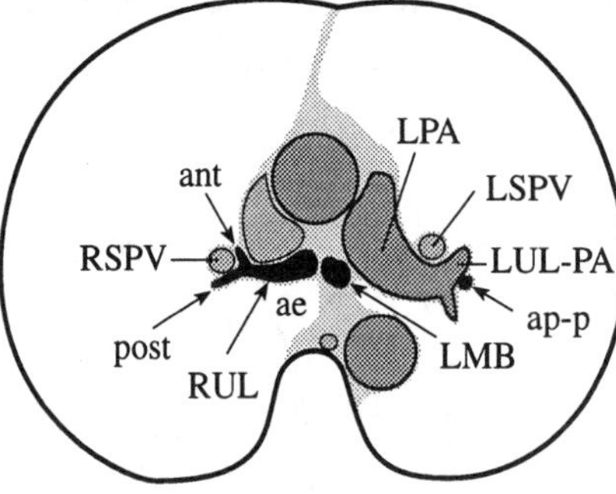

Level of right upper lobe bronchus

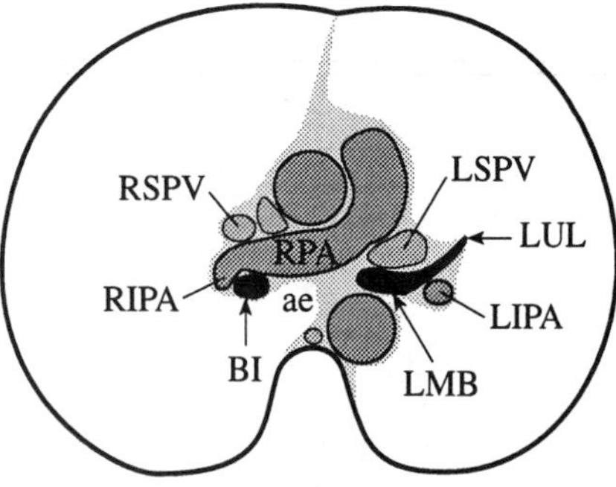

Level of bronchus intermedius

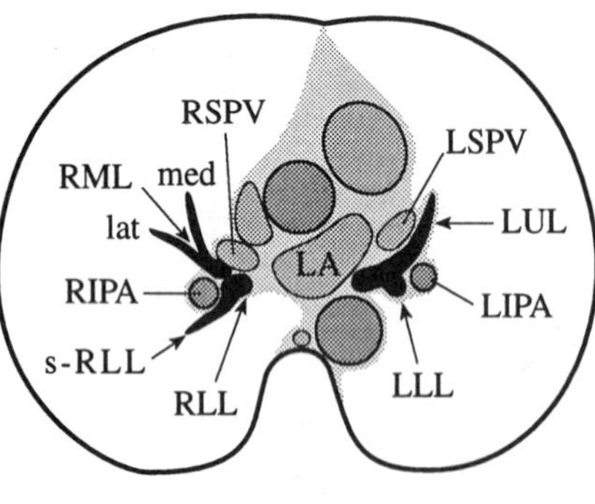

Level of right middle lobe bronchus

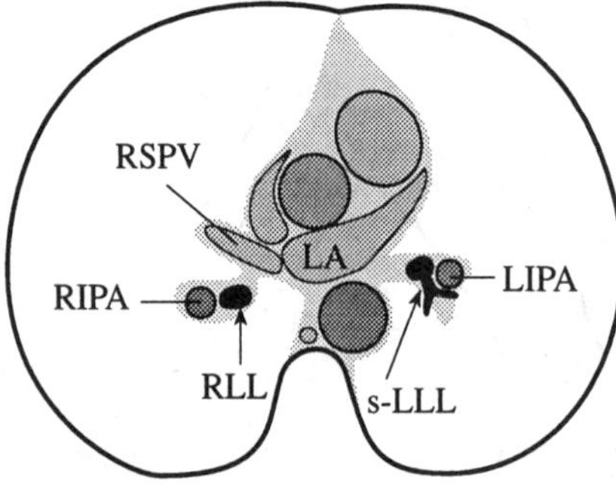

Level of left superior segmental bronchus

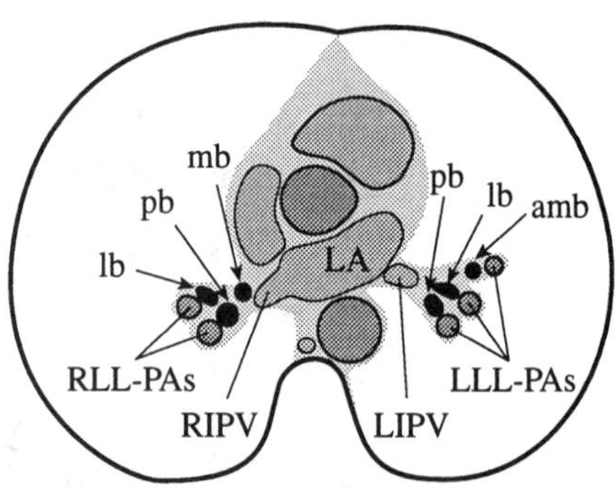

Level of lower lobe bronchi

Right

ant	= anterior RUL	pb	= posterobasal RLL
ap	= apical RUL	post	= posterior RUL
BI	= bronchus intermedius	RLL	= right lower lobe
lat	= lateral RML	RML	= right middle lobe
mb	= mediobasal RLL	RUL	= right upper lobe
med	= medial RML	s-RLL	= superior segment

Left

amb	= anteromediobasal LLL	ap-p	= apicoposterior LUL
lb	= laterobasal LLL	LLL	= left lower lobe
LMB	= left main bronchus	LUL	= left upper lobe
pb	= posterobasal LLL	s-LLL	= superior segment
ae	= azygoesophageal recess		

RIPV / LIPV	= right / left inferior pulmonary vein
RPA / LPA	= right / left pulmonary artery
RUL-PA / LUL-PA	= right / left upper lobe pulmonary artery
RIPA / LIPA	= right / left inferior pulmonary artery
RLL-PAs / LLL-PAs	= right / left lower lobe pulmonary arteries
RSPV / LSPV	= right / left superior pulmonary vein

Cross-sectional Anatomy of Bronchovascular Divisions

Embryology of airways

first 5 weeks GA	lung buds grow from ventral aspect of primitive foregut; *pulmonary agenesis*
5th week GA	trachea + esophagus separate
5–16 weeks	formation of tracheobronchial tree with bronchi, bronchioles, alveolar ducts, alveoli; *bronchogenic cyst* (= abnormal budding); *pulmonary hypoplasia* (= fewer than expected bronchi)
16–24 weeks	dramatic increase in number + complexity of airspaces and blood vessels; *small airways + reduction in number and size of acini*

Airway

= conducting branches for the transport of air; ~300,000 branching airways from trachea to bronchiole with an average of 23 airway generations

Definition:

bronchus = cartilage in wall

bronchiole = absence of cartilage

- membranous bronchiole = purely air conducting
- respiratory bronchiole = containing alveoli in their walls
- lobular bronchiole = supplies secondary pulmonary lobule; may branch into 3 or more terminal bronchioles
- terminal bronchiole = last generation of purely conducting bronchioles; each supplying one acinus

small airways = diameter <2 mm = small cartilaginous bronchi + membranous and respiratory bronchioles; account for 25% of airway resistance

large airways = diameter >2 mm; account for 75% of airway resistance

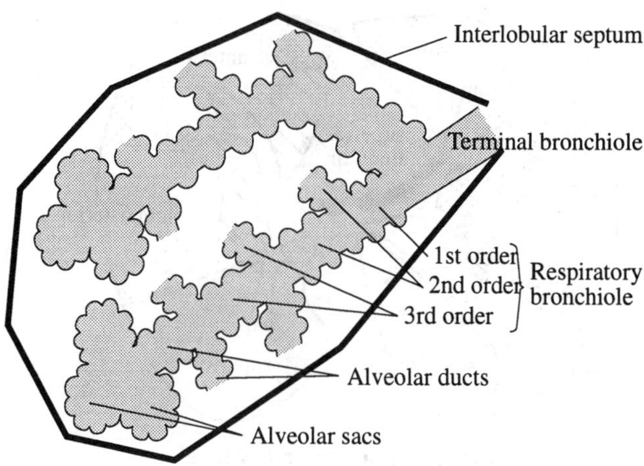

The Secondary Pulmonary Lobule

HRCT of normal lung (window level -700 HU, window width 1,000–1,500):
- √ -875 ± 18 HU at inspiration;
- √ -620 ± 43 HU at expiration

Acinus

= functionally most important subunit of lung = all parenchymal tissue distal to one terminal bronchiole comprising 2–5 generations of respiratory bronchioles + alveolar ducts + alveolar sacs + alveoli

√ radiologically not visible

[Primary Pulmonary Lobule]

= alveolar duct + air spaces connected with it

Secondary Pulmonary Lobule

= REID LOBULE

= smallest portion of lung surrounded by connective tissue septa = basic anatomic + functional pulmonary unit appearing as an irregular polyhedron measuring 10–25 mm on each side; separated from each other by thin fibrous interlobular septa (100 μm); supplied by 3–5 terminal bronchioles; contains 3–24 acini

Contents:
- — centrally = lobular core: branches of terminal bronchioles (0.1 mm wall thickness is below the resolution of HRCT) + pulmonary arterioles (1 mm)
- — peripherally (in interlobular septa): pulmonary veins + lymph vessels

HRCT:
- √ barely visible fine lines of increased attenuation in contact with pleura (= interlobular septa); best developed in subpleural areas of
  - — UL + ML: anterior + lateral + juxtamediastinal
  - — LL: anterior + diaphragmatic regions
- √ dotlike / linear / branching structures (= pulmonary arterioles) near center of secondary pulmonary lobule 3–5 mm from pleura

Surfactant

= surface-active material essential for normal pulmonary function

Substrate:
phospholipids (phosphatidylcholine, phosphatidylglycerol), other lipids, cholesterol, lung-specific proteins

Production:
type II pulmonary alveoli synthesize + transport + secrete lung surfactant; earliest production around 18th week of gestation (in amniotic fluid by 22nd week of gestation)

Action:
increases lung compliance, stabilizes alveoli, enhances alveolar fluid clearance, reverses surface tension, protects against alveolar collapse during respiration, protects epithelial cell surface, reduces opening pressure + precapillary tone

LUNG INTERSTITIUM

Division	*Components*
axial	bronchovascular sheaths lymphatics
middle (parenchymal)	alveolar wall (interalveolar septum)
peripheral	pleura subpleural connective tissue interlobular septa (enclosing pulmonary veins, lymphatics, walls of cortical alveoli)

LUNG FUNCTION

Lung Volumes & Capacities

1. Tidal volume (**TV**)
   = amount of gas moving in and out with each respiratory cycle
2. Residual volume (**RV**)
   = amount of gas remaining in the lung after a maximal expiration
3. Total lung capacity (**TLC**)
   = gas contained in lung at the end of a maximal inspiration

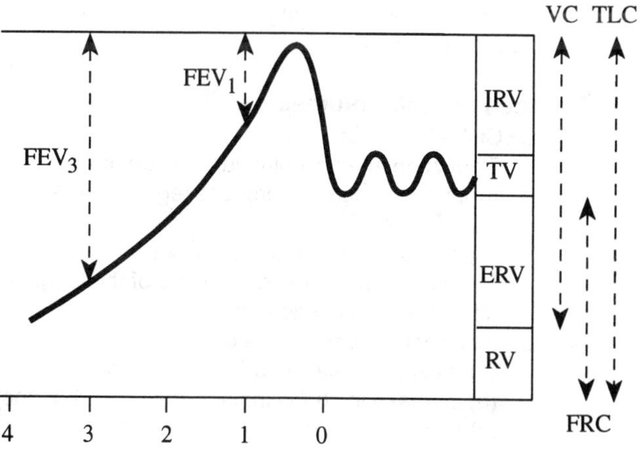

CHEST

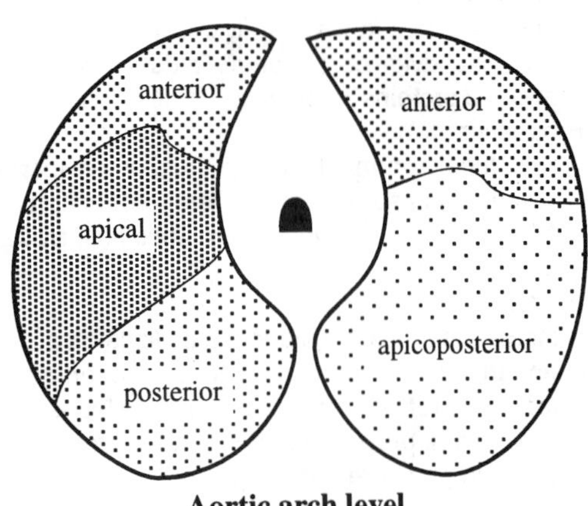

Aortic arch level

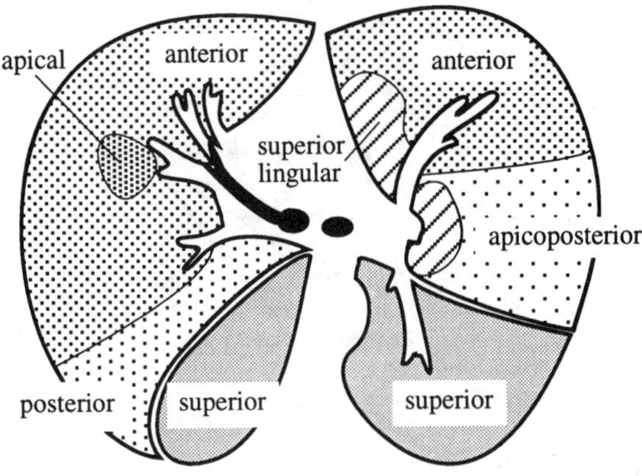

Left pulmonary artery level

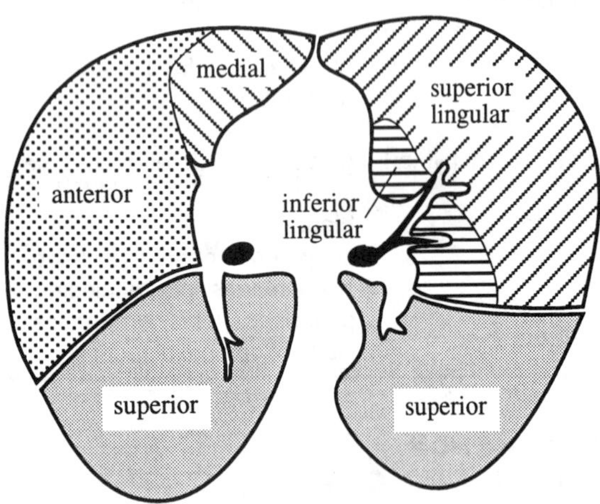

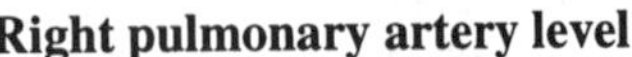

Right pulmonary artery level

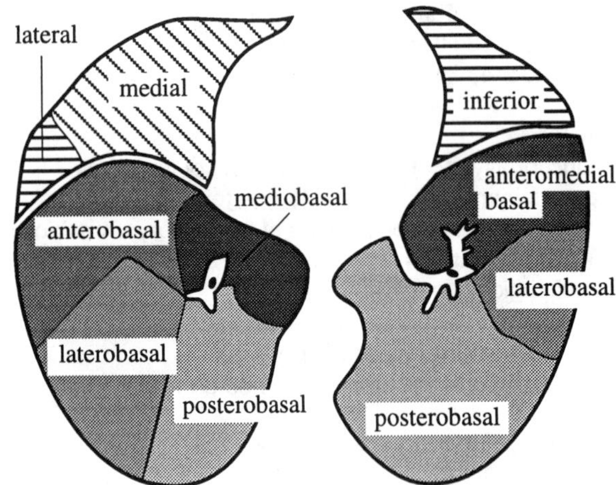

Cardiac ventricular level

Cross-sectional Anatomy of Lung Segments

4. Vital capacity (**VC**)
   = amount of gas that can be expired after a maximal inspiration without force
5. Functional residual capacity (**FRC**)
   = volume of gas remaining in lungs at the end of a quiet expiration

Changes in lung volumes

A. DECREASED VC:
   1. Reduction in functioning lung tissue due to
      (a) space-occupying process (eg, pneumonia, infarction)
      (b) surgical removal of lung tissue
   2. Process reducing overall volume of the lungs (eg, diffuse pulmonary fibrosis)
   3. Inability to expand lungs due to
      (a) muscular weakness (eg, poliomyelitis)
      (b) increase in abdominal volume (eg, pregnancy)
      (c) pleural effusion

B. INCREASED FRC and RV:
   characteristic of air trapping and overinflation (eg, asthma, emphysema)
   Associated with: increased TLC

C. DECREASED FRC and RV:
   1. Process reducing overall volume of lungs (eg, diffuse pulmonary fibrosis)
   2. Process that occupies volume within alveoli (eg, alveolar microlithiasis)
   3. Process that elevates diaphragm (eg, ascites, pregnancy), usually associated with decreased TLC

Flow rates

A. Spirometric measurements:
   1. Forced expiratory volume (FEV)
      = amount of air expired during a certain period (usually 1 + 3 sec);
      Normal values: $\mathbf{FEV_1}$ = 83%; $\mathbf{FEV_3}$ = 97%

2. Maximal midexpiratory flow rate (MMFR)
   = amount of gas expired during the middle half of forced expiratory volume curve (largely effort independent)
   Indicator of small airway resistance
3. Flow-volume loop
   = gas flow is plotted against the actual volume of lung at which this flow is occurring
   Useful in identifying obstruction in large airways

B. Resistance in small airways
   Closing volume = lung volume at which dependent lung zones cease to ventilate because of airway closure in small airway disease or loss of lung elastic recoil
   • decrease in FEV, MMFR, MBC:
     (a) expiratory airway obstruction (reversible as in spasmodic asthma / irreversible as in emphysema)
     (b) respiratory muscle weakness

Diffusing Capacity

= rate of gas transfer across the alveolocapillary membrane in relation to a constant pressure difference across it; measured by the carbon monoxide diffusion method

Reduction:

1. Ventilation / perfusion inequality: less CO is taken up by poorly ventilated or poorly perfused areas (eg, emphysema)
2. Reduction of total surface area (eg, emphysema, surgical resection)
3. Reduction in permeability from thickening of alveolar membrane (eg, cellular infiltration, edema, interstitial fibrosis)
4. Anemia with lack of hemoglobin

Arterial Blood Gas Abnormalities

• decreased pulmonary arterial O_2:
  1. alveolar hypoventilation
  2. impaired diffusion
  3. abnormal ventilation/perfusion ratios
  4. anatomic shunting

• elevated pulmonary arterial CO_2:
  1. alveolar hypoventilation
  2. impaired ventilation / perfusion ratios

V/Q Inequality

A. NORMAL
   (a) blood flow decreases rapidly from base to apex
   (b) ventilation decreases less rapidly from base to apex
   ◊ V/Q is low at base and high at apex
   ◊ Pulmonary arterial O_2 is substantially higher at apex
   ◊ Pulmonary arterial CO_2 is substantially higher at base

B. ABNORMAL
   chiefly resulting from non- / underventilated lung regions (non- / underperfused regions do not result in blood gas disturbances)

Compliance

= relationship of the change in intrapleural pressure to the volume of gas that moves into the lungs

A. DECREASED COMPLIANCE
   edema, fibrosis, granulomatous infiltration
B. INCREASED COMPLIANCE
   emphysema (faulty elastic architecture)

√ height of diaphragm at TLC can provide some indication of lung compliance, particularly valuable in sequential roentgenograms for comparison in:
  1. Diffuse interstitial pulmonary edema
  2. Diffuse interstitial pulmonary fibrosis

THYMUS

Origin: residual thymic tissue in neck in 1.8 – 21%

Embryogenesis:
dorsal + ventral wings of 3rd (and possibly 4th) branchial pouch begin to form the primordia of the inferior parathyroid and thymic glands at 4th–5th week of gestation; both glands separate from pharyngeal wall + migrate caudally and medially with the thymus pulling the inferior parathyroid glands along the thymopharyngeal tract; thymic primordium fuses with its contralateral counterpart inferior to thyroid gland; thymic tail thins + disappears by 8th week

Thymic weight:
increases from birth to age 11 – 12 years (22 ± 13 g in neonate, 34 ± 15 g at puberty); ratio of thymic weight to body weight decreases with age (involution after puberty, total fatty replacement after age 60)

√ measurement (perpendicular to axis of aortic arch): <18 mm before age 20; <13 mm after age 20
√ triangular shape like an arrowhead (62%), bilobed (32%), single lobe (6%)
√ muscular density of 30 HU (before puberty)
√ flat / concave borders with abundant fat (after puberty)
√ detected in 83% of subjects <50 years of age; in 17% of subjects >50 years of age
◊ atrophies under stress (due to increase in endogenous steroids)

Ectopic Tymus

√ solid mass
√ cystic mass (= endodermal-lined cavity of thymopharyngeal duct / cystic degeneration of Hassall corpuscles or glandular epithelium)

(1) Unilateral failure of thymic primordium to descend
  √ neck mass of thymic tissue on one side of neck
  √ ipsilateral absence of normal thymic lobe
  √ parathyroid tissue within ectopic thymus
(2) Small rest of thymus left behind within thymopharyngeal tract during migration
  √ neck mass
  √ normally positioned bilobed thymus
(3) Atypical location: trachea, skull base, intrathyroidal

CHEST DISORDERS

ACUTE EOSINOPHILIC PNEUMONIA

Etiology: idiopathic (no evidence of infection / exposure to potential antigens) with abrupt increase in lung cytokines

Age: 32 ± 17 years; M>F

Histo: eosinophilic infiltrates + pulmonary edema (from release of eosinophilic granules altering vascular permeability)

- acute respiratory failure in previously healthy individuals
- markedly elevated levels of eosinophils in bronchoalveolar lavage fluid
- no peripheral eosinophilia
- acute febrile illness of 1–5 days duration, myalgia

√ bilateral interstitial + air space opacities
√ pleural effusion

Rx: IV corticosteroids

Dx: bronchoscopy with bronchopulmonary lavage

DDx: chronic eosinophilic pneumonia (infiltrates with peripheral predominance)

AIDS

= Acquired immune deficiency syndrome
= ultimately fatal disease characterized by HIV seropositivity, specific opportunistic infections, specific malignant neoplasms (Kaposi sarcoma, Burkitt lymphoma, primary lymphoma of brain)
= patient with CD4 cell count <200 cells/μL (normal range, 800–1,200 cells/μL)

Incidence: 2 million Americans are infected with HIV + 270,000 have AIDS (estimate in 1993); >50% develop pulmonary disease

AIDS-related complex (ARC)
= GENERALIZED LYMPHADENOPATHY SYNDROME
= prodromal phase of HIV seropositivity, generalized lymphadenopathy, CNS diseases other than those associated with AIDS

Time interval: approximately 10 years between seroconversion + clinical AIDS

- weight loss, malaise, diarrhea
- fever, night sweats, lymphadenopathy
- lymphopenia with selective decrease in helper T-cells

Organism: human immunodeficiency virus (HIV) = human T-cell lymphotropic virus type III (HTLV III) = lymphadenopathy-associated virus (LAV)

Pathomechanism:
HIV retrovirus attaches to CD4 molecule on surface of T-helper lymphocytes + macrophages + microglial cells; after cellular invasion HIV genetic information is incorporated into cell's chromosomal DNA; virus remains dormant for weeks to years; after an unknown stimulus for viral replication CD4 lymphocytes are destroyed (normal range of 800–1,000 cells/mm^3) and others become infected leading to impairment of the immune system; CD4 lymphocyte number and function decreases (at an approximate rate of 50–80 cells/year)

CD4 lymphocyte count (cells/mm^3)	vs. HIV disease status
<300–400	thrush, hairy leukoplakia
<200–400	Pneumocystis pneumonia
<150	cerebral toxoplasmosis
<100	intestinal CMV + MAI infection
<50	AIDS-related lymphoma

Prognosis: median survival with CD4 lymphocyte count <50 cells/mm^3 is 12 months

Transmission by: intimate sexual contact, exposure to contaminated blood / bloody body secretions

Groups at risk:
1. Homosexual males (74%)
2. IV drug abusers (16%)
3. Recipients of contaminated blood products (3%)
4. Sexual partner of drug abuser + bisexual man
5. Infants born to woman infected with AIDS virus

◊ HIV antibodies present in >50% of homosexuals + 90% of IV drug abusers!
◊ Rate of heterosexual transmission is increasing!

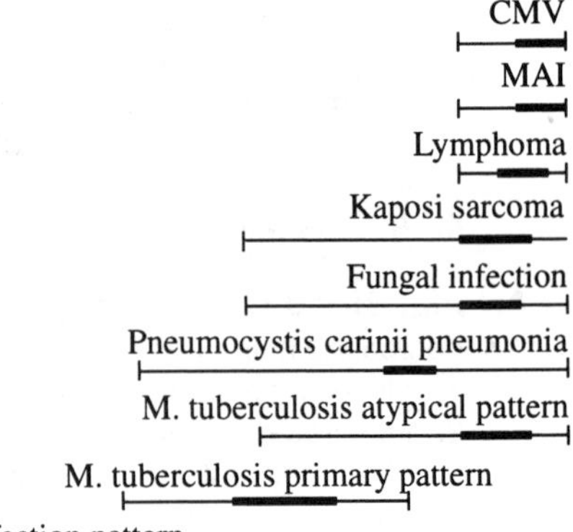

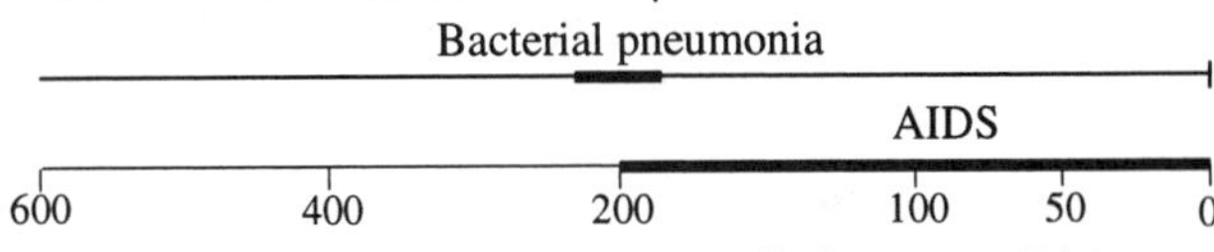

CD4 Lymphocyte Count versus Pulmonary Disease

Clinical classification:

group I	acute HIV infection with seroconversion
group II	asymptomatic HIV infection
group III	persistent generalized lymphadenopathy
group IV	other HIV disease
— subgroup A	constitutional disease
— subgroup B	neurologic disease
— subgroup C	secondary infectious disease
— subgroup D	secondary cancers
— subgroup E	other conditions

AIDS-defining pulmonary conditions (CDC, 1987):
(1) Tracheal / bronchial / pulmonary candidiasis
(2) Pulmonary CMV infection
(3) Herpes simplex bronchitis / pneumonitis
(4) Kaposi sarcoma
(5) Immunoblastic / Burkitt lymphoma
(6) Pneumocystis carinii pneumonia

A. LYMPHADENOPATHY
Cause:
reactive follicular hyperplasia = HIV adenopathy (50%), AIDS-related lymphoma (20%), mycobacterial infection (17%), Kaposi sarcoma (10%), metastatic tumor, opportunistic infection with multiple organisms, drug reaction
Location: mediastinum, axilla, retrocrural

B. OPPORTUNISTIC INFECTION
accounts for majority of pulmonary disease
◊ Pulmonary infection is often the first AIDS-defining illness!
1. Pneumocystis carinii pneumonia (60–80%)
20–40% develop >1 episode during disease
• CD4+ T helper lymphocyte cell count ≤200/mm^3
• subacute insidious onset with malaise, minimal cough
√ bilateral ground-glass infiltrates without effusion / adenopathy
√ bilateral perihilar interstitial infiltrates
√ diffuse bilateral alveolar infiltrates
Mortality: in 25% fatal

2. Fungal disease (<5%)
(a) Cryptococcus neoformans pneumonia (2–15%)
usually associated with brain / meningeal disease
√ segmental infiltrate + superimposed pulmonary nodules ± lymphadenopathy ± pleural effusion
(b) Histoplasma capsulatum
√ typically diffuse nodular / miliary pattern at time of diagnosis
√ normal CXR in up to 35%
(c) Coccidioides immitis
√ diffuse infiltrates + thin-walled cavities
(d) Candida albicans
(e) Aspergillus: less common + less invasive due to relative preservation of neutrophilic function

3. Mycobacterial infection (20%):
(a) M. tuberculosis (increasing frequency):
◊ AIDS patients are 500 times more likely to become infected than general population!
√ postprimary TB pattern with upper-lobe cavitating infiltrate (CD4 lymphocyte count of 200–500 cells/mm^3)
√ primary TB pattern with lung infiltrate / lung masses + hilar / mediastinal lymphadenopathy + pleural effusion (CD4 lymphocyte count of 50–200 cells/mm^3)
√ atypical TB pattern with diffuse reticular / nodular infiltrates (CD4 lymphocyte count of <50 cells/mm^3)
√ adenopathy of low attenuation with rim enhancement on CECT
(b) M. avium-intracellulare (5%)
√ adenopathy, pulmonary infiltrates, nodules, miliary disease
(c) M. kansasii and others
4. Bacterial pneumonia (5–30%):
(a) Haemophilus influenzae, Streptococcus pneumoniae, Staphylococcus aureus
(b) Nocardia pneumonia (<5%)
usually occurs in cavitating pneumonia
√ segmental / lobar alveolar infiltrate ± cavitation ± ipsilateral pleural effusion
5. CMV pneumonia
most frequent infection found at autopsy (49–81%), diagnosed before death in only 13–24%;
high combined prevalence with Kaposi sarcoma
6. Toxoplasmosis

C. TUMOR
1. Kaposi sarcoma (15%)
Location: lung involvement (20%) preceded by widespread skin + organ involvement
Site: peribronchovascular distribution (best appreciated on CT)
√ numerous fluffy ill-defined nodules / asymmetric clusters in a vague perihilar distribution
√ interlobular septal thickening
√ pleural effusion (30%)
√ lymphadenopathy (10–35%), late in disease
2. AIDS-related lymphoma of B-cell origin (2–5%)
primarily immunoblastic NHL / Burkitt lymphoma / non-Burkitt lymphoma; occasionally Hodgkin disease
Location: pulmonary involvement (9–31%), CNS, GI tract, liver, spleen, bone marrow
Site: primarily extranodal
√ solitary / multiple well-defined pulmonary nodules often coexistent with pleural effusion ± axillary / supraclavicular / cervical / hilar adenopathy
√ alveolar infiltrates, paraspinal masses

D. LYMPHOID INTERSTITIAL PNEUMONITIS
Age: in children <13 years of age

E. SEPTIC EMBOLI

F. PREMATURE DEVELOPMENT OF BULLAE (40%)
with disposition to spontaneous pneumothorax

ADULT RESPIRATORY DISTRESS SYNDROME

= SHOCK LUNG = POSTTRAUMATIC PULMONARY INSUFFICIENCY = HEMORRHAGIC LUNG SYNDROME = RESPIRATOR LUNG = STIFF LUNG SYNDROME = PUMP LUNG = CONGESTIVE ATELECTASIS = OXYGEN TOXICITY

= severe unexpected life-threatening acute respiratory distress characterized by abrupt onset of marked dyspnea, increased respiratory effort, severe hypoxemia associated with widespread airspace consolidation

Histo:
(a) up to 12 hours: fibrin + platelet microemboli
(b) 12–24 hours: interstitial edema
(c) 24–48 hours: capillary congestion, extensive interstitial + alveolar proteinaceous edema + hemorrhage, widespread microatelectasis, destruction of type I alveolar epithelial cells
(d) 5–7 days: extensive hyaline membrane formation, hypertrophy + hyperplasia of type II alveolar lining cells
(e) 7–14 days: extensive fibroblastic proliferation in interstitium + within alveoli, rapidly progressing collagen deposition + fibrosis; almost invariably associated with infection

Predisposed:
hemorrhagic / septic shock, massive trauma (pulmonary / general body), acute pancreatitis, aspiration of liquid gastric contents, heroine / methadone intoxication, massive viral pneumonia, traumatic fat embolism, near-drowning, conditions leading to pulmonary edema
mnemonic: "DICTIONARIES"
Disseminated intravascular coagulation
Infection
Caught drowning
Trauma
Inhalants: smoke, phosgene, NO_2
O$_2$ toxicity
Narcotics + other drugs
Aspiration
Radiation
Includes pancreatitis
Emboli: amniotic fluid, fat
Shock: septic, hemorrhagic, cardiogenic, anaphylactic

CXR:
√ NO cardiomegaly / pleural effusion
— up to 12 hours:
√ characteristic 12-hour delay between clinical onset of respiratory failure and CXR abnormalities
— 12–24 hours:
√ patchy ill-defined opacities throughout both lungs
— 24–48 hours:
√ massive airspace consolidation of both lungs
— 5–7 days:
√ consolidation becomes inhomogeneous (resolution of alveolar edema)
√ local areas of consolidation (pneumonia)
— >7 days:
√ reticular / bubbly lung pattern (diffuse interstitial + airspace fibrosis)

Complication of continuous positive pressure ventilation (= **barotrauma**)
Path:
(a) rupture of alveoli along margins of interlobular septa + vascular structures
(b) air dissection along interlobular septa + perivascular spaces (= interstitial emphysema)
(c) interstitial air rupturing into pleural space (= pneumothorax) / into mediastinum (= pneumomediastinum)
√ mottled air opacities often outlining bronchovascular bundles
√ large subpleural cysts without definable wall usually at diaphragmatic + mediastinal surface compressing adjacent lung

ALPHA-1 ANTITRYPSIN DEFICIENCY

= rare autosomal recessive disorder
Alpha-1 antitrypsin (glycoprotein) is synthesized in liver + released into serum
Action: proteolytic inhibitor of trypsin, chymotrypsin, elastase, plasmin, thrombin, kallikrein, leukocytic + bacterial proteases; neutralizes circulating proteolytic enzymes
Mode of injury from deficiency:
PMNs + alveolar macrophages sequester into lung during recurrent bacterial infections + release elastase, which digests basement membrane

Age: early age of onset (20–30 years); M:F = 1:1
• rapid + progressive deterioration of lung function
• chronic sputum production (50%)
√ severe panacinar emphysema with basilar predominance
√ reduction in size + number of pulmonary vessels in lower lobes
√ redistribution of blood flow to unaffected upper lung zones
√ bullae at both lung bases
√ marked flattening of diaphragm
√ minimal diaphragmatic excursion
√ multilobar cystic bronchiectasis (40%)
Cx: hepatic cirrhosis (in homozygotic individuals)

ALVEOLAR MICROLITHIASIS

= very rare disease of unknown etiology characterized by myriad of calcospherites (= tiny calculi) within alveoli
Age peak: 30–50 years; begins in early life; has been identified in utero; M:F = 1:1; in 50% familial (restricted to siblings)
• usually asymptomatic (70%)
• dyspnea on exertion (reduction in residual volume)
• cyanosis, clubbing of fingers
• striking discrepancy between striking radiographic findings and mild clinical symptoms
• NORMAL serum calcium + phosphorus levels
√ very fine, sharply defined, sandlike micronodulations (<1 mm)
√ diffuse involvement of both lungs
√ intense uptake on bone scan

CHEST

Prognosis:
(a) late development of pulmonary insufficiency secondary to interstitial fibrosis
(b) disease may become arrested
(c) microliths may continue to form / enlarge

DDx: "Mainline" pulmonary granulomatosis = IV abuse of talc-containing drugs such as methadone (rarely as numerous + scarring + loss of volume)

ALVEOLAR PROTEINOSIS

= PULMONARY ALVEOLAR PROTEINOSIS (PAP)
= accumulation of PAS positive phospholipid material in alveoli (= surfactant)

Etiology: ?; associated with dust exposure (eg, silicoproteinosis is histologically identical to PAP), immunodeficiency, hematologic + lymphatic malignancies, AIDS, chemotherapy

Pathophysiology:
(a) overproduction of surfactant by granular pneumocytes
(b) defective clearance of surfactant by alveolar macrophages

Histo: alveoli filled with proteinaceous material (the ONLY pure airspace disease), normal interstitium

Age peak: 30–50 years (age range 2–70 years); M:F = 3:1

• asymptomatic (10–20%)
• gradual onset of dyspnea + cough
• weight loss, weakness, hemoptysis
• defect in diffusing capacity

√ "bat-wing" consolidation of ground-glass pattern, predominant at bases
√ small acinar nodules + coalescence + consolidation
√ patchy peripheral / primarily unilateral infiltrates (rare)
√ reticular / reticulonodular / linear interstitial pattern with Kerley B lines (late stage)
√ slow clearing over weeks or months
√ slow progression (1/3), remaining stable (2/3)
√ NO adenopathy, NO cardiomegaly, NO pleural effusion

HRCT:
√ patchy ground-glass opacity
√ smooth septal thickening

Cx: infections (frequently secondary to poorly functioning macrophages + excellent culture medium): Nocardia asteroides (most common), mycobacterial, fungal, Pneumocystis, CMV

Prognosis:
highly variable course with clinical and radiologic episodes of exacerbation + remissions
(a) 50% improvement / recovery
(b) 30% death within several years under progression

Rx: bronchopulmonary lavage

DDx:
(a) during acute phase: pulmonary edema, diffuse pneumonia, ARDS
(b) in chronic stage:
1. Idiopathic pulmonary hemosiderosis (boys, symmetric involvement of mid + lower zones, progression to nodular + linear pattern)
2. Hemosiderosis (bleeding diathesis)
3. Pneumoconiosis
4. Hypersensitivity pneumonitis
5. Goodpasture syndrome (more rapid changes, renal disease)
6. Desquamative interstitial pneumonia ("ground glass" appearance, primarily basilar + peripheral)
7. Pulmonary alveolar microlithiasis (widespread discrete intraalveolar calcifications primarily in lung bases, rare familial disease)
8. Sarcoidosis (usually with lymphadenopathy)
9. Lymphoma
10. Bronchioloalveolar cell carcinoma (more focal, slowly enlarging with time)

AMNIOTIC FLUID EMBOLISM

= most common cause of maternal peripartum death
• dyspnea
• shock during / after labor + delivery

Pathogenesis: Amniotic debris enters maternal circulation resulting in (1) pulmonary embolization (2) anaphylactoid reaction (3) DIC

√ usually fatal before radiographs obtained
√ may demonstrate pulmonary edema

AMYLOIDOSIS

= disease characterized by an extracellular deposit of proteinaceous twisted ß-pleated sheet fibrils of great chemical diversity

Histo: protein (immunoglobulin) / polysaccharide complex; affinity for Congo red stain

@ Lung involvement
Incidence: 1° amyloidosis (in up to 70%), 2° amyloidosis (rare)

A. TRACHEOBRONCHIAL TYPE (most common)
• hemoptysis (most frequent complaint)
• stridor, cough, dyspnea, hoarseness, wheezing
√ multiple nodules protruding from wall of trachea / large bronchi
√ diffuse rigid narrowing of a long tracheal segment
√ prominent bronchovascular markings
√ destructive pneumonitis

B. NODULAR TYPE
Age: >60 years of age; M:F = 1:1
• usually asymptomatic
√ mediastinal / hilar adenopathy
√ solitary / multiple parenchymal nodules in a peripheral / subpleural location ± central calcification / ossification; slow growth over years
√ ± pleural effusion
DDx: metastatic disease, granulomatous disease, rheumatoid lung, sarcoidosis, mucoid impaction

C. DIFFUSE PARENCHYMAL TYPE (least common)
Age: >60 years of age
• usually asymptomatic with normal CXR
• cough + dyspnea with abnormal CXR
√ widespread small irregular densities (exclusively interstitial involvement) ± calcification
√ may become confluent ± honeycombing

CHEST

DDx: idiopathic interstitial fibrosis, pneumoconiosis (especially asbestosis), rheumatoid lung, Langerhans cell histiocytosis, scleroderma

ANKYLOSING SPONDYLITIS

Incidence: 1% of patients with ankylosing spondylitis
Histo: interstitial + pleural fibrosis with foci of dense collagen deposition, NO granulomas
- bone manifestations obvious + severe

Location: apices / upper lung fields
√ uni- / bilateral, coarse, linear shadows + cavities
√ bronchiectasis may be present
√ superinfection, especially with aspergillosis (mycetoma formation) / atypical mycobacteria
DDx: other causes of pulmonary apical fibrosis (primary infection by fungi / mycobacteria; cancer)

ASBESTOS-RELATED DISEASE

Substances:
aspect (length-to-diameter) ratio effects carcinogenicity:
eg, aspect ratio of 32 = 8 μm long, 0.25 μm wide
- commercial amphiboles: crocidolite, amosite
- commercial nonamphiboles / serpentines: chrysotile
- noncommercial contaminating amphiboles: actinolite, anthophyllite, tremolite

(a) relatively benign:
(1) Chrysotile (white asbestos) in Canada
(2) Anthophyllite in Finland, North America
(3) Tremolite
(b) relatively malignant:
(1) Crocidolite (blue / black asbestos) in South Africa, Australia
(2) Amosite (brown asbestos)
◊ Very fine fibers (crocidolite) associated with largest number of pleural disease!

Occupational exposure:
(a) asbestos mining + milling
(b) insulation, textile manufacturing, construction, ship building, gaskets, brake linings

Pulmonary asbestosis

= (term asbestosis reserved for) chronic progressive diffuse interstitial fibrosis
Incidence: in 49–52% of industrial asbestos exposure
Latency period: 40–45 years
Histo: interstitial fibrosis begins in peribronchiolar areas, then progresses to involve adjacent alveoli
Diagnostic criteria:
1. reliable history of exposure
2. appropriate time interval between exposure + detection
3. CXR evidence
4. restrictive pattern of lung impairment
5. abnormal diffusing capacity
6. bilateral crackles at posterior lung bases, not cleared by cough

- dyspnea
- restrictive pulmonary function tests

Location: more severe in lower subpleural zones (concentration of asbestos fibers under pleura)
√ small irregular opacities (NOT rounded as in coal / silica)
√ confined to lung bases, progressing superiorly
√ septal lines (= fibrous thickening around secondary lobules)
√ "shaggy" heart border = obscuration secondary to parenchymal + pleural changes
√ ill-defined outline of diaphragm
√ honeycombing (uncommon)
√ rarely massive fibrosis, predominantly at lung bases without migration toward hilum (DDx from silicosis / CWP)
√ NO hilar adenopathy
√ Ga-67 uptake gives a quantitative index of inflammatory activity
HRCT:
√ subpleural pulmonary arcades = branching linear structures most prominent posteriorly (initial finding) = centrilobular peribronchiolar fibrosis
√ curvilinear subpleural lines parallel to + within 1 cm of pleura (30%) = multiple subpleural dotlike reticulonodularities connected to the most peripheral branch of pulmonary artery
√ parenchymal band = linear <5 cm long + several mm wide opacity, often extending to pleura, which may be thickened + retracted at site of contact
√ reticulation = network of linear densities, usually <u>posteriorly</u> at lung bases
√ honeycombing = multiple cystic spaces <1 cm in diameter with thickened walls
√ thickened interlobular septal lines
√ thickened intralobular lines

Asbestos-related pleural disease

1. <u>Focal Pleural Plaques</u> (65%)
= hyalinized collagen in submesothelial layer of parietal pleura
Incidence: most common manifestation of exposure; 6% of general population will show plaques
Latent period: in 10% after 20 years; in 50% after 40 years
Histo: dense hypocellular undulating collagen fibers often arranged in a basket weave pattern ± focal / massive calcifications
Location: bilateral + multifocal; posterolateral midportion of chest wall between 7–10th rib; aponeurotic portion of diaphragm; mediastinum; following rib contours; visceral pleura + apices + costophrenic angles typically spared
- asymptomatic

√ usually focal area of pleural thickening (<1 cm thick) with edges thicker than central portions of plaque; in 48% only finding; in 41% with parenchymal changes; stable over time

√ no hilar adenopathy
√ usually not calcified
DDx: chest wall fat, rib fractures, rib companion shadows

2. Diffuse Pleural Thickening (17%)
= diffuse thickening of parietal pleura (visceral pleura involved in 90%, but difficult to demonstrate)
• may cause restriction of pulmonary function
May be associated with: rounded atelectasis
√ bilateral process with "shaggy heart" appearance (20%)
√ smooth; difficult to assess when viewed en face
√ thickening of interlobar fissures
√ focally thickened diaphragm
√ obliterated costophrenic angles (minority of cases)

3. Pleural Calcification (21–25–60%)
detected by radiography in 25%, by CT in 60%
Overall incidence: 20%
Latent period: >20 years to become visible; in 40% after 40 years
Histo: calcification starts in parietal pleura; calcium deposits may form within center of plaques
√ dense lines paralleling the chest wall, mediastinum, pericardium, diaphragm (bilateral diaphragmatic calcifications with clear costophrenic angles are (PATHOGNOMONIC)
√ advanced calcifications are leaflike with thick-rolled edges
DDx: talc exposure, hemothorax, empyema, therapeutic pneumothorax for TB (often unilateral, extensive sheetlike, on visceral pleura)

4. Pleural Effusion (21%)
Earliest asbestos-related pleural abnormality, frequently followed by diffuse pleural thickening + rounded atelectasis
Prevalence: 3% (increases with increasing levels of asbestos exposure)
Latent period: 8–10 years after exposure
• **benign asbestos pleurisy**
  • may be associated with chest pain (1/3)
  • usually small sterile, serous / hemorrhagic exudate
√ recurrent bilateral effusions
√ ± plaque formation
DDx: TB, mesothelioma

Atelectatic asbestos pseudotumor
= ROUNDED ATELECTASIS = "FOLDED LUNG"
= infolding of redundant pleura accompanied by segmental / subsegmental atelectasis
Location: posteromedial / posterolateral lower lobe (most common); frequently bilateral
√ 2.5–8 cm focal subpleural mass abutting a region of thickened pleura
√ size + shape show little progression, occasionally decrease in size
√ volume loss in adjacent lung
CT:
√ rounded / lentiform / wedge-shaped outline
√ contiguous to areas of diffuse pleural thickening ± calcification
√ partial interposition of lung between pleura + mass
√ "crow's feet" = linear bands radiating from mass into lung parenchyma (54%)
√ "vacuum cleaner" / "comet tail" sign = bronchovascular markings emanating from nodular subpleural mass + coursing toward ipsilateral hilum
√ "Swiss cheese" air bronchogram (18%)

Lung cancer in asbestos-related disease
Occurrence related to:
(a) cumulated dose of asbestos fibers
(b) smoking (synergistic carcinogenic effect)
◊ Increased risk by factor of up to 90 in smokers versus a factor of 5 in nonsmokers!
◊ Up to 25% of asbestos workers who smoke develop lung cancer!
(c) preexisting interstitial disease
(d) occupational exposure to known carcinogen
Latency period: 25–35 years
Associated with: increased incidence of gastric carcinoma
Histo: bronchioloalveolar cell carcinoma (most common); bronchogenic carcinoma (adenocarcinoma + squamous cell)
Location: at lung base / in any location if associated with smoking

ASPERGILLOSIS
Organism:
Aspergillus fumigatus = intensely antigenic ubiquitous soil fungus existing as
(a) conidiophores = reproductive form releasing thousands of spores
(b) hyphae (= matured spores) characterized by 45° dichotomous branching pattern
Occurrence:
commonly in sputum of normal persons, ability to invade arteries + veins facilitating hematogenous dissemination
M:F = 3:1
Predisposed:
(a) preexisting lung disease (tuberculosis, bronchiectasis)
(b) impairment of immune system (alcoholism, advanced age, malnutrition, concurrent malignancy, poorly controlled diabetes, cirrhosis, sepsis)
Cx: dissemination to heart, brain, kidney, GI tract, liver, thyroid, spleen
◊ Sputum cultures are diagnostically unreliable because of normal (saprophytic) colonization of upper airways!

CHEST

CHEST

Noninvasive Aspergillosis

= SAPROPHYTIC ASPERGILLOSIS

= noninvasive colonization of preexisting cavity / cyst in immunologically normal patients with cavitary disease [tuberculosis, sarcoidosis (common), bronchiectasis, bullous lung disease, carcinoma]

- sputum blood-streaked / severe hemoptysis (45–70%)
- elevated serum precipitins level for Aspergillus (50%)

√ solid round gravity-dependent mass within preexisting spherical / ovoid thin-walled cavity (= Mounod sign)

Histo: mycetoma = aspergilloma = **fungus ball** = masslike collection of intertwined hyphae matted together with fibrin, mucus, cellular debris colonizing a pulmonary cavity

√ crescent-shaped air space separates fungus ball from cavity wall

√ fungus ball may calcify in scattered / rimlike fashion

√ pleural thickening adjacent to preexisting cyst / cavity, commonly first sign before visualizing mycetoma

Semi-invasive Aspergillosis

= CHRONIC NECROTIZING ASPERGILLOSIS

= chronic cavitary slowly progressive disease in patients with preexisting lung injury (COPD, radiation therapy), mild immune suppression, or debilitation (alcohol, diabetes)

- symptoms mimicking pulmonary tuberculosis

√ progressive consolidation (usually upper lobe)

√ development of air crescent and fungus ball

Dx: pathologic examination demonstrating local tissue invasion

Invasive Pulmonary Aspergillosis

= often fatal form in severely immunocompromised patients (most commonly in lymphoma / leukemia patients with prolonged granulocytopenia) with absolute neutrophil count of <500

Path: endobronchial fungal proliferation followed by transbronchial vascular invasion eventually causes widespread hemorrhage + thrombosis of pulmonary arterioles + ischemic tissue necrosis + systemic dissemination; fungus ball = devitalized sequestrum of lung infiltrated by fungi

- Hx of series of bacterial infections + unremitting fever
- pleuritic chest pain (mimicking emboli)
- progression of pulmonary infiltrates despite broad-spectrum antibiotics

(a) early signs:

√ CT halo sign = single / multiple 1–3 cm peripheral nodules (= necrotic lung) with halo of ground-glass attenuation (= hemorrhagic edema)

√ patchy localized bronchopneumonia

(b) signs of progression

√ enlargement of nodules into diffuse bilateral consolidation

√ development into large wedge-shaped pleural-based lesions

√ air-crescent sign = cavitation of existing nodule (air crescent between sequestrum and lung) 1–3 weeks after granulocyte recovery

◊ has better prognosis than consolidation without cavitation (feature of resolution phase)

Dx: branching hyphae at tissue examination

Allergic Bronchopulmonary Aspergillosis

= hypersensitivity toward aspergilli in patients with long-standing asthma

Incidence: in 1–2% of patients with asthma, in 10% of patients with cystic fibrosis; most common + clinically important form

Age: mostly young patients (begins in childhood); may be undiagnosed for 10–20 years

A. ACUTE ALLERGIC BRONCHOPULMONARY ASPERGILLOSIS
Type I reaction = immediate hypersensitivity (IgE-mediated)
Histo: alveoli filled with eosinophils

B. CHRONIC ALLERGIC BRONCHOPULMONARY ASPERGILLOSIS
Type III reaction = delayed immune complex response = Arthus reaction (IgG-mediated)
Histo: bronchial damage secondary to Aspergillus antigen reacting with IgG antibodies, immune complexes activate complement leading to tissue injury

Pathophysiology:
inhaled spores are trapped in segmental bronchi of individuals with asthma, germinate, and form hyphae; immunologic response coupled with proteolytic enzymes causes pulmonary infiltrates + tissue damage + central bronchiectasis

Criteria:

(a) Primary diagnostic criteria:
acronym: ARTEPICS
Asthma (84–96%)
Roentgenographic transient or fixed pulmonary infiltrates
Test for A. fumigatus positive: immediate skin reaction
Eosinophilia in blood between 8% and 40%
Precipitating antibodies to A. fumigatus (70%)
IgE in serum elevated
Central bronchiectasis (late manifestation that proves diagnosis)
Serum-specific IgE and IgG A. fumigatus levels elevated

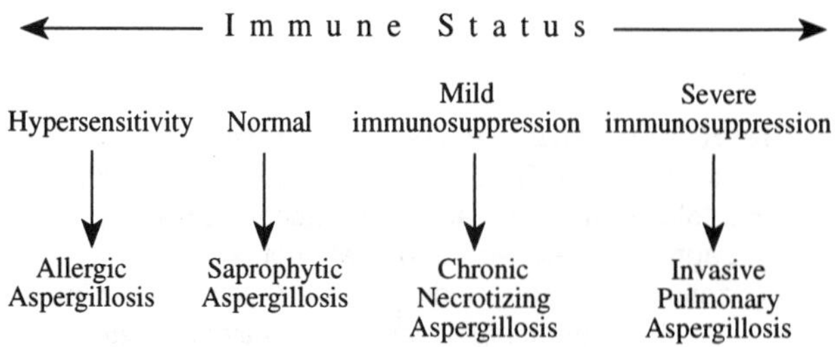

(b) Secondary diagnostic criteria (less common):
1. Aspergillus fumigatus mycelia in sputum
2. Expectoration of brown sputum plugs (54%)
3. Arthus reaction (= late skin reactivity with erythema + induration) to Aspergillus antigen

Staging:
I acute phase with all primary diagnostic criteria
II clearing of pulmonary infiltrates with declining IgE levels
III all criteria of stage I reappear after emission
IV corticosteroid dependency
V irreversible lung fibrosis

• flulike symptoms: fever, headache, malaise, weight loss, fleeting chest pain
√ migratory pneumonitis = transient recurrent "fleeting" alveolar patchy subsegmental / lobar infiltrates in upper lobes (50%), lower lobes (20%), middle lobe (7%), both lungs (65%); may persist for >6 months
√ central varicose / cystic bronchiectasis
√ "tramlike" bronchial walls (edema)
√ 1–2 cm ring shadows (= bronchus on end) around hilum + upper lobes (HALLMARK)
√ "finger-in-glove / toothpaste shadow" = V- or Y-shaped central mucus plugs in 2nd order bronchi of 2.5–6 cm in length remaining for months + growing in size
√ lobar consolidation (in 32%)
√ atelectasis (in 14%) with collateral air drift
√ cavitation (in 14%) secondary to postobstructive abscess
√ hyperinflation (due to bronchospasm)
√ pulmonary fibrosis + retraction
√ hilar elevation due to lobar shrinkage
√ emphysema
√ NORMAL peripheral bronchi
√ UNUSUAL are aspergilloma in cavity (7%), empyema, pneumothorax

DDx: hypersensitivity pneumonitis or allergic asthma (no hyphae in sputum, normal levels of IgE + IgG to A. fumigatus), tuberculosis, lipoid pneumonia, Löffler syndrome, bronchogenic carcinoma

Pleural aspergillosis
= Aspergillus empyema in patients with pulmonary tuberculosis, bacterial empyema, bronchopleural fistula
√ pleural thickening

ASPIRATION OF SOLID FOREIGN BODY
Age: in 50% <3 years
Source: in 85% vegetable origin (peanut, barley grass)
Location: almost exclusively in lower lobes; R:L = 2:1
√ obstructive overinflation (68%) + reflex vasoconstriction
√ collapse (14–53%)
√ infiltrate (11%)
√ radiopaque foreign body (9%)
√ air trapping (expiratory / lateral decubitus film)

NUC:
√ ventilation defect (initial breath) + retention (washout)

Cx: bronchiectasis (from long retention)
DDx: impacted esophageal foreign body

ASPIRATION PNEUMONIA
Predisposing conditions:
(1) CNS disorders / intoxication: alcoholism, mental retardation, seizure disorders, recent anesthesia
(2) Swallowing disorders: esophageal motility disturbances, head + neck surgery

• low-grade fever
• productive cough
• choking on swallowing

Location: gravity-dependent portions of lung, posterior segments of upper lobes + lower lobes in bedridden patients, frequently bilateral, right middle + lower lobe with sparing of left lung is common

A. ACUTE ASPIRATION PNEUMONIA
Cause: acid, food particles, anaerobic bacteria from GI tract provoke edema, hemorrhage, inflammatory cellular response, foreign-body reaction
√ segmental consolidation in dependent portion

B. CHRONIC ASPIRATION PNEUMONIA
Cause: repeated aspiration of foreign material from GI tract over long time / mineral oil (eg, in laxatives)
Associated with: Zenker diverticulum, esophageal stenosis, achalasia, TE fistula, neuromuscular disturbances in swallowing
√ recurring segmental consolidation
√ progression to interstitial scarring (= localized honeycomb appearance)
√ bronchopneumonic infiltrates of variable location over months / years
√ residual peribronchial scarring
Upper GI:
√ abnormal swallowing / aspiration

ASTHMA
= episodic reversible bronchoconstriction secondary to hypersensitivity to a variety of stimuli

A. INTRINSIC ASTHMA
Age: middle age
Pathogenesis:
probably autoimmune phenomenon caused by viral respiratory infection and often provoked by infection, exercise, pharmaceuticals; no environmental antigen

B. EXTRINSIC ASTHMA = ATOPIC ASTHMA
Pathogenesis:
secondary to antigens producing an immediate hypersensitivity response (type I); reagin sensitizes mast cells to release histamine followed by increased vascular permeability, edema, small muscle contraction; effects primarily bronchi causing airway obstruction

Nonoccupational allergens:
pollens, dog + cat fur, tamarind seed powder, castor bean, fungal spores, grain weevil
Occupational allergens:
(a) natural substances: wood dust, flour, grain, beans
(b) pharmaceuticals: antibiotics, ASA
(c) inorganic chemicals: nickel, platinum

Path: bronchial plugging with large amounts of viscid tenacious mucus (eosinophils, Charcot-Leyden crystals), edematous bronchial walls, hypertrophy of mucous glands + smooth muscle

ACUTE SIGNS:
- during asthmatic attack low values for FEV + MMFR and abnormal V/Q ratios
- increased resistance to airflow due to
  (a) smooth muscle contraction in airway walls
  (b) edema of airway wall caused by inflammation
  (c) mucus hypersecretion with airway plugging
- normal diffusing capacity

√ hyperexpansion of lungs = severe overinflation + air trapping
  √ flattened diaphragmatic dome
  √ deepened retrosternal air space
√ peribronchial cuffing (inflammation of airway wall)
√ bronchial dilatation
√ localized areas of hypoattenuation

CHRONIC CHANGES:
Normal chest x-ray in 73%, findings of abnormalities depend on
(a) age of onset (<15 years of age in 31%; >30 years of age in none)
(b) severity of asthma
√ central ring shadows = bronchiectasis
√ scars (from recurrent infections)

Cx:
(1) Pneumonia (2 x as frequent as in nonasthmatics)
  √ peripheral pneumonic infiltrates (secondary to blocked airways)
(2) Atelectasis (5–15%) from mucoid impaction
(3) Pneumomediastinum (5%), pneumothorax, subcutaneous emphysema; predominantly in children
(4) Emphysema
(5) Allergic bronchopulmonary aspergillosis with central bronchiectasis

ATYPICAL MEASLES PNEUMONIA

= clinical syndrome in patients who have been previously inadequately immunized with killed rubeola vaccine and are subsequently exposed to the measles virus (= type III immune complex hypersensitivity); noted in children who have received live vaccine before 13 months of age
- 2- to 3-day prodrome of headache, fever, cough, malaise
- maculopapular rash beginning on wrists + ankles (sometimes absent)
- postinfectious migratory arthralgias
- history of exposure to measles

√ extensive nonsegmental consolidation, usually bilateral
√ hilar adenopathy (100%)
√ pleural effusion (0–70%)
√ nodular densities of 0.5–10 cm in diameter in peripheral location, may calcify and persist up to 30 months

BARITOSIS

= inhalation of nonfibrogenic barium sulfate
- asymptomatic
- normal pulmonary function (benign course)

√ bilateral nodular / patchy opacities, denser than bone (high atomic number)
√ similar to calcified nodules
√ NO cor pulmonale, NO hilar adenopathy
√ regression if patient removed from exposure

BEHÇET SYNDROME

= rare multisystem disease of unknown origin characterized by
(1) aphthous stomatitis
(2) genital ulceration
(3) iritis
- positive pathergy test = unusual hypersensitivity to pricking with formation of pustules at site of needle prick within 24–48 hours
- skin changes: erythema nodosum, folliculitis, papulopustular lesions
- arthritis, encephalitis
- epididymitis

@ Chest (5%)
  √ multiple peripheral subpleural opacities (due to hemorrhage, necrotic pulmonary infarctions)
  √ increased radiopacity near hila (pulmonary artery aneurysm)
@ Veins (25%)
  √ large vein occlusion; may cause SVC syndrome
  √ subcutaneous thrombophlebitis
@ Arteries
  √ arterial occlusion / pulseless disease
  √ aneurysm of large arteries (in 2%)

BERYLLIOSIS

= chronic granulomatous disorder as a result of beryllium-specific cell-mediated immune response (= delayed hypersensitivity reaction after exposure to acid salts from extraction of beryllium oxide)
Substance: one of the lightest metals (atomic weight 9), marked heat resistance, great hardness, fatigue resistance, no corrosion
Occupational exposure: fluorescent lamp factories
Histo: noncaseating granulomas within interstitium + along vessels + in bronchial submucosa
- positive beryllium lymphocyte transformation test (blood test of T-lymphocyte response to beryllium)

A. ACUTE BERYLLIOSIS (25%)
  √ pulmonary edema following an overwhelming exposure

CHEST

B. CHRONIC BERYLLIOSIS
widespread systemic disease of liver, spleen, lymph nodes, kidney, myocardium, skin, skeletal muscle; removed from lungs + excreted via kidneys
Latent period: 5–15 years
√ fine nodularity (granulomas similar to sarcoidosis)
√ irregular opacities, particularly sparing apices + bases
√ hilar + mediastinal adenopathy (may calcify)
√ emphysema in upper lobes + interstitial fibrosis
√ pneumothorax in 10%
HRCT:
√ diffuse small parenchymal nodules (57%)
√ septal lines (50%)
√ patches of ground-glass attenuation (32%)
√ hilar adenopathy (21–35%), only in the presence of parenchymal abnormalities
√ bronchial wall thickening (46%)
√ pleural irregularities (25%)
DDx: (1) Nodular pulmonary sarcoidosis (indistinguishable)
(2) Asbestosis without hilar adenopathy

BLASTOMYCOSIS

= NORTH AMERICAN BLASTOMYCOSIS = GILCHRIST DISEASE = CHICAGO DISEASE
= rare systemic mixed pyogenic + granulomatous fungal infection
Organism: soil-born saprophytic dimorphic fungus Blastomyces dermatitidis, mycelial phase in soil + round thick-walled yeast form with broad-based budding in mammals
Geographic distribution:
worldwide; endemic in central + southeastern United States (Ohio + Mississippi river valleys, vicinity of Great Lakes), Africa, Canada (northern Ontario), Central + South America (acquired through activities in woods)
Age: several months of age to 80 years (peak between 25 and 50 years of age)
Mode of infection:
inhalation of fungal conidia (primary portal of entry); spread to extrapulmonary sites, eg, skin, bone (often direct extension from skin lesion resembling actinomycosis), joints
Predisposed: elderly, immunocompromised
Histo:
(a) exudative phase: accumulation of numerous neutrophils with infecting organism
(b) proliferative phase: proliferation of epitheloid granulomas + giant cells with central microabscesses containing neutrophils and yeast forms
• mouth ulcers
• fever, cough, weight loss, chest pain (majority)
• crusted verrucous lesions on exposed body areas
@ Lung
• Clinical patterns following pulmonary infection:
(a) severe pulmonary symptoms
(b) asymptomatic pulmonary infection with spontaneous resolution
(c) disseminated disease to single / multiple organs indolent for several years
(d) extrapulmonary manifestation involving male GU system, skeleton, skin
√ segmental / lobar airspace disease in lower lobes in acute illness (26–61%)
√ solitary / multiple irregular nodular masses / satellite lesions in paramediastinal location
√ air bronchogram in area of consolidation / mass (87%)
√ interstitial disease
√ cavitation if communicating with airway (13%)
√ hilar / mediastinal lymph node enlargement (<25%)
@ Bone
√ marked destruction ± surrounding sclerosis
√ periosteal reaction in long bones, but not in short bones
√ multiple osseous lesions are frequent
√ vertebral bodies + intervertebral disks are destroyed (similar to tuberculosis)
√ psoas abscess
√ lytic skull lesions + soft-tissue abscess
√ usually monarticular arthritis: knee > ankle > elbow > wrist > hand
@ GU tract (20%): prostate, epididymis

Dx: (1) culture of organism
(2) silver stain microscopy of tissues
Prognosis: spontaneous resolution of acute disease in up to 4 weeks; disease may reactivate for up to 3 years
Rx: (1) amphotericin B IV: 8–10 weeks for noncavitary + 10–12 weeks for cavitary lesions
(2) ketoconazole
DDx: other pneumonias (ie, bacterial, tuberculous, fungal), pseudolymphoma, malignant neoplasm (ie, alveolar cell carcinoma, lymphoma, Kaposi sarcoma)

BONE MARROW TRANSPLANTATION

= intravenous infusion of hematopoietic progenitor cells from patient's own marrow (autologous transplant) / HLA-matched donor (allogenic transplant) to reestablish marrow function after high-dose chemotherapy and total body irradiation for lymphoma, leukemia, anemia, multiple myeloma, congenital immunologic defects, solid tumors
Cx: pulmonary complications in 40–60%

Neutropenic phase pulmonary complications

Time: 2–3 weeks after transplantation
1. Angioinvasive aspergillosis
√ nodule surrounded by halo of ground-glass attenuation (= fungal infection spreading into lung parenchyma and surrounding area of hemorrhagic infarction)
√ segmental / subsegmental consolidation (= pulmonary infarction)
√ cavitation of nodule with air-crescent sign (during recovery phase with resolving neutropenia)

CHEST

√ <5 mm centrilobular nodules to 5 cm peribronchial consolidation (= airway invasion with surrounding zone of hemorrhage / organizing pneumonia)

2. Diffuse alveolar hemorrhage (20%)
   - hemosiderin-laden macrophages on lavage

   √ bilateral areas of ground-glass attenuation / consolidation
3. Pulmonary edema

   Cause: infusion of large volumes of fluid combined with cardiac + renal dysfunction

   √ prominent pulmonary vessels, interlobar septal thickening, ground-glass attenuation, pleural effusions
4. Drug toxicity

   Cause: bleomycin, busulfan, bischloronitrosurea (carmustine), methotrexate

   √ bilateral areas of ground-glass attenuation / consolidation / reticular attenuation (= fibrosis)

CHEST

Early phase pulmonary complications

Time: up to 100 days after transplantation

1. CMV pneumonia (23%)

   √ multiple small nodules + associated areas of consolidation + ground-glass attenuation (= hemorrhagic nodules)
2. Pneumocystis carinii pneumonia

   √ diffuse / predominantly perihilar / mosaic pattern of ground-glass attenuation with sparing of some secondary pulmonary lobules
3. Idiopathic interstitial pneumonia (12%)

   √ nonspecific findings (diagnosis of exclusion)

Late phase pulmonary complications

Time: after 100 days post transplantation

1. Bronchiolitis obliterans (in up to 10%)
2. BOOP
3. Chronic graft-versus-host disease

   infections, chronic aspiration, bronchiolitis obliterans, lymphoid interstitial pneumonia

BRONCHIAL ADENOMA

= misnomer secondary to locally invasive features, tendency for recurrence, and occasional metastasis to extrathoracic sites (10%) = low-grade malignancy

Incidence: 6–10% of all primary lung tumors

Age: mean age of 35–45 years (range 12–60 years); 90% occur <50 years of age; most common primary lung tumor under age 16; M:F = 1:1; Whites:Blacks = 25:1

Path: arises from duct epithelium of bronchial mucous glands (predominant distribution of Kulchitsky cells at bifurcations of lobar bronchi)

Types:

mnemonic: "CAMP"

Carcinoid	90%
Adenoid cystic carcinoma = Cylindroma	6%
Mucoepidermoid carcinoma	3%
Pleomorphic carcinoma	1%

Location: most commonly near / at bifurcation of lobar / segmental bronchi; central:peripheral = 4:1

— 48% on right : RLL (20%), RML (10%), RUL (7%), main right bronchus (8%), intermediate bronchus (3%)

— 32% on left : LLL (13%), LUL (12%), main left bronchus (6%), lingular bronchus (1%)

- hemoptysis (40–50%)
- atypical asthma
- persistent cough
- recurrent obstructive pneumonia
- asymptomatic (10%)

√ complete obstruction / air trapping in partial obstruction (rare) / nonobstructive (10–15%)

√ obstructive emphysema

√ recurrent postobstructive infection: pneumonitis, bronchiectasis, abscess

√ atelectasis / consolidation of a lung / lobe / segment (78%)

√ collateral air drift may prevent atelectasis

√ solitary round / oval slightly lobulated pulmonary nodule (19%) of 1–10 cm in size

√ hilar enlargement / mediastinal widening = central endo- / exobronchial mass

CT:

√ well-marginated sharply defined mass

√ in close proximity to an adjacent bifurcation with splaying of bronchus

√ coarse peripheral calcifications in 1/3 (cartilaginous / bony transformation)

√ may exhibit marked homogeneous enhancement

Biopsy: risky secondary to high vascularity of tumor

Prognosis: 95% 5-year survival rate, 75% 15-year survival rate after resection

Carcinoid

= NEUROENDOCRINE CARCINOMA

= slow-growing low-grade malignant tumor

Incidence: 12–15% of all carcinoid tumors in the body; 1–4% of all bronchial neoplasms

Age peak: 5th decade (range of 2nd–9th decade); 4% occur in children + adolescents; M:F = 2:1; very uncommon in Blacks

Path:

originates from neurosecretory cells of bronchial mucosa (= Kulchitsky cells = argentaffine cells) just as small cell cancer; part of APUD (amine precursor uptake and decarboxylation) system = chromaffin paraganglioma, which produces serotonin, ACTH, norepinephrine, bombesin, calcitonin, ADH, bradykinin

Pathologic classification:

(KCC = **Kulchitsky cell carcinoma**)

KCC I = **classic carcinoid** (least aggressive);
= bronchial adenoma (misnomer)
= central location with endobronchial growth; usually <2.5 cm in size + well-defined; younger patient; M:F = 1:10; lymph node metastases in 3%

KCC II = **atypical carcinoid** (25% of carcinoid tumors); mass usually >2.5 cm with well-defined margins; older patient; M:F = 3:1; lymph node metastases in 40–50%; metastases to brain, liver, bone (in 30%)

KCC III = **small cell carcinoma** (most aggressive); mediastinal lymphadenopathy; ill-defined tumor margins

◊ Rarely cause for carcinoid syndrome or Cushing syndrome!

- recurrent unifocal pneumonitis, hemoptysis
- wheezing, persistent cough, dyspnea, chest pain
- carcinoid syndrome (rare)
- endobronchial exophytic mass at endoscopy

Location: 58–90% central in lobar / segmental bronchi, 10–42% peripheral; located in submucosa; endobronchial / along bronchial wall / exobronchial

√ polypoid tumor with average size of 2.2 cm
√ most extend through bronchial wall thus involving bronchial lumen + parenchyma (= collar button lesion)
√ calcification / ossification (26–33%): central carcinoid (43%), peripheral carcinoid (10%)
√ vascular tumor supplied by bronchial circulation
√ cavitation (rare)
√ segmental / lobar atelectasis
√ obstructive pneumonitis
√ bronchiectasis + pulmonary abscess

Malignant potential: low

Metastases:
(a) regional lymph nodes in 25%
(b) distantly in 5% (adrenal, liver, brain, skin, osteoblastic bone metastases)

Prognosis:
95% 5-year survival rate for classic carcinoids;
57–66% 5-year survival rate for atypical carcinoids

Cylindroma

= ADENOID CYSTIC CARCINOMA (7%)

Second most common primary tumor of trachea

Path: mixed serous + mucous glands; resembles salivary gland tumor

Histo:
Grade 1: tubular + cribriform; no solid subtype
√ entirely intraluminal
Grade 2: tubular + cribriform; <20% solid subtype
√ predominantly intraluminal
Grade 3: solid subtype >20%
√ predominantly extraluminal

Age peak: 4–5th decade

- typical Hx of refractory "asthma"
- hemoptysis, cough, stridor, wheezing
- dysphagia, hoarseness

√ endotracheal mass with extratracheal extension

Malignant potential:
more aggressive than carcinoid with propensity for local invasion + distant metastases (lung, bone, brain, liver) in 25%

Rx: tracheal resection + adjunctive radiotherapy

Prognosis: 8.3 years mean survival

Mucoepidermoid carcinoma

Path: squamous cells + mucus-secreting columnar cells; resembles salivary gland tumor

√ may involve trachea = locally invasive tumor
√ sessile / polyploid endobronchial lesion

Pleomorphic adenoma

= MIXED TYPE = extremely rare

BRONCHIAL ATRESIA

= local obliteration of proximal lumen of a segmental bronchus

Proposed causes:
(a) local interruption of bronchial arterial perfusion >15 weeks GA (when bronchial branching is complete)
(b) tip of primitive bronchial bud separates from bud and continues to develop

Path: normal bronchial tree distal to obstruction patent and containing mucus plugs; alveoli distal to obstruction air-filled through collateral air drift

Associated with: lobar emphysema, cystic adenomatoid malformation

- minimal symptoms, apparent later in childhood (most by age 15) / adult life

Location: apicoposterior segment of LUL (>>RUL / ML)

√ decreased perfusion
√ overexpanded segment (collateral air drift with expiratory air-trapping)
√ fingerlike opacity lateral to hilum (= mucus plug distal to atretic lumen) is CHARACTERISTIC

OB-US (detected >24 weeks MA):
√ large echogenic fetal lung mass = fluid-filled lung distal to obstruction
√ dilated fluid-filled bronchus

Rx: no treatment because mostly asymptomatic

DDx: Congenital lobar emphysema (no mucus plug)

BRONCHIECTASIS

= localized mostly irreversible dilatation of bronchi often with thickening of the bronchial wall

Etiology:

A. Congenital
   1. Structural defect of bronchi: bronchial atresia, Williams-Campbell syndrome
   2. Abnormal mucociliary transport: Kartagener syndrome
   3. Abnormal secretions: mucoviscidosis = cystic fibrosis

B. Congenital / acquired immune deficiency (usually IgG deficiency):
chronic granulomatous disease of childhood, alpha 1-antitrypsin deficiency

C. Postinfectious: measles, whooping cough, Swyer-James syndrome, allergic bronchopulmonary aspergillosis, chronic granulomatous infection (TB)

D. Bronchial obstruction: neoplasm, inflammatory nodes, foreign body

E. Aspiration / inhalation: gastric contents / inhaled fumes (late complication)

F. Pulmonary fibrosis: **"traction bronchiectasis"** due to increased elastic recoil with bronchial dilatation + mechanical distortion of bronchi by fibrosis

Imaging definition on HRCT (modality of choice):
(1) lack of tapering of bronchi (in 80% = most sensitive finding)
(2) internal diameter of bronchus larger than adjacent pulmonary artery (in 60%)
(3) bronchi visible within 1 cm of pleura (in 45%)
(4) mucus-filled dilated bronchi (in 6%)

Classification:
1. **Cylindrical / tubular / fusiform bronchiectasis**
least severe type
reversible if associated with pulmonary collapse
√ 16 subdivisions of bronchi
√ square abrupt ending with lumen of uniform diameter and same width as parent bronchus
HRCT (study of choice):
√ "tram lines" (horizontal course)
√ "signet-ring sign" (vertical course) = cross-section of dilated bronchus + branch of pulmonary artery
2. **Varicose bronchiectasis**
Rare, associated with Swyer-James syndrome
√ 4–8 subdivisions of bronchi
√ beaded contour with normal pattern distally
3. **Saccular / cystic bronchiectasis**
most severe type
Associated with: severe bronchial infection
√ <5 subdivisions of bronchi
√ progressive ballooning dilatation toward periphery with diameter of saccules >1 cm
√ irregular constrictions may be present
√ dilatation of bronchi on inspiration, collapse on expiration
HRCT:
√ string of cysts = "string of pearls" (horizontal course) / cluster of cysts = "cluster of grapes"
√ air-fluid level (frequent)

Age: predominantly pediatric disease
• chronic cough
• recurrent infection with expectoration of purulent sputum
• shortness of breath
• hemoptysis (50%)

Associated with: obliterative + inflammatory bronchiolitis (in 85%)
Location: posterior basal segments of lower lobes, bilateral (50%), middle lobe / lingula (10%), central bronchiectasis in bronchopulmonary aspergillosis
√ normal radiograph in 7%
√ increase in size of lung markings (retained secretions)
√ loss of definition of lung markings (peribronchial fibrosis)
√ crowding of lung markings (if associated with atelectasis)
√ cystic spaces ± air-fluid levels <2 cm in diameter (dilated bronchi)
√ honeycomb pattern (in severe cases)
√ compensatory hyperinflation of uninvolved ipsilateral lung
√ increased background density
√ frequent exacerbations + resolutions (due to superimposed infections)

Cx: frequent respiratory infections
DDx of CT appearance:
(1) emphysematous blebs (no definable wall thickness, subpleural location)
(2) "reversible bronchiectasis" = temporary dilatation during pneumonia with return to normal within 4–6 months

BRONCHIOLITIS OBLITERANS

= CONSTRICTIVE BRONCHIOLITIS = OBLITERATIVE BRONCHIOLITIS
= inflammation of bronchioles leading to (sometimes reversible) obstruction of bronchiolar lumen

Etiology:
(1) Inhalation: 1–3 weeks after exposure to toxic fumes (isocyanates, phosgene, ammonia, sulfur dioxide, chlorine)
(2) Postinfectious: Mycoplasma (children), virus (older individual); *see* Swyer-James syndrome
(3) Drugs: penicillamine
(4) Connective tissue disorder: rheumatoid arthritis, scleroderma, systemic lupus erythematosus
(5) Chronic rejection: lung transplant, heart-lung transplant (30–50%)
(6) Chronic graft-versus-host disease: bone marrow transplant
(7) Cystic fibrosis (as a complication of repeated episodes of pulmonary infection)
(8) Idiopathic (in immunocompetent patients)

Path: submucosal and peribronchiolar fibrosis
= irreversible fibrosis of small airway walls with narrowing / obliteration of airway lumina by granulation tissue

Peak age: 40–60 years; M:F = 1:1
• insidious onset of dyspnea over many months
• obstructive pulmonary function tests
• no response to antibiotics
• persistent nonproductive cough
√ normal CXR (in up to 40%)
√ hyperinflated lungs = limited disease with connective tissue plugs in airways
√ bronchiectasis
√ decreased vascularity (reflex vasoconstriction)
HRCT (paired expiration-inspiration images:
√ "mosaic perfusion" of lobular air trapping (85–100%)
= patchy areas of decreased lung attenuation alternating with areas of normal attenuation
√ areas of decreased attenuation containing vessels of decreased caliber (due to alveolar hypoventilation + secondary vasoconstriction of alveoli distal to bronchiolar obstruction)
√ areas of increased attenuation containing vessels of increased caliber (uninvolved areas with compensatory increased perfusion)
√ bronchial wall thickening (87%)
√ bronchiectasis (66–80%)

CHEST

√ patchy air trapping on expiratory scans (due to collateral airdrift into postobstructive alveoli) = failure of volume / attenuation change between expiratory + inspiratory images
√ "tree-in-bud" appearance of bronchioles = centrilobular branching structures and nodules caused by peribronchiolar thickening + bronchiolectasis with secretions (the only direct, but uncommon sign)
√ centrilobular ground-glass opacities

Rx: steroids may stop progression

DDx: (1) Bacterial / fungal pneumonia (response to antibiotics, positive cultures)
(2) Chronic eosinophilic pneumonia (young female, eosinophilia in 2/3)
(3) Usual interstitial pneumonia (irregular opacities, decreased lung volume)

BRONCHIOLITIS OBLITERANS WITH ORGANIZING PNEUMONIA (BOOP)

= PROLIFERATIVE BRONCHIOLITIS
= CRYPTOGENIC ORGANIZING PNEUMONITIS (COP)

Prevalence: 20–30% of all chronic infiltrative lung disease

Cause: postobstructive pneumonia, organizing adult respiratory distress syndrome, lung cancer, extrinsic allergic alveolitis, pulmonary manifestation of collagen vascular disease, pulmonary drug toxicity, silo filler disease, idiopathic (50%)

Path: granulation tissue polyps filling the lumina of alveolar ducts and respiratory bronchioles (bronchiolitis obliterans) + variable degree of infiltration of interstitium and alveoli with macrophages (organizing pneumonia)
◊ Bronchiolitis obliterans component not present in up to 1/3!

Histo: plugs of immature fibroblasts (Masson bodies) covered with low cuboidal epithelium which may spread through collateral air drift pathways

Age: 40–70 years; M:F = 1:1

- clinical + functional + radiographic manifestation of organizing pneumonia
- nonproductive cough, dyspnea (1–4-month history), preceded by a brief flulike illness with sore throat, low-grade fever, malaise (in 33%)
- late respiratory crackles
- restrictive pulmonary function tests + diminished diffusing capacity on pulmonary function tests
- unresponsive to broad-spectrum antibiotics
- no organism identified

Location: mainly mid + lower lung zones; often subpleural (50%) and peribronchiolar distribution (30–50%)

CXR:
frequently mixture of:
√ uni- / bilateral patchy alveolar airspace consolidation (25–73%), often subpleural
√ 3–5 mm nodules (up to 50%)
√ irregular linear opacities (15–42%)
√ unilateral focal / lobar consolidation (5–31%)
√ pleural thickening (13%)
√ cavitation / pleural effusion (<5%)

HRCT:
√ patchy airspace consolidation (80%)
(a) bilateral in 90% involving all lung zones
(b) subpleural distribution in 50–60%
√ patchy ground-glass opacities (due to alveolitis) in 60%
√ 3–5 mm centrilobular nodules (30–50%) due to organized pneumonia
√ air bronchograms = cylindrical bronchial dilatation in areas of airspace consolidation (36–70%)
√ pleural effusion (28–35%)
√ adenopathy (27%)

Rx: improvement with corticosteroid therapy (in 84% of patients with idiopathic form)

Prognosis: persistent abnormalities (30%); 10% mortality due to progressive / recurrent disease

Dx: tissue examination from open lung biopsy

BRONCHIOLOALVEOLAR CARCINOMA

= ALVEOLAR CELL CARCINOMA = BRONCHIOLAR CARCINOMA

Incidence: 1.5–6% of all primary lung cancers (increasing incidence to ? 20–25%)

Etiology: development from type II alveolar epithelial cells, subtype of adenocarcinoma

Age: 40–70 years; M:F = 1:1 (strikingly high in women)

Path: peripheral neoplasm arising beyond a recognizable bronchus with tendency to spread locally using lung structure as a stroma (= **lepidic** growth)

Histo: cuboidal / columnar cells grow along alveolar walls + septa without disrupting the lung architecture or pulmonary interstitium (serving as "scaffolding" for tumor growth); subtype of adenocarcinoma

Subtypes:
(a) mucinous (80%): mucin-secreting tall columnar peglike bronchiolar cells; more likely multicentric; 26% 5-year survival rate
(b) nonmucinous (20%): cuboidal type II alveolar pneumocytes with production of surfactant / nonciliated bronchiolar (Clara) cells; more localized + solitary; 72% 5-year survival rate

Risk factors: localized pulmonary fibrosis (tuberculous scarring, pulmonary infarct) in 27%, diffuse fibrotic disease (scleroderma), previous exogenous lipid pneumonia

- history of heavy smoking (25–50%)
- often asymptomatic (even with disseminated disease)
- cough (35–60%), hemoptysis (11%)
- bronchorrhea = abundant white mucoid / watery expectoration (5–27%); can produce hypovolemia + electrolyte depletion; unusual + late manifestation only with diffuse bronchioloalveolar carcinoma
- shortness of breath (15%)
- weight loss (13%), fever (8%)

Location: peripherally, beyond a recognizable bronchus

Spread: tracheobronchial dissemination = cells detach from primary tumor + attach to alveolar septa elsewhere in ipsi- / contralateral lung; lymphogenous + hematogenous dissemination (in 50–60%)

A. LOCAL FORM (60–90%)
1. Ground-glass attenuation
   = early stage (due to lepidic growth pattern along alveolar septa with relative lack of acinar filling)
   √ ground-glass haziness
   √ bubblelike hyperlucencies / pseudocavitation
   √ airway dilatation
   √ lesion persists / progresses within 6–8 weeks
2. Single mass (43%)
   √ well-circumscribed focal mass in peripheral / subpleural location arising beyond a recognizable bronchus
   √ "rabbit ears" / pleural tags / triangular strand / "tail sign" (55%) = linear strands extending from nodule to pleura (desmoplastic reaction / scarring granulomatous disease / pleural indrawing)
   √ spiculated margin = sunburst appearance (73%)
   √ "open bronchus sign" = air bronchogram = tumor / mucus surrounding aerated bronchus ± narrowing / stretching / spreading of bronchi
   √ pseudocavitation (= dilatation of intact air spaces from desmoplastic reaction / bronchiectasis / focal emphysema) in 50–60%
   ◊ 2nd most common cell type associated with cavitation after squamous cell
   √ heterogeneous attenuation (57%)
   √ confined to single lobe
   √ rarely evolving into diffuse form
   √ slowly progressive growth on serial radiographs
   √ NO atelectasis
   √ negative FDG PET results in 55%
   Prognosis: 70% surgical cure rate for tumor <3 cm; 4–15 years survival time with single nodule

B. DIFFUSE FORM = Pneumonic form (10–40%)
1. Diffuse consolidation (30%)
   √ acinar airspace consolidation + air bronchogram + poorly marginated borders
   √ airspace consolidation may affect both lungs (mucus secretion)
   √ ± cavitation within consolidation
   √ "CT angiogram sign" = low-attenuation consolidation does not obscure vessels (mucin-producing subtype)
2. Lobar form
   √ ± expansion of a lobe with bulging of interlobar fissures
3. Multinodular form (27%)
   √ multiple bilateral poorly / well-defined nodules similar to metastatic disease
   √ multiple poorly defined areas of ground-glass attenuation / consolidation

√ pleural effusion (8–10%)

Prognosis: worse with extensive consolidation / multifocal / bilateral disease; death within 3 years with diffuse disease

BRONCHOGENIC CARCINOMA

= LUNG CANCER = LUNG CARCINOMA

Most frequent cause of cancer deaths in males (35% of all cancer deaths) and females (21% of all cancer deaths); most common malignancy of men in the world; 6th leading cancer in women worldwide

Prevalence: in 1991 161,000 new cases; 143,000 deaths

Age at diagnosis: 55–60 years (range 40–80 years); M:F = 1.4:1

- asymptomatic (10–50%) usually with peripheral tumors
- symptoms of central tumors:
  - cough (75%), wheezing, pneumonia
  - hemoptysis (50%), dysphagia (2%)
- symptoms of peripheral tumors:
  - pleuritic / local chest pain, dyspnea, cough
  - Pancoast syndrome, superior vena cava syndrome
  - hoarseness
- symptoms of metastatic disease (CNS, bone, liver, adrenal gland)
- paraneoplastic syndromes
  - cachexia of malignancy
  - clubbing + hypertrophic osteoarthropathy
  - nonbacterial thrombotic endocarditis
  - migratory thrombophlebitis
  - ectopic hormone production: hypercalcemia, syndrome of inappropriate secretion of antidiuretic hormone, Cushing syndrome, gynecomastia, acromegaly

Types:

1. **Adenocarcinoma** (50%)
   ◊ Most common cell type seen in women + nonsmokers!
   Intermediate malignant potential (slow growth, high incidence of early metastases)
   Histo: formation of glands / intracellular mucin
   Subtype: bronchioloalveolar carcinoma
   Location: almost invariably develops in periphery; frequently found in scars (tuberculosis, infarction, scleroderma, bronchiectasis) + in close relation to preexisting bullae
   √ solitary peripheral subpleural mass (52%) / alveolar infiltrate / multiple nodules
   √ may invade pleura + grow circumferentially around lung mimicking malignant mesothelioma
   √ upper lobe distribution (69%)
   √ air broncho- / bronchiologram on HRCT (65%)
   √ calcification in periphery of mass (1%)
   √ smooth margin / spiculated margin due to desmoplastic reaction with retraction of pleura

2. **Squamous cell carcinoma** = **epidermoid carcinoma** (30–35%)
   ◊ Strongly associated with cigarette smoking
   Histo: mimics differentiation of the epidermis by producing keratin ("epidermoid carcinoma"); central necrosis is common

Histogenesis: chronic inflammation with squamous metaplasia, progression to dysplasia + carcinoma in situ
- positive sputum cytology

◊ Most common cell type diagnosed that is radiologically occult!
- hypercalcemia from tumor-elaborated parathyroid hormonelike substance

◊ Slowest growth rate, lowest incidence of distant metastases

(a) Central location within main / lobar / segmental bronchus (2/3)
√ large central mass ± cavitation
√ distal atelectasis ± bulging fissure (due to mass)
√ postobstructive pneumonia
◊ All cases of pneumonia in adults should be followed to complete radiologic resolution!
√ airway obstruction with atelectasis (37%)

(b) Solitary peripheral nodule (1/3)
√ characteristic cavitation (in 7–10%)
◊ Squamous cell carcinoma is the most common cell type to cavitate!
√ invasion of chest wall
◊ Squamous cell carcinoma is the most common cell type to cause Pancoast tumor!

3. **Small cell undifferentiated carcinoma** (15%)
◊ Strongly associated with cigarette smoking
Rapid growth + high metastatic potential (early metastases in 60–80% at time of diagnosis); should be regarded as systemic disease regardless of stage; virtually never resectable
Path: arises from bronchial mucosa with growth in submucosa + subsequent invasion of peribronchial connective tissue
Histo: small uniform oval cells with scant cytoplasm; nuclei with stippled chromatin; numerous mitoses + large areas of necrosis; in 20% coexistent with non-small cell histologic types (most frequently squamous cell)
Subtype: oat cell cancer with hyperchromatic nuclei; ? related to Kulchitsky cell carcinomas
- smooth-appearing mucosal surface endoscopically
- ectopic hormone production: Cushing syndrome, inappropriate secretion of ADH

◊ Most common primary lung cancer causing superior vena caval obstruction (due to extrinsic compression / endoluminal thrombosis / invasion)!
Location: 90% central within lobar / mainstem bronchus (primary tumor rarely visualized)
√ typically large hilar / perihilar mass often associated with mediastinal widening (from adenopathy)
√ extensive necrosis + hemorrhage
√ small lung lesion (rare)
Staging evaluation:
CT of abdomen + head, bone scintigraphy, bilateral bone marrow biopsies

4. **Undifferentiated large cell carcinoma** (<5%)
◊ Strongly associated with smoking
Intermediate malignant potential; rapid growth + early distant metastases
Histo: tumor cells with abundant cytoplasm + large nuclei + prominent nucleoli; diagnosed per exclusion due to lack of squamous / glandular / small cell differentiation
Subtype: giant cell carcinoma with very aggressive behavior + poor prognosis
√ large bulky usually peripheral mass >6 cm (50%)
√ large area of necrosis
√ pleural involvement
√ large bronchus involved in central lesion (50%)

RISK FACTORS:
(1) cigarette smoking (squamous cell carcinoma + small cell carcinoma)
— related to number of cigarettes smoked, depth of inhalation, age at which smoking began
◊ 85% of lung cancer deaths are attributable to cigarette smoking!
◊ Passive smoking may account for 25% of lung cancers in nonsmokers!
(2) radon gas: may be the 2nd leading cause for lung cancer with up to 20,000 deaths per year
(3) industrial exposure: asbestos, uranium, arsenic, chlormethyl ether
(4) concomitant disease: chronic pulmonary scar + pulmonary fibrosis
Scar carcinoma
7% of lung tumors; 1% of autopsies
Origin: related to infarcts (>50%), tuberculosis scar (<25%)
Histo: adenocarcinoma (72%), squamous cell carcinoma (18%)
Location: upper lobes (75%)
◊ 45% of all peripheral cancers originate in scars!

PRESENTATION
√ solitary peripheral mass with corona radiata / pleural tail sign / satellite lesion
√ cavitation (16%): usually thick-walled with irregular inner surface; in 4/5 secondary to squamous cell carcinoma, followed by bronchioloalveolar carcinoma
√ central mass (38%): common in small cell carcinoma
√ unilateral hilar enlargement (secondary to primary tumor / enlarged lymph nodes)
Nodes on CT: 0–10 mm negative, 10–20 mm indeterminate, >20 mm positive
√ anterior + middle mediastinal widening (suggests small cell carcinoma)
√ segmental / lobar / lung atelectasis (37%) secondary to airway obstruction (particularly in squamous cell carcinoma)
√ "S sign of Golden" = incomplete lobar collapse with bulging contour produced by primary central tumor
√ rat tail termination of bronchus

√ bronchial cuff sign = focal / circumferential thickening of bronchial wall imaged end-on (early sign)
√ local hyperaeration (due to check-valve type endobronchial obstruction, best on expiratory view)
√ mucoid impaction of segmental / lobar bronchus (due to endobronchial obstruction)
√ persistent peripheral infiltrate (30%) = postobstructive pneumonitis
√ NO air bronchogram
√ pleural effusion (8–15%)
√ bone erosion of ribs / spine (9%)
√ involvement of main pulmonary artery (18%); lobar + segmental arteries (53%) may result in additional peripheral radiopacity (due to lung infarct)
√ calcification in 7% on CT (histologically in 14%) usually eccentric / finely stippled
(a) preexisting focus of calcium engulfed by tumor
(b) dystrophic calcium within tumor necrosis
(c) calcium deposit from secretory function of carcinoma (eg, mucinous adenocarcinoma)

Angio:
√ bronchogenic carcinoma supplied by bronchial circulation
√ distortion / stenosis / occlusion of pulmonary arterial circulation

MULTIPLE PRIMARY LUNG CANCERS
Incidence: 0.72–3.5%; in 1/3 synchronous, in 2/3 metachronous
◊ 10–32% of patients surviving resection of a lung cancer will develop a second primary!
Dx: biopsy mandatory for proper therapy because the tumor may have a different cell type

PARANEOPLASTIC MANIFESTATIONS
1. Carcinomatous neuromyopathy (4–15%)
2. Migratory thrombophlebitis
3. Hypertrophic pulmonary osteoarthropathy (3–5%)
4. Endocrine manifestations (15%) usually with small cell carcinoma: Cushing syndrome, inappropriate secretion of ADH, HPT, excessive gonadotropin secretion

LOCATION
60–80% arise in segmental bronchi
— central: small cell carcinoma, squamous cell carcinoma (sputum cytology positive in 70%); arises in central airway often at points of bronchial bifurcation, infiltrates circumferentially, extends along bronchial tree
— peripheral: adenocarcinoma, large cell carcinoma
— upper lobe: lower lobe = right lung : left lung = 3 : 2
— most common site: anterior segment of RUL
— **Pancoast tumor** (3%) = superior pulmonary sulcus tumor, frequently squamous cell carcinoma
• atrophy of muscles of ipsilateral upper extremity due to lower brachial plexus involvement
• Horner syndrome (enophthalmos, miosis, ptosis, anhidrosis) due to sympathetic chain + stellate ganglion involvement
√ apical pleural thickening / mass
√ ± soft-tissue invasion / bone destruction
— SVC obstruction (5%): often in small cell carcinoma

TNM STAGING
T1: <3 cm in diameter, surrounded by lung / visceral pleura
T2: >3 cm in diameter / invasion of visceral pleura / lobar atelectasis / obstructive pneumonitis / at least 2 cm from carina
T3: tumor of any size; less than 2 cm from carina / invasion of parietal pleura, chest wall, diaphragm, mediastinal pleura, pericardium; pleural effusion
T4: invasion of heart, great vessels, trachea, esophagus, vertebral body, carina / malignant effusion
N1: peribronchial / ipsilateral hilar nodes
N2: ipsilateral mediastinal nodes
N3: contralateral hilar / mediastinal nodes

STAGING FOR SMALL CELL LUNG CANCER
<u>Limited disease</u>:
1. Primary in one hemithorax
2. Ipsilateral hilar adenopathy
3. Ipsilateral supraclavicular adenopathy
4. Ipsi- and contralateral mediastinal adenopathy
5. Atelectasis
6. Paralysis of phrenic + laryngeal nerve
7. Small effusion without malignant cells

<u>Extensive disease</u> (60–80%):
1. Contralateral hilar adenopathy
2. Contralateral supraclavicular adenopathy
3. Chest wall infiltration
4. Carcinomatous pleural effusion
5. Lymphangitic carcinomatosis
6. Superior vena cava syndrome
7. Metastasis to contralateral lung
8. Extrathoracic metastases to bone (38%), liver (22–28%), bone marrow (17–23%), CNS (8–15%), retroperitoneum (11%), other lymph nodes

Prognosis: 7–11 months median survival; 15–20% 2-year disease-free survival rate

SPREAD
1. direct local extension
2. hematogenous (small cell ca.)
3. lymphatic spread (squamous cell ca.); tumor in 10% of normal-sized lymph nodes
4. transbronchial spread–least common

DISTANT METASTASES
@ Bone
(a) Marrow: in 40% at time of presentation
(b) Gross lesions in 10–35%:
Location: vertebrae (70%), pelvis (40%), femora (25%)
√ osteolytic metastases (3/4)
√ osteoblastic metastases (1/4): in small cell carcinoma / adenocarcinoma
√ occult metastases in 36% of bone scans

@ Adrenals: in 37% at time of presentation
@ Brain: asymptomatic metastases on brain scan in 7% (30% at autopsy), in 2/3 multiple
@ Kidney, GI tract, liver, abdominal lymph nodes
@ Lung-to-lung metastases (in up to 10%, usually in late stage)

Cx:
1. Diaphragmatic elevation (phrenic nerve paralysis)
2. Hoarseness (laryngeal nerve involvement, left > right)
3. SVC obstruction (5%): lung cancer is cause of all SVC obstructions in 90%
4. Pleural effusion (10%): malignant, parapneumonic, lympho-obstructive
5. Dysphagia: enlarged nodes, esophageal invasion
6. Pericardial invasion: pericardial effusion, localized pericardial thickening / nodular masses

Prognosis: mean survival time <6 months; 10–15% overall 5-year survival; survival at 40 months: squamous cell 30% > large cell 16% > adenocarcinoma 15% > oat cell 1%

Rx:
(1) Surgical resection for non-small cell histologic types
Unresectable: involvement of heart, great vessels, trachea, esophagus, vertebral body, malignant pleural effusion
(2) Adjuvant chemotherapy + radiation therapy in extensive resectable disease
(3) Chemotherapy for small cell carcinoma + radiation therapy for bulky disease, CNS metastases, spinal cord compression, SVC obstruction

BRONCHOGENIC CYST

= budding / branching abnormality of ventral diverticulum of primitive foregut (ventral segment = tracheobronchial tree; dorsal segment = esophagus) between 26 and 40 days of embryogenesis

Incidence: most common intrathoracic foregut cyst (54–63% in surgical series)

Histo: thin-walled cyst filled with mucoid material, lined with columnar respiratory epithelium, mucous glands, cartilage, elastic tissue, smooth muscle

• contains mucus / clear or turbid fluid
√ sharply outlined round / oval mass
√ may contain air-fluid level

CT:
√ cyst contents of water density (50%) / higher density (50%)

OB-US:
√ single unilocular pulmonary cyst
√ echogenic distended lung obstructed by bronchogenic cyst

A. MEDIASTINAL BRONCHOGENIC CYST (86%)
Associated with: spinal abnormalities
M:F = 1:1
• usually asymptomatic
• stridor, dysphagia
Location: pericarinal (52%), paratracheal (19%), esophageal wall (14%), retrocardiac (9%); usually on right
√ rarely communicate with tracheal lumen
√ may show esophageal compression

B. INTRAPULMONARY BRONCHOGENIC CYST (14%)
M > F
• infection (75%)
• dyspnea, hemoptysis (most common)
Location: lower:upper lobe = 2:1; usually medial third
√ 36% will eventually contain air
DDx: solitary pulmonary nodule, cavitated neoplasm, cavitated pneumonia, lung abscess

BRONCHOPULMONARY DYSPLASIA

= RESPIRATOR LUNG = complication of prolonged respirator therapy of intermittent PEEP with high oxygen concentration = oxygen toxicity + barotrauma

Stage I (2–3 days) : √ RDS pattern of hyaline membrane disease
Stage II (4–10 days) : √ complete opacification with air bronchogram;
associated with congestive failure from PDA
Stage III (10–20 days) : √ "spongy" / "bubbly" coarse linear densities, esp. in upper lobes
√ hyperaeration of lung
√ lower lobe emphysema
Stage IV (after 1 month) : √ same pattern;
40% mortality if not resolved by 1 month

Cx: (1) abnormal pulmonary function
(2) increased frequency of lower respiratory tract infections

Prognosis:
(1) complete clearing over months / years (1/3)
(2) retained linear densities in upper lobe emphysema (29%)

DDx: (1) Diffuse neonatal pneumonia (2) Meconium aspiration (3) Total anomalous pulmonary venous return (4) Congenital pulmonary lymphangiectasia (5) Cystic fibrosis (6) Idiopathic pulmonary fibrosis (7) Pulmonary interstitial emphysema (8) Wilson-Mikity syndrome

BRONCHOPLEURAL FISTULA

= BRONCHOPULMONARY FISTULA
= communication between the bronchial system / lung parenchyma + pleural space

Cause:
A. Trauma
1. Complication of resectional surgery (pneumonectomy, lobectomy, bullectomy)
2. Blunt / penetrating trauma
3. Barotrauma
B. Lung necrosis
1. Putrid lung abscess
2. Necrotizing pneumonia: Klebsiella, H. influenzae, Staphylococcus, Streptococcus; tuberculosis; fungus; Pneumocystis

CHEST

3. Infarction

C. Airway disease
1. Bronchiectasis (very rare)
2. Emphysema complicated by pneumonia / pneumothorax

D. Malignancy: lung carcinoma with postobstructive pneumonia / tumor necrosis following therapy

- large / persistent air leak
- acute / chronic empyema

HRCT:
√ direct visualization of bronchopleural fistula (in 50%)
√ peripheral air + fluid collection (indirect sign)

Dx: (1) Introduction of methylene blue into pleural space, in 65% dye appears in sputum
(2) Sinography (3) Bronchography

Rx: tube thoracostomy, open drainage, decortication, thoracoplasty, muscle-pedicle closure, transbronchial occlusions

BRONCHOPULMONARY SEQUESTRATION

= congenital malformation consisting of
(1) nonfunctioning lung segment
(2) no communication with tracheobronchial tree
(3) systemic arterial supply

Incidence: 0.15–6.4% of all congenital pulmonary malformations; 1.1–1.8% of all pulmonary resections

√ usually >6 cm in size
√ round / oval, smooth, well-defined solid homogeneous mass near diaphragm with mass effect
√ occasionally fingerlike appendage posteriorly + medially (anomalous vessel)
√ contrast enhancement of sequestration at the same time as thoracic aorta on rapid sequential CT scans
√ multiple / single air-fluid levels if infected
√ surrounded by recurrent pulmonary consolidation in a lower lobe that never clears completely
√ may communicate with esophagus / stomach
◊ Pulmonary sequestration with communication to GI tract is termed **bronchopulmonary foregut malformation**!

DDx: bronchiectasis, lung abscess, empyema, bronchial atresia, congenital lobar emphysema, cystic adenomatoid malformation, intrapulmonary bronchogenic cyst, Swyer-James syndrome, pneumonia, arteriovenous fistula, primary / metastatic neoplasm, hernia of Bochdalek

Bronchopulmonary Sequestrations

	INTRALOBAR	EXTRALOBAR
Prevalence	75%	25%
Pleural investment	visceral pleura	own pleura
Venous drainage	pulmonary veins	systemic veins
Symptomatic	adulthood	first 6 month
Etiology	acquired	developmental
Congen. anomalies	15%	50%

Intralobar sequestration *(75–86%)*

= enclosed by visceral pleura of affected pulmonary lobe but separated from bronchial tree

Etiology: controversial
(1) probably acquired in majority of patients
(2) early appearance of congenital accessory tracheobronchial bud leads to incorporation within one pleural investment

Path: chronic inflammation fibrosis: multiple irregular cordlike adhesions to mediastinum, diaphragm, parietal pleura; multiple cysts filled with fluid / thick gelatinous / purulent material; vascular sclerosis

Age at presentation: adulthood (50% >20 years); M:F = 1:1

Associated with congenital anomalies in 6–12%:
skeletal deformities (4%): scoliosis, rib + vertebral anomalies; esophagobronchial diverticula (4%); diaphragmatic hernia (3%); cardiac (including tetralogy of Fallot); renal: failure of ascent + rotation; cerebral anomalies; congenital pulmonary venolobar syndrome

- about 50% have symptoms by age 20; asymptomatic in 15%
- pain, repeated infection in same location (eg, recurrent acute lower lobe pneumonias)
- high-output congestive heart failure (in neonatal period) from L-to-L shunt
- cough + sputum production, hemoptysis

Location: posterobasal segments, rarely upper lung / within fissure; L:R = 3:2

CXR:
√ recurrent / persistent pneumonia localized to lower lobe
√ cavitation and cysts ± fluid levels
◊ Aeration of sequestered lung via Kohn pores / communication with tracheobronchial tree!

Bronchogram:
√ NO communication of rudimentary bronchial system of sequestration with tracheobronchial tree (rare exceptions)

Angio:
√ usually single large artery (mean diameter of 6 mm) coursing through inferior pulmonary ligament from
— distal thoracic aorta (73%)
— proximal abdominal aorta (22%)
— celiac / splenic artery
— intercostal artery (4%)
— anomalous branch of coronary artery
√ multiple aa. in 16% (with vessel diameter of <3 mm)
√ combined systemic + pulmonary arterial supply
√ venous drainage via
— normal pulmonary veins to L atrium (in 95%)
— azygos / hemiazygos vv. / intercostal vv. / SVC into R atrium (in 5%)

CT:
√ single / multiple thin-walled cysts containing fluid / mucus / pus / air-fluid level / air alone
√ mucus-impacted ectatic bronchi (= fat density) in sequestered lung

√ emphysema bordering normal lung (37%)
= postobstructive hyperinflation of sequestered lung
√ homogeneous / inhomogeneous soft-tissue mass with irregular borders
√ irregular enhancement (rare)
√ one / two anomalous systemic arteries arising from aorta (DDx: AVM, interrupted pulmonary artery, isolated anomaly, chronic infection / inflammation of lung or pleura, surgically created shunt)
√ premature atherosclerosis of anomalous arteries
◊ Mucoid impaction of bronchus surrounded by hyperinflated lung is CHARACTERISTIC!

OB-US:
√ spherical homogeneous highly echogenic mass
√ anomalous systemic artery seen by color Doppler

Cx: massive spontaneous nontraumatic pleural hemorrhage, chronic inflammation, fibrosis

DDx of mass: neurogenic tumor, lateral thoracic meningocele, extramedullary hematopoiesis, pleural tumor
DDx of cavity: lung abscess, necrotizing pneumonia, fungal / mycobacterial pneumonia, cavitating neoplasm, empyema
DDx of cysts: pulmonary abscess, empyema, bronchiectasis, emphysema, bronchogenic foregut cyst, pericardial cyst, eventration of diaphragm, congenital cystic malformation

Extralobar sequestration (14–25%)

= accessory lobe with its own pleural sheath (= "Rokitansky lobe"), which prevents collateral air drift resulting in an airless round mass

Etiology: development of an anomalous accessory / supernumerary tracheobronchial foregut bud
Path: single ovoid / rounded / pyramidal airless lesion between 0.5 and 15 cm (generally 3 to 6 cm) in size
Histo: resembles normal lung with diffuse dilatation of bronchioles + alveolar ducts + alveoli; dilatation of subpleural + peribronchiolar lymph vessels; covered by mesothelial layer overlying fibrous connective tissue; congenital cystic adenomatoid malformation type II is present in 15–25%
Incidence: 0.5–6% of all congenital lung lesions
Age: neonatal presentation; 61% within first 6 months of life; occasionally in utero; M:F = 4:1

Associated with congenital anomalies in 15–65%:
@ Lung: congenital diaphragmatic hernia (20–30%), eventration / diaphragmatic paralysis (up to 60%), cystic adenomatoid malformation (15–25%), lobar emphysema, bronchogenic cyst, pectus excavatum, congenital pulmonary venolobar syndrome
◊ May coexist / form part of spectrum with CAM
@ Heart: anomalous pulmonary venous return, cardiac / pericardial anomalies (8%)
@ GI tract: epiphrenic diverticula (2%), TE fistula (1.5%), duplication of GI tract, ectopic pancreas
@ Others: renal anomaly, vertebral anomaly

- respiratory distress + cyanosis + CHF in newborn (due to shunting of blood)
- feeding difficulties
- asymptomatic (rarely becomes infected) in 10%

Location: L:R = 4:1; typically within pleural space in posterior costodiaphragmatic sulcus between diaphragm + lower lobe (63–77%); mediastinum; within pericardium; within / below diaphragm (5–15%)

√ airless (NO communication with bronchial tree); in presence of air connection with GI tract is inferred
√ may contain cystic areas
√ mediastinal shift (if large)

Angio (diagnostic):
√ arterial supply from
— aorta as single / several small branches (80%)
— splenic, gastric, subclavian, intercostal branches (15%)
— pulmonary artery (5%)
√ venous drainage via
— systemic veins (80%) to R heart (IVC, azygos, hemiazygos, SVC, portal vein)
— pulmonary vein (25%)

CXR:
√ single well-defined homogeneous triangular mass (most commonly located adjacent to posterior medial hemidiaphragm)
√ NO air bronchograms
√ small "bump" on hemidiaphragm / inferior paravertebral region
√ opaque hemithorax ± ipsilateral pleural effusion (if sequestration large)
√ ± air-fluid level

CT:
√ homogeneous well-circumscribed soft-tissue density mass (no bronchial communication)

NUC (radionuclide angiography):
√ lack of perfusion during pulmonary phase followed by rapid perfusion in systemic phase
DDx: intrathoracic kidney, scimitar syndrome (with systemic supply to affected lung), hepatic herniation through diaphragm

OB-US:
◊ The vast majority in fetuses are extralobar!
√ conical / triangular homogeneous highly echogenic mass (many interfaces from multiple microscopically dilated structures)
√ color duplex may demonstrate vascular supply
√ polyhydramnios (? esophageal compression, excessive fluid secretion by sequestration)
√ fetal hydrops (? venous compression)
√ edema, ascites
√ hydrothorax (obstructed lymphatics + veins in torsed sequestration)

CHEST

DDx for chest lesion:
congenital cystic adenomatoid malformation, neuroblastoma, teratoma, diaphragmatic hernia
DDx for infradiaphragmatic lesion:
neuroblastoma, teratoma, adrenal hemorrhage, mesoblastic nephroma, foregut duplication
Cx: infection (in cases of communication with bronchus / GI tract)
Rx: resection (delineation of vascular supply helpful)
Prognosis: favorable (worse if pulmonary hypoplasia present); decreases in size / disappears in up to 65% before birth

Esophageal / Gastric Lung
= rare variant of pulmonary sequestration
Age: infancy (as it is symptomatic)
- cough related to feeding
- recurrent pulmonary infections

√ communication of bronchial tree of sequestered lung with esophagus / stomach

CANDIDIASIS
Organism: ubiquitous human saprophyte (Candida albicans most commonly) characterized by blastospheres (yeasts) admixed with hyphae / pseudohyphae (conventional stains)
At risk: patient with lymphoreticular malignancy
Entry: (a) aspiration
(b) hematogenous dissemination from GI tract / infected central venous catheter
- prolonged fever despite broad-spectrum antibacterial coverage
- cough, hemoptysis

√ patchy airspace consolidation in lower lobe distribution
√ interstitial pattern
√ diffuse micro- / macronodular disease
√ pleural effusion (25%)

CASTLEMAN DISEASE
= ANGIOFOLLICULAR LYMPH NODE HYPERPLASIA
= GIANT LYMPH NODE HYPERPLASIA
= ANGIOMATOUS LYMPHOID HAMARTOMA
= LYMPHOID HAMARTOMA
= benign masses of lymphoid tissue of unknown etiology
Size: up to 16 cm in diameter
CT:
√ well-defined mass of muscle density
√ spotty central calcification
√ enhancing rim (vascular capsule)
√ marked enhancement almost equal to aorta (in hyalin-vascular type)
√ slight enhancement (in plasma cell type)
Angio:
√ mass with multiple feeding vessels
√ dense homogeneous blush (hyalin-vascular type)
√ some hypervascularity (plasma cell type)
DDx: indistinguishable from lymphoma

Localized / Unicentric Angiofollicular Lymph Node Hyperplasia
A. HYALINE-VASCULAR TYPE (76–91%)
Cause: chronic antigenic stimulation / developmental abnormality of lymphoid tissue
Age: 4th decade; M:F = 1:1
Path: vascular proliferation + hyalinization with small follicle centers penetrated by capillaries, capillary proliferation in interfollicular areas
Location: mediastinal + cervical lymph nodes
- asymptomatic in 97%

B. PLASMA CELL TYPE (10–24%)
Cause: chronic viral antigenic stimulation
Average age: 22 years; M:F = 1:1
Path: sheets of plasma cells between normal / enlarged follicles
Location: mesenteric + retroperitoneal lymph nodes
- cough, dyspnea, hemoptysis
- lassitude, weight loss, fever
- growth retardation
- elevated sedimentation rate
- IgG, IgM, IgA hypergammaglobulinemia (50%)
- refractory microcytic anemia

Prognosis: treatment ~100% curative
Rx: (1) complete surgical resection
(2) radiation + steroid therapy

Generalized / Multicentric Angiofollicular Lymph Node Hyperplasia
A. HYPERPLASIA WITHOUT NEUROPATHY
Cause: disordered immunoregulation with polyclonal plasma cells from viral infection
Mean age: 57 years; M>F
- fatigue, anorexia, skin lesions, CNS disorders

√ peripheral multicentric adenopathy
√ hepatosplenomegaly
√ salivary gland enlargement
√ ± pulmonary lesions
Rx: systemic chemotherapy + corticosteroids + irradiation
Prognosis: mean survival of 27 months

B. HYPERPLASIA WITH NEUROPATHY
Cause: immunoregulatory deficits with uncontrolled B-cell proliferation + interleukin-6 dysregulation
Mean age: 40–60 years; M:F = 2:1
- skin lesions: hypertrichosis, hirsutism, sclerodermatous thickening, hyperpigmentation, hemangiomas
- distal symmetric sensorimotor neuropathy (50%)
- papilledema, pseudotumor cerebri (66%)
- monoclonal IgG (75%)

Rx: surgical resection, irradiation, chemotherapy
Prognosis: mean survival of 24–33 months

CHRONIC EOSINOPHILIC PNEUMONIA

= numerous eosinophils, macrophages, histiocytes, lymphocytes, PMNs within lung interstitium + alveolar sacs

Etiology: unknown

Age: middle-age; M < F

- common history of atopia (may occur during therapeutic desensitization procedure)
- adult onset asthma (wheezing)
- high fever, malaise, dyspnea (DDx to Löffler syndrome)
- peripheral blood eosinophilia (with rare exceptions)

√ homogeneous alveolar lung infiltrates with distribution at lung periphery = "photographic negative" of pulmonary edema

√ frequently bilateral nonsegmental

√ unchanged for many days / weeks (DDx to Löffler syndrome)

√ fast regression of infiltrates under steroids

Rx: dramatic response to steroid therapy (within 3–10 days)

CHRONIC MEDIASTINITIS

Etiology:

(1) Granulomatous infection: histoplasmosis (most frequent), tuberculosis, actinomycosis, Nocardia

(2) Mediastinal granuloma

(3) Fibrosing mediastinitis

(4) Radiation therapy

Mediastinal granuloma

= relatively benign massive coalescent adenitis with caseating / noncaseating lesions

Cause: primary lymph node infection (commonly tuberculosis / histoplasmosis)

Histo: thin fibrous capsule surrounding granulomatous lesion

√ lymphadenopathy

DDx: fibrosing mediastinitis (infiltrative, rare)

Fibrosing mediastinitis

= SCLEROSING MEDIASTINITIS = MEDIASTINAL COLLAGENOSIS

= diffuse fibrotic infiltration throughout mediastinum

Cause: abnormal host immune response to Histoplasma antigen (organisms recovered in 50%); autoimmune disease, methysergide-induced

May be associated with: retroperitoneal fibrosis, orbital pseudotumor, Riedel struma

Histo: infiltrative, often invasive fibrotic process with minimal / no apparent granulomatous foci

Age: 2nd–5th decade of life

- cough, dyspnea, hemoptysis
- dysphagia
- superior vena cava syndrome
- cor pulmonale (secondary to pulmonary arterial hypertension caused by compression of pulmonary arteries / veins)

Location: upper half of mediastinum in paratracheal region + anterior to trachea + near hilum

Site: right > left

√ widening of upper mediastinum

√ lobulated (in 86% calcified) paratracheal / hilar mass

NUC:

√ decreased / absent perfusion with normal ventilation

Cx:
(1) Compression of SVC (64%) + pulmonary veins (4%)
(2) Chronic obstructive pneumonia (narrowing of trachea / central bronchi) in 5%
(3) Esophageal stenosis (3%)
(4) Pulmonary infarcts + fibrosis (narrowing of pulmonary artery)
(5) Prominent intercostal arteries (narrowing of pulmonary artery)

DDx:
(1) Swyer-James syndrome
(2) Congenital absence of pulmonary artery
(3) Embolus to main pulmonary artery
(4) Bronchogenic carcinoma
(5) Lymphoma
(6) Metastatic carcinoma

CHURG-STRAUSS SYNDROME

= variant of polyarteritis nodosa

CLASSIC TRIAD:

(1) Allergic rhinitis and asthma

(2) Eosinophilic infiltrative disease
   (a) eosinophilic pneumonia
   (b) eosinophilic gastroenteritis

(3) Systemic small-vessel vasculitis with granulomatous inflammation
   usually develops within 3 years of onset of asthma

- ANCA (antineutrophil cytoplasmic autoantibodies) in 70%
- eosinophilia (almost 100%): peripheral eosinophilia in >30%

@ Kidney: less frequent + less severe renal disease compared with Wegener granulomatosis + microscopic polyangiitis

@ Heart: coronary arteritis, myocarditis (accounting for 50% of deaths)

@ CNS: neuropathy

CHYLOTHORAX

= leakage of chyle (= lymph containing chylomicrons = suspended fat) from thoracic duct or its branches into pleural space secondary to obstruction / disruption of thoracic duct (in 2%)

Route of thoracic duct:

Origin: arises from cisterna chyli anterior to L1/2 (10–15 mm in diameter and 5–7 cm long)

Course: enters thorax through aortic hiatus; ascends in right prevertebral location (between azygos vein + descending aorta); swings to left at T4–6 posterior to esophagus; ascends for a short distance along right of aorta; crosses behind aortic arch; runs ventrally at T3 between left common carotid artery + left subclavian artery

Termination: 3–5 cm above clavicle at venous angle (= junction of left subclavian + internal jugular veins)

CHEST

Variation: two (33%) or more (in up to 50%) main ducts each consisting of up to 8 separate channels

Etiology:

A. Developmental defects
   1. Thoracic duct atresia
   2. Lymphangiectasia
   3. Lymphangioma
   4. Lymphangiomatosis (rare): mediastinal / thoracic cystic hygroma of neck growing into mediastinum
   5. Lymphangioleiomyomatosis ± tuberous sclerosis

B. Trauma
   1. Closed / penetrating chest trauma / birth trauma (25%): latent period of 10 days
   2. Surgery (2nd most common cause): esophagectomy / cardiovascular surgery, esp. coarctation repair (0.5%), retroperitoneal surgery, neck surgery
   3. Subclavian venous catheter

C. Neoplasm (54%)
   1. Lymphoma (most common cause)
   2. Metastatic cancer

D. Fibrosing conditions
   1. Mediastinitis
   2. Tuberculosis
   3. Filariasis (rare)

E. Obstruction of central venous system / thoracic duct

F. Idiopathic / cryptogenic (15%): most common cause in neonatal period

G. Transdiaphragmatic passage of chylous ascites

Age: in full-term infants; may be present in utero; M:F = 2:1

Incidence: 1:10,000 deliveries

May be associated with:
Trisomy 21, TE-fistula, extralobar lung sequestration, congenital pulmonary lymphangiectasia

- high in neutral fat + fatty acid (low in cholesterol):
  - triglyceride level >110 mg/dL
- milky viscoid fluid (chylomicrons) after ingestion of milk / formula and clear during fasting

√ usually unilateral loculated pleural effusion
  (a) right chylothorax due to duct disruption inferior to T5–6 (more common)
  (b) left-sided chylothorax if duct disrupted above T5–6

√ low attenuation (fat) / high attenuation (protein content)

√ ± leakage of lymphangiographic contrast

√ polyhydramnios (? result of esophageal compression)

Cx: (1) Pulmonary hypoplasia
(2) Hydrops (congestive heart failure secondary to impaired venous return)

Rx: (1) Thoracentesis (leading to loss of calories, lymphocytopenia, hypogammaglobulinemia)
(2) Total parenteral nutrition
(3) Thoracic duct ligation (if drainage exceeds 1500 mL/day for adults or 100 mL/yr-age/day for children >5 years of age; drainage >14 days)
(4) Pleuroperitoneal shunt; tetracycline pleurodesis; mediastinal radiation; intrapleural fibrin glue; pleurectomy

COAL WORKER'S PNEUMOCONIOSIS

= CWP = ANTHRACOSIS = ANTHRACOSILICOSIS

= coal dust inhalation taken up by alveolar macrophages, in part cleared by mucociliary action (particle size >5 μ), in part deposited around bronchioles + alveoli, coal dust in itself is inert, but admixed silica is fibrogenic

Simple CWP

= aggregates of coal dust = coal macules (usually <3 mm)

NO progression in absence of further exposure

Histo: development of reticulin fibers associated with bronchiolar dilatation (focal emphysema) + bronchiolar artery stenosis (decreased capillary perfusion)

- poor correlation between symptoms, physiologic findings + roentgenogram

√ small round 1–5 mm opacities, frequently in upper lobes (radiographically only seen through superposition after an exposure of >10 years)

√ nodularity correlates with amount of collagen (NOT amount of coal dust)

Cx: (1) Chronic obstructive bronchitis
(2) Focal emphysema
(3) Cor pulmonale

COCCIDIOIDOMYCOSIS

Organism: dimorphic soil fungus Coccidioides immitis; arthrospores in desert soil spread by wind aerosolized in dry dust; highly infectious

Geographic distribution:
endemic in southwest desert of USA (San Joaquin Valley, central southern Arizona, western Texas, southern New Mexico) + northern Mexico + in parts of Central + South America; similar to histoplasmosis

Mode of infection: deposited in alveoli after inhalation + maturation into large thick-walled spherules with release of hundreds of endospores

Dx: (1) culture of organism
(2) spherules in pathologic material (demonstrated with Gomori-methenamine silver stain)
(3) positive skin test
(4) complement fixation titer

A. PRIMARY COCCIDIOIDOMYCOSIS
   = ACUTE RESPIRATORY COCCIDIOIDOMYCOSIS
   - 60–80% asymptomatic
   - "valley fever" = influenza-like symptoms
   - desert rheumatism (33%) = immune-complex–mediated arthritis (most commonly in ankle)
   - rash, erythema nodosum / multiforme (5–20%)

   √ segmental / lobar consolidation
   √ patchy infiltrates mainly in lower lobes (46–80%) frequently subpleural + abutting fissures
   √ peribronchial thickening
   √ hilar adenopathy (20%)
   √ pleural effusion (10%)

Chronic Respiratory Coccidioidomycosis

Prevalence: 5% of infected patients
- symptoms of postprimary tuberculosis
- hemoptysis in 50%

√ one / several well-defined nodules (= coccidioidomycoma) of 5–30 mm in size (in 5%)
√ persistent / progressive consolidation
√ "grape skin" thin-walled cavities (in 10–15%), in 90% solitary, 70% in anterior segment of upper lobes (DDx: TB), 3% rupture into pleural space due to subpleural location (pneumothorax / empyema / persistent bronchopleural fistula)
√ bronchiectasis
√ mediastinal adenopathy (10–20%)

Disseminated Coccidioidomycosis (in 1%)

= secondary phase of hematogenous spread to meninges, bones, skin, lymph nodes, subcutaneous tissue, joints (except GI tract)
- skin granulomas / abscesses

√ micronodular "miliary" lung pattern
√ pericardial effusion

CONGENITAL LOBAR EMPHYSEMA

= progressive overdistension of one / multiple lobes
M:F = 3 :1
Etiology:
(a) deficiency / dysplasia / immaturity of bronchial cartilage
(b) endobronchial obstruction (mucosal fold / web, prolonged endotracheal intubation, inflammatory exudate, inspissated mucus)
(c) bronchial compression (PDA, aberrant left pulmonary artery, pulmonary artery dilatation)
(d) polyalveolar / macroalveolar hyperplasia
Associated with: CHD in 15% (PDA, VSD)
- respiratory distress (90%) + progressive cyanosis within first 6 months of life

Location: LUL (42–43%), RML (32–35%), RUL (20%), two lobes (5%)
√ hazy masslike opacity immediately following birth (delayed clearance of lung fluid in emphysematous lobe over 1–14 days)
√ air trapping
√ hyperlucent expanded lobe (after clearing of fluid)
√ compression collapse of adjacent lobes
√ contralateral mediastinal shift
√ widely separated vascular markings
Mortality: 10%
Rx: surgical resection

CONGENITAL LYMPHANGIECTASIA

1. PRIMARY PULMONARY LYMPHANGIECTASIA (2/3)
   = abnormal development of lungs between 14–20th week of GA characterized by anomalous dilatation of pulmonary lymph vessels
   Path: subpleural cysts, ectatic tortuous lymph channels in pleura, interlobular septa + along bronchoarterial bundles; NO obstruction
   Age: usually manifest at birth; 50% stillborn; M = F
   May be associated with: total anomalous pulmonary venous return, hypoplastic left heart, Noonan syndrome
   - respiratory distress within few hours of birth

   Site: diffuse involvement of both lungs, occasionally only in one / two lobes (with good prognosis)
   √ marked prominence of coarse interstitial markings (simulating interstitial edema)
   √ hyperinflation
   √ scattered radiolucent areas (dilated airways)
   √ patchy areas of pneumonia + atelectasis
   √ pneumothorax
   Prognosis: in diffuse form invariably fatal at <2 months of age
2. GENERALIZED LYMPHANGIECTASIA
   = DIFFUSE LYMPHANGIOMA
   = proliferation of mainly lymphatic vascular spaces with relentless systemic progression
   Age: children, young adults
   Location: widespread visceral + skeletal involvement
   √ diffuse pulmonary interstitial disease
   √ chylous effusions in pleural + pericardial spaces
   √ ± lytic bone lesions
   √ lymphangiographic pooling of contrast material in dilated lymphatic channels / lymph nodes
3. LOCALIZED LYMPHANGIOMA
   = rare benign usually cystic lesion
   Histo: collection of dilated + proliferated lymph vessels (? hamartoma / benign neoplasm / focal sequestration of ectatic lymph tissue)
   Age: first 3 years of life; M = F
   - asymptomatic (33%)
   - dyspnea (from tracheal compression)

   Location: neck (80%), mediastinum, axilla, extremity
   √ discrete featureless mass
   √ may have chylous / pleural effusion
   √ may have lytic lesion in contiguous skeleton
   Prognosis: propensity for local recurrence
   DDx: hemangioma
4. SECONDARY LYMPHANGIECTASIA
   Secondary to elevated pulmonary venous pressure in CHD (TAPVR)

CONGENITAL PULMONARY VENOLOBAR SYNDROME

= unique form of lung hypoplasia / aplasia affecting one / more lobes in a constellation of distinctly different congenital anomalies of the thorax that often occur together; M:F = 1:1.4

A. MAJOR COMPONENTS
   1. Hypogenetic lung (69%): lobar agenesis / aplasia / hypoplasia
   2. Partial anomalous pulmonary venous return (31%)
      = scimitar syndrome
   3. Absence of pulmonary artery (14%)
   4. Pulmonary sequestration (24%)
   5. Systemic arterialization of lung without sequestration (10%)

CHEST

6. Absence / interruption of inferior vena cava (7%)
7. Duplication of diaphragm = accessory diaphragm (7%)
 = thin membrane in right hemithorax fused anteriorly with the diaphragm coursing posterosuperiorly to join with the posterior chest wall + trapping all / part of RML / RLL
 √ accessory fissurelike oblique line above right posterior costophrenic sinus (if trapped lung is aerated)
 √ solid mass along posterior right hemidiaphragm (if trapped lung is unaerated)
 CT:
  √ ovoid area of increased density in posterior right hemithorax (= dome of accessory diaphragm)

B. MINOR COMPONENTS
1. Tracheal trifurcation (extremely rare): 2 mainstem bronchi supply the right lung
2. Eventration of diaphragm
3. Partial absence of diaphragm
4. Phrenic cyst
5. Horseshoe lung
6. Esophageal / gastric lung
7. Anomalous superior vena cava
8. Absence of left pericardium

◊ The most constant components of the syndrome are hypogenetic lung + PAPVR!

Associated with:
(1) Vascular anomalies: hypoplastic artery, anomalous venous return, systemic arterial supply
(2) Anomalies of hemidiaphragm on affected side:
 √ retrosternal band on lateral CXR due to mediastinal rotation
 √ phrenic cyst
 √ diaphragmatic hernia
 √ accessory hemidiaphragm
(3) Hemivertebrae + scoliosis
(4) CHD (25–50%): secundum-type ASD, VSD, tetralogy of Fallot, PDA, coarctation of aorta, hypoplastic left heart, double-outlet right ventricle, double-chambered right atrium, endocardial cushion defect, persistent left SVC, pulmonary stenosis

• asymptomatic (40%)
• may have dyspnea / recurrent infections

Location: right-sided predominance; M:F = 1.0:1.4

√ hypoplasia / aplasia of one / more lobes of the lung with errors of lobation (bilateral left bronchial branching pattern / horseshoe lung)
√ "scimitar vein" (90%) = partial anomalous pulmonary venous return (commonly infradiaphragmatic into IVC / portal vein / hepatic vein / R atrium), on CXR seen only in 1/3
√ systemic arterial supply to abnormal segment my be present from thoracic aorta (bronchial, intercostal, transpleural) or abdominal aorta (celiac artery, transdiaphragmatic)
√ reticular densities (enlarged bronchial / transpleural arterial collaterals)
√ small hilus (absent / small pulmonary artery)
√ small right hemithorax + mediastinal shift
√ haziness of right heart border
√ cardiac dextroposition (in right lung hypoplasia)
√ anomalies of bony thorax / thoracic soft tissues
√ absent inferior vena cava
√ rib hypoplasia / malsegmentation
√ rib notching

CT:
 √ small hemithorax + mediastinal shift
 √ abnormalities of bronchial branching
 √ anomalously located pulmonary fissure
 √ discontinuity of hemidiaphragm
 √ pulmonary arterial hypoplasia
 √ hyparterial right bronchus (instead of eparterial)
 √ one / more vessels increasing in diameter toward diaphragm
 √ rind of subpleural fatty tissue in affected hemithorax
 √ lack of normal venous confluence of right lung

DDx: meandering pulmonary vein, dextrocardia, hypoplastic lung, Swyer-James syndrome

CRYPTOCOCCOSIS

= TORULOSIS = EUROPEAN BLASTOMYCOSIS

Organism: encapsulated unimorphic yeastlike fungus Cryptococcus neoformans; spherical single-budding yeast cell with thick capsule, stains with India ink; often in soil contaminated with pigeon excreta

Histo: granulomatous lesion with caseous necrotic center

Predisposed: opportunistic invader in diabetics + immunocompromised patients

• low-grade meningitis (affinity to CNS); M:F = 4:1

@ Lung
 √ well-circumscribed mass (40%) of 2–10 cm in diameter, usually peripheral location
 √ lobar / segmental consolidation (35%)
 √ cavitation (15%)
 √ hilar / mediastinal adenopathy (12%)
 √ calcifications (extremely rare)
 √ interstitial pneumonia (rare, in AIDS patients)

@ Musculoskeletal
 √ osteomyelitis (5–10%)
 √ arthritis (rare, usually from extension of osteomyelitis)

CYSTIC ADENOMATOID MALFORMATION

= CAM = congenital cystic abnormality of the lung characterized by an intralobar mass of disorganized pulmonary tissue communicating with bronchial tree + having normal vascular supply + drainage but delayed clearance of fetal lung fluid

Incidence: 25% of congenital lung disorders; 95% of congenital cystic lung lesions

Cause: arrest of normal bronchoalveolar differentiation between 5th–7th week of gestation with overgrowth of terminal bronchioles

Path: proliferation of bronchial structures at the expense of alveolar saccular development, modified by intercommunicating cysts of various size (adenomatoid overgrowth of terminal bronchioles, proliferation of smooth muscle in cyst wall, absence of cartilage)

TYPE I (50%):
Histo: single / multiple large cyst(s) >20 mm lined by ciliated pseudostratified columnar epithelium, mucus-producing cells in 1/3
Prognosis: excellent following resection

TYPE II (40%):
Histo: multiple cysts 5–12 mm lined by ciliated cuboidal / columnar epithelium
Prognosis: poor secondary to associated abnormalities

TYPE III (10%):
Histo: solitary large bulky firm mass of bronchuslike structures lined by ciliated cuboidal epithelium with 3–5 mm small microcysts
Prognosis: poor secondary to pulmonary hypoplasia / hydrops

In 25% associated with: cardiac malformation, pectus excavatum, renal agenesis, prune-belly syndrome, jejunal atresia, chromosomal anomaly, bronchopulmonary sequestration

Age of detection: children, neonates, fetus; M:F = 1:1

- respiratory distress + severe cyanosis in first week of life (66%) / within first year of life (90%) due to compression of normal lung + airways
- superimposed chronic recurrent infection (10%) after first year of life

Location: equal frequency in all lobes (middle lobe rarely affected); more than one lobe involved in 20%; mostly unilateral without side preference

CXR:
√ almost always unilateral expansile mass with well-defined margins (80%)
√ multiple air- / occasionally fluid-filled cysts
√ sometimes solid appearance (retained fetal lung fluid / type III lesion)
√ compression of adjacent lung
√ contralateral shift of mediastinum (87%)
√ hypoplastic ipsilateral lung
√ proper position of abdominal viscera
√ spontaneous pneumothorax (late sign)

CT:
◊ Postnatally becoming obstructed and filled with air
√ solitary / multiple fluid or air-fluid filled cysts with thin walls
√ surrounding focal emphysematous changes

OB-US:
√ single large cyst / multiple large cysts of 2–10 cm in diameter (Type I)
√ multiple small cysts of 5–12 mm in diameter (Type II)
√ large homogeneously hyperechoic mass compared to liver (Type III)
√ contralateral mediastinal shift (89%)
√ polyhydramnios (25–75%, ? from compression of esophagus or increased fluid production by abnormal lung) / normal fluid (28%) / oligohydramnios (6%)
√ fetal ascites (62–71%)
√ fetal hydrops in 33–81% (decreased venous return from compression of heart / vena cava)

Risk of recurrence: none

Cx: ipsi- / bilateral pulmonary hypoplasia

Prognosis: 50% premature, 25% stillborn
◊ Polyhydramnios, ascites, hydrops indicate a poor outcome!
◊ CAM becomes smaller in fetuses in many cases + occasionally almost disappears by birth!

DDx:
(1) Congenital lobar emphysema
(2) Diaphragmatic hernia
(3) Bronchogenic cyst (small solitary cyst near midline)
(4) Neurenteric cyst
(5) Bronchial atresia
(6) Bronchopulmonary sequestration (less frequently associated with polyhydramnios / hydrops)
(7) Mediastinal / pericardial teratoma

CYSTIC FIBROSIS

= MUCOVISCIDOSIS = FIBROCYSTIC DISEASE
= autosomal recessive multisystem disease characterized by mucous plugging of exocrine glands secondary to
(a) dysfunction of exocrine glands forming a thick tenacious material obstructing conducting system
(b) reduced mucociliary transport

Incidence: 1:2,000–1:2,500 livebirths; almost exclusively in Caucasians (5% carry a CF mutant gene allele); unusual in Blacks (1:17,000), Orientals, Polynesians
◊ The most common inherited disease among Caucasian Americans!

Cause: cystic fibrosis gene (= transmembrane conductance regulator gene) on long arm of chromosome 7 creates a defective transmembrane ion transport protein through deletion of an amino-acid; the normal product represents an epithelial chloride channel that supplies luminal water by osmosis; >230 different gene mutations (in 70% ΔF_{508})

Screening (for 6 most common mutations of CF gene): carrier detection rate of 85% of Northern Europeans, 90% of Ashkenazi Jews, 50% of American Blacks

Age at diagnosis: 1st year of life (70%), by age 4 years (80%), by age 12 years (90%); mean age of 2.9 years; M:F = 1:1

- elevated concentrations of sodium + chloride (>40 mmol/L for infants) in sweat
- decreased urinary PABA excretion
- infertility in males
- increased susceptibility to infection by Staphylococcus aureus + Pseudomonas aeruginosa

Prognosis: median survival of 28 years; pulmonary complications are the most predominant cause of morbidity and death (90%)

CHEST

@ Lung
- chronic cough
- recurrent pulmonary infections (reduced mucociliary clearance encourages Pseudomonas colonization)
- progressive respiratory insufficiency due to obstructive lung disease

Location: predilection for apical + posterior segments of upper lobes
√ "fingerlike" mucus plugging (mucoid impaction in dilated bronchi) within 1st month of life
√ subsegmental / segmental / lobar atelectasis with right upper lobe predominance (10%)
√ progressive cylindrical / cystic bronchiectasis (in 100% at >6 months of age) ± air-fluid levels due to prolonged mucus plugging preponderant in upper lobes
√ parahilar linear densities + peribronchial cuffing
√ focal peripheral / generalized hyperinflation secondary to collateral air drift into blocked airways)
√ hilar adenopathy
√ large pulmonary arteries (pulmonary arterial hypertension)
√ recurrent local pneumonitis (initiated by staphylococcus / Haemophilus influenza, succeeded by Pseudomonas)
√ allergic bronchopulmonary aspergillosis (with bronchial dilatation + mucoid impaction)

CT:
√ cylindrical (varicose / cystic) bronchiectasis
√ peribrochial thickening
√ bronchiectatic cyst (= bronchus directly leading into sacculation) in 56%
√ interstitial cysts in 32%
√ emphysematous bulla (= peripheral air space with long pleural attachment + without communication to bronchus) in 12%
√ periseptal emphysema
√ mucus plugs = tubular structures ± branching pattern
√ subsegmental / segmental collapse / consolidations

NUC:
√ matched patchy areas of decreased ventilation + perfusion

Cx: (1) Pneumothorax (rupture of bulla / bleb), common + recurrent
(2) Hemoptysis
(3) Cor pulmonale
(4) Hypertrophic pulmonary osteoarthropathy (rare)

Cause of death: massive mucus plugging (95%)

@ GI tract (85–90%)
- chronic obstipation
- failure to thrive

√ gastroesophageal reflux (21–27%) due to transient inappropriate lower esophageal sphincter relaxation
√ meconium plug syndrome (25%, most common cause of colonic obstruction in the infant)
√ distal intestinal obstruction syndrome (10–15–47%) = meconium ileus equivalent syndrome (in older child / young adult)
√ meconium ileus (10–16% at birth)
◊ Earliest clinical manifestation of cystic fibrosis!
√ fibrosing colonopathy = stricture of right colon with longitudinal shortening secondary to high-dose lipase supplementation
√ thickened nodular duodenal mucosal folds (due to unbuffered gastric acid, production of abnormal mucus, Brunner gland hypertrophy)
√ mild generalized small bowel dilatation with diffuse distortion + thickening of mucosal folds (at times involving colon + rectum)
√ large distended colon with mottled appearance (retained bulky dry stool)
√ pneumatosis intestinalis of colon (5%) from air block phenomena of obstructive pulmonary disease
√ "microcolon" = colon of normal length but diminished caliber
√ "jejunization of colon" = coarse redundant + hyperplastic colonic mucosa (distended crypt goblet cells)
√ Crohn disease
√ appendicitis
√ rectal prolapse between 6 months and 3 years in untreated patients (18–23%)

Cx: gastrointestinal perforation with meconium peritonitis (50%), volvulus of dilated segments, bowel atresia, intussusception at an average age of 10 years (1%)

@ Liver
√ steatosis (30%) due to untreated malabsorption, dietary deficiencies, hepatic dysfunction, medications
√ focal / multilobular biliary cirrhosis from inspissated bile
- signs of portal hypertension (clinically in 4–6%, autoptic in up to 50%)

√ portal hypertension (in 1% of biliary cirrhosis) + hepatosplenomegaly + hypersplenism

@ Biliary tree
Histo: mucus-containing cysts in gallbladder wall
- cholestasis (secondary to CBD obstruction)
- symptoms of gallbladder disease (3.6%)

√ sludge (33%)
√ cholelithiasis (12–24%): mostly cholesterol stones due to (1) interrupted enterohepatic circulation after ileal resection / (2) ileal dysfunction in distal intestinal obstruction syndrome
√ gallbladder atony
√ microgallbladder (25% at autopsy)
√ thickened trabeculated gallbladder wall
√ subepithelial cysts of gallbladder wall
√ atresia / stenosis of cystic duct

@ Pancreas

Histo: dilatation of acini + cyst formation due to obstruction from protein plugs as a result of precipitation of relatively insoluble proteins

Path: progressive ductectasia, pancreatic atrophy, increased pancreatic lobulation, fibrosis due to recurrent acute pancreatitis, replacement by fat

- steatorrhea + malabsorption + fat intolerance due to exocrine pancreatic insufficiency in 80–90% without affecting endocrine function (once 98% of entire pancreas is damaged)
  ◊ Cystic fibrosis is the most common cause of exocrine pancreatic insufficiency in patients <30 years of age!
- abdominal pain, bloating, flatulence, failure to thrive
- diabetes mellitus (secondary to pancreatic fibrosis) in 1% of children + 13% of adults
- acute pancreatitis (clinically rare)

√ diffuse pancreatic atrophy without fatty replacement
√ lipomatous pseudohypertrophy of pancreas
√ generalized increased echogenicity (70–100%)
√ complete / partial fatty replacement (-90 to -120 HU)
√ calcific chronic pancreatitis
√ pancreatic cystosis = microscopic / 1–3 mm small cysts replacing pancreas (common), occasionally macroscopic cysts up to 12 cm

@ Skull

√ sinusitis with opacification of well-developed maxillary, ethmoid, sphenoid sinuses
√ hypoplastic frontal sinuses

OB-US:

√ hyperechogenic bowel (in up to 60–70% of fetuses affected with cystic fibrosis)

Prognosis: median survival of 28 years; 2.3 deaths/100 patients from cardiorespiratory causes (78%), hepatic disease (4%)

DIAPHRAGMATIC HERNIA

Congenital diaphragmatic hernia

= absence of closure of the pleuroperitoneal fold by 9th week of gestational age

Embryology:

ventral component of diaphragm formed by septum transversum during 3rd–5th week GA; gradually extends posteriorly to envelop esophagus + great vessels; fuses with foregut mesentery to form the posteromedial portions of the diaphragm by 8th week GA; lateral margins of diaphragm develop from muscles of the thoracic wall; the posterolaterally located pleuroperitoneal foramina (Bochdalek) close last

Incidence: 1: 2,200–3,000 livebirths (0.04%); M:F = 2:1; most common intrathoracic fetal anomaly

◊ Delayed onset following group B streptococcal infection!

Etiology:

(1) delayed fusion of diaphragm (spontaneous self-correction may occur) / premature return of bowel from its herniated position within the umbilical coelom

(2) insult that inhibits / delays normal migration of the gut + closure of the diaphragm between 8–12th week of embryogenesis

Classification (Wiseman):

I. herniation early during bronchial branching leading to severe bilateral pulmonary hypoplasia; uniformly fatal

II. herniation during distal bronchial branching leading to unilateral pulmonary hypoplasia; survival possible

III. herniation late in pregnancy with compression of otherwise normal lung; excellent prognosis

IV. postnatal herniation with compression of otherwise normal lung; excellent prognosis

Associated anomalies in 20% of liveborn and in 90% of stillborn fetuses:

1. CNS (28%): neural tube defects
2. Gastrointestinal (20%): particularly malrotation, oral cleft, omphalocele
3. Cardiovascular (9–23%)
4. Genitourinary (15%)
5. Chromosomal abnormalities (4%): trisomy 18 + 21
6. Spinal defects
7. IUGR (with concurrent major abnormality in 90%)

Location: L:R = 5–9:1

◊ Right-sided hernias are frequently fatal!

(1) **Bochdalek hernia** (85–90%)

= posterolateral defect caused by maldevelopment / defective fusion of the cephalic fold of the pleuroperitoneal membranes

Incidence: 1:2,200–12,500 livebirths

Location: left (80%), right (15%), bilateral (5%)

Herniated organs:

(a) on left: omental fat (6%), bowel, spleen, left lobe of liver, stomach (rare), kidney, pancreas

(b) on right: part of liver, gallbladder, small bowel, kidney

mnemonic: "4 B's"

Bochdalek
Back (posterior location)
Babies (age at presentation)
Big (usually large)

(2) **Morgagni hernia** (1–2%)

= anteromedial parasternal defect (space of Larrey) caused by maldevelopment of septum transversum; R > L

Incidence: 1:100,000

Herniated organs: omental fat, transverse colon, liver

Often associated with:

chromosomal abnormality, mental retardation, heart defects, pericardial deficiency

CHEST

(a) abdominal viscera / fat may herniate into pericardial sac
(b) heart may herniate into upper abdomen

mnemonic: "4 M's"
Morgani
Middle (anterior + central location)
Mature (present in older children)
Minuscule (usually small)

(3) Septum transversum defect = defect in central tendon
(4) Hiatal hernia = congenitally large esophageal orifice
(5) **Eventration** (5%) = upward displacement of abdominal contents secondary to a congenitally thin hypoplastic diaphragm
Unilateral eventration may be associated with: Beckwith-Wiedemann syndrome, trisomy 13, trisomy 15, trisomy 18
Bilateral eventration may be associated with: toxoplasmosis, CMV, arthrogryposis
Location: anteromedial on right, total involvement on left side; R:L = 5:1
√ small diaphragmatic excursions
√ often lobulated diaphragmatic contour

- respiratory distress in neonatal period (life-threatening deficiency of small airways + alveoli)
- scaphoid abdomen

Herniated organs:
small bowel (90%), stomach (60%), large bowel (56%), spleen (54%), pancreas (24%), kidney (12%), adrenal gland, liver, gallbladder
√ bowel loops in chest
√ contralateral shift of mediastinum + heart
√ complete (1–2%) / partial absence of diaphragm
√ absence of stomach, small bowel in abdomen
√ passage of nasogastric tube under fluoroscopic control entering intrathoracic stomach
√ incomplete rotation + anomalous mesenteric attachment of bowel

OB-US (diagnosis possible by 18 weeks GA):
√ solid / multicystic / complex chest mass
√ mediastinal shift
√ nonvisualization of fetal stomach below diaphragm
√ fetal stomach at level of fetal heart
√ peristalsis of bowel within fetal chest (inconsistent)
√ paradoxical motion of diaphragm with fetal breathing (defect in diaphragm sonographically not visible)
√ scaphoid fetal abdomen with reduced abdominal circumference
√ herniated liver frequently surrounded by ascites
√ polyhydramnios (common, due to partial esophageal obstruction or heart failure) / normal fluid volume / oligohydramnios
√ swallowed fetal intestinal contrast appears in chest (CT amniography confirms diagnosis)

Cx: (1) Bilateral pulmonary hypoplasia
(2) Persistent fetal circulation (postsurgical pulmonary hypertension)

Prognosis: (1) Stillbirth (35–50%)
(2) Neonatal death (35%)
◊ Survival is determined by size of defect + time of entry + associated anomalies (34% survival rate if isolated, 7% with associated anomalies)

Indicators for poor prognosis:
large intrathoracic mass with marked mediastinal shift, IUGR, polyhydramnios, hydrops fetalis, detection <25 weeks MA, intrathoracic liver, dilated intrathoracic stomach, other malformations

Mortality: in 10% death before surgery;
40–50% operative mortality;
(a) stomach intrathoracic vs. intraabdominal = 60% vs. 6%
(b) polyhydramnios vs. normal amniotic fluid = 89% vs. 45%

DDx: Congenital adenomatoid malformation, mediastinal cyst (bronchogenic, neuroenteric, thymic)

Traumatic diaphragmatic hernia

Prevalence: 0.8–5.0% of all trauma patients; 5% of all diaphragmatic hernias, but 90% of all strangulated diaphragmatic hernias

Etiology of traumatic rupture of diaphragm:
(a) blunt trauma (5–50%) due to marked increase in intraabdominal pressure: motor vehicle accident, fall from height, bout of hyperemesis; L:R = 3:1, bilateral rupture in <3.6%
(b) penetrating trauma (50%): knife, bullet, repair of hiatus hernia
◊ usually <1 cm in diameter; detected at surgery

Herniated organs in order of frequency:
stomach, colon, small bowel, omentum, spleen, kidney, pancreas

- may be asymptomatic for months / years following trauma, onset of symptoms may be so long delayed that traumatic event is forgotten
- virtually all become ultimately symptomatic, most in <3 years
- **Bergqvist triad**:
(1) rib fractures (2) fracture of spine / pelvis
(3) traumatic rupture of diaphragm

Location: 90–98% on left side; posterolateral portion of diaphragm medial to spleen
Size: most tears are >10 cm in length
CXR:
◊ The first posttraumatic CXR is abnormal in only 28–64%!
√ nonvisualization of diaphragmatic contour
√ abnormally elevated contour of hemidiaphragm
Cave: cephalad margin of bowel may simulate an elevated diaphragm (look for haustra)
√ lower lobe mass / consolidation (herniated solid organ / omentum / airless bowel loop)
√ inhomogeneous mass with air-fluid level in left hemithorax
√ displacement of mediastinum + lung to contralateral side

√ mushroomlike mass of herniated liver in right hemithorax
√ "hourglass" constriction of afferent + efferent bowel loops at orifice
√ hydrothorax / hemothorax indicates strangulation
√ nasogastric tube above suspected level of hemidiaphragm
N.B.: tube first dips below diaphragm (rent spares esophageal hiatus with gastroesophageal junction remaining in its normal position)
√ location of diaphragm may be documented by
1. gas-filled bowel constricted at site of diaphragmatic laceration
2. barium study

CT (61% sensitive, 87% specific):
√ abrupt discontinuity of hemidiaphragm
√ herniation of omentum / abdominal viscera into thorax
√ "collar sign" = focal constriction of viscera at level of diaphragm
√ "absent diaphragm sign" = failure to see diaphragm

Associated injuries:
√ fractures of lower ribs
√ perforation of hollow viscus
√ rupture of spleen

Reasons fore diagnostic misses:
(1) left-sided defect covered by omentum
(2) right-sided defect sealed by liver
(3) positive pressure ventilation

Cx: life-threatening strangulation of bowel / stomach occurs in majority
◊ 90% of strangulated hernias are traumatic!

DDx: eventration, diaphragmatic paralysis

EMPHYSEMA

= group of pulmonary diseases characterized by permanently enlarged air spaces distal to terminal bronchioles accompanied by destruction of alveolar walls + local elastic fiber network

◊ The clinical term "chronic obstructive pulmonary disease (COPD)" should not be used in image interpretation! It encompasses: asthma, chronic bronchitis, emphysema!

Prevalence: 1.65 million people in United States

Cause: imbalance in elastase-antielastase system (due to increase in elastase activity in smokers / α_1-antiprotease deficiency) causing proteolytic destruction of elastin resulting in alveolar wall destruction

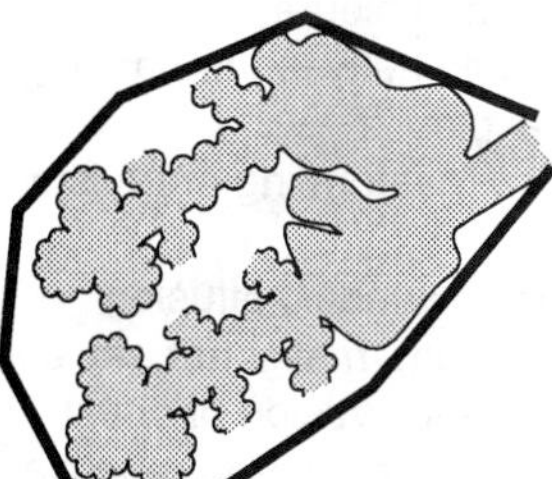
Centrilobar Emphysema

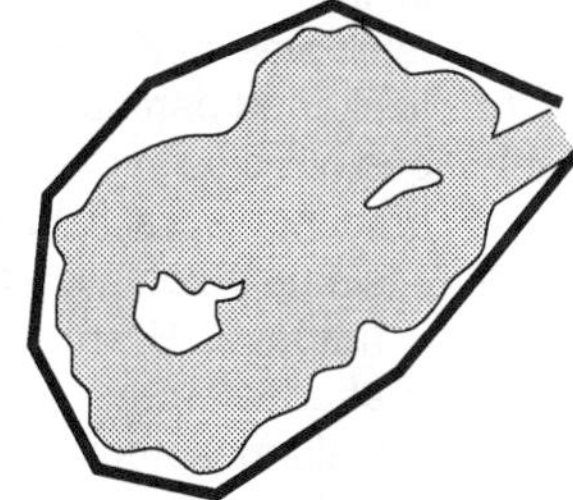
Panacinar Emphysema

• dyspnea on exertion
• irreversible expiratory airflow obstruction (due to decreased elastic recoil from parenchymal destruction)
• decreased carbon monoxide diffusing capacity

CXR (moderately sensitive, highly specific):
√ hyperinflated lung (most reliable sign)
√ low hemidiaphragm (= at / below 7th anterior rib)
√ flat hemidiaphragm (= <1.5 cm distance between line connecting the costo- and cardiophrenic angles + top of midhemidiaphragm)
√ retrosternal air space >2.5 cm
√ "barrel chest" = enlarged anteroposterior chest diameter
√ saber-sheath trachea
√ pulmonary vascular pruning + distortion (± pulmonary arterial hypertension)
√ right-heart enlargement
√ bullae

HRCT:
√ well-defined areas of abnormally decreased attenuation without definable wall (<-910 HU)

Rx: lung volume reduction surgery

CHEST

Centrilobular emphysema

= CENTRIACINAR EMPHYSEMA = PROXIMAL ACINAR EMPHYSEMA
= emphysematous change selectively affecting the acinus at the level of 1st + 2nd generations of respiratory bronchioles (most common form)

Path: normal + emphysematous alveolar spaces adjacent to each other

Histo: enlargement of respiratory bronchioles + destruction of centrilobular alveolar septa in the center of the secondary pulmonary lobule; CHARACTERISTICALLY surrounded by normal lung; distal alveoli spared; severity of destruction varies from lobule to lobule

Predisposed: smokers (in up to 50%), coal workers

Cause: excess protease with smoking (elastase is contained in neutrophils + macrophages found in abundance in lung of smokers)

• blue bloater

Site: apical and posterior segments of upper lobe + superior segment of lower lobe (relatively greater ventilation-perfusion ratio in upper lobes favors deposition of particulate matter and release of elastase in upper lungs)

CXR (80% sensitivity for moderate / severe stages):
√ irregular scattered area of radiolucency (best appreciated if lung opacified by edema / pneumonia / hemorrhage) = area of bullae, arterial depletion + increased markings
√ hyperinflated lung

HRCT:
√ "emphysematous spaces" (= focal area of air attenuation) >1 cm in diameter with central dot / line (representing the centrilobular artery of secondary pulmonary lobule) without definable wall and surrounded by normal lung

√ pulmonary vascular distortion + pruning with lack of juxtaposition of normal lung (advanced stage)

Panacinar emphysema

= PANLOBULAR EMPHYSEMA = DIFFUSE EMPHYSEMA = GENERALIZED EMPHYSEMA (rare)
= emphysematous change involving the entire acinus
= uniform nonselective destruction of all air spaces throughout both lungs

Path: uniform enlargement of acini from respiratory bronchioles to terminal alveoli (from center to periphery of secondary pulmonary lobule) secondary to destruction of lung distal to terminal bronchiole

Cause: autosomal recessive α-1-antitrypsin deficiency in 10–15% (proteolytic enzymes carried by leukocytes in blood gradually destroy lung unless inactivated by α-1-protease inhibitor)

Age: 6–7th decade (3rd–4th decade in smokers)

• pink puffer

Site: affects whole lung, but more severe at lung bases (due to greater blood flow)

CXR:
√ hyperinflated lung
√ decreased pulmonary vascular markings
√ lung destruction extremely uniform

HRCT:
√ diffuse simplification of lung architecture with pulmonary septal and vascular distortion + pruning (difficult to detect early, ie, prior to considerable lung destruction for lack of adjacent normal lung)
√ paucity of vessels
√ bullae

Paracicatricial emphysema

= PERIFOCAL / IRREGULAR EMPHYSEMA
= airspace enlargement + lung destruction developing adjacent to areas of pulmonary scarring

Usual cause: granulomatous inflammation, organized pneumonia, pulmonary infarction

Path: no consistent relationship to any portion of secondary lobule / acinus; frequently associated with bronchiolectasis producing "honeycomb lung"

• little functional significance

CXR (rarely detectable):
√ fine curvilinear reticular opacities + interposed radiolucent areas

HRCT:
√ low-attenuation areas adjacent to areas of fibrosis (diagnosable only in the absence of other forms of emphysema)

Paraseptal emphysema

= DISTAL ACINAR EMPHYSEMA = LOCALIZED EMPHYSEMA = LINEAR EMPHYSEMA
= focal enlargement + destruction of air spaces in one site in otherwise normal lung

Path: predominant involvement of alveolar ducts + sacs

Site: characteristically within subpleural lung and adjacent to interlobular septa + vessels

CXR:
√ area of lucency, frequently sharply demarcated from normal lung
√ bands of radiopacity (residual vessels / interstitium) may be present

HRCT:
√ peripheral low-attenuation area with remainder of lung normal

Cx: spontaneous pneumothorax; bullae formation

EMPYEMA

Stage

I "exudative" stage = inflamed pleura weeps proteinaceous fluid into pleural space = sterile exudate
  • elevated number of PMNs
  • pH >7.20; glucose >40 mg/dL (2.2 mmol/L); LDH <1000

II "fibropurulent" stage = accumulation of neutrophils + fibrin deposition on pleural surfaces
  — early stage II empyema
    • WBCs >5 x 10^9/mm^3, but no gross pus
    • pH between 7.0 and 7.2
    • glucose level >40 mg/dL
  — late stage II empyema
    • frank pus
    • pH <7.0
    • glucose level <40 mg/dL

  Cx: multiloculation
  Rx: chest tube drainage

III "organization" stage = fibroblast infiltration forming "pleural peel / pleural rind"
  Cx: limited expansion of lung
  Rx: decortication (with persistent sepsis despite appropriate antibiotic Rx + drainage / persistent thick pleural rind trapping underlying lung)

CT:
√ thickening of parietal pleura in 60% on NECT, in 86% on CECT
√ increased thickness + density of paraspinal subcostal tissue (inflammation of extrapleural fat)
√ curvilinear enhancement of chest wall boundary in 96% (inflammatory hyperemia of pleura)
√ "split pleura" sign = pleural fluid between enhancing thickened parietal + visceral pleura
√ gas bubbles in pleural space (gasforming organism / bronchopleural fistula)

DDx: simple / complicated parapneumonic effusion (negative Gram + culture stain), malignant effusion after sclerotherapy, malignant invasion of chest wall, mesothelioma, pleural tuberculosis, reactive mesothelial hyperplasia, pleural effusion of rheumatoid disease

EXTRAMEDULLARY PLASMACYTOMA

Uncommon form; relatively benign course (dissemination may be found months / ears later or not at all); questionable if precursor to multiple myeloma

Age: 35–40 years; M:F = 2:

Location: air passages (50%) predominantly in upper nose and oral cavity; conjunctiva (37%); lymph nodes (3%)

- usually not associated with increased immunoglobulin titer or amyloid deposition

√ mass of one to several cm in size with well-defined lobulated border

Classification:

1. Medullary plasmacytoma
2. Multiple myeloma:
   (a) scattered involvement of bone
   (b) myelomatosis of bone
3. Extramedullary plasmacytoma

DDx:

(1) MULTIPLE MYELOMA
= malignant course with soft-tissue involvement in 50–73%:
(a) microscopic infiltration
(b) enlargement of organs
(c) formation of tumor mass (1/3)
- usually associated with protein abnormalities
- may have amyloid deposition

Age incidence: 50–85 years

◊ tends to occur late in the course of the disease and indicates a poor prognosis (0–6% 5-year survival)

EXTRINSIC ALLERGIC ALVEOLITIS

= HYPERSENSITIVITY PNEUMONITIS
= characterized by an inappropriate host response to inhaled organic allergens that are often related to patient's occupation

Cause: exposure to organic dust of <5 μm particle size acting as antigen

Histo: diffuse predominantly mononuclear cell inflammation of bronchioles (bronchiolitis) + pulmonary parenchyma (alveolitis); ill-defined granulomas of <1 mm in diameter

- asymptomatic (10–40%)
- recurrent episodes of fever, chills, dry cough, dyspnea following exposure after 6-hour interval
- resolution of episodic symptoms after cessation of exposure, abate spontaneously over 1–2 days
- insidious onset of gradually progressive dyspnea
- reduction in vital capacity, diffusing capacity, arterial PO_2
- intracutaneous injection of antigen results in delayed hypersensitivity reaction
- presence of serum precipitins against antigen
- positive aerosol provocation inhalation test
- markedly increased cell count with often >50% T-lymphocytes on bronchoalveolar lavage

Location: predominantly midlung zones, occasionally lower lung zones, rarely upper lung zones

Specific antigens for immune complex disease (Type III = Arthus reaction):

1. **Farmer's lung** from moldy hay (Thermoactinomyces vulgaris or Micropolyspora faeni)
2. Hypersensitivity pneumonitis from forced-air equipment = **Pandora's pneumonitis** with heating / humidifying / air conditioning systems (thermophilic actinomycetes)
3. **Bird-fancier's lung**, pigeon breeder's lung from protein in bird serum / excrements / feathers
4. **Mushroom worker's lung** from mushroom compost (Thermoactinomyces vulgaris or Micropolyspora faeni)
5. **Bagassosis** from moldy sugar cane in sugar mill (contamination with Thermoactinomyces sacchari / vulgaris and Micropolyspora faeni)
6. **Malt worker's lung** from malt dust (Aspergillus clavatus)
7. **Maple bark disease** from moldy maple bark in saw mill (Cryptostroma corticale)
8. **Suberosis** from moldy cork dust (Penicillium frequentans)
9. **Sequoiosis** from redwood dust (Graphium species)

Thermophilic actinomycetes
= bacteria <1 μm in diameter with morphologic characteristics of fungi; found in soil, grains, compost, fresh water, forced-air heating, cooling system, humidifier, air-conditioning system

A. ACUTE EXTRINSIC ALLERGIC ALVEOLITIS
= heavy exposure to inciting antigen in domestic, occupational, atmospheric environment

Histo: filling of air spaces by polymorph neutrophils + lymphocytes

Onset of symptoms after exposure: 4–8 hours

- fever, chills, malaise, chest tightness, cough, dyspnea
- scanty mucoid expectoration
- frontal headache, arthralgia (common)

√ No CXR abnormalities in 30–95%
√ diffuse acinar consolidative pattern (edema + exudate filling alveoli) resolving within a few days
√ lymph node enlargement (unusual, more common with recurrence)

CT:
√ small + medium rounded opacities (large active granulomas)
√ diffuse dense airspace consolidation (confluent collections of intraalveolar histiocytes, interstitial + intraalveolar edema)

Dx: classical presentation of a known exposure history + typical symptoms + detection of serum precipitins to suspected antigen

B. SUBACUTE EXTRINSIC ALLERGIC ALVEOLITIS
= less intense but continuous exposure to inhaled antigens, usually in domestic environment

Histo: predominantly interstitial lymphocytic infiltrate, poorly defined granulomas, cellular bronchiolitis

Onset of symptoms after exposure: weeks – months

- recurrent respiratory / systemic symptoms: breathlessness upon exertion, fever + cough, weight loss, muscle + joint pain

√ changes may be completely reversible if present less than 1 year
√ interstitial nodular / reticulonodular pattern
CT:
√ poorly defined centrilobular micronodules <5 mm (cellular bronchiolitis + small granulomas)
√ widespread patchy ground-glass attenuation in 52% (obstructive pneumonitis, filling of alveoli by large mononuclear cell infiltrates)
√ areas of decreased attenuation + mosaic perfusion (86%)

C. CHRONIC EXTRINSIC ALLERGIC ALVEOLITIS
= prolonged insidious dust exposure
Onset of symptoms after exposure: months – years
- insidious progressive exertional dyspnea indistinguishable from idiopathic pulmonary fibrosis

Histo: proliferation of epithelial cells + predominantly peribronchiolar interstitial fibrosis
Location: usually in mid zones, relative sparing of lung apices + costophrenic sulci
√ irregular linear opacities (fibrosis)
√ loss of lung volume (cicatrization atelectasis)
√ pleural effusion (rare)
√ lymph node enlargement may occur
CT:
√ honeycombing without zonal predominance
√ focal air trapping / diffuse emphysema
√ coexistent subacute changes (due to continuing exposure)
Rx: mask, filter, industrial hygiene, alterations in forced-air ventilatory system, change in patient's habits / occupation / environment

CHEST

FAT EMBOLISM
= obstruction of pulmonary vessels by fat globules followed by chemical pneumonitis from unsaturated plasma fatty acids producing hemorrhage / edema
Incidence: in necropsy series in 67–97% of patients with major skeletal trauma, however, symptomatic fat embolism syndrome in <10% (M > F)
Onset: 24–72 hours after trauma
- dyspnea (progressive pulmonary insufficiency)
- fever
- systemic hypoxemia
- mentation changes: headaches, confusion
- petechiae (50%) from coagulopathy (release of tissue thromboplastin)

√ initial chest film usually negative (normal up to 72 hours)
√ platelike atelectasis
√ bilateral diffuse alveolar infiltrates
√ consolidation (may progress to ARDS)
NUC:
√ mottled peripheral perfusion defects (1–4 days after injury), later enlarging secondary to pneumonic infiltrates

FOCAL ORGANIZING PNEUMONIA
= unresolving pneumonia / pneumonia with incomplete resolution beyond 8 weeks
Prevalence: 5–10% of all pneumonias (87% of pneumonias resolve within 4 weeks, 12% within 4–8 weeks)
Predisposing factors: ? age, diabetes mellitus, chronic bronchitis, overuse of antibiotics
Histo: organization of intraalveolar exudate + thickening of alveolar septa / chronic inflammatory change of bronchial mucosa + obstructive lesion in bronchioles with organization
- cough, sputum, fever, hemoptysis (in 1/4)

√ ill-defined localized parenchymal abnormality with irregular margin
√ decrease in size of mass within 3–4 weeks
HRCT:
√ flat / ovoid lesion with irregular margin in subpleural location / along bronchovascular bundle
√ ± satellite lesions (44%) + air bronchogram (22%)

FRACTURE OF TRACHEA / BRONCHUS
Location: (a) mainstem bronchus 1–2 cm distal to carina (80%); R > L
(b) just above carina (20%)
√ fracture of first 3 ribs (53–91%), rare in children
√ pneumothorax (70%)
√ mediastinal ± subcutaneous emphysema
√ absence of pleural effusion
√ collapsed lung falling to dependent position (loss of anchoring support in bronchial transection)
√ atelectasis (may be late development)
√ inadequate reexpansion of lung despite chest tube (due to large air leak)
Prognosis: 30% mortality (in 15% within 1 hour)

GOODPASTURE SYNDROME
= autoimmune disease characterized by
(1) glomerulonephritis
(2) circulating antibodies against glomerular + alveolar basement membrane
(3) pulmonary hemorrhage
Pathogenesis:
cytotoxic antibody-mediated disease = Type II hypersensitivity; alveolar basement membrane becomes antigenic (perhaps viral etiology); IgG / IgM antibody with complement activation causes cell destruction + pulmonary hemorrhage, leads to hemosiderin deposition and pulmonary fibrosis
Age peak: 26 years (range 17–78 years); M:F = 7:1
- iron-deficiency anemia
- hepatosplenomegaly
- systemic hypertension

@ Lung
- preceding upper respiratory infection (in 2/3) + renal disease
- mild hemoptysis (72%) with hemosiderin-laden macrophages in sputum, commonly precedes the clinical manifestations of renal disease by several months

- cough, dyspnea, basilar rales
- √ patchy alveolar filling pattern with predominance in perihilar area + lung bases
- √ air bronchogram
- √ consolidation at lung bases + central lung fields
- √ gradually interstitial pattern (due to septal thickening) = organization of hemorrhage
- √ hilar lymph noes may be enlarged during acute episodes

@ Kidney
- glomerulonephritis with IgG deposits in characteristic linear pattern in glomeruli
- hematuria

Prognosis: death within 3 years (average 6 months) because of renal failure
Rx: cytotoxic chemotherapy, plasmapheresis, bilateral nephrectomy
DDx: idiopathic pulmonary hemosiderosis

GRANULOMA OF LUNG

Cause:
A. Sarcoidosis
B. Non-sarcoid granulomatous disease
(a) infectious
- bacterial: TB, gumma
- opportunistic: cryptococcosis
- parasitic: Dirofilaria immitis (dog heartworm)
- fungal: histoplasmosis, coccidioidomycosis, nocardiosis

(b) noninfectious
- foreign body: talc, beryllium, algae, pollen, cellulose, lipids, abuse of nasally inhaled drugs, aspiration of medication
- angiocentric lymphoproliferative disease
- vasculitides
- extrinsic allergic alveolitis
- Langerhans cell histiocytosis
- pulmonary hyalinizing granuloma
- peribronchial granuloma
- chronic granulomatous disease of childhood

Histo: epithelial cells, lymphocytes, macrophages, giant cells of Langhans type
Frequency: constitutes the majority of solitary pulmonary nodules
- nonproductive cough
- shortness of breath
- spontaneous pneumothorax

CXR:
◊ CXR detection requires multiple granulomas / clusters of granulomas (individual granuloma too small)!
√ central nidus of calcification in a laminated / diffuse pattern
√ absence of growth for at least 2 years

CT (most effective in nodules ≤3 cm of diameter with smooth discrete margins):
√ 50–60% of pulmonary nodules demonstrate unsuspected calcification by CT

DDx: Carcinoma (in 10% eccentric calcification in preexisting scar / nearby granuloma / true intrinsic stippled calcification in larger lesion)

HAMARTOMA OF CHEST WALL

= MESENCHYMOMA (incorrect as it implies neoplasm)
= focal overgrowth of normal skeletal elements with a benign self-limited course; extremely rare
Age: 1st year of life
√ moderate / large extrapleural well-circumscribed mass affecting one / more ribs
√ ribs near center of mass partially / completely destroyed
√ ribs at periphery deformed / eroded
√ significant amount of calcification / ossification (DDx: aneurysmal bone cyst)
√ mass compresses underlying lung
Rx: resection curative

HAMARTOMA OF LUNG

= composed of tissues normally found in this location in abnormal quantity, mixture, and arrangement
Incidence: 0.25% in population (autopsy); 6–8% of all solitary pulmonary lesions; most common benign lung tumor
Etiology:
1. Congenital malformation of a displaced bronchial anlage
2. Hyperplasia of normal structures
3. Cartilaginous neoplasm
4. Response to inflammation

Path: columnar, cuboidal, ciliated epithelium, fat (in 50%), bone, cartilage (predominates), muscle, vessels, fibrous tissue, calcifications, plasma cells originating in fibrous connective tissue beneath mucous membrane of bronchial wall
Age peak: 5th + 6th decade; M:F = 3:1
- mostly asymptomatic
- hemoptysis (rare)
- cough, vague chest pain, fever (with postobstructive pneumonitis)

Location: 2/3 peripheral; endobronchial in 10%; multiplicity (rare)
√ round smooth lobulated mass <4 cm (averages 2.5 cm)
√ calcification in 15% (almost pathognomonic if of chondroid "popcorn" type)
√ fat in 50% (detection by CT)
√ cavitation (extremely rare)
√ growth patterns: slow / rapid / stable with later growth
√ usually 5 mm increase in diameter per year
HRCT:
√ fat density detectable in 34% (-80 to -120 HU)
√ calcium + fat detectable in 19%
DDx: Lipoid pneumonia (ill-defined mass / lung infiltrate)

HEREDITARY HEMORRHAGIC TELANGIECTASIA

= RENDU-OSLER-WEBER SYNDROME
= hereditary multiorgan abnormality of vascular structure
Etiology: gene encoding a protein that binds transforming growth factor
Path: direct connections between arteries + veins with absence of capillaries (telangiectases are small AVMs)

CHEST

(a) small telangiectasis = focal dilatation of postcapillary venules with prominent stress fibers in pericytes along luminal borders
(b) fully developed telangiectasis = markedly dilated + convoluted venules with excessive layers of smooth muscle without elastic fibers directly connecting to dilated arterioles

@ Nose (telangiectasis of nasal mucosa)
- recurrent epistaxis: more severe over time in 66%; begins by age 10, present by age 21 in most cases

@ Skin (present in most cases by age 40)
telangiectases of lips, tongue, palate, fingers, face, conjunctiva, trunk, arms, nail beds

@ Lung (in 5–15%)
see PULMONARY ARTERIAL MALFORMATION

@ CNS (cerebral or spinal AVMs)
- subarachnoid hemorrhage
- seizure; paraparesis (less common)

@ GI tract (stomach, duodenum, small bowel, colon)
occasionally associated with AVMs / angiodysplasia
- recurrent GI bleeding (in 5th–6th decade)

@ Liver
presence of multiple AVMs / atypical cirrhosis
- high cardiac output failure (due to L-to-R shunt)

HISTOPLASMOSIS

Prevalence: nearly 100% in endemic area; up to 30% in Central + South America, Puerto Rico, West Africa, Southeast Asia

Organism: Histoplasma capsulatum = dimorphic fungus; worldwide most often in temperate climates; widespread in soil enriched by bird droppings of central North America (endemic in Ohio, Mississippi, St. Lawrence River valley; exists as a spore in soil + transforms into yeast form at normal body temperatures

Infection: inhalation of wind-borne spores (microconidia of 2–6 μm, macroconidia of 6–14 μm) which germinate within alveoli releasing yeast forms which are phagocytized but not killed by macrophages; invasion of pulmonary lymphatics with spread to hilar + mediastinal lymph nodes; hematogenous dissemination of parasitized macrophages throughout reticuloendothelial system (spleen!)

Path: spores incite formation of epitheloid granulomas, necrosis, calcification

Dx:
(1) Culture (sputum, lung tissue, urine, bone marrow, lymph node)
(2) Identification of yeast forms stained with PAS / Gomori methenamine silver
(3) Complement fixation test (absolute titer of 1:64 or 4-fold rise in convalescent titer suggest active / recent infection)
(4) Serum immunodiffusion: agar gel diffusion test (H precipitin band)

Rx: ketoconazole

Pulmonary histoplasmosis

A. ACUTE HISTOPLASMOSIS
- mostly asymptomatic and self-limiting illness (in 99.5%)
- fever, cough, malaise simulating viral upper respiratory infection 3 weeks after massive inoculum / in debilitated patients (infants, elderly)
- positive skin test for histoplasmosis

√ generalized lymphadenopathy
√ bilateral nonsegmental bronchopneumonic pattern with tendency to clear in one area + appear in another
√ multiple nodules changing into hundreds of punctate calcifications (usually >4 mm) after 9–24 months
√ "target lesion" = central calcification is PATHOGNOMONIC
√ hilar / mediastinal lymph node enlargement (DDx: acute viral / bacterial pneumonia)
√ "popcorn" calcification of mediastinal lymph nodes >10 mm
√ >5 splenic calcifications (40%)

CT:
√ paratracheal / subcarinal mass with regions of low attenuation (necrosis) + enhancing septa

B. CHRONIC HISTOPLASMOSIS (0.03%)

Predisposed: individuals with chronic obstructive pulmonary disease
Age: adult middle-aged white men
Pathophysiology: hyperimmune reaction
- cough, low-grade fever, night sweats simulating postprimary tuberculosis

√ segmental wedge-shaped peripheral consolidation of moth-eaten appearance from scattered foci of emphysematous lung
√ fibrosis in apical posterior segments of upper lobes (indistinguishable from postprimary TB) adjacent to emphysematous blebs

C. DISSEMINATED HISTOPLASMOSIS

Predisposed: impaired T-cell immunity; AIDS
Prevalence: 1:50,000 exposed individuals
Pathophysiology: progression of exogenous infection / reactivation of latent focus
- acute rapidly fatal infection
  - fever, weight loss, anorexia, malaise
  - cough (<50%)
  - abdominal pain, nausea, vomiting, diarrhea
- chronic intermittent illness
  - low-grade fever, weight loss, fatigue
  - adrenal insufficiency

√ normal CXR (>50%)
√ miliary / diffuse reticulonodular pattern rapidly progressing to diffuse airspace opacification
√ hilar + mediastinal adenopathy
√ hepatosplenomegaly

Cx: arthritis (most often knee), tenosynovitis, osteomyelitis

D. DELAYED MANIFESTATIONS
√ **histoplasmoma** (= continued growth of primary focus at 0.5–2.8 mm/year) adjacent to pleura + typically with laminated calcific rings;
in 20% associated with: mediastinal granulomas
√ broncholithiasis
√ **mediastinal granuloma** (more common)
= direct infection of mediastinal lymph nodes
Histo: involved nodes with varying degrees of central caseation ± calcification
• usually asymptomatic
Location: subcarinal / right paratracheal / hilar lymph nodes
√ widened mediastinum (enlarged nodes + veins)
√ lobulated mass of low-density lymph nodes 3–10 cm in thickness surrounded by a 2–5 mm thick fibrous capsule crisscrossed by irregularly shaped septa (CHARACTERISTIC)
√ displacement of SVC / esophagus
√ fibrosing mediastinitis (less common)
◊ Organism recovered in only 50%!

HYDATID DISEASE

= ECHINOCOCCOSIS
• asymptomatic
• eosinophilia (<25%)
• cough, expectoration, fever
• positive Casoni skin test in 60%
• hypersensitivity reaction (if cyst rupture occurs)
√ solitary (75%) / multiple (25%) sharply circumscribed spherical / ovoid masses
√ size of 1–10 cm in diameter (16–20 weeks doubling time)
√ cyst communicating with bronchial tree
√ "meniscus sign", "double arch sign," "moon sign," "crescent sign" (5%) = rupture of pericyst with air dissection between peri- and exocyst
√ "water lily sign," "sign of the Camalotte" = collapsed cyst membrane floating on the fluid
√ air-fluid level = rupture of all cyst walls
√ hydropneumothorax
√ calcification of cyst wall (<6%)
√ rib + vertebral erosion (rare)
√ mediastinal cyst: posterior (65%), anterior (26%), middle (9%) mediastinum

HYPOGENETIC LUNG SYNDROME

= collective name for congenital underdevelopment of one / more lobes of a lung separated into 3 forms:

1. **Pulmonary agenesis**
= complete absence of a lobe + its bronchus
CT:
√ missing bronchus + lobe(s)
2. **Pulmonary aplasia**
= rudimentary bronchus ending in blind pouch + absence of parenchyma + vessels
Incidence: 1:10,000; R:L = 1:1
CT:
√ absence of ipsilateral pulmonary artery
√ bronchus terminates in dilated blind pouch
√ absence of ipsilateral pulmonary tissue
3. **Pulmonary hypoplasia** (38%)
= completely formed but congenitally small bronchus with rudimentary parenchyma + small vessels
Developmental causes:
(a) Idiopathic
(b) Extrathoracic compression
1. Oligohydramnios
2. Fetal ascites
3. Membranous diaphragm
(c) Thoracic cage compression
1. Thoracic dystrophies
2. Muscular disease
(d) Intrathoracic compression
1. Diaphragmatic defect
2. Excess pleural fluid
3. Large intrathoracic cyst / tumor
CT:
√ small bronchus + lobe

◊ Hypogenetic lung is the most constant component of congenital pulmonary venolobar syndrome!
May be associated with: congenital tracheal stenosis, bronchitis, bronchiectasis
Location: R:L = 3:1; RML (65%) > RUL (40%) > RLL (20%) > LUL (20%) > LLL (15%); multiple lobes (45%)
• usually asymptomatic (in isolated hypogenetic lung)
• exertional dyspnea
√ small ipsilateral hemithorax + elevated hemidiaphragm
√ diminished pulmonary vascularity on involved side
√ small hilum on involved side (absent / small pulmonary artery)
√ mediastinum + heart shifted toward involved side
√ indistinct cardiomediastinal border on involved side
√ diminished radiolucency on involved side
√ large ipsilateral apical cap + blunted costophrenic angle
√ broad retrosternal band of opacity (LAT view)

HORSESHOE LUNG
= uncommon variant of hypogenetic lung syndrome in which RLL crosses midline between esophagus and heart + fuses with opposite lung
√ oblique fissure in left lower hemithorax (if both lungs separated by pleural layers)
√ pulmonary vessels + bronchi crossing midline

IDIOPATHIC INTERSTITIAL PNEUMONIA

Acute interstitial pneumonia

= AIP = [ACCELERATED INTERSTITIAL PNEUMONIA] = DIFFUSE ALVEOLAR DAMAGE = IDIOPATHIC ARDS = ACUTE DIFFUSE INTERSTITIAL FIBROSIS = HAMMAN-RICH SYNDROME
= rapidly progressive fulminant disease of unknown etiology that usually occurs in previously healthy subjects + produces diffuse alveolar damage
Path: temporally homogeneous organizing diffuse alveolar damage; little mature collagen deposition / architectural distortion / honeycombing (as opposed to UIP)

CHEST

Histo: thickening of alveolar wall due to alveolar edema + inflammatory cells; extensive alveolar damage with hyaline membrane formation; marked interstitial fibroblast proliferation with stabilizing nonprogressive scarring
Mean age: 50 years; M=F

- prodromal viral upper respiratory infection: cough, fever
- rapidly increasing dyspnea + acute respiratory failure
- requires ventilation within days to (1–4) weeks

Location: mainly lower lung zones
Site: predominantly central / subpleural (in 22%)
CXR:
√ progressive extensive bilateral airspace opacification: symmetric, bilateral, basilar
CT:
√ diffuse extensive bilateral airspace consolidation (in 67%) with basal predominance (similar to ARDS)
√ patchy (67%) / diffuse (38%) bilateral ground-glass opacities
√ anteroposterior lung attenuation gradient
Dx: negative bacterial / viral / fungal cultures; no inhalational exposure to noxious agents; no pulmonary drug toxicity
Prognosis: death within 1–6 months (60–90%); recovery in 12%

Subacute Interstitial Pneumonia

BOOP *see* BRONCHIOLITIS OBLITERANS

Nonspecific Interstitial Pneumonia With Fibrosis

= NONCLASSIFIABLE INTERSTITIAL PNEUMONIA
= interstitial pneumonia that cannot be classified as UIP / DIP / acute interstitial pneumonia / BOOP
Histo: temporal uniformity of
(a) cellular interstitial infiltrate with little / no fibrosis (48%)
(b) inflammation + fibrosis (38%)
(c) dense fibrosis dominant (14%);
occasionally intraalveolar accumulation of macrophages + focal areas of bronchiolitis obliterans organizing pneumonia
Cause: collagen vascular disease (16%), inhalational exposure to noxious agents (17%), recent surgery / severe pneumonia / ARDS (8%)
Mean age: 46 years; M<F

- dyspnea + dry cough (1-week to 5-year history)

Location: no zonal predominance
√ normal CXR in 14%
√ bibasilar irregular linear opacities + airspace consolidation
√ normal / slightly decreased lung volume
CT:
√ bilateral areas of scattered ground-glass opacities (100%)
√ bibasilar airspace consolidation (71%)
√ irregular linear opacities (29%)
√ bronchial dilatation in areas of consolidation (71%)
√ mediastinal lymphadenopathy (29%)
√ NO honeycombing
Prognosis: 11% overall mortality
Rx: corticosteroids (clinical + functional + radiographic improvement in 50–86%)
DDx: usual interstitial pneumonia (irregular reticular pattern + honeycombing involving subpleural + lower lung zones

Respiratory Bronchiolitis - Interstitial lung Disease

= interstitial pneumonia of smokers in which respiratory bronchiolitis is associated with limited peribronchiolar interstitial inflammation; ? early manifestation of DIP
Mean age: 36 years; M=F
Cause: heavy cigarette smoking
Histo: accumulation of brown-pigmented macrophages in respiratory bronchioles + surrounding air spaces

- mild dyspnea + cough
- pulmonary function test: mixed restrictive + obstructive

√ normal CXR (21%)
√ diffuse bibasilar small linear + nodular opacities (71%)
√ bibasilar atelectasis (12%)
√ bronchial wall thickening
CT:
√ scattered ground-glass opacities (66%)
√ centrilobular micronodules
√ centrilobular emphysema
Prognosis: excellent (after cessation of smoking / corticoid therapy)

Chronic Interstitial Pneumonia

= ORGANIZING INTERSTITIAL PNEUMONIA
= CHRONIC DIFFUSE SCLEROSING ALVEOLITIS

Usual Interstitial Pneumonia

= UIP = IDIOPATHIC PULMONARY FIBROSIS (IPF)
= MURAL TYPE OF FIBROSING ALVEOLITIS
= CRYPTOGENIC FIBROSING ALVEOLITIS
= commonest (90%) form of idiopathic interstitial pneumonia (may represent late stage of DIP)
Etiology: 50% idiopathic; 25% familial; drug exposure (bleomycin, cyclophosphamide (Cytoxan®), busulfan, nitrofurantoin); 20–30% associated with collagen vascular disease / immunologic disorder (mostly rheumatoid arthritis)
Pathophysiology:
repetitive episodes of lung injury to the alveolar wall causing alveoli to flood with proteinaceous fluid + cellular debris; incomplete lysis of intraalveolar fibrin; type II pneumocytes regenerate over the intraalveolar collagen incorporating the fibrous tissue into alveolar septa (= injury-inflammation-fibrosis sequence)

Mean age: 64 years; M>F
Path: simultaneous presence of inflammatory cell infiltration + fibrotic alveolar walls + honeycombing + areas of normal lung tissue (= temporal variegation)
Histo: proteinaceous exudate in interstitium + hyaline membrane formation in alveoli; necrosis of alveolar lining cells followed by cellular infiltration of mono- and lymphocytes + regeneration of alveolar lining; intraalveolar histiocytes; proliferation of fibroblasts + deposition of collagen fibers + smooth muscle proliferation; progressive disorganization of pulmonary architecture

- progressive dyspnea, dry cough, fatigue (over 1–3 years)
- "Velcro" rales = crepitations
- clubbing of fingers (83%)
- lymphocytosis on bronchoalveolar lavage (marker of alveolitis)
- pulmonary function tests: restrictive defects + decreased diffusing capacity for carbon monoxide

√ occasionally ground-glass pattern in early stage of alveolitis (alveolar wall injury, interstitial edema, proteinaceous exudate, hyaline membranes, infiltrate of monocytes + lymphocytes) in 15–62%
√ bilateral diffuse linear / small irregular reticulations (100%); basilar (85%) + peripheral (59%)
√ reticulonodular pattern = superimposition of linear opacities
√ heart border "shaggy"
√ honeycombing = numerous cystic spaces (up to 74%)
√ elevated diaphragm = progressive loss of lung volume (45–75%)
√ 1.5–3 mm diffusely distributed nodules (15–29%)
√ pleural effusion (4–6%), pleural thickening (6%)
√ pneumothorax in 7% (in late stages)
√ normal CXR (2–8%)

HRCT (88% sensitive):
Location: lung bases (68–80%)
Site: predominantly subpleural regions (79%)
√ patchy distribution with areas of normal parenchyma, active alveolitis, early + late fibrosis present at the same time (HALLMARK)
√ irregular linear opacities (82%) with architectural distortion of secondary pulmonary lobule
√ interlobular septal thickening (10%)
√ subpleural areas of honeycombing with cystic spaces outlined by thick fibrous walls (up to 96%)
√ subpleural lines (= fibrosis / functional atelectasis)
√ small peripheral convoluted cysts (= traction bronchiectasis) in 50%
√ ground-glass opacities (= diffuse inflammatory mononuclear cell infiltrates of active disease + fibroblast proliferation) in 65–76%

Cx: bronchogenic carcinoma (more frequent occurrence)
Rx: response to steroids in only 10–15%
Prognosis: average survival of 3–6 years; 45% 5-year mortality rate (overall 87%); no recovery

Desquamative Interstitial Pneumonia

= DIP = DESQUAMATIVE TYPE OF FIBROSING ALVEOLITIS
= second commonest (although rare) form of interstitial pneumonia with more benign course than UIP, may be self-limited disease or lead to UIP

Mean age: 42 years (approximately 8 years younger than in UIP); M>F
Path: filling of alveolar spaces with foamy histiocytes + relative preservation of lung architecture + mild fibrosis (temporally homogeneous)
Histo: alveoli lined by large cuboidal cells + filled with heavy accumulation of mononuclear cells (macrophages, NOT desquamated alveolar cells); relative preservation of alveolar anatomy; histologic uniformity from field to field
Predisposed: smokers (history in up to 90%)

- asymptomatic
- weight loss
- dyspnea + nonproductive cough (for 6–12 months)
- clubbing of fingers
- mild pulmonary function abnormalities

√ normal chest x-ray (3–22%)
√ "ground-glass" alveolar pattern sparing costophrenic angles (25–33%), diffuse ground-glass opacities (15%)
√ linear irregular opacities (60%), bilateral + basilar (46–73%)
√ lung nodules (15%)
√ honeycombing (13%)
√ preserved lung volume

HRCT:
Location: mainly middle + lower lung zones (73%); bilateral + symmetric (86%)
Site: predominantly subpleural distribution (59%)
√ patchy ground-glass attenuation
√ irregular linear opacities (= fibrosis) + architectural distortion (50%)
√ honeycombing + traction bronchiectasis (32%)
√ fibrosis of lower lung zones in late stage

Prognosis: better response to corticosteroid Rx than UIP (in 60–80%); median survival of 12 years; 5% 5-year mortality rate (overall 16–27%)

IDIOPATHIC PULMONARY HEMOSIDEROSIS

= IPH = probable autoimmune process with clinical + radiologic remissions + exacerbations characterized by eosinophilia + mastocytosis, immunoallergic reaction, pulmonary hemorrhage, iron deficiency anemia

Age: (a) Chronic form: most commonly <10 years of age
(b) Acute form (rare): in adults; M:F = 2:1

- iron deficiency anemia
- clubbing of fingers
- hepatosplenomegaly (25%)
- bilirubinemia

- recurrent episodes of severe hemoptysis
- √ bilateral patchy alveolar-filling pattern (= blood in alveoli); initially for 2–3 days with return to normal in 10–12 days unless episode repeated
- √ reticular pattern (= deposition of hemosiderin in interstitial space) later
- √ moderate fibrosis after repeated episodes
- √ hilar lymph nodes may be enlarged during acute episodes

Prognosis: death within 2–20 years (average survival 3 years)

DDx: SECONDARY PULMONARY HEMOSIDEROSIS caused by mitral valve disease
- √ septal lines (NOT in idiopathic form)
- √ lung ossifications (NOT in idiopathic form)

KARTAGENER SYNDROME

= IMMOTILE / DYSMOTILE CILIA SYNDROME

Incidence: 1:40,00; high familial incidence

Etiology: abnormal mucociliary function secondary to generalized deficiency of dynein arms of cilia affecting respiratory epithelium, auditory epithelium, sperm

Triad:
(1) Situs inversus (50%)
(2) Sinusitis
(3) Bronchiectasis

- deafness
- infertility (abnormal sperm tails)

Associated anomalies:
transposition of great vessels, tri- / bilocular heart, pyloric stenosis, postcricoid web, epispadia

KLEBSIELLA PNEUMONIA

Most common cause of Gram-negative pneumonias; community acquired

Incidence: responsible for 5% of adult pneumonias

Organism: Friedländer bacillus = encapsulated, nonmotile, Gram-negative rod

Predisposed: elderly, debilitated, alcoholic, chronic lung disease, malignancy

- bacteremia in 25%
- √ propensity for posterior portion of upper lobe / superior portion of lower lobe
- √ dense lobar consolidation
- √ bulging of fissure (large amounts of inflammatory exudate) CHARACTERISTIC but unusual
- √ empyema (one of the most common causes)
- √ patchy bronchopneumonia may be present
- √ uni- / multilocular cavities (50%) appearing within 4 days
- √ pulmonary gangrene = infarcted tissue (rare)

Cx: meningitis, pericarditis

Prognosis: mortality rate 25–50%

DDx: Acute pneumococcal pneumonia (bulging of fissures, abscess + cavity formation, pleural effusion / empyema frequent)

LANGERHANS CELL HISTIOCYTOSIS

= EOSINOPHILIC GRANULOMA

= HISTIOCYTOSIS X = LANGERHANS CELL GRANULOMATOSIS

= group of disorders of unknown origin characterized by granulomatous infiltration of lungs, bone, skin, lymph nodes, brain, endocrine glands

Manifestation:
(a) multisystem disease with poor prognosis
(b) confined to one system: most commonly eosinophilic granuloma of bone

Histo:
granuloma containing Langerhans cells, foamy histiocytes, lymphocytes, plasma cells, eosinophils

Langerhans cell
- — dendritic antigen-presenting cell found in basal layer of skin + in liver (Kupffer cell), lymph nodes, spleen, bone marrow, lung
- — contains unique mostly rod-shaped cytoplasmatic inclusion bodies known as Birbeck granules (identifiable only with electron microscopy)

Age: most frequently in 3rd–4th decade (range 3 months to 69 years); M:F = 4:1; Caucasians >> Blacks

@ Pulmonary Langerhans cell histiocytosis

Pathogenesis:
heavy cigarette smoking in young men with accumulation + activation of Langerhans cells (90% smokers) as a result of excess neuroendocrine cell hyperplasia + secretion of bombazine-like peptides

Path:
multifocal granulomatous infiltration centered on walls of bronchioles (= bronchiolitis) often extending into surrounding alveolar interstitium with subsequent bronchiolar destruction leading to thick-walled cysts presumably caused by check-valve bronchial obstruction + pneumothorax (no necrosis); in end-stage disease foci of LCG are replaced by fibroblasts forming CHARACTERISTIC stellate "starfish" scars with central remnants of persisting inflammatory cells

◊ CXR abnormalities more severe than clinical symptoms + pulmonary function tests!

- asymptomatic (up to 25%)
- nonproductive cough (75%)
- combination of obstructive + restrictive pulmonary function: presenting with pneumothorax in 15%
- fatigue, weight loss, fever (15–30%)
- dyspnea (40%)
- chest pain (25%) from pneumothorax / eosinophilic granuloma in rib
- diabetes insipidus (10–25%)
- lymphocytosis with predominance of T-suppressor cells on bronchoalveolar lavage (DDx: excess of T-helper cells in sarcoidosis)

Location: usually bilaterally symmetric, upper lobe predominance, sparing of costophrenic angles

Evolutionary sequence:
nodule – cavitated nodule – thick-walled cyst – thin-walled cyst
- √ ill-defined / stellate nodules 3–10 mm (granuloma stage)

√ diffuse fine reticular / reticulonodular pattern (cellular infiltrate)
√ "honeycomb lung" = multiple 1–5 cm cysts + subpleural blebs (fibrotic stage)
√ increased lung volumes in 1/3 (most other fibrotic lung diseases have decreased lung volumes!)
√ pleural effusion (8%), hilar adenopathy (unusual)
√ cavitation of large nodules (rare)
√ thymic enlargement

HRCT (combination virtually diagnostic):
√ complex / branching thin-walled cysts <5 mm in size equally distributed in central + peripheral lung zones
√ centrilobular peribronchiolar nodules
√ intervening lung appears normal

DDx for nodules:
sarcoidosis, hypersensitivity pneumonitis, berylliosis, TB, atypical TB, metastases, silicosis, coal worker's peumoconiosis

DDx for cysts:
emphysema, bronchiectasis, idiopathic pulmonary fibrosis, lymphangiomyomatosis

Cx:
1. Recurrent pneumothorax in 25% (from rupture of subpleural cysts) CHARACTERISTIC
2. Pulmonary hypertension
3. Superimposed Aspergillus fumigatus infection

Prognosis: improvement (50%), stable (33%), rapid progression (20%)

@ Bone involvement:
√ lytic bone lesions (skull, ribs, pelvis)
√ vertebra plana

Prognosis: poor with multisystem disease + organ dysfunction (especially with skin lesions); complete / partial regression (13–55%), progression (7–21%); 2–25% mortality

Rx: cessation of smoking, chemotherapy (vincristine sulfate, prednisone, methotrexate, 6-mercaptopurine)

DDx: sarcoidosis (equal sex distribution, always multisystem disease, not related to smoking, erythema nodosum, bilateral hilar lymphadenopathy, lung cavitation + pneumothorax rare, epitheloid cells)

LEGIONELLA PNEUMONIA

= LEGIONNAIRES' DISEASE

Organism: Legionella pneumophila, 1–2 μm, aerobic, gram-negative bacillus, weakly acid-fast, silver-impregnation stain

Predisposed: middle-aged / elderly, immunosuppressed, alcoholism, chronic obstructive lung disease, diabetes, cancer, cardiovascular disease, chronic renal failure, transplant recipients

Transmission: direct inhalation (air conditioning systems)

Prevalence: 6% of community-acquired pneumonias

Histo: leukocytoclastic fibrinopurulent pneumonia with histiocytes in intraalveolar exudate

- fever
- absence of sputum / lack of purulence (22–75%)

Clue: involvement of other organs with
- diarrhea (0–25%), myalgia, toxic encephalopathy
- liver + renal disease
- hyponatremia (20%)
- elevated serum transaminase / transpeptidase levels
- lack of quick response to penicillin / cephalosporin / aminoglycoside

Concomitant infection (in 5–10%):
Streptococcus pneumoniae, Chlamydia pneumoniae, Mycobacterium tuberculosis, Pneumocystis carinii

Location: unilateral / bilateral (less frequent); lobar / segmental
√ patchy bronchopneumonia (= multifocal consolidation)
√ moderate volume of pleural effusion (6–30–63%)
√ cavitation (rare)

Cx: progressive respiratory failure (most common cause of death; 6% mortality in healthy patients)

Rx: erythromycin

LIPOID PNEUMONIA

Etiology: aspiration of vegetable / animal / mineral oil (most common)

Predisposed: elderly, debilitated, neuromuscular disease, swallowing abnormalities (eg, scleroderma)

Mineral oil = inert pure hydrocarbon that does not initiate cough reflex

Path: pool of oil surrounded by giant cell foreign body reaction (mineral oil aspiration) / initially hemorrhagic bronchopneumonia (animal fat)

- mostly asymptomatic
- fever, constitutional symptoms
- lipid-laden macrophages in sputum / lavage fluid
- oil droplets in bronchial washing / needle aspirate

Location: predilection for RML + lower lobes
√ homogeneous segmental airspace consolidation (most common)
√ interstitial reticulonodular pattern (rare)
√ paraffinoma = circumscribed peripheral mass (granulomatous reaction + fibrosis often causing stellate appearance)
√ slow progression / no change

CT:
√ mass of low-attenuation approaching that of subcutaneous fat

LÖFFLER SYNDROME

= disorder of unknown etiology characterized by local areas of transient parenchymal consolidation associated with blood eosinophilia

Path: interstitial + alveolar edema containing a large number of lymphocytes

- no / mild symptoms
- eosinophilia
- history of atopia

√ single / multiple areas of homogeneous ill-defined consolidation
√ uni- or bilateral, nonsegmental distribution, predominantly in lung periphery
√ transient + shifting in nature (changes within one to several days)
Prognosis: may undergo spontaneous remission

LUNG TORSION

= rare complication of severe chest trauma
Mechanism: compression of lower thorax with lung twisted through 180°; usually in presence of a large amount of pleural air / fluid
Age: almost invariably in children
√ main lower lobe artery sweeping upward toward apex
√ lower lung vessels diminutive
√ unusual configuration of lobar collapse
√ lung infarction = opacification of involved lung (from edema + hemorrhage into air spaces)

LUNG TRANSPLANT

Indications:
emphysema, cystic fibrosis, CHD, idiopathic pulmonary fibrosis, α-1-antitrypsin deficiency, primary pulmonary hypertension, sarcoidosis, pneumoconiosis, malignancy
Survival rate: 90% 1-month survival, 70% 1-year survival

Acute rejection of lung transplant

Incidence: 60–80% with 2–3 significant episodes in first 3 months
Histo: mononuclear cell infiltrate around arteries, veins, bronchioles, alveolar septa with alveolar edema (initially) + fibrinous exudate (later)
Time of onset: first episode 5–10 days after transplantation; occasionally by 48 hours

- drop in arterial oxygen pressure WITHOUT infection / airway obstruction / fluid overload
- pyrexia, fatigue, decreased exercise tolerance

√ heterogeneous opacities in perihilar areas
√ ground-glass attenuation on HRCT
√ new increasing pleural effusion + septal thickening (most common, 90% specific, 68% sensitive) WITHOUT concomitant signs of LV dysfunction (increase in cardiac size / vascular pedicle width / vascular redistribution)
√ subpleural edema, peribronchial cuffing, airspace disease
Dx: (1) transbronchial biopsy
(2) rapid improvement of radiologic abnormalities after treatment with IV bolus of corticosteroids for 3 days
Rx: methylprednisolone, polyclonal T-cell antibody (antithymocyte globulin), monoclonal antibodies (CD3, OKT3), lymphoid irradiation

Anastomotic complications of lung transplant

1. Airway dehiscence (2–8%)
   √ presence of extraluminal air collections at anastomotic site (80%)
2. Airway stricture
   DDx: telescoped anastomosis
   Rx: laser resection, balloon bronchoplasty
3. Vascular stenosis
4. Diaphragmatic hernia from omentopexy
   Procedure: omental pedicle is harvested at time of transplantation through a small diaphragmatic incision + wrapped around anastomosis to prevent dehiscence

Chronic rejection of lung transplant

Prevalence: 24%
Path: obliterative bronchiolitis (36%), interstitial pneumonitis, rejection-mediated vasculopathy
Time of onset: 3–75 months after transplantation

- persistent coughing and wheezing
- slowly worsening exertional dyspnea

√ increased / diminished lung volumes
√ central + peripheral bronchiectasis
√ localized airspace disease
√ partial lobar atelectasis
√ thin irregular areas of increased opacity
√ pleural thickening
√ diminished peripheral lung markings
√ nodular / reticular opacities associated with peribronchial thickening

Hyperacute rejection

= rejection in cases of an immunoglobulin G donor-specific HLA antibody positive crossmatch
Path: acute diffuse alveolar damage

Posttransplantation infection

Cause: immunosuppression, reduced mucociliary clearance, interruption of lymphatic drainage, direct contact of transplant with environment via airways

A. INFECTION OF LUNG TRANSPLANT
Prevalence: 35–50%; major cause of morbidity + mortality in early postoperative period
Cause: ? absent cough reflex, impaired mucociliary transport in denervated lung
Organism: bacteria (23%) > CMV > Aspergillus > Pneumocystis
(1) within 1st month: gram-negative bacteria, fungi (candidiasis, aspergillosis)
(2) after 1st month: CMV, Pneumocystis carinii, bacteria, fungi

- fever, leukocytosis

√ lobar / multilobar consolidation (due to bacterial > fungal pathogens)
√ diffuse heterogeneous / ground-glass opacities (due to viral / disseminated fungal pathogens)
√ nodular opacities (due to fungal / unusual bacterial pathogens / CMV / septic emboli)
Cx: may progress rapidly to respiratory failure + death
Dx: transbronchial / open biopsy (80% accurate)

B. EXTRAPULMONARY INFECTION
thoracotomy wound infection, bacteremia, sepsis, empyema, central venous line infection

Posttransplantation lymphoproliferative disease

Incidence: 4%
Histo: spectrum from benign polyclonal proliferation of lymphoid tissue to non-Hodgkin lymphoma
Associated with: Epstein-Barr virus
Time of onset: 1 month to several years; related to immunosuppressive regimen
√ solitary / multiple discrete nodules
√ mediastinal / hilar lymphadenopathy

Reperfusion edema

= REIMPLANTATION RESPONSE
= infiltrate appearing within 48 hours after transplantation unrelated to fluid overload, LV failure, infection, atelectasis, or rejection; diagnosed by exclusion
Pathogenesis: permeability edema due to lymphatic disruption, pulmonary denervation, organ ischemia, trauma
Histo: fluid accumulation in interstitium consistent with noncardiogenic pulmonary edema
Time course: manifests within 24 hours, peaks at 2nd–4th postoperative day, resolves at variable rate ranging from days to 1–2 weeks to months
• increasing hypoxia before extubation; poor correlation between radiographic severity + physiologic parameters
Location: perihilar areas + basal regions
√ perihilar haze / rapid uni- or bilateral heterogeneously dense interstitial and/or air-space disease
Dx: per exclusion (radiographic changes not due to LV failure, hyperacute rejection, fluid overload, infection, atelectasis)

LYMPHANGIOMYOMATOSIS

= LYMPHANGIOLEIOMYOMATOSIS
= ? forme fruste of tuberous sclerosis
= rare disorder characterized by (1) gradually progressive diffuse interstitial lung disease (2) recurrent chylous pleural effusions (3) recurrent pneumothoraces
Etiology: unknown
Age: 17–50 years, exclusively in women of childbearing age
Histo: proliferation of atypical smooth muscle in pulmonary lymphatic vessels, blood vessels, and airways
Pathogenesis:
proliferated smooth muscle obstructs (a) bronchioles (trapping of air, overinflation, formation of cysts, pneumothorax), (b) venules (pulmonary edema, hemorrhage, hemosiderosis), (c) lymphatics (thickening of lymphatics, chylothorax)

May be associated with: Tuberous sclerosis (lung involvement in 1%)
• progressive exertional dyspnea + cough
• disease aggravated by pregnancy + oral contraceptives
• hemoptysis (30–40%), chyloptysis
• radiologic-physiologic discrepancy = severe airflow obstruction (reduced FEV_1, reduced ratio of FEV_1 to forced vital capacity) despite relatively normal findings on CXR
• combination of restrictive + obstructive ventilatory defects: hypoxia, markedly impaired diffusing capacity
• positive immunohistochemical staining of LAM cells with HMB-45 (monoclonal antibody for melanocytic lesion)

√ classic signs:
  √ coarse reticular interstitial pattern (caused by summation of multiple cyst walls)
  √ recurrent large chylothorax (20–50–75%)
  √ recurrent pneumothorax (40-50% at presentation; in 80% during course of disease)
√ normal / increased lung volume
  ◊ The only interstitial lung disease to develop increase in lung volume!
√ Kerley-B lines
√ pulmonary cysts + honeycombing
√ occasionally chylous ascites
√ mediastinal + retroperitoneal adenopathy (from smooth muscle proliferation)
HRCT:
  √ numerous randomly scattered thin-walled (<2 mm) cysts of various sizes (0.5–6 cm) surrounded by normal lung parenchyma
  √ bronchovascular bundles at periphery of cyst walls
  √ consolidations (due to hemorrhage following destruction of pulmonary microvasculature)

@ Kidney
  √ multiple hamartomas lacking fat (50%)
  √ simple cysts (occasionally large enough to lead to renal insufficiency)

Dx: open / transbronchial lung biopsy
Prognosis: 8.5-year survival rate of 38–78%; death within 10 years from progressive pulmonary insufficiency

DDx:
(1) Histiocytosis (cyst walls more variable in thickness and in upper lobes, nodules + septal thickening)
(2) Idiopathic pulmonary fibrosis = fibrosing alveolitis (small irregular thick-walled cysts + predominantly peripheral interstitial thickening
(3) Emphysema (lobular architecture preserved with bronchovascular bundle in central position, areas of lung destruction without arcuate contour)
(4) Bronchiectasis (bronchial wall thickening)
(5) Tuberous sclerosis (associated skin abnormalities, mental retardation, epilepsy)
(6) Neurofibromatosis (cystic air spaces predominantly in apical location)

LYMPHANGITIC CARCINOMATOSIS

= INTERSTITIAL CARCINOMA

= tumor cell accumulation within connective tissue (bronchovascular bundles, interlobular septa, subpleural space, pulmonary lymphatics) from tumor embolization of blood vessels followed by lymphatic obstruction, interstitial edema, and collagen deposition (fibrosis from desmoplastic reaction when tumor cells extend into adjacent pulmonary parenchyma)

Incidence: 7% of all pulmonary metastases

Tumor origin: bronchogenic carcinoma, carcinoma of breast (56%), stomach (46%), thyroid, pancreas, larynx, cervix

mnemonic: "**C**ertain **C**ancers **S**pread **B**y **P**lugging **T**he **L**ymphatics"

Cervix	**P**ancreas
Colon	**T**hyroid
Stomach	**L**arynx
Breast	

Path: (1) interstitial edema (2) interstitial fibrotic changes (3) lymphatic dilatation (4) tumor cells within connective tissue planes

- dyspnea (often preceding radiographic abnormalities)
- rarely dry cough + hemoptysis

Location: bilateral; unilateral if secondary to lung primary

CXR (accuracy 23%):

√ normal chest radiograph
√ reticular densities
√ coarsened bronchovascular markings
√ Kerley A + B lines
√ small lung volume
√ hilar adenopathy (20–50%)

HRCT:

√ well-defined smoothly thickened polygonal reticular network of 10–25 mm in diameter (= thickened interlobular septa)
√ irregular / nodular = "beaded" thickening of interlobular septa
√ central dot within secondary pulmonary lobule = thickened centrilobular bronchovascular bundle
√ subpleural thickening
√ pleural effusion (30–50%)
√ hilar / mediastinal lymphadenopathy (30–50%)

Prognosis: death within 1 year

DDx: (1) Fibrosing alveolitis (peripheral predominance)
(2) Extrinsic allergic alveolitis (no polygonal structures, pleural changes rare)
(3) Sarcoidosis (nodules of irregular outline more frequent in upper lobes, polygonal structures uncommon)

LYMPHOID INTERSTITIAL PNEUMONIA

= LYMPHOCYTIC INTERSTITIAL PNEUMONITIS

= LIP = lymphoproliferative disorder characterized by diffuse lymphocytic infiltration of pulmonary interstitium / diffuse lymphoid hyperplasia (probably immunologic disorder) with frequently chronic + progressive course

Histo: diffuse interstitial infiltrate of polyclonal lymphocytes + plasma cells; many cases reclassified as lymphoma

Associated with: Sjögren syndrome, systemic lupus erythematosus, myasthenia gravis, pernicious anemia, chronic active hepatitis, AIDS

◊ Indicative of AIDS when present in child under 13 years of age!

- dyspnea + cough
- cyanosis + clubbing (50%)
- enlargement of salivary glands (20%)
- NO lymphocytosis or history of atopia
- monoclonal gammopathy (usually IgM)

√ fine reticular changes in both lungs
√ resembling airspace disease (in severe form)
√ reticulonodular pattern

Rx: responsive to steroids

Localized form = PSEUDOLYMPHOMA

LYMPHOMA

7th leading cause of death from cancer in United States

Pathogenesis: ? viral cause

HD: contiguous spread requires scanning of abnormal area only

NHL: noncontiguous spread requires scanning of chest, abdomen, pelvis

@ Thorax

◊ Hodgkin disease more common in thorax than NHL at presentation (HD in 85%, NHL in 45%)

1. Lymphadenopathy
anterior mediastinal, pretracheal, hilar, subcarinal, axillary, periesophageal, paracardiac, superior diaphragmatic internal mammary lymph nodes
2. Lung parenchyma involvement (HD in 12%, NHL in 4%)
3. Pleural + subpleural lymphoma (up to 30%)

@ Abdomen

1. Periaortic adenopathy .... HD in 25%, NHL in 49%
2. Mesenteric adenopathy .... HD in 4%, NHL in 51%
3. Liver involvement .... HD in 8%, NHL in 14%
√ hepatomegaly with involvement .... HD in <30%, NHL in 57%
HD: commonly diffuse infiltrating process
NHL: diffuse infiltrating / discrete tumor nodules
4. Splenic involvement .... HD in 37%, NHL in 41%
HD: most common site of abdominal involvement
NHL: 3rd most common site of abdominal involvement; may be initial manifestation in large cell NHL
◊ Staging laparotomy necessary as 2/3 of tumor nodules <1 cm in size
5. Gastrointestinal involvement
in 10% of patients with abdominal lymphoma (uncommon in HD, common in histiocytic NHL); NHL accounts for 80% of all gastric lymphomas

CHEST

6. Renal involvement
   late manifestation, most commonly in NHL
7. Adrenal involvement
   more common in NHL
8. Extranodal involvement
   more frequent with histologically diffuse forms of NHL

Hodgkin Disease

40% of all lymphomas; disease of T cells

Age: bimodal distribution at 25–30 years + >70 years

• asymptomatic unilateral cervical adenopathy

Histo: Reed-Sternberg cell characteristic

1. nodular sclerosis: most common, localized, good prognosis; greatest adenopathy in anterior mediastinum
2. lymphocyte predominance: uncommon, localized, excellent prognosis, majority <35 years
3. mixed cellularity: more commonly abdominal than mediastinal, less favorable prognosis
4. lymphocyte depletion: uncommon, disseminated, older patients, rapidly fatal

Ann Arbor Staging Classification:

Stage I = limited to one / two contiguous anatomic regions on same side of diaphragm
I_E = single extralymphatic organ / site
Stage II = >2 anatomic regions / two noncontiguous regions on same side of diaphragm
II_E = with extralymphatic organ / site
Stage III = on both sides of diaphragm, not extending beyond lymph nodes, spleen (Stage III_S), Waldeyer's ring
III_E = with extralymphatic organ / site
Stage IV = organ involvement (bone marrow, bone, lung, pleura, liver, kidney, GI tract, skin) ± lymph node involvement
Substage A = absence of systemic symptoms
Substage B = fever, night sweats, pruritus, ≥10% weight loss

@ CHEST INVOLVEMENT

At presentation: 67% with intrathoracic disease

Sites of lymphoid aggregates:

1. Lymph nodes in mediastinum
2. Lymph nodes at bifurcation of 1st + 2nd order bronchi
3. Encapsulated lymphoid collections on thoracic surface deep to parietal pleura
4. Unencapsulated nodules at points of divisions of more distally situated bronchi, bronchioles, and pulmonary vessels
5. Unencapsulated lymphoid aggregates within peribronchial connective tissue
6. Small accumulations of lymphocytes in interlobular septa + lymphatic channels

A. INTRAPULMONARY MANIFESTATIONS
   in 15–30–40% during disease duration; most commonly in nodular sclerosing type; invariably subsequent to hilar adenopathy
   1. Bronchovascular form (most common type of involvement):
      √ coarse reticulonodular pattern contiguous with mediastinum = direct extension from mediastinal nodes along lymphatics
      √ nodular parenchymal lesions
      √ miliary nodules
      √ endobronchial involvement
      √ lobar atelectasis secondary to endobronchial obstruction (rare)
      √ cavitation secondary to necrosis (rare)
   2. Subpleural form
      √ circumscribed subpleural masses
      √ pleural effusion (20–50%) from lymphatic obstruction
   3. Massive pneumonic form (68%)
      √ diffuse nonsegmental infiltrate (pneumonic type)
      √ massive lobar infiltrates (30%)
      √ homogeneous confluent infiltrates with shaggy borders

Comparison of Histologic Classifications of Non-Hodgkin Lymphoma

International Working Formulation	*Rappaport Classification*
Low grade	
A. Small lymphocytic	Well-differentiated lymphocytic
B. Follicular, predominantly small cleaved cell	Nodular, poorly differentiated lymphocytic
C. Follicular, mixed small and large cell	Nodular, mixed
Intermediate grade	
D. Follicular, predominantly large cell	Nodular, histiocytic
E. Diffuse, small cleaved cell	Diffuse, poorly differentiated lymphocytic
F. Diffuse, mixed small and large cell	Diffuse, mixed
G. Diffuse, large cell, cleaved or noncleaved	...
High grade	
H. Diffuse large cell, immunoblastic	...
I. Small, noncleaved cell	...
J. Lymphoblastic	Undifferentiated

√ air bronchogram
4. Nodular form
√ multiple nodules <1 cm in diameter (DDx: metastatic disease)

B. EXTRAPULMONARY MANIFESTATIONS
1. Mediastinal + Hilar Lymphadenopathy
Most common manifestation, present in 90–99%, in thorax commonly multiple lymph node groups involved
Location:
anterior mediastinal + retrosternal nodes commonly involved (DDx: sarcoidosis); confined to anterior mediastinum in 40%; 20% with mediastinal nodes have hilar lymphadenopathy also; hilar lymph nodes involved bilaterally in 50%
Spread from anterior mediastinum to:
other mediastinal locations, pleura, pericardium, chest wall
◊ Involvement of multiple lymph node groups in 95%!
√ CXR: on initial film adenopathy identified in 50%
√ necrotic lymph nodes (commonly nodular sclerosing type)
√ lymph nodes may calcify following radiation / chemotherapy
2. Pleural Effusion (30%)
3. Pleural Masses + Plaques
(a) sternal erosion
(b) invasion of anterior chest wall

Cx:
1. Superimposed infection
√ consolidation with bulging borders: necrotizing bacterial pneumonia
√ multiple nodular foci: aspergillosis + nocardiosis
√ bilateral diffuse consolidation: Pneumocystis carinii
√ rapidly developing cavitation within consolidation: anaerobes / fungus
Dx: by culture, sputum cytology, lung biopsy
2. Drug toxicity

@ BONE INVOLVEMENT (15%)
√ frequently osteoblastic (28%), eg, ivory vertebrae
√ osteolysis of sternum / ribs (direct invasion)

Cx: increased risk for other malignancies from aggressive therapy (acute leukemia, NHL, radiation-induced sarcoma)

Non-Hodgkin Lymphoma

= NHL = disease of B cells

Incidence: 3% of all newly diagnosed cancers; 3rd most common cancer in childhood (behind leukemia + CNS neoplasms); 4 times more common than Hodgkin disease

Predisposed: (40–100 times greater risk) congenital immunodeficiency syndromes, organ transplant patients undergoing immunosuppression, patients with HIV infection, collagen vascular diseases

Age: all ages; median age of 55 years; M:F = 1.4:1

- chest / shoulder pain, dyspnea, dysphagia
- CHF, hypotension, SVC syndrome

Modified Rappaport Classification:
= categorization according to histologic distribution of lymphomatous cells
A. Nodular form = organized in clusters
1. Poorly differentiated lymphocytic (PDL)
2. Mixed lymphocytic / histiocytic (mixed cell)
3. Large cell (histiocytic)
B. Diffuse form = distortion of tissue architecture
1. well-differentiated lymphocytic (WDL)
2. intermediate-differentiated lymphocytic (IDL)
3. poorly differentiated lymphocytic (PDL)
4. mixed lymphocytic / histiocytic large cell (histiocytic) (DLCL); undifferentiated Burkitt lymphoma; undifferentiated non-Burkitt lymphoma (pleiomorphic); lymphoblastic (LBL); unclassified

Luke and Collins classification:
= categorization by morphologic characteristics of cell + cell of origin (T-cell, B-cell, non-B, non-T cell)

Working Formulation Classification (Kiel / Lennert):
= categorization by grade
A. Low grade
1. small lymphocytic (3.6%)
median age 61 years, 59% 5-year survival
2. follicular, small cleaved cell (22.5%)
median age 54 years, 70% 5-year survival
3. follicular, mixed (7.7%)
median age 56 years, 50% 5-year survival
B. Intermediate grade
1. follicular, large cell (3.8%)
median age 55 years, 45% 5-year survival
2. diffuse, small cleaved cell (6.9%)
median age 58 years, 33% 5-year survival
3. diffuse, mixed (6.7%)
median age 58 years, 38% 5-year survival
4. diffuse, large cell (19.7%)
median age 57 years, 35% 5-year survival
C. High grade
1. large cell, immunoblastic (7.9%)
median age 51 years, 32% 5-year survival
2. lymphoblastic (4.2%)
median age 17 years, 26% 5-year survival
3. small noncleaved cell (5%)
median age 30 years, 23% 5-year survival
D. Miscellaneous (12%)
composite, mycosis fungoides, histiocytic, extramedullary plasmacytoma

Staging: same Ann Arbor system as for Hodgkin disease

CHEST

Extranodal involvement:

@ GI tract:
stomach (3%), small bowel (5%), large bowel (2%), pancreas (0.7%), peritoneal nodules + ascites (1.4%)

@ Chest:
lung (6%), pleural fluid (3.3%), pericardial fluid (0.7%), heart (0.2%)

@ GU tract (10%):
kidneys (6%), testes (1.2%), ovaries (1.8%), uterus (1.2%)

@ Bone (3.8%)

@ CNS (2.4%)

@ Breast (1.2%)

@ Skin (6.4%)

@ Head and neck (1.7%)

@ Liver (14%)

@ Spleen (41%)

Nodal involvement:

@ Paraaortic lymph nodes (49%)

@ Mesenteric lymph nodes (51%):
predominantly in middle mediastinum, cardiophrenic angle

◊ Single lymph node involvement is often the only manifestation of intrathoracic disease!

@ Splenic hilar lymph nodes (53%)

◊ Lymphography 89% sensitive + 86% specific

Intrathoracic disease (40–50%):

√ hilar + mediastinal adenopathy (DDx: sarcoidosis; anterior nodes favor lymphoma)

◊ Nodes frequently not involved!

√ isolated lymph nodes may enhance (DDx: Castleman disease)

√ lung nodules + air bronchograms

√ pleural effusion

Prognosis: unfavorable

Non-Hodgkin lymphoma in childhood

Incidence: 3rd most common childhood malignancy (after leukemia + CNS tumors); 7% of all malignancies in children <15 years of age

Origin: B or T cell (in 90%) located outside marrow; (rarely) non-B and non-T cells located within bone marrow

Age: median age of 10 years; <15 years of age (most common); unusual <5 years of age; M > F

- chest pain, back pain, cough, dyspnea
- fever, anorexia, weight loss
- ± peripheral blood + bone marrow involvement (particularly in lymphoblastic NHL): with lymphoblastic bone marrow involvement of <25% patient is classified as having lymphoma

Staging (St. Jude):

I single extranodal tumor / single anatomic area

II (a) single extranodal tumor + regional nodes
(b) ≥2 nodal areas on same side of diaphragm
(c) 2 single extranodal tumors ± nodes on same side of diaphragm
(d) primary gastrointestinal tract tumor ± nodes

III (a) 2 single extranodal tumors on opposite sides of diaphragm
(b) ≥2 nodal areas on both sides of the diaphragm
(c) primary intrathoracic tumors (mediastinum, pleura, thymus)
(d) extensive primary intraabdominal disease
(e) paraspinal / epidural tumor

IV any of the above + initial CNS / bone marrow involvement

Differences between adult and childhood NHL:

Characteristics	Adult NHL	Childhood NHL
Primary site	nodal	extranodal
Histology	50% follicular, 50% diffuse	diffuse
Grade	low, intermediate, high	high
Histologic subtype	many	three
Sex predilection	none	70% male

Prognosis: 80% cure rate with multiple-agent chemotherapy

DDx:
1. Acute lymphocytic leukemia (>25% lymphoblasts within bone marrow)
2. Hodgkin disease (contiguous spread, nodes are site of origin)

1. **Undifferentiated / small noncleaved NHL** (39%);
Path: non-Burkitt lymphoma; Burkitt lymphoma
- abdominal mass ± ascites
- pain similar to appendicitis / intussusception

Primary site: abdomen (distal ileum, cecum, appendix); ovaries
Common site: mesenteric, inguinal, iliac nodes; CNS; bone marrow; kidney
Rare site: orbit, supradiaphragmatic paraspinal region, mediastinum, paranasal sinuses, bone, testes, pulmonary parenchyma
Cx: "leukemic transformation" (= extensive bone marrow involvement)

2. **Lymphoblastic (T-cell) NHL** (28%)
Primary site: mediastinum (66%)
Common site: neck, thymus, liver, spleen, CNS, bone marrow, gonads
Rare site: subdiaphragmatic (ileum, cecum, kidney, mesentery, retroperitoneum), orbit, paranasal sinus, thyroid, parotid
- respiratory distress, dysphagia
- SVC syndrome, pericardial tamponade

3. **Large cell (histiocytic) NHL** (26%)
Origin: B cell, T cells (small percentage)
Location: nodal + extranodal
Primary site: variable (Waldeyer ring, Peyer patches)

CHEST

Common site: peripheral lymph nodes, lung, bone, brain, skin
Rare site: hard palate, esophagus, trachea

MECONIUM ASPIRATION SYNDROME

= most common cause of neonatal respiratory distress in full term / postmature infants (hyaline membrane disease most common cause in premature infants)

Etiology: fetal circulatory accidents / placental insufficiency / postmaturity result in perinatal hypoxia + fetal distress with meconium defecated in utero

Pathogenesis: meconium produces bronchial obstruction + chemical pneumonitis

Incidence: 10% of all deliveries have meconium-stained amniotic fluid, 1% of all deliveries have respiratory distress

• cyanosis (rare)
√ large infant
√ bilateral diffuse grossly patchy opacities (atelectasis + consolidation)
√ hyperinflation with areas of emphysema (air trapping)
√ spontaneous pneumothorax + pneumomediastinum (25%) requiring no therapy
√ small pleural effusions (20%)
√ NO air bronchograms
√ rapid clearing usually within 48 hours

Cx: morbidity from anoxic brain damage is high

MEDIASTINAL LIPOMATOSIS

= excess unencapsulated fat deposition

Etiology:
(a) Exogenous steroids (average daily dose of >30 mg prednisone): (1) chronic renal disease, renal transplant (5%) (2) collagen vascular disease, vasculitis (3) hemolytic anemia (4) asthma (5) dermatitis (6) Crohn disease (7) myasthenia gravis
(b) Endogenous steroid elevation: (1) adrenal tumor (2) pituitary tumor / hyperplasia = Cushing disease (3) ectopic ACTH-production (carcinoma of the lung)
(c) Obesity

• moon facies
• buffalo hump
• supraclavicular + episternal fat

Location: upper mediastinum (common), cardiophrenic angles + paraspinal areas (less common)

√ upper mediastinal widening
√ paraspinal widening
√ increase in epicardial fat-pads
√ symmetric slightly lobulated extrapleural deposits extending from apex to 9th rib laterally

OTHER FEATURES:
√ osteoporosis
√ fractures
√ aseptic necrosis
√ increased rectosacral distance

MESOTHELIOMA

Benign mesothelioma

= LOCALIZED FIBROUS MESOTHELIOMA
= LOCALIZED FIBROUS TUMOR OF THE PLEURA
= SOLITARY FIBROUS TUMOR OF PLEURA
= BENIGN LOCALIZED MESOTHELIOMA
= BENIGN PLEURAL FIBROMA = FIBROSING MESOTHELIOMA = PLEURAL FIBROMYXOMA

Incidence: <5% of all pleural tumors
◊ No recognized association with asbestos exposure!

Age: 3rd–8th decade; mean age of 50–60 years; M:F = 1:1

Path: usually solitary mass arising from visceral pleura in 80% + parietal pleura in 20%

Histo: tumor originates from submesothelial fibroblasts, lined by layer of mesothelial cells
(a) relatively acellular fibrous tissue
(b) rounded spindle-shaped densely packed cells
(c) resembling hemangiopericytoma of lung

• asymptomatic in 50%
• cough, fever, dyspnea, chest pain (larger mass)
• digital clubbing (rare) + hypertrophic pulmonary osteoarthropathy in 20–35%
• episodic hypoglycemia (4%)
√ sharply circumscribed spherical / ovoid lobular mass of 2–
30 cm in diameter located near lung periphery / adjacent to pleural surface / within fissure
√ sessile with smooth tapered margin (common) / pedunculated with obtuse angle toward chest wall (rare, benign feature)
√ tumor may change in shape + location upon alteration of patient's position (if pedunculated)
√ areas of hemorrhage / necrosis may be present (favors malignancy)
√ ipsilateral pleural effusion (rare) containing hyaluronic acid

CT:
√ substantial contrast enhancement
√ heterogeneous enhancement due to myxoid degeneration + hemorrhage

MR:
√ hypointense on T1WI + hyperintense on T2WI

Cx: malignant degeneration in 37%

DDx: metastatic deposit

Rx: excision is curative (recurrence rate lower for pedunculated versus nodular tumor)

Malignant mesothelioma

= DIFFUSE MALIGNANT MESOTHELIOMA
= most common primary neoplasm of pleura

Prevalence: 7–13:1,000,000 persons/year; 2,000–3,000 cases/year in US

Etiology: asbestos exposure (13–100%); zeolite (nonasbestos mineral fiber); chronic inflammation (TB, empyema); irradiation

Carcinogenic potential:
proportional to aspect ratio (= length-to-diameter) of fiber and durability in human tissue:
crocidolite > amosite > chrysotile > actinolite, anthophyllite, tremolite
◊ Occupational exposure of asbestos found in only 40–80% of all cases!
◊ 5–10% of asbestos workers will develop mesothelioma (risk factor of 30 compared with general population)
◊ No relation to duration / degree of exposure or smoking history
Latency period: 20–35–45 years (earlier than asbestosis; later than asbestos-related lung cancer)
Peak age: 50–70 years (66%); M:F = 2–4–6:1
Path: multiple tumor masses involving predominantly the parietal pleura + to a lesser degree the visceral pleura; progression to thick sheetlike / confluent masses resulting in lung encasement
Histo: (a) epithelioid (60%) (b) sarcomatoid (15%) (c) biphasic (25%); intracellular asbestos fibers in 25%
Associated with: peritoneal mesothelioma; hypertrophic osteoarthropathy (10%)
Staging (Boutin modification of Butchart staging)
IA confined to ipsilateral parietal / diaphragmatic pleura
IB + visceral pleura, lung , pericardium
II invasion of chest wall / mediastinum (esophagus, heart, contralateral pleura) or metastases to thoracic lymph nodes
III penetration of diaphragm with peritoneal involvement or metastases to extrathoracic lymph nodes
IV distant hematogenous metastases
Stage at presentation: II in 50%, III in 28%, I in 18%, IV in 4%
- nonpleuritic (56%) / pleuritic chest pain (6%)
- dyspnea (53%)
- fever + chills + sweats (30%)
- weakness, fatigue, malaise (30%)
- cough (24%), weight loss (22%), anorexia (10%)
- expectoration of asbestos bodies (= fusiform segmented rodlike structures = iron-protein deposition on asbestos fibers [a subset of ferruginous bodies])

Spread:
(a) contiguous: chest wall, mediastinum, contralateral chest, pericardium, diaphragm, peritoneal cavity; lymphatics, blood
(b) lymphatic: hilar + mediastinal (40%), celiac (8%), axillary + supraclavicular (1%), cervical nodes
(c) hematogenous: lung, liver, kidney, adrenal gland
√ extensive irregular lobulated bulky pleural-based masses typically >5 cm / pleural thickening (60%)
√ exudative / hemorrhagic unilateral pleural effusion (30–60–80%) without mediastinal shift ("frozen hemithorax" = fixation by pleural rind of neoplastic tissue); effusion contains hyaluronic acid in 80–100%; bilateral effusions (in 10%)
√ distinct pleural mass without effusion (<25%)
√ associated with pleural plaques in 50% = pathologic HALLMARK of asbestos exposure
√ pleural calcifications (20%)
√ circumferential encasement = involvement of all pleural surfaces (mediastinum, pericardium, fissures) as late manifestation
√ extension into interlobar fissures (40–86%)
√ rib destruction in 20% (in advanced disease)
√ ascites (peritoneum involved in 35%)

CT:
√ pleural thickening (92%)
√ thickening of interlobar fissure (86%)
√ pleural effusion (74%)
√ contraction of affected hemithorax (42%):
√ ipsilateral mediastinal shift
√ narrowed intercostal spaces
√ elevation of ipsilateral hemidiaphragm
√ calcified pleural plaques (20%)

MR (best modality to determine resectability):
√ minimally hyperintense relative to muscle on T1WI
√ moderately hyperintense relative to muscle on T2WI

Metastases to:
ipsilateral lung (60%), hilar + mediastinal nodes, contralateral lung + pleura (rare), extension through chest wall + diaphragm
Prognosis: 10% of occupationally exposed individuals die of mesothelioma (in 50% pleural + in 50% peritoneal mesothelioma); mean survival time of 5–11 months
DDx: pleural fibrosis from infection (TB, fungal, actinomycosis), fibrothorax, empyema, metastatic adenocarcinoma (differentiation impossible)
Dx: video-assisted thoracoscopic surgery (postprocedural radiation therapy of all entry ports for tumor seeding of needle track [21%])

METASTASIS TO LUNG

Pulmonary metastases occur in 30% of all malignancies; mostly hematogenous
Age: >50 years (in 87%)
FREQUENCY:

	Origin of pulmonary mets		*Probability of pulmonary mets*	
1.	Breast	22%	Kidney	in 75%
2.	Kidney	11%	Osteosarcoma	in 75%
3.	Head and neck	10%	Choriocarcinoma	in 75%
4.	Colorectal	9%	Thyroid	in 65%
5.	Uterus	6%	Melanoma	in 60%
6.	Pancreas	5%	Breast	in 55%
7.	Ovary	5%	Prostate	in 40%
8.	Prostate	4%	Head and neck	in 30%
9.	Stomach	4%	Esophagus	in 20%

Incidence of pulmonary metastases:
mnemonic: "CHEST"

Choriocarcinoma	60%
Hypernephroma / Wilms tumor	30 / 20%
Ewing sarcoma	18%
Sarcoma (rhabdomyo- / osteosarcoma)	21 / 15%
Testicular tumor	12%

√ multiple nodules (in 75%) of varying sizes (most typical), 82% subpleural
√ fine micronodular pattern: highly vascular tumor (renal cell, breast, thyroid, prostate carcinoma, bone sarcoma, choriocarcinoma)
√ pneumothorax (2%): especially in children with bone tumors

CT:
√ noncalcified multiple (>10) round lesions >2.5 cm likely to be metastatic
√ connection to pulmonary arterial branches (75%)

Solitary Metastatic Lung Nodule

◊ A solitary lung nodule represents a primary lung tumor in 62% in patients with known Hx of neoplasm
◊ 5% of all solitary nodules are metastatic; most likely origin: colon carcinoma (30–40%), osteosarcoma, renal cell carcinoma, testicular tumor, breast carcinoma

Calcifying Lung Metastases (<1%)

mnemonic: "BOTTOM"
Breast
Osteo- / chondrosarcoma
Thyroid (papillary)
Testicular
Ovarian
Mucinous adenocarcinoma
+ lung metastases following radiation / chemotherapy

Cavitating Lung Metastases (4%)

mnemonic: "**S**quamous **C**ell **M**etastases **T**end to **C**avitate"
Squamous cell carcinoma, **S**arcoma
Colon
Melanoma
Transitional cell carcinoma
Cervix, under **C**hemotherapy

Hemorrhagic Lung Metastases

√ ill-defined nodules
1. Choriocarcinoma
2. Renal cell carcinoma
3. Melanoma
4. Thyroid carcinoma

Endobronchial Metastases

√ segmental / subsegmental atelectasis
1. Bronchogenic carcinoma
2. Lymphoma
3. Renal cell carcinoma
4. Breast cancer
5. Colon carcinoma

Lung Metastases In Childhood

mnemonic: "ROWE"
Rhabdomyosarcoma
Osteosarcoma
Wilms tumor
Ewing sarcoma

METASTASIS TO PLEURA

1. Lung (36%)
2. Breast (25%)
3. Lymphoma (10%)
4. Ovary (5%)
5. Stomach (2%)

MYCOPLASMA PNEUMONIA

= PRIMARY ATYPICAL PNEUMONIA (PAP)

Commonest cause of nonbacterial pneumonia with a mild course (only 2% require hospitalization), usually lasts 2–3 weeks; only 10% of infected subjects develop pneumonia

Incidence: 10–33% of all pneumonias; autumn peak
Organism: Eaton agent = pleuropneumonia-like organism (PPLO)
Age: most common in ages 5–20 years (esp. in closed populations

• mild symptoms of cough + low fever, malaise, otitis
• mild leukocytosis (20%)
• most common respiratory cause of cold agglutinin production (60%)

√ radiologic findings often diverge from clinical condition
√ pulmonary infiltrates show a significant lag time
√ fine interstitial infiltration from hilum into lower lobe (earliest change)
√ alveolar infiltrates: unilateral (L > R) airspace consolidation in segmental lower lobe in 50%, bilateral in 10–40%
√ small pleural effusions in 20%
√ hilar adenopathy (rare)

Cx: (1) Meningoencephalitis
(2) Erythema nodosum, erythema multiforme, Stevens-Johnson syndrome

Prognosis: 20% with recurrent symptoms of pharyngitis + bronchitis ± infiltrations

NEAR DROWNING

1. Sea-water drowning
   • hemoconcentration, hypovolemia
2. Fresh-water drowning
   • hemodilution, hypervolemia
   • hemolysis
3. Secondary drowning
   (a) pneumonia with toxic debris
   (b) progressive pulmonary edema
4. Dry drowning (20–40%)
   = laryngeal spasm prevents water from entering
   √ no roentgenographic abnormality

Similarities of all 4 types:
• hypoxemia
• metabolic acidosis
√ pulmonary edema
√ hyaline membrane formation = considerable loss of protein from blood

NEONATAL PNEUMONIA

Pathogenesis:
(a) in utero infection (ascending from premature rupture of membranes or prolonged labor / transplacental route)
(b) aspiration of infected vaginal secretions during delivery
(c) infection after birth

Organism:
(1) Group B streptococcus (GBS): in low–birth-weight premature infants; 50% mortality
√ radiographic picture may be identical to RDS (in 52%)
√ appearance suggesting retained lung fluid / focal infiltrates (35%)
√ normal CXR (13%)
√ cardiomegaly
√ pleural effusions (in 2/3, but RARE in RDS)
√ delayed onset diaphragmatic hernia (evidenced by clinical deterioration)
(2) Pneumococci: RDS-like
(3) Listeria: RDS-like
(4) Candida: progressive consolidation + cavitation
(5) Chlamydia: bronchopneumonic pattern

- afebrile
- lower ventilatory pressure requirements

√ bilateral focal / diffuse areas of opacities (may initially appear similar to fetal aspiration syndrome)
√ hyperaeration
√ may cause lobar atelectasis
√ may cause pneumothorax / pneumomediastinum
√ pleural effusion (exceedingly rare)

NOCARDIOSIS

Organism: Gram-positive acid-fast bacterium resembling fungus
Predisposed: immunocompromised
√ multiple poorly / well-defined nodules ± cavitation
√ lobar consolidation
√ empyema without sinus tracts
√ SVC obstruction (rare)

NONTUBERCULOUS MYCOBACTERIAL INFECTION OF LUNG

= ATYPICAL TUBERCULOSIS

Organisms:
M. kansasii: lung infection in subjects with good immune status
M. marinum: "swimming pool granuloma"
M. ulcerans: "Buruli ulcer" in tropical areas
M. scrofulaceum: cervical lymphadenitis in infants
M. avium intracellulare: esp. in AIDS

Organism causing pulmonary disease (Runyon classification):
ubiquitous organisms as part of normal environmental flora

1. Photochromogens
M. kansasii, M. simiae, M. asiaticum
• colonies turn yellow with exposure to light
◊ 70–80% of individuals from rural areas test positive on PPD-B (= antigen from M. kansasii)!
2. Scotochromogens
M. scrofulaceum, M. xenopi, M. szulgai, M. gordonae
• yellow colonies turn orange with exposure to light
3. Nonchromogens
M. avium-intracellulare, M. malmoense, M. terrae
• white / beige colonies without color change
4. Rapid growers
M. fortuitum-chelonei
• appear in culture in 3–5 days (all other groups appear in culture in 2–4 weeks)

Histo: lesions indistinguishable from M. tuberculosis
Source: soil, water, dairy products, bird droppings
Infection: inhalation of aerosolized water droplets (M. avium-intracellulare complex), food aspiration in patients with achalasia (M. fortuitum-chelonei), GI tract (in AIDS)

- cough (60–100%), hemoptysis (15–20%)
- asthma, dyspnea
- fever distinctly uncommon (10–13%)
- weakness + weight loss (up to 50%)
- weekly positive tuberculin skin test

A. CLASSICAL FORM
Age: 6th–7th decade, in Whites (80–90%), M>F
Predisposing factors:
COPD (25–72%), previous TB (20–24%), interstitial lung disease (6%), smoking >30 pack-years (46%), alcohol abuse (40%), cardiovascular disease (36%), chronic liver disease (32%), previous gastrectomy (18%)
Location: apical + anterior segments of upper lobes
√ chronic fibronodular / fibroproductive apical opacities (indistinguishable from reactivation TB)
√ cavitation in 80–95%
√ apical pleural thickening in 37–56%
√ additional patchy nodular alveolar opacities (due to bronchogenic spread) in ipsi- / contralateral lung in 40–70%
√ adenopathy (0–4%)
√ pleural effusion (5–20%)
√ typically NO hilar elevation

B. NONCLASSICAL FORM (20–30%)
Age: 7th–8th decade, 86% in Whites; M:F = 1:4
Predisposing factors: NONE
Location: predominantly in middle lobe + lingula
√ multiple bilateral nodular opacities throughout both lungs in random distribution
√ irregular curvilinear interstitial opacities (resembling bronchiectasis)

C. ASYMPTOMATIC GRANULOMAS
√ cluster of similar-sized nodules

D. ACHALASIA-RELATED INFECTION
with M. fortuitum-chelonei

CHEST

E. DISSEMINATED DISEASE
in immunocompromised patients: AIDS, transplant patients, lymphoproliferative disorders (esp., hairy cell leukemia), steroid + immunosuppressive therapy

CT:
√ multifocal bronchiectasis (79–94%), esp. middle lobe + lingula
√ centrilobular nodules of varying sizes, usually <1 cm (= micronodules) in 76–97%
√ bronchial wall thickening (97%)
√ airspace disease (76%)
√ cavitation (21%), esp. in upper lobes
√ interlobular septal thickening (12%)
◊ Unfavorable response to antituberculous therapy is suspicious for atypical TB!
DDx: M. tuberculosis (bronchiectasis less common + less extensive), bronchiolitis obliterans, sarcoidosis, fungal disease

PANBRONCHIOLITIS

= inflammatory lung disease, prevalent in Orientals but rare in Europeans + North Americans
Pathogenesis: unknown
HRCT:
√ centrilobular branching structures (segments of bronchiolectasis filled with secretions) + nodules surrounding respiratory bronchioles
√ mosaic perfusion
√ air trapping
√ bronchial dilatation
DDx: bronchiolitis obliterans

PARAGONIMIASIS OF LUNG

= parasitic disease caused by trematode Paragonimus (usually P. westermani = lung fluke) endemic to certain areas of East + Southeast Asia (China, Korea, Japan, Thailand, Laos, Philippines, India)
Infection: ingestion of raw / incompletely cooked freshwater crab / crayfish infected with metacercaria; larva exists in small intestine + penetrates the intestinal wall + enters peritoneal cavity; larva penetrates diaphragm + pleura to enter the lung
Cycle: from the final host (tiger, cat, dog, fox, weasel, opossum, human) eggs of worm pass to the outside with blood-streaked sputum; in fresh water a ciliated embryo (miracidium) develops; it becomes a tailed larva (cercaria) after invading a fresh water snail; when infected snail is eaten by crustacean, its tail detaches and it becomes a 300 μm encysted larva (metacercaria)

@ CNS
• meningoencephalitis (in 25%)
√ shell-like / soap–bubble-like calcifications of varying size (~50%)

CXR (pulmonary lesions in 83%, pulmonary + pleural lesions in 44%, pleural lesions in 17%):
<u>early findings</u> (lesions occur 3–8 weeks after ingestion):
√ uni- / bilateral pneumo- / hydropneumothorax (17%)
√ uni- / bilateral pleural effusion (3–54%)
√ focal patchy migrating airspace consolidation (= worm migration causing focal hemorrhagic pneumonia) (45%)
√ lobar / segmental collapse (airway obstruction from egg granuloma / intrusion of worm)
√ 2–4 mm thick and 2–7 cm long linear opacities abutting the pleura (41%) due to worm migration track
<u>later findings</u>:
√ lung cyst (cyst formation from infarction after arteriolar / venous obstruction by worm or egg; expansion of small airway by intraluminal parasite)
√ thick-walled cyst (due to fibrosis)
√ "eclipse effect" = eccentric thickening of cyst wall (due to intracystic one / two worms)
√ thin-walled cyst (when cyst connected to airway)
√ 10–15 mm nodules + masslike consolidation (24%) (due to cyst initially masked by pericystic airspace consolidation ± cyst filled with chocolate-colored necrotic fluid)
√ bronchiectasis (35%)

DDx: tuberculosis (nodular slowly changing lesion, residual fibrosis after treatment, no subpleural linear opacities)

PERICARDIAL CYST

Etiology:
(1) defect in embryogenesis of coelomic cavities
(2) sequela of pericarditis
Histo: lined by single layer of mesothelial cells
Age: 30–40 years; M:F = 3:2
• asymptomatic (50%)
Location: (a) cardiophrenic angle (75%), R:L = 3:1 / 3:2, 25% higher; may extend into major fissure
(b) mediastinum (rare)
√ sharply marginated round / ovoid / triangular mass usually 3–8 cm (range 1–28 cm) in diameter
√ change in size + shape with respiration / body position
√ attenuation values of 20–40 HU, occasionally higher

PNEUMATOCELE

= cystic air collection within lung parenchyma due to obstructive overinflation = regional obstructive emphysema
◊ does not indicate destruction of lung parenchyma
◊ occurs during healing phase
◊ appears to enlarge while patient improves
◊ frequently multiple
Developmental theories:
(1) small bronchioles undergo severe distension secondary to check-valve endobronchial / peribronchial obstruction

(2) focus of necrotic lung evacuates through a bronchus narrowed by edema / inflammation ; air space subsequently enlarges due to check-valve mechanism from enlarging pneumatocele / inflammatory exudate
(3) air from ruptured alveoli / bronchioles dissects along interstitial interlobular tissue and accumulates between visceral pleura and lung parenchyma = subpleural emphysematous bulla = subpleural air cyst

A. PNEUMATOCELE ASSOCIATED WITH INFECTION
Organism: Pneumococci, E. coli, Klebsiella, Staphylococcus (in childhood)
√ appears within 1st week, disappears within 6 weeks
√ thin-walled + completely air-filled cavity
√ ± air-fluid level + wall thickening (during infection)
√ pneumothorax
√ spontaneous resolution (in most)

B. TRAUMATIC PNEUMATOCELE = PNEUMATOCYST
Cause:
(a) air trapped within area of pulmonary laceration is initially obscured by surrounding contusion (hematoma); pneumatocyst appears within hours after blunt chest trauma
(b) intensive inflammatory response from hydrocarbon (furniture polish, kerosene) inhalation / ingestion
√ single / multiple pneumatoceles
√ spontaneous resolution over several weeks to months

PNEUMOCOCCAL PNEUMONIA

Most common Gram-positive pneumonia
90% community-acquired, 10% nosocomial
Incidence: 15% of all adulthood pneumonias, uncommon in child; peaks in winter + early spring; increased during influenza epidemics
Organism: Streptococcus pneumoniae (formerly Diplococcus pneumoniae), Gram-positive, in pairs / chains, encapsulated, capsular polysaccharide responsible for virulence + serotyping
Susceptible: elderly, debilitated, alcoholics, CHF, COPD, multiple myeloma, hypogammaglobulinemia, functional / surgical asplenia

- rusty blood-streaked sputum
- left-shift leukocytosis
- impaired pulmonary function

Location: usually involves one lobe only; bias for lower lobes + posterior segments of upper lobes (bacteria flow under gravitational influence to most dependent portions as in aspiration)
√ extensive airspace consolidation abutting against visceral pleura (lobar / beyond confines of one lobe through pores of Kohn) CHARACTERISTIC
√ slight expansion of involved lobes
√ prominent air bronchograms (20%)
√ patchy bronchopneumonic pattern (in some)
√ pleural effusion (parapneumonic transudate) uncommon with antibiotic therapy
√ cavitation (rare, with Type III)
Variations (modified by bronchopulmonary disease, eg, chronic bronchitis, emphysema):
√ bronchopneumonia-like pattern
√ effusion may be only presentation (esp. in COPD)
√ empyema (with persistent fever)
— in children:
√ round pneumonia = sharply defined round lesion
Prognosis: prompt response to antibiotics (if without complications); 5% mortality rate
Dx: blood culture (positive in 30%)
Cx: meningitis, endocarditis, septic arthritis, empyema (now rarely seen)

PNEUMOCYSTOSIS

= PNEUMOCYSTIS CARINII PNEUMONIA
◊ Most common cause of interstitial pneumonia in immunocompromised patients, which quickly leads to airspace disease
Organism:
ubiquitous obligate extracellular protozoan / fungus Pneumocystis carinii
(a) trophozoite develops into a cyst
(b) cyst produces up to eight daughter sporozoites which are released at maturity + develop into trophozoites
Pathomechanism:
trophozoite attaches to cell membrane of type I alveolar pneumocytes with subsequent cell death + leakage of proteinaceous fluid into alveolar space
Predisposed:
(1) debilitated premature infants, children with hypogammaglobulinemia (12%)
(2) AIDS (60–80%)
(3) other immunocompromised patients: congenital immunodeficiency syndrome, lymphoproliferative disorders, organ transplant recipients (renal transplant patients in 10%), patients on long-term corticosteroid therapy (nephrotic syndrome, collagen vascular disease), patients on cytotoxic drugs [under therapy for leukemia (40%), lymphoma (16%)]
◊ Often associated with simultaneous infection by CMV, Mycobacterium avium-intracellulare, herpes simplex

- severe dyspnea + cyanosis over 3–5 days
- subacute insidious onset of malaise + minimal cough (frequent in AIDS patients)
- respiratory failure (5–30%)
- WBC slightly elevated (PMNs)
- lymphopenia (50%) heralds poor prognosis

√ normal CXR in 10–39%
√ bilateral diffuse symmetric finely granular / reticular interstitial / airspace infiltrates (in 80%) with perihilar + basilar distribution (CHARACTERISTIC central location)
√ response to therapy within 5–7 days
√ rapid progression to diffuse alveolar homogeneous consolidation (DDx: pulmonary edema)
√ air bronchogram

CHEST

√ fine / coarse linear / reticular pattern = thickened coarse interstitial lung markings (in healing phase)
√ pleural effusion + hilar lymphadenopathy (uncommon)
√ atypical pattern (in 5%):
  √ isolated lobar disease / focal parenchymal opacities
  √ lung nodules ± cavitation
  √ hilar / mediastinal lymphadenopathy
  √ thin- / thick-walled regular / irregular cysts / cavities with predilection for upper lobes + subpleural regions
√ effect of prophylactic use of aerosolized pentamidine: redistribution of infection to upper lobes
  √ cystic lung disease
  √ spontaneous pneumothorax, frequently bilateral (6–7%)
  √ disseminated extrapulmonary disease (1%):
  √ punctate / rimlike calcifications within enlarged lymph nodes + abdominal viscera

CT:
  √ patchwork pattern (56%)
    = bilateral asymmetric patchy mosaic appearance with sparing of segments / subsegments of pulmonary lobe
  √ "ground-glass" pattern (26%)
    = bilateral diffuse air space disease (fluid + inflammatory cells in alveolar space) in symmetric distribution
  √ interstitial pattern (18%)
    = bilateral symmetric / asymmetric, linear / reticular markings (thickening of lobular septa)
  √ air-filled spaces (38%):
    (a) pneumatoceles = thin-walled spaces without lobar predilection resolving within 6 months
    (b) subpleural bullae (due to premature emphysema)
    (c) thin-walled cysts (? check-valve obstruction of small airways from aerosolized pentamidine)
    (d) necrosis of PCP granuloma
  √ pneumothorax (13%)
  √ lymphadenopathy (18%)
  √ pleural effusion (18%)
  √ pulmonary nodules
    usually due to malignancy (leukemia, lymphoma, Kaposi sarcoma, metastasis) / septic emboli
  √ pulmonary cavities
    usually due to superimposed fungal / mycobacterial infection

NUC:
  √ bilateral and diffuse Ga-67 uptake without mediastinal involvement prior to roentgenographic changes
    DDx: TB / MAI infection (with mediastinal involvement)

Dx: (1) sputum collection (2) bronchoscopy with lavage (3) transbronchial / transthoracic / open lung Bx

Prognosis: rapid fulminant disease; death within 2 weeks

Rx: co-trimoxazole IV, nebulized pentamidine

PNEUMONECTOMY CHEST

Early signs (within 24 hours):
  √ partial filling of thorax
  √ ipsilateral mediastinal shift + diaphragmatic elevation

Late signs (after 2 months):
  √ complete obliteration of space

N.B.: Depression of diaphragm / shift of mediastinum to contralateral side indicates a bronchopleural fistula / empyema / hemorrhage!

POSTOBSTRUCTIVE PNEUMONIA

= chronic inflammatory disease distal to bronchial obstruction

Cause:
1. Bronchogenic carcinoma (most commonly)
2. Bronchial adenoma
3. Granular cell myoblastoma (almost always tracheal lesion)
4. Bronchostenosis

Histo: "golden pneumonia" = cholesterol pneumonia endogenous lipid pneumonia = mixture of edema, atelectasis, round cell infiltration, bronchiectasis, liberation of lipid material from alveolar pneumocytes secondary to inflammatory reaction

√ frequently associated with some degree of atelectasis
√ persists unchanged for weeks
√ recurrent pneumonia in same region after antibiotic treatment

PROGRESSIVE MASSIVE FIBROSIS

= (PMF) = COMPLICATED PNEUMOCONIOSIS
= CONGLOMERATE ANTHRACOSILICOSIS

May develop / progress after cessation of dust exposure

Path: avascular amorphous central mass of insoluble proteins stabilized by cross-links + ill-defined bundles of coarse hyalinized collagen at periphery

Location: almost exclusively restricted to posterior segment of upper lobe / superior segment of lower lobe

√ large >1 cm opacities initially in middle + upper lung zones at periphery of lung
√ discoid contour (44%) = mass flat from front to back (thin opacity on lateral view, large opacity on PA view), medial border often ill-defined, lateral borders sharp + parallel to rib cage
√ migration toward hila starting at lung periphery; bilateral symmetry
√ apparent decrease in nodularity (incorporation of nodules from surroundings)
√ cavitation (occasionally) due to ischemic necrosis / superimposed TB infection
√ bullous scar emphysema
√ pulmonary hypertension

PSEUDOLYMPHOMA

= reactive benign lesion = localized form of lymphocytic interstitial pneumonitis (LIP); no progression to lymphoma

Histo: aggregates of plasma cells, reticulin cells, large + small lymphocytes with preserved lymphoid architecture resembling lymphoma histologically without lymph node involvement

Associated with: Sjögren syndrome

• mostly asymptomatic

√ well-demarcated dense infiltrate

CHEST

√ infiltrate typically in central location extending to visceral pleura
√ prominent air bronchogram
√ NO lymphadenopathy
Prognosis: occasionally progression to non-Hodgkin lymphoma
Rx: most patients respond well to steroids initially

PSEUDOMONAS PNEUMONIA

= most dreaded nosocomial infection because of resistance to antibiotics in patients with debilitating diseases on multiple antibiotics + corticosteroids; rare in community
Organism: Pseudomonas aeruginosa, Gram-negative
• bradycardia
• temperature with morning peaks
√ widespread patchy bronchopneumonia (secondary to bacteremia; unlike other Gram-negative pneumonias)
√ predilection for lower lobes
√ extensive bilateral consolidation
√ "spongelike pattern" with multiple nodules >2 cm (= extensive necrosis with formation of multiple abscesses)
√ small pleural effusions

PULMONARY ARTERIAL MALFORMATION

= PAVM = PULMONARY ARTERIOVENOUS ANEURYSM = PULMONARY ARTERIOVENOUS FISTULA = PULMONARY ANGIOMA = PULMONARY TELANGIECTASIA
= abnormal vascular communication between pulmonary artery and vein (95%) or systemic artery and pulmonary vein (5%)
Etiology:
(a) congenital defect of capillary structure (common)
(b) acquired in cirrhosis (hepatogenic pulmonary angiodysplasia), cancer, trauma, surgery, actinomycosis, schistosomiasis
Path: hemangioma of cavernous type
Pathophysiology:
low-resistance extracardiac R-to-L shunt (which may result in paradoxical embolism); quantification with Tc-99m–labeled albumin microspheres by measuring fraction of dose reaching kidneys
Age: 3rd–4th decade; manifest in adult life, 10% in childhood
Occurrence:
(a) isolated abnormality (40%)
(b) multiple (in 1/3)
associated with Rendu-Osler-Weber syndrome (in 30–60–88%) = hereditary hemorrhagic telangiectasia
◊ Only 5–15% of patients with Rendu-Osler-Weber disease have pulmonary AVMs!
Types:
1. Simple type (79%)
= single feeding artery empties into a bulbous nonseptated aneurysmal segment with a single draining vein
2. Complex type (21%)
= more than one feeding artery empties into septated aneurysmal segment with more than one draining vein

• asymptomatic in 56% (until 3rd–4th decade) if AVM single and <2 cm
• orthodeoxia (= increased hypoxemia with PaO_2 <85 mm Hg in erect position due to gravitational shift of pulmonary blood flow to base of lung)
• cyanosis with normal-sized heart (R-to-L shunt) in 25–50%, clubbing
• bruit over lesion (increased during inspiration)
• dyspnea on exertion (60–71%)
• epistaxis (79%)
• palpitation, chest pain
• No CHF
Location: lower lobes (65–70%) > middle lobe > upper lobes; bilateral (8–20%); medial third of lung
√ sharply defined, lobulated oval / round mass (90%) of 1 to several cm in size ("coin lesion")
√ cordlike bands from mass to hilum (feeding artery + draining veins)
√ in 2/3 single lesion, in 1/3 multiple lesions
√ enlargement with advancing age
√ change in size with Valsalva / Mueller maneuver / erect vs. recumbent position (decrease with Valsalva maneuver)
√ phleboliths (occasionally)
√ increased pulsations of hilar vessels
CT (98% detection rate):
√ homogeneous circumscribed noncalcified nodule / serpiginous mass up to several cm in diameter
√ vascular connection of mass with enlarged feeding artery + draining vein
√ sequential enhancement of feeding artery + aneurysmal part + efferent vein on dynamic CT
MR: (if contraindication to contrast / slow flow due to partial thrombosis / follow-up)
√ signal void on standard spin echo / high signal intensity on GRASS images
Angio (mostly obviated by MR / CT unless surgery or embolization contemplated)

Cx: CNS symptoms are commonly the initial manifestation
(1) Cerebrovascular accident: stroke (18%), transient ischemic attack (37%) secondary to paradoxical bland emboli
(2) Brain abscess (5–9%) secondary to loss of pulmonary filter function for septic emboli
(3) Hemoptysis (13%) secondary to rupture of PAVM into bronchus, most common presenting symptom
(4) Hemothorax (9%) secondary to rupture of subpleural PAVM
(5) Polycythemia
Prognosis: 26% morbidity, 11% mortality
DDx: solitary / multiple pulmonary nodules
Rx: embolization with coils / detachable balloons

PULMONARY CAPILLARY HEMANGIOMATOSIS

= bilateral pulmonary disease behaving like a low-grade nonmetastatic vascular neoplasm with slowly progressive pulmonary hypertension

Histo: sheets of thin-walled capillary blood vessels infiltrating pulmonary interstitium + invading pulmonary vessels, bronchioles, and pleura

Pathomechanism of pulmonary hypertension:
(a) veno-occlusive phenomenon secondary to invasion of small pulmonary veins
(b) progressive vascular obliteration secondary to in situ thrombosis + infarction
(c) pulmonary scar formation secondary to recurrent pulmonary hemorrhage

Age: 20–40 years

- dyspnea on exertion
- cor pulmonale: jugular venous distension, pedal edema, ECG-signs of RV failure (DDx: pulmonary veno-occlusive disease)
- elevated PA pressures + normal pulmonary wedge pressure
- hemoptysis + pleuritic chest pain in 1/3 (DDx: pulmonary thromboembolic disease)

CXR:
√ diffuse reticulonodular pattern
√ focal areas of interstitial fibrosis (recurrent episodes of pulmonary hemorrhage + thrombotic infarction)

CT:
√ thickening + nodularity of inter- and intralobular septa + walls of pulmonary veins
√ areas of ground-glass attenuation (= increased perfusion to extensive proliferating hemangiomatous tissue)

Angio:
√ combination of increased flow (to hemangiomatous areas) + decreased flow (to regions of thrombosis, infarction, and scarring)

Prognosis: death after 2- to 12-year interval from onset of symptoms

Rx: bilateral lung transplantation

DDx:
(1) Pulmonary veno-occlusive disease
(2) Idiopathic interstitial fibrosis
(3) Primary pulmonary hypertension (no increase in lung markings)
(4) Pulmonary hemangiomatosis (only in children, cavernous hemangiomas involving several organs)

PULMONARY CONTUSION

= most common manifestation of blunt chest trauma, esp. deceleration trauma

Path: exudation of edema + blood into air space + interstitium

Time of onset: apparent within 6 hours after trauma

- clinically inapparent
- hemoptysis (50%)

Location: posterior (in 60%)

Site: directly deep to site of impact / contrecoup

√ irregular patchy / diffuse homogeneous extensive consolidation (CT is more sensitive)
√ opacity may enlarge for 48–72 hours
√ rapid resolution beginning 24–48 hours, complete within 2–10 days
√ overlying rib fractures (frequent)

CT:
√ nonsegmental coarse ill-defined crescentic (50%) / amorphous (45%) opacification of lung parenchyma without cavitation
√ "subpleural sparing" = 1–2 mm rim of uniformly nonopacified subpleural portion of lung

Cx: pneumothorax

DDx: fat embolism (1–2 days after injury)

PULMONARY INTERSTITIAL EMPHYSEMA

= PIE = complication of respirator therapy with PEEP

Pathogenesis:
gas escapes from overdistended alveolus, dissects into perivascular sheath surrounding arteries, veins, and lymphatics, tracks into mediastinum forming clusters of blebs; **air-block** = compression + obstruction of pulmonary veins + mediastinal structures by interstitial pulmonary emphysema / pneumomediastinum / pneumothorax (obstruction esp. during expiration)

- sudden deterioration in patient's condition during respiratory therapy

√ elongated lucencies following distribution of bronchovascular tree
√ circular densities
√ bilateral, symmetrical distribution
√ lobar overdistension (occasionally)

Cx: pneumomediastinum, pneumothorax, subcutaneous emphysema, pneumopericardium, intracardiac air, pneumoperitoneum, pneumatosis intestinalis

PULMONARY LYMPHANGIOMATOSIS

= increased number of communicating lymphatic channels

√ smooth thickening of bronchovascular bundles + interlobular septa

CT:
√ diffuse increased attenuation of mediastinal fat
√ mild perihilar infiltration
√ pleural effusion
√ pleural thickening

PULMONARY MAINLINE GRANULOMATOSIS

= PULMONARY TALCOSIS
= microscopic pulmonary embolism in drug addicts from IV injection of talc-containing drugs (ground tablets)

Drugs: amphetamines, methylphenidate hydrochloride ("West coast"), tripelen amine ("blue velvet"), methadone hydrochloride, dilaudid, meperidine, pentazocine, propylhexedrine, hydromorphone hydrochloride

◊ added talc (= magnesium silicate) particles incite a granulomatous foreign-body reaction + subsequent fibrosis in perivascular distribution

- talc retinopathy (80%) = small glistening crystals
- angiothrombotic pulmonary hypertension + cor pulmonale

Early changes:
√ widespread micronodularity of "pinpoint" size (1–3 mm) with perihilar / basilar predominance
√ well-defined nodules predominantly in middle zones

Late changes:
√ loss of lung volume
√ coalescent opacities similar to progressive massive fibrosis (DDx: in silicosis away from hila)

DDx of late changes:
(1) Progressive massive fibrosis of silicosis / coal worker's pneumoconiosis
(2) Chronic sarcoidosis

Dx: lung biopsy

PULMONARY THROMBOEMBOLIC DISEASE

= PULMONARY EMBOLISM (PE)

Prevalence: 630,000 Americans/year with missed / delayed diagnosis in 400,000 causing death in 120,000; diagnosed in 1% of all hospitalized patients; in 12–64% at autopsy; in 9–56% of patients with deep venous thrombosis

Age: 60% >60 years of age

Cause: deep vein thrombosis (DVT) of LE in >90%; PE usually occurs within first 5–7 days of thrombus formation

Predisposing factors: immobilization (56%), surgery (54%)

Pathophysiology: A clot from the deep veins of the leg breaks off + fragments in right side of heart + showers lung with emboli varying in size

◊ On average >6–8 vessels are embolized!

Class 1 = <20% of pulmonary arteries occluded
- asymptomatic
- normal arterial blood gas levels
- normal pulmonary + systemic hemodynamics

Class 2 = 20–30% of pulmonary arteries occlude
- anxiety, hyperventilation
- arterial PO_2 <80 torr
- PCO_2 <35 torr

Class 3 = 30–50% of pulmonary arteries occluded
- dyspnea, collapse
- arterial PO_2 <65 torr
- arterial PCO_2 <30 torr
- elevated central venous pressure

Class 4 = >50% of pulmonary arteries occluded
- shock, dyspnea
- arterial PO_2 <50 torr
- arterial PCO_2 <30 torr
- elevated central venous pressure
- mean PA pressure >20 mm Hg
- systolic blood pressure <100 mm Hg

- Classic triad (<33%):
  (1) hemoptysis (25–34%) (2) pleural friction rub
  (3) thrombophlebitis
  ◊ only 10–33% of patients with fatal PE are symptomatic for DVT
  ◊ DVT diagnosed ante mortem in <30%
  ◊ clinically suspected diagnosis accurate in 26–45%
  ◊ 30% of patients with angiographically detected PE have negative bilateral venograms ("big bang" theory = clot embolizes in toto to lung leaving no residual in leg veins)
- may be asymptomatic
- false-positive clinical diagnosis in 62%
- acute dyspnea (81–86%)
- pleuritic chest pain (58–72%)
- apprehension (59%)
- cough (54–70%)
- tachycardia, tachypnea
- accentuated 2nd heart sound
- ECG changes (83%), mostly nonspecific: P-pulmonale, right-axis deviation, right bundle branch block, classic $S_1Q_3T_3$ pattern
- bronchospasm (histamine-mediated), bronchial plugging, rales (loss of surfactant)
- elevated levels of fibrinopeptide-A (FPA) = small peptide split off of fibrinogen during fibrin generation
- positive D-dimer assay (generated during clot lysis)

Location of PE: bilateral emboli (in 45%), RT lung only (36%), LT lung only (18%); multiple emboli [3–6 on average] in 65%

Distribution: RUL (16%), RML (9%), RLL (25%), LUL (14%), LLL (26%)

Site: central = segmental / larger (in 58%);
peripheral = subsegmental / smaller (in 42%);
in subsegmental branches exclusively (in 30%)

◊ Emboli are occlusive in 40%!

RESOLUTION OF PE
(through fibrinolysis + fragmentation):
in 8% by 24 hours, in 56% by 14 days, in 77% by 7 months; complete in 65%, partial in 23%, no resolution in 12%
◊ Resolution less favorable with increasing age + cardiac disease
◊ Resolution improved with urokinase > heparin within first week (after 1 year 80% for both)

A. EMBOLISM WITHOUT INFARCTION (90%)
Histo: hemorrhage + edema
√ normal chest film common (>29%), abnormal CXR in 40–93%
◊ A normal CXR has a negative predictive value of only 74%!
√ platelike atelectasis ± segmental / lobar consolidation in lower lung zones + pleural effusion (most common findings with the lowest positive predictive value)
√ Westermark sign = area of oligemia (due to vasoconstriction distal to embolus) in 2%
√ Fleischner sign = local widening of artery by impaction of embolus (due to distension by clot / pulmonary hypertension developing secondary to peripheral embolization)
√ "knuckle sign" = abrupt tapering of an occluded vessel distally

B. EMBOLISM WITH INFARCTION (10–60%)
= any opacity developing as a result of thromboembolic disease; more likely to develop in presence of cardiopulmonary disease with obstruction of pulmonary venous outflow (diagnosed in retrospect)
Histo: (1) incomplete infarction = reversible transient hemorrhagic congestion / edema usually resolving over several days to weeks
(2) complete infarction = hemorrhagic infarction with necrosis of lung parenchyma remaining permanently
√ segmentally distributed wedge-shaped consolidation (54%)
√ ± cavitation
√ Hampton hump = pleural-based shallow consolidation in form of a truncated cone with base against pleural surface + convex medial border
√ pleural effusion (54%)
√ thoracentesis: bloody (65%), predominantly PMNs (61%), exudate (65%)
√ NO air-bronchogram (hemorrhage into alveoli)
√ "melting sign" = within few days to weeks regression from periphery toward center
√ Fleischner lines = long-line shadows (fibrotic scar) from invagination of pleura at the base of the collapse resulting in pseudofissure
√ platelike atelectasis (27%)
√ cardiomegaly / CHF (17%)
√ elevated hemidiaphragm (17%)
√ subsequent nodular / linear scar

CT (spiral CT equal to angio in detection of emboli within proximal arteries of ≤5th / 6th generation):
◊ Subsegmental intraluminal filling defects (in 30%) usually not detectable!
◊ Detection poor in middle lobe + lingular branches (in 18%)!
√ peripheral wedge-shaped lung densities with the triangle base adjacent to pleural surface
√ vascular connection to a branch of pulmonary artery
√ peripheral rimlike contrast enhancement
√ intraluminal filling defect in pulmonary artery

NUC (VQ scan = guide for angiographic evaluation) interpreted in reference to Biello or PIOPED criteria (*see* page 788)
√ low- / intermediate-probability scans (73%): additional studies recommended
√ high-probability scan: in 12% normal angiogram

Angio (indicated within 24 hours of indeterminate NUC scan):
√ intraluminal defect (94%)
√ abrupt termination of pulmonary arterial branch
√ pruning + attenuation of branches
√ wedge-shaped parenchymal hypovascularity
√ absence of draining vein in affected segment
√ tortuous arterial collaterals

Cx of pulmonary angiography (1–2%):
arrhythmia, endocardial injury, cardiac perforation, cardiac arrest, contrast reaction
Mortality rate of pulmonary angiography: 0.2–0.5%
False-negative rate:
1–4–9% due to difficulty in visualizing subsegmental emboli (with only 30% interobserver agreement about presence of subsegmental emboli)

Acute thromboembolic pulmonary arterial hypertension

Hypertension disappears as emboli lyse
• sudden onset of chest pain
• acute dyspnea
• hemoptysis occasionally
Mortality:
3:1,000 surgical procedures; 200,000 deaths in 1975; 7–10% of all autopsies (death within first hour of PE in most patients); 26–30% if untreated; 8% if treated; fatal if >60% of pulmonary bed obstructed; healthy patients may survive obstruction of 50–60% of vascular bed
Rx:
1. Heparin IV: 10,000–15,000 units as initial dose; 8,000–10,000 units/hour during diagnostic evaluation; continued for 10–14 days
2. Streptokinase: better results with massive PE
3. Urokinase: slightly better than streptokinase
4. Coumadin: maintained for at least 3 months (15% complication rate)

Chronic thromboembolic pulmonary arterial hypertension

• history of previous embolic episodes
• dyspnea on exertion (DDx: interstitial lung disease)
• may be clinically silent
CT (77% sensitive):
√ vascular abnormalities:
√ direct visualization of thrombus (70%)
√ mural arterial irregularities ± abrupt narrowing / cutoff
√ decrease in caliber of small branches + narrowing of peripheral pulmonary vessels
√ main pulmonary artery diameter >28.6 mm
√ parenchymal abnormalities:
√ wedge-shaped pleura-based parenchymal bands with tip pointing to hila, often multiple, esp. involving lower lung (70%) = infarcted tissue replaced by scar
√ scattered geometric areas of low attenuation in 55% (due to oligemia) associated with vessels of small cross-sectional diameter
√ regional sharply demarcated areas of high attenuation (perfused lung on background of oligemic / nonperfused lung)
√ cylindric bronchial dilatation of segmental / subsegmental bronchi (64%)

PULMONARY VENOUS VARIX

= abnormal tortuosity + dilatation of pulmonary vein just before entrance into left atrium

Etiology: congenital / associated with pulmonary venous hypertension

- usually asymptomatic; may cause hemoptysis

Location: medial third of either lung below hila close to left atrium

√ well-defined lobulated round / oval mass
√ change in size during Valsalva / Mueller maneuver
√ opacification at same time as LA (on CECT)

Risk: (1) death upon rupture during worsening heart failure
(2) source of cerebral emboli

DDx: pulmonary arteriovenous fistula

RADIATION PNEUMONITIS

= damage to lungs after radiation therapy dependent on:
(a) irradiated lung volume
(b) radiation dose: unusual if <2000 R given in 2–3 weeks; common if >6000 R given in 5–6 weeks
(c) fractionation of dose
(d) concurrent / later chemotherapy

Pathologic phases:
(1) Exudative phase = edema fluid + hyaline membranes
(2) Organizing phase
(3) Fibrotic phase = interstitial fibrosis

Time of onset: usually 4–6 months after treatment

Location: confined to radiation port

1. ACUTE RADIATION PNEUMONITIS
(within 1–8 weeks after radiation therapy)

Path: depletion of surfactant (1 week to 1 month later), plasma exudation, desquamation of alveolar + bronchial cells

- asymptomatic (majority)
- nonproductive cough, shortness of breath, weakness, fever (insidious onset)
- acute respiratory failure (rare)

√ changes usually within portal entry fields
√ patchy / confluent consolidation, may persist up to 1 month (exudative reaction)
√ atelectasis + air bronchogram
√ spontaneous pneumothorax (rare)

CT:
√ homogeneous slight increase in attenuation (2–4 months after therapy)
√ patchy consolidation (1–12 months after therapy)
√ nonuniform discrete consolidation (most common; 3 months to 10 years after therapy)

Prognosis: recovery / progression to death / fibrosis

Rx: steroids

2. CHRONIC RADIATION DAMAGE
(9–12 months after radiation therapy)

Histo: permanent damage of endothelial + type I alveolar cells

May be associated with:
(1) thymic cyst
(2) calcified lymph nodes (in Hodgkin disease)
(3) pericarditis + effusion (within 3 years)

√ severe loss of volume
√ dense fibrous strands from hilum to periphery
√ thickening of pleura
√ pericardial effusion

CT:
√ solid consolidation (radiation fibrosis) + bronchiectasis (stabilized by 1 year after therapy)

RESPIRATORY DISTRESS SYNDROME OF NEWBORN

= RDS = HYALINE MEMBRANE DISEASE
= acute pulmonary disorder characterized by generalized atelectasis, intrapulmonary shunting, ventilation-perfusion abnormalities, reduced lung compliance

Cause: immature surfactant production (usually begins at 18–20 weeks of gestational age) causing acinar atelectasis + dilatation of terminal airways

Predisposed: perinatal asphyxia, cesarean section, infants of diabetic mothers, premature infants (<1000 g in 66%; 1000 g in 50%; 1500 g in 16%; 2000 g in 5%; 2500 g in 1%)

Onset: <2–5 hours after birth, increasing in severity from 24 to 48 hours, gradual improvement after 48–72 hours; M:F = 1.8:1

- abnormal retraction of chest wall
- cyanosis (carbon dioxide retention)
- expiratory grunting
- increased respiratory rate

√ hypoaeration with loss of lung volume (counteracted by respirator therapy)
√ reticulogranular pattern (coincides with onset of clinical signs)
√ prominent air bronchograms (distension of compliant airways)
√ bilateral + symmetrical distribution

Prognosis: spontaneous clearing within 7–10 days (mild course in untreated survivors); death in 18%

ACUTE COMPLICATIONS OF RDS
(a) Barotrauma with air-block phenomena
1. Parenchymal pseudocyst
2. Pulmonary interstitial emphysema
3. Pneumomediastinum, -thorax, -pericardium, -peritoneum,-retroperitoneum
4. Subcutaneous emphysema
5. Gas embolism

(b) Diffuse opacity
1. Worsening RDS
2. Superimposed pneumonia
3. Massive aspiration
4. Pulmonary hemorrhage
5. Congestive heart failure (PDA, fluid overload)

(c) Persistent patency of ductus arteriosus
oxygen stimulus is missing to close duct; gradual decrease in pulmonary resistance (by end of 1st week) leads to L-to-R shunt through PDA

(d) Hemorrhage
1. Pulmonary hemorrhage
2. Intracranial hemorrhage

(e) Necrotizing enterocolitis
(f) Acute renal failure

CHRONIC COMPLICATIONS OF RDS
1. Lobar emphysema
2. Localized interstitial emphysema
3. Delayed onset of diaphragmatic hernia
4. Recurrent inspiratory tract infections
5. Hyperinflation
6 Bronchopulmonary dysplasia (10–20%)
7. Retrolental fibroplasia
8. Subglottic stenosis (intubation)

Rx: exogenous surfactant intratracheally

RHEUMATOID LUNG

Incidence: 2–54% of patients with rheumatoid arthritis; M:F = 5:1 (although incidence of rheumatoid arthritis: M < F)

• rheumatoid arthritis

Stage 1: multifocal ill-defined alveolar infiltrates
Stage 2: fine interstitial reticulations (histio- and lymphocytes)
Stage 3: honeycombing

A. PLEURAL ABNORMALITIES (most frequent manifestation)
  • Hx of pleurisy (21%)
  √ pleural effusion (3%): unilateral (92%), with little change over months; M:F = 9:1; most often without other pulmonary changes, may antedate rheumatoid arthritis
    • exudate (with protein content >4 g/dL)
    • low in sugar content (<30 mg/dL) without rise during glucose infusion (75%)
    • low WBC high in lymphocytes
    • positive for rheumatoid factor, LDH, RA cells
  √ pleural thickening, usually bilateral
B. DIFFUSE INTERSTITIAL FIBROSIS (30%)
  • restrictive ventilatory defect
  Location: lower lobe predominance
  Histo: deposition of IgM in alveolar septa (DDx to IPF)
  √ punctate / nodular densities (mononuclear cell infiltrates in early stage)
  √ reticulonodular densities
  √ medium to coarse reticulations (mature fibrous tissue in later stage)
  √ honeycomb lung (uncommon in late stage)
C. NECROBIOTIC NODULES (rare)
  = well-circumscribed nodular mass in lung, pleura, pericardium identical to subcutaneous nodules associated with advanced rheumatoid arthritis
  Path: central zone of eosinophilic fibrinoid necrosis surrounded by palisading fibroblasts; nodule often centered on necrotic inflamed blood vessel (? vasculitis as initial lesion)
  • subcutaneous nodules (same histology)
  Associated with: interstitial lung disease
  √ well-circumscribed usually multiple nodules of 3–70 mm in size
  √ commonly located in lung periphery
  √ cavitation with thick symmetric walls + smooth inner lining (in 50%)
  √ NO calcification
D. CAPLAN SYNDROME
  = RHEUMATOID PNEUMOCONIOSIS
  = pneumoconiosis + rheumatoid arthritis in coal workers with rheumatoid disease;
  = hypersensitivity reaction to irritating dust particles in lungs of rheumatoid patients
  Incidence: 2–6% of all men affected by pneumoconioses (exclusively in Wales)
  Path: disintegrating macrophages deposit a pigmented ring of dust surrounding the central necrotic core + zone of fibroblasts palisading the zone of necrosis
  ◊ NOT necessarily evidence of long-standing pneumoconiosis
  • concomitant with joint manifestation (most frequent) / may precede arthritis by several years
  • concomitant with systemic rheumatoid nodules
  √ rapidly developing well-defined nodules of 5–50 mm in size with a tendency to appear in crops predominantly in upper lobes + in periphery of lung
  √ nodules may remain unchanged / increase in number / calcify
  √ background of pneumoconiosis
  √ pleural effusion (may occur)
E. BRONCHIAL ABNORMALITIES (30%)
  √ bronchiectasis
  √ bronchiolitis obliterans (may be transient + related to penicillamine therapy)
F. PULMONARY ARTERITIS
  = fibroelastoid intimal proliferation of pulmonary arteries
  • pulmonary arterial hypertension + cor pulmonale
G. CARDIAC ENLARGEMENT
  (pericarditis + carditis / congestive heart failure)
H. BONE ABNORMALITIES ON CXR
  √ arthritis of acromioclavicular joint, sternoclavicular joint, shoulder joint
  √ ankylosis of vertebral facet joints
  √ vertebral body collapse due to steroid use

ROUND PNEUMONIA

= NUMMULAR PNEUMONIA = fairly spherical pneumonia caused by pyogenic organisms

Organism: Haemophilus influenzae, Streptococcus, Pneumococcus

Age: children >> adults

• cough, chest pain, fever

Location: always posterior, usually in lower lobes

√ spherical infiltrate with slightly fluffy borders + air bronchogram
√ triangular infiltrate abutting a pleural surface (usually seen on lateral view)
√ rapid change in size and shape

SARCOIDOSIS

= BOECK SARCOID [*sarcoid* = sarcoma-like, Caesar Boeck describes skin lesions in 1899]
= immunologically mediated multisystem granulomatous disease of unknown etiology with variable presentation, progression, and prognosis

Prevalence: 10–40:100,000 in United States
Age peak: 20–40 years; M:F = 1:3 (female predominance only in Black population); American Blacks:American Whites = 10:1 (rare in African / South American Blacks); more common in blood group A
Immunology:
unknown antigen activates alveolar macrophages which release
— interleukin-1 (T-cell activator)
— fibronectin (fibroblast chemotactic factor)
— alveolar macrophage-derived growth factor (stimulates fibrosis)
and activates T lymphocytes which release
— interleukin-2 (stimulates growth of T-helper / cytolytic cells)
— immune interferon (polyclonal B-cell activator)
— monocyte chemotactic factor (attracts circulating monocytes and stimulates granuloma formation)

Histo: alveolitis (earliest changes); noncaseating epithelioid granulomas [composed of lymphocytes, peripheral fibroblasts, multinucleated giant cells] with occasional minimal central necrosis
Location: along course of lymphatic vessels: subpleural, septal, perivascular, peribronchial
DDx: indistinguishable from granulomas of berylliosis, treated TB, leprosy, fungal disease, hypersensitivity pneumonitis, Crohn disease, primary biliary cirrhosis

- angiotensin-converting enzyme (ACE) elevated in 70% [ACE is a product of macrophages and an indicator for the granuloma burden of the body]
  DDx: tuberculosis, leprosy, histoplasmosis, berylliosis, cirrhosis, hyperthyroidism, diabetes
- hypercalcemia + hypercalciuria in 2–15% [result of hydroxylation of 1,25-dihydroxy vitamin D in macrophages leading to increased intestinal resorption of calcium]
- Kveim-Stiltzbach test (positive in 70%) = intracutaneous injection of previously validated saline suspension of human sarcoid spleen / lymph nodes, rarely used
- functional pulmonary impairment (even with NO radiographic abnormality):
  — reduced VC + FRC + TLC [from generalized reduction in lung volume]
  — low lung compliance [from diffuse interstitial disease]
  — obstructive airway disease [from endobronchial lesions, peribronchial fibrosis]

Epidemiology:
found with varying frequency in every country in the world; higher prevalence in temperate climates compared to tropical regions (<10/100,000)

A. ACUTE FORM = **Löfgren Syndrome** (17%)
- fever + malaise + bilateral hilar adenopathy
- erythema nodosum
- arthralgia of large joints
- (occasionally) uveitis + parotitis

B. CHRONIC FORM
- asymptomatic (50%)
- fever, malaise, weight loss
- dry cough + shortness of breath (25%)
- hemoptysis in 4% (from endobronchial lesion / vascular erosion / cavitation)

Stage at presentation:

0	normal chest radiograph	5%
I	lymphadenopathy only	50%
II	lymphadenopathy + parenchymal disease	30%
III	parenchymal disease only	15%
IV	pulmonary fibrosis	20%

Prognosis:
75% complete resolution of hilar adenopathy
33% complete resolution of parenchymal disease
30% improve significantly
20% irreversible pulmonary fibrosis (may persist unchanged for >15 years)
10% mortality (cor pulmonale / CNS / lung fibrosis / liver cirrhosis)
25% relapse (in 50% detected by CXR)

@ Bone (6–20%):
√ phalangeal sclerosis of hands
√ lytic cystic lesions with lacelike trabecular pattern

@ Muscle (25%): myopathy
@ Eyes (5–25%): uveitis, photophobia, blurred vision, glaucoma (rare)
@ Myocardium (6–25%): ventricular arrhythmia, heart block, cardiomyopathy, congestive failure, angina, ventricular aneurysm
@ CNS (9%): hypothalamus, basal granulomatous meningitis, facial nerve palsy
@ Salivary gland (4%): bilateral parotid enlargement

@ Peripheral lymph node involvement (30%)

@ Skin disease (10–30%)
- erythema nodosum = multiple bilateral tender erythematous nodules mostly on anterior aspect of lower extremities
- lupus pernio = indurated bluish-purple elevations mainly on nose + digits
- skin plaques / scars

@ Thoracic disease (90%)
— adenopathy alone (43%)
— adenopathy + parenchymal disease (41%)
— parenchymal disease alone (16%)
Associated with: tuberculosis in up to 13%
√ <u>intrathoracic lymphadenopathy</u> (>85%)
Location:
(a) "1-2-3 sign" = Garland triad = bilateral hilar + right paratracheal groups (75–95%)
(b) isolated unilateral hilar enlargement (1–8%)
(c) mediastinal nodes are regularly enlarged on CT

Prognosis: adenopathy commonly decreases as parenchymal disease gets worse; subsequent parenchymal disease in 32%; adenopathy does not develop subsequent to parenchymal disease

√ eggshell calcification of lymph nodes (in 3% after 5 years, in 20% after 10 years)

√ parenchymal disease (60%); without adenopathy in 16–20%

◊ Parenchymal granulomas are invariably present on open lung biopsy!

Site: predominantly mid-zone involvement

√ reticulonodular pattern (46%)

√ acinar pattern (20%) = ill-defined 6–7 mm nodules / coalescent opacities

√ "alveolar / acinar sarcoidosis" (2–10%) = multiple large nodules >10 mm ± air bronchogram (= coalescence of numerous interstitial granulomas)

√ progressive fibrosis with upper lobe retraction + bullae (20%)

√ end-stage lung (11%)

√ airway disease

√ tracheal stenosis

√ bronchial stenosis (extrinsic compression by large lymph nodes / endobronchial granulomas)

√ bronchiectasis (scarring / fibrosis)

HRCT:

√ irregular septal thickening

√ perilymphatic nodules (= small nodules along bronchoarterial bundles and veins, in subpleural + interlobular septal lymphatics representing epitheloid cell granulomas)

√ traction bronchiectasis (TYPICAL)

√ ground-glass opacity (in alveolitis)

√ honeycombing

√ irregular / nodular bronchial wall thickening

Atypical manifestations (25%):

√ pleural effusion (2%) = exudate with predominance of lymphocytes, effusion clears in 2–3 months

√ focal pleural thickening

√ solitary / multiple pulmonary nodules

√ cavitation of nodules (0.6%)

√ isolated hilar / mediastinal nodal enlargement

√ bronchostenosis (2%) with lobar / segmental atelectasis

√ pulmonary arterial hypertension (periarterial granulomatosis without extensive pulmonary fibrosis)

Cx: √ pneumothorax secondary to chronic lung fibrosis (rare)

√ cardiomegaly from cor pulmonale (rare)

√ aspergilloma formation in apical bulla (in >50% of stage IV disease)

Diagnostic criteria:

(1) compatible clinical + radiologic picture

(2) noncaseous epitheloid granulomas on bronchial / transbronchial biopsy (diagnostic results in 60–95% and 80–95% respectively)

(3) negative results of special stains / cultures for other entities

ASSESSMENT OF ACTIVITY

(1) ACE titer (= angiotensin I converting enzyme)

(2) Bronchoalveolar lavage: 20–50% lymphocytes with number of T-suppressor lymphocytes 4–20 times above normal

(3) Gallium scan

√ uptake in lymph nodes + lung parenchyma + salivary glands (correlates with alveolitis + disease activity); monitor of therapeutic response (indicator of macrophage activity)

@ Abdominal disease

• strikingly elevated ACE levels in 91%

@ Liver (pathologic involvement in 24–79%):

√ hepatomegaly (18–29%)

√ nodular lesions in liver and spleen in 5–15% (= coalescent granulomata) occurring within 5 years of diagnosis

√ abdominal adenopathy (mean size of 2.6 cm)

@ Spleen (pathologic involvement in 24–59%):

√ splenomegaly (20–33%)

√ scattered nodular lesions (18%)

@ Lymphadenopathy (31%)

• frequently associated with thoracic adenopathy

√ mean lymph node size of 2.6 cm

@ Stomach (60 cases):

√ polypoid / nodular mass ± ulcer

√ loss of antral compliance

DDx: lymphoma

@ Genitourinary disease (0.2–5%)

@ Kidney:

√ renal calculi

@ Scrotum (0.5%)

√ hypoechoic lesions of epididymal + testicular sarcoidosis

SEPTIC PULMONARY EMBOLI

= lodgement of an infected thrombus in a pulmonary artery

Organism: S. aureus, Streptococcus

Predisposed: IV drug abusers, alcoholism, immunodeficiency, CHD, dermal infection (cellulitis, carbuncles)

Source:

(a) infected venous catheter / pacemaker wires, arteriovenous shunts for hemodialysis, drug abuse producing septic thrombophlebitis (eg, heroin addicts), pelvic thrombophlebitis, peritonsillar abscess, osteomyelitis

(b) tricuspid valve endocarditis (most common cause in IV drug abusers)

Age: majority <40 years

• sepsis, cough, dyspnea, chest pain

• shaking chills, high fever, severe sinus tachycardia

Location: predilection for lung bases

√ multiple nondescript pulmonary infiltrates (initially)
√ migratory infiltrates (old ones heal, new ones appear)
√ cavitation (frequent), usually thin-walled
√ pleural effusion (rare)
CT (more sensitive than CXR):
√ multiple peripheral parenchymal nodules ± cavitation / air bronchogram (83%)
√ wedge-shaped subpleural lesion with apex of lesion directed toward pulmonary hilum (50%)
√ feeding vessel sign = pulmonary artery leading to nodule (67%)
√ cavitation (50%), esp. in staphylococcal emboli
√ air bronchogram within pulmonary nodule (28%)
Cx: empyema (39%)

SIDEROSIS

= inert iron oxide / metallic iron deposits
Path: iron phagocytosed by macrophages in alveoli / respiratory bronchioles, elimination from lung by lymphatic circulation
Occupational exposure:
arc welding, cutting / burning of steel, foundry workers, grinders, fettlers, polishers (jewelry industry)
√ reticulonodular pattern (may disappear after exposure discontinued)
√ small round opacities (indistinguishable from silica / coal)
√ NO secondary fibrosis + NO hilar adenopathy (unless mixed dust inhalation as in siderosilicosis)

SILICOSIS

= inhalation of silicon dioxide; most prevalent silicosis of progressive nature after termination of exposure; similar to CWP (because of silica component in CWP)
Substance: Crystalline silica (quartz); one of the most widespread elements on earth
Occupational exposure: tunneling, mining, quarrying, sandblasting, ceramic industry
Path: small particles engulfed by macrophages; liberation of silica results in cell death; 2–3 mm nodules with layers of laminated connective tissue around smaller vessels
Cx: predisposes to tuberculosis

Acute Silicoproteinosis

= acute silicosis of sandblasters; exposure may be <1 year
Associated with: increased risk to develop autoimmune disease
√ diffuse airspace disease

Chronic Simple Silicosis

At least 10–20 years of dust exposure before appearance of roentgenographic abnormality
√ small 1–10 mm rounded opacities, beginning in upper + middle lung zones
√ may calcify centrally in 5–10% (rather typical for silicosis)
√ hilar lymphadenopathy, may calcify in 5% ("eggshell pattern")
√ ± reticulonodular pattern

HRCT:
√ nodules of 3–10 mm in size
√ thickened intra- and interlobular lines
√ subpleural curvilinear lines (peribronchiolar fibrosis)
√ ground-glass pattern = mild thickening of alveolar wall + interlobular septa (fibrosis / edema)
√ parenchymal fibrous bands
√ pleura-based nodular irregularities
√ traction bronchiectasis
√ honeycombing

Complicated Silicosis

√ conglomerate masses of nonsegmental distribution in middle + upper lung zones
√ progressive massive fibrosis = sausage-shaped masses with ill-defined margins (in advanced stages)
√ compensatory emphysema in unaffected portion
√ slow change over years
√ may cavitate

Silicotuberculosis

Doubtful synergistic relationship between silicosis + tuberculosis
√ little change over years with intermittently positive sputa

Caplan Syndrome

More common in coal worker's pneumoconiosis

SJÖGREN SYNDROME

= MYOEPITHELIAL SIALADENITIS
= probable autoimmune multisystem disorder (= collagen-vascular disease) characterized by dryness of mucous membranes affecting
(1) salivary + lacrimal glands
(2) mucosa + submucosa of pharynx
(3) tracheobronchial tree
(4) reticuloendothelial system
(5) joints

A. PRIMARY SJÖGREN SYNDROME
= autoimmune exocrinopathy
(a) recurrent parotitis in children
(b) SICCA SYNDROME = Mikulicz disease
= xerophthalmia + xerostomia
B. SECONDARY SJÖGREN SYNDROME
Associated with:
(a) connective tissue diseases
1. Rheumatoid arthritis (55%)
2. Systemic lupus erythematosus (2%)
3. Progressive systemic sclerosis (0.5%)
4. Psoriatic arthritis, primary biliary cirrhosis (0.5%)
(b) lymphoproliferative disorders
1. Lymphocytic interstitial pneumonitis (LIP)
2. Pseudolymphoma (25%)
3. Lymphoma (5%; 44 x increased risk): mostly B-cell lymphoma
4. Waldenström macroglobulinemia

Age: 35–70 (mean 57) years; M:F = 1:9
Path: benign lymphoepithelioma = lymphoid infiltrates in lacrimal + salivary glands, mucous glands of conjunctivae, nasal cavity, pharynx, larynx, trachea, bronchi

- xerophthalmia = dryness of eyes
  = keratoconjunctivitis sicca = desiccation of cornea + conjunctiva
- xerostomia = atrophy of salivary + parotid glands leading to diminished saliva production and dryness of mouth + lips
- xerorhinia = dryness of nose
- decreased sweating
- decreased vaginal secretions
- swelling of parotid gland: usually unilateral, recurrent
- rheumatoid factor (positive in up to 95%)
- ANA (positive in up to 80%)

CXR:
√ reticulonodular pattern (3–33–52%)
√ patchy consolidation
√ inspissated mucus:
√ atelectasis
√ recurrent pneumonia
√ bilateral lower lobe bronchiectasis
√ acute focal / lipoid pneumonia (secondary to oils taken to combat dry mouth)
√ ± pleural effusion
Sialogram:
√ nonobstructive punctate / globular / cavitary sialectasia (ducts + acini destroyed by lymphocytic infiltrates / infection)
US of parotid gland:
√ enlarged gland
√ multiple scattered cysts bilaterally (= cystic dilatation of intraparotid ducts + glands)
√ increased vascularity on color Doppler
MR of parotid gland:
√ inhomogeneous honeycomblike internal pattern (= areas of low intensity between nodular parenchyma of high signal intensity) on T2WI / Gd-enhanced T1WI
Cx: Lymphoma (occurs in significant number of patients)

STAPHYLOCOCCAL PNEUMONIA

Most common cause of bronchopneumonia
(a) common nosocomial infection (patients on antibiotic drugs most susceptible)
(b) accounts for 5% of community-acquired pneumonias (esp. in infants + elderly)
◊ secondary invader to influenza (commonest cause of death during influenza epidemics)
Organism: Staphylococcus aureus, Gram-positive, appears in clusters, coagulase-producing
√ rapid spread through lungs
√ empyema (esp. in children)
√ pneumothorax, pyopneumothorax
√ abscess formation
√ bronchopleural fistula

A. in CHILDREN:
√ rapidly developing lobar / multilobar consolidation
√ pleural effusion (90%)
√ pneumatocele (40–60%)
B. in ADULTS:
√ patchy often confluent bronchopneumonia of segmental distribution, bilateral in >60%
√ segmental collapse (air bronchograms absent)
√ late development of thick-walled lung abscess (25–75%)
√ pleural effusion / empyema (50%) (DDx from other pneumonias)

Cx: meningitis, metastatic abscess to brain / kidneys, acute endocarditis

STREPTOCOCCAL PNEUMONIA

Incidence: 1–5% of bacterial pneumonias (rarely seen); most common in winter months
Organism: Group A ß-hemolytic streptococcus = Streptococcus pyogenes, Gram-positive cocci appearing in chains
Predisposed: newborns, following infection with measles
Associated with: delayed onset of diaphragmatic hernia (in newborns)
- rarely follows tonsillitis + pharyngitis

√ patchy bronchopneumonia
√ lower lobe predominance (similar to staphylococcus)
√ empyema
Cx: (1) Residual pleural thickening (15%)
(2) Bronchiectasis
(3) Lung abscess
(4) Glomerulonephritis

SWYER-JAMES SYNDROME

= MACLEOD SYNDROME
= UNILATERAL LOBAR EMPHYSEMA
= IDIOPATHIC UNILATERAL HYPERLUCENT LUNG
Etiology: acute viral bronchiolitis in infancy / early childhood (adenovirus, RSV) preventing normal development of lung
Path: variant of postinfectious constrictive bronchiolitis with acute obliterative bronchiolitis, bronchiectasis, distal airspace destruction (developing in 7–30 months)
- asymptomatic
- cough, dyspnea on exertion, hemoptysis
- history of recurrent lower respiratory tract infections during childhood

Location: one / both lungs (usually entire lung, occasionally lobar / subsegmental)
√ unilateral hyperlucency of affected lung
√ small hemithorax with decreased / normal volume (collateral air drift)
√ air trapping during expiration
DDx: no air trapping with proximal interruption of pulmonary artery (no hilum), hypogenetic lung syndrome, pulmonary embolus

√ mild cylindrical bronchiectasis with paucity of bronchial subdivisions (cutoff at 4th–5th generation = "pruned tree" bronchogram)
√ small ipsilateral hilum (diminuted hilar vessels + attenuated arteries)
√ diminutive pulmonary vasculature

HRCT:
- √ bilateral areas of decreased attenuation
- √ areas of normal lung attenuation within hypoattenuating lung
- √ air trapping within hypoattenuating lung
- √ bronchiectasis

Angio:
- √ "pruned tree" appearance

NUC:
- √ decreased perfusion
- √ decreased ventilation + delayed washout

SYSTEMIC LUPUS ERYTHEMATOSUS

= most prevalent of the potentially grave connective tissue diseases characterized by involvement of vascular system, skin, serous + synovial membranes (type III immune complex phenomenon)

Incidence: 1:2,000; Blacks:Caucasians = 3:1; increased risk in relatives

Age: women of child-bear age; M:F = 1:10

- clinically heterogeneous due to different types of serum antibodies
- antinuclear DNA antibodies (87%)
- hypergammaglobulinemia (77%)
- LE cells (= antigen-antibody complexes engulfed by PMNs) in 78%
- chronic false-positive Wassermann test for syphilis (24%)
- Sjögren syndrome (frequent)
- anemia (78%)
- leukopenia (66%)
- thrombocytopenia (19%)

@ Skin changes (81%)
- "butterfly rash" (= facial erythema), discoid lupus erythematosus, alopecia, photosensitivity
- Raynaud phenomenon (15%)

@ Thoracic involvement (30–70%)
- ◊ affects respiratory system more commonly than any other connective tissue disease
- dyspnea, pleuritic chest pain (35%)
- respiratory dysfunction (>50%): single-breath diffusing capacity for carbon monoxide most sensitive indicator

(a) Pulmonary changes

Cause: chronic antibody damage to alveolar-capillary membrane

- √ lupus pneumonitis (acute form) = poorly defined patchy areas of increased density peripherally at lung bases (alveolar pattern) secondary to infection / uremia in 10%
- √ interstitial reticulations in lower lung fields (chronic form) in 3%
- √ fleeting platelike atelectasis in both bases (? infarction due to vasculitis)
- √ cavitating nodules (vasculitis)
- √ elevated sluggish diaphragms (progressive volume loss due to diaphragmatic dysfunction)
- √ hilar + mediastinal lymphadenopathy (extremely rare)

(b) Pleural changes (most common manifestation)
- √ recurrent bilateral pleural effusions (70%) from pleuritis
- √ pleural thickening

(c) Cardiovascular changes
- √ pericardial effusion (from pericarditis)
- √ cardiomegaly (primary lupus cardiomyopathy)

@ Joints
- arthralgia (95%)
- √ nonerosive arthritis of hands (characteristic) without deformity

@ Kidney

Incidence: kidneys involved in 100% with renal disease developing in 50%

Histo: focal membranous glomerulonephritis

- renal failure (fibrinoid thickening of basement membrane)
- √ aneurysms in interlobular + arcuate arteries (similar to polyarteritis nodosa)
- √ normal / decreased renal size

US:
- √ increased parenchymal echogenicity

Cx: (1) Nephrotic syndrome (common)
(2) Renal vein thrombosis (rare)

Prognosis: end-stage renal disease is common cause of death

@ GI tract (in up to 50%)
- buccal erosions / ulcerations
- GI tract bleeding
- √ motility disorder of lower esophagus (similar to scleroderma)
- √ esophagitis ± ulcers
- √ gastritis
- √ mesenteric ischemia: colitis, pseudoobstruction, ileus, thumbprinting, luminal narrowing
- √ nodularity of folds
- √ pneumatosis intestinalis, perforation
- √ painful ascites
- √ hepatomegaly, hepatitis, cirrhosis
- √ splenomegaly

Prognosis: 60–90% 10-year survival; death from renal failure / sepsis / CNS involvement / myocardial infarction

DRUG-INDUCED LUPUS ERYTHEMATOSUS = DIL (temporary phenomenon):

Agents: procainamide, hydralazine, isoniazid, phenytoin account for 90%

√ pulmonary + pleural disease more common than in SLE

TALCOSIS

= prolonged inhalation of magnesium silicate dust containing amphibole fibers (tremolite and anthophyllite) and silica

Talcosis resembles:
(1) Asbestosis (indistinguishable)
√ massive and bizarre pleural plaques
√ may encase lung with calcification
(2) Silicosis
√ small rounded + large opacities
√ fibrogenic process (NO regression after removal of patient from exposure)

TERATOID TUMOR OF MEDIASTINUM

= MEDIASTINAL GERM CELL TUMOR [= TERATOMA]
◊ The anterior mediastinum is the most common extragonadal site of primary germ cell tumors (1–3% of all germ cell tumors)!
Pathogenesis: "misplaced" multipotential primitive germ cells during migration from yolk endoderm to gonad
Incidence:
— adults: 15% of anterior mediastinal tumors
— children: 24% of anterior mediastinal tumors
◊ 16–28% of all mediastinal cysts!
◊ Occurs in same frequency as the usually larger thymoma!
◊ 1/3 of primary neoplasms in this area are in children

Classes: (1) Mature teratoma (solid)
(2) Cystic teratoma (dermoid cyst)
(3) Immature teratoma
(4) Malignant teratoma (teratocarcinoma)
(5) Mixed teratoma

Location: mediastinum is 3rd most common site for teratoid lesions (after gonadal + sacrococcygeal location); 5% of all teratomas occur in mediastinum, mostly anterosuperiorly (in only 1% posteriorly)
√ often inseparable from thymus gland

A. BENIGN TERATOID TUMOR (75–86%)
= MATURE TERATOMA
= most common histologic type
1. Epidermoid (52%) = ectodermal derivatives
2. Dermoid (27%) = ecto- + mesodermal derivatives
3. Teratoma (21%) = ecto- + meso- + endodermal derivatives

Path: spherical lobulated well-encapsulated tumor; typically multi- / unilocular cystic cavities with clear / yellow / brown liquid
Histo:
(a) ectoderm: skin, sebaceous material, hair, cysts lined by squamous epithelium
(b) mesoderm: bone, cartilage, muscle
(c) endoderm: GI + respiratory tissue, mucus glands
◊ Tumor capsule commonly has remnants of thymic tissue!
◊ Cyst formation is typical (usually lined by mucus-secreting tall epithelial cells)!
Age: young adults / children; M = F
• asymptomatic (in up to 53%)
• cough, dyspnea, chest pain, pulmonary infection, respiratory distress (due to compression by large tumor)
Location:
(a) anterior superior mediastinum near thymus / within thymic parenchyma
(b) posterior mediastinum (rare = 3–8%)
√ rounded mass bulging into right / left hemithorax sharply demarcated against adjacent lung
√ variations in density (may all be present):
√ fat-fluid level (rare but SPECIFIC)
√ water density
√ homogeneous soft-tissue density (indistinguishable from lymphoma / thymoma)
√ curvilinear peripheral / central calcification (20–43%, 4 x more common in benign lesions) in tumor wall / substance, ossification in mature bone
√ visualization of tooth (PATHOGNOMONIC)
√ often inseparable from thymic gland
√ enhancement of rim / tissue septa
Prognosis: approx. 100% 5-year survival rate
Rx: complete surgical excision

B. MALIGNANT TERATOID TUMOR (14–20%)
Histo: similar to mature teratoma but with primitive / immature tissue elements; commonly neural tissue arranged in rosettes / primitive tubules
◊ Teratocarcinoma / malignant teratoma = identical to teratoma with components of seminoma, endodermal sinus tumor, embryonal carcinoma, choriocarcinoma, sarcoma, carcinoma

1. **Seminoma** = germinoma = dysgerminoma
◊ 2nd most common mediastinal germ cell tumor!
◊ Most common primary malignant germ cell tumor of mediastinum!
Incidence: 2–6% of all mediastinal tumors; 5–13% of all malignant mediastinal tumors
Age: 3rd–4th decade; M >> F; white
Histo: uniform polyhedral / round cells arranged in sheets or forming small lobules separated by fibrous septa; varying amounts of mature lymphocytes
Path: large unencapsulated well-circumscribed mass
• asymptomatic (20–30%)
• chest pain / pressure, shortness of breath, weight loss, hoarseness, dysphagia, fever
• SVC obstruction (10%)
• elevated serum levels of HCG (7–18%)
• elevated serum levels of LDH (80%) correlate with tumor burden + rate of tumor growth
Metastases: to regional lymph nodes, lung, bone, liver
√ large bulky well-marginated lobulated mass
√ usually NO calcification
√ homogeneous soft-tissue density with slight enhancement
Prognosis: 75–100% 5-year survival rate; death from distant metastases

Rx: surgery + radiation therapy (very radiosensitive) ± cisplatin

2. **Nonseminomatous malignant germ cell tumor**
   (a) embryonic tissue
      (1) Embryonal carcinoma
   (b) extraembryonic tissue
      (1) Yolk sac = endodermal sinus tumor
      (2) Choriocarcinoma (least frequent)
   (c) combination = mixed germ cell tumor

   Path: large unencapsulated heterogeneous soft-tissue mass with tendency for invasion of adjacent structures

   Age: during 2nd to 4th decade M:F = 9:1; in children M = F

   Associated with: Klinefelter syndrome (in 20%), hematologic malignancy

   • chest pain, dyspnea, cough, weight loss, fever, SVC syndrome (90–100%)
   • elevated serum level of a-fetoprotein (80%) with endodermal sinus tumor / embryonal carcinoma
   • elevated serum level of LDH (60%)
   • elevated serum level of HCG (30%) [DDx: lung cancer; hepatocellular carcinoma; adenocarcinoma of pancreas, colon, stomach]

   Metastases to: lung, liver

   √ large tumor of heterogeneous texture with central hemorrhage / necrosis
   √ well circumscribed / with irregular margins
   √ enhancement of tumor periphery
   √ lobulation suggests malignancy
   √ invasion of mediastinal structures (SVC obstruction is ominous)
   √ pleural / pericardial effusion (from local invasion)
   ◊ Absence of primary testicular tumor / retroperitoneal mass proves primary!

   Rx: cisplatin-based chemotherapy + tumor resection

   Prognosis: 50% long-term survivors

Cx:
(1) Hemorrhage
(2) Pneumothorax (from bronchial obstruction with air trapping + alveolar rupture)
(3) Respiratory distress (rapid increase in size from fluid production) with compression of trachea / SVC (SVC syndrome)
(4) Fistula formation to aorta, SVC, esophagus
(5) Rupture into bronchus (expectoration of oily substance / trichoptysis in 5–14%, lipoid pneumonia)
(6) Rupture into pericardium (pericardial effusion), pleural cavity (pleural effusion)

DDx: thymoma

THORACIC PARAGANGLIOMA

= CHEMODECTOMA
= rare neural tumor arising from paraganglionic tissue

Age: 3rd–5th decade; M:F = 1:1

Path: extremely vascular well-marginated / irregular mass that may adhere to / envelop / invade adjacent mediastinal structures (bronchus, spinal canal)

Histo: anastomosing cords of granule-storing chief cells arranged in a trabecular pattern; identical appearance for benign and malignant tumors

May be associated with:
syn- / metachronous adrenal / extrathoracic paragangliomas; multiple endocrine neoplasia type 2; bronchial carcinoid tumor

• asymptomatic
• dyspnea, cough, chest pain, hemoptysis, neurologic deficits, SVC syndrome (if tumor large)
• signs of excessive catecholamine production: hypertension, headache, tachycardia, palpitations, tremor

Location: base of heart + great vessels (adjacent to pericardium / heart, within interatrial septum / left atrial wall); paravertebral sulci

CT:
√ sharply marginated 5–7 cm middle / posterior mediastinal mass
√ hypodense areas due to extensive cystic degeneration / hemorrhage
√ exuberant enhancement

MR:
√ heterogeneous intermediate signal intensity with areas of signal void from flowing blood on T1WI
√ high signal intensity on T2WI

NUC (I-123 / I-131 metaiodobenzylguanidine):
√ useful for localization as relatively specific

Angio (may precipitate cardiovascular crisis):
√ marked hypervascularity, multiple feeding vessels
√ homogeneous capillary blush

Rx: surgical excision with preoperative administration of α- or β-blockers (hypertensive crisis, tachycardia, dysrhythmia during manipulation)

THYMIC CYST

Incidence: 1–2% of mediastinal masses

Etiology:
(1) Congenital cyst (persistent tubular remnants of 3rd pharyngeal pouch = thymopharyngeal duct, develops during 5th–8th week of gestation)
(2) Acquired reactive multilocular cysts = cystic transformation of duct epithelial structures induced by an inflammatory process: eg, HIV
(3) Neoplastic cyst (cystic teratoma, cystic degeneration within a thymoma), S/P radiation therapy for Hodgkin disease

Associated with:
(1) Hodgkin disease (? thymic involvement / treatment-induced cystic degeneration)
(2) myasthenia gravis (rare)

• commonly asymptomatic
• symptomatic when hemorrhage occurs

Location: anterior mediastinum / lateral neck

√ unilocular cyst with thin walls containing clear fluid / multilocular cyst with thick walls containing turbid fluid or gelatinous material
√ may show partial wall calcification (rare)
√ low-density fluid (0–10 HU), may be higher depending on cyst contents

US:
√ typically anechoic
DDx: Benign thymoma, teratoma, dermoid cyst, Hodgkin disease, non-Hodgkin lymphoma, pleural fibroma

THYMIC HYPERPLASIA

Most common anterior mediastinal mass in pediatric age group through puberty
Age: particularly in young individual
Histo: numerous active lymphoid germinal centers
Etiology:
1. Hyperthyroidism (most common), Graves disease, treatment of primary hypothyroidism, idiopathic thyromegaly
2. Rebound hyperplasia in children recovering from severe illness (eg, from burns), after treatment for Cushing disorder, after chemotherapy
   √ thymus may regrow more than 50% (transient overgrowth and reducible with steroids)
3. Myasthenia gravis (65%)
4. Acromegaly
5. Addison disease

√ normal thymus visible in 50% of neonates 0–2 years of age
√ notch sign = indentation at junction of thymus + heart
√ sail sign = triangular density extending from superior mediastinum
√ wave sign = rippled border due to indentation from ribs
√ shape changes with respiration + position

THYMOLIPOMA

Incidence: 2–9% of thymic tumors
Age: 3–60 years (mean age of 22 years); M:F = 1:1
Path: lobulated pliable encapsulated tumor capable of growing to large size (in 68% >500 g, in 20% >2,000 g, the largest >16 kg)
Histo: benign adult adipose tissue interspersed with areas of normal / hyperplastic / atrophic thymus tissue (thymic tissue <33% of tumor mass)
• chest pain, dyspnea, cough (in 50%)
√ large lesions slump inferiorly from anterior mediastinum toward diaphragm
√ may drape around heart enlarging cardiac silhouette on frontal view
√ apparent elevation of diaphragm on lateral view
√ NO compression / invasion of adjacent structures
DDx: mediastinal lipoma (most common of intrathoracic fatty tumors), liposarcoma

THYMOMA

◊ Most common primary neoplasm of anterior superior mediastinum
Age: majority >40 years; 70% occur in 5th–6th decade; less frequent in young adults, rare in children; M:F = 1:1
Associated with: parathymic syndromes (40%) such as
• **Myasthenia gravis:**
  = autoimmune disorder characterized by antibodies against acetylcholine receptors of the postjunctional muscle membrane
  • progressive weakness, fatigue
  • fatigability of skeletal muscles innervated by cranial nerves, eg, ptosis, diplopia, dysphagia, dysarthria, drooling, difficulty with chewing
  • elevated serum level of anti-acetylcholine receptor antibodies
  ◊ 10–15–25% of patients with myasthenia gravis have a thymoma (in 65% due to thymic hyperplasia)
  ◊ 7–30–54% of patients with thymoma have myasthenia gravis; removal of thymic tumor often results in symptomatic improvement; myasthenia gravis may develop after surgical thymoma excision
  Rx: edrophonium chloride
• Pure red cell aplasia = aregenerative anemia
  = almost total absence of marrow erythroblasts + blood reticulocytes resulting in severe normochromic normocytic anemia
  ◊ 50% of patients with red cell aplasia have thymoma
  ◊ 5% of patients with thymoma develop red cell aplasia
• Acquired hypogammaglobulinemia
  ◊ 10% of patients with hypogammaglobulinemia have thymoma
  ◊ 6% of patients with thymoma have hypogammaglobulinemia
• Paraneoplastic syndromes occur with thymic carcinoid (10%): eg, Cushing syndrome (ACTH production)

• chest pain, dyspnea, cough (33%)
Path:
round / ovoid slow-growing primary epithelial neoplasm with smooth / lobulated surface divided into lobules by fibrous septa; areas of hemorrhage + necrosis may form cysts
(a) encapsulated = thick fibrous capsule ± calcifications
(b) locally invasive = microscopic foci outside capsule
(c) metastasizing = benign cytologic appearance with pleural + pulmonary parenchymal seeding
(d) thymic carcinoma
Histo:
(a) biphasic thymoma (most common)
  = epithelial + lymphoid elements in equal amounts
(b) predominantly lymphocytic thymoma
  = >2/3 of cells are lymphocytic
(c) predominantly epithelial thymoma
  = >2/3 of cells are epithelial
◊ Prognosis unrelated to cell type!
• asymptomatic (50% discovered incidentally)
• signs of mediastinal compression (25–30%): cough, dyspnea, chest pain, respiratory infection, hoarseness (recurrent laryngeal n.), dysphagia
• signs of tumor invasion (rare): SVC syndrome
Location: any anterior mediastinal location between thoracic inlet and cardiophrenic angle; rare in neck, other mediastinal compartments, lung parenchyma, or tracheobronchial tree
Size: 1–10 cm (up to 34 cm)

Noninvasive = benign thymoma

Age peak: 5th–6th decade, almost all are >25 years of age

√ oval / round lobulated sharply demarcated asymmetric homogeneous mass of soft-tissue density (equal to muscle), usually on one side of the midline
√ abnormally wide mediastinum
√ displacement of heart + great vessels posteriorly

CT:
- √ homogeneous soft-tissue mass with smooth / lobulated border partially / completely outlined by fat
- √ homogeneous enhancement
- √ areas of decreased attenuation (fibrosis, cysts, hemorrhage, necrosis)
- √ amorphous, flocculent central / curvilinear peripheral calcification (5–25%)

MRI:
- √ isointense to skeletal muscle on T1WI
- √ increased signal intensity (approaching that of fat) on T2WI
- √ fluid characteristics of cysts with high water content

Invasive [malignant] thymoma

◊ Malignancy defined according to extent of invasion into adjacent mediastinal fat + fascia!

Frequency: in 30–35% of thymomas

Stage I : intact capsule
Stage II : pericapsular growth into mediastinal fat
Stage III : invasion of surrounding organs such as lung, pericardium, SVC, aorta
Stage IVa : dissemination within thoracic cavity (metastases to pleura + lung in 6%)
Stage IVb : distant metastases (liver, bone, lymph nodes, kidneys, brain)

√ heterogeneous attenuation
√ spread by contiguity along pleural reflections, extension along aorta reaching posterior mediastinum / crus of diaphragm / retroperitoneum (transdiaphragmatic tumor extension)
√ irregular interface with lung
√ unilateral diffuse nodular pleural thickening / pleural masses encasing lung circumferentially
√ vascular encroachment
√ pleural effusion UNCOMMON

DDx: malignant mesothelioma, lymphoma, thymic carcinoma / malignant germ cell tumor (older male, no diffuse pleural seeding), peripheral lung carcinoma (no dominant mediastinal mass), metastatic disease (not unilateral)

Rx: radical excision ± adjuvant radiation therapy

Prognosis: 5-year survival of 93% for stage I, 86% for stage II, 70% for stage III, 50% for stage IV; 2–12% rate of recurrence for resected encapsulated thymomas

TORSION OF LUNG

Incidence: rare (<30 cases)

Cause: compression of lower thorax, tear on inferior pulmonary ligament, completeness of fissures

Associated with:
surgery (lobectomy), trauma, diaphragmatic hernia, pneumonia, pneumothorax, bronchus-obstructing tumor

Histo: ± hemorrhagic infarction + excessive air trapping

√ collapsed / consolidated lobe in unusual position
√ hilar displacement of atelectatic-appearing lobe in an inappropriate direction
√ alteration in normal course of pulmonary vasculature
√ rapid opacification of an ipsilateral lobe after trauma / thoracic surgery (DDx: pleural effusion)
√ change in position of opacified lobe on sequential radiographs
√ bronchial cutoff / distortion
√ lobar air trapping

TRACHEOBRONCHOMEGALY

= MOUNIER-KUHN SYNDROME = primary atrophy / dysplasia of supporting structures of trachea + major bronchi with abrupt transition to normal bronchi at 4th–5th division

Incidence: 0.5–1.5%

Age: discovered in 3rd–5th decade

- cough with copious sputum
- shortness of breath on exertion
- long history of recurrent pneumonias

May be associated with: Ehlers-Danlos syndrome

√ marked dilatation of trachea (>29 mm), right (>20 mm) + left (>15 mm) mainstem bronchi
√ sacculated outline / diverticulosis of trachea on lateral CXR (= protrusion of mucous membrane between rings of trachea)
√ may have emphysema, bullae in perihilar region

TRACHEOBRONCHOPATHIA OSTEOCHONDROPLASTICA

= rare benign disease characterized by cartilaginous / osseous nodules projecting from submucosa into tracheobronchial lumen

Cause: unknown; may be due to chronic inflammation, degenerative process, irritation by oxygen / chemical, metabolic disturbance, amyloidosis, tuberculosis, syphilis, heredity (high prevalence in Finland)

Pathogenetic theories:
(1) Ecchondrosis / exostosis of cartilage rings
(2) Cartilaginous / osseous metaplasia of internal elastic fibrous membrane of trachea

Histo: adipose tissue + calcified areas with foci of bone marrow; thinned normal overlying mucosa with inflammation + hemorrhage

Age: in 50% >50 years (11–72 years); M:F = 3:1

- usually asymptomatic (incidentally diagnosed)
- dyspnea, productive cough, hoarseness, hemoptysis, fever, recurrent pneumonia

Location: distal 2/3 of trachea, larynx, lobar / segmental bronchi, entire length of trachea; spares posterior membrane of trachea

CXR:
- √ scalloped / linear opacities surrounding + narrowing the trachea (best on lateral view)

CHEST

CT:
√ deformed thickened narrowed tracheal wall
√ irregularly spaced 1–3 mm calcific submucosal nodules of trachea + bronchi (similar to plaques)

Dx: bronchoscopy
DDx: relapsing polychondritis, tracheobronchial amyloidosis, sarcoidosis, papillomatosis, tracheobronchomalacia

TRANSIENT TACHYPNEA OF THE NEWBORN

= NEONATAL WET LUNG DISEASE = TRANSIENT RESPIRATORY DISTRESS OF THE NEWBORN = RETAINED FETAL LUNG FLUID

Incidence: 6%; most common cause of respiratory distress in newborn
Cause: cesarean section, precipitous delivery, breech delivery, prematurity, maternal diabetes
Pathophysiology:
delayed resorption of fetal lung fluid (normal clearance occurs through capillaries (40%), lymphatics (30%), thoracic compression during vaginal delivery (30%)
Onset: within 6 hours of life; peak at day 1 of age

- increasing respiratory rates during first 2–6 hours of life
- intercostal + sternal retraction
- normal blood gases during hyperoxygenation

√ linear opacities + perivascular haze + thickened fissures + interlobular septal thickening (interstitial edema)
√ mild hyperaeration
√ mild cardiomegaly
√ small amount of pleural fluid

Prognosis: resolving within 1–4 days (retrospective diagnosis)

DDx: (1) normal during first several hours of life
(2) diffuse pneumonitis / sepsis
(3) mild meconium aspiration syndrome
(4) "drowned newborn syndrome" = clear amniotic fluid aspiration
(5) alveolar phase of RDS (6) pulmonary venous congestion (7) pulmonary hemorrhage
(8) hyperviscosity syndrome = thick blood
(9) immature lung syndrome

TRAUMATIC LUNG CYST

Age: children + young adults are particularly prone
√ thin-walled air-filled cavity (50%) ± air-fluid level preceded by homogeneous well-circumscribed mass (hematoma)
√ oval / spherical lesion of 2–14 cm in diameter
√ single / multiple lesions; uni- or multilocular
√ usually subpleural under point of maximal injury
√ persistent up to 4 months + progressive decrease in size (apparent within 6 weeks)

TUBERCULOSIS

Prevalence: 10 million people worldwide, active TB develops in 5–10% of those exposed
Organism: Mycobacterium = acid-fast aerobic rods staining red with carbol-fuchsin; M. tuberculosis (95%), atypical types increasing: M. avium-intracellulare, M. kansasii, M. fortuitum
Susceptible: infants, pubertal adolescents, elderly, alcoholics, Blacks, diabetics, silicosis, measles, AIDS, sarcoidosis (in up to 13%)
Pathologic phases:
(a) exudative reaction (initial reaction, present for 1 month)
(b) caseous necrosis (after 2–10 weeks with onset of hypersensitivity)
(c) hyalinization = invasion of fibroblasts (granuloma formation in 1–3 weeks)
(d) calcification / ossification
(e) chronic destructive form in 10% (<1 year of age, adolescents, young adults)

Spread: regional lymph nodes, hematogenous dissemination, pleura, pericardium, upper lumbar vertebrae
Mortality: 1:100,000

- Positive PPD tuberculin test: 3 weeks after infection
- Negative PPD test:
  1. Overwhelming tuberculous infection (miliary TB)
  2. Sarcoidosis
  3. Corticosteroid therapy
  4. Pregnancy
  5. Infection with atypical Mycobacterium

ENDOBRONCHIAL (ACINAR) TUBERCULOSIS

Path: ulceration of bronchial mucosa followed by fibrosis leads to
(a) bronchial stenosis (lobar consolidation)
(b) bronchiectasis
(c) acinar nodules reflecting airway spread

HRCT:
√ airspace nodules
√ "tree-in-bud" appearance = nodular opacities along centrilobular artery + bronchiole
√ bronchiectasis

TUBERCULOMA

= manifestation of primary / postprimary TB
√ round / oval smooth sharply defined mass
√ 0.5–4 cm in diameter remaining stable for a long time
√ lobulated mass (25%)
√ satellite lesions (80%)
√ may calcify

CAVITARY TUBERCULOSIS

= hallmark of reactivation tuberculosis
= semisolid caseous material is expelled into bronchial tree after lysis
√ moderately thick-walled cavity with smooth inner surface

Cx:
(1) dissemination to other bronchial segments
√ multiple small acinar shadows remote from massive consolidation

(2) colonization with Aspergillus
√ aspergilloma

Primary pulmonary tuberculosis

Mode of infection: inhalation of infected airborne droplets
Age: usually in childhood, becoming commoner in adults
- asymptomatic (91%)
- symptomatic (5–10%)

Location: lower lobes, middle lobe, anterior segment of upper lobes
√ in children: massive hilar (60%) / paratracheal (40%) / subcarinal lymphadenopathy (in children), in 80% on right side;
in adults: mediastinal lymphadenopathy in 5–35–48%
√ one / more areas of homogeneous ill-defined airspace consolidation of 1–7 cm in diameter in 25–50–78% (requires several weeks for complete clearing with antituberculous therapy)
√ absent response to antibiotic Rx for "pneumonia"
√ atelectasis (8–18%), esp. in right lung (anterior segment of upper lobe / medial segment of middle lobe) secondary to
(a) endobronchial tuberculosis
(b) bronchial / tracheal compression by enlarged lymph nodes (68%)
√ pleural effusion (10% in childhood, 23–38% in adulthood) most commonly 3–7 months after initial exposure (from subpleural foci rupturing into pleural space)
√ pneumonic reaction (mid or lower lung zones) with segmental / lobar consolidation
√ calcified lung lesion (17%) / parenchymal scar <5 mm = **Ghon lesion**
√ calcified lymph node (36%) in hilus / mediastinum
√ **Ranke complex** = Ghon lesion + calcified lymph node (22%)
√ **Simon focus** = healed site of primary infection in lung apex
CT:
√ tuberculous adenopathy may demonstrate necrotic center with low attenuation after enhancement

Outcome of primary infection:
1. Immunity prevents multiplication of organism (containment of initial infection by delayed hypersensitivity response + granuloma formation in 1–3 weeks)
2. Progressive primary TB (inadequate immune mechanism with local progression) in 10%, most common in older children / teenagers
3. Miliary tuberculosis (uncontrolled massive hematogenous dissemination overwhelming host defense system)
4. Postprimary TB = reactivation TB (reactivation of dormant organisms after asymptomatic years)

Prognosis: 3.6% mortality rate
Cx: (1) Bronchopleural fistula + empyema
(2) Fibrosing mediastinitis

Postprimary pulmonary tuberculosis

= REACTIVATION TB = RECRUDESCENT TB
= infection under the influence of acquired hypersensitivity and immunity secondary to longevity of bacillus + impairment of cellular immunity
Incidence: 1% per year in persons with normal immunity, up to 10% in persons with deficient T-cell immunity
Etiology:
(a) reactivation of focus acquired in childhood
(b) initial infection in individual vaccinated with BCG
(c) continuation of initial infection
= progressive primary tuberculosis (rare)
Path: foci of caseous necrosis with surrounding edema, hemorrhage, mononuclear cell infiltration; formation of tubercles = accumulation of epithelioid cells + Langhans giant cells; bronchial perforation leads to intrabronchial dissemination (19–21%)
Age: predominantly in adulthood
Site: 85% in apical + posterior segments of upper lobe, 10% in superior segment of lower lobe, 5% in mixed locations (anterior + contiguous segments of upper lobe); R > L (DDx: histoplasmosis tends to affect anterior segment)

A. LOCAL EXUDATIVE TB
√ chronic patchy / confluent ill-defined areas of acinar consolidation (87–91%)
√ thin-walled cavitation with smooth inner surface (present in more advanced disease)
√ cavity under tension (air influx + obstructed efflux)
√ air-fluid level is strong evidence for superimposed bacterial / fungal infection
√ accentuated drainage markings toward ipsilateral hilum
√ acinar nodular pattern (20%) due to bronchogenic spread
√ pleural effusion (18%)
CT:
√ micronodules in centrilobular location (62%)
= solid caseation material in / surrounding the terminal / respiratory bronchioles
√ interlobular septal thickening (34–54%)
= increase in lymphatic flow as inflammatory response / impaired lymphatic drainage due to hilar lymphadenopathy

B. LOCAL FIBROPRODUCTIVE TB
√ sharply circumscribed irregular + angular masslike fibrotic lesion (in up to 7%)
√ thick-walled irregular cavitation (HALLMARK) secondary to expulsion of caseous necrosis into airways, esp. in apical / posterior segments of upper lobes (rare in children, in up to 45–51% in adults)
√ reticular pulmonary scars
√ cicatrization atelectasis = volume loss in affected lobe

√ bronchiectasis in apical / posterior segments of upper lobes
√ pleural thickening
√ apical cap = pleural rind = thickening of layer of extrapleural fat (3–25 mm) + pleural thickening (1–3 mm)
√ tuberculous lymphadenitis
√ calcified hilar / mediastinal nodes
√ Rasmussen aneurysm = aneurysm of terminal branches of pulmonary artery within wall of TB cavity secondary inflammatory necrosis of the vessel wall (4% at autopsies of cavitary TB)
  √ central cavity near hilum
  √ enlargement of central solid component of cavity
  √ opacification of pseudoaneurysm on CT / angio

Miliary Pulmonary Tuberculosis

= massive hematogenous dissemination of organisms any time after primary infection

Cause:
(1) severe immunodepression during postprimary state of infection
(2) impaired defenses during primary infection = PROGRESSIVE PRIMARY TB

Incidence: 2–3.5% of TB infections

√ chronic focus often not identifiable
√ radiographically recognizable after 6 weeks post hematogenous dissemination
√ generalized granulomatous interstitial small foci of pinpoint to 2–3 mm size
√ rapid complete clearing with appropriate therapy

HRCT (earlier detection than CXR):
  √ diffusely scattered discrete 1–2 mm nodules

Cx: dissemination via bloodstream affecting lymph nodes, liver, spleen, skeleton, kidneys, adrenals, prostate, seminal vesicles, epididymis, fallopian tubes, endometrium, meninges

UNILATERAL PULMONARY AGENESIS

= one-sided lack of primitive mesenchyme

Associated with:
anomalies in 60% (higher if right lung involved): PDA, anomalies of great vessels, tetralogy of Fallot (left-sided pulmonary agenesis), bronchogenic cyst, congenital diaphragmatic hernia, bone anomalies

- may be asymptomatic
- respiratory infections

√ complete opacity of hemithorax
√ ipsilateral absence of pulmonary artery + vein
√ absent ipsilateral mainstem bronchus
√ symmetrical chest cage with approximation of ribs
√ overdistension of contralateral lung
√ ipsilateral shift of mediastinum + diaphragm

VARICELLA-ZOSTER PNEUMONIA

Incidence: 14% overall; 50% in hospitalized adults

Age: >19 years (90%); 3rd–5th decade (75%); contrasts with low incidence of varicella in this age group

- vesicular rash

√ patchy diffuse airspace consolidation
√ tendency for coalescence near hila + lung bases
√ widespread nodules (30%) representing scarring
√ tiny 2–3 mm calcifications widespread throughout both lungs (2%)

Cx: unilateral diaphragmatic paralysis

Prognosis: 11% mortality rate

VIRAL PNEUMONIA

Organism: Rhinovirus (43%), respiratory syncytial virus (12%), Mycoplasma (10%), Parainfluenza virus, adenovirus, Influenza-virus

Path: necrosis of ciliated epithelial cells, goblet cells, bronchial mucous glands with frequent involvement of peribronchial tissues + interlobular septa

Age: most common cause of pneumonia in children under 5 years of age

Distribution: usually bilateral

√ hyperaeration + air trapping
√ "dirty chest" = peribronchial cuffing + opacification
√ perihilar linear densities (bronchial wall thickening)
√ interstitial pattern
√ airspace pattern (from hemorrhagic edema) in 50%
√ pleural effusion (20%)
√ hilar adenopathy (3%)
√ striking absence of pneumatoceles, lung abscess, pneumothorax
√ radiographic resolution lags 2–3 weeks behind clinical

Cx: bronchiectasis; unilateral hyperlucent lung

◊ Atypical measles pneumonia does NOT show the typical radiographic findings of viral pneumonias!

WEGENER GRANULOMATOSIS

= probable autoimmune disease characterized by systemic necrotizing granulomatous process with destructive angiitis

Path: peribronchial necrotizing granulomas + vasculitis not intimately related to arteries

Mean age of onset: 40 years (range of all ages); M:F = 2:1

CLASSIC TRIAD:
(1) respiratory tract granulomatous inflammation
(2) systemic small-vessel vasculitis
(3) necrotizing glomerulonephritis

@ Upper respiratory tract (100% involvement) (similar to midline granuloma)
(a) nasal cavity:
  - epistaxis from nasal mucosal ulceration
  - necrosis of nasal septum
  - saddle nose deformity
  √ progressive destruction of nasal cartilage + bone (DDx: relapsing polychondritis)
  √ granulomatous masses filling nasal cavities
(b) sinuses (maxillary antra most frequently):
  - sinus pain, purulent sinus drainage, rhinorrhea
  √ thickening of mucous membranes of paranasal sinuses

@ Pulmonary disease
- stridor (from tracheal inflammation + sclerosis)
- intractable cough, occasionally with hemoptysis

√ patchy alveolar infiltrates (with acute airspace pneumonia / pulmonary hemorrhage)
√ widely distributed multiple irregular masses / nodules of varying sizes (up to 9 cm), especially in lower lung fields
√ thick-walled cavities with irregular shaggy inner lining (25–50%)
√ pleural effusion in 25%
√ lymphadenopathy exceedingly rare

Cx: (1) dangerous airway stenosis (15% of adults, 50% of children)
(2) massive life-threatening pulmonary hemorrhage

@ Renal disease
focal glomerulonephritis in 20% at presentation, as disease progresses in 83%
Histo: focal necrosis, crescent formation, paucity/ absence of immunoglobulin deposits

@ Other organ involvement:
(a) Joints (56%): migratory polyarthropathy
(b) Skin + muscle (44%): inflammatory nodular skin lesions, cutaneous purpura
(c) Eyes + middle ear (29%): ocular inflammation, proptosis, otitis media
(d) Heart + pericardium (28%): myocardial infarction (vasculitis)
(e) CNS (22%): central / peripheral neuritis
(a) involvement of abdominal viscera

Cx: (1) Hypertension (2) Uremia (3) Facial nerve paralysis
Dx: lung / renal biopsy
Prognosis: death within 2 years from renal failure (83%) / respiratory failure
Rx: corticosteroids, cytotoxic drugs (cyclophosphamide), renal transplantation

Limited Wegener Granulomatosis
= Wegener granulomatosis WITHOUT renal involvement

Midline Granuloma
= mutilating granulomatous + neoplastic lesions limited to nose + paranasal sinuses with very poor prognosis; considered a variant of Wegener granulomatosis WITHOUT the typical granulomatous + cellular components

WILLIAMS-CAMPBELL SYNDROME
= congenital bronchial cartilage deficiency in the 4th to 6th bronchial generation either diffuse or restricted to focal area

HRCT:
√ cystic bronchiectasis distal to 3rd bronchial generation
√ emphysematous lung distal to bronchiectasis
√ inspiratory ballooning + expiratory collapse of dilated segments

WILSON-MIKITY SYNDROME
= PULMONARY DYSMATURITY
= similarity to bronchopulmonary dysplasia in patients breathing room air; rarely encountered anymore

Predisposed: premature infants <1500 g who are initially well
- gradual onset of respiratory distress between 10–14 days

√ hyperinflation
√ reticular pattern radiating from both hila
√ small bubbly lucencies throughout both lungs (identical to bronchopulmonary dysplasia)

Prognosis: resolution over 12 months

ZYGOMYCOSIS
= PHYCOMYCOSIS
= group of severe opportunistic sinonasal + pulmonary disease caused by a variety of Phycomycetes (soil fungi)

Organism: ubiquitous Mucor (most common), Rhizopus, Absidia with broad nonseptated hyphae of irregular branching pattern

At risk: immunoincompetent host with
1. lymphoproliferative malignancies and leukemia
2. acidotic diabetes mellitus
3. immunosuppression through steroids, antibiotics immunosuppressive drugs (rare)

Entry: inhalation / aspiration from sinonasal colonization
Path: angioinvasive behavior similar to aspergillosis

A. RHINOCEREBRAL FORM
= involvement of paranasal sinuses (frontal sinus usually spared) with extension into:
(a) orbit = orbital cellulitis
(b) base of skull = meningoencephalitis + cerebritis

B. PULMONARY FORM
√ segmental homogeneous consolidation
√ cavitary consolidation + air-crescent sign
√ nodules (from arterial thrombi + infarction)
√ rapidly progressive (often fatal) pneumonia

Dx: culture of fungus from biopsy specimen / demonstration within pathologic material
DDx: aspergillosis

DIFFERENTIAL DIAGNOSIS OF BREAST DISORDERS

BREAST DENSITY

Asymmetric Breast Density

A. OBVIOUS PATHOLOGIC LESION
  1. Stellate lesion
  2. Circular / ovoid lesion
  3. Calcifications
  4. Combination

B. PARENCHYMA
  1. Nodular densities + fat
     (a) normal TDLU
     (b) adenosis
  2. Linear densities + fat
  3. Fibrosis + fat
  4. Accessory breast

C. FIBROSIS
  1. Postinflammatory fibrosis
  2. Posttraumatic fibrosis
  3. Desmoplastic reaction

Diffuse Increase In Breast Density

√ generalized increased density
√ skin thickening
√ reticular pattern in subcutis

A. CANCER
  1. "Inflammatory" breast cancer (angiolymphatic spread)
     - rapid development of diffuse swelling, induration, skin redness + peau d'orange edema over 1/3 of breast surface

     Dx: skin biopsy
  2. Diffuse primary noninflammatory breast cancer
  3. Diffuse metastatic breast cancer
  4. Lymphoma / leukemia
     due to obstructive lymphedema of breast

B. INFECTIOUS MASTITIS
   usually in lactating breast

C. RADIATION
  (a) diffuse exudative edema within weeks after beginning of radiation therapy
  (b) indurational fibrosis months after radiation therapy

D. EDEMA
  1. Lymphatic obstruction: extensive axillary / intrathoracic lymphadenopathy, mediastinal / anterior chest wall tumor, axillary surgery
  2. Generalized body edema: congestive heart failure (breast edema may be unilateral if patient in lateral decubitus position), hypoalbuminemia (renal disease, liver cirrhosis), fluid overload

E. HEMORRHAGE
  1. Posttraumatic
  2. Anticoagulation therapy
  3. Bleeding diathesis

F. ACCIDENTAL INFUSION OF FLUID
   into subcutaneous tissue

OVAL-SHAPED BREAST LESION

Mammographic Evaluation Of Breast Masses

True mass or pseudomass?

A. SIZE
  — well-defined nodules <1.0 cm are of low risk for cancer
  — "most likely benign" nodules approaching 1 cm should be considered for ultrasound / aspiration / biopsy

B. SHAPE
  — increase in probability of malignancy: round < oval < lobulated < irregular < architectural distortion

C. MARGIN (most important factor)
  — well-circumscribed mass with sharp abrupt transition from surrounding tissue is almost always benign
  — "halo" sign of apparent lucency = optical illusion of Mach effect + true radiolucent halo is almost always (92%) benign but not pathognomonic for benignity
  — microlobulated margin worrisome for cancer
  — obscured margin may represent infiltrative cancer
  — irregular ill-defined margin has a high probability of malignancy
  — spiculated margin due to (a) fibrous projections extending from main cancer mass (b) previous surgery (c) sclerosing duct hyperplasia (radial scar)

D. LOCATION
  — intramammary lymph node typically in upper outer quadrant (in 5% of all mammograms)
  — large hamartoma + abscess common in retro- / periareolar location
  — sebaceous cyst in subcutaneous tissue

E. X-RAY ATTENUATION = DENSITY
  — fat-containing lesions are never malignant
  — high-density mass suspicious for carcinoma (higher density than equal volume of fibroglandular tissue due to fibrosis)

F. NUMBER
  — multiplicity of identical lesions decreases risk

G. INTERVAL CHANGE
  — enlarging mass needs biopsy

H. PATIENT RISK FACTORS
  — increasing age increases risk for malignancy
  — positive family history
  — history of previous abnormal breast biopsy
  — history of extramammary malignancy

Well-circumscribed Breast Mass

◊ Well-defined nonpalpable lesions have a 4% risk of malignancy!

A. BENIGN
1. Cyst (45%)
2. Fibroadenoma
3. Sclerosing adenoma
4. Intraductal papilloma (intracystic / solid)
5. Galactocele
6. Sebaceous cyst

B. MALIGNANT
1. Medullary carcinoma
2. Mucinous carcinoma
3. Intracystic papillary carcinoma
4. Invasive ductal cancer not otherwise specified (rare)
5. Pathologic intramammary lymph node
6. Metastases to breast: melanoma, lymphoma / leukemia, lung cancer, hypernephroma

Well-circumscribed De Novo Mass In Woman >40 Years Of Age

1. Cyst
2. Papilloma
3. Carcinoma
4. Sarcoma (rare)
5. Fibroadenoma (exceedingly rare)
6. Metastasis (extremely rare)

Fat-containing Breast Lesion

◊ Fat contained within a lesion proves benignity!

1. Lipoma
2. Galactocele
   = fluid with high lipid content (last phase)
   • during / shortly after lactation
3. Traumatic lipid cyst = fat necrosis = oil cyst
   • site of prior surgery / trauma
4. Focal collection of normal breast fat

Mixed Fat- And Water-density Lesion

1. Intramammary lymph node
2. Galactocele
3. Hamartoma = lipofibroadenoma = fibroadenolipoma
4. Small superficial hematoma

Breast Lesion With Halo Sign

A. HIGH-DENSITY LESION
   = vessels + parenchymal elements not seen in superimposed lesion
1. Cyst
2. Sebaceous cyst
3. Wart

B. LOW-DENSITY LESION
   = vessels + parenchyma seen superimposed on lesion
1. Fibroadenoma
2. Galactocele
3. Cystosarcoma phylloides

Stellate / Spiculated Breast Lesion

= mass / architectural distortion characterized by thin lines radiating from its margins

Risk of malignancy:
— 75% for nonpalpable spiculated masses
— 32% for nonpalpable irregular masses

A. PSEUDOSTELLATE STRUCTURE
   = SUMMATION SHADOWS
   caused by fortuitous superimposition of normal fibrous + glandular structures; unveiled by rolled views, spot compression views ± microfocus magnification technique

B. "BLACK STAR"
   √ groups of fine fibrous strands bunched together
   √ circular / oval lucencies within center
   √ change in appearance on different views
1. Radial scar = sclerosing duct hyperplasia
2. Posttraumatic fat necrosis

C. "WHITE STAR"
   √ individual straight dense spicules
   √ central solid tumor mass
   √ little change in different views
1. Invasive ductal carcinoma = scirrhous carcinoma
   = desmoplastic reaction + secondary retraction of surrounding structures
   • clinical dimensions larger than mammographic size
   √ distinct central tumor mass with irregular margins
   √ length of spicules increase with tumor size
   √ localized skin thickening / retraction when spiculae extend to skin
   √ commonly associated with malignant-type calcifications
2. Postoperative scar
   • correlation with history + site of biopsy
   √ scar diminishes in size + density over time
3. Postoperative hematoma
   • clinical information
   √ short-term mammographic follow-up confirms complete resolution
4. Breast abscess
   • clinical information
   √ high-density lesion with flamelike contour
5. Hyalinized fibroadenoma with fibrosis
   √ changing pattern with different projections
   √ may be accompanied by typical coarse calcifications of fibroadenomas
6. Granular cell myoblastoma
7. Fibromatosis
8. Extra-abdominal desmoid

mnemonic: "STARFASH"
Summation shadow
Tumor (malignant)
Abscess
Radial scar
Fibroadenoma (hyalinized), **F**at necrosis
Adenosis (sclerosing)

Scar (postoperative)
Hematoma (postoperative)

Tumor-mimicking Lesions

1. "Phantom breast tumor" = simulated mass
   (a) asymmetric density
      √ scalloped concave breast contour
      √ interspersed fatty elements
   (b) summation shadow = chance overlap of glandular breast structures
      √ failure to visualize "tumor" on more than one view
2. Silicone injections
3. Skin lesions
   (a) Dermal nevus
      √ sharp halo / fissured appearance
   (b) Skin calcifications
      √ lucent center (clue)
      √ superficial location (tangential views)
   (c) Sebaceous / epithelial inclusion cyst
   (d) Neurofibromatosis
   (e) Biopsy scar
4. Lymphedema
5. Lymph nodes
   Frequency: 5.4% for intramammary nodes
   Location: axilla, subcutaneous tissue of axillary tail, lateral portion of pectoralis muscle, intramammary (typically in upper outer quadrant)
   √ ovoid / bean-shaped mass(es) with fatty notch representing hilum
   √ central zone of radiolucency (fatty replacement of center) surrounded by "crescent" rim of cortex
   √ usually <1.5 cm (up to 4 cm) in size
   √ well-circumscribed with slightly lobulated margin
6. Hemangioma

Solid Breast Lesion By Ultrasound

Malignant Sonographic Characteristics

√ spiculation = alternating straight lines radiating perpendicularly from surface of nodule
   (a) hypoechoic relative to echogenic fibrous tissue
   (b) hyperechoic relative to surrounding fat
√ taller-than wide lesion = AP dimension greater than craniocaudal / transverse dimension
√ angular margin = contour of junction between hypo- or isoechoic solid nodule and surrounding tissue at acute / obtuse / 90° angles
√ acoustic shadowing behind all / part of nodule (= fibroelastic host response to scirrhous cancer)
√ central part of solid lesion very hypoechoic with respect to fat
√ punctate echogenic calcifications within hypoechoic mass (acoustic shadowing commonly not present)
√ radial extension / branch pattern (= intraductal component of breast cancer)
√ microlobulation = many small lobulations at surface of solid nodule

(according to data from A.T. Stavros)

Characteristic	Sens.	Specif.	PPV	Rel. risk
spiculation	36.0	99.4	91.8	5.5
taller than wide	41.6	98.1	81.2	4.9
angular margins	83.2	92.0	67.5	4.0
acoustic shadowing	48.8	94.7	64.9	3.9
branch pattern	29.6	96.6	64.0	3.8
markedly hypoechoic	68.8	60.1	60.1	3.6
calcifications	27.2	96.3	59.6	3.6
duct extension	24.8	95.2	50.8	3.0
microlobulation	75.2	83.8	48.2	2.9

◊ Approximately 5 malignant features are found per cancer. The combination of 5 findings increases the sensitivity to 98.4%!

Benign Sonographic Characteristics

√ absence of any malignant characteristics
   ◊ A single malignant feature prohibits classification of a nodule as benign!
√ marked hyperechogenic well-circumscribed nodule compared to fat = normal stromal fibrous tissue (may represent a palpable pseudomass / fibrous ridge)
√ smooth well-circumscribed ellipsoid shape
√ 2–3 smooth well-circumscribed gentle lobulations
√ thin echogenic capsule
√ kidney-shaped lesion = intramammary lymph node
◊ If specific benign features are not found the lesion is classified as indeterminate!

(according to data from A.T. Stavros)

Characteristic	Sens.	Specif.	NPV	Rel. risk
hyperechoic	100.0	7.4	100.0	0.00
≤3 lobulations	99.2	19.4	99.2	0.05
ellipsoid shape	97.6	51.2	99.1	0.05
thin echogenic capsule	95.2	76.0	98.8	0.07

BREAST CALCIFICATIONS

Indicative of focally active process; often requiring biopsy
◊ 75–80% of biopsied clusters of calcifications represent a benign process
◊ 10–30% of microcalcifications in asymptomatic patients are associated with cancers

Composition: hydroxyapatite / tricalcium phosphate / calcium oxalate

Results of breast biopsies for microcalcification:
(without any other mammographic findings)
(a) benign lesions (80%)
   1. Mastopathy without proliferation 44%
   2. Mastopathy with proliferation 28%
   3. Fibroadenoma 4%
   4. Solitary papilloma 2%
   5. Miscellaneous 2%
(b) malignant lesions (20%)
   1. Lobular carcinoma in situ 10%
      in 8% no spatial relationship to LCIS
   2. Infiltrating carcinoma 6%
   3. Ductal carcinoma in situ 4%

◊ Positive biopsy rate of >35% is desirable goal!

BREAST

A. LOCATION
(a) intramammary
1. **Ductal microcalcifications**
√ 0.1–0.3 mm in size, irregular, sometimes mixed linear + punctate
Occurrence: secretory disease, epithelial hyperplasia, atypical ductal hyperplasia, intraductal carcinoma
2. **Lobular microcalcifications**
√ smooth round, similar in size + density
Occurrence:
cystic hyperplasia, adenosis, sclerosing adenosis, atypical lobular hyperplasia, lobular carcinoma in situ, cancerization of lobules (= retrograde migration of ductal carcinoma to involve lobules), ductal carcinoma obstructing egress of lobular contents
N.B.: lobular and ductal microcalcifications occur frequently in fibrocystic disease + breast cancer!
(b) extramammary: arterial wall, duct wall, fibroadenoma, oil cyst, skin, etc.
B. SIZE
√ malignant calcifications usually <0.5 mm; rarely >1.0 mm
C. NUMBER
√ <4–5 calcifications per 1 cm^2 have a low probability for malignancy
D. MORPHOLOGY
(a) benign
1. smooth round calcifications: formed in dilated acini of lobules
2. solid / lucent-centered spheres: usually due to fat necrosis
3. crescent-shaped calcifications that are concave on horizontal beam lateral projection
= sedimented milk of calcium at bottom of cyst
4. lucent-centered calcifications: around accumulated debris within ducts / in skin
5. solid rod-shaped calcifications / lucent-centered tubular calcifications: formed within / around normal / ectatic ducts
6. eggshell calcifications in rim of breast cysts
7. calcifications with parallel track appearance
= vascular calcifications
(b) malignant
= calcified cellular secretions / necrotic cancer cells within ducts
√ calcifications of
- vermicular form
- varying in size
- linear / branching shape
E. DISTRIBUTION
1. clustered heterogeneous calcifications: adenosis, peripheral duct papilloma, hyperplasia, cancer
2. segmental calcifications within single duct network: suspect for multifocal cancer within lobe
3. regional / diffusely scattered calcifications with random distribution throughout large volumes of breast: almost always benign
F. TIME COURSE
malignant calcifications can remain stable for >5 years!
G. DENSITY

Malignant Calcifications
1. **Granular calcifications** = resembling fine grains of salt
√ amorphous, dotlike / elongated, fragmented
√ grouped very closely together
√ irregular in form, size, and density
2. **Casting calcifications** = fragmented cast of calcifications within ducts
√ variable in size + length
√ great variation in density within individual particles + among adjacent particles
√ jagged irregular contour
√ ± Y-shaped branching pattern
√ clustered (>5 per focus within an area of 1 cm^2)

Benign Calcifications
1. **Lobular calcifications** = arise within a spherical cavity of cystic hyperplasia, sclerosing adenosis, atypical lobular hyperplasia
√ sharply outlined, homogeneous, solid, spherical "pearl-like"
√ little variation in size
√ numerous + scattered
√ associated with considerable fibrosis
(a) adenosis
√ diffuse calcifications involving both breasts symmetrically
(b) periductal fibrosis
√ diffuse / grouped calcifications + irregular borders, simulating malignant process
2. Sedimented milk of calcium
Frequency: 4%
√ multiple, bilateral, scattered / occasionally clustered calcifications within microcysts
√ smudge-like particles at bottom of cyst on vertical beam
√ crescent-shaped on horizontal projection
= "teacup-like"
3. Plasma cell mastitis = periductal mastitis
√ sharply marginated calcifications of uniform density = intraductal form
√ sharply marginated hollow calcifications
= periductal form
4. Peripheral eggshell calcifications
(a) with radiolucent lesion
— liponecrosis micro- / macrocystica calcificans (= fatty acids precipitate as calcium soaps at capsular surface) as calcified fat necrosis / calcified hematoma
◊ May mimic malignant calcifications!
(b) with radiopaque lesion
— degenerated fibroadenoma
— macrocyst
√ high uniform density in periphery
√ usually subcutaneous
√ no associated fibrosis

5. Papilloma
   √ solitary raspberry configuration in size of duct
   √ central / retroareolar
6. Degenerated fibroadenoma
   √ bizarre, coarse, sharply outlined, "popcornlike" very dense calcification within dense mass (= central myxoid degeneration)
   √ eggshell type calcification (= subcapsular myxoid degeneration)
7. Arterial calcifications
   √ parallel lines of calcifications
8. Dermal calcifications
   Site: sebaceous glands
   √ hollow radiolucent center
   √ polygonal shape
   √ peripheral location (may project deep within breast even on 2 views at 90° angles)
   √ linear orientation when caught in tangent
   √ same size as skin pores
   Proof: superficial marking technique
9. Metastatic calcifications
   Cause: 2° hyperparathyroidism (in up to 68%)

NIPPLE AND SKIN

Nipple Retraction

1. Positional
2. Relative to inflammation / edema of periareolar tissue
3. Congenital
4. Acquired (carcinoma, ductal ectasia)

Nipple Discharge

◊ The most significant discharge comes from one breast + one orifice!

◊ The most common cause of bloody / serosanguinous discharge is intraductal papilloma!

Type of discharge:

A. Lactating breast: galactorrhea
B. Nonlactating breast:
   (a) normal: white, yellowish, greenish-gray
   (b) abnormal:
      1. <u>clear serous</u>: cancer 2–7%, papilloma 35%, fibrocystic change 36%, ductectasia 11%
      2. <u>bloody</u>: cancer 6–16%, papilloma 61%, fibrocystic change 12%, ductectasia 2%

• exfoliative cytology not helpful (true positive in 11%)

Site of origin:

A. Lobules + terminal duct lobular unit:
   1. Galactorrhea
   2. Fibrocystic changes
B. Larger lactiferous ducts (collecting duct, segmental duct, subsegmental duct)
   1. Solitary papilloma
   2. Papillary carcinoma
   3. Duct ectasia

Galactography:

injection of 0.1–0.3 cm^3 of water-soluble contrast material through blunt 27-gauge pediatric sialography needle (0.4–0.6 mm outer diameter, tip bent 90°)

DDx of intraductal defects:

gas bubble, clot, inspissated secretions, solitary intraductal papilloma, epithelial hyperplastic lesion, duct carcinoma

Galactographic filling defect		
	single	multiple
Multiple papilloma	5.6%	14.0%
Cancer	0.05%	9.7%

Secretory Disease

1. Retained lactiferous secretions
   result of incomplete / prolonged involution of lactiferous ducts
   √ branching pattern of fat density in dense breast (high lipid content)
2. Prolonged inspissation of secretion + intraductal debris
   √ duct dilatation
   √ calcifications with linear orientation toward subareolar area a few mm long: rod-shaped / sausage-shaped / spherical with hollow center
3. Galactocele
4. Plasma cell mastitis

Skin Thickening Of Breast

Normal skin thickness: 0.8–3 mm; may exceed 3 mm in inframammary region

A. LOCLAIZED SKIN THICKENING
   1. Trauma (prior biopsy)
   2. Carcinoma
   3. Abscess
   4. Nonsuppurative mastitis
   5. Dermatologic conditions
B. GENERALIZED SKIN THICKENING
   ◊ Skin is thickened initially and to the greatest extent in the lower dependent portion of breast!
   √ overall increased density with coarse reticular pattern (= dilated lymph vessels + interstitial fluid triggering fibrosis)
   (a) Axillary lymphatic obstruction
      1. Primary breast cancer
         — advanced breast cancer
         — invasive comedocarcinoma in large area
         ◊ Primary breast cancer not necessarily seen due to small size / hidden location (axillary tail, behind nipple)!
      2. Primary malignant lymphatic disease (eg, lymphoma)
   (b) Intradermal + intramammary obstruction of lymph channels
      1. Lymphatic spread of breast cancer from contralateral side
      2. Inflammatory breast carcinoma = diffusely invasive ductal carcinoma
   (c) Mediastinal lymphatic blockage
      1. Sarcoidosis
      2. Hodgkin disease

3. Advanced bronchial / esophageal carcinoma
4. Actinomycosis

(d) Advanced gynecologic malignancies from thoracoepigastric collaterals
1. Ovarian cancer
2. Uterine cancer

(e) Inflammation
1. Acute mastitis
2. Retromamillary abscess
3. Fat necrosis
4. Radiation therapy
5. Reduction mammoplasty

(f) Right heart failure
may be unilateral (R > L) / migrating with change in patient position (to avoid decubitus ulcer)

(g) Nephrotic syndrome, anasarca
1. Dialysis
2. Renal transplant

(h) Subcutaneous extravasation of pleural fluid following thoracentesis

Axillary Lymphadenopathy

= solid node >1.5 cm in size without fatty hilum

A. MALIGNANT
1. Metastasis from breast cancer in 26%
2. Metastases from non-breast primary (melanoma, ovary)
3. Lymphoma / chronic lymphocytic leukemia (17%)

B. BENIGN
1. Nonspecific benign lymphadenopathy (29%)
2. Sarcoidosis
3. Collagen vascular disease: rheumatoid arthritis, systemic lupus erythematosus
4. Psoriasis
5. HIV-related adenopathy
6. Reactive lymphadenopathy (breast infection / abscess / biopsy)

Radiographic features suspicious for malignancy:
- √ size increase of >100% over baseline
- √ size >3.3 cm
- √ change in shape
- √ spiculation of margins
- √ intranodal microcalcifications (without history of gold therapy)
- √ loss of radiolucent center / hilar notch
- √ increase in density

REPORTS

Breast Imaging Reporting And Data System (BIRD)

N = negative
there is nothing to comment on; breasts are symmetrical without masses, architectural disturbances / suspicious calcifications

B = benign finding
confidently labeled, eg, calcified fibroadenoma, multiple secretory calcifications, fat-containing lesion such as oil cyst, lipoma, galactocele, mixed-density hamartoma, intramammary lymph node, implant

P = probably benign finding – short interval follow-up
high probability of benign with radiologist's preference to establish its stability

S = suspicious abnormality – consider biopsy
lesion without characteristic morphology of cancer but definite probability of being malignant

M = highly suggestive of malignancy
biopsy is mandatory

Lexicon Descriptors For Reporting (ACR)

A. MASS

size	
shape	circular, oval, lobulated, irregular
margins	circumscribed, lobulated, obscured, indistinct, speculated
location	based on face of clock + depth in breast
associated findings	skin changes, calcifications, nipple retraction, trabecular thickening
attenuation	relative to an equal volume of breast tissue: high density, isodense, low density, fat density

B. CALCIFICATIONS

type	skin, vascular, coarse, rodlike, eggshell, punctate, pleomorphic
number	
size	
distribution	clustered, linear, segmental, regional, scattered, multiple groups
associated findings	skin changes, nipple retraction, architectural distortion, trabecular thickening

BREAST ANATOMY AND MAMMOGRAPHIC TECHNIQUE

BREAST ANATOMY

Lobes

15 – 20 lobes disposed radially around nipple, each lobe has a main lactiferous duct of 2.0–4,5 mm converging at the nipple with an opening in the central portion of nipple

Main duct: branches dichotomously eventually forming terminal ductal lobular units

Histo: epithelial cells, myoepithelial cells surrounded by extralobular connective tissue with elastic fibers

Terminal Duct Lobular Unit (TDLU)

(1) Extralobular terminal duct
  Histo: lined by columnar cells + prominent coat of elastic fibers + outer layer of myoepithelium

(2) Lobule
  (a) intralobular terminal duct
    Histo: lined by 2 layers of cuboidal cells + outer layer of myoepithelium
  (b) ductules / acini
  (c) intralobular connective tissue

Size: 1 – 8 mm (most 1 – 2 mm) in diameter

Change:
  (a) reproductive age: cyclic proliferation (up to time of ovulation) + cyclic involution (during menstruation)
  (b) post menopause: regression with fatty replacement

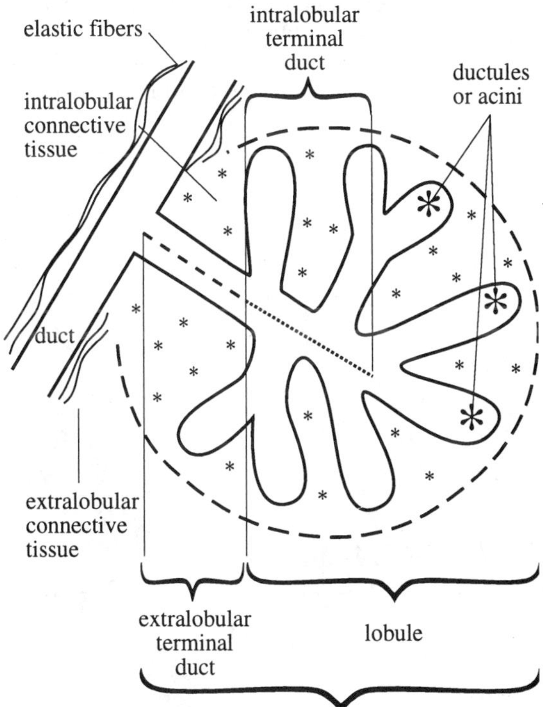

Significance:
  TDLU is site of fibroadenoma, epithelial cyst, apocrine metaplasia, adenosis (= proliferation of ductules + lobules), epitheliosis (= proliferation of mammary epithelial cells within preexisting ducts + lobules), ductal + lobular carcinoma in situ, infiltrating ductal + lobular carcinoma

Components Of Normal Breast Parenchyma

1. Nodular densities surrounded by fat
   (a) 1 – 2 mm = normal lobules
   (b) 3 – 9 mm = adenosis
2. Linear densities
   = ducts and their branches + surrounding elastic tissue
3. Structureless ground-glass density
   = stroma / fibrosis with concave contours

Parenchymal Breast Pattern (László Tabár)

Pattern I
named QDY = quasi dysplasia (for Wolfe classification)
√ concave contour from Cooper's ligaments
√ evenly scattered 1 – 2 mm nodular densities (= normal terminal ductal lobular units)
√ oval-shaped / circular lucent areas (= fatty replacement)

Pattern II
similar to N1 (Wolfe)
√ total fatty replacement
√ NO nodular densities

Pattern III
similar to P1 (Wolfe)
√ normal parenchyma occupying <25% of breast volume in retroareolar location

Pattern IV = adenosis pattern
similar to P2 (Wolfe)
Cause: hypertrophy + hyperplasia of acini within lobules
Histo: small ovoid proliferating cells with rare mitoses
√ scattered 3 – 7 mm nodular densities (= enlarged terminal ductal lobular units) = adenosis
√ thick linear densities (= periductal elastic tissue proliferation with fibrosis) = fibroadenosis
√ no change with increasing age (genetically determined)

Pattern V
similar to DY (Wolfe)
√ uniformly dense parenchyma with smooth contour (= extensive fibrosis)

MAMMOGRAPHIC FILM READING TECHNIQUE

1. Compare with earlier films
2. Scan "forbidden" areas
   (a) "Milky Way" = 2 – 3 cm wide area parallel with the edge of the pectoral muscle on MLO projection

BREAST

(b) "No man's land" = fatty replaced area between posterior border of parenchyma + chest wall on CC projection
(c) Medial half of breast on CC view
3. Look for increased retroareolar density
4. Look for parenchymal contour retraction
5. Look for architectural distortion
6. Look for straight lines superimposed on normal scalloped contour
7. Compare left with right side
8. Don't stop looking after one lesion is found

MAMMOGRAPHIC TECHNIQUE

BEAM QUALITY
Molybdenum target material with characteristic emission peaks of 17.9 + 19.5 keV (lower average energy than tungsten)
FOCAL SPOT
0.1 – 0.4 mm (0.1 mm for magnification views)
TUBE OUTPUT
80 – 100 mA
EXPOSURE
(a) without grid: 25 kV (optimum between contrast + penetration), exposure time of 1.0 seconds
(b) with grid: 26 – 27 kV; exposure time of 2.3 seconds
(c) microfocus magnification: 26 – 27 kV; 1.5 – 2.0 times magnification with 16 – 30 cm air gap
(d) specimen radiography: 22 – 24 kV
FILTER
(a) beryllium window (absorbs less radiation than glass tube)
(b) molybdenum filter (0.03 mm): allows more of lower energy radiation to reach breast
REDUCTION OF SCATTER RADIATION
(1) adequate compression (also improves contrast + decreases radiation dose)
(2) beam collimation to <8 – 10 cm
(3) air gap with microfocus magnification
(greater spatial resolution, 2 – 3-fold increase in radiation exposure)
(4) Moving grid
grid if compressed breast >5 cm / very dense breast (facilitates perception, 2 – 3-fold increase in radiation exposure)
SCREEN-FILM COMBINATION
(1) Intensifying screen phosphor
single screen systems
(2) Film-screen contact
(3) Mammography film with minimal base fog, sufficient maximum density + contrast
FILM PROCESSING
(1) Processing time of 3 minutes (42 – 45 seconds in developing fluid) superior to 90-second processor for double-emulsion film (which creates underdevelopment + compensatory higher radiation exposure)
(2) Developing temperature of 35° C (95° F)
(3) Developing fluid replenishment rate:
450 – 500 mL replenisher per square meter of film
QUALITY CONTROL
(1) Processor (daily)
with sensito- / densitometric measurements
(a) base fog <0.16 – 0.17
(b) maximum density >3.50
(c) contrast >1.9 – 2.0
(2) X-ray unit (semiannually)
(a) beam quality
(b) phototimer

Average glandular dose:
<0.6 mGy per breast for nonmagnification film-screen mammogram (ACR accreditation requirement)
Screen/film technique (molybdenum target; 0.03 mm molybdenum filter, 28 kVp):
mean absorbed dose: 0.05 rad for CC view
0.06 rad for LAT view

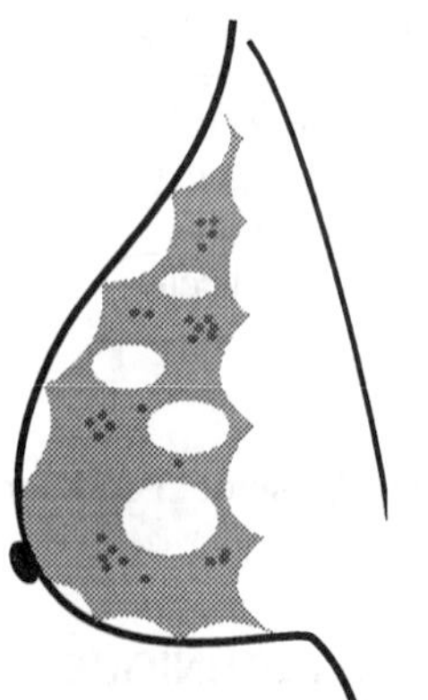
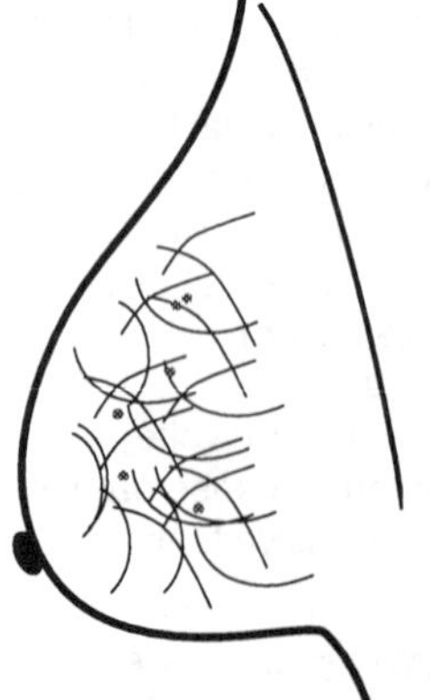
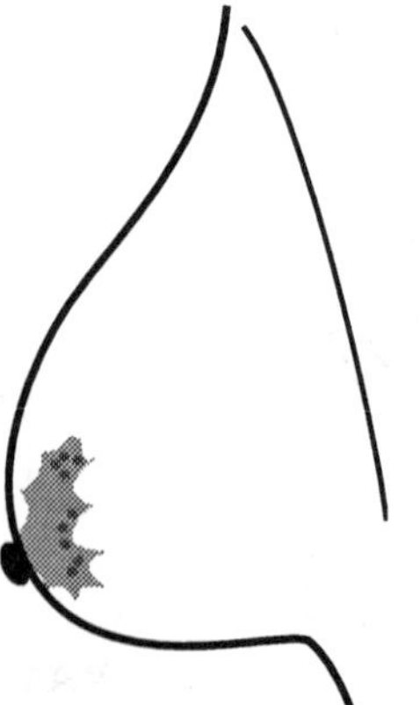
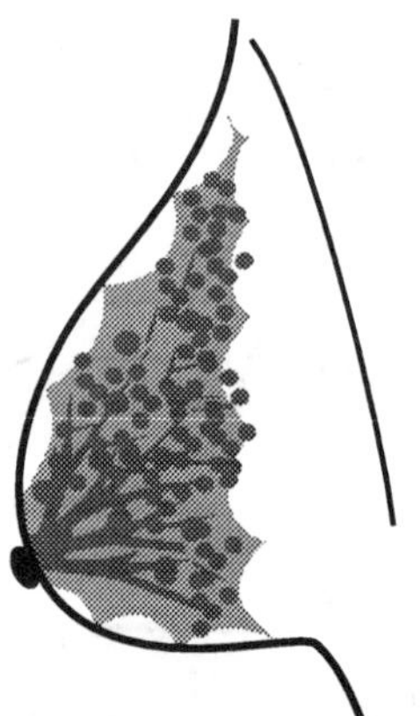
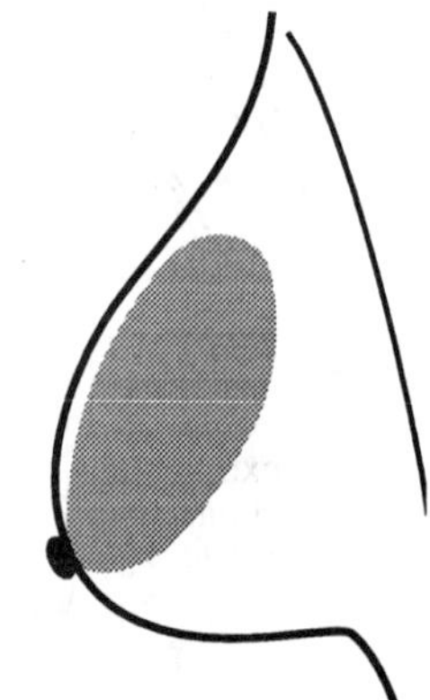

Parenchymal Breast Pattern
Pattern I **Pattern II** **Pattern III** **Pattern IV** **Pattern V**

BREAST

Effective dose equivalent H_E:
screen-film mammography .... 0.11 mSv
xeroradiographic mammography .... 0.78 mSv
chest .... 0.05 mSv
skull .... 0.15 mSv
abdomen .... 1.40 mSv
lumbar spine .... 2.20 mSv

Advantages of magnification mammography
1. Sharpness effect = increased resolution
2. Noise effect = noise reduced by a factor equal to the degree of magnification
3. Air-gap effect = increased contrast by reduction in scattered radiation
4. Visual effect = improved perception and analysis of small detail

Factors Affecting Mammographic Image Quality

A. RADIOGRAPHIC SHARPNESS
= subjective impression of distinctness / perceptibility of structure boundary / edge

1. **Radiographic contrast**
= magnitude of optical density difference between structure of interest + surroundings influenced by

(a) subject contrast
= ratio of x-ray intensity transmitted through one part of the breast to that transmitted through a more absorbing adjacent part affected by
— absorption differences in the breast (thickness, density, atomic number)
— radiation quality (target material, kilovoltage, filtration)
— scattered radiation (beam limitation, grid, compression)
(b) receptor contrast
= component of radiographic contrast that determines how the x-ray intensity pattern will be related to the optical density pattern in the mammogram

affected by
— film type
— processing (chemicals, temperature, time, agitation)
— photographic density
— fog (storage, safelight, light leaks)

2. **Radiographic blurring**
= lateral spreading of a structural boundary (= distance over which the optical density between the structure and its surroundings changes)
(a) motion
reduced by compression + short exposure time
(b) geometric blurring
affected by
— focal spot: size, shape, intensity distribution
— focus-object distance (= cone length)
— object-image distance
(c) receptor blurring
= light diffusion (= spreading of the light emitted by the screen) affected by
— phosphor thickness + particle size
— light-absorbing dyes + pigments
— screen-film contact

B. RADIOGRAPHIC NOISE
= unwanted fluctuation in optical density

1. **Radiographic mottle**
= optical density variations consist of
(a) receptor graininess
= optical density variation from random distribution of finite number of silver halide grains
(b) quantum mottle (principal contributor to mottle)
= variation in optical density from random spatial distribution of x-ray quanta absorbed in image receptor
affected by
— film speed + contrast
— screen absorption + conversion efficiency
— light diffusion
— radiation quality
(c) structure mottle
= optical density fluctuation from nonuniformity in the structure of the image receptor (eg, phosphor layer of intensifying screen)
2. **Artifacts**
= unwanted optical density variations in the form of blemishes on the mammogram
(a) improper film handling (static, crimp marks, fingerprints, scratches)
(b) improper exposure (fog)
(c) improper processing (streaks, spots, scratches)
(d) dirt + stains

BREAST DISORDERS

BREAST CANCER

Origin: terminal ductal lobular unit

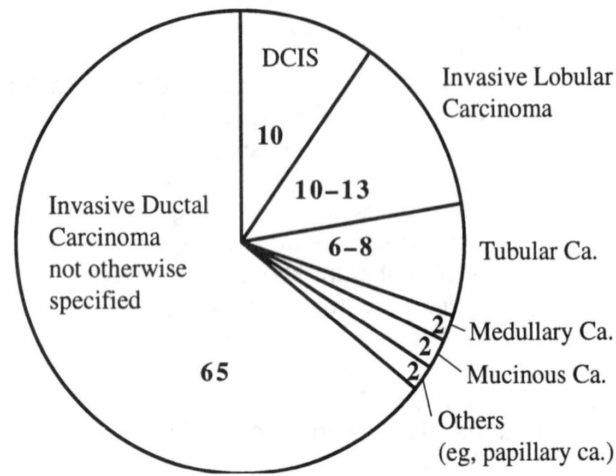

Distribution of Breast Cancers in Screening Population
(numbers are in percentage)

A. NONINVASIVE BREAST CANCER (15%)
= malignant transformation of epithelial cells lining mammary ducts + lobules confined within boundaries of basement membrane
Rx: little data is available to provide insight into proper treatment

1. **Ductal carcinoma in situ** (DCIS)
= intraductal carcinoma
Incidence: 10–25–40% in screening population; 70% of noninvasive carcinomas
Age: most >55 years
Histo: heterogeneous group of malignancies originating within extralobular terminal duct + without invasion of basement membrane
Subgroups: comedocarcinoma, non-comedocarcinomas (solid, micropapillary, cribriform)
• may persist for years without palpable abnormality (in screening population)
• palpable mass / Paget disease of nipple / nipple discharge (in symptomatic patients)
◊ 50% of DCIS are >5 cm in size
◊ Histologic size of DCIS is independent of histologic subgroup
◊ Almost all "comedo" type DCIS contain significant microcalcifications
◊ DCIS often involves the nipple + subareolar ducts
Spectrum of mammographic findings:
√ calcifications only (72%)
√ soft-tissue abnormality + calcification (12%)
√ soft-tissue abnormality only (10%)
√ nonvisible (6%)

Prognosis: 20–50% develop invasive disease 5–10 years after initial diagnosis of DCIS
Rx:
(1) Simple / modified mastectomy: cure rate of almost 100%
(2) Local excision alone: 25% rate of recurrence within 26 months in immediate vicinity of biopsy site
(3) Local excision + radiotherapy: 2–17% rate of recurrence

Treatment problems:
1. Occult invasion in 5–20% of patients
2. Multifocality
(= >1 focus in same quadrant of breast)
3. Multicentricity
(= >1 focus in different quadrants of breast) in 14% of lesions <25 mm, in 100% of lesions >50 mm
4. Axillary metastases in 1–2%

(a) High nuclear grade DCIS ("**comedo type**")
Prevalence: 60% of all DCIS
Precursor: none; one stage development
Path: "comedo" = pluglike appearance of necrotic material that can be expressed from the cut surface
Characteristics:
} nuclear grade: large / intermediate nuclei, numerous mitoses, aneuploidy
} growth pattern: predominantly solid cell proliferation; atypically micropapillary / cribriform
} necrosis: extensive (HALLMARK)
} calcifications (90%): dystrophic / amorphous within necrosis in center of dilated ductal system outlining most of the lobe in classic solid growth pattern
• estrogen- + progesterone-receptor negative
• overexpression of c-erb B-2 oncogene product and P53 suppressor gene mutation
• often symptomatic lesion with nipple discharge
√ ductal system enlarged to 300–350 μ
√ linear / branching pattern of calcifications scattered in a large part of lobe / whole lobe
√ large solid high-density casting calcifications (fragmented, coalesced, irregular) in solid growth pattern
√ "snake skin–like" / "birch tree flowerlike" dotted casting calcifications within necrosis of micropapillary / cribriform growth pattern
√ palpable dominant mass without calcifications (very unusual)
√ nipple discharge (rare)
Prognosis: higher recurrence rate than noncomedo-group

BREAST

(b) Low nuclear grade DCIS ("**noncomedo** type")
Prevalence: 40% of all DCIS
Precursor lesion:
atypical ductal hyperplasia (ADH) with slight / moderate / severe atypia
◊ 52–56% of ADH at core biopsy are associated with malignancy at excision!
Characteristics:
} nuclear grade: monomorphic small round nuclei, few / no mitoses
} growth pattern: predominantly micropapillary / cribriform; atypically solid cell proliferation (often coexist)
} necrosis: not present in classic micropapillary / cribriform growth pattern
} calcifications (50%): laminated / psammoma-like due to active secretion by malignant cells into duct lumen
√ fine granular "cotton ball" calcifications in micropapillary / cribriform growth pattern
√ coarse granular "crushed stone" / "broken needle tip" / "arrowhead" calcifications in less common solid growth pattern
◊ Size of "noncomedo" DCIS often underestimated mammographically (? due to lower density of calcifications at periphery of lesion)!
√ palpable dominant mass without calcifications (intracystic papillary carcinoma, multifocal papillary carcinoma in situ)
√ nonpalpable asymmetric density with architectural distortion
√ occasionally serous / bloody nipple discharge + ductal filling defects on galactography
Risk of recurrence: 2%
Prognosis: 30% eventually develop into invasive cancer
Dx: surgical biopsy
◊ Core needle biopsy could result in diagnosis of only proliferative breast disease that is usually intermixed!

2. **Lobular carcinoma in situ** (LCIS)
= arises in epithelium of blunt ducts of mammary lobules
Incidence: 0.8–3.6% in screening population; 3–6 % of all breast malignancies; 25% of noninvasive carcinomas; high incidence during reproductive age but decreasing with age
Age: most 40–54 years (earlier than DCIS / invasive tumors)
Histo: monomorphous small cell population filling + expanding ductules of the lobule
◊ Synchronous invasive cancer in 5%!
• not palpable
√ mammographically occult
√ may atypically present as a noncalcified mass (in 7%), calcifications + mass (in 10%), asymmetric opacity (2%)
◊ High frequency of multicentricity (70%) + bilaterality (30%)!
Dx: incidental microscopic finding depending on accident of biopsy (performed for unrelated reasons + findings)
Prognosis:
20–30% develop invasive ductal > lobular carcinoma within 20 years after initial diagnosis
◊ 1% per year lifetime risk for invasive malignancy
◊ LCIS serves as a marker of increased risk for developing invasive carcinoma in either breast!
Rx: recommendations range from observation (with follow-up examinations every 3–6 months + annual mammograms) to unilateral / bilateral simple mastectomy

3. **Intracystic papillary carcinoma in situ** (0.5–2%)
= rare variant of noncomedo DCIS
Age: average of 51 years
• well-circumscribed + freely movable
• aspiration may yield bloody fluid (cytology negative in 80%)
√ intracystic mass on pneumocystography
√ solid intracystic mass on US
√ round benign appearing mass on mammography
Prognosis: favorable

B. INVASIVE BREAST CANCER (85%)

1. **Infiltrating / invasive ductal carcinoma** (65%) of no special type / otherwise not specified (NOS)
10% false-negative ratio
Histo:
grade I = well-differentiated
grade II = moderately differentiated
grade III = poorly differentiated
• palpable in 70%
• larger by palpation than on mammogram
√ spiculated mass (36%) is PRINCIPAL FINDING
√ malignant calcifications (45–60%)

2. **Infiltrating / invasive lobular carcinoma** (5–10%)
◊ 2nd most common type of breast cancer; 30–50% of patients will develop a second primary in same / opposite breast within 20 years
◊ Most frequently missed breast cancer (difficult to detect mammographically + clinically) with 19–43% false-negative rate (occult in dense breast)
Median age: 45–56 years; 2% of all ILC occur in women <35 years
Path: multicentricity + bilaterality (in up to 1/3); tendency to grow around ducts, vessels, and lobules without destruction of anatomic structures (targetoid growth); no substantial connective tissue reaction
Histo: 20% grade I, 64% grade II, 16% grade III
Metastases: GI tract, gynecologic organs, peritoneum, retroperitoneum, carcinomatous meningitis

BREAST

- palpable in 69%
  - area of subtle skin thickening / induration
  - large hard mass / fine nodularity

N.B.: may be seen on CC view only in many cases

√ architectural distortion (= retraction of normal glandular tissue with thickening + disturbance of fibrous septa) in 18–30% is MOST COMMON MAMMOGRAPHIC FINDING
Histo: straight single file of uniform small cells with round oval nuclei ("Indian files") growing around ducts resulting in subtle changes in architecture
√ irregular spiculated mass >1 cm (16–28%)
√ poorly defined mass ± spicules <1 cm (22%)
√ asymmetric opacity (= ill-defined area of increased opacity without central tumor nidus) in 8–19%
√ round / ovoid mass with regular borders (1%)
√ microcalcifications (0–24%)
√ retraction of skin (25%) + nipple (26%)
√ skin thickening

3. **Tubular carcinoma** (6–8%)
= well-differentiated form of ductal carcinoma
(a) low grade: bilateral in 1:3
(b) high grade: bilateral in 1:300
Associated with: lobular carcinoma in situ in 40%
Mean age: 40–49 years
- positive family history in 40%
- nonpalpable

√ high-opacity nodule with spiculated margins
√ <17 mm in diameter; mean diameter of 8 mm
DDx: radial scar

4. **Medullary carcinoma** (2%)
= SOLID CIRCUMSCRIBED CARCINOMA
◊ Fastest growing breast cancer!
Path: well-circumscribed mass with nodular architecture + lobulated contour; central necrosis is common in larger tumors; reminiscent of medullary cavity of bone
Histo: intense lymphoplasmocytic reaction (reflecting host resistance); propensity for syncytial growth; no glands
Incidence: 11% of breast cancers in women <35 years of age; 40–50% of medullary cancers in women <50 years of age
Mean age: 46–54 years
- softer than average breast cancer

√ well-defined round / oval noncalcified uniformly dense mass (hemorrhage) with lobulated margin
√ may have partial / complete halo sign
US:
√ hypoechoic mass with some degree of through transmission
√ distinct / indistinct margins
√ large central cystic component
DDx: fibroadenoma
Prognosis: 92% 10-year survival rate

5. **Mucinous / colloid carcinoma** (1.5–2%)
Path:
(a) pure form: aggregates of tumor cells surrounded by abundant pools of extracellular mucin (gelatinous / colloid fluid)
(b) mixed form: contains areas of infiltrating ductal carcinoma not surrounded by mucin
Age: 1% in women <35 years; 7% of carcinomas in women >75 years
- slow growth rate of pure form
- "swish" / "crush" sensation during palpation
- 60% estrogen-receptor positive

√ well-circumscribed usually lobulated mass of round / ovoid shape
√ pleomorphic clustered / clumped amorphous / punctate calcifications (rare)
√ may enlarge fast (through mucin production)
√ solid mass on US
Prognosis: favorable

6. **Papillary carcinoma** (1–2–4%)
= rare ductal carcinoma forming papillary structures
N.B.: Do not confuse with micropapillary / cribriform growth pattern of ductal carcinoma
Histo: multilayered papillary projections extending from vascularized stalks; no myoepithelial layer (as in benign lesions); neurosecretory granules + positive CEA-reactivity in 85% (absent in benign lesions)
Types:
(a) multiple intraductal carcinomas with papillary configuration
(b) Intracystic papillary carcinoma
= in situ malignancy
(c) invasive carcinoma with papillary growth pattern (microscopic frond formation)
Age: 25–89 (mean 50–60) years; peak age of 40–75 years
- palpable mass (67%)
- nipple discharge (22–35%) often tinged with blood
- rich in estrogen and progesterone receptors

Location: single nodule in central portion of breast; multiple nodules extending from subareolar area to periphery of breast
√ multinodular pattern (55%) = lobulated mass / cluster of well-defined contiguous nodules
√ solitary well-circumscribed round / ovoid nodule with average diameter of 2–3 cm
√ usually confined to single quadrant
√ associated microcalcifications in 60%
√ multiple filling defects / disruption of an irregular duct segment / complete obstruction of duct system at galactography
US:
√ solid hypoechoic mass with lobulated smooth margins + acoustic enhancement
√ ± blood flow on color Doppler
Prognosis: 90% 5-year survival after simple mastectomy + axillary node dissection

DDx: solitary central duct papilloma; multiple peripheral benign papillomas

C. PAGET DISEASE OF THE NIPPLE (5%)

D. INFLAMMATORY BREAST CARCINOMA
= tumor emboli within dermal lymphatics
Prevalence: 1–4% of breast cancers
Age: 52 years (on average)
Histo: infiltrating ductal carcinoma
Location: L > R breast; bilaterality in 30–55%
- palpable tumor (63%)
- erythema of skin (13–64%)
- edema of skin (13%)
- nipple retraction (13%)
- palpable axillary adenopathy (up to 91%)

√ tumor mass ± malignant-type calcifications
√ diffusely increased breast density
√ stromal coarsening (50%)
√ thickening of Cooper ligaments
√ extensive skin thickening (71%)

Prognosis: 2% 5-year survival; median survival time of 7 months (untreated) + 18 months (after radical mastectomy)
DDx: breast abscess

Epidemiology Of Breast Cancer

Incidence:
2–5 breast cancers/1,000 women; in USA >142,000 new cases per year (of which 25,000 are in situ); 25% of all female malignancies
◊ One of 9 women will develop breast cancer during her life!
Age: 0.3–2% in women <30 years of age;
15% in women <40 years of age;
85% in women >30 years of age
Mortality: 43,000 deaths per year
◊ Death rate has remained stable for past 60 years!

Risk Factors (increasing risk):

A. DEMOGRAPHIC FACTORS
- increasing age (66% of cancers in women >50 years):

Age	Prevalence of Cancer	
25	5:100,000	1:19,608
40	80:100,000	1:1,250
45	1075:100,000	1:93
50	180:100,000	1:555
55	3030:100,000	1:33
60	240:100,000	1:416

Relative risk compared with woman of age 60:

30 years of age	0.07	60 years of age	1.00
35 years of age	0.19	70 years of age	1.27
40 years of age	0.35	80 years of age	1.45
50 years of age	0.71		

- Whites > Blacks after age 40
- Jewish women + nuns
- upper > lower social class
- unmarried > married women

B. REPRODUCTIVE VARIABLES
- nulliparous > parous

Relative risk compared with nulliparous:

age at 1st pregnancy	<19 years	0.5
age at 1st pregnancy	20–30 years	—
age at 1st pregnancy	30–34 years	1.0
age at 1st pregnancy	>35 years	>1.0

- first full-term pregnancy after age 35: 2 x risk
- low parity > high parity

- early age at menarche (<12 years)

Relative risk compared with onset of regular ovulatory cycle:

	menarche <12	menarche >12
immediately	3.7	1.6
1–4 years	2.3	1.6
>5 years	1.6	1.0

PREDICTIVE VALUES OF RADIOGRAPHIC SIGNS FOR MALIGNANCY	
1. Classic mammographic findings of malignancy + palpable abnormality (only 3% of cancers present this way)	100%
2. Classic mammographic findings of malignancy + NO palpable finding (only 6% of cancers present this way)	74%
3. Indeterminate mammographic features + palpable mass	11%
4. Indeterminate mass + no palpable finding	5%
5. Mammographically benign mass	2%
6. Asymmetric density (mass questionable) + clinical finding	4%
7. Asymmetric density (mass questionable) + NO clinical finding	0%
8. Microcalcifications + clinical abnormality	25%
9. Microcalcifications + NO clinical abnormality (>3 punctate irregular microcalcifications in area <1 cm^2)	21%
10. Vein dilatation	0%
11. Skin thickening	0%
12. Duct dilatation	0%

- late age at menopause
  Relative risk compared with menopause before age 44 years:
  natural menopause >55 years of age 2.0
- early bilateral oophorectomy
  Relative risk compared with menopause between ages 45–49 years:
  artificial menopause at 50–54 years 1.34
  artificial menopause before age 45 0.77

C. MULTIPLE PRIMARY CANCERS
- 4–5 x increase in risk for cancer in contralateral breast
- increased risk after ovarian + endometrial cancer

D. FAMILY HISTORY
- breast cancer in first-degree relative
  Relative risk compared with negative family Hx:
  (+) for mother 1.8
  (+) for sister 2.5
  (+) for mother + sister 5.6
- 25% of patients with carcinoma have a positive family history
- carcinoma tends to affect successive generations approx. 10 years earlier

E. BENIGN BREAST DISEASE
- 2–4 x increased risk with atypical hyperplasia
  Relative risk compared with no biopsy:
  benign breast disease in all patients 1.5
  nonproliferative disease 0.9
  proliferative disease without atypia 1.6
  fibroadenoma + hyperplasia 3.5
  atypical duct hyperplasia (ADH)
  no family history of breast cancer 4.4
  family history of breast cancer 8.9

F. MAMMOGRAPHIC FEATURES
- prominent duct pattern + extremely dense breasts according to Wolfe classification N1 (0.14%), P1 (0.52%), P2 (1.95%), DY (5.22%)

G. RADIATION EXPOSURE
excess risk of 3.5–6 cases per 1,000,000 women per year per rad after a minimum latent period of 10 years (atomic bomb, fluoroscopy during treatment of tuberculosis, irradiation for postpartum mastitis)

H. GEOGRAPHY
- Western + industrialized nations (highest incidence)
- Asia, Latin America, Africa (decreased risk)

Breast cancer evaluation

A. PRIMARY = LOCALIZING SIGNS OF BREAST CANCER
1. Dominant mass seen on two views with
   (a) *spiculation* = stellate / star-burst appearance (= fine linear strands of tumor extension + desmoplastic response); "scirrhus" caused by:
   (1) infiltrating ductal carcinoma (75% of all invasive cancers)
   (2) invasive lobular carcinoma (occasionally)
   √ mass feels larger than its mammographic / sonographic size
   DDx: prior biopsy / trauma / infection
   (b) *smooth border*
   (1) intracystic carcinoma (rare): subareolar area; bloody aspiration
   (2) medullary carcinoma: soft tumor
   (3) mucinous / colloid carcinoma: soft tumor
   (4) papillary carcinoma
   √ "telltale" signs: lobulation, small comet tail, flattening of one side of the lesion, slight irregularity
   √ halo sign (= Mach band) may be present
   DDx: cyst (sonographic evaluation)
   (c) *lobulation*
   Appearance similar to fibroadenoma (only characteristic calcifications may exclude malignancy)
   ◊ the likelihood of malignancy increases with number of lobulations
   - clinical size of mass > radiographic size (Le Borgne's law)

2. Asymmetric density = star-shaped lesion
   √ distinct central tumor mass with volumetric rather than planar appearance (additional coned compression views!)
   √ denser relative to other areas (= vessels + trabeculae cannot be seen within high-density lesion)
   √ fat does not traverse density
   √ corona of spicules
   √ in any quadrant (but fatty replacement occurs last in upper outer quadrant)
   DDx: postsurgical fibrosis, traumatic fat necrosis, sclerosing duct hyperplasia
3. Microcalcifications
   Associated with malignant mass by mammogram in 40%, pathologically with special stains in 60%, on specimen radiography in 86%
   ◊ 20% of clustered microcalcifications represent a malignant process!
   (a) *shape:* fragmented, irregular contour, polymorphic, casting rod-shaped without polarity, Y-shaped branching pattern, granular "salt and pepper" pattern, reticular pattern
   (b) *density:* various densities
   (c) *size:* 100–300 μ (usually); rarely up to 2 mm
   (d) *distribution:* tight cluster over an area of 1 cm^2 or less is most suggestive; coursing along ductal system seen in ductal carcinoma with comedo elements
4. Architectural distortion
   due to desmoplastic reaction
   √ ragged irregular border
   DDx: postsurgical fibrosis
5. Interval change
   (a) neodensity = de novo developing density (in 6% malignant)
   (b) enlarging mass (malignant in 10–15%)

BREAST

6. Enlarged single duct
   (low probability for cancer in asymptomatic woman with normal breast palpation)
   √ solitary dilated duct >3 cm long
   DDx: inspissated debris / blood, papilloma
7. Diffuse increase in density (late finding)
   Cause: (1) plugging of dermal lymphatics with tumor cells
   (2) less flattening of sclerotic + fibrous elements of neoplasm in comparison with more compressible fibroglandular breast tissue

B. SECONDARY = NONLOCALIZING SIGNS OF BREAST CANCER
1. Asymmetric thickening
2. Asymmetric ducts, especially if discontinuous with subareolar area
3. Skin changes
   (a) retraction = dimpling of skin from desmoplastic reaction causing shortening of Cooper ligaments / direct extension of tumor to skin
   DDx: trauma, biopsy, abscess, burns
   (b) skin thickening secondary to blocked lymphatic drainage / tumor in lymphatics
   • peau d'orange
   DDx: normal in inframammary region
4. Nipple / areolar abnormalities
   (a) retraction / flattening of nipple
   DDx: normal variant
   (b) Paget disease = eczematoid appearance of nipple + areola in ductal carcinoma
   √ associated with ductal calcifications toward the nipple
   DDx: nipple eczema
   (c) nipple discharge
   • spontaneous persistent discharge
   • need not be bloody
   DDx: lactational discharge
5. Abnormal veins
   venous diameter ratio of >1.4:1 in 75% of cancers; late sign + thus not very important
6. Axillary nodes (sign of advanced / occult cancer)
   √ >1.5 cm without fatty center
   DDx: reactive hyperplasia

LOCATION OF BREAST MASSES
benign + malignant masses are of similar distribution
@ upper outer quadrant (54%)
@ upper inner quadrant (14%)
@ lower outer quadrant (10%)
@ lower inner quadrant (7%)
@ retroareolar (15%)
◊ Mediolateral oblique view is important part of screening because it includes largest portion of breast tissue + considers most common location of cancers!

METASTATIC BREAST CANCER
@ Axillary lymph adenopathy
Incidence: 40–74%
Risk for positive nodes: 30% if primary >1 cm, 15% if primary <1 cm
@ Bone
@ Liver
Incidence: 48–60%
US: √ hypoechoic (83%) / hyperechoic (17%) masses

Screening Of Asymptomatic Patients

Definition of screening (World Health Organization):
A screening test must
(a) be adequately sensitive and specific
(b) be reproducible in its results
(c) identify previously undiagnosed disease
(d) be affordable
(e) be acceptable to the public
(f) include follow-up services

Guidelines of American Cancer Society, American College of Radiology, American Medical Association, National Cancer Institute:
1. Breast self-examination to begin at age 20
2. Breast examination by physician every 3 years between 20–40 years, in yearly intervals after age 40
3. Baseline mammogram between age 35–40; follow-up screening based upon parenchymal pattern + family history
4. Initial screening at 30 years if patient has first-degree relative with breast cancer in premenopausal years; follow-up screening based upon parenchymal pattern
5. Mammography at yearly intervals after age 40
6. All women who have had prior breast cancer require annual follow-up

Additional recommendations:
1. Baseline mammogram 10 years earlier than age of mother / sister when their cancer was diagnosed
2. Screening at 2-year intervals for women >70 years

Rate of detected abnormalities
30 abnormalities in 1,000 screening mammograms:
20–23 benign lesions
7–10 cancers

VALUE OF SCREENING MAMOGRAPHY
Indication:
decrease in cancer mortality through earlier detection + intervention when tumor size small + lymph nodes negative; tumor grade of no prognostic significance in tumors <10 mm in size

1. Health Insurance Plan (HIP) 1963–1969 randomized controlled study of 62,000 women aged 40–64
   - 25–30% reduction in mortality in women >50 years (followed for 18 years)
   - 25% reduction in mortality in women 40–49 years (followed for 18 years); no significant effect at 5- and 10-year follow-up
   - 19% of cancers found by mammography alone
   - 61% of cancers found at physical examination
   - effectiveness of screening <50 years of age is uncertain
2. Breast Cancer Detection Demonstration Project (BCDDP) 1973–1980
   4,443 cancers found in 283,000 asymptomatic volunteers
   - 41.6% of cancers found by mammography alone (77% with negative nodes)
   - 8.7% of cancers found by physical examination alone
   - 59% of noninfiltrating cancers found by mammography alone
   - 25% of cancers were intraductal (vs. 5% in previous series)
   - 21% of cancers found in women aged 40–49 years (mammography alone detected 35.4%)
3. Two-county Swedish trial 1977–1990
   randomized controlled study of 78,000 women in study group + 56,700 in control group aged 40–74 years
   (a) single MLO mammogram at 2-year intervals for women <50 years of age
   (b) single MLO mammogram at 3-year intervals for women ≥50 years of age
   - 40% reduction in mortality at 7 years in women 50–74 years
   - 0% reduction in mortality at 7 years in women 40–49 years

OCCULT VERSUS PALPABLE CANCERS

27% are occult cancers (NO age difference)

Positive axillary nodes: occult cancers (19%); palpable cancers (44%)

10-year survival: occult cancers (65%); palpable cancers (25%)

Role Of Mammography

Overall detection rate:

58–69%; 8% if <1 cm in size

Mammographic accuracy:

88% correctly diagnosed by radiologist
27% detected only by mammography
8% misinterpretations
4% not detected
15–30% positive predictive value (national average)

Mammographically Missed Cancers

False-negative screening mammogram = pathologic diagnosis of breast cancer within 1 year after negative mammogram with the following types of misses:

(a) lesion could not be seen in retrospect (25–33%) = "acute cancer" = cancer surfacing in screening interval
(b) cancer undetected by first reader but correctly identified by second reader (14%)
(c) visible in retrospect on prior mammogram (61%)

Incidence: approx. 10–25–30% of all cancers; approx. 3 cancers:2000 mammograms; 5–15–22% of palpable breast cancers

Cause:

1. Misinterpretation (52%):
   (a) benign appearance (18%): medullary carcinoma, colloid carcinoma, intracystic papillary carcinoma, some infiltrating ductal carcinomas
   (b) present on previous mammogram (17%)
   (c) seen on one view only (9%)
   (d) site of previous biopsy (8%)
2. Observer error (30–43%):
   overlooked, presence of obvious finding = "satisfied search" phenomenon, rushed interpretation, heavy caseload, extraneous distraction, eye fatigue
3. Technical error (5%):
   (a) poor image quality
   (b) failure to image region of interest
4. Tumor biology:
   (a) small tumor size
   (b) failure to incite desmoplastic reaction (eg, invasive lobular carcinoma)
   (c) masked by dense breast parenchyma
   (d) no associated microcalcifications (approx. 50% of cancers)
   (e) developing soft-tissue radiopacity

Location of missed cancers:

retroglandular area (33%), lateral parenchyma (31%), central (18%), medial (13%), subareolar (4%)

Radiation-induced Breast Carcinoma

◊ Lifetime risk with cumulative carcinogenic effect related to age!

(a) women age <35: 7.5 additional cancers per 1 million irradiated women per year per rad
(b) women age >35: 3.5 additional cancers per 1 million irradiated women per year per rad

Role Of Breast Ultrasound

Indications:

◊ Ultrasound is no screening tool!

A. TARGETED EXAM
   (1) initial study of palpable lump in patient <30 years of age / pregnant / lactating
   ◊ Ultrasound will not add useful information in an area that contains only fatty tissue on a mammogram!

BREAST

(2) characterization of mammographic / palpable mass as fluid-filled / solid
◊ Ultrasound will add useful information if there is water-density tissue in the area of palpable abnormality!
◊ Differentiation of cystic from solid lesion is the principal role of ultrasound!
(3) additional evaluation of nonpalpable abnormality with uncertain mammographic diagnosis
(4) search for focal lesion as cause for mammographic asymmetric density
(5) confirmation of lesion seen in one mammographic projection only

B. WHOLE-BREAST EXAM
(1) Breast secretions
(2) Suspected leaks from silicone implant
(3) Follow-up of multiple known mammographic / sonographic lesions
(4) Radiographically dense breast with strong family history of breast cancer
(5) Metastases thought to be of breast origin, but with negative clinical + mammographic exam
(6) Mammography not possible: "radiophobic" patient, bedridden patient, after mastectomy

C. INTERVENTINAL PROCEDURE
(1) Ultrasound-guided cyst aspiration
(2) Ultrasound-guided core biopsy
(3) Ultrasound-guided ductography, if
(a) secretions cannot be expressed
(b) duct cannot be cannulated

Accuracy: 98% accuracy for cysts; 99% accuracy for solid masses; small carcinomas have the least characteristic features

Role Of Breast MRI

Indications: ambiguous mammographic findings; positive clinical examination + negative mammographic/sonographic findings
Sensitivity: 72–93–100%
√ rapid enhancement reaching a markedly higher amplitude than parenchymal tissue
DDx: fibroadenoma in premenopausal patient, ductal hyperplasia ± atypia, lobular neoplasia, inflammatory disease, scar <6 months old in nonirradiated breast, scar <18 months old in irradiated breast, fibrocystic change (apocrine metaplasia, sclerosing adenosis)
√ intense early rim / peripheral enhancement (± central necrosis)
√ malignant mass margination

Role Of Stereotaxic Biopsy

Indications: obviously malignant nonpalpable lesion, indeterminate likely benign lesion, anxiety over lesion
Types: well-defined solid mass, indistinct / spiculated mass, clustered microcalcifications
Advantage: single-stage surgical procedure
Problematic: 3–5 mm small lesion, fine scattered microcalcifications, indistinct density, area of architectural distortion
Excision:
radial scar suspected (in up to 28% associated with tubular carcinoma), lesion close to chest wall, lesion in axillary tail, very superficial lesion, atypia / atypical hyperplasia (in 49–61% associated with malignancy), carcinoma in situ (in 9–20% associated with invasion), branching microcalcifications suggestive of DCIS with comedo necrosis
Sensitivity: 85–99% with core needle biopsy (100% specific), 68–93% with fine-needle aspiration (88–100% specific)
Miss rate: 3–8% for stereotaxic biopsy, 3% for surgery

BREAST CYST

Incidence: most common single cause of breast lumps between 35 and 55 years of age
Age: any; most common in later reproductive years + around menopause
Histo: cyst wall lined by single layer of
(a) flattened epithelial cells; cyst fluid with Na^+/K^+ ratio ≥3
(b) epithelial cells with apocrine metaplasia (secretory function); cyst fluid with Na^+/K^+ ratio <3
Cause: fluid cannot be absorbed due to obstruction of extralobular terminal duct by fibrosis / intraductal epithelial proliferation
• size changes over time

Simple Breast Cyst

√ well-defined flattened oval / round (if under pressure) mammographic mass + surrounding halo
(DDx: well-defined solid mass)
√ solitary / multiple
√ needle aspiration of fluid (proof) + postaspiration mammogram as new baseline

US (98–100% accuracy):
◊ Correlate with palpation / mammogram as to size, shape, location, surrounding tissue density!
√ spherical / ovoid lesion with anechoic center
√ well-circumscribed thin echogenic capsule
√ posterior acoustic enhancement (may be difficult to demonstrate in small / deeply situated cysts)
√ thin edge shadows
√ occasionally multilocular ± thin septations / cluster of cysts

PNEUMOCYSTOGRAPHY (for symptomatic cysts):
√ air remains mammographically detectable for up to 3 weeks
√ therapeutic effect of air insufflation (equal to 60–70% of aspirated fluid volume): no cyst recurrence in 85–94% (40–45% cyst recurrence without air insufflation)

Complex breast cyst

= any cyst that does not meet criteria of simple cyst

Cause: fibrocystic changes (vast majority), infection, malignancy (extremely rare)
◊ 0.3% of all breast cancers are intracystic

◊ Patients with apocrine cysts are at greater risk to develop breast cancer!

√ uniformly thick wall + tenderness = inflammation / infection

√ diffuse low-level internal echoes (= "foam" cyst)
(a) with mobility upon increase in power output = subcellular material like protein globs, floating cholesterol crystals, cellular debris
(b) without mobility upon increase in power output = cells like foamy macrophages, apocrine metaplasia, epithelial cells, pus, blood

√ fluid-debris level
Rx: aspiration to rule out blood / pus

√ thick septation / eccentric wall thickening further characterized by protruding ill-defined outer margin, convex microlobulated inner margin ("mural nodule"), nonmobile mass with coarse heterogeneous echotexture, CD flow within thickening
Rx: treated like solid nodule

√ spongelike cluster of microcysts
Rx: treated like solid nodule

Rx: complete aspiration (assures benign cause), core needle biopsy (if partially / nonaspiratable)

DDx: artifactual scatter in superficial / deep small cysts, fibroadenoma, papilloma, carcinoma

CYST ASPIRATION
- inspection of cyst fluid:
(a) normal: turbid greenish / grayish / black fluid
(b) abnormal: straw-colored clear fluid / dark blood

√ needle moves within nonaspiratable complex cyst
√ fluid without blood should be discarded
√ bloody fluid should be examined cytologically

CARCINOMA OF MALE BREAST

Incidence: 0.2%; 1,400 new cases/year with 300 deaths;
◊ 3.7% of male breast carcinomas occur in men with Klinefelter syndrome!

Peak age: 60–69 years

At risk: (males with increased estrogen levels)
1. Klinefelter syndrome (20-fold risk over normals): XXY chromosomes
2. Liver disease: cirrhosis, schistosomiasis, malnutrition
3. Radiation therapy to chest
4. Occupational heat exposure (diminished testicular function)
5. Testicular atrophy: injury, mumps-orchitis, undescended testis
6. Jewish background
7. Family history

◊ Gynecomastia is NOT a risk factor!

Histo: infiltrating ductal carcinoma

- firm painless retroareolar / upper-outer-quadrant mass
- breast swelling, bloody nipple discharge, retraction

Location: L >R breast; bilaterality is uncommon

√ resembles scirrhous carcinoma of female breast
√ usually located eccentrically
√ calcifications fewer + more scattered + more round + larger
√ enlarged axillary nodes (in 50% at time of presentation)
√ metastases to pleura, lung, bone, liver

Delay in diagnosis from onset of symptoms: 6–18 months

Rx: surgery, hormonal manipulation (85% estrogen receptor and 75% progesterone receptor positive)

Prognosis: 5-year survival rate for stage 1 = 82–100% for stage 2 = 44–77%, for stage 3 = 16–45%, stage 4 = 4–8% (not worse than for women!)

DDx: breast abscess, gynecomastia, epidermal inclusion cyst

CHRONIC ABSCESS OF BREAST

= COLD ABSCESS usually seen in lactating women
- fever, pain, increased WBC (clinical diagnosis)
- rapid response to antibiotics

Location: most commonly in central / subareolar area

√ ill-defined mass of increased density with flamelike contour
√ secondary changes common: architectural distortion, nipple + areolar retraction, lymphedema, skin thickening, pathologic axillary nodes
√ liquefied center can be aspirated

US:
√ anechoic / nearly anechoic area with posterior enhancement

CYSTOSARCOMA PHYLLODES

= GIANT FIBROADENOMA = ADENOSARCOMA
= PHYLLODE TUMOR
= usually benign giant form of intracanalicular fibroadenoma

Incidence: 1: 6,300 examinations; 0.3–1.5% of all breast tumors; 3% of all fibroadenomas

Age: 5th–6th decade (mean age of 45 years, occasionally in women <20 years of age

Histo: similar to fibroadenoma but with increased cellularity + pleomorphism (wide variations in size, shape, differentiation) of its stromal elements; fibroepithelial tumor with leaflike (phyllodes) growth pattern = branching projections of tissue into cystic cavities; cavernous structures contain mucus; cystic degeneration + hemorrhage

- rapidly enlarging breast mass; periods of remission
- sense of fullness
- huge, firm, mobile, discrete, lobulated, smooth mass
- discoloration of skin, wide veins, shining skin

√ large noncalcified mass with smooth polylobulated margins mimicking fibroadenoma
√ rapid growth to large size (>6–8 cm), may fill entire breast

US:
√ fluid-filled clefts in large tumors

Prognosis: limited invasion frequently seen; 15–20% recurrence rate if not completely excised

Cx: in 5–10% degeneration into malignant fibrous histiocytoma / fibrosarcoma / liposarcoma / chondrosarcoma / osteosarcoma with local invasion + hematogenous metastases to lung, pleura, bone (axillary metastases quite rare)

DERMATOPATHIC LYMPHADENOPATHY

= benign reactive lymphadenopathy within breast associated with cutaneous rashes

Cause: exfoliative dermatitis, erythroderma, psoriasis, atopic dermatitis, skin infection)

Histo: follicular pattern retained, germinal centers enlarged, enlarged paracortical area with pale-staining cells (lymphocytes, Langerhans cells, interdigitating reticulum cells)

• mobile nontender firm subcutaneous nodules

Location: often bilateral

Site: predominantly upper outer quadrant

√ regional subcentimeter masses with central / peripheral radiolucent notches

EPIDERMAL INCLUSION CYST

= benign cutaneous / subcutaneous lesion

Cause: congenital, metaplasia, trauma (needle biopsy, reduction mammoplasty), obstructed hair follicle

Path: cyst filled with keratin

Histo: stratified squamous epithelium

• smooth round nodule attached to skin with blackened pore, movable against underlying tissue

√ circumscribed round / oval iso- / high-density mass of 0.8–10.0 cm in diameter

√ may contain heterogeneous microcalcifications

US:

√ circumscribed hypoechoic solid mass extending into dermis

DDx: sebaceous cyst (epithelial cysts containing sebaceous glands)

FAT NECROSIS OF BREAST

= TRAUMATIC LIPID CYST = OIL CYST = aseptic saponification of fat by tissue lipase after local destruction of fat cells with release of lipids + hemorrhage + fibrotic proliferation

Etiology: direct external trauma, breast biopsy, reduction mammoplasty, irradiation, nodular panniculitis (Weber-Christian disease), ductal ectasia of chronic mastitis

Incidence: 0.5% of breast biopsies

Histo: cavity with oily material surrounded by "foam cells" (= lipid-laden macrophages)

• history of trauma in 40% (eg, prior surgery, radiation >6 months ago, reduction mammoplasty, lumpectomy)

• firm, slightly fixed mass

• skin retraction (50%)

• yellowish fatty fluid on aspiration

Location: anywhere; more common in areolar region; near biopsy site / surgical scar

√ ill-defined irregular spiculated dense mass (indistinguishable from carcinoma if associated with distortion, skin thickening, retraction)

√ well-circumscribed mass with translucent areas at center (= homogeneous fat density of oil cyst) surrounded by thin pseudocapsule (in old lesions)

√ calcifies in 4–7% (= **liponecrosis macrocystica calcificans**)

√ occasionally curvilinear / eggshell calcification in wall

√ fine spicules of low density vary with projection

√ localized skin thickening / retraction possible

US:

√ hypo- / anechoic mass with ill- / well-defined margins ± acoustic shadowing

√ complex cyst with mural nodules / echogenic bands

Weber-Christian disease

= nonsuppurative panniculitis with recurrent bouts of inflammation = areas of fat necrosis, involving subcutaneous fat + fat within internal organs

• accompanied by fever + nodules over trunk and limbs

FIBROADENOMA

= ADULT-TYPE FIBROADENOMA

= estrogen-induced benign tumor originating from TDLU; forms during adolescence; pregnancy + lactation are growth stimulants; regression after menopause (mucoid degeneration, hyalinization, involution of epithelial components, calcification)

Incidence: 3rd most common type of breast lesion after fibrocystic disease + carcinoma; most common benign solid tumor in women of childbearing age

Age: mean age of 30 years (range 13–80 years); median age 25 years; most common breast tumor under age 25 years

Hormonal influence:

slight enlargement at end of menstrual cycle + during pregnancy; regresses after menopause; may occur in postmenopausal women receiving estrogen replacement therapy

Histo: mixture of proliferated fibrous stroma + epithelial ductal structures

(a) intracanalicular fibroadenoma compressing ducts

(b) pericanalicular fibroadenoma without duct compression

(c) combination

• firm, smooth, sometimes lobulated, freely movable mass

• in 35% not palpable

• NO skin fixation

• rarely tender / painful

• clinical size = radiographic size

Size: 1–5 cm (in 60%); multiple in 15–25%; bilateral in 4%

√ circular / oval-shaped lesion of low density

√ nodular / lobulated contour when larger (areas with different growth rates)

√ smooth, discrete margins (indistinguishable from cysts when small)

√ often with "halo" sign

√ smoothly contoured calcifications of high + fairly equal density in 3% due to necrosis from regressive changes in older patients:
  (a) peripheral subcapsular myxoid degeneration
    √ peripheral marginal ringlike calcifications
  (b) central myxoid degeneration
    √ "popcorn" type of calcification (PATHOGNOMONIC)
  (c) calcifications within ductal elements
    √ pleomorphic linear ± branching pattern
  ◊ Calcifications enlarge as soft-tissue component regresses!

US:
  √ round (3%) / oval mass (96%) with length-to-depth ratio of >1.4 (in carcinomas usually <1.4)
  √ hypoechoic similar to fat lobules (80–96%) / hyperechoic / mixed pattern / anechoic / isoechoic compared with adjacent fibroglandular tissue
  √ homogeneous (48–89%) / inhomogeneous (12–52%) texture
  √ regular (57%) / lobulated (15–31%) / irregular (6–58%) contour
  √ "hump and dip" sign = small focal contour bulge immediately contiguous with a small sulcus (57%)
  √ intratumoral bright echoes (10%) = macrocalcifications

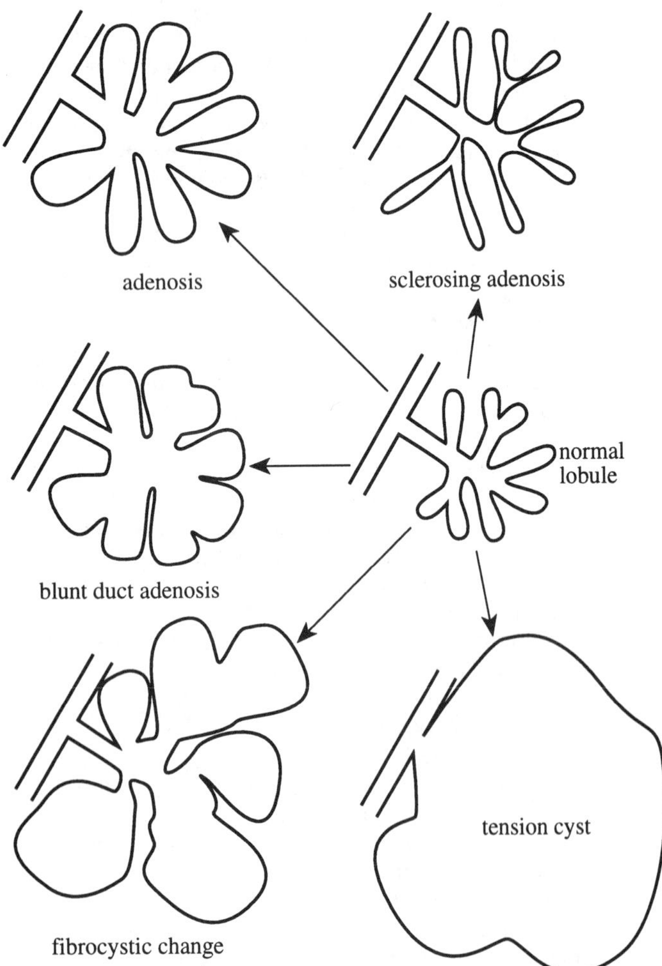

  √ posterior acoustic enhancement (17–25%) / acoustic shadow without calcifications (9–11%)
  √ echogenic halo (capsule) with lateral shadowing

Juvenile / Giant / Cellular Fibroadenoma

= fibroadenoma >5 cm in diameter / weighing >500 g

Cause: hyperplasia + distortion of normal breast lobules secondary to hormonal imbalances between estradiol + progesterone levels

Age: any (mostly in adolescent girls)

Histo: more glandular + more stromal cellularity than adult type of fibroadenoma; ductal epithelial hyperplasia

• rapidly enlarging well-circumscribed nontender mass
• dilated superficial veins, stretched skin

√ discrete mass with rounded borders

DDx: medullary / mucinous / papillary carcinoma / carcinoma within fibroadenoma

FIBROCYSTIC CHANGES

= Mazoplasia = mastitis fibrosa cystica = chronic cystic mastitis = cystic disease = generalized breast hyperplasia = desquamated epithelial hyperplasia = fibroadenomatosis = mammary dysplasia = Schimmelbusch disease = fibrous mastitis = mammary proliferative disease

◊ Not a disease since found in 72% of screening population >55 years of age

◊ The College of American Pathologists suggests to use the term "fibrocystic changes / condition" in mammography reports!

Incidence: most common diffuse breast disorder; in 51% of 3,000 autopsies

Age: 35–55 years

Etiology: exaggeration of normal cyclical proliferation + involution of the breast with production + incomplete absorption of fluid by apocrine cells

• asymptomatic in macrocystic disease
• fullness, tenderness, pain in microcystic disease
• palpable nodules + thickening
• symptoms occur with ovulation; regression with pregnancy + menopause

Histo:
  (1) overgrowth of fibrous connective tissue = stromal fibrosis, fibroadenoma
  (2) cystic dilatation of ducts + cyst formation (in 100% microscopic, in 20% macroscopic)
  (3) hyperplasia of ducts + lobules + acini = adenosis; ductal papillomatosis

√ individual round / ovoid cysts with discrete smooth margins
√ lobulated multilocular cyst
√ enlarged nodular pattern (= fluid-distended lobules + extensive extralobular fibrous connective tissue overgrowth)
√ "teacup-like" curvilinear thin calcifications with horizontal beam + low-density round calcifications in craniocaudal projection = milk of calcium (4%)

√ "oyster pearl–like" / psammoma-like calcifications
√ "involutional type" calcifications = very fine punctate calcifications evenly distributed within one / more lobes against a fatty background (from mild degree of hyperplasia in subsequently atrophied glandular tissue)

US:
√ ductal pattern, ductectasia, cysts, ill-defined focal lesions

Risk for Invasive Breast Carcinoma

A. NO INCREASED RISK
   1. Nonproliferative lesions: adenosis, florid adenosis, apocrine metaplasia without atypia, macro- / microcysts, duct ectasia, fibrosis, mild hyperplasia (more than 2 but not more than 4 epithelial cells deep), mastitis, periductal mastitis, squamous metaplasia
   2. Fibroadenoma
B. SLIGHTLY INCREASED RISK (1.5–2 times):
   1. Moderate + florid solid / papillary hyperplasia
   2. Papilloma with fibrovascular core
   3. Sclerosing adenosis
C. MODERATELY INCRAESED RISK (5 times): Ductal / lobular atypical hyperplasia (borderline lesion with some features of carcinoma in situ)
D. HIGH RISK (8–11 times):
   1. Atypical hyperplasia + family history of breast cancer
   2. Ductal / lobular carcinoma in situ

Adenosis

= hyperplasia + hypertrophy of glandular elements
√ increase in size of lobules to 3–7 mm
√ "snowflake pattern" of widespread ill-defined nodular densities
√ adenosis lobules are sonographically iso- to mildly hypoechoic compared with fat

Sclerosing Adenosis

= adenosis + reactive fibrosis = proliferating acinar structure maintaining a lobular configuration
√ adenosis + diffusely scattered calcifications (calcifications in cystically dilated acinar structure)
√ diffusely dense breast
√ focally dense breast appearing as a nodule / spiculated lesion

Fibrosis

√ round / oval clustered microcalcifications with smooth contours + associated fine granular calcifications filling lobules

Atypical Lobular Hyperplasia

= proliferation of round cells of LCIS type growing along terminal ducts in permeative fashion (pagetoid growth) between benign epithelium + basal myoepithelium BUT NOT completely obliterating terminal ductal lumina / distending lobules (as in lobular carcinoma in situ)
√ no mammographic correlate

Atypical Ductal Hyperplasia

= low-grade intraductal proliferation with partial / incompletely developed features of noncomedo DCIS
√ frequent calcifications

Intraductal Papillomatosis

= hyperplastic polypoid lesions within a duct
Age: perimenopausal
• spontaneous bloody / serous / serosanguinous nipple discharge (most common cause of nipple discharge)
√ small retroareolar opacity (= dilated duct) extending 2–3 cm into breast
√ intraluminal filling defect on galactography

GALACTOCELE

= retention of fatty material in areas of cystic duct dilatation appearing during / shortly after lactation
Cause: ? abrupt suppression of lactation
Age: occurs during / shortly after lactation
• thick inspissated milky fluid (colostrum)
Location: retroareolar area
√ large radiopaque lesion of water density (1st phase)
√ smaller lesion of mixed density + fat-water level with horizontal beam (2nd phase)
√ small radiolucent lesion resembling lipoma
√ ± fluid-calcium level

GRANULAR CELL TUMOR

= GRANULAR CELL MYOBLASTOMA OF BREAST
= benign tumor, occasionally locally invasive + metastasizing
Origin: ? Schwann cell, smooth muscle, or undifferentiated mesenchymal cell
Prevalence: 1:1,000 primary breast carcinomas
Age : 20–59 (mean 35) years; more common in Blacks
Histo: rounded groups of large cells with small dark regular nuclei + abundant eosinophilic granular cytoplasm; not immunoreactive to cytokeratin + epithelial membrane antigen BUT to S-100 protein
DDx: carcinoma, lymphoma, metastasis
◊ Fine-needle aspirate may be difficult to interpret!
Location: tongue, skin, bronchial wall, subcutaneous breast tissue (6–8%)
Site: more commonly <u>other than</u> upper outer quadrant
• asymmetric lump with slow growth, hardness, skin fixation / retraction, ulceration
• often fixed to pectoralis fascia
√ well-circumscribed spiculated mass 1–3 cm in diameter
√ stellate extensions (tumor insinuating itself into surrounding breast tissue)
√ may exhibit acoustic shadow
Rx: wide local excision

GYNECOMASTIA

Cause:
(1) Hormonal
   (a) puberty: high estradiol levels
   (b) older men: decline in serum testosterone levels

(c) hypogonadism (Klinefelter syndrome, testicular neoplasm)
(d) tumors: adrenal carcinoma, pituitary adenoma, testicular tumor, hyperthyroidism
(2) Systemic disorders
advanced alcoholic cirrhosis, hemodialysis in chronic renal failure, chronic pulmonary disease (emphysema, TB), malnutrition
(3) Drug-induced
estrogen treatment for prostate cancer, digitalis, cimetidine, thiazide, spironolactone, reserpine, isoniazid, ergotamine, marijuana
(4) Neoplasm: hepatoma (with estrogen production)
(5) Idiopathic
mnemonic: "CODES"
Cirrhosis
Obesity
Digitalis
Estrogen
Spironolactone

Incidence: 85% of all male breast masses
Age: adolescent boys (40%), men >50 years (32%)
Histo: increased number of ducts, proliferation of duct epithelium, periductal edema, fibroplastic stroma, adipose tissue
• palpable firm mass >2 cm in subareolar region
Location: bilateral (63%), left-sided (27%), right-sided (10%)
√ mild prominence of subareolar ducts in flame-shaped distribution (focal type)
√ homogeneously dense breast (diffuse type)
DDx: pseudogynecomastia (= fatty proliferation)

HAMARTOMA OF BREAST

= FIBROADENOLIPOMA = LIPOFIBROADENOMA
= ADENOLIPOMA
Incidence: 2–16:10,000 mammograms
Mean age: 45 (27–88) years
Histo: normal / dysplastic mammary tissue composed of dense fibrous tissue + variable amount of fat, delineated from surrounding tissue without a true capsule
• soft, often nonpalpable (60%)
Location: retroareolar (30%),
upper outer quadrant (35%)
√ round / ovoid well-circumscribed mass usually > 3 cm
√ mixed density with mottled center (secondary to fat) = "slice of sausage" pattern
√ thin smooth pseudocapsule (= thin layer of surrounding fibrous tissue)
√ peripheral radiolucent zone
√ may contain calcifications
DDx: liposarcoma, Cowden disease

HEMATOMA OF BREAST

Cause: (1) surgery / biopsy (most common)
(2) blunt trauma
(3) coagulopathy (leukemia, thrombocytopenia)
(4) anticoagulant therapy

√ well-defined ovoid mass (= hemorrhagic cyst)
√ ill-defined mass with diffuse increased density (edema + hemorrhage)
√ adjacent skin thickening / prominence of reticular structures
√ regression within several weeks leaving (a) no trace (b) architectural distortion (c) incomplete resolution
√ calcifications (occasionally)
US:
√ hypoechoic mass with internal echoes

JUVENILE PAPILLOMATOSIS

Path: many aggregated cysts with interspersed dense stroma
Histo: cysts lined by flat duct epithelium / epithelium with apocrine metaplasia, sclerosing adenosis, duct stasis; marked papillary hyperplasia of duct epithelium with often extreme atypia
Mean age: 23 years (range of 12–48 years)
• localized palpable tumor
• family history of breast cancer in 28% (affected first-degree relative in 8%; in one / more relatives in 28%)
Prognosis: development of synchronous (4%) / metachronous (4%) breast cancer after 8–9 years.
DDx: fibroadenoma

LACTATING ADENOMA

= newly discovered painless mass during 3rd trimester of pregnancy / in lactating woman
Etiology: ? variant of fibroadenoma / tubular adenoma / lobular hyperplasia or de novo neoplasm
Path: well-circumscribed yellow spherical mass with lobulated surface + rubbery firm texture and without capsule
Histo: secretory lobules lined by granular and foamy to vacuolated cytoplasm + separated by delicate connective tissue
• firm freely movable painless mass
√ homogeneously hypoechoic / isoechoic mass
√ posterior acoustic enhancement (most) / shadowing
√ fibrous septa
Prognosis: regression after completion of breast feeding
DDx: breast carcinoma (1:1,300–1:6,200 pregnancies)

LIPOMA OF BREAST

= usually solitary asymptomatic slow-growing lesion
Mean age: 45 years + postmenopause
• soft, freely movable, well delineated
√ usually >2 cm
√ radiolucent lesion easily seen in dense breast; almost invisible in fatty breast
√ discrete thin radiopaque line (= capsule), seen in most of its circumference
√ displacement of adjacent breast parenchyma
√ calcification with fat necrosis (extremely rare)
DDx: fat lobule surrounded by trabeculae / suspensory ligaments

LYMPHOMA OF BREAST

A. Primary lymphoma: 0.05–0.53% prevalence
B. Metastatic lymphoma

Histo: large cell type NHL (majority), Hodgkin disease, leukemia, plasmacytoma
Age: 50–60 years; M < F
Location: right-sided predominance; 13% bilateral
√ round / oval mass
√ infiltrate with poorly defined borders
√ skin thickening
√ axillary nodes involved in 35%

PSEUDOLYMPHOMA
= lymphoreticular lesion as an overwhelming response to trauma

MAMMARY DUCT ECTASIA

= PLASMA CELL MASTITIS = VARICOCELE TUMOR OF BREAST = MASTITIS OBLITERANS
= COMEDOMASTITIS = PERIDUCTAL MASTITIS
= SECRETORY DISEASE OF BREAST
= rare aseptic inflammation of subareolar area

Pathogenesis (speculative):
(1) Stasis of intraductal secretion leads to duct dilatation + leakage of inspissated material into parenchyma giving rise to an aseptic chemical mastitis (periductal mastitis); the extravasated material is rich in fatty acids = nontraumatic fat necrosis
(2) Periductal inflammation causes damage to elastic lamina of duct wall resulting in duct dilatation

Histo: ductal ectasia, heavily calcified ductal secretions; infiltration of plasma cells + giant cells + eosinophils
Mean age: 54 years
• often asymptomatic
• breast pain, nipple discharge, nipple retraction, mamillary fistula, subareolar breast mass

Location: subareolar, often bilateral + symmetric; may be unilateral + focal
√ dense triangular mass with apex toward nipple
√ distended ducts connecting to nipple
√ periphery blending with normal tissue
√ multiple often bilateral dense round / oval calcifications with lucent center + polarity (= orientation toward nipple)
(a) periductal
√ oval / elongated calcified ring around dilated ducts with very dense periphery (surrounding deposits of fibrosis + fat necrosis)
(b) intraductal
√ fairly uniform linear, often "needle-shaped" calcifications of wide caliber, occasionally branching (within ducts / confined to duct walls)
√ nipple retraction / skin thickening may occur
Sequela: cholesterol granuloma
DDx: breast cancer

MAMMOPLASTY

= COSMETIC BREAST SURGERY

Augmentation Mammoplasty

Most frequently performed plastic surgery in U.S.
Frequency: 150,000 procedures in 1993 (80% for cosmesis, 20% for reconstruction); 2 million American women have breast implants (estimate)

Methods:
1. Injection augmentation (no longer practiced): paraffin, silicone, fat from liposuction
   Cx: tissue necrosis resulting in dense, hard, tender breast masses
2. Implants
   (a) spongelike masses of Ivalon, Etrheron, Teflon
   (b) Silicone elastomer (silastic) smooth / textured shell containing silicone gel / saline: >100 varieties
   — single lumen of polymerized methyl polysiloxane with smooth / textured outer silicone shell / polyurethane coating
   — double lumen with inner core of silicone + outer chamber of saline
   — triple lumen
   (c) expandable implant ± intraluminal valves = saline injection into port with gradual tissue expansion for breast reconstruction
   Location: retroglandular / subpectoral
3. Autogenous tissue transplantation (for breast reconstruction) with musculocutaneous flaps: transverse rectus abdominis muscle (TRAM), latissimus dorsi, tensor fascia lata, gluteus maximus

Mammographic technique for implants:
1. Two standard views (CC and MLO views) for most posterior breast tissue
   ◊ 22–83% of fibroglandular breast tissue obscured by implant depending on size of breast + location of implant + degree of capsular contraction on standard views!
   ◊ The false-negative rate of mammography increases from 10–20% to 41% in patients with implants!
2. Two Eklund (= implant displacement) views (CC and 90° LAT views) for compression views of anterior breast tissue = "push-back" view = breast tissue pulled anteriorly in front of implant while implant is pushed posteriorly + superiorly thus excluding most of the implant

Cx of silicone-gel–filled implant:
1. Capsular fibrosis, calcification, contracture (15–50%): more frequent with retroglandular implants
   • distortion of breast contour with hard capsule
   √ crenulated contour (US helpful)
   √ capsular calcifications at periphery of prosthesis
   √ fibrous capsule delineated by US (unleaked silicone is echolucent)

2. Implant migration
   Cause: overdistension of implant pocket at surgery

3. Rupture of prosthesis
   Prevalence: >50% after 12 years
   • change in contour / location of implant
   • flattening of implant
   • breast pain

   A. INTRACAPSULAR RUPTURE (more common)
   = broken implant casing with silicone leakage contained by intact fibrous capsule
   Mammo (11–23% sensitive, 89–98% specific):
   √ bulging / peaking of implant contour

   US (59–70% sensitive, 57–92% specific, 49% accurate):
   √ "stepladder" sign = series of parallel horizontal echogenic straight / curvilinear lines inside implant (= collapsed implant shell floating within silicone gel)
   √ heterogeneous aggregates of low- to medium-level echogenicity (65% sensitive, 57% specific)
   N.B.: visualization of internal lumen within anechoic space in double-lumen implants can be confused on US with intracapsular rupture

   MR (81–94% sensitive, 93–97% specific, 84% accurate):
   √ "linguine" sign = multiple hypointense wavy lines within implant (= pieces of free-floating collapsed envelope surrounded by silicone gel)
   √ "inverted teardrop" / "noose" / "keyhole" / "lariat (= lasso)" sign = loop-shaped hypointense structure contiguous with implant envelope (= small focal invagination of shell with silicone on either side)
   √ = infolded polyurethane coat of a single lumen prosthesis
   √ hypointense subcapsular lines paralleling the fibrous capsule (= minimally displaced ruptured shell as early sign) (DDx: phase-encoding artifact caused by motion)

   B. EXTRACAPSULAR RUPTURE
   = extrusion + migration of silicone droplets through tear in both implant + overlying fibrous capsule
   • palpable breast masses
   • paresthesia of arm (from nerve impingement secondary to fibrosis surrounding silicone migrated to axilla / brachial plexus)
   • silicone nipple discharge (rare)
   √ silicone droplets in breast
   √ axillary silicone lymphadenopathy
   US:
   √ "snowstorm" pattern = markedly hyperechoic nodule with well-defined anterior but indistinct posterior margin and intense shadowing echogenic noise (= free silicone droplets mixing with breast tissue)
   √ occasionally "dirty" complex cyst (= larger collection of free silicone)

   (c) "gel bleed" = leakage of silicone through porous but intact implant gel

4. Localized pain / paresthesia
5. ? development of autoimmune disorders (eg, scleroderma, lupus erythematosus)
6. Infection / hematoma formation

Reduction Mammoplasty
√ swirled architectural distortion (in inferior breast best seen on mediolateral view)
√ postsurgical distortion
√ residual isolated islands of breast tissue
√ fat necrosis
√ dystrophic calcifications
√ asymmetric tissue oriented in nonanatomic distribution

MASTITIS

Puerperal Mastitis
= usually interstitial infection during lactational period
  (a) through infected nipple cracks
  (b) hematogenous
  (c) ascending via ducts = galactophoritis

Organism: staphylococcus, streptococcus
• tender swollen red breast (DDx: inflammatory carcinoma)
• enlarged painful axillary lymph nodes
• ± febrile, elevated ESR, leukocytosis
√ diffuse increased density
√ diffuse skin thickening
√ swelling of breast
√ enlarged axillary lymph nodes
√ rapid resolution under antibiotic therapy

Nonpuerperal Mastitis
1. Infected cyst
2. Purulent mastitis with abscess formation
3. Plasma cell mastitis
4. Nonspecific mastitis

Granulomatous Mastitis
1. Foreign-body granuloma
2. Specific disease (TB, sarcoidosis, leprosy, syphilis, actinomycosis, typhus)
3. Parasitic disease (hydatid disease, cysticercosis, filariasis, schistosomiasis)

METASTASES TO BREAST
Incidence: 1%
Mean age: 43 years

Primaries: leukemia / lymphoma > malignant melanoma > ovarian carcinoma > lung cancer > sarcoma
◊ In up to 40% no known history of primary cancer!

√ solitary mass (85%), esp. in upper outer quadrant
√ multiple masses
√ skin adherence (25%) ± skin thickening
√ axillary node involvement (40%)

PAGET DISEASE OF THE NIPPLE

= uncommon manifestation of breast cancer

• eczemalike scaling + excoriation of nipple and areola
• nipple discharge + itching

Histo: Paget cell = large pleomorphic cells with pale cytoplasm invading the epidermis; histologically + biologically similar to comedocarcinoma

Associated with:
extensive invasive / noninvasive ductal carcinoma limited to one duct in subareolar area / remote + multicentric

√ negative mammogram in 50%
√ nipple / areolar thickening
√ dilated duct
√ linearly distributed microcalcifications
√ retroareolar soft-tissue mass

Prognosis: similar to infiltrating duct carcinoma

PAPILLOMA OF BREAST

= usually benign proliferation of ductal epithelial tissue

Age: 30–77 years (juvenile papillomatosis = 20–26 years)

Histo: hyperplastic proliferation of ductal epithelium; lesion may be pedunculated / broad-based; connective tissue stalk covered by epithelial cells proliferating in the form of apocrine metaplasia / solid hyperplasia may cause duct obstruction + distension to form an intracystic papilloma

DDx: invasive papillary carcinoma

Central solitary papilloma

Location: subareolar within major duct

NOT premalignant

• spontaneous bloody / serous / clear nipple discharge (52–100%)
◊ Most common cause of serous / sanguinous nipple discharge!
• "trigger point" = nipple discharge produced upon compression of area with papilloma
• intermittent mass disappearing with discharge

√ negative mammogram / intraductal nodules in subareolar area
√ asymmetrically dilated single duct
√ subareolar amorphous coarse calcifications
√ dilated duct with obstructing / distorting intraluminal filling defect on ductography (= galactography)

Cx: 0–14% frequency of carcinoma development

Peripheral multiple papillomas

Location: within terminal ductal lobular unit; bilateral in up to 14%

In 10–38% associated with:
atypical ductal hyperplasia, lobular carcinoma in situ, papillary + cribriform intraductal cancers, radial scar

• nipple discharge (20%)

√ round / oval / slightly lobulated well-circumscribed nodules
√ segmental distribution with dilated ducts extending from beneath the nipple (20%)
√ may be associated with coarse microcalcifications

Cx: 5% frequency of carcinoma development; increased risk dependent on degree of cellular atypia

Prognosis: in 24% recurrence after surgical treatment

RADIAL SCAR

= SCLEROSING DUCT HYPERPLASIA = INDURATIVE MASTOPATHY = FOCAL FIBROUS DISEASE
= BENIGN SCLEROSING DUCTAL PROLIFERATION
= NONENCAPSULATED SCLEROSING LESION
= INFILTRATING EPITHELIOSIS

= benign proliferative breast lesion (malignant potential is controversial); "scar" = fibroelastic center with surrounding stellate proliferation of contracted ducts + lobules

Incidence: 1–2/1,000 screening mammograms; in 2–16% of mastectomy specimens

Path: entrapped tubules in sclerotic center surrounded by a corona of contracted ducts + lobules (sclerosing adenosis) and papillomatosis

Histo: central core of elastosis (= acellular connective tissue and abundant deposits of elastin); one / more ducts obliterated by connective tissue

May be associated with: tubular carcinoma, comedo carcinoma, invasive lobular carcinoma + contralateral breast cancer

◊ Avoid frozen section!

• rarely palpable

√ mean diameter of 0.33 cm (range, 0.1–0.6 cm)
√ irregular noncalcified mass often with architectural distortion
√ variable appearance in different projections
√ oval / circular translucent areas at center
√ very thin long spicules, clumped together centrally
√ radiolucent linear structures paralleling spicules
√ no skin thickening / retraction

Rx: surgical excision required for definite diagnosis

DDx: carcinoma, postsurgical scar, fat necrosis, fibromatosis, granular cell myoblastoma

SARCOMA OF BREAST

Incidence: 1% of malignant mammary lesions

Age: 45–55 years

Histo: fibrosarcoma, rhabdomyosarcoma, osteogenic sarcoma, mixed malignant tumor of the breast, malignant fibrosarcoma and carcinoma, liposarcoma

• rapid growth
√ smooth / lobulated large dense mass
√ well-defined outline
√ palpated size similar to mammographic size

Angiosarcoma

= highly malignant vascular breast tumor

Incidence: 200 cases in world literature; 0.04% of all malignant breast tumors; 8% of all breast sarcomas

Age: 3rd–4th decade of life

Histo: hyperchromatic endothelial cells; network of communicating vascular spaces
- stage I: cells with large nucleoli
- stage II: endothelial lining displaying tufting + intraluminal papillary projections
- stage III: mitoses, necrosis, marked hemorrhage

Metastasis: hematogenous spread to lung, skin, subcutaneous tissue, bone, liver, brain, ovary; NOT lymphatic

• rapidly enlarging painless immobile breast mass
√ skin thickening + nipple retraction
√ large solitary mass with ill-defined nonspiculated border

US:
√ well-defined multilobulated hypoechoic mass with hyperechoic areas (from hemorrhage)

Prognosis: 1.9–2.1 years mean survival; 14% overall 3-year survival rate

Rx: simple mastectomy without axillary lymph node dissection

DDx: phyllodes tumor, lactating breast, juvenile hypertrophy
◊ Frequently misdiagnosed as lymphangioma / hemangioma!

DIFFERENTIAL DIAGNOSIS OF CARDIOVASCULAR DISORDERS

CONGENITAL HEART DISEASE

Classification of CHD

	Acyanotic	Cyanotic
Increased PBF + increased CT ratio	*L-R shunts* VSD ASD PDA ECD PAPVR	*T-lesions* Transposition Truncus arteriosus TAPVR "Tingles" (single ventricle / atrium) Tricuspid atresia (without RVOT obstruction)
Normal PBF + normal CT ratio	*LV outflow obstruction* AS Coarctation Interrupted aortic arch Hypoplastic left heart PS *LV inflow obstruction* Obstructed TAPVR Cor triatriatum Pulmonary vein atresia Congenital MV stenosis *Muscle disease* Cardiomyopathy Myocarditis Anomalous LCA	
Decreased PBF + normal CT ratio Cardiomegaly		*VSD present* Tetralogy of Fallot Tricuspid atresia (with PS + nonrestrictive ASD) Pulmonary atresia + VSD *Intact ventricular septum*

Incidence of CHD in liveborn infants

Overall incidence: 8–9:1000 livebirths

- most common CHD: mitral valve prolapse (5–20%), bicuspid aortic valve (2%) [usually not recognized before late infancy / childhood]
- ASD + VSD + PDA account for 45% of all CHD
- 12 lesions account for 89% of all CHD

Ventricular septal defect	30.3%
Patent ductus arteriosus	8.6%
Pulmonary stenosis	7.4%
Septum secundum defect	6.7%
Coarctation of aorta	5.7%
Aortic stenosis	5.2%
Tetralogy of Fallot	5.1%
Transposition	4.7%
Endocardial cushion defect	3.2%
Hypoplastic right ventricle	2.2%
Hypoplastic left heart	1.3%
TAPVR	1.1%
Truncus arteriosus	1.0%
Single ventricle	0.3%
Double outlet right ventricle	0.2%

High-risk pregnancy:
(1) Previous sibling with CHD: 2– 5%
(2) Previous 2 siblings with CHD: 10–15%
(3) One parent with CHD: 2–10%

Most common causes for CHF + PVH in neonate:
1. Left ventricular failure due to outflow obstruction
2. Obstruction of pulmonary venous return

CHD With Relatively Long Life

Congenital lesions compatible with a relative long life are:
1. Mild tetralogy: mild pulmonic stenosis + small VSD
2. Valvular pulmonic stenosis: with relatively normal pulmonary circulation
3. Transposition of great vessels: some degree of pulmonic stenosis + large VSD
4. Truncus arteriosus: delicate balance between systemic + pulmonary circulation
5. Truncus arteriosus type IV: large systemic collaterals
6. Tricuspid atresia + transposition + pulmonic stenosis
7. Eisenmenger complex
8. Ebstein anomaly
9. Corrected transposition without intracardiac shunt

Juxtaposition Of Atrial Appendages

1. Tricuspid atresia with transposition
2. Complete transposition
3. Corrected transposition of great arteries
4. DORV

Continuous Heart Murmur

1. PDA
2. AP window
3. Ruptured sinus of Valsalva aneurysm
4. Hemitruncus
5. Coronary arteriovenous fistula

Congestive Heart Failure & Cardiomegaly

mnemonic: "Ma McCae & Co."

Myocardial infarction
anemia
Malformation
cardiomyopathy
Coronary artery disease
aortic insufficiency
effusion
Coarctation

Congenital Cardiomyopathy

mnemonic: "CAVE G"

Cystic medial necrosis of coronary arteries
Aberrant left coronary artery
Viral
Endocardial fibroelastosis
Glycogen storage disease (Pompe)

Neonatal Cardiac Failure

A. OBSTRUCTIVE LESIONS
   1. Coarctation of the aorta
   2. Aortic valve stenosis
   3. Asymmetrical septal hypertrophy / hypertrophic obstructive cardiomyopathy
B. VOLUME OVERLOAD
   1. Congenital mitral valve incompetence
   2. Corrected transposition with left (= tricuspid) AV valve incompetence
   3. Congenital tricuspid insufficiency
   4. Ostium primum ASD
C. MYOCARDIAL DYSFUNCTION / ISCHEMIA
   1. Nonobstructive cardiomyopathy
   2. Anomalous origin of LCA from pulmonary trunk
   3. Primary endocardial fibroelastosis
   4. Glycogen storage disease (Pompe disease)
   5. Myocarditis
D. NONCARDIAC LESIONS
   1. AV fistulas: hemangioendothelioma of liver, AV fistula of brain, vein of Galen aneurysm, large pulmonary AV fistula

Presenting Age In CHD

AGE	SEVERE PVH	PVH + SHUNT VASCULARITY
0 – 2 days	Hypoplastic left heart Aortic atresia TAPVR below diaphragm Myocardiopathy in IDM	Hypoplastic left heart TAPVR above diaphragm Complete transposition
3 – 7 days		PDA in preterm infant
7 – 14 days	CoA + VSD / PDA Aortic valve stenosis Peripheral AVM Endocardial fibroelastosis Anomalous left coronary artery	Coarctation of aorta (CoA) AVM

2. Transient tachypnea of the newborn
3. Intraventricular / subarachnoid hemorrhage
4. Neonatal hypoglycemia (low birth weight, infants of diabetic mothers)
5. Thyrotoxicosis (transplacental passage of LATS hormone)

Syndromes With CHD

5 p – (Cri-du-chat) Syndrome
Incidence of CHD: 20%

DiGeorge Syndrome
= congenital absence of thymus + parathyroid glands
1. Conotruncal malformation
2. Interrupted aortic arch

Down Syndrome = MONGOLISM = TRISOMY 21
1. Endocardial cushion defect (25%)
2. Membranous VSD
3. Ostium primum ASD
4. AV communis
5. Cleft mitral valve
6. PDA
7. 11 rib pairs (25%)
8. Hypersegmented manubrium (90%)

Ellis-van Creveld Syndrome
Incidence of CHD: 50%
- polydactyly
- √ single atrium

Holt-Oram Syndrome
= UPPER LIMB-CARDIAC SYNDROME
Incidence of CHD: 50%
1. ASD
2. VSD
3. Valvular pulmonary stenosis
4. Radial dysplasia

Hurler Syndrome
Cardiomyopathy

Ivemark Syndrome
Incidence of CHD: 100%
- asplenia
- √ complex cardiac anomalies

Klippel-Feil Syndrome
Incidence of CHD: 5%
1. Atrial septal defect
2. Coarctation

Marfan Syndrome = ARACHNODACTYLY
1. Aortic sinus dilatation
2. Aortic aneurysm
3. Aortic insufficiency
4. Pulmonary aneurysm

Noonan Syndrome
1. Pulmonary stenosis
2. ASD
3. Hypertrophic cardiomyopathy

Osteogenesis Imperfecta
1. Aortic valve insufficiency
2. Mitral valve insufficiency
3. Pulmonic valve insufficiency

Postrubella Syndrome
- low birth weight
- deafness
- cataracts
- mental retardation

1. Peripheral pulmonic stenosis
2. Valvular pulmonic stenosis
3. Supravalvular aortic stenosis
4. PDA

Trisomy 13–15
VSD, tetralogy of Fallot, DORV

Trisomy 16–18
VSD, PDA, DORV

Turner Syndrome (XO) = OVARIAN DYSGENESIS
Incidence of CHD: 35%
1. Coarctation of the aorta (in 15%)
2. Bicuspid aortic valve
3. Dissecting aneurysm of aorta

Williams Syndrome = IDIOPATHIC HYPERCALCEMIA
- peculiar elfinlike facies
- mental + physical retardation
- hypercalcemia (not in all patients)

1. Supravalvular aortic stenosis (33%)
2. ASD, VSD
3. Valvular + peripheral pulmonary artery stenosis
4. Aortic hypoplasia, stenoses of more peripheral arteries

SHUNT EVALUATION

Evaluation Of L-to-R Shunts
A. AGE
- Infants:
  (1) Isolated VSD
  (2) VSD with CoA / PDA / AV canal
  (3) PDA
  (4) Ostium primum
- Children / adults:
  (1) ASD
  (2) Partial AV canal with competent mitral valve
  (3) VSD / PDA with high pulmonary resistance
  (4) PDA without murmur

B. SEX
99% chance for ASD / PDA in female patient

HEART

C. CHEST WALL ANALYSIS
   √ 11 pair of ribs + hypersegmented manubrium: Down syndrome
   √ pectus excavatum + straight back: prolapsing mitral valve
D. CARDIAC SILHOUETTE
   √ absent pulmonary trunk: corrected transposition with VSD; pink tetralogy
   √ left-sided ascending aorta: corrected transposition with VSD
   √ tortuous descending aorta: aortic valve incompetence + ASD
   √ huge heart: persistent complete AV canal (PCAVC); VSD + PDA; VSD + mitral valve incompetence
   √ enlarged left atrium: intact atrial septum; mitral regurgitation (endocardial cushion defect, prolapsing mitral valve + ASD)

DIFFERENTIAL DIAGNOSIS OF L-R SHUNTS

	RA	RV	PA	LA	LV	Prox. Ao
ASD	inc	inc	inc	nl	nl	nl
VSD	nl	inc	inc	inc	inc	nl
PDA	nl	nl	inc	inc	inc	often inc

Shunt With Normal Left Atrium

A. PRECARDIAC SHUNT
   1. Anomalous pulmonary venous connection
B. INTRACARDIAC SHUNT
   1. ASD (8%)
   2. VSD (25%)
C. POSTCARDIAC SHUNT
   1. PDA (12%)

Aortic Size In Shunts

A. EXTRACARDIAC SHUNTS
   √ aorta enlarged + hyperpulsatile
   1. PDA
B. PRE- AND INTRACARDIAC SHUNTS
   √ aorta small but not hypoplastic
   1. Anomalous pulmonary venous return
   2. ASD
   3. VSD
   4. Common AV canal

Abnormal Heart Chamber Dimensions

A. LEFT VENTRICULAR VOLUME OVERLOAD
   1. VSD
   2. PDA
   3. Mitral incompetence
   4. Aortic incompetence
B. LEFT VENTRICULAR HYPERTROPHY
   1. Coarctation
   2. Aortic stenosis
C. RIGHT VENTRICULAR VOLUME OVERLOAD
   1. ASD
   2. Partial APVR / total APVR
   3. Tricuspid insufficiency
   4. Pulmonary insufficiency
   5. Congenital / acquired absence of pericardium
   [6. Ebstein anomaly] – not truly RV
D. RIGHT VENTRICULAR HYPERTROPHY
   1. Pulmonary valve stenosis
   2. Pulmonary hypertension
   3. Tetralogy of Fallot
   4. VSD
E. FIXED SUBVALVULAR AORTIC STENOSIS
F. HYPOPLASTIC LEFT / RIGHT VENTRICLE, COMMON VENTRICLE
G. CONGESTIVE CARDIOMYOPATHY

Cardiomegaly In Newborn

A. NONCARDIOGENIC
   1. Metabolic:
      (a) ion imbalance in serum levels of sodium, potassium, and calcium
      (b) hypoglycemia
   2. Decreased ventilation
      (a) asphyxia
      (b) transient tachypnea
      (c) perinatal brain damage
   3. Erythrocyte function
      (a) anemia
      (b) erythrocythemia
   4. Endocrine
      (a) glycogen storage disease
      (b) thyroid disease: hypo- / hyperthyroidism
   5. Infant of diabetic mother
   6. Arteriovenous fistula
      (a) vein of Galen aneurysm
      (b) hepatic angioma
      (c) chorioangioma
B. CARDIOGENIC
   1. Arrhythmia
   2. Myo- / pericarditis
   3. Cardiac tumor
   4. Myocardial infarction
   5. Congenital heart disease

CYANOTIC HEART DISEASE

Chemical cyanosis = $PaO_2 \leq 94\%$
Clinical cyanosis = $PaO_2 \leq 85\%$
◊ Decrease in hemoglobin delays detectability!
Most common cause of cyanosis
— in newborn is transposition of great vessels
— in child is tetralogy of Fallot!

A. OVERCIRCULATION VASCULARITY
   mnemonic: "5 T's + CAD"
   1. **T**ransposition, complete
   2. **T**ricuspid atresia with transposition
   3. **T**runcus arteriosus
   4. **T**APVR above diaphragm
   5. **T**ingle ventricle
   6. **C**ommon atrium
   7. **A**ortic atresia
   8. **D**ORV

B. DECREASED VASCULARITY (with R-to-L shunt)
 (a) at ATRIAL LEVEL
  1. Isolated pulmonary stenosis / atresia
  2. Tricuspid atresia without transposition with pulmonary stenosis
  3. Ebstein / Uhl malformation
  4. Congenital tricuspid regurgitation
  5. Pericardial effusion
 (b) at VENTRICULAR LEVEL
  1. Tetralogy of Fallot
  2. Single ventricle
  3. Tricuspid atresia without transposition without pulmonary stenosis
  4. DORV
  5. Asplenia syndrome
  6. Corrected transposition + VSD

C. PULMONARY VENOUS HYPERTENSION
  1. Atresia of common pulmonary vein
  2. TAPVR below diaphragm
  3. Aortic atresia

N.B.: tricuspid atresia = the great mimicker

Increased pulmonary blood flow with cyanosis

= ADMIXTURE LESIONS = bidirectional shunt with 2 components:
(a) mixing of saturated blood (L-R shunt) and unsaturated blood (R-L shunt)
(b) NO obstruction to pulmonary blood flow

Evaluation process:
√ PA segment absent = transposition
√ PA segment present:
 (a) L atrium normal (= extracardiac shunt) = TAPVR
 (b) L atrium enlarged (= intracardiac shunt) = truncus arteriosus

N.B.: Overcirculation + cyanosis = complete transposition until proven otherwise!

ADMIXTURE LESIONS = T-LESIONS
mnemonic: "5 **T**'s + **CAD**"
Transposition of great vessels = complete TGV ± VSD (most common cause for cyanosis in neonate)
Tricuspid atresia with or without transposition + VSD (2nd most common cause for cyanosis in neonate)
Truncus arteriosus
Total anomalous pulmonary venous return (TAPVR) above diaphragm
 (a) supracardiac
 (b) cardiac (coronary sinus / right atrium)
"**T**ingle" = single ventricle
Common atrium
Aortic atresia
Double-outlet right ventricle (DORV type I) / Taussig-Bing anomaly (DORV type II)

Clues:
√ skeletal anomalies: Ellis-van Creveld syndrome (truncus / common atrium)
√ polysplenia: common atrium
√ R aortic arch: persistent truncus arteriosus
√ ductus infundibulum: aortic atresia
√ pulmonary trunk seen: supracardiac TAPVR; DORV; tricuspid atresia; common atrium
√ ascending aorta with leftward convexity: single ventricle
√ dilated azygos vein: common atrium + polysplenia + interrupted IVC; TAPVR to azygos vein
√ left-sided SVC: vertical vein of TAPVR
√ "waterfall" right hilum: single ventricle + transposition
√ large left atrium (rules out TAPVR)
√ prominent L heart border: single ventricle with inverted rudimentary R ventricle; levoposition of R atrial appendage (tricuspid atresia + transposition)
√ age of onset ≤2 days: aortic atresia

Decreased pulmonary blood flow with cyanosis

= two components of (a) impedance of blood flow through right heart due to obstruction / atresia at pulmonary valve / infundibulum (b) R-to-L shunt; pulmonary circulation maintained through systemic arteries / PDA

mnemonic: "P2 TETT"
Pulmonic stenosis with ASD
Pulmonic atresia
Tetralogy of Fallot
Ebstein anomaly
Tricuspid atresia with pulmonic stenosis
Transposition of great vessels with pulmonic stenosis

A. SHUNT AT VENTRICULAR LEVEL
 1. Tetralogy of Fallot
 2. Tetralogy physiology (associated with pulmonary obstruction):
  — Complete / corrected transposition
  — Single ventricle
  — DORV
  — Tricuspid atresia (PS in 75%)
  — Asplenia syndrome
 √ prominent aorta with L / R aortic arch; inapparent pulmonary trunk
 √ NORMAL R atrium (without tricuspid regurgitation)
 √ NORMAL-sized heart (secondary to escape mechanism into aorta)
 Clues:
  1. Skeletal anomaly (eg, scoliosis): tetralogy (90%)
  2. Hepatic symmetry: asplenia
  3. Right aortic arch: tetralogy, complete transposition, tricuspid atresia
  4. Aberrant right subclavian artery: tetralogy
  5. Leftward convexity of ascending aorta: single ventricle with inverted right rudimentary ventricle, corrected transposition, asplenia, JAA (tricuspid valve atresia)

HEART

B. SHUNT AT ATRIAL LEVEL
1. **P**ulmonary stenosis / atresia with intact ventricular septum
2. **E**bstein malformation + Uhl anomaly
3. **T**ricuspid atresia (ASD in 100%)
√ moderate to severe cardiomegaly
√ R atrial dilatation
√ R ventricular enlargement (secondary to massive tricuspid incompetence)
√ inapparent aorta
√ left aortic arch

ACYANOTIC HEART DISEASE

Increased Pulmonary Blood Flow Without Cyanosis

= indicates L-R shunt with increased pulmonary blood flow (shunt volume >40%)

A. WITH LEFT ATRIAL ENLARGEMENT
Indicates shunt distal to mitral valve = increased volume without escape defect
1. VSD (25%): small aorta in intracardiac shunt
2. PDA (12%): aorta + pulmonary artery of equal size in extracardiac shunt
3. Ruptured sinus of Valsalva aneurysm (rare)
4. Coronary arteriovenous fistula (very rare)
5. Aortopulmonary window (extremely rare)

B. WITH NORMAL LEFT ATRIUM
Indicates shunt proximal to mitral valve = volume increased with escape mechanism through defect
1. ASD (8%)
2. Partial anomalous pulmonary venous return (PAPVR) + sinus venosus ASD
3. Endocardial cushion defect (ECD) (4%)

Normal Pulmonary Blood Flow Without Cyanosis

A. OBSTRUCTIVE LESION
(a) Right ventricular outflow obstruction
1. at level of pulmonary valve: subvalvular / valvular / supravalvular pulmonic stenosis
2. at level of peripheral pulmonary arteries: peripheral pulmonary stenosis

(b) Left ventricular inflow obstruction
1. at level of peripheral pulmonary veins: pulmonary vein stenosis / atresia
2. at level of left atrium: cor triatriatum
3. at level of mitral valve: supravalvular mitral stenosis, congenital mitral stenosis / atresia, “parachute” mitral valve

(c) Left ventricular outflow obstruction
1. at level of aortic valve: anatomic subaortic stenosis, functional subaortic stenosis (IHSS), valvular aortic stenosis, hypoplastic left heart, supravalvular aortic stenosis
2. at level of aorta: interruption of aortic arch, coarctation of aorta

B. CARDIOMYOPATHY
1. Endocardial fibroelastosis
2. Hypertrophic cardiomyopathy
3. Glycogen storage disease

C. HYPERDYNAMIC STATE
1. Noncardiac AVM (cerebral AVM, vein of Galen aneurysm, large pulmonary AVM, hemangioendothelioma of liver)
2. Thyrotoxicosis
3. Anemia
4. Pregnancy

D. MYOCARDIAL ISCHEMIA
1. Anomalous left coronary artery
2. Coronary artery disease (CAD)

PULMONARY VASCULARITY

Increased Pulmonary Vasculature

A. OVERCIRCULATION
= shunt vascularity = arterial + venous overcirculation
(a) Congenital heart disease (most common)
(1) L-R shunts (2) Admixture cyanotic lesions
(b) High-flow syndromes
(1) Thyrotoxicosis (2) Anemia (3) Pregnancy (4) Peripheral arteriovenous fistula
√ diameter of right descending pulmonary artery larger than trachea just above aortic knob
√ increased size of veins + arteries with size larger than accompanying bronchus (= “kissing cousin” sign), best seen just above hila on AP view
√ enlarged hilar vessels (lateral view)
√ visualization of vessels below 10th posterior rib

B. PULMONARY VENOUS HYPERTENSION
√ redistribution of flow (not seen in younger children)
√ indistinctness of vessels with Kerley lines (= interstitial edema)
√ alveolar edema
√ fine reticulated pattern

C. PRECAPILLARY HYPERTENSION
√ enlarged main + right and left pulmonary arteries
√ abrupt tapering of pulmonary arteries

D. PROMINENT SYSTEMIC / AORTOPULMONARY COLLATERALS
1. Tetralogy of Fallot with pulmonary atresia (= pseudotruncus)
2. VSD + pulmonary atresia (single ventricle, complete transposition, corrected transposition)
3. Pulmonary-systemic collaterals
√ coarse vascular pattern with irregular branching arteries (from aorta / subclavian arteries)
√ small central vessels despite apparent increase in vascularity

Decreased Pulmonary Vascularity

= obstruction to pulmonary flow
√ vessels reduced in size and number
√ hyperlucent lungs
√ small pulmonary artery segment + hilar vessels

Normal Pulmonary Vascularity & Normal-sized Heart

mnemonic: “MAN”
Myocardial ischemia
Afterload (= pressure overload problems)
Normal

Pulmonary Arterial Hypertension

= PAH = sustained pulmonary arterial pressure in systole >30 mm Hg, in diastole >15 mm Hg, mean pressure >20 mm Hg secondary to reduction in cross-sectional area of pulmonary vascular bed with concomitant increase in pulmonary vascular resistance

Pathogenesis:

A. PRIMARY PAH (rare) = plexogenic pulmonary arteriopathy = unknown cause / mechanism
B. SECONDARY PAH (more common)
   (a) primary pleuropulmonic disease
      1. Parenchymal pulmonary disease
         = **cor pulmonale**:
         COPD, emphysema, chronic bronchitis, asthma, bronchiectasis, malignant infiltrate, granulomatous disease, cystic fibrosis, end-stage fibrotic lung, S/P lung resection, idiopathic hemosiderosis, alveolar proteinosis, alveolar microlithiasis
      2. Alveolar hypoventilation
         = hypoxic pulmonary arterial hyperperfusion: chronic high altitude, sleep apnea, hypoventilation due to neuromuscular disease / obesity
      3. Pleural disease + chest deformity
         fibrothorax, thoracoplasty, kyphoscoliosis
   (b) primary vascular disease
      1. Congenital heart disease
         — increased flow: large L-R shunt (Eisenmenger syndrome)
         — decreased flow: tetralogy of Fallot
      2. Capillary obliteration: chronic pulmonary thromboembolism, persistent fetal circulation, arteritides (eg, Takayasu)
      3. Venous obliteration: pulmonary venoocclusive disease
   (c) pulmonary venous hypertension

Histo:

Grade I = hypertrophy of media of muscular pulmonary arteries + arterioles
Grade II = hypertrophy of muscle cells + proliferation of intima cells in small muscular arteries + arterioles
Grade III = muscular hypertrophy + intimal thickening + subendothelial fibrosis
Grade IV = occlusion of vessels with progressive dilatation of small arteries nearby; muscular hypertrophy less apparent
Grade V = tortuous channels within proliferation of endothelial cells (= plexiform + angiomatoid lesions) + intraalveolar macrophages
Grade VI = thrombosis + necrotizing arteritis

√ "pruning" of pulmonary arteries = disproportionate increase in caliber of central fibrous arteries + decrease in caliber of smaller muscular arteries (from sustained increase in pressure)
√ increase in vessel caliber of central + peripheral arteries (from sustained increase in flow by a factor of >2)
√ calcification of central pulmonary vessels (PATHOGNOMONIC)
√ NO increase of pulsations in middle third of lung
√ normal-sized heart / right heart enlargement

Cor Pulmonale

mnemonic: "TICCS BEV"

Thoracic deformity
Idiopathic
Chronic pulmonary embolism
COPD
Shunt (ASD, VSD, etc)
Bronchiectasis
Emphysema
Vasculitis

Pulmonary Venous Hypertension

= INCREASED VENOUS PULMONARY PRESSURE
= VENOUS CONGESTION
= pulmonary capillary wedge pressure (PCWP) >15 mm Hg

Cause:

A. LEFT VENTRICULAR INFLOW TRACT OBSTRUCTION
   √ normal-sized heart with right ventricular hypertrophy
   √ prominent pulmonary trunk
   @ proximal to mitral valve:
      √ normal-sized left atrium
      1. TAPVR below the diaphragm
      2. Primary pulmonary veno-occlusive disease
      3. Stenosis of individual pulmonary veins
      4. Atresia of common pulmonary vein
      5. Cor triatriatum
      6. Left atrial tumor / clot
      7. Supravalvular ring of left atrium
      8. Fibrosing mediastinitis
      9. Constrictive pericarditis
   @ at mitral valve level
      √ enlarged left atrium
      1. Rheumatic mitral valve stenosis ± regurgitation (99%)
         √ enlarged left atrial appendage
      2. Congenital mitral valve stenosis
      3. Parachute mitral valve (= single bulky papillary muscle)
B. LEFT VENTRICULAR FAILURE
   (a) ABNORMAL PRELOAD with secondary mitral valve incompetence (= volume overload)
      1. Aortic valve regurgitation
      2. Eisenmenger syndrome (= R-to-L shunt in VSD)
      3. High-output failure:
         noncardiac AVM (cerebral AVM, vein of Galen aneurysm, large pulmonary AVM, hemangioendothelioma of liver, iatrogenic), thyrotoxicosis, anemia, pregnancy

HEART

(b) ABNORMAL AFTERLOAD
(= pressure overload)
= LV outflow tract obstruction
1. Hypoplastic left heart syndrome
2. Aortic stenosis (supravalvular, valvular, anatomic subaortic)
3. Interrupted aortic arch
4. Coarctation of the aorta

(c) DISORDERS OF CONTRACTION AND RELAXATION
1. Endocardial fibroelastosis
2. Glycogen storage disease (Pompe disease)
3. Cardiac aneurysm
4. Cardiomyopathy
   (a) congestive (alcohol)
   (b) hypertrophic obstructive cardiomyopathy (HOCM), particularly in IDM
   — asymmetric septal hypertrophy (ASH)
   — idiopathic hypertrophic subaortic stenosis (IHSS)

(d) MYOCARDIAL ISCHEMIA
1. Anomalous left coronary artery
2. Coronary artery disease (CAD)

√ moderate redistribution (PCWP 13–15 mm Hg)
√ redistribution (PCWP 15–18 mm Hg)
√ indistinct vessel margins due to interstitial edema (PCWP 18–25 mm Hg)
√ alveolar pulmonary edema (PCWP >30 mm Hg)

Pulmonary Artery-Bronchus Ratios

= ratio of diameters of end-on segmental pulmonary artery + accompanying end-on bronchus

A. ERECT CHEST FILM
1. Normal (effect of gravity):
   upper lung zone .... 0.85 ± 0.15
   lower lung zone .... 1.34 ± 0.25
2. Pulmonary plethora (balanced engorgement):
   upper lung zone .... 1.62 ± 0.31
   lower lung zone .... 1.56 ± 0.28
3. Decompensated CHF (redistribution from left-sided CHF):
   upper lung zone .... 1.50 ± 0.25
   lower lung zone .... 0.87 ± 0.20

B. SUPINE CHEST FILM
1. Normal (gravitational effect lost):
   upper lung zone .... 1.01 ± 0.13
   lower lung zone .... 1.05 ± 0.13
2. Decompensated CHF (inverted pattern / plethora pattern):
   upper lung zone .... 1.49 ± 0.31
   lower lung zone .... 0.96 ± 0.31

AORTA

Enlarged Aorta

A. INCREASED VOLUME LOAD
1. Aortic insufficiency
2. PDA

B. POSTSTENOTIC DILATATION
1. Valvular aortic stenosis

C. INCREASED INTRALUMINAL PRESSURE
1. Coarctation
2. Systemic hypertension

D. MURAL WEAKNESS / INFECTION
1. Cystic media necrosis: Marfan / Ehlers-Danlos syndrome
2. Congenital aneurysm
3. Syphilitic aortitis
4. Mycotic aneurysm
5. Atherosclerotic aneurysm (compromised vasa vasorum)

E. LACERATION OF AORTIC WALL
1. Traumatic aneurysm
2. Dissecting hematoma

Aortic Wall Thickening

1. Intramural hematoma
   = aortic dissection without intimal tear
2. Aortitis
   segments of aortic arch + branch vessels
3. Atherosclerotic plaque
   √ irregular narrowing of aortic lumen
4. Adherent thrombus

Double Aortic Arch

Common cause of vascular ring; usually isolated condition

Incidence: 55% of all vascular rings

Age: usually detected in infancy

• usually asymptomatic
• stridor, dyspnea, recurrent pneumonia
• dysphagia (less common than respiratory symptoms, more common after starting baby on solids)

Location: descending aorta in 75% on left, in 25% on right side; smaller arch anterior in 80%; right arch larger + more cephalad than left in 80%

√ two separate arches arise from single ascending aorta
√ each arch joins to form a single descending aorta
√ impressions may be present on both sides of trachea: usually R > L
√ small anterior tracheal impression
√ broad posterior + bilateral esophageal indentations

CT:
√ "four-artery sign" = each arch gives rise to 2 dorsal subclavian + 2 ventral carotid arteries evenly spaced around trachea on section cephalad to aortic arch

DDx: right arch with aberrant left subclavian artery (indistinguishable by esophagram when dominant arch on right side)

Right Aortic Arch

Incidence: 1–2%

INCIDENCE OF RIGHT AORTIC ARCH IN CONGENITAL HEART DISEASE
1. Truncus arteriosus 35%
2. Tetralogy of Fallot 25%
3. TGV.................................. 10%
4. Tricuspid atresia................. 5%

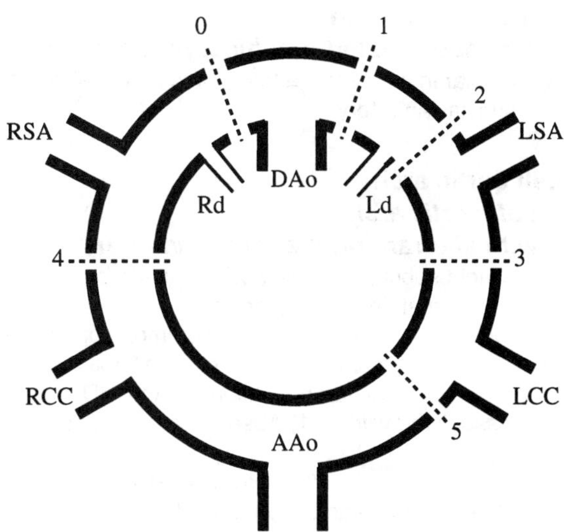

Edwards' Hypothetical Aortic Arch Development

RSA = right subclavian a. AAo = ascending aorta
LSA = left subclavian a. DAo = descending aorta
RCC = right common carotid a. Rd = right ductus
LCC = left common carotid a. Ld = left ductus

0 = normal left aortic arch
1 = right aortic arch with mirror-image branching; ductus from pulmonary a. to left brachiocephalic / subclavian a. = no vascular ring
2 = right aortic arch with mirror-image branching; ductus from pulmonary a. to descending aorta = complete vascular ring
3 = right aortic arch with aberrant left subclavian a.; ductus from pulmonary a. to descending aorta (most common complete vascular ring)
4 = left aortic arch with aberrant right subclavian a.
5 = right aortic arch with aberrant left brachiocephalic artery; ductus from pulmonary a. to descending aorta (very uncommon)
2 + 3 = right aortic arch with isolated left subclavian a. (very uncommon)

5. Large VSD 2%

Rare anomalies:
1. Corrected transposition 50%
2. Pseudotruncus 50%
3. Asplenia 30%
4. Pink tetralogy 15%

mnemonic: "TRU TETRA TRIC"
- **TRU**ncus arteriosus
- **TE**tralogy of Fallot
- **TRA**nsposition
- **TRIC**uspid atresia

Right aortic arch with aberrant left subclavian artery

= RAA with ALSA
= interruption of embryonic left arch between left CCA and left subclavian artery; most common type of right aortic arch anomaly: 35–72%; 2nd most common cause of vascular ring after double aortic arch

Incidence: 1:2,500
Associated with: congenital heart disease in 5–12%:
1. Tetralogy of Fallot (2/3 = 8%)
2. ASD ± VSD (1/4 = 3%)
3. Coarctation (1/12 = 1%)

• usually asymptomatic (loose ring around trachea + esophagus)
• may be symptomatic in infancy / early childhood provoked by bronchitis + tracheal edema
• may be symptomatic in adulthood provoked by torsion of aorta

√ left common carotid artery is first branch of ascending aorta
√ left subclavian artery arises from descending aorta via the remnant of the left dorsal aortic root
√ bulbous configuration of origin of LSA (= remnant of embryonic left arch) = retroesophageal aortic diverticulum = **diverticulum of Kommerell** (N.B.: originally described as diverticular outpouching at origin of right subclavian artery with left aortic arch)
  √ small rounded density left lateral to trachea
  √ impression on left side of esophagus simulating a double aortic arch (aortic diverticulum / ligamentum arteriosum)
√ vascular ring (= left ductus extends from aortic diverticulum to left pulmonary artery)
  √ right aortic arch impression on tracheal air shadow
  √ right-sided esophageal indentation (right arch)
  √ masslike density silhouetting top of aortic arch just posterior to trachea on LAT CXR
  √ broad posterior impression on esophagus (left subclavian artery / aortic diverticulum)
  √ small anterior impression on trachea
  √ aorta descends on right side

Right aortic arch with mirror-image branching

2nd most common aortic arch anomaly: 24–60%
= interruption of embryonic left arch between left subclavian artery and descending aorta; dorsal to left ductus arteriosus

(a) Type 1 = interruption of left aortic arch distal to ductus arteriosus (common)
Associated with: cyanotic congenital heart disease in 98%:
1. Tetralogy of Fallot (87%)
2. Multiple defects (7.5%)
3. Truncus arteriosus (2–6%)
4. Transposition (1–10%)
5. Tricuspid atresia (5%)
6. ASD ± VSD (0.5%)

◊ 25% of patients with tetralogy have right aortic arch!
◊ 37% of patients with truncus arteriosus have right aortic arch!

√ NO vascular ring, NO retroesophageal component
√ NO structure posterior to trachea
√ R arch impression on tracheal air shadow
√ NORMAL barium swallow

HEART

(b) Type 2 = interruption of left aortic arch proximal to ductus arteriosus (rare)
true vascular ring (if duct persists);
rarely associated with CHD

Right aortic arch
with isolated left subclavian artery

3rd most common right aortic arch anomaly: 2%
= interruption of embryonic left arch between
(a) left CCA and left subclavian artery and
(b) left ductus and descending aorta
resulting in a connection of left subclavian artery with left pulmonary artery

Associated with: tetralogy of Fallot

√ left common carotid artery arises as the first branch
√ left subclavian artery attaches to left pulmonary artery through PDA
√ NO vascular ring, NO retroesophageal component
• congenital subclavian steal syndrome

Right aortic arch
with aberrant left brachiocephalic artery

Similar in appearance to R aortic arch + aberrant L subclavian artery

Left aortic arch

Left aortic arch
with aberrant right subclavian artery

= right subclavian artery arises as 4th branch from proximal descending aorta

Incidence: 0.4–2.3%; most common congenital aortic arch anomaly; in 37% of Down syndrome children with CHD

Associated with: (1) Absent recurrent pharyngeal nerve
(2) CHD in 10–15%

Course: (a) behind esophagus (80%)
(b) between esophagus + trachea (15%)
(c) anterior to trachea (5%)

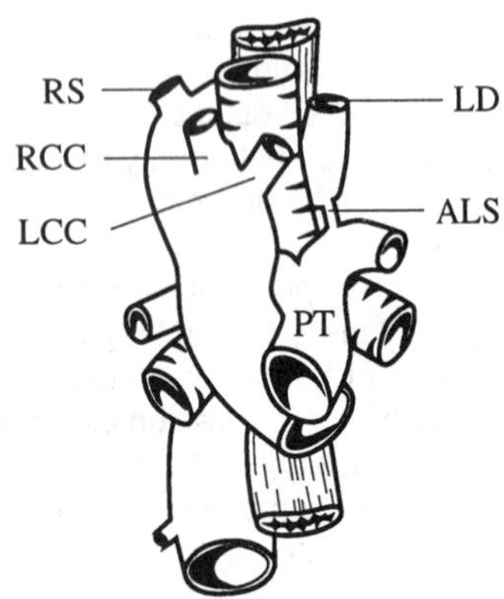

Right Aortic Arch with Aberrant Left Subclavian Artery

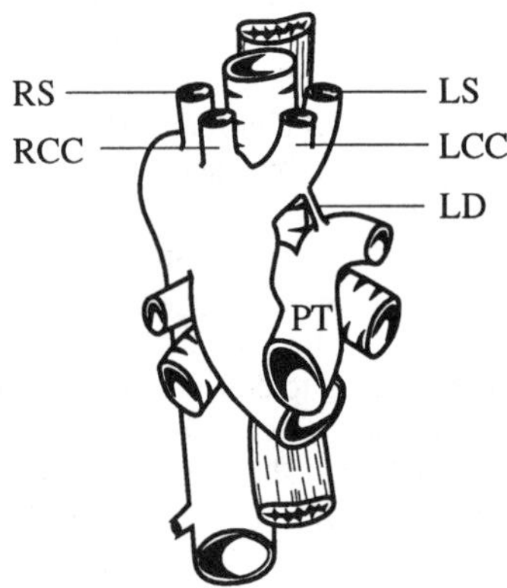

Right Aortic Arch with Mirror-image Branching

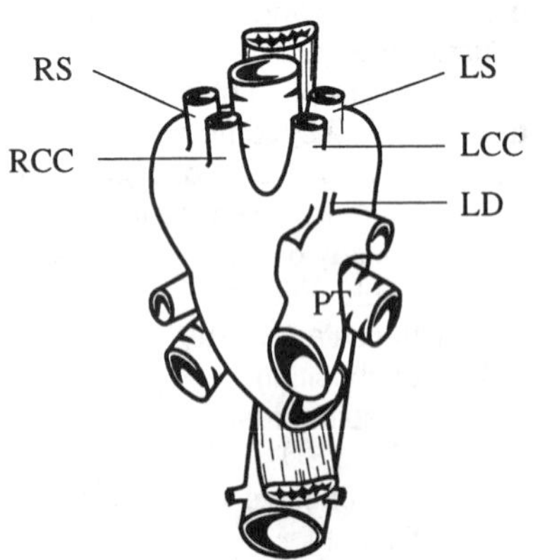

Double Aortic Arch

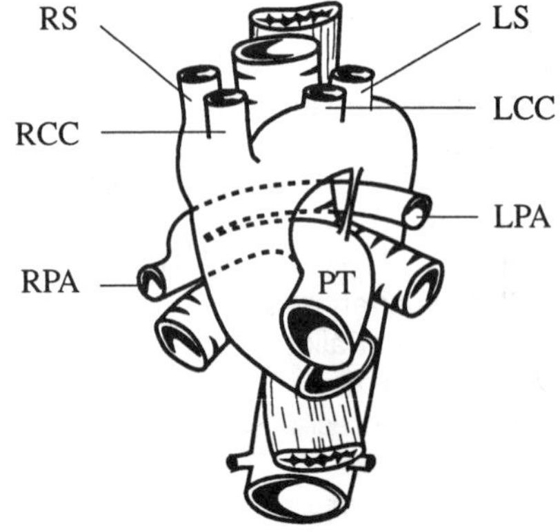

Aberrant Left Pulmonary Artery

ALS = aberrant left subclavian a.
LS = left subclavian a.
LCC = left common carotid a.
LD = left ductus arteriosus
LPA = left pulmonary a.
PT = pulmonary trunk
RCC = right common carotid a.
RPA = right pulmonary a.
RS = right subclavian a.

- asymptomatic / dysphagia lusoria (rare)
- √ soft-tissue opacity crossing the esophagus obliquely upward toward the right shoulder
- √ masslike opacity in right paratracheal region
- √ rounded opacity arising from superior aortic margin posterior to trachea + esophagus on LAT CXR
- √ dilated origin of aberrant subclavian artery (in up to 60%) = diverticulum of Kommerell = remnant of embryonic right arch
- √ unilateral L-sided rib notching (if aberrant right subclavian artery arises distal to coarctation)

Anomalous innominate artery compression syndrome

= origin of R innominate artery to the left of trachea coursing to the right

√ anterior tracheal compression

Bovine aortic arch

= common origin of brachiocephalic trunk + left common carotid artery

Cervical aortic arch

Associated with: right aortic arch (in 2/3)

- pulsatile neck mass
- upper airway obstruction
- dysphagia
- √ mediastinal widening
- √ absence of normal aortic knob
- √ aortic arch near lung apex
- √ tracheal displacement to opposite side + anteriorly
- √ apparent cutoff of tracheal air column (secondary to crossing of descending aorta to side opposite of arch)

DDx: carotid aneurysm

Pattern of vascular compression of esophagus and trachea

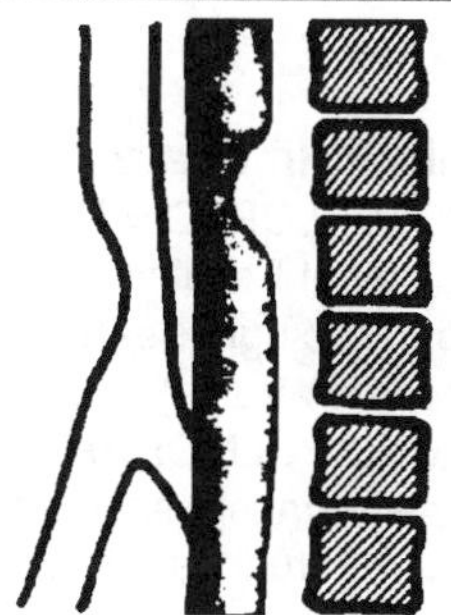

A. Anterior tracheal indentation + large posterior esophageal impression:
1. Double aortic arch
2. Right aortic arch with aberrant left subclavian + left ductus / ligamentum arteriosus
3. Left aortic arch with aberrant right subclavian + right ductus / ligamentum (extremely rare)

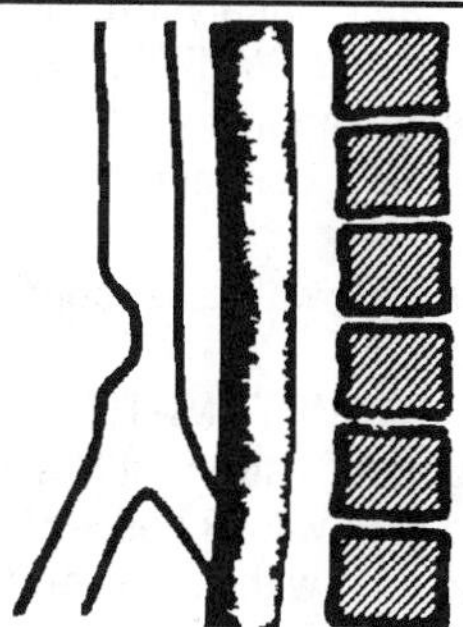

B. Anterior tracheal indentation
1. Compression by innominate artery with origin more distal along arch
2. Compression by left common carotid with origin more proximal on arch
3. Common origin of innominate and left common carotid artery

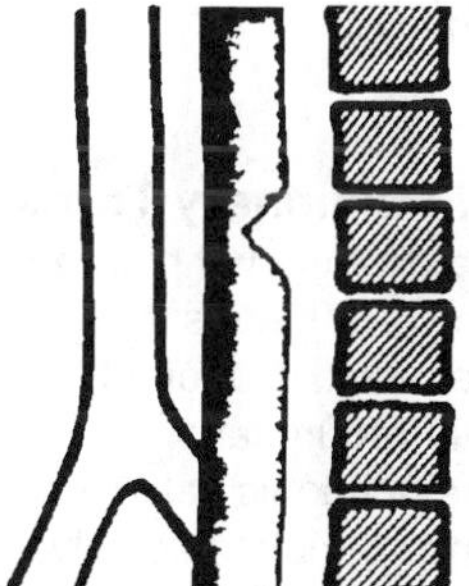

C. Small posterior esophageal impression
- dysphagia lusoria (lusorius, *Latin* = playful)
1. Left aortic arch with aberrant right subclavian artery
2. Right aortic arch with aberrant left subclavian artery (very rare)

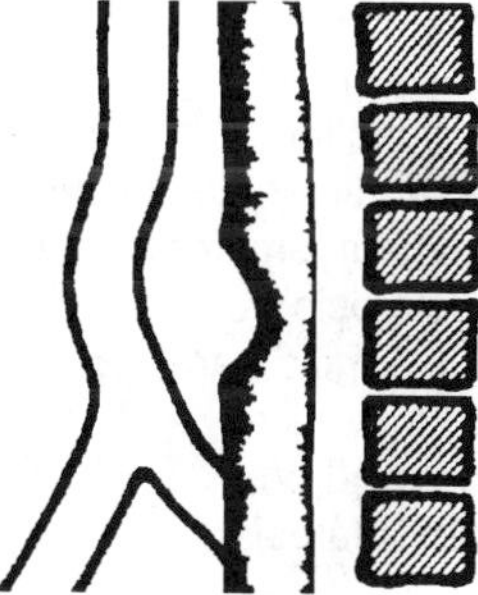

D. Posterior tracheal indentation + anterior esophageal impression
1. Aberrant left pulmonary artery

Vascular Rings

= anomaly characterized by encirclement of trachea + esophagus by aortic arch + branches

A. USUALLY SYMPTOMATIC LESIONS
- chronic stridor, wheezing, recurrent pneumonia
- dysphagia, failure to thrive

1. Double aortic arch with R descending aorta + L ductus arteriosus
2. R aortic arch with R descending aorta + aberrant L subclavian artery + persistent L ductus / ligamentum teres
3. L arch with L descending aorta + R ductus / ligamentum
4. Aberrant L pulmonary artery = "pulmonary sling"

Frequency of CXR findings:
— frontal CXR:
√ right aortic arch (85%)
√ focal indentation of distal trachea (73%)
– lateral CXR:
√ anterior tracheal bowing (92%)
√ increased retrotracheal opacity (79%)
√ focal tracheal narrowing (77%)

B. OCCASIONALLY SYMPTOMATIC LESIONS
1. Anomalous innominate
2. Anomalous L common carotid artery / common trunk
3. R aortic arch with L descending aorta + L ductus / ligamentum

C. USUALLY ASYMPTOMATIC LESIONS
1. L aortic arch + aberrant R subclavian artery
2. L aortic arch with R descending aorta
3. R aortic arch with R descending aorta + mirror-image branching
4. R aortic arch with R descending aorta + aberrant L subclavian artery
5. R aortic arch with R descending aorta + isolation of L subclavian artery
6. R aortic arch with L descending aorta + L ductus / ligamentum

Aortic Stenosis

A. ACQUIRED
1. Takayasu aortitis
2. Radiation aortitis
3. Aortic dissection
4. Infected aortic aneurysm with abscess
5. Pseudoaneurysm from laceration
6. Atherosclerosis (rare)
7. Syphilitic aortitis (rare)

B. CONGENITAL
1. Williams syndrome
2. Neurofibromatosis
3. Rubella
4. Mucopolysaccharidosis
5. Hypoplastic left heart syndrome

Abnormal Left Ventricular Outflow Tract

LVOT = area between IVS + aML from aortic valve cusps to mitral valve leaflets

1. Membranous subaortic stenosis
= crescent-shaped fibrous membrane extending across LVOT + inserting at aML
√ diffuse narrowing of LVOT
√ abnormal linear echoes in LVOT space (occasionally)
2. Prolapsing aortic valve vegetation
3. Narrowed LVOT (<20 mm)
(a) Long-segment subaortic stenosis
√ aortic valve closure in early systole with coarse fluttering
√ high-frequency flutter of mitral valve in diastole (aortic regurgitation)
√ symmetric LV hypertrophy
(b) ASH / IHSS
√ asymmetrically thickened septum bulging into LV + LVOT
√ systolic anterior motion of aML (SAM)
(c) Mitral stenosis
(d) Endocardial cushion defect

PULMONARY ARTERY

Invisible Main Pulmonary Artery

A. UNDERDEVELOPED = RVOT OBSTRUCTION
1. Tetralogy of Fallot
2. Hypoplastic right heart syndrome (tricuspid / pulmonary atresia)

B. MISPLACED PULMONARY ARTERY
1. Complete transposition of great vessels
2. Persistent truncus arteriosus

Unequal Pulmonary Blood Flow

1. Tetralogy of Fallot
√ diminished flow on left side (hypoplastic / stenotic pulmonary artery in 40%)
2. Persistent truncus arteriosus (esp. Type IV)
√ diminished / increased blood flow to either lung
3. Pulmonary valvular stenosis
√ increased flow to left lung secondary to jet phenomenon

Dilatation Of Pulmonary Trunk

1. Idiopathic dilatation of pulmonary artery
2. Pulmonic valve stenosis
√ poststenotic dilatation of trunk + left pulmonary a.
3. Pulmonary regurgitation
(a) severe pulmonic valve insufficiency
(b) absence of pulmonic valve (may be associated with tetralogy)
4. Congenital L-to-R shunts
5. Pulmonary arterial hypertension
6. Aneurysm: mycotic / traumatic

SITUS

= term describing the position of atria, tracheobronchial tree, pulmonary arteries, thoracic + abdominal viscera

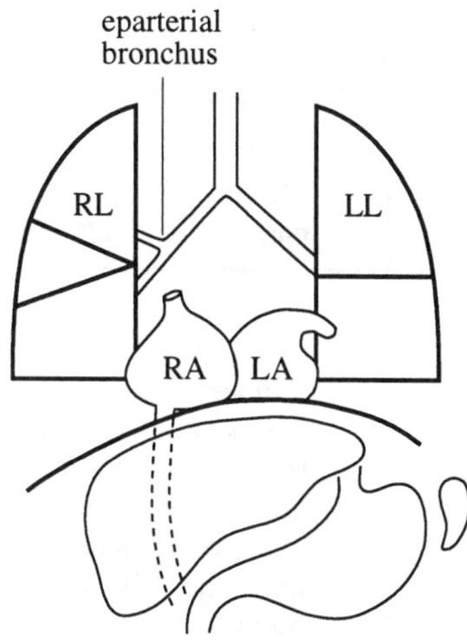

SITUS SOLITUS
anterior view

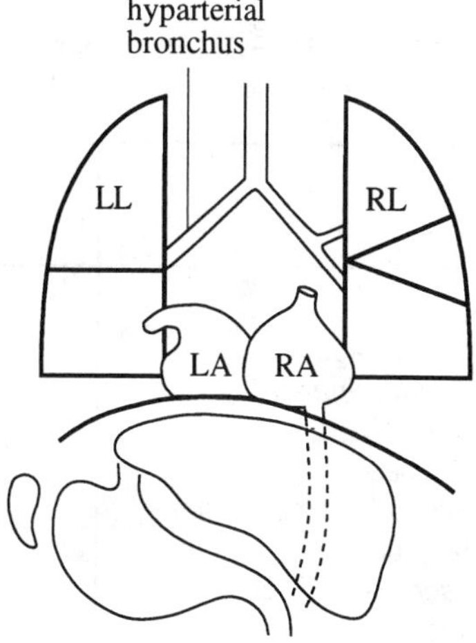

SITUS INVERSUS
anterior view

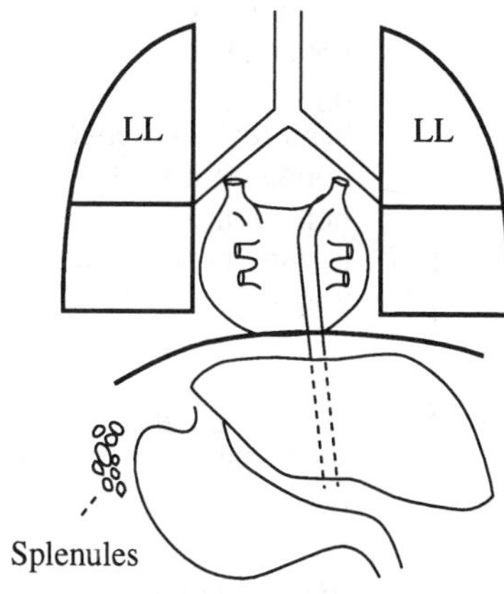

LEFT ISOMERISM
posterior view

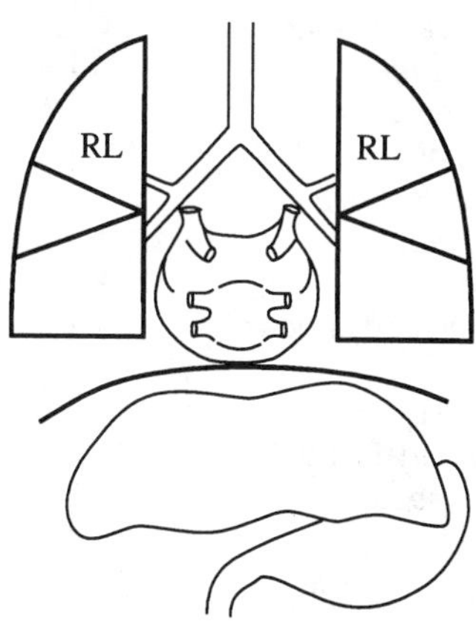

RIGHT ISOMERISM
posterior view

A. SITUS SOLITUS = normal situs
   = position of morphologic LA is the same as that of the aortic arch + stomach bubble + hyparterial bronchus + bilobed lung; the position of the morphologic RA is the same as that of the eparterial bronchus + trilobed lung
   1. Abdominal situs solitus
      √ liver + IVC are right-sided
      √ stomach, spleen, abdominal aorta are left-sided
   2. Cardiac situs solitus
      √ morphologic right atrium is right-sided
      √ morphologic left atrium is left-sided

   Associated with:
   (a) levocardia : <1% chance for CHD
   (b) dextrocardia : 95% chance for CHD
B. SITUS INVERSUS
   = mirror-image position of normal
   1. Abdominal situs inversus
      √ mirror-image position of abdominal organs
   2. Cardiac situs inversus
      √ morphologic right atrium is left-sided
      √ morphologic left atrium is right-sided

   Associated with:
   (a) dextrocardia = situs inversus totalis (usual variant): 3–5% chance for CHD, eg, Kartagener syndrome
   (b) levocardia (extremely rare): 95% chance for CHD

C. SITUS INDETERMINATUS / INDETERMINUS / AMBIGUUS
   = ambiguous relationship
   1. Abdominal situs ambiguus
      √ liver may be midline + symmetric
      √ bowel malrotations are typical
   2. Cardiac situs ambiguus
      √ atrial morphology indeterminate / bilateral right atria (right atrial isomerism) / bilateral left atria (left atrial isomerism)

   Associated with:
   (a) bilateral right isomerism / sidedness = asplenia syndrome
   (b) bilateral left isomerism / sidedness = polysplenia syndrome

HETEROTAXIA

= CARDIOSPLENIC SYNDROMES = sporadic disorders with abnormal relationship between abdominal organs + tendency toward symmetric development of organs within trunk + associated cardiac anomalies

	Asplenia bilateral R sidedness	**Polysplenia** bilateral L sidedness
CLINICAL		
Presenting age	newborn / infant	infant / adult
Sex predominance	male	female
Cyanosis	severe	usually absent
Heart disease	severe	moderate / none (5 – 10%)
Howell-Jolly / Heinz bodies	present	absent
Spleen scan	no spleen	multiple small spleens
Characteristic ECG	none	abnormal P wave vector
Prognosis	poor	good
Mortality	high	low
PLAIN FILM		
Lung vascularity	decreased	normal / increased
Aortic arch	right / left	right / left
Cardiac apex	right / left / midline	right / left
Bronchi	bilateral eparterial	bilateral hyparterial
Minor fissure	possibly bilateral	none / normal
Stomach	midline / right / left	right / left
Liver	symmetrical / R / L	in various positions
Malrotation of bowel	yes (microgastria)	yes
CARDIOGRAPHY		
Coronary sinus	usually absent	sometimes absent
Atrial septum	common atrium (100%)	ASD (84%)
AV valve	atresia / common valve	normal / abnormal MV
Single ventricle	44%	infrequent
IVS	VSD	VSD common
Great vessels	d- / l-transposition (72%)	normal relationship
Pulmonary stenosis	the rule	frequent
Pulmonary veins	TAPVR	PAPVR (42%) TAPVR (6%)
Single coronary artery	19%	
SVC	bilateral (53%)	bilateral (33%)
IVC-aorta relationship	same side of spine	normal
IVC	normal	interrupted (84%) / normal
Azygos vein	inapparent	continuation R / L

Cardiac position

= determined by base-apex axis; no assumption is made regarding cardiac chamber / vessel arrangement

A. POSITION OF CARDIAC APEX
   1. Levocardia = apex directed leftward
   2. Dextrocardia = apex directed rightward
   3. Mesocardia = vertical / midline heart (usually with situs solitus)

   √ atrial septum characteristically bowed into left atrium in cardiac situs solitus with dextrocardia + cardiac situs inversus with levocardia (DDx: juxtapositioned atrial appendages)

B. CARDIAC DISPLACEMENT
   by extracardiac factors (eg, lung hypoplasia, pulmonary mass)
   1. Dextroposition
      suggests hypoplasia of ipsilateral pulmonary artery (PAPVR implies scimitar syndrome)
   2. Levoposition
   3. Mesoposition

C. CARDIAC INVERSION
   = alteration of normal relationship of chambers
   1. D-bulboventricular loop
   2. L-bulboventricular loop

D. TRANSPOSITION
   = alteration of anterior-posterior relationship of great vessels

HEART

CARDIAC TUMOR

Prevalence: 0.017–0.08–0.3%
- weight loss, fever, malaise
- congestive heart failure, palpitations, heart murmur
- syncope
- dyspnea, cough, chest pain

Location: pericardial, intramural, intracavitary

Malignant Heart Tumors

Prevalence: 25% of all cardiac tumors in adults
10% of all cardiac tumors in children

1. Sarcoma: undifferentiated sarcoma, angiosarcoma, rhabdomyosarcoma
2. Malignant fibrous histiocytoma
   Prevalence: 1–2% of all primary cardiac tumors
   Age: more common in adults than children
3. Metastatic disease
   most commonly lung, melanoma, breast
   ◊ 20–40 times more frequent than primary tumor!
4. Lymphoma
   Incidence: cardiac involvement in 29% on autopsy; pericardial involvement more frequent
   - intractable congestive heart failure
   - chest pain

   √ SVC obstruction
5. Malignant teratoma
6. Multiple cardiac myxomas

Benign Heart Tumor In Adults

1. Myxoma (most common cardiac tumor)
2. Papillary fibroelastoma
3. Lipoma
4. Hydatid cyst (uncommon):
   √ localized bulge of left cardiac contour
   √ curvilinear / spotty calcifications (resembling myocardial aneurysm)
   Cx: may rupture into cardiac chamber / pericardium

Congenital Cardiac Tumor

Incidence: 1:10,000

1. Rhabdomyoma (58%): usually multiple masses
2. Teratoma (20%): intrapericardiac, extracardiac
   √ multicystic mass
3. Fibroma (12%): intramural
   may be associated with: Gorlin syndrome
   Location: free LV wall / interventricular septum
   √ may be pedunculated
   √ calcification and cystic degeneration centrally
   √ tendency for slow growth
   Cx: fetal hydrops secondary to obstruction, pericardial effusion, fetal arrhythmia, fetal death
4. Hemangioma (arise from RT atrium, pericardial effusion, skin hemangiomas), lymphangioma, neurofibroma, myxoma, mesothelioma:
   √ mass-occupying lesion impinging upon cardiac cavities

PERICARDIUM

Pericardial Effusion

= pericardial fluid >50 mL

Etiology:

A. SEROUS FLUID = transudate
   congestive heart failure, hypoalbuminemia, irradiation
B. BLOOD = hemopericardium
   (a) iatrogenic: cardiac surgery / catheterization, anticoagulants, chemotherapy
   (b) trauma: penetrating / nonpenetrating
   (c) acute myocardial infarction / rupture
   (d) rupture of ascending aorta / pulmonary trunk
   (e) coagulopathy
   (f) neoplasm: mesothelioma, sarcoma, teratoma, fibroma, angioma, metastasis (lung, breast, lymphoma, leukemia, melanoma)
C. LYMPH
   neoplasm, congenital, cardiothoracic surgery, obstruction of hilum / SVC
D. FIBRIN = exudate
   (a) infection: viral, pyogenic, TB
   (b) uremia: 18% in acute uremia; 51% in chronic uremia; dialysis patient
   (c) collagen disease: rheumatoid arthritis, SLE, acute rheumatic fever
   (d) hypersensitivity

mnemonic: "CUM TAPPIT RV"
Collagen vascular disease
Uremia
Metastasis
Trauma
Acute myocardial infarction
Purulent infection
Post MI syndrome
Idiopathic
Tuberculosis
Rheumatoid arthritis
Virus

CXR:
√ normal with fluid <250 mL / in acute pericarditis
√ "water bottle configuration" = symmetrically enlarged cardiac silhouette
√ loss of retrosternal clear space
√ "fat-pad sign" = separation of retrosternal from epicardial fat line >2 mm (15%)
√ rapidly appearing cardiomegaly + normal pulmonary vascularity
√ "differential density sign" = increase in lucency at heart margin secondary to slight difference in contrast between pericardial fluid + heart muscle
√ diminished cardiac pulsations

ECHO:
√ separation of epi- and pericardial echoes extending into diastole (rarely behind LA)
√ volume estimates by M-mode:
(a) separation only posteriorly = <300 mL
(b) separation throughout cardiac cycle = 300–500 mL
(c) plus anterior separation = >1000 mL

HEART

Pneumopericardium

Etiology: shearing mechanism of injury of the heart during blunt trauma

Path: tear in fibrous pericardium, usually along the course of the phrenic nerve, allows pneumomediastinal air to enter

√ thick shaggy soft-tissue density of fibrous pericardium separated by air from cardiac density
√ air limited to distribution of pericardial reflection

VENA CAVA

Vena cava anomalies

1. Retrocaval ureter = circumcaval ureter
2. Duplicated IVC
   Incidence: 0.2–3%
   Etiology: persistence of right + left supracardinal veins
   √ small / equal-sized left IVC formed by left iliac vein
   √ crossover to right IVC via left renal vein / or more inferiorly
   √ crossover usually anterior / rarely posterior to aorta
   DDx: left gonadal v./ a., inferior mesenteric v.
3. Transposition of IVC = solitary left IVC
   Incidence: 0.2–0.5%
   Etiology: persistence of left + regression of right supracardinal vein
   √ left IVC usually crosses over via left renal vein / or more inferiorly
   √ crossover usually anterior / rarely posterior to aorta
4. Retroaortic left renal vein
   Incidence: 1.8–2.4%
   Etiology: persistence of posterior intersupracardinal anastomosis + regression of anterior intersubcardinal anastomosis
   √ crossover usually below / occasionally at level of right renal vein
5. Circumaortic left renal vein
   Incidence: 1.5–8.7%
   Etiology: persistence of anterior intersubcardinal + posterior intersupracardinal anastomosis
   √ venous collar encircling aorta
6. Interrupted IVC with azygos / hemiazygos continuation *see* AZYGOS CONTINUATION p. 517
7. Persistent left SVC = Bilateral SVCs
   Incidence: 0.3% of general population; 4.3–11% of patients with CHD
   Etiology: failure of regression of left anterior + common cardinal veins + left sinus horn
   May be associated with: ASD, azygos continuation of IVC
   Course: lateral to aortic arch, anterior to left hilum
   √ left SVC drains into enlarged coronary sinus (common)
   √ left SVC drains into LA (rare) creating a R-to-L shunt (increased prevalence of CHD)
   √ hemiazygos arch formed by left superior intercostal vein + persistent left SVC (20%)
   √ absent / small left brachiocephalic vein (65%)
   √ absence of right SVC (10–18%)
   √ anastomosis between right + left anterior cardinal veins (in 35%)

IVC Obstruction

A. INTRINSIC OBSTRUCTION
   (a) neoplastic (most frequent)
      1. Renal cell carcinoma (in 10%), Wilms tumor
      2. Adrenal carcinoma, pheochromocytoma
      3. Pancreatic carcinoma, hepatic adenocarcinoma
      4. Metastatic disease to retroperitoneal lymph nodes (carcinoma of ovary, cervix, prostate)
   (b) nonneoplastic
      1. Idiopathic
      2. Proximally extending thrombus from femoroiliac veins
      3. Systemic disorders: coagulopathy, Budd-Chiari syndrome, dehydration, infection (pelvic inflammatory disease), sepsis, CHF
      4. Postoperative / traumatic phlebitis, ligation, plication, clip, cava filter, severe exertion
B. INTRINSIC CAVAL DISEASE
   (a) neoplastic
      1. Leiomyoma, leiomyosarcoma, endothelioma
   (b) nonneoplastic
      1. Congenital membrane
C. EXTRINSIC COMPRESSION
   (a) neoplastic
      1. Retroperitoneal lymphadenopathy (adults) due to metastatic disease, lymphoma, granulomatous disease (TB)
      2. Renal + adrenal tumors (children)
      3. Hepatic masses
      4. Pancreatic tumor
      5. Tumor-induced desmoplastic reaction (eg, metastatic carcinoid)
   (b) nonneoplastic
      1. Hepatomegaly
      2. Tortuous aorta / aortic aneurysm
      3. Retroperitoneal hematoma
      4. Massive ascites
      5. Retroperitoneal fibrosis
D. FUNCTIONAL OBSTRUCTION
   1. Pregnant uterus
   2. Valsalva maneuver
   3. Straining / crying (in children)
   4. Supine position with large abdominal mass

E. COLLATERAL PATHWAYS
   1. Deep pathway: ascending lumbar veins to azygos vein (right) + hemiazygos vein (left) + intravertebral, paraspinal, extravertebral plexus (Batson plexus)
   2. Intermediate pathway: via periureteric plexus + left gonadal vein to renal vein
   3. Superficial pathway: external iliac vein to inferior epigastric vein + superior epigastric vein + internal mammary vein into subclavian vein

HEART

4. Portal pathway: retrograde flow through internal iliac vein + hemorrhoidal plexus into inferior mesenteric vein + splenic vein into portal vein

SURGERY

Surgical Procedures

A. AORTICOPULMONARY WINDOW SHUNT
= side-to-side anastomosis between ascending aorta and left pulmonary artery (reversible procedure)
◊ Tetralogy of Fallot

B. BLALOCK-HANLON PROCEDURE
= surgical creation of ASD
◊ Complete transposition

C. BLALOCK-TAUSSIG SHUNT
= end-to-side anastomosis of subclavian artery to pulmonary artery, performed ipsilateral to innominate artery / opposite to aortic arch
Modified Blalock-Taussig shunt uses synthetic graft material such as polytetrafluoroethylene (Gore-Tex®) in an end-to-side anastomosis between subclavian artery + ipsilateral branch of pulmonary artery
◊ Tetralogy of Fallot, Tricuspid atresia with pulmonic stenosis

D. FONTAN PROCEDURE
= (1) external conduit from right atrium to pulmonary trunk (= venous return enters pulmonary artery directly) (2) closure of ASD: floor constructed from flap of atrial wall and roof from piece of prosthetic material
◊ Tricuspid atresia

E. GLENN SHUNT
= end-to-side shunt between distal end of right pulmonary artery and SVC; reserved for patients with cardiac defects in which total correction is not anticipated
◊ Tricuspid atresia

F. POTT SHUNT
= side-to-side anastomosis between descending aorta + left pulmonary artery
◊ Tetralogy of Fallot

G. MUSTARD PROCEDURE
(a) removal of atrial septum (b) pericardial baffle placed into common atrium such that systemic venous blood is rerouted into left ventricle and pulmonary venous return into right ventricle and aorta
◊ Complete transposition

H. RASHKIND PROCEDURE = balloon atrial septostomy
◊ Complete transposition

I. RASTELLI PROCEDURE
external conduit (Dacron) with porcine valve connecting RV to pulmonary trunk
◊ Transposition

J. WATERSTON-COOLEY SHUNT
= side-to-side anastomosis between ascending aorta and right pulmonary artery; (a) extrapericardial (WATERSTON) (b) intrapericardial (COOLEY)
◊ Tetralogy of Fallot

Postoperative Thoracic Deformity

A. ON RIGHT SIDE
1. Systemic-PA shunt: Blalock-Taussig shunt, Waterston-Cooley shunt, Glenn shunt, Central conduit shunt
2. Atrial septectomy: Blalock-Hanlon procedure
3. VSD repair: through RA
4. Mitral valve commissurotomy

B. ON LEFT SIDE
1. PDA
2. Coarctation
3. PA banding
4. Mitral valve commissurotomy
5. Systemic-PA shunt: Blalock-Taussig shunt, Pott shunt

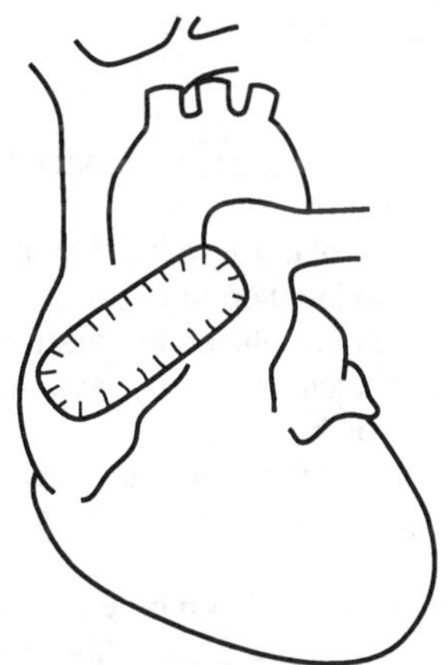
Fontan Procedure

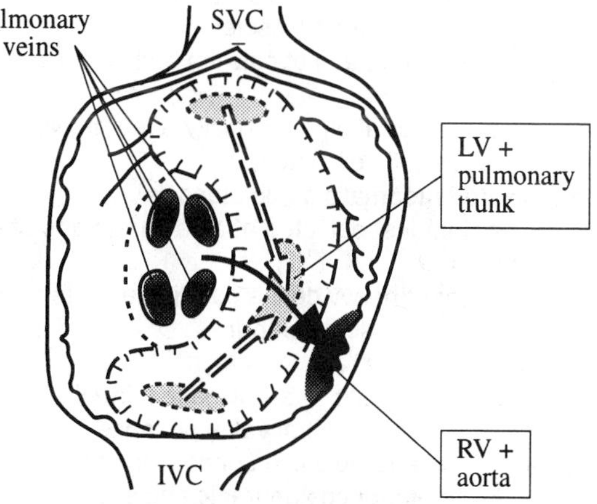

Mustard Procedure
(lateral view into opened right atrium)

HEART

Heart valve prosthesis

1. Starr-Edwards
   √ caged ball
   ◊ predictable performance from large long-term experience
2. Bjørk-Shiley / Lillehei-Kaster / St. Jude
   √ tilting disk
   ◊ excellent hemodynamics, very low profile, durable
3. Hancock / Carpentier-Edwards (= porcine xenograft)
   Ionescu-Shiley (= bovine xenograft)
   ◊ low incidence of thromboembolism, no hemolysis, central flow, inaudible

CARDIAC CALCIFICATIONS

Detected by:
fluoroscopy (at low-beam energies ≤75 kVp; 57% sensitivity) < digital subtraction fluoroscopy < conventional CT < ultrafast CT (96% sensitivity)

@ Coronary arteries
see below

@ Cardiac valves
◊ Valvar calcification means stenosis — its amount is proportionate to degree and duration of stenosis!

1. **Aortic valve**
   • usually indicates significant aortic stenosis
   Cause:
   congenital bicuspid valve (70–85%) > atherosclerotic degeneration > rheumatic aortic stenosis (rare), syphilis, ankylosing spondylitis
   Location: above + anterior to a line connecting carina + anterior costophrenic angle (lateral view)
   (a) Stenotic congenital bicuspid valve
   • calcium first detected at an average age of 28 years
   √ usually extensive cluster of heavy dense calcific deposits assuming a nodular contour
   √ poststenotic dilatation of ascending aorta
   (b) Degenerative aortic stenosis
   • calcium first detected at an average age of 54 years
   ◊ In patients >65 years aortic valve calcification in 90% due to atherosclerosis!
   √ curvilinear shape of calcium outlining tricuspid leaflets
   √ diffuse dilatation + tortuosity of aorta (NO poststenotic dilatation)
   (c) Isolated rheumatic aortic stenosis
   • calcium first detected at an average age of 47 years
   √ cluster of heavy dense calcific deposits without bicuspid contour
2. **Mitral valve leaflet**
   Cause: rheumatic heart disease (virtually always), mitral valve prolapse
   Location: inferior to a line connecting carina + anterior costophrenic angle (on lateral view)
   • calcium first detected in early thirties when patients become overtly symptomatic
   √ delicate calcification similar to coronary arteries (DDx: calcium in RCA / LCX)
   √ superior-to-inferior motion
3. **Pulmonic valve**
   Cause: tetralogy of Fallot, pulmonary stenosis, atrial septal defect
   √ calcific pattern similar to calcified mitral valve
4. **Tricuspid valve** (extremely rare)
   Cause: rheumatic heart disease, septal defect, tricuspid valve defect, infective endocarditis

@ Annulus
= valve rings serve as fibrous skeleton of the heart for attachment of myocardial fibers + cardiac valves

1. **Mitral annulus**
   Cause: degenerative (physiologic in elderly)
   Age: >65 years
   May be associated with: mitral valve prolapse
   Commonly associated with: aortic valve calcium
   √ dense bandlike calcification starting at posterior aspect + progressing laterally frequently forming a "reversed C" / "U" / "J"
   Cx: mitral insufficiency, atrial fibrillation, heart block
2. **Aortic annulus**
   √ usually in combination with degenerative aortic valve calcification
3. **Tricuspid annulus**
   Associated with: long-standing RV hypertension
   Location: right AV groove
   √ bandlike C-shaped configuration

@ Pericardium
Cause: idiopathic pericarditis, rheumatoid arthritis (5%), tuberculosis, viral, chronic renal failure, radiotherapy of mediastinum
Location: calcification over less pulsatile right-sided chambers, atrioventricular grooves, pulmonary trunk
◊ 50% of patients with constrictive pericarditis show pericardial calcifications!
Cx: constrictive pericarditis

@ Myocardium
Cause: infarction, aneurysm, rheumatic fever, myocarditis
Location: apex / anterolateral wall of LV (coincides with typical location of LV aneurysms)
√ fine curvilinear contour outlines the aneurysm
√ shaggy laminated calcification suggests associated calcification of mural thrombus
√ coarse amorphous calcifications are caused by trauma, cardioversion, infection, endocardial fibrosis

@ Interventricular septum
Location: triangular fibrous area between mitral + tricuspid annuli (= trigona fibrosa) representing the basal segment of interventricular septum, closely related to bundle of His

Always associated with:
heavy calcification of mitral annulus / aortic valve
Cx: heart block

@ Left atrial wall
Cause: rheumatic mitral valve disease
(a) diffuse form
• patient usually in bilateral CHF + atrial fibrillation
√ diffuse sheetlike calcification starting in the appendage sparing posterolateral wall on right side
Cx: mural thrombus formation + emboli
(b) localized form
√ nodular calcific scar in posterior wall (= McCallum patch) due to injury from a forceful jet in mitral valve insufficiency

@ Cardiac tumor
atrial myxoma (in 10% calcified), rhabdomyoma, fibroma, angioma, osteosarcoma, osteoclastoma

@ Endocardium
Cause: cardiac aneurysm, thrombus, endocardial fibroelastosis

@ Pulmonary artery
Cause: severe precapillary pulmonary arterial hypertension, syphilis

@ Ductus arteriosus
(a) in adults: indicates patency of ductus with associated long-standing precapillary pulmonary hypertension
(b) in children: ductus likely closed
√ calcium deposition in ligament of Botallo

Coronary Artery Calcification

= due to (1) arteriosclerosis of intima (2) Mönckeberg medial sclerosis (exceedingly rare)
Histo: calcified subintimal plaques
◊ Calcium is deposited in hemorrhagic areas within atheromatous plaques!
CXR (detection rate up to 42%):
◊ indicating more severe coronary artery disease
Fluoroscopy: (promoted as inexpensive screening test)
(a) asymptomatic population
— calcifications in 34% in asymptomatic male individuals
— in 35% of patients with calcifications exercise test will be positive (without calcifications only in 4% positive)
— calcifications indicate >50% stenosis with 72–76% sensitivity, 78% specificity); frequency of coronary artery calcifications with normal angiogram increases with age; predictive values in population <50 years as good as exercise stress test
(b) symptomatic population
— in 54% of symptomatic patients with ischemic heart disease
◊ In symptomatic patients 94% specificity for obstructive disease (>75% stenosis) of at least one of the three major vessels!

Location:
"coronary artery calcification triangle" = triangular area along mid left heart border, spine, and shoulder of LV containing left main coronary artery, proximal portions of LAD + LCX calcifications at autopsy:
LAD (93%), LCX (77%), left main CA (70%), RCA (69%)
√ parallel calcified lines (lateral view)
Prognosis: 58% 5-year survival rate with and 87% without calcifications

Vasculitis

A. LARGE-VESSEL VASCULITIS
1. Giant cell (temporal) arteritis
2. Takayasu disease
B. MEDIUM-SIZED–VESSEL VASCULITIS
1. Polyarteritis nodosa
2. Kawasaki disease
C. SMALL-VESSEL VASCULITIS
(a) ANCA-associated small-vessel vasculitis (= antineutrophil cytoplasmic autoantibodies)
1. Wegener granulomatosis
2. Churg-Strauss syndrome
3. Microscopic polyangiitis
(b) immune-complex small-vessel vasculitis
1. Henoch-Schönlein purpura
2. Essential cryoglobulinemic vasculitis
3. Cutaneous leukocytoclastic angiitis
others: lupus, rheumatoid, Sjögren, Behçet, Goodpasture, serum sickness, drug-induced, hypocomplementemic urticaria
(c) inflammatory bowel disease vasculitis

PULSUS ALTERNANS

= alternating arterial pulse height with regular cardiac rhythm
1. Intrinsic myocardial abnormality
severe left ventricular dysfunction (CHF, aortic valvular disease, hypothermia, hypocalcemia, hyperbaric stress, ischemia)
2. Alternating end-diastolic volumes
abnormalities in venous filling + return (obstructed venous return, IVC balloon)

ARTERIAL HYPERTENSION

A. ESSENTIAL (85–90%)
B. RENAL PARENCHYMAL DISEASE (5–10%)
C. POTENTIALLY CURABLE(1–2%)
(a) vascular
1. Renovascular disease
2. Coarctation
(b) hormonal
1. Pheochromocytoma
2. Cushing syndrome
3. Primary aldosteronism
4. Hyperthyroidism
5. Myxedema
(c) renal
1. Unilateral renal disease

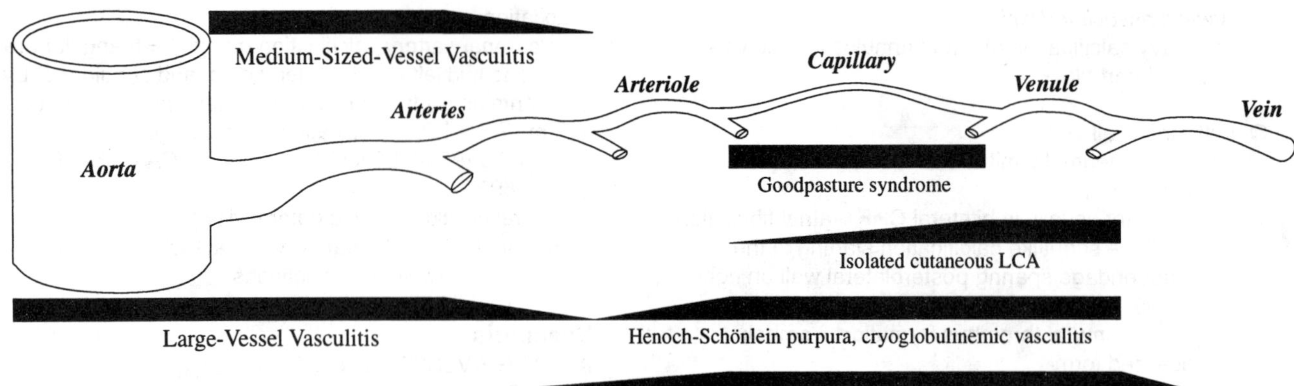

Noninfectious Vasculitides

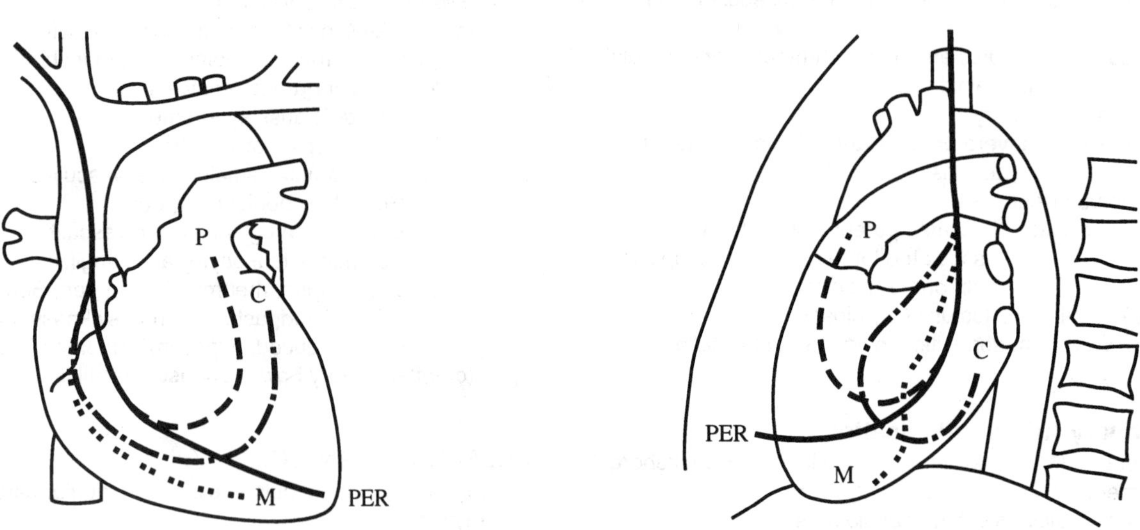

Central Venous Line Positions

C = coronary sinus, M = middle cardiac vein, P = main pulmonary artery, PER = perforation

CARDIOVASCULAR ANATOMY AND ECHOCARDIOGRAPHY

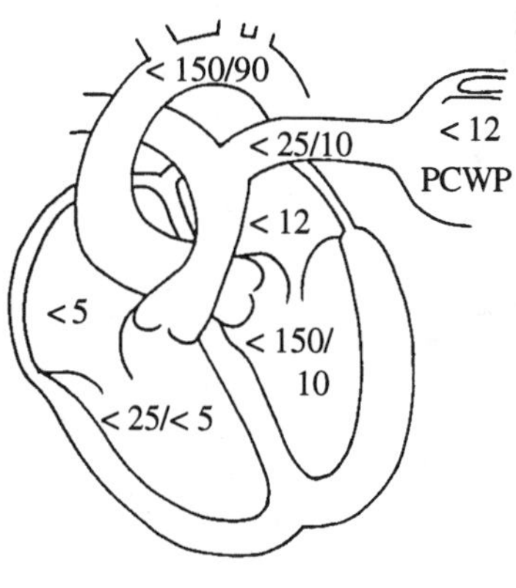

Normal Blood Pressures
PCWP = pulmonary capillary wedge pressure

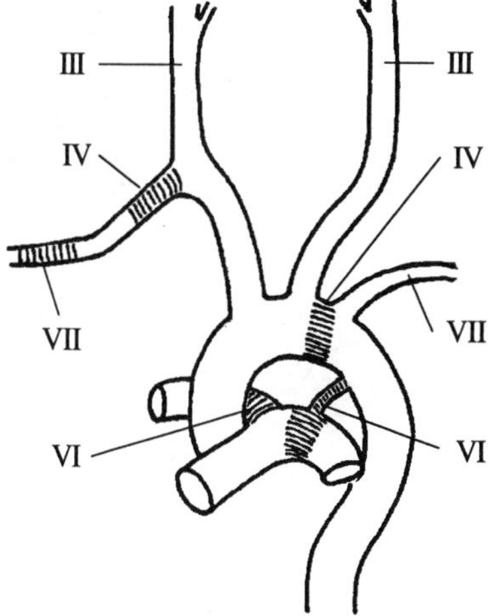

Development of Major Blood Vessels
numbers refer to embryologic aortic arches
most portions of aortic arches I, II, V regress

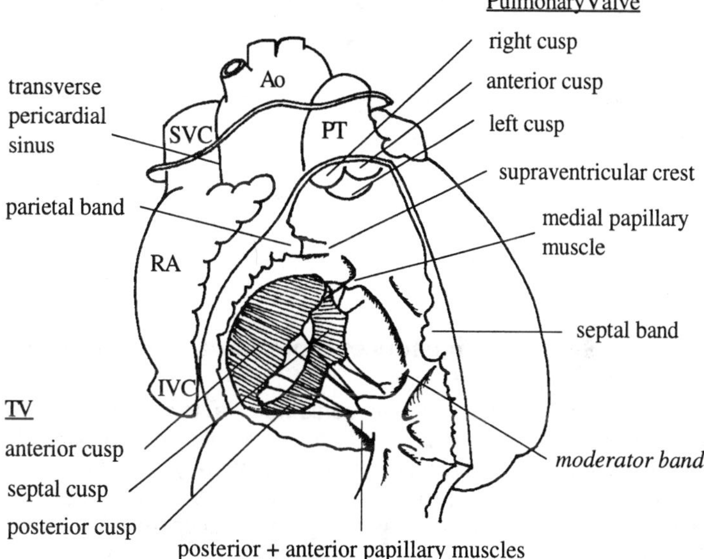

Right Ventricle Viewed From Front
Demarcation between posteroinferior inflow portion and anterosuperior outflow portion by prominent muscular bands forming an almost circular orifice

— parietal band
— crista supraventricularis
— septomarginal trabeculae (= septal band + moderator band)

Anterior papillary muscle originates from moderator band!

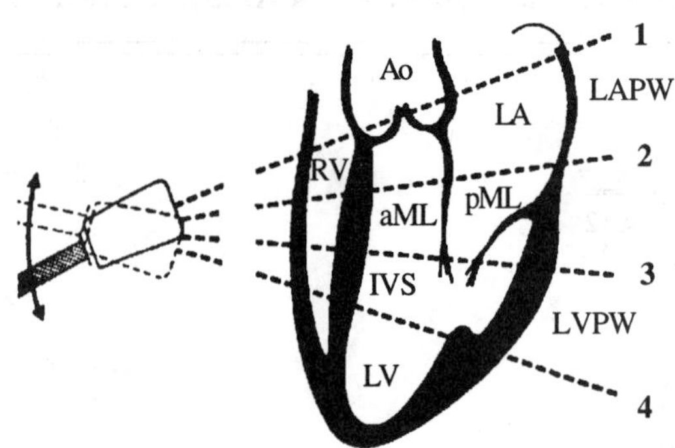

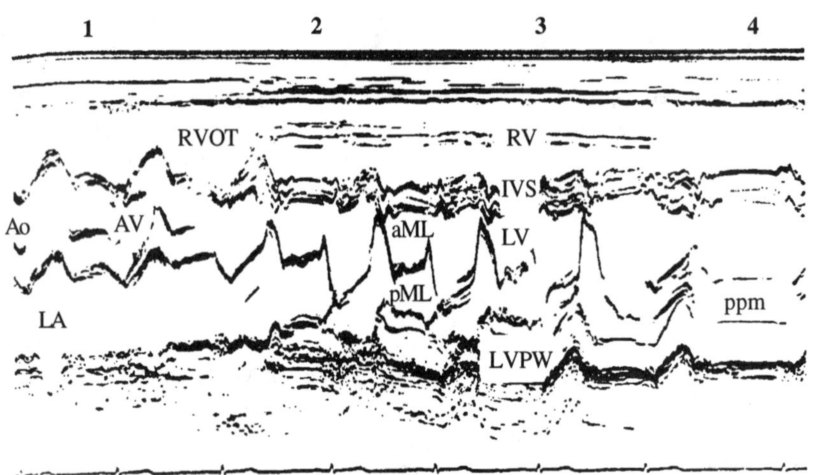

Sweep of Transducer From Aorta Toward Apex

Area 1: recognized by parallel motion of both aortic walls (a) toward the transducer during systole (b) away from the transducer during diastole. Left atrial posterior wall (LAPW) does not move because of mediastinal attachment by pulmonary veins.
Aortic valve cusps (right coronary + noncoronary / left cusps) are positioned in middle of aorta during diastole, open abruptly during systole at onset of ventricular ejection in a "box-like" fashion.
Aortic + LA dimension are similar in most cases.

Area 2: Aortic-septal continuity = anterior aortic wall becomes interventricular septum
Aortic-mitral continuity = posterior aortic wall becomes anterior mitral valve leaflet
Mitral valve with typical "M" configuration during diastole; motion of aML toward transducer during systole secondary to movement of whole mitral valve apparatus

Area 3: posterior mitral valve leaflet (pML) = reciprocal "W-shaped" configuration; left ventricular posterior wall (LVPW) shows anterior motion during systole.

Area 4: Chordae tendineae in continuity with mitral valve leaflets merge with a thick posterior band of echoes representing the posteromedial papillary muscle (ppm).

HEART

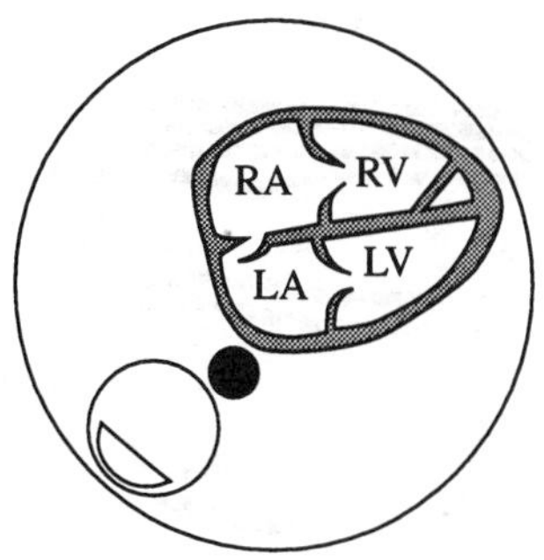

Fetal Four-Chamber View

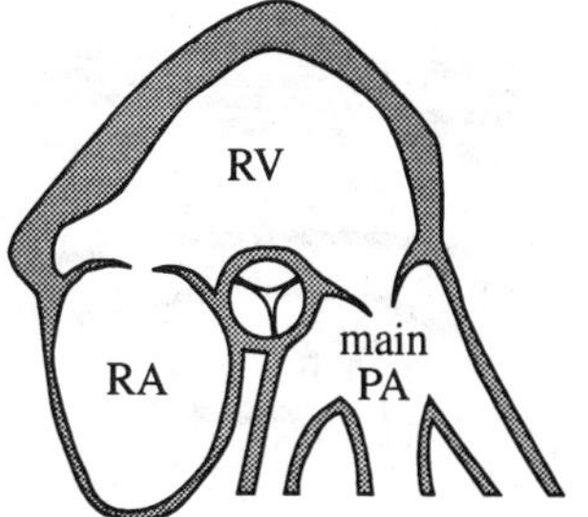

Fetal Short-axis View

Fetal echocardiographic views

A. FOUR-CHAMBER VIEW
   1. Position of heart within thorax
   2. Number of cardiac chambers
   3. Ventricular proportion
   4. Integrity of atrial + ventricular septa
   5. Position + size + excursion of AV valves

B. PARASTERNAL LONG-AXIS VIEW
   = LEFT VENTRICULAR OUTFLOW TRACT
   1. Continuity between ventricular septum + anterior aortic wall
   2. Caliber of aortic outflow tract
   3. Excursion of aortic valve leaflets

C. SHORT-AXIS VIEW OF OUTFLOW TRACTS
   1. Spatial relationship between aorta + pulmonary artery
   2. Caliber of aortic + pulmonary outflow tracts

D. AORTIC ARCH VIEW

Identification of fetal RV
- √ RV lies closest to anterior chest wall
- √ foramen ovale flap seen within LA
- √ prominent moderator band + papillary muscles in RV

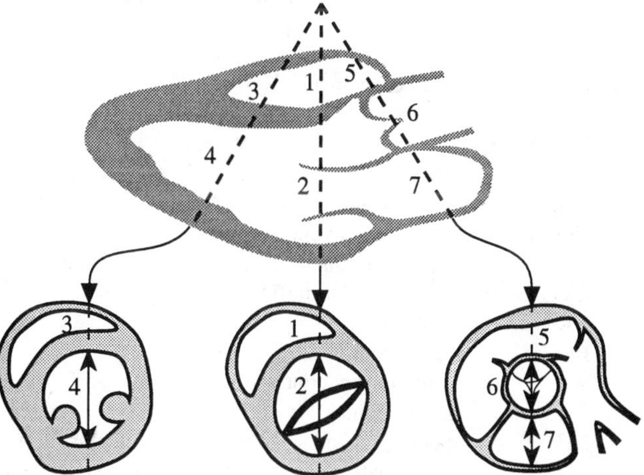

Parasternal Long- And Short-Axis Views

1, 3, 5 = RV dimension
6 = aortic root
7 = LA
2 = LV dimension at mitral level
4 = LV dimension at papillary muscle level

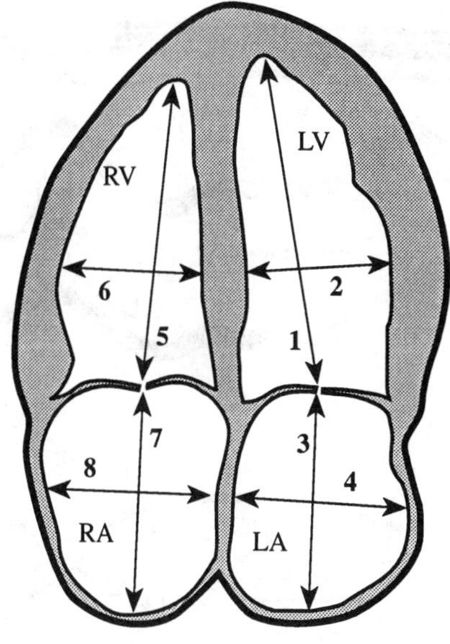

Apical 4-Chamber View

1 = LV long axis
2 = LV short axis
3 = LA major axis
4 = LA minor axis
5 = RV long axis
6 = RV short axis
7 = RA major axis
8 = RA minor axis

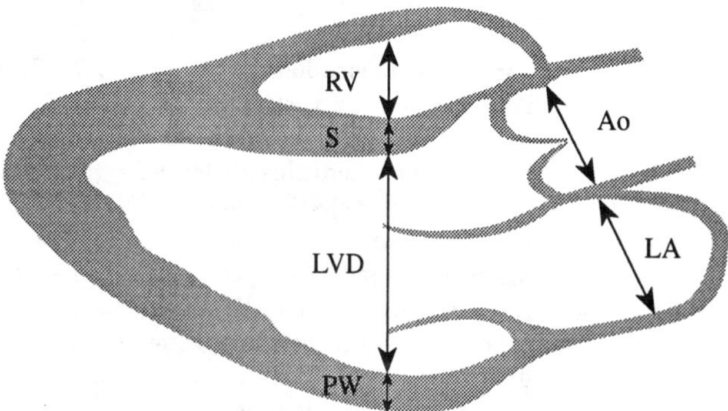

Parasternal Long-Axis View

Ao = aorta
LA = left atrium
LVD = left ventricular diameter
PW = posterior wall
RV = right ventricle
S = spetum

HEART

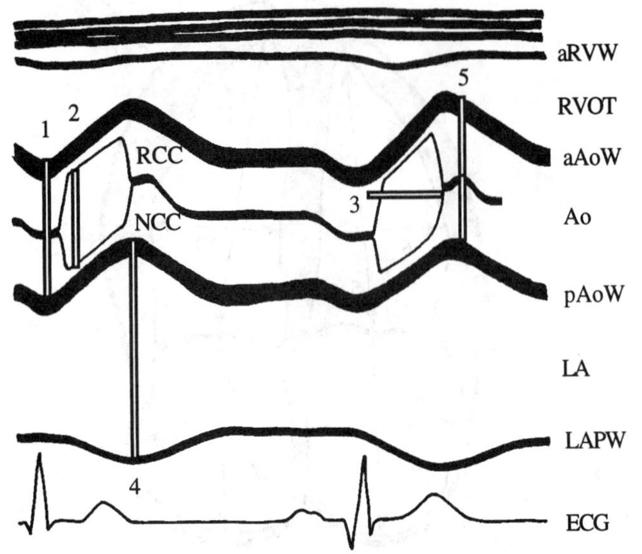

Echocardiogram of Aortic Root

1 = **aortic root dimension**, measured at end-diastole at R-wave of ECG .... 2.1 – 4.3 cm
increased in: aneurysm of aorta, aortic insufficiency

2 = **aortic cusp separation**: .... 1.7 – 2.5 cm
decreased in: aortic stenosis, low stroke volume
increased in: aortic insufficiency

3 = **left ventricular ejection time**

4 = **left atrial diameter**, measured at moment of mitral valve opening.......... 2.3 – 4.4 cm

5 = **eccentricity index of aortic valve cusps** = ratio of anterior to posterior dimension (rarely used) .... <1.3

4 ÷ 1 = **ratio of LA-to-aortic root dimension** .... 0.87 – 1.11

aRVW = anterior right ventricular wall
RVOT = right ventricular outflow tract
aAoW = anterior aortic wall
Ao = aorta
pAoW = posterior aortic wall
LA = left atrium
LAPW = left atrial posterior wall
NCC = noncoronary cusp
RCC = right coronary cusp
ECG = electrocardiogram

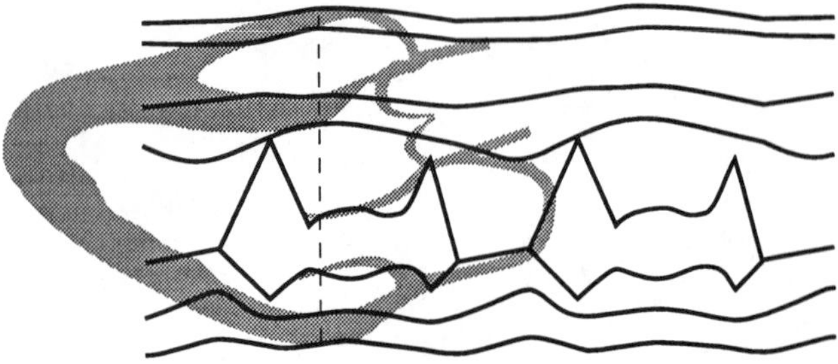

Mitral Valve in Mid-Diastole

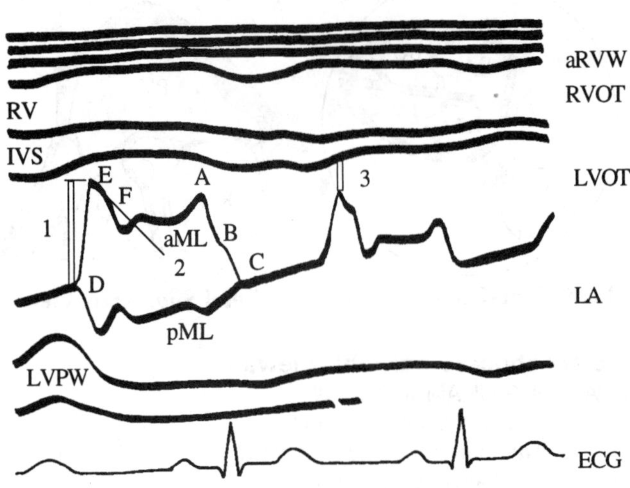

Echocardiogram of Mitral Valve

1 = **mitral valve excursion** = opening amplitude of anterior leaflet of mitral valve (DE amplitude) .... 2 – 3 cm
decreased in: nonpliable MV stenosis, low cardiac output, low compliance of LV
increased in: MV prolapse, high flow through MV

2 = **E to F slope** = early diastolic posterior motion of anterior leaflet .... 7 – 15 cm/sec
decreased in: mitral valve stenosis, low compliance of LV

3 = **septal-mitral valve distance** = E point septal separation..................... 2.9 – 4.1 mm
decreased in: ostium primum ASD, IHSS
increased in: dilated LV

RV = right ventricle
IVS = interventricular septum
LVPW = left ventricular posterior wall
aML = anterior mitral valve leaflet
pML = posterior mitral valve leaflet
aRVW = anterior right ventricular wall
RVOT = right ventricular outflow tract
LVOT = left ventricular outflow tract
LA = left atrium
ECG = electrocardiogram
A = point of atrial contraction
C = closure point
DE = opening secondary to passive ventricular filling
CD = systole with steady anterior drift of coapted leaflets (passive movement secondary to movement of

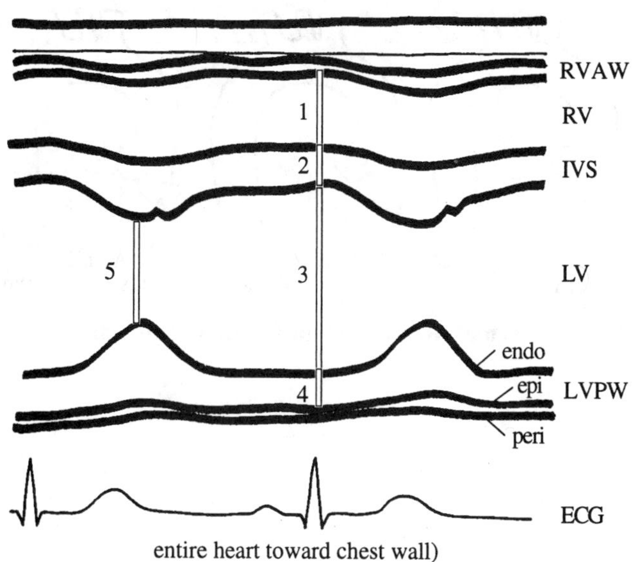

entire heart toward chest wall)

Echocardiogram of Right and Left Ventricle

1 = **RV end-diastolic dimension** (RVEDD) at R-wave of ECG .... 0.7 – 2.3 cm
increased in: RV volume overload

2 = **septal thickness** = end-diastolic IVS thickness at R-wave of ECG .... 0.9 ± 0.06 cm
decreased in: CAD
increased in: asymmetric septal hypertrophy, IHSS

3 = **LV end-diastolic dimension** (LVEDD) at R-wave of ECG .... 4.6 ± 0.54 cm

4 = **LVPW thickness**, measured at end-diastole at peak of R-wave of ECG: 0.94 ± 0.09 cm
increased in: LV hypertrophy

5 = **LV end-systolic dimension** (LVESD) .... 2.9 ± 0.5 cm

3 and 5 = **fractional shortening of internal diameter**
= (EDD - ESD)/EDD x 100 .... 0.25 - 0.42

IVS:LVPW thickness .... <1.3

RVAW = right ventricular anterior wall
RV = right ventricle
IVS = interventricular septum
LV = left ventricle
LVPW = left ventricular posterior wall
endo = endocardium
epi = epicardium
peri = pericardium

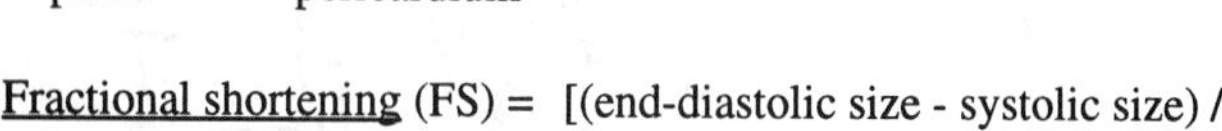

Fractional shortening (FS) = [(end-diastolic size - systolic size) / end-diastolic size] x 100
— for LV = 25 – 42%
— for IVS = 28 – 62%
— for LVPW = 36 – 70%

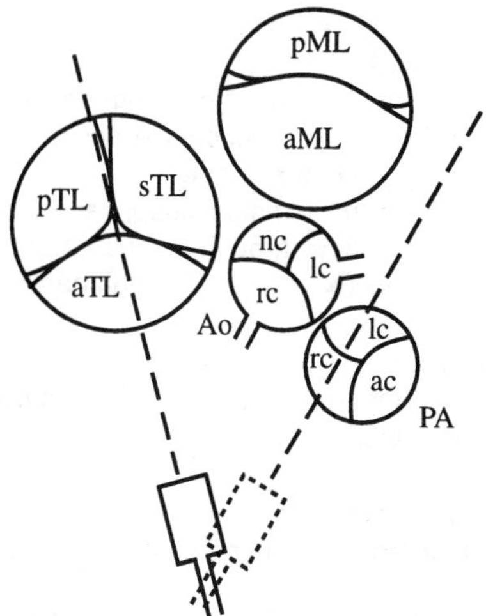

Diagram Showing the Relationship of the Four Cardiac Valves in Cross Section

aTL, pTL, sTL = anterior, posterior, septal tricuspid valve leaflets
aML, pML = anterior, posterior mitral valve leaflets
rc, lc, nc (Ao) = right, left, noncoronary cusps of aorta
rc, lc, ac (PA) = right, left, anterior cusps of pulmonary artery

HEART

Aortic isthmus variants

Aortic isthmus

= narrowing of the aorta in newborn between left subclavian artery and ductus arteriosus

Age: up to 2 months of age

Prognosis: aortic isthmus disappears due to cessation of flow through ductus arteriosus + increased flow through narrowed region

Aortic spindle

= normal variant of circumferential aortic bulge below isthmus region

Ductus diverticulum

= focal bulge along anteromedial aspect of aortic isthmus

Frequency: in 33% of infants, in 9% of adults

√ focal bulge with smooth uninterrupted margins
- √ gently sloping symmetric shoulders (classic ductus diverticulum)
- √ shorter steeper slope superiorly + more gentle slope inferiorly (atypical ductus diverticulum)

DDx: posttraumatic false aneurysm

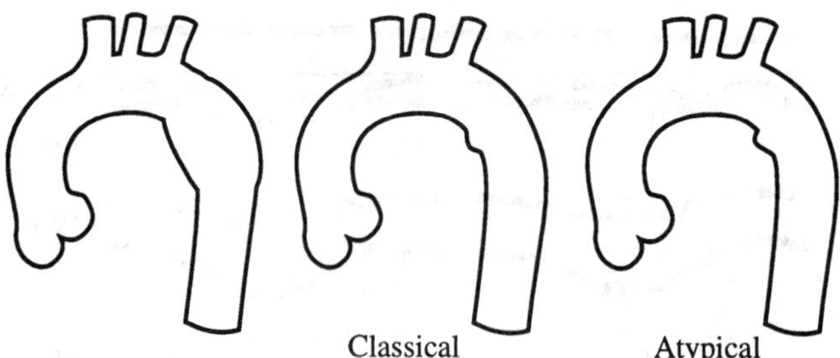

Normal Aortic Arch in 45° LAO Projection

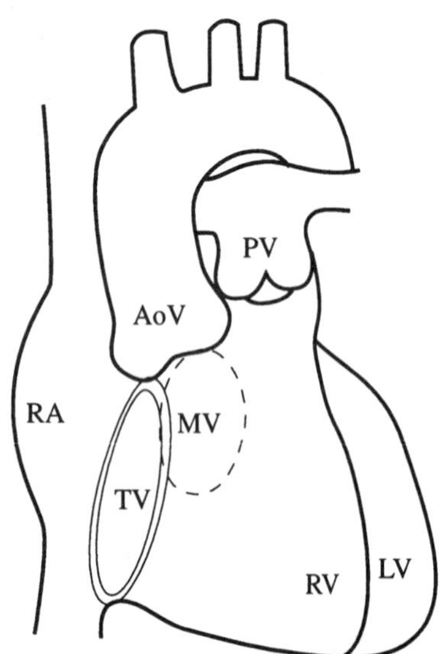

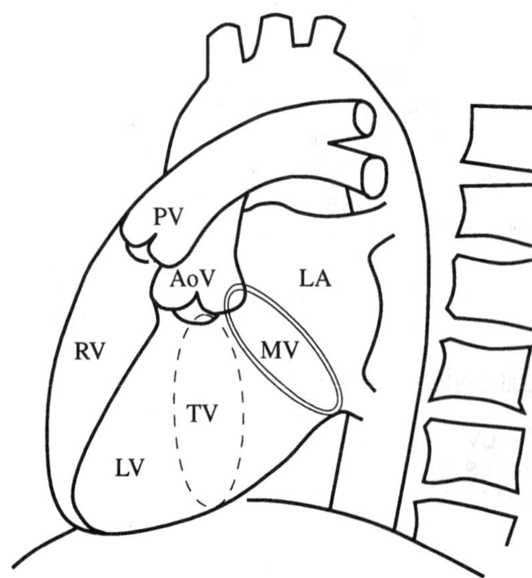

Heart Valve Positions

AoV = aortic valve, LA = left atrium, LV = left ventricle, MV = mitral valve, PV = pulmonic valve, RA = right atrium, RV = right ventricle, TV = tricuspid valve

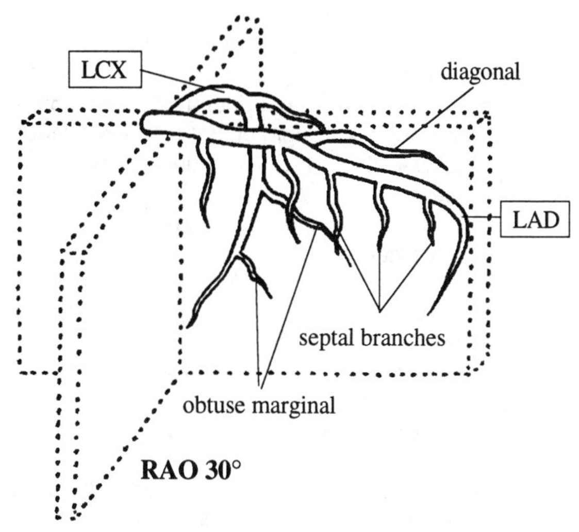

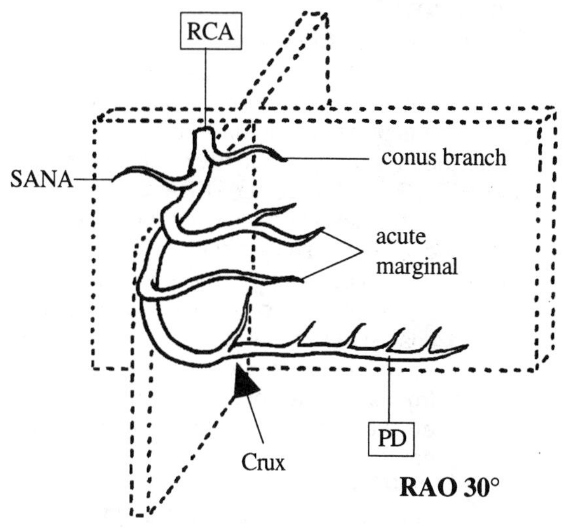

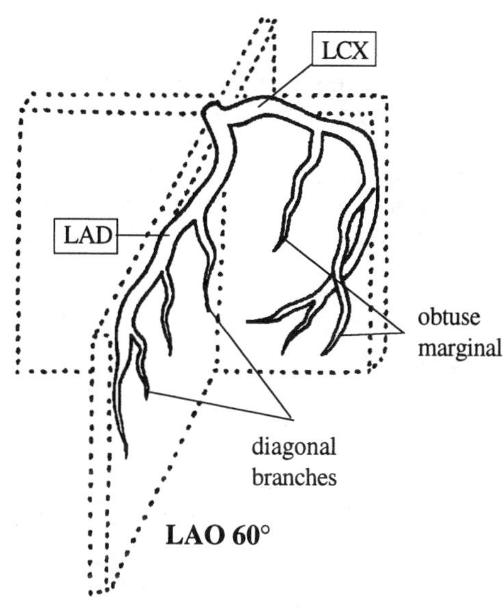

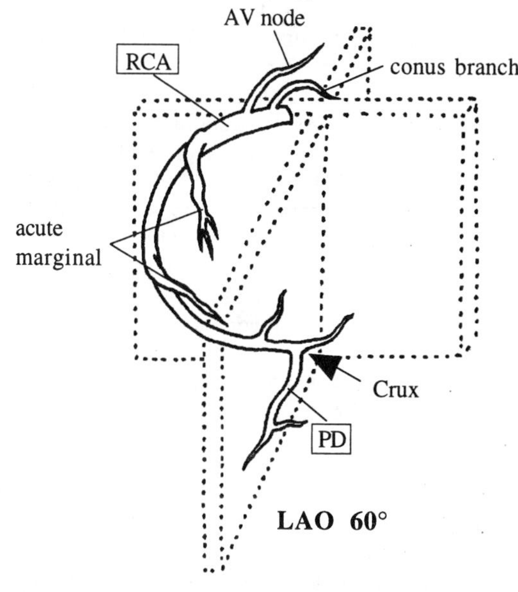

Anatomy of Left Coronary Artery

Marginals emanate from vessels in the AV groove (RCA, LXR)
- — on left side called obtuse marginal arteries
- — on right side called acute marginal arteries

Diagonals emanate from vessel in the interventricular groove (LAD)
Note: **D**iagonals from LA**D**

Coronary dominance
the dominant vessel is the one that supplies the inferolateral wall of LV

AV-node branch from RCA (in 90%) = conus branch (1st branch in 50%)

SA-node branch from RCA (in >50%)

Anatomy of Right Coronary Artery

Arteries in atrioventricular plane:
- RCA = right coronary artery
- LCX = left circumflex artery, gives blood supply to anterolateral papillary muscle

Arteries in interventricular plane:
- LAD = left anterior descending artery, gives blood supply to anterolateral papillary muscle
- PD = posterior descending artery, gives blood supply to posteromedial papillary muscle
- SANA = sinoatrial node artery

HEART

CORONARY ARTERIES

Coronary Artery Collaterals

A. INTRACORONARY COLLATERALS
   = filling of a distal portion of an occluded vessel from the proximal portion
   √ tortuous course outside the normal path

B. INTERCORONARY COLLATERALS
   = between different coronary arteries / between branches of the same artery
   Location: on epicardial surface, in atrial / ventricular septum, in myocardium
   1. proximal RCA to distal RCA
      (a) by way of acute marginal branches
      (b) from sinoatrial node artery (SANA) to atrioventricular node artery (AVNA) = Kugel collateral
   2. RCA to LAD
      (a) between PDA and LAD through ventricular septum / around apex
      (b) conus artery (1st branch of RCA) to proximal part of LAD
      (c) acute marginals of RCA to right ventricular branches of LAD
   3. distal RCA to distal LCX
      (a) posterolateral segment artery of RCA to distal LCX (in AV groove)
      (b) AVNA of RCA to LCX (through atrial wall)
      (c) posterolateral branch of RCA to obtuse marginal branches of LCX (over left posterolateral ventricular wall)
   4. proximal LAD to distal LAD
      (a) proximal diagonal to distal diagonal artery of LAD
      (b) proximal diagonal to LAD directly
   5. LAD to obtuse marginal of LCX

Coronary Artery Dominance

= vessel that supplies the inferior portion of left ventricle
RCA in 80%
LCA in 10%
RCA + LCA (codominance with balanced supply) in 10%

Coronary Arteriography

Contrast agents:
1. Monomeric ionic contrast material:
   (a) negative inotropic = depression of myocardial contractility due to hyperosmolality of sodium + decrease in total calcium
   (b) peripheral vasodilatation
2. Meglumine diatrizoate (contains small quantities of sodium citrate + EDTA)
3. Nonionic contrast material = slight increase in LV contractility

Mortality: 0.05%

Risk factors associated with death:
1. multiple ventricular premature contractions
2. congestive heart failure
3. systemic hypertension
4. severe triple-vessel coronary artery disease (highest risk)
5. LV ejection fraction <30%
6. Left main coronary artery stenosis

Projections:
(a) LAO + 20 – 30° caudocranial angulation proximal 1/3 of LAD + origin of first diagonal branch
(b) LAO + 20 – 30° craniocaudal angulation = "spider view"
    Left main coronary artery, proximal LCX, first marginal / diagonal branches
(c) RAO + 20 – 30° craniocaudal angulation
    Proximal 1/3 of LCX + origin of its branches
(d) RAO + 20 – 30° caudocranial angulation
    Separation of LAD from diagonal branches

False-negative interpretation:
(1) eccentric lesion in 75%
(2) foreshortening of vessel
(3) overlap of other vessels remedied by angulated projections: improved diagnosis (50%), upgrade to more significant stenosis (30%), lesion unmasked (20%)

PULSATILITY

= assessment of vascular resistance (increased resistance reduces diastolic flow)
◊ Can be assessed in vessels too small / tortuous to be imaged (Doppler angle unnecessary)!
◊ Index should be calculated for each of several cardiac cycles (5 heartbeats adequate) an average value taken

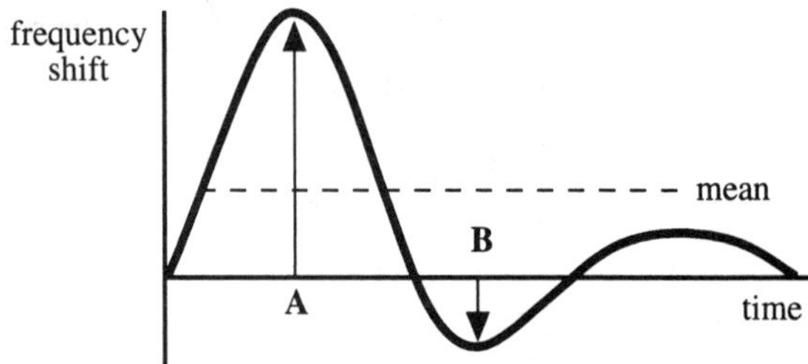

S = A = maximal systolic shift
D = B = end-diastolic frequency shift

1. Full pulsatility index of Gosling (PI_F) = $1/A_0^2\ SA_i^2$
2. Simplified pulsatility index (PI) = (S - D)/mean
3. Resistance index (RI) = Pourcelot index
   = (S - D)/S or 1 - (D/S)
4. Stuart index = A/B ratio = S/D ratio
5. B/A ratio = B(100%)/A

DECREASE IN LUMEN DIAMETER VS. CROSS-SECTIONAL AREA

decrease in lumen diameter	decrease in cross-sectional area
20%	36%
40%	64%
60%	84%
80%	96%

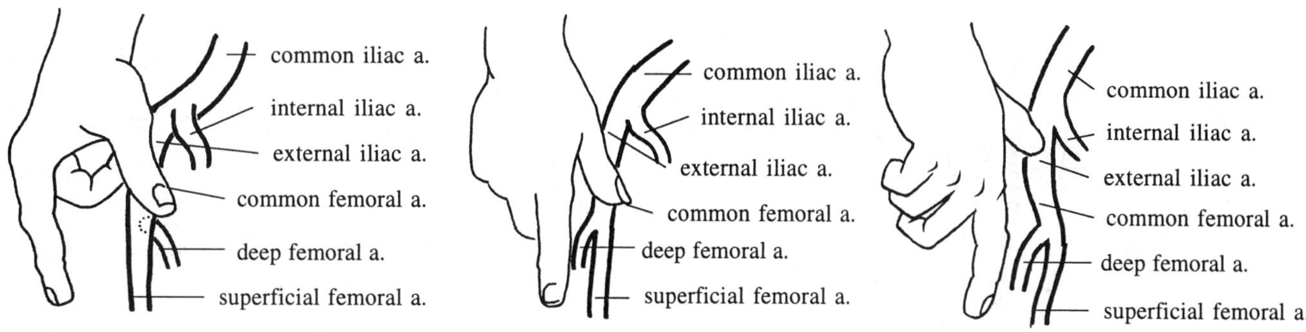

Pelvic Arterial Anatomy (right side)

Contents of femoral triangle

mnemonic: "NAVEL" (from lateral to medial)

- **N**erve
- **A**rtery
- **V**ein
- **E**mpty space
- **L**ymphatics

VENOUS SYSTEM OF LOWER EXTREMITY

Deep veins of lower extremity

3 paired stem veins of the calf accompany the arteries as venae commitantes + anastomose freely with each other:

1. **Anterior tibial veins**
   draining blood from dorsum of foot, running within extensor compartment of lower leg close to interosseous membrane
2. **Posterior tibial veins**
   formed by confluence of superficial + deep plantar veins behind ankle joint

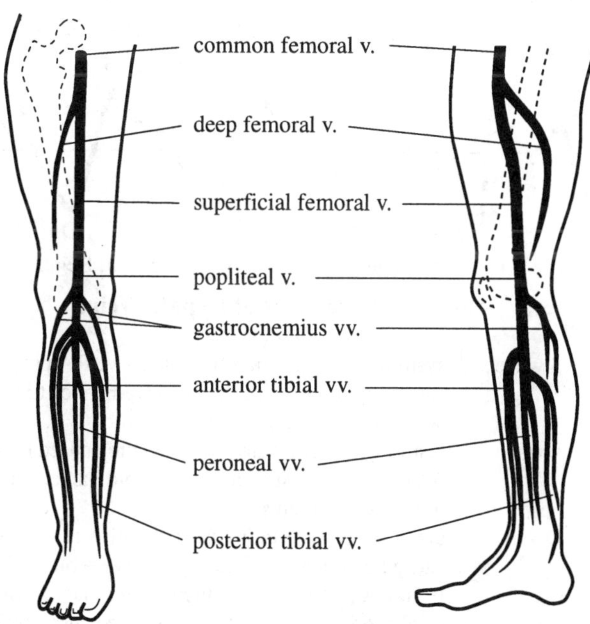

Deep Venous System of Lower Extremity

3. **Peroneal veins**
   directly behind + medial to fibula
4. Calf veins
   (a) **Soleal muscle veins**
   baggy valveless veins in soleus muscle (= sinusoidal veins); draining into posterior tibial + peroneal veins or lower part of popliteal vein
   (b) **Gastrocnemius veins**
   thin straight veins with valves; draining into lower + upper parts of popliteal vein
5. **Popliteal vein**
   formed by stem veins of lower leg
6. **Femoral / superficial femoral vein**
   continuation of popliteal vein; receives deep femoral vein about 9 cm below inguinal ligament
7. **Deep femoral vein**
   draining together with superficial femoral vein into common femoral vein; may connect to popliteal vein (38%)
8. **Common femoral vein**
   formed by confluence of deep + superficial femoral vein; becomes external iliac vein as it passes beneath inguinal ligament

Superficial veins of lower extremity

1. **Greater saphenous vein**
   formed by union of veins from medial side of sole of foot with medial dorsal veins; ascends in front of medial malleolus; passes behind medial condyles of tibia + femur
   (a) Posterior arch vein
   connected to deep venous system by communicating veins
   (b) **Anterior superficial tibial vein**
   (c) **Posteromedial superficial thigh vein**
   often connects with upper part of lesser saphenous vein
   (d) **Anterolateral superficial thigh vein**
   (e) Tributaries in fossa ovalis
   — superficial inferior epigastric vein
   — superficial external pudendal vein
   — superficial circumflex iliac vein

HEART

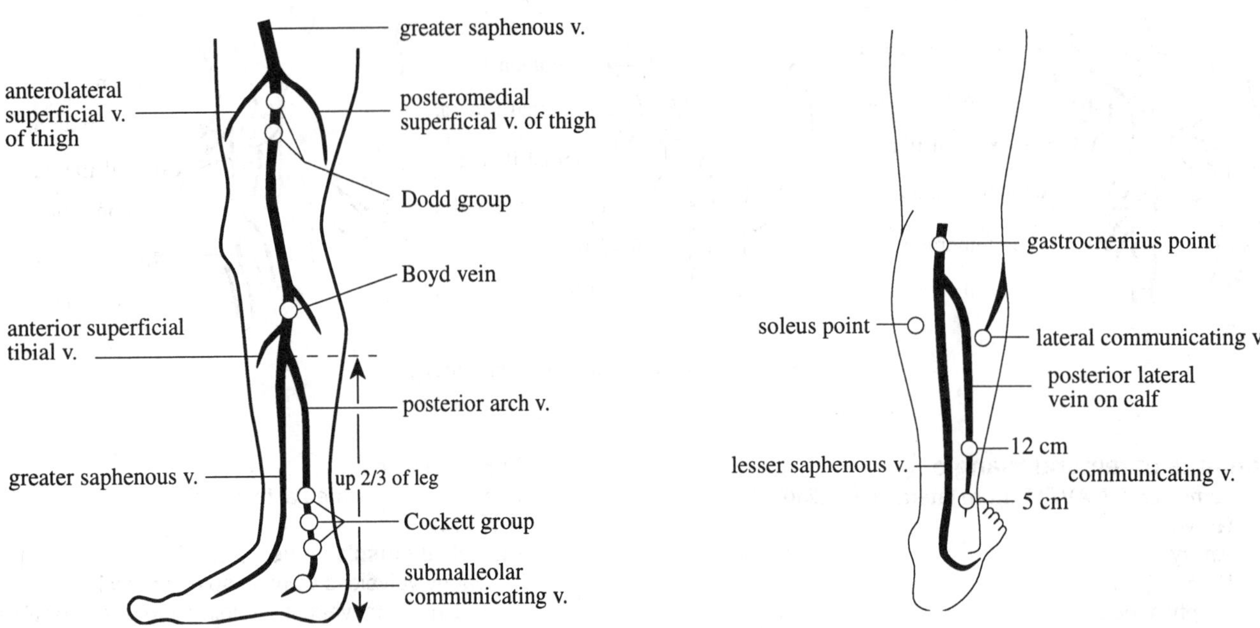

Superficial Venous System of Lower Extremity

2. **Lesser saphenous vein**
originates at outer border of foot behind lateral malleolus as continuation of dorsal venous arch; enters popliteal vein between heads of gastrocnemius in popliteal fossa within 8 cm of knee joint (60%) or joins with greater saphenous vein via posteromedial / anterolateral superficial thigh veins (20%)

Communicating = perforating veins

>100 veins in each leg

(a) medial
1. Submalleolar communicating vein
2. **Cockett group**
group of 3 veins located 7, 12, 18 cm above the tip of medial malleolus connecting posterior arch vein with posterior tibial vein
3. **Boyd vein**
located 10 cm below knee joint connecting main trunk of greater saphenous vein to posterior tibial veins
4. **Dodd group**
group of 1 or 2 veins passing through Hunter canal (= subsartorial canal) to join greater saphenous vein with superficial femoral vein

(b) lateral
1. **Lateral communicating vein**
located from just above lateral malleolus to junction of lower-to-mid thirds of calf connecting lesser saphenous vein with peroneal veins
2. **Posterior mid-calf communicating veins**
located posteriorly 5 + 12 cm above os calcis joining lesser saphenous vein to peroneal veins
3. **Soleal + gastrocnemius points**
joining short saphenous vein to soleal / gastrocnemius veins

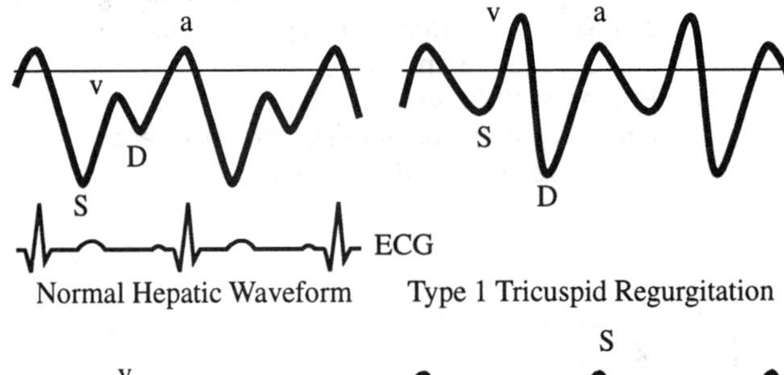

Normal Hepatic Waveform Type 1 Tricuspid Regurgitation

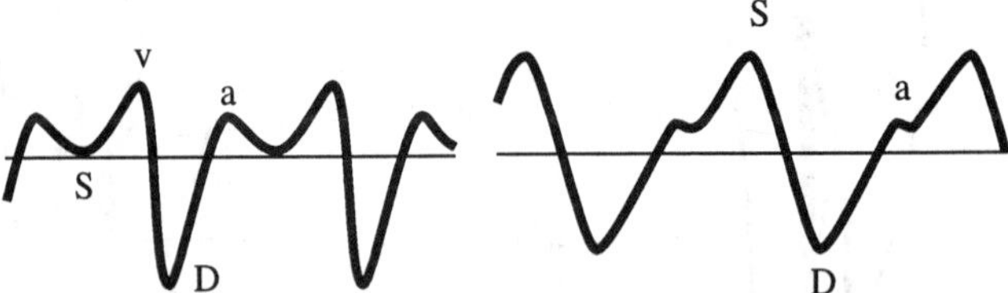

Type 2 Tricuspid Regurgitation Type 3 Tricuspid Regurgitation

Doppler Waveforms of Hepatic Veins

S wave = systolic wave resulting from negative RA pressure caused by atrial relaxation + movement of tricuspid anulus toward cardiac apex

v wave = resulting from elevated RA pressure caused by RA overfilling against a closed tricuspid valve; occurs in <50% of patients

D wave = diastolic wave resulting from negative RA pressure caused by opening of tricuspid valve + blood flow from RA into RV; equal to / smaller than S wave

a-wave = resulting from elevated RA pressure caused by RA contraction; in 66% of patients

CARDIOVASCULAR DISORDERS

ABERRANT LEFT PULMONARY ARTERY

= PULMONARY SLING = failure of development / obliteration of left 6th aortic arch followed by development of a collateral branch of right pulmonary artery to supply the left lung

Site: left PA passes above right mainstem bronchus + between trachea and esophagus on its way to left lung

Age at presentation: neonate / infant / child

Associated with:

(1) "napkin-ring trachea" = absent pars membranacea (50%)

(2) PDA (most common), ASD, persistent left SVC

- stridor (most common), wheezing, apneic spells, cyanosis
- respiratory infection
- feeding problems

√ deviation of trachea to left

√ "inverted-T" appearance of mainstem bronchi = horizontal course secondary to lower origin of right mainstem bronchus

√ anterior bowing of right mainstem bronchus

√ "carrot-shaped trachea" = narrowing of tracheal diameter in caudad direction resulting in functional tracheal stenosis

√ obstructive emphysema / atelectasis of RUL + LUL

√ low left hilum

√ separation of trachea + esophagus at hilum by soft-tissue mass

√ anterior indentation on esophagram

AMYLOIDOSIS

= extracellular deposits of insoluble fibrillar protein

- asymptomatic / CHF (restrictive cardiomyopathy), arrhythmia

CXR:

√ normal / generalized cardiomegaly

√ pulmonary congestion

√ pulmonary deposits of amyloid

NUC:

√ striking uptake of Tc-99m pyrophosphate greater than bone (50–90%)

ECHO:

√ granular sparkling appearance of myocardium

√ LV wall thickening

√ decreased LV systolic + diastolic function

ANOMALOUS LEFT CORONARY ARTERY

= left coronary artery arises from pulmonary trunk (left sinus of Valsalva)

Hemodynamics:

with postnatal fall in pulmonary arterial pressure perfusion of LCA drops (ischemic left coronary bed), collateral circulation from RCA with flow reversal in LCA

— adequate collateral circulation = lifesaving

— inadequate collateral circulation = myocardial infarction

— large collateral circulation = L-to-R shunt with volume overload of heart

- episodes of sweating, ashen color (angina symptomatology)
- ECG: anterolateral infarction
- continuous murmur (if collaterals large)

√ dilatation of LV

√ enlargement of LA

√ normal pulmonary vascularity / redistribution

Rx:

(1) Ligation of LCA at its origin from pulmonary trunk

(2) Ligation of LCA + graft of left subclavian artery to LCA

(3) Creation of an AP window + baffle from AP window to ostium of LCA

DDx: Endocardial fibroelastosis, viral cardiomyopathy (NO shocklike symptoms)

ANOMALOUS PULMONARY VENOUS RETURN

Total anomalous pulmonary venous return

= TAPVR = anomalous connection between pulmonary veins and systemic veins secondary to embryologic failure of the common pulmonary vein to join the posterior wall of the left atrium

Prevalence: 2% of CHD

Age: symptomatic in 1st year of life

Associated with:

ASD / patent foramen ovale (necessary for survival), bronchopulmonary sequestration, pulmonary arteriovenous malformation, cystic adenomatoid malformation

A. <u>SUPRADIAPHRAGMATIC TAPVR</u>

Type I = SUPRACARDIAC TAPVR (52%)
= drainage into left brachiocephalic vein / right + left persistent SVC / azygos vein; <10% obstructed

Type II = CARDIAC TAPVR (30%)
= drainage into coronary sinus (80%) / RA

Hemodynamics:

— functional L-to-R shunt from pulmonary veins to right atrium

— increased pulmonary blood flow (= overcirculation)

— ASD restores oxygenated blood to left side

— normal systemic venous pressure with increased flow through widened SVC

— after birth CHF secondary to

(a) mixture of systemic + pulmonary venous blood in RA

(b) volume overload of RV

- cyanosis
- neck veins undistended (shunt level distally)
- R ventricular heave (= increased contact of enlarged RV with sternum)

- cyanosis
- neck veins undistended (shunt level distally)
- R ventricular heave (= increased contact of enlarged RV with sternum)
- systolic ejection murmur (large shunt volume)

√ "figure of 8" / "snowman" configuration of cardiac silhouette (= dilated SVC + left vertical vein)
√ pretracheal density on lateral film (= left vertical vein)
√ enlargement of RA + RV (= volume overload)
√ normal LA (= ASD acts as escape valve)
√ increased pulmonary blood flow (= overcirculation)
√ absent connection of pulmonary veins to LA

Sub- / Infradiaphragmatic TAPVR (12%)

= Type III
= drainage into portal vein / IVC / ductus venosus / left gastric vein with constriction of descending pulmonary vein by diaphragm en route through esophageal hiatus leading to pulmonary venous hypertension + RV pressure overload; >90% obstructed

- intense cyanosis + respiratory distress (R-to-L shunt through ASD)

Prognosis: death within a few days of life
Associated with: asplenia syndrome (80%), polysplenia
√ unique appearance of pulmonary edema + pulmonary venous congestion with normal-sized heart (DDx: hyaline membrane disease)
√ low anterior indentation on barium-filled esophagus

Mixed Type Of TAPVR (6%) = Type IV

= with various connections to R side of heart (6%)

HEART

Partial Anomalous Pulmonary Venous Return

= PAPVR
May occur in isolation
Prevalence: 0.3–0.5% of patients with CHD
May be associated with:
(1) Atrial septal defect (25%)
 (a) RUL pulmonary vein enters SVC / RA (2/3)
  frequently associated with: sinus venosus type ASD (90%)
  √ RUL vein courses in a horizontal direction
 (b) LUL pulmonary vein enters brachiocephalic vein (1/3)
  frequently associated with: ostium secundum type ASD
  √ vertical mediastinal density lateral to aortic knob extending upward and medially with smooth curvilinear border (DDx: persistent left SVC)
(2) Hypogenetic lung as a component of congenital pulmonary venolobar syndrome
 = SCIMITAR SYNDROME
 = part / all of the hypogenetic lung is drained by an anomalous vein

Anomalous vein drains into:
— IVC below right hemidiaphragm (33%)
— suprahepatic portion of IVC (22%)
— hepatic veins
— portal vein (11%)
— azygos vein
— coronary sinus
— right atrium (22%)
— left atrium = "meandering pulmonary vein"
 ◊ Drainage into suprahepatic portion of IVC / right atrium may be a clue for interruption of intrahepatic portion of IVC!

May be associated with: systemic arterialization of the lung without sequestration
Location: almost exclusively on right side
√ tubular structure paralleling the right heart border in the configuration of a Turkish sword = "scimitar" (PA view)

- ASD symptomatology

CECT:
√ nodular / tubular opacity (= anomalous vein), which opacifies in phase with pulmonary vein

AORTIC ANEURYSM

Cause:
1. Atherosclerosis (73–80–90%):
2. Traumatic (15–20%): following transection
3. Congenital (2%): aortic sinus, post coarctation, ductus diverticulum
4. Syphilis (19%): ascending aorta + arch
5. Mycotic = bacterial dissection
6. Cystic media necrosis (Marfan / Ehlers-Danlos syndrome, annuloaortic ectasia)
7. Inflammation of media + adventitia: Takayasu arteritis, giant cell arteritis, relapsing polychondritis, rheumatic fever, rheumatoid arthritis, ankylosing spondylitis, Reiter syndrome, psoriasis, ulcerative colitis, systemic lupus erythematosus, scleroderma, Behçet disease, radiation
8. Increased pressure: systemic hypertension, aortic valve stenosis
9. Abnormal volume load: severe aortic regurgitation

TRUE ANEURYSM
= permanent dilatation of all layers of weakened but intact wall

FALSE ANEURYSM
= focal perforation with all layers of wall disrupted; escaped blood contained by adventitia / perivascular connective tissue + organized blood

FUSIFORM ANEURYSM (80%)
= circumferential involvement

SACCULAR ANEURYSM
= involvement of portion of wall

Abdominal Aortic Aneurysm (AAA)

◊ There is no consensus regarding the definition of an atherosclerotic AAA!

= focal widening >3 cm (ultrasound literature); twice the size of normal aorta / >4 cm (Bergan, Ann Surg 1984)
Normal size of abdominal aorta >50 years of age: 12–19 mm in women; 14–21 mm in men

Prevalence: 1.4–8.2% in unselected population; in 6% >80 years of age; in 6–20% of patients with signs of atherosclerotic disease; M>F; Whites:Blacks = 3:1

Cause: ? genetic (10-fold increase in risk as first-degree relative of patient with AAA); structural defect of aortic wall caused by increased proteolysis; copper deficiency

Risk factors: male sex, age >75 years, white race, prior vascular disease, hypertension, cigarette smoking, family history, hypercholesterolemia

Age: >60 years; M:F = 5–9:1

Associated with:
(a) visceral + renal artery aneurysm (2%)
(b) isolated iliac + femoral artery aneurysm (16%): common iliac (89%), internal iliac (10%), external iliac (1%)
(c) stenosis / occlusion of celiac trunk / SMA (22%)
(d) stenosis of renal artery (22–30%)
(e) occlusion of inferior mesenteric artery (80%)
(f) occlusion of lumbar arteries (78%)

Growth rate of aneurysm of 3–6 cm in diameter: 0.39 cm / year

- asymptomatic (30%)
- abdominal mass (26%)
- abdominal pain (37%)

◊ Imaging should provide information about
(a) the proximal extent of the aneurysm which determines the site of clamping of the aorta (origin of renal arteries)
(b) the course of the left renal vein (retroaortic?)!

Location: infrarenal (91–95%) with extension into iliac arteries (66–70%)
Plain film: √ mural calcification (75–86%)
US: √ >98% accuracy in size measurement
NCCT:
√ perianeurysmal fibrosis (10%), may cause ureteral obstruction
√ "crescent sign" = peripheral high-attenuating crescent in aneurysm wall (= acute intramural hematoma) = **sign of impending rupture**

CECT:
(a) ruptured aneurysm:
√ anterior displacement of kidney
√ extravasation of contrast material
√ fluid collection / hematoma within posterior pararenal + perirenal spaces
√ free intraperitoneal fluid
√ perirenal "cobwebs"
(b) contained leak
√ laminated mural calcification
√ periaortic mass of mixed / soft-tissue density
√ lateral "draping" of aneurysm around vertebral body
√ focal discontinuity of calcifications (unreliable)
√ indistinct aortic wall (unreliable)

Angio:
√ focally widened aortic lumen >3 cm
√ apparent normal size of lumen secondary to mural thrombus (11%)
√ mural clot (80%)
√ slow antegrade flow of contrast medium
Contained rupture = extraluminal hematoma / cavity
√ absent parenchymal stain = avascular halo
√ displacement + stretching of aortic branches

Cx:
(1) Rupture (25%)
(a) into retroperitoneum: commonly on left
(b) into GI tract: massive GI hemorrhage
(c) into IVC: rapid cardiac decompensation
Incidence: aneurysm <4 cm in 10%, 4–5 cm in 23%, 5–7 cm in 25%, 7–10 cm in 46%, >10 cm in 60%
- sudden severe abdominal pain ± radiating into back
- faintness, syncope, hypotension

Prognosis: 64–94% die before reaching hospital
Increased risk: size >6 cm, growth >5 mm / 6 months, pain + tenderness
◊ The exact moment of rupture is unpredictable!
◊ Cause of death in 1.3% of men >65 years!
(2) Peripheral embolization
(3) Infection
(4) Spontaneous occlusion of aorta

Prognosis: 17% 5-year survival without surgery, 50–60% 5-year survival with surgery

Rx: surgery recommended if >5 cm in diameter; 4–5% surgical mortality for nonruptured, 30–80% for ruptured aneurysm

Postoperative Cx:
(1) Left colonic ischemia (1.6%) with 10% mortality
(2) Renal failure (14%)
(3) 0–8% mortality rate for elective surgery

Atherosclerotic aneurysm

Incidence: leading cause of thoracic aortic aneurysm
Histo: diseased intima with secondary degeneration + fibrous replacement of media; ultimately wall of aneurysm composed of acellular + avascular connective tissue
Pathophysiology:
progressive weakening of media results in vessel dilatation + increased tension of vessel wall (law of Laplace = tensile stress varies with product of blood pressure and radius of vessel); compromise of mural vascular nutrition (vasa vasorum) causes further degeneration + progressive dilatation
Age: elderly; M > F
Location: distal abdominal aorta > iliac a. > popliteal a. > common femoral a. > aortic + descending thoracic aorta > carotid a.
Site: (1) infrarenal aorta (associated with thoracic aneurysm in 29%)

(2) descending thoracic aorta distal to left subclavian artery
(3) thoracoabdominal

√ fusiform (80%), saccular (20%)

Cx: rupture (cause of death in 50%): usually unrestrained + fatal in thoracic location

Degenerative aneurysm

= medial degeneration

Most common cause of aneurysm in ascending aorta

Cause: (1) genetically transmitted metabolic disorder: Marfan syndrome, Ehlers-Danlos syndrome
(2) acquired: result of repetitive aortic injury + repair associated with aging

Inflammatory aortic aneurysm

= defined as triad of
(1) thickened aneurysm wall
(2) extensive perianeurysmal + retroperitoneal fibrosis
(3) dense adhesions of adjacent abdominal organs

Frequency: 3–10% of all AAAs; M:F = 6:1 to 30:1

Mean age: 62–68 years

- abdominal / back pain
- weight loss + anorexia (20–41%)
- elevated ESR (40–88%)
- tender pulsatile abdominal mass (15–30%)

Comorbidities: arterial hypertension (34–69%), arterial occlusive disease (10–47%), diabetes mellitus (3–13%), coronary artery disease (33–55%)

√ entrapment of ureters (10–21%)

√ sonolucent halo around aorta

Cx: enlargement + rupture (lower rate than in noninflammatory aneurysm)

Mycotic aneurysm

Incidence: 2.6% of all abdominal aneurysms

A. PRIMARY MYCOTIC ANEURYSM (rare)
unassociated with any demonstrable intravascular inflammatory process

B. SECONDARY MYCOTIC ANEURYSM
= aneurysm due to nonsyphilitic infection

Predisposing factors:
(1) IV drug abuse (2) bacterial endocarditis (12%) (3) immunocompromise (malignancy, alcoholism, steroids, chemotherapy, autoimmune disease, diabetes) (4) atherosclerosis (5) aortic trauma caused by accidents / aortic valve surgery / coronary artery bypass surgery / arterial catheterization

Mechanism:
(a) septicemia with abscess formation via vasa vasorum
(b) septicemia with abscess formation via vessel lumen
(c) direct extension of contiguous infection
(d) preexisting intima laceration (trauma, atherosclerosis, coarctation)

Organism: S. aureus (53%), Salmonella (33-50%), nonhemolytic Streptococcus, Pneumococcus, Gonococcus, Mycobacterium (contiguous spread from spine / lymph nodes)

Histo: loss of intima + destruction of internal elastic lamella; varying degrees of destruction of muscularis of media + adventitia

- frequently insidious, fever
- positive blood culture in 50%

Site: ascending aorta > abdominal visceral artery > intracranial artery > lower / upper extremity artery

√ true aneurysm (majority)

√ saccular structure arising eccentrically from aortic wall with rapid enlargement

√ interrupted ring of aortic wall calcification

√ periaortic gas collection

√ adjacent vertebral osteomyelitis

√ adjacent reactive lymph node enlargement

Cx: (1) life-threatening rupture + hemorrhage (75%)
(2) uncontrolled sepsis if untreated

Prognosis: 67% overall mortality

Syphilitic aneurysm

Spectrum:
1. Uncomplicated syphilitic aortitis
2. Syphilitic aortic aneurysm (mostly saccular)
3. Syphilitic aortic vasculitis (aortic regurgitation)

Incidence: 12% of patients with untreated syphilis

Onset: 10–30 years after initial spirochete infection

Histo: chronic inflammation of aortic adventitia + media beginning at vasa vasorum + leading to obstruction of vasa vasorum followed by nutritional impairment of media + loss of elastic fibers + smooth muscle fibers

- positive venereal disease research laboratory (VDRL) test
- positive microhemagglutination assay - Treponema pallidum (MHA-TP) test

Location: ascending aorta (36%), aortic arch (34%), proximal descending aorta (25%), distal descending aorta (5%), aortic sinuses (<1%)

√ asymmetric enlargement of aortic sinuses (DDx to medial degeneration with symmetric enlargement)

√ saccular (75%) / fusiform (25%) aneurysm

√ pencil-thin dystrophic aortic wall calcification (up to 40%) most severe in ascending aorta, frequently obscured by thick coarse irregular calcifications of secondary atherosclerosis

Prognosis: death in 2%, rupture in up to 40%; death within months of onset of symptoms if untreated

Thoracic aortic aneurysm

Most common vascular cause of mediastinal mass!

◊ 10% of mediastinal masses are of vascular origin!

Average diameter of thoracic aorta (<4–5 cm wide):
— aortic root: 3.6 cm
— ascending aorta 1 cm proximal to arch: 3.5 cm
— proximal descending aorta: 2.6 cm

HEART

— middle descending aorta: 2.5 cm
— distal descending aorta: 2.4 cm

Associated with: hypertension, coronary artery disease, abdominal aneurysm

Mean age: 65 years; M:F = 3:1

• substernal / back / shoulder pain (26%)
• SVC syndrome (venous compression)
• dysphagia (esophageal compression)
• stridor, dyspnea (tracheobronchial compression)
• hoarseness (recurrent laryngeal nerve compression)

√ mediastinal mass with proximity to aorta
√ wide tortuous aorta
√ curvilinear peripheral calcifications (75%)
√ circumferential / crescentic mural thrombus
√ Angio: may show normal caliber secondary to mural thrombus

Cx: (1) Rupture into mediastinum, pericardium, either pleural sac, extrapleural space
√ high-attenuation fluid
(2) Aortobronchopulmonary fistula
√ consolidation of lung adjacent to aneurysm
◊ Most aneurysms rupture when >10 cm in size

Prognosis: 1-year survival 57%, 3-year survival 26%, 5-year survival 19% (60% die from ruptured aneurysm, 40% die from other causes)

Surgical mortality: 10%

Traumatic aortic pseudoaneurysm

= CHRONIC AORTIC PSEUDOANEURYSM

◊ 2nd most common form of thoracic aortic aneurysm;
◊ most common type occurring in young patients

Incidence: 2.5% of patients who survive initial trauma of acute aortic transection

√ usually calcified
√ may contain thrombus

Cx: (1) progressive enlargement
(2) rupture (even years after insult)

AORTIC DISSECTION

= spontaneous longitudinal separation of aortic intima + adventitia by circulating blood having gained access to the media of the aortic wall splitting it in two

Path: (a) transverse tear in weakened intima (95–97%)
(b) no intimal tear (3–5%) = INTRAMURAL HEMATOMA OF AORTA

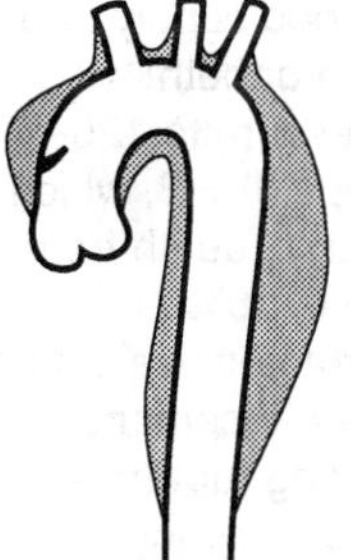
DeBakey Type I
Stanford Type A

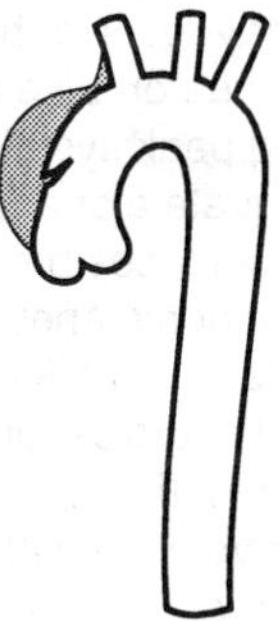
DeBakey Type II
Stanford Type A

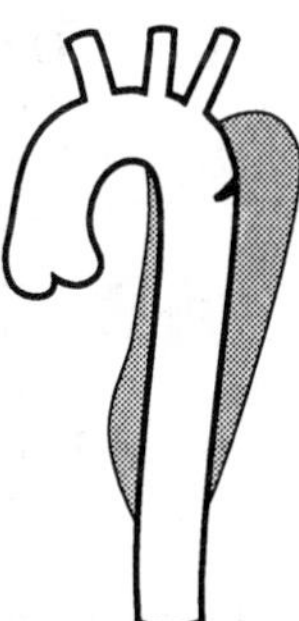
DeBakey Type III
Stanford Type B

Aortic Dissection

Pathogenesis:
intimal tear results from combination of following factors:
(1) medial degeneration decreases cohesiveness within aortic wall
(2) persistent aortic motion secondary to beating heart results in stress within aortic wall
(3) hydrodynamic forces accentuated by hypertension

Incidence: 3:1,000 (more common than all ruptures of thoracic + abdominal aorta combined); 1:205 autopsies; 2,000 cases/year in United States

Peak age: 60 years (range 13–87 years); M:F = 3:1

Predisposed: (cystic medial necrosis / disease of aortic wall)
◊ Starts in fusiform aneurysms in 28%
◊ Does not occur in aneurysms <5 cm in diameter

1. Hypertension (60–90%)
2. Marfan syndrome (16%)
3. Ehlers-Danlos syndrome
4. Relapsing polychondritis
5. Valvular aortic stenosis
6. Turner syndrome
7. Behçet disease
8. Coarctation
9. Bicuspid aortic valve
10. S/P prosthetic valve
11. Trauma (rare)
12. Catheterization
13. Pregnancy
14. Aortitis (eg, SLE)
15. Cocaine abuse

NOT syphilis

◊ In women 50% of dissections occur during pregnancy!

• sharp tearing intractable anterior / posterior chest pain (75–95%) radiating to jaw, neck, low back (DDx: myocardial infarction)
• murmur ± bruit (65%) from aortic regurgitation
• asymmetric peripheral pulses + blood pressures (59%)
• absent femoral pulses (25%), reappearing after reentry
• pulse deficit: in up to 50% of type A dissection, in 16% of type B dissection
• hemodynamic shock (25%)
• neurologic deficits (25%): hemiplegia, paraparesis (due to compromise of anterior spinal artery of Adamkiewicz)
• persistent oliguria
• congestive heart failure (rare) due to acute aortic insufficiency
• recurrent arrhythmias / right bundle branch block
• signs of pericardial tamponade: clouded sensorium, extreme restlessness, dyspnea, distended neck veins

Types:

DeBakey Type I (29–34%) = ascending aorta + portion distal to arch
DeBakey Type II (12–21%) = ascending aorta only
DeBakey Type III (50%) = descending aorta only
Subtype IIIA = up to diaphragm
Subtype IIIB = below diaphragm

Stanford Type A (70%) = ascending aorta ± arch in first 4 cm in 90%
Stanford Type B (20–30%) = descending aorta only

mnemonic: **A** **a**ffects **a**scending aorta and **a**rch;
B **b**egins **b**eyond **b**rachiocephalic vessels!

Clinical classification:
(1) Acute aortic dissection: <2 weeks old
(2) Chronic aortic dissection: >2 weeks old

Location of dissection (following helical flow pattern):
- — on anterior + right lateral wall of ascending aorta just distal to aortic valve (65%)
- — on superior + posterior wall of transverse aortic arch (10%)
- — on posterior + left lateral wall of upper descending aorta distal to left subclavian artery (20%)
- — more distal aorta (5%) usually terminating in left iliac artery (80%) / right iliac artery (10%) [involvement of left renal artery in 50%]

◊ An exit / distal tear / reentry occurs in 10%!

CXR (best assessment from comparison with serial films):
- √ normal CXR in 25%
- √ "calcification sign" = inward displacement of atherosclerotic plaque by >4–10 mm from outer aortic contour (7%), can only be applied to contour of descending aorta secondary to projection, may be misleading in presence of periaortic soft-tissue mass / hematoma
- √ disparity in size between ascending + descending aorta
- √ irregular wavy contour / indistinct outline of aorta
- √ widening of superior mediastinum to >8 cm due to hemorrhage / large false channel (40–80%)
- √ cardiac enlargement (LV hypertrophy / hemopericardium)
- √ left pleural effusion (27%)
- √ atelectasis of lower lobe
- √ rightward displacement of trachea / endotracheal tube

ECHO:
- (a) transthoracic US: 59–85% sensitive + 63–96% specific for type A dissection; poorer for type B
- (b) transesophageal US: up to 99% sensitive + 77–97% specific
- (c) intravascular in conjunction with aortography to differentiate true from false lumen
- √ intimal flap (seen in more than one view)
- √ pericardial fluid
- √ aortic insufficiency

False-positives: reverberation echoes from aneurysmal ascending aorta / calcified atheromatous plaque, postoperative periaortic hematoma

Angio (86–88% sensitive, 75–94% specific):

◊ Aortography 1st choice for final confirmation + staging because of contrast limitation!

Superior to any other technique in demonstrating
- — entry + reentry points (in 50%)
- — branch vessel involvement + coronary arteries
- — aortic insufficiency

- √ visualization of intimal / medial flap (75–79%) = linear radiolucency within opacified aorta
- √ "double barrel aorta" (87%) = opacification of two aortic lumens
- √ abnormal catheter position outside anticipated aortic course
- √ compression of true lumen by false channel (72–85%)
- √ aortic valvular regurgitation (30%)
- √ increase in aortic wall thickness >6–10 mm
- √ obstruction of aortic branches: left renal artery (25–30%)
- √ ulcerlike projections caused by truncated branches
- √ slower blood flow in false lumen

False-negative: complete thrombosis of false channel (10%), intimal flap not tangential to x-ray beam

False-positive: thickening of aortic wall due to aneurysm, aortitis, adjacent neoplasm / hemorrhage

CECT (87–94% sensitive, 87–100% specific):
within 4 hours (if patient responds rapidly to medical Rx); detection as accurate as angio with single-level dynamic scanning
- √ crescentic high-attenuation clot within false lumen
- √ internally displaced intimal calcification (DDx: calcification of thrombus on luminal surface or within)
- √ intimal flap separating two aortic channels (may be seen without contrast in anemic patients)

False-negative: inadequate contrast opacification, thrombosed lumen misinterpreted as aortic aneurysm with mural thrombus

False-positive: streak artifacts secondary to cardiac / aortic motion, opacified normal sinus of Valsalva, normal pericardial recess mistaken for thrombus

MR (95–100% sensitive, 90–100% specific):
- √ intimal flap of medium intensity outlined by signal voids of rapidly flowing blood
- √ intimal flap more difficult to detect in presence of slow flow / thrombus
- √ "cobwebs" (= bands of medial elastic lamellae spanning the junction of the dissecting septum with the outer wall of the false lumen) mark the false lumen in 80%

Cx:
- (1) Retrograde dissection
  - (a) aortic insufficiency
  - (b) occlusion of coronary artery (8%)
  - (c) rupture into pericardial sac / pleural space: 70% mortality
  - (d) rupture into RV, LA, vena cava, pulmonary artery producing large L-to-R shunt
- (2) occlusion / transient obstruction of major aortic branches (30%)
- (3) rupture of aorta
- (4) development of saccular aneurysm requiring surgery (15%)

◊ Organs may receive their blood supply through either the true or false lumen or both!

Rx:
- (1) Reducing peak systolic pressure to 120–70 mm Hg (adequate alone for Type III = B, which rarely progresses proximally): death from rupture of aortic aneurysm in 46% of hypertensive + 17% of normotensive patients
- (2) Immediate surgical graft reinforcement of aortic wall (Type I, II = A) preventing rupture + progressive aortic valve insufficiency

Prognosis without Rx:
immediate death (3%); death within: 1 day (20–30%), 1 week (50–62%), 3 weeks (60%), 1 month (75%), 3 months (80%), 1 year (80–95%)

HEART

Prognosis with Rx:
5–10% mortality rate following timely surgery;
40% 10-year survival rate after leaving hospital
DDx: Penetrating ulcer of thoracic aorta (= atherosclerotic lesion of mid-descending aorta with ulceration extending through intima into aortic media)

AORTIC GRAFT INFECTION

Classification:
(1) PERIGRAFT INFECTION (2–6%)
- fever, chills, leukocytosis
- groin swelling / drainage

(2) AORTOENTERIC FISTULA (0.6–2%)
- acute / chronic GI bleeding (may be occult)
- sepsis

Normal postoperative course:
◊ complete resolution of hematoma by 2–3 months
◊ disappearance of ectopic gas by 3–4 weeks

CT (94% sensitive, 85% specific, 91% accurate):
√ perigraft soft tissue
√ ectopic gas (fistulous communication with bowel / gas-producing organism)
√ focal bowel wall thickening (indicates fistula)
√ >5 mm soft tissue between graft + surrounding wrap (beyond 7th postoperative week)
√ focal discontinuity of calcified aneurysmal wrap

False positives:
perigraft hematoma in early postoperative period, pseudoaneurysm (in 15–20%)
Prognosis: 17–75% mortality; 30–50% morbidity

AORTIC REGURGITATION

= AORTIC INSUFFICIENCY
Cause:
A. INTRINSIC AORTIC VALVE DISEASE
1. Congenital bicuspid valve
2. Rheumatic endocarditis
3. Bacterial endocarditis (perforation / prolapse of cusp)
4. Myxomatous valve associated with cystic medial necrosis
5. Aortic valve prolapse
6. Prosthetic valve: mechanical break, thrombosis, paravalvular leak

B. PRIMARY DISEASE OF ASCENDING AORTA
(a) Dilatation of aortic annulus
1. Syphilitic aortitis
2. Ankylosing spondylitis (5–10%)
3. Reiter disease
4. Rheumatoid arthritis
5. Cystic medial necrosis: Marfan syndrome

(b) Laceration = aortic dissection
1. Deceleration trauma
2. Hypertension

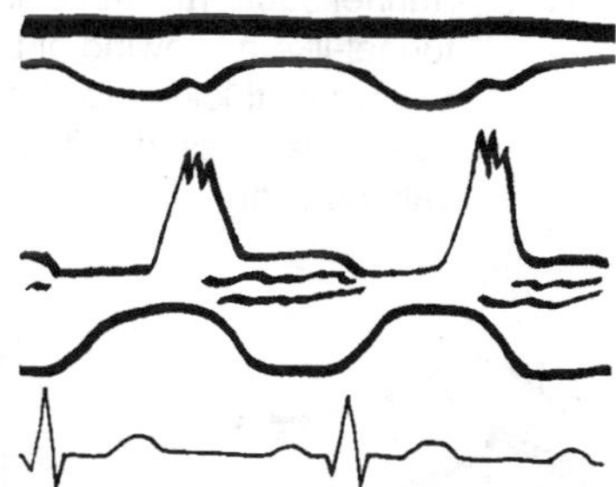

Mitral Valve in Severe Aortic Regurgitation
The valve is almost completely closed before onset of ventricular systole. Atrial contraction has little effect in reopening the valve. Complete closure occurs with ventricular systole. A high-velocity flutter of aML is present in diastole.

Pathogenesis: progressive enlargement of diastolic + systolic LV dimensions result in increase in myocardial fiber length + increase in stroke volume; decompensation occurs if critical limit of fiber length is reached
- "water-hammer pulse" = twin-peaked pulse
- systolic ejection murmur + high-pitched diastolic murmur
- Austin Flint murmur = soft mid-diastolic or presystolic bruit

√ LV enlargement (cardiothoracic ratio >0.55) + initially normal pulmonary vascularity (DDx: congestive cardiomyopathy, pericardial effusion)
√ normal aorta (in intrinsic valve disease)
√ dilatation ± calcification of ascending aorta (in aortic wall disease)
√ tortuous descending aorta
√ increased pulsations along entire aorta

ECHO:
√ aortic root dilatation
√ high frequency flutter of aML (occasionally pML) during first 2/3 of diastole (CHARACTERISTIC)
√ high frequency diastolic flutter of IVS (uncommon)
√ diastolic flutter of aortic valve (SPECIFIC, but rare)
√ premature aortic valve opening (high diastolic LV pressure)
√ decreased MV opening (aML pushed posteriorly by regurgitant aortic jet)
√ premature closure of mitral valve (high diastolic LV pressure produces MV closure before beginning of systole in severe acute aortic insufficiency)
√ LV dilatation + large amplitude of LV wall motion (volume overload, increased ejection fraction):

End-systolic LV diameter	Action
<50 mm	yearly follow-up
50–54 mm	4- to 6-month follow-up
>55 mm	valve replacement

Doppler:
√ slope of peak diastolic to end-diastolic velocity decrease >3 m/sec^2 in severe aortic regurgitation
√ area of color Doppler regurgitant flow
√ ratio of width of regurgitant beam to width of aortic root is good predictor of severity (color Doppler)

HEART

AORTIC RUPTURE

= blood leakage through aneurysmatic aortic wall

Pathogenesis: small clefts occur at a fragile site within inner thrombus gradually expanding to outer layer of thrombus with gradual seepage of flowing blood into mural thrombus and aneurysmal wall

CT:
- √ high-attenuation crescent sign (71%)

AORTIC STENOSIS

Aortic valve area decreased to <0.8 cm^2 = 0.4 cm^2/m^2 BSA (normal 2.5–3.5 cm^2)

A. ACQUIRED AORTIC STENOSIS
   1. Rheumatic valvulitis (almost invariably associated with mitral valve disease)
   2. Fibrocalcific senile aortic stenosis (degenerative)

B. CONGENITAL AORTIC STENOSIS (most common)
   = most frequent CHD associated with IUGR
   1. Subvalvular AS (30%)
   2. Valvular AS (70%): degeneration of bicuspid valve most common cause
   3. Supravalvular AS

Pathogenesis: increased gradient across valve produces LV hypertrophy and diminished LV compliance; increased muscle mass may outstrip coronary blood supply (subendocardial myocardial ischemia with angina); LV decompensation leads to LV dilatation + pulmonary venous congestion

- asymptomatic for many years
- angina, syncope, heart failure
- systolic murmur
- carotid pulsus parvus et tardus
- diminished aortic component of 2nd heart sound
- sudden death in severe stenosis (20%) after exercise (diminished flow in coronary arteries causes ventricular dysrhythmias + fibrillation)

√ poststenotic dilatation of ascending aorta (in 90% of acquired, in 70% of congenital AS)
√ normal-sized / enlarged LV (small LV chamber with thick walls)

@ in adults >30 years
  √ calcification of aortic valve (best seen on RAO); indicates gradient >50 mm Hg
  √ discrete enlargement of ascending aorta (NO correlation with severity of stenosis)
  √ calcification of mitral annulus
  √ "left ventricular configuration" = concavity along mid left lateral heart border + increased convexity along lower left lateral heart border

@ in children / young adults
  √ prominent ascending aorta
  √ left ventricular heart configuration

@ in infancy:
  √ left ventricular stress syndrome

ECHO:
  √ thickened + calcified aortic valve with multiple dense cusp echoes throughout cardiac cycle (right > noncoronary > left coronary cusp)
  √ decreased separation of leaflets in systole with reduced opening orifice (13–14 mm = mild AS; 8–12 mm = moderate AS; <8 mm = severe AS)
  √ ± doming in systole
  √ dilated aortic root
  √ increased thickness of LV wall (= concentric LV hypertrophy)
  √ hyperdynamic contraction of LV (in compensated state)
  √ decreased mitral EF slope (reduced LV compliance)
  √ LA enlargement
  √ increased aortic valve gradient (Doppler)
  √ decreased aortic valve area (unreliable)

  DDx: calcification of aortic annulus in elderly / calcified coronary artery ostium (thickened cusp echoes only in diastole)

Prognosis: depends on symptomatology (angina, syncope, CHF)

Subvalvular Aortic Stenosis

= SUBAORTIC STENOSIS

(a) Anatomic / fixed subaortic stenosis

Associated with: cardiac defects in 50% (usually VSD)

Type I : thin 1–2 mm membranous diaphragmatic stenosis, usually located within 2 cm or less of valve annulus
Type II : thick collarlike stenosis
Type III : irregular fibromuscular stenosis
Type IV : "tunnel subaortic stenosis" = fixed tunnel-like narrowing of LVOT = excessive thickening of only upper ventricular septum with normal mitral valve motion

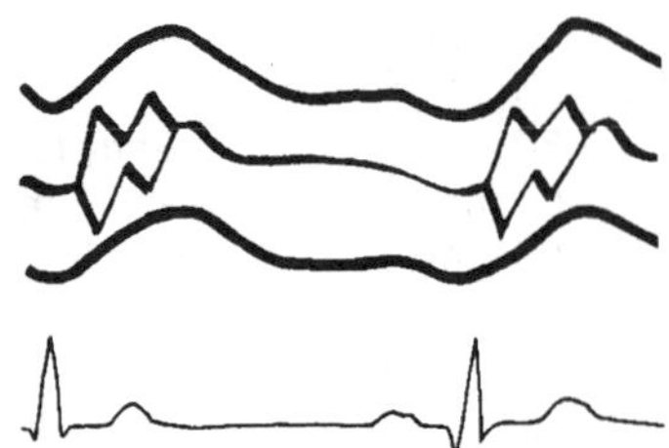

Aortic Valve in Hypertrophic Subaortic Stenosis
during midsystole the aortic valve closes secondary to subvalvular obstruction

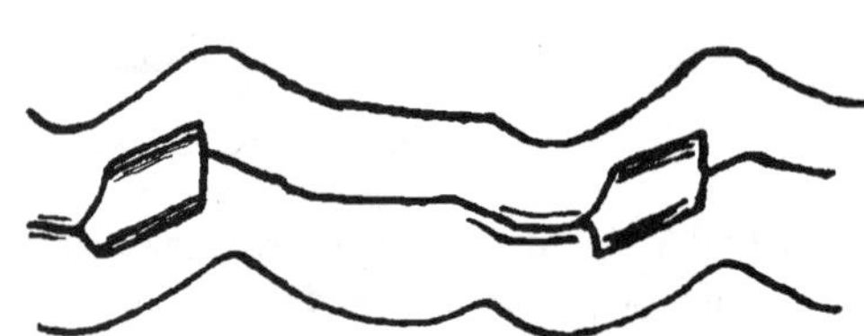

Aortic Valvular Stenosis
decreased separation of thickened deformed leaflets

HEART

(b) Functional / dynamic subaortic stenosis
1. Asymmetric septal hypertrophy (ASH)
2. Idiopathic hypertrophic subaortic stenosis (IHSS)
3. Hypertrophic obstructive cardiomyopathy (HOCM) may occur in infants of diabetic mothers

√ asymmetrically thicker ventricular septum than free wall of LV (95%)
√ normal / small left + right ventricular cavities (95%)
√ systolic anterior motion of mitral valve
√ lucent subaortic filling defect in systole
ECHO:
√ coarse systolic flutter of valve cusps
√ opening of leaflets followed by rapid inward move in mid systole, leaflets may remain in partially closed position through latter portion of systole (to appose borders of the flow jet)
Cx: mitral regurgitation (secondary to abnormal position of anterolateral papillary muscle preventing complete closure of MV in systole)

Valvular aortic stenosis
= fusion of commissures between cusps
Congenital types:
(a) bicuspid / unicuspid (in 95%): in 1–2% of population; M > F; commonly associated with coarctation of the aorta
(b) tricuspid (5%)
(c) dysplastic thickened aortic cusps
√ valvular calcifications (in 60% of patients >24 years of age)
@ IN INFANT with critical aortic stenosis:
• intractable CHF in first days / weeks of life with severe dyspnea
• may simulate neonatal sepsis
Associated with: L-to-R shunts (ASD, VSD)
√ marked cardiomegaly (thickened wall of LV)
√ pulmonary venous hypertension
√ decreased ejection fraction
√ doming of thickened valve cusps
√ dilated ascending aorta
Rx: emergency surgical dilatation
@ IN CHILD:
• asymptomatic until late in life
√ normal pulmonary vascularity
√ LV configuration with normal size of heart
√ large posterior noncoronary cusp, smaller fused right + left cusps
√ doming of thickened valve cusps
√ eccentric jet of contrast
√ poststenotic dilatation of ascending aorta
ECHO:
√ increase in echoes from thickened deformed leaflets (maximal during diastole)
√ decrease in leaflet separation

Supravalvular aortic stenosis
Types:
(a) localized hourglass narrowing just above aortic sinuses
(b) discrete fibrous membrane above sinuses of Valsalva
(c) diffuse tubular hypoplasia of ascending aorta + branching arteries
Associated with: peripheral PS, valvular + discrete subvalvular AS, Marfan syndrome, Williams syndrome
√ dilatation + tortuosity of coronary arteries (may undergo early atherosclerotic degeneration secondary to high pressure)
ECHO:
√ narrowing of supravalvular aortic area (normal root diameter: 20–37 mm)
√ normal movement of cusps

AORTIC TRANSECTION
= TRAUMATIC AORTIC RUPTURE = aortic tear from rapid horizontal deceleration / blunt chest trauma
Pathophysiology:
1. Incomplete rupture (15%)
(a) intimal hemorrhage without tear
(b) transverse tear of intima
(c) tear into media with subadventitial accumulation of blood (40–60%) = false aneurysm
◊ Aorta goes on to rupture completely within 24 hours in 50% of patients!
2. Complete rupture (85%) with exsanguination before reaching a hospital
3. Periaortic hemorrhage ± aortic injury
• interscapular severe chest pain, dyspnea, dysphagia
• hypertension of upper extremities = acute traumatic coarctation
• bilateral femoral pulse deficit
• systolic murmur in 2nd left parasternal interspace
Site: (a) Aortic isthmus just distal to left subclavian artery (88–95%): brachiocephalic arteries + ligamentum arteriosum fix aorta in this region
(b) Aortic arch with avulsion of brachiocephalic trunk (4.5%)
(c) Ascending aorta immediately above aortic valve (1%)
Cx: aortic valve rupture, coronary artery laceration, hemopericardium + cardiac tamponade; NO mediastinal hematoma
(d) Descending aorta (1.8%)
CXR:
N.B.: There are no plain CXR findings of aortic injury (since aortic integrity is maintained by intact adventitia)! The source of <u>mediastinal hematoma</u> are frequently the azygos, hemiazygos, paraspinal and intercostal vessels!
◊ Aortic injury is the cause of mediastinal hematoma in only 12.5%!
√ normal admission CXR in 28% (radiographic signs may not develop until 6–36 hours): 96% NPV for supine CXR

<u>Most specific signs</u>:
√ deviation of nasogastric tube to the right of T4 spinous process (67%)

HEART

√ depression of left mainstem bronchus anteroinferiorly >40° below the horizontal + toward right (53%)
√ mediastinal width >8 cm at level of aortic knob (75%): 53–100% sensitive, 1–60% specific
√ mediastinal width to chest width >0.25
√ obscuration / irregularity of aortic arch contour (75%)
√ leftward displacement of left mediastinal stripe abnormally extending above the level of aortic arch forming a left apical cap
√ thickening of right paratracheal stripe >4–5 mm (= hematoma between pleura + trachea)
√ left / right "apical cap" sign in 37% (= extrapleural hematoma along brachiocephalic vessels)
√ opacification of aortopulmonary window
√ loss of contour of descending aorta
√ widening of left paraspinal interface >5 mm
√ tracheal compression + displacement toward right (61%)
√ rapidly accumulating commonly left-sided hemothorax without evident rib fracture (break in mediastinal pleura)
√ fractures of 1st + 2nd rib (17%)

mnemonic: "BAD MEAT"
Bronchus depression (left main)
Aortic silhouette shaggy
Death in 80–90%
Mediastinal widening
Enteric (nasogastric) tube displacement
Apical cap
Tracheal shift

NECT screening (55% sensitive, 65% specific):
√ obliteration of aorta-fat interface with increased attenuation (= mediastinal hematoma)
◊ A negative CT examination for mediastinal hemorrhage has an almost 100% NPV for aortic injury!
◊ All patients with periaortic / middle / superior mediastinal hemorrhage require aortography! Save your contrast for that study!

CECT:
√ abrupt change in aortic contour at inner aortic wall
√ aortic pseudoaneurysm
√ intimal flap
√ pseudocoarctation = diminished caliber of the descending aorta
√ extravasation of contrast material

False positive:
residual thymic tissue, atelectatic lung, pericardial recess, patient motion, streak artifacts, partial volume effect with pulmonary artery

Angio (definitive means for diagnosis):
True positive:
In 20% of patients with mediastinal hematoma angio demonstrates acute traumatic aortic injury!
√ traumatic false aneurysm
√ tear of intima (5–10%) / media
√ rupture with extravasation of contrast material
√ posttraumatic dissection (11%)
√ posttraumatic coarctation

DDx: ductus diverticulum (in 10% of normals), aortic spindle, infundibula of brachiocephalic arterial branches, atherosclerotic aortic ulceration

Recommendation for work-up:
(1) normal well-defined mediastinal contours on CXR: no further imaging
(2) unequivocally abnormal mediastinum on CXR: angiography (± CT for other reasons)
(3) Clinically stable patient with equivocal CXR: CECT of thorax

Prognosis:
(1) 70–85% fatal at scene of trauma
(2) 15–30% reach hospital (due to formation of periaortic hematoma + false aneurysm contained by adventitia ± surrounding connective tissue)
(a) with surgical repair: 60–70% survive
(b) no intervention: 80% dead within 1 hour; 85% dead within 24 hours, 98% dead within 10 weeks; chronic false aneurysm may develop in 2–5% at isthmus / descending aorta

Chronic posttraumatic aortic pseudoaneurysm

= aneurysm existing for >3 months (amount of wall fibroplasia following rupture usually not sufficient to prevent subsequent rupture until at least 3 months after initial traumatic episode)

Incidence: 2–5% of patients surviving aortic transection >24–48 hours

- symptom-free period of months to years (in 11% >10 years)
- delayed clinical symptoms (42% within 5 years, 85% within 20 years): chest pain, back pain, dyspnea, cough, hoarseness, dysphagia, systolic murmur

Location: descending aorta at level of lig. arteriosum filling the aorticopulmonary window (most commonly)

√ well-defined rounded mass in left paramediastinal region
√ ± inferior displacement of left mainstem bronchus

Cx: CHF, partial obstruction of aortic lumen, bacterial endocarditis, aortoesophageal fistula, aortic dissection, obstruction of tracheobronchial tree, systemic emboli

Prognosis: enlargement + eventual rupture;
10-year survival rate: 85% with surgical repair, 66% without surgical repair

AORTOPULMONIC WINDOW

= defect in septation process characterized by large round / oval communication between left wall of ascending aorta + right wall of pulmonary trunk

- clinically resembles PDA

CXR:
√ shunt vascularity
√ cardiomegaly (LA + LV enlarged)
√ diminutive aortic knob
√ prominent pulmonary trunk

Angio (left ventriculogram / aortogram in AP / LAO projection):
√ defect several mm above aortic valve
√ pulmonary valve identified (DDx to truncus arteriosus)

ARTERIOSCLEROSIS OBLITERANS

= ASO = hardening of the arteries

Prevalence: 2.4 million people in U.S.; in 1978 12% of autopsies had ASO as leading cause of death (excluding MI)

Etiology: unknown

Contributing factors:
aging, diabetes (16–44%), hypertension, atherosclerosis
Effect of hyperlipidemia:
(a) High-density lipoproteins (HDL) have a protective effect: carry 25% of blood cholesterol
(b) Low-density lipoproteins (LDL): carry 60% of blood cholesterol

Histo: deposition of lipids, blood products, carbohydrates, begins as disruption of intimal surface; fatty streaks (as early as childhood); fibrous plaques (as early as 3rd decade); thrombosis, ulceration, calcification, aneurysm

Age: 50–70 years; M > F (after menopause)

Clinical classification:
(1) intermittent claudication = ischemic symptoms with exercise: calf, thigh, hip, buttock
(2) ischemic symptoms at rest (indicative of multisegment disease)

- cramping / burning / aching pain
- cold extremity
- paresthesia
- trophic changes: hair loss, thickened nails
- ulcer, gangrene
- decreased / absent pulses

Location: medium + large arteries; frequently at bifurcations; most frequent:
— superficial femoral artery in adductor canal (diabetics + nondiabetics)
— aortoiliac segment (nondiabetics)
— tibioperoneal trunk (diabetics)

Prognosis:
accelerated by diabetes (34% will require amputation), hypertension, lipoprotein abnormalities, heart disease (decreased cardiac output resulting in increased blood viscosity from polycythemia), chronic addiction to tobacco (11.4% will require amputation), intermittent claudication (5–7% require amputation if nondiabetic = 1–2% per year), ischemic ulcer / rest pain (19.6% require amputation)

ASPLENIA SYNDROME

= BILATERAL RIGHT-SIDEDNESS
= IVEMARK SYNDROME

Incidence: 1:1,750 to 1:40,000 livebirths; M > F

Associated with:
(a) CHD (in 50%):
TAPVR (almost 100%), endocardial cushion defect (85%), single ventricle (51%), TGA (58%), pulmonary stenosis / atresia (70%), dextrocardia (42%), mesocardia, VSD, ASD, absent coronary sinus, common atrium, common hepatic vein
(b) GI anomalies:
Partial / total situs inversus, annular pancreas, agenesis of gallbladder, ectopic liver, esophageal varices, duplication + hypoplasia of stomach, Hirschsprung disease, hindgut duplication, imperforate anus
(c) GU anomalies (15%):
Horseshoe kidney, double collecting system, hydroureter, cystic kidney, fused / horseshoe adrenal, absent left adrenal, bilobed urinary bladder, bicornuate uterus
(d) Cleft lip / palate, scoliosis, single umbilical artery, lumbar myelomeningocele

- cyanosis in neonatal period / infancy (if severe cyanotic CHD)
- Howell-Jolly bodies = RBC inclusions in patients with absent spleen

√ absent spleen

@ Lung
√ bilateral trilobed lungs = bilateral minor fissures (SPECIFIC)
√ bilateral eparterial bronchi (tomogram) = pulmonary arteries inferior to bronchi on PA view + projecting anterior to trachea on LAT view
√ diminished pulmonary vascularity / pulmonary venous hypertension (TAPVR below diaphragm)
√ bilateral SVC
√ bilateral right atrial appendages

@ Abdomen
√ absent spleen
√ centrally located liver = hepatic symmetry
√ stomach on right / left side / in central position
√ juxtaposed IVC ("piggybacked") to aorta = abdominal aorta + IVC located on same side of spine (aorta usually posterior) (NEARLY PATHOGNOMONIC)

Prognosis: 80% mortality by end of 1st year of life

ATRIAL SEPTAL DEFECT

Most common congenital cardiac defect in subjects >20 years of age

Incidence: 8–14% of all CHD; M:F = 1:4

Age: presentation frequently > age 40 secondary to benign course
(a) mildly symptomatic (60%): dyspnea, fatigue, palpitations
(b) severely symptomatic (30%): cyanosis, heart failure

Embryology:
1. Septum primum = membrane growing from atrial walls toward endocardial cushion
2. Ostium primum = temporary orifice between septum primum + endocardial cushion, which becomes obliterated by 5th week
3. Ostium secundum = multiple small coalescing perforations in septum primum
4. Septum secundum = membrane developing on right side of septum primum + covering part of ostium secundum

HEART

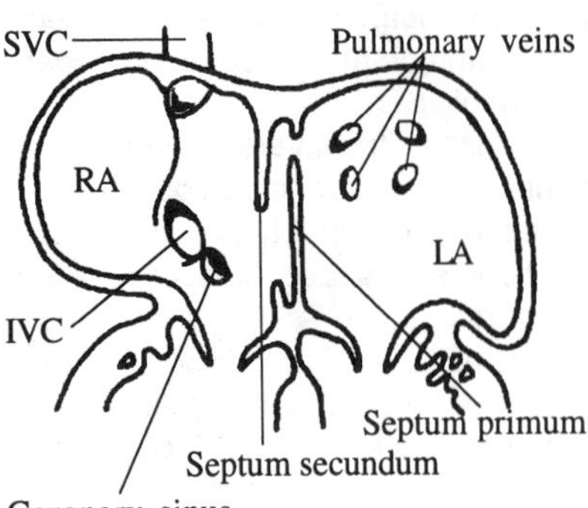

Normal Newborn Heart

Atrial septum consists of two components

(a) right side: septum secundum (muscular, firm) with posterior opening = foramen ovale

(b) left side: septum primum (fibrous, thin) with anterior opening = ostium secundum

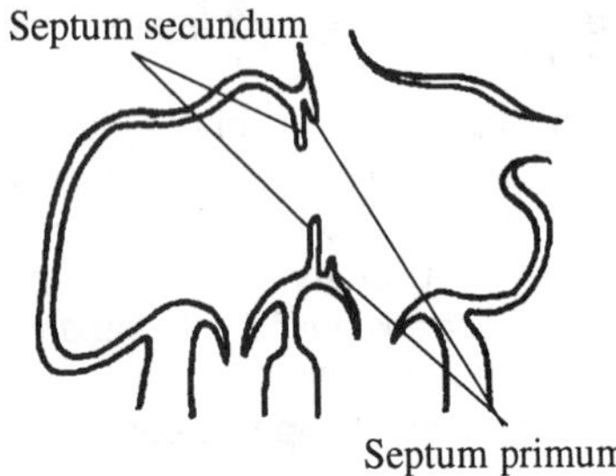

Ostium Secundum Defect

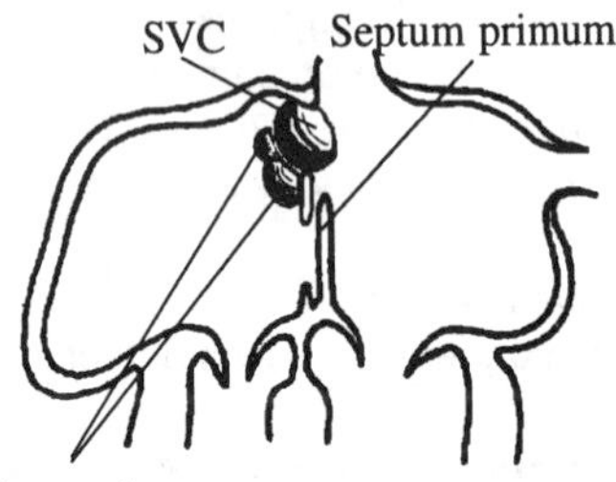

Sinus Venosus Defect

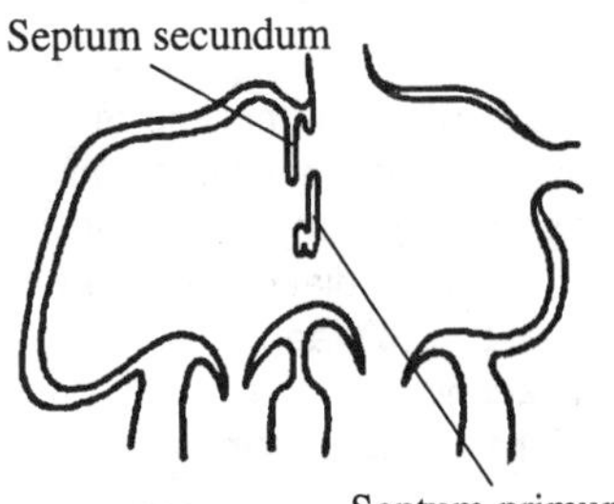

Ostium Primum Defect

5. Foramen ovale = orifice limited by septum secundum + septum primum
6. Foramen ovale flap = lower edge of septum primum (foramen ovale patent in 6%, probe-patent in 25%; not considered an ASD)

A. OSTIUM SECUNDUM ASD (60–70%)

= exaggerated resorptive process of septum primum leads to absence / fenestration of the foramen ovale flap

Location: in the body of the atrial chamber at fossa ovalis

Size: large defect of 1–3 cm in diameter

May be associated with:

prolapsing mitral valve, pulmonary valve stenosis, tricuspid atresia, TAPVR, hypoplastic left heart, interrupted aortic arch

B. OSTIUM PRIMUM ASD (30%)

= defect of atrioventricular endocardial cushion

Location: inferior to fossa ovalis at outlet portion of atrial septum

Almost always associated with:

endocardial cushion defects, cleft mitral valve, anterior fascicular block

C. SINUS VENOSUS ASD (5%)

= defect of the superior inlet portion of the atrial septum

Location: superior to fossa ovalis near entrance of superior vena cava (SVC straddles ASD)

Associated with: partial anomalous pulmonary venous return in 90% (RUL pulmonary veins connect to SVC / right atrium), Holt-Oram syndrome, Ellis-van Creveld syndrome

D. LUTEMBACHER SYNDROME = ASD + mitral stenosis

Hemodynamics:

no hemodynamic perturbance in the fetus; after birth physiologic increase in LA pressure creates a L-to-R shunt (shunt volume may be 3–4 times that of systemic blood flow) with volume overload of RV leading to RV dilatation, right heart failure, pulmonary hypertension; diastolic pressure differences in atria determine direction of shunt; pulmonary pressure remains normal for decades before Eisenmenger syndrome sets in; pulmonary hypertension in young adulthood (6%)

- repeated respiratory infections
- feeding difficulties
- arrhythmias
- thromboembolism
- asymptomatic; occasionally discovered by routine CXR
- right ventricular heave
- fixed splitting of second heart sound with accentuation of pulmonary component
- ECG: right axis deviation + some degree of right bundle branch block

HEART

- exertional dyspnea after development of pulmonary arterial hypertension (= Eisenmenger syndrome)
- cyanosis may occur (shunt reversal to R-to-L shunt), typically during 3rd–4th decade
- right heart failure in patients >40 years

CXR:
- √ normal (if shunt <2 x systemic blood flow)
- √ "hilar dance" = increased pulsations of central pulmonary arteries (DDx: other L-to-R shunts)
- √ overcirculation (if pulmonary-to-systemic blood flow ≥2:1)
- √ loss of visualization of SVC (= clockwise rotation of heart due to RV hypertrophy)
- √ small appearing aorta with normal aortic knob
  - √ normal size of LA after shunt reversal (due to immediate decompression into RA) in EISENMENGER SYNDROME
  - √ enlargement of pulmonary trunk + arteries
  - √ RV enlargement

ECHO:
- √ paradoxical interventricular septal motion (due to volume overload of RV)
- √ direct visualization of ASD (= lack of echoes of atrial septum) in subcostal view
- √ diastolic blood flow from interatrial septum crossing RA + tricuspid valve observed by color Doppler

Angio:
- √ RA fills with contrast shortly after LA is opacified (on levophase of pulmonary angio in AP or LAO projection)
- √ injection into RUL pulmonary vein to visualize exact size + location of ASD (LAO 45° + C-C 45°)

Prognosis:
(1) Mortality: 0.6% in 1st decade; 0.7% in 2nd decade; 2.7% in 3rd decade; 4.5% in 4th decade; 5.4% in 5th decade; 7.5% in 6th decade; median age of death is 37 years
(2) Spontaneous closure: 22% in infants <1 year; 33% between ages 1 and 2 years; 3% in children >4 years

Cx: (1) Tricuspid insufficiency (secondary to dilatation of AV ring)
(2) Mitral valve prolapse
(3) Atrial fibrillation (in 20% 1st presenting symptom in patients > age 40)

Rx: (if vascular changes still reversible = resistance of pulmonary-to-systemic system ≤0.7); 1% surgical mortality
1. Surgical patch closure
2. Rashkind foam + stainless steel prosthesis

BENEFICIAL ASD
= secundum type ASD serves an essential compensatory function in:
1. Tricuspid atresia
   RA blood reaches pulmonary vessels via ASD + PDA; improvement through Rashkind procedure
2. TAPVR
   significant shunt volume only available through ASD (VSD / PDA much less reliable)
3. Hypoplastic left heart
   systemic circulation maintained via RV with oxygenated blood from LA through ASD into RA

AZYGOS CONTINUATION OF IVC
= INTERRUPTED IVC WITH AZYGOS / HEMIAZYGOS CONTINUATION

Incidence: 0.2–0.6–2% of CHD

Etiology: failure of right subcardinal vein to anastomose with hepatic vein resulting in drainage of suprarenal IVC to heart via cranial portion of supracardinal vein (ie, azygos vein)

May be associated with:
polysplenia syndrome (more common), asplenia syndrome (rare), indeterminate situs (= situs ambiguus), persistent left SVC, dextrocardia, transposed abdominal viscera, duplicated IVC, retroaortic left renal vein, congenital pulmonary venolobar syndrome
- √ enlargement of azygos arch to >7 mm
- √ widening of right paraspinal stripe contiguous with azygos arch (= enlarged paraspinal + retrocrural azygos veins)
- √ widening of left paraspinal stripe (= enlarged hemiazygos vein)
- √ absence of hepatic ± infrahepatic IVC
- √ drainage of hepatic veins directly into right atrium via suprahepatic segment of IVC (N.B.: IVC shadow present on LAT CXR!)
- √ drainage of iliac + renal veins via azygos / hemiazygos vein

BACTERIAL ENDOCARDITIS
Predisposed:
1. Rheumatic valve disease
2. Mitral valve prolapse with mitral regurgitation
3. Aortic stenosis, mitral stenosis, aortic regurgitation, mitral regurgitation
4. Most CHD (VSD, TOF) except ostium secundum ASD
5. Previous endocarditis
6. Drug addicts:
   endocarditis of tricuspid valve causes multiple septic pulmonary emboli
7. Bicuspid aortic valve:
   responsible for 50% of aortic valvular bacterial endocarditis
8. Prosthetic valve:
   4% incidence of bacterial endocarditis
   - √ exaggerated valve motion (= disintegration of suture line + regurgitation)

Valve vegetations
ECHO:
- √ usually discrete focal echodensities with sharp edges; may show fuzzy / shaggy nonuniform thickening of cusps (vegetations) in systole + diastole
- √ may appear as shaggy echoes that prolapse when the valve is closed (DDx to mitral valve prolapse)

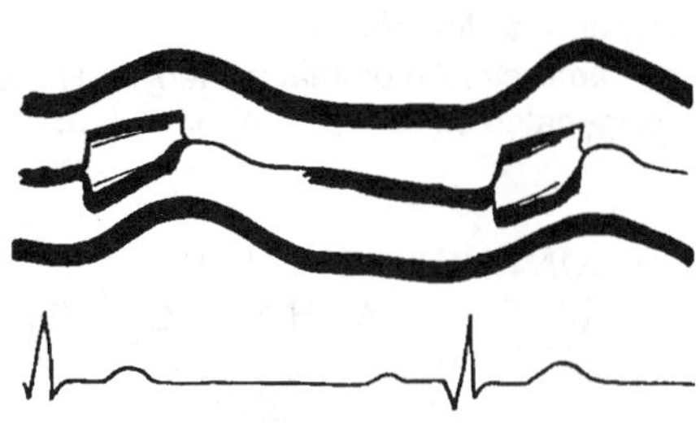

Aortic Valve Endocarditis

BUERGER DISEASE

= THROMBANGITIS OBLITERANS
= idiopathic recurrent segmental obliterative vasculitis of small + medium-sized peripheral arteries + veins (panangiitis)

Incidence: <1% of all chronic vascular diseases; more common in Israel, Orient, India

Etiology: unknown

Histo:
(a) acute stage: multiple microabscesses within fresh / organizing thrombus; all layers of vessel wall inflamed but intact; internal elastic lamina may be damaged; multinucleated giant cells within microabscesses (PATHOGNOMONIC)
(b) subacute stage: thrombus organization with little residual inflammation
(c) chronic stage: lumen filled with organized recanalized thrombus, fibrosis of adventitia binds together artery, vein, and nerve

Associated with: cigarette smoking (95%)

- instep claudication ± distal ulceration (symptoms abate on cessation of smoking + return on its resumption)
- Raynaud phenomenon (33%)

Location: legs (80%), arms (10–20%)

Site: starts in palmar + plantar vessels with proximal progression

√ superficial + deep migratory thrombophlebitis (20–33%)
√ arterial occlusions, tapered narrowing of arteries
√ abundant corkscrew-shaped collaterals
√ direct collateral following the path of the original artery (Martorell sign) in 80%
√ skip lesions = multiple segments involved with portions of arterial wall remaining unaffected
√ absence of generalized arteriosclerosis / arterial calcifications (90%)

CARDIAC TAMPONADE

= significant compression of heart by fluid contained within pericardial sac resulting in impaired diastolic filling of ventricles

Cause: *see* Pericardial effusion (page 459)

- tachycardia
- pulsus paradoxus = exaggeration of normal pattern = drop in systolic arterial pressure >10 mm Hg during inspiration (secondary to increase in right heart filling during inspiration at the expense of left heart filling)
- elevated central venous pressure with distended neck veins
- falling blood pressure
- distant heart sounds / friction rub
- ECG: reduced voltage, ST elevation, PR depression, nonspecific T-wave abnormalities

√ normal lung fields + normal pulmonary vascularity
√ rapid enlargement of heart size
√ distension of SVC, IVC, hepatic + renal veins
√ periportal edema
√ hepatomegaly

Doppler-US:
√ episodes of high-velocity hepatopetal flow separated by long intervals of minimal flow

ECHO:
√ diastolic collapse of RV
√ cyclical collapse of either atrium

Rx: pericardiocentesis / pericardial drainage

CARDIOMYOPATHY

Congestive cardiomyopathy

= DILATED CARDIOMYOPATHY

Etiology:
(a) Myocarditis: viruses, bacteria
(b) Endocardial fibroelastosis = thickened endocardium + reduced contractility
(c) Infants of diabetic mothers
(d) Inborn error of metabolism: glycogenosis, mucolipidosis, mucopolysaccharidosis
(e) Coronary artery disease: myocardial infarction, anomalous origin of left coronary artery, coronary calcinosis
(f) Muscular dystrophies

- tendency for CHF

√ cardiomegaly + poor contractility of ventricular wall
√ global heart enlargement
√ LA enlargement without enlargement of LA appendage

ECHO:
√ enlarged LV with global hypokinesis
√ IVS and LVPW of equal thickness with decreased amplitude of motion
√ low-profile / "miniaturized" mitral valve
√ mildly enlarged LA (elevated end-diastolic LV pressure)
√ enlarged hypokinetic right ventricle

Hypertrophic cardiomyopathy

= OBSTRUCTIVE CARDIOMYOPATHY
= characterized by nondilated hypertrophy of left ventricle in the absence of cardiac / systemic disease that would cause LV hypertrophy

1. SYMMETRIC / CONCENTRIC HYPERTROPHY (2–20%)
   (a) midventricular (b) diffuse (c) apical
2. ASYMMETRIC SEPTAL HYPERTROPHY (ASH)
   = IDIOPATHIC HYPERTROPHIC SUBAORTIC STENOSIS (IHSS) = SUBAORTIC STENOSIS
   = HYPERTROPHIC OBSTRUCTIVE CARDIOMYOPATHY
   = basal septum of LV disproportionately thickened
3. APICAL HYPERTROPHY (2–3%)
   = myocardial wall thickening confined to apical portion of LV

HEART

- usually clinically benign
- giant inverted T wave

Left ventriculography:

√ spade-shaped deformity of LV cavity

Pathophysiology:

— LV hypertrophy leads to subaortic stenosis, abnormal diastolic function, myocardial ischemia

— rapid blood flow through narrow outflow tract causes the anterior leaflet of mitral valve to displace anteriorly toward septum during systole (Venturi effect)

— mitral regurgitation (from displaced MV leaflet)

Etiology: autosomal dominant transmission

- exertional angina + dyspnea, fatigue
- syncope, arrhythmia, sudden death

√ prominent left midheart border (septal hypertrophy)

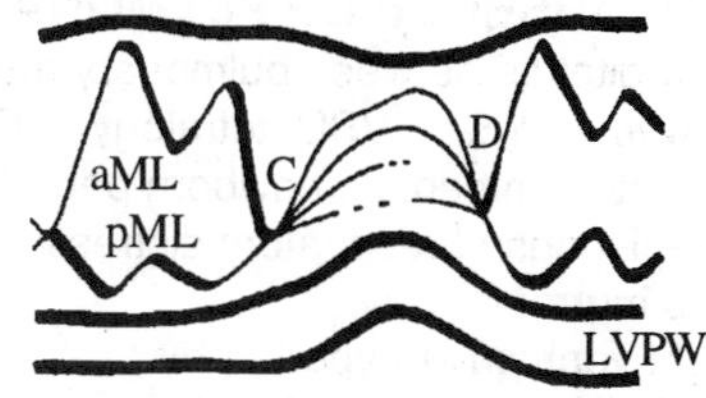

Systolic Anterior Motion (SAM) of MV in IHSS
mitral valve leaflets move abruptly toward septum at a rate greater than the endocardium of the posterior wall; responsible for obstruction to blood ejected from LV

ECHO:

√ IVS >14 mm thick; posterolateral wall >11 mm thick; IVS:LVPW thickness >1.3:1

√ systolic anterior motion of mitral valve (SAM) causing narrowed LVOT in systole

√ midsystolic closure of aortic valve

√ increased LVOT gradient with late systolic peaking on Doppler

Restrictive Cardiomyopathy

Etiology: (a) infiltrative disease: amyloid, glycogen, hemochromatosis
(b) constrictive pericarditis

CHRONIC VENOUS STASIS DISEASE

= CHRONIC VENOUS INSUFFICIENCY

= insufficiency / incompetence of venous valves in deep venous system of lower extremity

Cause:

(a) postphlebitic valvular incompetence: destruction of valve apparatus results in short thickened valves secondary to scar formation

(b) primary valvular incompetence: shallow elongated redundant valve cusps prevent effective closure

Associated with: incompetent venous valves in the calf (secondary to pressure dilatation from stasis in deep venous system) leading to superficial vein varicosities

- edema, induration (= fluid exudation from increased capillary pressure)
- ulceration (from minor trauma + decreased diffusion of oxygen secondary to fibrin deposits around capillaries)
- skin hyperpigmentation (= breakdown products of exudated RBCs)
- aching pain

√ venous reflux on descending venography with Valsalva
(a) 82% in deep venous system alone
(b) 2% in saphenous vein alone
(c) 16% in both

bilateral in 75%

Grade:

1 = minimal incompetence = to level of upper thigh
2 = mild incompetence = to level of lower thigh
3 = moderate incompetence = to level of knee
4 = severe incompetence = to level of calf veins

COARCTATION OF AORTA

M:F = 4:1; rare in Blacks

A. LOCALIZED COARCTATION [former classification = ADULT / POSTDUCTAL / JUXTADUCTAL TYPE] (most common type)

= short discrete narrowing close to ligamentum arteriosum

◊ Coexistent cardiac anomalies uncommon!

Location: most frequent in juxtaductal portion of arch

- incidental finding late in life
- ductus usually closed

√ shelflike lesion at any point along the aortic arch

√ narrow isthmus above the lesion

√ poststenotic aortic dilatation distally

B. TUBULAR HYPOPLASIA [former classification = INFANTILE / PREDUCTAL / DIFFUSE TYPE]

= hypoplasia of long segment of aortic arch after origin of innominate artery

◊ Coexistent cardiac anomalies common!

- CHF in neonatal period (in 50%)

Hemodynamics:

fetus : no significant change because only 10% of cardiac output flows through aortic isthmus

neonate : determined by how rapidly the ductus closes; without concurrent VSD overload of LV leads to CHF in 2nd / 3rd week of life

Collateral circulation: via subclavian artery and its branches:

— intercostals
— anterior spinal artery
— lateral thoracic
— internal mammary
— scapular artery
— transverse cervical artery

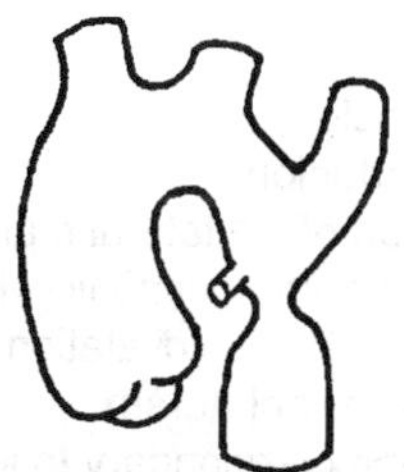

Localized Coarctation

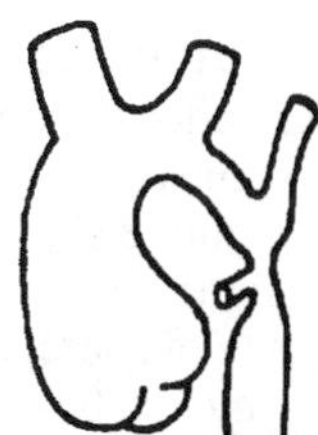

Tubular Hypoplasia

HEART

Associated with: (in 50%):
1. Bicuspid aortic valve (in 25–50%), which may result in calcific aortic valve stenosis (after 25 years of age) + bacterial endocarditis
2. Intracardiac malformations:
   PDA (33%), VSD (15%), aortic stenosis, aortic insufficiency, ASD, TGV, ostium primum defect, truncus arteriosus, double-outlet right ventricle
3. Noncardiac malformations (13%):
   Turner syndrome (13–15%)
4. Cerebral berry aneurysms
5. Mycotic aneurysm distal to CoA

Prognosis: 11% mortality prior to 6 months of age

Rx: ages 3–5 years are ideal time for operation (late enough to avoid restenosis + early enough before irreversible hypertension occurs); surgical correction past 1 year of age decreases operative mortality drastically; 3–11% perioperative mortality

Procedures:
1. Resection + end-to-end anastomosis
2. Patch angioplasty
3. Subclavian flap (Waldhausen procedure) using left subclavian artery as a flap

Postsurgical Cx:
1. Residual coarctation (in 32%)
2. Subsequent obstruction (rare)
3. Mesenteric arteritis: 2–3 days after surgery secondary to paradoxical hypertension from increased plasma renin
   • abdominal pain, loss of bowel control
4. Chronic persistent hypertension

HEART

Symptomatic CoA

◊ Second most common cause of CHF in neonate (after hypoplastic left heart)

Time: (a) toward the end of 1st week of life in "critical stenosis"
(b) more commonly presents in older child

• lower extremity cyanosis (in tubular hypoplasia)
• left ventricular failure (usually toward end of 1st week of life)
√ generalized cardiomegaly
√ increased pulmonary vascularity (L-to-R shunt through PDA / VSD)
√ pulmonary venous hypertension / edema
√ "figure 3 sign" hidden by thymus

Asymptomatic CoA

• headaches (from hypertension)
• claudication (from hypoperfusion)
√ "figure 3 sign" = indentation of left lateral margin of aortic arch in the region of aortic-pulmonic window (at site of coarctation and poststenotic dilatation)
√ "reverse 3 sign" on barium esophagram
√ elevated left ventricular apex (secondary to left ventricular hypertrophy)
√ scalloped contouring of soft-tissues posterior to sternum (= dilated tortuous internal mammary arteries) on LAT CXR (in 28%)
√ dilatation of brachiocephalic vessels + aorta proximal to stenosis
√ obscuration of superior margin of aortic arch
√ rib notching (in 75%; mostly in adults over age 20; unusual before age 6)

Location: ribs 3–8 (most pronounced in 3rd + 4th ribs, less pronounced in lower ribs)

Site: central + lateral thirds of posterior rib
(a) bilateral
(b) unilateral on left side: left aortic arch with aberrant right subclavian artery below CoA
(c) unilateral on right side: right aortic arch with anomalous left subclavian artery below CoA

CONGENITAL ABSENCE OF PULMONARY VALVE

Massive regurgitation between pulmonary artery and RV

Associated with in 90%: VSD, tetralogy of Fallot (50%)

• cyanosis (not in immediate newborn period)
• repeated episodes of respiratory distress
• continuous murmur
• ECG: right ventricular hypertrophy
√ prominent main, right, and left pulmonary artery
√ RV dilatation (increased stroke volume)
√ partial obstruction of right / left mainstem bronchus (compression by vessel)
√ right-sided aorta (33%)

CONGESTIVE HEART FAILURE

= elevation of microvascular pressure of lung; most common cause of interstitial + airspace edema of lungs

Cause:
(a) back pressure from LV: long-standing systemic hypertension, aortic valve disease, coronary artery disease, cardiomyopathy, myocardial infarction
(b) obstruction proximal to LV: mitral valve disease, LA myxoma, cor triatriatum

Histo:
(a) Interstitial phase: fluid in loose connective tissue around conducting airways and vessels + engorgement of lymphatics
(b) Alveolar phase: increase in alveolar wall thickness
(c) Alveolar airspace phase: alveoli filled with fluid + loss of alveolar volume; pulmonary fibrosis upon organization of intra-alveolar fibrin (if chronic)

√ large heart
√ vascular congestion

1. **Interstitial pulmonary edema** (invariably precedes alveolar edema)
   • NO abnormal physical finding
   • hypoxemia (ventilation-perfusion inequality)
   √ loss of sharp definition of vascular markings
   √ thickening of interlobular septa (pulmonary venous wedge pressure 17–20 mm Hg)
   √ poorly defined increased bronchial wall thickness
   √ thickening of interlobar fissures (due to fluid in subpleural connective tissue layer)

2. **Airspace edema** (when volume of capillary filtration exceeds that of lymphatic drainage)
   - severe dyspnea / orthopnea
   - tachypnea + cyanosis
   - dry cough / copious frothy sputum
   - hypoxemia (vascular shunting)
   - √ poorly defined patchy acinar opacities
   - √ coalescence of acinar consolidation, particularly in medial third of lung
   - √ butterfly / bat-wing distribution of consolidation (= consolidated hilum + uninvolved lung cortex)

CONSTRICTIVE PERICARDITIS

= fibrous thickening of pericardium interfering with filling of ventricular chambers through restriction of heart motion

Age: 30–50 years; M:F = 3:1

Etiology:

1. Idiopathic (most common)
2. Viral (Coxsackie B)
3. Tuberculosis (formerly most common)
4. Chronic renal failure
5. Rheumatoid arthritis
6. Neoplastic involvement
7. Radiotherapy to mediastinum

Causes of acute pericarditis:

mnemonic: "MUSIC"

Myocardial infarction (acute)
Uremia
Surgery (cardiac)
Infection
Cancer

- dyspnea
- abdominal enlargement (ascites + hepatomegaly)
- peripheral edema
- pericardial knock sound = loud early-diastolic sound
- neck vein distension
- Kussmaul sign = failure of venous pressure to fall with inspiration
- prominent X and Y descent on venous pressure curve
- √ linear / plaquelike pericardial calcifications (50%): predominantly over RV, posterior surface of LV, in atrioventricular groove
- √ dilatation of SVC, azygos vein
- √ small atria
- √ normal / small-sized heart (enlargement only due to preexisting disease)
- √ normal pulmonary vascularity / pulmonary venous hypertension
- √ straightening of right + left heart borders
- √ increase in ejection fraction (small EDV)

CT:
- √ epicardium = visceral pericardium >2 mm thick
- √ dilatation of SVC + IVC
- √ reflux of contrast into coronary sinus
- √ flattening of right ventricle + curvature of interventricular septum toward left
- √ pleural effusion + ascites

ECHO (nonspecific features):
- √ thickening of pericardium
- √ rapid early filling motion followed by flat posterior wall motion during diastasis period (= period between early rapid filling and atrial contraction)

Cx: protein-losing enteropathy (increased pressure in IVC + portal vein)

DDx: Cardiac tamponade, restrictive cardiomyopathy (eg, amyloid)

CORONARY ARTERY FISTULA

= single / multiple fistulous connections between a coronary artery (R > L) and other heart structures

Abnormal communication with (>90% right heart):
RV > RA > pulmonary trunk > coronary sinus > SVC

Hemodynamics: L-to-R shunt; pulmonary:systemic blood flow = <1.5:1 (usually)

- √ may have normal CXR (in small shunts)
- √ cardiomegaly + shunt vascularity (in large shunts)

Angio:
- √ dilated tortuous coronary artery with anomalous connection

COR TRIATRIATUM

= rare congenital anomaly in which a fibromuscular septum with a single stenotic / fenestrated / large opening separates the embryologic common pulmonary vein from the left atrium:

(1) proximal / accessory chamber lies posteriorly receiving pulmonary veins
(2) distal / true atrial chamber lies anteriorly connected to left atrial appendage + emptying into LV through mitral valve

Etiology: failure of common pulmonary vein to incorporate normally into left atrium

Associated with: ASD, PDA, anomalous pulmonary venous drainage, left SVC, VSD, tetralogy of Fallot, atrioventricular canal

- dyspnea, heart failure, failure to thrive
- clinically similar to mitral valve stenosis
- √ pulmonary venous distention + interstitial edema + dilatation of pulmonary trunk and pulmonary arteries (in severe obstruction)
- √ enlarged RA + RV
- √ mild enlargement of LA

Angio:
- √ dividing membrane on levophase of pulmonary arteriogram

Prognosis (if untreated):
usually fatal within first 2 years of life; 50% 2-year survival; 20% 20-year survival

Rx: surgical excision of obstructing membrane

DEEP VEIN THROMBOSIS

= DVT

Incidence: 140,000–250,000 new cases per year in United States with an estimated sole / major cause of 50,000–200,000 deaths per year (15% of in-hospital deaths); 6–7 million stasis skin changes; in 0.5% cause of skin ulcers

HEART

Pathogenetic factors:
1. Hypercoagulability
2. Decreased blood flow / stasis
3. Intimal injury
4. Decreased fibrinolytic potential of veins
5. Platelet aggregation

Risk factors:
1. Surgery, esp. on legs / pelvis: orthopedic (45–50%) especially total hip replacement >50%), gynecologic (7–35%), neurosurgery (18–20%), urologic (15–35%), general surgery (20–25%)
2. Severe trauma
3. Prolonged immobilization: hemiplegic extremity, paraplegia + quadriplegia, casting / orthopedic appliances
4. Malignancy (risk factor 2.5) = Trousseau syndrome
5. Obesity (risk factor 1.5)
6. Diabetes
7. Pregnancy (risk factor 5.5) and for 8–12 weeks postpartum
8. Medication: birth control pills, estrogen replacement, tamoxifen (risk factor 3.2)
9. Decreased cardiac function: congestive heart failure, myocardial infarction (20–50%; risk factor 3.5)
10. Age >40 years (risk factor 2.2)
11. Varicose veins
12. Previous DVT (risk factor 2.5)
13. Patients with blood group A > blood group 0
14. Polycythemia
15. Smoking

Location:
1. Dorsal veins of calf (± ascending thrombosis)
2. Iliofemoral veins (± descending thrombosis)
3. Peripheral + iliofemoral veins simultaneously
4. rare: internal iliac v., ovarian v., ascending lumbar vv.

L:R = 7:3 due to compression of left common iliac v. by left common iliac a. (arterial pulsations lead to chronic endothelial injury with formation of intraluminal spur, which is present in 22% of autopsies + in 90% of patients with DVT)

- Local symptoms due to obstruction / phlebitis usually only when (a) thrombus occlusive (b) clot extends into popliteal / more proximal vein (14–78% sensitivity, 4–21% specificity)
  - warmth
  - swelling (measurement of circumference)
  - blanching of skin (phlegmasia dolens alba) / blue leg with complete obstruction (phlegmasia cerulea dolens)
  - deep crampy pain in affected extremity, worse in erect position, improved while walking
  - tenderness along course of affected vein
  - Homans sign = calf pain with dorsal flexion of foot
  - Payr sign = pain upon compression of sole of foot

◊ 2/3 of deep vein thromboses are clinically silent
◊ Clinically suspected DVT only in 50% confirmed
◊ DVT symptomatology due to other causes in 15–35% of patients
◊ Negative bilateral venograms in 30% of patients with angiographically detected pulmonary emboli (big bang theory = clot embolizes in toto to the lung leaving no residual in vein)

Venography (89% sensitivity, 97% specificity):
false negative in 11%, false positive in 5%;
study aborted / nondiagnostic in 5%
Risk: postvenography phlebitis (1–2%), contrast reaction, contrast material-induced skin slough, nephropathy
√ intraluminal filling defect constant on all images
√ nonfilling of calf veins
√ inadequate filling of common femoral vein + external + common iliac veins

B-Mode US (88–100% sensitivity, 92–100% specificity, >90% accuracy for DVT in thigh and popliteal veins):
√ lack of complete luminal collapse with venous compression (DDx: deformity + scarring from prior DVT; technical difficulties in adductor canal + distal deep femoral vein)
  √ visualization of clot within vein (DDx: slow flowing blood; machine noise)
√ <75% increase in diameter of common femoral vein during Valsalva
√ venous diameter at least twice that of adjacent artery suggests thrombus <10 days old

Doppler US:
√ absence of spontaneity (= any waveform recording), not reliable in peripheral veins
√ continuous venous signal = absence of phasicity (= no cyclic variation in flow velocity with respiration, ie, decrease in expiration + increase in inspiration) is suspicious for proximal obstruction
√ attenuation / absence of augmentation (= no increase in flow velocity with distal compression) indicates venous occlusion / compression in intervening venous segments
√ pulsatile venous flow is a sign of congestive heart failure / pericardial effusion / cardiac tamponade / pulmonary embolism with pulmonary hypertension

Venous Occlusion Plethysmography :
— 87–95–100% sensitivity, 92–100% specificity for above-knee DVT
— 17–33% sensitivity for below-knee DVT
= temporary obstruction of venous outflow by pneumatic cuff around mid-thigh inflated above venous pressure leads to progressive increase in blood volume in lower leg; upon release of cuff limb quickly returns to resting volume with prompt venous runoff; limb blood volume changes are measured by *impedance plethysmography* in which a weak alternating current is passed through the leg; the electrical resistance varies inversely with blood volume; the current strength is held constant and voltage changes directly reflect blood volume changes

HEART

√ initial rise in venous volume (= venous capacitance) diminished
√ delay in venous outflow = "fall" measured at 3 seconds
False positives (6%): severe cardiopulmonary disease, pelvic mass, reduced arterial inflow
False negatives: calf vein thrombosis, small thrombus

I-125–Labeled Fibrinogen:
— 90% sensitive for calf vein thrombus
— 60–80% sensitive for femoral vein thrombus
— insensitive for thrombus in upper thigh / pelvis
Risk: results not available for several days, transmission of viral infection
False positives: hematoma, inflammation, wound, old small thrombus isolated in common femoral / iliac vein

Cx:
(1) Pulmonary embolism (50%): in 90% from lower extremity / pelvis; in 60% with proximal "free-floating" / "widow-maker" thrombus; occurs usually between 2nd to 4th (7th) day of thrombosis
Source of pulmonary emboli:
multiple sites (1/3), cryptogenic in 50%;
(a) lower extremity (46%)
(b) inferior vena cava (19%)
(c) pelvic veins (16%)
(d) mural heart thrombus (4.5%)
(e) upper extremity (2%)
Likelihood of pulmonary embolism:
77% for iliac veins, 35–67% for femoropopliteal vein, 0–46% for calf veins
(2) Postphlebitic syndrome (PPS) in 20% of cases with DVT (= recanalization to a smaller lumen, focal wall changes) due to valvular incompetence
(3) Phlegmasia cerulea / alba dolens (= severely impaired venous drainage resulting in gangrene)

Prognosis: tibial / peroneal venous thrombi resolve spontaneously in 40%, stabilize in 40%, propagate into popliteal vein in 20%
Prophylaxis: intermittent compression of legs, heparin, warfarin
Rx:
(1) Heparin IV
(2) Systemic anticoagulation (warfarin) for ≥3 months decreases risk of recurrent DVT in initial 3 months from 50% to 3% + fatal pulmonary embolism from 30% to 8%; necessity for anticoagulation in DVT of calf veins is controversial
(3) Caval filter (10–15%) in patients with contraindication / complication from anticoagulation or progression of DVT / PE despite adequate anticoagulation
DDx: pseudothrombophlebitis (= signs + symptoms of DVT produced by popliteal cyst / traumatic hematoma)

DOUBLE-OUTLET RIGHT VENTRICLE
= DORV = TAUSSIG-BING HEART = most of the aorta + pulmonary artery arise from the RV secondary to maldevelopment of conotruncus
Type 1 = aorta posterior to pulmonary artery + spiraling course (most frequent)
Type 2 = Taussig-Bing heart = aorta posterior to pulmonary artery + parallel course
Type 3 = aorta anterior to pulmonary artery + parallel course
Hemodynamics:
fetus : no CHF in utero (in absence of obstructing other anomalies)
neonate: ventricular work overload leads to CHF
Associated with: VSD (100%), pulmonary stenosis (50%), PDA
√ aorta overriding the interventricular septum with predominant connection to RV
√ aorta posterior / parallel / anterior to pulmonary artery
√ LV enlargement (volume overload)

DUCTUS ARTERIOSUS ANEURYSM
= fusiform aneurysm of ductus arteriosus, usually patent toward aorta + completely / incompletely occluded toward pulmonary artery
Incidence: <100 cases
Classification:
(a) according to age: infantile, childhood, adult type
(b) according to cause: congenital, infectious, traumatic
Pathogenesis: ? delay in closure, ? myxoid degeneration of ductus wall, ? abnormal elastic fibers
Age: most <2 months of age
• dyspnea, tachypnea, hoarseness
√ pulmonary artery displaced anteromedially
√ distal aortic arch displaced laterally
CXR:
√ left-sided upper mediastinal mass in aorticopulmonary window
√ tracheal displacement to right + anteriorly / posteriorly
√ consolidation of adjacent lung (compression, fibrosis, hemorrhage)
CT: √ contrast-enhancing mass in classic location
ECHO: √ cystic mass with pulsatile flow
Cx: rupture, dissection, infection, thromboembolic disease, phrenic nerve compression
Prognosis: usually fatal (without prompt surgery)

EBSTEIN ANOMALY
= downward displacement of septal + posterior leaflets of dysplastic tricuspid valve with ventricular division into
(a) a large superior atrialized portion and
(b) a small inferior functional chamber
Etiology: chronic maternal lithium intake (10%)
Hemodynamics: tricuspid valve insufficiency leads to tricuspid regurgitation ("Ping-Pong" volume); may be followed by CHF in utero / in neonate (50%); survival into adulthood if valve functions normally
Associated with: PDA, ASD (R-to-L shunt)

HEART

- cyanosis in neonatal period (R-to-L shunt), may improve / disappear postnatally with decrease in pulmonary arterial pressure
- systolic murmur (tricuspid insufficiency)
- Wolff-Parkinson-White syndrome (10%) = paroxysmal supraventricular tachycardia / right bundle branch block (responsible for sudden death)

√ "boxlike / funnel-like" cardiomegaly (enlargement of RA + RV)
√ extreme RA enlargement (secondary to insufficient tricuspid valve)
√ IVC + azygos dilatation (secondary to tricuspid regurgitation)
√ hypoplastic aorta + pulmonary trunk (the ONLY cyanotic CHD to have this feature)
√ normal LA
√ calcification of tricuspid valve may occur

ECHO:
√ large "sail-like" tricuspid valve structure within dilated right heart
√ tricuspid regurgitation identified by Doppler ultrasound

Prognosis: 50% infant mortality; 13% operative mortality

Rx: 1. Digitalis + diuretics
2. Tricuspid valve prosthesis

EISENMENGER COMPLEX

= EISENMENGER DEFECT
= (1) high VSD ± overriding aorta with hypoplastic crista supraventricularis
(2) RV hypertrophy
and as consequence of increased pulmonary blood flow:
(3) dilatation of pulmonary artery + branches
(4) intimal thickening + sclerosis of small pulmonary arteries + arterioles

- cyanosis appears in 2nd + 3rd decade with shunt reversal

EISENMENGER SYNDROME

= EISENMENGER REACTION
= development of high pulmonary vascular resistance after many years of increased pulmonary blood flow secondary to L-to-R shunt (ASD, PDA, VSD), which leads to a bidirectional (= balanced) shunt and ultimately to R-to-L shunt

Etiology:
pulmonary microscopic vessels undergo reactive muscular hypertrophy, endothelial thickening, in situ thrombosis, tortuosity + obliteration; once initiated, pulmonary hypertension accelerates the vascular reaction, thus increasing pulmonary hypertension in a vicious cycle with RV failure + death

√ pronounced dilatation of central pulmonary arteries (pulmonary trunk, main pulmonary artery, intermediate branches)
√ pruning of peripheral pulmonary arteries
√ enlargement of RV
√ LA + LV return to normal size (with decrease of L-to-R shunt)
√ pulmonary veins NOT distended (NO increase in pulmonary blood flow)
√ NO redistribution of pulmonary veins (normal venous pressure)

Dx: measurement of pulmonary artery pressure + flow via catheter

ENDOCARDIAL CUSHION DEFECT

= ECD = ATRIOVENTRICULAR SEPTAL DEFECT
= PERSISTENT OSTIUM ATRIOVENTRICULARE COMMUNE = PERSISTENT COMMON ATRIOVENTRICULAR CANAL
= persistence of primitive atrioventricular canal + anomalies of AV valves

Associated with:
(1) Down syndrome:
in 25% of trisomy 21 an ECD is present;
in 45% of ECD trisomy 21 is present
(2) Asplenia, polysplenia

A. INCOMPLETE / PARTIAL ECD
= (1) Ostium primum ASD
(2) Cleft in anterior mitral valve leaflet / trileaflet
(3) Accessory short chordae tendineae arising from anterior MV leaflet insert directly into crest of deficient ventricular septum
√ left atrioventricular valve usually has 3 leaflets with a wide cleft between anterior + septal leaflet
√ "gooseneck" deformity secondary to downward attachment of anterior MV leaflet close to interventricular septum by accessory chordae tendineae
√ communication between LA–RA or LV–RA, occasionally LV–RV
√ right atrioventricular valve usually normal

B. TRANSITIONAL / INTERMEDIATE ATRIOVENTRICULAR CANAL (uncommon)
= (1) Ostium primum ASD
(2) High membranous VSD
(3) Wide clefts in septal leaflets of both AV valves
(4) Bridging tissue between anterior + posterior common leaflet of both AV valves

C. COMPLETE ECD = AV COMMUNIS = COMMON AV CANAL
= (1) Ostium primum ASD above
(2) Posterior VSD below
(3) One AV valve common to RV + LV with 5–6 leaflets
(a) anterior common "bridging" leaflet
(b) two lateral leaflets
(c) posterior common "bridging" leaflet

Type 1 = chordae tendineae of anterior bridging leaflet attached to both sides of ventricular septum
Type 2 = chordae tendineae of anterior leaflet attached medially to anomalous papillary muscle within RV, but unattached to septum
Type 3 = free-floating anterior leaflet with chordae attachments to septum; only type becoming symptomatic in infancy!

√ common atrioventricular orifice
√ oval septal defect consisting of a low ASD + high VSD
√ atrial septum secundum usually spared ("common atrium" if absent)
√ frequently associated with mesocardia / dextrocardia

Hemodynamics:
fetus : atrioventricular valves frequently incompetent leading to regurgitation + CHF
neonate: L-to-R shunt after decrease of pulmonary vascular resistance resulting in pulmonary hypertension
• incomplete right bundle branch block (distortion of conduction tissue)
• left-anterior hemiblock

CXR:
√ increased pulmonary vascularity (= shunt vascularity)
√ redistribution of pulmonary blood flow (mitral regurgitation)
√ enlarged pulmonary artery
√ diminutive aorta (secondary to L-to-R shunt)
√ cardiac enlargement out of proportion to pulmonary vascularity (L-to-R shunt + mitral insufficiency)
√ enlarged RV + LV
√ enlarged RA (LV blood shunted to RA)
√ normal-sized LA (secondary to ASD)
ECHO:
√ visualization of ASD + VSD + valve + site of insertion of chordae tendineae
√ paradoxical anterior septal motion (secondary to ASD)
√ atrioventricular insufficiency + shunts identified by Doppler ultrasound
Angio:
AP projection:
√ gooseneck deformity of LVOT (in diastole)
√ cleft in anterior leaflet of mitral valve (in systole)
√ mitral regurgitation
Hepatoclavicular projection in 45° LAO + C-C 45° (= 4-chamber view):
√ best view to demonstrate LV-RA shunt
√ best view to demonstrate VSD (inflow tract + posterior portion of interventricular septum in profile)
LAT projection:
√ irregular appearance of superior segment of anterior mitral valve leaflet over LVOT

Prognosis: 54% survival rate at 6 months, 35% at 12 months, 15% at 24 months, 4% at 5 years; 91% long-term survival with primary intracardiac repair, 4–17% operative mortality

ENDOCARDIAL FIBROELASTOSIS
= diffuse endocardial thickening of LV + LA from deposition of collagen + elastic tissue
Etiology:
(1) ? viral infection
(2) Secondary endocardial fibroelastosis
= subendocardial ischemia in critical LVOT obstruction: aortic stenosis, coarctation, hypoplastic left heart syndrome
• sudden onset of CHF during first 6 months of life
√ mitral insufficiency:
(a) involvement of valve leaflets
(b) shortening + thickening of chordae tendineae
(c) distortion + fixation of papillary muscles
√ enlarged LV = dilatation of hypertrophied LV from mitral regurgitation
√ restricted LV motion
√ enlarged LA
√ pulmonary venous congestion + pulmonary edema
√ LLL atelectasis (= compression of left lower lobe bronchus by enlarged LA)
Prognosis: mortality almost 100% by 2 years of age

FLAIL MITRAL VALVE
Cause:
(1) ruptured chordae tendineae in rheumatic heart disease, ischemic heart disease, bacterial endocarditis
(2) rupture of head of papillary muscle in acute myocardial infarction, chest trauma
Location: chordae to leaflet from posteromedial papillary muscle (single vessel blood supply)
√ deep holosystolic posterior movement
√ random anarchic motion pattern of flail parts in diastole
√ excessively large amplitude of opening of aML

HYPOPLASTIC LEFT HEART SYNDROME
= SHONE SYNDROME = AORTIC ATRESIA
= underdevelopment of left side of heart characterized by (a) aortic valve atresia (b) hypoplastic ascending aorta (c) hypoplastic / atretic mitral valve (d) endocardial fibroelastosis giving rise to small LA + small LV + small ascending aorta
Incidence: most common cause of CHF in neonate; responsible for 25% of all cardiac deaths in 1st week of life
Hemodynamics:
pulmonary venous return is diverted from LA to RA through herniated foramen ovale / ASD (L-to-R shunt); RV supplies (a) pulmonary artery (b) ductus arteriosus (c) descending aorta (antegrade flow) (d) aortic arch + ascending aorta + coronary circulation (retrograde flow) leading to RV work overload + CHF
• characteristically presents within first few hours of life
• ashen gray color (inadequate atrial L-to-R shunt with systemic underperfusion)
• myocardial ischemia (decreased perfusion of aorta + coronary arteries)
• cardiogenic shock, metabolic acidosis
• CHF (RV volume + pressure overload)
OB-US:
√ small left ventricular cavity (apex of LV and RV should be at same level)
√ hypoplastic ascending aorta + aortic arch
√ aortic coarctation (in 80%)

ECHO:
- √ normal / enlarged LA
- √ small LV
- √ enlarged RA
- √ herniation + prolapse of foramen ovale flap into RA
- √ small / absent aortic root
- √ absent / grossly distorted mitral valve echoes

Angio:
- √ retrograde flow in ascending aorta + aortic arch + coronary arteries via PDA
- √ stringlike ascending aorta <6 mm in diameter
- √ massive enlargement of RV + RVOT

Prognosis: almost 100% fatal by 6 weeks

Rx: (1) Norwood procedure = palliative attempt
(2) Cardiac transplant

HYPOPLASTIC RIGHT VENTRICLE

= PULMONARY ATRESIA WITH INTACT VENTRICULAR SEPTUM

= underdeveloped right ventricle due to pulmonary atresia in the presence of an intact interventricular septum

Type I = small RV secondary to competent tricuspid valve (more common)

Type II = normal / large RV secondary to incompetent tricuspid valve

Hemodynamics:
- fetus : L-to-R atrial shunt through foramen ovale; retrograde flow through ductus arteriosus into pulmonary vascular bed
- neonate : closure of ductus results in cyanosis, acidosis, death

- √ small right ventricular cavity (apex of RV + LV should be at same level)
- √ atresia of pulmonary valve
- √ hypoplastic proximal pulmonary artery
- √ secundum atrial septal defect (frequently associated)

Rx: prostaglandin E1 infusion + valvotomy + systemic-pulmonary artery shunt

IDIOPATHIC DILATATION OF PULMONARY ARTERY

= CONGENITAL ANEURYSM OF PULMONARY ARTERY

Age: adolescence; M < F

- • systolic ejection murmur (in most cases)
- √ dilated main pulmonary artery
- √ normal peripheral pulmonary vascularity
- √ normal pulmonary arterial pulsations
- √ NO lateralization of pulmonary flow

Dx per exclusion:
1. Absence of shunts, CHD, acquired disease
2. Normal RV pressure
3. No significant pressure gradient across pulmonic valve

DDx: (1) Marfan syndrome
(2) Takayasu arteritis

INTERRUPTION OF AORTIC ARCH

= rare congenital anomaly as a common cause of death in the neonatal period

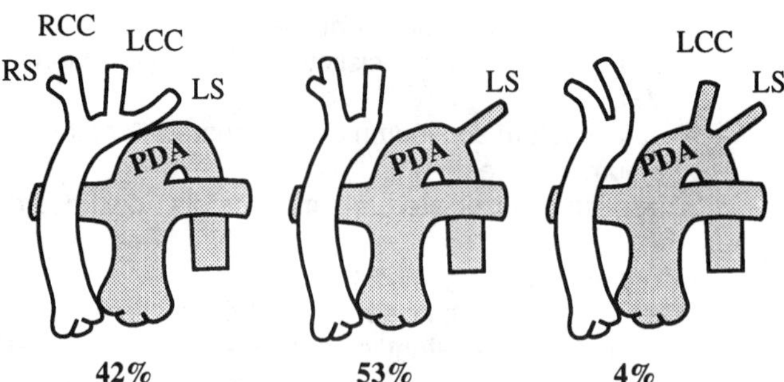

Interruption of Aortic Arch

Trilogy: (1)Interrupted aortic arch
(2) VSD
(3) PDA (pulmonary blood supplies lower part of body)

Associated with (in 1/3):
1. Bicuspid aortic valve
2. Muscular subaortic stenosis
3. ASD
4. Truncus arteriosus
5. Transposition
6. Complete anomalous pulmonary venous return

- • presents with CHF

Location:
- Type A: distal to left subclavian artery (42%)
- Type B: between left CCA and subclavian artery (53%) associated with: DiGeorge syndrome
- Type C: between innominate and left CCA (4%)

- √ dilatation of right atrium + ventricle
- √ dilatation of pulmonary artery
- √ ascending aorta much smaller than pulmonary artery
- √ arch formed by pulmonary artery + ductus arteriosus gives the appearance of a low aortic arch
- √ aortic knob absent
- √ trachea in midline
- √ NO esophageal impression
- √ retrosternal clear space increased (small size of ascending aorta)
- √ increased pulmonary vascularity (L-to-R shunt)

Prognosis: 76% dead at end of 1st month

INTERRUPTION OF PULMONARY ARTERY

= pulmonary trunk continues only as one large artery to one lung while systemic aortic collaterals supply the other side

Associated with: CHD (particularly if interruption on left side):
1. Tetralogy of Fallot
2. Scimitar syndrome = congenital pulmonary venolobar syndrome
3. PDA, VSD
4. Pulmonary hypertension

Collateral supply:
1. Arteries arising from arch + ascending aorta
2. Bronchial vessels
3. Intercostal vessels

4. Branches from subclavian artery

Location: usually opposite from aortic arch; R + L pulmonary artery equally involved

CXR:
- √ hypoplastic ipsilateral lung
- √ mediastinal shift toward involved lung
- √ hemidiaphragm may be elevated
- √ small hyperlucent ipsilateral chest with narrowed intercostal spaces
- √ "comma-shaped" small distorted hilar shadow
- √ asymmetry of pulmonary vascularity
- √ normal respiratory motion (normal aeration of hypoplastic lung)

NUC: √ absent perfusion with normal aeration

Angio: √ absent pulmonary artery

Rx: surgical anastomosis between proximal + distal pulmonary artery (to prevent progressive pulmonary hypertension with dyspnea, cyanosis, hemoptysis, death)

DDx: (1) Hemitruncus
(2) Swyer-James syndrome (ipsilateral air trapping, reduced ventilation + perfusion)

INTRAVENOUS DRUG ABUSE

Complications secondary to:
- (a) direct toxic effects of drugs or drug combinations (eg, heroin + cocaine / Talwin)
- (b) direct toxic effects of adulterants [eg, heroin is mixed ("cut") with quinine, baking soda, sawdust]
- (c) septic preparation
- (d) injection technique
- (e) choice of injection site (eg, "groin hit" into femoral vein; "pocket shot" into jugular, subclavian, brachiocephalic vein)

A. Cardiovascular complications
1. Arterial pseudoaneurysm
   may be followed by rupture with exsanguination / loss of limb
2. Arteriovenous fistula
3. Arterial occlusion
   - (a) at injection site due to intimal damage, thrombosis, spasm
   - (b) distal to injection site due to embolization, spasm
4. Venous thrombosis
5. Intravenous migration of needle to heart / lungs
6. Embolization of infectious agent / foreign body / air through inadvertent arterial injection ("hit the pink")
7. Endocarditis (most commonly S. aureus)

B. Soft-tissue complications
1. Hematoma / abscess
2. Foreign bodies
3. Lymphadenopathy
4. Cellulitis

C. Skeletal complications
1. Osteomyelitis
   - (a) direct contamination: eg, pubic bone ("groin hit") / clavicle ("pocket shot")
   - (b) hematogenous: spine most commonly affected
2. Septic arthritis: sacroiliac, sternoclavicular, symphysis pubis, hip, knee, wrist

D. Pleuropulmonary complications
1. Pneumothorax ("pocket shot")
2. Hemo- / pyothorax
3. Septic pulmonary emboli

E. Gastrointestinal complications
1. Severe colonic ileus
2. Colonic pseudoobstruction
3. Necrotizing enterocolitis
4. Liver abscess

F. Genitourinary complications
1. Focal / segmental glomerulosclerosis (heroin abuser)
2. Amyloidosis

G. CNS complications
1. Spinal epidural abscess in 5–18% (from vertebral osteomyelitis)
2. Cord compression (from collapsed vertebral body)
3. Cerebral infarction (from subacute bacterial endocarditis, toxic effect of drug, spasm, intimal damage from "pocket shot")
4. Intracranial hemorrhage (from trauma, hypertension, injection of anticholinergic drugs, vasculitis, rupture of mycotic aneurysm)
5. Meningitis, cerebral abscess

ISCHEMIC HEART DISEASE

= CORONARY ARTERY DISEASE (CAD)

Incidence: 1.5 million/year; leading cause of death in industrial nations

Morbidity: 28.7 cases per 1,000 men per year

Mortality: 3.1 deaths per 1,000 men per year

Noninvasive testing:
1. Noninvasive testing is of marginal benefit when disease prevalence is <0.2 / >0.7
2. Concordant thallium-201 and stress ECG are greater predictors of disease probability than either one used alone and/or when discordant
3. Sequential thallium-201 and stress ECG are most useful to establish the diagnosis of CAD when pretest prevalence is intermediate + test results are concordant

CXR:
- √ often normal
- √ coronary artery calcification
- √ pulmonary venous hypertension following acute infarction (40%)
- √ LV aneurysm

ECHO:
- √ region of dilatation with disturbance of wall movement
  - (1) Akinesis = no wall motion
  - (2) Hypokinesis = reduced wall motion
  - (3) Dyskinesis = paradoxical systolic expansion
  - (4) Asynchrony = disturbed temporal sequence of contraction

Coronary angiography: 1.2 million procedures per year

HEART

KAWASAKI SYNDROME

= MUCOCUTANEOUS LYMPH NODE SYNDROME

= acute febrile multisystem vasculitis of unknown cause involving large + medium-sized + small arteries with a predilection for the coronary arteries

Incidence: average of 1.1:100,000 population per year

Histo: panvasculitis

Age: <5 years of age (in 85%); peak age of 1–2 years; M:F = 1.5:1

Associated with: polyarthritis (30–50%), aseptic meningitis (25%), hepatitis (5–10%), pneumonitis (5–10%)

- fever >5 days
- mucosal reddening (injected fissured lips, injected pharynx, strawberry tongue) in 99%
- nonpurulent cervical lymphadenopathy (82%)
- maculopapular rash on extensor surfaces (99%)
- bilateral nonpurulent conjunctivitis (96%)
- erythema of palms + soles with desquamation (88%)

@ Cardiovascular system (1/3)

1. Coronary artery abnormality (15–25%)
   √ coronary artery aneurysm: LCA (2/3), RCA (1/3); proximal segment in 70%; 48% regress, 37% diminish in size
   √ coronary artery stenosis (39%) due to thrombus formation in aneurysm + intimal thickening
   √ coronary artery occlusion (8%) in aneurysms >9 mm
2. Myocarditis (25%)
3. Pericarditis
4. Valvulitis
5. Atrioventricular conduction disturbance

√ intestinal pseudoobstruction

√ transient gallbladder hydrops

Prognosis: 0.4–3% mortality (from myocardial infarction / myocarditis with congestive heart failure / rupture of coronary artery aneurysm)

Rx: aspirin (100 mg/kg per day) + gamma globulin

DDx: infantile polyarteritis

MICROSCOPIC POLYANGIITIS

= pauci-immune necrotizing small-vessel angiitis without granulomatous inflammation

Path: necrotizing arteritis identical to polyarteritis nodosa but with vasculitis in arterioles, venules and capillaries

- ANCA (antineutrophil cytoplasmic autoantibodies) in >80%
- negative serologic tests for hepatitis B

◊ Most common cause of the pulmonary-renal syndrome!

√ pulmonary infiltrates

√ glomerulonephritis (90%)

MITRAL REGURGITATION

= MITRAL INSUFFICIENCY

Cause:

1. Rheumatic heart disease
   (a) isolated: frequently seen in children
   (b) uncommon in adults (mostly combined with stenosis)
2. Bacterial endocarditis
3. Myocardial infarction with involvement of papillary muscle (posteromedial > anterolateral papillary m.)
4. Congenital (short / abnormally inserted chordae tendineae)
5. Marfan syndrome
6. Corrected transposition with Ebstein-like anomaly
7. Idiopathic hypertrophic subaortic stenosis (IHSS)
8. Persistent ostium primum ASD with cleft mitral valve
9. Mitral valve prolapse syndrome
10. Functional / secondary (from dilatation of mitral ring in any condition with dilatation of LV)

Pathogenesis: backward flow of blood from LV into LA during LV systole; increased volume of blood under elevated pressure causes dilatation of LA; marked increase in LV diastolic volume with little increase in LV diastolic pressure

√ mild pulmonary venous hypertension (less than with mitral stenosis)

√ LA + LV enlargement (cardiothoracic ratio >0.55)

√ enlarged LA appendage (with history of previous rheumatic heart disease)

√ mitral annular calcification (frequent)

ECHO:

√ LV volume overload
   √ normal-sized / enlarged LV
   √ increased septal + posterior wall motion

√ increased EF slope

√ early closure of aortic valve (LV stroke volume partially lost to LA)

√ LA enlargement (in chronic MV insufficiency)

√ bulging of interatrial septum to the right during systole

√ Doppler is only diagnostic tool + allows assessment of severity

MITRAL STENOSIS

Acquired causes:

principal cause: rheumatic heart disease

rare cause: mass obstructing LV inflow (tumor, myxoma, thrombus)

M:F = 1:8

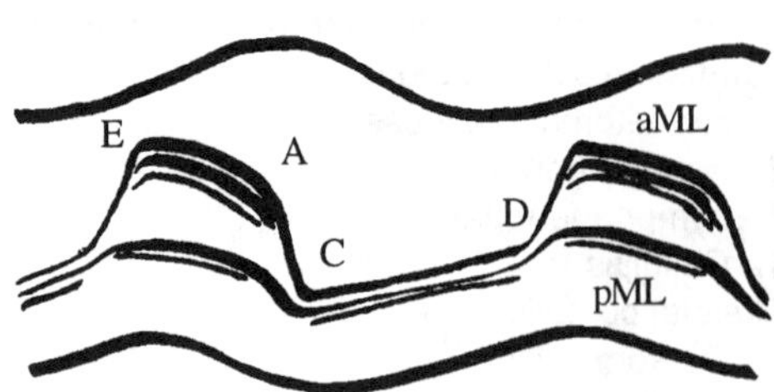

Classic Mitral Valve Stenosis

Pathogenesis:
rise in left atrial + pulmonary vascular pressure throughout systole and into diastole; development of medial hypertrophy + intimal sclerosis in pulmonary arterioles leads to pulmonary arterial hypertension, RV hypertrophy, tricuspid regurgitation, RV dilatation, right heart failure

- history of rheumatic fever (in 50%)
- atrial fibrillation
- systemic embolization from thrombosis of atrial appendage

Stages (according to degree of pulmonary venous hypertension):
Stage 1 : loss of hilar angle, redistribution
Stage 2 : interstitial edema
Stage 3 : alveolar edema
Stage 4 : hemosiderin deposits + ossification

√ calcification of valve leaflets (calcification of mitral annulus is a feature of age)
√ prominent pulmonary artery segment (precapillary hypertension)
√ small aorta (if forward cardiac output decreased)
√ enlarged LA ± wall calcification
  √ "double density" seen through right upper cardiac border (AP view)
  √ bulge of superior posterior cardiac border below carina (lateral view)
  √ esophagus displaced toward right + posteriorly
√ dilated left atrial appendage (not present with retracting clot)
√ hypertrophy of RV
√ dilatation of RV (tricuspid insufficiency / pulmonary hypertension)
  √ increase in cardiothoracic ratio
  √ diminution of retrosternal clear space
  √ IVC pushed backward (lateral view)
√ redistribution of pulmonary blood flow to upper lobes (postcapillary pressure 16–19 mm Hg)
√ interstitial pulmonary edema (postcapillary pressure 20–25 mm Hg)
√ alveolar edema (postcapillary pressure 25–30 mm Hg)
ECHO:
  √ thickening of leaflets toward free edge (fibrosis, calcification)
  √ flattening of EF slope = MV remains open throughout diastole due to persistently high LA pressure (crude index of severity of MV stenosis)
  √ diastolic anterior tracking of pML in 80% (secondary to diastolic anterior pull by larger + more mobile aML)
  √ diastolic doming of MV leaflets
  √ commissure fusion = increased echodensity + decreased leaflet motion at level of commissure
  √ <u>area reduction of MV orifice</u>: normal within 4–6 cm^2; mild narrowing with <2 cm^2; severe narrowing with <1 cm^2 (reproducible to within 0.3 cm^2)
  √ shortening + fibrosis of chordae tendineae
  √ abnormal septal motion = early diastolic dip of IVS due to rapid filling of RV (in severe MV stenosis)
  √ slowed LV filling pattern of small LV
  √ dilatation of LA (>5 cm increases risk of atrial fibrillation + left atrial thrombus)
  √ DE opening amplitude reduced to <20 mm indicating loss of valve pliability (DDx: low cardiac output state)
  √ absent A-wave common (atrial fibrillation)
  √ increase in valve gradient + pressure halftime on Doppler

Rx: (1) Commissurotomy if valves pliable + calcium absent + MV regurgitation absent
(2) Valve replacement for symptomatic patients with severely stenotic valves

DDx:
(1) Pseudomitral stenosis in decreased LV compliance (decreased EF slope, normal leaflet thickness + motion)
(2) Rheumatic mitral insufficiency (indistinguishable findings + evidence of LV volume overload)
(3) LA myxoma (mass behind MV + in LA)
(4) Low cardiac output (apparent small valve orifice)

LUTEMBACHER SYNDROME = rheumatic mitral valve stenosis + ASD

MITRAL VALVE PROLAPSE

Incidence: 2–6% of general population; 5–20% of young women; ? autosomal dominant inheritance
Age: commonly 14–30 years
Cause:
(1) "Floppy mitral valve" = elongation of cusps + chordae leading to redundant valve tissue, which prolapses into LA during systole
Associated with:
(a) Skeletal abnormalities: scoliosis, straightening of thoracic spine, narrow anteroposterior chest dimension, pectus excavatum deformity of sternum
(b) Barlowe syndrome = straight back syndrome
(c) Marfan syndrome
(d) Tricuspid valve prolapse
(e) Long-standing ASD
(2) Secondary MV prolapse:
papillary muscle dysfunction, rupture chordae tendineae, rheumatic mitral insufficiency, primary pulmonary hypertension, ostium secundum ASD

- arrhythmias, palpitation, chest pain, light-headedness, syncope
- responsible for midsystolic click + late systolic murmur (when associated with mitral regurgitation)

√ LA not enlarged (unless associated with significant mitral regurgitation)
ECHO:
  √ interruption of CD line with bulge toward left atrium
    √ abrupt midsystolic posterior buckling of both leaflets (classic pattern)
    √ "hammocklike" pansystolic posterior bowing of both leaflets
  √ multiple scallops on mitral valve leaflets (short-axis parasternal view)

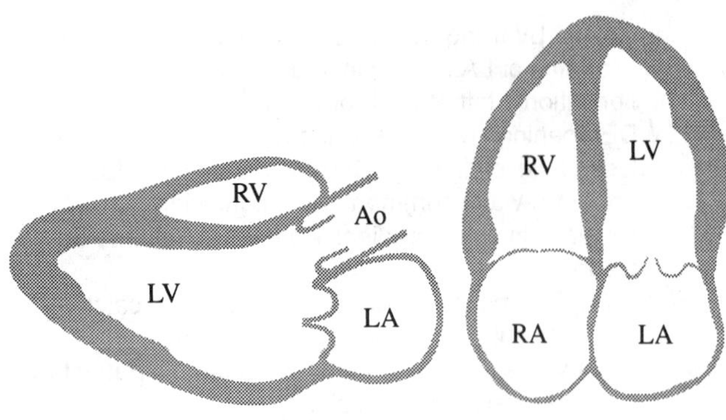

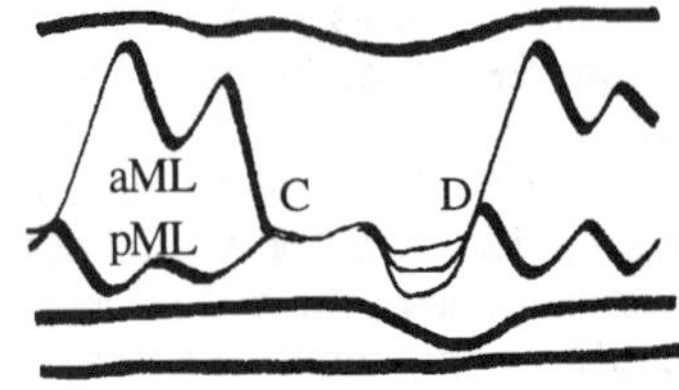

Mid systolic Mitral Valve Prolapse

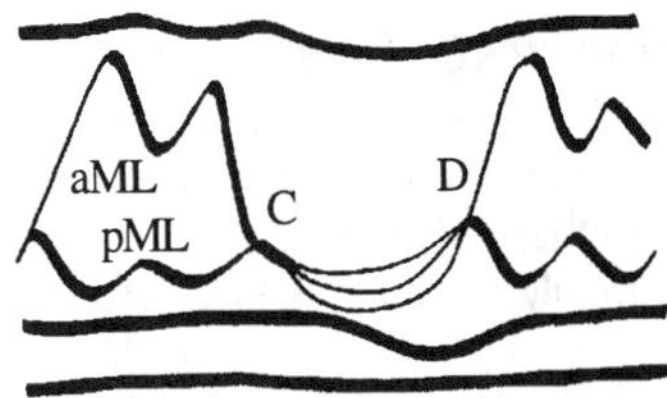

Holosystolic Mitral Valve Prolapse

- √ valve leaflets may appear thickened (myxomatous degeneration + valve redundancy)
- √ mitral valve leaflets passing >2 mm posterior to plane of mitral annulus (apical 4-chamber view)
- √ hyperactive atrioventricular groove
- √ mitral annulus may be dilated >4.7 cm^2

DDx: (1) Pericardial effusion (systolic posterior displacement of MV leaflets + entire heart)
(2) Bacterial endocarditis (mimicked by locally thickened + redundant leaflets)

MYOCARDIAL INFARCTION

Incidence: 1,500,000 per year in United States resulting in 500,000 deaths (50% occur in asymptomatic individuals)

- • atrioventricular block (common with inferior wall infarction as AV nodal branch originates from RCA); complete heart block has worse prognosis because it indicates a large area of infarction

CXR:
- √ normal-sized heart (84–95%) in acute phase if previously normal
- √ cardiomegaly: high incidence of congestive heart failure in anterior wall infarction, multiple myocardial infarctions, double- and triple-vessel CAD, LV aneurysm

CECT:
- √ perfusion defect within 60–90 seconds after bolus injection
- √ delayed enhancement of infarcted tissue peaking at 10–15 minutes (due to accumulation of iodine in ischemic cells), size of enhanced area correlates well with size of infarct

Cx: (myocardium is prone to rupture during 3rd–14th day post infarction)

A. LEFT VENTRICULAR FAILURE (60–70%)
- • "cardiac shock" = systolic pressure <90 mm Hg
- ◊ Signs of pulmonary venous hypertension are a good predictor of mortality (>30% if present, <10% if absent)
- √ progressive enlargement of heart
- √ haziness + indistinctness of pulmonary arteries
- √ increase in size of right descending pulmonary artery >17 mm
- √ pleural effusion
- √ septal lines
- √ perihilar ± peripheral parenchymal clouding
- √ alveolar pulmonary edema

Mortality: 30–50% with mild LV failure; 44% with pulmonary edema; 80–100% with cardiogenic shock; 8% in absence of LV failure

B. ANEURYSM (12–15% of survivors)

C. MYOCARDIAL RUPTURE (3.3%)
- • occurs usually on 3rd–5th day post MI
- √ enlargement of heart (slow leakage of blood into pericardium)

Prognosis: cause of death in 13% of all infarctions; almost 100% mortality

D. RUPTURE OF PAPILLARY MUSCLE (1%)
from infarction of posteromedial papillary muscle in inferior MI (common) / anterolateral papillary muscle in anterolateral MI (uncommon)
- • sudden onset of massive mitral insufficiency
- • unresponsive to medical management
- √ abrupt onset of severe persistent pulmonary edema
- √ minimal LV enlargement / normal-sized heart
- √ NO dilatation of LA (immediate decompression into pulmonary veins)

Prognosis: 70% mortality within 24 hours; 80–90% within 2 weeks

E. RUPTURE OF INTERVENTRICULAR SEPTUM (0.5–2%)
- • occurs usually within 4–21 days with rapid onset of L-to-R shunt
- • Swan-Ganz catheterization: increase in oxygen content of RV, capillary wedge pressure may be within normal limits
- √ right-sided cardiac enlargement
- √ engorgement of pulmonary vasculature
- √ NO pulmonary edema (DDx to ruptured papillary muscle)

Prognosis: 24% mortality within 24 hours; 87% within 2 months; >90% in 1 year

F. DRESSLER SYNDROME (<4%)
= POSTMYOCARDIAL INFARCTION SYNDROME
Etiology: autoimmune reaction
Onset: 2–3 weeks (range 1 week–several months) following infarction
• relapses occur as late as 2 years after initial episode
• fever
√ pericarditis + pericardial effusion
√ pleuritis + pleural effusion
√ pneumonitis

Right Ventricular Infarction

Right ventricle involved in 33% of left inferior myocardial infarction
√ decreased RV ejection fraction
√ accumulation of Tc-99m pyrophosphate
Prognosis: in 50% RV ejection fraction returns to normal within 10 days
Cx: (1) cardiogenic shock (unusual)
(2) elevation of RA pressure
(3) decrease of pulmonary artery pressure

MYXOMA

Most common benign primary intracardiac tumor (true neoplasm) in adults, 40–50% of all cardiac tumors
Age: 30–60 years; M<F
Classification: sporadic (most frequent);
familial type (mean age of 24 years);
complex type = Carney syndrome
Path: (a) gelatinous, friable, papillary / villous pedunculated tumor
(b) round / polypoid sessile tumor
Histo: hypocellular amorphous acid mucopolysaccharide matrix covered by a monolayer of endothelial cells
• short history + rapid progression
• dyspnea, chest pain
• constitutional symptoms:
  • fever, myalgia, arthralgia, weight loss
  • leukocytosis, anemia, elevated ESR,
  • hypergammaglobulinemia

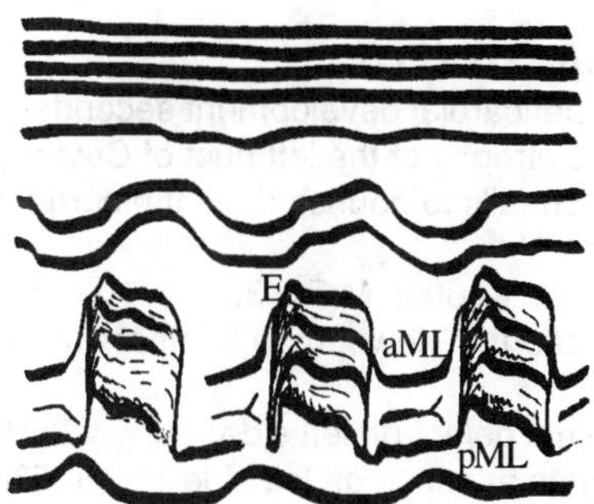

Atrial Myxoma Prolapsing Into Mitral Valve Orifice
Note the interval between the opening of aML and pML and the moment that the tumor reaches its maximal anterior excursion at point E when a slight additional opening of the aML results; aML stays open during entire diastole as a result of obstruction to left atrial emptying.

• positional symptoms (ie, change with position):
  • tachyarrhythmia, murmur
  • syncope
Location: LA:RA = 4:1; ventricles (exceptional); attached to atrial septum by small stalk near fossa ovalis (75%); may protrude into ventricle causing partial obstruction of atrioventricular valve
√ generalized cardiac enlargement
√ atrial obstruction (mimicking valvular stenosis)
√ persistent defect in atrium / diastolic defect in ventricle

A. LEFT ATRIAL MYXOMA
with obstruction of mitral valve:
√ enlargement of LA
√ pulmonary venous hypertension / edema
√ ossific lung nodules
√ NO enlargement of atrial appendage
Cx: systemic emboli (27%) in 50% to CNS (stroke / "mycotic" aneurysm)

B. RIGHT ATRIAL MYXOMA
with obstruction of tricuspid valve:
√ enlargement of RA
√ prominent SVC, IVC, azygos vein
√ decreased pulmonary vascularity
Cx: pulmonary emboli

ECHO: (2D-ECHO is study of choice)
√ hyperechoic mass ± mobile
◊ M-mode findings of only historical interest!
√ dense echoes appearing posterior to aML soon after onset of diastole
√ pML obscured
√ tumor echoes can be traced into LA
√ dilated LA
√ reduced E-F slope
CT:
√ intraluminal filling defect
MR:
√ hypointense on T1WI, hyperintense on T2WI
Rx: surgical excision ± valvuloplasty / valve replacement
Prognosis: 5–14% recurrence rate
DDx: (1) Thrombus (most commonly in LA + LV)
(2) Other cardiac tumors: sarcoma, malignant mesenchymoma, metastasis

Carney Syndrome

= COMPLEX MYOMA
(1) multiple myxomas recurring at an increased rate
(2) pigmented + myxomatous skin lesions
(3) myxoid fibroadenomas of the breast
(4) pituitary adenoma + testicular tumors
(5) adrenocortical disease (Cushing disease)

PATENT DUCTUS ARTERIOSUS

= PDA = persistence of left 6th aortic arch
Incidence: 9% of all CHD; M:F = 1:2
Associated with: prematurity, birth asphyxia, high-altitude births, rubella syndrome, coarctation, VSD, trisomy 18 + 21

HEART

Normal physiology in mature infant:
increase in arterial oxygen pressure leads to constriction + closure of duct
◊ functional closure due to muscular contraction within 10–15 hours
◊ anatomic closure due to subintimal fibrosis + thrombosis: in 35% by 2 weeks; in 90% by 2 months; in 99% by 1 year
• mostly asymptomatic
• congestive heart failure (rare) usually by 3 months of age if L-to-R shunt is large
• continuous murmur
• bounding peripheral pulses (intraaortic pressure runoff through PDA)

CXR (mimics VSD):
√ LA enlargement
√ enlarged pulmonary artery segment
√ increase of pulmonary vasculature (less flow directed to LUL)
√ enlarged RV + LV
√ enlarged ascending aorta + aortic arch (thymus may obscure this)
√ prominent ductus infundibulum (diverticulum) = prominence between aortic knob + pulmonary artery segment
√ obscured aortopulmonary window
√ "railroad track" = calcified ductus arteriosus

ECHO:
√ LA:Ao ratio ≥1.2:1 (signalizes significant L-to-R shunt)

Angio:
√ catheter course from RA to RV, main pulmonary artery, PDA, descending aorta
√ communication from aorta (distal to left subclavian artery) to left pulmonary artery on AP / LAT / LAO aortogram

PDA In Premature Infant

Premature infant not subject to medial muscular hypertrophy of small pulmonary artery branches (which occurs in normal infants subsequent to progressive hypoxia in 3rd trimester)
• CHF
Cause:
(a) pulmonary artery pressure remains low without opposing any L-to-R shunts (PDA / VSD)
(b) ductus arteriosus remains open secondary to hypoxia in RDS
√ recurrence of alveolar airspace filling after resolution of RDS
√ granular pattern of hyaline membrane disease becomes more opaque
√ enlargement of heart (masked by positive pressure ventilation)

Rx:
(a) Medical therapy:
(1) supportive oxygen, diuretics, digitalis
(2) avoid fluid overload (not to increase shunt volume)
(3) antiprostaglandins = indomethacin opposes prostaglandins, which are potent duct dilators
(b) Surgical ligation

Beneficial PDA

= compensatory effect of PDA in:
1. Tetralogy of Fallot
cyanosis usually occurs during closure of duct shortly after birth
2. Eisenmenger pulmonary hypertension
PDA acts as escape valve shunting blood to descending aorta
3. Interrupted aortic arch
supply of lower extremity via PDA

Nonbeneficial PDA

in L-to-R shunts (VSD, aortopulmonic window) a PDA increases shunt volume

PENETRATING AORTIC ULCER

= characterized by ulceration of atheromatous plaque that disrupts the internal elastic lamina + results in hemorrhage into media / rupture through wall of aorta

Location: middle of descending thoracic aorta

Angio:
√ ulcerated atherosclerotic plaque
√ aortic wall thickening

CECT:
√ focally ulcerated plaque
√ intramural hematoma cannot be differentiated from intraluminal thrombus / atherosclerotic plaque

MR:
√ deeply ulcerated aortic plaque
√ subacute hematoma in aortic wall indicated by high signal intensity on T1WI + T2WI (methemoglobin) either localized or mimicking type 3 dissection
√ aortic rupture with contained hematoma

DDx: (1) Aortic dissection (intimal flap, patent false lumen)
(2) Atheroma / thrombus (low signal intensity on T1WI + T2WI)

PERICARDIAL DEFECT

= failure of pericardial development secondary to premature atrophy of the left duct of Cuvier (cardinal vein), which fails to nourish the left pleuropericardial membrane

Incidence: 1:13,000; M:F = 3:1

Age at detection: newborn to 81 years (mean 21 years)

Location:
(a) foraminal defect on left side (35%)
(b) complete absence on left side (35%)
(c) diaphragmatic pericardial aplasia (17%)
(d) total bilateral absence (9%)
(e) foraminal defect on right side (4%)

Associated with (in 30%):
(1) Bronchogenic cyst (30%)
(2) VSD, PDA, mitral stenosis
(3) Diaphragmatic hernia, sequestration

- mostly asymptomatic
- ECG: right axis deviation, right bundle branch block
- palpitations, tachycardia, dyspnea, dizziness, syncope
- positional discomfort while lying on left side
- nonspecific intermittent chest pain (lack of pericardial cushioning, torsion of great vessels, tension on pleuropericardial adhesions, pressure on coronary arteries by rim of pericardial defect)

√ size:

— small foraminal defect	=	no abnormality
— large defect	=	herniation of cardiac structures / lung
— complete absence	=	levoposition of heart

√ absence of left pericardial fat-pad
√ levoposition of heart with lack of visualization of right heart border
√ prominence / focal bulge in the area of RVOT, main pulmonary artery, left atrial appendage
√ sharp margination + elongation of left heart border
√ insinuation of lung between heart + left hemidiaphragm
√ insinuation of lung between aortic knob + pulmonary a.
√ increased distance between heart + sternum secondary to absence of sternopericardial ligament (cross-table lateral projection)
√ pneumopericardium following pneumothorax
√ NO tracheal deviation

Rx: foraminal defect requires surgery because of (a) herniation + strangulation of left atrial appendage (b) herniation of LA / LV
(1) closure of defect with pleural flap
(2) resection of pericardium

PERSISTENT FETAL CIRCULATION

= PERSISTENT PULMONARY HYPERTENSION OF THE NEWBORN
= delay in transition from intra- to extrauterine pulmonary circulation

Cause: primary disorder related to birth asphyxia, concurrent parenchymal lung disease (meconium aspiration, pneumonia, pulmonary hemorrhage, hyaline membrane disease, pulmonary hypoplasia), concurrent cardiovascular disease, hypoxic myocardial injury, hyperviscosity syndromes)

- labile PO_2

√ structurally normal heart

POLYARTERITIS NODOSA

= PERIARTERITIS NODOSA = systemic necrotizing inflammation of medium-sized + small muscular arteries <u>without</u> glomerulonephritis or vasculitis in arterioles, capillaries, venules

Incidence: rare (2 new cases/million/year); M > F
Etiology: ? deposition of immune complexes
Path: mucoid degeneration + fibrinoid necrosis begins within media; absence of vasculitis in vessels other than arteries (DDx: necrotizing angiitis, mycotic aneurysm)
Histo: polymorphonuclear cell infiltrate in all layers of arterial wall + perivascular tissue (acute phase), mononuclear cell infiltrate, intimal proliferation, thrombosis, perivascular inflammation (chronic stage)
Associated with: hepatitis B antigenemia

- low-grade fever, myalgia, arthralgias
- malaise, abdominal pain, weight loss
- tender subcutaneous nodules (15%)
- elevated ESR, thrombocytosis, anemia
- peripheral neuropathy
- painless hematuria

Location: all organs may be involved, kidney (85%), heart (65%), liver (50%), pancreas, bowel, CNS (cerebrovascular accident, seizure)

@ Kidney (most frequently affected organ)
√ multiple small intrarenal aneurysms (interlobar, arcuate, interlobular arteries)
√ aneurysms may disappear (thrombosis) or appear in new locations
√ arterial narrowing + thrombosis (chronic stage / healing stage)
√ multiple small cortical infarcts
Cx: perinephric / subcapsular hemorrhage (rupture of aneurysm)

@ Chest (involved in 70%)
√ cardiac enlargement / pericardial effusion (14%)
√ pleural effusion (14%)
√ pulmonary venous engorgement (21%)
√ massive pulmonary edema (4%)
√ linear densities / platelike atelectasis (10%)
√ wedge-shaped / round peripheral infiltrates of nonsegmental distribution (14%) (simulating thromboembolic disease with infarction)
√ cavitation may occur
√ interstitial lower lung field pneumonitis

@ Liver (66%)
@ Mesenteric vessels (50%)
- abdominal pain, ulcer formation, GI bleeding, intestinal infarction

@ Skeletal muscle (39%)
@ Skin (20%)

Angiography (61% sensitivity, 80% true-positive rate):
√ 1–5 mm saccular aneurysms of small + medium-sized arteries in 60–75% as a result of necrosis of the internal elastic lamina (HALLMARK)
√ luminal irregularities + stenoses of arteries
√ arterial occlusions + small tissue infarctions

Cx: hypertension, renal failure, hemorrhage secondary to aneurysm rupture, organ infarction due to vessel thrombosis, gangrene of fingers / toes
Rx: steroids (50% 5-year survival rate)

POLYSPLENIA SYNDROME

= BILATERAL LEFT-SIDEDNESS

Age: presentation in infancy / adulthood; M < F

HEART

Associated with:
(a) CHD (90–95%):
APVR (70%), dextrocardia (37%), ASD (37%), ECCD (43–65%), pulmonic valvular stenosis (23%), TGA (13–17%), DORV (13–20%)
(b) GI abnormalities:
esophageal atresia, TE fistula, gastric duplication, preduodenal portal vein, duodenal webs + atresia, short bowel, mobile cecum, malrotation, semiannular pancreas, biliary atresia, absent gallbladder
(c) GU anomalies (15%):
renal agenesis, renal cysts, ovarian cysts
(d) Vertebral anomalies, common celiac trunk–SMA

- heart murmur, CHF, occasional cyanosis
- leftward / superiorly directed P-wave vector
- heart block (due to ECCD)
- extrahepatic biliary obstruction

√ bilateral morphologic LA appendages: pointed, tubular, narrow-based

@ Lung
√ bilateral morphologic left lungs (68%), normal (18%), bilateral R-sided lungs (7%)
√ bilateral hyparterial bronchi (= arteries projecting superior to bronchi on PA view + posterior to tracheobronchial tree on LAT view)
√ normal / increased pulmonary vascularity
√ bilateral SVC (50%)
√ large azygos vein (MOST SPECIFIC sign) may mimic aortic arch
√ absence of middle lobe fissure
√ cardiac apex on R / in midline

@ Abdomen
√ presence of ≥2 spleens (usually two major + indefinite number of splenules) located on both sides of the mesogastrium (esp. greater curvature of stomach)
√ hepatic symmetry
√ absence of gallbladder (50%)
√ stomach on right (40%) / left side
√ malrotation of bowel (80%)
√ azygos / hemiazygos continuation with interruption of hepatic segment of IVC (65–70%)
√ preduodenal portal vein

OB-US:
√ absence of intrahepatic IVC
√ aorta anterior to spine in midline
√ "double vessel" sign = 2 vessels of similar size in paraspinous location posterior to heart = aorta + azygos vein on left / right side of spine

Prognosis: 50% mortality by 4 months;
75% mortality by 5 years;
90% mortality by midadolescence

POPLITEAL ARTERY ENTRAPMENT SYNDROME

= popliteal artery classically winding medially and then inferiorly to the tendinous insertion of the medial head of the gastrocnemius

Incidence: 35 cases in American surgical literature; bilateral in up to 66%

Cause: anomalous development and course of medial head of gastrocnemius muscle, which attaches to medial femoral condyle after development of primitive popliteal artery in 20 mm embryo slinging around lateral aspect of popliteal a.

Pathophysiology:
flow unimpeded when muscle relaxed; increased arterial angulation with muscle contraction (early); progressive intimal hyperplasia ("atheroma" = misnomer) due to microtrauma in area of repeated arterial compression; ultimately occlusion / thrombosis within aneurysm (late)

Age: <35 years in 68%; age peaks at 17 and 47 years; M:F = 9:1

- slowly progressive intermittent unilateral calf claudication (early) esp. during periods of prolonged standing
- acute ischemia of leg with permanent occlusion of popliteal a. (late)

√ posterior tibial pulse obliterated during active plantar flexion against resistance
√ PVR has 40% false-positive results
√ ankle-arm index reduced during active muscle contraction
√ Doppler waveforms of posterior tibial a. diminished during muscle contractions

Angio (biplanar views with hyperextended knee):
√ medial deviation of artery (29%), popliteal stenosis (11%), poststenotic dilatation (8%)

Dx:
√ arteriography with typical medial deviation of popliteal a. before + after gastrocnemius contraction
√ popliteal a. thrombosis / occlusion

Cx: popliteal a. aneurysm

DDx: cystic adventitial disease of popliteal a., arterial embolism, premature arteriosclerosis, popliteal aneurysm with thrombosis, popliteal a. trauma, popliteal a. thrombosis, Buerger disease, spinal cord stenosis (= neurogenic claudication)

PRIMARY PULMONARY HYPERTENSION

= PLEXOGENIC PULMONARY ARTERIOPATHY

Diagnosis per exclusion:
clinically unexplained progressive pulmonary arterial hypertension without evidence for thromboembolic disease + pulmonary venoocclusive disease

Histo: plexiform + angiomatoid lesions = tortuous channels within proliferation of endothelial cells

Age: 3rd decade; M < F

- dyspnea on exertion, syncope
- easy fatigability
- hyperventilation
- chest pain
- hemoptysis

PSEUDOCOARCTATION

= AORTIC KINKING = elongated redundant thoracic aorta with acute kink / anterior buckling just distal to origin of left subclavian artery at lig. arteriosum
= variant of coarctation without a pressure gradient

Age: 12–64 years

Associated with:
hypertension, bicuspid aortic valve, PDA, VSD, aortic / subaortic stenosis, single ventricle, ASD, anomalies of aortic arch branches
- asymptomatic
- ejection murmur
- NO pressure gradient across the buckled segment

√ anteromedial deviation of aorta
√ "chimney-shaped" high aortic arch (in children)
√ rounded / oval soft-tissue mass in left paratracheal region + superior to presumed normally positioned aortic arch [secondary to elongation of ascending aorta + aortic arch] (in adults)
√ anterior displacement of esophagus
√ NO rib notching / dilatation of brachiocephalic arteries / LV enlargement / poststenotic dilatation

Angio:
√ high position of aortic arch
√ "figure 3 sign" = notch in descending aorta at attachment of short ligamentum arteriosum

DDx: true coarctation, aneurysm, mediastinal mass

PULMONARY ATRESIA

= CONGENITAL ABSENCE OF PULMONARY ARTERY
= atretic pulmonary valve with underdeveloped pulmonary artery distally

May be associated with: hypogenetic lung

CXR:
√ small hemithorax of normal radiodensity
√ mediastinal shift to affected side
√ elevation of ipsilateral diaphragm
√ reticular network of vessels on affected side (due to systemic collateral circulation from bronchial arteries)
√ rib notching from prominence of intercostal arteries (due to large transpleural collateral vessels)

OB-US:
√ small / enlarged / normal right ventricle
√ progressive atrial enlargement (tricuspid regurgitation)
√ flow reversal in ductus arteriosus + main pulmonary artery (most reliable)

PULMONARY ATRESIA WITH INTACT INTERVENTRICULAR SEPTUM

Associated with: ASD (R-to-L shunt)

Type I : no remaining RV, no tricuspid regurgitation
√ moderately enlarged RA (depending on size of ASD)

Type II : normal RV with tricuspid regurgitation
√ massive enlargement of RA

√ cardiomegaly (LV, RA)
√ concave / small pulmonary artery segment
√ diminished pulmonary vascularity

PULMONARY VENOOCCLUSIVE DISEASE

= fibrous narrowing of intrapulmonary veins in the presence of a normal left heart characterized by pulmonary arterial hypertension, pulmonary edema, normal wedge pressures

Age: children, adolescents; M:F = 1:1

Histo: fibrous narrowing + thrombosis in up to 95% of pulmonary veins

√ pulmonary edema
√ pleural effusions
√ delayed filling of normal main pulmonary veins + left heart

Prognosis: poor (no effective therapy)

PULMONIC STENOSIS

Pulmonary artery stenosis without VSD = 8% of all CHD

- mostly asymptomatic
- cyanosis / heart failure
- loud systolic ejection murmur

√ systolic doming of pulmonary valve (= incomplete opening)
√ normal / diminished / increased pulmonary vascularity (depending on presence + nature of associated malformations)
√ enlarged pulmonary trunk + left pulmonary artery (poststenotic dilatation)
√ prominent left pulmonary artery + normal right pulmonary artery
√ hypertrophy of RV with reduced size of RV chamber
√ elevation of cardiac apex
√ increased convexity of anterior cardiac border on LAO
√ diminution of retrosternal clear space
√ cor pulmonale
√ mild enlargement of LA (reason unknown)
√ calcification of pulmonary valves in older adults (rare)

Prognosis: death at mean age of 21 years if untreated

Subvalvular pulmonic stenosis

A. INFUNDIBULAR PULMONIC STENOSIS
typically in tetralogy of Fallot

B. SUBINFUNDIBULAR PULMONIC STENOSIS
= hypertrophied anomalous muscle bundles crossing portions of RV
Associated with: VSD (73–85%)
(a) low type:
courses diagonally from low anterior septal side to crista posteriorly
(b) high type:
horizontal defect across RV below infundibulum

Valvular pulmonic stenosis

1. CLASSIC / TYPICAL PULMONIC VALVE STENOSIS (95%)
= commissural fusion of pulmonary cusps
Age of presentation: childhood
- pulmonic click
- ECG: hypertrophy of RV

√ thickened dome-shaped valve
√ dilated main + left pulmonary artery
√ jet of contrast
Rx: balloon valvuloplasty

2. DYSPLASTIC PULMONIC VALVE STENOSIS (5%)
= thickened redundant distorted cusps, immobile secondary to myxomatous tissue
- NO click

HEART

√ NO poststenotic dilatation
Rx: surgical resection of redundant valve tissue

CXR:
- √ normal pulmonary vascularity
- √ normal-sized heart

Angio:
- √ increase in trabecular pattern of RV
- √ hypertrophied crista supraventricularis (lateral projection)

TRILOGY OF FALLOT (infantile presentation)
(1) severe pulmonic valvular stenosis
(2) hypertrophy of RV
(3) ASD with R-to-L shunt (increased pressure in RA forces foramen ovale open)

Supravalvular pulmonic stenosis

60% of all pulmonary valve stenoses

Site of narrowing: pulmonary trunk, pulmonary bifurcation, one / both main pulmonary arteries, lobar pulmonary artery, segmental pulmonary artery

Shape of narrowing:
(a) localized with poststenotic dilatation
(b) long tubular hypoplasia

May be associated with:
(1) Valvular pulmonic stenosis, supravalvular aortic stenosis, VSD, PDA, systemic arterial stenoses
(2) Familial peripheral pulmonic stenoses + supravalvular aortic stenosis
(3) Williams-Beuren syndrome: PS, supravalvular AS, peculiar facies
(4) Ehlers-Danlos syndrome
(5) Postrubella syndrome: peripheral pulmonic stenoses, valvular pulmonic stenosis, PDA, low birth weight, deafness, cataract, mental retardation
(6) Tetralogy of Fallot / critical valvular pulmonic stenosis

RAYNAUD SYNDROME

= episodic digital ischemia in response to cold / emotional stimuli

Pathogenesis:
(1) increase in vasoconstrictor tone
(2) low blood pressure
(3) slight increase in blood viscosity
(4) immunologic factors (4–81%)
(5) cold provocation

- exaggerated response of digit to cold / emotional stress:
  - numbness + loss of tactile perception
  - demarcated pallor / cyanosis
- hyperemic throbbing during rewarming
- sclerodactyly
- small painful ulcers at tip of digit

Raynaud disease

= PRIMARY VASOSPASM = SPASTIC FORM
= exaggerated cold-induced constriction of smooth muscle cells in otherwise normal artery

Cause: ? acquired adrenoreceptor hypersensitivity
May be associated with: early stages of autoimmune disorders
Age: most common in young women

- usually affects all fingers of both hands equally

√ normal segmental arm + digit pressures at room temperature
√ peaked digit volume pulse = rapid rise in systole, anacrotic notch just before the peak, dicrotic notch high on the downslope

PPG:
- √ flat-line tracing at low temperatures (10°–22°C) with sudden reappearance of normal waveform at 24–26°C = "threshold phenomenon"

Raynaud phenomenon

= SECONDARY VASOSPASM WITH OBSTRUCTION
= OBSTRUCTIVE FORM
= digital artery occlusion due to stenotic process in normally constricting artery / associated with an abnormally high blood viscosity

Cause:
1. Atherosclerosis (most frequent)
   (a) embolization from an upstream lesion
   (b) occlusion of major arteries supplying arm
2. Arterial trauma
3. End stage of many autoimmune disorders: eg, scleroderma, rheumatoid arthritis, systemic lupus erythematosus
4. Takayasu disease
5. Buerger disease
6. Drug intoxication (ergot, methysergide)
7. Dysproteinemia
8. Primary pulmonary hypertension
9. Myxedema

- normal vasoconstrictive response to cold

√ reduced segmental arm + digit pressures at room temperature

PPG (76% sensitivity, 92% specificity):
- √ flat-line / barely detectable tracing at low temperature with gradual increase of amplitude upon rewarming

Hand magnification angiography:
1. Baseline angiogram with ambient temperature
2. Stress angiogram immediately following immersion of hand in ice water for 20 seconds

RHABDOMYOMA OF HEART

= benign hamartoma arising from myocardium

Prevalence: most common cardiac tumor in infancy + childhood
Histo: "spider cell" = central nucleus surrounded by clear cytoplasm and radial extensions
Associated with: tuberous sclerosis (in 50–86%)

- asymptomatic (incidental detection)
- obstructed blood flow, murmur, arrhythmia
- heart failure
- supraventricular tachycardia (accessory conductive pathways within tumor)

Location: usually multiple; ventricular wall with intramural growth + tendency to involve interventricular septum; atrial wall (rare)

US:
- √ fetal nonimmune hydrops
- √ solid echogenic sessile mass ± intracavitary component bulging into ventricular outflow tract / atrioventricular valve

MR:
- √ tumor hyperintense to myocardium on T1WI

Prognosis: may regress spontaneously in patients <4 years of age

DDx: fibroma (solitary centrally calcified + cystic tumor, in ventricular myocardium, associated with Gorlin syndrome), teratoma (single intrapericardial multicystic mass), hemangioma (arise from RT atrium, pericardial effusion, skin hemangiomas)

SINGLE VENTRICLE

= UNIVENTRICULAR HEART
= DOUBLE INLET SINGLE VENTRICLE
= failure of development of interventricular septum ± absence of one atrioventricular valve (mitral / tricuspid atresia) ± aortic / pulmonic stenosis

- • conduction defect (aberrant anatomy of conduction system)
- √ two atrioventricular valves connected to a main ventricular chamber
- √ the single ventricle may be a LV (85%) / RV / undetermined
- √ a second rudimentary ventricular chamber may be present, which is located anteriorly (in left univentricle) / posteriorly (in right univentricle)
- √ rudimentary chamber ± connection to one great artery
- √ may be associated with tricuspid / mitral atresia

SINUS OF VALSALVA ANEURYSM

= deficiency between aortic media + annulus fibrosis of aortic valve resulting in distension + eventual aneurysm formation

Age: puberty to 30 years of age

Site: right sinus / noncoronary sinus (>90%)
- ◊ Right sinus usually ruptures into RV, occasionally into RA
- ◊ Noncoronary sinus ruptures into RA

- • sudden retrosternal pain, dyspnea, continuous murmur
- √ shunt vascularity
- √ cardiomegaly
- √ prominent ascending aorta

SPLENIC ARTERY ANEURYSM

= most frequent of visceral artery aneurysms

Etiology: medial degeneration with superimposed atherosclerosis, congenital, mycotic, pancreatitis, trauma, portal hypertension

Predisposed: women with ≥2 pregnancies (88%)

May be associated with: fibromuscular disease (in 20%)

M:F = 1:2
- • usually asymptomatic
- • pain, GI bleeding

Location: intra- / extrasplenic
- √ calcified wall of aneurysm (2/3)

Cx: rupture of aneurysm (6–9%, higher during pregnancy) with up to 76% mortality

DDx: renal artery aneurysm, tortuous splenic artery

SUBCLAVIAN STEAL SYNDROME

= stenosis / obstruction of subclavian artery near its origin with flow reversal in ipsilateral vertebral artery at the expense of the cerebral circulation

Incidence: 2.5% of all extracranial arterial occlusions

Etiology:
- (a) congenital: interruption of aortic arch, preductal infantile coarctation, hypoplasia of left aortic arch, hypoplasia / atresia / stenosis of an anomalous left subclavian artery with right aortic arch, coarctation with aberrant subclavian artery arising distal to the coarctation
- (b) acquired: atherosclerosis (94%), dissecting aneurysm, chest trauma, embolism, tumor thrombosis, inflammatory arteritis (Takayasu, syphilitic), ligation of subclavian artery in Blalock-Taussig shunt, complication of coarctation repair, radiation fibrosis

Age: average 59–61 years; M:F = 3:1; Whites:Blacks = 8:2

Associated with: additional lesions of extracranial arteries in 81%

- • lower systolic blood pressure by >20–40 mm Hg on affected side
- • delayed weak / absent pulse in ipsilateral extremity
- • Signs of vertebrobasilar insufficiency (40%):
  - • syncopal episodes initiated by exercising the ischemic arm
  - • headaches, nausea, vertigo, ataxia
  - • mono-, hemi-, para-, quadriparesis, paralysis
  - • diplopia, dysphagia, dysarthria, paresthesias around mouth
  - • uni- / bilateral homonymous hemianopia
- • Signs of brachial insufficiency (3–10%):
  - • intermittent / constant pain in affected arm precipitated by increased activity of that arm
  - • paresthesia, weakness, coolness, numbness, burning in fingers + hand
  - • fingertip necrosis

Location: L:R = 3:1

Color Doppler:
- √ reversal of vertebral artery flow, augmented by reactive hyperemia (blood pressure cuff inflated above systolic pressure for 5 minutes) / arm exercise

Angio:
- √ subclavian stenosis / occlusion (aortic arch injection)
- √ reversal of vertebral artery flow (selective injection of contralateral subclavian / vertebral artery)
  - CAVE: "false steal" = transient retrograde flow in contralateral vertebral artery caused by high-pressure injection

Rx: bypass surgery, PTA (good long-term results)

HEART

Partial Subclavian Steal Steal Syndrome
= retrograde flow in systole + antegrade flow in diastole

Occult Subclavian Steal Syndrome
= reverse flow seen only after provocative maneuvers, ie, ipsilateral arm exercise of 5 minutes / 5 minutes inflation of sphygmomanometer > systolic blood pressure levels

SUPERIOR VENA CAVA SYNDROME
= obstruction of SVC with development of collateral pathways

Etiology:
- (a) Malignant lesion (80–90%)
  1. Bronchogenic carcinoma (>50%)
  2. Lymphoma
- (b) Benign lesion
  1. Granulomatous mediastinitis (usually histoplasmosis, sarcoidosis, TB)
  2. Substernal goiter
  3. Ascending aortic aneurysm
  4. Pacer wires / central venous catheters (23%)
  5. Constrictive pericarditis

Collateral routes:
1. Esophageal venous plexus = "downhill varices" (predominantly upper 2/3)
2. Azygos + hemiazygos veins
3. Accessory hemiazygos + superior intercostal veins = "aortic nipple" (visualization in normal population in 5%)
4. Lateral thoracic veins + umbilical vein
5. Vertebral veins

- • head and neck edema (70%)
- • cutaneous enlarged venous collaterals
- • headache, dizziness, syncope
- • with benign etiology: slower onset + progression, both sexes, 25–40 years of age
- • with malignancy: rapid progression within weeks, mostly males, 40–60 years of age
- • proptosis, tearing
- • dyspnea, cyanosis, chest pain
- • hematemesis (11%)
- √ superior mediastinal widening (64%)
- √ encasement / compression / occlusion of SVC
- √ dilated cervical + superficial thoracic veins (80%)
- √ SVC thrombus

NUC:
- √ increased tracer uptake in quadrate lobe + posterior aspect of medial segment of left lobe (umbilical pathway toward liver when injected in upper extremity)

SYPHILITIC AORTITIS
= LUETIC AORTITIS

Incidence: in 10–15% of untreated patients (accounts for death in 1/3)

Path: periaortitis (via lymphatics), mesaortitis (via vasa vasorum) = primarily disease of media leading to secondary injury of intima, which predisposes the intima to premature calcific atherosclerosis

Age: between 40 and 65 years

Site: ascending aorta (36%), aortic arch (24%), descending aorta (5%), sinus of Valsalva (1%), pulmonary artery

- √ thick aortic wall (fibrous + inflammatory tissue)
- √ saccular (75%) / fusiform (25%) dilatation of ascending aorta
- √ small saccular aneurysms often protrude from fusiform aneurysm
- √ fine pencil-like <u>calcifications of intima</u> (15–20%) in ascending aorta, late in disease

Cx:
- (1) stenosis of coronary ostia (intimal thickening)
- (2) aortic regurgitation (syphilitic valvulitis), rare

DDx: degenerative calcification of ascending aorta (older population, no aneurysm, no aortic regurgitation)

TAKAYASU ARTERITIS
= PULSELESS DISEASE = AORTITIS SYNDROME = AORTOARTERITIS = IDIOPATHIC MEDIAL AORTOPATHY = AORTIC ARCH SYNDROME

= granulomatous inflammation of unknown pathogenesis affecting segments of aorta + major aortic branches + pulmonary arteries limited to persons usually <50 years of age

◊ The only form of aortitis that produces stenosis / occlusion of the aorta!

Etiology: probably cell-mediated inflammation

Incidence: 2.6 new cases/million/year; 2.2% (at autopsy)

Age: 12–66 years; M:F = 1:8; especially in Orientals

Histo:
- (a) Acute stage: granulomatous infiltrative process focused on elastic fibers of media of arterial wall consisting of multinucleate giant cells, lymphocytes, histiocytes, plasma cells
- (b) Fibrotic stage (weeks to years): progressive fibrosis of vessel wall resulting in constriction from intimal proliferation / thrombotic occlusion / aneurysm formation (from extensive destruction of elastic fibers in the media); ultimately leads to fibrosis of intima + adventitia

  ◊ Morphologically indistinguishable from temporal arteritis!

- • prepulseless / systemic phase of a few months to a year = nonspecific systemic signs + symptoms of fever, night sweats, weakness, weight loss, myalgia, arthralgia
  ◊ Mean interval of 8 years between onset of symptoms and diagnosis
- • pulseless phase = signs + symptoms of ischemia of limb (claudication, pulse deficit, bruits) + renovascular hypertension
- • erythrocyte sedimentation rate (ESR) >20 mm/hour in 80%

Location:
- Type I : <u>classic pulseless type</u> = brachiocephalic trunk + carotid arteries + subclavian arteries
- Type II : combination of type I + III
- Type III : <u>atypical coarctation type</u> = thoracic and abdominal aorta distal to arch + its major branches

Type IV : dilated type = extensive dilatation of the length of the aorta + its branches

Commonly involved: left subclavian artery (<50%), left common carotid artery (20%), brachiocephalic trunk, renal arteries, celiac trunk, superior mesenteric artery, pulmonary arteries (>50%)

Infrequently involved: axillary, brachial, vertebral, iliac arteries (usually bilaterally), coronary arteries

√ arterial wall thickening + contrast enhancement
√ full-thickness calcification (chronic disease)

@ Aorta
- √ long + diffuse / short + segmental irregular stenosis / occlusion of major branches of aorta near their origins
- √ stenotic lesions of thoracic aorta > abdominal aorta
- √ frequent skipped lesions
- √ abundant collateralization (late phase)
- √ aneurysmal dilatation of aorta = diffusely dilated lumen with irregular contours (common in ascending aorta + arch)
- √ fusiform / saccular aortic aneurysms (10–15%) (common in descending thoracic + abdominal aorta)

@ Brachiocephalic arteries
- √ multisegmented dilatation of carotid artery producing segmental septa
- √ diffuse homogeneous circumferential thickening of vessel wall in proximal common carotid artery
- √ increase in flow velocity + turbulence
- √ distal CCA, ICA, ECA spared with dampened waveforms

@ Pulmonary arteries (50–80%)
- √ pulmonary arterial lesions specific for Takayasu arteritis : dilatation of pulmonary trunk (19%), nodular thrombi (3%), "pruned tree" appearance of pulmonary arteries (66%)
- √ systemic-pulmonary artery shunts

CXR:
- √ widened supracardiac shadow >3.0 cm
- √ wavy / scalloped appearance of lateral margin of descending aorta
- √ aortic calcification (15%) commonly in aortic arch + descending aorta
- √ focal decrease of pulmonary vascularity

Cx: (1) Cerebrovascular accidents
(2) Heart failure due to aortic regurgitation

DDx: atherosclerosis, temporal arteritis (CCA not involved), fibromuscular dysplasia (in ICA not CCA), idiopathic carotid dissection (ICA), syphilitic aortitis (calcification of ascending aorta)

Rx: steroids, angioplasty after decline of active inflammation

TEMPORAL ARTERITIS

= CRANIAL / GRANULOMATOUS ARTERITIS
= POLYMYALGIA RHEUMATICA = GIANT CELL ARTERITIS (poor choice because Takayasu disease is also a giant cell arteritis)
= systemic granulomatous vasculitis limited to persons usually >50 years of age

Incidence: 1.7 new cases/million/year

Histo:
(a) acute stage: granulomatous infiltrative process focused on elastic fibers of arterial wall consisting of multinucleate giant cells, lymphocytes, histiocytes, plasma cells
(b) fibrotic stage (weeks to years): progressive fibrosis of vessel wall resulting in constriction from intimal proliferation / thrombotic occlusion / aneurysm formation

◊ Morphologically indistinguishable from Takayasu arteritis!

Age peak: 65–75 years; M:F = 1:3

- prodromal phase of flulike illness of 1–3 weeks:
  - malaise, low-grade fever, weight loss, myalgia
  - unilateral headache (50–90%)
- chronic stage:
  - jaw claudication (while chewing + talking)
  - palpable tender temporal artery
  - neuro-ophthalmic manifestations: visual impairment / diplopia / blindness
  - polymyalgia rheumatica (50%) = intense myalgia of shoulder + hip girdles
- erythrocyte sedimentation rate (ESR) of 40–140 mm/hour (HALLMARK)

Location: any artery of the body; mainly medium-sized branches of aortic arch (10%), external carotid artery branches (particularly temporal artery); extracranial arteries below neck (9%): subclavian > axillary > brachial > profunda femoris > forearm > calf; commonly bilateral + symmetric

√ long smooth stenotic arterial segments with skip areas
√ smooth tapered occlusions with abundance of collateral supply
√ absence of atherosclerotic changes
√ aortic root dilatation + aortic valve insufficiency

Dx: biopsy of palpable temporal artery

Prognosis: disease may be self-limiting (1–2 years); 10% mortality within 2–3 years

TETRALOGY OF FALLOT

= underdevelopment of pulmonary infundibulum secondary to unequal partitioning of the conotruncus

Incidence: 8% of all CHD; most common CHD with cyanosis after 1 year of life

TETRAD:
1. Obstruction of right ventricular outflow tract: usually at pulmonary infundibulum, occasionally at pulmonic valve
2. VSD
3. Right ventricular hypertrophy
4. Aorta overriding the interventricular septum

Hemodynamics:
fetus : pulmonary blood flow supplied by retrograde flow through ductus arteriosus with absence of RV hypertrophy / IUGR

HEART

neonate : R-to-L shunt bypassing pulmonary circulation with decrease in systemic oxygen saturation (cyanosis); pressure overload + hypertrophy of RV secondary to pulmonic-infundibular stenosis

Associated with:

1. Bicuspid pulmonic valve (40%)
2. Stenosis of left pulmonary artery (40%)
3. Right aortic arch (25%)
4. TE fistula
5. Down syndrome
6. Forked ribs, scoliosis
7. Anomalies of coronary arteries in 10% (single RCA / LAD from RCA)

- cyanosis by 3–4 months of age (concealed at birth by PDA)
- dyspnea on exertion, clubbing of fingers and toes
- "squatting position" when fatigued (increases pulmonary blood flow)
- "episodic spells" = loss of consciousness
- polycythemia, lowered PO_2 values, systolic murmur in pulmonic area

√ pronounced concavity in region of pulmonary artery trunk (small / absent PA)
√ coeur en sabot (boot-shaped heart) = enlargement of right ventricle
√ right-sided aortic arch in 25%
√ marked reduction in caliber + number of pulmonary vessels
√ asymmetric pulmonary vascularity
√ reticular pattern with horizontal course usually in periphery (= prominent collateral circulation of pleuropulmonary connections)

OB-US:
√ dilated aorta overriding the interventricular septum
√ usually perimembranous VSD
√ mildly stenotic RV outflow tract
√ NO RV hypertrophy in midtrimester

ECHO:
√ discontinuity between anterior aortic wall + interventricular septum (= overriding of the aorta)
√ small left atrium
√ RV hypertrophy with small right ventricular outflow tract
√ widening of the aorta
√ thickening of right ventricular wall + interventricular septum

Prognosis: spontaneous survival without surgical correction in 50% up to age 7; in 10% up to age 21

Rx: surgery in early childhood
(a) palliative
1. Blalock-Taussig shunt = end-to-side anastomosis of subclavian to pulmonary artery opposite aortic arch (64% survival rate at 15 years, 55% at 20 years)
2. Pott operation on left = anastomosis of left PA with descending aorta
3. Waterston-Cooley procedure = anastomosis between ascending aorta + right pulmonary artery
4. Central shunt = Rastelli procedure = tubular synthetic graft between ascending aorta + pulmonary artery

(b) corrective open cardiac surgery = VSD-closure + reconstruction of RV outflow tract by excision of obstructing tissue (82% survival rate at 15 years)

Operative mortality: 3–10%

Pink Tetralogy
= infundibular hypertrophy in VSD (3%)

Pentalogy Of Fallot
= tetralogy + ASD

Trilogy Of Fallot
= pulmonary stenosis + RV hypertrophy + patent foramen ovale

THORACIC OUTLET SYNDROME
= compression of nerves, veins, and arteries between chest and arm

Cause:

A. CONGENITAL
1. Cervical rib
   = elevation of floor of scalene triangle with decrease of costoclavicular space
   Incidence: 0.5–1% of population
   ◊ 5–10% of complete cervical ribs cause symptoms
   ◊ 10–20% of symptomatic patients have a responsible cervical rib
   Cx: aneurysmal dilatation of subclavian a.
2. Scalenus minimus muscle (rare)
   extending from transverse process of 7th cervical vertebra to 1st rib with insertion between brachial plexus + subclavian artery
3. Anterior scalene muscle = scalenus anticus syndrome (most common) = wide / abnormal insertion / hypertrophy of muscle
4. Anomalous 1st rib = unusually straight course with narrowing of costoclavicular space

B. ACQUIRED
1. Muscular body habitus
   = arterial compression in pectoralis minor tunnel
2. Slender body habitus
   with long neck, sagging shoulders
3. Fracture of clavicle / 1st rib (34%)
   with nonanatomic alignment / exuberant callus
4. Supraclavicular tumor / lymphadenopathy

- pain in forearm + hand which increases upon elevation of arm
- paresthesias of hand + fingers (numbness, "pins and needles") in 95%
- decreased skin temperature, discoloration of hand
- intermittent claudication of fingers (from ischemia)
- hyperabduction maneuver with obliteration of radial pulse (34%)

HEART

- Raynaud phenomenon (40%): episodic constriction of small vessels
- supraclavicular bruit (15–30%)

Bidirectional Doppler:
1. Adson maneuver (for scalenus anticus muscle) = hold deep inspiration while neck is fully extended + head turned toward ipsilateral and opposite side
2. Costoclavicular maneuver (compression between clavicle + 1st rib) = exaggerated military position with shoulders drawn back and downward
3. Hyperabduction maneuver (compression by humeral head / pectoralis minor muscle) = extremity monitored through range of 180° abduction

√ complete cessation of flow in one position

Photoplethysmography:
1. Photo pulse transducer secured to palmar surface of one fingertip of each hand
2. Arterial pulsations recorded with arm in
   (a) neutral position
   (b) extended 90° to side
   (c) 180° over the head
   (d) in "military" position with arms at 90° + shoulders pressed back

√ complete disappearance of pulse in one position

Angio:
√ abnormal course of distal subclavian artery
√ focal stenosis / occlusion
√ poststenotic dilatation of distal subclavian artery
√ aneurysm
√ stress test: bandlike / concentric constriction
√ mural thrombus ± distal embolization
√ venous thrombosis / obstruction

DDx: Cervical disk disease, radiculopathy, spinal cord tumor, trauma to brachial plexus, arthritis, carpal tunnel syndrome, Pancoast tumor, peripheral arterial occlusive disease, aneurysm, causalgia, thromboembolism, Raynaud disease, vasculitis

TRANSPOSITION OF GREAT ARTERIES

Complete transposition of great arteries

= TGA = D-TRANSPOSITION = failure of the aorticopulmonary septum to follow a spiral course characterized by (1) aorta originating from RV (2) pulmonary artery originating from LV (3) normal position of atria + ventricles

Incidence: 10% of all CHD

VARIATIONS:
1. Complete TGA + intact interventricular septum
2. Complete TGA + VSD: CHF due to VSD
3. Complete TGA + VSD + PS: PS prevents CHF = longest survival

Hemodynamics:
- fetus : no hemodynamic compromise with normal birth weight
- neonate : mixing of the 2 independent circulations necessary for survival

Admixture of blood from both circulations via:
(1) PDA + patent foramen ovale (when PDA closes worst prognosis)
(2) VSD (in 50%)

- cyanosis (most common cause for cyanosis in neonate) 2nd most common cause of cyanosis after tetralogy of Fallot
- symptomatic 1–2 weeks following birth

CXR:
√ "egg-on-its-side" appearance of heart = narrow superior mediastinum secondary to hypoplastic thymus + hyperaeration + abnormal relationship of great vessels
√ cardiac enlargement beginning 2 weeks after birth
√ right heart enlargement
√ enlargement of LA (with VSD)
√ absent pulmonary trunk (99%) = PA located posteriorly in midline
√ increased pulmonary blood flow (if not associated with PS)
√ midline aorta (30%) / ascending aorta with convexity to the right
√ right aortic arch in 3% (difficult assessment due to midline position + small size)

OB-US:
√ great arteries arise from ventricles in a parallel fashion
√ aorta anterior + to right of pulmonary artery (in 60%; rarely side by side)

Prognosis: overall 70% survival rate at 1 week, 50% at 1 month, 11% at 1 year by natural history

Rx:
(1) Prostaglandin E1 administration to maintain ductal patency
(2) Rashkind procedure = balloon septostomy to create ASD
(3) Blalock-Hanlon procedure = surgical creation of ASD

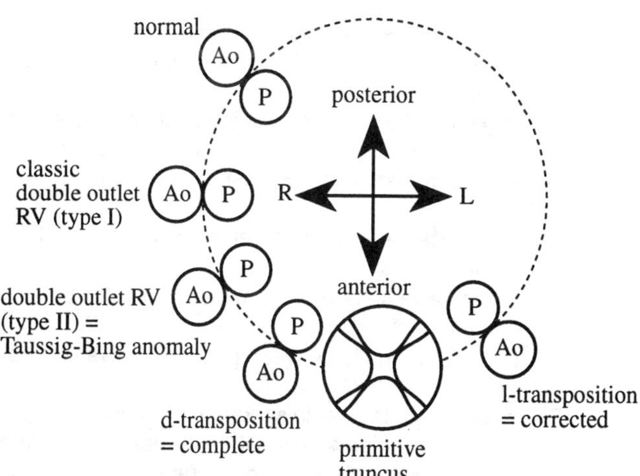

HEART

(4) Mustard operation (corrective) = removal of atrial septum + creation of intraatrial baffle directing the pulmonary venous return to RV + systemic venous return to LV; 79% 1-year survival rate; 64–89% 5-year survival

Corrected transposition of great arteries

= CONGENITALLY CORRECTED TRANSPOSITION
= L-TRANSPOSITION
= anomalous looping of the primordial ventricles associated with lack of spiral rotation of conotruncal septum characterized by
(1) Transposition of great arteries
(2) Inversion of ventricles (LV on right side, RV on left side):
(a) RA connected to morphologic LV
(b) LA connected to morphologic RV
(3) AV valves + coronary arteries follow their corresponding ventricles

Hemodynamics: functionally corrected abnormality

Associated with:
(1) usually perimembranous VSD (in >50%)
(2) pulmonic stenosis (in 50%)
(3) anomaly of left (= tricuspid) atrioventricular valves (Ebstein-like)
(4) dextrocardia (high incidence)

• atrioventricular block (malalignment of atrial + ventricular septa)

CXR:
√ abnormal convexity / straightening in upper portion of left heart border (ascending aorta arising from inverted RV)
√ inapparent aortic knob + descending aorta (overlying spine)
√ inapparent pulmonary trunk (rightward posterior position) = PREMIER SIGN
√ humped contour of lower left heart border with elevation above diaphragm (anatomic RV)
√ apical notch (= septal notch)
√ increased pulmonary blood flow (if shunt present)
√ pulmonary venous hypertension (if left-sided AV valve incompetent)
√ LA enlargement

Angio:
√ original LV on right side: smooth-walled, cylinder- / cone-shaped with high recess emptying into aorta (= venous ventricle)
√ original RV on left side: bulbous, triangular shape, trabeculated chamber with infundibular outflow tract into pulmonary trunk (= arterial ventricle)

OB-US:
√ great arteries arise from ventricles in a parallel fashion
√ aortic valve separated from tricuspid valve by a complete infundibulum
√ fibrous continuity between pulmonic valve + mitral valve

Prognosis: (unfavorable secondary to additional cardiac defects) 40% 1-year survival rate, 30% 10-year survival rate

TRICUSPID ATRESIA

2nd most common cause of pronounced neonatal cyanosis (after transposition) characterized by absent tricuspid valve, ASD, and small VSD (in most patients)

Incidence: 1.5% of all CHD

1. TRICUSPID ATRESIA WITHOUT TRANSPOSITION (80%)
(a) without PS (b) with PS (c) with pulmonary atresia
2. TRICUSPID ATRESIA WITH TRANSPOSITION
(a) without PS (b) with PS [most favorable combination] (c) with pulmonary atresia

◊ Usually small VSD + PS (75%) restrict pulmonary blood flow

• progressive cyanosis from birth on, increasing with crying = OUTSTANDING FEATURE (inverse relationship between degree of cyanosis + volume of pulmonary blood flow)
• pansystolic murmur (VSD)
• ECG: left-axis deviation

CXR (typical cardiac contour):
√ left rounded contour = enlargement + hypertrophy of LV
√ right rounded contour = enlarged RA
√ flat / concave pulmonary segment
√ normal / decreased pulmonary vascularity
√ typical flattening of right heart border with transposition (in 15%)

Prognosis: may survive well into early adulthood

Rx:
1. Blalock-Taussig procedure (if pulmonary blood flow decreased in infancy)
2. Glenn procedure = shunt between IVC + right PA (if total correction not anticipated)
3. Fontan procedure = external conduit from RA to pulmonary trunk + closure of ASD (if pulmonary vascular disease has not developed)

TROUSSEAU SYNDROME

= PARANEOPLASTIC THROMBOEMBOLISM

Incidence: 1–11%; higher in terminally ill cancer patients

Tumors: mucin-secreting adenocarcinoma of GI tract and pancreas (most common), lung, breast, ovary, prostate

Pathogenesis: (?)
(a) tumors activate coagulation + depress anticoagulant function
(b) cancer cells cause injury to endothelial lining, activate platelets + coagulation

Type of lesion: (1) Venous thrombosis
(2) Arterial thromboembolism
(3) Nonbacterial thrombotic endocarditis

◊ Patients with thromboembolism have an increased incidence of occult malignancy!

Prevalent criteria:
— absence of apparent cause for thromboembolism
— age >50 years
— multiple sites of venous thrombosis
— simultaneous venous + arterial thromboembolism
— resistance to oral anticoagulant therapy

— associated other paraneoplastic syndromes
— regression of thromboembolism with successful treatment of cancer
• disorders of consciousness (cerebral emboli)
• muscular pain + weakness (emboli to skeletal muscle)
• decompensated disseminated intravascular coagulation
√ deep vein thrombosis
√ pulmonary embolism
√ nonbacterial thrombotic endocarditis (echocardiography)
Rx: (1) Heparin (more successful than warfarin)
(2) Greenfield filter

TRUNCUS ARTERIOSUS

= PERSISTENT TRUNCUS ARTERIOSUS
= SINGLE OUTLET OF THE HEART
= abnormal septation of the conotruncus characterized by
(1) one great artery arising from the heart giving rise to the coronary, pulmonary, and systemic arteries, straddling
(2) large VSD

Incidence: 2% of all CHD

Types:

Type I	(50%) =	main PA + aorta arise from common truncal valve
Type II	(25%) =	both pulmonary arteries arise from back of trunk
Type III	(10%) =	both pulmonary arteries arise from side of trunk
Type IV	=	"Pseudotruncus" = absence of pulmonary arteries; pulmonary supply from systemic collaterals arising from descending aorta
Subtype A	=	infundibular VSD present
Subtype B	=	VSD absent

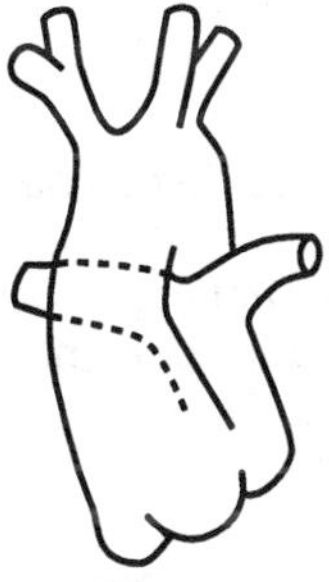
Type I

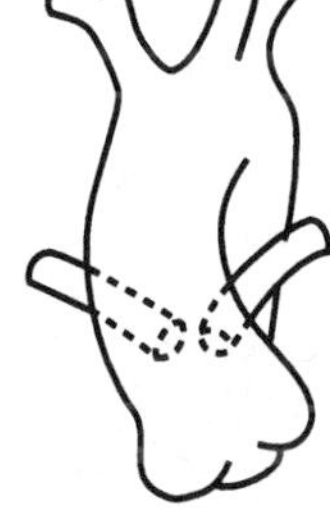
Type II

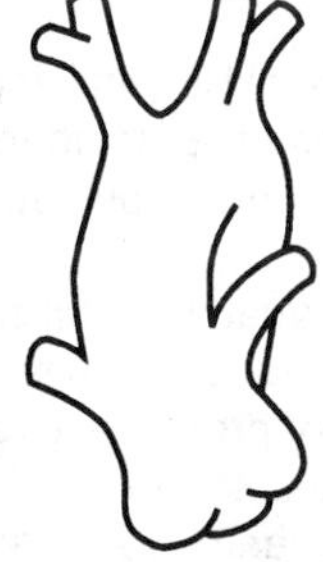
Type III

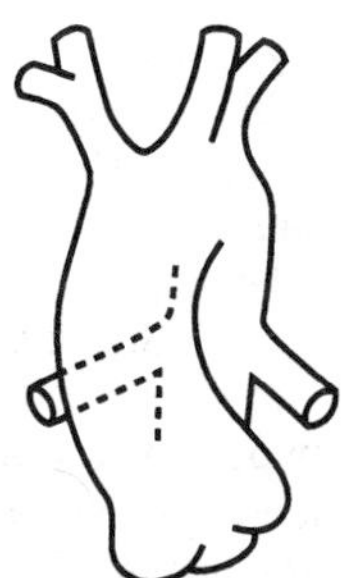
Type IV

Associated with:
(1) Right aortic arch (in 35%)
cyanosis + shunt vascularity + right aortic arch = TRUNCUS
(2) Forked ribs

Hemodynamics:
fetus : CHF only with incompetent valve secondary to massive regurgitation from truncus to ventricles
neonate: L-to-R shunt after decrease in pulmonary resistance (massive diversion of flow to pulmonary district) leads to CHF (ventricular overload) / pulmonary hypertension with time

• moderate cyanosis, apparent with crying
• severe CHF within first days / months of life (in large R-to-L shunt)
• systolic murmur

CXR:
√ cardiomegaly (increased LV volume)
√ enlarged LA (50%) secondary to increased pulmonary blood flow
√ large "aortic shadow" = truncus arteriosus
√ "waterfall / hilar comma sign" = elevated right hilum (30%); elevated left hilum (10%)
√ concave pulmonary segment (50%) (type I has left convex pulmonary segment)
√ markedly increased pulmonary blood flow, may be asymmetric

ECHO:
√ single arterial vessel overriding the interventricular septum (DDx: tetralogy of Fallot)
√ frequently dysplastic + incompetent single semilunar valve with 3–6 leaflets (most commonly 3 leaflets)

Prognosis: 40% 6-months survival rate,
20% 1-year survival rate

Rx: Rastelli procedure (30% no longer operable at 4 years of age) = (a) artificial valve placed high in RVOT and attached via a Dacron graft to main pulmonary artery (b) closure of VSD

Hemitruncus

= rare anomaly characterized by
(a) one pulmonary artery (commonly right PA) arising from trunk
(b) one pulmonary artery arising from RV / supplied by systemic collaterals

Associated with: PDA (80%), VSD, tetralogy (usually isolated to left PA)

• acyanotic

Pseudotruncus arteriosus

= TRUNCUS TYPE IV = severe form of tetralogy of Fallot with atresia of the pulmonary trunk; entire pulmonary circulation through bronchial collateral arteries (NOT a form of truncus arteriosus in its true sense); characterized by (1) pulmonary atresia (2) VSD with R-to-L shunt (3) RV hypertrophy

Associated with: right aortic arch in 50%

HEART

• cyanosis
√ concavity in area of pulmonary segment
√ commalike abnormal appearance of pulmonary artery
√ absent normal right and left pulmonary artery (lateral chest film)
√ esophageal indentation posteriorly (due to large systemic collaterals)
√ prominent hilar + intrapulmonary vessels (= systemic collaterals)
√ "coeur en sabot" = RV enlargement
√ prominent ascending aorta with hyperpulsations

VENTRICULAR ANEURYSM

A. CONGENITAL LEFT VENTRICULAR ANEURYSM
rare, young Black adult
(a) Submitral type:
√ bulge at left middle / upper cardiac border
(b) Subaortic type:
√ small + not visualized
√ heart greatly enlarged (from aortic insufficiency)

B. ACQUIRED LEFT VENTRICULAR ANEURYSM
= complication of myocardial infarction, Chagas disease
• may be asymptomatic + well tolerated for years
• occasionally associated with persistent heart failure, arrhythmia, peripheral embolization

True Ventricular Aneurysm

= circumscribed noncontractile outpouching of ventricular cavity with broad mouth + localized dyskinesis
Cause: sequela of transmural myocardial infarction
Location:
(a) left anterior + anteroapical: readily detected (anterior + LAO views)
(b) inferior + inferoposterior: less readily detected (steep LAO + LPO views)
Detection rate: 50% by fluoroscopy; 96% by radionuclide ventriculography; frequently not visible on CXR
√ localized bulge of heart contour = "squared-off" appearance of mid left lateral margin of heart border
√ localized paradoxical expansion during systole (CHARACTERISTIC)
√ rim of calcium in fibrotic wall (chronic), rare
√ akinetic / severely hypokinetic segment
√ left ventriculography in LAO, RAO is diagnostic
√ wide communication with heart chamber (no neck)
Cx: wall thrombus with embolization
Prognosis: rarely ruptures

Pseudoaneurysm Of Ventricle

= FALSE ANEURYSM = left ventricular rupture contained by fused layers of visceral + parietal pericardium / extracardiac tissue
(a) cardiac rupture with localized hematoma contained by adherent pericardium; typically in the presence of pericarditis
(b) subacute rupture with gradual / episodic bleeding

Etiology: trauma, myocardial infarction
Location: typically at posterolateral / diaphragmatic wall of LV
√ left retrocardiac double density
√ diameter of mouth smaller than the largest diameter of the globular aneurysm
√ delayed filling
Cx: high risk of delayed rupture (infrequent in true aneurysms)

VENTRICULAR SEPTAL DEFECT

Most common CHD (25–30%): (a) isolated in 20%
(b) with other cardiac anomalies in 5%;
◊ Acyanotic L-to-R shunt + right aortic arch (in 2–5%) = VSD

1. MEMBRANOUS = PERIMEMBRANOUS VSD (75–80%)
Location: posterior + inferior to crista supraventricularis near commissure between right and posterior (= noncoronary) aortic valve cusps
May be associated with:
small aneurysms of membranous septum commonly leading to decrease in size of membranous VSD (their presence does not necessarily predict eventual complete closure)
2. SUPRACRISTAL = CONAL VSD (5–8%)
◊ Crista supraventricularis = inverted U-shaped muscular ridge posterior + inferior to pulmonary valve
(a) RV view = VSD just beneath pulmonary valve with valve forming part of superior margin of defect
(b) LV view = VSD just below commissure between R + L aortic valve cusps
Cx: right aortic valve cusp may herniate into VSD (= aortic insufficiency)
3. MUSCULAR VSD (5–10%)
May consist of multiple VSDs; bordered entirely by myocardium
Location: (a) inlet portion (b) trabecular portion (c) infundibular / outlet portion
4. ATRIOVENTRICULAR CANAL TYPE
= ENDOCARDIAL CUSHION TYPE
= POSTERIOR VSD (5–10%)
Location: adjacent to septal + anterior leaflet of mitral valve; rare as isolated defect

Hemodynamics:
small bidirectional shunt during fetal life (similar pressures in RV + LV); after birth a decrease in pulmonary arterial pressure + increase in systemic arterial pressure occurs with development of L-to-R shunt
(a) small VSD: little / no hemodynamic significance
(b) large VSD: pulmonary vascular disease + hypertension will increase RV pressure; eventually leads to shunt reversal (R-to-L shunt)
(c) very large VSD: gross right ventricular overload creates CHF soon after birth

NATURAL HISTORY OF VSD causing reduction in pulmonary blood flow:

1. Spontaneous closure
   in 40% within first 2 years of life; 60% by 5 years (65% with muscular VSD, 25% with membranous VSD); with large VSD in 10%; with small VSD in 50%
2. Eisenmenger syndrome
   = progressive increase in pulmonary vascular resistance through intima + medial hyperplasia; occurs in 10% of large VSDs by 2 years of age
3. RVOT obstruction
   infundibular hypertrophy in 3% = pink tetrad
4. Prolapse of right aortic valve cusp
   = aortic valve insufficiency

CLASSIFICATION:

Group I: "maladie de Roger" = small shunt with defect <1 cm; normal pulmonary artery pressure, normal pulmonary vascular resistance; spontaneous closure
- asymptomatic
- heart murmur
- √ normal plain film

Group II: moderate shunt with defect of 1–1.5 cm; intermediate pulmonary artery pressure; normal pulmonary vascular resistance; spontaneous closure in large percentage
- respiratory infections, mild dyspnea
- √ slight prominence of pulmonary vessels (45% shunt)
- √ slight enlargement of LA

Group III: nonrestrictive large shunt with size equal to aortic valve orifice; pulmonary artery pressure approaching systemic levels; slightly increased pulmonary vascular resistance; pulmonary blood flow 2–4 x systemic flow
- bouts of respiratory infections
- feeding problems, failure to thrive
- √ prominent pulmonary segment + vessels (= shunt vascularity)
- √ enlargement of LA + LV
- √ normal / small aorta

Group IV: Eisenmenger syndrome with shunt reversal into R-to-L shunt; irreversible increase in pulmonary vascular resistance (when pulmonary vascular resistance >0.75 of systemic vascular resistance)
- cyanotic, but less symptomatic; CHF rare
- √ decrease of pulmonary vessel caliber
- √ decrease in size of LA + LV

CXR (with increase in size of VSD):
- √ enlargement of LA
- √ enlargement of pulmonary artery segment
- √ enlargement of LV
- √ RV hypertrophy
- √ increase in pulmonary blood flow (>45% of pulmonary blood flow from systemic circulation)
- √ Eisenmenger reaction

ECHO:
- √ lack of echoes in region of interventricular septum with sharp edges (DDx: artifactual dropout with sound beam parallel to septum); muscular VSD difficult to see
- √ LA enlargement
- √ prolapse of aortic valve cusp (in supracristal VSD)
- √ deformity of aortic cusp (in membranous VSD)

Angio:

Projections:
- (a) LAO 60° C-C 20° for membranous + anterior muscular VSD
- (b) LAO 45° C-C 45° (hepatoclavicular) for posterior endocardial cushion + posterior muscular VSD
- (c) RAO for supracristal VSD + assessment of RVOT

√ RVOT / pulmonary valve fill without filling of RV chamber (in supracristal VSD)

Rx:

(a) large VSD + left heart failure at 3 months of age: aim is to delay closure until child is 18 months of age; pulmonary-to-systemic blood flow >2:1 requires surgery before pulmonary hypertension becomes manifest
   1. Digitalis + diuretics
   2. Pulmonary artery banding
   3. Patching of VSD: surgical approach through RA / through RV for supracristal VSD

(b) small VSDs without increase in pulmonary arterial pressure are followed

HEART

LIVER, BILE DUCTS, PANCREAS, AND SPLEEN

DIFFERENTIAL DIAGNOSIS OF HEPATIC, BILIARY, PANCREATIC, AND SPLENIC DISORDERS

RIGHT UPPER QUADRANT PAIN

A. BILE DUCTS
1. Biliary colic / bile duct obstruction
2. Acute cholecystitis / cholangitis

B. LIVER
1. Acute hepatitis: alcoholic, viral, drug-related, toxic
2. Hepatic abscess
3. Hepatic tumor: metastases, hepatocellular carcinoma, hemangioma, focal nodular hyperplasia, hepatic adenoma
4. Hemorrhagic cyst
5. Hepatic congestion: acute hepatic congestion, Budd-Chiari syndrome
6. Perihepatitis from gonococcal / chlamydial infection (Fitz-Hugh-Curtis syndrome)

C. PANCREAS
1. Acute pancreatitis

D. INTESTINES
1. Acute appendicitis
2. Peripyloric ulcer
3. Small bowel obstruction
4. Irritable bowel
5. Colitis / ileitis
6. Intestinal tumor

E. LUNG
1. Pneumonia
2. Pulmonary infarction

F. KIDNEY
1. Acute pyelonephritis
2. Ureteral calculus
3. Renal / perirenal abscess
4. Renal infarction
5. Renal tumor

G. OTHERS
1. Costochondritis
2. Herpes zoster

LIVER

Diffuse Hepatic Enlargement

A. METABOLIC
1. Fatty infiltration
2. Amyloid
3. Wilson disease
4. Gaucher disease
5. Von Gierke disease
6. Niemann-Pick disease
7. Weber-Christian disease
8. Galactosemia

B. MALIGNANCY
1. Lymphoma
2. Diffuse metastases
3. Diffuse HCC
4. Angiosarcoma

C. INFLAMMATION / INFECTION
1. Hepatitis
2. Mononucleosis
3. Miliary TB, histoplasmosis, sarcoid
4. Malaria
5. Syphilis
6. Leptospirosis
7. Chronic granulomatous disease of childhood
8. Sarcoidosis

D. VASCULAR
1. Passive congestion

E. OTHERS
1. Early cirrhosis
2. Polycystic liver disease

Increased Liver Attenuation

Abnormal deposits of substances with high atomic numbers

A. IRON
(a) diffuse iron accumulation
1. Genetic / primary hemochromatosis
2. Erythropoietic hemochromatosis
3. Bantu siderosis
4. Transfusional iron overload

(b) focal iron accumulation
1. Hemorrhagic metastases: choriocarcinoma, melanoma
2. Hepatic adenoma
3. Siderotic regenerative nodules of cirrhosis
   ◊ An iron-poor focus within a siderotic nodule on T2WI is suspect of HCC!
4. Focal hemochromatosis

B. COPPER
Wilson disease = hepatolenticular degeneration = increased copper deposits in liver + basal ganglia

C. IODINE
Amiodarone (= antiarrhythmic drug with 37% iodine by weight)
√ 95–145 HU (range of normal for liver 30–70 HU)

D. GOLD
Colloidal form of gold for therapy of rheumatoid arthritis

E. THOROTRAST
Alpha-emitter with atomic number of 90

F. THALLIUM
Accidental / suicidal ingestion of rodenticides (lethal dose is 0.2–1.0 gram)

G. ACUTE MASSIVE PROTEIN DEPOSITS

H. GLYCOGEN STORAGE DISEASE

mnemonic: "GG CHAT"
Gold therapy
Glycogen storage disease
Cyclophosphamide
Hemochromatosis / hemosiderosis
Amiodarone
Thorotrast

Generalized Increase In Liver Echogenicity

1. Fatty liver
2. Steatohepatitis
3. Cirrhosis (fibrosis + fatty liver)
4. Chronic hepatitis
5. Vacuolar degeneration

Primary Benign Liver Tumor

A. EPITHELIAL TUMORS
  (a) hepatocellular
    1. Regenerative nodules
    2. Adenomatous hyperplastic nodules
    3. Focal nodular hyperplasia
    4. Hepatocellular adenoma
  (b) cholangiocellular
    1. Bile duct adenoma
    2. Biliary cystadenoma

B. MESENCHYMAL TUMORS
  (a) tumor of adipose tissue
    1. Lipoma
    2. Myelolipoma
    3. Angiomyolipoma
  (b) tumor of muscle tissue
    1. Leiomyoma
  (c) tumor of blood vessels
    1. Infantile hemangioendothelioma
    2. Hemangioma
    3. Peliosis hepatis
  (d) mesothelial tumor
    1. Benign mesothelioma

C. MIXED TISSUE TUMOR
  1. Mesenchymal hamartoma
  2. Benign teratoma

D. MISCELLANEOUS
  1. Adrenal rest tumor
  2. Pancreatic rest

Primary Malignant Liver Tumor

A. EPITHELIAL TUMOR
  (a) hepatocellular
    1. Hepatoblastoma (7%)
    2. Hepatocellular carcinoma (75%)
  (b) cholangiocellular (6%)
    1. Cholangiocarcinoma
    2. Biliary cystadenocarcinoma

B. MESENCHYMAL TUMOR
  (a) tumor of blood vessels
    1. Angiosarcoma
    2. Epithelioid hemangioendothelioma
    3. Kaposi sarcoma
  (b) other tumor
    1. Embryonal sarcoma
    2. Fibrosarcoma

C. TUMOR OF MUSCLE TISSUE
  1. Leiomyosarcoma
  2. Rhabdomyosarcoma

D. MISCELLANEOUS
  1. Carcinosarcoma
  2. Teratoma
  3. Yolk sac tumor
  4. Carcinoid
  5. Squamous carcinoma
  6. Primary lymphoma

Focal Liver Lesion

A. SOLITARY
  (a) benign
    1. Simple cyst / echinococcal cyst
    2. Cavernous hemangioma
    3. Abscess
    4. Hematoma / traumatic cyst
    5. Adenoma
    6. Focal nodular hyperplasia
    7. Fatty change
  (b) malignant
    1. Hepatoma
    2. Metastasis
    3. Peripheral cholangiocarcinoma

B. MULTIPLE
  (a) benign
    1. Simple cysts
    2. Cavernous hemangioma
    3. Polycystic disease
    4. Multiple abscesses
    5. Caroli disease
    6. Adenoma
    7. Regenerating hepatic nodules
    8. Sarcoidosis
  (b) malignant
    1. Metastases (most common malignant liver tumor)
    2. Multifocal hepatoma
    3. Lymphoma

Solitary Echogenic Liver Mass

mnemonic: "**H**yperechoic **F**ocal **M**asses **A**ffecting the **L**iver"

Hematoma, **H**epatoma, **H**emangioma, **H**emochromatosis
Fatty infiltration, **F**ocal nodular hyperplasia, **F**ibrosis
Metastasis
Adenoma
Lipoma

Bull's-eye Lesions Of Liver

1. Candidiasis (in immunocompromised)
2. Metastases
3. Lymphoma, leukemia
4. Sarcoidosis
5. Septic emboli
6. Other opportunistic infections
7. Kaposi sarcoma

Cystic Liver Lesion

A. NONNEOPLASTIC
  1. Congenital hepatic cyst
  2. Hematoma
  3. Echinococcal cyst
  4. Abscess

5. Cystic liver disease
6. Autosomal dominant polycystic disease

B. NEOPLASTIC
1. Mesenchymal hamartoma
2. Undifferentiated sarcoma (embryonal sarcoma)
3. Malignant mesenchymoma
4. Biliary cystadenoma / cystadenocarcinoma <5% of intrahepatic cysts of biliary origin
5. Lymphangioma
6. Necrotic neoplasm
7. Cystic metastasis (ovarian / gastric carcinoma)

Vascular "Scar" Tumor Of Liver
1. Focal nodular hyperplasia
2. Hepatic adenoma
3. Giant cavernous hemangioma
4. Fibrolamellar hepatocellular carcinoma
5. Well-differentiated hepatocellular carcinoma
6. Hypervascular metastasis
7. Intrahepatic cholangiocarcinoma

Low-density Mass In Porta Hepatis
1. Choledochal cyst
2. Hepatic cyst
3. Pancreatic pseudocyst
4. Enteric duplication
5. Hepatic artery aneurysm
6. Biloma

Low-density Hepatic Mass With Enhancement
1. Hepatoma
2. Hypervascular metastases (lesions that may be obscured after contrast injection: pheochromocytoma, carcinoid, melanoma)
3. Cavernous hemangioma
4. Focal nodular hyperplasia with central fibrous scar
5. Hepatic adenoma

Fat-containing Liver Mass
1. Hepatoma
2. Angiomyolipoma

Hepatic Calcification
A. INFECTION
1. Tuberculosis (48%), histoplasmosis, gumma, brucellosis
2. Echinococcal cyst (in 33%)
3. Chronic granulomatous disease of childhood
4. Old pyogenic / amebic abscess

B. VASCULAR
1. Hepatic artery aneurysm
2. Portal vein thrombosis
3. Hematoma

C. BILIARY
1. Intrahepatic calculi

D. BENIGN TUMORS
1. Congenital cyst
2. Cavernous hemangioma
3. Capsule of regenerating nodules
4. Infantile hemangioendothelioma

E. PRIMARY MALIGNANT TUMOR
1. Hepatoblastoma (10–20%)
2. Cholangiocellular carcinoma

F. METASTATIC TUMOR
1. Mucinous carcinoma of colon, breast, stomach
2. Ovarian carcinoma (psammomatous bodies)
3. Melanoma, pleural mesothelioma, osteosarcoma, carcinoid, leiomyosarcoma

mnemonic: "4H TAG MAP"
Hepatoma
Hemochromatosis
Hemangioma
Hydatid disease
Thorotrast
Abscess
Granulomas (healed)
Metastases
Absent mnemonic
Porcelain gallbladder

Portal Venous Gas
◊ Should be considered a life-threatening event and sign of bowel infarction + gangrene until proved otherwise!

Etiology:

A. INTESTINAL NECROSIS (in 74% of adults)
1. Bowel infarction secondary to arterial and venous occlusions (vascular accidents, superior mesenteric artery syndrome)
2. Ulcerative colitis
3. Necrotizing enterocolitis associated with mesenteric arterial thrombosis
4. Perforated gastric ulcer

B. GI OBSTRUCTION
1. Small bowel obstruction (duodenal atresia)
2. Imperforate anus
3. Esophageal atresia

C. MISCELLANEOUS
1. Hemorrhagic pancreatitis
2. Sigmoid diverticulitis
3. Intraabdominal abscess
4. Pneumonia
5. Iatrogenic injection of air during endoscopy
6. Dead fetus
7. Diabetes, diarrhea

mnemonic: "BE NICE"
BE (air embolism during double contrast barium enema)
Necrotizing enterocolitis
Infarction (mesenteric)
Catheterization of umbilical vein
Erythroblastosis fetalis

Pathogenesis:
1. Luminal bacterial overgrowth with gas-forming organisms invading the submucosa and veins of the intestinal wall

2. Intestinal necrosis with gas infiltrating directly through damaged intestinal wall into intestinal venules (bowel obstruction, ulcer)
3. Elevated intraluminal pressure in conjunction with mucosal ulceration

Composition of colonic gas:
methane, carbon dioxide, oxygen, nitrogen, hydrogen
√ branching linear gas densities in periphery of liver
√ gas in mesenteric vessels
√ pneumatosis of intestinal wall

US:
√ intensely hyperechoic foci within lumen of portal vein + liver parenchyma

Doppler:
√ tall sharp bidirectional spikes (overloading of Doppler receiver from strong reflection of gas bubble in bloodstream) superimposed on normal portal vein spectrum

Prognosis: often fatal within 1 week of diagnosis
DDx: pneumobilia (central bile ducts close to liver hilum)

Hyperperfusion Abnormalities Of Liver

= areas of early enhancement on arterial-dominant phase due to decreased portal blood flow / formation of intrahepatic arterioportal shunts / increased aberrant drainage through hepatic veins

A. LOBAR / SEGMENTAL
1. Portal venous thrombosis
2. Obstruction by malignant neoplasm
3. Ligation of portal vein
4. Cirrhosis with arterioportal shunt
5. Hypervascular gallbladder disease

B. SUBSEGMENTAL
1. Obstruction of peripheral portal branches
2. Percutaneous needle biopsy / ethanol ablation
3. Acute cholecystitis

C. SUBCAPSULAR of unknown origin

D. EARLY-ENHANCING PSEUDOLESIONS IN LEFT HEPATIC LOBE
1. Aberrant venous drainage: gastric v., cystic v., capsular v.

E. GENERALIZED HETEROGENEOUS
1. Cirrhosis

Dampening Of Hepatic Vein Doppler Waveform

= "portalization" of hepatic vein flow pattern
1. Liver cirrhosis
2. Budd-Chiari syndrome
3. Inferior vena cava obstruction
4. Extrinsic compression of hepatic veins
5. Various parenchymal abnormalities of liver

Aberrant Hepatic Artery

= hepatic artery coursing between IVC + portal vein
1. Replaced right hepatic artery (50%)
2. Right hepatic artery with early bifurcation of common hepatic artery into right + left hepatic arteries (20%)
3. Accessory right hepatic artery (15%)
4. Replacement of entire hepatic trunk to SMA (15%)

LIVER

GALLBLADDER

Nonvisualization Of Gallbladder On OCG

Peak opacification of gallbladder: 14–19 hours (13–35% of dose excreted in urine)

A. EXTRABILIARY CAUSES
1. Failure to ingest contrast
2. Fasting
3. Failure to reach absorptive surface of bowel
   (a) vomiting, nasogastric suction
   (b) esophageal / gastric obstruction
   (c) hiatal, umbilical, inguinal hernias
   (d) Zenker, epiphrenic, gastric, duodenal, jejunal diverticulum
   (e) gastric ulcer, gastrocolic fistula
   (f) malabsorption, diarrhea
   (g) postoperative ileus, severe trauma
   (h) inflammation: acute pancreatitis, acute peritonitis
4. Deficiency of bile salts
   Crohn disease, surgical resection of terminal ileum, liver disease, cholestyramine therapy, abnormal communication between biliary system and gastrointestinal tract

B. INTRINSIC GALLBLADDER DISEASE
1. Cholecystectomy
2. Anomalous position
3. Obstruction of cystic duct
4. Chronic cholecystitis

Oral Cholecystogram (OCG)

Dose: 6 x 0.5 g tablets 2 hours after evening meal

A. PATIENT SELECTION
- bilirubin <5 mg% (not necessary if due to hemolysis)
- ◊ Contraindicated in serious liver disease!
- ◊ Relative contraindications in peritonitis, postoperative ileus, acute pancreatitis!

B. TOXICITY
1. Nausea + vomiting (also noted in 29% on placebo)
2. Immediate anaphylactic response
3. Delayed hypotensive reaction (increased risk in cirrhosis)
4. Renal failure
5. Precipitation of hyperthyroidism

Nonvisualization Of Gallbladder On US

1. Contracted gallbladder
2. Chronic cholecystitis
3. Gallbladder carcinoma
4. Perforation of gallbladder
5. Congenital absence

High-density Bile

1. Hemorrhagic cholecystitis
2. Hemobilia
3. Prior contrast administration
   (a) vicarious excretion of urographic agent
   (b) cholecystopaque
4. Milk of calcium bile

Displaced Gallbladder

A. NORMAL IMPRESSION
by duodenum / colon (positional change)
B. HEPATIC MASS
hepatoma, hemangioma, regenerating nodule, metastases, intrahepatic cyst, polycystic liver, hydatid disease, hepar lobatum (tertiary syphilis), granuloma, abscess
C. EXTRAHEPATIC MASS
1. Retroperitoneal tumor (renal, adrenal)
2. Polycystic kidney
3. Lymphoma
4. Lymph node metastasis to porta hepatis
5. Pancreatic pseudocyst

Alteration In Gallbladder Size

NORMAL MEASUREMENTS
Size: 7–10 cm in length; 2–3.5 cm in width
Capacity: 30–50 mL
Wall thickness: 2–3 mm

Enlarged Gallbladder

= CHOLECYSTOMEGALY
A. OBSTRUCTION
1. Cystic duct obstruction (40%)
(a) Hydrops: chronic cystic duct obstruction + distension with clear sterile mucus (white bile)
(b) Empyema: acute / chronic obstruction with superinfection of bile
2. Cholelithiasis causing obstruction (37%)
3. Cholecystitis with cholelithiasis (11%)
4. Courvoisier phenomenon (10%) = secondary to neoplastic process in pancreas / duodenal papilla / ampulla of Vater / common bile duct
5. Pancreatitis
B. UNOBSTRUCTED (mostly neuropathic)
1. S/P vagotomy
2. Diabetes mellitus
3. Alcoholism
4. Appendicitis (in children)
5. Narcotic analgesia
6. WDHA syndrome
7. Hyperalimentation
8. Acromegaly
9. Kawasaki syndrome
10. Anticholinergics
11. Bedridden patient with prolonged illness
12. AIDS (in 18%)
C. NORMAL (2%)

Small Gallbladder

1. Chronic cholecystitis
2. Cystic fibrosis: in 25% of patients
3. Congenital hypoplasia / multiseptated gallbladder

Diffuse Gallbladder Wall Thickening

= anterior wall of gallbladder >3 mm
A. INTRINSIC
1. Acute cholecystitis
2. Chronic cholecystitis (10–25%)
3. Xanthogranulomatous cholecystitis
4. Hyperplastic cholecystosis (in 91% diffuse)
5. Gallbladder perforation
6. Sepsis
7. Gallbladder carcinoma (in 41% diffuse)
8. AIDS cholangiopathy (average of 9 mm in up to 55%)
9. Sclerosing cholangitis
10. Gallbladder varices
B. EXTRINSIC
1. Hepatitis (in 80%)
2. Hypoalbuminemia
3. Renal failure
4. Right heart failure
5. Systemic venous hypertension
6. Hepatic venous obstruction
7. Ascites
8. Multiple myeloma
9. Portal node lymphatic obstruction
10. Cirrhosis
11. Acute myelogenous leukemia
12. Brucellosis
13. Graft-versus-host disease
C. PHYSIOLOGIC
= contracted gallbladder after eating

Focal Gallbladder Wall Thickening

A. METABOLIC
1. Metachromatic sulfatides
2. Hyperplastic cholecystoses
B. BENIGN TUMOR
1. Adenoma: glandular elements (0.2%)
2. Papilloma: fingerlike projections (0.2%)
3. Villous hyperplasia
4. Fibroadenoma
5. Cystadenoma: ? premalignant
6. Neurinoma, hemangioma
7. Carcinoid tumor
C. MALIGNANT TUMOR
1. Carcinoma of gallbladder: adenocarcinoma / squamous cell carcinoma (in 59% focal)
2. Leiomyosarcoma
3. Metastases: from malignant melanoma (15%), lung, kidney, esophagus, breast, carcinoid, Kaposi sarcoma, lymphoma, leukemia
D. INFLAMMATION / INFECTION
1. Inflammatory polyp: in chronic cholecystitis
2. Parasitic granuloma: Ascaris lumbricoides, Paragonimus westermani, Clonorchis, filariasis, Schistosoma, Fasciola
3. Intramural epithelial cyst / mucinous retention cyst
4. Xanthogranulomatous cholecystitis (in 9% focal)
E. WALL-ADHERENT GALLSTONE = embedded stone
F. HETEROTOPIC MUCOSA
1. Ectopic pancreatic tissue
2. Ectopic gastric glands

3. Ectopic intestinal glands
4. Ectopic hepatic tissue
5. Ectopic prostatic tissue

Fixed Filling Defects In Gallbladder

mnemonic: "PANTS"

Polyp
Adenomyomatosis
Neurinoma
Tumor, primary / secondary
Stone, wall-adherent

Mobile Intraluminal Mass In Gallbladder

1. Tumefactive sludge
2. Blood clot
3. Nonshadowing stone

Comet-tail Artifact In Liver And Gallbladder

A. LIVER
   1. Foreign metallic body (eg, surgical clip)
   2. Intrahepatic calcification
   3. Pneumobilia
   4. Multiple bile duct hamartoma = von Meyenburg complex

B. GALLBLADDER
   1. Rokitansky-Aschoff sinus
   2. Intramural stone
   3. Cholesterolosis of gallbladder

Echogenic Fat In Hepatoduodenal Ligament

= sign of pericholecystic inflammation

1. Cholecystitis
2. Perforated duodenal ulcer
3. Pancreatitis
4. Diverticulitis

BILE DUCTS

Gas In Biliary Tree

mnemonic: "I GET UP"

Incompetent sphincter of Oddi (after sphincterotomy / passage of a gallstone)
Gallstone ileus
Emphysematous cholecystitis (actually in gallbladder)
Trauma
Ulcer (duodenal ulcer perforating into CBD)
Postoperative (eg, cholecystoenterostomy)

Obstructive Jaundice In Adult

Etiology:

A. BENIGN DISEASE (76%)
   1. Traumatic / operative stricture (44%)
   2. Calculi (21%)
   3. Pancreatitis (8%)
   4. Sclerosing cholangitis (1%)
   5. Recurrent pyogenic cholangitis
   6. Parasitic disease (ascariasis)
   7. Liver cysts
   8. Aortic aneurysm

B. MALIGNANCY (24%)
   1. Pancreatic carcinoma (18%)
   2. Ampullary / duodenal carcinoma (8%)
   3. Cholangiocarcinoma (3%)
   4. Metastatic disease (2%)
      from stomach, pancreas, lung, breast, colon, lymphoma

Level and cause of obstruction:

A. INTRAPANCREATIC
   1. Choledocholithiasis
      ◊ Most common cause of biliary obstruction (in 15% of patients with cholelithiasis)!
   2. Chronic pancreatitis
   3. Pancreatic carcinoma

B. SUPRAPANCREATIC (5%)
   = between pancreas + porta hepatis
   1. Cholangiocarcinoma
   2. Metastatic adenopathy

C. PORTA HEPATIS (5%)
   1. Klatskin tumor
   2. Spread from adjacent tumor (GB, liver)
   3. Surgical stricture

D. INTRAHEPATIC
   1. Cystadenoma, cystadenocarcinoma
   2. Mirizzi syndrome
   3. Caroli disease
   4. Cholangitis: recurrent pyogenic ~, sclerosing ~, AIDS cholangitis

Incidence of infected bile in bile duct obstruction:

(a) incomplete / partial obstruction in 64%
(b) complete obstruction in 10%
◊ Infection twice as high with biliary calculi than with malignant obstruction!

Organism: E. coli (21%), Klebsiella (21%), Enterococci (18%), Proteus (15%)

Test Sensitivity For Common Bile Duct Obstruction

1. Intravenous cholangiography
   depends on level of bilirubin: <1 mg/dL in 92%; <2 mg/dL in 82%; <3 mg/dL in 40%; >4 mg/dL in <10%
   False-negative rate: 45%
   Cx: adverse reactions in 4–10%
2. US
   88–90% sensitivity for dilatation of CBD
   ◊ in 27–95% correct level of obstruction determined by US
   ◊ in 23–81% correct cause of obstruction determined by US
   √ CBD >4–8 mm / 10% of patient's age in years
   √ increase in CBD size after fatty meal
   √ "Swiss cheese sign" = abundance of fluid-filled structures on liver sections
   √ intrahepatic "double channel" / "shotgun" sign = two parallel tubular structures composed of portal vein + dilated intrahepatic bile ducts

√ intrahepatic bile duct >2 mm / >40% of adjacent portal vein

False-negative: not dilated in acute obstruction (in 70%), sclerosing cholangitis, intermittent obstruction from choledocholithiasis

False-positive: dilated hepatic artery in cirrhosis / portal hypertension / hepatic neoplasm, patients after cholecystectomy

3. CT
   100% visualization in tumorous obstruction, 60% in nontumorous obstruction
4. NUC
   √ delayed / nonvisualization of biliary system (93% specificity)
   √ vicarious excretion of tracer through kidneys
   DDx: Hepatocellular dysfunction (delayed clearance of cardiac blood pool)

Neonatal Obstructive Jaundice

= severe persistent jaundice in a child beyond 3–4 weeks of age

Cause:

A. INFECTION
   (a) bacterial: E. coli, syphilis, Listeria monocytogenes
   (b) viral: TORCH, hepatitis B, Coxsackie, echovirus, adenovirus
B. METABOLIC
   (a) inherited: alpha-1-antitrypsin deficiency, cystic fibrosis, galactosemia, hereditary tyrosinemia
   (b) acquired: inspissated bile syndrome (= cholestasis due to erythroblastosis); cholestasis due to total parenteral nutrition
C. BILIARY TRACT ABNORMALITIES
   (a) extrahepatic: biliary obstruction / hypoplasia / atresia, choledochal cyst, spontaneous perforation of bile duct, "bile plug" syndrome
   (b) intrahepatic: ductular hypoplasia / atresia
D. IDIOPATHIC NEONATAL HEPATITIS

mnemonic: "CAN"
Choledochal cyst
Atresia
Neonatal hepatitis

NUC–imaging regimen:

(1) Premedication with phenobarbital (5 mg/kg/day) over 5 days to induce hepatic microsomal enzymes which enhance uptake and excretion of certain compounds and increase bile flow
(2) IDA scintigraphy (50 µCi/kg; minimum of 1 mCi)
(3) Imaging at 5-minute intervals for 1 hour + at 2, 4, 6, 8, 24 hours

Large Nonobstructed CBD

1. Passage of stone (return to normal after days to weeks)
2. Common duct surgery (return to normal in 30–50 days)
3. Postcholecystectomy dilatation (in up to 16%)
4. Intestinal hypomotility
5. Normal variant (aging)

Fatty-meal sonography (to differentiate from obstruction with 74% sensitivity, 100% specificity)

Method: peroral Lipomul (1.5 mL/kg) followed by 100 mL of water [cholecystokinin causes contraction of gallbladder, relaxation of sphincter of Oddi, increase in bile secretion], CBD measured before and 45 / 60 minutes after stimulation

√ little change / decrease in size = normal response
√ increase in size >2 mm = partial obstruction

Filling Defect In Bile Ducts

A. ARTIFACT
   1. Pseudocalculus = contracted sphincter of Boyden + Oddi with smooth arcuate contour
   2. Air bubble: confirmed by positional changes
   3. Blood clot: spheroid configuration, spontaneous resolution with time
B. BILIARY CALCULI
C. MIRIZZI SYNDROME
D. NEOPLASM
   1. Cholangiocarcinoma: irregular stricture, intraluminal polypoid mass
   2. Others: ampullary carcinoma, hepatoma, villous tumor, hamartoma, carcinoid, adenoma, papilloma, fibroma, lipoma, neuroma, cystadenoma, granular cell myoblastoma, sarcoma botryoides
E. PARASITES
   1. Ascaris lumbricoides: long linear filling defect / discrete mass if coiled
   2. Liver fluke (Clonorchis sinensis, Fasciola hepatica): intrahepatic epithelial hyperplasia, periductal fibrosis, cholangitis, liver abscess, hepatic duct stones, common duct obstruction
   3. Hydatid cyst: after erosion into biliary tree

Bile Duct Narrowing

A. BENIGN STRICTURE (44%)
   (a) trauma
      1. Postoperative stricture (95–99%) associated with cholecystectomy
      2. Blunt / penetrating trauma
      3. Hepatic artery embolization
      4. Infusion of chemotherapeutic agents
   (b) inflammation
      1. Sclerosing cholangitis
      2. Recurrent pyogenic cholangitis
      3. Acute / chronic pancreatitis
      4. Pancreatic pseudocyst
      5. Perforated duodenal ulcer

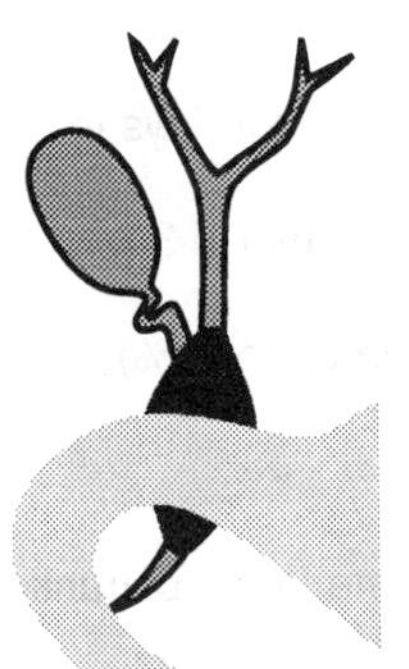
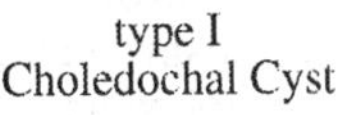
type I
Choledochal Cyst

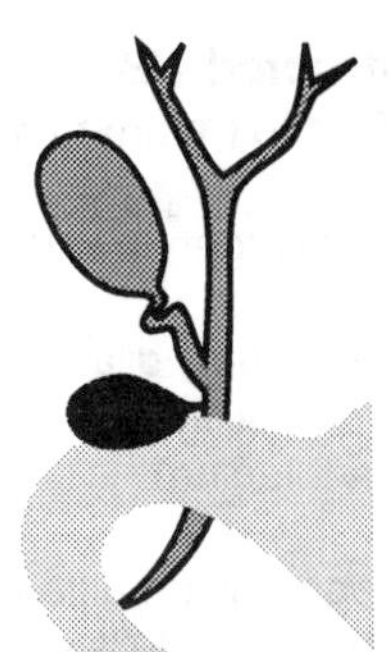
type II
Diverticulum

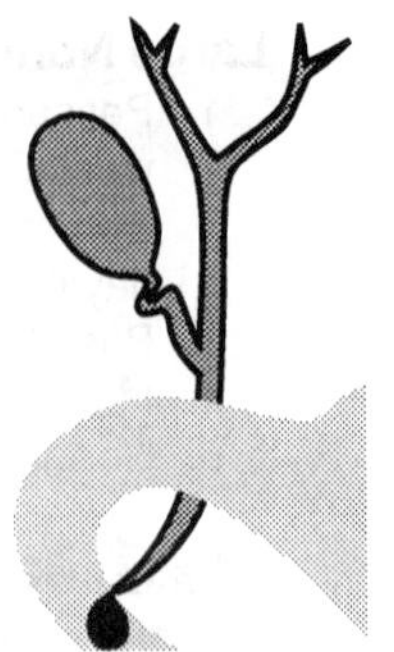
type III
Choledochocele

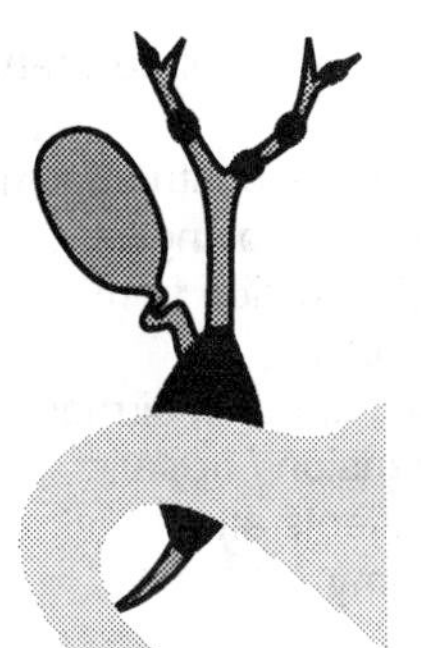
type IVa
saccular dilatation of CBD + intrahepatic ducts

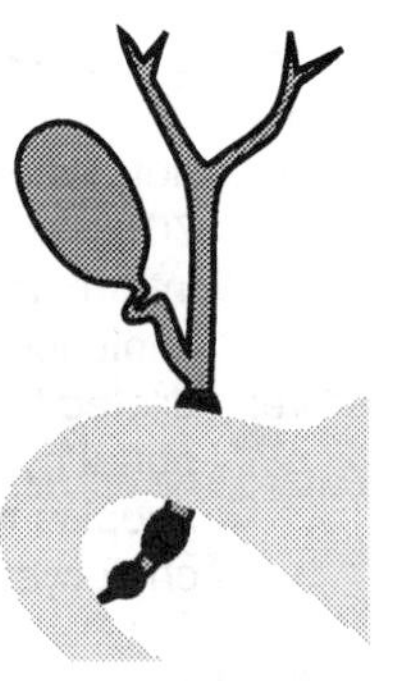
type IVb
saccular dilatation of CBD

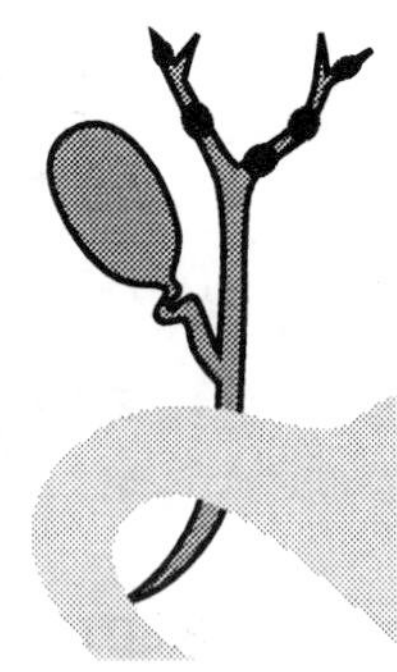
type V
Caroli disease

Classification of Congenital Biliary Cysts

6. Erosion by biliary calculus
7. Gallstones + cholecystitis
8. Abscess
9. Radiation therapy
10. Papillary stenosis

(c) congenital
1. Choledochal cyst

B. MALIGNANT STRICTURE
1. Pancreatic carcinoma
2. Ampullary carcinoma
3. Cholangiocarcinoma
4. Compression by enlarged lymph node

Papillary Stenosis

Etiology:

A. PRIMARY PAPILLARY STENOSIS (10%)
1. Congenital malformation of papilla
2. Sequelae of acute / chronic inflammation
3. Adenomyosis

B. SECONDARY PAPILLARY STENOSIS (90%)
1. Mechanical trauma of stone passage (choledocholithiasis in 64%; cholecystolithiasis in 26%)
2. Functional stenosis: associated with pancreas divisum, history of pancreatitis
3. Reflex spasm
4. Previous surgical manipulation
5. Periampullary neoplasm

√ prestenotic dilatation of CBD
√ increase in pancreatic duct diameter (83%)
√ long smooth narrowing / beak (fibrotic stenosis)
√ prolonged bile-to-bowel transit time >45 minutes on Tc-IDA scintigraphy

Periampullary Tumor

1. Pancreatic carcinoma (85%)
2. Cholangiocarcinoma of distal common bile duct (6%)
3. Ampullary tumor (4%)
4. Duodenal wall tumor
   adenocarcinoma, adenoma, carcinoid, smooth muscle tumor

Double-duct Sign

= dilatation of common bile duct + pancreatic duct
1. Ampullary tumor (most common)
2. Other periampullary tumor
3. Papillary stenosis
4. Stone impacted in ampulla of Vater

Congenital Biliary Cysts

(Todani classification)

I. Common bile duct cyst = choledochal cyst (77–87%)
   a. marked cystic dilatation of CBD + CHD
   b. focal segmental dilatation of CBD distally
   c. cylindric dilatation of CBD + CHD
II. Diverticulum of extrahepatic ducts (1.2–3%) originating from CBD / CHD
III. Choledochocele (1.4–6%)
IV. Multiple segmental cysts
   a. in intra- and extrahepatic ducts (19%)
   b. in extrahepatic ducts only (rare)
V. Intrahepatic cysts = Caroli disease

PANCREAS

Congenital Pancreatic Anomalies

1. Pancreas divisum
2. Annular pancreas
3. Agenesis of dorsal pancreas
   May be associated with:
   abnormal situs, polysplenia, intestinal malrotation

Pancreatic Calcification

1. CHRONIC PANCREATITIS
   Numerous irregular stippled calcifications of varying size; predominantly intraductal
   (a) Alcoholic pancreatitis (in 20–50%):
   √ calcifications limited to head / tail in 25%
   (b) Biliary pancreatitis (in 2%)
   (c) Hereditary pancreatitis (in 35–60%):
   √ round calcifications throughout gland
   (d) Idiopathic pancreatitis
   (e) Pancreatic pseudocyst

2. NEOPLASM
   (a) Microcystic adenoma (in 33%):
      √ "sunburst" appearance of calcifications
   (b) Macrocystic cystadenoma In 15%):
      √ amorphous peripheral calcifications
   (c) Adenocarcinoma (in 2%): with "sunburst" pattern
   (d) Cavernous lymphangioma / hemangioma:
      √ multiple phleboliths
   (e) Metastases from colon cancer
3. INTRAPARENCHYMAL HEMORRHAGE
   (a) Old hematoma / abscess / infarction
   (b) Rupture of intrapancreatic aneurysm
4. HYPERPARATHYROIDISM (in 20%):
   50% of patients develop chronic pancreatitis, concomitant nephrocalcinosis
   ◊ indistinguishable from alcoholic pancreatitis
5. CYSTIC FIBROSIS
   Fine granular calcifications imply advanced pancreatic fibrosis
6. HEMOCHROMATOSIS
7. KWASHIORKOR = tropical pancreatitis:
   ◊ indistinguishable from alcoholic pancreatitis

Fatty Replacement & Atrophy Of Pancreas

1. Main pancreatic duct obstruction
2. Cystic fibrosis
3. Schwachman syndrome
4. Hemochromatosis
5. Viral infection
6. Malnutrition

Pancreatic Mass

A. NEOPLASTIC
   1. Adenocarcinoma
   2. Islet cell tumor
   3. Cystadenoma / -carcinoma
   4. Solid and papillary neoplasm
   5. Lymphoma

B. INFLAMMATORY
   1. Acute pancreatitis
   2. Pseudocyst
   3. Pancreatic abscess

Pancreatic Neoplasm

Origin: — in 99% exocrine ductal epithelium
— in 1% acinar portion of pancreatic glands
— in 0.1% malignant ampullary tumor with better prognosis

A. EXOCRINE NEOPLASM
   (a) Ductal cell origin
      1. Ductal adenocarcinoma (90%)
      2. Ductectatic mucinous tumor
         = mucin-hypersecreting carcinoma
      3. Cystic neoplasm (10–15%)
         — serous microcystic neoplasm
         — mucinous macrocystic neoplasm
      4. Solid and papillary epithelial neoplasm (rare)
      5. Cystic changes of von Hippel-Lindau disease
   (b) Acinar cell origin
      1. Acinar cell carcinoma (1%)
   (c) Indeterminate origin
      1. Pancreaticoblastoma = infantile pancreatic carcinoma

B. ENDOCRINE NEOPLASM
   (a) Nonfunctioning islet cell tumor
   (b) Functioning islet cell tumor
      1. Insulinoma
      2. Glucagonoma
      3. Gastrinoma
      4. Somatostatinoma
      5. VIPoma
      6. "PP-oma" = pancreatic polypeptide
      7. Carcinoid

C. NONEPITHELIAL ORIGIN
   1. Lymphoma
      (a) Primary lymphoma:
         <1% of pancreatic neoplasms
      (b) Secondary lymphoma
         √ large homogeneous solid mass, infrequently with central cystic area
         √ peripancreatic nodal masses
         √ peripancreatic vessels displaced + stretched
   2. Metastases
      renal cell carcinoma, melanoma, lung cancer, breast cancer, ovarian cancer, hepatocellular carcinoma, sarcoma

Hypervascular Pancreatic Tumors

A. PRIMARY
   Islet cell tumor, microcystic adenoma, solid and papillary epithelial neoplasm
B. METASTASES from
   angiosarcoma, leiomyosarcoma, melanoma, carcinoid, renal cell carcinoma, adrenal carcinoma, thyroid carcinoma

Pancreatic Cyst

1. Pseudocyst (85%): secondary to obstructive tumor / trauma / acute pancreatitis (in 2–4%), chronic pancreatitis (in 10–15%) [develop within 10–20 days, consolidated after 6–8 weeks]
2. Congenital cyst (rare)
   (a) solitary
   (b) multiple (when associated with cystic disease of the liver / other organs):
      adult polycystic kidney disease (hepatic cysts in 90% at autopsy); von Hippel-Lindau disease (pancreatic cysts in 72% at autopsy; in only 25% on CT)
3. Acquired cyst:
   (a) retention cyst (= exudate within bursa omentalis)
   (b) parasitic cyst: Echinococcus multilocularis, amebiasis
   (c) **mucinous ductal ectasia** (= obstruction of pancreatic duct as a result of filling with mucus)
      √ massive ductal dilatation
      √ intraluminal filling defects on ERCP

4. Cystic pancreatic neoplasm (5–15%):
   <5% of all pancreatic tumors
   (a) microcystic adenoma = serous cystadenoma
   (b) macrocystic adenoma = mucinous cystic neoplasm
   (c) solid and cystic papillary epithelioid neoplasm
   (d) cystic islet cell tumor (rare)
   (e) Variants of pancreatic ductal adenocarcinoma (rare): mucinous colloid adenocarcinoma = ductectatic mucinous tumor of pancreas = mucin-hypersecreting carcinoma; papillary intraductal adenocarcinoma; adenosquamous carcinoma; anaplastic adenocarcinoma
   (f) pancreatic sarcoma (extremely rare)
5. Cystic metastases (3–12% at autopsy): renal cell carcinoma, melanoma, lung tumors, breast carcinoma, hepatocellular carcinoma, ovarian carcinoma
6. Retroperitoneal lymphangioma / hemangioma

Hyperamylasemia

A. PANCREATIC
   1. Acute / chronic pancreatitis
   2. Pancreatic trauma
   3. Pancreatic carcinoma
B. GASTROINTESTINAL
   1. Perforated peptic ulcer
   2. Intestinal obstruction
   3. Peritonitis
   4. Acute appendicitis
   5. Afferent loop syndrome
   6. Mesenteric ischemia / infarction
   7. Portal vein thrombosis
C. TRAUMA
   1. Burns
   2. Cerebral trauma
   3. Postoperative
D. OBSTETRICAL
   1. Pregnancy
   2. Ruptured ectopic pregnancy
E. RENAL
   1. Transplantation
   2. Renal insufficiency
F. METABOLIC
   1. Diabetic ketoacidosis
   2. Drugs
G. PNEUMONIA
H. SALIVARY GLAND LESION
   1. Facial trauma
   2. Mumps

SPLEEN

Nonvisualization of spleen

1. Asplenia syndrome
2. Polysplenia syndrome
3. Traumatic fragmentation of spleen
4. Wandering spleen

Small spleen

1. Hereditary hypoplasia
2. Irradiation
3. Infarction
4. Polysplenia syndrome
5. Atrophy

Splenomegaly

√ inferior tip of spleen extends below tip of right lobe of liver
√ AP diameter of spleen >2/3 of abdominal diameter

A. CONGESTIVE SPLENOMEGALY
   heart failure, portal hypertension, cirrhosis, cystic fibrosis, portal / splenic vein thrombosis, acute splenic sequestration crisis of sickle cell disease
B. NEOPLASM
   leukemia, lymphoma, metastases, primary neoplasm
C. STORAGE DISEASE
   Gaucher disease, Niemann-Pick disease, gargoylism, amyloidosis, diabetes mellitus, hemochromatosis, histiocytosis
D. INFECTION
   hepatitis, malaria, infectious mononucleosis, kala azar, leishmaniosis, brucellosis, TB, typhoid, syphilis, echinococcosis, subacute bacterial endocarditis
E. HEMOLYTIC ANEMIA
   hemoglobinopathy, hereditary spherocytosis, primary neutropenia, thrombotic thrombocytopenic purpura
F. EXTRAMEDULLARY HEMATOPOIESIS
   osteopetrosis, myelofibrosis
G. COLLAGEN VASCULAR DISEASE
   systemic lupus erythematosus, rheumatoid arthritis, Felty syndrome
H. SPLENIC TRAUMA
I. OTHERS
   1. Sarcoidosis
      √ splenomegaly in up to 60%
      √ inhomogeneous enhancement after bolus injection (multiple 2–3 cm nodular lesions)
      √ necrotic mass with focal calcifications
   2. Hemodialysis

Splenic lesion

mnemonic: "L'CHAIM"

Lymphoma
Cyst
Hematoma
Abscess
Infarct
Metastasis

Solid splenic lesion

A. MALIGNANT TUMOR
   1. Lymphoma (Hodgkin disease, non-Hodgkin lymphoma, primary splenic lymphoma)
      — spleen involved in 70%
      ◊ splenomegaly in non-Hodgkin lymphoma indicates involvement in most patients

LIVER

◊ 30% of patients with splenomegaly have no involvement from non-Hodgkin lymphoma
◊ 30% of patients with lymphoma of any kind have splenic involvement without splenomegaly
√ homogeneous splenomegaly (from diffuse infiltration)
√ miliary nodules
√ large 2–10 cm nodules (10–25%)
√ nodes in splenic hilum (50%) in NHL; uncommon in Hodgkin disease

2. Metastasis (7%)
melanoma (6–34%), breast carcinoma (12–21%), bronchogenic carcinoma (9–18%), colon carcinoma (4%), renal cell carcinoma (3%), ovary (8%), prostate (6%), stomach (7%), pancreas, endometrial cancer
3. Angiosarcoma
4. Malignant fibrous histiocytoma, leiomyosarcoma, fibrosarcoma

B. BENIGN TUMOR
1. Hamartoma = **Splenoma**
√ solid / cystic splenic mass of low attenuation
2. Hemangioma
3. Hematopoietic
4. Sarcoidosis
√ nodular lesions in liver and spleen in 5–15% (= coalescent granulomata) occurring within 5 years of diagnosis
√ hepatosplenomegaly
√ abdominal adenopathy (mean size of 2.6 cm)
5. Gaucher disease (islands of RES cells laden with glucosylceramide)
6. Inflammatory pseudotumor
7. Lymphangioma

C. SPLENIC INFARCTION

Cystic splenic lesion

A. CONGENITAL
1. Epidermoid cyst = true cyst = congenital cyst

B. VASCULAR
1. Splenic laceration / fracture
2. Hematoma
3. **False cyst** = posttraumatic cyst = nonpancreatic pseudocyst of the spleen
◊ 80% of all splenic cysts are pseudocysts (= secondary cysts)
Cause: cystic end stage of old trauma, infection, infarction!
√ internal echoes from debris
√ calcifications within cyst wall may resemble eggshell
√ smaller size than true cyst
4. Cystic degeneration of infarct
(a) occlusion of splenic a. / branches (hemolytic anemia, endocarditis, SLE, arteritides, pancreatic cancer)
(b) venous thrombosis of splenic sinusoids (massive splenomegaly)
5. Peliosis
Associated with:
Hodgkin disease, myeloma, disseminated cancer, TB, anabolic + contraceptive steroids, thorium dioxide injection, viral infection

C. INFECTION / INFLAMMATION
1. Pyogenic abscess
Prevalence: 0.1–0.7%
Cause: hematogenous spread (75%), penetrating trauma (15%), infarction (10%)
Predisposed: endocarditis, drug abuse, penetrating trauma, neoplasm, sickle cell disease
• fever, chills, LUQ pain (in <50%)
√ irregular borders without capsule
√ gas within abscess
Rx: 76% success rate for percutaneous drain
2. Microabscesses
Organism: fungus (especially Candida, Aspergillus, Cryptococcus)
Prevalence: 26% of splenic abscesses
Predisposed: immunocompromised patient
√ splenomegaly
√ multiple hypoattenuating "target" lesions of 5–10 mm often associated with hepatic + renal involvement
3. Granulomatous infection
(a) Mycobacterium tuberculosis: miliary TB
√ mild splenomegaly uncommon
(b) M. avium-intracellulare
√ marked splenomegaly in 20%
4. Pneumocystis carinii infection
√ splenomegaly + multiple hypoattenuating foci
5. Parasitic cyst (Echinococcus)
Prevalence: in <2% of patients with hydatid disease
6. Pancreatic pseudocyst
Prevalence: in 1.1–5% of patients with pancreatitis

D. CYSTIC NEOPLASM
1. Cavernous hemangioma
◊ Most common primary neoplasm of the spleen!
2. Lymphangioma / lymphangiomatosis
3. Lymphoma (most common malignant neoplasm!)
4. Necrotic metastasis:
◊ In 7% of patients with widespread metastasis!
malignant melanoma (in 50%); breast, lung, ovarian, pancreatic, endometrial, colonic, prostatic, carcinoma; chondrosarcoma

Increased splenic density

1. Sickle cell anemia (in 5% of sicklers)
2. Hemochromatosis
3. Thorotrast exposure
4. Lymphangiography

Splenic calcification

A. DISSEMINATED
   1. Phlebolith: visceral angiomatosis
   2. Granuloma (most common): histoplasmosis, TB, brucellosis
B. CAPSULAR & PARENCHYMAL
   1. Pyogenic / tuberculous abscess
   2. Pneumocystis carinii infection
   2. Infarction (multiple)
   3. Hematoma
C. VASCULAR
   1. Splenic artery calcification
   2. Splenic artery aneurysm
   3. Splenic infarct
D. CALCIFIED CYST WALL
   1. Congenital cyst
   2. Posttraumatic cyst
   3. Echinococcal cyst
   4. Cystic dermoid
   5. Epidermoid

mnemonic: "HITCH"
- **H**istoplasmosis (most common)
- **I**nfarct (sickle cell disease)
- **T**uberculosis
- **C**yst (Echinococcus)
- **H**ematoma

Iron accumulation

A. DIFFUSE
   1. Multiple blood transfusions
   2. Sickle cell anemia
B. FOCAL
   1. Gamna Gandy bodies
   2. Angiosarcoma

Hyperechoic splenic spots

1. Granulomas: miliary tuberculosis, histoplasmosis
2. Phleboliths
3. Lymphoma / leukemia
4. Myelofibrosis
5. Gamna-Gandy nodules (in portal hypertension)

ANATOMY OF LIVER, BILE DUCTS, AND PANCREAS

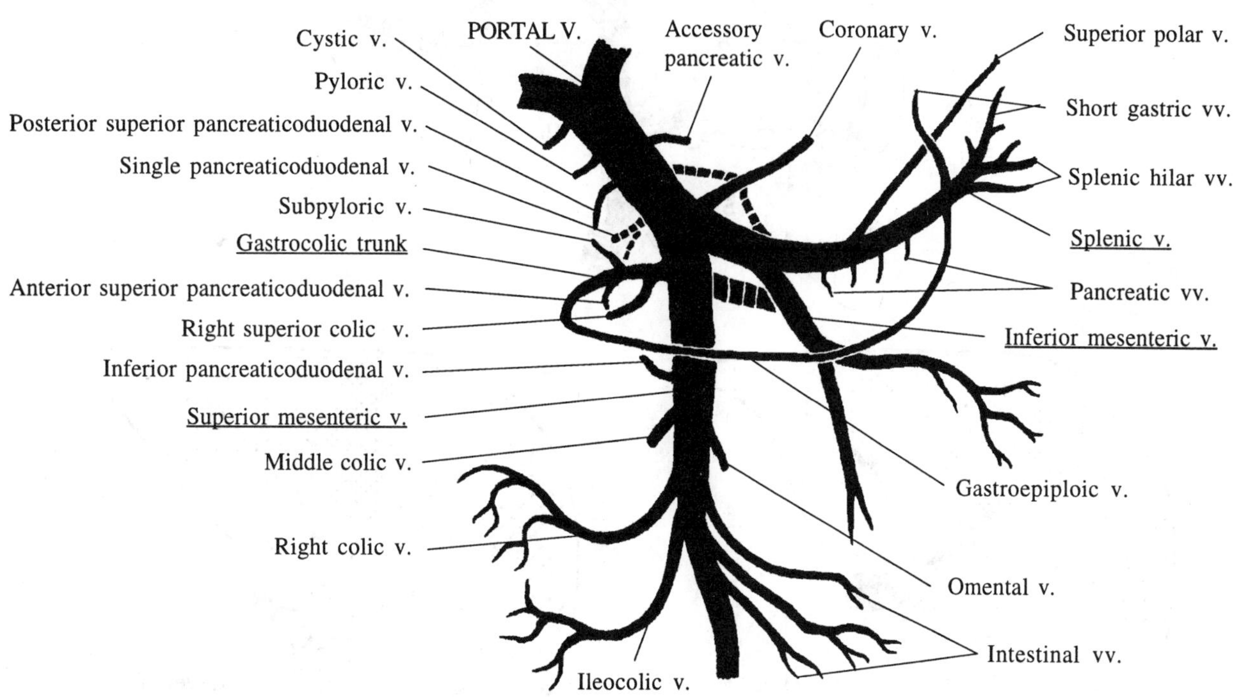

Extrahepatic Portal Vein Tributaries

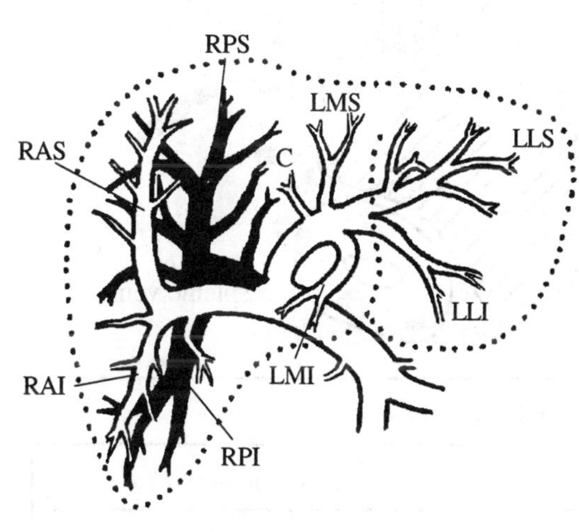

Intrahepatic Portal Vein Branches

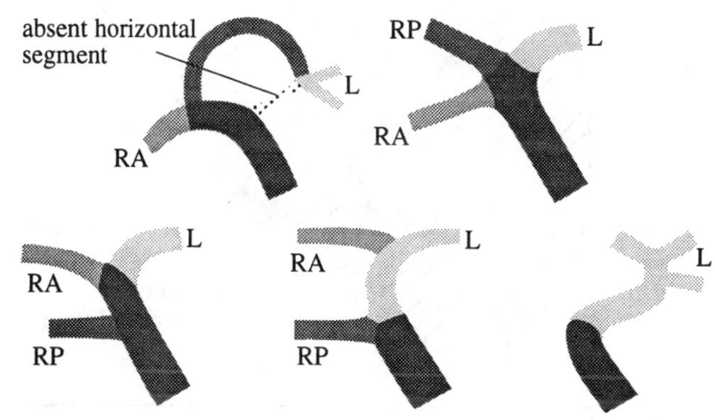

Variations of Intrahepatic Portal Venous System (20%)

A. LEFT PORTAL VEIN
   1. Absence of horizontal segment (0.2%)
B. RIGHT PORTAL VEIN
   1. Trifurcation of main portal vein (11%)
   2. Origin of RP segment from main portal vein (5%)
   3. Origin of RA segment from left portal vein (4%)
   4. Absence of main right, RA, and RP portal segments

RA = right anterior segment
RAI = right anterior inferior
RAS = right anterior superior
RP = right posterior segment
RPI = right posterior inferior
RPS = right posterior superior
C = caudate lobe
L = left portal vein
LMI = left median inferior
LMS = left median superior
LLI = left lateral inferior
LLS = left lateral superior

LIVER

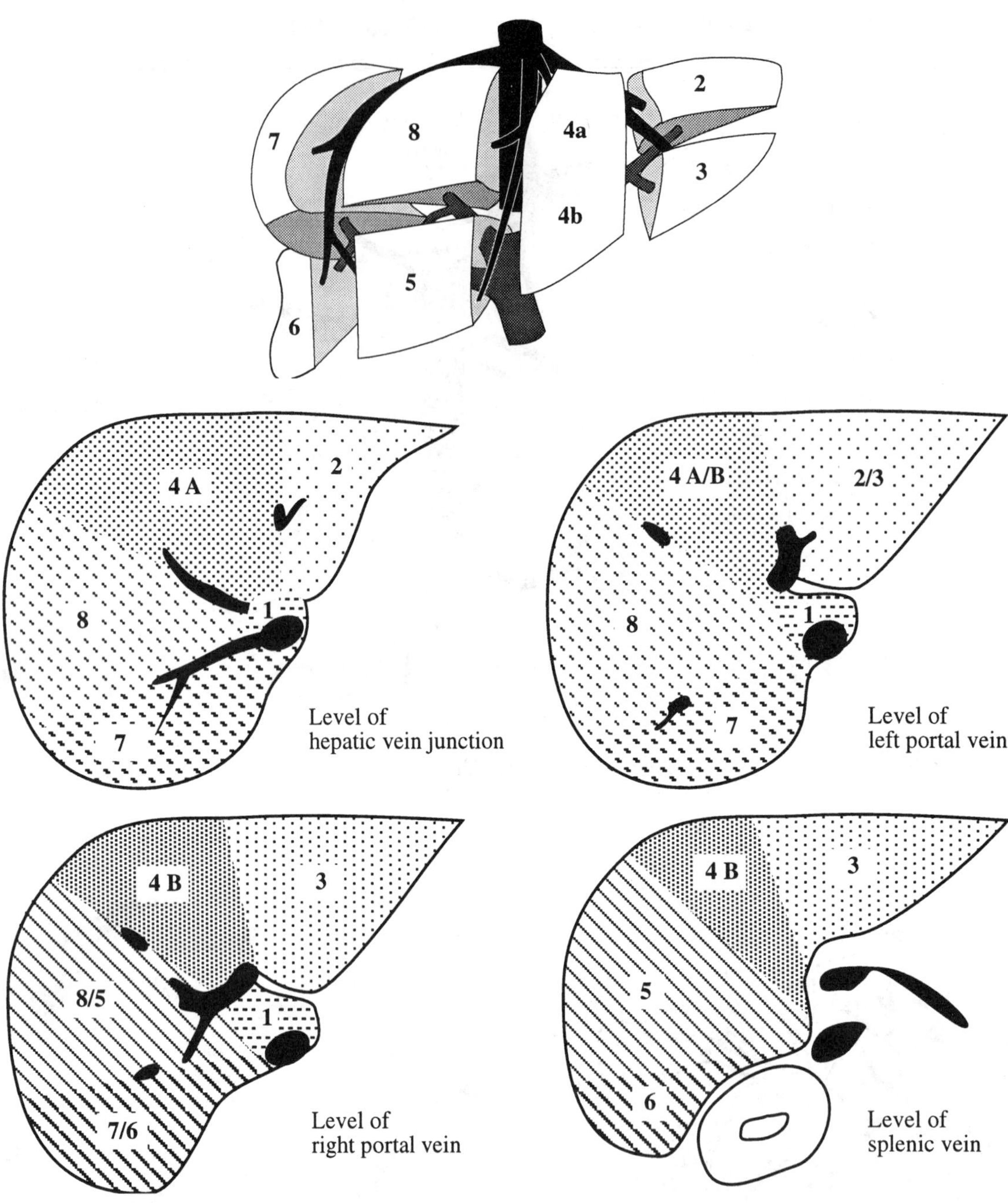

<table>
<tr><th colspan="3">Functional Segmental Liver Anatomy</th></tr>
<tr><th colspan="2">(Goldsmith & Woodburne)</th><th colspan="2">(Couinaud & Bismuth)</th></tr>
<tr><td>CAUDATE LOBE</td><td></td><td></td><td>1</td></tr>
<tr><td>LEFT LOBE</td><td>Left lateral segment</td><td>Left lateral superior subsegment</td><td>2</td></tr>
<tr><td></td><td></td><td>Left lateral inferior subsegment</td><td>3</td></tr>
<tr><td></td><td>Left medial segment</td><td>Left medial superior subsegment</td><td>4 a</td></tr>
<tr><td></td><td></td><td>Left medial inferior subsegment</td><td>4 b</td></tr>
<tr><td>RIGHT LOBE</td><td>Right anterior segment</td><td>Right anterior inferior subsegment</td><td>5</td></tr>
<tr><td></td><td></td><td>Right anterior superior subsegment</td><td>8</td></tr>
<tr><td></td><td>Right posterior segment</td><td>Right posterior inferior subsegment</td><td>6</td></tr>
<tr><td></td><td></td><td>Right posterior superior subsegment</td><td>7</td></tr>
</table>

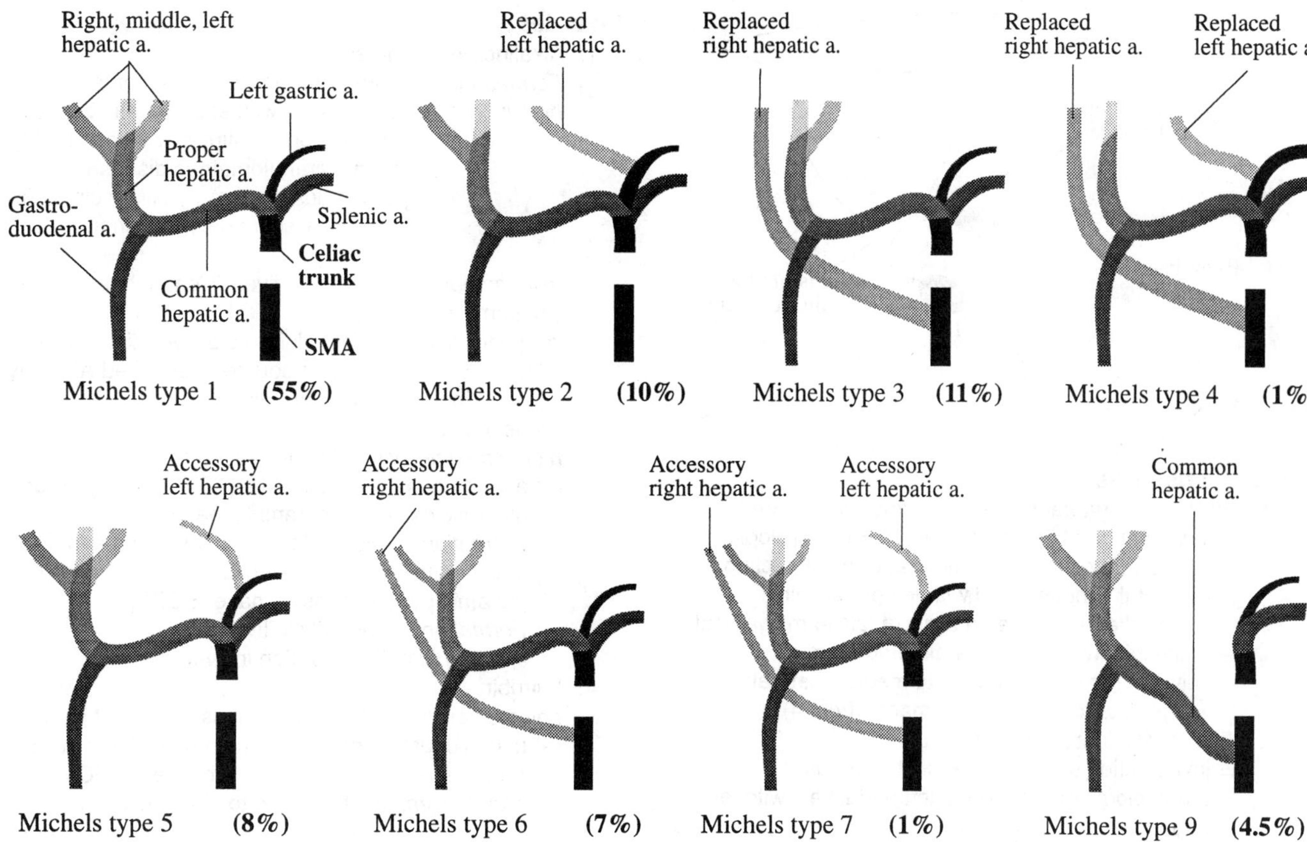

Functional Segmental Liver Anatomy

based on distribution of 3 major hepatic veins:

(a) middle hepatic vein
divides liver into right and left lobe
also separated by main portal vein scissura (Cantlie line) passing through IVC + long axis of gallbladder)

(b) left hepatic vein
divides left lobe into medial + lateral sectors

(c) right hepatic vein
divides right lobe into medial + lateral sectors

Each of the four sections is further divided by an imaginary transverse line drawn through the right + left portal vein into anterior + posterior segments; the segments are numbered counterclockwise from IVC

Hepatic arterial anatomy (Michels classification)

Type I (55%):
- celiac trunk trifurcates into LT gastric a. + splenic a. + common hep. a.
- common hep. a. divides into gastroduodenal a. + proper hep. a.
- RT hep. a. + LT hep. a. arise from proper hep. a.
- middle hep. a. (supplying caudate lobe) arises from
  (a) LT / RT hep. a.
  (b) proper hep. a. (in 10%)

Type II (10%):
- common hep. a. divides into gastroduodenal + RT hep. a.
- LT hep. a. replaced to LT gastric a.
- middle hep. a. from RT hep. a.

Type III (11%):
- common hep. a. divides into gastroduodenal + LT hep. a.
- RT hep. a. replaced to superior mesenteric a.
- middle hep. a. from LT hep. a.

Type IV (1%):
- common hep. a. divides into middle hep. a. + gastroduodenal a.
- RT hep. a. + LT hep. a. are both replaced

Type V (8%):
- accessory LT hep. a. arises from LT gastric a.

Type VI (7%):
- accessory RT hep. a. arises from superior mesenteric a.

Type VII (1%):
- accessory RT + LT hepatic a.

Type VIII (2%):
- combinations of accessory + replaced hepatic aa.

Type IX (4.5%):
- hepatic trunk replaced to superior mesenteric a.

Type X (0.5%):
- hepatic trunk replaced to LT gastric a.

LIVER

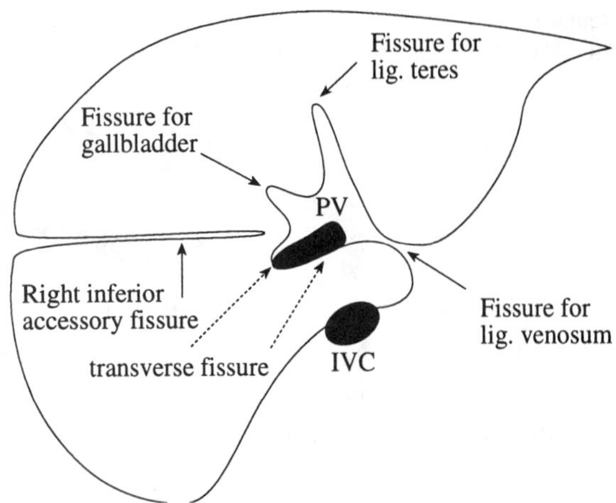

Hepatic fissures

1. Fissure for ligamentum teres = umbilical fissure
   = invagination of ligamentum teres = embryologic remnant of obliterated umbilical vein connecting placental venous blood with left portal vein
   — located at dorsal free margin of falciform ligament
   — runs into liver with visceral peritoneum
   — divides left hepatic lobe into medial + lateral segments (divides subsegment 3 from 4)
2. Fissure for ligamentum venosum
   = invagination of obliterated ductus venosus
   = embryologic connection of left portal vein with left hepatic vein
   — separates caudate lobe from left lobe of liver
   — lesser omentum within fissure separates the greater sac anteriorly from lesser sac posteriorly
3. Fissure for gallbladder
   = shallow peritoneal invagination containing the gallbladder
   — divides right from left lobe of liver
4. Transverse fissure
   = invagination of hepatic pedicle into liver
   — contains horizontal portion of left + right portal veins
5. Accessory fissures
   (a) Right inferior accessory fissure
   = from gallbladder fossa / just inferior to it to lateroinferior margin of liver
   (b) others (rare)

Normal size of liver

Sonographic measurements along vertical (craniocaudad) axis:

(a) midclavicular line
- <13 cm = normal
- 13.0–15.5 cm = indeterminate (in 25% of patients)
- >15.5 cm = hepatomegaly (87% accuracy)

(b) preaortic line >10 cm
(c) prerenal line >14 cm

Normal hemodynamics parameter of liver

Portal vein velocity: >11 cm/sec
Congestion index (= cross-sectional area of portal vein divided by average velocity): 0.070 ± 0.09
Hepatic artery resistive index: 0.60–0.64 ± 0.06

Liver tests

1. Alkaline phosphatase (AP)
   Formation: bone, liver, intestine, placenta
   high increase: cholestasis with extrahepatic biliary obstruction (confirmed by rise in γGT), drugs, granulomatous disease (sarcoidosis), primary biliary cirrhosis, primary + secondary malignancy of liver
   mild increase: all forms of liver disease, heart failure
2. γ-glutamyl transpeptidase (GGT)
   very sensitive in almost all forms of liver disease
   Utility: confirms hepatic source of elevated AP, may indicate significant alcohol use
3. Transaminases
   high increase: viral / toxin-induced acute hepatitis
   (a) aspartate aminotransferase (AST; formerly serum glutamic oxaloacetic transaminase [SGOT])
   Formation: liver, muscle, kidney, pancreas, RBCs
   (b) alanine aminotransferase (ALT; formerly serum glutamic pyruvic transaminase [SGPT])
   Formation: primarily in liver
   • rather specific elevation in liver disease
4. Bilirubin
   helps differentiate between various causes of jaundice
   (a) unconjugated / indirect bilirubin = insoluble in water
   Formation: breakdown of senescent RBCs
   Metabolism: tightly bound to albumin in vessels, actively taken up by liver, cannot be excreted by kidneys
   (b) conjugated / direct bilirubin = water-soluble
   Formation: conjugation in liver cells
   Metabolism: excretion into bile; not reabsorbed by intestinal mucosa + excreted in feces
   Elevation:
   - overproduction: hemolytic anemia, resorption of hematoma, multiple transfusions
   - decreased hepatic uptake: drugs, sepsis
   - decreased conjugation: Gilbert syndrome, neonatal jaundice, hepatitis, cirrhosis, sepsis
   - decreased excretion into bile: hepatitis, cirrhosis, drug-induced cholestasis, sepsis, extrahepatic biliary obstruction
5. Lactic dehydrogenase (LDH)
   nonspecific and therefore not helpful
   high increase: primary or metastatic liver involvement
6. Alpha fetoprotein (AFP)
   >400 ng/mL strongly suggests that focal mass represents a hepatocellular carcinoma

Normal size of bile ducts

@ CBD at point of maximum diameter:
≤5 mm = normal; 6–7 mm = equivocal;
≥8 mm = dilated
@ CHD at porta hepatis + CBD in head of pancreas: 5 mm
@ right intrahepatic duct just proximal to CHD: 2–3mm

@ CHD at porta hepatis + CBD in head of pancreas: 5 mm
@ right intrahepatic duct just proximal to CHD: 2–3mm
@ Cystic duct diameter: 1.8 mm
average length of 1–2 cm
distal cystic duct posterior to CBD (in 95%), anterior to CBD (in 5%)

Bile Duct Variants

Incidence: 2.4% of autopsies;
13% of operative cholangiograms

A. ABERRANT INTRAHEPATIC DUCT
may join CHD, CBD, cystic duct, right hepatic duct, gallbladder
— anomalous right hepatic duct entering CHD / cystic duct (4–5%)
Cx: (1) postoperative bile leak if severed
(2) segmental biliary obstruction if ligated

B. CYSTIC DUCT ENTERING RIGHT HEPATIC DUCT

C. DUCTS OF LUSCHKA
= small ducts from hepatic bed draining directly into gallbladder

D. DUPLICATION OF CYSTIC DUCT / CBD

E. CONGENITAL TRACHEOBILIARY FISTULA
= fistulous communication between carina and left hepatic duct
• infants with respiratory distress
• productive cough with bilious sputum
√ pneumobilia

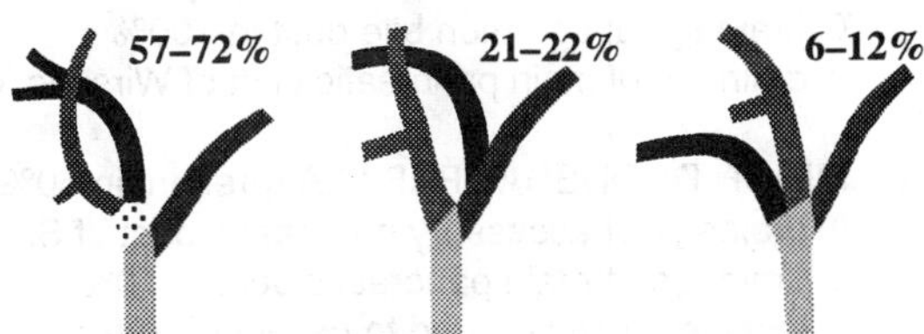

Bile Duct Variants

right posterior segmental duct
right anterior segmental duct
common hepatic duct
right hepatic duct
left hepatic duct

Pancreaticobiliary Junction Variants

A. Angle between CBD + pancreatic duct:
(a) usually acute at 5°–30°
(b) occasionally abnormal at up to 90°

B. Sphincter of Oddi
= muscle fibers encircling the CBD + pancreatic duct at choledochoduodenal junction
(a) choledochal sphincter = encircles distal CBD
(b) pancreatic duct sphincter (in 33% separate)

C. Types of union between CBD + pancreatic duct:
(a) 2–10 (mean 5) mm short common channel (85%) with a diameter of 3–5 mm
(b) separate entrances into duodenum
(c) 8–15 mm long common channel
(d) pancreatic duct inserting into CBD >15 mm from entrance into duodenum
(e) CBD inserting into pancreatic duct

CONGENITAL GALLBLADDER ANOMALIES

Agenesis Of Gallbladder

Incidence: 0.04 - 0.07 % (autopsy)
Associated with:
common: rectovaginal fistula, imperforate anus, hypoplasia of scapula + radius, intracardiac shunt
rare: absence of corpus callosum, microcephaly, atresia of external auditory canal, tricuspid atresia, TE fistula, dextroposition of pancreas + esophagus, absent spleen, high position of cecum, polycystic kidney

Hypoplastic Gallbladder

(a) congenital
(b) associated with cystic fibrosis

Septations Of Gallbladder

A. LONGITUDINAL SEPTA
1. Duplication of gallbladder
= two separate lumens + two cystic ducts
Incidence: 1:3,000 to 1:12,000
2. Bifid gallbladder = double gallbladder
= two separate lumens with one cystic duct
3. Triple gallbladder (extremely rare)

B. TRANSVERSE SEPTA
1. Isolated transverse septum
2. PHRYGIAN CAP (2–6% of population)
= kinking / folding of fundus ± septum
3. Multiseptated gallbladder (rare)
= multiple cystlike compartments connected by small pores
Cx: stasis + stone formation

C. GALLBLADDER DIVERTICULUM
= persistence of cystohepatic duct

Gallbladder Ectopia

Most frequent locations:
(1) beneath the left lobe of the liver > (2) intrahepatic > (3) retrohepatic
Rare locations:
(4) within falciform ligament (5) within interlobar fissure (6) suprahepatic (lodged between superior surface of right hepatic lobe + anterior chest wall) (7) within anterior abdominal wall (8) transverse mesocolon (9) retrorenal (10) near posterior spine + IVC (11) intrathoracic GB (inversion of liver)
Associated with: eventration of diaphragm

"Floating GB"
= gallbladder with loose peritoneal reflections, may herniate through foramen of Winslow into lesser sac

"Torqued GB"
= results in hydrops

PANCREAS

Pancreatic Development & Anatomy

A. DORSAL ANLAGE (in mesoduodenum)
Origin: arises from dorsal wall of duodenum
◊ forms cranial portion of head + isthmus + body + tail of pancreas

LIVER

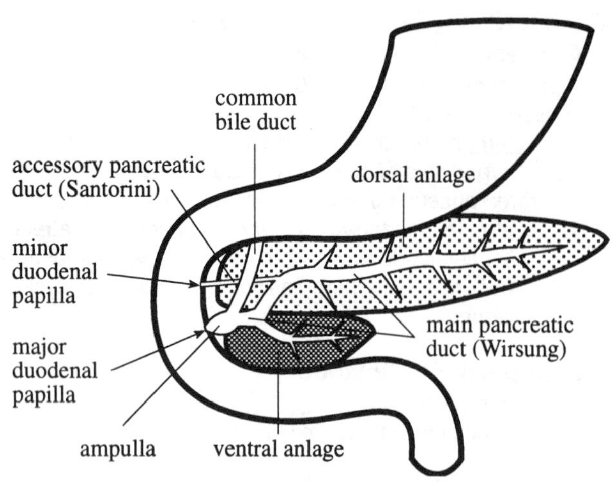

Anatomy of Pancreatic Ducts

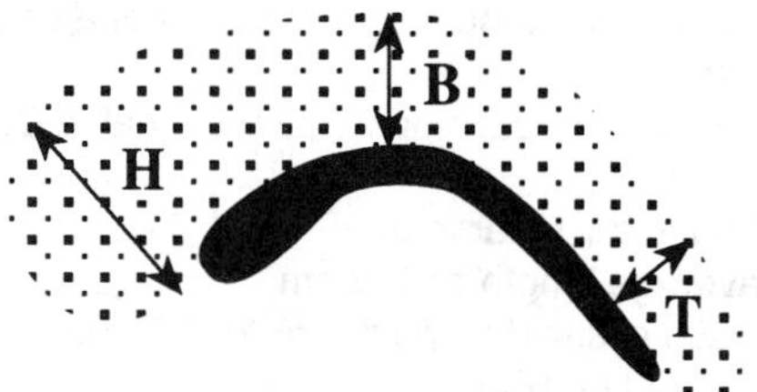

Pancreatic diameters (on TRV image)

H	=	head	=	1.5 – 3.0 cm
B	=	body	=	1.2 – 2.5 cm
T	=	tail	=	1.0 – 2.5 cm

– prone to atrophy (poor in polypeptides)
√ drains to the minor papilla through accessory duct of Santorini

B. VENTRAL ANLAGE (below primordial liver bud)
Origin: ventral bud arises from ventral wall of duodenum and is composed of right + left lobes (the left ventral bud regresses completely), migrates to opposite side of duodenum + fuses with dorsal anlage during 6th week GA
◊ forms caudal portion of the pancreatic head + uncinate process + CBD
– not prone to atrophy (rich in polypeptides)
√ the ventral duct of Wirsung drains with the CBD through ampulla of Vater and becomes the major drainage pathway for the entire pancreas after fusion with the duct of Santorini

C. MAIN PANCREATIC DUCT OF WIRSUNG
distal portion of dorsal duct connects with ventral duct; proximal portion of dorsal duct may disappear

D. ACCESSORY PANCREATIC DUCT OF SANTORINI
= proximal portion of dorsal duct which has not atrophied

E. AMPULLA OF VATER
= space within medial wall of second portion of duodenum below surface of papilla of Vater

F. MAJOR DUODENAL PAPILLA = papilla of Vater
◊ drainage of common bile duct in 100%
◊ drainage of main pancreatic duct of Wirsung in 90%

G. MINOR DUODENAL PAPILLA (present in 60%)
◊ drainage of accessory pancreatic duct of Santorini
◊ drainage of main pancreatic duct in 10%
√ located a few cm orad to papilla of Vater

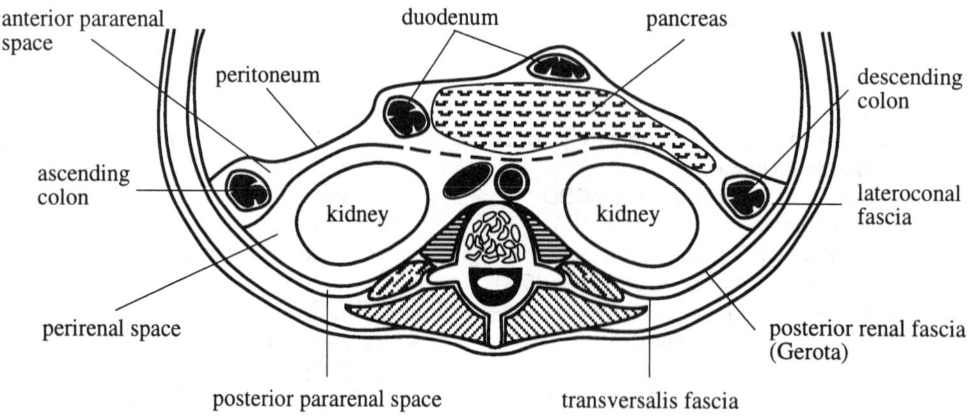

Extraperitoneal Spaces

SPLEEN

A. NORMAL SIZE
   in adults : 12 cm length, 7–8 cm anteroposterior diameter, 3–4 cm thick; splenic index (LxWxH) of <480
   in children : formula for length = 5.7 + 0.31 x age (in years)

B. NORMAL WEIGHT 150 (100–265) g
   estimated weight = splenic index x 0.55

C. CT ATTENUATION
   (a) without enhancement:
      40–60 HU; 5–10 HU less than liver
   (b) with enhancement:
      normal heterogeneous enhancement during parenchymal phase after bolus injection (due to varying blood flow rates through the cords of the red pulp)

D. MR SIGNAL INTENSITY
   (a) on T1WI : liver > spleen > muscle
   (b) on T2WI : spleen > liver

IRON METABOLISM

Total body iron: 5 g
  (a) functional iron: 4 g
     Location: hemoglobin of RBCs, myoglobin of muscle, various enzymes
  (b) stored iron: 1 g
     Location: hepatocytes, reticuloendothelial cells of liver (Kupffer cells) + spleen + bone marrow

Absorption: 1–2 mg/day through gut
Transport: bound to transferrin intravascularly

Deposition:
  (a) transferrin-transfer to:
     hepatocytes, RBC precursors in erythron, parenchymal tissues (eg, muscle)
  (b) phagocytosis by:
     reticuloendothelial cells phagocytize senescent erythrocytes (= extravascular hemolysis); RBC iron stored as ferritin / released and bound to transferrin

DISORDERS OF LIVER, BILIARY TRACT, PANCREAS, AND SPLEEN

ACCESSORY SPLEEN

= failure of coalescence of several small mesodermal buds in the dorsal mesogastrium which comprise the spleen

Incidence: 10–30% of population; multiple in 10%

◊ undergoes hypertrophy after splenectomy and is responsible for recurrence of hematologic disorders (idiopathic thrombocytopenic purpura, hereditary spherocytosis, acquired autoimmune hemolytic anemia, hypersplenism)

Location: splenic hilum (most common), gastrosplenic ligament, other suspensory ligaments of spleen, rare in pancreas / pelvis

NUC (Tc-99m sulfur colloid scan / spleen-specific Tc-99m denatured RBCs):
- √ usually <1 cm in diameter
- √ <10% identified when normal spleen present

AMPULLARY TUMOR

= benign / malignant tumors arising from glandular epithelium of ampulla of Vater

Age: 6th + 7th decade; M:F = 2:1

Path: average diameter of <3 cm

Histo: (a) dysplastic epithelium in glandular / villous structures of tubular / villous adenoma
(b) carcinoma in situ
(c) invasive carcinoma often with desmoplastic reaction

Associated with: familial adenomatous polyposis syndromes (eg, familial polyposis coli, Gardner syndrome) [100–200-fold risk], colon carcinoma

- malaise, epigastric pain, weight loss
- intestinal bleeding (tumor ulceration)
- intermittent jaundice (ductal obstruction)
- gray "aluminum / silver colored" stools (3%)
- chills, fever, RUQ pain (ascending cholangitis) in up to 20%
- endoscopy: tumor extending through orifice (63%), prominent papilla / submucosal mass (25%), not visualized (9%)

TNM staging:
- T1 : tumor confined to ampulla
- T2 : tumor extending into duodenal wall
- T3 : invasion of pancreas <2 cm deep
- T4 : invasion of pancreas >2 cm deep

International Union against Cancer staging:
- I = tumor confined to ampulla
- II = tumor extension into duodenal wall / pancreas
- III = regional lymph node involvement (Lnn stations around head + body of pancreas, anterior + posterior pancreaticoduodenal, pyloric, common bile duct, proximal mesenteric)
- IV = invasion of pancreas >2 cm deep

√ tumor often inapparent due to small size

UGI:
- √ indentation of duodenal lumen at papilla of Vater with filling defect >1.5 cm
- √ surface irregularity + deep barium-filled crevices in villous tumor

Biliary imaging:
- √ dilatation of most distal segment of common bile duct
- √ stenosis (circumferential tumor growth around ampulla / desmoplastic reaction)
- √ irregular predominantly polypoid filling defect
- √ ± pancreatic dilatation = double-duct sign (may be absent if tumor small / accessory pancreatic duct decompresses pancreatic system / main pancreatic duct drains into minor papilla)

Endoscopic US (most sensitive technique):
87% staging accuracy

Rx: Whipple procedure (= pancreaticoduodenectomy)

Prognosis: 28–70% 5-year survival for ampullary carcinomas (depending on stage)

DDx:
1. Periampullary duodenal adenoma / adenocarcinoma (usually larger lesion with significant intraduodenal extension)
2. Choledochocele (cystic lesion filling with biliary contrast)
3. Brunner gland tumor, pancreatic rest ("myoepithelial hamartoma"), leiomyoma, carcinoid (often produce somatostatin)
4. Duodenitis, pancreatitis
5. Stone impaction in ampulla

ANNULAR PANCREAS

= uncommon congenital anomaly wherein a ring of normal pancreatic tissue encircles the duodenum secondary to abnormal migration of ventral pancreas (head + uncinate); most common congenital anomaly of pancreas

Age at discovery: childhood (50%); adulthood (50%)

Associated with: other congenital anomalies (in 75%): esophageal atresia, TE fistula, duodenal atresia / stenosis, duodenal diaphragm, imperforate anus, malrotation, Down syndrome

Location: 2nd portion of duodenum (85%); 1st / 3rd portion of duodenum (15%)

- mostly asymptomatic with incidental discovery
- neonate: persistent vomiting (duodenal obstruction)
- adult : nausea, vomiting (60%), abdominal pain (70%), hematemesis (10%), jaundice (50%)

√ polyhydramnios (in utero)
√ "double bubble" = dilated duodenal bulb + stomach
√ enlargement of pancreatic head

UGI:
- √ eccentric narrowing with lateral notching + medial retraction of 2nd part of duodenum
- √ concentric narrowing of mid-descending duodenum

√ reverse peristalsis, pyloric incompetency
ERCP (most specific):
√ normally located main duct in pancreatic body + tail
√ small duct originating on anterior left + passing posteriorly around duodenum communicates with main duct (in 85%)
Cx: increased incidence of
(1) periampullary peptic ulcers
(2) pancreatitis (15–20%) usually confined to pancreatic head and annulus
Rx: gastrojejunostomy / duodenojejunostomy

ASCARIASIS

Most frequent helminthic infection in humans
Organism: Ascaris lumbricoides, 25–35 cm long as adult worm; life span of 1 year
Country: 644 million humans harbor the roundworm; 70– 90% in America; in United States endemic in: Appalachian range, southern + Gulf coast states
Prevalence: 25% of world population infected
(a) in United States: 12% in blacks, 1% in whites
(b) in parts of Africa, Asia, South America: 90%
Cycle:
ingestion of contaminated water / soil / vegetable; larvae penetrate intestinal wall; migrate into mesenteric lymphatics + veins into liver; reach lung via right heart + pulmonary artery; mature in pulmonary capillary bed to 2–3 mm length; burrow into alveoli; ascend in respiratory tract; are swallowed and again reach small intestine, where they become adult worms whose eggs leave the body by the fecal route

- abnormal liver function tests + biliary colic
- hypereosinophilia only present during acute stage of larval migration

√ barium study
√ cholangiography (49%)
US:
√ tubular echogenic filling defect with 2–4 mm wide central sonolucent line (= worm with digestive tract) within dilated common bile duct
Cx: (1) Intestinal obstruction
(2) Intermittent biliary obstruction with acute cholangitis, cholecystitis, pancreatitis
(3) Liver abscess (rare)
(4) Granulomatous stricture of extrahepatic bile ducts (rare)
Rx: Mebendazole

BANTI SYNDROME

= NONCIRRHOTIC IDIOPATHIC PORTAL HYPERTENSION = NONCIRRHOTIC PORTAL FIBROSIS = HEPATOPORTAL SCLEROSIS
= syndrome characterized by (1) splenomegaly (2) hypersplenism (3) portal hypertension
Etiology: increased portal vascular resistance possibly due to portal fibrosis + obliterative venopathy of intrahepatic portal branches
Histo: slight portal fibrosis, dilatation of sinusoids, intimal thickening with eccentric sclerosis of peripheral portal vein walls
Age: middle-aged women; rare in America + Europe but common in India + Japan

- elevated portal vein pressure (without cirrhosis, parasites, venous occlusion)
- normal liver function tests
- cytopenia (due to hypersplenism)
- normal / slightly elevated hepatic venous wedge pressure

√ esophageal varices
√ patent hepatic veins
√ patent extrahepatic portal vein + multiple collaterals
Prognosis: 90% 5-year survival; 55% 30-year survival

BILIARY CYSTADENOCARCINOMA

= BILE DUCT CYSTADENOCARCINOMA
= rare malignant multilocular cystic tumor originating from biliary cystadenoma
Histo: (a) with ovarian stroma (good prognosis), in females only
(b) without ovarian stroma (bad prognosis)

- hemorrhagic internal fluid

√ nodularity with septations are suggestive of malignancy
√ coarse calcifications
DDx: no image differentiation from biliary cystadenoma

BILIARY CYSTADENOMA

= BILE DUCT CYSTADENOMA
= rare benign premalignant multilocular cystic tumor originating in bile ducts; probably deriving from ectopic nests of primitive biliary tissue
Incidence: 4.6% of all intrahepatic cysts of bile duct origin
Age: >30 years (82%), peak incidence in 5th decade; M:F = 1:4; predominantly Caucasian
Path: multiloculated cystic tumor with well-defined thick capsule containing proteinaceous fluid
Histo: single layer of cuboidal / tall columnar biliary-type epithelium with papillary projections, subepithelial stroma resembling that of the ovary
◊ Similar to mucinous cystic tumors of pancreas + ovary
Location: intrahepatic bile ducts (85%); extrahepatic bile ducts (15%); right lobe (48%); left lobe (20–35%); both lobes (15–30%); gallbladder (rare)

- abdominal swelling with palpable mass (90%)
- dyspepsia, anorexia, nausea + vomiting
- jaundice

√ mass of 1.5–35 cm in size
√ up to 11 liters of clear / cloudy, serous / mucinous / gelatinous, purulent / hemorrhagic / bilious fluid containing hemosiderin / cholesterol / necrosis
√ papillary excrescences + mural nodules
√ septations between cysts
US:
√ ovoid multiloculated anechoic mass with highly echogenic septations / papillary growths

LIVER

√ may contain fluid-fluid levels

CT:

√ multiloculated mass of near water density

√ contrast enhancement in wall + internal septa

MR:

√ locules with variable signal intensity on T1WI + T2WI depending on their protein content

Angio:

√ avascular mass with small clusters of peripheral abnormal vessels

√ stretching + displacement of vessels

√ thin subtle blush of neovascularity in septa + wall

Cx: malignant transformation into cystadenocarcinoma (indicated by invasion of capsule); rupture into peritoneum / retroperitoneum

Rx: surgical resection (recurrence common)

DDx: liver abscess, echinococcal cyst, cystic mesenchymal hamartoma (children + young adults), undifferentiated sarcoma (children + young adults), necrotic hepatic metastasis, cystic primary hepatocellular carcinoma

BILIARY-ENTERIC FISTULA

Incidence: 5% at cholecystectomy; 0.5% at autopsy

Etiology: cholelithiasis (90%), acute / chronic cholecystitis, biliary tract carcinoma, regional invasive neoplasm, diverticulitis, inflammatory bowel disease, peptic ulcer disease, echinococcal cyst, trauma, congenital communication

Communication with:

duodenum (70%), colon (26%), stomach (4%), jejunum, ileum, hepatic artery, portal vein (caused death of Ignatius Loyola), bronchial tree, pericardium, renal pelvis, ureter, urinary bladder, vagina, ovary

A. CHOLECYSTODUODENAL FISTULA (51–70%)
   1. Perforated gallstone (90%): associated with gallstone ileus in 20%
   2. Perforated duodenal ulcer (10%)
   3. Surgical anastomosis
   4. Gallbladder carcinoma

B. CHOLECYSTOCOLIC FISTULA (13–21%)

C. CHOLEDOCHODUODENAL FISTULA (13–19%) due to perforated duodenal ulcer disease

D. MULTIPLE FISTULAE (7%)

√ branching tubular radiolucencies, more prominent centrally

√ barium filling of biliary tree

√ multiple hyperechoic foci with dirty shadowing

DDx: patulous sphincter of Oddi, ascending cholangitis, surgery (choledochoduodenostomy, cholecystojejunostomy, sphincterotomy)

BUDD-CHIARI SYNDROME

= HEPATIC VENO-OCCLUSIVE DISEASE

= global / segmental obstruction of hepatic venous outflow

Cause:

A. IDIOPATHIC (66%)

B. THROMBOSIS
   (a) Hypercoagulable state: polycythemia rubra vera (1/3), oral contraceptives, pregnancy + postpartum state, paroxysmal nocturnal hemoglobulinuria (successive thrombosis of small veins), sickle cell disease
   mnemonic: "5 P's"
   Paroxysmal nocturnal hemoglobulinuria
   Platelets (thrombocytosis)
   Pill (birth control pills)
   Pregnancy
   Polycythemia rubra vera
   (b) Injury to vessel wall: phlebitis, trauma, hepatic radiation injury, chemotherapeutic + immunosuppressive drugs in patients with bone marrow transplants, venoocclusive disease from pyrrolizidine alkaloids (senecio) found in medicinal bush teas in Jamaica

C. NONTHROMBOTIC OBSTRUCTION
   (a) Tumor growth into IVC / hepatic veins (renal cell carcinoma, hepatoma, adrenal carcinoma, metastasis, primary leiomyosarcoma of IVC)
   (b) Membranous obstruction of suprahepatic IVC = IVC diaphragm (believed to be a congenital web or an acquired lesion from long-standing IVC thrombosis); common cause in Oriental + Indian population (South Africa, India, Japan, Korea); very rare in Western countries
   (c) Right atrial tumor
   (d) Constrictive pericarditis
   (e) Right heart failure

Pathophysiology: hepatic venous thrombosis leads to elevation of sinusoidal pressure which causes delayed / reversed portal venous inflow, ascites, alteration in hepatic morphology

M < F

Location:

Type I : occlusion of IVC ± hepatic veins

Type II : occlusion of major hepatic veins ± IVC

Type III : occlusion of small centrilobar veins

√ hepatosplenomegaly (early sign)

√ hypertrophy of caudate lobe (88%) [DDx: cirrhosis]

√ ascites

√ gallbladder wall thickening >6 mm

√ nonvisualization of hepatic veins (75%) / vein diameter <3 mm (measured 2 cm from IVC)

√ communications between right / middle hepatic vein and inferior right hepatic vein

√ enlarged inferior right hepatic vein (18%)

√ portal vein diameter >12 mm (in adults), >8 mm (in children)

√ visualization of paraumbilical vein

√ hypodensity in atrophic areas / periphery (82%) with inversion of portal blood flow

√ patchy enhancement (85%) with normal portal blood flow

√ ± narrowing / obstruction of intrahepatic IVC

CT:

√ enhancement of enlarged caudate lobe

LIVER

√ hypodense nonenhancing peripheral zones of liver (= reversed portal venous blood flow due to increased postsinusoidal pressure produced by hepatic venous obstruction)
√ failure to identify hepatic veins
√ hepatic vein thrombi (18–53%)

MRI:
√ reduction in caliber / complete absence of hepatic veins
√ multiple comma-shaped intrahepatic flow voids (= intrahepatic collaterals)

US:
√ hepatic veins not visualized / reduced in size / filled with thrombus
√ communicating collateral vessels
√ reversed flow in hepatic veins
√ absent / sluggish blood flow within IVC

Doppler:
— hepatic veins:
 √ absent / reversed / flat flow / loss of cardiac modulation in hepatic veins
 √ reversed flow in IVC
— portal vein:
 √ flow demodulation = disappearance of portal vein velocity variations with breathing
 √ slow flow (<11 cm/sec) / hepatofugal flow in portal vein
 √ congestion index >0.1
 √ portal vein thrombosis (20%)
— hepatic artery:
 √ resistive index >0.75

NUC (Tc-99m sulfur colloid):
√ central region of normal activity (hot caudate lobe) surrounded by greatly diminished activity (venous drainage of hypertrophied caudate lobe into IVC by separate vein)
√ colloid shift to spleen + bone marrow
√ wedge-shaped focal peripheral defects

Angio (inferior venocavography, hepatic venography):
√ absence of main hepatic veins
√ spider weblike appearance of collaterals + small hepatic veins
√ stretching + draping of intrahepatic arteries with hepatomegaly
√ inhomogeneous prolonged intense hepatogram with fine mottling
√ large lakes of sinusoidal contrast accumulation

Portography:
√ central hepatic enhancement (normal hepatopetal flow)
√ reversed portal flow in liver periphery (supplied only by hepatic artery)
√ bidirectional / hepatofugal main portal vein flow

Acute Budd-Chiari Syndrome (1/3)

◊ Caudate lobe has not had time to hypertrophy!
• rapid onset of abdominal pain (liver congestion)
• insidious onset of intractable ascites
√ hepatomegaly without derangement of liver function
√ ascites (97%)

CT:
√ diffuse hypodensity on NECT
√ early enhancement of caudate lobe + central portion around IVC with decreased enhancement peripherally
√ hypodense lumina of hepatic veins on CECT
√ decreased attenuation of enhancing areas with patchy inhomogeneous enhancement in liver periphery on delayed scans

Chronic Budd-Chiari Syndrome (2/3)

• insidious onset of jaundice, intractable ascites
• portal hypertension, variceal bleeding
√ enlargement of central region (= caudate lobe + adjacent central part of right lobe + medial segment of left lobe
√ nonsegmental / lobar atrophy of affected liver (due to extensive fibrosis) with diminished attenuation before + after contrast administration
√ progressive patchy enhancement radiating outward from major portal vessels (on dynamic bolus CT)
√ "reticulated mosaic" enhancement = diffuse patchy lobular enhancement separated by irregular linear areas of low density in central area
√ delayed homogeneous enhancement of entire liver after several minutes

Color Doppler:
√ "bicolored" hepatic veins (due to intrahepatic collateral pathways) are PATHOGNOMONIC

Dx: liver biopsy
Rx: anticoagulants, surgery / balloon dilatation (depending on etiology); portosystemic shunt; liver transplantation (for advanced cases)

CANDIDIASIS OF LIVER

= almost exclusively seen in immunocompromised patients (leukemia, chronic granulomatous disease of childhood, renal transplant, chemotherapy for myeloproliferative disorders)
◊ Most common systemic fungal infection in immunocompromised patients!
• abdominal pain
• persistent fever in neutropenic patient whose leukocyte count is returning to normal
• elevated alkaline phosphatase
√ hepatomegaly
√ "target" / "bull's-eye" sign = multiple small hypoechoic / hypoattenuating masses with centers of increased echogenicity / attenuation
 ◊ Bull's-eye lesion becomes visible only when neutropenia resolves!

NUC:
√ uniform uptake / focal photopenic areas
√ diminished Ga-67 uptake

Dx: biopsy evidence of yeast / pseudohyphae in central necrotic portion of lesion
DDx: metastases, lymphoma, leukemia, sarcoidosis, septic emboli, other infections, Kaposi sarcoma

LIVER

CAROLI DISEASE

= COMMUNICATING CAVERNOUS ECTASIA OF INTRAHEPATIC DUCTS

= rare probably autosomal recessive disorder characterized by congenital segmental saccular cystic dilatation of major intrahepatic bile ducts

Etiology: (a) ? perinatal hepatic artery occlusion
(b) ? hypoplasia / aplasia of fibromuscular wall components

Age: childhood + 2nd–3rd decade, occasionally in infancy; M:F = 1:1

Associated with:
medullary sponge kidney (in 80%), infantile polycystic kidney disease, renal tubular ectasia, choledochal cyst (rare), congenital hepatic fibrosis

- recurrent cramplike upper abdominal pain
- NO cirrhosis / portal hypertension

√ multiple cystic structures converging toward porta hepatis as either localized / diffusely scattered cysts communicating with bile ducts (DDx: polycystic liver disease)
√ segmental saccular / beaded appearance of intrahepatic bile ducts extending to periphery of liver
√ portal radicles completely surrounded by dilated bile ducts = central dot sign on CT
√ bridge formation across dilated lumina
√ intraluminal bulbar protrusions
√ frequent ectasia of extrahepatic ducts + CBD
√ sludge / calculi in dilated ducts

Cx: (1) bile stasis with recurrent cholangitis (2) biliary calculi (3) liver abscess (4) septicemia (5) increased risk for cholangiocarcinoma

CHOLANGIOCARCINOMA

Intrahepatic cholangiocarcinoma

= CHOLANGIOCELLULAR CARCINOMA

Incidence: 1/3 of all malignancies originating in the liver; 8–13% of all cholangiocarcinomas; 2nd most common primary hepatic tumor after hepatoma

Types:
(1) Massive / nodular type
(2) Diffuse (sclerosing cholangitis) type
◊ Cannot be depicted by cross-sectional imaging!

Histo: adenocarcinoma arising from the epithelium of a small intrahepatic bile duct with prominent desmoplastic reaction (fibrosis); ± mucin and calcifications

Average age: 50–60 years; M > F

- abdominal pain (47%)
- palpable mass (18%)
- weight loss (18%)
- painless jaundice (12%)

Spread: (a) local extension along duct
(b) local infiltration of liver substance
(c) metastatic spread to regional lymph nodes (in 15%)

√ mass of 5–20 cm in diameter
√ satellite nodules in 65%
√ punctate / chunky calcifications in 18%
√ calculi in biliary tree

NUC:
√ cold lesion on sulfur colloid / IDA scans
√ segmental biliary obstruction
√ may show uptake on gallium scan

US:
√ dilated biliary tree
√ predominantly homo- / heterogeneous mass
√ hyper- (75%) / iso- / hypoechoic (14%) mass

CT:
√ single predominantly homogeneous round / oval hypodense mass with irregular borders
√ "peripheral washout sign" = early minimal / moderate rim enhancement with progressive concentric filling and clearing of contrast material in rim of lesion on delayed images
√ marked homogeneous delayed enhancement (74%)

MR:
√ large central heterogeneous hypointense mass on T1WI
√ hyperintense periphery (viable tumor) + large central hypointensity (fibrosis) on T2WI

Angiography:
√ avascular / hypo- / hypervascular mass
√ stretched / encased arteries (frequent)
√ neovascularity in 50%
√ lack of venous invasion

Prognosis: <20% resectable; 30% 5-year survival

Extrahepatic cholangiocarcinoma

= BILE DUCT CARCINOMA

Age peak: 6–7th decade, M:F = 3:2

Incidence: <0.5% of autopsies; 90% of all cholangiocarcinomas; more frequent in Far East

Histo: well-differentiated sclerosing adenocarcinoma (2/3), anaplastic carcinoma (11%), cystadenocarcinoma, adenoacanthoma, malignant adenoma, squamous cell = epidermoid carcinoma, leiomyosarcoma

Predisposed:
(1) Inflammatory bowel disease (10 x increased risk); incidence of 0.4–1.4% in ulcerative colitis; latent period of 15 years; tumors usually multicentric + predominantly in extrahepatic sites; GB involved in 15% (simultaneous presence of gallstones is rare)
(2) Sclerosing cholangitis (10%)
(3) Caroli disease (due to chronic biliary stasis)
(4) Clonorchis sinensis infestation (Far East); most common cause worldwide
(5) Thorotrast exposure
(6) History of other malignancy (10%)
(7) Previous surgery for choledochal cyst / congenital biliary atresia
(8) Alpha-1-antitrypsin deficiency
(9) Autosomal dominant polycystic disease
(10) Cholecystolithiasis (20–50%), probably coincidental
(11) Papillomatosis of bile ducts

• gradual onset of fluctuating painless jaundice
• cholangitis (10%)
• weight loss, fatigability
• intermittent epigastric pain
• elevated bilirubin + alkaline phosphatase
• enlarged tender liver

Growth pattern:
(1) Obstructive type (70–85%)
√ U- / V-shaped obstruction with nipple, rattail, smooth / irregular termination
(2) Stenotic type (10–25%)
√ strictured rigid lumen with irregular margins + prestenotic dilatation
(3) Polypoid / papillary type (5–6%)
√ intraluminal filling defect with irregular margins

Spread: (a) lymphatic spread: cystic + CBD nodes (>32%), celiac nodes (>16%), peripancreatic nodes, superior mesenteric nodes
(b) infiltration of liver (23%)
(c) peritoneal seeding (9%)
(d) hematogenous (extremely rare): liver, peritoneum, lung

Location:

left / right hepatic duct	in 8–13%
confluence of hepatic ducts (Klatskin tumor)	in 10–26%
common hepatic duct	in 14–37%
proximal CBD	in 15–30%
distal CBD	in 30–50%
cystic duct	in 6%

UGI:
√ infiltration / indentation of stomach / duodenum

Cholangiography (PTC or ERC best modality to depict bile duct neoplasm):
√ exophytic intraductal tumor mass (46%), 2–5 mm in diameter
√ frequently long / rarely short concentric focal stricture in infiltrating sclerosing cholangitic type with wall irregularities
√ prestenotic diffuse / focal biliary dilatation (100%)
√ progression of ductal strictures (100%)

US / CT:
√ dilatation of intrahepatic ducts without extrahepatic duct dilatation
√ failure to demonstrate the confluence of L + R hepatic ducts
√ mass within / surrounding the ducts at point of obstruction (21% visible on US, 40% visible on CT)
√ infiltrating tumor visible as highly attenuating lesion in 22% on CT, in 13% on US
√ exophytic tumor visible in 100% on CT as low-attenuation mass, in 29% on US
√ polypoid intraluminal tumor visible as isoechoic mass within surrounding bile in 100% on US, in 25% on CT

Angiography:
√ hypervascular tumor with neovascularity (50%)
√ arterioarterial collaterals along the course of bile ducts associated with arterial obstruction
√ poor / absent tumor stain
√ displacement / encasement / occlusion of hepatic artery + portal vein

Cx: (1) Obstruction leading to biliary cirrhosis
(2) Hepatomegaly
(3) Intrahepatic abscess (subdiaphragmatic, perihepatic, septicemia)
(4) Biliary peritonitis
(5) Portal vein invasion

Prognosis: median survival of 5 months; 1.6% 5-year survival; 39% 5-year survival for carcinoma of papilla of Vater

DDx: benign stricture, chronic pancreatitis, sclerosing cholangitis, edematous papilla, idiopathic inflammation of CBD

CHOLANGITIS

Acute Cholangitis

Cause:
(a) benign disease:
(1) stricture from prior surgery (36%) (2) calculi (30%) (3) sclerosing cholangitis (4) obstructed drainage catheter (5) parasitic infestation
(b) malignant disease: ampullary carcinoma

Types:
A. ACUTE NONSUPPURATIVE ASCENDING CHOLANGITIS
• bile remains clear
• patient nontoxic
B. ACUTE SUPPURATIVE ASCENDING CHOLANGITIS (14%)
Associated with: obstructing biliary stone or malignancy
• septicemia, CNS depression, lethargy, mental confusion, shock (50%)
√ purulent material fills biliary ducts

Organism: E. coli > Klebsiella > Pseudomonas > Enterococci
• recurrent episodes of sepsis + RUQ pain
• Charcot triad (70%): fever + chills + jaundice
• bile cultures in 90% positive for infection

Cx: miliary hepatic abscess formation

Prognosis: 100% mortality if not decompressed; 40–60% mortality with treatment; 13–16% overall mortality rate

AIDS Cholangitis

Organism: CMV, Cryptosporidium
• RUQ pain, fever, jaundice
• elevated WBC count
• abnormal LFT (esp. serum alkaline phosphatase)
√ irregular mild dilatation of intra- and extrahepatic bile ducts similar to sclerosing cholangitis
√ stricture of distal CBD / papillary stenosis
√ mural thickening of gallbladder + bile ducts
√ ± pericholecystic fluid

LIVER

Primary sclerosing cholangitis

= insidious progressive inflammatory disease causing multifocal strictures of intra- and extrahepatic bile ducts

Etiology: idiopathic, ? hypersensitivity reaction (speculative)

Prevalence: 1% as common as alcoholic liver disease

Age: <45 years (2/3); range 21–39–67 years; M:F = 7:3

Histo:

Stage 1: degeneration of epithelial bile duct cells + infiltration with lymphocytes ± neutrophils; inflammation + scarring + enlargement of periportal triads (pericholangitis)

Stage 2: fibrosis + inflammation infiltrating periportal parenchyma with piecemeal necrosis of hepatocytes; enlargement of portal triads; bile ductopenia

Stage 3: portal-to-portal fibrous septa; severe degenerative changes + disappearance of bile ducts; cholestasis in periportal + paraseptal hepatocytes

Stage 4: frank cirrhosis

Associated with:

(1) Inflammatory bowel disease (ulcerative colitis in 50–74%, Crohn disease in 13%)
◊ 1–4% of patients with inflammatory bowel disease develop sclerosing cholangitis!
(2) Cirrhosis, chronic active hepatitis, pericholangitis, fatty degeneration
(3) Pancreatitis
(4) Retroperitoneal / mediastinal fibrosis
(5) Peyronie disease
(6) Riedel thyroiditis, hypothyroidism
(7) Retroorbital pseudotumor

• abnormal liver function tests: serum alkaline phosphatase, γ-glutamyltransferase
• progressive chronic / intermittent obstructive jaundice (most frequent)
• history of previous biliary surgery (53%) + chronic / recurrent pancreatitis (14%)
• fever, night sweats, chills, RUQ pain, itching (10–15%)

Location:

1. CBD almost always involved
2. Intra- and extrahepatic ducts (68–89%)
3. Cystic duct involved in 15–18%
4. Intrahepatic ducts only (1–11–25%)
5. Extrahepatic ducts only (2–3%)

√ intrahepatic bile duct calculi (8%): soft black crushable stones / sandlike grit

US:
√ brightly echogenic portal triads
√ echogenic biliary casts / punctate coarse calcifications along portal vein branches

CT:
√ dilatation, stenosis, pruning, beading of intrahepatic bile ducts (80%)
√ dilatation, stenosis, wall nodularity, duct wall thickening, mural contrast enhancement of extrahepatic bile ducts (100%)
√ hepatic metastases + lymph nodes in porta hepatis
√ subtle foci of high attenuation in intrahepatic bile ducts

Cholangiography:
√ multifocal strictures with predilection for bifurcations + skip lesions (uninvolved duct segments of normal caliber) involving intra- and extrahepatic bile ducts
√ "pruned tree" appearance (= opacification of central ducts + diffuse obstruction of peripheral smaller radicles)
√ "cobblestone" appearance (= coarse nodular mural irregularities) in 50%
√ small saccular outpouchings (diverticula / pseudodiverticula) = PATHOGNOMONIC
√ CLASSIC "beaded appearance" (= alternating segments of dilatation and focal circumferential stenoses)
√ new strictures + lengthening of strictures between 6 months and 6 years (<20%)
√ marked ductal dilatation (24%)
√ polypoid mass (7%)
√ gallbladder irregularities uncommon

NUC (Tc-99m-IDA scan):
√ multiple persistent focal areas of retention in distribution of intrahepatic biliary tree
√ marked prolongation of hepatic clearance
√ gallbladder visualized only in 70%

Cx: (1) Biliary cirrhosis
(2) Portal hypertension
(3) Cholangiocarcinoma (6–12–15%)

Rx: 4th leading indication for liver transplantation

DDx:
(1) Sclerosing cholangiocarcinoma (progressive cholangiographic changes within 0.5–1.5 years of initial diagnosis, marked ductal dilatation upstream from a dominant stricture, intraductal mass >1 cm in diameter)
(2) Acute ascending cholangitis (history)
(3) Primary biliary cirrhosis (disease limited to intrahepatic ducts, strictures less pronounced, pruning + crowding of bile ducts, normal AMA titer)

Recurrent pyogenic cholangitis

= PRIMARY CHOLANGITIS = RECURRENT PYOGENIC HEPATITIS = ORIENTAL CHOLANGIOHEPATITIS = ORIENTAL CHOLANGITIS = HONG KONG DISEASE = INTRAHEPATIC PIGMENT STONE DISEASE

Etiology: ? clonorchis infestation; endemic to South China, Indochina, Taiwan, Japan, Korea

Incidence: 3rd most common cause of an acute abdomen in Hong Kong after appendicitis and perforated ulcer

Age: 20–50 years; M:F = 1:1

Associated intrabiliary infestation:
Clonorchis sinensis, Ascaris lumbricoides, Escherichia coli

• recurrent attacks of fever, chills, abdominal pain, jaundice

Location: particularly in lateral segment of L lobe + posterior segment of R lobe
√ marked dilatation of proximal intrahepatic ducts (3–4 mm) in 100%
√ decreased arborization of intrahepatic radicles
√ intrahepatic bile ducts filled with nonshadowing soft mudlike pigment (calcium bilirubinate) stones (64%)
√ dilatation of CBD (68%) + choledocholithiasis (30%)
√ bile duct strictures (22%)
√ pneumobilia (3–52%)
√ segmental hepatic atrophy (36%)
Cx: liver abscess (18%), splenomegaly (14%), biloma (4%), pancreatitis (4%)
DDx: complication of Caroli disease

Secondary sclerosing cholangitis

Cause:
(1) chronic bacterial cholangitis from bile duct stricture / choledocholithiasis
(2) ischemic bile duct damage from treatment with floxuridine
(3) infectious cholangiopathy in AIDS
(4) previous biliary tract surgery
(5) congenital biliary tree anomalies
(6) bile duct neoplasm

CHOLECYSTITIS

Acute cholecystitis

Etiology: (a) in 80–95% cystic duct obstruction by impacted calculus; 85% disimpact spontaneously
(b) in 10% acalculous cholecystitis
Pathogenesis: chemical irritation from concentrated bile, bacterial infection, reflux of pancreatic secretions
Age peak: 5–6th decade; M:F = 1:3
• persisting (>6 hours) RUQ pain radiating to right shoulder / scapula / interscapular area (DDx: biliary colic usually <6 hours)
• nausea, vomiting, chills, fever
• RUQ tenderness + guarding
• ± leukocytosis, elevated levels of alkaline phosphatase and transaminase and amylase
• mild hyperbilirubinemia (20%)
• Murphy sign = inspiratory arrest upon palpation of GB area (falsely positive in 6% of patients with cholelithiasis)

Oral cholecystography:
√ nonvisualization / poor visualization of gallbladder
US (81–100% sensitivity, 60–100% specificity):
√ GB wall thickening >3 mm (45–72% sensitive, 76–88% specific)
√ hazy delineation of GB wall
√ "halo sign" = GB wall lucency (in 8%) = 3-layered configuration with sonolucent middle layer (edema)
√ striated wall thickening (62%) = several alternating irregular discontinuous lucent + echogenic bands within GB wall (100% PPV)
√ GB hydrops = distension with AP diameter >5 cm or enlargement of greater than 4 x 10 cm
√ positive sonographic Murphy sign (in 85–88%) = focal tenderness over gallbladder (63–94% sensitive, 85–93% specific, 72% NPV)
false-negative Murphy sign:
lack of patient responsiveness, pain medication, inability to press directly on GB (position deep to liver / protected by ribs), GB wall necrosis
√ crescent-shaped / loculated pericholecystic fluid (in 20%) = inflammatory intraperitoneal exudate / abscess
√ gallstones (83–98% sensitive, 52–77% specific)
√ impacted gallstone in GB neck / cystic duct
√ echogenic shadowing fat within hepatoduodenal ligament ± conspicuous color Doppler flow (due to inflammation)
Color Doppler US:
√ visualization of cystic artery >50% of the length of the gallbladder (30% sensitive, 98% specific)
NUC (86–97% sensitivity, 73–100% specificity , 95–98% accuracy):
√ visualization of biliary tract + bowel
√ nonvisualization of GB during 1st hour (in 83%)
√ nonvisualization of GB by 4 hours (99% specificity)
√ nonvisualization of GB + CBD (in 13%)
√ rim sign (34%) = increased activity in GB fossa conforming to inferior hepatic edge (= sign of hyperemia); predictive value of 57% for gangrenous GB + 94% for acute cholecystitis
√ increased perfusion to GB fossa during "arterial phase" (in up to 80%)

False-positive scans (10–12%) = nonvisualization of GB in absence of acute cholecystitis:
congenital absence of GB, carcinoma of GB, chronic cholecystitis, acute pancreatitis, alcoholic liver disease, hepatocellular disease, severe intercurrent illness, total parenteral nutrition, hyperalimentation, prolonged fasting, recent feeding <4–6 hours prior to study
Reduction to 2% false-positive scans through:
(1) delayed images up to 4 hours
(2) cholecystokinin (Sincalide®) injection 15 minutes prior to study
(3) morphine IV (0.04 mg/kg) at 40 minutes + reimaging after 20 minutes (contraction of sphincter of Oddi + rise in intrabiliary pressure)
False-negative scans (4.8%): dilated cystic duct

Cx:
(1) Gangrene of gallbladder
√ shaggy, irregular, asymmetric wall (mucosal ulcers, intraluminal hemorrhage, necrosis)
√ hyperechoic foci within GB wall (microabscesses in Rokitansky-Aschoff sinuses)
√ intraluminal pseudomembranes (gangrene)
√ coarse nonshadowing nondependent echodensities (= sloughed necrotic mucosa / sludge / pus / clotted blood within gallbladder)

LIVER

(2) Perforation of gallbladder (in 2–20%)
  (a) acute free perforation with peritonitis causing pericholecystic abscess in 33%
  (b) subacute localized perforation causing pericholecystic abscess in 48%
  (c) chronic perforation resulting in internal biliary fistula causing pericholecystic abscess in 18%
  Location: most commonly perforation of fundus
  √ gallstone lying free in peritoneal cavity
  √ sonolucent / complex collection surrounding GB
(3) Empyema of gallbladder
  √ multiple medium / coarse highly reflective intraluminal echoes without shadowing / layering / gravity dependence (purulent exudate / debris)

mnemonic: "GAME BEG"
Gangrene
Abscess (pericholecystic)
Mirizzi syndrome
Emphysematous cholecystitis
Bouveret syndrome (= gallstone erodes into duodenum leading to duodenal obstruction)
Empyema
Gallstone ileus

Acute acalculous cholecystitis

Frequency: 5–15% of all acute cholecystitis cases
Etiology: probably caused by decreased blood flow within cystic artery
(1) depressed motility / starvation in trauma, burns, surgery, total parenteral nutrition, anesthesia, mechanical ventilation, narcotics, shock, congestive heart failure, arteriosclerosis, polyarteritis nodosa, SLE, diabetes mellitus
(2) obstruction of cystic duct by extrinsic inflammation, lymphadenopathy, metastases
(3) infection from Salmonella, cholera, Kawasaki syndrome

√ thickened gallbladder wall >4–5 mm
√ echogenic bile sludge
√ gallbladder distension
√ pericholecystic fluid in absence of ascites
√ subserosal edema
√ sloughed mucosal membrane
√ Murphy sign = pain + tenderness with transducer pressure over the gallbladder

Cx: gallbladder perforation
Prognosis: 6.5% mortality rate

Chronic cholecystitis

Most common form of gallbladder inflammation
√ gallstones
√ smooth / irregular GB wall thickening (mean of 5 mm)
√ mean volume of 42 mL
NUC:
  √ normal GB visualization in majority of patients
  √ delayed GB visualization (1–4 hours)
  √ visualization of bowel prior to GB (sensitivity 45%, specificity 90%)
  √ noncontractility / decreased response after CCK injection (decreased GB ejection fraction)

Emphysematous cholecystitis

= ischemia of gallbladder wall + infection with gas-producing organisms
Etiology: calculous (70–80%) / acalculous cystic duct obstruction with inflammatory edema resulting in cystic artery occlusion
Organism: Clostridium perfringens, Clostridium welchii, E. coli, staphylococcus, streptococcus
Age: >50 years; M:F = 5:1
Predisposed: diabetics (20–50%), debilitating diseases
- WBC count may be normal (1/3)
- point tenderness rare (diabetic neuropathy)

Plain film:
  √ gas appears 24–48 hours after onset of symptoms
  √ air-fluid level in GB lumen, air in GB wall within 24–48 hours after acute episode
  √ pneumobilia (rare)
US:
  √ high-level echoes outlining GB wall

Cx: gangrene (75%); gallbladder perforation (20%)
Mortality: 15%
DDx:
1. Enteric fistula
2. Incompetent sphincter of Oddi
3. Air-containing periduodenal abscess
4. Periappendiceal abscess in malpositioned appendix
5. Lipomatosis of gallbladder

Xanthogranulomatous cholecystitis

= FIBROXANTHOGRANULOMATOUS INFLAMMATION
= CEROID GRANULOMAS OF THE GALLBLADDER
= uncommon inflammatory disease of gallbladder characterized by presence of multiple intramural nodules

Etiology:
rupture of occluded Rokitansky-Aschoff sinuses with subsequent intramural extravasation of inspissated bile + mucin attracting histiocytes to phagocytose the insoluble cholesterol
Incidence: 1–2%
Age: 7th + 8th decade
Histo: mixture of ceroid (waxlike) xanthogranuloma with foamy histiocytes + multinucleated foreign body giant cells + lymphocytes + fibroblasts containing areas of necrosis (in newer lesions)
May be associated with: gallbladder carcinoma (11%)

√ preservation of 2–3 mm thick mucosal lining (in 82%)
√ thickened gallbladder wall: 91% diffuse, 9% focal
√ infiltration of pericholecystic fat: in 45% focal, in 54% diffuse
√ hepatic extension (45%)
√ biliary obstruction (36%)
√ lymphadenopathy (36%)
US:
  √ intramural hypoechoic nodules
CT:
  √ 5–20 mm small intramural hypoattenuating nodules
  √ poor / heterogeneous contrast enhancement

DDx: gallbladder carcinoma (in 59% focal, in 41% diffuse thickening of gallbladder wall, multiple masses within liver)

CHOLEDOCHAL CYST

= CYSTIC DILATATION OF EXTRAHEPATIC BILE DUCT

= segmental aneurysmal dilatation of common bile duct without involvement of gallbladder / cystic duct; most common congenital lesion of bile ducts

Etiology: anomalous junction of pancreatic duct and CBD proximal to duodenal papilla, higher pressure in pancreatic duct and absent ductal sphincter allows free reflux of enzymes into CBD resulting in weakening of CBD wall

Classification:

malunion of pancreaticobiliary duct

- Kimura Type I = pancreatic duct enters the proximal / mid CBD
- Kimura Type II = CBD drains into pancreatic duct

Prevalence: 1:13,000 admissions; high prevalence in Japanese

Age: <10 years (50%) + young adulthood, 80% diagnosed in childhood, 7% during pregnancy, occasionally detected up to 7th decade; M:F = 1:4

Histo: fibrous cyst wall without epithelial lining

Associated with:

(1) dilatation, stenosis or atresia of other portions of the biliary tree (2%)
(2) gallbladder anomaly (aplasia, double GB)
(3) failure of union of left + right hepatic ducts
(4) pancreatic duct + accessory hepatic bile ducts may drain into cyst
(5) polycystic liver disease

- Classic triad (20–30% of adult patients):
  (1) intermittent obstructive jaundice (33–50%)
  (2) recurrent RUQ colicky pain (>75–90%), back pain
  (3) intermittent palpable RUQ abdominal mass (<25%)
- recurrent fever, chills, weight loss, pruritus

Types:

(a) marked cystic dilatation of CBD + CHD
(b) focal segmental dilatation of CBD distally
(c) cylindric dilatation of CBD + CHD

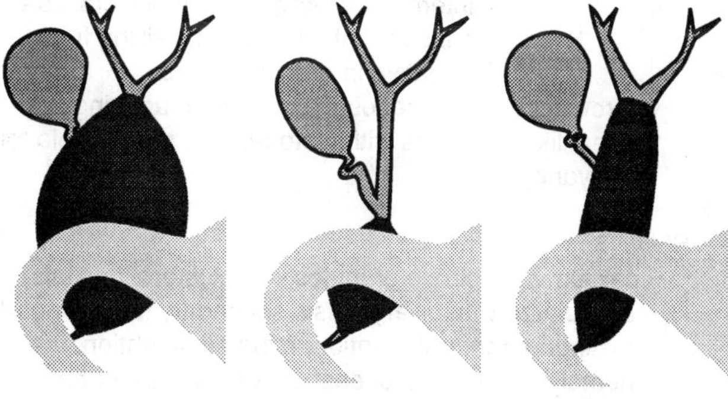

Choledochal Cysts

√ size: diameter of 2 cm up to 15 cm (largest contained 13 liters)

√ NO / mild peripheral intrahepatic bile duct dilatation

√ may contain stones / sludge

UGI:

√ soft-tissue mass in RUQ

√ anterior displacement of 2nd portion of duodenum + distal portion of stomach / widening of C-loop with inferior displacement of duodenum

US:

√ ballooned / fusiform cyst beneath porta hepatis separate from gallbladder

◊ Communication with common hepatic / intrahepatic ducts needs to be demonstrated!

√ abrupt change of caliber at junction of dilated segment to normal ducts

√ intrahepatic bile duct dilatation (16%) secondary to stenosis

OB-US (earliest diagnosis at 25 weeks MA):

√ right-sided cyst in fetal abdomen + adjacent dilated hepatic ducts

DDx: duodenal atresia; cyst of ovary, mesentery, omentum, pancreas, liver

NUC with HIDA:

(excludes effectively DDx of hepatic cyst, pancreatic pseudocyst, enteric duplication, spontaneous loculated biloma)

√ photopenic area within liver that fills within 60 minutes + stasis of tracer within cyst

√ prominent hepatic ductal activity (dilatation of ducts)

Cx:

1. Stones in gallbladder, within cyst, in intrahepatic biliary tree, in pancreatic duct (8–50%)
2. Recurrent pancreatitis (33%)
3. Cholangitis (20%)
4. Malignant transformation into bile duct carcinoma + gallbladder carcinoma (increasing with age, <1% in 1st decade, 7–14% > age 20)
5. Cyst rupture with bile peritonitis (1.8%)
6. Bleeding
7. Biliary cirrhosis + portal hypertension

Rx: excision of cyst + Roux-en-Y hepaticojejunostomy

DDx: mesenteric, omental, ovarian, renal, adrenal, hepatic, pancreatic cyst, gastrointestinal duplication, hydronephrotic kidney

CHOLEDOCHOCELE

= DUODENAL DUPLICATION CYST

= ENTEROGENOUS CYST OF AMPULLA OF VATER / DUODENUM = INTRADUODENAL CHOLEDOCHAL CYST = DIVERTICULUM OF COMMON BILE DUCT

= cystic dilatation of the distal / intramural duodenal portion of the CBD with herniation of CBD into duodenum (similar to ureterocele)

Etiology:

(1) congenital:
  (a) originates from tiny bud / diverticulum of distal CBD (found in 5.7% of normal population)
  (b) stenosis of ductal orifice / weakness of ductal wall

LIVER

(2) acquired: stone passage followed by stenosis + inflammation

Age: 33 years (manifestation usually in adulthood)

Types: (a) CBD terminates in cyst, cyst drains into duodenum (common)
(b) cyst drains into adjacent intramural portion of CBD (less common)

• biliary colic, episodic jaundice, nausea, vomiting
√ stones / sludge are frequently present

UGI:
√ smooth well-defined intraluminal duodenal filling defect in region of papilla
√ change in shape with compression / peristalsis

Cholangiography (diagnostic):
√ smooth clublike / saclike dilatation of intramural segment of CBD

Cx: choledocholithiasis, pancreatitis
Rx: sphincterotomy / sphincteroplasty
DDx: choledochal cyst (involves more than only terminal portion of CBD)

CHOLELITHIASIS

Predisposing factors: "female, forty, fair, fat, fertile, flatulent"

(a) Hemolytic disease
sickle cell disease (7–37%), hereditary spherocytosis (43–85%), thalassemia, pernicious anemia (16–20%), prosthetic cardiac valves + mitral stenosis (hemolysis), cirrhosis (hemolysis secondary to hypersplenism), Rhesus / ABO blood group incompatibility (perinatal period)

(b) Metabolic disorder = disruption of biliary lithogenic index
diabetes mellitus, obesity, pancreatic disease, cystic fibrosis, hypercholesterolemia, hemosiderosis (20%), hyperparathyroidism, hypothyroidism, prolonged use of estrogens / progesterone, pregnancy

(c) Cholestasis
— hepatic dysfunction: hepatitis, neonatal sepsis
— biliary tree malformation: Caroli disease
— biliary obstruction: parasitic infection, benign / malignant strictures, foreign bodies (sutures, ascariasis)
— prolonged fasting (total parenteral nutrition)
— Methadone intake

(d) Inflammatory bowel disease
intestinal malabsorption has a 10 x increased risk of stone formation
— Crohn disease (28–34%)

(e) Genetic predisposition = familial
Navaho, Pima, Chippewa Indians

(f) Others
muscular dystrophy

GALLSTONES IN NEONATE

◊ rare without predisposing factors

Associated with: total parenteral nutrition, furosemide, GI dysfunction, prolonged fasting, phototherapy

Composition:

A. CHOLESTEROL STONE (70%)
= main component of most calculi (70%)
√ lucent (93%), calcified (7%)
√ slightly hypodense compared with bile
(a) pure cholesterol stones (10%): yellowish, soft
√ buoyancy in contrast-enhanced bile
√ density of <100 HU
(b) mixture of cholesterol + calcium carbonate / bilirubinate (70%)
√ laminated appearance
√ radiopaque on plain film (15–20%)

B. PIGMENT STONE (30%)
• black = compact "lacquer" of bilirubin derivatives with a high affinity for calcium carbonate
• brown = granular precipitate of calcium bilirubinate (in inflamed / infected gallbladders) contains <25% cholesterol
√ multiple tiny faceted / spiculated homogeneously radiopaque stones
CT:
√ usually denser than bile

Radioopacity:
√ lucent stones (84%):
cholesterol (85%), pigment (15%)
√ calcified stones (16% on plain film, 60% on CT):
cholesterol (33%), pigment (67%)

Location of calcium:
√ <u>calcium phosphate</u> deposited centrally within cholesterol stones
√ <u>calcium carbonate</u> deposited radially within aging cholesterol / peripherally around cholesterol + pigmented stones

FLOATING GALLSTONES (20–25%)

(a) relatively pure cholesterol stones
(b) gas-containing stones
(c) rise in specific gravity of bile (1.03) from oral cholecystopaques (1.06) causing stones (1.05) to float

GAS-CONTAINING GALLSTONES

Mechanism: dehydration of older stones leads to internal shrinkage + dendritic cracks + subsequent nitrogen gas–filling from negative internal pressure

√ "crow-foot" = "Mercedes-Benz" sign = radiating streaklike lucencies within stone, also responsible for buoyancy

SLUDGE

= calcium-bilirubinate granules + cholesterol crystals associated with biliary stasis secondary to prolonged fasting, parenteral nutrition, hyperalimentation, hemolysis, cystic duct obstruction, acute + chronic cholecystitis

√ nonshadowing echogenic homogeneous mass shifting position slowly

√ "sludge ball" = tumefactive sludge (DDx: gallbladder cancer)

DDx: hemobilia, blood clot, parasitic infestation, mucus

Cholecystolithiasis

Incidence: 2% of children;
10% of population; M:F = 1:3;
in 3rd decade M:F = 2%:4%;
in 7th decade M:F = 10%:25%

Peak age: 5th–6th decade

- asymptomatic (60–65%); become symptomatic at a rate of 2% per year
- **biliary colic** (misnomer) due to obstruction of cystic duct / common bile duct develops in 33% (18% overall risk in 20 years)
  = acute RUQ / epigastric / LUQ / precordial / lower abdominal pain increasing over seconds / minutes + remaining fairly steady for 4–6 hours
  - no tenderness upon palpation

Abdominal plain film (10–16% sensitive)
√ calcified gallstones

OCG (65–90% sensitive)
√ filling defect in contrasted gallbladder lumen
√ nonvisualization of gallbladder (25%) = inconclusive

CT (80% sensitive):
√ hyperdense calcified gallstones in 60%
√ hypodense cholesterol stones ≤140 HU = pure cholesterol stone (= ≥80% cholesterol content)
◊ Inverse relationship between CT attenuation number + cholesterol content
√ gallstones isointense to bile in 21–24% and thus undetectable by CT (<30 HU)

US (91–98% sensitive; in 5% falsely negative):
√ mobile echogenic structure + acoustic shadowing within gallbladder (100% PPV)
√ reverberation artifact
√ nonvisualization of GB + collection of echogenic echoes with acoustic shadowing (15–25%)
√ "double-arc shadow" = 2 echogenic curvilinear parallel lines separated by sonolucent rim (ie, GB wall + GB lumen + stone with acoustic shadowing)
√ focal nonshadowing opacities <5 mm in diameter (in 70% gallstones)
√ infrequently adherent to wall

FALSE-NEGATIVE US (5%):
contracted GB, GB in anomalous / unusual location, small gallstone, gallstone impacted in GB neck / cystic duct, immobile patient, obese patient, extensive RUQ bowel gas

Cx: cholangitis, pancreatitis, fistula; cancer of GB + bile ducts (2–3 x more frequent)

Cholangiolithiasis

A. CHOLEDOCHOLITHIASIS

◊ Most common cause of bile duct obstruction!

Etiology: (a) passed stones originating in GB
(b) primary development in intra- / extrahepatic ducts

Incidence: in 12–15% of cholecystectomy patients; in 3–4% of postcholecystectomy patients; in 75% of patients with chronic bile duct obstruction

Risk indicators for CBD stone:
(1) recent history of jaundice
(2) recent history of pancreatitis
(3) elevated serum bilirubin >17 μmol/L
(4) elevated serum amylase >120 IU/L
(5) dilated CBD >6 mm (16%)
(6) obscured bile duct

- recurrent episodes of jaundice, chills, fever (25–50%)
- elevated transaminase (75%)
- spontaneous passage with stones <6 mm size

Cholangiography (most specific technique):
√ stone visualization in 92%

Peroperative cholangiography:
prolongs operation by 30 minutes;
4% false-negatives; 4–10% false-positives

US (22–82% sensitive):
√ stone visualization in 13–75% (more readily with CBD dilatation + good visibility of pancreatic head)
√ dilated ducts in 64–77% / normal-sized duct in 36%
√ dilatation of CBD with administration of fatty meal / cholecystokinin
√ no stone in gallbladder (11%)

CT:
√ stone visualization in 75–85% (isoattenuating to bile in 15–25%)
√ target sign = intraluminal mass with crescentic ring (= stone of soft-tissue density) in 85%

NUC:
√ delayed bowel activity beyond 2 hours
√ persistent hepatic + common bile duct activity to 24 hours
√ prominent ductal activity beyond 90 minutes with visualization of secondary ducts

B. STONE IN CYSTIC DUCT REMNANT:
retained in 0.4% after surgery for choledocholithiasis

CHRONIC GRANULOMATOUS DISEASE OF CHILDHOOD

= recessive sex-linked immunodeficiency disorder resulting in purulent infections + granuloma formation primarily involving lymph nodes, skin, lungs

Etiology: polymorphonuclear leukocyte dysfunction characterized by inability to generate hydrogen peroxide causing prolonged intracellular survival of phagocytized catalase-positive bacteria

Organism: most commonly staphylococcus, Serratia marcescens, gram-negative enterococci

Path: chronic infection with granuloma formation / caseation / suppuration

Age: onset in childhood; M > F (more severe in boys)

- recurrent chronic infections: suppurative lymphadenitis, pyoderma
- chronic diarrhea
- perianal fistula + abscess

@ Chest
- √ chronic pneumonia
- √ hilar lymphadenopathy
- √ pleural effusions

@ Liver
- √ hepatosplenomegaly
- √ hepatic abscess
- √ liver calcifications

@ GI tract
- √ esophageal dysmotility, esophagitis, stricture
- √ gastric antral narrowing ± gastric outlet obstruction

@ Bone
- √ osteomyelitis

CIRRHOSIS

= chronic liver disease characterized by diffuse parenchymal necrosis, regeneration and scarring with abnormal reconstruction of preexisting lobular architecture

Etiology:

A. TOXIC
(1) Alcoholic liver disease in 75% (2) Drug-induced (prolonged methotrexate, oxyphenisatin, alpha-methyldopa, nitrofurantoin, isoniazid) (3) Iron overload (hemochromatosis, hemosiderosis)

B. INFLAMMATION: Viral hepatitis, Schistosomiasis

C. BILIARY OBSTRUCTION
(1) Cystic fibrosis (2) Inflammatory bowel disease (3) Primary biliary irrhosis (4) Obstructive infantile cholangiopathy

D. VASCULAR
(1) Prolonged CHF = cardiac cirrhosis
(2) Hepatic venoocclusive disease

E. NUTRITIONAL
(1) Intestinal bypass (2) Severe steatosis
(3) Abetalipoproteinemia

F. HEREDITARY
(1) Wilson disease (2) Alpha-1-antitrypsin deficiency
(3) Juvenile polycystic kidney disease
(4) Galactosemia (5) Type IV glycogen storage disease (6) Hereditary fructose intolerance
(7) Tyrosinemia (8) Hereditary tetany (9) Osler-Weber-Rendu syndrome (10) Familial cirrhosis

G. IDIOPATHIC / CRYPTOGENIC

Cirrhosis in children: biliary atresia, hepatitis, α-1–antitrypsin deficiency, tyrosinemia, hemochromatosis, Wilson disease, schistosomiasis

Morphology:

(a) micronodular cirrhosis (<3 mm): usually due to alcoholism, biliary obstruction, hemochromatosis, venous outflow obstruction, previous small-bowel bypass surgery, Indian childhood fibrosis
(b) macronodular cirrhosis (3–15 mm, up to several cm): usually due to chronic viral hepatitis, Wilson disease, α-1–antitrypsin deficiency
(c) mixed cirrhosis

Nodular lesions:

(a) **regenerative nodules** = localized proliferation of hepatocytes + supporting stroma
(b) cirrhotic nodule = regenerative nodule largely / completely surrounded by fibrous septa
(c) dysplastic nodule [adenomatous hyperplasia] = cluster of hepatocytes >1 mm in diameter with evidence of dysplasia; common in hepatitis B and C, α-1–antitrypsin deficiency, tyrosinemia
(d) hepatocellular carcinoma

Associated with: anemia, coagulopathy, hypoalbuminemia, cholelithiasis, pancreatitis, peptic ulcer disease, diarrhea, hypogonadism

- anorexia, weakness, fatigue, weight loss
- jaundice, continuous low-grade fever
- ascites, bleeding from esophageal varices, hepatic encephalopathy

√ enlarged (early stage) / normal / shrunken liver
√ shrinkage of right lobe (segments 5–8) and medial segment of left lobe (segments 4a + 4b) with concomitant hypertrophy of lateral segment of left lobe (segments 2 +3) and caudate lobe (segment 1):
- √ ratio of caudate to right lobe >0.65 on transverse images [sensitivity 43–84%, least sensitive in alcoholic cirrhosis, most sensitive in cirrhosis caused by hepatitis B; specificity 100%; 26% sensitivity; 84–96% accuracy] (DDx: Budd-Chiari syndrome)
- √ diameter of quadrate lobe (segment 4) <30 mm (= distance between left wall of gallbladder and ascending portion of left portal vein) due to selective atrophy (95% specific)

√ widened porta hepatis + interlobar fissure
√ surface nodularity + indentations (regenerating nodules)
√ signs of portal hypertension
√ splenomegaly
√ ascites (failure of albumin synthesis, overproduction of lymph due to increased hydrostatic pressure in sinusoids / decreased splanchnic output due to portal hypertension)
√ associated with fatty infiltration (in early cirrhosis)

US (sensitivity 65–80%; DDx: chronic hepatitis, fatty infiltration):

Hepatic signs:
- √ hepatomegaly (63%)
- √ hypertrophy of caudate lobe (26%)
  - √ ratio of width of caudate lobe to width of right hepatic lobe >0.65 (43–84% sensitive, 100% specific)
- √ surface nodularity (88% sensitive, 82–95% specific)
- √ increased hepatic parenchymal echogenicity in 66% (as a sign of superimposed fatty infiltration)
- √ increased sound attenuation (9%)
- √ heterogeneous coarse (usually) / fine echotexture (7%)
- √ decreased / normal definition of walls of portal venules (sign of associated fatty infiltration NOT of fibrosis)
- √ occasional depiction of isoechoic regenerative nodules

LIVER

√ dilatation of hepatic arteries (increased arterial flow) with demonstration of intrahepatic arterial branches (DDx: dilated biliary radicals)
√ increase in hepatic artery resistance after meal ingestion
√ "portalization" of hepatic vein waveform = dampened oscillations of hepatic veins resembling portal vein flow

Extrahepatic signs:
√ splenomegaly
√ ascites
√ signs of portal hypertension

CT:
√ native + enhanced parenchymal inhomogeneity
√ decreased attenuation (steatosis) in early cirrhosis
√ isodense / hyperdense (siderotic) regenerative nodules
√ nodular / lobulated liver contour
√ predominantly portal venous supply to dysplastic nodules
√ hypodense area adjacent to portal vein (= peribiliary cysts from obstructed extramural peribiliary glands)

MR (problem-solving tool):
√ no alteration of liver parenchyma
√ regenerating nodules = hypointense lesions (due to iron deposits within nodules) with hyperintense septa (due to vascularity) on T2WI
√ dysplastic nodule = iso- / hyperintense on T1WI + iso- / hypointense on T2WI
√ HCC nodule = hypo- / iso- / hyperintense on T1WI + usually hyperintense on T2WI with marked enhancement during arterial phase

Angio:
√ stretched hepatic artery branches (early finding)
√ enlarged tortuous hepatic arteries = "corkscrewing" (increase in hepatic arterial flow)
√ shunting between hepatic artery and portal vein
√ mottled parenchymal phase
√ delayed emptying into venous phase
√ pruning of hepatic vein branches (normally depiction of 5th order branches) = postsinusoidal compression by developing nodules

NUC (Tc-99m–labeled sulfur colloid):
√ high blood pool activity secondary to slow clearance
√ colloid shift to bone marrow + spleen + lung
√ shrunken liver with little or no activity + splenomegaly
√ mottled hepatic uptake (pseudotumors) on colloid scan (normal activity on IDA scans!)
√ displacement of liver + spleen from abdominal wall by ascites

Cx: (1) Ascites: cause / contributor to death in 50%
(2) Portal hypertension
(3) Hepatocellular carcinoma (in 7–12%)
(4) Cholangiocarcinoma

Fatality from:
esophageal variceal bleeding (in 25%), hepatorenal syndrome (10%), spontaneous bacterial peritonitis (5–10%), complications from treatment of ascites (10%)

Primary Biliary Cirrhosis

= CHRONIC NONSUPPURATIVE DESTRUCTIVE CHOLANGITIS

Histo: idiopathic progressive destructive cholangitis of interlobar and septal bile ducts, portal fibrosis, nodular regeneration, shrinkage of hepatic parenchyma

Age: 35–55 years; M:F = 1:9

- fatigue, pruritus
- xanthelasma / xanthoma (25%)
- hyperpigmentation (50%)
- insidious onset of pruritus (60%)
- IgM increased (95%)
- positive antimitochondrial antibodies (AMA) in 85–100%

√ normal extrahepatic ducts
√ cholelithiasis in 35–39%
√ hepatomegaly (50%)
√ tortuous intrahepatic ducts with narrowing + caliber variation / decreased arborization = "tree-in-winter" appearance

NUC:
√ marked prolongation of hepatic Tc-99m IDA clearance
√ uniform hepatic isotope retention
√ normal visualization of GB and major bile ducts in 100%

DDx: (1) Sclerosing cholangitis (young men)
(2) CBD obstruction

Prognosis: mean survival 6 (range 3–11) years after onset of cholestatic symptoms

CLONORCHIASIS

Rarely of clinical significance

Country: Japan, Korea, Central + South China, Taiwan, Indochina

Organism: Chinese liver fluke = Clonorchis sinensis

Cycle: parasite cysts digested by gastric juice, larvae migrate up the bile ducts, remain in small intrahepatic ducts until maturity (10–30 mm in length), travel to larger ducts to deposit eggs

Infection: snail + freshwater fish serve as intermediate hosts; infection occurs by eating raw fish; hog, dog, cat, man are definite hosts

Path: (a) desquamation of epithelial bile duct lining with adenomatous proliferation of ducts + thickening of duct walls (inflammation, necrosis, fibrosis)
(b) bacterial superinfection with formation of liver abscess

- remittent incomplete obstruction + bacterial superinfection

√ multiple crescent- / stiletto-shaped filling defects within bile ducts

Cx: (1) Bile duct obstruction (conglomerate of worms / adenomatous proliferation)
(2) Calculus formation (stasis / dead worms / epithelial debris)
(3) Jaundice in 8% (stone / stricture / tumor)
(4) Generalized dilatation of bile ducts (2%)

CONGENITAL BILIARY ATRESIA

Etiology: ? variation of same infectious process as in neonatal hepatitis with additional component of sclerosing cholangitis or vascular injury

Histo: proliferation of bile ducts in all portal triads

In 15% associated with: polysplenia, trisomy 18

NUC [phenobarbital-augmented cholescintigraphy] (90–97% sensitivity, 63–94% specificity, 90% accuracy):

} preparation of patient with 5 ng/kg/d phenobarbital twice a day for 3–7 days to stimulate biliary secretion (via induction of hepatic enzymes + increase in conjugation + excretion of bilirubin)

√ good hepatic activity within 5 min
√ delayed clearance from cardiac blood pool
√ NO biliary excretion
√ NO visualization of bowel on delayed images at 6 and 24 hours
√ increased renal excretion

DDx: severe hepatocellular dysfunction

US:

√ normal (visualization of gallbladder in 20%)

Rx: Kasai procedure (= portoenterostomy)
(a) child <60 days of age: 90% success rate
(b) child between 60 and 90 days of age: 50% success rate
(c) child >90 days of age: 17% success rate

CONGENITAL HEPATIC FIBROSIS

= congenital cirrhosis with rapid + fatal progression

Histo: fibrous tissue within hepatic parenchyma with excess numbers of distorted terminal interlobular bile ducts + cysts which rarely communicate with bile ducts

Age: usually present in childhood resulting in early death

Associated with: autosomal recessive type of polycystic kidney disease, medullary sponge kidney (80%)

• hepatosplenomegaly, portal hypertension
• predisposed to cholangitis + calculi

√ "lollipop-tree" = ectasia of peripheral biliary radicles
√ hepatosplenomegaly
√ periportal fibrosis + portosystemic collaterals

Cx: portal hypertension, hepatocellular carcinoma, cholangiocellular carcinoma

DUCTECTATIC MUCINOUS TUMOR OF PANCREAS

= MUCIN-HYPERSECRETING CARCINOMA
= rare intraductal tumor typified by voluminous mucin secretions

Site: (a) main duct tumor causes diffuse segmental dilatation of the entire main pancreatic duct
(b) branch duct tumor causes focal dilatation of affected branches; mainly in uncinate process

• endoscopy: inspissated mucus spilling out of a dilated hepatopancreatic ampulla

√ mass usually in uncinate portion of pancreatic head
√ cystic dilatation of pancreatic duct surrounded by thin rim of normal pancreatic parenchyma
√ grapelike clusters of cysts containing thick mucinous secretions

Prognosis: better than pancreatic adenocarcinoma

ECHINOCOCCAL DISEASE

Echinococcus Granulosus

= HYDATID DISEASE
= E. cysticus (more common); man is accidental host
(a) pastoral (European) form: dog is definite host; intermediate hosts are cattle, sheep, horses, hogs; endemic in sheep-raising countries: Australia, New Zealand, North + East Africa, USSR, Mediterranean countries, Near + Middle East countries, Japan, Argentina, Chile, Uruguay
(b) sylvatic (northern) form: wolf is definite host; intermediate hosts are deer, moose; endemic in northwestern Canada, Alaska

Cycle: ingestion of contaminated material (eggs passed in feces of dog / other carnivore); eggs hatch in duodenum; larvae penetrate intestinal wall + mesenteric venules; larvae carried into portal circulation; larvae are filtered in capillaries of liver > lung > other organs

Organs: liver (73%); lung (14%); peritoneum (12%); kidney (6%); spleen (4%); spinal cord; brain; bladder; thyroid; prostate; heart; orbit (1–20%); bone

Histo:

A. ENDOCYST (parasitic component of capsule)
= inner GERMINATIVE LAYER (resembling wet tissue paper) giving rise to brood capsules which may remain attached to cyst wall harboring up to 400,000 scolices / may detach + form sediment in cyst fluid = "hydatid sand" / may break up into numerous self-contained daughter cysts

B. ECTOCYST = CYST MEMBRANE = laminated chitinlike substance secreted by parasite

C. PERICYST = highly vascularized adventitial layer (resembling egg white), organized host granulation tissue replaces tissue necrosis (due to compression of expanding cyst), marginal vascular rim of 0.5–4 mm

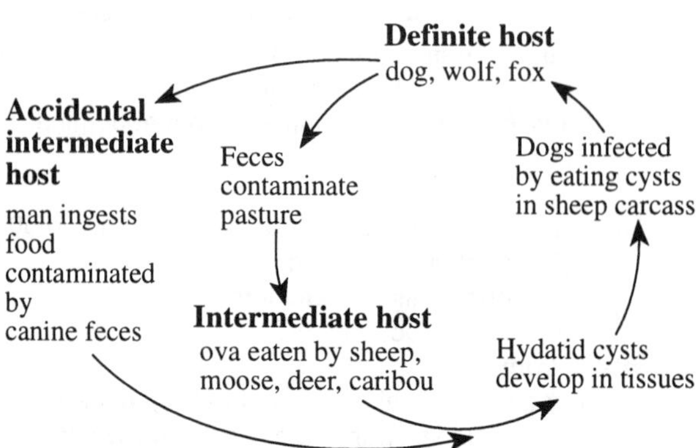

Parasitic Cycle of Echinococcus Granulosus

LIVER

- pain / asymptomatic
- recurrent jaundice + biliary colic (transient obstruction by membrane fragments + daughter cysts expelled into biliary tree)
- blood eosinophilia (20–50%)
- urticaria + anaphylaxis (following rupture)
- Tests:
  1. Casoni intradermal test (60% sensitivity; may be falsely positive)
  2. Complement fixation double diffusion (65% sensitivity)
  3. Immunoelectrophoresis (most specific)
  4. Indirect hemagglutination (85% sensitivity)

Time to diagnosis: 11–81 (mean 51) years

Location: right lobe > left lobe of liver; multiple cysts in 20%

Size: up to 50 cm (average size of 5 cm), up to 16 liters of fluid

Plain film:
- √ may have peripheral crescentic / curvilinear / polycyclic calcifications (10–33%), located in pericyst
  - ◊ The presence of calcifications does not imply death of parasite!
- √ pneumohydrocyst (infection / communication with bronchial tree)

US:
- √ complex heterogeneous mass (most common)
- √ well-defined anechoic cyst (common)
- √ "racemose" appearance = multiseptated cyst = daughter cysts internally and tangent to mother cyst (characteristic, but rare)
- √ floating undulating membrane / vesicles = separation of laminated membrane from pericyst (characteristic, but rare)
  - ◊ Floating membrane does not indicate death of parasite!
- √ mass with eggshell calcification (least common)

CT:
- √ well-demarcated low-density round masses of fluid attenuation ± internal septations
- √ enhancement of cyst wall + septations

MR:
- √ hypointense rim surrounding multiloculated cyst

Angio:
- √ avascular area with splaying of arteries
- √ halo of increased density around cyst (inflammation / compressed liver)

Cholangiography:
- √ cyst may communicate with bile ducts: right hepatic duct (55%), left hepatic duct (29%), CHD (9%), gallbladder (6%), CBD (1%)

Percutaneous aspiration:
- fluid analysis positive for hydatid disease in 70% (fragments of laminated membrane in 54%; scolices in 15%; hooklets in 15%)
- ◊ Risk of anaphylactic shock (0.5%), asthma (3%), implantation of spilled protoscoleces

Cx: (1) Compression of vital structures
(2) Infection
(3) Rupture (25–90%)
  (a) contained = rupture of laminated membrane with cyst contents contained within pericyst
  (b) communicating = cyst contents escapes through biliary / bronchial tree
  (c) direct = tear of endocyst + ectocyst + pericyst with cyst contents spilling into pleural / peritoneal cavity (anaphylaxis, metastatic hydatidosis)

Rx: (1) Surgery (in 10% recurrence)
(2) Anthelmintics (albendazole, medendazole)
(3) Injection of scolecidal agents (silver nitrate, 20 / 30% hypertonic saline solution, 0.5% cetrimide solution, 95% ethanol)

Echinococcus multilocularis

= E. alveolaris = less common but more aggressive form of echinococcal disease

Primary host: fox, wolf

Secondary host: rodents (moles, lemmings, wild mice); domestic cat; dog

Endemic to: eastern France, southern Germany, western Austria, much of Soviet Union, Japan, Alaska, Canada, some areas in Turkey

Infection: eating wild fruits contaminated with fox / wolf feces; direct contact with fox / wolf; contact with dogs / cats that have ingested infested rodents

Path: larvae proliferate by exogenous extension + penetration of surrounding tissue (= diffuse + infiltrative process resembling malignancy); chronic granulomatous reaction with central necrosis, cavitation, calcification

Histo: daughter cysts with thick lamellar wall arising on outer surface of original cyst, rarely containing scolices

Location: liver (access via portal vein); widespread hematogenous dissemination is not uncommon

- clinical manifestation 5–20 years after ingestion
- abdominal discomfort, jaundice, hepatomegaly
- eosinophilia

- √ aggressive growth pattern
  - √ geographic infiltrating lesion with ill-defined margins
  - √ invasion of IVC, diaphragm
  - √ metastases to lung, heart, brain (in 10%)
- √ faint / dense amorphous / nodular / flame-shaped calcifications (dystrophic calcifications scattered throughout necrotic + granulomatous tissue)

US:
- √ echogenic geographic ill-defined single / multiple solid masses
- √ ± irregular cystic areas
- √ propensity of spread to liver hilum

CT:
- √ heterogeneous hypodense poorly marginated infiltrating masses
- √ pseudocystic necrotic regions of near water density surrounded by hyperdense solid component
- √ little / no enhancement

Angio:
- √ intrahepatic arterial tapering + obstruction

Cx: Budd-Chiari syndrome, IVC thrombosis, portal hypertension

Prognosis: fatal within 10–15 years (if left untreated)

DDx: hepatocellular carcinoma (biopsy!), large hemangioma (characteristic enhancement pattern), metastasis, epithelial hemangioendothelioma

EPIDERMOID CYST OF SPLEEN

= EPITHELIAL CYST = PRIMARY CYST OF SPLEEN

Cause: infolding of peritoneal mesothelium / collection of peritoneal mesothelial cells trapped within splenic sulci

Histo: (1) mesothelial lining (2) squamous epithelial lining = epidermoid cyst = squamous metaplasia from embryonic inclusions within preexisting mesothelial surface epithelium

Age: 2nd–3rd decade (average age of 18 years)

May be associated with: polycystic kidney disease

(a) unilocular + solitary (80%)
(b) multiple + multilocular (20%)

- √ average size of 10 cm
- √ peripheral septations / cyst wall trabeculations (in 86%)
- √ curvilinear calcification in wall (9–25%)
- √ may contain cholesterol crystals, fat, blood

Cx: trauma, rupture, infection

EPITHELIOID HEMANGIOENDOTHELIOMA

= primary malignant vascular tumor of liver (soft tissue, bone, lung)

Age: average age of 45 years; M:F = 1:2

Possibly associated with: oral contraceptives, exposure to vinyl chloride

Path: multifocal nodules varying in size from a few mm to several cm involve both lobes of the liver (due to rapid perivascular extension); nodules may coalesce in liver periphery

Histo: dendritic spindle-shaped cells + epithelioid round cells in a matrix of myxoid + fibrous stroma; neoplastic endothelial cells invade sinusoids + terminal hepatic veins + portal veins cutting off the tumor's blood supply

- • in 80%: abdominal pain, weakness, anorexia, jaundice

Metastases to: spleen, mesentery, lymph nodes, lung, bone

- √ multiple nodules (nodular form)
- √ peripheral subcapsular growth (diffuse form) without deforming liver contour
- √ increased tumor vascularity
- √ hypertrophy of uninvolved liver

Plain film:
- √ hepatic calcifications (15%)

US:
- √ typically hypoechoic lesions (due to central core of myxoid stroma)

CT:
- √ low-attenuation masses on NECT, may become isoattenuating with rest of liver on CECT (due to vasoformative growth + compensatory hepatic arterial flow with portal vein occlusion)

Angio:
- √ hyper- and hypovascularity (dependent upon degree of sclerosis + hyalinization)
- √ invasion ± occlusion of portal + hepatic veins

NUC:
- √ decreased perfusion to central myxoid tumor portion + increased perfusion to cellular areas on sulfur colloid scan
- √ photopenic defect on static sulfur colloid scan
- √ NOT gallium avid

Prognosis: 20% die within 2 years, 20% survive for 5–28 years ± treatment

DDx of multiple nodules: metastatic disease

DDx of diffuse form: sclerosing carcinoma, vaso-occlusive disease

FATTY LIVER

= FATTY INFILTRATION OF THE LIVER = HEPATIC STEATOSIS

Cause:

A. METABOLIC DERANGEMENT
poorly controlled diabetes mellitus (50%), obesity, hyperlipidemia, acute fatty liver of pregnancy, protein malnutrition, parenteral hyperalimentation, malabsorption (jejunoileal bypass), glycogen storage disease, glycogen synthetase deficiency, cystic fibrosis, Reye syndrome, corticosteroids, severe hepatitis, trauma, congestive heart failure

B. HEPATOTOXINS
alcohol (>50%), carbon chlorides, phosphorus, amiodarone, chemotherapy

Histo: hepatocytes with large cytoplasmatic fat vacuoles containing triglycerides; >5% fat of total liver weight

- • NO abnormal liver function tests
- √ rapid change with time (few days to >10 months) depending on clinical improvement (abstinence from alcohol, improved nutrition) + degree of severity

Diffuse Fatty Infiltration

- √ hepatomegaly (75–80%) / normal sized liver

Plain film:
- √ radiolucent liver sign = enlarged radiolucent liver

US (sensitivity >90%, accuracy 85–97%):
- √ increased sound attenuation (scattering of sound beam) = poor definition of posterior aspect of liver
- √ fine (more typical) / coarsened hyperechogenicity (compared with kidney)
- √ impaired visualization of borders of hepatic vessels
- √ attenuation of sound beam (feature of fat, NOT fibrosis)

LIVER

CT:
- √ areas of lower attenuation than normal portal vein / IVC density
- √ reversal of liver-spleen density relationship (spleen is normally 6–12 HU below liver density)
- √ hyperdense intrahepatic vascular structures

NUC:
- Tc-99m sulfur colloid scan:
  - √ diffuse heterogeneous uptake (68%)
  - √ reversal of liver-spleen uptake (41%)
  - √ increased bone marrow uptake (41%)
- Xe-133 ventilation scan:
  - √ increased activity during washout phase (38%)

MR:
- √ slightly increased signal on T1WI + T2WI; relatively insensitive (10% fat by weight will alter SE signal intensities only by 5–15%)
- √ fat turns black with Dixon technique

FAT-SPARED AREA in diffuse fatty infiltration

Cause: direct drainage of systemic blood into liver

Location: (a) posterior edge of segment 4 = anterior to portal vein bifurcation (drainage of aberrant gastric vein)
(b) next to gallbladder bed (drainage of cystic vein)
(c) subcapsular skip areas

- √ hypoechoic ovoid / spherical / sheetlike mass
- √ NO mass effect (undisplaced course of vessels)

DDx: tumor mass

Focal fatty infiltration

Etiology: ? vascular origin, focal tissue hypoxia

Distribution: (a) lobar / segmental uniform lesions
(b) lobar / segmental nodular lesions
(c) perihilar lesions
(d) diffuse nodular lesions
(e) diffuse patchy lesions
predominantly in centrilobar + periportal regions, subcapsular distribution may be due to variants of blood supply (direct connections between peripheral portal radicles + perforating capsular / accessory cystic veins)

Location: right lobe, caudate lobe, perihilar region

- √ fan-shaped lobar / segmental distribution with angulated / interdigitating geographic margins
- √ lesions extend to periphery of liver
- √ NO mass effect (undisplaced course of vessels, no bulging of liver contour)

US:
- √ hyperechoic area with poorly defined / sharp margins
- √ multiple / rarely single echogenic nodules simulating metastases (rare)

CT:
- √ patchy areas of decreased attenuation ranging from -40 to +10 HU (DDx: liver tumor)
- √ NO contrast enhancement

MR (not sensitive for fat):
- √ high signal on T1WI + low / isointense signal on T2WI

NUC with colloid:
- √ no significant changes on sulfur colloid images (SPECT imaging may detect focal fatty infiltration)

DDx: primary / secondary hepatic tumor

FOCAL NODULAR HYPERPLASIA

= FNH = rare benign congenital hamartomatous malformation or reparative process in areas of focal injury; SPECIFIC DIAGNOSIS RARELY POSSIBLE

Cause: (?) congenital arteriovenous malformation triggers focal hepatocellular hyperplasia owing to a regional increase in blood flow
◊ Oral contraceptives DO NOT cause FNH, but exert a trophic effect on its growth!

Incidence: only 357 cases reported; 2nd most common benign tumor of liver; 4% of all primary hepatic tumors in pediatric population, 3–8% in adult population; twice as common as hepatocellular adenoma

Path: localized, well-delineated, usually solitary (80–95%), subcapsular mass of numerous small lobules within an otherwise normal liver; no true capsule; frequently central fibrous scar in area of interconnection of fibrous bands (HALLMARK) containing centrally an arterial malformation with spiderlike branches supplying the component nodules

Histo: composed of multiple spherical aggregates of hepatocytes often containing increased amounts of fat + triglycerides + glycogen; thick-walled arteries within fibrous septa radiating from the center toward the periphery; absent portal triads + central veins; bile duct proliferation within fibrous septa without connection to biliary tree; Kupffer cells; difficult differentiation from regenerative nodules of cirrhosis + hepatocellular adenoma

Age peak: 3rd–4th decade (range: 7 months to 75 years); M:F = 1:2–4

Associated with: hepatic hemangioma (in 23%), meningioma, astrocytoma, arterial dysplasia of other organs in case of multiple FNH

- • initially often asymptomatic (in 50–90% incidental finding)
- • vague abdominal pain (10–15%) due to mass effect
- • normal liver function
- • hepatomegaly / abdominal mass

- √ size <5 cm (in 85%); right lobe:left lobe = 2:1
- √ well-circumscribed, nonencapsulated nodular cirrhotic-like mass in an otherwise normal liver
- √ NO calcifications
- √ pedunculated mass (in 5–20%)
- √ multiple masses (in 20%)

NECT:
- √ iso- / slightly hypoattenuating homogeneous mass

LIVER

CECT:
- √ transient intense hyperdensity (after 30–60 sec) on bolus injection followed rapidly by isodensity
  - ◊ Lesion may be missed without precontrast study!
- √ hypodense central stellate scar = central fibrous core with radiating fibrous septa (15–33%) (DDx: fibrolamellar HCC)
- √ ± early enhancement of vessels traversing central scar
- √ hypodense mass during peak portal venous phase
- √ isodense mass following portal venous phase
- √ hyperdense central scar on delayed images (delayed washout of contrast from myxomatous scar tissue)

US:
- √ iso- / hypo- / hyperechoic (33%) homogeneous mass
- √ hyperechoic central scar in 18%
- √ displacement of hepatic vessels

Doppler:
- √ enlarged afferent blood vessel with central arterial hypervascularity + centrifugal filling to the periphery in "spoke-wheel" pattern
- √ large draining veins at tumor margins
- √ may show high-velocity Doppler signals with arterial pulsatility from arteriovenous shunts

NUC:

Sulfur colloid scan:
- √ normal uptake (50–70%), hot spot (7–10%)
  - ◊ Only FNH contains sufficient Kupffer cells to cause normal / increased uptake (almost PATHOGNOMONIC)!
- √ cold spot (30–50%) (DDx: hepatic adenoma, hemangioma, hepatoblastoma, liver herniation, hepatocellular carcinoma)

Tc-HIDA:
- √ normal / increased uptake (40–70%), cold spot (60%)

Tc-99m–tagged RBCs:
- √ increased uptake during early phase
- √ defect relative to liver on delayed images

MR:
- √ usually homogeneous signal intensity of lesion
- √ iso- to hypointense on T1WI (94–100%)
- √ slightly hyper- to isointense on T2WI (94–100%)
- √ atypically hyperintense lesion on T1WI in 6%
- √ central scar hypointense on T1WI
- √ central scar hyperintense on T2WI in 75% (due to vascular channels + edema) / hypointense in 25% (absent or minimal edema)

CEMR:
- √ dense enhancement in arterial phase
- √ isointense during portal venous phase
- √ hyperintense on delayed images
- √ late + prolonged enhancement of central scar
- √ occasionally prolonged enhancement (due to entrapment of Gd-DTPA by functioning hepatocytes inside tumor followed by 1% excretion into biliary tree)
- √ less uptake of IV superparamagnetic iron oxide than surrounding liver (uptake mechanism similar to that of sulphur colloid)

Angio:
- √ discretely marginated hypervascular mass (90%) with intense capillary blush / hypovascular (10%)
- √ enlargement of main feeding artery with central blood supply (= "spoke-wheel" pattern in 33%)
- √ homogeneous parenchymal stain
- √ decreased vascularity in central stellate fibrous scar

Rx: (1) Discontinuation of oral contraceptives
(2) Resection of pedunculated mass
(3) Diagnostic excisional biopsy for extensive tumor (FNH seldom requires surgery)

Cx: rarely rupture with hemoperitoneum (increased incidence in patients on oral contraceptives — 14%)

DDx:
1. Fibrolamellar carcinoma (scar calcified, metastases, retroperitoneal adenopathy, tumor hemorrhage + necrosis causing pain, hypointense scar on T2WI)
2. Hepatic adenoma (10 cm large tumor, symptomatic due to propensity for hemorrhage in 50%, central scar atypical)
3. Well-differentiated hepatocellular carcinoma (internal necrosis + hemorrhage, vascular invasion, metastases, rim-enhancement of pseudocapsule)
4. Giant cavernous hemangioma (larger tumor, may calcify, globular peripheral enhancement followed by centripetal filling, retention of contrast on delayed images, CSF-like behavior on MRI)
5. Hypervascular metastasis (hypovascular during portal venous phase, older patient)
6. Intrahepatic cholangiocarcinoma (less vascular, dominant large central scar, metastases)

GALLBLADDER CARCINOMA

Most common biliary cancer (9 x more common than extrahepatic bile duct cancer);
5th most common gastrointestinal malignancy (after colorectal, pancreatic, gastric, esophageal carcinoma);
3% of all intestinal neoplasms

Incidence: 0.4–4.6% of biliary tract operations; 6,500 deaths/year in United States

Peak age: 6–7th decade; M:F = 1:3–1:4
◊ 85% occur in 6th decade or later!

Histo: (a) well differentiated adenocarcinoma of scirrhous type (80–90%)
(b) anaplastic carcinoma, squamous cell carcinoma, adenoacanthoma (10–20%)
(c) carcinoid, sarcoma, basal cell carcinoma, lymphoma (extremely rare)

Staging:
- I mucosa only
- II mucosa + muscularis
- III mucosa + muscularis + serosa
- IV gallbladder wall + lymph nodes
- V hepatic / distant metastases

Predisposed: patients with porcelain gallbladder (22%); gallbladder polyp >2 cm is likely malignant

Associated with:
(1) Gallstones in 64–98%
◊ Gallbladder carcinoma occurs in only 1% of all patients with gallstones!
(2) Porcelain gallbladder (in 4–60%): prevalence of gallbladder carcinoma in 11–22% of autopsies
(3) Inflammatory bowel disease (predominantly ulcerative colitis, less common in Crohn disease)
(4) Familial polyposis coli
(5) Chronic cholecystitis
- history of past GB disease (50%)
- malaise, vomiting, weight loss
- RUQ pain (54–76%)
- obstructive jaundice (35–74%)
- abnormal liver function tests (20–75%)

Location: usually in body / fundus; rarely in cystic duct
Growth types:
√ focal (59%) / diffuse (41%) thickening of GB wall
√ polypoid / fungating intraluminal mass with wide base (14–25%)
√ replacement of gallbladder by mass (37–70%)
√ pericholecystic infiltration: in 76% focal, in 24% diffuse
√ dilatation of biliary tree (38–70%)
√ fine granular / punctate flecks of calcification (mucinous adenocarcinoma)
OCG:
√ nonvisualization of gallbladder (2/3)
Metastases: in 75–77% at time of diagnosis
(a) direct invasion of liver (34–89%), duodenum (12%), colon (9%), stomach, bile duct, pancreas, right kidney, abdominal wall
(b) lymphatic spread (26–41–75%): porta hepatis, portacaval, lesser omental, superior + posterior pancreaticoduodenal, paraaortic nodes
(c) intraperitoneal seeding (common)
(d) hematogenous spread (less common): liver, lung, bones
(e) neural spread (frequent): associated with more aggressive tumors
(f) intraductal spread (least common): particularly in papillary adenocarcinoma

Cx: perforation of gallbladder + abscess formation
√ gallstones located within abscess
Prognosis: 75% unresectable at presentation; average survival is 6 months; 5% 1-year survival rate; 6% 5-year survival rate

DDx: (1) Xanthogranulomatous cholecystitis (lobulated mass filling gallbladder + stones)
(2) Acute / chronic cholecystitis (generalized gallbladder wall thickening <10 mm)
(3) Liver tumor invading gallbladder fossa
(4) Tumors from adjacent organs (pancreas, duodenum)
(5) Metastases (melanoma, leukemia, lymphoma)
(6) Polyps: cholesterol polyp, hyperplastic polyp, granulation polyp
(7) Adenomyomatosis

GLYCOGEN STORAGE DISEASE

= autosomal recessive diseases with varying severity and clinical syndromes

A. VON GIERKE DISEASE (TYPE I)
Etiology: defect in glucose-6-phosphatase with excess deposition of glycogen in liver, kidney, intestines
Dx: failure of rise in blood glucose after glucagon administration
Age at presentation: infancy
√ hepatomegaly
US:
√ increased echogenicity (glycogen / fat)
CT:
√ increased (glycogen) / normal / decreased (fat) parenchymal attenuation
Prognosis: death in infancy, may survive into adulthood with early therapy
Cx: (1) Hepatic adenoma
(2) Hepatocellular carcinoma

B. POMPE DISEASE (TYPE II)
= abnormal metabolism with enlargement of myocardial cells due to glycogen deposition; similar to endocardial fibroelastosis
Etiology: defect in lysosomal glucosidase
√ massive cardiomegaly with CHF
√ hepatomegaly
Prognosis: sudden death in 1st year of life (due to conduction abnormalities); survival rarely beyond infancy

C. CORI DISEASE (TYPE III)
D. ANDERSEN DISEASE (TYPE IV)
E. McARDLE DISEASE (TYPE V)
F. HERS DISEASE (TYPE VI)

HEMOCHROMATOSIS

= excess iron deposition in various parenchymal organs (liver, pancreas, spleen, kidneys, heart) leading to cirrhosis with portal hypertension [HEMOSIDEROSIS
= increased iron deposition without organ damage]

Cause: excess iron deposition from
(a) increased GI absorption:
1. Genetic hemochromatosis
2. Erythropoietic hemochromatosis
3. Bantu siderosis
(b) IV blood transfusion
(c) intravascular (extrasplenic) hemolysis

Genetic hemochromatosis

= IDIOPATHIC / PRIMARY HEMOCHROMATOSIS
= excessive absorption + parenchymal retention of dietary iron that favors accumulation within non-RES organs (liver, pancreas, heart, pituitary gland)

Cause: autosomal recessive disorder (human-leukocyte antigen[HLA]-linked abnormal gene located on short arm of chromosome 6) with mucosal defect in intestinal wall / increased absorption of intestinal iron

Prevalence: 1:220 whites of northern European ancestry; homozygote frequency up to 0.25–0.50%; heterozygote carriers >10%

Pathophysiology:
absorbed iron is selectively bound to transferrin; increased transferrin saturation in portal circulation favors selective iron uptake by periportal hepatocytes as initial site of iron accumulation; RES cells are incapable of storing excess iron

Path: excess iron stored as crystalline iron oxide (ferric oxyhydroxide) within cytoplasmic ferritin + lysosomal hemosiderin; iron overload affects parenchymal cells (liver, pancreas, heart) NOT Kupffer cells / RE cells of bone marrow + spleen (abnormal function of RES)

- asymptomatic during 1st decade of disease
- hyperpigmentation (90%)
- hepatomegaly (90%)
- arthralgias (50%)
- diabetes mellitus (30%) secondary to insulin resistance by hepatocytes + pancreatic b-cell damage from iron deposition
- CHF + arrhythmia (15%)
- loss of libido, impotence, amenorrhea, testicular atrophy, loss of body hair
- liver iron index > 2 (= liver iron concentration [micromoles per gram of dry weight] per patient's age)

CT (60% sensitivity for iron):
√ diffuse / rarely focal increase in liver density (up to 75–130 HU)
√ depiction of hepatic veins on NECT
√ dual energy CT (at 80 + 120 kVp) can quantitate amount of iron deposition

MR:
(skeletal muscle = good signal intensity reference)
√ significant signal loss in liver on T2WI with signal intensity equal to background noise
√ normal pancreatic signal intensity in noncirrhotics
√ pancreatic signal intensity equal to / less than muscle (in 90% of cirrhotic patients)
√ normal signal intensity of spleen (in 86%) due to abnormal RES function

Dx: liver biopsy

Cx: (1) Periportal fibrosis resulting in cirrhosis (if iron concentration >22,000 µg/g of liver tissue)
(2) Hepatocellular carcinoma (14–30%)
(3) Insulin-dependent diabetes mellitus (30–60%)
(4) Congestive cardiomyopathy (15%)

Rx: phlebotomies in precirrhotic stage

Prognosis: normal life expectancy with early diagnosis and treatment

Secondary hemochromatosis

Cause:
(1) Erythrogenic hemochromatosis = increased absorption of iron secondary to erythroid hyperplasia in ineffective erythropoiesis (eg, thalassemia, NOT in sickle cell anemia)
Path: no excess Kupffer cell iron
(2) Bantu siderosis = excessive dietary iron from food preparation in iron containers (Kaffir beer)
(3) Transfusional iron overload = patients receiving > 40 units of blood (iron storage capacity of RES = 10 g of iron)

Path: iron deposition initially in RES (phagocytosis of intact RBC) with sparing of parenchymal cells of pancreas; after saturation of RES storage capacity parenchymal cells of other organs accumulate iron (liver, pancreas, myocardium)

Age: 4–5th decade; M:F = 10:1

- little clinical significance

MR:
√ signal loss in liver on T2WI with signal intensity greater than background noise (iron in Kupffer cells)
√ splenic signal intensity less than muscle

HEPATIC ABSCESS

= localized collection of pus in the liver resulting from any infectious process with destruction of the hepatic parenchyma + stroma

Types: pyogenic (88%), amebic (10%), fungal (2%)

Location: multiple in 50%

√ hepatomegaly
√ elevation of right hemidiaphragm
√ pleural effusion
√ right lower lobe atelectasis / infiltration
√ gas within abscess (esp. Klebsiella)

MR:
√ hypointense on T1WI + hyperintense on T2WI (72%)
√ perilesional edema (35%)
√ "double target sign" on T2WI = hyperintense center (fluid) + hypointense sharply marginated inner ring (abscess wall) + hyperintense poorly marginated ring (perilesional edema)
√ rim enhancement (86%)

Pyogenic liver abscess

Organisms: E. coli, aerobic streptococci, St. aureus, anaerobic bacteria (45%)

Incidence: 0.016%

Etiology: (1) Ascending cholangitis from obstructive biliary tract disease (malignant / benign)
(2) Portal phlebitis (suppurative appendicitis, colitis, diverticular disease)
(3) Infarction from embolism / septicemia
(4) Indwelling arterial catheters
(5) Direct spread from contiguous infection (cholecystitis, peptic ulcer, subphrenic sepsis)
(6) Trauma (rupture, penetrating wounds, biopsy, surgery)
(7) Cryptogenic in 45% (invasion of cysts / dead tissue by pyogenic intestinal flora)

Age: 6–7th decade; M > F

- pyrexia (79%)
- abdominal pain (68%)
- nocturnal sweating (43%)
- vomiting / malaise (39%)
- jaundice (0–20%)

- positive blood culture (50%)

Location: solitary abscess in right lobe (40–75%), in left lobe (2–10%); multiple abscesses in 10–34–73% (more often of biliary than hematogenous origin)

US:
- √ hypoechoic round lesion with well-defined mildly echogenic rim
- √ distal acoustic enhancement
- √ coarse clumpy debris / low-level echoes / fluid-debris level
- √ intensely echogenic reflections with reverberations (from gas) in 20–30%

CT:
- √ inhomogeneous hypodense single / multiloculated cavity
- √ "double target sign" = wall-enhancement + surrounding hypodense zone (6–30%)
- √ "cluster sign" = several abnormal foci within the same anatomic area; suggestive of biliary origin

NUC:
- √ photon-deficient area on sulfur colloid + IDA scan
- √ Ga-67 citrate uptake in 80%
- √ In-111 tagged WBC uptake is highly specific (since WBCs normally go to liver, may need sulfur colloid test for correlation)

Cx: (1) Septicemia
(2) Rupture into right subphrenic space
(3) Rupture into abdominal cavity
(4) Rupture into pericardium
(5) Empyema
(6) Common hepatic duct obstruction

Mortality: 20–80%; 100% if unrecognized / untreated

Amebic abscess

Organism: Entamoeba histolytica

Etiology: spread of viable amebae from colon to liver via portal system

Incidence: in 1–25% of intestinal amebiasis

Age: 3rd–5th decade; M:F = 4:1
- amebic dysentery
- amebic hepatitis (15%)

Location: liver abscess (right lobe) in 2–25%; systemic dissemination by invasion of lymphatics / portal system (rare); liver:lung:brain = 100:10:1

Size: 2–12 cm; multiple liver abscesses in 25%
- √ nodularity of abscess wall (60%)
- √ internal septations (30%)
- √ not gas-containing (unless hepatobronchial / hepatoenteric fistula present)

NUC:
- √ sensitivity of sulfur colloid scan is 98%
- √ photon-deficient area surrounded by rim of uptake on Ga-67 scan

Aspiration:
typically opaque reddish / dirty brown / pink material ("anchovy paste" / "chocolate sauce"), usually sterile, parasite confined to margin of abscess

Cx: (1) Diaphragmatic disruption (rare) is strongly suggestive of amebic abscess
(2) Fistulization into colon, right adrenal gland, bile ducts, pericardium

Rx: conservative treatment with chloroquine / metronidazole (Flagyl®)

HEPATIC ADENOMA

= HEPATOCELLULAR ADENOMA = LIVER CELL ADENOMA

= rare benign neoplasm, most frequent hepatic tumor in young women after use of contraceptive steroids

Path: no true capsule; pseudocapsule due to compression of liver tissue containing multiple large vessels; high incidence of hemorrhage + necrosis + fatty change; no scar

Histo: solitary spherical benign growth of hepatocytes; sheets of hepatocytes without portal veins or central veins; scattered thin-walled vascular channels + bile canaliculi; decrease in number of abnormally functioning Kupffer cells; hepatocytes contain increased amounts of glycogen ± fat

Age: young women in childbearing age; not seen in males unless on anabolic steroids

Associated with: oral contraceptives (2.5 x risk after 5-year use, 7.5 x risk after 9-year use, 25 x risk >9-year use), steroids, pregnancy, diabetes mellitus, type Ia glycogen storage disease (von Gierke) in 60%

◊ Pregnancy may increase tumor growth rate + lead to tumor rupture!

◊ Tumor remission may occur with dietary therapy leading to normal insulin, glucagon, and serum glucose levels

- asymptomatic (20%)
- RUQ pain as sign of mass effect (40%) / intratumoral or intraperitoneal hemorrhage (40%)
- hepatomegaly

Location: right lobe of liver in subcapsular location (75%)
- √ round well-circumscribed mass; between 6–30 cm in size (average size of 8–10 cm)
- √ intraparenchymal / pedunculated (in 10%)
- √ unusual "nodule-in-nodule" appearance in large tumors (DDx: hepatocellular carcinoma)

CT:
- √ round mass of decreased density; areas of necrosis (30–40%)
- √ hyperdense areas of fresh intratumoral hemorrhage (22–50%)
- √ transiently enhancing on arterial-phase images
- √ iso- / hypoattenuating on delayed-phase images

US:
- √ usually small well-demarcated solid echogenic / complex hyper- and hypoechoic heterogeneous mass with anechoic areas (if large)

MR:
- √ inhomogeneous on all pulse sequences (indistinguishable from HCC)
- √ often hyperintense areas on T1WI (due to presence of fat-laden hepatocytes / hemorrhage)

√ isointense (sheets of hepatocytes) and hyperintense areas (necrosis, hemorrhage) on T2WI

NUC:
- √ focal photopenic lesion on sulfur colloid scan (because lesion composed of hepatocytes + nonfunctioning Kupffer cells) surrounded by rim of increased uptake (due to compression of adjacent normal liver containing Kupffer cells); may show uptake equal to / slightly less than liver (23%)
- √ usually increased activity on HIDA scan
- √ NO gallium uptake

Angio:
- √ usually hypervascular mass
- √ homogeneous but not intense stain in capillary phase
- √ enlarged hepatic artery with feeders at tumor periphery (50%)
- √ hypo- / avascular regions (secondary to hemorrhage / necrosis)
- √ neovascularity

CAVE: percutaneous biopsy carries high risk of bleeding!

Cx: (1) Spontaneous hemorrhage with subcapsular hematoma / hemoperitoneum (41%)
(2) Malignant transformation (? contiguous development of hepatocellular carcinoma)
(3) Recurrence after resection

Rx: surgical resection (to prevent rupture)

DDx: hepatocellular carcinoma

HEPATIC ANGIOSARCOMA

= HEMANGIOENDOTHELIAL SARCOMA = KUPFFER CELL SARCOMA = HEMANGIOSARCOMA

Prevalence: 0.14–0.25 per million; <2% of all primary liver neoplasms; most common sarcoma of liver (followed by fibrosarcoma > malignant fibrohistiocytoma > leiomyosarcoma)

Etiology: (a) thorotrast = thorium dioxide (7–10%) with latent period of 15–24 years
(b) arsenic
(c) polyvinyl chloride (latent period of 4–28 years)

Associated with: hemochromatosis, von Recklinghausen disease

Path: (a) multifocal / multinodular lesions (71%) of up to >5 cm in size
(b) large solitary mass with hemorrhage + necrosis

Histo:
(a) vessels lined with malignant endothelial cells (eg, sinusoids) causing atrophy of surrounding liver
(b) vasoformative = forming poorly organized vessels
(c) forming solid nodules of malignant spindle cells

Age: 6–7th decade; M:F = 4:1

- abdominal pain, weakness, fatigue, weight loss
- spontaneous hemoperitoneum (27%)
- jaundice
- NO elevation of a-fetoprotein

Early metastases to:
lung, spleen (16%), porta hepatis nodes, portal vein, thyroid, peritoneal cavity, bone marrow (rapid metastatic spread)

- √ portal vein invasion
- √ hemorrhagic ascites

Plain film:
- √ circumferential displacement of residual thorotrast

NUC:
- √ single / multiple photopenic areas on sulfur colloid scan
- √ increased gallium uptake
- √ perfusion blood pool mismatch (initial decrease followed by slow increase in RBC concentration) as in hemangioma on 3-phase red blood cell scan

US:
- √ solid / mixed mass with anechoic areas (hemorrhage / necrosis)
- √ multiple nodules

CT:
- √ hypodense masses with high-density regions (hemorrhage) / low-attenuation regions (old hemorrhage / necrosis)
- √ striking peripheral enhancement on dynamic CT as in large hemangioma

MR:
- √ hypointense on T1WI + hyperintense on T2WI
- √ peripheral Gd-pentetate enhancement on T1WI

Angio:
- √ hypervascular stain around tumor periphery in late arterial phase with puddling; NO arterial encasement

CAVE: Biopsy may lead to massive bleeding in 16%! Opt for open rather than percutaneous biopsy!

Prognosis: rapid deterioration with median survival of 6 months (13 months under chemotherapy)

DDx for multiple lesions: metastases

DDx for single lesion: cavernous hemangioma

HEPATIC CYST

= second most common benign hepatic lesion

Prevalence: 2–7%; increasing with age

A. ACQUIRED HEPATIC CYST
secondary to trauma, inflammation, parasitic infestation, neoplasia

B. CONGENITAL HEPATIC CYST
= defective development of aberrant intrahepatic bile ducts

Incidence: liver cysts detected at autopsy in 50%; in 22% detected during life

Age of detection: 5th–8th decade

Histo: cysts surrounded by fibrous capsule + lined by columnar epithelium, related to bile ducts within portal triads; no communication with bile ducts

Associated with:
(1) Tuberous sclerosis
(2) Polycystic kidney disease (25–33% have liver cysts)
(3) Polycystic liver disease: autosomal dominant; M:F = 1:2; (50% have polycystic kidney disease)

LIVER

- hepatomegaly (40%); pain (33%); jaundice (9%)

Size of cyst: range from microscopic to huge (average 1.2 cm; in 25% largest cyst <1 cm; in 40% largest cyst >4 cm; maximal size of 20 cm); multiple cysts spread throughout liver (in 60%) / solitary cyst

√ "cold spot" on IDA, Ga-68, Tc-99m sulfur colloid scans
√ echo-free cyst, may show fluid-fluid interface

Rx: sclerosing with minocycline hydrochloride (Dose: 1 mg per 1-mL cyst content up to 500 mg in 10 mL of 0.9% saline + 10 mL 1% lidocaine) following contrast opacification of cyst to confirm absence of communication with biliary tree / leakage into peritoneal cavity

HEPATIC HEMANGIOMA

Cavernous hemangioma of liver

most common benign liver tumor (78%); second most common liver tumor after metastases

Incidence: 1–4%; autopsy incidence 0.4–7.3%; increased with multiparity

Cause: ? enlarging hamartoma present since birth, ? true vascular neoplasm

Age: rarely seen in young children; M:F = 1:5

Histo: large vascular channels filled with slowly circulating blood; lined by single layer of mature flattened endothelial cells separated by thin fibrous septa; no bile ducts; thrombosis of vascular channels common resulting in fibrosis + hemorrhage + myxomatous degeneration + calcifications

Associated with: (1) Hemangiomas in other organs
(2) Focal nodular hyperplasia
(3) Rendu-Osler-Weber disease

- asymptomatic if tumor small (50–70%)
- may present with spontaneous life-threatening hemorrhage if large (5%)
- hepatomegaly
- may enlarge during pregnancy
- abdominal discomfort + pain (from thrombosis in large hemangioma)
- Kasabach-Merritt syndrome (= hemangioma + thrombocytopenia) rare

Location: frequently peripheral / subcapsular in posterior right lobe of liver; 20% are pedunculated; multiple in 10–20%

Size: <4 cm (90%);
>10 cm = giant cavernous hemangioma

√ may have central area of fibrosis = areas of nonenhancement / nonfilling / cystic space (occurrence increases with age)
√ calcifications (phleboliths / septal calcifications) are extremely uncommon

US:
√ uniformly hyperechoic (60–70%) mass due to multiple interfaces created by blood-filled spaces separated by fibrous septa
√ inhomogeneous hypoechoic mass (up to 40%) in larger hemangiomas with well-defined thick / thin echogenic lobulated border due to hemorrhagic necrosis, scarring, myxomatous change centrally
√ homogenous (58–73%) / heterogeneous (fibrosis, thrombosis, hemorrhagic necrosis)
√ hypoechoic center possible
√ may show acoustic enhancement (37–77%)
√ unchanged in size / appearance (82%) on 1-to-6-year follow-up
√ no Doppler signals / signals with peak velocity of <50 cm/sec

CT (combination of precontrast images, good bolus, dynamic scanning):
√ well-circumscribed spherical / ovoid low-density mass
√ may have areas of higher / lower density within mass
√ typical pattern of low density on NECT + peripheral enhancement + complete fill-in on delayed images 3–30 minutes post IV bolus (55–89%)
√ peripheral (72%) / central (in 8%) / diffuse dense (in 8%) enhancement
√ complete (75%) / partial (24%) / no (2%) fill-in to isodensity in delayed phase

Angio (historical gold standard):
√ dense opacification of well-circumscribed, dilated, irregular, punctate vascular lakes / puddles in late arterial + capillary phase starting at periphery in ring- / C-shaped configuration
√ normal-sized feeders; AV shunting (very rare)
√ contrast persistence late into venous phase

NUC (95% accuracy with SPECT):
Indication: lesions >2 cm (detectable in 70–90%)
√ delayed filling on Tc-99m labeled RBC scans (dose of 15–20 mCi) with increased activity on delayed images at 1–2 hours
√ cold defect on sulfur colloid scans

MR (90–95% accuracy):
√ spheroid / ovoid (87%) mass with smooth well-defined lobulated margins (87%); no capsule
√ homogeneous internal architecture if <4 cm, hypointense internal inhomogeneities if >4 cm (due to fibrosis)
√ hypo- / isointense on T1WI; hyperintense "light bulb" appearance on T2WI (due to slow flowing blood) (DDx: hepatic cyst, hypervascular tumor, necrotic tumor, cystic neoplasm)
√ uniform enhancement at 1 second in 40% of small hemangiomas <1.5 cm after gadolinium-DTPA
√ peripheral nodular enhancement progressing centripetally with centrally uniform enhancement (50%) / persistent hypointensity (30%)

Bx: may be biopsied safely provided normal liver is present between tumor + liver capsule
√ nonpulsatile blood (73%)

√ endothelial cells without malignancy (27%)

Prognosis: no growth when <4 cm in diameter; giant cavernous hemangiomas may enlarge

LIVER

Cx (rare): (1) Spontaneous rupture (4.5%)
(2) Abscess formation
(3) Kasabach-Merritt syndrome (platelet sequestration)

DDx: hypervascular malignant neoplasm / metastasis (quick homogeneous filling during arterial phase of small hemangiomas)

Infantile hemangioendothelioma of liver

= INFANTILE HEPATIC HEMANGIOMA = CAPILLARY / CAVERNOUS HEMANGIOMA
= most common benign hepatic tumor during first 6 months of life

Histo: multiple anastomosing thick-walled vascular spaces similar to cavernous hemangioma lined by plump endothelial cells in single or (less often) multiple cell layers; areas of extramedullary hematopoiesis / thrombi; scattered bile ducts; involutional changes (infarction, hemorrhage, necrosis, scarring)

Classification:
(a) Hemangioendothelioma type 1 (more common): orderly proliferation of small blood vessels
(b) Hemangioendothelioma type 2: more aggressive histologic pattern
DDx: angiosarcoma
(c) Cavernous hemangioma: dilated vascular spaces lined by flat endothelial cells
◊ Relationship to adult cavernous hemangioma unknown!

Age at presentation: <6 months in 85%, during 1st month in 33%, >1 year in 5%; M:F = 1:1.4–1:2

- abdominal mass secondary to hepatomegaly
- cutaneous hemangiomas (9–45–87%) occur with multinodular form
- may present with high-output CHF secondary to AV shunts within tumor (8 –15–25%)
- **Kasabach-Merritt syndrome** (in 11%)
  = hemorrhagic diathesis due to platelet sequestration by tumor / disseminated intravascular coagulopathy; characterized by an association of hemangioma, or hemangioendothelioma, or angiosarcoma with thrombocytopenia and purpura)
- hemolytic anemia

Size: several mm up to 20 cm (average size of 3 cm)

√ diffuse involvement of entire liver, rarely focal
√ single mass (50%) / multiple masses (50%)
√ enlargement of celiac + hepatic arteries + proximal aorta
√ rapid decrease in aortic caliber below celiac trunk
√ enlarged hepatic veins (increased venous flow)

Plain film:
√ fine speckled / fibrillary calcifications in 16% (DDx: hepatoblastoma, hamartoma, metastatic neuroblastoma)

US:
√ predominantly hypoechoic / complex / hyperechoic lesion
√ multiple sonolucent areas (= enlarging vascular channels secondary to initial rapid growth) (DDx: mesenchymal hamartoma)

OB-US:
√ polyhydramnios + fetal hydrops

CT:
√ focal areas of low attenuation
√ early peripheral enhancement (72%)
√ variable delayed central enhancement (similar to cavernous hemangioma)

MR:
√ heterogeneous hypointense multinodular lesion on T1WI ± hyperintense areas of hemorrhage
√ varying degrees of hyperintensity on T2WI (resembling adult hemangioma)
√ decreasing signal intensity with fibrotic replacement on T2WI

NUC (sulfur colloid, tagged RBC):
√ increased flow in viable portions of lesion during angiographic phase
√ increased activity mixed with central photopenic areas (hemorrhage, necrosis, fibrosis) on delayed tagged RBC images
√ photopenic defect on delayed sulfur colloid images

Angio:
√ enlarged, tortuous feeding arteries and stretched intrahepatic vessels
√ hypervascular tumor with inhomogeneous stain; clusters of small abnormal vessels
√ pooling of contrast material in sinusoidal lakes with rapid clearing through early draining veins (AV shunting)

Prognosis: rapid growth in first 6 months followed by tendency to involute within 6–8 months; 32–75% survival rate in complicated cases

Cx: (1) Congestive heart failure
(2) Hemorrhagic diathesis
(3) Obstructive jaundice
(4) Hemoperitoneum (rupture of tumor)

Rx: (1) No treatment if asymptomatic
(2) Reduction in size with steroids / radiotherapy / chemotherapy
(3) Embolization
(4) Surgical resection / liver transplantation

DDx: (1) Hepatoblastoma (>1 year of age, elevated α-fetoprotein, more heterogeneous)
(2) Mesenchymal hamartoma (usually multilocular cystic mass)
(3) Metastatic neuroblastoma (elevated catecholamines in urine, adrenal mass, nonenhancing multiple liver masses)

HEPATITIS

Acute hepatitis

- markedly elevated AST + ALT
- increase in serum-conjugated bilirubin

Viral Markers of Hepatitis

Virus	Tests	Interpretation
HAV	Anti-HAV IgM	acute hepatitis (can remain positive for >1 year)
	Anti-HAV IgG	past hepatitis, lifelong immunity
HBV	HBsAg	acute / chronic disease
	Anti-HBc IgM	acute infection (if titer high); chronic infection (if titer low)
	Anti-HBc IgG	past / recent HBV contact (may be only serum indicator of past infection)
	HBe	active viral replication
	Anti-HBe	low / absent replicative state (typically present in long-standing HBV carriers)
	Anti-HBs	imunity after vaccination
	HBV-DNA	active viral replication
HCV	Anti-HCV	past / current infection
	RIBA	test for various viral components
	HCV-RNA	active viral replication
HDV	Anti-HDV IgM	acute / chronic infection
	Anti-HDV IgG	chronic infection (if titer high + IgM positive); past infection if titer low + IgM negative)
	HDV-RNA	active viral replication
HEV	Anti-HEV IgM	acute hepatitis
	Anti-HEV IgG	past hepatitis
	HEV-RNA	viral replication

US:
- √ diffusely decreased parenchymal echogenicity
- √ increased brightness of portal triads ("starry sky" pattern) = centrilobular pattern (DDx: leukemic infiltrate, diffuse lymphomatous involvement, toxic shock syndrome)
- √ edema of gallbladder fossa
- √ thickening + increase in echogenicity of fat within falciform ligament, ligamentum venosum, porta hepatis, periportal connective tissue

Chronic hepatitis

= process present for at least 6 months

Diseases: autoimmune hepatitis; hepatitis B, C, D; cryptic hepatitis; chronic drug hepatitis; primary biliary cirrhosis; primary sclerosing cholangitis; Wilson disease; α-1-antitrypsin deficiency

US:
- √ increased liver echogenicity
- √ coarsening of parenchymal texture
- √ silhouetting of portal vein walls = loss of definition of portal venules
- √ NO sound attenuation

Cx: cirrhosis (10% for hepatitis B; 20–50% for hepatitis C)

HEPATOBLASTOMA

Incidence: 3rd most common abdominal tumor in children; most frequent malignant hepatic tumor in children (51%)

Incidence increased with: hemihypertrophy, Beckwith syndrome

Histo: (a) epithelial type = small cells resembling embryonal / fetal liver
(b) mixed type = epithelial cells + mesenchymal cells (osteoid, cartilaginous, fibrous tissue)

Age: <3 years; <18 months (in 50%); peak age between 18 and 24 months; range from newborn to 15 years; M:F = 2:1

- upper abdominal mass, weight loss, nausea, vomiting
- precocious puberty (production of endocrine substances)
- persistently + markedly elevated α-fetoprotein (66%)

Metastases to: lung (frequent)

Location: right lobe of the liver

- √ usually solitary mass with an average size of 10–12 cm
- √ coarse calcifications / osseous matrix (12–30%)

US:
- √ large heterogeneous echogenic mass, sometimes with calcifications, occasionally cystic areas (necrosis / extramedullary hematopoiesis)

CT:
- √ hypointense tumor with peripheral rim enhancement

MR:
- √ inhomogeneously hypointense on T1WI with hyperintense foci (hemorrhage)
- √ inhomogeneously hyperintense with hypointense bands (fibrous septa) on T2WI

NUC:
- √ photopenic defect

Angio:
- √ hypervascular mass with dense stain
- √ marked neovascularity; NO AV-shunting
- √ vascular lakes may be present
- √ avascular areas (secondary to tumor necrosis)
- √ may show caval involvement (= unresectable)

Prognosis: 60% resectable; 75% mortality; better prognosis than hepatoma; better prognosis for epithelial type than mixed type

DDx: hemangioendothelioma (fine granular calcifications), metastatic neuroblastoma, mesenchymal hamartoma, hepatocellular carcinoma (>5 years of age, no calcifications)

HEPATOCELLULAR CARCINOMA

= HEPATOMA = most frequent primary visceral malignancy in the world; 80–90% of all primary liver malignancies; 2nd most frequent malignant hepatic tumor in children (39%) after hepatoblastoma

Incidence: (a) in industrialized world: 0.2–0.8%
(b) in sub-Saharan Africa, Southeast Asia, Japan, Greece, Italy: 5.5–20%

Peak age: (a) industrialized world: 6th–7th decade; M:F = 2.5:1; fibrolamellar subtype (in 3–10%) below age 40 years

LIVER

(b) high incidence areas: 30–40 years; M:F = 5:1
(c) in children: >5 years of age; M:F = 4:3

Etiology:
1. Cirrhosis (60–90%)
   Latent period: 8 months to 14 years from onset of cirrhosis
   Incidence of HCC:
   — 44% in macronodular (= postnecrotic) cirrhosis due to hepatitis B virus, alcoholism, hemochromatosis
   — 6% in micronodular cirrhosis due to alcoholism
   ◊ 5% of alcoholic cirrhotics develop HCC!
   (a) alcohol (c) cardiac
   (b) hemochromatosis (d) biliary atresia
2. Chronic hepatitis B / C; 12% develop HCC
3. Carcinogens
   (a) aflatoxin (b) siderosis (c) thorotrast
   (d) oral contraceptives / anabolic androgens
4. Inborn errors of metabolism
   (a) α-1-antitrypsin deficiency
   (b) galactosemia
   (c) type I glycogen storage disease (von Gierke)
   (d) Wilson disease
   (e) tyrosinosis

mnemonic: "WHAT causes HCC?"
Wilson disease
Hemochromatosis
Alpha-1-antitrypsin deficiency
Tyrosinosis
Hepatitis
Cirrhosis (alcoholic, biliary, cardiac)
Carcinogens (aflatoxin, sex hormones, thorotrast)

Histo: HCC cells resemble hepatocytes in appearance + structural pattern (trabecular, pseudoglandular = acinar, compact, scirrhous);
(a) expansive encapsulated HCC: collapsed portal vein branches at capsule
(b) infiltrative nonencapsulated HCC: portal venules communicate with tumoral sinusoids = often invasion of portal ± hepatic veins

GROWTH PATTERN:
(a) solitary massive (27–50–59%): bulk in one (most often right) lobe with satellite nodules
(b) multicentric small nodular (15–25%): small foci of usually <2 cm (up to 5 cm) in both hepatic lobes
(c) diffuse microscopic (10 - 15–26%): tiny indistinct nodules closely resembling cirrhosis

Vascular supply: hepatic artery, portal vein in 6%

• elevated a-fetoprotein (75–90%), negative in cholangiocarcinoma
• elevated liver function tests
• persistent RUQ pain, hepatomegaly, ascites
• fever, weight loss, malaise
• Paraneoplastic syndromes:
  (a) sexual precocity / gynecomastia
  (b) hypercholesterolemia
  (c) erythrocytosis (tumor produces erythropoietin)
  (d) hypoglycemia
  (e) hypercalcemia
  (f) carcinoid syndrome

Metastases to: lung (most common = 8%), adrenal, lymph nodes, bone

√ portal vein invasion (25–33–48%)
√ arterioportal shunting (4–63%)
√ invasion of hepatic vein (16%) / IVC (= Budd-Chiari syndrome)
√ occasionally invasion of bile ducts
√ calcifications in ordinary HCC (2–9–25%); however, common in fibrolamellar (30–40%) and sclerosing HCC
√ hepatomegaly and ascites
√ tumor fatty metamorphosis (2–17%)

NUC:
√ Sulfur colloid scan: single cold spot (70%), multiple defects (15–20%), heterogeneous distribution (10%)
√ Tc-HIDA scan: cold spot / atypical uptake in 4% (delayed images)
√ Gallium-scan: avid accumulation in 70–90% (in 63% greater, in 25% equal, in 12% less uptake than liver)

CT (sensitivity of 63% in cirrhosis, 80% without cirrhosis):
√ hypodense mass / rarely isodense / hyperdense in fatty liver
  √ dominant mass with satellite nodules
  √ mosaic pattern = multiple nodular areas with differing attenuation on CECT (up to 63%)
  √ diffusely infiltrating neoplasm
√ encapsulated HCC = circular zone of radiolucency surrounding the mass (12–32–67%)

False-positive: confluent fibrosis, regenerative nodule

Biphasic CECT:
√ enhancement during hepatic arterial phase (80%)
√ decreased attenuation during portal venous phase with inhomogeneous areas of contrast accumulation
√ isodensity on delayed scans (10%)
√ thin contrast-enhancing capsule (50%) due to rapid washout
√ wedge-shaped areas of decreased attenuation (segmental / lobar perfusion defects due portal vein occlusion by tumor thrombus)

CT with intraarterial ethiodol injection:
√ hyperdense mass detectable as small as 0.5 cm US (86–99% sensitivity, 90–93% specificity, 50–94% accuracy):
√ hyperechoic HCC (13%) due to fatty metamorphosis or marked dilatation of sinusoids
√ hypoechoic HCC (26%) due to solid tumor
√ HCC of mixed echogenicity (61%) due to nonliquefactive tumor necrosis
√ Doppler peak velocity signals >250 cm/sec

MR:
√ hypointense (50%) / iso- to hyperintense (with fatty metamorphosis) on T1WI
√ ring sign = well-defined hypointense capsule on T1WI (24–44%), double layer of inner hypointensity (fibrous tissue) + outer hyperintensity (compressed blood vessels + bile ducts) on T2WI in expansive type of HCC

√ mildly hyperintense on T2WI
√ Gd-DTPA enhancement peripherally (21%) / centrally (7%) / mixed (10%) / no enhancement (21%)
√ improved lesion detectability after intravenous administration of superparamagnetic iron oxide

Angio:
√ "thread and streaks" = linear parallel vascular channels coursing along portal venous radicles seen with portal venous involvement
√ in differentiated HCC: enlarged arterial feeders, coarse neovascularity, vascular lakes, dense tumor stain, arterioportal shunts
√ in anaplastic HCC: vascular encasement, fine neovascularity, displacement of vessels + corkscrew-like vessels of cirrhosis

Prognosis: >90% overall mortality; 17% resectability rate; 6 months average survival time; 30% 5-year survival time
Cx: spontaneous rupture (in 8%)
Rx: (1) Resection (2) I-131 antiferritin IgG (remission rate >40% up to 3 years)
DDx: hepatocarcinoma, cholangiocarcinoma, focal nodular hyperplasia, hemangioma, hepatic adenoma

Fibrolamellar Hepatocellular Carcinoma

NO underlying cirrhosis or known risk factors
• α-fetoprotein negative
Age: 5–35 (mean 23) years; M:F = 1:1
Path: well-circumscribed strikingly desmoplastic tumor with calcifications + fibrous central scar
Histo: hepatocyte-like cells with granular eosinophilic cytoplasm growing in sheets / cords / trabeculae separated by broad bands of fibrous stroma arranged in parallel lamellae
√ partially / completely encapsulated solitary mass 4–17 cm in diameter
√ prominent central fibrous scar (45–60%)
√ central stellate / trabecular calcifications (30–55%)

CT:
√ mass of low attenuation + varying degrees of enhancement

MRI:
√ homogeneous mildly hypointense tumor on T1WI; slightly hyperintense on T2WI
√ hypointense central scar on T1WI + T2WI

Angio:
√ dense tumor stain without arterioportal shunting / neovascularity

Prognosis: 48% resectability rate; 32 months average survival time; 63% 5-year survival time
DDx: focal nodular hyperplasia (hyperintense central scar on T2WI)

HYPERPLASTIC CHOLECYSTOSIS

= variety of degenerative + proliferative changes of gallbladder wall characterized by hyperconcentration, hyperexcitability, and hyperexcretion
Incidence: 30–50% of all cholecystectomy specimens; M:F = 1:6

Cholesterolosis

= abnormal deposits of cholesterol esters in macrophages within lamina propria (foam cells) + in mucosal epithelium

1. STRAWBERRY GALLBLADDER
   = LIPID CHOLECYSTITIS = CHOLESTEROSIS
   = planar form = seedlike patchy / diffuse thickening of the villous surface pattern (disseminated micronodules)
   Associated with: cholesterol stones in 50–70%
   • not related to serum cholesterol level
   √ radiologically not demonstrable
2. CHOLESTEROL POLYP (90%)
   = polypoid form
   = abnormal deposit of cholesterol ester producing a villouslike structure covered with a single layer of epithelium and attached via a delicate stalk
   ◊ Most common fixed filling defect of GB
   Location: commonly in middle 1/3 of gallbladder
   √ multiple small filling defects <10 mm in diameter
   DDx: papilloma, adenopapilloma, inflammatory granuloma

Adenomyomatosis Of Gallbladder

= increase in number + height of mucosal folds
Histo: hyperplasia of epithelial + muscular elements with mucosal outpouching of epithelium-lined cystic spaces into (46%) or all the way through (30%) a thickened muscular layer as tubules / crypts / saccules (= intramural diverticula = Rokitansky-Aschoff sinus); develop with increasing age
Incidence: 5% of all cholecystectomies
Age: >35 years; M:F = 1:3
Associated with: (1) Gallstones in 25–75%
(2) Cholesterolosis in 33%

A. GENERALIZED FORM
   = **Adenomyomatosis**
   √ "pearl necklace gallbladder" = tiny extraluminal extensions of contrast on OCG (enhanced after contraction)
B. SEGMENTAL FORM
   compartmentalization most often in neck / distal 1/3
C. LOCALIZED FORM IN FUNDUS
   = **Adenomyoma**
   √ smooth sessile mass in GB fundus
   = solitary adenomyoma + extraluminal diverticula-like formation
D. ANNULAR FORM
   √ "hourglass" configuration of GB with transverse congenital septum

HYPOSPLENISM

= no uptake of Tc-99m sulfur colloid

A. ANATOMIC ABSENCE OF SPLEEN
   1. Congenital asplenia = Ivemark syndrome
   2. Splenectomy
B. FUNCTIONAL ASPLENIA
   = spleen anatomically present without uptake of Tc-99m sulfur colloid

1. Circulatory disturbances:
   occlusion of splenic artery / vein, hemoglobinopathies (sickle cell disease, hemoglobin-SC disease, thalassemia), polycythemia vera, idiopathic thrombocytopenic purpura
2. Altered RES activity:
   thorotrast irradiation, combined splenic irradiation + chemotherapy, replacement of RES by tumor / infiltrate, splenic anoxia (cyanotic congenital heart disease), sprue
3. Autoimmune disease
   Cx: children at risk for pneumococcal pneumonia (liver partially takes over immune response later in life)

C. FUNCTIONAL ASPLENIA + SPLENIC ATROPHY
Ulcerative colitis, Crohn disease, celiac disease, tropical sprue, dermatitis herpetiformis, thyrotoxicosis, idiopathic thrombocytopenic purpura, thorotrast

D. FUNCTIONAL ASPLENIA + NORMAL / LARGE SPLEEN
Sarcoidosis, amyloidosis, sickle cell anemia (if not infarcted)

• RBC (acanthocytes, siderocytes)
• lymphocytosis, monocytosis
• Howell-Jolly bodies (intraerythrocytic inclusions)
• thrombocytosis
√ spleen not visualized on Tc-99m sulfur colloid
√ Tc-99m heat-damaged RBCs / In-111 labeled platelets may demonstrate splenic tissue if Tc-99m sulfur colloid does not
Cx: increased risk of infection (pneumococcus, meningococcus, influenza)

LIPOMA OF LIVER

Extremely rare
• asymptomatic
May be associated with: tuberous sclerosis
US:
√ echogenic mass
√ striking acoustic refraction (sound velocity in soft tissue 1,540 m/sec, in fat 1,450 m/sec)
Prognosis: no malignant potential

LIVER TRANSPLANT

Indication: (a) in childhood: biliary atresia (52%), acute fulminant hepatic failure (11%), α-1-antitrypsin deficiency (9%), cryptogenic cirrhosis (6%), chronic active hepatitis (4%)

NORMAL POSTTRANSPLANT FINDINGS
(1) Periportal edema (21%)
Cause: ? lymphedema in early posttransplantation period, occasionally associated with acute rejection
√ "periportal collar" of low attenuation on CT + hyperechogenicity on US
(2) Fluid collection around falciform ligament (11%)

Vascular complications in liver transplant

1. Anastomotic narrowing of IVC / portal vein
   ◊ Discrepancies in caliber between donor + recipient vessel have no pathologic significance!
   • venous hypertension of lower part of body
   • portal hypertension
2. Thrombosis of IVC / portal vein
3. Hepatic artery stenosis (11–13%)
   Location: at / near anastomotic site
   √ marked focal increase in velocity >200–300 cm/sec + poststenotic turbulence
   √ intrahepatic tardus et parvus waveform = slowed systolic acceleration time (SAT >0.08 sec) distal to stenosis (73% sensitive)
   √ diminished pulsatility (RI <0.5) due to ischemia
4. Hepatic artery thrombosis (3–9–16% in adults, 9–19–42% in children)
   Time of onset: usually within first 2 months
   • Three types of clinical presentation:
   (1) fulminant hepatic necrosis + rapid deterioration
   (2) bile leak, bile peritonitis, bacteremia, sepsis
   (3) relapsing bacteremia
   √ absence of hepatic artery flow
   FP Doppler (10%):
   low flow state, small vessel size, severe liver edema (in first 72 hours after transplantation, viral hepatitis, rejection)
   FN Doppler: arterial collaterals
   √ multiple hypoechoic lesions in liver periphery (= infarcts)
   Mortality: 50–58%
5. Hepatic artery pseudoaneurysm

Parenchymal complications in liver transplant

1. Rejection
   ◊ Can ONLY be diagnosed with liver biopsy!
2. Infarction (10%)
   √ may calcify
   √ may liquefy developing into intrahepatic biloma
3. Graft infection

Biliary complications in liver transplant

Incidence: 13–25%
1. Biliary obstruction
   (a) stricture at anastomosis
   (b) tension mucocele of allograft cystic duct remnant
   √ extrinsic mass compressing CHD
   √ fluid collection adjacent to CHD
   (c) intrahepatic stricture
   as complication of arterial ischemia
2. Bile leak
   (a) anastomotic site: 70% within 1st month
   (b) T-tube exit site: 50% within 10 days
   (c) bile duct necrosis (hepatic artery occlusion)
   ◊ The intrahepatic biliary epithelium is perfused solely by the hepatic artery!
   (d) after liver biopsy
   (e) common hepatic duct leak
   Incidence: 4.3–23%

LYMPHOMA OF LIVER

A. Primary lymphoma (rare)
  √ solid solitary mass
B. Secondary lymphoma (common)
  autoptic incidence of liver involvement:
    60% in Hodgkin disease
    50% in non-Hodgkin lymphoma

Pattern:
  (a) infiltrative diffuse (most common): no alteration in hepatic architecture
  (b) focal nodular: detectable by cross-sectional imaging
  (c) combination of diffuse + nodular (3%)

Detection rate (for CT, MRI): <10%

MACROCYSTIC ADENOMA OF PANCREAS

= MUCINOUS CYSTIC NEOPLASM = MUCINOUS CYSTADENOMA / CYSTADENOCARCINOMA
= thick-walled uni- / multilocular low-grade malignant tumor composed of large mucin-containing cystic spaces

Frequency: 10% of pancreatic cysts; 1% of pancreatic neoplasms
Mean age: 50 years (range of 20–95 years); in 50% between 40–60 years;
M:F = 1:19
Path: large smooth round / lobulated multiloculated cystic mass encapsulated by a layer of fibrous connective tissue
Histo: similar to biliary and ovarian mucinous tumors; cysts lined by tall columnar, mucin-producing cells subtended by a densely cellular mesenchymal stroma (reminiscent of ovarian stroma), often in papillary arrangement, lack of cellular glycogen
  (a) mucinous cystadenoma
  (b) mucinous cystadenocarcinoma = stratified papillary epithelium
  ◊ All mucinous cystic neoplasms should be considered as malignant neoplasms of low-grade malignant potential

Location: often in pancreatic tail (90%) / body, infrequently in head

• asymptomatic
• abdominal pain, anorexia

√ well-demarcated thick-walled mass of 2–36 (mean 10–12) cm in diameter
√ multi- / unilocular large cysts >2 cm with thin septa <2 mm
  ◊ A tumor with <6 cysts of >2 cm in diameter is in 93–95% a mucinous cystic neoplasm!
√ solid papillary excrescences protrude into the interior of tumor (sign of malignancy)
√ amorphous discontinuous peripheral mural calcifications (10–15%)
√ hypovascular mass with sparse neovascularity
√ vascular encasement and splenic vein occlusion may be present
√ great propensity for invasion of adjacent organs

US:
  √ cysts may contain low-level echoes

CT:
  √ internal septations may not be visualized without contrast enhancement
  √ cysts with attenuation values of water; may have different levels of attenuation within different cystic cavities
  √ enhancement of cyst walls

Angio:
  √ predominantly avascular mass
  √ cyst wall + solid components may demonstrate small areas of vascular blush + neovascularity
  √ displacement of surrounding arteries + veins by cysts

Metastases:
  √ round thick-walled cystic lesions in liver

Prognosis: invariable transformation into cystadenocarcinoma
Rx: complete surgical excision (5-year survival rate of 74–90%)
DDx:
  (1) Pseudocyst: inflammatory changes in peripancreatic fat, pancreatic calcifications, temporal evolution, history of alcoholism, elevated levels of amylase
  (2) Lymphangioma / hemangioma
  (3) Variants of ductal adenocarcinoma:
    (a) mucinous colloid adenocarcinoma / ductectatic mucinous tumor of pancreas = mucin-hypersecreting carcinoma
    (b) papillary intraductal adenocarcinoma
    (c) adenosquamous carcinoma: squamous component predisposes to necrosis + cystic degeneration
    (d) anaplastic adenocarcinoma: lymphadenopathy + metastases at time of presentation
  (4) Solid and cystic papillary epithelioid neoplasm: hemorrhagic cystic changes in 20%
  (5) Cystic islet cell tumor: hypervascular component
  (6) Cystic metastases: history of malignant disease
  (7) Atypical serous cystadenoma: smaller tumor with greater number of smaller cysts
  (8) Sarcoma
  (9) Infection: amebiasis, Echinococcus multilocularis

MESENCHYMAL HAMARTOMA OF LIVER

= rare developmental cystic liver tumor

Histo: disordered arrangement of primitive fluid-filled mesenchyme, bile ducts, hepatic parenchyma; stromal / cystic predominance with cysts of a few mm up to 14 cm in size; no capsule
Age peak: 15–24 months (range from newborn to 19 years); M:F = 2:1

• slow progressive abdominal enlargement
• ± respiratory distress and lower extremity edema

Location: right lobe:left lobe = 6:1; 20% pedunculated

√ 16 cm average tumor size (range of 5–29 cm)
√ grossly discernible cysts in 80%

US:
  √ multiple rounded cystic areas on an echogenic background

√ may appear solid in younger infant (when cysts are still small)
CT:
√ multiple lucencies of variable size + attenuation
MR:
√ varying signal intensity (varying concentrations of protein in cystic predominance type) / hypointense on T1WI (mesenchymal predominance type)
√ marked hyperintensity of cystic locules / hypointense fibrosis on T2WI
NUC:
√ one / more areas of diminished uptake on sulfur colloid scan
Angio:
√ hypovascular mass
√ may show patchy areas of neovascularity
√ enlarged irregular tortuous feeding vessels

METASTASES TO LIVER

Incidence:
liver is most common metastatic site after regional lymph nodes; incidence of metastatic carcinoma 20 x greater than primary carcinoma; metastases represent 22% of all liver tumors in patients with known malignancy; most common malignant lesion of the liver

Enhancement characteristics compared with normal liver:
√ lesion enhancement during arterial phase (metastases are supplied by hepatic artery)
√ less enhancement during portal venous phase (metastases have a negligible portal venous supply)
√ extracellular space agents accumulate more in tumor tissue (metastases have a larger interstitial space)

Organ of origin: colon (42%), stomach (23%), pancreas (21%), breast (14%), lung (13%)
- hepatomegaly (70%)
- abnormal liver enzymes (50–75%)

Location: both lobes (77%), right lobe (20%), left lobe (3%)
Number: multiple (50–98%), solitary (2%)
Size: >33% smaller than 2 cm

√ involvement of liver + spleen typical in lymphoma + melanoma

NUC: 80–95% sensitivity in lesions >1.5 cm; lesions <1.5 cm are frequently missed; sensitivity increases with metastatic deposit size, peripheral location, and use of SPECT

NECT: important for hypervascular tumors (eg, renal cell carcinoma, carcinoid, islet cell tumors) which may be obscured by CECT

CECT:
Technique:
optimal is bolus technique with dynamic incremental scanning; sensitivity is decreased relative to NCCT if scans are obtained during equilibrium phase of contrast administration
√ circumferential bead- or bandlike enhancement during arterial phase + peripheral washout on delayed images
√ no (35%), peripheral (37%), mixed (20%), central (8%) enhancement
√ complete isodense fill-in on delayed scans in 5% (DDx: hemangioma)
◊ CT-sensitivity 88–90%; specificity 99%; lesions of approx. 1 cm can usually be detected!

CT-Angiography (most sensitive imaging modality):
Indication: patients with potentially resectable isolated liver metastases / preoperative to partial hepatectomy for detection of additional metastases (additional lesions detected in 40–55%)
(1) CT arteriography = angiography catheter in hepatic artery, detects lesions by virtue of increased enhancement
(2) CT arterial portography = angiography catheter in SMA, detects hypodense lesions on a background of increased enhancement of normal surroundings in portal venous phase

CT-delayed iodine scanning:
= CT performed 4–6 hours following administration of 60 mg iodine results in detection of additional lesions in 27%

Calcified Liver Metastases

Incidence: 2–3%
1. Mucinous carcinoma of GI tract (colon, rectum, stomach)
2. Endocrine pancreatic carcinoma
3. Leiomyosarcoma, osteosarcoma
4. Malignant melanoma
5. Papillary serous ovarian cystadenocarcinoma
6. Lymphoma
7. Pleural mesothelioma
8. Neuroblastoma
9. Breast cancer
10. Medullary carcinoma of the thyroid
11. Renal cell carcinoma
12. Lung carcinoma
13. Testicular carcinoma

mnemonic for mucinous adenocarcinoma: "COBS"
Colon carcinoma
Ovarian carcinoma
Breast carcinoma
Stomach carcinoma

Hypervascular Liver Metastases

1. Renal cell carcinoma
2. Carcinoid tumor
3. Colonic carcinoma
4. Choriocarcinoma
5. Breast carcinoma
6. Melanoma
7. Pancreatic islet cell tumor
8. Ovarian cystadenocarcinoma
9. Sarcomas
10. Pheochromocytoma

mnemonic: "CHIMP"
Carcinoid, **C**olon cancer
Hypernephroma
Islet cell carcinoma
Melanoma
Pheochromocytoma

Hemorrhagic Liver Metastases
mnemonic: "CT BeComes MR"
Colon carcinoma
Thyroid carcinoma
Breast carcinoma
Choriocarcinoma
Melanoma
Renal cell carcinoma

Echogenic Liver Metastases
Incidence: 25%
1. Colonic carcinoma (mucinous adenocarcinoma) 54%
2. Hepatoma 25%
3. Treated breast carcinoma 21%

Liver Metastases of Mixed Echogenicity
Incidence: 37.5%
1. Breast cancer 31%
2. Rectal cancer 20%
3. Lung cancer 17%
4. Stomach cancer 14%
5. Anaplastic cancer 11%
6. Cervical cancer 5%
7. Carcinoid 1%

Cystic Liver Metastases
1. Mucinous ovarian carcinoma
2. Colonic carcinoma
3. Sarcoma
4. Melanoma
5. Lung carcinoma
6. Carcinoid tumor

mnemonic: "LC GOES"
Leiomyosarcoma (and other sarcomas)
Choriocarcinoma
Gastric carcinoma
Ovarian carcinoma
Endometrial carcinoma
Small cell carcinoma

Echopenic Liver Metastases
Incidence: 37.5%
1. Lymphoma 44%
2. Pancreas 36%
3. Cervical cancer 20%
4. Lung (adenocarcinoma)
5. Nasopharyngeal cancer

Rx: Exclusion criteria for metastasectomy:
(1) advanced stage of primary tumor
(2) >4 metastases
(3) extrahepatic disease
(4) <30% normal liver tissue / function available after resection

METASTASES TO PANCREAS
Frequency: 3–10% (autopsy)
Organ of origin: renal cell carcinoma (30%), bronchogenic carcinoma (23%), breast carcinoma (12%), soft-tissue sarcoma (8%), colonic carcinoma (6%), melanoma (6%)
√ solitary (78%) / multiple (17%) ovoid masses with discrete smooth margins
√ diffuse pancreatic enlargement (5%)
CECT:
√ heterogeneously (60%) / homogeneously (17%) hyperattenuating relative to pancreas
√ hypoattenuating relative to pancreas (20%)
√ isoattenuating relative to pancreas (5%)
Concomitant intraabdominal metastases to:
liver (36%), lymph nodes (30%), adrenal glands (30%)

DDx: ductal pancreatic adenocarcinoma (uniformly nonenhancing mass, encasement of vessels)

MICROCYSTIC ADENOMA OF PANCREAS
= SEROUS CYSTADENOMA = GLYCOGEN-RICH CYSTADENOMA
= benign lobulated neoplasm composed of innumerable small cysts (1–20 mm) containing proteinaceous fluid separated by thin connective tissue septa
Incidence: approximately 50% of all cystic pancreatic neoplasms
Histo: cyst walls lined by cuboidal / flat glycogen-rich epithelial cells derived from centroacinar cells of pancreas (DDx: lymphangioma), thin fibrous pseudocapsule
Age: 34–88 years; mean age 65 years; 82% over 60 years of age; M:F = 1:4

Associated with: von Hippel-Lindau syndrome
• pain, weight loss, jaundice
• palpable mass

Location: any part of pancreas affected, slight predominance for head
√ well-demarcated lobulated mass 1–25 (mean 5) cm in diameter with smooth / nodular contour
√ innumerable small <2 cm cysts; uncommonly few large cysts (in <5%) / cyst up to 8 cm in diameter
√ prominent central stellate scar (CHARACTERISTIC)
√ amorphous central calcifications (in 33% on plain film) in dystrophic area of stellate central scar ("sunburst")
√ pancreatic duct + CBD may be displaced, encased, or obstructed
US:
√ solid predominantly echogenic mass with mixed hypoechoic + echogenic areas
CT:
√ attenuation values close to water
√ contrast enhancement
MR:
√ delayed enhancement of scar on contrast-enhanced FLASH images

LIVER

Angio:
- √ hypervascular mass with dilated feeding arteries, dense tumor blush, prominent draining veins, neovascularity, occasional AV shunting, NO vascular encasement

Prognosis: no malignant potential
Rx: surgical excision / follow-up examinations

MILK OF CALCIUM BILE

= LIMY BILE = CALCIUM SOAP = precipitation of particulate material with high concentration of calcium carbonate, calcium phosphate, calcium bilirubinate

Associated with: chronic cholecystitis + gallstone obstruction of cystic duct

√ diffuse opacification of GB lumen with dependent layering
√ usually functionless GB on oral cholecystogram

US:
- √ intermediate features between sludge + gallstones

MIRIZZI SYNDROME

= extrinsic right-sided compression of common hepatic duct by large gallstone impacted in cystic duct / gallbladder neck / cystic duct remnant; accompanied by chronic inflammatory reaction

Frequently associated with: formation of fistula between gallbladder and common hepatic duct

- • jaundice

√ normal CBD below level of impacted stone
√ TRIAD:
(1) gallstone impacted in GB neck
(2) dilatation of bile ducts above level of cystic duct
(3) smooth curved segmental stenosis of CHD

Cholangiography:
- √ partial obstruction of CHD due to external compression on lateral side of duct / eroding stone

DDx: lymphadenopathy, neoplasm of GB / CHD

MULTIPLE BILE DUCT HAMARTOMA

= VON MEYENBURG COMPLEX

Incidence: 0.15–2.8% of autopsies
Etiology: failure of involution of embryonic bile ducts
Histo: cluster of proliferated bile ducts lined by single layer of cuboidal cells embedded in fibrocollagenous tissue with single ramified lumen, communication with biliary system usually obliterated
Associated with: polycystic liver disease
Size: 0.1–10 mm

CT:
- √ multiple irregular hypodense lesions of up to 10 mm

US:
- √ multiple small cysts / echogenic areas (if size not resolved) up to 10 mm ± comet-tail artifact

Angio:
- √ multiple areas of abnormal vascularity in form of small grapelike clusters persisting into venous phase

DDx: metastatic liver disease

MULTIPLE ENDOCRINE NEOPLASIA

= MEN = MULTIPLE ENDOCRINE ADENOMAS (MEA)
= familial autosomal dominant adenomatous hyperplasia characterized by neoplasia of more than one endocrine organ

Theory: cells of involved principal organs originate from neural crest and produce polypeptide hormones in cytoplasmic granules which allow **a**mine **p**recursors **u**ptake and **d**ecarboxylation = APUD cells

		reminder:
Type I	= Wermer syndrome	PPP
Type II	= Sipple syndrome (Type IIA)	PMP
Type III	= Mucosal neuroma syndrome (Type IIB)	MPM

MEA	Type I	Type II	Type III
Pituitary adenoma	+		
Parathyroid adenoma	+	+	
Medullary thyroid carcinoma		+	+
Pancreatic island cell tumor	+		
Pheochromocytoma		+	+
Ganglioneuromatosis			+

MEN I syndrome

= WERMER SYNDROME
= autosomal dominant trait with high penetrance; M:F = 1:1

Cause: genetic defect in chromosome 11
Organ involvement:
1. Parathyroid hyperplasia (97%): multiglandular
2. Pancreatic islet cell tumor (30–80%):
   - ◊ Likely multiple + behaving malignant!
   - ◊ Primary cause of morbidity + mortality!
   - (a) gastrinoma = Zollinger-Ellison syndrome (most common type, in 50%), usually multicentric
   - (b) insulinoma
   - (c) VIPoma = WDHH-syndrome (watery diarrhea, hypokalemia, hypochlorhydria)
3. Anterior pituitary gland tumor (15–50%):
   - (a) nonfunctioning
   - (b) prolactin, growth hormone, corticotropin, TSH
4. Combination of parathyroid + pancreas + pituitary involvement (40%)
5. Adrenocortical hyperplasia (up to 33–40%)
6. Carcinoid
7. Lipoma

- • usually asymptomatic

May be associated with:
thyroid tumor (20%), thymoma, buccal mucosal tumor, colonic polyposis, Ménétrier disease

MEN II syndrome

= SIPPLE DISEASE = MEN Type IIA

Organ involvement:
1. Medullary carcinoma of thyroid
2. Pheochromocytoma: bilateral in 50%; malignant in 3%
   diagnosed before (in 10%) / after detection (in 17%) of medullary thyroid carcinoma

3. Parathyroid neoplasia
   • ± hyperparathyroidism

May be associated with: carcinoid tumors, Cushing disease

MEN III syndrome

= MUCOSAL NEUROMA SYNDROME = MEN Type IIB

Organ involvement:
1. Medullary carcinoma of thyroid
2. Pheochromocytoma
3. Oral + intestinal neuroganglioneuromatosis
   ◊ Usually precedes the appearance of thyroid carcinoma + pheochromocytoma!

• long slender extremities (Marfanoid appearance)
• thickened lips (due to submucosal nodules)
• nodular deformity of tongue (mucosal neuromas of tongue often initially diagnosed by dentists)
• prognathism
• corneal limbus thickening
• constipation alternating with diarrhea

@ GI tract
√ thickened / plaquelike colonic wall
√ dilated colon with abnormal haustral markings
√ alternating areas of colonic spasm + dilatation
√ multiple submucosal neuromas throughout small bowel, may act as lead point for intussusception

NEONATAL HEPATITIS

Etiology: CMV, hepatitis A/B, rubella, toxoplasmosis, spirochetes, idiopathic

Path: multinucleated giant cells, bile ducts relatively free of bile

NUC:

Technique: often performed after pretreatment with phenobarbital (5 mg/kg x 5 days) to maximize hepatic function

√ normal / decreased hepatic tracer accumulation
√ prolonged clearance of tracer from blood pool
√ bowel activity faint / delayed usually by 24 hours (best seen on lateral view; covering liver activity with lead shielding is helpful)
√ gallbladder may not be visualized

Prognosis: spontaneous remission

DDx: biliary atresia

PANCREAS DIVISUM

= most common anatomic variant of pancreas due to failure of fusion of the ventral and dorsal anlage at 8th week of fetal life with dorsal pancreatic duct (Santorini) draining through minor (accessory) papilla + ventral pancreatic duct (Wirsung) with CBD draining through major papilla

Prevalence: 4–9–14% in autopsy series;
2–8% in ERCP series;
3–7% in normal population;
12–26% in patients with idiopathic recurrent pancreatitis

Hypothesis: relative / actual stenosis of minor papilla predisposes to nonalcoholic recurrent pancreatitis in dorsal segment

• clinical relevance continues to be debated

Pancreatography: ONLY reliable means for diagnosis
√ contrast injection into major papilla demonstrates only short ventral pancreatic duct with early arborization
√ contrast injection into minor papilla fills dorsal pancreatic duct
√ no communication between ventral + dorsal ducts

CT:
√ oblique fat cleft between ventral + dorsal pancreas (25%)
√ failure to see union of dorsal + ventral pancreatic ducts (rare)

PANCREATIC ACINAR CELL CARCINOMA

= rare neoplasm of exocrine origin

Age: 40–81 (mean 62) years; M:F = 86:14; 87% Caucasian

• increased serum lipase ± amylase
• syndrome of elevated lipase =
  • disseminated subcutaneous + intraosseous fat necrosis (usually distal to knees / elbows)
  • polyarthropathy
  • skin lesions resembling erythema nodosum
• biliary obstruction distinctly uncommon

√ lobulated well-defined mass of 2–15 cm in diameter
√ thin enhancing capsule
√ tumor necrosis usually present
√ moderately vascular tumor + neovascularity + arterial and venous encasement

Prognosis: median survival of 7–9 months

DDx:
(1) pancreatic adenocarcinoma (small, irregular, locally invasive, without capsule, biliary obstruction if located in head of pancreas)
(2) Nonfunctioning islet-cell tumor
(3) Microcystic cystadenoma
(4) Solid and papillary epithelial neoplasm
(5) Oncocytic tumor of pancreas

PANCREATIC DUCTAL ADENOCARCINOMA

= DUCT CELL ADENOCARCINOMA (duct cells comprise only 4% of pancreatic tissue)

Incidence: 80 - 95% of nonendocrine pancreatic neoplasms; 5th leading cause of cancer death in the United States (27,000 per year)

Etiology: alcohol abuse (4%), diabetes (2 x more frequent than in general population, particularly in females), hereditary pancreatitis (in 40%); cigarette smoking (risk factor 2 x)

Path: scirrhous infiltrative adenocarcinoma with a dense cellularity + sparse vascularity

Mean age at onset: 55 years; peak age in 7th decade; M:F = 2:1

STAGE I = confined to pancreas
II = + regional lymph node metastases
III = + distant spread

◊ At presentation
— 65% of patients have advanced local disease / distant metastases

— 21% of patients have localized disease with spread to regional lymph nodes
— 14% of patients have tumor confined to pancreas

Extension:
(a) local extension beyond margins of organ (68%): posteriorly (96%), anteriorly (30%), into porta hepatis (15%), into splenic hilum (13%)
(b) invasion of adjacent organs (42%): duodenum > stomach > left adrenal gland > spleen > root of small bowel mesentery

Metastases: liver (30–36%), regional lymph nodes >2 cm (15–28%), ascites from peritoneal carcinomatosis (7–10%), lungs (pulmonary nodules / lymphangitic), pleura, bone

- weight loss, anorexia, fatigue
- pain in hypochondrium radiating to back
- obstructive jaundice (75%): most frequent cause of malignant biliary obstruction
- new onset diabetes (25–50%), steatorrhea
- thrombophlebitis

Location: pancreatic head (56–62%); body (26%); tail (12%)
Size: 2–10 cm (in 60% between 4–6 cm)

UGI:
√ "antral padding" = extrinsic indentation of the posteroinferior margin of antrum
√ "Frostberg 3" sign = inverted 3 contour to the medial portion of the duodenal sweep
√ spiculated duodenal wall + traction + fixation (neoplastic infiltration of duodenal mucosa / desmoplastic response)
√ irregular / smooth nodular mass with ampullary carcinoma

BE:
√ localized haustral padding / flattening / narrowing with serrated contour at inferior aspect of transverse colon / splenic flexure
√ diffuse tethering throughout peritoneal cavity (intraperitoneal seeding)

CT (99% detection rate for dynamic CT scan; 89% in predicting nonresectability):
√ pancreatic mass (95%) / diffuse enlargement (4%) / normal scan (1%)
√ mass with central zone of diminished attenuation (75–83%)
√ pancreatic + bile duct obstruction without detectable mass (4%)
√ duct dilatation (58%): 3/4 biductal, 1/10 isolated to one duct; dilated pancreatic duct (67%); dilated bile ducts (38%)
√ atrophy of pancreatic body + tail (20%)
√ calcifications (2%)
√ postobstructive pseudocyst (11%)
√ obliteration of retropancreatic fat (50%)
√ thickening of celiac axis / SMA (invasion of perivascular lymphatics) in 60%
√ dilated collateral veins (12%)
√ thickening of Gerota fascia (5%)
√ local tumor extension posteriorly, into splenic hilum, into porta hepatis (68%)
√ contiguous organ invasion (duodenum, stomach, mesenteric root) in 42%

US:
√ hypoechoic pancreatic mass
√ focal / diffuse (10%) enlargement of pancreas
√ contour deformity of gland; rounding of uncinate process
√ dilatation of pancreatic ± biliary duct

MR (no diagnostic improvement over CT):
√ hypointense lesion on fat-suppressed T1WI
√ diminished enhancement on dynamic contrast images

Angiography (70% accuracy):
√ hypovascular tumor / neovascularity (50%)
√ arterial encasement: SMA (33%), splenic artery (14%), celiac trunk (11%), hepatic artery (11%), gastroduodenal artery (3%), left renal artery (0.6%)
√ venous obstruction: splenic vein (34%), SMV (10%)
√ venous encasement: SMV (23%), splenic vein (15%), portal vein (4%)

Cholangiography:
√ "rattail / nipplelike" occlusion of CBD
√ nodular mass / meniscuslike occlusion in ampullary tumors

Pancreatography (abnormal in 97%):
√ irregular, nodular, rat-tailed, eccentric obstruction
√ localized encasement with prestenotic dilatation
√ acinar defect

Prognosis:
10% 1-year survival, 2% 3-year survival, <1% 5-year survival; 14 months medial survival after curative resection, 8 months after palliative resection, 5 months without treatment; tumors resectable in only 8–15% at presentation, 5% 5-year survival rate after surgery

DDx: focal pancreatitis, islet cell carcinoma, metastasis, lymphoma, normal variant

PANCREATIC ISLET CELL TUMORS

Origin: embryonic neuroectoderm, derivatives of APUD (amine precursor uptake and decarboxylation) cell line arising from islet of Langerhans (APUDoma)
Prevalence: 1:1,000,000 population/year; isolated or part of MEN I syndrome (= Wermer syndrome)
Path: (a) small tumor: solid well-demarcated
(b) large tumor: cystic changes + necrosis + calcifications
Histo: sheets of small round cells + numerous stromal vessels

Average time from onset of symptoms to diagnosis is 2.7 years

Classification: (a) functional (85%)
(b) nonfunctional (below threshold of detectability) / hypofunctional

Metastases: in 60–90% to liver ± regional lymph nodes
◊ Hyperechoic liver metastasis is suggestive of islet cell tumor rather than pancreatic adenocarcinoma!

√ calcifications highly suggestive of malignancy

NUC:
√ somatostatin receptor imaging with octreotide

DDx:
1. Pancreatic ductal adenocarcinoma (hypovascular, smaller, encasement of SMA + celiac trunk)
2. Microcystic adenoma (benign tumor, small cysts, older women)
3. Metastatic tumor: renal cell carcinoma (clinical Hx)
4. Solid and papillary epithelial neoplasm (young female, hemorrhagic areas)
5. Paraganglioma
6. Sarcoma (rare)

ACTH-producing tumor

rare cause of Cushing syndrome
- increased level of serum cortisol
- impaired glucose tolerance > central obesity > hypertension, oligomenorrhea > osteoporosis > purpura > striae > muscle atrophy

Prognosis: almost all malignant with metastases at time of diagnosis

Gastrinoma

2nd most common islet cell tumor; in a cells / d cells
Age: 8% in patients <20 years; M > F
Path: (a) islet cell hyperplasia (10%)
(b) benign adenoma (30%): in 50% solitary, in 50% multiple (especially in MEN I)
(c) malignant (50–60%) with metastases to liver, spleen, lymph nodes, bone

Associated with: MEN Type I (in 10–40%)
- Zollinger-Ellison syndrome: severe recurrent peptic ulcer disease (>90%), malabsorption, hypokalemia, gastric hypersecretion, hyperacidity / occasionally hypoacidity, diarrhea (from gastric hypersecretion)
  ◊ Only 1:1,000 patients with peptic ulcer disease has a gastrinoma!
- GI bleeding
- elevated serum levels of gastrin

Location:
(a) 87% in pancreas (50% solitary in head / tail)
(b) ectopic (7–33%):
— duodenal wall (13% in medial wall of duodenum = gastrinoma triangle)
— peripancreatic nodes / spleen
— stomach, jejunum
— omentum, retroperitoneum
— ovary

frequently in "gastrinoma triangle" (= triangle defined by porta hepatis as apex of triangle + 2nd and 3rd parts of duodenum as the base)

√ average tumor size 3.4 cm (up to 15 cm)
√ occasionally calcifications
√ homogeneous hypoechoic mass

Angio:
√ hypervascular lesion (70%)
√ hepatic venous sampling after intraarterial stimulation with secretin

CT:
√ transiently hyperdense on dynamic CT (majority)
√ thickening of gastric rugal folds

MR:
√ low-intensity mass on fat-suppressed T1WI
√ diminished central + peripheral ring enhancement
√ high-intensity mass on fat-suppressed T2WI

Sensitivity of preoperative localization:
25% for US, 35% for CT, 20% for MRI, 42–63% for transhepatic portal venous sampling for gastrin, 68–70% for selective angiography, 77% for arteriography combined with intra-arterial injection of secretin

Rx: surgery curative in 30%

Glucagonoma

Uncommon tumor; derived from a cells; M < F
Associated with: MEN
- necrolytic erythema migrans (erythematous macules / papules on lower extremity, groin, buttocks, face) in >70% of patients
- diarrhea, diabetes, painful glossitis, weight loss, anemia
- plasma glucagon level > 1,000 ng/L

Location: predominantly in pancreatic body / tail
√ tumor size 2.5–25 cm (mean 6.4 cm) with solid + necrotic components
√ hypervascular in 90%; successful angiographic localization in 15%

Cx: deep vein thrombosis + pulmonary embolism
Prognosis: in 60–80% malignant transformation (liver metastases at time of diagnosis in 50%); 55% 5-year survival rate

Insulinoma

Most common functioning islet cell tumor
Age: 4th–6th decade; M:F = 2:3
Associated with: MEN Type I
Path: (a) single benign adenoma (80–90%)
(b) multiple adenomas / microadenomatosis (5–10%)
(c) islet cell hyperplasia (5–10%)
(d) malignant adenoma (5–10%)
- Whipple triad: starvation attack + hypoglycemia (fasting glucose <50 mg/dL) + relief by IV dextrose
- neuroglycopenic symptoms: headaches, confusion, coma
- hypoglycemia exacerbated by fasting results in frequent meals to avoid symptoms
- sweating, palpitations, tremor (secondary to catecholamine release in response to hypoglycemia)
- obesity
- firm rubbery palpable mass at surgery (in >90%)

Location: no predilection for any part of pancreas, 2–5% in ectopic location; 10% multiple (especially in MEN I)
√ average tumor size 1–2 cm; <1.5 cm in 70%

US (20–75% preoperative and 75–100% endoscopic + intraoperative sensitivity)
√ round / oval smoothly marginated solid homogeneously hypoechoic mass

Angio:
√ hypervascular tumor (66%): accurate angiographic localization in 50–90%
√ transhepatic portal venous sampling (correct localization in 95%)
√ hepatic venous sampling after intraarterial stimulation with calcium gluconate

CECT (30–75% sensitivity):
√ hypo- / iso- / hyperattenuating lesion

MR:
√ low signal intensity on fat-suppressed T1WI
√ hyperintense on T2WI + dynamic contrast-enhanced + suppressed inversion recovery images

Prognosis: malignant transformation in 5–10%

Rx: surgery curative

Nonfunctioning islet cell tumor

Incidence: 3rd most common islet cell tumor after insulinoma + gastrinoma; 15–25% of all islet cell tumors

Derived from either alpha or beta cells

Age: 24–74 (mean 57) years

- mostly asymptomatic (hormonally quiescent)
- abdominal pain, jaundice, gastric variceal bleeding
- palpable mass, gastric outlet obstruction

Location: predominantly in pancreatic head

√ tumor size 6–20 cm (>5 cm in 72%) with solid + necrotic components
√ coarse nodular calcifications (20–25%)
√ CT contrast enhancement in 83%
√ hypoechoic mass
√ late dense capillary stain
√ large irregular pathologic vessels with early venous filling

Prognosis: in 80–100% malignant transformation with metastases to liver + regional nodes; 60% 3-year survival; 44% 5-year survival

Rx: may respond to systemic chemotherapy

LIVER

Somatostatinoma

Derived from delta cells

- inhibitory syndrome = inhibitory action of somatostatin on other pancreatic + bowel peptides (growth hormone, TSH, insulin, glucagon, gastric acid, pepsin, secretin)
- diabetes, cholelithiasis, steatorrhea
- elevated level of somatostatin

Location: predominantly in pancreatic head

√ tumor size 0.6–20 cm (average >4 cm)
√ hypervascular

Prognosis: 50–90% malignant transformation; metastatic disease in 70% at time of initial diagnosis

VIPoma

= solitary tumor liberating **V**asoactive **I**ntestinal **P**eptides acting directly on cyclic adenosine monophosphate within epithelial cells of bowel relaxing vascular smooth muscle; sporadic occurrence

Histo: adenoma / hyperplasia

M:F = 1:2

- **WDHA syndrome** = **w**atery **d**iarrhea + **h**ypokalemia + **a**chlorhydria (more recently + more accurately described as) **WDHH syndrome** = **w**atery **d**iarrhea + **h**ypokalemia + **h**ypochlorhydria = "pancreatic cholera" = **Verner-Morrison syndrome**
- dehydration due to massive diarrhea (>1 L/day)

Location:
(1) pancreas: from delta cells predominantly in pancreatic body / tail
(2) extrapancreatic: retroperitoneal ganglioblastoma, pheochromocytoma, lung, neuroblastoma (in children)

√ average size 5–10 cm with solid + necrotic tissue
√ mostly hypervascular tumor
√ dilatation of gallbladder

Prognosis: in 50–80% malignant transformation

DDx: small cell carcinoma of lung / neuroblastoma may also cause WDHH syndrome

PANCREATIC LIPOMATOSIS

= FATTY REPLACEMENT = FATTY INFILTRATION
= deposition of fat cells in pancreatic parenchyma

Predisposing factors:
1. Atherosclerosis of elderly
2. Obesity
3. Steroid therapy
4. Diabetes mellitus
5. Cushing syndrome
6. Chronic pancreatitis
7. Main pancreatic duct obstruction
8. Cystic fibrosis
9. Malnutrition / dietary deficiency
10. Hepatic disease
11. Hemochromatosis
12. Viral infection
13. Schwachman-Diamond syndrome

√ fatty replacement often uneven
√ increase in AP diameter of pancreatic head with focal fatty replacement = lipomatous pseudohypertrophy
√ prominently lobulated external contour

US: √ increased pancreatic echogenicity

CT: √ "marbling" of pancreatic parenchyma / total fatty replacement / lipomatous pseudohypertrophy

PANCREATIC FATTY SPARING

= sparing of fatty change in pancreatic head + uncinate process (ventral pancreatic anlage) as initial stage in pancreatic lipomatosis

Histo: ventral pancreatic anlage has smaller + more densely packed acini with scanty / absent interacinar fat

US:
√ rounded / triangular hypoechoic area within pancreatic head / uncinate process + diffusely increased echogenicity in remainder of gland

CT:
√ higher-density region of pancreatic head + uncinate process with diffusely decreased attenuation of pancreatic body + tail

PANCREATIC PSEUDOCYST

= collection of pancreatic fluid encapsulated by fibrous tissue

Etiology: (1) Acute pancreatitis ; pseudocysts mature in 6–8 weeks
(2) Chronic pancreatitis
(3) Posttraumatic
(4) Pancreatic cancer

Incidence: 2–4% in acute pancreatitis; 10–15% in chronic pancreatitis

Location: 2/3 within pancreas

Atypical location (may dissect along tissue planes in 1/3):
(a) intraperitoneal: mesentery of small bowel / transverse colon / sigmoid colon
(b) retroperitoneal: along psoas muscle; may present as groin mass / in scrotum
(c) intraparenchymal: liver, spleen, kidney
(d) mediastinal (through esophageal hiatus > aortic hiatus > foramen of Morgagni > erosion through diaphragm): may present as neck mass

Plain film / contrast radiograph:
- √ smooth extrinsic indentation of posterior wall of stomach / inner duodenal sweep (80%)
- √ indentation / displacement of splenic flexure / transverse colon (40%)
- √ downward displacement of duodenojejunal junction
- √ gastric outlet obstruction
- √ splaying of renal collecting system / ureteral obstruction

US (pseudocyst detectable in 50–92%; 92–96% accuracy):
- √ usually single + unilocular cyst
- √ multilocular in 6%
- √ fluid-debris level / internal echoes (may contain sequester, blood clot, cellular debris from autolysis)
- √ septations (rare; sign of infection / hemorrhage)
- √ may increase in size (secondary to hypertonicity of fluid, communication with pancreatic duct, hemorrhage, erosion of vessel)
- √ obstruction of pancreatic duct / CBD

CT:
- √ fluid in pseudocyst (0–30 HU)
- √ cyst wall calcification (extremely rare)

Pancreatography:
- √ communication with pancreatic duct in up to 70%

Cx (in 40%):
1. Rupture into abdominal cavity, stomach, colon, duodenum
2. Hemorrhage / formation of pseudoaneurysm
3. Infection
   - √ gas bubbles (DDx: fistulous communication to GI tract)
   - √ increase in attenuation of fluid contents
4. Intestinal obstruction

Prognosis: spontaneous resolution (in 20–50%) secondary to rupture into GI tract / pancreatic / bile duct

DDx: pancreatic cystadenoma, cystadenocarcinoma, necrotic pancreatic carcinoma, fluid-filled bowel loop, fluid-filled stomach, duodenal diverticulum, aneurysm

PANCREATIC TRANSPLANTATION

Complications: sepsis, rejection, pancreatitis, pseudocyst, pancreatic abscess (22%), anastomotic leak

Prognosis: 40% survival rate >1 year

Graft-vessel Thrombosis in Pancreatic Transplant (2–19%)

A. EARLY THROMBOSIS
<1 month after transplantation
Cause: technical error in fashioning anastomosis, microvascular damage due to preservation injury

B. LATE THROMBOSIS
>1 month after transplantation
Cause: alloimmune arteritis with gradual occlusion of small blood vessels

Acute Rejection of Pancreatic Transplant

- focal tenderness over transplant
- measurement of urinary + serum amylase, blood glucose (nonspecific for diagnosis of rejection)

US:
- √ poor margination of transplant
- √ acoustic inhomogeneity
- √ dilated pancreatic duct

PANCREATITIS

Cause:

A. IDIOPATHIC (20%)

B. ALCOHOLISM: acute pancreatitis (15%); chronic pancreatitis (70%)

C. CHOLELITHIASIS: acute pancreatitis (75%); chronic pancreatitis (20%)

D. METABOLIC DISORDERS
1. Hypercalcemia in hyperparathyroidism (10%), multiple myeloma, amyloidosis, sarcoidosis
2. Hereditary pancreatitis: autosomal dominant, only Caucasians affected, most common cause of large spherical pancreatic calcifications in childhood, recurrent episodes of pancreatitis, development into pancreatic carcinoma in 20–40%; pronounced dilatation of pancreatic duct; pseudocyst formation (50%); associated with type I hypercholesterolemia
3. Hyperlipidemia Types I and V
4. Kwashiorkor = Tropical pancreatitis

E. INFECTION / INFESTATION
1. Viral infection (mumps, hepatitis, mononucleosis)
2. Parasites (ascariasis, clonorchis)

F. TRAUMA
1. Penetrating ulcer
2. Blunt / penetrating trauma
3. Surgery (in 0.8% of Billroth-II resections, 0.8% of splenectomies, 0.7% of choledochal surgery, 0.4% of aortic graft surgery)

G. STRUCTURAL ABNORMALITIES
1. Pancreas divisum
2. Choledochocele

H. DRUGS
Azathioprine, thiazide, furosemide, ethacrynic acid, sulfonamides, tetracycline, phenformin, steroids (eg, renal transplant), asparaginase, procainamide

I. MALIGNANCY
Pancreatic carcinoma (in 1%), metastases, lymphoma

Theories of pathogenesis:
Reflux of bile / pancreatic enzymes / duodenal succus
(a) terminal duct segment shared by common bile duct + pancreatic duct
(b) obstruction at papilla of Vater from inflammatory stenosis, edema / spasm of sphincter of Oddi, tumor, periduodenal diverticulum
(c) incompetent sphincter of Oddi

Acute pancreatitis

= inflammatory disease of pancreas producing temporary changes with restoration of normal anatomy + function following resolution

Path:
1. EDEMATOUS PANCREATITIS:
   edema, congestion, leukocytic infiltrates; mortality rate of 4%
2. NECROTIZING PANCREATITIS:
   proteolytic destruction of pancreatic parenchyma; mortality rate of 80–90%
   (a) HEMORRHAGIC PANCREATITIS:
       + fat necrosis and hemorrhage
   (b) SUPPURATIVE PANCREATITIS:
       + bacterial infection

A. Diffuse pancreatitis (52%)
B. Focal pancreatitis (48%): location of head:tail = 3:2

Clinical stages:
I = EDEMATOUS PANCREATITIS (75%)
- rapid improvement following conservative therapy
- gradual decrease of elevated enzymes

Mortality: 1–5%

II = PARTIALLY NECROTIZING PANCREATITIS
- delayed / no response to conservative therapy
- delayed / no normalization of enzymes
  - leukocytosis of <16,000
  - hyperglycemia of <200 mg/100 mL
  - hypocalcemia of >4 mval/L
- base deficit of <4 mval/L

Mortality: 30–75%

III = TOTALLY NECROTIZING PANCREATITIS
- deterioration under conservative therapy
  - leukocytosis of >16,000
  - hyperglycemia of >200 mg/100 mL
  - hypocalcemia of <4 mval/L
  - base deficit of >4 mval/L

Mortality: 100% (40% by 2nd day, 75% by 5th day, 100% by 10th day)

- acute abdominal pain (peaking after a few hours, resolving in 2–3 days), nausea, vomiting
- raised pancreatic amylase + lipase in blood + urine
- increased amylase-creatinine clearance ratio
- signs of hemorrhagic pancreatitis:
  - Cullen sign = periumbilical ecchymosis
  - Grey-Turner sign = flank ecchymosis
  - Fox sign = infrainguinal ecchymosis

√ NO findings on US / CT in 29%

Abdominal film:
√ "colon cutoff" sign = dilated transverse colon with abrupt change to a gasless descending colon (inflammation via phrenicocolic ligament causes spasm + obstruction at the splenic flexure impinging on a paralytic colon)
√ "sentinel loop" (10–55%) = localized segment of gas-containing bowel in duodenum (in 20–45%) / terminal ileum / cecum
√ "renal halo" sign = water-density of inflammation in anterior pararenal space contrasts with perirenal fat; more common on left side
√ mottled appearance of peripancreatic area (secondary to fat necrosis in pancreatic bed, mesentery, omentum)
√ intrapancreatic gas bubbles (from acute gangrene / suppurative pancreatitis)
√ "gasless abdomen" = fluid-filled bowel associated with vomiting
√ ascites

CXR (findings in 14–71%):
√ pleural effusion (in 5%), usually left-sided, with elevated amylase levels (in 85%)
√ left-sided diaphragmatic elevation
√ left-sided subsegmental atelectasis (20%)
√ parenchymal infiltrates, pulmonary infarction
√ pulmonary edema, ARDS
√ pleural empyema, pericardial effusion
√ mediastinal abscess, mediastinal pseudocyst
√ pancreatico-bronchial / -pleural / -pulmonary fistula

UGI:
√ esophagogastric varices (from splenic vein obstruction)
√ enlarged tortuous edematous rugal folds along antrum + greater curvature (20%)
√ widening of retrogastric space (from pancreatic enlargement / inflammation in lesser sac)
√ diminished duodenal peristalsis + edematous folds
√ widening of duodenal sweep + downward displacement of ligament of Treitz
√ Poppel sign = edematous swelling of papilla
√ Frostberg inverted-3 sign = segmental narrowing with fold thickening of duodenum
√ jejunal + ileal fold thickening (proteolytic spread along mesentery)

BE:
√ narrowing, nodularity, fold distortion along inferior haustral row of transverse colon ± descending colon

Cholangiography:
√ long gently tapered narrowing of CBD

√ prestenotic biliary dilatation
√ smooth / irregular mucosal surface

Bone films (findings in 6%):
secondary to metastatic intramedullary lipolysis + fat necrosis
√ punched out / permeative destruction of cancellous bone + endosteal erosion
√ aseptic necrosis of femoral / humeral heads
√ metaphyseal infarcts, predominantly in distal femur + proximal tibia

US (pancreatic visualization in 62–78%):
√ hypoechoic diffuse / focal enlargement of pancreas
√ dilatation of pancreatic duct (if head focally involved)
√ perivascular cloaking = spread of inflammatory exudate along perivascular spaces
√ extrapancreatic hypoechoic mass with good acoustic transmission (= phlegmonous pancreatitis)
√ fluid collection: lesser sac (60%), L > R anterior pararenal space (54%), posterior pararenal space (18%), around left lobe of liver (16%), in spleen (9%), mediastinum (3%), iliac fossa, along transverse mesocolon / mesenteric leaves of small intestine
Fate of fluid collection:
(a) complete resolution
(b) pseudocyst formation
(c) bacterial infection = abscess
√ pseudocyst formation (52%): extension into lesser sac, transverse mesocolon, around kidney, mediastinum, lower quadrants of abdomen

CT (pancreatic visualization in 98%):
√ no detectable change in size / appearance (29%)
√ hypodense (5–20 HU) mass in phlegmonous pancreatitis; may persist long after complete recovery
√ hyperdense areas (50–70 HU) in hemorrhagic pancreatitis for 24–48 hours
√ enlargement with convex margins + indistinctness of gland with parenchymal inhomogeneity
√ thickening of anterior pararenal fascia
√ non–contrast-enhancing parenchyma during bolus injection (= pancreatic necrosis)

Angiography:
√ may be normal
√ hypovascular areas (15–56%)
√ hypervascularity + increased parenchymal stain (12– 45%)
√ venous compression secondary to edema
√ formation of pseudoaneurysms (in 10% with chronic pancreatitis): splenic artery (50%), pancreatic arcades, gastroduodenal artery

Cx:
1. Phlegmon (18%) = solid mass characterized by edema, infiltration of inflammatory cells + necrosis: extension into lesser sac, anterior pararenal space, transverse mesocolon, small bowel mesentery, retroperitoneum, pelvis
2. Pseudocyst formation (10%)
3. Hemorrhage (3%)
4. Abscess (2–10%): 2–4 weeks after severe acute pancreatitis; most commonly due to E. coli
√ may contain gas within pancreatic bed
DDx: air secondary to intestinal fistula
5. Pancreatic ascites
6. Biliary duct obstruction
7. Thrombosis of splenic vein / SMV
8. Pseudoaneurysm
(a) rupture into preexisting pseudocyst
(b) digestion of arterial wall by enzymes
Incidence: in up to 10% of severe pancreatitis
Location: splenic artery (most common), gastroduodenal, pancreatico-duodenal, hepatic artery
Mortality: 37% for rupture, 16–50% for surgery

Therapy:
1. Conservative (NPO, gastric tube, atropine, analgesics, sedation, prophylactic antibiotics) for stage I
2. Early surgery in stages II and III

Chronic pancreatitis

= continuing inflammatory disease of pancreas characterized by irreversible damage to anatomy + function
A. CHRONIC CALCIFYING PANCREATITIS:
√ protein plugs / calculi within ductal system
B. CHRONIC OBSTRUCTIVE PANCREATITIS:
secondary to slow growing tumor / surgical duct ligation / ampullary stenosis
√ dilatation of pancreatic duct
√ normal sized / focally or diffusely enlarged / small atrophic gland
√ calcifications uncommon

• acute exacerbation of epigastric pain (93%): decreasing with time due to progressive destruction of gland, usually painless after 7 years
• jaundice (42%) from common bile duct obstruction
• steatorrhea (80%)
• diabetes mellitus (58%)
• secretin test with decreased amylase + bicarbonate in duodenal fluid

Plain film:
√ numerous irregular calcifications (in 20–50% of alcoholic pancreatitis) PATHOGNOMONIC

UGI:
√ displacement of stomach / duodenum by pseudocyst
√ shrinkage / fold induration of stomach (DDx: linitis plastica)
√ stricture of duodenum

Cholangiopancreatography (most sensitive imaging modality):
√ slight ductal ectasia / clubbing of side branches (minimal disease)
√ "nipping" = narrowing of the origins of side branches

LIVER

√ dilatation >2 mm, tortuosity, wall rigidity, main ductal stenosis (moderate disease)
√ "beading, chain of lakes, string of pearls" = dilatation, stenosis, obstruction of main pancreatic duct + side branches (severe disease)
√ intraductal protein plugs / calculi
√ prolonged emptying of contrast material
√ may have stenosis / obstruction + prestenotic dilatation of CBD

US / CT:
√ irregular (73%) / smooth (15%) / beaded (12%) pancreatic ductal dilatation (in 41–68%)
√ small atrophic gland (in 10–54%)
√ pancreatic mostly intraductal calcifications (4–68%)
√ inhomogeneous gland with increased echogenicity (62%)
√ irregular pancreatic contour (45–60%)
√ focal (12–32%) / diffuse (27–45%) pancreatic enlargement
√ mostly mild biliary ductal dilatation (29%)
√ intra- / peripancreatic pseudocysts (20–34%)
√ segmental portal hypertension (= splenic vein thrombosis + splenomegaly) in 11%
√ arterial pseudoaneurysm formation
√ peripancreatic fascial thickening + blurring of organ margins (16%)
√ ascites / pleural effusion (9%)

MR:
√ loss of signal intensity on fat-suppressed T1WI (from loss of aqueous protein in pancreatic acini secondary to fibrosis)
√ diminished contrast enhancement (from loss of normal capillary network replaced by fibrous tissue)

Angiography:
√ increased tortuosity + angulation of pancreatic arcades + intrahepatic arteries (88%)
√ luminal irregularities / focal fibrotic arterial stenoses (25–75%) / smooth beaded appearance
√ irregular parenchymal stain
√ venous compression / occlusion (20–50%)
√ portoportal shunting + gastric varices without esophageal varices

Cx: pancreatic carcinoma (2–4%), jaundice, pseudocyst formation, pancreatic ascites, thrombosis of splenic / mesenteric / portal vein

Rx: surgery for infected pseudocyst, GI-bleeding from portal hypertension, common bile duct obstruction, gastrointestinal obstruction

PASSIVE HEPATIC CONGESTION

Cause: CHF, constrictive pericarditis

Pathophysiology: chronic central venous hypertension transmitted to hepatic sinusoids results in centrilobular congestion + eventually hepatic atrophy, necrosis, fibrosis

• abnormal liver function tests

CT:
√ globally delayed enhancement (36%)
√ enhancement of portal veins + hepatic arteries + immediately adjacent parenchyma (56%)
√ "reticulated mosaic" pattern = lobular patchy areas of enhancement separated by coarse linear regions of diminished attenuation (100%)
√ diminished periportal attenuation (24%)
√ diminished attenuation around intrahepatic IVC (8%)
√ prominent IVC + hepatic vein enhancement (due to contrast reflux from right atrium into dilated IVC)

DDx: Budd-Chiari syndrome (regional / lobular distribution of reticulated mosaic pattern, caudate lobe hypertrophy)

PELIOSIS HEPATIS

[*pelios* , Greek = purple]

= rare benign disorder characterized by multiple blood-filled cavities randomly distributed throughout liver

Cause: (a) ? acquired: chronic infection (TB), hepatotoxic drugs (androgen-anabolic steroids, chemotherapeutic agents) diabetes mellitus, chronic renal failure
(b) ? congenital: angiomatous malformation

Histo: (1) **Phlebectatic** peliosis hepatis (early stage) = endothelial-lined cysts (= ? dilatation of central veins) communicating with dilated hepatic sinusoids + compression of surrounding liver
(2) **Parenchymal** peliosis hepatis (late stage) = irregularly shaped cysts without lining communicating with dilated hepatic sinusoids + areas of liver cell necrosis

Associated with: hormonally induced benign / malignant tumors

Age: fetal life (rare) to adult life

√ hepatomegaly

Angio:
√ multiple small (several mm to 1.5 cm) round collections of contrast medium scattered throughout liver in late arterial phase of hepatic arteriogram
√ ± simultaneous opacification of hepatic veins

Prognosis: reversible after drug withdrawal / progression to hepatic failure / intraperitoneal hemorrhage leading to death

PERICHOLECYSTIC ABSCESS

Cause: subacute perforation of gallbladder wall subsequent to gangrene + infarction due to acute cholecystitis

Prevalence: 2–20%

Location: (a) gallbladder bed (most common)
√ area of low-level echoes in liver adjacent to gallbladder
(b) intramural
√ small area of low-level echoes within thickened gallbladder wall
(c) intraperitoneal
√ area of low-level echoes within peritoneal cavity adjacent to gallbladder

Rx: (1) Emergency operation
(2) Antibiotic treatment + elective operation
(3) Percutaneous abscess drainage

PORCELAIN GALLBLADDER

= calcium incrustation of gallbladder wall

Incidence: 0.6–0.8% of cholecystectomy patients; M:F = 1:5

Histo: (a) flakes of dystrophic calcium within chronically inflamed + fibrotic muscular wall
(b) microliths scattered diffusely throughout mucosa, submucosa, glandular spaces, Rokitansky-Aschoff sinuses

Associated with: gallstones in 90%

- minimal symptoms

√ curvilinear (muscularis) / granular (mucosal) calcifications in segment of wall / entire wall
√ nonfunctioning GB on oral cholecystogram
√ highly echogenic shadowing curvilinear structure in GB fossa (DDx: stone-filled contracted GB)
√ echogenic GB wall with little acoustic shadowing (DDx: emphysematous cholecystitis)
√ scattered irregular clumps of echoes with posterior acoustic shadowing

Cx: 10–20% develop carcinoma of gallbladder

PORTAL HYPERTENSION

- normal hepatic blood flow of 550–900 mL/min (= 25% of cardiac output) passes through portal system (2/3) + through hepatic artery (1/3)

Classification:

A. DYNAMIC / HYPERKINETIC PORTAL HYPERTENSION
congenital / traumatic / neoplastic arterioportal fistula

B. INCREASED PORTAL RESISTANCE

@ Prehepatic
— portal vein thrombosis (portal phlebitis, oral contraceptives, coagulopathy, neoplastic invasion, pancreatitis, neonatal omphalitis)
— portal vein compression (tumor, trauma,lymphadenopathy, portal phlebosclerosis, pancreatic pseudocyst)

@ Intrahepatic (= obstruction of portal venules)
— presinusoidal
1. Congenital hepatic fibrosis
2. Idiopathic noncirrhotic fibrosis
3. Primary biliary cirrhosis
4. a-1–antitrypsin deficiency
5. Wilson disease
6. Sarcoid liver disease
7. Toxic fibrosis (arsenic, copper, PVC)
8. Reticuloendotheliosis
9. Myelofibrosis
10. Felty syndrome
11. Schistosomiasis
12. Cystic fibrosis
13. Chronic malaria

— sinusoidal
1. Hepatitis
2. Sickle cell disease

— postsinusoidal
1. Cirrhosis (most frequent): Laennec cirrhosis, postnecrotic cirrhosis from hepatitis
2. Venoocclusive disease of liver

@ Posthepatic
1. Budd-Chiari syndrome
2. Constrictive pericarditis
3. CHF (tricuspid incompetence)

Pathophysiology:
continued elevated pressure despite formation of portal venous collateral vessels may be explained by
(a) backward flow theory = hypodynamic flow theory
= continuing increase in intrahepatic resistance + inadequate collateralization
- low / stagnant portal venous flow rates

(b) forward flow theory = hyperdynamic flow theory
= splanchnic flow increases secondary to splanchnic vasodilatation + increase in cardiac output to preserve hepatic perfusion
- increased portal venous flow rates >15 mL/min/kg

- elevated hepatic wedge pressure (HWP) = portal venous pressure (normal <10 mm Hg); normal values seen in presinusoidal portal hypertension
- **caput medusae** = drainage from paraumbilical + omental veins through superficial veins of chest (lateral thoracic vein to axillary vein; superficial epigastric vein to internal mammary vein and subclavian vein) + abdominal wall (circumflex iliac vein and superficial epigastric vein to femoral vein; inferior epigastric vein to external iliac vein)
- hemorrhaging esophageal varices (50%)

@ Splanchnic system:
√ portal vein >13 mm (57% sensitivity, 100% specificity)
√ SMV + splenic vein >10 mm; coronary vein >4 mm; recanalized umbilical vein >3 mm (size of vessels not related to degree of portal hypertension or presence of collaterals)
√ loss of respiratory increase of splanchnic vein diameters (80% sensitivity, 100% specificity)
√ portal vein aneurysm
√ portal vein thrombosis
√ cavernous transformation of portal vein
√ increased echogenicity + thickening of portal vein walls

Doppler US:
√ continuous portal vein flow without respiratory changes
√ reduction of mean portal vein velocities to 7–12 cm/sec (normally 12–30 cm/sec)
√ loss of flow increase in portal venous system during expiration
√ may have hepatofugal flow within spontaneous splenorenal shunts (indicates high incidence of hepatic encephalopathy)
√ dilated hepatic artery may demonstrate elevated resistive index >0.78

@ Portosystemic collaterals:

Type of Varices	Frequency (%)
Coronary venous	80–86
Esophageal	45–65
Paraumbilical	10–43
Abdominal wall	30
Perisplenic	30
Retrogastric / gastric	2–27
Paraesophageal	22
Omental	20
Retroperitoneal-paravertebral	18
Mesenteric	10
Splenorenal	10
Gastrorenal	7

√ varices = serpentine tubular rounded structures
√ coronary (left gastric) vein >5–6 mm (in 26%)
√ esophageal varices (= subepithelial + submucosal veins) supplied by anterior branch of left gastric vein
√ paraesophageal varices (endoscopically not visible) supplied by posterior branch of coronary (= left gastric) vein draining into azygos + hemiazygos vv. + vertebral plexus
◊ NOT connected to esophageal varices!
√ mediastinal / lung mass on CXR in 5–8%
√ gallbladder wall varices in thickened gallbladder wall (in 80% associated with portal vein thrombosis)

@ Cruveilhier-von Baumgarten syndrome (20–35%)
= recanalized paraumbilical veins (NOT recanalized umbilical veins)
√ hypoechoic channel in ligamentum teres
(a) size <2 mm (in 97% of normal subjects; in 14% of patients with portal hypertension)
(b) size ≥2 mm (86% sensitivity for portal hypertension)

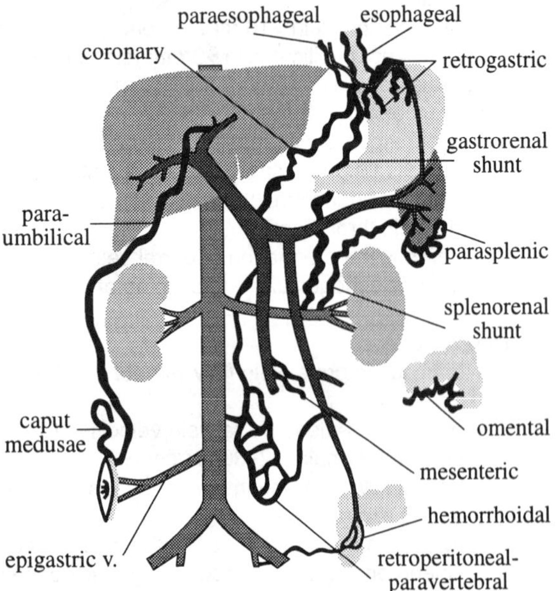

Portosystemic Collateral Vessels in Portal Hypertension

√ arterial signal on Doppler US in 38%
√ hepatofugal venous flow (82% sensitivity, 100% specificity for portal hypertension)

@ Spontaneous portosystemic shunts
• high frequency of hepatic encephalopathy
1. Splenorenal / splenoadrenorenal shunt
2. Gastrorenal shunt
3. Mesenterorenal shunt (between SMV + right renal v.)
4. Splenocaval shunt (between splenic v. + left hypogastric v.)
5. Gastropulmonary shunt (between gastric / esophageal vv. and pericardiophrenic / inferior pulmonary vv.)
6. Intrahepatic shunt (portal v. to hepatic v.)

@ Spleen
√ splenomegaly (absence does not rule out portal hypertension)
√ siderotic Gamna-Gandy nodules in 13% (= small foci of perifollicular + trabecular hemorrhage)
√ multiple 3–8 mm low-intensity spots on FLASH / GRASS images
√ multiple hyperechoic spots on US
√ multiple faint calcifications on CT

√ ascites

Cx: Acute gastrointestinal bleeding (mortality of 30–50% during 1st bleeding)

Segmental Portal Hypertension

= splenic vein occlusion / superior mesenteric vein occlusion

Portosystemic Surgical Connections

1. Portacaval shunt
= portal vein to IVC end-to-side / side-to-side
2. Distal splenorenal shunt = Warren shunt (popular)
= splenic vein to left renal vein
3. Mesocaval shunt
= synthetic graft between SMV and IVC
(a) short "H-graft" to posterior wall of SMV
(b) long "C-graft" to anterior wall of SMV
(c) direct mesocaval shunt dividing IVC (rare)
4. Mesoatrial shunt
= polytetrafluoroethylene (PTFE) graft between anterior wall of SMV superior to pancreas and right atrium coursing through abdomen + diaphragm into right thoracic cavity

Doppler criteria for shunt patency:
√ increased local velocities
√ turbulence + severe spectral broadening
√ dilatation of recipient vein at shunt site
√ phasic flow pattern in portal tributaries
√ hepatofugal flow in intrahepatic portal vein branches
√ reduction in size + number of portosystemic collaterals
√ reduction / absence of ascites or splenomegaly

LIVER

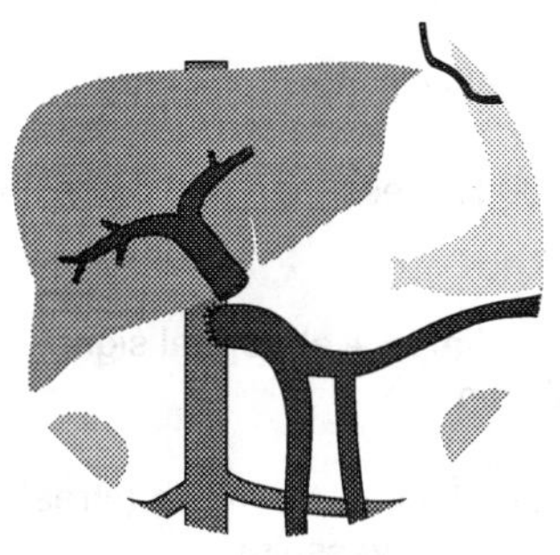
End-to-side portocaval shunt

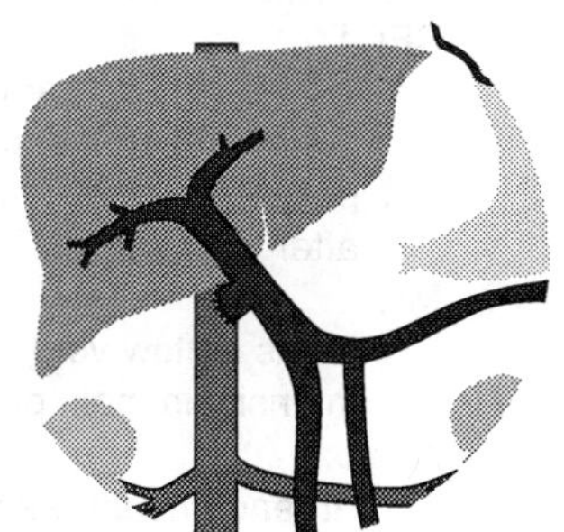
Side-to-side portocaval shunt

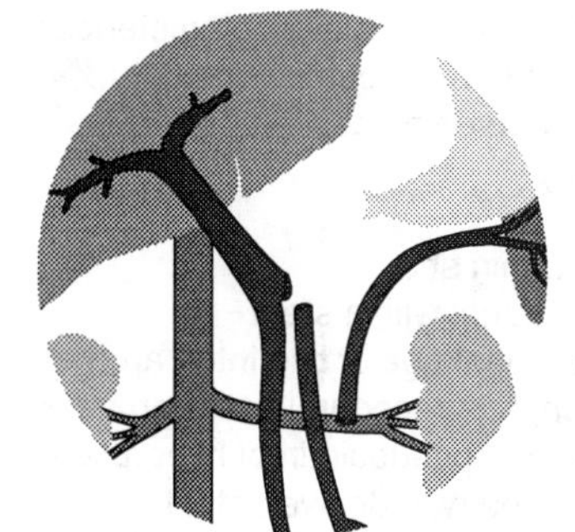
Splenorenal (Warren) shunt

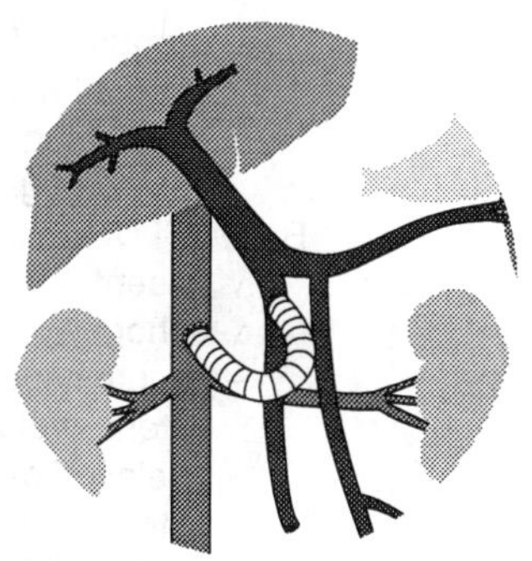
Mesocaval shunt

Surgical Portosystemic Shunts

Transjugular Intrahepatic Portosystemic Shunt (TIPS)

= portal decompression through percutaneously established shunt with expandable metallic stent between hepatic + portal veins within the liver

Indication: patients with esophageal + gastric variceal hemorrhage / refractory ascites due to advanced liver disease with portal hypertension, hepatorenal syndrome

Type of stent: 10-mm Wall stent (curved), Palmaz stent (straight), Strecker stent, spiral Z stent

Shunt surveillance: at regular 3–6 months intervals for

A. MORPHOLOGY
1. Ascites
2. Portosystemic collaterals
3. Size of spleen
4. Diameter of stent (usually 8–10 mm)
5. Configuration of stent: areas of narrowing
6. Extension of stent into portal + hepatic veins

B. HEMODYNAMICS
1. Direction of flow in: extrahepatic portal vein, RT + LT portal vein, SMV, splenic vein, all 3 hepatic veins, intrahepatic IVC, paraumbilical vein, coronary vein
2. Peak blood flow velocity within main portal vein
3. Peak blood flow velocity within proximal + mid + distal aspects of stent
4. Hepatic artery: PSV, EDV, RI

Pre- and post-TIPS baseline study under stable fasting conditions!

	Pre-TIPS	Post-TIPS
Portal vein velocity (cm/s)	10–30	40–60
Mean portal vein velocity (cm/s)	18 ± 6	55 ± 7
Portal pressure (mm Hg)	37 ± 8	22 ± 6
Shunt peak velocity (cm/s)		95 ± 58

√ high-velocity turbulent flow (50–270 cm/sec) at least double that of pre-TIPS values
√ superimposed cardiac + respiratory variations
√ increase in hepatic artery velocities from 77 cm/sec (pre-TIPS) to 119 cm/sec (post-TIPS)

Cx:
1. Shunt obstruction
2. Hepatic vein stenosis
3. Vascular injury: hepatic artery pseudoaneurysm, arterioportal fistula
4. Intrahepatic / subcapsular hematoma
5. Hemoperitoneum (due to penetration of liver capsule)
6. Transient bile duct dilatation (due to hemobilia)
7. Bile collection
8. stent dislodgment with embolization to right atrium, pulmonary artery, internal jugular vein

Mortality: <2% (intraperitoneal hemorrhage)

TIPS failure

Cause: acute thrombosis, improper stent placement, intimal hyperplasia, hepatic vein stenosis, change in stent configuration, bulging of liver parenchyma into shunt

1. Shunt obstruction (38%)
   Prevalence: 31% at 1 year, 42% at 2 years
   • recurrent bleeding = shunt abnormality in 100%
   A. >50% STENOSIS
      Time of onset: in 30–80% within 12 months
      √ irregular filling defects along wall of shunt on color Doppler
         ◊ pseudointimal hyperplasia is isoechoic to blood!
      √ gradual decrease in shunt velocity over 1–6 months (due to intimal hyperplasia)
      √ maximal shunt velocity of <60 cm/sec (>95% sensitive + specific)
      √ in- / decrease in peak flow velocity in similar location within stent >50 cm/sec relative to initial baseline study
      √ velocity transition zone within stent with flow acceleration by a factor of 2
      √ decrease in maximal portal vein velocity >33% from baseline
      √ reversal of portal venous flow direction (100% sensitive, 92% specific, 71% PPV, 100% NPV)
      √ loss of pulsatility of portal / shunt flow
      √ change in flow direction in collateral veins from baseline

√ retrograde flow in RHV (developing stenosis of right hepatic venous outflow tract)
√ developing / worsening ascites / splenomegaly

B. OCCLUSION
√ absent flow within shunt
√ echogenic material within stent
- acute cause: leakage of bile into / around stent, prolonged procedural catheterization
- delayed cause: pseudointimal hyperplasia, stent shortening with delayed stent expansion

PORTAL VEIN THROMBOSIS

Etiology:

A. IDIOPATHIC (mostly): ? neonatal sepsis
B. SECONDARY:
(1) Tumor invasion by HCC, cholangiocarcinoma, pancreatic carcinoma, gastric carcinoma / extrinsic compression by tumor
(2) Trauma; umbilical venous catheterization
(3) Blood dyscrasia; clotting disorder; estrogen therapy; severe dehydration; Cx of splenectomy (7%, higher in patients with myeloproliferative disorders)
(4) Intraabdominal sepsis with phlebitis; perinatal omphalitis; pancreatitis; ascending cholangitis
(5) Cirrhosis + portal hypertension (5%)

Age: predominantly children, young persons

• abdominal pain
• portal systemic encephalopathy
• hematemesis (esophageal varices)

√ nonvisualization of portal vein
√ calcification within clot / wall of portal vein
√ splenomegaly
√ ascites

Plain film:
√ hepatosplenomegaly
√ enlarged azygos vein
√ paraspinal varices

UGI:
√ esophageal varices
√ thickening of bowel wall

US:
√ echogenic material within vessel lumen (67%)
√ increase in portal vein diameter (57%)
◊ Malignant thrombus tends to distend vein + exhibit pulsatile flow, a bland thrombus does not!
√ portosystemic collateral circulation (48%)
√ enlargement of thrombosed segment >15 mm (38%)
√ no flow on postprandial Doppler color scans
√ cavernous transformation = **cavernoma** (19%)
√ failure to visualize the extrahepatic portal vein
√ presence of a racemose conglomerate of collateral veins with portal venous flow linking pancreas + duodenum + gallbladder fossa
√ decrease in hepatic artery resistive index
√ RI <0.50 (in acute occlusive portal vein thrombosis)
√ minimal decrease / normal RI (in chronic portal vein thrombosis / nonocclusive thrombosis)
√ thickening of lesser omentum

CECT:
√ low-density center in portal vein surrounded by peripheral enhancement
√ portal vein density 20–30 HU less than aortic density after contrast

MR:
√ areas of flow void in portal area + abnormal signal intensity in main portal vein

Angio:
√ "thread and streaks" sign of tumor thrombus (streaky contrast opacification of tumor vessels)

Cx: (1) Hepatic infarction
(2) Bowel infarction

POSTCHOLECYSTECTOMY SYNDROME

= symptoms recurring / persisting after cholecystectomy

Incidence:
mild recurrent symptoms in 9–25%; severe symptoms in 2.6–32% (result of 1,930 cholecystectomies):
— completely cured (61%)
— satisfactory improvement with
(a) persistent mild dyspepsia (11%)
(b) mild attacks of pain (24%)
— failure with
(a) occasional attacks of severe pain (3%)
(b) continuous severe distress (1.7%)
(c) recurrent cholangitis (0.7%)

Cause:

A. BILIARY CAUSES
(a) Incomplete surgery
1. Gallbladder / cystic duct remnant
2. Retained stone in cystic duct remnant
3. Overlooked CBD stone
(b) Operative trauma
1. Bile duct stricture
2. Bile peritonitis
(c) Bile duct pathology
1. Fibrosis of sphincter of Oddi
2. Biliary dyskinesia
3. Biliary fistula
(d) Residual disease in neighboring structures
1. Pancreatitis
2. Hepatitis
3. Cholangitis
(e) Overlooked bile duct neoplasia

B. EXTRABILIARY CAUSES (erroneous preoperative diagnosis)
(a) Other GI tract disease:
1. Inadequate dentition
2. Hiatus hernia
3. Peptic ulcer
4. Spastic colon
(b) Anxiety state, air swallowing
(c) Abdominal angina
(d) Carcinoma outside gallbladder
(e) Coronary artery disease

RICHTER SYNDROME

= development of large cell / diffuse histiocytic lymphoma in patients with CLL

Etiology: transformation / dedifferentiation of CLL lymphocytes

Incidence in CLL patients: 3–10%

Median age: 59 years

Medium time interval after diagnosis of CLL: 24 months

- fever (65%) without evidence of infection
- increasing lymphadenopathy + hepatosplenomegaly (46%)
- weight loss (26%)
- abdominal pain (26%)

Location: bone marrow, lymph nodes, liver, spleen, bowel, lung, pleura, kidney, dura

Prognosis: median survival time: 4 months from diagnosis of lymphoma; 14% rate of remission rate

SCHISTOSOMIASIS

Worldwide major cause of portal hypertension: 200 million people affected

Types:

A. SCHISTOSOMA HAEMATOBIUM
in Africa, Mediterranean, Southwest Asia

B. SCHISTOSOMA MANSONI
occurs in >70 million inhabitants of parts of Africa, Caribbean, Arabic peninsula, West Indies, northern part of South America

C. SCHISTOSOMA JAPONICUM
coastal areas of China, Japan, Formosa, Philippines, Celebes

Cycle:
cercariae enter lymphatics + blood system via thoracic duct; larvae are transported into mesenteric capillaries; mature in portal system + liver into worms; worms live in pairs in copula within portal vein + tributaries for 10–15 years; female swims against bloodflow to reach venules of urinary bladder (S. haematobium) or intestine + rectum (S. mansoni, S. japonicum); deposits eggs in wall of urinary bladder or intestines, eggs pass with urine + feces; hatch within water to release miracidia which infect snail hosts; cercariae emerge after maturation from snails

Infection: cercariae penetrate human skin / buccal mucosa from contaminated water (slow-moving streams, irrigation canals, paddy fields, lakes)

Histo: granulomatous reaction + fibrosis along portal vein branches

- clinically mild infection with chronic course

@ Liver
- √ marked diffuse thickening of echogenic walls of portal venules = periportal fibrosis
  - ◊ Schistosoma infection is the most frequent cause of liver fibrosis worldwide!
- √ hepatosplenomegaly
- √ portal vein dilatation in 73% (= portal hypertension)
- √ normal parenchymal echogenicity + small peripheral hyperechoic foci in 50% (= fibrosis of portal radicles)
- √ hyperechoic gallbladder bed
- √ thickened gallbladder wall

@ GI tract
- √ gastric + esophageal varices
- √ polypoid bowel wall masses (esp. in sigmoid)
- √ granulomatous colitis
- √ strictures with extensive pericolic inflammation

Cx: ileus

SCHWACHMAN-DIAMOND SYNDROME

= rare congenital absence of pancreatic exocrine tissue, 2nd most frequent cause of exocrine pancreatic insufficiency in childhood

- pancreatic insufficiency
- recurrent respiratory and skin infections (secondary to bone marrow hypoplasia)
- dwarfism (metaphyseal dysostosis)
- normal electrolytes in sweat
- tends to improve with time

√ total fatty replacement of pancreas

SOLID AND PAPILLARY NEOPLASM OF PANCREAS

= SOLID AND CYSTIC TUMOR = PAPILLARY-CYSTIC NEOPLASM = SOLID AND PAPILLARY EPITHELIAL NEOPLASM

= rare, low-grade malignant tumor; often misclassified as nonfunctioning islet cell tumor, cystadenoma, cystadenocarcinoma of pancreas

Prevalence: 0.17–2.7% of all nonendocrine pancreatic tumors

Mean age: 25 (range 10–74) years ; M:F = 1:9; especially in black and East Asian patients

Path: large well-encapsulated mass with considerable hemorrhagic necrosis + cystic degeneration

Histo: sheets + cords of cells arranged around a fibrovascular stroma

- vague upper abdominal discomfort and pain
- gradually enlarging abdominal mass

Location: tail of pancreas (most frequently)

- √ well-encapsulated inhomogeneous round / lobulated pancreatic mass with solid + cystic portions
- √ may be completely cystic (when complicated by extensive necrosis + internal hemorrhage)
- √ fluid-debris level (20%)
- √ mean diameter of 9 cm (range 3–15 cm)
- √ ± stippled / punctate / amorphous dystrophic calcification (33%)
- √ hypovascular with no contrast enhancement / enhancement of solid tissue projecting toward center of mass

US:
- √ echogenic mass with necrotic center

MR:
- √ high signal intensity on T1WI (consistent with hemorrhagic necrosis)

Prognosis: (1) excellent after excision
(2) metastases (in 4%): omentum, lymph nodes, liver

LIVER

DDx: (1) Microcystic adenoma (innumerable tiny cysts, older age group)
(2) Mucinous cystic neoplasm (large uni- / multilocular cysts, older age group)
(3) Nonfunctioning islet cell tumor (hypervascular)
(4) Pleomorphic carcinoma of pancreas (smaller tumor in older patient)
(5) Pancreaticoblastoma (childhood tumor)
(6) Calcified hemorrhagic pseudocyst

SPLENIC ANGIOSARCOMA

Incidence: rare, <100 cases in literature
Cause: usually not due to thorotrast or toxic exposure to vinyl chloride / arsenic as in liver angiosarcoma
Age: 50–60 years
• splenomegaly, abdominal pain
√ multiple nodules of varying size usually enlarging the spleen
√ solitary complex mass with variable contrast enhancement
√ metastasizes to liver (70%)
√ spontaneous rupture (33%)
MR:
√ focal / diffuse hypointense foci on T1WI + T2WI (iron deposition from hemorrhage)
Prognosis: 20% survival rate after 6 months

SPLENIC HAMARTOMA

= rare nonneoplastic tumor composed of a mixture of normal splenic elements
Etiology: congenital
May be associated with: hamartomas elsewhere as in tuberous sclerosis
Histo: (a) white pulp subtype = aberrant lymphoid tissue
(b) red pulp subtype = aberrant complex of sinusoids
(c) mixture (most common)
• asymptomatic
CT:
√ attenuation equal to splenic tissue
√ prolonged enhancement
MR:
√ heterogeneously hyperintense on T2WI
√ diffuse heterogeneous enhancement, more homogeneous on delayed images

SPLENIC HEMANGIOMA

Cause: congenital, arising from sinusoidal epithelium
Prevalence: 0.03–14% (autopsy); M > F
◊ Most common primary splenic tumor!
Age: 20–50 years
Histo: proliferation of vascular channels lined by single layer of endothelium; mostly of cavernous type; may contain areas of infarction, hemorrhage, thrombosis, fibrosis
May be associated with: Klippel-Trénaunay-Weber syndrome (multiple hemangiomas)
• asymptomatic / pain + fullness in LUQ
√ usually small single lesion <4 cm, up to 17 cm in size
√ foci of speckled / snowflakelike calcifications
MR:
√ hyperintense on T2WI
√ progressive centripetal enhancement with persistent uniform enhancement on delayed images
Prognosis: slow growth, thus becoming symptomatic in adulthood
Cx: (1) Spontaneous splenic rupture (in up to 25%)
(2) Kasabach-Merritt syndrome (= anemia, thrombocytopenia, coagulopathy) with large hemangioma
(3) Malignant degeneration

SPLENIC INFARCTION

◊ Most common cause of focal defects!
Cause:
1. Embolic: bacterial endocarditis (responsible in 50%), atherosclerosis with plaque emboli, cardiac thrombus (atrial fibrillation, left ventricular thrombus), metastatic carcinoma
2. Local thrombosis: sickle cell disease (leading to functional asplenia), myelo- / lymphoproliferative disorders (CML most common), polycythemia vera, myelofibrosis with myeloid metaplasia + splenomegaly, Gaucher disease
3. Vasculitis: periarteritis nodosa
4. Vascular compromise of splenic artery: focal inflammatory process (eg, pancreatitis), thrombus from splenic artery aneurysm, splenic torsion
5. Therapeutic complication: transcatheter hepatic arterial embolization

mnemonic: "PSALMS"
Pancreatic carcinoma, **P**ancreatitis
Sickle cell disease / trait
Adenocarcinoma of stomach
Leukemia
Mitral stenosis with emboli
Subacute bacterial endocarditis

• LUQ pain, fever
• elevated erythrocyte sedimentation rate, leukocytosis
• abnormal lactate dehydrogenase levels

√ single / multiple focal wedge-shaped peripheral defects
CT phases:
(a) hyperacute phase (day 1)
√ mottled area of increased attenuation on NECT (hemorrhage)
√ large focal hyperattenuating lesion on CECT
√ mottled pattern of contrast enhancement
(b) acute (days 2–4) + subacute phase (days 4–8)
√ focal progressively more well-demarcated areas of decreased attenuation without enhancement
(c) chronic phase (2–4 weeks)
√ size decreases + attenuation returns to normal
√ complete resolution / residual contour defect
√ areas of calcification
Cx: superimposed infection, splenic rupture

SPLENIC TRAUMA

◊ Most frequently injured intraperitoneal organ in blunt abdominal trauma

Associated with: other solid visceral / bowel injuries (29%); lower rib fractures in 44%, injury to left kidney in 10%, injury to left diaphragm in 2%

Technique: scanning delay of 60–70 sec to avoid the phase of heterogeneous splenic enhancement

CT sensitivity: >95% for splenic injury, but not reliable to determine need for surgical intervention

◊ Attenuation of active extravasation (80–370 HU) exceeds that of splenic parenchyma / clotted blood

Prognosis: high PPV for surgery

1. Intrasplenic laceration
   √ linear parenchymal defect
   √ almost always associated with hemoperitoneum
2. Splenic fracture
   √ laceration traverses two capsular surfaces
3. Subcapsular hematoma
   √ crescentic lesion along splenic margin flattening / indenting the normally convex lateral margin
4. Perisplenic hematoma
   √ "sentinel clot" (= area of >60 HU adjacent to spleen) sensitive predictor of splenic injury
5. Delayed splenic rupture
   = hemorrhage >48 hours after trauma
   Prevalence: 0.3–20% of blunt splenic injuries
   Time of onset: in 70% within 2 weeks of injury, in 90% within 4 weeks of injury

Rx: 52% surgery (splenectomy (8%), splenorrhaphy), 48% nonsurgical management

SPLENOSIS

= autotransplantation of splenic tissue to other sites following trauma

Age: young men with history of trauma / splenectomy

Time of detection: mean of 10 years (range of 6 months – 32 years) after trauma

Location: diaphragmatic surface, liver, omentum, mesentery, peritoneum, pleura

√ multiple small encapsulated sessile implants (few mm – 3 cm)

√ demonstrated by Tc-99m sulfur colloid; In-111 labeled platelets; Tc-99m heat-damaged RBC (best detection rate)

DDx: accessory spleen

SPONTANEOUS PERFORATION OF COMMON BILE DUCT

Pathogenesis: unknown (? CBD obstruction, localized mural malformation, ischemia, trauma)

Age: 5 weeks to 3 years of age

• vague abdominal distension
• mild persistent hyperbilirubinemia
• varying acholic stools

US:
   √ biliary ascites / loculated subhepatic fluid
   √ localized pseudocholedochal cyst in porta hepatis

Hepatobiliary scintigraphy:
   √ radioisotope diffusely throughout peritoneal cavity

THOROTRASTOSIS

Thorotrast = 25% colloidal suspension of thorium dioxide; used as contrast agent between late 1920s and mid 1950s, in particular for cerebral angiography and liver spleen imaging; chemically inert with high atomic number of 90; >100,000 people injected

Thorium dioxide = consists of 11 radioactive isotopes (thorium-232 is major isotope); decay by means of alpha, beta, and gamma emission; biologic half-life of 1.34×10^{10} years; hepatic dose of 1000–3000 rads in 20 years

Distribution: phagocytosed by RES + deposited in liver (70%), spleen (30%), bone marrow, abdominal lymph nodes (20%)

√ linear network of metallic density contrast material in spleen, lymph nodes, liver

√ spleen may be shrunken / nonfunctional

Cx: hepatic fibrosis, angiosarcoma (50%), cholangiocarcinoma, hepatocellular carcinoma (latency period of 3–40 years; mean 26 years)

UNDIFFERENTIATED SARCOMA OF LIVER

= EMBRYONAL SARCOMA

Incidence: 4th / 5th most common liver tumor in pediatric population

Age: <2 months (in 5%); 6–10 years (in 52%); by 15 years (in 90%); up to 49 years; M:F = 1:1

Histo: primitive undifferentiated stellate / spindle-shaped sarcomatous cells closely packed in whorls + sheets / scattered loosely in a myxoid ground substance with foci of hematopoiesis (50%)

• painful RUQ mass and fever
• mild anemia + leukocytosis (50%)
• elevated liver enzymes (33%)
• fever (5%)

Location: right lobe (75%); left lobe (10%); both lobes (15%)

√ 7–14–21 cm in size

√ well-defined margins (fibrous pseudocapsule)

NUC:
   √ photodefect on sulfur colloid scan

US / CT:
   √ large intrahepatic mass with cystic areas up to 4 cm in diameter (myxoid stroma + necrosis + hemorrhage)
   √ discordant finding between US (solid) + CT (cystlike)

Angio:
   √ hypo- / hypervascular with stretching of vessels
   √ scattered foci of neovascularity

Prognosis: mostly results in death within 12 months

DDx: mesenchymal hamartoma
   (a) solid lesion + cystic degeneration: hepatocellular carcinoma, fibrolamellar carcinoma, intrahepatic cholangiocarcinoma, angiosarcoma, epithelioid hemangioendothelioma, other sarcomas, lymphoma, metastatic disease, hepatocellular adenoma

LIVER

(b) solitary cystic lesion:
biliary cystadenoma / ~carcinoma, cystic degeneration of hepatocellular carcinoma, bacterial / parasitic abscess, metastatic disease, posttraumatic resolving hematoma

WANDERING SPLEEN

= ABERRANT / FLOATING / PTOTIC / DRIFTING / DYSTOPIC / DISPLACED / PROLAPSED SPLEEN
= excessively mobile spleen on an elongated pedicle displaced from its usual position in LUQ

Cause: embryologically absent / malformed gastrosplenic + splenorenal ligaments; lax abdominal musculature during pregnancy

Age: any (higher frequency in women of childbearing age)

- asymptomatic mobile abdominal / pelvic mass
- chronic vague lower abdominal / back pain
- nausea, vomiting, eructation, flatulence
- acute abdomen (with splenic infarction)

√ empty splenic fossa
√ inverted malpositioned stomach
√ displaced large spleen (congestion during torsion)

Cx:
1. Torsion with prolonged venous occlusion: perisplenitis, localized peritonitis, adhesions, venous thrombosis, hypersplenism
2. Torsion with arterial occlusion: hemorrhagic infarction, subcapsular / intrasplenic hemorrhage, gangrene, degenerative cysts, functional asplenism
3. GI complications:
   @ Stomach: compression, distension, volvulus, traction diverticulum, varices
   @ Small bowel: dilatation, obstruction
   @ Colon: compression, volvulus, laxity, ptosis

Rx:
1. Splenectomy (4% postsplenectomy sepsis)
2. Splenopexy
3. Conservative treatment (if asymptomatic)

GASTROINTESTINAL TRACT

DIFFERENTIAL DIAGNOSIS OF GASTROINTESTINAL DISORDERS

ABNORMAL INTRA-ABDOMINAL AIR

Abnormal Air Collection

1. Abnormally located bowel
   Chilaiditi syndrome (= colon interposed between liver and chest wall), inguinal hernia
2. Pneumoperitoneum
3. Retropneumoperitoneum
   perforation of duodenum / rectum / ascending + descending colon, diverticulitis, ulcerative disease, endoscopic procedure
4. Gas in bowel wall
   gastric pneumatosis, phlegmonous gastritis, endoscopy, rupture of lung bulla
5. Gas within abscess
   located in subphrenic, renal, perirenal, hepatic, pancreatic space, lesser sac
6. Gas in biliary system
   hepatobiliary fistula, surgery, duodenal ulcer, duodenal diverticulum, cancer, stone, patulous ampulla, emphysematous cholecystitis
   √ gas outlines choledochus ± gallbladder
   √ peripheral branches of bile ducts not filled
   mnemonic: "SITS"
   Stone
   Inflammation (emphysematous cholecystitis)
   Tumor with fistula
   Surgery
7. Gas in portal venous system
   √ branching air within 2 cm of liver periphery

Pneumoperitoneum

Etiology:

A. DISRUPTION OF WALL OF HOLLOW VISCUS
   (a) blunt / penetrating trauma
      1. Perforating foreign body (eg, thermometer injury to rectum, vaginal stimulator in rectum)
      2. Compressor air directed toward anus
   (b) iatrogenic perforation
      1. Laparoscopy / laparotomy (58%): absorbed in 1–24 days dependent on initial amount of air introduced and body habitus (80% in asthenic, 25% in obese patients)
         ◊ After 3 days free air should be followed with suspicion!
      2. Leaking surgical anastomosis
      3. Endoscopic perforation
      4. Enema tip injury
      5. Diagnostic pneumoperitoneum
   (c) diseases of GI tract
      1. Perforated gastric / duodenal ulcer
      2. Perforated appendix
      3. Ingested foreign-body perforation
      4. Diverticulitis (ruptured Meckel diverticulum / sigmoid diverticulum, jejunal diverticulosis)
      5. Necrotizing enterocolitis with perforation
      6. Inflammatory bowel disease (eg, toxic megacolon)
      7. Obstruction† (gas traversing intact mucosa): neoplasm, imperforate anus, Hirschsprung disease, meconium ileus
      8. Ruptured pneumatosis cystoides intestinalis† with "balanced pneumoperitoneum" (= free intraperitoneal air acts as tamponade of pneumatosis cysts thus maintaining a balance between intracystic air + pneumoperitoneum)
      9. Idiopathic gastric perforation = spontaneous perforation in premature infants (congenital gastric muscular wall defect)

B. THROUGH PERITONEAL SURFACE
   (a) transperitoneal manipulation
      1. Abdominal needle biopsy / catheter placement
      2. Mistaken thoracentesis / chest tube placement
      3. Endoscopic biopsy
   (b) extension from chest†
      1. Dissection from pneumomediastinum (positive pressure breathing, rupture of bulla / bleb, chest surgery)
      2. Bronchopleural fistula
   (c) rupture of urinary bladder
   (d) penetrating abdominal injury

C. THROUGH FEMALE GENITAL TRACT†
   (a) iatrogenic
      1. Perforation of uterus / vagina
      2. Culdocentesis
      3. Rubin test = tubal patency test
      4. Pelvic examination
   (b) spontaneous
      1. Intercourse, orogenital insufflation
      2. Douching
      3. Knee-chest exercise, water skiing, horseback riding

D. INTRAPERITONEAL
   1. Gasforming peritonitis
   2. Rupture of abscess

Note † = asymptomatic spontaneous pneumoperitoneum without peritonitis

√ air in lesser peritoneal sac
√ gas in scrotum (through open processus vaginalis)

<u>Large collection of gas</u>:
√ abdominal distension, no gastric air-fluid level
√ "football sign" = large pneumoperitoneum outlining entire abdominal cavity
√ "double wall sign" = "Rigler sign" = "bas-relief sign"
= air on both sides of bowel as intraluminal gas + free air outside (usually requires >1,000 mL of free intraperitoneal gas + intraperitoneal fluid)

√ "telltale triangle sign" = triangular air pocket between 3 loops of bowel
√ depiction of diaphragmatic muscle slips = two or three 6–13 cm long and 8–10 mm wide arcuate soft-tissue bands directed vertically inferiorly + arching parallel to diaphragmatic dome superiorly
√ outline of ligaments of anterior inferior abdominal wall:
√ "inverted V sign" = outline of both lateral umbilical ligaments (containing inferior epigastric vessels)
√ outline of medial umbilical ligaments (obliterated umbilical arteries)
√ "urachus sign" = outline of middle umbilical ligament

RUQ gas (best place to look for small collections):
√ single large area of hyperlucency over the liver
√ oblique linear area of hyperlucency outlining the posteroinferior margin of liver
√ doge's cap sign = triangular collection of gas in Morison pouch (posterior hepatorenal space)
√ outline of falciform ligament = long vertical line to the right of midline extending from ligamentum teres notch to umbilicus; most common structure outlined
√ ligamentum teres notch = inverted V-shaped area of hyperlucency along undersurface of liver
√ ligamentum teres sign = air outlining fissure of ligamentum teres hepatis (= posterior free edge of falciform ligament) seen as vertically oriented sharply defined slitlike / oval area of hyperlucency between 10th and 12th rib within 2.5–4.0 cm of right vertebral border 2–7 mm wide and 6–20 mm long
√ "saddlebag / mustache / cupola sign" = gas trapped below central tendon of diaphragm
√ parahepatic air = gas bubble lateral to right edge of liver

Pseudopneumoperitoneum

= process mimicking free air

A. ABDOMINAL GAS
   (a) gastrointestinal gas
      1. Pseudo-wall sign = apposition of gas-distended bowel loops
      2. Chilaiditi syndrome
      3. Diaphragmatic hernia
      4. Diverticulum of esophagus / stomach / duodenum
   (b) extraintestinal gas
      1. Retroperitoneal air
      2. Subdiaphragmatic abscess
B. CHEST
   1. Pneumothorax
   2. Empyema
   3. Irregularity of diaphragm
C. FAT
   1. Subdiaphragmatic intraperitoneal fat
   2. Interposition of omental fat between liver + diaphragm

Pneumoretroperitoneum

Cause: (1) Traumatic rupture (usually duodenum)
(2) Perforation of duodenal ulcer
(3) Gas abscess of pancreas (usually extends into lesser sac)
(4) Urinary tract gas (trauma, infection)
(5) Dissected mediastinal air

√ kidney outlined by gas
√ outline of psoas margin ± gas streaks in muscle bundles

Pneumatosis Intestinalis

= PNEUMATOSIS CYSTOIDES INTESTINALIS = BULLOUS EMPHYSEMA OF THE INTESTINE = INTESTINAL GAS CYSTS = PERITONEAL LYMPHOPNEUMATOSIS

◊ Attributed to at least 58 causative factors!

A. BOWEL NECROSIS / GANGRENE
   ◊ Most common + life-threatening cause!
   Pathogenesis: damage + disruption of mucosa with entry of gasforming bacteria into bowel wall (cysts contain 50% hydrogen = evidence of bacterial origin)
   necrotizing enterocolitis, ischemia + infarction (mesenteric thrombosis), neutropenic colitis, sepsis, volvulus, emphysematous gastritis, caustic ingestion
B. MUCOSAL DISRUPTION
   Pathogenesis: increased intestinal gas pressure leads to overdistension and dissection of gas into bowel wall
   (a) intestinal obstruction:
      pyloric stenosis, annular pancreas, imperforate anus, Hirschsprung disease, meconium plug syndrome, obstructing neoplasm
   (b) intestinal trauma:
      endoscopy ± biopsy, biliary stent perforation, sclerotherapy, bowel surgery, postoperative bowel anastomosis, penetrating / blunt abdominal trauma, trauma of child abuse, intracatheter jejunal feeding tube, barium enema
   (c) infection / inflammation:
      peptic ulcer disease, intestinal parasites, tuberculosis, peritonitis, inflammatory bowel disease (Crohn disease, ulcerative colitis, pseudomembranous colitis), ruptured jejunal diverticula, Whipple disease, systemic amyloidosis
D. INCREASED MUCOSAL PERMEABILITY
   Pathogenesis: defects in lymphoid tissue of bowel wall allows bacterial gas to enter bowel wall
   (a) immunotherapy:
      graft-versus-host disease, organ transplantation, bone marrow transplantation
   (b) others:
      AIDS enterocolitides, steroid therapy, chemotherapy, radiation therapy, collagen vascular disease (scleroderma, systemic lupus erythematosus, periarteritis dermatomyositis), intestinal bypass enteropathy, diabetes mellitus

C. PULMONARY DISEASE

Pathogenesis: alveolar rupture with air dissecting interstitially along bronchovascular bundles to mediastinum + retroperitoneally along vascular supply of viscera

Chronic obstructive pulmonary disease (chronic bronchitis, emphysema, bullous disease of lung), asthma, cystic fibrosis, chest trauma (barotrauma from artificial ventilation, chest tube), increased intrathoracic pressure associated with retching + vomiting

Path: (a) microvesicular type = 10–100 mm cysts / bubbles within lamina propria
(b) linear / curvilinear type = streaks of gas oriented parallel to bowel wall

Location: any part of GI tract; may be discontinuous with spread to distant sites along mesentery

Site: subserosa > submucosa > muscularis > mesentery; mesenteric side >> antimesenteric side

√ radiolucent clusters of cysts along contour of bowel wall (best demonstrated on CT)
√ segmental mucosal nodularity (DDx: polyposis)
√ ± pneumoperitoneum / pneumoretroperitoneum (asymptomatic large pneumoperitoneum may persist for months / years)
√ ± gas in mesenteric + portal vein

Prognosis:
wide spectrum from innocuous to fatal; clinical outcome impossible to predict based on x-ray findings
◊ linear gas collections have probably a more severe connotation
◊ pneumatosis of the colon is likely clinically insignificant
◊ extent of pneumatosis is inversely related to severity of disease

Soap-bubble Appearance In Abdomen Of Neonate

1. Feces in infant fed by mouth
2. Meconium ileus:
   gas mixed with meconium, usually RLQ
3. Meconium plug:
   gas in and around plug, in distribution of colon
4. Necrotizing enterocolitis: submucosal pneumatosis
5. Atresia / severe stenosis: pneumatosis
6. Hirschsprung disease:
   impacted stool, sometimes pneumatosis

ABDOMINAL CALCIFICATIONS & OPACITIES

Opaque Material In Bowel

mnemonic: "CHIPS"
Chloral hydrate
Heavy metals (lead)
Iron
Phenothiazines
Salicylates

Diffuse Abdominal Calcifications

1. Cystadenoma of ovary
   √ granular, sandlike psammomatous calcifications
2. Pseudomyxoma peritonei
   (a) pseudomucinous adenoma of ovary
   (b) mucocele of appendix
3. Undifferentiated abdominal malignancy
4. Tuberculous peritonitis
   √ mottled calcifications, simulating residual barium
5. Meconium peritonitis
6. Oil granuloma
   √ annular, plaquelike

Focal Alimentary Tract Calcifications

A. ENTEROLITHS
   1. Appendicolith: in 10–15% of acute appendicitis
   2. Stone in Meckel diverticulum
   3. Diverticular stone
   4. Rectal stone
   5. Proximal to partial obstruction (eg, tuberculosis, Crohn disease)
B. MESENTERIC CALCIFICATIONS
   1. Dystrophic calcification of omental fat deposits + appendices epiploicae (secondary to infarction / pancreatitis / TB)
   2. Cysts: mesenteric cyst, hydatid cyst
   3. Calcified mesenteric lipoma
C. INGESTED FOREIGN BODIES
   trapped in appendix, diverticula, proximal to stricture
   1. Calcified seeds + pits (bezoar)
   2. Birdshot
D. TUMOR
   1. Mucocele of appendix
      √ crescent-shaped / circular calcification
   2. Mucinous adenocarcinoma of stomach / colon
      = COLLOID CARCINOMA
      √ small mottled / punctate calcifications in primary site ± in regional lymph node metastases, adjacent omentum, metastatic liver foci
   3. Gastric / esophageal leiomyoma: calcifies in 4%
   4. Lipoma

Abdominal Wall Calcifications

A. IN SOFT TISSUES
   1. Hypercalcemic states
   2. Idiopathic calcinosis
B. IN MUSCLE
   (a) parasites:
      1. Cysticercosis = Taenia solium
         √ round / slightly elongated calcifications
      2. Guinea worm = dracunculiasis
         √ stringlike calcifications up to 12 cm long
   (b) injection sites
      from quinine, bismuth, calcium gluconate, calcium penicillin
   (c) myositis ossificans
C. IN SKIN
   1. Soft-tissue nodules: papilloma, neurofibroma, melanoma, nevi
   2. Scar: √ linear density

GI

3. Colostomy / ileostomy
4. Tattoo markings

Abdominal Vascular Calcifications

A. ARTERIES
1. Atheromatous plaques
2. Arterial calcifications in diabetes mellitus

B. VEINS
phleboliths = calcified thrombus, generally seen below interspinous line
1. normal / varicose veins
2. hemangioma

C. LYMPH NODES
1. Histoplasmosis / tuberculosis
2. Chronic granulomatous disease
3. Residual lymphographic contrast
4. Silicosis

ABNORMAL INTRA-ABDOMINAL FLUID

Ascites

A. TRANSUDATE:
(1) Cirrhosis (75%): poor prognostic sign
(2) Hypoproteinemia, (3) CHF, (4) Constrictive pericarditis, (5) Chronic renal failure, (6) Budd-Chiari syndrome

B. EXUDATE:
(1) Carcinomatosis, (2) Polyserositis, (3) TB peritonitis, (4) Pancreatitis, (5) Meigs syndrome

C. HEMORRHAGIC / CHYLOUS FLUID

Early signs (accumulation in pelvis):
√ round central density in pelvis + ill-defined bladder top
√ thickening of peritoneal flank stripe
√ space between properitoneal fat and gut >3 mm

Late signs:
√ Hellmer sign = medial displacement of lateral liver margins
√ medial displacement of ascending + descending colon
√ obliteration of hepatic + splenic angles
√ bulging flanks
√ gray abdomen
√ floating centralized loops
√ separation of loops

High-density Ascites

1. Tuberculosis: 20–45 HU; may be lower
2. Ovarian tumor
3. Appendiceal tumor

Neonatal Ascites

A. GASTROINTESTINAL
(a) perforation of hollow viscus
meconium peritonitis
(b) inflammatory lesions
Meckel diverticulum, appendicitis
(c) cyst rupture
mesenteric / omental / choledochal cyst
(d) bile leakage
biliary obstruction / perforation

B. PORTOHEPATIC
(a) extrahepatic portal vein obstruction
atresia of veins, compression by mass
(b) intrahepatic portal vein obstruction
portal cirrhosis (neonatal hepatitis), biliary cirrhosis (biliary atresia)

C. URINARY TRACT
◊ Urine ascites (most common cause) from lower urinary tract obstruction + upper urinary tract rupture: posterior / anterior urethral valves, ureterovesical / ureteropelvic junction obstruction, renal / bladder rupture, anterior urethral diverticulum, bladder diverticula, neurogenic bladder, extrinsic bladder mass

D. GENITAL
ruptured ovarian cyst, hydrometrocolpos

E. HYDROPS FETALIS
immune hydrops, nonimmune hydrops (usually cardiac causes)

F. MISCELLANEOUS
chylous ascites, lymphangiectasia, congenital syphilis, trauma, idiopathic

Chylous Ascites

IN ADULTS:	1. Inflammatory process	(35%)
	2. Tumor	(30%)
	3. Idiopathic	(23%)
	4. Trauma	(11%)
	5. Congenital	(1%)
IN CHILDREN:	1. Congenital	(39%)
	2. Inflammatory process	(15%)
	3. Trauma	(12%)
	4. Tumor	(3%)
	5. Idiopathic	(33%)

Fluid Collections

mnemonic: "BLUSCHINGS"
Biloma
Lymphocele, **L**ymphangioma, **L**ymphoma (almost anechoic by US)
Urinoma
Seroma
Cyst (pseudocyst, peritoneal inclusion cyst)
Hematoma (aneurysm, AVM)
Infection, **I**nfestation (empyema, abscess, Echinococcus)
Neoplasm (necrotic)
GI tract (dilated loops, ileus, duplication)
Serosa (ascites, pleural fluid, pericardial effusion)

Intra-abdominal Cyst In Childhood

1. Omental cyst (greater omentum / lesser sac, multilocular)
2. Mesenteric cyst (between leaves of small bowel mesentery)
3. Choledochal cyst
4. Intestinal duplication
5. Ovarian cyst

GI

6. Pancreatic pseudocyst
7. Cystic renal tumor
8. Abscess
9. Meckel diverticulum (communicates with GI tract)
10. Lymphangioma
11. Mesenteric lymphoma
12. Intramural tumor

MECHANICAL INTESTINAL OBSTRUCTION

= occlusion / constriction of bowel lumen

Common causes of obstruction in children

Nursery	Intestinal atresia, midgut volvulus, meconium ileus, Hirschsprung disease, small bowel atresia with meconium ileus, meconium plug syndrome, small left colon syndrome, imperforate anus, obstruction from duplication cyst
First 3 months	Inguinal hernia, Hirschsprung disease, midgut volvulus
6 — 24 months	Ileocolic intussusception
Childhood	Appendicitis

Gastric outlet obstruction

A. CONGENITAL LESION
   1. Antral mucosal diaphragm = antral web
   2. Gastric duplication: usually along greater curvature, abdominal mass in infancy
   3. Hypertrophic pyloric stenosis

B. INFLAMMATORY NARROWING
   1. Peptic ulcer disease: cause in adults in 60–65%
   2. Corrosive gastritis
   3. Crohn disease, sarcoidosis, syphilis, tuberculosis

C. MALIGNANT NARROWING
   1. Antral carcinoma: cause in adults in 30–35%
   2. Scirrhous carcinoma of pyloric channel

D. OTHERS
   1. Prolapsed antral polyp / mucosa
   2. Bezoar
   3. Gastric volvulus
   4. Postoperative stomal edema

Abdominal plain film:
- √ large smoothly marginated homogeneous mass displacing transverse colon + small bowel inferiorly
- √ one / two air-fluid levels

Duodenal obstruction

A. CONGENITAL
   1. Annular pancreas
   2. Peritoneal bands = Ladd bands
   3. Aberrant vessel

B. INFLAMMATORY NARROWING
   1. Chronic duodenal ulcer scar
   2. Acute pancreatitis: phlegmon, abscess, pseudocyst
   3. Acute cholecystitis: perforated gallstone

C. INTRAMURAL HEMATOMA
   1. Blunt trauma (accident, child abuse)
   2. Anticoagulant therapy
   3. Blood dyscrasia

D. TUMORAL NARROWING
   1. Primary duodenal tumors
   2. Tumor invasion from pancreas, right kidney, lymph node enlargement

E. EXTRINSIC COMPRESSION
   1. Aortic aneurysm
   2. Pseudoaneurysm

F. OTHERS
   1. Superior mesenteric artery syndrome from extensive burns, body cast, rapid weight loss, prolonged bed rest
   2. Bezoar (in gastrectomized patient)

mnemonic: "VA BADD TU BADD"

<u>child</u>	<u>adult</u>
Volvulus	**T**umor
Atresia	**U**lcer
Bands	**B**ands
Annular pancreas	**A**nnular pancreas
Duplication	**D**uplication
Diverticulum	**D**iverticulum

Abdominal plain film:
- √ double-bubble sign = air-fluid levels in stomach + duodenum
- √ frequently normal due to absence of gas from vomiting

Jejunal and ileal obstruction

= SMALL BOWEL OBSTRUCTION (SBO)

Technique: best evaluated by CT (95% accurate, 94% sensitive, 96% specific)

A. CONGENITAL
   1. Ileal atresia / stenosis
   2. Enteric duplication: located on antimesenteric side, mostly in ileum
   3. Midgut volvulus from arrest in rotation + fixation of small bowel during fetal life
   4. Mesenteric cyst from meconium peritonitis: located on mesenteric side
   5. Meckel diverticulum

B. EXTRINSIC BOWEL LESIONS
   1. Fibrous adhesions from previous surgery / peritonitis (in 75%)
   2. Hernias (inguinal, femoral, umbilical, paraduodenal, foramen of Winslow, incisional, Spigelian, obturator)
   3. Volvulus
   4. Masses: neoplasm, abscess

C. LUMINAL OCCLUSION
   1. Swallowed foreign body, bezoar, gallstone, bolus of Ascaris lumbricoides, inspissated milk
   2. Meconium ileus:
      √ microcolon in cystic fibrosis
   3. Meconium ileus equivalent
   4. Intussusception (tumor, Meckel diverticulum, chronic ulcer, adhesion)
   5. Tumor (rare): eg, lipoma

D. INTRINSIC BOWEL WALL LESION
1. Strictures from neoplasm, Crohn disease, tuberculous enteritis, parasitic disease, potassium chloride tablets, surgical anastomosis, irradiation, massive deposition of amyloid
2. Intramural hemorrhage: blunt trauma, Henoch-Schönlein purpura
3. Vascular insufficiency: arterial / venous occlusion

Acquired Small Bowel Obstruction In Childhood

mnemonic: "AAIIMM"
Adhesions
Appendicitis
Intussusception
Incarcerated hernia
Malrotation
Meckel diverticulum

Small Bowel Obstruction In Adulthood

mnemonic: "SHAVIT"
Stone (gallstone ileus)
Hernia
Adhesion
Volvulus
Intussusception
Tumor

Plain abdominal radiograph (50–66% sensitive):
√ "candy cane" appearance in erect position = >3 distended small bowel loops >3 cm with gas-fluid levels (>3–5 hours after onset of obstruction)
√ disparity in size between obstructed loops and contiguous small bowel loops of normal caliber beyond site of obstruction
√ small bowel positioned in center of abdomen
√ little / no gas + stool in colon with complete mechanical obstruction after 12–24 hours
√ "stretch sign" = erectile valvulae conniventes completely encircle bowel lumen
√ "stepladder appearance" in low obstruction (the greater the number of dilated bowel loops, the more distal the site of obstruction)
√ "string-of-beads" indicate peristaltic hyperactivity to overcome mechanical obstruction
√ hyperactive peristalsis / aperistalsis = fatigued small bowel
CAVE: little / no gas in small bowel from fluid-distended loops may lead one to overlook obstruction

Plain abdominal radiographic categories:
1. Normal
= absence of small intestinal gas / gas within 3–4 variably shaped loops <2.5 cm in diameter
2. Mild small bowel stasis
= single / multiple loops of 2.5–3 cm in diameter with ≥3 air-fluid levels
3. Probable SBO pattern
= dilated multiple gas- / fluid-filled loops with air-fluid levels + moderate amount of colonic gas
4. Definite SBO pattern
= clearly disproportionate gaseous / fluid distension of small bowel relative to colon

UGI:
√ "snake head" appearance = active peristalsis forms bulbous head of barium column in an attempt to overcome obstruction
√ barium appears in colon >12 hours

Enteroclysis for adhesive obstruction:
√ abrupt change in caliber of bowel with normal caliber / collapsed bowel distal to obstruction
√ stretched folds of normal pattern
√ angulated + fixed bowel segment
Enteroclysis categories of SBO (Shrake):
(a) low-grade partial SBO
= sufficient flow of contrast material through point of obstruction so that fold pattern beyond obstruction is readily defined
(b) high-grade partial SBO
= stasis + delay in arrival of contrast so that contrast material is diluted in distended prestenotic loop with minimal contrast in postobstructive loop leading to difficulty in defining fold pattern after transition point
(c) complete SBO
= no passage of contrast material 3–24 hours after start of examination

CT (poor sensitivity for low-grade partial obstruction)
US:
√ small bowel loops dilated >3 cm
√ length of dilated segment >10 cm
√ increased peristalsis of dilated segment (may become paralytic in prolonged obstruction)
√ colon collapsed

Location of obstruction:
(a) valvulae conniventes high + frequent = jejunum
(b) valvulae conniventes sparse / absent = ileum

Closed Loop Obstruction

= bowel obstruction at two points
Cause: adhesion (75%), volvulus, incarcerated hernia
√ U-shaped distended loop
√ increasing intraluminal fluid
√ fixation of bowel loop = no change in position
√ "coffee bean sign" = gas-filled loop
√ "pseudotumor" = fluid-filled loop
√ U- or C-shaped dilated bowel loop on CT
√ "beak sign" = point of obstruction on CT / UGI
√ "whirl sign" = twisting of bowel + mesentery on CT
√ stretched mesenteric vessels converging toward torsion

GI

Strangulated Obstruction

= triad of (1) mechanical obstruction proximal to the involved segment (2) closed-loop obstruction of the involved segment (3) venous congestion of the involved segment

CT:
- √ slight circumferential thickening of bowel wall
  - √ increased wall attenuation
  - √ target / halo sign
- √ serrated beak at site of obstruction (32–100% specific)
- √ unusual course of mesenteric vasculature
- √ mesenteric haziness due to edema (95% specific)
- √ diffuse engorgement of mesenteric vasculature
- √ poor / no enhancement of bowel wall (100% specific)
- √ delayed prolonged enhancement of bowel wall
- √ large amount of ascites
- √ pneumatosis intestinalis

Colonic Obstruction

Incidence: 25% of all intestinal obstructions

A. NEONATAL COLONIC OBSTRUCTION
1. Meconium plug syndrome
2. Colonic atresia
3. Anorectal malformation: rectal atresia, imperforate anus

B. LUMINAL OBTURATION
1. Fecal impaction
   - √ bubbly pattern of large mass of stool
2. Fecaloma
3. Gallstone (in sigmoid narrowed by diverticulitis)
4. Intussusception

C. BOWEL WALL LESION

(a) malignant (60–70% of obstructions): predominantly in sigmoid

(b) inflammatory
1. Crohn disease
2. Ulcerative colitis
3. Mesenteric ischemia
4. Sigmoid diverticulitis (15%)
   - √ stenotic segment >6 cm
5. Acute pancreatitis

(c) infectious:
infectious granulomatous process (actinomycosis, tuberculosis, lymphogranuloma venereum), parasitic disease (amebiasis, schistosomiasis)

(d) wall hematoma:
blunt trauma, coagulopathy

D. EXTRINSIC

(a) mass impression
1. Endometriosis
2. Large tumor mass: prostate, bladder, uterus, tubes, ovaries
3. Pelvic abscess
4. Hugely distended bladder
5. Mesenteritis
6. Poorly formed colostomy

(b) severe constriction
1. Volvulus (3rd most common cause): sigmoid colon, cecum, transverse colon, compound volvulus (= ileosigmoid knot)
2. Hernia: transverse colon in diaphragmatic hernia, sigmoid colon in left inguinal hernia
3. Adhesion

Abdominal plain-film patterns:

(a) dilated colon only = competent ileocecal valve

(b) dilated small bowel (25%) = incompetent ileocecal valve

(c) dilated colon + dilated small bowel = ileocecal valve obstruction secondary to cecal overdistension

- √ gas-fluid levels distal to hepatic flexure (fluid is normal in cecum + ascending colon); sign not valid with diarrhea / saline catharsis / enema
- √ cecum most dilated portion (in 75% of cases); critical at 10 cm diameter (high probability for impending perforation)
- ◊ The lower the obstruction, the more proximal the distension!

BE: emergency barium enema of unprepared colon in suspected obstruction!
contraindicated in toxic megacolon, pneumatosis intestinalis, portal vein gas, extraluminal gas

ILEUS

[ileus = stasis / inability to push fluid along (term does not distinguish between mechanical and nonmechanical causes)]

= ADYNAMIC / PARALYTIC / NONOBSTRUCTIVE ILEUS

= derangement impairing proper distal propulsion of intestinal contents

Cause:

— in neonate:
1. Hyperbilirubinemia
2. Intracranial hemorrhage
3. Aspiration pneumonia
4. Necrotizing enterocolitis
5. Aganglionosis

— in child / adult:
1. Postoperative ileus
   - usually resolves by 4th postoperative day
2. Visceral pain: obstructing ureteral stone, common bile duct stone, twisted ovarian cyst, blunt abdominal / chest trauma
3. Intra-abdominal inflammation / infection: peritonitis, appendicitis, cholecystitis, pancreatitis, salpingitis, abdominal abscess, hemolytic-uremic syndrome, gastroenteritis
4. Ischemic bowel disease
5. Anticholinergic drugs: atropine, propantheline, morphine + derivatives, tricyclic antidepressants, dilantin, phenothiazines, hexamethonium bromide

GI

6. Neuromuscular disorder: diabetes, hypothyroidism, porphyria, lead poisoning, uremia, hypokalemia, amyloidosis, urticaria, sprue, scleroderma, Chagas disease, vagotomy, myotonic dystrophy, CNS trauma, paraplegia, quadriplegia
7. Systemic disease: septic / hypovolemic shock, urticaria
8. Chest disease: lower lobe pneumonia, pleuritis, myocardial infarction, acute pericarditis, congestive heart failure
9. Retroperitoneal disease: hemorrhage (spine trauma), abscess

mnemonic: "Remember the P's"
Pancreatitis
Pendicitis
Peptic ulcer
Perforation
Peritonitis
Pneumonia
Porphyria
Postoperative
Potassium deficiency
Pregnancy
Pyelonephritis

- intestinal sounds decreased / absent
- abdominal distension

√ large + small bowel ± gastric distension
√ decreased small bowel distension on serial films
√ delayed but free passage of contrast material
Rx: not amenable to surgical correction

Localized Ileus

= isolated distended loop of small / large bowel
= SENTINEL LOOP
Often associated with an adjacent acute inflammatory process
Etiology:

1. Acute pancreatitis:	duodenum, jejunum, transverse colon
2. Acute cholecystitis:	hepatic flexure of colon
3. Acute appendicitis:	terminal ileum, cecum
4. Acute diverticulitis:	descending colon
5. Acute ureteral colic:	GI tract along course of ureter

Intestinal Pseudoobstruction

A. TRANSIENT PSEUDOOBSTRUCTION
1. Electrolyte imbalance
2. Renal failure
3. Congestive heart failure

B. CHRONIC PSEUDOOBSTRUCTION
1. Scleroderma
2. Amyloidosis

C. IDIOPATHIC PSEUDOOBSTRUCTION
1. Chronic intestinal pseudoobstruction syndrome
   - persistently decreased peristalsis + clinical obstruction

   Age: neonatal period / delayed for months + years
2. Megacystis-microcolon-intestinal-hypoperistalsis syndrome

ESOPHAGUS

Esophageal Contractions

◊ Esophageal motor activity needs to be evaluated in recumbent position without influence of gravity!
PERISTALTIC EVENT = coordinated contractions of esophagus
PERISTALTIC SEQUENCE = aboral stripping wave clearing esophagus

A. PRIMARY PERISTALSIS
= orderly peristaltic sequence with progressive aboral stripping traversing entire esophagus with complete clearance of barium; centrally mediated (medulla) swallow reflex via glossopharyngeal + vagal nerve; initiated by swallowing
√ rapid wave of inhibition followed by slower wave of contraction
◊ Normal peristaltic sequence will be interrupted by repetitive swallowing before peristaltic sequence is complete!

B. SECONDARY PERISTALSIS
= local peristaltic wave identical to primary peristalsis but elicited through esophageal distension = sensorimotor stretch reflex
◊ Esophageal motility can be evaluated with barium injection through nasoesophageal tube despite patient's inability to swallow!

C. TERTIARY CONTRACTIONS
= nonpropulsive esophageal motor event characterized by disordered up-and-down movement of bolus without clearing of esophagus
Cause:
1. Presbyesophagus
2. Diffuse esophageal spasm
3. Hyperactive achalasia
4. Neuromuscular disease: diabetes mellitus, Parkinsonism, amyotrophic lateral sclerosis, multiple sclerosis, thyrotoxic myopathy, myotonic dystrophy
5. Obstruction of cardia: neoplasm, distal esophageal stricture, benign lesion, S/P repair of hiatal hernia

◊ Tertiary activity does not necessarily imply a significant motility disturbance!
Age: in 5–10% of normal adults during 4th–6th decade

(a) nonsegmental = partial luminal indentation
Location: in lower 2/3 of esophagus
√ spontaneous repetitive nonpropulsive contraction
√ "yo-yo" motion of barium
√ "corkscrew" appearance = scalloped configuration of barium column

√ "rosary bead" / "shish kebab" configuration
= compartmentalization of barium column
√ no lumen-obliterating contractions
(b) segmental = luminal obliteration (rare)
√ "curling" = erratic segmental contractions
√ "rosary-bead" appearance

Abnormal Esophageal Peristalsis

A. PRIMARY MOTILITY DISORDERS
1. Achalasia
2. **Diffuse esophageal spasm**
   - severe intermittent pain while swallowing

   √ compartmentalization of esophagus by numerous tertiary contractions

   Dx: extremely high pressures on manometry
3. Presbyesophagus
4. Chalasia
5. Congenital TE fistula
6. Intestinal pseudoobstruction

B. SECONDARY MOTILITY DISORDERS
(a) Connective tissue disease
1. Scleroderma
2. SLE
3. Rheumatoid arthritis
4. Polymyositis
5. Dermatomyositis
6. Muscular dystrophy

(b) Chemical / physical injury
1. Reflux / peptic esophagitis
2. S/P vagotomy
3. Caustic esophagitis
4. Radiotherapy

(c) Infection
Fungal: candidiasis
Parasitic: Chagas disease
Bacterial: TB, diphtheria
Viral: herpes simplex

(d) Metabolic disease
1. Diabetes mellitus
2. Amyloidosis
3. Alcoholism
4. Electrolyte disturbances

(e) Endocrine disease
1. Myxedema
2. Thyrotoxicosis

(f) Neoplasm
(g) Drug-related
atropine, propantheline, curare
(h) Muscle disease
1. Myotonic dystrophy
2. Muscular dystrophy
3. Oculopharyngeal dystrophy
4. Myasthenia gravis (disturbed motility only in striated muscle of upper 1/3 of esophagus)
   √ persistent collection of barium in upper third of esophagus
   √ findings reversed by cholinesterase inhibitor edrophonium (Tensilon®)

(i) Neurologic disease
1. Parkinsonism
2. Multiple sclerosis
3. CNS neoplasm
4. Amyotrophic lateral sclerosis
5. Bulbar poliomyelitis
6. Cerebrovascular disease
7. Huntington chorea
8. Ganglioneuromatosis
9. Wilson disease
10. Friedreich ataxia
11. Familial dysautonomia (Riley-Day)
12. Stiff-man syndrome

Diffuse Esophageal Dilatation

= ACHALASIA PATTERN = MEGAESOPHAGUS

A. ESOPHAGEAL MOTILITY DISORDER
1. Idiopathic achalasia
2. Chagas disease: patients commonly from South America; often associated with megacolon + cardiomegaly
3. Postvagotomy syndrome
4. Scleroderma
5. Systemic lupus erythematosus
6. Presbyesophagus
7. Ehlers-Danlos syndrome
8. Diabetic / alcoholic neuropathy
9. Anticholinergic drugs
10. Idiopathic intestinal pseudoobstruction = degeneration of innervation
11. Amyloidosis: associated with macroglossia, thickened small bowel folds
12. Esophagitis

B. DISTAL OBSTRUCTION
1. Infiltrating lesion of distal esophagus / gastric cardia (eg, carcinoma) = pseudoachalasia
2. Benign stricture
3. Extrinsic compression

mnemonic: "MA'S TACO in a SHell"
Muscular disorder (eg, myasthenia gravis)
Achalasia
Scleroderma
Trypanosomiasis (Chagas disease)
Amyloidosis
Carcinoma
Obstruction
Stricture (lye, potassium, tetracycline)
Hiatal hernia

Air Esophagogram

1. Normal variant
2. Scleroderma
3. Distal obstruction: tumor, stricture, achalasia
4. Thoracic surgery
5. Mediastinal inflammatory disease
6. S/P total laryngectomy (esophageal speech)
7. Endotracheal intubation + PEEP

Abnormal Esophageal Folds

A. TRANSVERSE FOLDS
   1. **Feline esophagus**
      frequently seen with gastroesophageal reflux; normally found in cats
      √ transient contraction of longitudinally oriented muscularis mucosae
   2. Fixed transverse folds
      due to scarring from reflux esophagitis
      √ stepladder appearance in distal esophagus

B. LONGITUDINAL FOLDS
   normally 1–2 mm wide in collapsed esophagus; >3 mm with submucosal edema / inflammation
   1. Gastroesophageal reflux
   2. Opportunistic infection
   3. Caustic ingestion
   4. Irradiation

DDx: 1. Varices
      √ tortuous / serpentine folds that can be effaced by esophageal distension
   2. Varicoid carcinoma
      √ fixed rigid folds with abrupt demarcation due to submucosal spread

Esophageal Inflammation

A. CONTACT INJURY
   (a) reflux related
      1. Peptic ulcer disease
      2. Barrett esophagus
      3. Scleroderma (patulous LES)
      4. Nasogastric intubation
   (b) caustic
      1. Foreign body
      2. Corrosives
   (c) thermic
      Habitual ingestion of excessively hot meals / liquids

B. RADIATION INJURY

C. INFECTION
   1. Candidiasis
   2. Herpes simplex virus / CMV
   3. Diphtheria

D. SYSTEMIC DISEASE
   (a) dermatologic disorders
      pemphigoid, epidermolysis bullosa
   (b) others:
      1. Crohn disease
      2. Graft-versus-host disease
      3. Behçet disease
      4. Eosinophilic gastroenteritis

Esophageal Ulceration

A. PEPTIC
   1. Reflux esophagitis: scleroderma
      √ shallow / deep ulcers in distal esophagus
   2. Barrett esophagus
   3. Crohn disease
      √ aphthous ulcers in variable location
   4. Dermatologic disorders: benign mucous membrane pemphigoid, epidermolysis bullosa dystrophica, Behçet disease

B. INFECTIOUS
   1. Herpes
      √ discrete superficial ulcers in midesophagus
   2. Cytomegalovirus
      √ large flat ulcer in mid- or distal esophagus

C. CONTACT INJURY / EXTERNAL INJURY
   1. Corrosives: alkali, strictures in 50%
   2. Alcohol-induced esophagitis
   3. Drug-induced = "pill esophagitis":
      (a) antibiotics (tetracyclines), quinidine, potassium chloride
         √ discrete superficial ulcers in midesophagus
      (b) alendronate (= inhibitor of osteoclastic activity)
         √ long-segment involvement with severe ulceration
   4. Radiotherapy: smooth stricture >4500 rads
      √ shallow / deep ulcers conforming to radiation portal
   5. Nasogastric tube
      √ elongated stricture in middle + distal 1/3
   6. Endoscopic sclerotherapy

D. MALIGNANT
   1. Esophageal carcinoma

Location:
   @ Upper esophagus
      1. Barrett ulcer in islets of gastric mucosa
   @ Midesophagus
      1. Herpes esophagitis
      2. CMV esophagitis
      3. Drug-induced esophagitis
   @ Distal esophagus
      1. Reflux esophagitis
      2. CMV esophagitis

DDx:
   1. Sacculation
      = outpouching in distal esophagus due to asymmetric scarring in reflux esophagitis
   2. Esophageal intramural pseudodiverticula
   3. Artifact
      (a) tiny precipitates of barium
      (b) transient mucosal crinkling in inadequate distension
      (c) irregular Z-line

Double-barrel Esophagus

1. Dissecting intramural hematoma from emetogenic injury
2. Mallory-Weiss tear
   trauma, esophagoscopy (in 0.25%), bougienage (in 0.5%), ingestion of foreign bodies, spontaneous (bleeding diathesis)
3. Intramural abscess
4. Intraluminal diverticulum
5. Esophageal duplication (if communication with esophageal lumen present)

GI

Esophageal Diverticulum

1. ZENKER DIVERTICULUM (pharyngoesophageal)
2. INTERBRONCHIAL DIVERTICULUM
   = traction diverticulum
   response to pull from fibrous adhesions following lymph node infection (TB), contains all 3 esophageal layers
   Location: usually on right anterolateral wall of interbronchial segment
   √ calcified mediastinal nodes
3. INTERAORTICOBRONCHIAL DIVERTICULUM
   = thoracic pulsion diverticulum
   Location: on left anterolateral wall between inferior border of aortic arch + upper margin of left main bronchus
4. EPIPHRENIC DIVERTICULUM (rare)
   Location: usually on lateral esophageal wall, right > left, in distal 10 cm
   √ often associated with hiatus hernia
5. INTRAMURAL ESOPHAGEAL PSEUDODIVERTICULOSIS
   √ outpouching from mucosal glands

Tracheobronchoesophageal Fistula

A. CONGENITAL
   1. Congenital tracheoesophageal fistula

B. MALIGNANT
   1. Lung cancer
   2. Metastases to mediastinal lymph nodes
   3. Esophageal cancer

   Often following radiation treatment of these tumors!

C. TRAUMATIC
   1. Instrumentation (esophagoscopy, bougienage, pneumatic dilatation)
   2. Blunt ("crush injury") / penetrating chest trauma
   3. Surgery
   4. Foreign-body perforation
   5. Corrosives
   6. Postemetic rupture = Boerhaave syndrome

D. INFECTIOUS / INFLAMMATORY
   1. TB, syphilis, histoplasmosis, actinomycosis, Crohn disease
   2. Perforated diverticulum
   3. Pulmonary sequestration / cyst

Long Smooth Esophageal Narrowing

1. Congenital esophageal stenosis
   √ at junction between middle + distal third
   √ weblike / tubular stenosis of 1 cm in length
2. Surgical repair of esophageal atresia
   √ interruption of primary peristaltic wave at anastomosis
   √ secondary contractions may produce retrograde flow with aspiration
   √ impaction of food
3. Caustic burns = alkaline burns
4. Alendronate (= inhibitor of osteoclastic activity)
5. Gastric acid: reflux, hyperemesis gravidarum
6. Intubation: reflux + compromise of circulation
7. Radiotherapy for esophageal carcinoma; tumor of lung, breast, or thymus; lymphoma; metastases to mediastinal lymph nodes
   Onset of stricture: usually 4–8 months post Rx
   Dose: 3000–5000 rad
8. Postinfectious: moniliasis (rare)

Lower Esophageal Narrowing

mnemonic: "SPADE"

Scleroderma
Presbyesophagus
Achalasia; **A**nticholinergics
Diffuse esophageal spasm
Esophagitis

Focal Esophageal Narrowing

1. **Web**
   = 1- to 2-mm thick (vertical length) area of complete / incomplete circumferential narrowing
2. **Ring**
   = 5- to 10-mm thick (vertical length) area of complete / incomplete circumferential narrowing
3. **Stricture**
   = >10 mm in vertical length
   mnemonic: "LETTERS MC"
   Lye ingestion
   Esophagitis
   Tumor
   Tube (prolonged nasogastric intubation)
   Epidermolysis bullosa
   Radiation
   Surgery, **S**cleroderma
   Moniliasis
   Congenital

Esophageal Filling Defect

A. BENIGN TUMORS
   <1% of all esophageal tumors
   (a) Submucosal tumor (75%)
   = nonepithelial, intramural
   1. Leiomyoma (50% of all benign tumors)
   2. Lipoma, fibroma, lipoma, fibrolipoma, myxofibroma, hamartoma, hemangioma, lymphangioma, neurofibroma, schwannoma, granular cell myoblastoma
      √ primary wave stops at level of tumor
      √ proximal esophageal dilatation + hypotonicity
      √ rigid esophageal wall at site of tumoral implant
      √ disorganized / altered / effaced mucosal folds around defect
      √ tumor shadow on tangential view extending beyond esophageal margin

   (b) Mucosal tumor (25%) = epithelial, intraluminal
   1. Fibrovascular / inflammatory polyp; adenomatous polyp
   2. Squamous papilloma, fibropapilloma

GI

3. Villous adenoma, fibroadenoma
   √ no interruption of primary peristaltic wave
   √ well-circumscribed central radiolucent defect
   √ symmetric ampullary distension of esophagus around defect
   √ no change of mucosal pattern at periphery of defect

B. MALIGNANT TUMORS
1. Esophageal cancer, varicoid squamous cell carcinoma
2. Gastric cancer
3. Leiomyosarcoma, carcinosarcoma, pseudosarcoma
4. Metastases: malignant melanoma, lymphoma (<1% of gastrointestinal lymphomas), stomach, lung, breast

C. VASCULAR
varices

D. INFECTION / INFLAMMATION
Candida / herpes esophagitis, drug-induced inflammatory reaction

E. CONGENITAL / NORMAL VARIANT
1. Prolapsed gastric folds
2. Esophageal duplication cyst (0.5–2.5% of all esophageal tumors)

F. FOREIGN BODIES
retained food particles (chicken bone, fish bone, pins, coins, small toys, meat), undissolved effervescent crystals, air bubbles

Esophageal Mucosal Nodules / Plaques

1. Candida esophagitis
   √ diffuse / localized discrete plaques
2. Reflux esophagitis (early stage)
   √ tiny poorly defined nodules in distal esophagus
3. Barrett esophagus
   √ localized reticular pattern often adjacent to distal aspect of high stricture
4. Glycogen acanthosis
   √ diffuse / localized nodules / plaques
5. Superficial spreading carcinoma
   √ localized coalescent nodules / plaques
6. Artifacts (undissolved effervescent agent, air bubbles, debris)

Extrinsic Esophageal Impression

Cervical Causes Of Esophageal Impression

A. OSSEOUS LESIONS
1. Anterior marginal osteophyte / DISH
2. Anterior disk herniation
3. Cervical trauma + hematoma
4. Osteomyelitis
5. Bone neoplasm

B. ESOPHAGEAL WALL LESIONS
(a) muscle
1. Cricopharyngeus
2. Esophageal web

(b) vessel
1. Pharyngeal venous plexus
2. Lymph node enlargement

C. ENDOCRINE ORGANS
1. Thyroid / parathyroid enlargement (benign / malignant)
2. Fibrotic traction after thyroidectomy

D. Retropharyngeal / mediastinal abscess

Thoracic Causes Of Esophageal Impression

A. NORMAL INDENTATIONS
aortic arch, left mainstem bronchus, left inferior pulmonary vein, diaphragmatic hiatus

B. ABNORMAL VASCULATURE
right-sided aortic arch, cervical aortic arch, aortic unfolding, aortic tortuosity, aortic aneurysm, double aortic arch ("reverse S"), coarctation of aorta ("reverse figure 3"), aberrant right subclavian artery
= arteria lusoria (semilunar / bayonet-shaped imprint upon posterior wall of esophagus), aberrant left pulmonary artery (between trachea + esophagus), anomalous pulmonary venous return (anterior), persistent truncus arteriosus (posterior)

C. CARDIAC CAUSES
(a) enlargement of chambers
left atrial / left ventricular enlargement: mitral disease (esophageal displacement backward + to the right)
(b) pericardial masses
pericardial tumor / cyst / effusion

D. MEDIASTINAL CAUSES
mediastinal tumor, lymphadenopathy (metastatic, tuberculous), inflammation, cyst

E. PULMONARY CAUSES
pulmonary tumor, bronchogenic cyst, atypical pulmonary fibrosis (retraction)

F. ESOPHAGEAL ABNORMALITIES
1. Esophageal diverticulum
2. Paraesophageal hernia
3. Esophageal duplication

STOMACH

Widened Retrogastric Space

A. PANCREATIC MASSES (most common cause)
1. Acute + chronic pancreatitis
2. Pancreatic pseudocyst
3. Pancreatic cystadenoma + carcinoma

B. OTHER RETROPERITONEAL MASSES
sarcoma, renal tumor, adrenal tumor, lymph node enlargement, abscess, hematoma

C. GASTRIC MASSES
1. Leiomyoma, leiomyosarcoma

D. OTHERS
1. Aortic aneurysm
2. Choledochal cyst
3. Obesity
4. Postsurgical disruptions + adhesions

GI

5. Ascites
6. Gross hepatomegaly + enlarged caudate lobe
7. Hernia involving omentum

Gastric Pneumatosis

A. INFECTION
  1. Emphysematous gastritis
B. ISCHEMIA
  1. Gastric ulcer disease with intramural perforation
  2. Severe necrotizing gastroenteritis
  3. Gastric carcinoma
  4. Volvulus
  5. Gastric infarction
C. TRAUMA
  (a) Iatrogenic = gastric manipulation
    1. Recent gastroduodenal surgery
    2. Endoscopy (1.6%)
  (b) Ingested material:
    1. Corrosive gastritis
    2. Acid ingestion
D. OVERDISTENSION (increased intraluminal pressure)
  1. Gastric outlet obstruction
  2. Volvulus
  3. Overinflation during gastroscopy
  4. Profuse severe vomiting
E. DISSECTING AIR
  1. Rupture + dissection of subpleural blebs in bullous emphysema along esophageal wall / mediastinum
F. IDIOPATHIC
  1. (Intramural / nonbacterial) gastric emphysema
    = cystic pneumatosis
    = benign idiopathic submucosal air lucencies

√ thin discrete sharply defined streaks of gas in submucosa ± subserosa
√ irregular radiolucent band of innumerable small bubbles with constant relationship to each other
√ bulging of mucosa
√ gas within portal venous system

Gastric Atony

= gastric retention in the absence of mechanical obstruction

Pathophysiology: reflex paralysis

A. ACUTE GASTRIC ATONY
  (may develop within 24–48 hours)
  1. Acute gastric dilatation: secondary to decreased arterial perfusion (ischemia, congestive heart failure) in old patients, usually fatal
  2. Postsurgical atony, ureteral catheterization
  3. Immobilization: body cast, paraplegia, postoperative state
  4. Abdominal trauma: especially back injury
  5. Severe pain: renal / biliary colic, migraine headaches, severe burns
  6. Infection: peritonitis, pancreatitis, appendicitis, subphrenic abscess, septicemia
B. CHRONIC GASTRIC ATONY
  1. Neurologic abnormalities: brain tumor, bulbar poliomyelitis, vagotomy, tabes
  2. Muscular abnormalities: scleroderma, muscular dystrophy
  3. Drug-induced atony: atropine, morphine, heroin, ganglionic blocking agents
  4. Electrolyte imbalance: diabetic ketoacidosis, hypercalcemia, hypocalcemia, hypokalemia, hepatic coma, uremia, myxedema
  5. Diabetes mellitus = gastroparesis diabeticorum (0.08% incidence)
  6. Emotional distress
  7. Lead poisoning
  8. Porphyria

• abdominal distension
• vascular collapse (decreased venous return)
• vomiting

√ large stomach filled with air + fluid (up to 7,500 mL)
√ retention of barium
√ absent / diminished peristaltic activity
√ patulous pylorus
√ frequently dilated duodenum

DDx: gastric volvulus, pyloric stenosis

Narrowing Of Stomach

= **linitis plastica** type of stenosis

A. MALIGNANCY
  1. Scirrhous gastric carcinoma (involving portion / all of stomach)
  2. Hodgkin lymphoma, NHL
  3. Metastatic involvement (carcinoma of breast, pancreatic carcinoma, colonic carcinoma)
B. INFLAMMATION
  1. Chronic gastric ulcer disease with intense spasm
  2. Pseudo-Billroth-I pattern of Crohn disease
  3. Sarcoidosis
    √ polypoid appearance, pyloric hypertrophy
    √ gastric ulcers, duodenal deformity
  4. Eosinophilic gastritis
  5. Polyarteritis nodosa
  6. Stenosing antral gastritis / hypertrophic pyloric stenosis
C. INFECTION
  1. Tertiary stage of syphilis
    √ absent mucosal folds + peristalsis
    √ no change over years
  2. Tuberculosis (rare)
    √ hyperplastic nodules / ulcerative lesion / annular lesion
    √ pyloric obstruction, may cross into duodenum
  3. Histoplasmosis
  4. Actinomycosis
  5. Strongyloidiasis
  6. Phlegmonous gastritis
  7. Toxoplasmosis
D. TRAUMA
  1. Corrosive gastritis

GI

2. Radiation injury
3. Gastric freezing
4. Hepatic arterial chemotherapy infusion

E. OTHERS
1. Perigastric adhesions (normal mucosa, no interval change, normal peristalsis)
2. Amyloidosis
3. Pseudolymphoma
4. Exogastric mass (hepatomegaly, pancreatic pseudocyst)

mnemonic: "SLIMRAGE"
Scirrhous carcinoma of stomach
Lymphoma
Infiltration from adjacent neoplasm
Metastasis (breast carcinoma)
Radiation therapy
Acids (corrosive ingestion)
Granulomatous disease (TB, sarcoidosis, Crohn)
Eosinophilic gastroenteritis

Antral Narrowing

mnemonic: "SPICER"
Sarcoidosis, **S**yphilis
Peptic ulcer disease
Infection (tuberculosis)
Cancer, **C**rohn disease, **C**austic
Eosinophilic granuloma
Radiation

Intramural-extramucosal Lesions Of Stomach

√ sharply delineated marginal / contour defect
√ stretched folds over intact mucosa
√ acute angle at margins
√ may ulcerate centrally
√ may become pedunculated and acquire polypoid appearance over years

A. NEOPLASTIC
1. Leiomyoma (48%)
2. Neurogenic tumors (14%)
3. Heterotopic pancreas (12%)
4. Fibrous tumor (11%)
5. Lipoma (7%)
6. Hemangioma (7%)
7. Glomus tumor (rare)
8. Carcinoid
9. Metastatic tumor

B. INFLAMMATION / INFECTION
1. Granuloma:
(1) Foreign-body granuloma (2) Sarcoidosis (3) Crohn disease (4) Tuberculosis (5) Histoplasmosis
2. Eosinophilic gastritis
3. Tertiary syphilis: infiltrative / ulcerative / tumorous type
4. Echinococcal cyst

C. PANCREATIC ABNORMALITIES
1. Ectopic pancreas
2. Annular pancreas
3. Pancreatic pseudocyst

D. DEPOSITS
1. Amyloid
2. Endometriosis
3. Localized hematoma

E. OTHERS
1. Varices (ie, fundal)
2. Duplications (4% of all GI tract duplications)

Gastric Filling Defects

A. INTRINSIC WALL LESIONS
(a) benign (most common)
1. Polyps: hyperplastic, adenomatous, villous, hamartomatous (Peutz-Jeghers syndrome, Cowden disease)
2. Leiomyoma
3. Granulomatous lesions:
(a) Eosinophilic granuloma, (b) Crohn disease, (c) Tuberculosis ,(d) Sarcoidosis
4. Pseudolymphoma = benign reactive proliferation of lymphoid tissue
5. Extramedullary hematopoiesis
6. Ectopic pancreas
7. Gastric duplication cyst
8. Intramural hematoma
9. Esophagogastric herniation

(b) malignant
1. Gastric carcinoma, lymphoma
2. Gastric sarcoma: leiomyosarcoma, liposarcoma, leiomyoblastoma
3. Gastric metastases: melanoma, breast, pancreas, colon

B. EXTRINSIC IMPRESSIONS ON STOMACH
in 70% nonneoplastic (extrinsic pseudotumors in 20%)
(a) normal organs: organomegaly, tortuous aorta, heart, cardiac aneurysm
(b) benign masses:
cysts of pancreas, liver, spleen, adrenal, kidney; gastric duplication, postoperative deformity (eg, Nissen fundoplication)
(c) malignant masses: enlarged celiac nodes
(d) inflammatory lesion:
left subphrenic abscess / hematoma
— lateral displacement: enlarged liver, aortic aneurysm, enlarged celiac nodes
— medial displacement: splenomegaly, mass in colonic splenic flexure, cardiomegaly, subphrenic abscess

C. INTRALUMINAL GASTRIC MASSES
1. Bezoar
2. Foreign bodies: food, pills, blood clot, gallstone

D. TUMORS OF ADJACENT ORGANS
pancreatic carcinoma + cystadenoma, liver carcinoma, carcinoma of gallbladder, colonic carcinoma, renal carcinoma, adrenal carcinoma, lymph node involvement

E. THICKENED GASTRIC FOLDS

Filling defect of gastric remnant

A. IATROGENIC
surgical deformity / plication defect, suture granuloma
B. INFLAMMATORY
bile reflux gastritis, hyperplastic polyps
C. INTUSSUSCEPTION
1. **Jejunogastric intussusception**
(efferent loop in 75%, afferent loop in 25%)
(a) acute form: high intestinal obstruction, left hypochondriac mass, hematemesis
(b) chronic / intermittent form: may be self-reducing
√ "coil spring" appearance of gastric filling defect
2. Gastrojejunal / gastroduodenal mucosal prolapse
• often asymptomatic
• bleeding, partial obstruction
D. NEOPLASTIC
1. Gastric stump carcinoma: >5 years after resection for benign disease; 15% within 10 years; 20% after 20 years
2. Recurrent carcinoma (10%) secondary to incomplete removal of gastric cancer
3. Malignancy at anastomosis (incomplete resection)
E. INTRALUMINAL MATTER: bezoar

mnemonic: "PUBLICS"
Polyp (hyperplastic polyp due to bile reflux)
Ulcer (anastomotic)
Bezoar, **B**lind loop syndrome
Loop (afferent loop syndrome)
Intussusception at gastrojejunostomy
Cancer (recurrent, residual, de novo)
Surgical deformity, **S**uture granuloma

Thickened gastric folds

A. INFLAMMATION / INFECTION
1. Inflammatory gastritis:
alcoholic, hypertrophic, antral, corrosive, postirradiation, gastric cooling
2. Crohn disease
3. Sarcoidosis
4. Infectious gastritis:
bacterial invasion, bacterial toxins from botulism, diphtheria, dysentery, typhoid fever, anisakiasis, TB, syphilis
5. Pseudolymphoma
B. MALIGNANCY
1. Lymphoma
2. Gastric carcinoma
C. INFILTRATIVE PROCESS
1. Eosinophilic gastritis
2. Amyloidosis
D. PANCREATIC DISEASE
1. Pancreatitis
2. Direct extension from pancreatic carcinoma
E. OTHERS
1. Zollinger-Ellison syndrome
2. Ménétrièr disease
3. Gastric varices

mnemonic: "ZEAL VOLUMES C^3P^3"
Zollinger-**E**llison syndrome
Amyloidosis
Lymphoid hyperplasia
Varices
Operative defect
Lymphoma
Ulcer disease (peptic)
Ménétrièr disease
Eosinophilic gastroenteritis
Syphilis
Crohn disease, **C**arcinoma, **C**orrosive gastritis
Pancreatitis, **P**ancreatic carcinoma,
Postradiation gastritis

Gastric ulcer

A. HORMONAL
1. Zollinger-Ellison syndrome
2. Hyperparathyroidism (in 1.3–24%)
duodenum:stomach = 4:1; M:F = 3:1
◊ Duodenal ulcers predominate in females!
◊ Gastric ulcers predominate in males!
• absence of gastric hypersecretion
3. Steroid-induced ulcer
gastric > duodenal location;
frequently multiple + deep ulcers;
commonly associated with erosions
• bleeding (in 1/3)
4. Curling ulcer (burn) (in 0.09–2.6%)
5. Retained gastric antrum
B. INFLAMMATION
1. Peptic ulcer disease
2. Gastritis
3. Radiation-induced ulcer
C. BENIGN MASS
1. Leiomyoma
2. Granulomatous disease
3. Pseudolymphoma (lymphoid hyperplasia)
D. MALIGNANT MASS
1. Gastric carcinoma
2. Lymphoma (2% of all gastric neoplasms)
√ multiple ulcers with aneurysmal appearance
3. Leiomyosarcoma, neurogenic sarcoma, fibrosarcoma, liposarcoma
4. Metastases
(a) hematogenic: malignant melanoma, breast cancer, lung cancer
(b) per continuum: pancreas, colon, kidney
E. DRUGS
ASA: greater curvature

Bull's-eye lesions

A. PRIMARY NEOPLASMS
1. Leiomyoma, leiomyosarcoma
2. Lymphoma
3. Carcinoid
4. Primary carcinoma
B. HEMATOGENOUS METASTASES
1. Malignant melanoma
√ usually spares large bowel

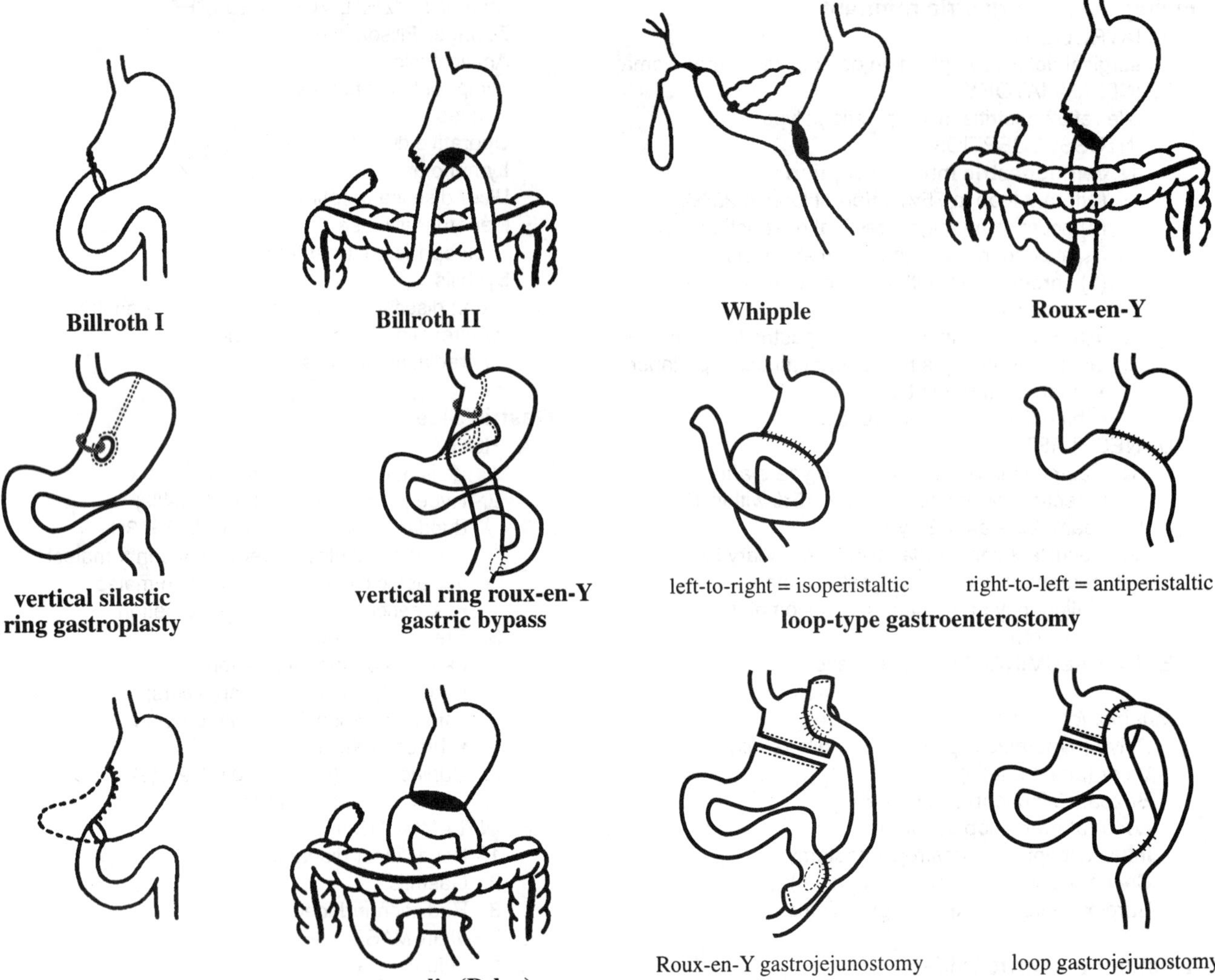

Gastric Surgical Procedures

2. Breast cancer (15%)
   √ scirrhous appearance in stomach
3. Cancer of lung
4. Renal cell carcinoma
5. Kaposi sarcoma
6. Bladder carcinoma

C. ECTOPIC PANCREAS
   in duodenum / stomach

D. EOSINOPHILIC GRANULOMA
   most frequently in stomach

Complications of postoperative stomach

1. Filling defect of gastric remnant
2. Retained gastric antrum
3. Dumping syndrome
4. Afferent loop syndrome
5. Stomal obstruction
   (a) temporary reversible: edema of suture line, abscess / hematoma, potassium deficiency, inadequate electrolyte replacement, hypoproteinemia, hypoacidity
   (b) late mechanical: stomal ulcer (75%)

mnemonic: "LOBULATING"

Leaks (early)
Obstruction (early)
Bezoar
Ulcer (especially marginal)
Loop (afferent loop syndrome)
Anemia (macrocytic secondary to decreased intrinsic factor)
Tumor (? increased incidence)
Intussusception
Not feeling well after meals (dumping syndrome)
Gastritis (bile reflux)

Lesions Involving Stomach And Duodenum

1. Lymphoma: in <33% of patients with lymphoma
2. Gastric carcinoma: in <5%, but 50 x more common than lymphoma
3. Peptic ulcer disease
4. Tuberculosis: in 10% of gastric TB
5. Crohn disease: pseudo-Billroth-I pattern
6. Strongyloidiasis
7. Eosinophilic gastroenteritis

DUODENUM

Extrinsic Pressure Effect On Duodenum

A. BILE DUCTS
normal impression, dilated CBD, choledochal cyst

B. GALLBLADDER
normal impression, gallbladder hydrops, Courvoisier phenomenon, gallbladder carcinoma, pericholecystic abscess

C. LIVER
hepatomegaly, hypertrophied caudate lobe, anomalous hepatic lobe, hepatic cyst, hepatic tumor

D. RIGHT KIDNEY
bifid collecting system, hydronephrosis, multiple renal cysts, polycystic kidney disease, hypernephroma

E. RIGHT ADRENAL
adrenal carcinoma, enlargement in Addison disease

F. COLON
duodenocolic apposition due to anomalous peritoneal fixation, carcinoma of hepatic flexure

G. VESSELS
lymphadenopathy, duodenal varices, dilated arterial collaterals, aortic aneurysm, intramural / mesenteric hematoma

Widened duodenal sweep

A. NORMAL VARIANT

B. PANCREATIC LESION
1. Acute pancreatitis
2. Chronic pancreatitis
3. Pancreatic pseudocyst
4. Pancreatic carcinoma
5. Metastasis to pancreas
6. Pancreatic cystadenoma

C. VASCULAR LESION
1. Lymph node enlargement: lymphoma, metastasis, inflammation
2. Cystic lymphangioma of the mesentery

D. RETROPERITONEAL MASS
1. Aortic aneurysm
2. Choledochal cyst

Thickened Duodenal Folds

A. INFLAMMATION
(a) within bowel wall:
peptic ulcer disease, Zollinger-Ellison syndrome, regional enteritis, lymphoid hyperplasia, uremia
(b) surrounding bowel wall:
pancreatitis, cholecystitis

B. INFECTION
giardiasis, TB, strongyloidiasis, celiac disease

C. NEOPLASIA
lymphoma, metastases to peripancreatic nodes

D. DIFFUSE INFILTRATIVE DISORDER
Whipple disease, amyloidosis, mastocytosis, eosinophilic enteritis, intestinal lymphangiectasia

E. VASCULAR DISORDER
duodenal varices, mesenteric arterial collaterals, intramural hemorrhage (trauma, Schönlein-Henoch purpura), chronic duodenal congestion (congestive heart failure, portal venous hypertension); lymphangiectasia

F. HYPOPROTEINEMIA
nephrotic syndrome, Menetrier disease, protein-losing enteropathy

G. GLANDULAR ENLARGEMENT
Brunner gland hyperplasia, cystic fibrosis

mnemonic: "BAD HELP"
Brunner gland hyperplasia
Amyloidosis
Duodenitis (Z-E syndrome, peptic)
Hemorrhage
Edema, **E**ctopic pancreas
Lymphoma
Pancreatitis, **P**arasites

Duodenal Filling Defect

A. EXTRINSIC
gallbladder impression, CBD impression, gas-filled diverticulum

B. INTRINSIC TO WALL
(a) benign neoplastic mass
adenoma, leiomyoma, lipoma, hamartoma (Peutz-Jeghers syndrome), prolapsed antral polyp, Brunner gland adenoma, villous adenoma, islet cell tumor, gangliocytic paraganglioma
(b) malignant neoplastic mass
carcinoid tumor, adenocarcinoma, ampullary carcinoma, lymphoma, sarcoma, metastasis (stomach, pancreas, gallbladder, colon, kidney, melanoma), retroperitoneal lymph node involvement
(c) nonneoplastic mass
papilla of Vater, choledochocele, duplication cyst, pancreatic pseudocyst, duodenal varix, mesenteric artery collaterals, intramural hematoma, adjacent abscess, stitch abscess, ectopic pancreas, heterotopic gastric mucosa, prolapsed antral mucosa, Brunner gland hyperplasia, benign lymphoid hyperplasia

C. INTRALUMINAL
blood clot, foreign body (fruit pit, gallstone, feeding tube)

Duodenal Tumor

Benign Duodenal Tumors

1. Leiomyoma (27%)
2. Adenomatous polyp (21%)
3. Lipoma (21%)
4. Brunner gland adenoma (17%)
5. Angiomatous tumor (6%)
6. Ectopic pancreas (2%)
7. Duodenal cyst (2%)
8. Neurofibroma (2%)
9. Hamartoma (2%)

Malignant Duodenal Tumors

1. Adenocarcinoma (73%)
   Location: 40% in duodenum, most often in 2nd + 3rd portion = periampullary neoplasm
   (a) suprapapillary: apt to cause obstruction + bleeding
   (b) peripapillary: extrahepatic jaundice
   (c) intrapapillary: GI bleeding
   May be associated with: Peutz-Jeghers syndrome
   √ annular / polypoid / ulcerative
   Metastases: regional lymph nodes (2/3)
   DDx: (1) Primary bile duct carcinoma
   (2) Ampullary carcinoma
2. Leiomyosarcoma (14%)
   most often beyond 1st portion of duodenum
   √ up to 20 cm in size
   √ frequently ulcerated exophytic mass
3. Carcinoid (11%)
4. Lymphoma (2%)
   √ marked wall thickening
   √ bulky periduodenal lymphadenopathy

Enlargement Of Papilla Of Vater

A. Normal variant
   identified in 60% of UGI series; atypical location in 3rd portion of duodenum in 8%; 1.5 cm in diameter in 1% of normals
B. Papillary edema
   1. Impacted stone
   2. Pancreatitis (Poppel sign)
   3. Acute duodenal ulcer disease
   4. Papillitis
C. Perivaterian neoplasms
   = tumor mass + lymphatic obstruction
   1. Adenocarcinoma
   2. Adenomatous polyp (premalignant lesion)
   √ irregular surface + erosions
D. Lesions simulating enlarged papilla
   1. Benign spindle cell tumor
   2. Ectopic pancreatic tissue

Duodenal Narrowing

A. DEVELOPMENTAL ANOMALIES
   1. Duodenal atresia
   2. Congenital web / duodenal diaphragm
   3. Intraluminal diverticulum
   4. Duodenal duplication cyst
   5. Annular pancreas
   6. Midgut volvulus, peritoneal bands (Ladd bands)
B. INTRINSIC DISORDERS
   (a) inflammation / infection
   1. Postbulbar ulcer
   2. Crohn disease
   3. Sprue
   4. Tuberculosis
   5. Strongyloidiasis
   (b) tumor
   duodenal / ampullary malignancy
C. DISEASE IN ADJACENT STRUCTURES
   1. Pancreatitis, pseudocyst, pancreatic carcinoma
   2. Cholecystitis
   3. Contiguous abscess
   4. Metastases to pancreaticoduodenal nodes (lymphoma, lung cancer, breast cancer)
D. TRAUMA
   1. Duodenal rupture
   2. Intramural hematoma
E. VASCULAR
   1. Superior mesenteric artery syndrome
   2. Aorticoduodenal fistula
   3. Preduodenal portal vein (anterior to descending duodenum)

Dilated Duodenum

Megaduodenum = marked dilatation of entire C-loop
Megabulbus = dilatation of duodenal bulb only

A. VASCULAR COMPRESSION
   superior mesenteric artery syndrome, abdominal aortic aneurysm, aorticoduodenal fistula
B. PRIMARY DUODENAL ATONY
   (a) scleroderma, dermatomyositis, SLE
   (b) Chagas disease, aganglionosis, neuropathy, surgical / chemical vagotomy
   (c) focal ileus: pancreatitis, cholecystitis, peptic ulcer disease, trauma
   (d) altered emotional status, chronic idiopathic intestinal pseudoobstruction
C. INFLAMMATORY / NEOPLASTIC INDURATION OF MESENTERIC ROOT
   Crohn disease, tuberculous enteritis, pancreatitis, peptic ulcer disease, strongyloidiasis, metastatic disease
D. FLUID DISTENSION
   celiac disease, Zollinger-Ellison syndrome

Postbulbar Ulceration

1. Benign postbulbar peptic ulcer
   √ medial aspect of upper 2nd portion
   √ incisura pointing to ulcer
   √ occasionally barium reflux into common bile duct
   √ ring stricture
   √ stress- and drug-induced ulcers heal without deformity
2. Zollinger-Ellison syndrome
   √ multiple ulcers distal to duodenal bulb
   √ thickening of folds + hypersecretion
3. Leiomyoma

GI

4. Malignant tumors:
   (a) primaries
   adenocarcinoma, lymphoma, sarcoma
   (b) contiguous spread
   pancreas, colon, kidney, gallbladder
   (c) hematogenous spread
   melanoma, Kaposi sarcoma
   (d) lymphogenic spread
   metastases to periduodenal lymph nodes
5. Granulomatous disease: Crohn disease, TB
6. Aorticoduodenal fistula
7. Mimickers: ectopic pancreas, diverticulum

SMALL BOWEL

Small Bowel Diverticula

A. TRUE DIVERTICULA
   (a) Duodenal diverticula
      1. Racemose diverticula: bizarre, lobulated
      2. Giant diverticula
      3. Intraluminal diverticula: result of congenital web / diaphragm
   (b) Jejunal diverticulosis
   (c) Meckel diverticulum
B. PSEUDODIVERTICULA
   1. Scleroderma
   2. Crohn disease
   3. Lymphoma
   4. Mesenteric ischemia
   5. Communicating ileal duplication
   6. Giant duodenal ulcer

Small Bowel Ulcer

Aphthous Ulcers Of Small Bowel

A. INFECTION
   1. Yersinia enterocolitis (25%)
   2. Salmonellosis
   3. Tuberculosis
   4. Rickettsiosis
B. INFLAMMATION
   1. Crohn disease (22%)
   2. Behçet syndrome
   3. Reiter syndrome
   4. Ankylosing spondylitis

Large Nonstenotic Ulcers Of Small Bowel

1. Primary nonspecific ulcer	47% incidence
2. Yersiniosis	33%
3. Crohn disease	30%
4. Tuberculosis	18%
5. Salmonellosis / shigellosis	7%
6. Meckel diverticulum	5%

Multiple Small Bowel Ulcers

A. DRUGS
   1. Potassium tablets
   2. Steroids
   3. Nonsteroidal anti-inflammatory drugs
B. INFECTION / INFLAMMATION
   1. Bacillary dysentery
   2. Ischemic enteritis
   3. Ulcerative jejunoileitis as complication of celiac disease
C. TUMOR
   1. Neoplasms
   2. Intestinal lymphoma

Cavitary Small Bowel Lesions

1. Lymphoma (exoenteric form)
2. Leiomyosarcoma (exoenteric form)
3. Primary adenocarcinoma
4. Metastases (especially malignant melanoma)

Separation Of Bowel Loops

A. INFILTRATION OF BOWEL WALL / MESENTERY
   (a) inflammation / infection
      1. Crohn disease
      2. TB
      3. Radiation injury
      4. Retractile mesenteritis
      5. Intraperitoneal abscess
   (b) deposits
      1. Intestinal hemorrhage / mesenteric vascular occlusion
      2. Whipple disease
      3. Amyloidosis
   (c) tumor
      1. Carcinoid tumor: local release of serotonin responsible for muscular thickening + fibroplastic proliferation = desmoplastic reaction
      2. Primary carcinoma of small bowel (unusual presentation)
      3. Lymphoma
      4. Neurofibromatosis
B. ASCITES
   hepatic cirrhosis (75%), peritonitis, peritoneal carcinomatosis, congestive heart failure, constrictive pericarditis, primary / metastatic lymphatic disease
C. EXTRINSIC MASS
   1. Peritoneal mesothelioma, mesenteric tumors (fibroma, lipoma, fibrosarcoma, leiomyosarcoma, malignant mesenteric lymphoid tumor, metastases)
   2. Intraperitoneal abscess
   3. Retractile mesenteritis (fibrosis, fatty infiltration, panniculitis)

Normal Small Bowel Folds & Diarrhea

1. Pancreatic insufficiency
2. Lactase deficiency
3. Lymphoma / pseudolymphoma

Dilated Small Bowel & Normal Folds

mnemonic: "SOS"
Sprue
Obstruction
Scleroderma

A. EXCESSIVE FLUID
(a) mechanical obstruction
due to adhesion, hernia, neoplasm
√ "string-of-beads sign" = air bubbles between mucosal folds in a fluid-filled small bowel
√ "pseudotumor sign" = closed-loop obstruction
(b) malabsorption syndromes
1. Celiac disease, tropical + nontropical sprue
2. Lactase deficiency

B. BOWEL WALL PARALYSIS
= functional ileus = adynamic ileus
1. Surgical vagotomy
2. Chemical vagotomy from drug effects: atropine-like substances, morphine, L-dopa, glucagon
3. Chagas disease
4. Metabolic: hypokalemia, diabetes
5. Intrinsic + extrinsic intra-abdominal inflammation
6. Chronic idiopathic pseudoobstruction

C. VASCULAR COMPROMISE
1. Mesenteric ischemia (atherosclerosis)
2. Acute radiation enteritis
3. Amyloidosis
4. SLE

D. BOWEL WALL DESTRUCTION
1. Lymphoma
2. Scleroderma (smooth muscle atrophy)
3. Dermatomyositis

Abnormal Small Bowel Folds

Thickened Folds Of Stomach & Small Bowel

1. Lymphoma
2. Crohn disease
3. Eosinophilic gastroenteritis
4. Zollinger-Ellison syndrome
5. Ménétrièr disease
6. Cirrhosis = gastric varices + hypoproteinemia
7. Amyloidosis
8. Whipple disease

Thickened Smooth Folds ± Dilatation

A. EDEMA
(a) hypoproteinemia
cirrhosis, nephrotic syndrome, protein-losing enteropathy (celiac disease, Whipple disease)
(b) increased capillary permeability
angioneurotic edema, gastroenteritis
(c) increased hydrostatic pressure
portal venous hypertension
(d) Zollinger-Ellison syndrome

B. HEMORRHAGE
(a) vessel injury
ischemia, infarction, trauma
(b) vasculitis
connective tissue disease, Henoch-Schönlein purpura, thrombangitis obliterans, irradiation
(c) hypocoagulability
hemophilia, anticoagulant therapy, hypofibrinogemia, circulating anticoagulants, fibrinolytic system activation, idiopathic thrombocytopenic purpura, coagulation defects (leukemia, lymphoma, multiple myeloma, metastatic carcinoma), hypoprothrombinemia

C. LYMPHATIC BLOCKAGE
1. Tumor infiltration: lymphoma, pseudolymphoma
2. Irradiation
3. Mesenteric fibrosis
4. Intestinal lymphangiectasia
5. Whipple disease

D. DEPOSITS
1. Eosinophilic enteritis
2. Pneumatosis intestinalis
3. Amyloidosis
4. Abetalipoproteinemia
5. Crohn disease
6. Graft-versus-host disease
7. Immunologic deficiency: hypo- / dysgammaglobulinemia

Thickened Irregular Folds ± Dilatation

A. INFLAMMATION
1. Crohn disease
B. NEOPLASTIC
1. Lymphoma, pseudolymphoma
C. INFECTION
(a) protozoan
giardiasis, strongyloidiasis, hookworm
(b) bacterial
Yersinia enterocolitica, typhoid fever, tuberculosis
(c) fungal: histoplasmosis
(d) AIDS-related infection
D. IDIOPATHIC
(a) lymphatic dilatation
1. Lymphangiectasia
2. Inflammatory process, tumor growth, irradiation fibrosis
3. Whipple disease
(b) cellular infiltration
1. Eosinophilic enteritis
2. Mastocytosis
(c) deposits
1. Zollinger-Ellison syndrome
2. Amyloidosis
3. Alpha chain disease: defective secretory IgA system
4. A-b-lipoproteinemia: recessive, retinitis pigmentosa, neurologic disease
5. A-a-lipoproteinemia
6. Fibrocystic disease of the pancreas
7. Polyposis syndrome

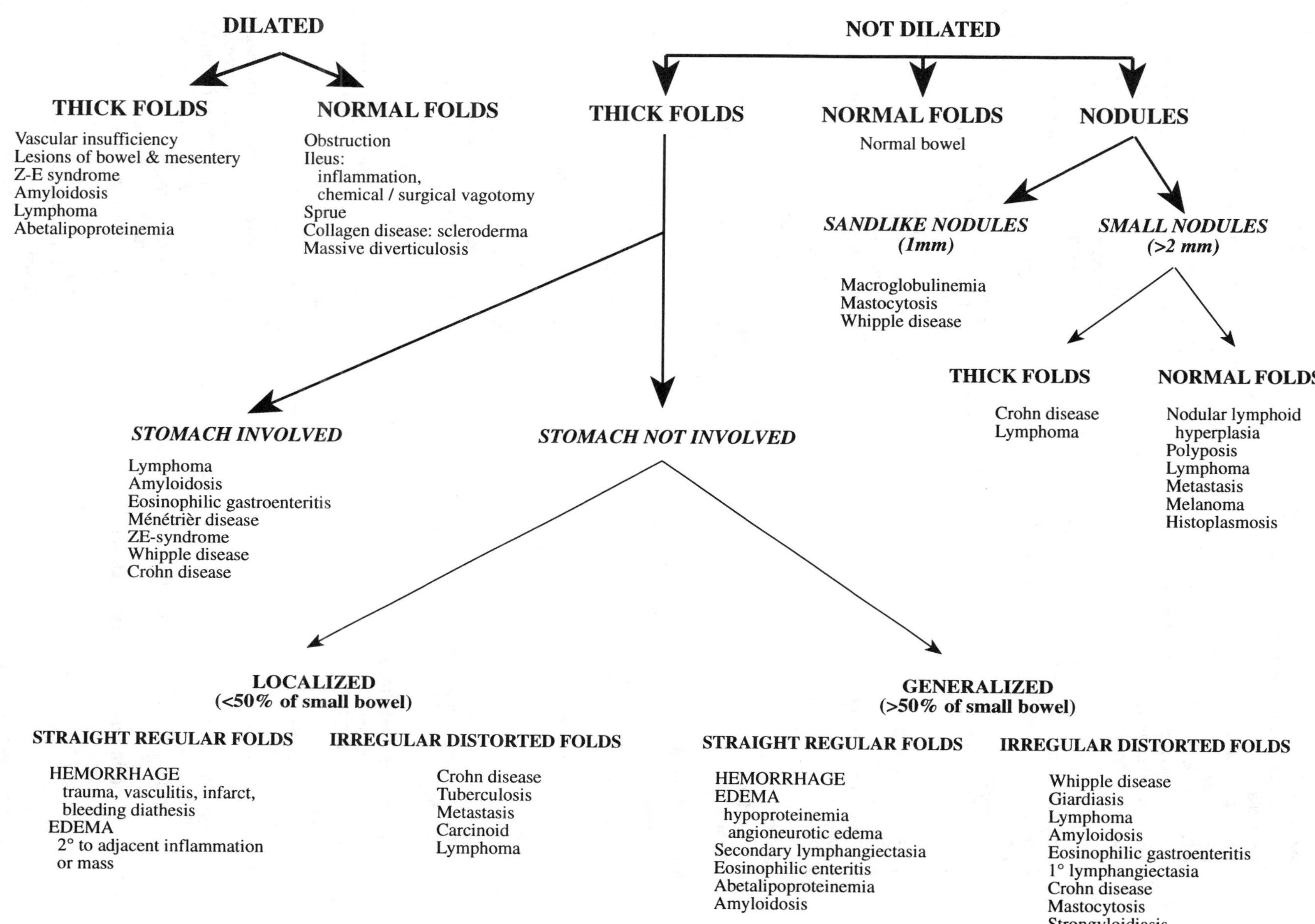
ABNORMAL SMALL BOWEL CALIBER & CONTOUR
DILATED
THICK FOLDS
Vascular insufficiency
Lesions of bowel & mesentery
Z-E syndrome
Amyloidosis
Lymphoma
Abetalipoproteinemia
NORMAL FOLDS
Obstruction
Ileus:
inflammation,
chemical / surgical vagotomy
Sprue
Collagen disease: scleroderma
Massive diverticulosis
NOT DILATED
THICK FOLDS
STOMACH INVOLVED
Lymphoma
Amyloidosis
Eosinophilic gastroenteritis
Ménétrièr disease
ZE-syndrome
Whipple disease
Crohn disease
STOMACH NOT INVOLVED
LOCALIZED
(<50% of small bowel)
STRAIGHT REGULAR FOLDS
HEMORRHAGE
trauma, vasculitis, infarct,
bleeding diathesis
EDEMA
2° to adjacent inflammation
or mass
IRREGULAR DISTORTED FOLDS
Crohn disease
Tuberculosis
Metastasis
Carcinoid
Lymphoma
GENERALIZED
(>50% of small bowel)
STRAIGHT REGULAR FOLDS
HEMORRHAGE
EDEMA
hypoproteinemia
angioneurotic edema
Secondary lymphangiectasia
Eosinophilic enteritis
Abetalipoproteinemia
Amyloidosis
IRREGULAR DISTORTED FOLDS
Whipple disease
Giardiasis
Lymphoma
Amyloidosis
Eosinophilic gastroenteritis
1° lymphangiectasia
Crohn disease
Mastocytosis
Strongyloidiasis
NORMAL FOLDS
Normal bowel
NODULES
SANDLIKE NODULES
(1mm)
Macroglobulinemia
Mastocytosis
Whipple disease
SMALL NODULES
(>2 mm)
THICK FOLDS
Crohn disease
Lymphoma
NORMAL FOLDS
Nodular lymphoid
hyperplasia
Polyposis
Lymphoma
Metastasis
Melanoma
Histoplasmosis

mnemonic: "G. WILLIAMS"
Giardiasis
Whipple disease, **W**aldenström macroglobulinemia
Ischemia
Lymphangiectasia
Lymphoma
Inflammation
Amyloidosis, **A**gammaglobulinemia
Mastocytosis, **M**alabsorption
Soft-tissue neoplasm (carcinoid, lipoma)

Tethered Folds

= indicative of desmoplastic reaction
√ kinking, angulation, tethering, separation of bowel loops

1. Carcinoid
2. Postoperative in Gardner syndrome
3. Retractile mesenteritis
4. Hodgkin disease
5. Peritoneal implants
6. Endometriosis
7. Tuberculous peritonitis
8. Mesothelioma
9. Postoperative adhesions

Atrophy Of Folds

1. Celiac disease
2. Chronic radiation injury

Ribbonlike Bowel

= featureless / tubular nature of small bowel with effacement of folds

1. Graft-versus-host disease
2. Celiac disease
3. Small bowel infection
4. Injury from radiation / corrosive medication
5. Allergy
6. Ischemia
7. Amyloid, mastocytosis
8. Lymphoma, pseudolymphoma
9. Crohn disease

Delayed Small Bowel Transit

= transit time >6 hours
mnemonic: "SPATS DID"
Scleroderma
Potassium (hypokalemia)
Anxiety
Thyroid (hypothyroidism)
Sprue
Diabetes (poorly controlled)
Idiopathic
Drugs (opiates, atropine, phenothiazine)

Multiple Stenotic Lesions Of Small Bowel

1. Crohn disease
2. End-stage radiation enteritis
3. Metastatic carcinoma
4. Endometritis
5. Eosinophilic gastroenteritis
6. Tuberculosis
7. Drug-induced (eg, potassium chloride tablets, NSAIDs)

Small Bowel Filling Defects

Solitary Filling Defect

A. INTRINSIC TO BOWEL WALL
 (a) benign neoplasm: leiomyoma (97%), adenoma, lipoma, hemangioma, neurofibroma
 (b) malignant primary: adenocarcinoma, lymphoma (desmoplastic response), sarcoma, carcinoid
 (c) metastases: from melanoma, lung, kidney, breast
 (d) inflammation: inflammatory pseudotumor
 (e) infection: parasites

B. EXTRINSIC TO BOWEL WALL
 1. Duplication cyst
 2. Endometrioma

C. INTRALUMINAL
 1. Gallstone ileus
 2. Parasites (ascariasis, strongyloidiasis)
 3. Inverted Meckel diverticulum
 4. Blood clot
 5. Foreign body, bezoar, pills, seeds

Multiple Filling Defects Of Small Bowel

A. POLYPOSIS SYNDROMES
 1. Peutz-Jeghers syndrome
 2. Gardner syndrome
 3. Disseminated gastrointestinal polyposis
 4. Generalized gastrointestinal juvenile polyposis
 5. Cronkhite-Canada syndrome

B. BENIGN TUMORS
 1. Multiple simple adenomatous polyps
 2. Hemangioma
 3. Leiomyoma, neurofibroma
 4. Nodular lymphoid hyperplasia
  = normal terminal ileum in children + adolescents; may be associated with dysgammaglobulinemia
  √ symmetric fairly sharply demarcated filling defects
 5. Varices (= multiple phlebectasia in jejunum, oral mucosa, tongue, scrotum)

C. MALIGNANT TUMORS
 1. Carcinoid tumor
 2. Lymphoma
  (a) primary lymphoma (rarely multiple)
  (b) secondary lymphoma: gastrointestinal involvement in 63% of disseminated disease; 19% in small intestine
 3. Metastases: melanoma > lung > breast > choriocarcinoma > kidney > stomach, uterus, ovary, pancreas

D. INTRALUMINAL
 1. Gallstones
 2. Foreign bodies, food particles, seeds, pills
 3. Parasites: ascariasis, strongyloidiasis, hookworm, tapeworm

Sandlike lucencies of small bowel

1. Waldenström macroglobulinemia
2. Mastocytosis
3. Histoplasmosis
4. Nodular lymphoid hyperplasia
5. Intestinal lymphangiectasia
6. Eosinophilic gastroenteritis
7. Lymphoma
8. Crohn disease
9. Whipple disease
10. Yersinia enterocolitis
11. Cronkhite-Canada syndrome
12. Cystic fibrosis
13. Food particles / gas bubbles
14. Strongyloides stercoralis

Small bowel tumors

Incidence: 1:100,000; 1.5–6% of all GI neoplasms
Malignant:benign = 1:1
Symptomatic malignant:symptomatic benign = 3:1
Location of small bowel primaries:
ileum (41%), jejunum (36%), duodenum (18%)

ROENTGENOGRAPHIC APPEARANCE:

(1) pedunculated intraluminal tumor, usually originating from mucosa
 √ smooth / irregular surface without visible mucosal pattern
 √ moves within intestinal lumen twice the length of the stalk

(2) sessile intraluminal tumor without stalk, usually from tissues outside mucosa
 √ smooth / irregular surface without visible mucosal pattern

(3) intra- / extramural tumor
 √ base of tumor greater than any part projecting into the lumen
 √ mucosal pattern visible, may be stretched

(4) serosal tumor
 √ displacement of adjacent loops
 √ small bowel obstruction (rare)
 √ coil-spring pattern of intussusceptum

CT: small bowel wall >1.5 cm thick
Cx: small-bowel obstruction (in up to 10%)

Benign small bowel tumors

- asymptomatic (80%)
- melena, pain, weakness
- palpable abdominal mass (20%)

Types:

1. Leiomyoma (36–49%)
 Location: any segment
2. Lipoma (14–16%)
 Location: duodenum (32%), jejunum (17%), ileum (51%)
 √ fat-density on CT
3. Adenoma (15–20%)
4. Hemangioma (13–16%)
5. Lymphangioma (5%)
 Location: duodenum > jejunum > ileum
6. Neurogenic tumor (1%)

Malignant small bowel tumors

At risk: Crohn disease, celiac disease, polyposis syndromes, history of small-bowel diverting surgery

- asymptomatic (10–30%)
- pain due to intermittent obstruction (80%)
- weight loss (66%)
- gastrointestinal blood loss (50%)
- palpable abdominal mass (50%)

1. Carcinoid (25–41%)
 Location: predominantly distal ileum
 √ calcified mesenteric mass on CT
2. Adenocarcinoma (25–26%)
 Location: duodenum (48%), jejunum (44%), ileum (8%)
3. Lymphoma (16–17%)
 √ aneurysmal dilatation
4. Gastrointestinal stromal tumor (GIST) = leiomyosarcoma (9–10%)
 Location: ileum (50%)
5. Vascular malignancy (1%)
6. Fibrosarcoma (0.3%)
7. Metastatic tumor

CECUM

Ileocecal valve abnormalities

A. Lipomatosis: >40 years of age, female
 √ stellate / rosette pattern

B. NEOPLASM
 1. Lipoma, adenomatous polyp, villous adenoma
 2. Carcinoid tumor
 3. Adenocarcinoma: 2% of all colonic cancers
 4. Lymphoma: often involving terminal ileum

C. INFLAMMATION
 1. Crohn disease
 2. Ulcerative colitis
  √ patulous valve, fixed in open position
 3. Tuberculosis
 4. Amebiasis
  √ terminal ileum not involved (in United States)
 5. Typhoid fever, anisakiasis, schistosomiasis, actinomycosis
 6. Cathartic abuse

D. PROLAPSE
 (a) antegrade: indistinguishable from lipomatosis / prolapsing mucosa / neoplasm
 (b) retrograde

E. INTUSSUSCEPTION

F. LYMPHOID HYPERPLASIA

Coned cecum

A. INFLAMMATION
 1. Crohn disease
  √ involvement of ascending colon + terminal ileum
 2. Ulcerative colitis
  √ backwash ileitis (in 10%)
  √ gaping ileocecal valve

3. Appendicitis
4. Typhlitis
5. Perforated cecal diverticulum

B. INFECTION
1. Tuberculosis
   √ colonic involvement more prominent than that of terminal ileum
2. Amebiasis
   √ involvement of cecum in 90% of amebiasis
   √ thickened ileocecal valve fixed in open position
   √ reflux into normal terminal ileum
   √ skip lesions in colon
3. Actinomycosis
   • palpable abdominal mass
   • indolent sinus tracts in abdominal wall
4. Blastomycosis
5. **Anisakiasis**
   from ingestion of raw fish with ascaris-like nematode
6. Typhoid, Yersinia

C. TUMOR
1. Carcinoma of the cecum
2. Metastasis to cecum

Cecal filling defect

A. ABNORMALITIES OF THE APPENDIX
1. Acute appendicitis / appendiceal abscess
2. Crohn disease
3. Inverted appendiceal stump / appendiceal intussusception
4. Mucocele
5. Myxoglobulosis
6. Appendiceal neoplasm: carcinoid tumor (90%), leiomyoma, neuroma, lipoma, adenocarcinoma, metastasis

B. COLONIC LESION
1. Ameboma
2. Primary cecal neoplasm
3. Ileocolic intussusception
4. Lipomatosis of ileocecal valve

C. UNUSUAL ABNORMALITIES
1. Ileocecal diverticulitis (in 50% < age 30 years)
2. Solitary benign ulcer of the cecum
3. Adherent fecolith (eg, in cystic fibrosis)
4. Endometriosis
5. Burkitt lymphoma

mnemonic: "CECUM TIPSALE"
Carcinoma
Enteritis
Carcinoid
Ulcerative colitis
Mucocele of appendix
Tuberculosis
Intussusception
Periappendiceal abscess
Stump of the appendix
Ameboma
Lymphoma
Endometriosis

COLON

Colon cutoff sign

= abrupt cutoff of gas column at splenic flexure
1. Acute pancreatitis (inflammatory exudate along transverse mesocolon)
2. Colonic obstruction
3. Mesenteric thrombosis
4. Ischemic colitis

Colonic thumbprinting

= sharply defined fingerlike marginal indentations at contours of wall
1. ISCHEMIA = Ischemic colitis
   occlusive vascular disease, hypercoagulability state, hemorrhage into bowel wall (bleeding diathesis, anticoagulants), traumatic intramural hematoma
2. INFLAMMATION
   ulcerative colitis, Crohn colitis
3. INFECTION
   acute amebiasis, schistosomiasis, strongyloidiasis, cytomegalovirus (in renal transplant recipients), pseudomembranous colitis
4. MALIGNANT LESIONS
   localized primary lymphoma, hematogenous metastases
5. MISCELLANEOUS
   endometriosis, amyloidosis, pneumatosis intestinalis, diverticulosis, diverticulitis, hereditary angioneurotic edema

mnemonic: "PSALM II"
Pseudomembranous colitis
Schistosomiasis
Amebic colitis
Lymphoma
Metastases (to colon)
Ischemic colitis
Inflammatory bowel disease

Colonic urticaria pattern

A. OBSTRUCTION
1. Obstructing carcinoma
2. Cecal volvulus
3. Colonic ileus

B. ISCHEMIA

C. INFECTION / INFLAMMATION
1. Yersinia enterocolitis
2. Herpes
3. Crohn disease

D. URTICARIA

Colonic ulcers

A. IDIOPATHIC
1. Ulcerative colitis
2. Crohn colitis

B. ISCHEMIC
1. Ischemic colitis

C. TRAUMATIC
1. Radiation injury
2. Caustic colitis

D. NEOPLASTIC
   1. Primary colonic carcinoma
   2. Metastases (prostate, stomach, lymphoma, leukemia)
E. INFLAMMATORY
   1. Pseudomembranous colitis
   2. Pancreatitis
   3. Diverticulitis
   4. Behçet syndrome
   5. Solitary rectal ulcer syndrome
   6. Nonspecific benign ulceration
F. INFECTION
   (a) protozoan
      1. Amebiasis
      2. Schistosomiasis
      3. Strongyloidiasis
   (b) bacterial
      1. Shigellosis, salmonellosis
      2. Staphylococcal colitis
      3. Tuberculosis
      4. Gonorrheal proctitis
      5. Yersinia colitis
      6. Campylobacter fetus colitis
   (c) fungal
      histoplasmosis, mucormycosis, actinomycosis, candidiasis
   (d) viral
      1. Lymphogranuloma venereum
      2. Herpes proctocolitis
      3. Cytomegalovirus (transplants)

Aphthous Ulcers

1. Crohn disease
2. Amebic colitis
3. **Yersinia enterocolitis**
   Organism: Gram-negative
   • fever, diarrhea, RLQ pain
   Location: terminal ileum
   √ thickened folds + ulceration
   √ lymphoid nodular hyperplasia
4. Salmonella, shigella infection
5. Herpes virus infection
6. Behçet syndrome
7. Lymphoma
8. Ischemia

Multiple Bull's-eye Lesions Of Bowel Wall

mnemonic: "MaCK CLaN"
Melanoma and
Carcinoma
Kaposi sarcoma
Carcinoid
Lymphoma and
Neurofibromatosis

Double-tracking Of Colon

= longitudinal extraluminal tracks paralleling the colon
1. Diverticulitis: generally 3–6 cm in length
2. Crohn disease: generally >10 cm
3. Primary carcinoma: wider + more irregular

Colonic Narrowing

A. CHRONIC STAGE OF ANY ULCERATING COLITIS
   (a) inflammatory:
      ulcerative colitis, Crohn colitis, solitary rectal ulcer syndrome, nonspecific benign ulcer
   (b) infectious:
      amebiasis, schistosomiasis, bacillary dysentery, TB, fungal disease, lymphogranuloma venereum, herpes zoster, cytomegalovirus, strongyloides
   (c) ischemic: ischemic colitis
   (d) traumatic:
      radiation injury, cathartic colon, caustic colitis
B. MALIGNANT LESION
   (a) primary: colonic carcinoma (annular / scirrhous); complication of ulcerative colitis + Crohn colitis
   (b) metastatic:
      from prostate, cervix, uterus, kidney, stomach, pancreas, primary intraperitoneal sarcoma
      — hematogenous (eg, breast)
      — lymphangitic spread
      — peritoneal seeding
C. EXTRINSIC PROCESS
   (a) inflammation:
      retractile mesenteritis, diverticulitis, pancreatitis
   (b) deposits:
      amyloidosis, endometriosis, pelvic lipomatosis
D. POSTSURGICAL
   adhesive bands, surgical anastomosis
E. NORMAL
   Cannon point

Localized Colonic Narrowing

mnemonic: "SCARED CELL-MATE"
Schistosomiasis
Carcinoid
Actinomycosis
Radiation
Endometriosis
Diverticulitis
Colitis
Extrinsic lesion
Lymphoma
Lymphogranuloma venereum
Metastasis
Adenocarcinoma
Tuberculosis
Entamoeba histolytica

Microcolon

mnemonic: "MI MCA"
Meconium ileus
Ileal atresia
Megacystis-microcolon-hypoperistalsis syndrome
Colonic atresia (distal to atretic segment)
Aganglionosis (Hirschsprung disease)

Colonic Filling Defects

Submucosal Tumor

1. Lipoma
2. Carcinoid

3. Leiomyoma
4. Lymphangioma, hemangioma

Single Colonic Filling Defect

A. BENIGN TUMOR
1. Polyp
(hyperplastic, adenomatous, villous adenoma, villoglandular); most common benign tumor
2. Lipoma
Most common intramural tumor; 2nd most common benign tumor; M < F
Location: ascending colon + cecum > left side of colon
3. Carcinoid: 10% metastasize
4. Spindle cell tumor
(leiomyoma, fibroma, neurofibroma); 4th most common benign tumor; rectum > cecum
5. Lymphangioma, hemangioma

B. MALIGNANT TUMOR
(a) primary tumor:
carcinoma, sarcoma
(b) secondary tumor:
metastases (breast, stomach, lung, pancreas, kidney, female genital tract), lymphoma, invasion by adjacent tumors

C. INFECTION
1. Ameboma
2. Polypoid granuloma: schistosomiasis, TB

D. INFLAMMATION
1. Inflammatory pseudopolyp: ulcerative colitis, Crohn disease
2. Periappendiceal abscess
3. Diverticulitis
4. Foreign-body perforation

E. NONSESSILE INTRALUMINAL BODY
1. Fecal impaction
2. Foreign body
3. Gallstone
4. Bolus of Ascaris worms

F. MISCELLANEOUS
1. Endometriosis
3rd most common benign tumor
Location: sigmoid colon, rectosigmoid junction (at level of cul-de-sac)
• may cause bleeding (after invasion of mucosa)
2. Localized amyloid deposition
3. Suture granuloma
4. Intussusception
5. Pseudotumor (adhesions, fibrous bands)
6. Colitis cystica profunda

Multiple Colonic Filling Defects

A. NEOPLASMS
(a) polyposis syndrome:
familial polyposis, Gardner syndrome, Peutz-Jeghers syndrome, Turcot syndrome, juvenile polyposis syndrome, disseminated gastrointestinal polyps, multiple adenomatous polyps
(b) hematogenous metastases:
from breast, lung, stomach, ovary, pancreas, uterus
(c) multiple tumors
- benign:
neurofibromatosis, colonic lipomatosis, multiple hamartoma syndrome (Cowden disease)
- malignant:
lymphoma, leukemia, adenocarcinoma

B. INFLAMMATORY PSEUDOPOLYPS
ulcerative colitis, Crohn colitis, ischemic colitis, amebiasis, schistosomiasis, strongyloidiasis, trichuriasis

C. ARTIFACTS
feces, air bubbles, oil bubbles, mucous strands, ingested foreign body (eg, corn kernels)

D. MISCELLANEOUS
nodular lymphoid hyperplasia, lymphoid follicular pattern, hemorrhoids, diverticula, pneumatosis intestinalis, colitis cystica profunda, colonic urticaria, submucosal colonic edema secondary to obstruction, cystic fibrosis, amyloidosis, ulcerative pseudopolyps, proximal to obstruction

mnemonic: "MILL P^3"
Metastases (to colon)
Ischemia (thumbprinting)
Lymphoma
Lymphoid hyperplasia
Polyposis
Pseudopolyposis (with inflammatory bowel disease); **P**neumatosis cystoides

Carpet Lesions Of Colon

= flat lobulated lesions with alteration of surface texture + little / no protrusion into lumen
Location: rectum > cecum > ascending colon
Cause:
A. NEOPLASMS
1. Tubular / tubulovillous / villous adenoma
2. Familial polyposis
3. Adenocarcinoma
4. Submucosal tumor spread (from adjacent carcinoma)

B. MISCELLANEOUS
1. Nonspecific follicular proctitis
2. Biopsy site
3. Endometriosis
4. Rectal varices
5. Colonic urticaria

Colonic Polyp

Terminology:
1. **Polyp**
= mass projecting into the lumen of a hollow viscus above the level of the mucosa; usually arises from mucosa, may derive from submucosa / muscularis propria

	Single Polyp	Multiple Polyps
Neoplastic (10 %)		
— epithelial	1. Tubular adenoma 2. Tubulovillous adenoma 3. Villous adenoma 4. Turcot syndrome	1. Familial adenomatosis coli 2. Adenomatosis of GI tract 3. Gardner syndrome
— nonepithelial	1. Carcinoid 2. Leiomyoma 3. Lipoma 4. Hem-, lymphangioma 5. Fibroma, neurofibroma	
Nonneoplastic (90%)		
— unclassified	1. Hyperplastic polyp	1. Hyperplastic polyposis
— hamartomatous	1. Juvenile polyp 2. Peutz-Jeghers syndrome	1. Juvenile polyposis
— inflammatory	1. Ulcerative colitis 2. Benign lymphoid polyp 3. Fibroid granulation polyp	1. Cronkhite-Canada syndrome 2. Ulcerative colitis

(a) neoplastic: adenoma / carcinoma
(b) nonneoplastic: hamartoma / inflammatory polyp

2. **Pseudopolyp**
   = scattered island of inflamed edematous mucosa on a background of denuded mucosa
   (a) pseudopolyposis of ulcerative colitis
   (b) "cobblestoning" of Crohn disease
3. **Postinflammatory (filiform) polyp**
   = fingerlike projection of submucosa covered by mucosa on all sides following healing + regeneration of inflammatory (most common in ulcerative colitis) / ischemic / infectious bowel disease

Histologic classification:

A. ADENOMATOUS POLYPS
   = **Familial adenomatous polyposis syndrome**
   1. Familial polyposis
   2. Gardner syndrome
   3. Turcot syndrome

B. HAMARTOMATOUS POLYPS
   = HAMARTOMATOUS POLYPOSIS SYNDROMES
   1. Peutz-Jeghers syndrome (most in small bowel)
   2. Cowden disease
   3. Juvenile polyposis
   4. Cronkhite-Canada syndrome
   5. Bannayan-Riley-Ruvalcaba syndrome

C. POLYPOSIS LOOK-ALIKES
   1. Inflammatory polyposis
   2. Lymphoid hyperplasia
   3. Lymphoma
   4. Metastases
   5. Pneumatosis coli

Polyposis Syndromes

= more than 100 polyps in number

Mode of transmission:

A. HEREDITARY
   (a) autosomal dominant
      1. Familial (multiple) polyposis
      2. Gardner syndrome
      3. Peutz-Jeghers syndrome
   (b) autosomal recessive
      1. Turcot syndrome

B. NONHEREDITARY
   1. Cronkhite-Canada syndrome
   2. Juvenile polyposis

RECTUM AND ANUS

Rectal Narrowing

1. Pelvic lipomatosis + fibrolipomatosis
2. Lymphogranuloma venereum
3. Radiation injury of rectum
4. Chronic ulcerative colitis

Enlarged Presacral Space

Normal width <5 mm in 95%; abnormal width >10 mm

A. RECTAL INFLAMMATION / INFECTION
   ulcerative colitis, Crohn colitis, idiopathic proctosigmoiditis, radiation therapy

B. RECTAL INFECTION
   1. Proctitis (TB, amebiasis, lymphogranuloma venereum, radiation, ischemia)
   2. Diverticulitis

C. BENIGN RECTAL TUMOR
1. Developmental cyst (dermoid, enteric cyst, tailgut cyst)
2. Lipoma, neurofibroma, hemangioendothelioma
3. Epidermal cyst
4. Rectal duplication

D. MALIGNANT RECTAL TUMOR
1. Adenocarcinoma, cloacogenic carcinoma
2. Lymphoma, sarcoma, lymph node metastases
3. Prostatic carcinoma, bladder tumors, cervical cancer, ovarian cancer

E. BODY FLUIDS / DEPOSITS
1. Hematoma: surgery, sacral fracture
2. Pus: perforated appendix, presacral abscess
3. Serum: edema, venous thrombosis
4. Deposit of fat: pelvic lipomatosis, Cushing disease
5. Deposit of amyloid: amyloidosis

F. SACRAL TUMOR
1. Sacrococcygeal teratoma, anterior sacral meningocele
2. Chordoma, metastasis to sacrum

G. MISCELLANEOUS
1. Inguinal hernia containing segment of colon
2. Colitis cystica profunda
3. Pelvic lipomatosis

Lesions Of Ischiorectal Fossa

A. Congenital and developmental anomalies
1. Gartner duct cyst
2. Klippel-Trénaunay syndrome
3. Tailgut cyst

B. Inflammatory and hemorrhagic lesions
1. Fistula in ano
2. Ischiorectal / perirectal abscess
3. Extraperitoneal pelvic hematoma
4. Rectal perforation

C. Secondary neoplasm
per direct extension / hematogenous spread: anorectal / prostatic / pelvic / sacral tumor; lung cancer; melanoma; lymphoma

D. Primary neoplasm
1. Aggressive angiomyxoma
2. Lipoma
3. Plexiform neurofibroma
4. Anal adenocarcinoma
5. Squamous cell carcinoma

PERITONEUM

Peritoneal Mass

A. SOLID MASS
1. Peritoneal mesothelioma
2. Peritoneal carcinomatosis

B. INFILTRATIVE PATTERN
1. Peritoneal mesothelioma

C. CYSTIC MASS
1. Cystic mesothelioma
2. Pseudomyxoma peritonei
3. Bacterial / mycobacterial infection

MESENTERY & OMENTUM

Omental Mass

◊ 33% of primary omental tumors are malignant!
◊ Secondary neoplasms are more frequent than primary!

A. SOLID MASS
(a) benign: leiomyoma, lipoma, neurofibroma
(b) malignant: leiomyosarcoma, liposarcoma, fibrosarcoma, lymphoma, peritoneal mesothelioma, hemangiopericytoma, metastases
(c) Infection: tuberculosis

B. CYSTIC MASS
hematoma

Mesenteric Mass

A. ROUND SOLID MASSES
◊ Benign primary tumors are more common than malignant primary tumors!
◊ Secondary neoplasms are more frequent than primary!
◊ Cystic are more common than solid tumors!
◊ Malignant solid tumors have a tendency to be located near root of mesentery, benign solid tumors in periphery near bowel!
1. Metastases especially from colon, ovary (most frequent neoplasm of mesentery)
2. Lymphoma
3. Leiomyosarcoma (more frequent than leiomyoma)
4. Neural tumor (neurofibroma, ganglioneuroma)
5. Lipoma (uncommon), lipomatosis, liposarcoma
6. Fibrous histiocytoma
7. Hemangioma
8. Desmoid tumor (most common primary)

B. ILL-DEFINED MASSES
metastases (ovary), lymphoma, fibromatosis, fibrosing mesenteritis (associated with Gardner syndrome), lipodystrophy, mesenteric panniculitis

C. STELLATE MASSES
peritoneal mesothelioma, retractile mesenteritis, fibrotic reaction of carcinoid, radiation therapy, desmoid tumor, Hodgkin disease, tuberculous peritonitis, ovarian metastases, diverticulitis, pancreatitis
◊ A mesenteric mass with calcifications suggests carcinoid tumor !

D. LOCULATED CYSTIC MASSES (2/3)
cystic lymphangioma (most common), pseudomyxoma peritonei, cystic mesothelioma, mesenteric cyst, mesenteric hematoma, benign cystic teratoma, cystic spindle cell tumor (= centrally necrotic leiomyoma / leiomyosarcoma)

Mesenteric / Omental Cysts

= "BUBBLES OF THE BELLY"
◊ The first step is to determine the organ of origin!
1. Lymphangioma

2. Nonpancreatic pseudocyst
   = sequelae of mesenteric / omental hematoma / abscess
   Path: thick-walled, usually septated cystic mass with hemorrhagic / purulent contents
3. Duplication cyst
4. Mesothelial cyst
5. Enteric cyst

Umbilical Tumor

A. PRIMARY (38%)
   benign / malignant neoplasm, skin tumor
B. METASTASES (30%)
   = "Sister Joseph nodule"
   • firm painful nodule
   • ± ulceration with serosanguinous / purulent discharge
   Cause: gastrointestinal cancer (50%), undetermined (25%), ovarian cancer, pancreatic cancer, small cell carcinoma of lung (very rare)
   Spread:
   (a) direct extension from anterior peritoneal surface
   (b) extension along embryonic remnants: falciform, median umbilical, omphalomesenteric ligaments
   (c) hematogenous
   (d) retrograde lymphatic flow from inguinal, axillary, paraaortic nodes
   (e) iatrogenic: laparoscopic tract, tract of percutaneous needle biopsy
C. NONNEOPLASTIC
   1. Endometriosis (32%)
   2. Granuloma
   3. Incarcerated hernia

ABDOMINAL LYMPADENOPATHY

Regional Patterns Of Lymphadenopathy

@ Retrocrural nodes
   Abnormal size: >6 mm
   Common cause: lung carcinoma, mesothelioma, lymphoma
@ Gastrohepatic ligament nodes
   = superior portion of lesser omentum suspending stomach from liver
   Abnormal size: >8 mm
   Common cause: carcinoma of lesser curvature of stomach, distal esophagus, lymphoma, pancreatic cancer, melanoma, colon + breast cancer
   DDx: coronary varices
@ Porta hepatis nodes
   = in porta hepatis extending down hepatoduodenal ligament, anterior + posterior to portal vein
   Abnormal size: >6 mm
   Common cause: carcinoma of gallbladder + biliary tree, liver, stomach, pancreas, colon, lung, breast
   Cx: high extrahepatic biliary obstruction
@ Pancreaticoduodenal nodes
   = between duodenal sweep + pancreatic head anterior to IVC
   Abnormal size: >10 mm
   Common cause: lymphoma, pancreatic head, colon, stomach, lung, breast cancer
@ Perisplenic nodes
   = in splenic hilum
   Abnormal size: >10 mm
   Common cause: NHL, leukemia, small bowel neoplasm, ovarian cancer, carcinoma of right / transverse colon
@ Retroperitoneal nodes
   = periaortic, pericaval, interaortocaval
   Abnormal size: >10 mm
   Common cause: lymphoma, renal cell, testicular, cervical, prostatic carcinomas
@ Celiac and superior mesenteric artery nodes
   = preaortic nodes
   Abnormal size: >10 mm
   Common cause: any intra-abdominal neoplasm
@ Pelvic nodes
   = along common, external + internal iliac vessels
   Abnormal size: >15 mm
   Common cause: carcinoma of bladder, prostate, cervix, uterus, rectum

Enlarged Lymph Node With Low-density Center

1. Tuberculosis, Mycobacterium avium-intracellulare
2. Pyogenic infection
3. Whipple disease
4. Lymphoma
5. Metastatic disease after radiation + chemotherapy

GASTROINTESTINAL HEMORRHAGE

Mortality: approx. 10%
◊ Barium examination should be avoided in acute bleeders!

Source:
A. UPPER GASTROINTESTINAL HEMORRHAGE
   = bleeding site proximal to ligament of Treitz
   @ Esophagogastric junction
      1. Esophageal varices (17%): 50% mortality
      2. Mallory-Weiss syndrome (7–14%): very low mortality
   @ Stomach
      1. Acute hemorrhagic gastritis (17–27%)
      2. Gastric ulcer (10%)
      3. Pyloroduodenal ulcer (17–25%)
      Mortality: <10% if under age 60; >35% if over age 60
   @ Other causes (14%): visceral artery aneurysm, vascular malformation, neoplasm, vascular-enteric fistula
      Average mortality: 8–10%

B. LOWER GASTROINTESTINAL HEMORRHAGE
@ Small intestine
tumor (eg, leiomyoma, metastases), ulcers, diverticula (eg, Meckel diverticulum), inflammatory bowel disease (eg, Crohn disease), vascular malformation, visceral artery aneurysm, aortoenteric fistula
@ Colorectal (70%)
1. Diverticula (most common): hemorrhage in 25% of patients with diverticulosis; spontaneous cessation of bleeding in 80%; recurrent bleeding in 25%
2. Colonic angiodysplasia = dilated submucosal arteries + veins overlying mucosal thinning (? secondary to mucosal ischemia)
3. Colitis, tumors, mesenteric varices

INFANTILE GASTROINTESTINAL BLEEDING
(1) Peptic ulcer
(2) Varices
(3) Ulcerated Meckel diverticulum

Intramural Hemorrhage
A. VASCULITIS
1. Henoch-Schönlein purpura
B. TRAUMA
C. COAGULATION DEFECT
1. Anticoagulant therapy
2. Thrombocytopenia
3. Disseminated intravascular coagulation
D. DISEASES WITH COAGULATION DEFECT
1. Hemophilia
2. Leukemia, lymphoma
3. Multiple myeloma
4. Metastatic carcinoma
5. Idiopathic thrombocytopenic purpura
E. ISCHEMIA (often fatal)
• abdominal pain
• melena
Site: submucosal / intramural / mesenteric
√ "stacked coin" / "picket fence" appearance of mucosal folds (due to symmetric infiltration of submucosal blood)
√ "thumbprinting" = rounded polypoid filling defect (due to focal accumulation of hematoma in bowel wall)
√ separation + uncoiling of bowel loops
√ narrowing of lumen + localized filling defects (asymmetric hematoma)
√ no spasm / irritability
√ mechanical obstruction + proximal distension of loops
Prognosis: resolution within 2–6 weeks

GI ABNORMALITIES IN CHRONIC RENAL FAILURE AND RENAL TRANSPLANTATION
@ Esophagus
1. Esophagitis: candida, CMV, herpes
@ Stomach & duodenum
1. Gastritis
√ thickened gastric folds (38%)
√ edema + erosions
Cause:
(a) imbalance of gastrin levels + gastric acid secretion due to (1) reduced removal of gastrin from kidney with loss of cortical mass (2) impaired acid feedback mechanism (3) hypochlorhydria
(b) opportunistic infection (eg, CMV)
2. Gastric ulcer (3.5%)
3. Duodenal ulcer (2.4%)
4. Duodenitis (47%)
@ Colon
More severely + frequently affected after renal transplantation
1. Progressive distention + pseudoobstruction
Contributing factors: dehydration, alteration of diet, inactivity, nonabsorbable antacids, high-dose steroids
2. Ischemic colitis
(a) primary disease responsible for end-stage renal disease (eg, diabetes, vasculitis)
(b) trauma of renal transplantation
3. Diverticulitis
Contributing factors: chronic obstipation, steroids, autonomic nervous dysfunction
4. Pseudomembranous colitis
5. Uremic colitis = nonspecific colitis
6. Spontaneous colonic perforation
Cause: nonocclusive ischemia, diverticula, duodenal + gastric ulcers
@ Pancreas
1. Pancreatitis
Cause: hypercalcemia, steroids, infection, immunosuppressive agents, trauma
@ General
1. GI hemorrhage
Cause: gastritis, ulcers, colonic diverticula, ischemic bowel, infectious colitis, pseudomembranous colitis, nonspecific cecal ulceration
2. Bowel perforation (in 1–4% of transplant recipients)
3. Opportunistic infection
Organism: Candida, herpes, CMV, strongyloides
4. Malignancy
(a) skin tumors
(b) lymphoma

ENTEROPATHY

Protein-losing Enteropathy
A. DISEASE WITH MUCOSAL ULCERATION
1. Carcinoma
2. Lymphoma
3. Inflammatory bowel disease
4. Peptic ulcer disease
B. HYPERTROPHIED GASTRIC RUGAE
1. Ménétrièr disease
C. NONULCERATIVE MUCOSAL DISEASE
1. Celiac disease
2. Tropical sprue

GI

3. Whipple disease
4. Allergic gastroenteropathy
5. Gastrocolic fistula
6. Villous adenoma of colon

D. LYMPHATIC OBSTRUCTION
1. Intestinal lymphangiectasia

E. HEART DISEASE
1. Constrictive pericarditis
2. Tricuspid insufficiency

Malabsorption

= deficient absorption of any essential food materials within small bowel

(1) PRIMARY MALABSORPTION
= the digestive abnormality is the only abnormality present
1. Celiac disease = nontropical sprue
2. Tropical sprue
3. Disaccharidase deficiencies

(2) SECONDARY MALABSORPTION
= occurring during course of gastrointestinal disease

(a) enteric
1. Whipple disease
2. Parasites: hookworm, Giardia, fish tapeworm
3. Mechanical defects: fistulas, blind loops, adhesions, volvulus, short circuits
4. Neurologic: diabetes, functional diarrhea
5. Inflammatory: enteritis (viral, bacterial, fungal, nonspecific)
6. Endocrine: Zollinger-Ellison syndrome
7. Drugs: neomycin, phenindione, cathartics
8. Collagen disease: scleroderma, lupus, polyarteritis
9. Lymphoma
10. Benign + malignant small bowel tumors
11. Vascular disease
12. CHF, agammaglobulinemia, amyloid, abetalipoproteinemia, intestinal lymphangiectasia

(b) gastric
vagotomy, gastrectomy, pyloroplasty, gastric fistula (to jejunum, ileum, colon)

(c) pancreatic
pancreatitis, pancreatectomy, pancreatic cancer, cystic fibrosis

(d) hepatobiliary
intra- and extrahepatic biliary obstruction, acute + chronic liver disease

Roentgenographic Signs In Malabsorption

√ SMALL BOWEL WITH NORMAL FOLDS + FLUID
1. Maldigestion (deficiency of bile salt / pancreatic enzymes)
2. Gastric surgery
3. Alactasia

√ SMALL BOWEL WITH NORMAL FOLDS + WET
1. Sprue
2. Dermatitis herpetiformis

√ DILATED DRY SMALL BOWEL
1. Scleroderma
2. Dermatomyositis
3. Pseudoobstruction: no peristaltic activity

√ DILATED WET SMALL BOWEL
1. Sprue
2. Obstruction
3. Blind loop

√ THICKENED STRAIGHT FOLDS + DRY SMALL BOWEL
1. Amyloidosis (malabsorption is unusual)
2. Radiation
3. Ischemia
4. Lymphoma (rare)
5. Macroglobulinemia (rare)

√ THICKENED STRAIGHT FOLDS + WET SMALL BOWEL
1. Zollinger-Ellison syndrome
2. Abetalipoproteinemia: rare inherited disease characterized by CNS damage, retinal abnormalities, steatorrhea, acanthocytosis

√ THICKENED NODULAR IRREGULAR FOLDS + DRY SMALL BOWEL
1. Lymphoid hyperplasia
2. Lymphoma
3. Crohn disease
4. Whipple disease
5. Mastocytosis

√ THICKENED NODULAR IRREGULAR FOLDS + WET SMALL BOWEL
1. Lymphangiectasia
2. Giardiasis
3. Whipple disease (rare)

Small Bowel Nodularity With Malabsorption

mnemonic: "**W**hat **I**s **H**is **M**ain **A**im? **L**ay **E**ggs, **B**y **G**od"

Whipple disease
Intestinal lymphangiectasia
Histiocytosis
Mastocytosis
Amyloidosis
Lymphoma, **L**ymph node hyperplasia
Edema
Blood
Giardiasis

GI

ANATOMY AND FUNCTION OF GASTROINTESTINAL TRACT

GASTROINTESTINAL HORMONES

Cholecystokinin

= CCK = 33 amino acid residues (former name: Pancreozymin); the 5 C-terminal amino acids are identical to those of gastrin, causing similar effects as gastrin

Produced in: duodenal + upper intestinal mucosa
Released by: fatty acids, some amino acids (phenylalanine, methionine), hydrogen ions

Effects:

@ Stomach
- (1) weakly stimulates HCl secretion
- (2) given alone: inhibits gastrin, which leads to decrease in HCl production
- (3) stimulates pepsin secretion
- (4) stimulates gastric motility

@ Pancreas
- (1) stimulates secretion of pancreatic enzymes (= Pancreozymin)
- (2) stimulates bicarbonate secretion (weakly by direct effect; strongly through potentiating effect on secretin)
- (3) stimulates insulin release

@ Liver
- (1) stimulates water + bicarbonate secretion

@ Intestine
- (1) stimulates secretion of Brunner glands
- (2) increases motility

@ Biliary tract
- (1) strong stimulator of gallbladder contraction
- (2) relaxation of sphincter of Oddi

Gastrin

= 17 amino acid peptide amide;
PENTAGASTRIN
= acyl derivative of the biologic active C-terminal tetrapeptide amide

Produced in: antral cells + G-cells of pancreas
Released by:
- (a) vagal stimulation, gastric distension
- (b) short-chain alcohol (ethanol, propanol)
- (c) amino acids (glycine, ß-alanine)
- (d) caffeine
- (e) hypercalcemia

mediated by neuroendocrine cholinergic reflexes

Inhibited by: drop in pH of antral mucosa to <3.5

Effects:

@ Stomach:
- (1) stimulation of gastric HCl secretion from parietal cells, which in turn:
- (2) increases pepsinogen production by chief cells through local reflex
- (3) increase in antral motility
- (4) trophic effect on gastric mucosa (parietal cell hyperplasia)

@ Pancreas
- (1) strong increase in enzyme output
- (2) weakly stimulates fluid + bicarbonate output
- (3) stimulates insulin release

@ Liver
- (1) water + bicarbonate secretion

@ Intestine
- (1) stimulates secretion of Brunner glands
- (2) increases motility

@ Gallbladder
- (1) stimulates contraction

@ Esophagus
- (1) increases resting pressure of LES

Glucagon

Produced in: α-cells (and β-cells) of pancreas
Released by: low blood glucose levels

Effects:

@ Intestines
- (1) lowers pressure of GE sphincter
- (2) hypotonic effect on duodenum > jejunum > stomach > colon

@ Hormones
- (1) releases catecholamines from the adrenal gland that paralyze intestinal smooth muscle
- (2) increases serum insulin + glucose levels (mobilization of hepatic glycogen)

@ Biliary tract
- (1) increases bile flow
- (2) relaxes gallbladder + sphincter of Oddi

Dose for radiologic imaging: 1 mg maximum
- ◊ IV administration causes a quick response + rapid dissipation of action!
- ◊ IM administration prolongs onset + increases length of action!

Half-life: 3–6 minutes
Side effects: nausea + vomiting, weakness, dizziness (delayed onset of 1.5–4 hours after IM administration)

Contraindication:
- (1) hypersensitivity / allergy to glucagon: urticaria, periorbital edema, respiratory distress, hypotension, coronary artery spasm (?), circulatory arrest
- (2) known hypertensive response to glucagon
- (3) pheochromocytoma: glucagon stimulates release of catecholamines
- (4) insulinoma: insulin-releasing effect may result in hypoglycemia
- (5) glucagonoma
- (6) poorly controlled diabetes mellitus

Secretin

Produced in: duodenal mucosa
Released by: hydrogen ions providing a pH <4.5

Effects:
@ Stomach
(1) inhibits gastrin activity, which leads to decrease in HCl secretion
(2) stimulates pepsinogen secretion by chief cells (potent pepsigogue)
(3) decreases gastric and duodenal motility + contraction of pyloric sphincter
@ Pancreas
(1) increases alkaline pancreatic secretions ($NaHCO_3$)
(2) weakly stimulates enzyme secretion
(3) stimulates insulin release
@ Liver
(1) stimulates water + bicarbonate secretion (most potent choleretic)
@ Intestine
(1) stimulates secretion of Brunner glands
(2) inhibits motility
@ Esophagus
(1) opens LES

ESOPHAGUS

Lower Esophageal Anatomy

A. **Esophageal Vestibule**
= saccular termination of lower esophagus with upper boundary at tubulovestibular junction + lower boundary at esophagogastric junction
√ collapsed during resting state
√ assumes bulbous configuration with swallowing
(a) tubulovestibular junction = A level = junction between tubular and saccular esophagus
(b) phrenic ampulla = bell-shaped part above diaphragm (term should be discarded because of dynamic changes of configuration)
(c) submerged segment = infrahiatal part of esophagus
√ widening / disappearance is indicative of gastroesophageal reflux disease (GERD)

B. **Gastroesophageal Junction**
Site: at upper level of gastric sling fibers, straddles cardiac incisura demarcating the left lateral margin of GE junction

C. **Z line** = B level = squamocolumnar junction line not acceptable criterion for locating GE junction
Site: 1–2 cm above gastric sling fibers

D. **Lower Esophageal Sphincter**
= physiologic 2–4 cm high pressure zone corresponding to esophageal vestibule
√ tightly closed during resting state
√ assumes bulbous configuration with swallowing

Muscular Rings Of Esophagus

A Ring

= contracted / hypertrophied muscles in response to incompetent GE sphincter
• rarely symptomatic / dysphagia
Location: at tubulovestibular junction = superior aspect of vestibule
√ usually 2 cm proximal to GE junction at upper end of vestibule
√ varies in caliber during the same examination, may disappear on maximum distension
√ broad smooth narrowing with thick rounded margins
√ visible only if tubular esophagus above + vestibule below are distended

B Ring

= sling fibers representing a U-shaped thickening of inner muscle layers with open arm of U toward lesser curvature = inferior aspect of vestibule
Location: < 2 cm from hiatal margins
√ only visible when esophagogastric junction is above hiatus
√ thin ledge-like ring just below the mucosal junction (Z line)

STOMACH

Gastric Cells

1. Chief cells
= peptic / zymogenic cells
Location: body + fundus
produce: pepsinogen
2. Parietal cells
= oxyntic cells
Location: body + fundus
produce: H^+, Cl^-, intrinsic factor, prostaglandins
3. Mucous neck cells
produce: mucoprotein, mucopolysaccharide, aminopolysaccharide sulfate
4. Argentaffine cells
= enteroendocrine cells
Location: body + fundus
produce: glucagon-like substance (A-cells), somatostatin (D-cells), vasoactive intestinal polypeptide (D_1-cells), 5-hydroxytryptamine (EC-cells)
5. G-cells
Location: pylorus
produce: gastrin

Effect Of Bilateral Vagotomy

= cholinergic denervation
(1) decreased MOTILITY of stomach + intestines
(2) decreased GASTRIC SECRETION
(3) decreased TONE OF GALLBLADDER + bile ducts
(4) increased TONE OF SPHINCTERS (Oddi + lower esophageal sphincter)

Pylorus

= fan-shaped specialized circular muscle fibers with:
(a) distal sphincteric loop = right canalis loop
√ corresponds to radiologic pyloric sphincter
(b) proximal sphincteric loop = left canalis loop
√ 2 cm proximal to distal sphincteric loop on greater curvature (seen during complete relaxation)

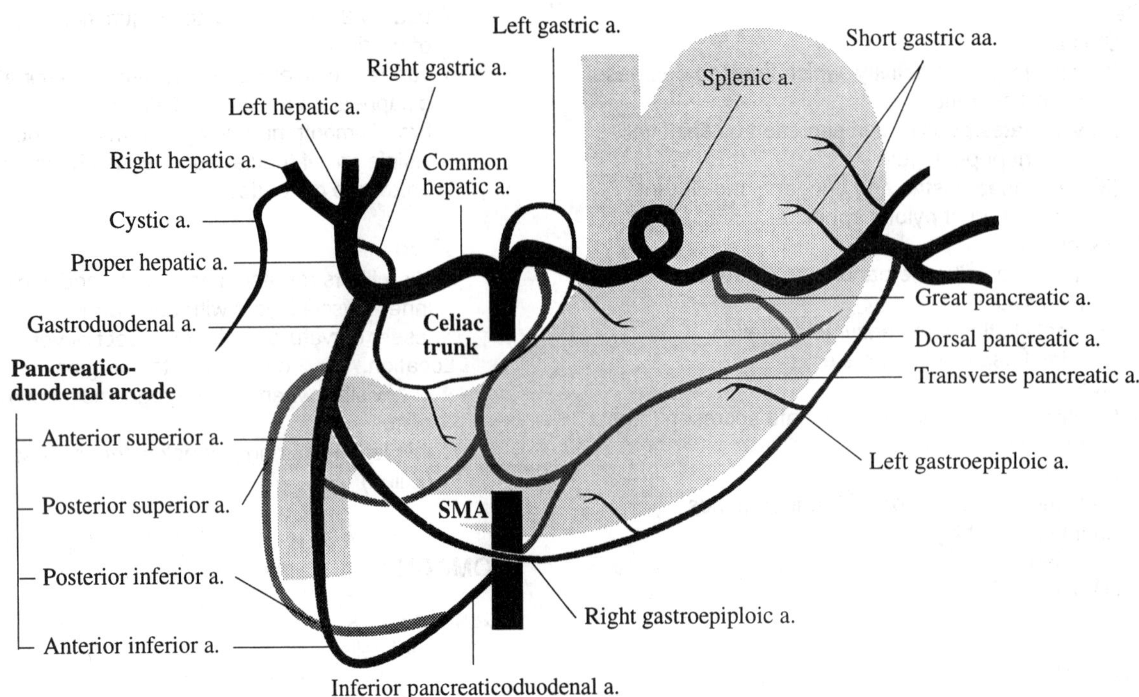

Blood Supply of Stomach, Duodenum, and Pancreas

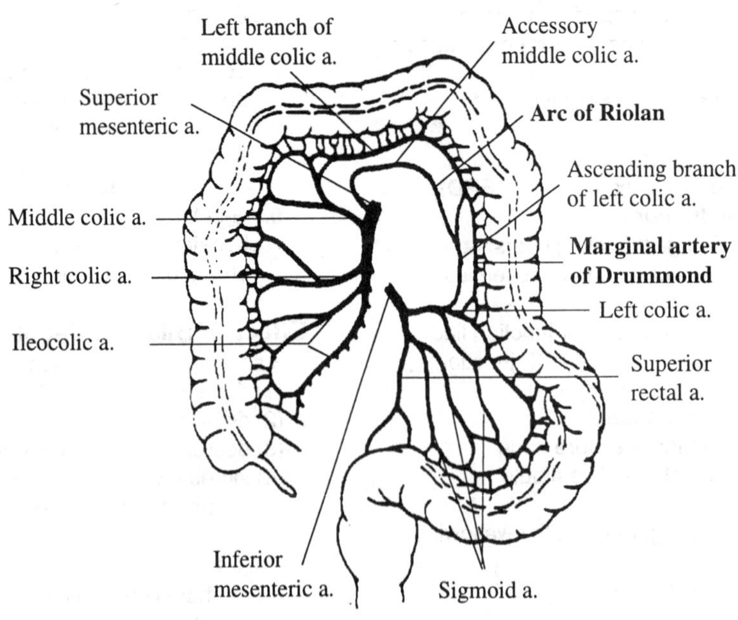

Blood Supply of Large Intestine

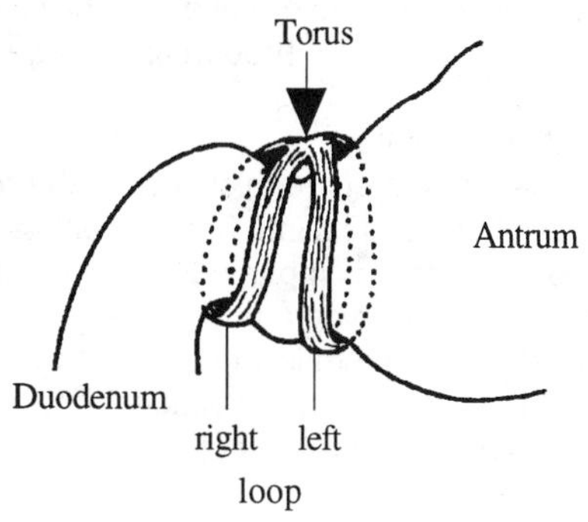

(c) torus
= fibers of both sphincters converge on the lesser curvature side to form a muscular prominence; prolapse of mucosa between sphincteric loops produces a niche simulating ulcer

√ pyloric channel 5–10 mm long, wall thickness of 4–8 mm

√ concentric indentation of the base of the duodenal bulb

SMALL BOWEL

Duodenal segments

(1) duodenal bulb + short postbulbar segment: intraperitoneal + freely movable
(2) descending duodenum: retroperitoneal attached to head of pancreas
(3) horizontal = transverse segment: retroperitoneal crossing the spine
(4) ascending portion retroperitoneal ascending to level of duodenojejunal junction

VARIATIONS:
(1) "mobile duodenum" / "water-trap duodenum"
= long postbulbar segment with undulation / redundancy
(2) duodenum inversum / duodenum reflexum
= distal duodenum ascends to the right of spine to the level of duodenal bulb + then crosses spine horizontally + fixated in normal location

Small bowel folds

A. NORMAL FOLD THICKNESS

@ jejunum	1.7–2.0 mm	>2.5 mm pathologic
@ ileum	1.4–1.7 mm	>2.0 mm pathologic

B. NORMAL NUMBER OF FOLDS

@ jejunum	4–6 / inch
@ ileum	3–5 / inch

C. NORMAL FOLD HEIGHT

@ jejunum	3.5–7.0 mm
@ ileum	2.0–3.5 mm

D. NORMAL LUMEN DIAMETER

@ upper jejunum	3.0–4.0 cm	>4.5 cm pathologic
@ lower jejunum	2.5–3.5 cm	>4.0 cm pathologic
@ ileum	2.0–2.8 cm	>3.0 cm pathologic

RULE OF 3's:
◊ wall thickness <3 mm
◊ valvulae conniventes <3 mm
◊ diameter <3 cm
◊ air-fluid levels <3

Normal bowel caliber

mnemonic: "3-6-9-12"

3 cm	maximal size of small bowel
6 cm	maximal size of transverse colon
9 cm	maximal size of cecum
12 cm	maximal caliber of cecum before it may burst

Small bowel peristalsis

A. INCREASED
1. Vagal stimulation
2. Acetylcholine
3. Anticholinesterase (eg, neostigmine)
4. Cholecystokinin

B. DECREASED
1. Atropine (eg, Pro-Banthine®)
2. Bilateral vagotomy

INTESTINAL FUNCTION

Intestinal gas

A. INFLUX
1. Aerophagia .... 2 L
2. Liberation from intestinal tract
   (a) neutralization of bicarbonate in secretions (CO_2) .... 8 L
   (b) bacterial fermentation (CO_2, H_2, CH_4, H_2S) .... 15 L
3. Diffusion from blood (N_2, O_2, CO_2)

B. EFFLUX
1. Diffusion from intestines into blood and expulsion from lung .... 50 L
2. Expulsion from anus .... 2 L

Intestinal fluid

A. INFLUX
1. Oral ingestion .... 2.5 L
2. Intestinal secretions .... 8.2 L
   saliva .... 1.5 L
   bile .... 0.5 L
   gastric secretions .... 2.5 L
   pancreatic secretions .... 0.7 L
   intestinal secretions .... 3.0 L

B. EFFLUX
1. Peranal .... 0.1 L
2. Intestinal resorption (primarily in ileum + ascending colon) .... 10.6 L

GI

Defecography / Evacuation Proctography

evacuation time = 15 (range 5–40) seconds

anorectal angle = angle formed between central axis of anal canal + line parallel to posterior wall of rectum
- √ 90° at rest and during voluntary contraction (squeeze maneuver)
- √ more obtuse during defecation straining (void)

anorectal junction = point of taper of distal rectal ampulla as it merges with the anal canal; position of anorectal junction referenced to plane of ischial tuberosities = 0–3.5 cm; elevation during squeeze of 0–4.5 cm; elevation during void of -3.0–0 cm

rectovaginal space = space between vagina and rectum

perineum = area between external genital organs and anal verge

rectocele = measurement of anteroposterior depth of convex wall protrusion extending beyond expected margin of normal rectal wall
small <2 cm;
moderate = 2–4 cm;
large >4 cm

peritoneocele = extension of rectouterine excavation to below upper third of vagina; containing liquid / bowel / omentum

enterocele = bowel present in peritoneocele

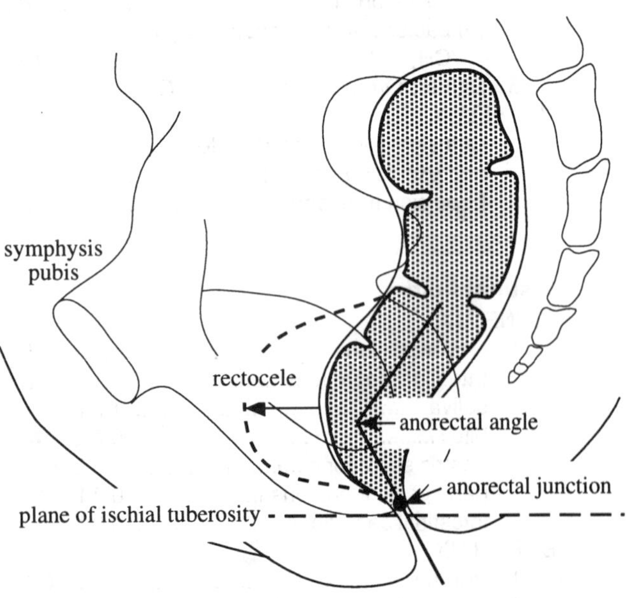

Defecographic Measurements

rectal prolapse = descent of entire thickness of rectal wall through anal verge

rectal intussusception
= descent of the entire thickness of the rectal wall possibly extending into anal canal; starting 6–11 cm above anus; accompanied by formation of a circular indentation forming a ring pocket
- √ infolding of <3 mm in width / > 3 mm in width / intraluminal narrowing / descent into anal canal / external prolapse

PERITONEUM

Peritoneal Spaces

Definitions:

Ligament = formed by two folds of peritoneum supporting a structure within the peritoneal cavity

Omentum = specialized structure connecting stomach to an additional structure

Mesentery = two peritoneal folds connecting a portion of bowel to the retroperitoneum

Embryology:

above transverse mesocolon:

A. RIGHT PERITONEAL SPACE
forms perihepatic space + lesser sac:
1. Right subphrenic space:
   - — located between right hepatic lobe + diaphragm
   - — limited posteriorly by right superior reflection of coronary lig. + right triangular ligament
2. Right subhepatic space:
   - — divided into
     - • anterior right subhepatic space: located just posterior to porta hepatis, communicating with lesser sac via epiploic foramen (= foramen of Winslow)
     - • posterior right subhepatic space = Morison pouch = hepatorenal fossa
       - ◊ Most dependent portion of the abdomen in supine patient!
3. Bare area of liver
   - — situated between reflections of right + left coronary ligaments
   - — continuous with right anterior pararenal space
4. Lesser sac:
   - • superior recess:
     - — surrounds medial aspect of caudate lobe
     - — separated from splenic recess by gastropancreatic fold
   - • splenic recess:
     - — extends across midline to splenic hilum
   - • inferior recess:
     - — separates stomach from pancreas + transverse mesocolon
     - — anteriorly covered by lesser omentum

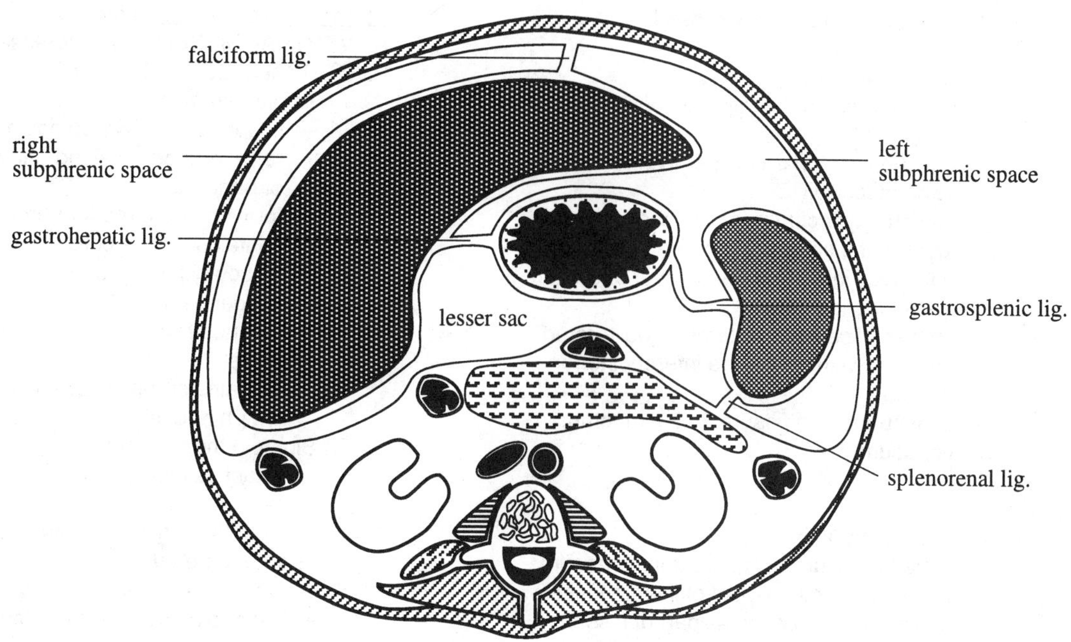

Ligaments and Peritoneal Spaces in Upper Abdomen

5. Lesser omentum = combination of gastrohepatic ligament + hepatoduodenal ligament
6. Right triangular ligament:
   — forms from coalescence of superior + inferior reflections of right coronary ligament
   — divides posterior aspect of right perihepatic space into right subphrenic space + posterior right subhepatic space

B. LEFT PERITONEAL SPACE
forms left subphrenic space
1. Left subphrenic space:
   — artificially divided into
      • immediate subphrenic space: between diaphragm + gastric fundus
      • perisplenic space: bounded inferiorly by phrenicocolic lig.
      • subhepatic space = gastrohepatic recess: located between lateral segment of left hepatic lobe + stomach
   — separated from right subphrenic space by falciform ligament
2. Left triangular ligament:
   — forms from coalescence of superior + inferior reflections of left coronary ligament
   — located along superior aspect of left hepatic lobe

C. DORSAL MESENTERY gives rise to:
1. Gastrophrenic ligament
   — courses through immediate subphrenic space
   — suspends stomach from dome of diaphragm
2. Gastropancreatic ligament
   — formed by proximal left gastric artery
   — attaches posterior aspect of gastric fundus to retroperitoneum
   - partially separates superior recess of lesser sac from splenic recess

3. Phrenicocolic ligament
   — major suspensory ligament of spleen
   — attaches proximal descending colon to left hemidiaphragm
   — separates left subphrenic space from left paracolic gutter

4. Gastrosplenic ligament
   — remnant of dorsal mesentery
   — connects greater curvature of stomach with splenic hilum
   — contains short gastric vessels

5. Splenorenal ligament
   — connects posterior aspect of spleen to anterior pararenal space
   — contributes to left lateral + posterior border of lesser sac
   — encloses tail of pancreas + distal splenic artery + proximal splenic vein

6. Gastrocolic ligament
   — forms portion of anterior border of lesser sac
   — forms superior aspect of greater omentum
   — connects greater curvature of stomach with superior aspect of transverse colon
   — contains gastroepiploic vessels

GI

D. VENTRAL MESENTERY gives rise to:

1. Falciform ligament
   = sickle-shaped fold composed of two layers of peritoneum
   — attaches ventral surface of liver to anterior abdominal wall
   — its right layer continues into the superior layer of the coronary ligament, its left layer continues into the anterior layer of the left triangular ligament
   — contains ligamentum teres (= obliterated umbilical vein) in its free inferoposterior margin
   — continuous with fissure for ligamentum venosum

2. Gastrohepatic ligament:
   — arises in fissure of ligamentum venosum
   — connects medial aspect of liver to lesser curvature of stomach as part of lesser omentum
   — contains left gastric artery, coronary vein, lymph nodes

3. Hepatoduodenal ligament:
   — forms inferior edge of gastrohepatic ligament
   — forms anterior margin of epiploic foramen
   — extends from proximal duodenum to porta hepatis
   — contains common hepatic duct, common bile duct, hepatic artery, portal vein

<u>below transverse mesocolon</u>:

A. VENTRAL MESENTERY regresses

B. DORSAL MESENTERY forms:

1. Tansverse mesocolon:
   — suspends transverse colon from retroperitoneum along anteroinferior edge of pancreas
   — forms posteroinferior border of lesser sac
   — contains middle colic vessels
2. Small bowel mesentery:
   — suspends small bowel from retroperitoneum
   — extends from ligament of Treitz to ileocecal valve
   — contains superior mesenteric vessels + lymph nodes
3. Sigmoid mesocolon:
   — attaches sigmoid colon to posterior pelvic wall
   — contains sigmoid + hemorrhoidal vessels
4. Greater omentum:
   — inferior continuation of gastrocolic ligament
   — formed by double reflection of dorsal mesogastrium thus composed of 4 layers of peritoneum
5. Superior + inferior ileocecal recesses:
   — located above + below terminal ileum
6. Retrocecal space:
   — present only if peritoneum reflects posterior to cecum
7. Right + left paracolic gutters:
   — located lateral to ascending + descending colon
8. Intersigmoid recess:
   — located along undersurface of sigmoid mesocolon

GASTROINTESTINAL DISORDERS

ACHALASIA

= failure of organized peristalsis + relaxation at level of lower esophageal sphincter

Etiology: (a) idiopathic: abnormality of Auerbach plexus / medullary dorsal nucleus; ? neurotropic virus, ? gastrin hypersensitivity
(b) Chagas disease

√ megaesophagus = dilatation of esophagus beginning in upper 1/3, ultimately entire length
√ absence of primary peristalsis below level of cricopharyngeus
√ nonperistaltic contractions
√ "bird-beak" / "rattail" deformity = V-shaped conical + symmetric tapering of stenotic segment with most marked narrowing at GE junction
√ Hurst phenomenon = temporary transit through cardia when hydrostatic pressure of barium column is above tonic LES pressure
√ sudden esophageal emptying after ingestion of carbonated beverage (eg, Coke)
√ "vigorous achalasia" = numerous tertiary contractions in nondilated distal esophagus of early achalasia
√ prompt relaxation of LES upon amyl nitrate inhalation (smooth-muscle relaxant)

CXR:
√ right convex opacity behind right heart border; occasionally left convex opacity if thoracic aorta tortuous
√ right convex opacity may be tethered by azygos arch allowing for greater dilatation above + below
√ air-fluid level (stasis in thoracic esophagus filled with retained secretions + alimentary residue)
√ small / absent gastric air bubble
√ anterior displacement + bowing of trachea (LAT view)
√ patchy bilateral alveolar opacities resembling acute / chronic aspiration pneumonia (M. fortuitum-chelonei infection)

Cx: esophageal carcinoma in 2–7% (usually midesophagus)

Rx: pneumatic dilatation / surgical myotomy

DDx: (1) Neoplasm (separation of gastric fundus from diaphragm; normal peristalsis; asymmetric tapering)
(2) Peptic stricture of esophagus

ADENOMA OF SMALL BOWEL

Location: duodenum (21%), jejunum (36%), ileum (43%) esp. ileocecal valve

Histo: (1) Hamartomatous polyp (77%), multiple in 47%, 1/3 of multiple lesions associated with Peutz-Jeghers syndrome
(2) adenomatous polyp (13%), may have malignant potential
(3) polypoid gastric heterotopic tumor (10%)

ADENOMATOUS COLONIC POLYP

= EPITHELIAL POLYP
Most common benign colonic tumor (68–79%)

Predisposed: previously detected polyp / cancer; family history of polyps / cancer; idiopathic inflammatory bowel disease; Peutz-Jeghers syndrome; Gardner syndrome; familial polyposis

Prevalence: 3% in 3rd decade; 10% in 7th decade; 26% in 9th decade

Location: rectum (21–34%); sigmoid (26–38%); ascending colon (9–12%); transverse colon (12–13%); descending colon (6–18%); multiple in 35–50% (usually <5–10 in number)

Histo:
1. Tubular adenoma (75%)
   = cylindrical glandular structure lined by stratified columnar epithelium + nests of epithelium within lamina propria
   √ usually < 10 mm in diameter
   √ often pedunculated if >10 mm
   malignant potential: <10 mm in 1%; 10–20 mm in 10%; >20 mm in 35%
2. Tubulovillous adenoma (15%)
   = mixture between tubular + villous adenoma
   malignant potential: <10 mm in 4%; 10–20 mm in 7%; >20 mm in 46%
3. Villous adenoma (10%)
   = thin frondlike projections from surface with epithelium outlining their margins ("villous fronds")
   • potassium depletion
   √ often >20 mm in diameter with papillary surface
   √ often broad-based sessile lesion
   √ heterogeneous low attenuation on CT (due to capacious mucin becoming trapped within papillary projections + crevices)
   malignant potential: <10 mm in 10%; 10–20 mm in 10%; >20 mm in 53%

Size & malignancy:
<5 mm in 0%; 5–9 mm in 1%; 10–20 mm in 10%; >20 mm in 46% malignant
◊ All polyps >10 mm should be removed!
◊ Time for adenoma-carcinoma sequence probably averages 10–15 years!

Probability of coexistent colonic growth:
— synchronous adenoma in 50%
— metachronous adenoma in 30–40%
— synchronous adenocarcinoma in 1.5–5%
— metachronous adenocarcinoma in 5–10%

• asymptomatic (75%)
• diarrhea, abdominal pain
• peranal hemorrhage (67%)

Colonoscopy (incomplete in 16–43%)

GI

BE (rate of detection of polyps <10 mm higher with double than single contrast; false-negative rate of 7%):
√ sessile flat / round polyp
√ pedunculated polyp: stalk >2 cm in length almost always indicative of a benign polyp
√ suggestive of malignancy: irregular lobulated surface, broad base = width of the base greater than height, retraction of colonic wall = dimpling / indentation / puckering at base of tumor, interval growth
√ lacelike / reticular surface pattern CHARACTERISTIC for villous adenoma (occasionally in tubular adenoma)

DDx: (1) Nonneoplastic: hyperplastic polyp, inflammatory pseudopolyp, lymphoid tissue, ameboma, tuberculoma, foreign-body granuloma, malacoplakia, heterotopia, hamartoma
(2) Neoplastic subepithelial: lipoma, leiomyoma, neurofibroma, hemangioma, lymphangioma, endothelioma, myeloblastoma, sarcoma, lymphoma, enteric cyst, duplication, varix, pneumatosis, hematoma, endometriosis

ADENOCARCINOMA OF SMALL BOWEL

Frequency: about 50 times less common than colonic carcinoma
Risk factors: Crohn disease, sprue, Peutz-Jeghers syndrome, Lynch syndrome II, congenital bowel duplication, ileostomy, duodenal / jejunal bypass surgery
Histo: mostly moderately to well differentiated; may arise in villous tumors / de novo; no correlation between size and invasiveness
Location: duodenum (~50%, especially near ampulla), jejunum > ileum
√ annular stricture with "overhanging edges" (60%)
√ lobulated / ovoid polypoid sessile mass (41%)
◊ Duodenal tumors tend to be papillary / polypoid!
√ ulcerated mass (27%)
CT:
√ soft-tissue mass with heterogeneous attenuation
√ moderate contrast enhancement
Cx: intussusception
DDx: lymphoma (lymphadenopathy more bulky)

AFFERENT LOOP SYNDROME

= PROXIMAL LOOP / BLIND LOOP SYNDROME
= partial intermittent obstruction of afferent loop leading to overdistension of loop by gastric juices after Billroth-II gastrojejunostomy
Cause: gastrojejunostomy with left-to-right anastomosis (= proximal jejunal loop attached to greater curvature instead of lesser curvature), mechanical factors (intussusception, adhesion, kinking), inflammatory disease, neoplastic infiltration of local mesentery or anastomosis, idiopathic motor dysfunction
• postprandial epigastric fullness relieved by bilious vomiting
• vitamin B_{12} deficiency with megaloblastic anemia
• afferent loop with abnormal bacterial flora (Gram negative, resembling colon in quality + quantity)

Abdominal plain film:
√ normal in 85% (no air in lumen of afferent loop)
UGI:
√ preferential emptying of stomach into proximal loop
√ proximal loop stasis
√ regurgitation
CT:
√ rounded water-density masses adjacent to head + tail of pancreas forming a U-shaped loop
√ oral contrast material may not enter loop
√ may result in biliary obstruction (increased pressure at ampulla)
Rx: antibiotic therapy

AIDS

◊ Gastrointestinal involvement due to opportunistic infections + AIDS-associated neoplasms!
◊ Pathologic abnormalities at multiple sites with single / several opportunistic organisms are frequent!

AIDS-defining illness related to CD4 T-lymphocyte count [cells/μL]:
<400 extrapulmonary Mycobacterium tuberculosis, Kaposi sarcoma
<200 Candida albicans, Histoplasma capsulatum, Cryptosporidium species, Pneumocystis carinii, Non-Hodgkin lymphoma
<100 Cytomegalovirus, Herpes simplex virus, Mycobacterium avium complex

A. VIRAL PATHOGENS
1. **Cytomegalovirus infection**
◊ Most common cause of life-threatening opportunistic viral infection in AIDS patients!
Organism: double-stranded DNA virus of the herpes family
Infection: ubiquitous among humans occurring at an early age in populations with poor sanitation + crowded living conditions
◊ Result of reactivation of latent virus in previously infected host!
Prevalence: 13% of all gastrointestinal diseases in AIDS patients
Path: infection of endothelial cells leads to small vessel vasculitis resulting in hemorrhage, ischemic necrosis, ulceration
Histo: large mononuclear epithelial / endothelial cells that contain intranuclear / cytoplasmatic inclusions with surrounding inflammation
Location: colon > small bowel (terminal ileum) > esophagus > stomach
@ Esophagus
√ single / multiple large superficial ulcers
@ Small bowel
√ luminal narrowing secondary to marked bowel wall thickening
√ thickened irregular folds (vasculitis leading to thrombosis + ischemia)

GI

√ penetrating ulcer ± perforation
√ CMV pseudotumor (uncommon)
@ Colon (CMV colitis)
• hematochezia, crampy abdominal pain, fever
√ findings of toxic megacolon
√ discrete small well-defined nodules (similar to lymphoid nodular hyperplasia) throughout entire colon
√ aphthous ulcers on background of normal mucosa
√ marked bowel wall thickening
√ double-ring / target sign on CT (due to increased submucosal edema)
√ ascites
√ inflammation of pericolonic fat + fascia
Rx: ganciclovir (effective in 75%)

2. **Herpes simplex virus infection**
◊ Result of reactivation of latent virus in previously infected host
Organism: neurotropic DNA virus of herpes family
Prevalence: 70% for type 1, 16% for type 2 (endemic in United States); type 2 much more common in AIDS
Infection: direct inoculation through mucous membrane contact; from dormant state in root ganglia reactivated + transported via efferent nerves to mucocutaneous surface
Location: oral cavity, esophagus, rectum, anus
√ multiple small discrete ulcers

3. **HIV infection**
◊ Not an AIDS-defining illness!
Infection: acute HIV-infection with transient immunosuppression / during AIDS
√ >2 cm large solitary ulcer in the mid- or distal esophagus (HIV-infected cells cause alterations in cytokines resulting in infiltration of inflammatory cells into submucosa + destruction of mucosa)
Rx: corticosteroids

B. FUNGAL PATHOGENS

1. **Candidiasis**
◊ The absence of thrush does not exclude the diagnosis of candidal esophagitis!
Organism: commensal fungus Candida albicans
Prevalence: 10–20% (in United States); up to 80% in developing countries
Location: oral cavity, esophagus
√ discrete linear / irregular longitudinally oriented filling defects in esophagus
Cx: disseminated systemic candidiasis (rare + indicative of granulocytopenia from chemotherapy / direct inoculation via catheter)

2. **Histoplasmosis**
Organism: dimorphic opportunistic fungus
Prevalence: 10% GI involvement with disseminated histoplasmosis in AIDS patients
Location: colon > terminal ileum
√ segmental inflammation / applecore lesion / bowel stricture
√ hepatosplenomegaly
√ mesenteric lymphadenopathy
√ diffuse hypoattenuation of spleen

C. PROTOZOAN PATHOGENS

1. **Cryptosporidiosis**
◊ One of the most common causes of enteric disease in AIDS patients!
Organism: intracellular parasite Cryptosporidium
Prevalence: 16% (in United States) + up to 48% (in developing countries) in patients with diarrhea
• severe diarrhea with fluid loss of 10–17 L/day
Location: jejunum > other small bowel > stomach > colon
√ Cryptosporidium antritis (= area of focal gastric thickening + ulceration)
√ small bowel dilatation (increased secretions)
√ regular fold thickening + effacement (atrophy, blunting, fusion, loss of villi)
√ "toothpaste" appearance of small bowel (mimicking sprue)
√ dilution of barium (hypersecretion)
√ marked antral narrowing (extensive inflammation)
Dx: microscopic identification in stool / biopsy

2. **Pneumocystosis**
◊ Likely to occur inpatients treated with aerosolized pentamidine!
Organism: eukaryotic microbe Pneumocystis carinii
Prevalence: pulmonary infection in 75% of AIDS patients; in <1% dissemination
Location: liver, spleen, lymph nodes
√ hepatic + splenic + nodal punctate calcifications
√ multiple tiny echogenic foci in spleen
√ multiple low-attenuation lesions of varying size in spleen (foamy eosinophilic material) with subsequently progressive rimlike / punctate calcifications

D. BACTERIAL PATHOGENS

1. **Tuberculosis**
◊ Most common cause of serious HIV-related infection worldwide with tendency to occur earlier than other AIDS-defining opportunistic infections!
Prevalence: 4% (in United States) + 43% (in developing countries) of HIV-infected persons
Infection: swallowing of infected sputum; hematogenous spread from pulmonary focus; direct extension from lymph node
Location: lymph nodes, liver, spleen, peritoneum, GI tract (especially ileum, colon, ileocecal valve)
√ low-attenuation mesenteric lymphadenopathy (suggestive of necrosis)

√ segmental ulceration
√ inflammatory stricture
√ hypertrophic lesion resembling polyp or mass

2. **Mycobacterium avium complex infection**
= PSEUDO-WHIPPLE DISEASE
◊ Most common opportunistic infection of bacterial origin in AIDS patients!
◊ Most common nontuberculous mycobacterial infection in AIDS patients!
Organism: facultative intracellular acid-fast bacillus M. avium / M. intracellulare
Infection: invasion of Peyer patches + adjacent mesenteric lymph nodes
Histo: true granulomas with Langhans giant cells and caseous necrosis are rare because infection occurs in patients with advanced disease and a CD4 cell count of <100/μL
• diarrhea, malabsorption
Location: jejunum (most common)
√ mild dilatation of middle + distal small bowel
√ diffuse irregular mucosal fold thickening and nodularity without ulceration
√ mesenteric + retroperitoneal lymphadenopathy (1.0–1.5 cm in size) with homogeneous soft-tissue attenuation causing segmental separation of small bowel loops
√ hepatosplenomegaly
√ multiple tiny echogenic foci in liver + spleen (occasionally large hypoechoic / low-attenuation lesions)
Dx: (1) visualization of large numbers of intracellular acid-fast bacilli in foamy histiocytes of tissue specimens
(2) tissue culture
DDx: Whipple disease (positive with periodic acid-Schiff stain just like M. avium, but not with acid-fast stain, responsive to tetracyclines)

E. OTHER INFECTIONS

1. **Bacillary angiomatosis**
Organism: Rickettsiales Bartonella henselae
Histo: characteristic pattern of vascular proliferation with bacilli
Location: cutis (mimicking Kaposi sarcoma), liver, spleen, lymph nodes
√ peliosis (blood-filled cystic spaces) of liver / spleen
√ abdominal lymphadenopathy with contrast enhancement

2. **Isospora belli**
◊ Infection resembles cryptosporidiosis
Organism: protozoan pathogen
Histo: oval oocysts within bowel lumen / epithelial cells; localized inflammation; fold atrophy
Location: small intestine
• severe watery diarrhea
√ fold thickening

F. AIDS-ASSOCIATED NEOPLASMS

1. Kaposi sarcoma
2. **Non-Hodgkin lymphoma**
◊ 2nd most common AIDS-associated neoplasm
Prevalence: in 4–10% of AIDS patients (60 times higher risk compared with general population); occurs in all AIDS risk groups
Histo: multiclonal B-cell lymphoma of high or intermediate grade
• at initial presentation widely disseminated disease often with extranodal involvement
Location: CNS, bone marrow, GI tract (stomach, small bowel)
@ Stomach
√ circumferential / focal wall thickening
√ mural mass ± ulceration
@ Small bowel
√ diffuse / focal wall thickening
√ excavated mass
√ solitary / multiple liver lesions

Differential diagnostic considerations:

1. Splenomegaly (31–45%)
Cause: nonspecific (most), lymphoma, infection (M. avium-intracellulare, P. carinii)
2. Lymphadenopathy (21–60%)
Cause: reactive hyperplasia (most), Kaposi sarcoma, lymphoma, infections
Size: <3 cm in diameter (in 95%)
3. Hepatomegaly (20%)
Cause: nonspecific, hepatitis, fatty infiltration, lymphoma, Kaposi sarcoma
4. AIDS-related cholangiopathy:
Organism: CMV, Cryptosporidium
√ papillary stenosis of CBD
√ dilatation of extra- and intrahepatic bile ducts
√ periductal fibrosis
√ strictures + irregularities of bile ducts resembling primary sclerosing cholangitis
√ intraluminal polypoid filling defects
5. AIDS-related esophagitis:
Organism: Candida, herpes simplex, CMV
√ giant esophageal ulcer: HIV (76%), CMV (14%)
√ esophageal fistula / perforation: tuberculosis, actinomycosis
6. Gastritis
Organism: CMV (GE junction + prepyloric antrum), Cryptosporidium (antrum)
7. AIDS enteritis
Organism: Cryptosporidium, M. avium complex
8. AIDS colitis
— ischemic bowel
— acute appendicitis
— neutropenic colitis
— pseudomembranous colitis
— infectious colitis / ileitis
9. Bowel obstruction
(a) infection
(b) intussusception: Kaposi sarcoma, lymphoma

AMEBIASIS

= primary infection of the colon by protozoan Entamoeba histolytica

Countries: worldwide distribution, most common in warm climates; South Africa, Egypt, India, Asia, Central + South America (20%); United States (5%)

Route: contaminated food / water (human cyst carriers); cyst dissolves in small bowel; trophozoites settle in colon; proteolytic enzymes + hyaluronidase lyse intestinal epithelium; may embolize into portal venous + systemic blood system

Histo: amebic invasion of mucosa + submucosa causing tiny ulcers, which spread beneath mucosa + merge into larger areas of necrosis; mucosal sloughing; secondary bacterial infection

- asymptomatic for months / years
- acute attacks of diarrhea (loose mucoid bloodstained stools)
- fever, headache, nausea

Location: (areas of relative stasis) right colon + cecum (90%) > hepatic + splenic flexures > rectosigmoid

√ loss of normal haustral pattern with granular appearance (edema, punctate ulcers)
√ "collarbutton" ulcers
√ cone-shaped cecum
√ several cm long stenosis of bowel lumen in transverse colon, sigmoid colon, flexures (result of healing + fibrosis); in multiple segments
√ ameboma = hyperplastic granuloma with bacterial invasion of amebic abscess; usually annular + constricting / intramural mass / cavity continuous with bowel lumen; shrinkage under therapy in 3–4 weeks
√ ileocecal valve thickened + fixed in open position with reflux
√ involvement of distal ileum (10%)

Dx: stool examination / rectal biopsy

Cx:
(1) Toxic megacolon with perforation
(2) Amebic abscess in liver (2%), brain, lung (transdiaphragmatic spread of infection), pericolic, ischiorectal, subphrenic space
(3) Intussusception in children (due to ameboma)
(4) Fistula formation (colovesical, rectovesical, rectovaginal, enterocolic)

AMYLOIDOSIS

= group of heterogeneous disorders caused by interstitial deposits of a protein-polysaccharide in various organs leading to hypoxia, mucosal edema, hemorrhage, ulceration, mucosal atrophy, muscle atrophy

Histo: amorphous eosinophilic hyaline material deposited around terminal blood vessels, stains with Congo red + crystal violet; amyloid fibrils have β-pleated sheet structure (= β fibrilloses)

Biochemical classification (1979):

1. AL amyloidosis
   (A = amyloidosis, L = light chain immunoglobulin)
   - monoclonal protein in serum + urine
   - occurs in primary amyloidosis + myeloma-associated amyloidosis

   Histo: massive deposits in muscularis mucosae + submucosa

   √ thickening of folds with polyps / large nodules
2. SAA amyloidosis (S = serum, AA = amyloid A)
   - occurs in secondary = reactive amyloidosis

   Histo: expansion of lamina propria

   √ coarse mucosal pattern + innumerable fine granular elevations
3. AF amyloidosis (A = amyloid, F = familial)
   - AF prealbumin as precursor of fibrils
   - occurs in familial amyloidosis
4. AS amyloidosis (A = amyloid, S = senile)
   - AS prealbumin as precursor of fibrils
   - occurs in senile amyloidosis

   √ massive amyloid deposition
5. AH amyloidosis (A = amyloid, H = hemodialysis)
   - β_2 microglobulin as precursor of fibrils
6. AE amyloidosis (A = amyloid, E = endocrine)
   - calcitonin produced by medullary thyroid carcinoma is precursor of fibrils

Reimann classification (1935):

1. Primary = idiopathic amyloidosis
   = probably autosomal dominant inheritance with immunologically determined dysfunction of plasma cells
   - absence of discernible preceding / concurrent disease

   Location: (predominant involvement of connective tissues + mesenchymal organs) heart (90%), lung (30–70%), liver (35%), spleen (40%), kidneys (35%), adrenals, tongue (40%), GI tract (70%), skin + subcutis (25%)

   √ tendency to nodular deposition
2. Secondary amyloidosis (most common form)
   - following / coexistent with prolonged infectious / inflammatory processes

   Cause: rheumatoid arthritis (in 20%), Still disease, tuberculosis, osteomyelitis, leprosy, chronic pyelonephritis, bronchiectasis, ulcerative colitis, Waldenström macroglobulinemia, familial Mediterranean fever, lymphoreticular malignancy, paraplegia

   Location: spleen, liver, kidneys (>80%), breast, tongue, GI tract, connective tissue

   √ small amyloid deposits
3. Amyloidosis associated with multiple myeloma
   - may precede development of multiple myeloma

   Incidence: 10–15%

   √ primary amyloidosis with osteolytic lesions in myelomatous disease
4. Tumor-forming / organ-limited amyloidosis
   - related to primary type

   (a) hereditary = familial amyloidosis
   (b) senile amyloidosis (limited to heart / brain / pancreas / spleen)

   √ large localized masses

GI

◊ GI involvement in primary more common than in secondary amyloidosis!
• malabsorption (diarrhea, protein loss)
• occult GI bleeding
• obstruction
• macroglossia
@ Esophagus (11%)
  √ loss of peristalsis
  √ megaesophagus
@ Stomach (37%)
  • postprandial epigastric pain + heartburn
  • acute erosive hemorrhagic gastritis
  (a) diffuse infiltrative form
    √ small-sized stomach with rigidity + loss of distensibility simulating linitis plastica (from thickening of gastric wall)
    √ effaced rugal pattern
    √ diminished / absent peristalsis
    √ marked retention of food
  (b) localized infiltration (often located in antrum)
    √ irregularly narrowed + rigid antrum
    √ thickened rugae
    √ superficial erosions / ulcerations
  (c) amyloidoma = well-defined submucosal mass
@ Small bowel (74%)
  (a) diffuse form (more common)
    √ diffuse uniform thickening of valvulae conniventes in entire small bowel
    √ broadened flat undulated mucosal folds (mucosal atrophy)
    √ "jejunalization" of ileum
    √ impaired intestinal motility
    √ small bowel dilatation
  (b) localized form (less common)
    √ multiple pea- / marble-sized deposits
    √ pseudoobstruction = physical + plain-film findings suggesting mechanical obstruction with patent large + small bowel on barium examination (involvement of myenteric plexus)
  Cx: small bowel infarction
@ Colon (27%):
  √ pseudopolyps in colon
@ Bone:
  √ bone cysts
@ Spleen:
  Histo: (a) nodular form involving lymph follicles
  (b) diffuse form infiltrating red pulp
  √ discrete masses
  √ splenomegaly (4–13%)
  Cx: spontaneous splenic rupture (from vascular fragility + acquired coagulopathy)
Dx: by rectal / gingival biopsy
DDx: Whipple disease, intestinal lymphangiectasia, lymphosarcoma

ANGIODYSPLASIA OF COLON

= VASCULAR ECTASIA = ARTERIOVENOUS MALFORMATION
Cause: ?; acquired lesion
Associated with: aortic stenosis (20%)
Incidence at autopsy: 2%
Age: majority >55 years
Location: (a) cecum + ascending colon (majority)
(b) descending + sigmoid colon (25%)
• chronic intermittent low-grade bleeding
• occasionally massive bleeding
√ "vascular tufts" = cluster of vessels during arterial phase along antimesenteric border
√ early opacification of ileocolic vein
√ densely opacified dilated tortuous ileocolic vein into late venous phase
√ contrast extravasation (unusual)

ANISAKIASIS

= parasitic disease of GI tract
Cause: ingestion of Anisakis larvae present in raw / undercooked fish (mackerel, cod, pollack, herring, whiting, bonito, squid) consumed as sashimi, sushi, ceviche, lomi-lomi
Organism: worm with straight / serpentine / circular threadlike appearance
◊ Site of penetration by larvae determines clinical form!
@ Gastric anisakiasis
  • acute gastric pain, nausea, vomiting a few hours after ingestion (DDx: acute gastritis, peptic ulcer, food poisoning, neoplasia)
  • eosinophilia
  √ mucosal edema
  √ about 3-cm-long threadlike filling defects (= larvae)
@ Intestinal anisakiasis
  • diffuse abdominal tenderness / colicky abdominal pain, nausea, vomiting (DDx: acute appendicitis, regional enteritis, intussusception, ileus, diverticulitis, neoplasia)
  • leukocytosis without eosinophilia (frequent)
  Histo: marked edema, eosinophilic infiltrates, granuloma formation
  √ thickened folds
  √ disappearance of Kerckring folds
  √ thumbprinting / saw-tooth appearance
  √ irregular luminal narrowing
  √ eosinophilic ascites (DDx: eosinophilic gastroenteritis, hypereosinophilic syndrome)
  Cx: ileus
@ Colonic anisakiasis (rare)
  DDx: colonic tumor

ANORECTAL MALFORMATION

(1) Imperforate anus
(2) Cloacal malformation
(3) Cloacal exstrophy
Embryology:
during weeks 3 and 4 the dorsal part of the yolk sac folds are incorporated into embryo forming the *primitive hindgut* consisting of distal part of transverse + descending + sigmoid colon, rectum, superior portion of anal canal, epithelium of urinary bladder, and most of the urethra; at 4 weeks the transverse *rectovesical septum* descends caudally between allantois and hindgut dividing the *cloaca* into *urogenital sinus*

GI

ventrally + *anorectal canal* dorsally; by 7th week the rectovaginal septum fuses with cloacal membrane creating a *urogenital membrane* ventrally + anal membrane dorsally; perineum is formed by fusion of rectovesical septum + cloacal membrane; *anal membrane* ruptures by 9th week

In 48% associated with: (part of VACTERL syndrome)

(1) GU anomalies (20%): renal agenesis / ectopia, vesicoureteral reflux, obstruction, hypospadia (3.1%); M > F;
(2) Lumbosacral segmentation anomalies (30%): dysplasia, agenesis, hemivertebrae
(3) GI anomalies (11%): esophageal atresia ± tracheoesophageal fistula (4%), duodenal atresia / stenosis
(4) Cardiovascular anomalies (8%)
(5) Abdominal wall (2%)
(6) Cleft lip–cleft palate (1.6%)
(7) Down syndrome (1.5%)
(8) Meningomyelocele (0.5%) + occult myelodysplasia
(9) Others (8%)

Caudal regression syndrome: anorectal atresia, sacral agenesis, renal agenesis / dysplasia, lower limb hypoplasia, sirenomelia

ANTRAL MUCOSAL DIAPHRAGM

= antral web

Age range: 3 months to 80 years

Associated with: gastric ulcer (30–50%)

• symptomatic if opening <1 cm

Location: usually 1.5 cm from pylorus (range 0–7 cm)

√ constant symmetric band of 2–3 mm thickness traversing the antrum perpendicular to long axis of stomach
√ "double bulb" appearance (in profile)
√ concentric / eccentric orifice
√ normal peristaltic activity

APPENDICITIS

Incidence: 7–12% in Western world population

Etiology: obstruction of appendiceal lumen by lymphoid hyperplasia (60%), fecolith (33%), foreign bodies (4%), stricture, tumor, parasite; Crohn disease (in 25%)

Peak age: 2nd–3rd decade

• fever (56%)
• nausea + vomiting (40%)
• RLQ pain over appendix = McBurney sign (72%)
• leukocytosis (88%)

False positive: 7–45% (average 20%)

False negative: 7–33% (average 20%)

◊ 32–45% rate of misdiagnosis in women between ages 20–40!

Atypical location: within pelvis (30%), extraperitoneal (5%)

Abdominal plain film (abnormalities seen in <50%):

◊ Plain-film findings become more distinctive after perforation, while clinical findings subside / simulate other diseases!

√ usually laminated calcified appendicolith in RLQ (in 7–15%)
  ◊ Appendicolith + abdominal pain = 90% probability of acute appendicitis!
  ◊ Appendicolith in acute appendicitis means a high probability for gangrene / perforation!
√ "cecal ileus" = gas-fluid level in cecum in gangrene (= local paralysis)
√ thickening of cecal wall
√ small bowel obstruction pattern = small bowel dilatation with air-fluid levels (in 43% of perforations)
√ colon cutoff sign = amputation of gas at the hepatic flexure (in 20% of perforations) due to spastic ascending colon
√ water-density mass + paucity / absence of intestinal gas in RLQ (in 24% of perforations)
√ extraluminal gas (in 33% of perforations)
  √ gas loculation
  √ mottled bacteriogenic gas
  √ pneumoperitoneum (rare)
√ focal increase in thickness of lateral abdominal wall in 32% (= edema between properitoneal fat line + cecum)
√ loss of properitoneal fat line
√ loss of pelvic fat planes around the bladder / right obturator (= fluid / pus in cul-de-sac)
√ loss of definition of right inferior hepatic outline (= free peritoneal fluid)
√ distortion of psoas margin + flank stripes

BE / UGI (accuracy 50–84%):

√ failure to fill appendix with barium (normal finding in up to 35%)
√ indentation along medial wall of cecum (= edema at base of appendix / matted omentum / periappendiceal abscess)

US (77–94% sensitive, 90% specific, 78–96% accurate; nondiagnostic study in 4% due to inadequate compression of RLQ); useful in ovulating women (false-negative appendectomy rate in males 15%, in females 35%):

√ visualization of noncompressible appendix as a blind-ending tubular aperistaltic structure (seen only in 2% of normal adults, but in 50% of normal children)
√ target appearance of ≥6 mm in total diameter on cross section (81%) / mural wall thickness ≥2 mm
√ diffuse hypoechogenicity (associated with higher frequency of perforation)
√ lumen may be distended with anechoic / hyperechoic material
√ loss of wall layers
√ visualization of appendicolith (6%)
√ localized periappendiceal fluid collection
√ prominent hyperechoic mesoappendix / pericecal fat

Color Doppler US:

√ increased conspicuity (= increase in size + number) of vessels in and around the appendix = hyperemia
√ decreased resistance of arterial waveforms
√ continuous / pulsatile venous flow

CT (87–98% sensitive, 83–97% specific, 93% accurate):

√ abnormal appendix

√ distended lumen
√ circumferentially thickened ± enhancing wall
√ appendicolith = homogeneous / ringlike calcification (25%)
√ periappendicular inflammation
√ linear streaky densities in periappendicular / pericecal / mesenteric / pelvic fat
√ phlegmon = pericecal soft-tissue mass
√ pericecal / mesenteric / pelvic abscess = poorly encapsulated single / multiple fluid collection with air / extravasated contrast material
√ focal cecal apical thickening (80%)
√ "arrowhead" sign = funnel of contrast medium in cecum centering about occluded orifice of appendix

Cx: perforation (13–30%)

DDx: colitis, diverticulitis, epiploic appendagitis, small bowel obstruction, infectious enteritis, duodenal ulcer, pancreatitis, intussusception, Crohn disease, mesenteric lymphadenitis, ovarian torsion, pelvic inflammatory disease

Rx: finding of appendicolith is sufficient evidence to perform prophylactic appendectomy in asymptomatic patients (50% have perforation / abscess formation at surgery)

ASCARIASIS

= most common parasitic infection in world; cosmopolitan occurrence; endemic along Gulf Coast, Ozark Mountains, Nigeria, Southeast Asia

Organism: Ascaris lumbricoides = roundworm parasite, 15–35 cm in length; production of 200,000 eggs daily

Cycle: infection by contaminated soil, eggs hatch in duodenum, larvae penetrate into venules / lymphatics, carried to lungs, migrate to alveoli and up the bronchial tree, swallowed, maturation in jejunum within 2.5 months

Age: children age 1–10 years

• colic
• eosinophilia
• appendicitis
• hematemesis / pneumonitis
• jaundice (if bile ducts infested)

Location: jejunum > ileum (99%), duodenum, stomach, CBD, pancreatic duct

√ 15- to 35-cm-long tubular filling defects
√ barium-filled enteric canal outlined within Ascaris
√ whirled appearance, occasionally in coiled clusters ("bolus of worms")

Cx: (1) Perforation of bowel
(2) Mechanical obstruction

BANNAYAN-RILEY-RUVALCABA SYNDROME

= RUVALCABA-MYHRE-SMITH SYNDROME

Cause: autosomal dominant transmission

• pigmented genital lesions

√ hamartomatous intestinal polyps (in 45%): usually in distal ileum + colon
√ macrocephaly
√ subcutaneous and visceral lipomas + hemangiomas

BARRETT ESOPHAGUS

= BARRETT SYNDROME
= replacement of stratified squamous epithelium by metaplastic columnar epithelium (Barrett epithelium) containing goblet cells

Cause: chronic gastroesophageal reflux with epithelial injury from esophagitis

Contributing factors:
genetic influence, reduced LES pressure, transient LES relaxation, hiatal hernia, delayed acid clearance, reduced acid sensitivity, duodenogastroesophageal reflux, alcohol, tobacco, chemotherapy, scleroderma (37%), S/P repair of esophageal atresia / esophagogastric resection / Heller esophagomyotomy

Histo: (1) specialized columnar epithelium (proximal)
(2) junctional-type epithelium (distal to above)
(3) fundic-type epithelium (most distally)

Incidence: in general 0.3–4%; 7–10–20% of patients with symptoms of reflux

Associated with: moderate + severe esophagitis (94%), no / mild esophagitis (6%)

Age: 0–15 years and 40–88 years (mean of 55 years); M > F; mainly among Whites

• dysphagia (due to esophageal stricture)
• heartburn, substernal chest pain, regurgitation
• low-grade upper intestinal bleeding
• asymptomatic

Location: middle to lower esophagus
N.B.: the squamocolumnar junction does not coincide with the GE junction, is irregular and lies >2–3 cm orad from the gastroesophageal junction

Distribution: circumferential / focal

√ several-cm-long stricture (71%) in midesophagus (40%) or lower esophagus (60%; DDx: peptic stricture without Barrett esophagus)
√ large deep wide-mouthed peptic ulcer (= Barrett ulcer) at upwardly displaced squamocolumnar junction / within columnar epithelium
√ fine reticular mucosal pattern (3–30%) located distally from stricture (DDx: gastroesophageal reflux, monilial + viral esophagitis, superficial spreading carcinoma)
√ thickened irregular mucosal folds (28–86%)
√ fine granular mucosal pattern (DDx: reflux esophagitis, acanthosis, leukoplakia, superficial spreading carcinoma, moniliasis / herpes simplex / CMV esophagitis)
√ gastroesophageal reflux (45–63%)
√ distal esophageal widening (34–66%; due to abnormal motility)
√ hiatal hernia (75–94%)
√ uptake of Tc-99m pertechnetate by columnar epithelium

Dx: velvety pinkish red appearance of gastric-type mucosa extending from gastric mucosa into distal esophagus (endoscopy with biopsy)

Cx: 1. Ulceration ± penetration into mediastinum
2. Stricture

GI

3. Adenocarcinoma (0–10–46%;) 40-fold higher risk than general population
   √ plaquelike / focal irregularity / nodularity / sessile polyps

Rx: (1) stop smoking, avoid bedtime snacks + foods that lower LES pressure, lose excess weight
(2) suppress gastric acidity: antacids, H_2-receptor antagonists (cimetidine, ranitidine, famotidine), H^+K^+-adenosintriphosphatase inhibitor (omeprazole)
(3) improve LES pressure: metoclopramide, bethanechol
(4) esophageal resection in high-grade dysplasia

BEHÇET SYNDROME

= uncommon chronic multisystem inflammatory disorder of unknown etiology with relapsing course characterized by mucocutaneous-ocular symptoms as a triad of aphthous stomatitis, genital ulcers, ocular inflammation

Age at onset: 3rd decade; M:F = 2:1

Major criteria: buccal + genital ulceration, ocular inflammation, skin lesions

Minor criteria: thrombophlebitis, GI + CNS lesions, arthritis, family history

• abdominal pain + diarrhea (50%)

@ Mucocutaneous: aphthous stomatitis, papules, pustules, vesicles, folliculitis, erythema nodosum–like lesions
@ Genital: ulcers on penis + scrotum / vulva + vagina
@ Ocular: relapsing iridocyclitis, hypopyon, choroiditis, papillitis, retinal vasculitis
@ Articular: mild nondestructive arthritis
@ Vascular: migratory thrombophlebitis
@ CNS: chronic meningoencephalitis
@ Esophagus: ulceration, stenosis, perforation
@ Small bowel: ulceration, perforation
@ Colon: multiple discrete deep ulcers in normal mucosa (DDx: granulomatous / ulcerative colitis)

INTESTINAL BEHÇET DISEASE

= presence of intestinal ulcers

Incidence: <1%

Location: terminal ileum, cecum

√ deep round ulcers similar in appearance to peptic ulcers of stomach / duodenum
√ multiple shallow / longitudinal / aphthoid ulcers

Cx: panperitonitis with high mortality due to tendency for perforation at multiple sites

DDx: Reiter syndrome, Steven-Johnson syndrome, SLE, ulcerative colitis, ankylosing spondylitis

BEZOAR

= persistent concretions of foreign matter composed of accumulated ingested material in intestines (from Persian word padzahr = antidote, counterpoison)

Incidence: 0.4% (large endoscopic series)

Etiology: material unable to exit stomach because of large size, indigestibility, gastric outlet obstruction, poor gastric motility (diabetes, mixed connective tissue disease, myotonic dystrophy, hypothyroidism)

Predisposition:
previous gastric surgery (vagotomy, pyloroplasty, antrectomy, partial gastrectomy), inadequate chewing, missing teeth, dentures, massive overindulgence of food with high fiber contents

• anorexia, bloating, early satiety / may be asymptomatic

(a) **Phytobezoar** (55% of all bezoars):
= poorly digested fibers, skin + seeds of fruits and vegetables usually forming in stomach, may become impacted in small bowel
• history of recent ingestion of pulpy foods
Food: oranges, persimmons (most common, unripe persimmons contain the tannin shibuol that forms a gluelike coagulum after contact with dilute acid)
Site of impaction: stomach, jejunum, ileum
√ intraluminal filling defect without constant site of attachment to bowel wall
√ interstices filled with barium
√ coiled-spring appearance (rare)
√ partial / complete obstruction
Cx: decubitus ulceration + pressure necrosis of bowel wall, perforation, peritonitis
DDx: lobulated / villous adenoma, leiomyosarcoma, metastatic melanoma, intussusception

(b) **Trichobezoar** (hair):
80% are < age 30, almost exclusively in females;
Associated with: gastric ulcer in 24–70%

BLUNT ABDOMINAL TRAUMA

CT is imaging method of choice for evaluation of stable patients

Hemoperitoneum

ATTENUATION VALUES OF BLOOD

during IV contrast administration and assuming an initially normal hematocrit without significant dilution from intraperitoneal fluid (ascites, urine, succus, lavage fluid)

— serum (after hematocrit effect) 0–20 HU
— fresh unclotted blood 30– 45 HU
— clotted blood 60–100 HU
— active arterial extravasation >180 HU

Location: paracolic gutters, pelvis

√ "sentinel clot" sign = the highest attenuation value of blood clot marks the anatomic site of visceral injury
√ high-density active arterial extravasation always surrounded by lower-density hematoma
(DDx: extravasated oral contrast is not surrounded by lower-density material)

Hypovolemia

√ "collapsed cava" sign = persistent flattening of IVC (due to decreased venous return)
N.B.: abort CT examination as shock is imminent!

GI

√ small hypodense spleen (decreased enhancement)
√ small aorta + mesenteric arteries (due to intense vasoconstriction)
√ shock nephrogram = lack of renal contrast excretion
√ "shock bowel" = generalized thickening of small bowel folds + increased enhancement + luminal fluid dilatation (due to vasoconstriction of mesenteric vessels)
√ marked enhancement of adrenal gland

Blunt trauma to spleen

◊ The spleen is the most frequently injured solid parenchymal organ within the abdomen!

Cause: blunt trauma (most frequent)

Associated with: rib fractures (in 40%), left renal injury
◊ 20% of patients with left rib fractures have a splenic injury!
◊ 25% of patients with left renal injury have a splenic injury!

CECT (95% accuracy):
√ mottled parenchymal enhancement = contusion
√ hypoattenuating hematoma complete separation of splenic fragments (= fracture)
√ crescentic region of low attenuation compressing normal parenchyma = subcapsular hematoma
√ round hypodense inhomogeneous region ± hyperdense clot = intrasplenic hematoma
√ hypoattenuating line connecting opposing visceral surfaces + perisplenic fluid = splenic laceration
√ multiple lacerations = "shattered spleen"
√ high-attenuation area = contrast extravasation / pseudoaneurysm
√ hemoperitoneum (= disruption of splenic capsule)

Sequelae: splenic pseudocyst (20–30 HU)

Cx: delayed rupture up to 10 days later

Rx: up to 91% of stable patients can be treated conservatively with observation; transcatheter embolization

DDx:
(1) Normal lobulation / splenic cleft (smoothly contoured, medially located)
(2) Adjacent unopacified jejunum simulating splenic tissue
(3) Early differential enhancement of red and white pulp (scan obtained within 20–50 sec)
(4) Perisplenic fluid from ascites / urine / succus / bile / lavage

Blunt trauma to liver (20%)

◊ Second most frequently injured intraabdominal viscus

Associated with: splenic injury in 45%

Location: R > L lobe

Site: perivascular, paralleling right + middle hepatic arteries + posterior branches of right portal vein, avulsion of right hepatic vein from IVC (13%)
◊ Left lobe injury more often associated with damage to duodenum, pancreas, transverse colon

CECT:
√ hypoattenuating hematoma
√ lenticular configuration (= subcapsular hematoma) usually resolving within 6–8 weeks
√ irregular linear branching / round regions of low attenuation = laceration
√ focal / diffuse periportal tracking (in up to 22%) due to dissecting hemorrhage / bile / dilated periportal lymphatics (secondary to elevated central venous pressure / injury to lymphatics)
√ alteration in distribution of vessels + ducts
√ hypodense wedge extending to liver surface = focal hepatic devascularization
√ focal hyperdense (80–350 HU) area = active hemorrhage / pseudoaneurysm
√ hemoperitoneum (inability of liver veins to contract)
√ intrahepatic / subcapsular gas (usually due to necrosis)

Cx: in up to 20%
(1) delayed rupture (rare)
(2) hemobilia
(3) arteriovenous fistula / pseudoaneurysm
(4) biloma ± infection
(5) superinfection of hematoma / devascularized hepatic parenchyma

Rx: conservative treatment in up to 80% in adults + 97% in children; transcatheter embolization

Healing: 1–6–15 months

DDx:
(1) beam-hardening artifact from adjacent ribs / from air-contrast level in stomach
(2) Focal fatty infiltration

Blunt trauma to gallbladder (2%)

Associated with: injury to liver , duodenum
√ pericholecystic fluid (extraperitoneal location of GB)
√ free intraperitoneal fluid

CECT:
√ blurred contour of GB
√ focal thickening / discontinuity of GB wall
√ intraluminal enhancing mucosal flap
√ hyperattenuating blood within GB lumen
√ mass effect on adjacent duodenum
√ collapsed GB = GB rupture
√ focal periportal tracking = GB rupture

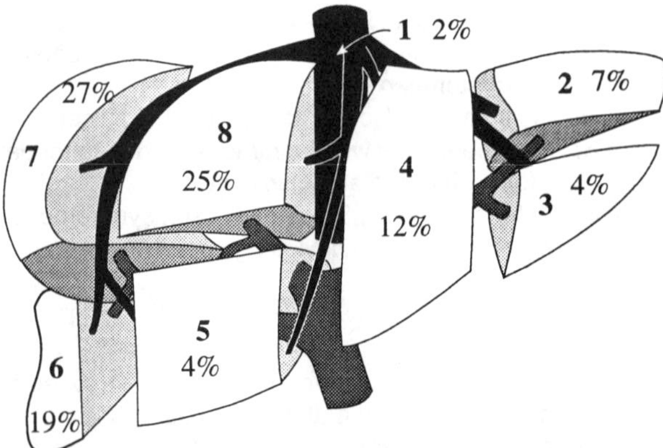

Distribution of Traumatic Hepatic Lesions

US:
- √ focal hypoechoic thickening
- √ echogenic mass within GB lumen

Blunt trauma to GI tract (5%)

Location: jejunum distal to ligament of Treitz > duodenum > ascending colon at ileocecal valve > descending colon

CECT (88–92% sensitive):
- √ hypodense free fluid (85%), particularly in interloop location due to perforation
- √ focal bowel wall thickening > 3 mm = intramural hematoma (75%) ± intestinal obstruction
- √ focal discontinuity of bowel wall
- √ sentinel clot sign adjacent to bowel
- √ streaky hyperattenuating mesentery
- √ mesenteric hematoma (39%)
- √ hyperdense contrast enhancement of injured bowel wall = delayed venous transit time (20%)
- √ pneumoperitoneum (15–32%)
- √ extravasation of oral contrast material + gas

N.B.: clinical signs + symptoms may be delayed for 24 hours (increasing mortality to 65%)

Blunt trauma to pancreas (3%)

Mechanism: compression against vertebral column with shear across pancreatic neck

Associated with: injury to liver, duodenum

Classification:
- I minor contusion / hematoma, capsule + major duct intact
- II parenchymal injury without major duct injury
- III major ductal injury
- IV severe crush injury

Location: junction of body + tail
- √ posttraumatic pancreatitis
  - √ edema / fluid in peripancreatic fat
  - √ focal / diffuse pancreatic enlargement
  - √ irregularity of pancreatic contour
- √ area of low-attenuation laceration (actual site of laceration difficult to visualize)
- √ fluid around superior mesenteric artery
- √ fluid in transverse mesocolon / lesser sac
- √ fluid between pancreas and splenic vein
- √ thickening of anterior pararenal fascia

N.B.: 24–48 hours delayed scans uncover findings not present earlier

Rx: I + II conservative management;
III + IV need surgery within 24 hours

Cx: recurrent pancreatitis, pseudocyst, pseudoaneurysm, fistula, abscess (attendant mortality of 20%)

Blunt trauma to kidney

Incidence: 10% of injuries in emergency room

Cause: motor vehicle accident, contact sports, falls, fights, assaults

Mechanism: direct blow (>80%) often lacerated by lower ribs, acceleration-deceleration (renal artery tear)

Associated with: other organ injury in 20%
- • >95% hematuria
  - ◊ 25% of patients with gross hematuria have significant injuries!
  - ◊ 24% of patients with renal pedicle injury have no hematuria!
  - ◊ Only 1–2% with microhematuria (<35 RBCs per high-power field) have a severe renal injury!

Classification:
- I contusion + corticomedullary laceration (up to 85%)
- II deep laceration generally communicating with collecting system (10%)
- III catastrophic injury: shattered kidney, renal artery pedicle injury (5%)
- IV UPJ avulsion / laceration (rare)

Location: simultaneous upper + lower GU tract injury in <5%
- √ focal patchy areas of decreased enhancement / striated nephrogram = contusion
- √ irregular linear hypodense parenchymal areas = renal laceration
- √ laceration connecting two cortical surfaces = fracture
- √ multiple separated renal fragments ± perfusion = shattered kidney
- √ superficial crescentic hypodense area compressing adjacent parenchyma = subcapsular hematoma
  - ◊ Subcapsular / perinephric hematoma usually proportional to extent of injury
- √ wedge-shaped perfusion defect = segmental arterial injury
- √ diffuse nonperfusion of kidney = devascularized kidney
- √ persistent nephrogram on delayed scans = renal vein thrombosis

N.B.: Delayed images to check for urine leak!

Rx:
1. Blunt trauma I: expectant
2. Blunt trauma II: controversial
3. Blunt trauma III + IV: surgery
4. Penetrating injury (stab wound, gunshot wound): surgery depending on location

Blunt trauma to ureteropelvic junction (rare)

= laceration (60%) / avulsion of ureter at UPJ

Mechanism: tension on renal pedicle by sudden deceleration

Age: usually young boys

Associated with: fracture of transverse process (30%)
- • gross / microscopic hematuria (53–60%)
- √ massive extravasation of contrast material medially in the region of UPJ
- √ nonfilling of affected ureter (with avulsion)
- √ ± circumferential perinephric urinoma

Blunt trauma to bladder

Associated with: pelvic fracture in 70%

Indications for urethrogram:
- • blood at urethral meatus
- • "floating" prostate
- • inability to pass Foley catheter
- √ symphysis diastasis

CT cystogram:
√ focal thickening of bladder wall = contusion
√ contrast extravasation = *see* BLADDER RUPTURE

BOERHAAVE SYNDROME

= complete transmural disruption of esophageal wall with extrusion of gastric content into mediastinum / pleural space secondary to food bolus impaction
- forceful vomiting with sudden onset of pain (substernal, left chest, in neck, pleuritic, abdominal)
- dyspnea
- NO hematemesis (blood escapes outside esophageal lumen)

√ rent of 2–5 cm in length, 2–3 cm above GE junction, predominantly on left posterolateral wall
√ pleural effusion on left >> right side / hydropneumothorax
√ pneumomediastinum (single most important plain-film finding), pneumopericardium, subcutaneous air
√ "V-sign of Naclerio" = localized mediastinal emphysema with air between lower thoracic aorta + diaphragm
√ mediastinal widening
√ air-fluid level within mediastinum
√ extravasation of contrast medium into mediastinum / pleura

BRUNNER GLAND HYPERPLASIA

Etiology: hyperplasia secondary to hyperacidity
Physiology: secrete a clear viscous alkaline substance into crypts of Lieberkühn
MORPHOLOGIC TYPES:
1. Diffuse nodular hyperplasia
2. Circumscribed nodular hyperplasia: in suprapapillary portion
3. Single adenomatous hyperplastic polyp: in duodenal bulb

Location: duodenal glands begin in vicinity of pylorus extending distally within proximal 2/3 of duodenum
√ multiple nodular filling defects (usually limited to 1st portion of duodenum
√ "cobblestoning" (most common finding)
√ occasionally single large mass ± central ulceration

BURKITT LYMPHOMA

= most common type of non-Hodgkin lymphoma in children; initially described in Africa
Etiology: tumor from undifferentiated B-cell–derived lymphocytes; associated with Epstein-Barr virus
Age: children + young adults
Path: resemblance to Hodgkin disease
Histo: characteristic "starry sky" pattern
Location: mandible (first), maxilla; multifocal (10%)
- jaw mass
- abdominal mass
- paraplegia
- NO peripheral leukemia

√ usually intraabdominal extranodal involvement with sparing of spleen

A. ENDEMIC FORM OF BURKITT LYMPHOMA
endemic in areas with malaria: tropical Africa, New Guinea
50% of all childhood cancers in central Africa
Age: 6–8 years
@ Mandible / maxilla
√ grossly destructive lesion, spicules of bone growing at right angles
√ large soft-tissue mass
@ Other skeleton
√ reminiscent of Ewing tumor / reticulum cell sarcoma
√ lamellated periosteal reaction around major long bones

B. NONENDEMIC FORM OF BURKITT LYMPHOMA
Age: 10–12 years
Location: abdominal involvement (69%): tumors of small bowel (terminal ileum), mesentery, retroperitoneum, ovary, uterus, salivary glands, thyroid, kidneys, bone marrow
√ well-defined sharply marginated homogeneous tumors (75%)
√ ascites (13%)
√ renal masses / enlargement (5%)
√ hydronephrosis (28%)
√ conspicuous absence of lymph node disease
√ pleural effusion (most common chest abnormality)
Rx: dramatic response to chemotherapy
Prognosis: long-term survival in 50%

CARCINOID

= most common primary tumor of small bowel + appendix (>95% of all carcinoids); belongs to APUDomas; M:F = 2:1
Path: firm yellow submucosal nodule arising from argentophil Kulchitsky cells in the crypts of Lieberkühn (= argentaffinoma); invasion into mesentery incites an intense fibrotic reaction
Histo: low-grade malignancy = resemble adenocarcinomas but do not have their aggressive behavior; malignant through invasion of muscularis
Biochemistry:
tumor elaborates (1) ACTH (2) histamine (3) bradykinin (4) kallikrein (5) serotonin = 5-hydroxytryptamine (from tryptophan over 5-hydroxytryptophan), which is metabolized in liver by monamine oxidase into 5-hydroxyindole acetic acid (5-HIAA) and excreted in urine; 5-hydroxytryptophan is destroyed in pulmonary circulation
- asymptomatic (66%)
- pain / obstruction (19%)
- weight loss (16%)
- palpable mass (14%)

- **Carcinoid syndrome** (7% of small bowel carcinoids) caused by excess serotonin levels, requires that serotonin metabolism (to 5-HIAA in liver) is bypassed

(a) with liver metastases
(b) with primary pulmonary / ovarian carcinoids
- recurrent diarrhea (70%)
- right-sided endocardial fibroelastosis (35%) resulting in tricuspid regurgitation + pulmonary valve stenosis + right heart failure
- attacks precipitated by ingestion of food / alcohol
- asthmatic wheezing from bronchospasm (15%)
- desquamative skin lesions (5%)
- nausea & vomiting, fever
- hypotension
- cutaneous flushing (rare)

Metastases:
to lymph nodes, liver (in 90% of patients with carcinoid syndrome), lung, bone (osteoblastic)
(a) incidence versus tumor size

tumor of <1 cm	(in 75%)	metastasizes in	2%
tumor of 1–2 cm	(in 20%)	metastasizes in	50%
tumor of >2 cm	(in 5%)	metastasizes in	85%

(b) incidence versus location

tumor in ileum	(in 28%)	metastasizes in	35%
tumor in appendix	(in 46%)	metastasizes in	3%
tumor in rectum	(in 17%)	metastasizes in	1%

Liver metastases seen:	best /	(only) on:
(a) NECT	35%	(3%)
(b) CECT in HAP	35%	(14%)
(c) CECT in PVP	30%	(3%)

HAP = hepatic arterial-dominant phase of triple phase CT
PVP = portal venous-dominant phase of triple phase CT

RULE OF 1/3:
◊ 1/3 occur in small bowel
◊ 1/3 have metastases
◊ 1/3 are multiple
◊ 1/3 have a second malignancy

Location: between gastric cardia and anus
@ Appendix (30–45%)
commonly benign; surgical incidence of 0.03–0.7%
Site: tip (70%), middle (20%), base (10%) of appendix
@ Small bowel (25–35%)
Location: ileum (91%); jejunum (7%), duodenum (2%); multiple in 15–35%
@ Rectum (10–15%): metastasize in 10%
@ Colon (5%): ascending colon, often malignant
@ Stomach (rare)
@ Other organs (5%): bronchus, thyroid, pancreas, biliary tract, teratomas (ovarian, sacrococcygeal, testicular)
@ may be multicentric

UGI:
√ small smooth submucosal mass (usually <2 cm) impinging eccentrically on lumen
√ angulation + kinking of loops leading to obstruction (DIAGNOSTIC)
√ spiculated / tethered appearance of mucosal folds (desmoplastic reaction)
√ separation of loops due to large mesenteric metastases

CT:
√ stellate radiating pattern + beading of mesenteric neurovascular bundles (desmoplastic reaction)
√ retraction + shortening of mesentery
√ displacement + kinking + separation of adjacent bowel loops
√ segmental thickening of adjacent bowel loops (encasement of mesenteric vessels leads to chronic ischemia)
√ calcification of mesenteric mass
√ low-density lymphadenopathy (due to necrosis)
√ liver metastases may become isodense following slow contrast infusion

Angio:
√ thickening + foreshortening of mesenteric vessels
√ kinking of small- and medium-sized vessels with stellate configuration
√ venous occlusion / mesenteric varices
√ encasement of medium-sized vessels
√ simulated hypervascularity secondary to fibrotic retraction of mesenteric vessels

NUC (I-123 MIBG imaging):
√ uptake in 44–63% (higher frequency of radiotracer uptake in midgut carcinoids + with elevated serotonin levels)

US:
√ persistent fluid-distended appendix without typical signs of appendicitis

Cx: second primary malignant neoplasm in other location (36% at necropsy)
Rx: Somatostatin / SMS 201-995
DDx: oat-cell carcinoma, pancreatic carcinoma, medullary thyroid carcinoma, retractile mesenteritis, desmoplastic carcinoma / lymphoma

CATHARTIC COLON

= prolonged use of stimulant-irritant cathartics (>15 years) resulting in neuromuscular incoordination from chronically increased muscular activity + tonus

Agents: castor oil, senna, phenolphthalein, cascara, podophyllum, aloin
Location: involvement of colon proximal to splenic flexure
√ effaced mucosa with flattened smooth surface
√ diminished / absent haustrations
√ "pseudostrictures" = smoothly tapered areas of narrowing are typical (sustained tonus of circular muscles)
√ poor evacuation of barium
√ flattened + gaping ileocecal valve
√ shortened but distensible ascending colon
DDx: "burned-out" ulcerative colitis with right-sided predominance (very similar)

CHAGAS DISEASE

= damage of ganglion cells by neurotoxin liberated from protozoa Trypanosoma cruzi resulting in aperistalsis of GI tract + dilatation

Endemic to Central + South America (esp. eastern Brazil)
Histo: decreased number of cells in medullary dorsal motor nucleus + Wallerian degeneration of vagus + decrease / loss of argyrophilic cells in myenteric plexus of Auerbach

Peak age: 30–50 years; M:F = 1:1
• intermittent / persistent dysphagia
• odynophagia (= fear of swallowing)
• foul breath, regurgitation, aspiration
• Mecholyl test: abnormal response indicative of deficient innervation; 2.5–10 mg methacholine subcutaneously followed by severe tetanic nonperistaltic contraction 2–5 minutes after injection, commonly in distal half of esophagus, accompanied by severe pain
@ Dilatative cardiomyopathy (myocarditis)
@ Megacolon (bowels move at intervals of 8 days to 5 months)
Cx: impacted feces, sigmoid volvulus
@ Esophagus: changes as in achalasia

CHALASIA

= continuously relaxed sphincter with free reflux in the absence of a sliding hernia
Etiology: elevated submerged segment
Causes: (1) Delayed development of esophagogastric region in newborns
(2) Scleroderma, Raynaud disease
(3) S/P forceful dilatation / myotomy for achalasia
√ free / easily induced reflux

CHRONIC IDIOPATHIC INTESTINAL PSEUDOOBSTRUCTION

= nonpropulsive intestine characterized by impaired response to intestinal dilatation without definable cause; ? autosomal dominant
Age: all ages, M:F = 1:1
• recurrent attacks of abdominal distension, periumbilical pain, nausea, vomiting, constipation
√ mild to marked gaseous distension of duodenum + proximal small bowel
√ esophageal dilation + hypoperistalsis (lower third)
√ excessive duodenal dilation (DDx: megaduodenum, superior mesenteric artery syndrome)
√ ligament of Treitz may be placed lower than usual
√ delayed transit of barium through affected segments
√ disordered motor activity (fluoroscopy)

COLITIS CYSTICA PROFUNDA

= rare benign condition characterized by submucosal mucus-containing cysts lined by normal colonic epithelium
Etiology: probably related to chronic inflammation
Age: primarily disease of young adults
• brief periods of bright red rectal bleeding
• mucous / bloody discharge
• intermittent diarrhea
Location: (a) localized to rectum (most commonly) / sigmoid
(b) generalized colonic process (less common)
√ nodular polypoid / cauliflower-like lesions <2 cm in size, containing no gas
√ spiculations mimicking ulcers (barium-filled clefts between nodules)
DDx: pneumatosis (rarely affects rectum)

COLORECTAL CARCINOMA

Most common cancer of GI tract; 2nd most frequently diagnosed malignancy; 2nd most common cause of death from malignancy after lung cancer (in men) + breast cancer (in women)
Predisposed: socioeconomic status; diet low in fiber + high in fat and animal protein; obesity (in men); asbestos worker
Syndromes (6% of colorectal carcinomas):
familial adenomatous polyposis syndrome (= familial polyposis, Gardner syndrome, Turcot syndrome), Peutz-Jeghers syndrome, hereditary nonpolyposis colon cancer syndrome

Risk factors:
1. Colonic adenoma
— malignancy in 5% of tubular adenomas
— malignancy in 40% of villous adenomas
Proof of adenoma-carcinoma sequence:
(a) frequent coexistence of adenoma + carcinoma
(b) similar distribution within colon
(c) consistent proportional prevalence in population having varied magnitudes of colon cancer risk
(d) increased frequency of carcinoma in patients with adenomas
(e) reduction of cancer incidence following endoscopic removal of polyps
(f) all patients with familial adenomatous polyposis syndrome develop colon carcinoma if colon not removed
(g) similarity of DNA + chromosomal constitution
◊ 93% of colorectal carcinomas arise from adenomatous polyp!
◊ A patient with one adenoma has a 9% chance of having a colorectal carcinoma in next 15 years!
◊ It takes about 7 years for a 1-cm adenoma to become an invasive cancer!
◊ 5% of adenomas 5 mm in size develop into invasive cancers (5 mm is considered critical mass of intraepithelial neoplasia)!
2. Dysplasia of colon within flat mucosa
3. Family history of benign / malignant colorectal tumors, 3–5 x risk in first-degree relatives
4. Chronic ulcerative colitis (3–5% incidence; cumulative incidence of 26% after 25 years of colitic symptoms)
5. Prominent lymphoid follicular pattern
6. History of endometrial / breast cancer
7. Crohn disease (particularly in bypassed loops / in vicinity of chronic fistula)
8. Pelvic irradiation
9. Ureterosigmoidostomy

Screening recommendations:
as / more effective than mammographic screening
(a) for persons >50 years of age: annual fecal occult-blood test + sigmoidoscopy / BE every 3 to 5 years
(b) for first-degree relatives of patients with colon cancer screening should start at age 40

Incidence: 15% of all newly diagnosed cancers; 13% of all cancer deaths; 156,000 new cases/year with 61,300 deaths; 6.5% lifetime probability of any White person to develop colorectal cancer; 3/100,000 in 30- to 34-year-olds; 532/100,000 for >85-year-olds

Age: median age of 71 years for colon cancer; median age of 69 years for rectal cancer; M:F = 3:2

Histo: (1) Adenocarcinoma with varied degrees of differentiation
(2) Mucinous carcinoma (uncommon)
(3) Squamous cell carcinoma + adenoacanthoma (rare)

Staging (modified Dukes = Astler-Coller classification):

- A limited to mucosa
- B involvement of muscularis propria
  - B_1 extension into muscularis propria
  - B_2 extension through muscularis propria into serosa / mesenteric fat (35%)
- C lymph node metastases (50%)
  - C_1 + growth limited to bowel wall
  - C_2 + growth extending into adipose tissue
- D distant metastases

Staging (UICC-AJCC Colorectal Cancer Staging System):

Stage	Grouping			5-year survival
0	Tis	N0	M0	>95%
I	T1	N0	M0	
	T2	N0	M0	75–100%
II	T3	N0	M0	
	T4	N0	M0	50–75%
III	any T	N1	M0	
	any T	N2,3	M0	30–50%
IV	any T	any N	M1	<10%

Legend:
- Tis carcinoma in situ
- T1 invasion of submucosa
- T2 invasion of muscularis propria
- T3 invasion of subserosa / pericolic tissue
- T4 invasion of other organs
- N1 1 to 3 pericolic Lnn
- N2 >4 pericolic Lnn
- N3 any Lnn along course of a vascular trunk

Metastases (lymphatic / hematogenous venous):
1. liver (75%; 15–20% at time of surgery)
2. retroperitoneal + mesenteric nodes (10–15%)
3. adrenal (10–14%)
4. lung (5–50%)
5. ovary (3–8%)
6. psoas muscle tumor deposit
7. malignant ascites
8. bone (5%)
9. brain (5%)

◊ Because of absence of lymphatics in lamina propria colon cancer will not metastasize until it penetrates the muscularis mucosa!

- rectal bleeding, iron deficiency anemia
- change in caliber of stools
- obstruction (poor prognostic indicator)
- hydronephrosis (13%)
- positive fecal occult blood testing (2–6% positive-result rate ; 5–10% positive predictive value; fails to detect 30 –50% of colorectal carcinomas + up to 75% of adenomas): Hemoccult (hematein), Hemoquant (porphyrins), Haemselect (hemoglobin)
- progressive elevation of carcinoembryonic antigen (CEA) >10 μg/L indicative of recurrent / metastatic disease

Location: rectum (15–33 –41%), sigmoid (20–37%), descending colon (10–11%), transverse colon (12%), ascending colon (8–16%), cecum (8–10%); "aging gut" = number of right-sided lesions increasing with age

Colonoscopy: cecum not visualized in 10–36%; fails to detect 12% of colonic polyps (10% in areas never reached by colonoscope)
Cx: perforation in 0.2% (0.02% for BE); death in 1:5,000 (1:50,000 for BE)

BE (sensitivities for polyps >1 cm: single contrast 77–94%, double contrast 82–98%; for polyps <1 cm: single contrast 18–72%, double contrast 61–83%):
√ fungating polypoid carcinoma;
- chronic bleeding, intussusception

√ annular ulcerating carcinoma = "applecore lesion";
= annular constriction is a result of tumor growing along the lymphatic channels which parallel the circular muscle fibers of the inner layer of the muscularis propria; longitudinal growth is limited with abrupt transition to normal mucosa
- colonic obstruction

√ "saddle lesion" = growth characteristics between polypoid mass + annular constricting lesion
√ scirrhous carcinoma = rare variant of diffusely infiltrating adenocarcinoma (signet-ring type); often seen in ulcerative colitis
= circumferential + longitudinal tumor spread within the loose submucosal tissue between muscularis mucosa + muscularis propria
- long-segment stricture similar to linitis plastica

√ curvilinear / mottled calcifications (rare) are CHARACTERISTIC of mucinous adenocarcinoma

CT: staging accuracy of 48–90%, for lymph node metastases of 25–73%
CT staging (poor accuracy compared with modified Duke classification):
- Stage 1 intramural polypoid mass
- Stage 2 thickening of bowel wall
- Stage 3 slight invasion of surrounding tissues
- Stage 4 massive invasion of surrounding tissue + adjacent organs / distant metastases

√ low-density mass + low-density lymph nodes in mucinous adenocarcinoma (= >50% of tumor composed of extracellular mucin)
√ psammomatous calcifications in mucinous adenocarcinoma

√ signs of Lnn involvement: single lymph node >1 cm in diameter / cluster of ≥3 nodes <1 cm / node of any size within mesentery

MR (staging accuracy of 73%, 40% sensitivity for lymph node metastases)

Prognosis:

Survival rate of 40–50% overall in 5 years (unchanged over past 40 years); 80–90% with Duke A; 70% with Duke B; 33% with Duke C; 5% with Duke D

Recurrence in 1/3 of patients:
(a) local recurrence at line of anastomosis (60%) within 1 year after resection in 50%, within 2 years after resection in 70–80%
(b) distant metastases (26%)
(c) local recurrence + metastases (14%)

Risk after detection of colon cancer:
of 5% for synchronous colon cancer
of 14% for synchronous cancer with "sentinel polyp"
of 35% for additional adenomatous polyp
of 3% for metachronous colon cancer
of 4% for extracolonic malignancy

Cx: (1) Obstruction (frequently in descending + sigmoid colon)
(2) Perforation
(3) Intussusception
(4) Pneumatosis cystoides intestinalis
(5) Pseudomyxoma peritonei (from low-grade adenocarcinoma of colon)

DDx: (1) Prolapsing ileocecal valve (change on palpation)
(2) Spasm (intact mucosa, released by propantheline bromide)
(3) Diverticulitis

Lynch Syndrome

= HEREDITARY NONPOLYPOSIS COLORECTAL CANCER SYNDROME
= families with high incidence of colorectal cancers + increased incidence of synchronous and metachronous colorectal cancers

A. Lynch I = no associated extracolonic cancer
B. Lynch II = associated with extracolonic malignancy: transitional cell carcinoma of ureter + renal pelvis, adenocarcinoma of endometrium, stomach, small bowel, pancreas, biliary tract, brain, hematologic malignancy, carcinoma of skin + larynx

Etiology: autosomal dominant abnormality of chromosome 2 with defect in DNA replication-repair process
(a) accelerated adenoma-carcinoma sequence
(b) dysplasia in flat mucosa of colon

Prevalence: 5–10% of patients with colon cancer; 5 times more common than familial adenomatous polyposis syndrome

Mean age: 45 years

Location: 70% proximal to splenic flexure

Prognosis: better stage for stage than in other cancers (5-year survival rate of 65% versus 44% in sporadic cases)

Surveillance: colonoscopy every 1–2 years from ages 22–35 years

Rectal Cancer

Incidence: 45,000 rectal cancers/year in United States

Pathologic staging of rectal cancer:

Astler-Coller/TNM		Description	5-year survival
A	T1,N0,M0	limited to submucosa	80%
B1	T2,N0,M0	limited to muscularis propria	70%
B2	T3,N0,M0	transmural extension	60–65%
C1	T2,N1,M0	nodes (+), into muscularis	35–45%
C2	T3,N1,M0	nodes (+), transmural	25%
	T4	invasion of adjacent organs	
D	M1	distant metastasis	<25%

Risk of recurrence:
5% for T1
10% for T2 33% for T1,N1 + T2N1
25% for T3 66% for T3N1
50% for T4

Staging accuracy:
(1) Digital rectal examination: 68–75–83%; limited to lesions within 10 cm of anal verge
(2) CT: 48–72–92%, better for more extensive regional spread; 25–73% for lymph node involvement
(3) MR: 74–84–93% with tendency for overstaging
(4) Transrectal ultrasound: 64–77–94% with tendency for overstaging; limited to lesions <14 cm from anal verge + nonstenotic lesions; 50–83% sensitivity for lymph node involvement

Transrectal US (81% accuracy):

Normal layers: (a) hyperechoic interface of balloon + mucosa (b) hypoechoic mucosa + muscularis mucosa (c) hyperechoic submucosa (d) hypoechoic muscularis propria (e) hyperechoic serosa

√ hypoechoic mass disrupting rectal wall
  √ no interruption of hyperechoic submucosa = tumor confined to mucosa + submucosa
  √ no interruption of hyperechoic serosa = tumor confined to rectal wall
  √ break in outermost hyperechoic layer = tumor penetrates into perirectal fat
  √ irregular serrated outer border of muscularis propria (pseudopodia through serosa)

√ hypoechoic perirectal lymph nodes (= tumor involvement)

COLONIC VOLVULUS

= most common form of volvulus

A. VOLVULUS OF CECUM
Associated with: malrotation + long mesentery
Age peak: 20–40 years; M > F
√ "kidney-shaped" distended cecum, usually positioned in LUQ
√ tapered end of barium column points toward torsion

B. VOLVULUS OF SIGMOID
= sigmoid twists on mesenteric axis
Usually in elderly / psychiatrically disturbed
Degree of torsion: 360° (50%), 180° (35%), 540° (10%)

√ greatly distended paralyzed loop with fluid-fluid levels, mainly on left side, extending toward diaphragm (erect film)
√ "coffee-bean sign" = distinct midline crease corresponding to mesenteric root in largely gas-distended loop (supine)
√ "bird-of-prey sign" = tapered hooklike end of barium column

CT:
√ "whirl sign" = tightly torsioned mesentery formed by twisted afferent + efferent loop

CONGENITAL INTESTINAL ATRESIA

Incidence: 1:300 livebirths
Cause: usually sporadic vascular accidents (primary / secondary to volvulus or gastroschisis)
Location: jejunum + ileum (70%), duodenum (25%), colon (5%); may involve multiple sites
√ "triple bubble sign" = intraluminal gas in stomach + duodenal bulb + proximal jejunum as pathognomonic sign for jejunal atresia
√ bulbous bowel segment sign = dilated loop of bowel just proximal to site of atresia (due to prolonged impaction of intestinal contents) with curvilinear termination
√ gasless lower abdomen (gut usually air-filled by 4 hours after birth)
√ meconium peritonitis (6%)
√ polyhydramnios (in 50% with duodenal / proximal jejunal atresia; rarely in ileal / colonic atresia)
Prognosis: 88% survival for isolated atresia

CRICOPHARYNGEAL ACHALASIA

= hypertrophy of cricopharyngeus muscle (= upper esophageal sphincter) with failure of complete relaxation
Etiology:
1. Normal variant without symptoms: seen in 5–10% of adults
2. Compensatory mechanism to gastroesophageal reflux
3. Neuromuscular dysfunction of deglutition
   (a) primary neural disorders:
   brainstem disorder (bulbar poliomyelitis, syringomyelia, multiple sclerosis, amyotrophic lateral sclerosis); central / peripheral nerve palsy; cerebrovascular occlusive disease; Huntington chorea
   (b) primary muscle disorder:
   myotonic dystrophy; polymyositis; dermatomyositis; sarcoidosis; myopathies secondary to steroids / thyroid dysfunction; oculopharyngeal myopathy
   (c) myoneural junction disorder:
   myasthenia gravis; diphtheria; tetanus

- mostly asymptomatic
- dysphagia

◊ Cineradiography / videotape recording required for demonstration!
√ distension of proximal esophagus + pharynx
√ smoothly outlined shelf- / liplike projection posteriorly at level of cricoid (= pharyngoesophageal junction) = level of C5/6
√ barium may overflow into larynx + trachea
Cx: Zenker diverticula
Rx: cricopharyngeal myotomy

COWDEN DISEASE

= MULTIPLE HAMARTOMA SYNDROME
= autosomal dominant disease with high penetrance characterized by multiple hamartomas + neoplasms of endodermal, ectodermal, mesodermal origin
Incidence: 160 cases reported
Age: 2nd decade
@ Mucocutaneous tumors
- facial papules
- oral papillomas (lips, gingiva, tongue)
- palmoplantar keratosis, acral keratosis

@ Breast lesions (in 50%):
√ fibrocystic disease + fibroadenomas
√ breast cancer (20–30%): often bilateral + ductal
@ GI tract
√ multiple hamartomatous polyps (in 30–60%, commonly in rectosigmoid)
@ Thyroid abnormalities (in 60–70%):
√ adenomas + goiter
√ follicular thyroid adenocarcinoma (3–4%)
@ Genitourinary lesions
@ Skeletal abnormalities

CROHN DISEASE

= REGIONAL ENTERITIS = disease of unknown etiology with prolonged + unpredictable course characterized by discontinuous + asymmetric involvement of entire GI tract
Prevalence: 2–3:100,000 white adults
Path: transmural inflammation (noncaseating granuloma with Langhans giant cells and epitheloid cells, edema, fibrosis); obstructive lymphedema + enlargement of submucosal lymphoid follicles; ulceration of mucosa overlying lymphoid follicles
Age: onset between 15–30 years; M:F = 1:1
- recurrent episodes of diarrhea
- colicky / steady abdominal pain
- low-grade fever
- weight loss, anorexia
- occult blood + anemia
- perianal abscess / fistula (40%)
- malabsorption (30%)

Associated with: erythema nodosum, pyoderma gangrenosum

INTESTINAL MANIFESTATIONS
@ Esophagus (rare)
@ Stomach (1–2%) = granulomatous gastritis
√ pseudo–post Billroth-I appearance
√ "rams horn sign" = poorly distensible smooth tubular narrowed antrum + widened pylorus + narrow duodenal bulb

GI

√ aphthous ulcers (= pinpoint erosions)
√ cobblestone mucosa
√ antral-duodenal fistula

@ Duodenum (4–10%)
almost always associated with gastric involvement
Location: duodenal bulb + proximal half of duodenum
√ superficial erosions / aphthoid ulcers (early lesion)
√ thickened duodenal folds

@ Small bowel (80%) = regional enteritis
terminal ileum (alone / in combination in 95%); jejunum / ileum (15–55%)
√ thickening + slight nodularity of circular folds
√ aphthous ulcers
√ cobblestone mucosa / ulceration
√ commonly associated with medial cecal defect

@ Colon (22–55%) = granulomatous colitis
particularly on right side with rectum + sigmoid frequently spared
√ tiny 1- to 2-mm nodular filling defects (lymphoid follicular pattern)
√ aphthous ulcers with "target / bull's-eye" appearance
√ "transverse stripe sign" = 1-cm-long straight stripes representing contrast medium within deep grooves of coarse mucosal folds
√ long fistulous tracts parallel to bowel lumen

@ Appendicitis (20%)

@ Rectum (14–50%)
√ deep / collarbutton ulcers
√ rectal sinus tracts

Phases:

(a) Earliest changes
√ nodular enlargement of lymphoid follicles
√ blunting / flattening / distortion / straightening / thickening of valvulae conniventes (obstructive lymphedema, usually first seen in terminal ileum)
√ aphthous ulcers = nodules with shallow central barium collection up to 5 mm in diameter
Location: duodenal bulb, second portion of duodenum, terminal ileum

(b) Advanced nonstenotic phase
√ skip lesions (90%) = discontinuous involvement with intervening normal areas
√ cobblestone appearance = serpiginous longitudinal + transverse ulcers separated by areas of edema
√ thick + blunted small bowel folds (inflammatory infiltration of lamina propria + submucosa)
√ straightening + rigidity of small bowel loops with luminal narrowing (spasm + submucosal edema)
√ separation + displacement of small bowel loops (from lymphedematous wall thickening / increase in mesenteric fat / enlarged mesenteric lymph nodes / perforation with abscess formation)
√ pseudopolyps = islands of hyperplastic mucosa between denuded mucosa
√ inflammatory polypoid masses
√ sessile / pedunculated / filiform postinflammatory polyps
√ diffuse mucosal granularity due to 0.5- to 1-mm round lucencies (= blunted + fused villi seen en face)
√ pseudodiverticula = pseudosacculations = bulging area of normal wall opposite affected scarred wall on antimesenteric side

(c) Stenotic phase
√ "string sign" = strictures (in 21%, most frequently in terminal ileum) / marked narrowing of rigid loops
√ normal proximal loops may be dilated with stasis ulcers + fecoliths

CT:
√ homogeneous density of thickened bowel wall (DDx: ulcerative colitis with inhomogeneous attenuation)
√ "double halo configuration" (50%) = intestinal lumen surrounded by inner ring of low attenuation (= edematous mucosa) + outer ring of soft-tissue density (= thickened fibrotic muscularis + serosa) (DDx: radiation enteritis, ischemia, mesenteric venous thrombosis, acute pancreatitis)
√ luminal narrowing + proximal dilatation
√ skip areas of asymmetric bowel wall thickening of 10–20 mm in 82% (DDx: ulcerative colitis with a mean thickness of 8 mm)
√ "creeping fat" = massive proliferation of mesenteric fat (40%) with mass effect separating small bowel loops
√ mesenteric adenopathy (18%)
√ abscess (DDx: postoperative blind loop)

US:
√ "pseudokidney" / target sign = thickening of bowel wall (22–65–89%) of 5–20 mm (DDx: ulcerative colitis)
√ circumferential diffusely hypoechoic bowel wall with loss of normal layering (due to transmural edema, inflammation, fibrosis)
√ rigid + noncompressible bowel segment with reduction / loss of peristalsis
√ hyperemia of gut wall + adjacent fat on color Doppler
√ inflammatory mass = phlegmon (14%), abscess (4%)
√ distended fluid-filled loops (12%)
√ hypoechoic fistulous tract

Prognosis: recurrence rate of up to 39% after resection (commonly at the site of the new terminal ileum, most frequently during first 2 years after resection); mortality rate of 7% at 5 years, 12% at 10 years after 1st resection

Cx: (1) Fistula (33%):
(a) enterocolic:
most frequently between ileum and cecum
(b) enterocutaneous (8–21%):
rectum-to-skin; rectum-to-vagina
(c) perineal fistula + sinus tracts
◊ Crohn disease is 3rd most common cause of fistula / sinus tracts (*DDx:* iatrogenic [most common cause], diverticula [2nd most common cause])!
(2) Intramural sinus tracts
(3) Abscess (DDx: acute appendicitis)
(4) Free perforation (1–2%)

(5) Toxic megacolon
(6) Small bowel obstruction (15%)
(7) Hydronephrosis (from ureteric compression, generally on right side)
(8) Adenocarcinoma in ileum / colon (particularly in bypassed loops / in vicinity of chronic fistula)
◊ 4–20 x increased risk of colonic adenocarcinoma compared with general population with a latency period of 25–30 years!
(9) Lymphoma in large + small bowel

DDx: (1) Yersinia (in terminal ileum, resolution within 3–4 months)
(2) Tuberculosis (more severe involvement of cecum, pulmonary TB)
(3) Actinomycosis, histoplasmosis, blastomycosis, anisakiasis
(4) Segmental infarction (acute onset, elderly patient)
(5) Radiation ileitis (appropriate history)
(6) Lymphoma (no spasm, luminal narrowing is uncommon, tumor nodules)
(7) Carcinoid tumor (tumor nodules)
(8) Eosinophilic gastroenteritis
(9) Potassium stricture

EXTRAINTESTINAL MANIFESTATIONS

@ Hepatobiliary
1. Fatty infiltration of liver (steroid therapy, hyperalimentation)
2. Hepatic abscess
3. Gallstones (28–34%)
3–5 x higher risk than expected; stone formation caused by interrupted enterohepatic circulation with malabsorption of bile salts in terminal ileum; risk correlates with length of diseased ileum / resected ileum / duration of disease
4. Acute cholecystitis
5. Sclerosing cholangitis (10%) + hepatoma
6. Bile duct + gallbladder carcinoma

@ Genitourinary
1. Urolithiasis: oxalate (frequent) / urate stones
2. Hydronephrosis
3. Renal amyloidosis
4. Focal cystitis
5. Ileoureteral / ileovesical fistula (5–20%)

@ Musculoskeletal
• digital clubbing (11–40%)
• mild self-limiting seronegative peripheral migratory arthritis (15–22%): may precede bowel disease in 10%; severity + course correlates well with severity of intestinal disease; resection of diseased bowel leads to regression of symptoms
1. Hypertrophic osteoarthropathy
2. Ankylosing spondylitis (in 3–16%)
◊ Axial skeletal involvement usually precedes onset of GI symptoms!
• unrelated in severity / course to activity level of bowel disease
√ symmetric bilateral sacroiliitis
√ spondylitis with syndesmophytes
3. Peripheral erosive arthritis
√ small marginal erosions
√ periostitis
√ propensity for osseous ankylosis
4. Avascular necrosis of femoral head (steroid Rx)
5. Pelvic osteomyelitis (contiguous involvement)
6. Septic arthritis
7. Muscle abscess
8. Retarded skeletal growth + maturation

@ Erythema nodosum, uveitis

CRONKHITE-CANADA SYNDROME

= nonneoplastic nonhereditary inflammatory polyps (as in juvenile polyposis) associated with ectodermal abnormalities; no familial predisposition

Incidence: >100 cases described

Histo: hamartomatous polyps resembling juvenile / retention polyps = multiple cystic spaces filled with mucin secondary to degenerative changes; expansion + inflammation of lamina propria

Age: 62 years (range 42–75 years); M < F

• exudative protein-losing enteropathy
• diarrhea (disaccharidase deficiency, bacterial overgrowth in small intestine)
• severe weight loss, anorexia
• abdominal pain
• nail atrophy
• brownish macules of hand + feet
• alopecia

√ multiple polyps
√ thickened gastric rugae
Location: stomach (100%); small bowel (>50%); colon (100%)

Prognosis: rapidly fatal in women within 6–18 months (cachexia); tendency toward remission in men

DESMOID TUMOR

= uncommon benign tumor consisting of fibrous tissue with insidious growth [desmos = "band / tendon"]
= subgroup of fibromatoses

Types:
1. ABDOMINAL DESMOID
Location: mesentery (most common mesenteric primary), musculoaponeurosis of rectus, internal oblique muscle; occasionally external oblique muscle
2. EXTRA-ABDOMINAL DESMOID
= musculoaponeurotic fibromatosis
Location: pelvis, chest wall, mediastinum

Age: peak age in 3rd decade, 70% between 20 and 40 years of age; M:F = 1:3

Path: poorly circumscribed coarsely trabeculated tumor resembling scar tissue, confined to musculature + overlying aponeurosis

Histo: elongated spindle-shaped cells of uniform appearance, septated by dense bands of collagen, infiltration of adjacent tissue (DDx: low-grade fibrosarcoma, reactive fibrosis)

Associated with: Gardner syndrome, multiple pregnancies, prior trauma
- firm slowly growing deep-seated mass

Size: 5–20 cm in diameter
MR:
√ hypointense to muscle on T1WI + variable intensity on T2WI
CT:
√ ill-defined / well-circumscribed mass
√ usually higher attenuation than muscle
√ ± enhancement
√ retraction, angulation, distortion of small / large bowel with mesenteric infiltration
US:
√ sharply defined + smoothly marginated mass of low / medium / high echogenicity
Cx: compression / displacement of bowel / ureter, intestinal perforation
Prognosis: locally aggressive growth; 25–65% recurrence rate
Rx: local resection + radiotherapy, antiestrogen therapy
DDx: (1) Malignant tumor: metastasis, fibrosarcoma, rhabdomyosarcoma, synoviosarcoma, liposarcoma, fibrous histiocytoma, lymphoma,
(2) Benign tumor: neurofibroma, neuroma, leiomyoma
(3) Acute hematoma

DIAPHRAGM DISEASE

= small bowel webs due to NSAIDs
Effect of NSAID: gastric irritation, ulceration of small intestines
Frequency: in 10% of patients receiving long-term NSAID therapy
Path: foci of submucosal fibrosis with interruption of adjacent muscularis mucosae
- blood + protein loss
- intermittent intestinal obstruction

Location: ileum > jejunum
Enteroclysis:
√ multiple concentric diaphragm-like strictures
DDx: Crohn disease

GI

DISACCHARIDASE DEFICIENCY

= enzyme deficiencies for any of the disaccharides (maltose, lactose, etc.)
A. PRIMARY
B. SECONDARY to other diseases (eg, Crohn disease)
Pathophysiology:
(a) unabsorbed disaccharides produce osmotic diarrhea
(b) bacterial fermentation produces short-chain volatile fatty acids causing further osmotic + irritant diarrhea
√ normal small bowel series without added lactose
√ abnormal small bowel series done with lactose (50 g added to 600 cm^3 of barium suspension)
√ small + large bowel distension
√ dilution of barium
√ shortening of transit time

DISTAL INTESTINAL OBSTRUCTION SYNDROME

= MECONIUM ILEUS EQUIVALENT
= impaction of inspissated stool in distal part of ileum + proximal part of colon
Prevalence: 7–15–41% of children / adolescents with cystic fibrosis; 2% in patients <5 years of age
Cause: tenacious intestinal mucus, steatorrhea due to pancreatic insufficiency, undigested food residue, disordered intestinal motility with increase in intestinal transit time, fecal stasis, dehydration
Age: 2nd–3rd decade of life
- recurrent bouts of colicky abdominal pain (from fecal impaction / constipation) in RLQ
- palpable cecal mass

√ bubbly granular ileocecal soft-tissue mass in RLQ
√ partial / complete small bowel obstruction (due to puttylike fecal material in terminal ileum / right colon)
√ thickening of mucosal folds
√ cystic fibrosis of lung
CT:
Location: cecum > ascending colon > transverse colon > descending colon (contiguous involvement)
√ diffuse colonic thickening
√ mural striation (50%)
√ mesenteric soft-tissue infiltration (100%)
√ increased pericolonic fat (60%)
Cx: intussusception, volvulus
Rx: stool softeners, oral polyethylene glycol-electrolyte solution (Go-lytely®), increasing dose of pancreatic enzyme supplements, mucolytic agents (N-acetylcysteine) orally / with Gastrografin® enema
DDx: appendicitis, partial intestinal obstruction (adhesion / stricture from previous bowel surgery)

DIVERTICULAR DISEASE OF COLON

= overactivity of smooth muscle causing herniation of mucosa + submucosa through muscle layers
Incidence: 5–10% in 5th decade; 33–48% over age 50; 50% past 7th decade; M:F = 1:1; most common affliction of colon in developed countries
Cause: decreased fecal bulk (diet high in refined fiber + low in roughage)
Location: in 80% in sigmoid (= narrowest colonic segment with highest pressure); in 17% distributed over entire colon; in 4–12% isolated to cecum / ascending colon

Prediverticular disease of colon

= longitudinal + circular smooth muscle thickening with redundancy of folds secondary to myostatic contracture
√ "saw-tooth sign" = crowding + thickening of haustral folds (shortening of colonic segment)
√ plump marginal indentations
√ superimposed muscle spasm (relieved by antispasmodics)

DDx: hemorrhage; ischemia; radiation changes; pseudomembranous colitis

Colonic diverticulosis

= acquired herniations of mucosa + muscularis mucosae through the muscularis propria with wall components of mucosa, submucosa, serosa = false diverticula of pulsion type

Site:
- (a) lateral diverticula arise between mesenteric + antimesenteric teniae on opposite sides
- (b) antimesenteric intertaenial diverticula opposite of mesenteric side

Intramural type vasa recta (= nutrient arteries) pass through the circular muscle (weakness in muscular wall) and are carried over the fundus of the diverticula as it enlarges

- √ size: initially tiny (3- to 10-mm) V-shaped protrusions increasing up to several cm in diameter
- √ bubbly appearance of air-containing diverticula
- √ residual barium within diverticula from previous study
- √ spiky irregular outline (antimesenteric intertaenial ridge is typical site for intramural diverticula)
- √ smooth dome-shaped appendages with a short neck
- √ may be pointed, attenuated, irregular with variable filling
- √ circular line with sharp outer edge + fuzzy blurred inner edge (en face view in double contrast BE)
- √ **Giant sigmoid diverticulum** = large gas-containing cyst (air entrapment secondary to ball-valve mechanism) arising in left iliac fossa

CT:
- √ diverticula
- √ distorted luminal contour + muscular hypertrophy

Colonic diverticulitis

= perforation of diverticulum with intramural / localized pericolic abscess

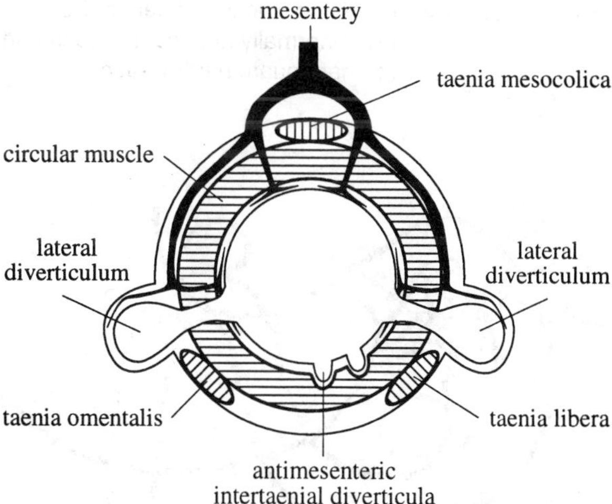

Cross Section through Colon

Incidence: 5% of population; in 10–35% of diverticular disease; increasing frequency with age

Pathogenesis: mucosal abrasion from inspissated fecal material leads to perforation of thin wall

- pain + local tenderness + mass in LLQ
- fever (25%), leukocytosis (36%)

Location: sigmoid colon (most commonly)
- √ localized ileus
- √ ± pattern of small bowel obstruction (kinking / edema if small bowel adheres to abscess)
- √ gas in abscess / fistula
- √ pneumoperitoneum (rare)

BE (77–86% sensitive):
- √ focal area of eccentric luminal narrowing caused by pericolic / intramural inflammatory mass
- √ marked thickening + distortion of mucosal folds
- √ mucosal tethering
- √ extraluminal contrast = PERIDIVERTICULITIS
  - √ "double-tracking" = pericolonic longitudinal sinus tract
  - √ pericolonic collection = peridiverticular abscess
  - √ fistula to bladder / small bowel / vagina

CT (79–93% sensitive, 77% specific):
- √ poorly marginated hazy area of increased attenuation ± fine linear strands within pericolic fat (98%)
- √ diverticula (84%) = flask-shaped structures projecting through colonic wall + filled with air / barium / fecal material
- √ circumferential bowel wall thickening of >4 mm (70%)
- √ frank abscess (47%) = central liquid / gas
- √ fluid ± air of peritonitis (16%)
- √ fluid at root of mesentery
- √ fistula formation (14%): most commonly colovesical, also colovaginal, coloenteric, colocutaneous
- √ colonic obstruction (12%)
- √ intramural sinus tracts (9%)
- √ ureteral obstruction (7%)

US (85–98% sensitive, 80–97% specific):
- √ thickening of bowel wall = >4 mm distance between echogenic lumen interface and serosa
- √ diverticula = round / oval hypo- / hyperechoic foci protruding from colonic wall with focal disruption of normal layer continuity ± internal acoustic shadowing
- √ inflammatory pericolic fat = regionally increased echogenicity adjacent to colonic wall ± ill-defined hypoechoic zones
- √ pericolic abscess

Prognosis:
- (a) self-limiting (usually)
- (b) transmural perforation
- (c) superficial ulceration
- (d) chronic abscess

DDx:
- (1) Colonic neoplasm (shorter segment, heaped-up margins, ulcerated mucosa)
- (2) Crohn colitis (double-tracking longer than 10 cm)

Rx: antibiotics, surgery (in 25%), percutaneous abscess drainage

Colonic diverticular hemorrhage

Not related to diverticulitis

Incidence: in 3–47% of diverticulosis

Location: 75% located in ascending colon (larger neck + dome of diverticula)

- massive rectal hemorrhage without pain

√ extravasation of radionuclide tracers

√ angiographic contrast pooling in bowel lumen

Rx: (1) transcatheter infusion of vasoconstrictive agents (Pitressin®)
(2) embolization with Gelfoam®

DUMPING SYNDROME

= early postprandial vascular symptomatology of sweating, flushing, palpitation, feeling of weakness and dizziness

Pathophysiology: rapid entering of hypertonic solution into jejunum resulting in fluid shift from blood compartment into small bowel

Incidence: 1–5%; M:F = 2:1

◊ Roentgenologic findings not diagnostic!

√ rapid emptying of barium into small bowel (= loss of gastric reservoir function)

Rx: lying down, diet

DDx: late postprandial hypoglycemia (90–120 minutes after eating)

DUODENAL ATRESIA

= most common cause of congenital duodenal obstruction; second most common site of gastrointestinal atresias after ileum

Incidence: 1:10,000; M:F = 1:1

Etiology: defective vacuolization of duodenum between 6th–11th weeks of fetal life; rarely from vascular insult (extent of obstruction usually involves larger regions with vascular insult)

Age at presentation: first few days of life

- persistent bilious vomiting a few hours after birth / following 1st feeding
- rapid deterioration secondary to loss of fluids + electrolytes

Isolated sporadic anomaly (30–52%)

Associated anomalies (in 60%):

(1) Down syndrome (20–33%);
◊ 25% of fetuses with duodenal atresia have Down syndrome!
◊ <5% of fetuses with Down syndrome have duodenal atresia!

(2) CHD (8–30–50%): endocardial cushion defect, VSD

(3) Gastrointestinal anomalies (26%): esophageal atresia, biliary atresia, duodenal duplication, imperforate anus, small bowel atresia, intestinal malrotation, Meckel diverticulum, transposed liver, annular pancreas (20%)

(4) Urinary tract anomalies (8%)

(5) Vertebral + rib anomalies (37%)

Location: (a) usually distal to ampulla of Vater (80%)
(b) proximal duodenum (20%)

√ "double bubble sign" = gas-fluid levels in duodenal bulb + gastric fundus

√ total absence of intestinal gas in small / large bowel

√ colon of normal caliber

OB-US (usually not identified prior to 24 weeks GA):

- ± elevated AFP

√ "double bubble sign" = simultaneous distension of stomach + 1st portion of duodenum, continuity of fluid between stomach + duodenum must be demonstrated

√ increased gastric peristalsis

√ polyhydramnios in 3rd trimester (100%)

Prognosis: 36% mortality in neonates

DDx: (1) Prominent incisura angularis causing bidissection of stomach
(2) Choledochal cyst
(3) Annular pancreas
(4) Peritoneal bands
(5) Intestinal duplication

Cx: prematurity (40%) secondary to preterm labor related to polyhydramnios

DUODENAL DIVERTICULUM

Incidence: 1–5% of GI studies; 22% of autopsies

A. PRIMARY DIVERTICULUM
= mucosal prolapse through muscularis propria
Location: 2nd portion (62%), 3rd portion (30%), 4th portion (8%)
Site: medial wall in region of papilla (88%), posteriorly (8%), lateral wall (4%)

B. SECONDARY DIVERTICULUM
= all layers of duodenal wall = true diverticulum as complication of duodenal / periduodenal inflammation
Location: almost invariably in 1st portion of duodenum

- mostly asymptomatic

Cx: (1) Perforation + peritonitis (2) Bowel obstruction (3) Biliary obstruction (4) Bleeding (5) Diverticulitis

DUODENAL ULCER

Incidence: 200,000 cases/year; 2–3 x more frequent than gastric ulcers; M:F = 3:1

Pathophysiology: too much acid in duodenum from
(a) abnormally high gastric secretion
(b) inadequate neutralization

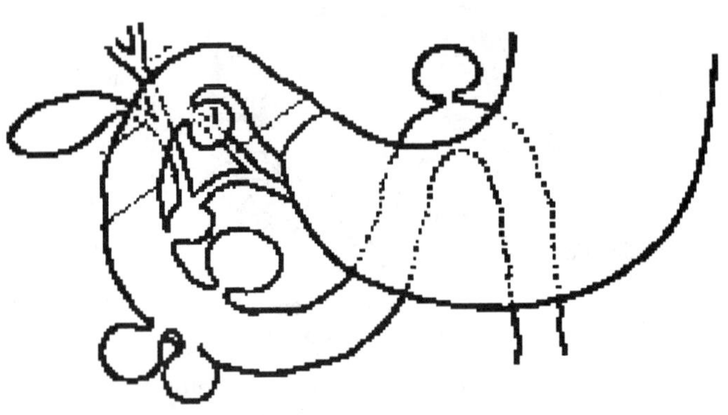

GI

Predisposed: cortisone therapy, severe cerebral injury, after surgery, chronic obstructive pulmonary disease
Location: (a) bulbar (95%):
anterior wall (50%), posterior wall (23%), inferior wall (22%), superior wall (5%)
(b) postbulbar (3–5%):
majority on medial wall of supraampullary region; tendency for hemorrhage in 66%; M:F = 7:1
√ frequently small round / ovoid / linear ulcer niche
√ "kissing ulcers" = ulcers opposite from each other on anterior + posterior wall
√ giant duodenal ulcer >3 cm (rare) with higher morbidity + mortality; may be overlooked by simulating a normal / deformed duodenal bulb
√ "cloverleaf deformity, hourglass stenosis" (healed stage) with prestenotic dilatation of recesses
Cx: (1) Obstruction (5%)
(2) Perforation (<10%): anterior > posterior wall; fistula to gallbladder
(3) Penetration (<5%) = sealed perforation
(4) Hemorrhage (15%): melena > hematemesis
Rx: antral resection (Billroth I) + vagotomy

DUODENAL VARICES
= dilated collateral veins secondary to portal hypertension (posterior superior pancreaticoduodenal vein)
√ lobulated filling defects (best demonstrated in prone position, maximal luminal distension will obliterate them)
√ commonly associated with fundal + esophageal varices

DUPLICATION CYST
= uncommon congenital anomaly found anywhere along alimentary tract from tongue to anus
Incidence: 15% of pediatric abdominal masses are gastrointestinal duplication cysts
Theories of formation:
(1) Abortive twinning
(2) Persistent embryologic diverticula
(3) Split notochord
(4) Aberrant luminal recanalization
(5) Intrauterine vascular accident
associated with alimentary tract atresia in 9%
Age: presentation often in infancy / early childhood
Path: spherical cyst / tubular structure located in / immediately adjacent to gastrointestinal tract; shares a common muscle wall + blood supply; has a separate mucosal lining; cyst contents are usually serous
Histo: smooth muscle wall + lined with alimentary tract mucosa; ectopic mucosa squamous, transitional, ciliated mucosa; lymphoid aggregates; ganglion cells
◊ Gastric mucosa + pancreatic tissue are the only ectopic tissues of clinical importance!
• respiratory distress (with esophageal duplication)
• palpable abdominal mass
• nausea, emesis

Location: ileum (30–33%), esophagus (17–20%), colon (13–30%), jejunum (10–13%), stomach (7%), pylorus (4%), duodenum (4–5%), ileocecal junction (4%), rectum (4%);
◊ In 7–15% concomitant duplications elsewhere in the alimentary tract!
Site: on mesenteric aspect of alimentary canal
Morphology:
(a) large spherical / saccular cyst (82%)
(b) small intramural cyst
(c) tubular sausage-shaped cyst (18%): commonly along small + large bowel; frequently communicates with lumen of adjacent gut
√ elongated tubular / spherical cystic mass
√ muscular rim sign (= echogenic inner mucosal lining + hypoechoic outer rim) in 47%
√ cyst paralleling normal bowel lumen
Cx: bowel obstruction, intussusception, bleeding (due to presence of gastric mucosa / pressure necrosis of adjacent mucosa by cyst expansion / from intussusception)
DDx:
(1) Omental cyst (greater omentum / lesser sac, multilocular)
(2) Mesenteric cyst (between leaves of small bowel mesentery)
(3) Choledochal cyst
(4) Ovarian cyst
(5) Pancreatic pseudocyst
(6) Cystic renal tumor
(7) Abscess
(8) Meckel diverticulum (communicates with GI tract)
(9) Lymphangioma
(10) Mesenteric lymphoma
(11) Intramural tumor

Colonic duplication cyst
Incidence: 13% of all alimentary tract duplications
A. CYSTIC COLONIC DUPLICATION (7%)
Path: closed spherical cyst; contains gastric mucosa in 2% + ectopic pancreatic tissue in 5%
• abdominal mass, bowel obstruction, GI hemorrhage
Location: cecum (40%) ± intussusception
B. COLORECTAL TUBULAR DUPLICATION (6%)
= DUPLICATION OF THE HINDGUT
= double-barreled duplication involving part / all of large bowel with "twin" segment on mesenteric / antimesenteric side
Symptomatic age: neonatal period / infancy; M:F = 1:2
May be associated with:
rectogenital / rectourinary fistula, duplication of internal / external genitalia, vertebral anomalies, multisystem congenital anomaly complex
• bowel obstruction
• passage of feces through vagina
√ simultaneous opacification of true + twin colon

GI

√ duplication may terminate at
(a) 2nd functional anus
(b) imperforate perineal orifice
(c) fistulous communication with GU tract

C. DOUBLE APPENDIX

Duodenal Duplication Cyst

Incidence: 5% of all alimentary tract duplications
Path: noncommunicating spherical cyst; may contain ectopic gastric mucosa in 21%, small bowel mucosa, pancreatic tissue

- obstruction, palpable abdominal mass
- hemorrhage (due to peptic ulceration)
- jaundice (due to biliary obstruction)
- pancreatitis (due to ectopic pancreatic tissue)

Site: on mesenteric side of anterior wall of 1st + 2nd portion of duodenum
√ mass in concavity of duodenal C-loop
√ compression + displacement of 1st / 2nd portion of duodenum superiorly + anteriorly
Cx: pancreatitis from perforation of duplication cyst
DDx: pancreatic cyst, pancreatic pseudocyst, choledochal cyst, choledochocele, duodenal intramural tumor, pancreatic tumor

Esophageal Duplication Cyst

arises from foregut
Incidence: 10–20% of all alimentary tract duplications; 0.5–2.5% of all esophageal masses; M:F = 2:1
Path: contains ectopic gastric mucosa in 43%
Histo: contains no cartilage, lined by gastrointestinal tract epithelium
Associated with: vertebral anomalies, esophageal atresia, small bowel duplication (18%)
Location: adjacent to esophagus / within esophageal musculature at any level, paraspinal position; R:L = 2:1; in right pleural space detached from esophagus (rare)

A. CERVICAL ESOPHAGUS (23%)
- asymptomatic enlarging lateral neck mass
- upper airway obstruction in newborn

DDx: thyroglossal duct cyst, branchial cleft cyst, cystic hygroma, cervical tumor, cervical lymphadenopathy

B. MIDESOPHAGUS (17%)
- severe upper airway obstruction in early infancy

DDx: bronchogenic cyst, neurenteric cyst, intramural esophageal tumor

C. DISTAL ESOPHAGUS (60%)
- frequently asymptomatic

Location: paraspinal
DDx: bronchogenic cyst, neurenteric cyst, intramural esophageal tumor

√ closed spherical cyst, almost never communicating
CXR:
√ posterior mediastinal mass ± air-fluid level
√ lobar consolidation + central cavitation (from autodigestion of lung tissue by gastric secretions)
√ thoracic vertebral anomalies
UGI:
√ displacement of esophagus by paraesophageal mass
√ intramural extramucosal mass
US:
√ hypoechoic fluid-filled cyst + inner mucosal lining
Cx: (1) Peptic ulceration (secondary to gastric mucosa)
(2) Perforation (secondary to penetrating ulcer)
(3) Hematemesis (from erosion into esophagus)
(4) Hemoptysis + autodigestion of pulmonary tissue (from erosion into tracheobronchial tree)

Gastric Duplication Cyst

= intramural gastric cyst lined with secretory epithelium
Incidence: 7% of all alimentary tract duplications
Path: noncommunicating spherical cyst (majority); may communicate with aberrant pancreatic duct; ectopic pancreatic tissue found in 37%
Symptomatic age: infancy; in 75% detected before age 12; M:F = 1:2

- pain (from overdistension of cyst, rupture with peritonitis, peptic ulcer formation, internal pancreatitis)
- vomiting, anemia, fever
- symptoms mimicking congenital hypertrophic pyloric stenosis (if duplication in antrum / pylorus)

Most common site: greater curvature (65%)
√ paragastric cystic mass up to 12 cm in size, indenting greater curvature
√ seldom communicates with main gastric lumen at one or both ends
√ may enlarge + ulcerate
√ Tc-99m uptake
US:
√ cyst with two wall layers (inner echogenic layer of mucosa, outer hypoechoic layer of muscle)
√ clear / debris-containing fluid
Cx: (1) Partial / complete small bowel obstruction
(2) Relapsing pancreatitis (with ductal communication)
(3) Ulceration, perforation, fistula formation
DDx: pancreatic cyst, pancreatic pseudocyst, mesenteric cyst, leiomyoma, adenomatous polyp, hamartoma, lipoma, neurofibroma, teratoma

Rectal Duplication Cyst

Incidence: 4% of all alimentary tract duplications
Path: spherical fluid-filled cyst; may contain duodenal / gastric mucosa + pancreatic tissue
Site: posterior to rectum / anus
√ communication with rectum / perianal fistula (in 20%)
Symptomatic age: childhood

- constipation + fecal soiling
- palpable retrorectal / retroanal mass
- intractable excoriation of perianal skin (with chronic perianal fistula)

√ cystic mass; may be echogenic (due to solid material ± gas from communication with rectum)

DDx: anterior meningocele, sacrococcygeal teratoma, retrorectal abscess, pilonidal cyst, sacral bone tumor

Small bowel duplication cyst

Incidence: most common of all alimentary tract duplications

Symptomatic age: neonatal period (1/3); <2 years of age (in 72%)

Path: contains ectopic gastric mucosa in 24%; ectopic pancreatic tissue in jejunum (8%)

May be associated with: small bowel atresia

- neonatal bowel obstruction
- intussusception, palpable mass
- acute abdominal pain, hemorrhage

Location: ileum (33%), jejunum (10%), ileocecal (4%)

√ low small bowel obstruction ± soft-tissue mass
√ cyst may serve as lead point for intussusception

DDx: mesenteric cyst, pancreatic pseudocyst, omental cyst, exophytic hepatic cyst, ovarian cyst

Thoracoabdominal duplication

= FOREGUT DUPLICATION
= long tubular cyst closed at its cranial end, passing through diaphragm through its own hiatus, in 60% communicating with normal duodenum / jejunum / ileum

Incidence: 2% of all alimentary tract duplications

Associated with: thoracic vertebral anomalies

Histo: gastric mucosa in 29%

Symptomatic age: 50% during neonatal period; 80% within 1st year of life

- severe respiratory distress
- chest pain, GI bleeding, anemia

√ tubular right posterior mediastinal mass ± air
√ thoracic vertebral anomaly
√ contrast material may enter through distal connection

ECTOPIC PANCREAS

= PANCREATIC REST

Incidence: 2–10% of autopsies; M:F = 2:1

- asymptomatic

Location: distal greater curvature of antrum / pylorus (80%), duodenal bulb, jejunum, ileum, Meckel diverticulum; lesions may be multiple

√ smooth cone- / nipple-shaped submucosal nodule 1–5 cm in size
√ central umbilication representing orifice of filiform duct

ENTERIC CYST

= cyst lined by gastrointestinal mucosa without bowel wall

Etiology: migration of small bowel / colonic diverticulum into mesentery / mesocolon

Path: unilocular thin smooth-walled cyst with serous contents lined by enteric epithelium + thin fibrous wall

US:
√ hypoechoic cystic mass, occasionally with septations

DDx: duplication cyst (reduplication of bowel wall)

EOSINOPHILIC GASTROENTERITIS

= uncommon self-limited form of gastroenteritis with remissions + exacerbations characterized by infiltration of eosinophilic leukocytes into stomach / small bowel wall + usually marked peripheral eosinophilia

Cause: unknown

Histo: fibrous tissue + eosinophilic infiltrate of gastrointestinal mucosa

Age: in children + young adults with allergy + eosinophilia

A. EOSINOPHILIC GRANULOMA
   = FIBROUS POLYPOID LESION
   = INFLAMMATORY PSEUDOTUMOR
   = localized form / circumscribed type
   Location: almost exclusively in stomach (most common in antrum + pylorus)
   √ submucosal polypoid mass / pedunculated polyp
B. EOSINOPHILIC GASTROENTERITIS
   = diffuse type
   = eosinophilic infiltration of mucosa, submucosa, and muscular layers of small intestine ± stomach by mature eosinophils (? gastric pendant to Löffler syndrome)

- recurrent episodes of abdominal pain, diarrhea, vomiting
- weight loss
- hematemesis (from ulceration)
- peripheral eosinophilia, anemia
- history of systemic allergy / food allergy

Location: entire small bowel (particularly jejunum), distal stomach, omentum, mesentery

Site: (a) mucosal (b) muscular (c) serosal (rare)

@ Stomach (almost always limited to antrum)
  √ "wet stomach"
  √ ulcers are rare
  (a) mucosal type
    √ enlarged gastric rugae / cobblestone nodules / polyps
  (b) muscular type
    √ thickened + rigid wall with narrowed gastric antrum / pylorus
    √ bulky intraluminal mass up to 9 cm in size
  Cx: pyloric obstruction
  DDx: hypertrophic gastritis, lymphoma, carcinoma

@ Small bowel (involved in 50%)
  √ separation of small bowel loops
  (a) mucosal type
    • malabsorption + hypoproteinemia
    √ thickening + distortion of folds predominantly in jejunum
  (b) submucosal / muscular type
    √ motility disturbance
    √ small-bowel obstruction
    √ effacement of mucosal pattern + narrowing of lumen
  (c) serosal type
    √ ascites

Prognosis: tendency toward spontaneous remission

Rx: steroids / removal of sensitizing agent

GI

EPIPLOIC APPENDAGITIS

= rare inflammation of one of the 100 epiploic appendages

Cause: (a) primary: torsion (exercise), venous thrombosis
(b) secondary: inflammation of adjacent organ (eg, diverticulitis, appendicitis)

Histo: acute infarction with fat necrosis, inflammation, thrombosed vessels with hemorrhagic suffusion

- abrupt onset of localized abdominal pain, gradually resolving over 3–7 days

◊ Almost never suspected preoperatively!

Location: anterolaterally / (occasionally) anteromedially to ascending / descending / sigmoid colon

US:
√ solid hyperechoic noncompressible ovoid mass
√ hypoechoic margin (93%)

CT:
√ pericolonic oval-shaped pedunculated mass, 1–4 cm in diameter, with fat attenuation (approx. -60 HU)
√ hyperattenuating peripheral rim + fat stranding
√ thickening of adjacent visceral peritoneal lining (93%)

Prognosis: spontaneous resolution
Rx: conservative management
DDx: torsion / infarction of greater omentum, diverticulitis, appendicitis

ESOPHAGEAL ATRESIA & TRACHEOESOPHAGEAL FISTULA

= incomplete division of primitive foregut into respiratory + digestive tracts characterized by failure of formation of tubular esophagus + abnormal communication between esophagus + trachea; occurring at 3rd–5th week of intrauterine life

Incidence: 1:2,000–4,000 livebirths; most common sporadic congenital anomaly diagnosed in childhood

Risk of recurrence in sibling: 1%

Associated anomalies (17–56–70%):
1. Cardiac (15–39%): patent ductus arteriosus, ASD, VSD, right-sided aortic arch (5%)
2. Musculoskeletal (24%): radial ray hypoplasia, vertebral anomalies
3. Gastrointestinal (20%): anorectal anomalies, duodenal atresia
4. Genitourinary (12%): unilateral renal agenesis
5. Chromosomal (3–19%): trisomy 18, 21, 13
   ◊ Trisomy 18 is present in 75–100% of fetuses + in 3–4% of neonates with esophageal atresia!

mnemonic: "ARTICLES"
Anal atresia
Renal anomalies
TE fistula
Intestinal atresia / malrotation
Cardiac anomaly (PDA, VSD)
Limb anomalies (radial ray hypoplasia, polydactyly)
Esophageal atresia
Spinal anomalies

mnemonic: "VACTERL"
Vertebral anomalies
Anorectal anomaly
Cardiovascular anomalies
Tracheo-
Esophageal fistula
Renal anomalies
Limb anomalies

- drooling from excessive accumulation of pharyngeal secretions (esophageal atresia = EA)
- obligatory regurgitation of ingested fluids (EA)
- coughing + choking during feeding (TEF)
- recurrent pneumonia + progressive respiratory distress of variable severity (tracheoesophageal fistula = TEF)

Location: between upper 1/3 + lower 1/3 of esophagus just above carina

√ "coiled tube" = inability to pass feeding tube into stomach (esophageal atresia)
√ retrotracheal air-filled pouch causing compression / displacement of esophagus

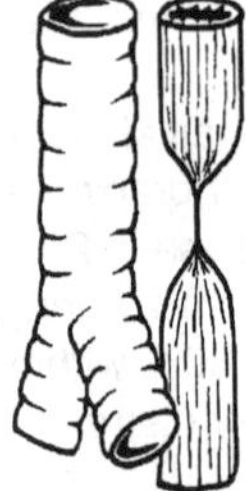

Esophageal atresia **9%**

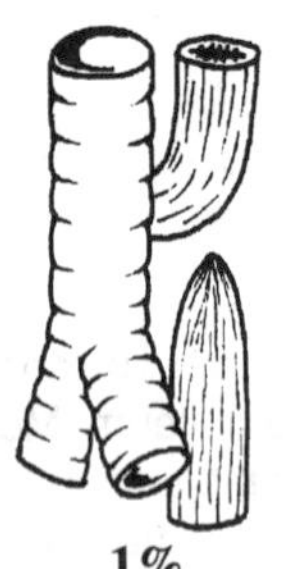

1%

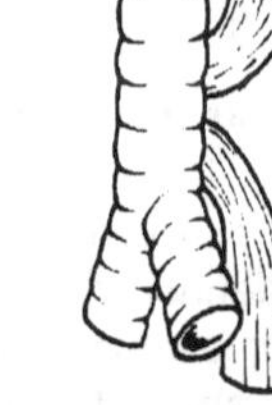

2%

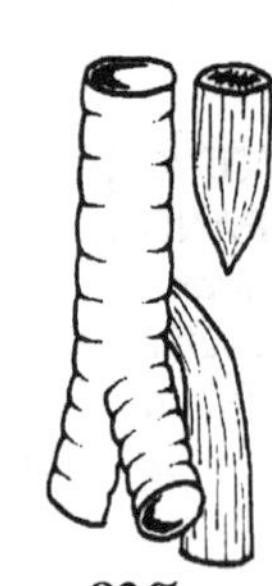

82%

Esophageal atresia + TE fistula

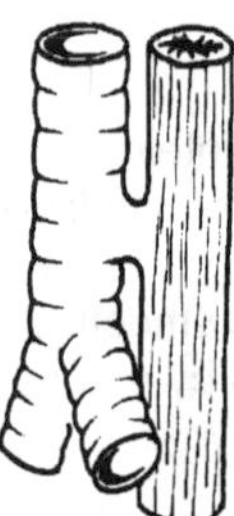

TE fistula without esophageal atresia **6%**

GI

√ gasless abdomen (esophageal atresia ± proximal TE fistula)
√ bowel gas present in 90% (distal TE fistula / H-type fistula)
√ non- / hypoperistaltic esophageal segment (6–15 cm) in midesophagus
√ aspiration pneumonia, esp. in dependent upper lobes

OB-US (anomalies not identified before 24 weeks GA):
- √ polyhydramnios in 33–60%
  - ◊ TE-fistula with esophageal atresia is cause of polyhydramnios in only 3%!
- √ absence of fluid-distended stomach (in 10–41%; in remaining cases TE-fistula / gastric secretions allow some gastric distension)
- √ small abdomen (birth weight <10th percentile in 40%)
- √ distended proximal pouch of atretic esophagus

Cx after repair:
(1) Anastomotic leak
(2) Recurrent TE fistula
(3) Aspiration pneumonia secondary to
  (a) esophageal stricture
  (b) disordered esophageal motility distal to TE fistula
  (c) gastroesophageal reflux

DDx: pharyngeal pseudodiverticulum (traumatic perforation of posterior pharynx from finger insertion into oropharynx during delivery / tube insertion)

Esophageal Atresia Without Fistula (8–9%)
Associated anomalies in 17% (mostly Down syndrome + other atresias of GI tract)

Esophageal Atresia With Fistula
1. Proximal TE fistula (1%)
2. Distal TE fistula (82–86%)
3. Proximal + distal TE fistula (1–2%)

Associated anomalies in 30% (mostly cardiovascular)

Tracheo-esophageal Fistula Without Atresia (6%)
Associated anomalies in 23% (mostly cardiovascular)

ESOPHAGEAL CANCER
Incidence: <1% of all cancers; 4–10% of all GI malignancies; 11,000 cases/year (United States in 1994); M:F = 4:1; Blacks:Whites = 2:1

High-risk regions: Iran, parts of Africa, Italy, China

Predisposing factors:
achalasia (risk factor of 1000 x), asbestosis, Barrett esophagus, celiac disease, ionizing radiation, caustic stricture (risk factor of 1000 x), Plummer-Vinson syndrome, tannins, alcohol, tobacco, history of oral / pharyngeal cancer, tylosis palmaris et plantaris

mnemonic: "BELCH SPAT"
Barrett esophagus
EtOH abuse
Lye stricture
Celiac disease
Head and neck tumor
Smoking
Plummer-Vinson syndrome
Achalasia
Tylosis

Cancer Staging:
TNM system:
- T1 tumor invades lamina propria / submucosa
- T2 tumor invades muscularis propria
- T3 tumor invades adventitia
- T4 tumor invades adjacent structures

Stage I = T1,N0,M0
Stage IIA = T2/3,N0,M0
Stage IIB = T1/2,N1,M0
Stage III = T3,N1,M0 or T4,N0/1,M0
Stage IV = T1-4,N0/1,M1

CT staging (Moss):
- Stage 1 intraluminal tumor / localized wall thickening of 3–5 mm
- Stage 2 localized / circumferential wall thickening >5 mm
- Stage 3 contiguous spread into adjacent mediastinum (trachea, bronchi, aorta, pericardium)
  - √ loss of fat planes (nonspecific due to cachexia, often still resectable)
  - √ mass in contact with aorta >90° arc (in 20–70% still resectable)
  - √ displacement / compression of airway (90–100% accuracy for invasion)
  - √ esophagotracheal / -bronchial fistula (unresectable)
- Stage 4 distant metastases
  - √ enlarged abdominal lymph nodes >10 mm (12–85% accuracy)
  - √ hepatic, pulmonary, adrenal metastases
  - √ direct erosion of vertebral body
  - √ tumor >3 cm wide = high frequency of extra-esophageal spread

Histo:
(1) Squamous cell carcinoma (81–95%)
(2) Adenocarcinoma (4–19%) arising from mucosal / submucosal glands or heterotopic gastric mucosa or columnar-lined epithelium (Barrett)
  (a) in 70% from Barrett esophagus
  (b) at gastroesophageal junction
(3) Mucoepidermoid carcinoma, adenoid cystic carcinoma
(4) Carcinosarcoma = pseudosarcoma = spindle-cell squamous carcinoma
  Age: in men >45 years
  Location: usually middle third of esophagus
  √ large bulky polypoid smooth, lobulated, scalloped intraluminal mass, may be pedunculated

(5) Leiomyosarcoma, rhabdomyosarcoma, fibrosarcoma, malignant lymphoma

- dysphagia (87–95%) of <6 months' duration
- weight loss (71%)
- retrosternal pain (46%)
- regurgitation (29%)

Location: upper 1/3 (15–20%); middle 1/3 (37–44%); lower 1/3 (38–43%)

Radiologic types:
(1) Polypoid / fungating form (most common)
√ sessile / pedunculated tumor with lobulated surface
√ protruding, irregular, polycyclic, overhanging, steplike "apple core" lesion
(2) Ulcerating form
√ large ulcer niche within bulging mass
(3) Infiltrating form
√ gradual narrowing with smooth transition (DDx: benign stricture)
(4) Varicoid form = superficial spreading carcinoma
Histo: longitudinal extension within wall without invasion beyond mucosa / submucosa
√ tiny confluent nodules / plaques
DDx: Candida esophagitis

Metastases:
(a) lymphogenic: anterior jugular chain + supraclavicular nodes (primary in upper 1/3); paraesophageal + subdiaphragmatic nodes (primary in middle 1/3); mediastinal + paracardial + celiac trunk nodes (primary in lower 1/3)
(b) hematogenous: lung, liver, adrenal gland

CXR:
√ widened azygoesophageal recess with convexity toward right lung (in 30% of distal + midesophageal cancers)
√ thickening of posterior tracheal stripe + right paratracheal stripe >4 mm (if tumor located in upper third of esophagus)
√ widened mediastinum
√ tracheal deviation
√ posterior tracheal indentation / mass
√ retrocardiac mass
√ esophageal air-fluid level
√ lobulated mass extending into gastric air bubble
√ repeated aspiration pneumonia (with tracheoesophageal fistula)

Cx: fistula formation to trachea (5–10%) / bronchi / mediastinum

Prognosis: 3–5–20% 5-year survival rate

Mean survival time:
90 days with subdiaphragmatic lymphadenopathy
180 days with local invasion + abdominal metastases
480 days without evidence of invasion / metastases

Rx: (1) chemotherapy (fluorouracil, cisplatin, bleomycin sulfate, mitomycin) + surgery
(2) chemotherapy + irradiation (~4,000 cGy)
(3) chemotherapy + irradiation + surgery

Operative mortality: 3–8%

ESOPHAGEAL INTRAMURAL PSEUDODIVERTICULOSIS

= dilated excretory ducts of deep esophageal adnexal mucous glands
Etiology: uncertain
Incidence: about 100 cases in world literature
Site: diffuse / segmental involvement
In 90% associated with:
any severe esophagitis (most often reflux / Candida), esophageal stricture
√ multiple tiny rounded / flask-shaped barium collections in longitudinal rows parallel to long axis of esophagus
√ appear to "float" outside esophagus without apparent communication with lumen
√ commonly associated with strictures in distal esophagus

ESOPHAGEAL PERFORATION

Cause:
(1) Iatrogenic injury (most common cause, 55%): complication of endoscopy, dilatation of stricture, bougie, disruption of suture line following surgical anastomosis, attempted intubation
(2) Spontaneous rupture = Boerhaave syndrome (15%): emetogenic injury of the esophagus from sudden increase in intra-abdominal pressure + relaxation of distal esophageal sphincter in the presence of a moderate to large amount of gastric contents
(3) Closed chest trauma (10%)
(4) Esophageal carcinoma
(5) Retained foreign body (14%): coin, aluminum pop-tops, metallic button, safety pin, invisible plastic toy) leading to perforation (in pediatric age group)
(6) Barrett ulcer

- pain, dysphagia, odynophagia
- rapid onset of overwhelming sepsis: fever, tachycardia, hypotension, shock

Plain film (normal in 9–12%):
√ pneumomediastinum
√ subcutaneous emphysema of the neck
√ delayed widening of the mediastinum (secondary to mediastinitis)
√ hydrothorax (after rupture into pleural cavity), usually unilateral
√ hydropneumothorax (often not initially seen)
√ confirmation with contrast study (90% of contrast esophagrams are positive)

CT:
√ extraluminal air (92%; most useful sign)
√ periesophageal / mediastinal fluid (92%)
√ pleural effusion (75%)
√ esophageal thickening
√ extravasation of oral contrast material

Esophagography with:
(1) water-soluble contrast material (10% false-negative results)
(2) barium (if result with water-soluble material negative)

A. UPPER / MID-ESOPHAGEAL PERFORATION
Location: at level of cricopharyngeus muscle (most frequent)
√ widening of upper mediastinum
√ right-sided hydrothorax

B. DISTAL ESOPHAGEAL PERFORATION (more common)
Cause: biopsy, dilatation of stricture, Boerhaave syndrome
√ left-sided hydrothorax
√ little mediastinal changes

Cx: (1) Acute mediastinitis (2) Obstruction of SVC (3) Mediastinal abscess
Prognosis: 20–60% mortality

ESOPHAGEAL VARICES

= dilated submucosal veins due to increased collateral blood flow from portal venous system to azygos system

A. UPHILL VARICES
= collateral blood flow from portal vein via azygos vein into SVC (usually lower esophagus drains via left gastric vein into portal vein)
Cause:
(a) intrahepatic obstruction from cirrhosis
(b) splenic vein thrombosis (usually gastric varices)
(c) obstruction of hepatic veins
(d) IVC obstruction below hepatic veins
(e) IVC obstruction above hepatic vein entrance / CHF
(f) marked splenomegaly / splenic hemangiomatosis (rare)
√ varices in lower half of esophagus

B. DOWNHILL VARICES
= collateral blood flow from SVC via azygos vein into IVC / portal venous system (upper esophagus usually drains via azygos vein into SVC)
Cause: obstruction of superior vena cava distal to entry of azygos vein most commonly due to lung cancer, lymphoma, retrosternal goiter, thymoma, mediastinal fibrosis
√ varices in upper 1/3 of esophagus

EXAMINATION TECHNIQUE
(a) small amount of barium (not to obscure varices)
(b) relaxation of esophagus (not to compress varices): refrain from swallowing because succeeding swallow initiates a primary peristaltic wave that lasts for 10–30 seconds; sustained Valsalva maneuver precludes from swallowing
(c) in LAO projection with patient recumbent / in Trendelenburg position ± Valsalva maneuver / deep inspiration

Plain film:
√ lobulated masses in posterior mediastinum (visible in 5–8% of patients with varices)
√ silhouetting of descending aorta
√ abnormal convex contour of azygoesophageal recess

UGI:
√ thickened sinuous interrupted mucosal folds (earliest sign)
√ tortuous radiolucencies of variable size + location
√ "worm-eaten" smooth lobulated filling defects
√ findings may be accentuated after sclerotherapy

CT:
√ thickened esophageal wall + lobulated outer contour
√ scalloped esophageal luminal masses
√ right- / left-sided soft-tissue masses (= paraesophageal varices)
√ marked enhancement following dynamic CT

Cx: bleeding in 28% within 3 years; exsanguination in 10–15%
DDx: varicoid carcinoma of esophagus

ESOPHAGEAL WEB

= ringlike esophageal constriction caused by thin mucosal membrane projecting into lumen; covered by squamous epithelium on superior + inferior surfaces
Age: middle-aged females
? association with:
Plummer-Vinson syndrome = Paterson-Kelly syndrome (iron deficiency anemia, stomatitis, glossitis, dysphagia, thyroid disorder, spoon-shaped nails)
Cause: *mnemonic:* "BIEP"
B-ring (Schatzki ring)
Idiopathic (= transverse mucosal fold)
Epidermolysis bullosa
Plummer-Vinson disease
Path: hyperkeratosis + chronic inflammation of submucosa
• mostly asymptomatic (unless severely stenosing)
Location: in cervical esophagus near cricopharyngeus (most common) > thoracic esophagus; occasionally multiple
√ visualized during maximal distension (in one tenth of a second)
√ arises at right angles from anterior esophageal wall
√ thin delicate membrane of uniform thickness of <3 mm
Cx: high risk of upper esophageal + hypopharyngeal carcinoma
Rx: (1) balloon dilatation
(2) bougienage during esophagoscopy
DDx: stricture (circumferential + thicker = 1- to 2-mm thick [vertical length] area of complete / incomplete circumferential narrowing

ESOPHAGITIS

Acute esophagitis

mnemonic for cause: "CRIER"
Corrosives, **C**rohn disease
Reflux
Infection, **I**ntubation
Epidermolysis bullosa
Radiation therapy
√ thickened >3-mm-wide folds with irregular lobulated contour
√ mucosal nodularity (= multiple ulcerations + intervening edema)

√ erosions
√ vertically oriented ulcers usually 3–10 mm in length
√ inflammatory esophagogastric polyp = proximal gastric fold extending across esophagogastric junction (rare)
√ abnormal motility

Candida esophagitis

= MONILIASIS = CANDIDIASIS

√ Most common cause of infectious esophagitis!

Organism: C. albicans, C. tropicalis; endogenous (majority) / transmitted by another human / animal; often discovered in diseased skin, GI tract, sputum, female genital tract, urine with an indwelling Foley catheter

Predisposed:

(a) individuals with depressed immunity: hematologic disease, renal transplant, leukemia, chronic debilitating disease, diabetes mellitus, steroids, chemotherapy, radiotherapy, AIDS
◊ Most common type of fungi found with opportunistic infections!
(b) delayed esophageal emptying: scleroderma, strictures, achalasia, S/P fundoplication
(c) antibiotics

Path: patchy, creamy-white plaques covering a friable erythematous mucosa

Histo: mucosal plaques = necrotic epithelial debris + fungal colonies

- dysphagia (= difficulty swallowing)
- severe odynophagia (= painful swallowing from segmental spasm)
- intense retro- / substernal pain
- associated with thrush (= oropharyngeal moniliasis) in 20–50–80%

Location: predilection for upper 1/2 of esophagus

√ involvement of long esophageal segments
√ longitudinal plaques = grouping of tiny 1–2 mm nodular filling defects with linear orientation (= heaped-up areas of mucosal plaques)
√ "cobblestone" appearance = mucosal nodularity in early stage (from growth of colonies on surface)
√ **shaggy** / fuzzy / serrated contour (from coalescent plaques, pseudomembranes, erosions, ulcerations, intramural hemorrhage) in fulminant candidiasis
√ narrowed lumen (from spasm, pseudomembranes, marked edema)
√ "intramural diverticulosis" = multiple tiny indentations + protrusions
√ sluggish / absent primary peristalsis
√ strictures (rare)
√ mycetoma resembling large intraluminal tumor (rare)

Diagnostic sensitivity: endoscopy (97%), double contrast (88%), single contrast (55%)

Cx: (1) systemic candidiasis ("microabscesses" in liver, spleen, kidney)
(2) gastric bezoar due to large fungus ball (after long-standing esophageal candidiasis)

Rx: Mycostatin®

DDx: glycogen acanthosis, reflux esophagitis, superficial spreading carcinoma, artifacts (undissolved effervescent crystals, air bubbles, retained food particles), herpes esophagitis, acute caustic ingestion, intramural pseudodiverticulosis, squamous papillomatosis, Barrett esophagus, epidermolysis bullosa, varices

Caustic esophagitis

= CORROSIVE ESOPHAGITIS

Corrosive agents:
lye (sodium hydroxide), washing soda (sodium carbonate), household cleaners, iodine, silver nitrate, household bleaches, Clinitest® tablets (tend to be neutralized by gastric acid)

◊ Severity of injury dependent on contact time + concentration of corrosive material!

Associated with: injury to pharynx + stomach (7–8%): antral burns more common with acid (buffering effect of gastric acid on alkali)

Location: middle + lower thirds of esophagus

Stage I : acute necrosis from protein coagulation
√ mucosal blurring (edema)
√ diffusely atonic + dilated esophagus
√ tertiary contractions

Stage II : frank ulceration in 3–5 days
√ ulceration + pseudomembranes

Stage III: scarring + stricture from fibroblastic activity
√ long segmental stricture after 10 days when acute edema subsides (7–30%)

Cx: (1) Esophageal / gastric perforation during ulcerative stage
(2) Squamous cell carcinoma in injured segment

Chronic esophagitis

√ luminal narrowing with tapered transition to normal + proximal dilatation
√ circumferential / eccentric stricture
√ sacculations = pseudodiverticula

Cytomegalovirus esophagitis

Organism: member of herpesvirus group

Associated with: AIDS

- severe odynophagia

√ diffusely normal mucosal background
√ one / more **large ovoid flat ulcers** (up to several cm in size) near gastroesophageal junction
√ discrete small superficial ulcers indistinguishable from herpes esophagitis (uncommon)

Rx: ganciclovir (relatively toxic)

Dx: endoscopic brushings, biopsy specimen, cultures

Drug-induced esophagitis

Agents: tetracycline, doxycycline, potassium chloride, quinidine, aspirin, ascorbic acid, alprenolol chloride, emepronium bromide

- severe odynophagia
- history of taking medication with little / no water immediately before going to bed

Location: midesophagus at site of compression by aortic arch / left mainstem bronchus
√ superficial solitary / several discrete / localized clusters of tiny ulcers distributed circumferentially
√ dramatic healing of lesion 7–10 days after withdrawal of offending agent
DDx: herpes esophagitis (less localized)

Herpes Esophagitis

◊ 2nd most common cause of opportunistic infection!
Organism: Herpes simplex virus type I (DNA core virus) secreted in saliva of 2% of healthy population
Age: 15–30 years; usually males
- history of recent exposure to sexual partners with herpetic lesions on lips / buccal mucosa
- flulike prodrome of 3–10 days (headaches, fever, sore throat, upper respiratory symptoms, myalgia)
- severe acute dysphagia / odynophagia

May be associated with: oropharyngeal herpetic lesions / oropharyngeal candidiasis
Location: midesophagus (level of left main bronchus)
√ initially vesicles / blisters that subsequently rupture
√ **multiple small** discrete superficial punctate / linear / stellate (often "diamond shaped") **ulcers** surrounded by radiolucent halos of edematous mucosa
√ intervening mucosa normal (without plaques)
√ multiple plaquelike lesions (only with severe infection)
Rx: oral / intravenous acyclovir
Dx: rising serum titer for HSV type 1, viral culture, biopsy (immunofluorescent staining for HSV antigen, demonstration of intranuclear inclusions)
DDx: drug-induced esophagitis, Crohn disease, esophageal intramural pseudodiverticulosis

Human Immunodeficiency Virus Esophagitis

- maculopapular rash + ulcers of soft palate

√ one / more **giant flat** ovoid / diamond-shaped **ulcers** (at time of seroconversion) indistinguishable from CMV esophagitis
Dx: ONLY per exclusion
DDx: CMV esophagitis, mycobacterial esophagitis, actinomycosis, potassium chloride, quinidine, caustic ingestion, nasogastric intubation, radiation therapy, endoscopic sclerotherapy

Reflux Esophagitis

= esophageal inflammation secondary to reflux of acid-peptic contents of the stomach; reflux occurs if resting pressure of LES <5 mm Hg (may be normal event if followed by rapid clearing)
Histo: basal cell hyperplasia with wall thickening + thinning of epithelium, mucosal edema + erosions, inflammatory infiltrate
Determinants: (1) Frequency of reflux
(2) Adequacy of clearing mechanism
(3) Volume of refluxed material
(4) Potency of refluxed material
(5) Tissue resistance

Reflux preventing features:
(1) Lower esophageal sphincter
(2) Phrenoesophageal membrane
(3) Length of subdiaphragmatic esophagus
(4) Gastroesophageal angle of His (70–110°)

May be associated with: sliding hiatal hernia (in most patients), scleroderma, nasogastric intubation
- heartburn, epigastric discomfort
- choking, globus hystericus
- retrosternal pain
- thoracic / cervical dysphagia

Site: usually lower 1/3 / lower 1/2 with continuous disease extending proximally from GE junction
√ segmental esophageal narrowing (edema / spasm / stricture)
√ granular / finely nodular appearance of thickened longitudinal mucosal folds with poorly defined borders (mucosal edema + inflammation) in early stages
√ single marginal ulcer / erosion at or adjacent to gastroesophageal junction
√ multiple areas of superficial ulceration in distal esophagus
√ prominent mucosal fold ending in polypoid protuberance within hiatal hernia / cardia
√ interruption of primary peristalsis at inflamed segment
√ nonperistaltic waves in distal esophagus following deglutition (85%)
√ incomplete relaxation of LES (75%), incompetent sphincter (33%)
√ acid test = abnormal motility elicited by acid barium (pH 1.7)
√ "felinization" = transverse ridges of esophagus secondary to contraction of muscularis mucosae (similar to cat esophagus)
NUC (pertechnetate):
√ esophageal activity (Barrett esophagus similar to ectopic gastric mucosa)

Reflux tests:
1. Reflux of barium in RPO position, may be elicited by coughing / deep respiratory movements / swallowing of saliva + water / anteflexion in erect position: only in 50% accurate
2. Water-siphon test: in 5% false negative; large number of false positives
3. Tuttle test = measurement of esophageal pH: 96% accurate
4. Radionuclide gastroesophageal reflux test (typically combined with gastric emptying test):
   Technique: ROI drawn over distal esophagus + compared with time-activity curve over stomach, scaled to 4%
   √ esophageal activity >4% stomach activity

Cx of reflux:
(a) from acid + pepsin acting on esophageal mucosa:
1. Motility disturbance
2. Stricture

3. Schatzki ring
4. Barrett esophagus
5. Iron-deficiency anemia
6. Reflux / peptic esophagitis

(b) from aspiration of gastric contents
1. Acute aspiration pneumonia
2. Mendelson syndrome
3. Pulmonary fibrosis

Viral esophagitis

Predisposed: immunocompromised, eg, underlying malignancy, debilitating illness, radiation treatment, steroids, chemotherapy, AIDS

FAMILIAL ADENOMATOUS POLYPOSIS

= FAMILIAL MULTIPLE POLYPOSIS = autosomal dominant disease with 80% penetrance (gene for familial polyposis localized on chromosome 5); sporadic occurrence in 1/3

Incidence: 1:7,000 to 1:24,000 livebirths

Histo: tubular / villotubular adenomatous polyps; usually about 1,000 adenomas

Age: polyps appear around puberty

- family history of colonic polyps (66%)
  ◊ Screening of family members after puberty!
- clinical symptoms begin during 3rd–4th decade (range 5–55 years)
- vague abdominal pain, weight loss
- diarrhea, bloody stools
- protein-losing enteropathy (occasionally)

Associated with: (1) Hamartomas of stomach in 49%
(2) Adenomas of duodenum in 25%
(3) Periampullary carcinoma

√ "carpet of polyps" = myriad of 2–3 mm (up to 2 cm) polypoid lesions

@ Colon (100%): more numerous in distal colon; always affecting rectum
√ normal haustral pattern

@ Stomach (5%)

@ Small bowel (<5%)

Cx: malignant transformation: colon > stomach > small bowel (in 12% by 5 years; in 30% by 10 years; in 100% by 20 years after diagnosis; age at carcinomatous development usually 20–40 years; multiple carcinomas in 48%)
◊ Periampullary carcinoma is the most common cause of death after prophylactic colectomy!

Rx: prophylactic total colectomy in late teens / early twenties before symptoms develop +
(1) Permanent ileostomy
(2) Continent endorectal pull-through pouch
(3) Kock pouch (= distal ileum formed into a one-way valve by invaginating the bowel at skin site)

DDx: other polyposes, lymphoid hyperplasia, lymphosarcoma, ulcerative colitis with inflammatory pseudopolyps

GALLSTONE ILEUS

Incidence: 0.4–5% of all intestinal obstructions (20% of obstruction in patients >65 years; 24% of obstructions in patients >70 years); develops in <1% of patients with cholelithiasis; in 1 of 6 perforations; risk increases with age

Age: average 65–75 years; M:F = 1:4 –7

- previous history of gallbladder disease
- intermittent episodes of acute colicky abdominal pain (20–30%)
- nausea, vomiting, fever, distension, obstipation

√ **Rigler triad** on plain film:
1. Partial / complete intestinal obstruction (usually small bowel), "string of rosary beads" = multiple small amounts of air trapped between dilated + stretched valvulae conniventes (in 86%)
2. Gas in biliary tree (in 69%)
3. Ectopic calcified gallstone (in 25%): stones are commonly >2.5 cm in diameter

√ change in position of previously identified gallstone

UGI / BE:
√ well-contained localized barium collection lateral to first portion of duodenum (barium-filled collapsed GB + possibly biliary ducts)
Fistulous communication:
CHOLECYSTODUODENAL (60%), choledochoduodenal, cholecystocolic, choledochocolic, cholecystogastric
√ identification of site of obstruction: terminal ileum (60–70%), proximal ileum (25%), distal ileum (10%), pylorus, sigmoid, duodenum (Bouveret syndrome)

Cx: recurrent gallstone ileus in 5–10% (additional silent calculi more proximally)

Prognosis: high mortality

GANGLIOCYTIC PARAGANGLIOMA

= rare benign tumor of the GI tract

Frequency: <100 cases reported

Origin: pancreatic endocrine rest that remained when the ventral primordium rotated around the duodenum

Age: 50–60 years of age; M:F = 2:1

Location: almost exclusively in 2nd portion of duodenum near the ampulla of Vater on the medial / lateral wall of duodenum

- GI hemorrhage, abdominal pain

√ polypoid smooth-surfaced intraluminal mass
√ homogeneously enhancing mural / extrinsic solid mass of soft-tissue attenuation
√ well-circumscribed hypoechoic mass contiguous with bowel
√ no biliary duct dilatation

DDx: adenocarcinoma (biliary duct dilatation, hypovascular), leiomyosarcoma (cystic internal hemorrhage / necrosis), hemangioma, duplication cyst, choledochal cyst, lipoma, hamartoma, inflammatory fibroid polyp (distal small bowel), lymphoma (isolated in stomach and ileum)

GARDNER SYNDROME

= autosomal dominant disease (? variant of familial polyposis) characterized by a triad of (1) colonic polyposis (2) osteomas (3) soft-tissue tumors

Histo: adenomatous polyps

Age: 15–30 years

Associated with: ? MEA complex
(1) periampullary / duodenal carcinoma (12%)
(2) thyroid carcinoma
(3) adrenal adenoma / carcinoma
(4) parathyroid adenoma
(5) pituitary chromophobe adenoma
(6) carcinoid, adenoma of small bowel
(7) retroperitoneal leiomyoma

• skin pigmentation

◊ Familial polyposis + Gardner syndrome may occur in the same family!

◊ Extraintestinal manifestations occur usually earlier than in intestinal polyposis!

@ Polyposis
Location: colon (100%), stomach (5–68%), duodenum (90%), small bowel (<5%)
√ multiple colonic polyps appearing during puberty, increasing in number during 3rd–4th decade
√ lymphoid hyperplasia of terminal ileum
√ hamartomas of stomach

@ Soft-tissue tumors
(a) sebaceous / epidermoid inclusion cysts (scalp, back, face, extremities)
(b) fibroma, lipoma, leiomyoma, neurofibroma
(c) desmoid tumors (3–29%); peritoneal adhesions (desmoplastic tendency); mesenteric fibrosis, retroperitoneal fibrosis, mammary fibromatosis, marked keloid formation, hypertrophied scars (anterior abdominal wall) arise 1–3 years after surgery
• GI / urinary tract obstruction

@ Osteomatosis of membranous bone (50%)
Location: calvarium, mandible (81%), maxilla, ribs, long bones

@ Long bones
√ localized wavy cortical thickening / exostoses
√ slight shortening + bowing

@ Teeth
√ odontoma, unerupted supernumerary teeth, hypercementosis
√ tendency toward numerous caries (dental prosthesis at early age)

Cx: malignant transformation in 100% (average age at death is 41 years if untreated)

Rx: prophylactic total colectomy at about 20 years of age

GASTRIC CARCINOMA

3rd most common GI malignancy after colorectal + pancreatic cancer, 6th leading cause of cancer deaths

Prevalence: declining; 24,000 cases/year in USA

Risk factors: smoking, nitrites, nitrates, pickled vegetables

Predisposed: pernicious anemia (risk factor of 2), chronic atrophic gastritis, adenomatous + villous polyp (7–27% are malignant), gastrojejunostomy, Billroth II > Billroth I

Histo: adenocarcinoma (95%); rarely squamous cell carcinoma / adenoacanthoma

Staging:
T1 tumor limited to mucosa / submucosa
T2 tumor involves muscle / serosa
T3 tumor penetrates through serosa
T4a invasion of adjacent contiguous tissues
T4b invasion of adjacent organs, diaphragm, abdominal wall
N1 involvement of perigastric nodes within 3 cm of primary along greater / lesser curvature
N2 involvement of regional nodes >3 cm from primary along branches of celiac axis
N3 paraaortic, hepatoduodenal, retropancreatic, mesenteric nodes
M1 distant metastases

Location: mostly distal third of stomach + cardia; 60% on lesser curvature, 10% on greater curvature; esophagogastric junction in 30%

Probability of malignancy of an ulcer: at lesser curvature 10–15%, at greater curvature 70%, in fundus 90%

Morphology:
1. Polypoid / fungating carcinoma
2. Ulcerating / penetrating carcinoma (70%)
3. Infiltrating / scirrhous carcinoma (5–15%)
   = linitis plastica
   Histo: frequently signet ring cell type + increase in fibrous tissue
   Location: antrum, fundus + body (38%)
   √ firmness, rigidity, reduced capacity of stomach, aperistalsis in involved area
   √ granular / polypoid folds with encircling growth
4. Superficial spreading carcinoma
   = confined to mucosa / submucosa; 5-year survival of 90%
   √ patch of nodularity
   √ little loss of elasticity
5. Advanced bulky carcinoma

• GI bleeding, abdominal pain, weight loss

UGI:
√ rigidity
√ filling defect
√ amputation of folds ± ulceration ± stenosis
√ calcifications (mucinous adenocarcinoma)

CT:
√ irregular nodular luminal surface
√ asymmetric thickening of folds
√ mass of uniform density / varying attenuation
√ wall thickness >6 mm with gas distension + 13 mm with positive contrast material distension

GI

Prognostic Parameters of Gastric Carcinoma

Tumor Size	Metastases	Limited to Submucosa	5-Year Survival Rate
1 cm	11%		87%
2 cm	25%	70%	67%
3 cm	45%		35%
4 cm	59%	60%	33%
>4 cm	72%	33%	

√ increased density in perigastric fat
√ enhancement exclusively in linitis plastica type
√ nodules of serosal surface (= dilated surface lymphatics)
√ diameter of esophagus at gastroesophageal junction larger than adjacent aorta (DDx: hiatal hernia)
√ lymphadenopathy below level of renal pedicle (3%)

Metastases:

1. along peritoneal ligaments
   (a) gastrocolic lig.: transverse colon, pancreas
   (b) gastrohepatic + hepatoduodenal lig.: liver
2. local lymph nodes
3. hematogenous: liver (most common), adrenals, ovaries, bone (1.8%), lymphangitic carcinomatosis of lung (rare)
4. peritoneal seeding:
   on rectal wall = Blumer shelf
   on ovaries = Krukenberg tumor
5. left supraclavicular lymph node = Virchow node

Prognosis:
overall 5-year survival rate of 5–18%, mean survival time of 7–8 months;
— 85% 5-year survival in stage T1
— 52% 5-year survival in stage T2
— 47% 5-year survival in stage T3
— 17% 5-year survival in stage N1-2
— 5% 5-year survival in stage N3

Early Gastric Cancer (20%)

= invasion limited to mucosa + submucosa (T1 lesion)
Classification of Japan Research Society for Gastric Cancer:

Type I Protruded type = >0.5 cm height with protrusion into gastric lumen (10–20%)
Type II Superficial type = <0.5 cm height
IIa slightly elevated surface (10–20%)
IIb flat / almost unrecognizable (2%)
IIc slightly depressed surface (50–60%)
Type III Excavated type (5–10%)

Advanced Gastric Cancer (T_2 lesion and higher)

Bormann classification:
Type 1 broad-based elevated polypoid lesion
Type 2 elevated lesion + ulceration + well-demarcated margin
Type 3 elevated lesion + ulceration + ill-defined margin
Type 4 ill-defined flat lesion
Type 5 unclassified, no apparent elevation

GASTRIC DIVERTICULUM

stomach is least common site of diverticula
Incidence: 1:600–2,400 of UGI studies
Etiology: (a) traction secondary to scarring / periantral inflammation = true diverticulum
(b) pulsion (less common) = false diverticulum
Age: beyond 40 years
Often associated with: aberrant pancreas in antral location
Location: juxtacardiac on posterior wall (75%), prepyloric (15–22%), greater curve (3%)
√ pliability + varying degrees of distension
√ NO mass, edema or rigidity of adjacent folds

DDx: small ulcer in intramural-extramucosal mass

GASTRIC POLYP

Incidence: 1.5–5%, most common benign gastric tumor

Associated with: hyperacidity + ulcers, chronic atrophic gastritis, gastric carcinoma

A. NONNEOPLASTIC
1. INFLAMMATORY POLYP (75–90%)
   = HYPERPLASTIC POLYP = REGENERATIVE POLYP
   Histo: cystically dilated glands lined by gastric epithelium + acute and chronic inflammatory infiltrates in lamina propria
   Associated with: chronic atrophic gastritis, pernicious anemia
   Location: random distribution within stomach; usually multiple
   √ sharply delineated polyp with smooth circular border
   √ "Mexican hat sign" = stalk seen en face overlying the head of polyp
   √ sessile / pedunculated
   √ usually <2 cm in diameter without progression
   √ no contour defect of stomach
   Prognosis: no malignant potential
2. HAMARTOMATOUS POLYP (rare)
   Histo: densely packed gastric glands + bundles of smooth muscle
   Associated with: Peutz-Jeghers syndrome
   √ sessile / pedunculated
   √ usually <2 cm in diameter
3. RETENTION POLYP (rare)
   Histo: dilated cystic glands + stroma
   Associated with: Cronkhite-Canada syndrome

GI

B. NEOPLASTIC

1. ADENOMATOUS POLYP (10–20%)
   = true neoplasm with malignant potential (10–80%, increasing with size)
   Age: increasing incidence with age; M:F = 2:1
   Histo: intestinal metaplasia (common) + marked cellular atypism
   Associated with: Gardner syndrome; coexistent with gastric carcinoma in 35%
   Location: more commonly in antrum (antrum spared in Gardner syndrome)
   √ broad-based elliptical / mushroom-shaped ± pedicle; often single
   √ usually >2 cm in diameter (in 80%)
   √ smooth / irregular lobulated contour
2. VILLOUS POLYP (rare)
   √ trabeculated / lobulated slightly irregular contour
   Cx: malignant transformation

DDx: (1) Ménétrièr disease (antrum spared)
(2) Eosinophilic polyp (peripheral eosinophilia, linitis plastica appearance, small bowel changes)
(3) Lymphoma
(4) Carcinoma

GASTRIC ULCER

Benign Gastric Ulcer

95% of all gastric ulcers

Cause:

1. Stress
2. Burns = curling ulcer
3. Cerebral disease = Cushing ulcer
4. Uremia
5. Severe prolonged illness
6. Gastritis
7. Steroid therapy
8. Intubation
9. Stasis ulcer proximal to pyloric / duodenal obstruction
10. HPT (25% with ulcer disease)

Pathophysiology:
disrupted mucosal barrier (Helicobacter pylori) with vulnerability to acid + secretion of large volume of gastric juice containing little acid

Incidence: 5:10,000; 100,000/year (United States)
Age peak: 55–65 years; M:F = 1:1
Multiplicity:
(a) multiple in 2–8% (17–24% at autopsy), especially in patients on Aspirin®
(b) coexistent duodenal ulcer in 5–64%; gastric:duodenal = 1:3 (adults) = 1:7 (children)

• abdominal pain: in 30% at night, in 25% precipitated by food

Location: lesser curvature at junction of corpus + antrum within 7 cm from pylorus; proximal half of stomach in older patients (geriatric ulcer); adjacent to GE junction within hiatal hernia

√ ulcer size usually <2 cm (range 1–250 mm); in 4% >40 mm
√ Haudek niche = conical / collar button-shaped barium collection projecting outside gastric contour (profile view)
√ Hampton line = 1-mm thin straight lucent line traversing the orifice of the ulcer niche (seen on profile view + with little gastric distension) = ledge of touching overhanging gastric mucosa of undermined benign ulcer
√ ulcer collar = smooth thick lucent band interposed between the niche and gastric lumen (thickened rim of edematous gastric wall) in well-distended stomach
√ ulcer mound = smooth, sharply delineated, gently sloping extensive tissue mass surrounding a benign ulcer (edema + lack of wall distensibility) in well-distended stomach
√ ulcer crater = round / oval barium collection with smooth border on dependent side (en face view)
√ halo defect = wide lucent band symmetrically surrounding ulcer resembling extensive ulcer mound (viewed en face)
√ ring shadow: ulcer on nondependent side (en face view)
√ radiating thick folds extending directly to crater edge fusing with the effaced marginal fold of the ulcer collar / halo of ulcer mound
√ incisura defect = smooth, deep, narrow, sharp indentation on greater curvature opposite a niche on lesser curvature at / slightly below the level of the ulcer (spastic contraction of circular muscle fibers)

Prognosis: healing in 50% by 3 weeks, in 100% by 6–8 weeks; slower healing in older patients; only complete healing proves benignancy
Cx: bleeding, perforation

Malignant Gastric Ulcer

Incidence: 5% of ulcers are malignant
Prognosis: partial healing may occur
Location: anywhere within stomach; fundal ulcers above level of cardia are usually malignant

√ ulcer location within gastric lumen, ie, not projecting beyond expected margin of stomach (profile view)
√ eccentrically located ulcer within the tumor
√ irregularly shaped ulcer
√ shallow ulcer with width greater than depth
√ nodular ulcer floor
√ abrupt transition between normal mucosa + abnormal tissue at some distance (usually 2–4 cm) from ulcer edge
√ rolled / rounded / shouldered edges surrounding ulcer
√ nodular irregular folds approaching ulcer with fused / clubbed / amputated tips
√ rigidity / lack of distensibility
√ associated large irregular mass
√ **Carman meniscus sign** = curvilinear lens-shaped intraluminal form of crater with convexity of crescent toward gastric wall and concavity toward gastric lumen (profile view, usually under compression) found in specific type of ulcerating carcinoma, seen only infrequently; wall aspect can also be concave / flat

GI

√ **Kirklin meniscus complex** = Carman sign (appearance of crater) + radiolucent slightly elevated rolled border

GASTRIC VARICES

Cause: portal hypertension (varices seen in 2–78%)
Location: (a) esophagogastric junction (most common)
(b) along lesser curvature (in 11–75% of patients with portal hypertension / cirrhosis)
Feeding vessels:
1. Left gastric vein (between splenic vein + stomach)
2. Short gastric veins (between spleen + fundus)
3. Retrogastric vein (between splenic vein + esophagogastric junction)

• increased prevalence of portosystemic encephalopathy
√ barium study: 65–89% rate of detection
√ endoscopy: most practical method
√ splenic portography
√ hepatofugal blood flow along SMV into left gastric + splenic vein
Cx: variceal bleeding in 3–10–36%
◊ Gastric varices bleed less frequently but more severely than esophageal varices!

GASTRIC VOLVULUS

= abnormal degree of rotation of one part of stomach around another part, usually requires >180° twisting to produce complete obstruction
Etiology: (a) abnormality of suspensory ligaments (hepatic, splenic, colic, phrenic)
(b) unusually long gastrohepatic + gastrocolic mesenteries
Usually associated with: diaphragmatic abnormality:
1. Paraesophageal hiatus hernia in 33%
2. Eventration

Types:
A. ORGANOAXIAL VOLVULUS
rotation around a line extending from cardia to pylorus
B. MESENTEROAXIAL VOLVULUS
rotation around an axis extending from lesser to greater curvature

• severe epigastric pain
• vigorous attempts to vomit without results
• inability to pass tube into stomach
√ massively distended stomach in LUQ extending into chest
√ incomplete / absent entrance of barium into stomach
√ barium demonstrates area of twist
Cx: intramural emphysema, perforation
DDx: gastric atony, acute gastric dilatation, pyloric obstruction

GASTRITIS

Corrosive Gastritis

Agents:
(a) acid, formaldehyde
• clinically usually silent
Location: esophagus usually unharmed, severe gastric damage, duodenum may be involved (newer potent materials cause atypical distribution)
(b) alkaline
Location: pylorus + antrum most frequently involved

A. ACUTE CHANGES (edema + mucosal sloughing)
√ marked enlargement of gastric rugae + erosions / ulceration
√ complete cessation of motor activity
√ gas in portal venous system
Cx: perforation
B. CHRONIC CHANGES
√ firm thick nonpliable wall
√ stenotic / incontinent pylorus (if involved)
√ gastric outlet obstruction (cicatrization) after 3–10 weeks

Emphysematous Gastritis

= rare but severe form of widespread phlegmonous gastritis subsequent to mucosal disruption characterized by gas in wall of stomach
Cause of mucosal disruption:
ingestion of toxic / corrosive substances (most common), alcohol abuse, trauma, gastric infarction, necrotizing enterocolitis, ulcer
Histo: bacterial invasion of submucosa + subserosa
Organism: hemolytic streptococcus, Clostridium welchii, E. coli, S. aureus
• explosive onset of abdominal pain, nausea, chills, fever, leukocytosis
• bloody foul-smelling emesis
√ linear small gas bubbles within grossly thickened gastric wall
√ may be associated with gas in portal vein
Cx: cicatricial stenosis / sinus tract formation
Prognosis: 60–80% mortality

Erosive Gastritis

= HEMORRHAGIC GASTRITIS
Incidence: 0.5–10% of GI studies
Etiology (in 50% without causative factors):
(1) Peptic disease: emotional stress, alcohol, acid, corrosives, severe burns, anti-inflammatory agents (aspirin, steroids, phenylbutazone, indomethacin)
(2) Infection: herpes simplex virus, CMV, Candida
(3) Crohn disease: aphthoid ulcers identical in appearance to varioliform erosions
Histo: epithelial defect not penetrating beyond muscularis mucosae
• 10–20% of all GI hemorrhages (usually without significant blood loss)
• vague dyspepsia, ulcerlike symptoms
Location: antrum, rarely extending into fundus; aligned on surface of gastric rugal folds

GI

√ varioliform erosion = tiny fleck of barium surrounded by radiolucent halo ("target lesion") <5 mm, usually multiple
√ incomplete erosion = linear streaks / dots of barium without surrounding mound of edema / inflammation
√ nodularity / scalloping of prominent antral folds
√ contiguous duodenal disease may be present
√ limited distensibility, poor peristalsis / atony, delayed gastric emptying

Phlegmonous Gastritis

Etiology: septicemia, local abscess, postoperative stomach, complication of gastric ulcer / cancer
Organism: Streptococcus
Path: multiple gastric wall abscesses, which may communicate with lumen
- severe fulminating illness
- patient may vomit pus

Location: usually limited to stomach not extending beyond pylorus; submucosa is the most severely affected gastric layer
√ barium dissection into submucosa + serosa

GIARDIASIS

= overgrowth of commensal parasite Giardia lamblia
Organism:
Giardia lamblia (flagellated protozoan); often harmless contaminant of duodenum + jejunum in motile form (= trophozoite) attached to mucosa by suction disk, nonmotile form (= cyst) shed in feces; capable of pathogenic behavior with invasion of gut wall
Incidence: 1.5–2% of population in United States, infests 4–16% of inhabitants of tropical countries, found in 3–20% of children in parts of southern United States
Predisposed: altered immune mechanism (dysgammaglobulinemia, nodular lymphoid hyperplasia of ileum)
Histo: blunted villi (may be misdiagnosed as celiac disease especially in children), cellular infiltrate of acute + chronic inflammation in lamina propria
- abdominal pain, weight loss, failure to thrive (especially in children)
- spectrum from asymptomatic to severe debilitating diarrhea, steatorrhea (related to number of organisms)
- reduced fat absorption (simulating celiac disease)

Location: most pronounced in duodenum + jejunum

√ thickened distorted mucosal folds in duodenum + jejunum (mucosal edema) with normal ileum
√ marked spasm + irritability with rapid change in direction + configuration of folds
√ hypersecretion with blurring + indistinctness of folds
√ hyperperistalsis with rapid transit time
√ segmentation of barium (from motility disturbance + excess intraluminal fluid)
√ ± lymphoid hyperplasia (associated with immunoglobulin deficiency state)

Dx: (1) Detection of Giardia lamblia cysts in formed feces or trophozoites in diarrheal stools
(2) Trophozoites in duodenal aspirate / jejunal biopsy
DDx: Strongyloides / hookworm infection
Rx: quinacrine (Atabrine®)

GLYCOGEN ACANTHOSIS

= benign degenerative condition with accumulation of cellular glycogen within squamous epithelial lining of esophagus; etiology unknown
Incidence: in up to 15% of endoscoped patients
Age: middle-aged / elderly individuals
Histo: hyperplasia + hypertrophy of squamous mucosal cells secondary to increased glycogen; no malignant potential
- asymptomatic
- white oval mucosal plaques of 2–15 mm in diameter on otherwise normal appearing mucosa

Location: middle (common) / distal esophagus
√ multiple 1–3 mm rounded nodules / plaques
Dx: biopsy
DDx: Candida esophagitis (lesions disappear under treatment in contrast to glycogen acanthosis)

GRAFT-VERSUS-HOST DISEASE

= T lymphocytes from donor bone marrow cause selected epithelial damage of recipient target organs
Bone marrow transplantation for treatment of:
leukemia, lymphoma, aplastic anemia, immunologic deficit, metabolic disorders of hematopoietic system, some metastatic disease
Incidence: 30–70% of patients with allogeneic (= donor genetically different from host) transplant
Target organs: GI tract (small bowel), skin, liver

@ Skin
- maculopapular rash on face, trunk, extremities

@ Liver
- elevation of hepatic enzymes ± liver failure

@ GI tract
- profuse secretory diarrhea
- abdominal cramping, fever, nausea, vomiting

Path: severe mucosal atrophy / destruction
√ shaggy fold thickening
√ "ribbon bowel" = small bowel fold effacement with tubular appearance (DDx: viral enteritis, ischemia, celiac disease, radiation, soybean allergy)
√ loss of haustration, spasm, edema, ulceration, granular mucosal pattern of colon (simulating ulcerative colitis)
√ small bowel "cast" = prolonged coating of abnormal bowel for hours to days
√ circular collections of contrast material on cross section + parallel tracks on longitudinal section
√ severely decreased transit time
CT:
√ abnormally enhancing thin layer of mucosa diffusely involving small + large bowel

GI

√ fluid-filled distended poorly opacified bowel (oral contrast material not given!)

Cx: infection with opportunistic organisms, eg, Candida albicans, herpes virus, invasive fungal organisms, CMV, varicella-zoster virus, Epstein-Barr virus, hepatitis viruses, rotavirus, adenovirus, Coxsackie virus A and B, P. carinii, pneumococcus

Prognosis: fatal in up to 15% (due to opportunistic infections)

Rx: steroids + cyclosporine

DDx: superinfection with enteroviruses

HELICOBACTER PYLORI INFECTION

Organism: worldwide gram-negative spiral-shaped bacillus [formerly Campylobacter pylori]

Prevalence: increasing with age; >50% of Americans >60 years of age

Path: surface epithelial damage + inflammation with mucosal infiltration by neutrophils, plasma cells, and lymphoid nodules

Location: gastric antrum > proximal half of stomach

Site: beneath mucus layer on surface epithelial cells

- asymptomatic (vast majority)
- dyspepsia, epigastric pain

√ gastritis
- √ thickened gastric folds
- √ polypoid gastritis mimicking malignant tumor
- √ enlarged areae gastricae

√ gastric ulcer (60–80% prevalence of H. pylori)

√ duodenal ulcer (90–100% prevalence of H. pylori)

Dx: (1) Endoscopic brushings + biopsy
(2) Breath test measuring urease activity after ingestion of carbon-14–labeled urea
(3) Serologic test for IgG antibodies

Rx: triple therapy (= bismuth + metronidazole + tetracycline / amoxicillin) results in 95% cure rate after 2 weeks of therapy

HEMANGIOMA OF SMALL BOWEL

Increased incidence in: Turner syndrome, tuberous sclerosis, Osler-Weber-Rendu disease

Location: duodenum (2%), jejunum (55%), ileum (42%)

√ multiple sessile compressible intraluminal filling defects

√ nodular segmental mucosal abnormality

√ phleboliths in intestinal wall

HENOCH-SCHÖNLEIN PURPURA

= most common systemic allergic vasculitis in children precipitated by bacterial / viral infection, allergies, insect sting, drugs (eg, penicillin, sulfonamides, aspirin)

Cause: deposition of IgA-dominant immune complexes in venules, capillaries, and arterioles

Age: children (peak age of 5 years) + adults

- most frequent manifestations:
  - purpuric skin rash on legs + extensor surfaces on arms
  - colicky abdominal pain + GI bleeding
  - microscopic hematuria + proteinuria in 50% (from proliferative glomerulonephritis with IgA deposits demonstrated by immunofluorescence)
- often begins as an upper respiratory tract infection
- arthralgias

√ thickened valvulae conniventes (due to hemorrhage + edema)

Cx: renal insufficiency (10–20%), end-stage renal disease (5%)

Rx: high doses of corticosteroids + azathioprine

HERNIA

External Hernia

= bowel extending outside the abdominal cavity

Incidence: 95% of all hernias

Location:

1. Inguinal hernia
2. Femoral hernia
3. **Spigelian hernia**
   Frequency: 2% of anterior abdominal hernias
   = acquired ventrolateral hernia through defect in aponeurosis between transverse and rectus muscle of abdomen at junction of semilunar + arcuate lines below umbilicus
   √ hernia sac dissects laterally to rectus abdominis muscle through a fibrous groove (= semicircular / spigelian line)
   √ hernia sac lies beneath an intact external oblique aponeurosis
4. Petit lumbar triangle
5. Obturator foramen
6. Sciatic notch
7. Diaphragmatic hernia (foramen of Bochdalek + Morgagni)
8. Richter hernia = entrapment of antimesenteric border of bowel in hernia orifice, usually seen in older women with femoral hernias
9. Perineal hernia (rare)
   (a) anterior perineal hernia = defect of urogenital diaphragm anterior to superficial transverse perineal m. + lateral to bulbocavernosus m. + medial to ischiocavernosus m. (only in females)
   (b) posterior perineal hernia = defect in levator ani m. / between levator ani m. and coccygeus m. posterior to superficial transverse perineal m.
   √ defecating proctography

Internal Hernia

Incidence: 5% of all hernias, responsible for <1% of mechanical small bowel obstruction

Classification of hernias:

(a) retroperitoneal: usually congenital containing a hernial sac
1. paraduodenal (ligament of Treitz)
2. foramen of Winslow
3. intersigmoid
4. pericecal / ileocolic
5. supravesical

GI

(b) anteperitoneal:
small group of hernias without a peritoneal sac
1. transmesenteric (transverse / sigmoid mesocolon)
2. transomental
3. pelvic (including broad ligament)

A. PARADUODENAL HERNIA (53%)
(a) through fossa of Landzert on left side (3/4)
√ lateral to 4th portion of duodenum and behind descending + transverse mesocolon
(b) through fossa of Waldeyer on right side (1/4)
√ caudal to SMA and inferior to 3rd portion of duodenum

B. LESSER SAC HERNIA (<10%)
through foramen of Winslow in retrogastric location
Invaginated gut:
ileum > jejunum, cecum, appendix, ascending colon, Meckel diverticulum, gallbladder, greater omentum

C. HERNIA THROUGH BROAD LIGAMENT (very rare)
after laceration / fenestration from surgery or during pregnancy

Hiatal Hernia

Associated with: diverticulosis (25%), reflux esophagitis (25%), duodenal ulcer (20%), gallstones (18%)

Sliding Hiatal Hernia (99%)

= AXIAL HERNIA = CONCENTRIC HERNIA
= esophagogastric junction remains in chest with portion of peritoneal sac forming part of wall of hernia

Etiology: rupture of phrenicoesophageal membrane due to repetitive stretching with swallowing
Incidence: increasing with age

√ reducible in erect position
√ epiphrenic bulge = entire vestibule + sleeve of stomach are intrathoracic
√ distance between B ring (if visible) and hiatal margin >2 cm
√ peristalsis ceases above hiatus (end of peristaltic wave delineates esophagogastric junction)
√ tortuous esophagus having an eccentric junction with hernia
√ numerous coarse thick gastric folds within suprahiatal pouch (>6 longitudinal folds)
√ ± gastroesophageal reflux

CT:
√ dehiscence of diaphragmatic crura >15 mm
√ pseudomass within / above esophageal hiatus
√ increase in fat surrounding distal esophagus (= herniation of omentum through phrenicoesophageal ligament)

DDx: normal temporary cephalad motion of esophagogastric junction by 1–2 cm into chest due to contraction of longitudinal muscle during esophageal peristalsis

Paraesophageal Hernia (1%)

= ROLLING HIATAL HERNIA = PARAHIATAL HERNIA = portion of stomach superiorly displaced into thorax with esophagogastric junction remaining in subdiaphragmatic position

√ cardia in normal position
√ herniation of portion of stomach anterior to esophagus
√ frequently nonreducible
√ may be associated with gastric ulcer of lesser curvature at level of diaphragmatic hiatus

Totally Intrathoracic Stomach

= defect in central tendon of diaphragm in combination with slight volvulus in transverse axis of stomach behind heart

√ cardia may be intrathoracic (usually) / subdiaphragmatic
√ great gastric curvature either on right / left side

Congenitally Short Esophagus

(not true hernia, very rare)
= gastric ectopy by lack of lengthening of esophagus

√ nonreducible intrathoracic gastric segment (in erect / supine position)
√ cylindrical / round intrathoracic segment with large sinuous folds
√ short straight esophagus
√ circular narrowing at gastroesophageal junction, frequently with ulcer
√ gastroesophageal reflux

Umbilical Hernia

= protrusion of abdominal contents / fat into anterior abdominal wall via umbilical ring

Prevalence: 4% of all hernias; M<F
Cause: failed closure of umbilical ring, obesity, multiple pregnancies, intra-abdominal masses, liver failure, increased intra-abdominal pressure, weak abdominal wall

√ may contain fat / small bowel / colon
√ herniation of antimesenteric border of intestine (Richter hernia)
√ Meckel diverticulum in hernial sac (Littré hernia)

Cx: strangulation, incarceration
DDx: paraumbilical, spigelian, epigastric, incisional hernia

HIRSCHSPRUNG DISEASE

= AGANGLIONOSIS OF THE COLON = AGANGLIONIC MEGACOLON
= absence of parasympathetic ganglia in muscle (Meissner plexus) + submucosal layers (Auerbach plexus) secondary to an arrest of craniocaudal migration of neuroblasts along vagal trunks before 12th week leading to relaxation failure of the aganglionic segment

Incidence: 1:5,000–8,000 livebirths; usually sporadic; familial in 4%
Age: full-term infant during first 6 weeks of life (70–80%); M:F = 4–9:1; extremely rare in premature infants

GI

Associated with: trisomy 21 (2%)
Location: at varying distances proximal to anus, usually rectosigmoid
(a) short segment disease .... (80%)
(b) long segment disease .... (15%)
(c) total colonic aganglionosis .... (5%)
(d) skip aganglionosis = sparing of rectum (very rare)

- failure to pass meconium within first 24 hours of life
- intermittent constipation + paradoxical diarrhea (25%)
- rectal manometry with absence of spike activity

√ "transition zone" = aganglionic segment appears normal in size
√ dilatation of large + small bowel aborally from transition zone
√ marked retention of barium on delayed films after 24 hours
√ normal-appearing rectum in 33%
√ 10- to 15-cm segment of persistent corrugated / convoluted rectum (= abnormal uncoordinated contractions of the aganglionic portion of colon) in 31% (DDx: colitis, milk allergy, normal intermittent spasm of rectum)

N.B.: avoid digital exam / cleansing enema prior to radiographic studies!

OB-US:
√ dilated small bowel / dilated colon

Cx: (1) Necrotizing enterocolitis
(2) Cecal perforation (secondary to stasis, distension, ischemia)
(3) Obstructive uropathy

Dx: suction mucosal biopsy of rectum (increased acetylcholinesterase activity)

Rx: (1) Swenson pull-through procedure
(2) Duhamel operation
(3) Soave procedure

HODGKIN DISEASE

Incidence: 0.75% of all cancers diagnosed each year
Age: bimodal peaks at age 25–30 years and 75–80 years
Histo: Reed-Sternberg cell = binucleate cell with prominent centrally located nucleolus

(1) Lymphocyte predominance (5%)
= abundance of normal-appearing lymphocytes + relative paucity of abnormal cells; often diagnosed in younger people; frequently early stage; systemic symptoms are uncommon; most favorable natural history

(2) Nodular sclerosis (78%)
= lymph nodes traversed by broad bands of birefringent collagen separating nodules, which consist of normal lymphocytes, eosinophils, plasma cells, and histiocytes; most common subtype; typically mediastinal involvement; 1/3 with systemic symptoms

(3) Mixed cellularity (17%)
= diffuse effacement of lymph nodes with lymphocytes, eosinophils, plasma cells + relative abundance of atypical mononuclear and Reed-Sternberg cells; more commonly advanced stage at presentation and older age

(4) Lymphocyte depletion (1%)
= paucity of normal-appearing lymphocytes + abundance of abnormal mononuclear and Reed-Sternberg cells; least common subtype with worst prognosis; associated with advanced stage and systemic symptoms

STAGE
I involvement of single lymph node region
II involvement of ≥ 2 lymph node regions on same side of diaphragm
III lymph node involvement on both sides of diaphragm
IV diffuse / disseminated involvement of ≥ 1 extralymphatic organs / tissues ± associated lymph node involvement
E = extralymphatic site
S = splenic involvement
A = absence of fever, night sweats, >10% weight loss in past 6 months
B = presence of fever, night sweats, >10% weight loss in past 6 months

- painless lymphadenopathy
- alcohol-induced pain
- unexplained fevers, night sweat, weight loss
- generalized pruritus

Location: intestinal involvement uncommon (10–15%); duodenum + jejunum (67%); terminal ileum (20%)
√ narrow rigid obstructive lesion
√ abundance of desmoplastic reaction (DDx from NHL)
√ infiltrating (60%); polypoid (26%); ulcerated (14%)
Prognosis: excellent for isolated / localized disease

HYPERPLASTIC POLYP OF COLON

= intestinal metaplasia consisting of mucous glands lined by a single layer of columnar epithelium; NO malignant potential
Path: infolding of epithelium into the glandular lumen
Location: rectum
√ usually <5 mm in diameter

HYPERTROPHIC PYLORIC STENOSIS

= idiopathic hypertrophy and hyperplasia of circular muscle fibers of pylorus with proximal extension into gastric antrum
Incidence: 3:1,000; M:F = 4–5:1
Etiology: inherited as a dominant polygenic trait; increased incidence in firstborn boys; acquired rather than congenital condition

Infantile Form Of Hypertrophic Pyloric Stenosis

Age: manifestation at 2–8 weeks of life

- nonbilious projectile vomiting (sour formula / clear gastric contents) with progression over a period of several weeks after birth (15–20%)
- positive family history

- palpable olive-shaped mass (80% sensitive in experienced hands, up to 14% false positive)
- nasogastric aspirate >10 mL (92% sensitive, 86% specific)

UGI (95% sensitivity):

Precautions: (1) empty stomach via nasogastric tube before study
(2) remove contrast at end of study

√ pyloric wall thickness >10 mm
√ elongation + narrowing of pyloric canal (2–4 cm in length)
√ "double / triple track sign" = crowding of mucosal folds in pyloric channel
√ "string sign" = passing of small barium streak through pyloric channel
√ Twining recess = "diamond sign" = transient triangular tentlike cleft / niche in midportion of pyloric canal with apex pointing inferiorly secondary to mucosal bulging between two separated hypertrophied muscle bundles on the greater curvature side within pyloric channel
√ "pyloric teat" = outpouching along lesser curvature due to disruption of antral peristalsis
√ "antral beaking" = mass impression upon antrum with streak of barium pointing toward pyloric channel
√ Kirklin sign = "mushroom sign" = indentation of base of bulb (in 50%)
√ gastric distension with fluid
√ active gastric hyperperistalsis
√ "caterpillar sign" = gastric hyperperistaltic waves

US:

√ "target sign" = hypoechoic ring of hypertrophied pyloric muscle around echogenic mucosa centrally on cross-section
√ "cervix sign" = indentation of muscle mass on fluid-filled antrum on longitudinal section
√ "antral nipple sign" = redundant pyloric channel mucosa protruding into gastric antrum
√ pyloric volume >1.4 cm^3 (= 1/4 Π x [maximum pyloric diameter]^2 x pyloric length); most criteria independent of contracted or relaxed state (33% false negative)
√ pyloric length (mm) + 3.64 x muscle thickness (mm) > 25
√ pyloric muscle wall thickness ≥3 mm

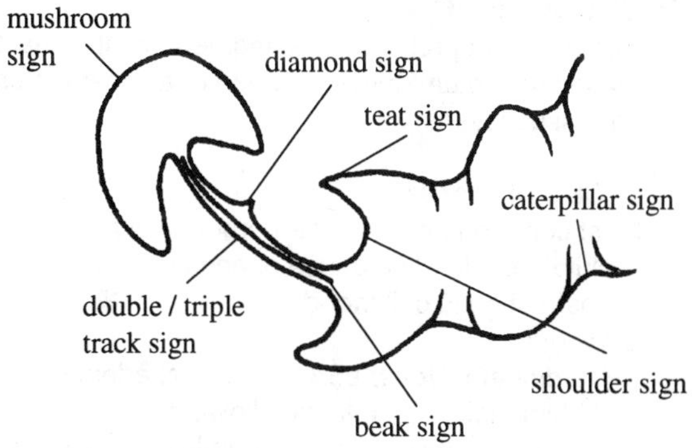

mushroom sign
diamond sign
teat sign
caterpillar sign
double / triple track sign
shoulder sign
beak sign

√ pyloric transverse diameter ≥13 mm with pyloric channel closed
√ elongated pyloric canal ≥17 mm in length
√ exaggerated peristaltic waves
√ delayed gastric emptying of fluid into duodenum

Cx: hypochloremic metabolic alkalosis

DDx:

1. **Infantile pylorospasm**
   √ muscle thickness between 1.5 and 3 mm
   √ variable caliber of antral narrowing
   √ antral peristalsis
   √ delayed gastric emptying
   √ elongation of pylorus
   Prognosis: resolves in several days / ? early stage of evolving pyloric stenosis
   Rx: effective with metoclopramide hydrochloride
2. Milk allergy
3. Eosinophilic gastroenteritis

Adult Form Of Hypertrophic Pyloric Stenosis

(secondary to mild infantile form)

- acute obstructive symptoms uncommon
- nausea, intermittent vomiting
- postprandial distress, heartburn

Associated with:
(1) peptic ulcer disease (in 50–74%) (prolonged gastrin production secondary to stasis of food)
(2) chronic gastritis (54%)

√ persistent elongation (2–4 cm) + concentric narrowing of pyloric channel
√ parallel + preserved mucosal folds
√ antispasmodics show no effect on narrowing
√ proximal benign ulcer (74%), usually near incisura

Focal Pyloric Hypertrophy

= TORUS HYPERPLASIA
= localized muscle hypertrophy on the lesser curvature
= milder atypical form of HPS
√ flattening of distal lesser curvature

IMPERFORATE ANUS

Prevalence: 1:5,000 live births

A. LOW ANOMALY (55%)
   = bowel has passed through levator sling
   - fistula to perineum / vulva

   Rx: readily reparable
B. INTERMEDIATE DEFECT (least common)
   = bowel ends within levator muscle as a result of abnormality in posterior migration of rectum
   - fistula opening low in vagina / vestibule

   Rx: 2- / 3-stage operation
C. HIGH ANOMALY
   = bowel ends above levator sling; M > F
   - fistulous connection to perineum / vagina / posterior urethra (air in bladder in males; air in vagina in females)

GI

Cx: associated malformations more common + more severe
Rx: multiple surgical procedures

√ distance between rectal air and skin will not accurately outline the extent of atretic rectum and anus (varying length during crying with increase in abdominal pressure + contraction of levator ani muscle)

US:
√ ≤15 mm distance between anal dimple + distal rectal pouch on transperineal images indicates low lesion

OB-US (earliest detection by 20–29 weeks GA):
• absent / low disaccharidase level in amniotic fluid
√ dilated colon in lower pelvis with U- / S-shaped configuration ± intraluminal calcifications
√ normal amniotic fluid (unless also TE fistula)
√ absence of anal characteristics (= hypoechoic circular rim with central echogenic stripe)

INTESTINAL LYMPHANGIECTASIA

A. CONGENITAL LYMPHANGIECTASIA = PRIMARY PROTEIN-LOSING ENTEROPATHY
= generalized congenital malformation of lymphatic system with atresia of the thoracic duct + gross dilatation of small bowel lymphatics; usually sporadic; may be inherited
Age: presentation before 30 years
• asymmetric generalized lymphedema (due to protein-losing enteropathy with hypoproteinemia)
• chylous pleural effusions (45%)
• diarrhea (60%), steatorrhea (20%)
• vomiting (15%)
• abdominal pain (15%) + distension
• decreased albumin + globulin
• lymphocytopenia (90%)
• decreased serum fibrinogen, transferrin, ceruloplasmin

B. ACQUIRED LYMPHANGIECTASIA
Causes leading to dilatation of intestinal lymphatics:
1. Mesenteric adenitis
2. Retroperitoneal fibrosis
3. Diffuse small bowel lymphoma
4. Pancreatitis
5. Pericardial effusion with obstruction of thoracic duct

• peripheral edema / anasarca (KEY SYMPTOM)
• chylous + serous effusion
• diarrhea, vomiting, abdominal pain, malabsorption, steatorrhea
• hypoproteinemia secondary to protein loss into intestinal lumen

Path: dilatation of lymph vessels in mucosa + submucosa + abundance of foamy fat-staining macrophages (negative for PAS)
√ diffuse symmetric marked enlargement of folds in jejunum + ileum (due to dilated intestinal lymphatics + hypoproteinemic edema)
√ slight separation + rigidity of folds
√ dilution of barium column (considerable increase in intestinal secretions from malabsorption)
√ no / mild dilatation of bowel

Lymphangiogram (not always diagnostic):
√ hypoplasia of lower extremity lymphatics
√ occlusion of thoracic duct / large tortuous thoracic duct
√ obstruction of cisterna chyli with backflow into mesenteric + intestinal lymphatics
√ hypoplastic lymph nodes

Dx: small bowel biopsy (dilated lymphatics in lamina propria + vascular core)
Rx: low-fat diet with medium-chain triglycerides (direct absorption into portal venous system)
DDx: (1) Whipple disease (more segmentation + fragmentation, wild folds)
(2) Amyloidosis (edema + secretions usually absent)
(3) Hypoalbuminemia (less pronounced symmetric thickening of folds, less prominent secretions)

INTRALUMINAL DUODENAL DIVERTICULUM

= congenital lesion secondary to elongation of an incomplete duodenal diaphragm
Age at presentation: in young adult
• easy satiety
• vomiting
• upper abdominal cramping pain

Location: 2nd–3rd portion of duodenum
√ barium-filled sac within duodenal lumen (pathognomonic picture) = "windsock, comma, teardrop" appearance
√ anchored to the lateral wall of the duodenum
√ "halo" sign = duodenal mucosa covers outer + inner wall of diverticulum

INTRAMURAL ESOPHAGEAL RUPTURE

= DISSECTING INTRAMURAL HEMATOMA
= mucosal tear with dissecting hemorrhage into submucosa and involvement of venous plexus
• hematemesis
√ intramural hematoma simulates retained solid material within lumen
√ "mucosal stripe sign" = dissected mucosa floating within lumen

INTUSSUSCEPTION

= invagination or prolapse of a segment of intestinal tract (= intussusceptum) into the lumen of adjacent intestine (= intussuscipiens)

A. IN CHILDREN (94%)
Most common abdominal emergency of early childhood, leading cause of acquired bowel obstruction in childhood
Etiology:
(1) idiopathic (over 95%): mucosal edema + lymphoid hyperplasia following viral gastroenteritis; predominantly at ileocecal valve

(2) lead point (5%): Meckel diverticulum (most common), lymphosarcoma, polyp, enterogenous cyst, duplication cyst, suture granuloma, appendiceal inflammation, Henoch-Schönlein purpura, inspissated meconium; usually >6 years of age

Age: peak incidence between 6 months and 2 years; 3–9 months (40%); <1 year (50%); <2 years (75%); >3 years (<10%); M:F = 2:1

- abrupt onset of violent crampy pain (90%), vomiting (85%)
- abdominal mass (60%)
- "currant jelly" bloody stools (60%)

Location: ileocolic (75–95%) > ileoileal (4%) > colocolic

Cx: vascular compromise secondary to incorporation of mesentery (hemorrhage, infarction, acute inflammation)

B. IN ADULTS (6%)

Etiology:

(1) specific cause (80%): benign tumor (1/3), malignant tumor (1/5), lipoma, Meckel diverticulum, prolapsed gastric mucosa, aberrant pancreas, adhesions, foreign body, feeding tube, chronic ulcer (TB, typhoid), prior gastroenteritis, gastroenterostomy, trauma

without anatomic lead point:
celiac disease, scleroderma, Whipple disease, fasting, anxiety, agonal state

(2) idiopathic (20%)

- recurrent episodes of colicky pain, nausea, vomiting

Location: ileoileal (40%) > ileocolic (13%)

Plain film (no abnormality in 25%):
√ abdominal soft-tissue mass (50–60%), usually in RUQ
√ loss of inferior hepatic margin
√ small bowel obstruction (25%) with nipplelike termination of gas shadow

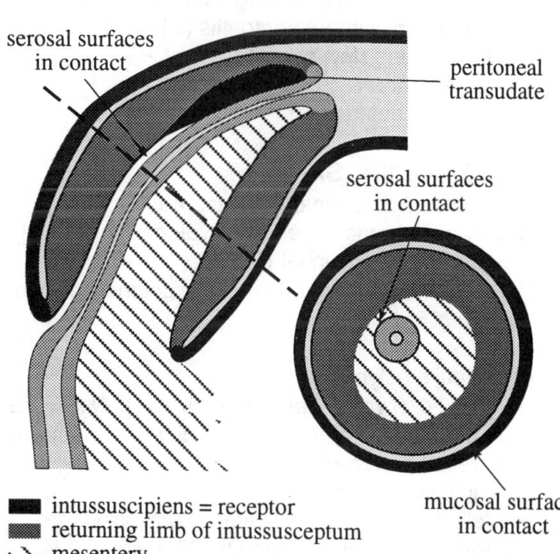

Antegrade barium study:
√ "coil spring" appearance
√ beaklike abrupt narrowing of barium column demonstrating a central channel

Retrograde barium study:
√ convex intracolic mass + "coiled spring" pattern

US (close to 100% sensitive):
√ "doughnut / target / bull's eye sign" (on transverse scan) = concentric rings of alternating hypoechoic + hyperechoic layers (= intussuscipiens) with central hyperechoic portion (= mesentery of intussusceptum)
√ "pseudokidney / sandwich / hay fork sign" (on longitudinal scan) = hypoechoic layers on each side of echogenic center of mesenteric fat
√ peritoneal fluid trapped inside intussusception (associated with irreducibility + ischemia)
√ color Doppler demonstrates mesenteric vessels dragged between entering + returning wall of intussusceptum
◊ Absence of blood flow suggests bowel necrosis!

CT:
√ "multiple concentric rings" = 3 concentric cylinders (central cylinder = canal + wall of intussusceptum; middle cylinder = crescent of mesenteric fat; outer cylinder = returning intussusceptum + intussuscipiens)
√ proximal obstruction

HYDROSTATIC / PNEUMATIC REDUCTION

◊ <1% mortality if reduction occurs <24 hours after onset!

Overall success rate: 70–85%

Contraindications: pneumoperitoneum, peritonitis, hypovolemic shock

Technique:

(1) Sedation with morphine sulfate (0.2 mg/kg IM) / fentanyl citrate IV (straining increases intraluminal pressure of distended colon)
(2) Anal seal with 24-F Foley catheter + balloon inflation to size equal to interpediculate distance of L5; balloon pulled down to levator sling; taped to buttocks; both buttocks firmly taped together
(3) 60% wt/vol barium sulfate with container between 24–36 inches above level of anus
(4) Maximally 3 attempts for 3 minutes each
(5) Manual manipulation increases colonic pressure
(6) Reduction should be accomplished within 10 minutes
(7) Extensive reflux into small bowel desirable to exclude residual ileoileal intussusception

"Rule of 3s":
(1) 3.5 feet (105 cm) above table (=120 mm Hg)
(2) 3 attempts
(3) 3 minutes between attempts (delay allows venous congestion + edema to subside)

Alternative medium:
(1) 1:4 Gastrografin®-water solution raised to a height of 5 feet (150 cm)
(2) air: delivers higher intracolonic pressures, faster, less fluoroscopic time, smaller tears, less contamination of peritoneal cavity

GI

Cx: perforation (0.4–2%; colonic bursting pressure ~200 mm Hg); reduction of nonviable bowel; incomplete reduction; missed lead point
Prognosis: 3.5–10% rate of recurrence

ISCHEMIC COLITIS

= nonocclusive vascular disease within the territory of the inferior mesenteric artery characterized by acute onset + rapid clinical and radiographic evolutionary changes

Etiology: diminished blood flow within bowel wall (mucosa + submucosa most sensitive to ischemia); major mesenteric vessels usually patent

Precipitating factors:
(a) bowel obstruction: volvulus, carcinoma (proximal bowel segment affected)
(b) thrombosis: cardiovascular disease, collagen vascular disease, sickle cell disease, hemolytic-uremic syndrome, oral contraceptives
(c) trauma: history of aortoiliac reconstruction (2%) with ligation of IMA

mnemonic: "VINTS"
Vasculitis
Incarceration (hernia, volvulus)
Nonocclusive ischemia (shock, CHF)
Thrombosis (atherosclerosis, emboli, polycythemia vera, hyperviscosity)
Spontaneous

Age: >50 years
• abrupt onset of lower abdominal pain + rectal bleeding
• abdominal tenderness, diarrhea

Location: left colon (90%), splenic flexure = Griffith point (80%) + sigmoid ("watershed areas"), rectum spared

Plain film (usually normal):
√ segmental thumbprinting = marginal indentations on mesenteric side (rare finding on plain film)

BE (in 90% abnormal):
◊ Single contrast may efface thumbprinting, but double contrast overall is more sensitive!
√ thumbprinting (75%) due to submucosal hemorrhage + edema
√ transverse ridging = markedly enlarged mucosal folds (spasm), some wall pliability is preserved
√ serrated mucosa = inflammatory edema + superficial longitudinal / circumferential ulceration
√ deep penetrating ulcers (late)

CT:
√ symmetric / lobulated segmental thickening of colonic wall
√ irregular narrowed atonic lumen (= thumbprinting)
√ curvilinear collection of intramural gas
√ portal + mesenteric venous air
√ blood clot in SMA / SMV

US:
√ absence / barely visible color flow
√ absence of arterial signals
√ nonstratified (= indistinct layers) thickened bowel wall >3 mm

Angio (findings similar to inflammatory disease):
√ normal / slightly attenuated arterial supply
√ mild acceleration of arteriovenous transit time
√ small tortuous ectatic draining veins

Prognosis:
(1) Transient ischemia = complete resolution within 1–3 months
(2) Stricturing ischemia = incomplete delayed healing
√ narrowed foldless segment of several cm in length with smooth tapering margins
(3) Gangrene with necrosis + perforation (extremely uncommon)

JEJUNOILEAL DIVERTICULAR DISEASE

= JEJUNAL DIVERTICULOSIS
= rarest form of gastrointestinal diverticular disease

Cause: acquired mucosal herniation (= pulsion diverticulum)
Incidence: 0.5–2.3% on UGI; 0.3–4.5% of autopsy series; M > F
Age: 6th–7th decades
Location: 80% in jejunum, 15% in ileum (usually solitary), 5% in jejunum + ileum
Site: on mesenteric border near entrance of vasa recti
• intermittent upper abdominal pain, flatulence, episodes of diarrhea (30%)

Plain film:
√ air-fluid levels in multiple diverticula
√ slight dilatation of intestinal loops in area of diverticula

BE:
√ may not fill (narrow neck / stagnant secretions)
√ trapped barium on delayed film after 24 hours

Cx:
(1) Blind loop syndrome with bacterial overgrowth
• steatorrhea, diarrhea, malabsorption, weight loss
• megaloblastic anemia (overgrowth of coliform bacteria leads to deconjugation of bile acids + intraluminal metabolism of vitamin B12)
(2) Free perforation = leading cause of pneumoperitoneum without peritonitis (21–40% mortality)
(3) Hemorrhage (few cases)
(4) Diverticulitis
(5) Intestinal obstruction

JUVENILE POLYPOSIS

= rare autosomal dominant disease with variable penetrance characterized by development of multiple (>5) juvenile polyps in GI tract
◊ Most common familial / nonfamilial colonic polyp in children (75%)!

Categories:
A. Juvenile polyposis of infancy
Age: 4–6 years (range 1–10 years); M:F = 3:2
• protein-losing enteropathy, diarrhea, hemorrhage
• rectal prolapse
√ intussusception
B. Colonic & generalized juvenile polyposis
Age: in 85% manifested by 20 years of age
• prolapse of polyp / rectum
• rectal bleeding, anemia

Path: hamartomatous polyps; adenomas may coexist
Histo: little / no smooth muscle; hyperplasia of mucous glands; retention cysts develop with obstruction of gland orifices (multiple mucin-filled spaces); edematous inflamed expanded lamina propria
DDx: familial adenomatous polyposis, Peutz-Jeghers syndrome

- rectal bleeding (95%) most commonly as intermittent bright red hematochezia
- anemia, pain
- diarrhea, constipation
- abdominal pain (from intussusception)
- rectal prolapse (rare)

Location: rectosigmoid (80%); rare in small bowel + stomach; not in esophagus

√ solitary polyp (75%); multiple polyps (1/3) of smooth round contour
√ lesion of pinpoint size / up to several cm in diameter
√ invariably on stalk of variable length

Dx: (1) any number of polyps with family history
(2) polyps throughout the GI tract
(3) >5–10 polyps in colon
Cx: colorectal cancer by 35 years of age (in 15%)
DDx: solitary juvenile polyps (<5 polyps, 1% prevalence in children)

KAPOSI SARCOMA

= multicentric malignant neoplasm originating from endothelial cells of lymphatic / blood vessels
Cause: HIV regulatory protein (trans-activator target [TAT]) important for viral replication is thought to cause proliferation of Kaposi sarcoma cells
Incidence: most common AIDS-related neoplasm (10–20–34%); in 51% of homosexual / bisexual men with AIDS; rare in hemophiliacs; M:F = 50:1
Histo: proliferation of spindle cells with numerous extravasated RBCs located in clefts between stromal cells

@ Skin (most frequent site)
@ Lymph nodes (2nd most frequent site):
√ abdominal + pelvic lymphadenopathy with high contrast-enhancement (secondary to vascularity)
Associated with high frequency of GI tract involvement
@ GI tract (40%, 3rd most frequent site):
- usually clinically silent
- concurrent with / after cutaneous disease

◊ GI tract is the only site of involvement in <5%!
Location: anywhere within GI tract; often multifocal
√ thickened nodular folds
√ multiple submucosal nodules ± central umbilication
√ polypoidal mass
√ infiltrating lesion
@ Liver (34% at autopsy)
infrequently contributes to morbidity + mortality
√ multiple 5–12 mm nodules hyperechoic on US, hypoattenuating on NECT/CECT indistinguishable from multiple hemangiomas
DDx: metastatic disease, fungal microabscesses, multiple areas of bacillary angiomatosis (= swollen venous lakes in liver)
@ Lung (18–47% of patients with cutaneous sarcoma):
= late complication of AIDS
Site: peribronchial + perivascular axial interstitium (91%); middle / lower lung zones (92%)
√ coarsening of bronchovascular bundles
√ tram track opacities
√ peribronchial cuffing
√ septal lines (38–71%)
√ central perihilar coalescent consolidation ± air bronchograms in 45% (= confluent tumor)
√ small (50%) / large (28%) pulmonary nodules (= tumor proliferation extending into parenchyma)
√ pleural effusion (33–67%), chylothorax (rare)
√ moderate lymphadenopathy (16%)
@ Lower extremities
√ lytic cortical lesion
√ subcutaneous nodules
Dx: visualization + biopsy of mass with red-purple color

LADD BANDS

= congenital peritoneal bands extending from cecum / hepatic flexure over anterior surface of 2nd / 3rd portion of duodenum causing duodenal obstruction at its 2nd portion (even without volvulus)
Associated with: malrotation

LEIOMYOMA

Location: 2/3 occur in stomach
Path: arising from muscularis propria / submucosa / muscularis mucosae / smooth muscle of blood vessels within wall of viscus
Histo: intersecting bands of muscle + fibrous tissue in a well-defined capsule
DDx: fibroma, neurofibroma, hemangioma

Esophageal leiomyomatosis

Age: 6–18 (mean of 11) years; M >F
Cause: (1) sporadic (50%)
(2) familial disease (20%): leiomyomas of uterus, vulva, tracheobronchial tree, small bowel, rectum
(3) Alport syndrome (30%) = nephritis, high-frequency sensorineural hearing loss, congenital cataract
Site: distal third / half of esophagus ± extension into proximal stomach

- slowly progressive dysphagia over years

√ smooth tapered narrowing of distal esophagus over an average length of 6 cm
√ decreased / absent esophageal peristalsis
√ smooth relatively symmetric defect at cardia (from thickened muscle bulging into gastric fundus)
CT:
√ marked circumferential wall thickening of up to 4 cm from mass with relatively low soft-tissue attenuation

GI

DDx: (1) primary achalasia (shorter narrowed segment)
(2) secondary achalasia (older individual, recent onset of dysphagia)
(3) stricture from reflux esophagitis
(4) idiopathic muscular hypertrophy of the esophagus (in late adulthood, corkscrew appearance of esophagus with nonperistaltic contractions, cardia rarely involved)

Leiomyoma of esophagus

◊ Most common benign tumor of esophagus!

Incidence: 1:1,119 (autopsy study); 50% of all benign esophageal tumors

Age: young adults; 3% in children; M > F

- usually asymptomatic (due to slow growth)
- dysphagia, odynophagia, dyspepsia
- hematemesis if large (rare)

Site: frequently lower + mid 1/3 of esophagus; intramural; multiple leiomyomas in 3–4%

√ 2–15 cm large smooth well-defined intramural mass causing eccentric thickening of wall + deformity of lumen
√ may have coarse calcifications
◊ Leiomyoma is the only calcifying esophageal tumor!
√ ulceration uncommon

CT:
√ uniform soft-tissue density
√ diffuse contrast enhancement

CAVE: high percentage misdiagnosed as extrinsic lesion!

Leiomyoma of small bowel

Most common benign tumor of small bowel

Location: duodenum (21%), jejunum (48%), ileum (31%); single in 97%

Site: mainly serosal (50%), mainly intraluminal (20%), intramural (10%)

Size: <5 cm (50%), 5–10 cm (25%), >10 cm (25%)

√ small ulcer + large barium-filled cavity (central necrosis + communication with lumen)
√ hypervascular

Leiomyoma of stomach

2nd most common benign gastric tumor (after gastric polyp), most common of calcified benign tumors

Location: pars media (39%), antrum (26%), pylorus (12%), fundus (12%), cardia (10%)

Site: intraluminal submucosal (60%), exophytic subserosal (35%), combined intramural-extramural dumbbell type mass (5%)

√ average size of 4.5 cm
√ ovoid mass with smooth margin + smooth surface (most frequently)
√ forms right angle with gastric wall
√ ulcerated in 50%
√ pedunculated intraluminal tumor in submucosal growth (rare)
√ "iceberg phenomenon" = large extraluminal component in subserosal growth
√ calcifies in 4%

Cx: (1) Hemorrhage (acute / chronic)
(2) Obstruction (tumor bulk / intussusception)
(3) Infection
(4) Fistulization / perforation
(5) Malignant degeneration (benign:malignant = 3:1)

LEIOMYOSARCOMA

Leiomyosarcoma of small bowel

Location: duodenum (26%), jejunum (34%), ileum (40%)

√ usually >6 cm in size
√ nodular mass: intraluminal (10%), intraluminal pedunculated (5%), intramural (15%), chiefly extrinsic (66%)
√ mucosa may be stretched + ulcerated (50%)
√ may show central ulcer pit / fistula communicating with a large necrotic center
√ intussusception

Leiomyosarcoma of stomach

Incidence: 0.1–3% of all gastric malignancies

Age: 10–73 years; M > F

Histo: pleomorphism, hypercellularity, mitotic figures, cystic degeneration, necrosis

- GI bleeding (from ulceration)
- obstruction

Metastases:
(a) hematogenous to liver, lung, peritoneum; rarely to bone + soft tissue
(b) direct extension into omentum, retroperitoneum
(c) lymph nodes (rare)

Location: anterior / posterior wall of body of stomach

√ average size of 12 cm
√ intramural mass
√ may be pedunculated
√ large masses tend to be exogastric
√ very frequently ulcerated

CT:
√ lobulated irregular outline
√ central zones of low density (necrosis with liquefaction)
√ air / positive contrast within tumor (= ulceration)
√ dystrophic calcifications

Carney syndrome

Triad of (1) Gastric epitheloid leiomyosarcoma
(2) Functioning extraadrenal paraganglioma
(3) Pulmonary chondromas

Incidence: 24 patients reported; M:F = 1:11

LIPOMA

Most common submucosal tumor in colon

Incidence: in colon in 0.25% (autopsy)

Location: colon (particularly cecum + ascending colon) > duodenum > ileum > stomach > jejunum > esophagus

- asymptomatic
- crampy pain, hemorrhage (rare)

GI

√ smooth, sharply outlined, round / ovoid globular mass of 1–3 cm in diameter
√ short thick pedicle in 1/3 caused by repeated peristaltic activity (prone to intussuscept)
√ marked radiolucency
√ change in shape + size on compression due to softness
  √ "squeeze sign" = sausage-shaped mass on postevacuation radiographs

CT:
  √ sharply defined intramural mass of fat density

Cx: intussusception (rare) / ulceration (rare)
Prognosis: NO liposarcomatous degeneration

LYMPHANGIOMA

= congenital malformation of lymphatic vessels
Path: usually multiloculated large thin-walled cystic mass with chylous / serous / hemorrhagic fluid contents
Location: mesentery
√ proximal bowel dilatation (in partial bowel obstruction)
US:
  √ multiseptated cystic mass with lobules
  √ fluid anechoic / with internal echoes / sedimentation
CT:
  √ cystic mass with contents of water- to fat-density
MR:
  √ serous contents: hypointense on T1WI + hyperintense on T2WI
  √ hemorrhage / fat: hyperintense on T1WI + T2WI
Rx: surgery (difficult due to intimate attachment to bowel wall)

LYMPHOGRANULOMA VENEREUM

= LGV = sexually transmitted disease caused by virus Chlamydia trachomatis producing a nonspecific granulomatous inflammatory response in infected mucosa (mononuclear cells + macrophages), perirectal lymphatic invasion
Location: rectum, may extend to sigmoid + descending colon
M:F = 3.4:1
√ narrowing + shortening + straightening of rectosigmoid
√ widening of retrorectal space
√ irregularity of mucosa + ulcerations
√ paracolic abscess
√ fistula to pericolic area, rectum, vagina (common)
Rx: tetracyclines effective in acute phase before scarring has occurred

LYMPHOID HYPERPLASIA

Incidence: normal variant in 13% of BE examinations
Histo: hyperplastic lymph follicles in lamina propria (Peyer patches), probably compensatory attempt for immunoglobulin deficiency
Etiology:
  (1) Normal in child / young adult
  (2) Self-limiting local / systemic inflammation / infection / allergy
  (3) May be related to immunodeficiency / dysgammaglobulinemia with small bowel involvement

Age: (a) generally in children <2 years
  (b) in adults invariably associated with late onset immunoglobulin deficiency (IgA, IgM)
Associated with: splenomegaly, large tonsils, eczematous dermatitis, achlorhydria, pernicious anemia, acute pancreatitis, colonic carcinoma
At risk for:
  (1) **Good syndrome** (10%)
    = gastric carcinoma + benign thymoma + lymphoid hyperplasia
  (2) Respiratory infections
  (3) Giardia lamblia infection (90%)
  (4) Functional thyroid abnormalities

Location: primarily jejunum, may involve entire small bowel, ascending colon + hepatic flexure, seldom in sigmoid / rectum
• malabsorption (diarrhea + steatorrhea)
• low serum concentrations of IgA, IgG, IgM
√ mucosa studded with innumerable 1–3 mm small uniform polypoid lesions
√ lesions may be umbilicated (uncommon)

LYMPHOMA OF GASTROINTESTINAL TRACT

Classification:
  A. PRIMARY LYMPHOMA OF BOWEL
    (a) localized (b) diffuse
    Predisposed: Arabs + Middle Eastern Jews
    Associated with: celiac disease
  B. SECONDARY INTESTINAL LYMPHOMA
    as part of generalized systemic process

Incidence: 4–20% of all NHL; 10% of patients with abdominal lymphoma have bowel involvement
At risk: long-standing celiac disease, AIDS, systemic lupus erythematosus, Crohn disease, history of chemotherapy
Median age: 60 years
Histo:
  (1) T-cell malignant lymphoma (in celiac disease)
  (2) B-cell lymphoma
  (3) Immunoproliferative small intestinal disease (= Mediterranean lymphoma)
  (4) Low-grade B-cell lymphoma (= lymphoma of mucosa-associated lymphoid tissue)
  (5) Follicular lymphoma
  (6) Burkitt lymphoma (in children)
  (7) Mantle cell lymphoma
  (8) Hodgkin disease (<15%)

May be associated with: enlargement of extra-abdominal lymph nodes, malabsorption
Radiographic types:
  1. Polypoid / nodular (47%)
    √ enlarged nodular folds
  2. Ulcerative (42%)
    √ ulcerative lesions, may be complicated by perforation
    √ aneurysmal configuration

3. Diffusely infiltrating (11%)
   √ diffuse hoselike thickening of bowel wall
   √ decreased / absent peristalsis

CT staging:
- Stage I — tumor confined to bowel wall
- Stage II — limited to local nodes
- Stage III — widespread nodal disease
- Stage IV — disseminated to bone marrow, liver, other organs

Location: 10–25% of NHL are extranodal; stomach > small bowel > colon > esophagus; multicentric in 10–50%

√ enlargement of spleen
√ bulky enlargement of regional lymph nodes

@ Esophagus
least common site of GI involvement (in <1%)

@ Stomach
1–5% of all gastric malignancies; most common site of extranodal Hodgkin disease; 25% of extranodal lymphoma; mostly NHL with histiocytic cell type; isolated primary gastric malignancy in 10%
Site: arises in lymphoid tissue of lamina propria; no predilection for any particular region of stomach
Direct extension into: pancreas, spleen, transverse colon, liver
√ flexibility of gastric wall preserved
√ duodenum often affected when antrum involved
√ circumscribed mass with endogastric / exogastric (25%) growth
√ broad tortuous mucosal folds over large portions of stomach (diffuse form)
√ large irregular ulcers
CT:
   √ diffuse involvement of entire stomach (50%), typically more than half of gastric circumference
   √ segmental involvement (15%)
   √ ulcerated mass (8%)
   √ average wall thickness of 4–5 cm
   √ luminal irregularity (66%)
   √ hyperrugosity (58%)
Prognosis: 55% 5-year survival rate after resection

@ Small bowel
1/5 of all small bowel malignancies; most common malignant small bowel tumor; multiple sites of involvement in 1/5; most common cause of intussusception in children >6 years
Location: ileum (51%), jejunum (47%), duodenum (2%),
Site: arising from lymphoid patches of Peyer
Types:
1. Infiltrating lymphoma with plaquelike involvement of wall >5 cm in length (80%) / >10 cm in length (20%) (DDx: Crohn disease)
   √ ± ulceration (considerable excavation)
   √ desmoplastic response
   √ thickened valvulae with corrugated appearance
   √ aneurysmal dilatation (secondary to destruction of autonomic nerve plexus + muscle / tumor necrosis)
2. Single / multiple polypoid mucosal / submucosal masses
   √ cobblestone defects due to lymphomatous polyps
   √ nodules may ulcerate
   √ may cause intussusception
   √ sprue pattern
3. Endoexoenteric mass
   √ large mass with only small intramural component
   √ ± ulcer + fistulae + aneurysmatic dilatation
4. Mesenteric / retroperitoneal adenopathy
   √ single / multiple extraluminal masses displacing bowel
   √ ill-defined confluent mass engulfing + encasing multiple loops of adjacent bowel
   √ "sandwich configuration" = mass surrounding mesenteric vessels that are separated by perivascular fat
   √ conglomerate mantle of retroperitoneal + mesenteric mass

@ Colon
Less commonly involved than stomach / small bowel; 1.5% of all abdominal lymphomas
Location: cecum most commonly involved (85%)
√ single mass > diffuse infiltration > polypoid lesion
√ paradoxical dilatation
√ gross mural circumferential / focal soft-tissue thickening (average size of 5 cm)
√ slight enhancement
√ massive regional + distant mesenteric + retroperitoneal adenopathy
DDx: frequently resembles inflammatory disease / polyposis

Prognosis: (a) 71–82% 2-year survival rate in isolated bowel lymphoma
(b) 0% 2-year survival rate in stage IV disease with bowel involvement

Cx during chemotherapy: perforation (9–40%), hemorrhage

MALIGNANT MELANOMA

= develops from melanocytes derived from neural crest cells, arising in preexisting benign nevi

Incidence: 1% of all cancers

@ Skin primary
Clark staging:
- Level I — all tumor cells above basement membrane (in situ lesion)
- Level II — tumor extends to papillary dermis
- Level III — tumor extends to interface between papillary + reticular dermis
- Level IV — tumor extends between bundles of collagen of reticular dermis
- Level V — tumor invasion of subcutaneous tissue (in 87% metastatic)

Breslow staging:

thin	<0.75 mm depth of invasion
intermediate	0.76–3.99 mm depth of invasion
thick	>4 mm depth of invasion

METASTASES:
latent period of 2–20 years after initial diagnosis (most commonly 2–5 years)
Primary site: head + neck (79%), eye (77%), GU system (67%), GI tract (in up to 60%)

@ Lymphadenopathy
— in 23% with level II + IV
— in 75% with level V

@ Bone (11–17%)
• often initial manifestation of recurrence
• poor prognosis
Location: axial skeleton (80%), ribs (38%)

@ Lung (70% at autopsy)
most common site of relapse;
respiratory failure most common cause of death

@ Liver (17–23%; 58–66% at autopsy)
√ single / multiple lesions 0.5–15 cm in size
√ larger lesion often necrotic
√ may be partially calcified

@ Spleen (1–5%; 33% at autopsy)
√ single / multiple lesions of variable size
√ solid / cystic

@ GI tract + mesentery (4–8%)
• abdominal pain, GI bleeding
Location: small intestine (35–50%), colon (14–20%), stomach (7–20%)
√ multiple submucosal nodules ± "bull's-eye / target" appearance = central ulceration
√ irregular amorphous cavity (exoenteric growth)
√ intussusception (10–20%)

@ Kidney (up to 35% at autopsy)

@ Adrenal (11%, up to 50% at autopsy)

@ Subcutis

Prognosis: 30–40% eventually die from this tumor

MALLORY-WEISS SYNDROME

= mucosal + submucosal tear with involvement of venous plexus

Pathophysiology: violent projection of gastric contents against lower esophagus

Age: 30–60 years; M > F

Predisposed: alcoholics

• history of repeated vomiting prior to hematemesis
• massive painless hematemesis

Location: at / above / below (76%) esophagogastric junction
√ longitudinal single tear in 77%, in 23% multiple tears
√ extravasation of barium

Angio:
√ bleeding site at gastric cardia

DDx: peptic ulcer / ulcerative gastritis

MALROTATION

= abnormal position of gut secondary to a narrow mesenteric attachment as a result of arrest in the embryologic development of gut rotation + fixation

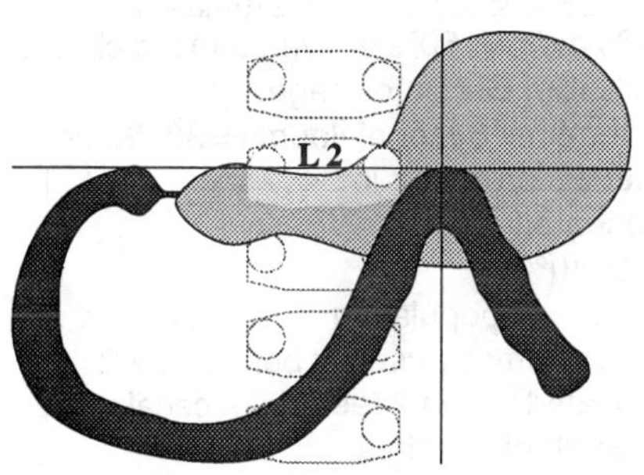

normal duodenal position

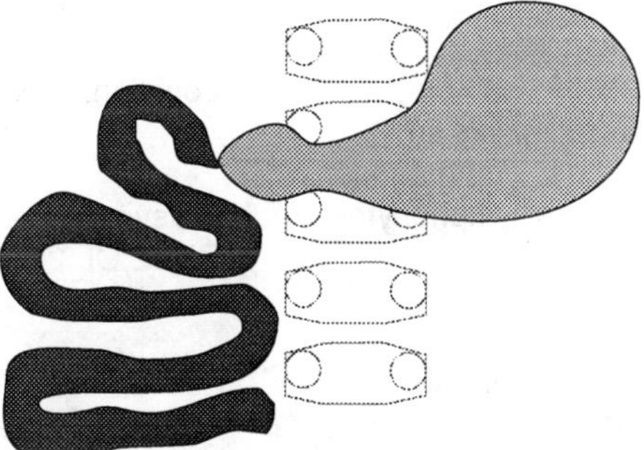
nonrotation of duodenum

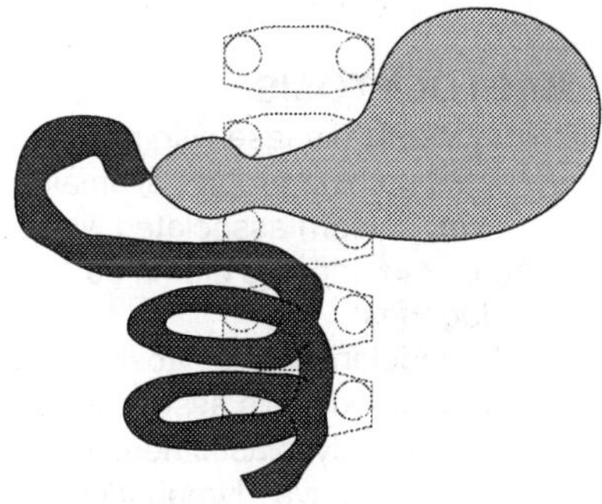
corkscrew duodenum + jejunum

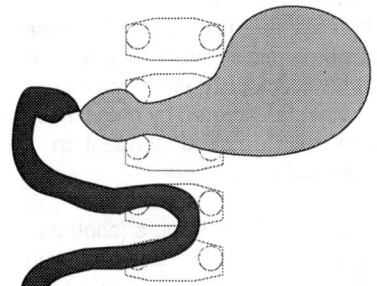

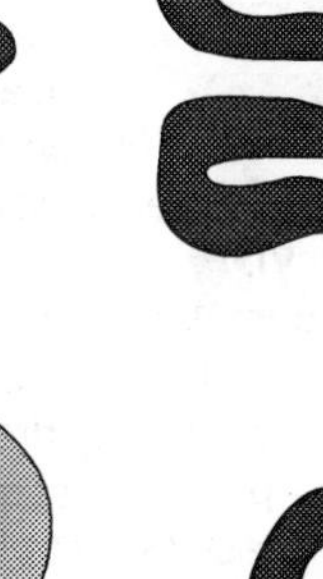
partial duodenal rotation with jejunum in right upper quadrant

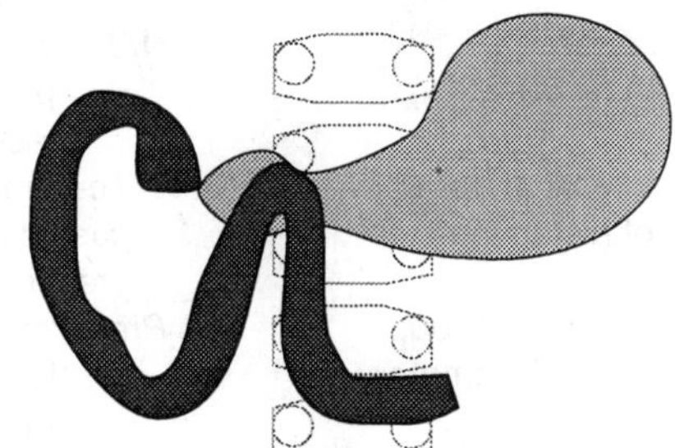
partial duodenal rotation with duodenojejunal junction over right pedicle

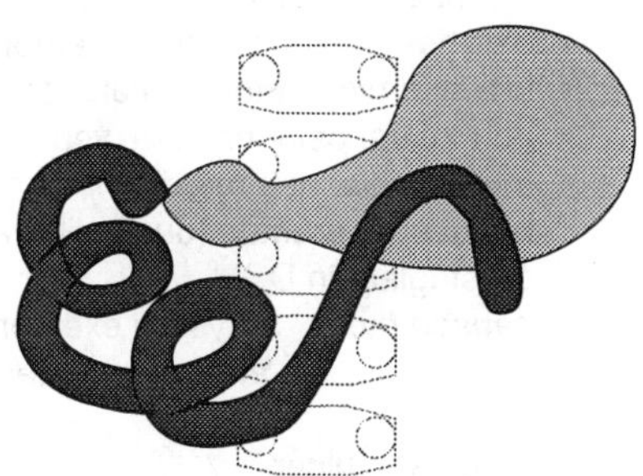
redundant-duodenum malrotation to right of spine

Embryology:
duodenojejunal + ileocolic segments of primitive digestive tube rotate by 270° in a counterclockwise direction about the omphalomesenteric vessels to cross beneath the vessels (future SMA + SMV); LUQ fixation at ligament of Treitz (an extension of the right crus of diaphragm) + fibrous tissue around celiac artery, located to left of L2) + RLQ fixation of cecum
Definition: nonrotation ≤ 90°; malrotation = 90–270°
Associated with: urinary pseudoobstruction, prune-belly syndrome, cloacal exstrophy
Barium meal & barium enema:
Purpose: guess the location of abnormal peritoneal fixation from position of bowel!
√ clearly abnormal position of duodenum (81%):
√ duodenum + jejunum to the right of spine (30%)
√ corkscrew duodenum + jejunum (29%)
√ duodenojejunal junction low + in midline (22%)
√ unusual abnormal position of duodenum (16%):
√ duodenojejunal junction over right pedicle
√ duodenojejunal junction to left of spine but low
√ duodenal redundancy to right of spine
√ Z-shape configuration of duodenum + jejunum
√ nonrotation = small bowel on right + colon on left (in 0.2% incidental finding in adults)
√ abnormal position of duodenum + cecum (84%)
√ normal position of duodenum (3%)
√ normal position of cecum (in 5–20%)
DDx: mobile cecum (15%)
CT:
√ SMV positioned to left of SMA (80%)
√ aplastic / hypoplastic uncinate process of pancreas
Cx: midintestinal volvulus, duodenal obstruction, internal herniation

MASTOCYTOSIS

= systemic disease with mast cell proliferation in skin + RES (lamina propria of small bowel; bone; lymph nodes; liver; spleen) associated with eosinophils + lymphocytes
Age: <6 months old (in 50%)
Categories:
I indolent mastocytosis (most frequent)
II mastocytosis associated with myeloproliferative / myelodysplastic hematologic disorder
III aggressive / lymphadenopathic mastocytosis with eosinophilia
IV mast cell leukemia (rare)
• diarrhea, malabsorption, steatorrhea, anorexia
• urticaria pigmentosa = cutaneous form (in 80–90%)
• abdominal pain, nausea, vomiting
• tachycardia, asthma, flushing, gastrointestinal upset, headache, pruritus (due to liberation of histamine / prostaglandin D_2)
caused by: physical exertion, heat, certain foods, alcohol, nonsteroidal anti-inflammatory drugs
@ Stomach ulcer
@ Small bowel
√ generalized irregular distorted thickened folds ± wall thickening
√ diffuse pattern of 2–3 mm sandlike mucosal nodules
√ urticaria-like lesions of gastric + intestinal mucosa
@ Reticuloendothelial system
√ hepatomegaly
√ Budd-Chiari hepatic veno-occlusive disease
√ reversed portal venous flow
√ cavernous transformation of portal vein
√ splenomegaly (43–61%)
√ ascites: (a) transudative secondary to liver disease
(b) exudative from mast cell proliferation of peritoneum
@ Bone
√ sclerotic bone lesions
Dx: skin / bone marrow biopsy; jejunal biopsy demonstrates an excess of mast cells
Cx: (1) Peptic ulcer disease (histamine-mediated acid secretion)
(2) Leukemia
Rx: antihistamines, histamine decarboxylase inhibitors, sodium chromoglycase; steroids; splenectomy (for symptomatic splenomegaly / hypersplenism)
DDx: carcinoid, pheochromocytoma

MECKEL DIVERTICULUM

= persistence of the omphalomesenteric duct (= vitelline duct), which usually obliterates by 5th embryonic week
◊ Most common congenital abnormality of the GI tract!
Incidence: 0.3–2–3% of population (at autopsy)
Age: majority in children <10 years of age; M:F = 3:1
Histo: contains ectopic mucosa in 50%: gastric / pancreatic / colonic mucosa
◊ <u>Frequency of ectopic gastric mucosa</u>: 15–34% overall; 60% in symptomatic children; in >95% with GI hemorrhage
Location: within terminal 6 feet of ileum (= 30–90 cm from ileocecal valve); in 94% on antimesenteric border
• asymptomatic (20–40%)
RULE OF 2s: (1) in 2% of population
(2) symptomatic usually before age 2
(3) located within 2 feet of ileocecal valve
(4) length of 2 inches
NUC (>85% sensitivity, >95% specificity, >83–88% accuracy):
√ accumulation of radiotracer in right lower quadrant coinciding with uptake of tracer in stomach
N.B.: sensitivity drops after adolescence, because patients asymptomatic throughout childhood are less likely to have ectopic gastric mucosa
◊ Tc-99m pertechnetate is excreted by mucoid cells of gastric mucosa, excretion is not dependent on presence of parietal cells
Preparation:
(1) No irritative measures for 48 hours (contrast studies, endoscopy, cathartics, enemas, drugs irritating GI tract)
(2) Fasting for 3–6 hours (results in decreased gastric secretion + diminished bowel peristalsis)
(3) Evacuation of bowel + bladder prior to study

Dose: 5–20 mCi (100 μCi/kg) Tc-99m pertechnetate
Radiation dose: 0.54 rad/2 mCi for thyroid;
0.3 rad/2 mCi for large intestine;
0.2 rad/2 mCi for stomach
Imaging: serial images in 5- to 10-minute intervals for 1 hour
√ improved visualization through
(a) pentagastrin = stimulates uptake (6 μg/kg SC 20 min prior to pertechnetate)
(b) cimetidine = inhibits secretion (maximum 300 mg/dose IV 1 hour prior)
(c) glucagon = decreases peristalsis (50 μg/kg IM 5–10 minutes prior)
√ poor visualization with use of perchlorate + atropine (= depressed uptake)

False-positive results:
(1) Ectopic gastric mucosa in gastrogenic cyst, enteric duplication, normal small bowel, Barrett esophagus
(2) Increased blood pool in AVM, hemangioma, hypervascular tumor, aneurysm
(3) Duodenal ulcer, ulcerative colitis, Crohn disease, appendicitis, laxative abuse
(4) Intussusception, intestinal obstruction, volvulus
(5) Urinary tract obstruction, caliceal diverticulum
(6) Anterior meningomyelocele
(7) Poor technique

mnemonic: "HA GUIDI"
Hemangioma
Appendicitis
Gastric ectopia
Urinary obstruction
Intussusception
Duplication of bowel
Inflammatory bowel disease

False-negative results:
(1) Insufficient mass of ectopic gastric mucosa
(2) Dilution of intraluminal activity (hemorrhage / hypersecretion)

mnemonic: "MIS"
Malrotation of ileum
Irritable bowel in RLQ (rapid transit)
Small amount of ectopic gastric mucosa

Enteroclysis:
√ elongated, smoothly marginated, clublike, intraluminal mass parallel to long axis of distal ileum = inverted Meckel diverticulum (20%)
√ 0.5–20-cm-long blind pouch on the antimesenteric border of ileum with junctional fold pattern

Angio (59% accuracy):
√ presence of vitelline artery (= anomalous end branch of superior mesenteric artery) is PATHOGNOMONIC

Cx (in 20%):
(1) GI bleeding secondary to ulceration (in 95% due to ectopic gastric mucosa)
(2) Acute diverticulitis
(3) Intestinal obstruction secondary to intussusception (diverticulum acts as lead point) / volvulus (when omphalomesenteric diverticulum attached to umbilicus by fibrous band)
(4) Malignant tumor (rare): carcinoma, sarcoma, carcinoid
(5) Chronic abdominal pain

MECONIUM ILEUS

= small bowel obstruction secondary to desiccated meconium pellets impacted in distal ileum

Age: may develop in utero (in 15%)

Associated with:
cystic fibrosis with thick + sticky meconium due to deficiency of pancreatic secretions (in almost 100%)
◊ Earliest clinical manifestation of cystic fibrosis!
◊ Virtually all infants with meconium ileus prove to have cystic fibrosis
◊ 10–15% of infants with cystic fibrosis present with meconium ileus!

• abdominal distension, bilious emesis
• failure to pass meconium within 48 hours

√ numerous dilated small bowel loops without air-fluid levels (fluid not present)
√ "bubbly" / "frothy" appearance of intestinal contents
√ "soap-bubble" / "applesauce" appearance in RLQ (in 50–66%)
√ multiple round / oval filling defects in distal ileum + colon
√ microcolon (unused colon in antenatal obstruction)

OB-US:
√ unusual echogenic intraluminal areas in small bowel (DDx: normal transient inspissated meconium)
√ usually polyhydramnios
√ fluid-filled dilated small bowel

Cx (in 40–50%): volvulus, ischemia, necrosis, stenosis, atresia, perforation, meconium peritonitis, pseudocyst

Rx: (1) Nonionic contrast media enema (because of risk of bowel perforation)
(2) 17% Hypaque / Conray enema mixed with acetylcysteine (Mucomyst®)
(3) Gastrografin® enema with Tween 80 (attention to fluid + electrolyte balance)

DDx: Hirschsprung disease, small bowel atresia with meconium ileus, meconium plug syndrome, small left colon syndrome, imperforate anus, obstruction from duplication cyst

MECONIUM PERITONITIS

= sterile chemical peritonitis secondary to perforation of bowel proximal to high-grade / complete obstruction that seals in utero due to inflammatory response

Incidence: 1:35,000 livebirths

Age: antenatal perforation after 3rd month of gestation

Cause:
(1) Atresia (secondary to ischemic event) (50%)
(a) of small bowel (usually ileum or jejunum)
(b) of colon (uncommon)
(2) Bowel obstruction (46%)
(a) meconium ileus
(b) volvulus, internal hernia
(c) intussusception, congenital bands, Meckel diverticulum

GI

(3) Hydrometrocolpos
  ◊ Meconium peritonitis due to cystic fibrosis diagnosed in utero in 8% + at birth in 15–40%!
  ◊ Intraperitoneal meconium may calcify within 24 hours!

Types:
(a) fibroadhesive type (most common):
  = intense chemical reaction of peritoneum, which seals off the perforation
  • no evidence for active leak at birth
  √ dense mass with calcium deposits
  √ calcific plaques scattered throughout peritoneal cavity
(b) cystic type:
  = cystic cavity formed by fixation of bowel loops surrounding the perforation site, which continues to leak meconium
  √ cyst outlined by calcific rim
(c) generalized type:
  • perforation occurs immediately antenatally
  • active leakage of bowel contents
  √ complicated ascites

√ intraabdominal calcifications (conspicuously absent in cystic fibrosis)
  √ peripherally calcified pseudocysts
  √ small flecks of calcifications scattered throughout abdomen
  √ larger aggregates of calcifications along inferior surface of liver / flank / processus vaginalis / scrotum
√ obstructive roentgen signs following birth
√ separation of bowel loops by fluid
√ microcolon = "unused colon"
√ meconium hydrocele producing labial mass
OB-US:
  √ polyhydramnios (64–71%)
  √ fetal ascites (54–57%)
  √ bowel dilatation (27–29%)
  √ intraabdominal bright echogenic mass
  √ multiple linear / clumped foci of calcifications (84%); may develop within 12 hours after perforation
  √ meconium pseudocyst = well-defined hypoechoic mass surrounded by an echogenic calcified wall (= contained perforation)
  DDx: (1) Intraabdominal teratoma
  (2) Fetal gallstones
  (3) Isolated liver calcifications
Mortality: up to 62%
Prognosis: generally good; surgery may not be required when perforation site is completely healed

MECONIUM PLUG SYNDROME
= local inspissation of meconium leading to low colonic obstruction
Age: newborn infant (symptomatic within first 24 hours of life)
Cause: cystic fibrosis (25%), Hirschsprung disease, prematurity, maternal magnesium sulfate treatment
• abdominal distension
• vomiting
• failure to pass meconium
√ distended transverse + ascending colon + dilated small bowel (proximal to obstruction)
√ occasionally bubbly appearance in colon (DDx: submucosal air in necrotizing enterocolitis)
√ presacral pseudotumor (no gas in rectum)
√ double-contrast effect = barium between meconium plug + colonic wall
Rx: water-soluble enema
DDx: Hirschsprung disease

MELANOSIS COLI
= benign brown-black discoloration of colonic mucosa
Incidence: 10% of autopsies
Cause: ? chronic anthracene cathartic usage
• asymptomatic
Prognosis: no malignant potential

MÉNÉTRIÈR DISEASE
= GIANT HYPERTROPHIC GASTRITIS
= HYPERPLASTIC GASTROPATHY
= characterized by excessive mucus production and TRIAD of (1) Giant mucosal hypertrophy
(2) Hypoproteinemia
(3) Hypochlorhydria
Histo: hyperplasia of glandular tissue + microcyst formation, mucosal thickness up to 6 mm (normal range: 0.6–1.0 mm)
Age: 20–70 years; M:F = 2:1
Associated with: benign gastric ulcer (13–72%)
• protein-losing enteropathy with hypoproteinemia + peripheral edema
• weight loss
• gastrointestinal bleeding
• absent / decreased acid secretion (>50%) epigastric pain vomiting
Location: throughout fundus + body, particularly prominent along greater curvature, antrum usually spared (DDx to lymphoma: usually in antrum)
√ markedly enlarged + tortuous gastric folds in spite of adequate gastric distension
√ relatively abrupt demarcation between normal + abnormal areas
√ marked hypersecretion (mucus)
√ preserved pliability
CT:
  √ wall thickening of proximal stomach
  √ nodular symmetric folds
DDx: lymphoma, polypoid variety of gastric carcinoma, acute gastritis, chronic gastritis, gastric varices

MESENTERIC LYMPHADENITIS
= clinical entity whose symptoms relate to benign inflammation of lymph nodes in the bowel mesentery
Cause: Yersinia enterocolitica, Y pseudotuberculosis, viral infection

Age: children, young adults
• nausea, vomiting, diarrhea, fever
• diffuse / RLQ pain + tenderness
Location: usually RLQ (immediately anterior to right psoas muscle in 78%, small bowel mesentery in 56%)
√ enlarged mesenteric lymph nodes
√ isolated ileal wall thickening (33%)
√ colonic wall thickening (18%)
N.B.: visualization of entire normal appendix is necessary to differentiate from acute appendicitis!
DDx: appendicitis (enlarged nodes immediately anterior to right psoas muscle in 40–82%, nodes less numerous + smaller), Crohn disease

MESENTERIC ISCHEMIA

Acute mesenteric ischemia

Etiology:
(a) arterial: atheromatous disease, embolic disease, dissecting aortic aneurysm, fibromuscular hyperplasia, arteritis, endotoxin shock, hypoperfusion (shock, hypovolemia), disseminated intravascular coagulation, direct trauma, radiation
— **occlusive mesenteric infarction** (90% mortality)
1. embolus (40–50%) just distal to middle colic a.
2. SMA thrombosis (20–40%) at origin + site of atherosclerotic narrowing (ostium stenosis)
— **nonocclusive mesenteric ischemia** (10% mortality)
= preexisting atherosclerosis with systemic low-flow state (cardiac failure / intraoperative hypotension, bowel vasospasm)
(b) venous (<10%): young patient, often following abdominal surgery
Location: superior mesenteric vein > inferior mesenteric vein > portal vein
(c) incarceration of hernia, volvulus, constriction by adhesive bands, intussusception
Prevalence: 5% for SMA; 4% for celiac artery; 11% for inferior mesenteric artery
Pathophysiology: mucosa is most sensitive area to anoxia from arterial / venous occlusion with early ulcerations leading to formation of strictures
• first crampy, then continuous abdominal pain with acute event
• cardiac disease predisposing to embolization
• gut emptying (vomiting / diarrhea)
• WBC >12,000/μl with left shift (80%)
• gross rectal bleeding
Location: (a) any segment of small bowel
(b) distal transverse colon, splenic flexure, cecum (most common)
Consequences:
dependent on magnitude of insult, duration of process, adequacy of collaterals
(a) reversible ischemia
1. Complete restitution of bowel wall secondary to abundant collaterals
2. Healing with fibrosis + stricture formation
(b) irreversible ischemia
1. Transmural infarction with bowel perforation

Plain film:
√ gasless abdomen (= fluid-filled loops from exudation) (21%)
√ bowel distension to splenic flexure (= perfusion territory of SMA) in 43%
√ "thumbprinting" (36%) = thickening of bowel wall + valvulae (edema)
√ small bowel pseudoobstruction (most frequently in thrombosis)
√ pneumatosis = dissection of luminal gas into bowel wall (28%)
√ mesenteric + portal vein gas (14%)
√ ascites (14%)
Barium:
√ "scalloping / thumbprinting" = thickening of wall + valvulae
√ "picket fencing"
√ separation + uncoiling of loops
√ narrowed lumen
√ circumferential ulcer
CT (26–73–82% sensitive):
√ focal / diffuse bowel dilatation (10–56–71%) with gas (43%) / fluid (29%)
√ portal venous gas (5–13–36%) / mesenteric vein gas (28%)
√ pneumoperitoneum (7%)
√ ascites (43%)
√ mesenteric edema
(a) arterial occlusion:
√ thrombosis of SMA (4–18%)
√ pneumatosis intestinalis (22–30%)
√ thumbprinting (26%) = thickening of bowel wall
√ lack of bowel wall enhancement with arterial occlusion
(b) venous thrombosis:
√ SMV / portal vein thrombosis (15%)
√ thickened intestinal wall (64%)
√ marked contrast enhancement
Angio:
√ occlusion / vasoconstriction / vascular beading
√ embolus lodged at major branching points distal to first 3 cm of SMA

NUC:
(a) IV / IA Tc-99m sulfur colloid / labeled leukocytes, Ga-citrate, Tc-99m pyrophosphate:
√ tracer accumulation 5 hours after onset of ischemia (more intense uptake with transmural infarcts)
(b) intraperitoneal injection of Xe-133 in saline is absorbed by intestine:
√ decreased washout with abnormal perfusion of strangulated bowel

Prognosis:
(1) Massive infarction of small + large bowel if mesenteric embolization occurs proximal to middle colic artery (= limited collateral flow)
(2) Focal segments of intestinal ischemia if mesenteric embolization occurs distal to middle colic artery (= good collateral flow)

Mortality: 70–80–92% for intestinal infarction

Chronic mesenteric ischemia

= ABDOMINAL ANGINA
= intermittent mesenteric ischemia in severe arterial stenosis with inadequate collateralization provoked by food ingestion

- postprandial abdominal pain 15–20 minutes after food intake (due to "gastric steal" diverting blood flow away from intestine)
- fear of eating large meals
- weight loss, malabsorption
- reflex emptying of bowel after eating

Barium:
(a) Subacute:
√ flattening of one border
√ pseudosacculation / pseudodiverticula on antimesenteric border
(b) Chronic:
√ 7- to 10-cm-long smooth pliable strictures
√ dilatation of gut between strictures
√ thinned + atrophic valvulae
Cx: obstruction

Duplex US:
√ celiac trunk occlusion + retrograde perfusion of hepatic artery through SMA
√ PSV >300 cm/sec and EDV >45 cm/sec in SMA
√ peak systolic velocity >160 cm/sec in celiac trunk for >50% stenosis (57% sensitivity, 100% specificity) during fasting state

MESOTHELIAL CYST

= MESENTERIC / OMENTAL CYST

Etiology: failure of mesothelial peritoneal surfaces to coalesce
Path: unilocular thin-walled cyst usually with serous, occasionally chylous / hemorrhagic fluid contents
Histo: lined by mesothelial cells + surrounded by thin layer of fibrous tissue
Location: small bowel, mesentery (78%), mesocolon

- asymptomatic

√ single cyst up to several cm in size
√ omental cysts may be pedunculated

CT:
√ near-water density / soft-tissue density
√ ± fluid levels related to fat + water components

Cx: torsion, hemorrhage, intestinal obstruction
DDx: lymphangioma (septations)

METASTASES TO SMALL BOWEL

Origin: colon > stomach > breast > ovary > uterine cervix > melanoma > lung > pancreas

Spread:
(1) Intraperitoneal seeding: primary mucinous tumor of ovary, appendix, colon; breast cancer
(2) Hematogenous dissemination with submucosal deposits: malignant melanoma, breast carcinoma, lung carcinoma, Kaposi sarcoma
(3) Direct extension from adjacent neoplasm: ovary, uterus, prostate, pancreas, colon, kidney

√ fixation + tenting + transverse stretching (= across long axis) of folds secondary to mesenteric + peritoneal infiltration (most common form)

UGI:
√ single mass protruding into lumen resembling annular carcinoma
√ "bull's-eye" lesions = multiple polypoid masses with sizable ulcer craters
√ obstruction from kinking / annular constriction / large intraluminal mass
√ compression by direct extension of primary tumor / involved nodes

CT:
√ soft-tissue density nodules / masses
√ sheets of tissue causing thickening of bowel wall + mesenteric leaves
√ fixation + angulation of bowel loops (in tumors with desmoplastic response)
√ ascites

METASTASES TO STOMACH

Organ of origin: malignant melanoma, breast, lung, colon, prostate, leukemia, secondary lymphoma

- GI bleeding + anemia (40%)
- epigastric pain

√ solitary mass (50%)
√ multiple nodules (30%)
√ linitis plastica (20%): especially breast
√ multiple umbilicated nodules: melanoma

MIDGUT VOLVULUS

= torsion of entire gut around SMA due to a short mesenteric attachment of small intestine in malrotation

Age: neonate / young infant; occasionally older child / adult

In 20% associated with: (1) Duodenal atresia
(2) Duodenal diaphragm
(3) Duodenal stenosis
(4) Annular pancreas

Pathophysiology:
degree of twisting can change due to natural movement of bowel + determines symptomatology; severe volvulus (= twist of 3 and a half turns) causes bowel necrosis

- acute symptoms in newborn (medical emergency): bile-stained vomiting (intermittent, postprandial, projectile); abdominal distension; shock
- intermittent obstructive symptoms in older child: recurring attacks of nausea, vomiting, and abdominal pain
- failure to thrive (hypoproteinemic gastroenteropathy as a result of lymphatic + venous obstruction)

GI

Plain film:
- √ dilated air-filled duodenal bulb + paucity of gas distally
- √ "double bubble sign" = air-fluid levels in stomach + duodenum
- √ isolated collection of gas-containing bowel loops distal to obstructed duodenum = gas-filled volvulus = closed-loop obstruction (from nonresorption of intestinal gas secondary to obstruction of mesenteric veins)

Barium studies:
- √ duodenojejunal junction (ligament of Treitz) located lower than duodenal bulb + to the right of expected position
- √ spiral course of midgut loops = "apple-peel / twisted ribbon / corkscrew" appearance (in 81%)
- √ duodenal-fold thickening + thumbprinting (mucosal edema + hemorrhage)
- √ abnormally high position of cecum

CT:
- √ whirl-like pattern of small bowel loops + adjacent mesenteric fat converging to the point of torsion (during volvulus)
- √ SMV to the left of SMA (NO volvulus)
- √ chylous mesenteric cyst (from interference with lymphatic drainage)

US:
- √ clockwise whirlpool sign = color Doppler depiction of mesenteric vessels moving clockwise with caudal movement of transducer
- √ distended proximal duodenum with arrowhead-type compression over spine
- √ superior mesenteric vein to the left of SMA
- √ thick-walled bowel loops below duodenum + to the right of spine associated with peritoneal fluid

Angio:
- √ "barber pole sign" = spiraling of SMA
- √ tapering / abrupt termination of mesenteric vessels
- √ marked vasoconstriction + prolonged contrast transit time
- √ absent venous opacification / dilated tortuous superior mesenteric vein

Cx: intestinal ischemia + necrosis in distribution of SMA (bloody diarrhea, ileus, abdominal distension)

DDx: pyloric stenosis (same age group, no bilious vomiting)

MUCOCELE OF APPENDIX

Mucocele

= distension of appendix with sterile mucus

Etiology:
- (a) (perhaps) cystic dilatation of lumen secondary to obstruction by fecolith, foreign body, carcinoid, endometriosis, adhesions, volvulus
- (b) mucosal hyperplasia
- (c) mucinous cystadenoma
- (d) mucinous cystadenocarcinoma

Incidence: 0.07–0.3% of appendectomies

Mean age: 55 years; M:F = 1:4

Associated with: colonic adenocarcinoma (6-fold risk), mucin-secreting tumor of ovary

- • asymptomatic (25%)
- • acute / chronic right lower quadrant pain
- √ globular, smooth-walled, broad-based mass invaginating into cecum
- √ nonfilling of the appendix on BE
- √ peripheral rimlike calcifications frequent

CT:
- √ round sharply defined mass with homogeneous content of near-water / soft-tissue attenuation

US:
- √ purely cystic / cystic with fine internal echoes / complex cystic mass with high-level echoes
- √ gravity-dependent echoes = layering of protein macroaggregates / inspissated mucoid material

NUC:
- √ intense early gallium uptake (affinity to acid mucopolysaccharides of mucus)

Cx:
(1) Rupture with pseudomyxoma peritonei
(2) Torsion with gangrene + hemorrhage
(3) Herniation into cecum with bowel obstruction

Myxoglobulosis

= rare variant of mucocele of the appendix characterized by clusters of pearly white mucous balls intermixed with mucus
- • usually asymptomatic
- • may appear as acute appendicitis
- √ multiple 1- to 10-mm small rounded annular, nonlaminated calcified spherules (PATHOGNOMONIC)

DDx: inverted appendiceal stump, acute appendicitis, carcinoma of the cecum

NECROTIZING ENTEROCOLITIS

= NEC = ischemic bowel disease secondary to hypoxia, perinatal stress, infection (endotoxin), congenital heart disease

Incidence: most common GI emergency in premature infants

Age: develops >48–72 hours after birth; in 90% within first 10 days of life

Path: acute inflammation + mucosal ulceration + widespread transmural necrosis

Organism: not yet isolated; often occurs in miniepidemics within nursery

Predisposed: premature infant (50–80%), Hirschsprung disease, bowel obstruction (small bowel atresia, pyloric stenosis, meconium ileus, meconium plug syndrome)

- • blood-streaked stools (in 50%); explosive diarrhea
- • bile emesis
- • mild respiratory distress
- • generalized sepsis

Location: usually in terminal ileum (most commonly involved), cecum, right colon; rarely in stomach, upper bowel

- √ disarrayed bowel gas pattern (no longer normal array of polygons)
- √ distension of small bowel and colon (loops wider than vertebral body L1) ± air-fluid levels, commonly in RLQ (1st sign)

GI

√ tubular loops of bowel
√ bowel wall thickening + "thumbprinting"
√ "fixed" bowel = persistent abnormal loop of bowel without change on supine vs. prone films / for >24 hours
√ pneumatosis intestinalis (80%)
  — in curvilinear shape (= subserosal) or
  — bubbly / cystic (= submucosal gas collection from gasforming organisms / dissection of intraluminal gas)
√ "bubbly" appearance of bowel due to gas in wall / intraluminal gas / fecal matter (intraluminal contents are composed of blood, sloughed colonic mucosa, intraluminal gas, some fecal material)
√ gas in portal venous system (frequently transient, does not imply hopeless outcome)
√ ascites
√ pneumoperitoneum (immediate surgery required)

N.B.: Barium enema is contraindicated! May be used judiciously in selected cases with radiologic + clinical doubt!

Cx: (1) Inflammatory stricture after healing (BE follow-up in survivors)
(2) Bowel perforation in 12–32%

PELVIC LIPOMATOSIS + FIBROLIPOMATOSIS

= nonmalignant overgrowth of adipose tissue with minimal fibrotic + inflammatory components compressing soft-tissue structures within pelvis

Age: 9–80 years (peak 25–60 years); M:F = 10:1; NO racial predominance for Blacks; obesity NOT contributing factor

• often incidental finding
• urinary frequency, flank pain, suprapubic tenderness
• recurrent urinary tract infections
• low back pain, fever

√ elongation + narrowing of rectum
√ elevation of rectosigmoid + sigmoid colon out of pelvis
√ increase in sacrorectal space >10 mm
√ stretching of sigmoid colon
√ elongation + elevation of urinary bladder with symmetric inverted pear shape
√ elongation of posterior urethra
√ pelvic lucency; CT confirmatory
√ medial / lateral displacement of ureters

Cx of fibrolipomatosis:
(1) Ureteral obstruction (40% within 5 years)
(2) IVC obstruction

PERITONEAL MESOTHELIOMA

= only primary tumor of peritoneum arising from mesothelial cells lining peritoneal cavity

Age: 55–66 years; M >> F

Associated with: asbestos exposure

Spread: intraperitoneal along serosal surfaces; direct invasion of liver, pancreas, bladder, bowel

Location: pleura (67%), peritoneum (30–40%), pericardium (2.5%), processus vaginalis (0.5%)

√ thickening of mesentery, omentum, peritoneum, bowel wall
√ nodular masses in anterior parietal peritoneum becoming confluent cakelike
√ disproportionately small amount of ascites
√ areas of calcification (rare)

CT:
  √ nodular irregular thickening of peritoneal surfaces
  √ localized masses
  √ infiltrating sheets of tissue
  √ foci of calcifications
  √ ascites of near-water density
  √ stellate configuration of neurovascular bundles
  √ pleated thickening of mesenteric leaves

NUC:
  √ diffuse uptake of gallium-67

Prognosis: extremely poor due to advanced disease at presentation (most patients die within 1 year)

Cystic mesothelioma

= rare benign neoplasm without metastatic potential but tendency for local recurrence (in 27–50%)

Path: multiple thin-walled cysts lined by mesothelial cells + filled with watery fluid; intermediate form between benign adenomatoid tumor + malignant peritoneal mesothelioma

◊ Not associated with asbestos exposure!

Median age: 37 years; M << F

Location: any peritoneal / omental surface, most frequently in pelvis

• contains watery fluid

√ uni- / multilocular cystic tumor (cysts of 1 mm to 6 cm) without calcifications

DDx: lymphangioma, ovarian carcinoma

PERITONEAL METASTASES

= PERITONEAL CARCINOMATOSIS
= intraabdominal spread of malignant tumors

Origin: (a) common: ovary, stomach, colon
(b) less common: pancreas, uterus, bladder

√ massive ascites
√ desmoplastic reaction at (a) anterior border of rectum (Blumer shelf) (b) mesenteric side of terminal ileum

CT:
  √ increased density of linear network in mesenteric fat
  √ loculated fluid collections in peritoneal cavity
  √ apparent thickening of mesenteric vessels (= fluid within leaves of mesentery)
  √ adnexal mass of cystic / soft-tissue density (= Krukenberg tumor)
  √ small nodular densities on peritoneal surface
  √ "omental cake" = thickening of greater omentum
  √ lobulated mass in pouch of Douglas
  √ calcified peritoneal implants in serous cystadenocarcinoma of ovary (in up to 40% with stage III / IV disease)

PEUTZ-JEGHERS SYNDROME

= rare autosomal dominant disease with incomplete penetrance characterized by intestinal polyposis + mucocutaneous pigmentation (= hamartomatosis); often spontaneous mutation

Incidence: 1:7,000 livebirths; in 50% familial, in 50% sporadic; most frequent of polyposis syndromes to involve small intestines
Age: 25 years at presentation (range 10–30 years); M:F = 1:1
Path: multiple small sessile / large pedunculated polyps
Histo: benign hamartomatous polyp with smooth muscle core arising from muscularis mucosae + extending treelike into lamina propria of polyp; misplaced epithelium in submucosa, muscularis propria, subserosa frequently surrounding mucin-filled spaces

• mucocutaneous pigmentation (similar to freckles)
  = 1–5 mm small elongated melanin spots on mucous membranes (lower lips, gums, palate) + facial skin (nose, cheeks, around eyes) + volar aspects of toes and fingers (100%), becoming noticeable in first few years of life
• cramping abdominal pain (small bowel intussusception in 47%)
• rectal bleeding, melena (30%)
• prolapse of polyp through anus
• chronic hypochromic microcytic anemia

Location: small bowel (jejunum + ileum > duodenum) > colon > stomach; mouth + esophagus spared

@ Small bowel (>95%)
  √ multiple usually broad-based polyps separated by wide areas of intervening flat mucosa
  √ multilobulated surface of larger polyps
  √ myriad of 1- to 2-mm nodules of up to several cm = carpet of polyps
  √ intussusception usually confined to small bowel
@ Colon + rectum (30%)
  √ multiple scattered 1- to 30-mm polyps; NO carpeting
@ Stomach + duodenum (25%)
  √ diffuse involvement with multiple polyps
@ Respiratory + urinary tract
  √ adenoma of bronchus + bladder

Cx:
(1) Transient intussusception (pedunculated polyp)
(2) Carcinoma of GI tract (2–3%)
(3) Carcinoma of pancreas (13%)
(4) Carcinoma of breast (commonly bilateral + ductal)
(5) Ovarian tumor (5%): ovarian sex cord tumor, mucinous cystic tumor, cystadenoma, granulosa cell tumor
(6) Endometrial cancer: adenoma malignum of cervix
(7) Testicular tumor: feminizing Sertoli cell tumor

Rx:
(1) Endoscopic removal of all polyps >5 mm
(2) Surgery is reserved for obstruction, severe bleeding, malignancy

Prognosis: decreased life expectancy (risk of cancer approaching 40% by 40 years of age)
DDx: familial adenomatous polyposis, juvenile polyposis (similar age), Cowden syndrome, Cronkhite-Canada syndrome

POSTCRICOID DEFECT

= variable defect seen commonly in the fully distended cervical esophagus; no pathologic value

Etiology: redundancy of mucosa over rich postcricoid submucosal venous plexus
Incidence: in 80% of normal adults
Location: anterior aspect of esophagus at level of cricoid cartilage

√ tumor- / weblike lesion with variable configuration during swallowing

DDx: submucosal tumor, esophageal web (persistent configuration)

POSTINFLAMMATORY POLYPOSIS

= PSEUDOPOLYPOSIS
= reepithelialized inflammatory polyps as sequelae of mucosal ulceration

Etiology: ulcerative colitis (10–20%); granulomatous colitis (less frequent); schistosomiasis (endemic); amebic colitis (occasionally); toxic megacolon
Location: most common in left hemicolon, may occur in stomach / small intestine

√ sessile + frondlike appearance (often)
√ filiform polyposis = multiple wormlike projections only attached at their bases (CHARACTERISTIC)

Pathogenesis: ulcerative undermining of strips of mucosa with reepithelialization of denuded surfaces of tags + bowel wall
Prognosis: NO malignant potential
DDx: familial polyposis (polyps terminate in bulbous heads)

PRESBYESOPHAGUS

= defect in primary peristalsis + LES relaxation associated with aging

Incidence: 15% in 7th decade; 50% in 8th decade; 85% in 9th decade
Associated with: hiatus hernia, reflux

• usually asymptomatic

√ impaired / no primary peristalsis
√ often repetitive nonperistaltic tertiary contractions in distal esophagus
√ mild / moderate esophageal dilatation
√ poor LES relaxation

DDx: diabetes, diffuse esophageal spasm, scleroderma, esophagitis, achalasia, benign stricture, carcinoma

PROGRESSIVE SYSTEMIC SCLEROSIS

= PSS = multisystem connective tissue disorder (collagen-vascular disease) of unknown etiology characterized by widespread disorder of the microvasculature causing exuberant interstitial fibrosis with atrophy + sclerosis of many organ systems
= SCLERODERMA = variety of skin disorders associated with hardening of skin;

by extent of cutaneous involvement divided into:
(a) DIFFUSE SCLERODERMA
  tends to involve older women;
  interstitial pulmonary fibrosis more severe;
  organ failure more likely

(b) SYSTEMIC SCLEROSIS WITH LIMITED SCLERODERMA (formerly CREST syndrome) CREST features more common; pulmonary arterial hypertension more common + more severe)

May be associated with:
other connective tissue diseases (especially SLE and polymyositis/dermatomyositis)

Cause: autoimmune condition with genetic predisposition, may be initiated by environmental antigen (eg, toxic oil syndrome in Spain through ingestion of adulterated rape seed oil / ingestion of L-tryptophan)
Peak age: 30–50 years; M:F = 1:3
Histo: vasculitis + submucosal fibrosis extending into muscularis, smooth muscle atrophy (initially hypertrophy and finally atrophy of collagen fibers)

- CREST: **C**alcinosis of skin
  Raynaud phenomenon
  Esophageal dysmotility
  Sclerodactyly
  Telangiectasia
- antinuclear antibodies (30–80%):
  - centromere antibody (ACA) specific for limited disease
  - anti–topoisomerase-1 (= antiScl-70) identifies patients with diffuse cutaneous disease
- antibodies to extracellular matrix proteins and type I + IV collagen
- rheumatoid factor (35%)
- LE cells (5%)
- weakness, generalized debility

Prognosis: 50–67% 5-year survival rate

Gastrointestinal scleroderma (in 40–45%)

◊ Third most common manifestation of scleroderma (after skin changes + Raynaud phenomenon)
◊ May precede other manifestations!
- abdominal pain, diarrhea
- multiple episodes of pseudoobstruction

√ hepatomegaly

@ Esophagus (in 42–95%)
◊ First GI tract location to be involved!
- dysphagia (50%)
- heartburn (30%)

√ normal peristalsis above aortic arch (striated muscle in proximal 1/3 of esophagus)
√ hypotonia / atony + hypokinesia / aperistalsis in lower 2/3 of esophagus (>50%)
√ deficient emptying in recumbent position
√ thin / vanished longitudinal folds
√ mild to moderate dilatation of esophagus
√ chalasia (= patulous lower esophageal sphincter)
√ gastroesophageal reflux (70%)
√ erosions + superficial ulcers (from asymptomatic reflux esophagitis: NO protective esophageal contraction)
√ fusiform stricture usually 4–5 cm above gastroesophageal junction (from reflux esophagitis)
√ esophageal shortening + sliding hiatal hernia
Cx: peptic stricture, aspiration, Barrett esophagus, adenocarcinoma

@ Stomach (less frequent involvement)
√ gastric dilatation
√ decreased motor activity + delayed emptying

@ Small bowel (in up to 45%)
◊ PSS is rapidly progressing once small intestine is involved!
- malabsorption (delayed intestinal transit time + bacterial overgrowth)

√ marked dilatation of small bowel (in particular duodenum = megaduodenum, jejunum) simulating small bowel obstruction
CAVE: misdiagnosis of obstruction may lead to exploratory surgery!
√ abrupt cutoff at SMA level (atrophy of neural cells with hypoperistalsis)
√ prolonged transit time with barium retention in duodenum up to 24 hours
√ "hidebound / accordion" pattern (60%) = sharply defined folds of normal thickness with decreased intervalvular distance (tightly packed folds) within dilated segment (due to predominant involvement of circular muscle)
√ pseudodiverticula (10–40%) = asymmetric sacculations with squared tops + broad bases on mesenteric side (due to eccentric smooth muscle atrophy)
√ pneumatosis cystoides intestinalis + pneumoperitoneum (occasionally)
√ excess fluid with bacterial overgrowth (= "pseudo–blind loop syndrome")
√ normal mucosal fold pattern
Cx: intussusception without anatomic lead point

@ Colon (up to 40–50%)
- constipation (common), may alternate with diarrhea

√ pseudosacculations + wide-mouthed "diverticula" on antimesenteric side (formed by repetitive bulging through atrophic areas) in transverse + descending colon
√ eventually complete loss of haustrations (simulating cathartic colon)
√ marked dilatation (may simulate Hirschsprung disease)
√ stercoral ulceration (from retained fecal material)
Cx: life-threatening barium impaction

DDx: (1) Dermatomyositis (similar radiographic findings)
(2) Sprue (increased secretions, segmentation, fragmentation, dilatation most significant in midjejunum, normal motility)

GI

(3) Obstruction (no esophageal changes, no pseudodiverticula)
(4) Idiopathic intestinal pseudoobstruction (usually in young people)

Pulmonary scleroderma (in 10–25%)

Path: almost 100% involvement in autopsy series
Histo: thickening of basement membrane of alveoli + small arteries and veins

- slightly productive cough + progressive dyspnea
- hematemesis
- pulmonary function abnormalities in the absence of frank roentgenographic changes (typical dissociation of clinical, functional, and radiologic evidence)
- pericarditis

Location: most prominent at both lung bases (where blood flow greatest)

√ fine / coarse reticulations / diffuse interstitial infiltrates
√ subpleural fibrocystic spaces (honeycombing)
√ low lung volumes from progressive volume loss
√ alveolar changes (secondary to aspiration of refluxed gastric contents with disturbed esophageal motility / mineral oil taken to combat constipation)
√ air esophagram (DDx: achalasia, mediastinitis)
√ pleural reaction / effusion distinctly uncommon

Cx: (1) Pulmonary arterial hypertension (6–60%)
(2) Increased incidence of lung cancer

@ Heart: sclerosis of cardiac muscle ± cor pulmonale

Renal scleroderma (25%)

Onset: common within 3 years
Histo: fibrinoid necrosis of afferent arterioles (also seen in malignant hypertension)

√ renal cortical necrosis
√ spotty inhomogeneous nephrogram (constriction + occlusion of arteries)
√ concomitant arterial ectasia

Cx: renal failure (from nephrosclerosis)

Musculoskeletal scleroderma

- edema of distal portion of extremities
- thickened inelastic waxy skin most prominent about face + extremities
- symmetrical polyarthralgias (50–80%)
- Raynaud phenomenon (may proceed other symptoms by months / years)
- atrophy + thickening of skin and musculature (78%)

@ Fingers
- "sausage digit" = edema of digits associated with loss of transverse skin folds + lack of definition of subcutaneous fat

√ "tapered fingers" = sclerodactyly = atrophy + resorption of soft tissues of fingertips + soft-tissue calcifications
√ acroosteolysis = "penciling" / "autoamputation" = resorption of distal phalanges of hand (63%) beginning at volar aspect of terminal tufts with proximal progression
√ calcinosis (25%) = punctate soft-tissue calcifications of fingertips, axilla, ischial tuberosity, forearm, elbow (over pressure area), lower leg, face
√ calcifications around tendons. bursae, within joints

@ Arthritis
- stiffness in small joints, occasionally in knee, shoulder, wrist
- lack of motility, eventually contractures

√ arthritis of interphalangeal joints of hands (25%)
Location: 1st CMC, MCP, DIP, PIP
√ central / marginal erosions (50%)
√ resorption of palmar aspect of terminal phalanges (most frequent sign)
√ bony erosions of carpal bones (trapezium), distal radius + ulna, mandible, ribs, lateral aspect of clavicle, humerus, acromion, mandible, cervical spine
√ joint-space narrowing (late)
DDx: rheumatoid, psoriatic, erosive arthritis
√ soft-tissue swelling ± periarticular osteoporosis
√ NO significant osteoporosis
√ ± flexion contractures of fingers (from tendon sheath inflammation + fibrosis)

√ erosion of superior aspect of ribs
√ widening of periodontal membrane

PROLAPSED ANTRAL MUCOSA

= prolapse of hypertrophic + inflammatory mucosa of gastric antrum into duodenum resulting in pyloric obstruction

√ mushroom- / umbrella- / cauliflower-shaped filling defect at duodenal base
√ filling defect varies in size + shape
√ redundant gastric rugae can be traced from pyloric antrum through pyloric channel
√ gastric hyperperistalsis

PSEUDOMEMBRANOUS COLITIS

= CLOSTRIDIUM DIFFICILE DISEASE (more appropriate name because pseudomembranes are uncommon)

Cause: overgrowth of Gram-positive Clostridium difficile in response to a decrease in normal intestinal flora
Etiologic agent: cytotoxin produced by C. difficile
Predisposed:
(a) complication of antibiotic therapy with tetracycline, penicillin, ampicillin, clindamycin, lincomycin, amoxicillin, chloramphenicol, cephalosporins
(b) complication of some chemotherapeutic agents: methotrexate, fluorouracil
(c) following surgery / renal transplantation / irradiation; intestinal vascular insufficiency
(d) shock, uremia
(e) proximal to large bowel obstruction
(f) debilitating diseases: lymphosarcoma, leukemia
(g) immunosuppressive therapy with actinomycin D

Histo: pseudomembranes (exudate composed of leukocytes, fibrin, mucin, sloughed necrotic epithelium held in columns by strands of mucus) on a partially denuded colonic edematous mucosa (mucosa generally intact); reactive edema in lamina propria, submucosa, and eventually subserosa

- profuse watery diarrhea, abdominal cramps, tenderness
- fever, fecal blood, leukocytosis
- less common: chronic diarrhea, toxic megacolon, hyperpyrexia, leukemoid reaction, hypoalbuminemia with anasarca
- confluent small yellow plaques (= pseudomembranes) adherent to mucosal surface seen on endoscopy (50%)

Location: rectum (95%); confined to right + transverse colon (5–27%)

Plain film:
- √ adynamic ileus pattern = moderate gaseous distension of small bowel + colon
- √ "transverse banding" = marked thickening + distortion of haustral folds
- √ "thumbprinting" most prominent in transverse colon
- √ diffusely shaggy + irregular surface (confluent pseudomembranes)

BE (CONTRAINDICATED in severe cases):
- √ "accordion-like" haustral thickening = contrast material trapped between distorted thickened closely spaced transverse edematous folds (simulating intramural tracts)
- √ pseudoulcerations = barium filling clefts between pseudomembranes
- √ irregular ragged polypoid contour of colonic wall
- √ discrete multiple plaquelike lesions of 2–4 mm in size (DDx: polyposis, nodular form of lymphoma)
  N.B.: Risk of colonic perforation!

CT (85% sensitive, 48% specific):
- √ colonic wall thickening of 4–22 mm (61–88%)
- √ smooth circumferential thickening (44%)
- √ accordion sign (51–70%) = alternating bands of edematous haustral folds separated by intraluminal contrast material
- √ nodular thickening (17%)
- √ homogeneous enhancement due to hyperemia
- √ pericolonic stranding (42%)
- √ ascites (15–25%)
- √ NO colonic abnormality (12–39%)

Dx: (1) Stool assay for Clostridium difficile cytotoxin (detects toxin B): cumbersome to perform
(2) Enzyme immunoassay test (up to 33% false-negative results): detects toxin A + B
(3) Stool culture (95% sensitive): not available for 2 days
(4) Pseudomembranes on proctosigmoidoscopy

Cx: peritonitis

Prognosis: 15% mortality; most patients recover within 2 weeks

Rx: discontinuation of suspected antibiotic + administration of vancomycin / metronidazole with attention to fluid and electrolyte balance

PSEUDOMYXOMA PERITONEI

= "jelly belly" = "gelatinous ascites" = slow insidious accumulation of large amounts of intraperitoneal gelatinous material

Etiology: rupture of mucinous cystadenoma / cystadenocarcinoma of appendix (male) / ovary (female); rarely associated with malignancy of colon (<5%), stomach, uterus, pancreas, common bile duct, urachal duct, omphalomesenteric duct

- slowly progressive massive abdominal distension
- recurrent abdominal pain
- √ thickening of peritoneal + omental surfaces
- √ omental cake
- √ posterior displacement of bowel loops + mesentery
- √ voluminous septated / loculated pseudoascites
- √ several thin-walled cystic masses of different size throughout abdominal cavity
- √ scalloped contour of liver margins
- √ annular / semicircular calcifications (rare but highly suggestive)

CT:
- √ tumor collection of very low attenuation (common) / soft-tissue density (rare)

US:
- √ hypoechoic collection (common) / more solid appearance (rare)

DDx: peritoneal metastases, pancreatitis with pseudocysts, pyogenic peritonitis, widespread echinococcal disease, ascites

Prognosis: 50% 5-year survival rate

RADIATION INJURY

= obliterative endarteritis with irradiation in excess of 4,000–4,500 rads

Incidence: 5%; increased risk after pelvic surgery

√ radiographic changes within field of radiation only

Radiation gastritis

Permanent radiographic findings of radiation injury appear 1 month to 2 years after therapy
- √ gastric ulceration + deformity (pylorus)
- √ enlargement + effacement of gastric folds
- √ antral narrowing + rigidity (similar to linitis plastica)

Radiation enteritis

Permanent radiographic findings of radiation injury appear >1–2 years following irradiation

Predisposed: women (cancer of cervix, endometrium, ovary), patients with bladder cancer

- crampy abdominal pain (from intermittent obstruction)
- persistent diarrhea
- occult intestinal hemorrhage

Location: ileum; concomitant radiation damage to colon / rectum
- √ irregular nodular thickening of folds with straight transverse course ± ulcerations
- √ serrated bowel margin
- √ thickened bowel wall with luminal narrowing
- √ multiple strictures + partial mechanical obstruction

GI

√ separation of adjacent bowel loops by >2 mm
√ shortening of small bowel
√ fixation + immobilization of bowel loops with similar radiographic appearance between examinations (from dense desmoplastic response to irradiation)
CT: √ increased attenuation of mesentery
DDx: Crohn disease, lymphoma, ischemia, hemorrhage

Radiation injury of rectum

Manifestation of radiation colitis can occur up to 15 years following irradiation
Predisposed: 90% in women (carcinoma of cervix)
• tenesmus, diarrhea, bleeding, constipation
√ ridgelike appearance of mucosa (submucosal fibrosis)
√ irregularly outlined ulcerations (rare)
CT:
√ narrowed partially distensible rectum
√ thick homogeneous rectal wall
√ "target sign" = submucosal circumferential lucency
√ proliferation of perirectal fat >10 mm
√ thickening of perirectal fascia
√ "halo effect" = increase in pararectal fibrosis
Cx: (1) Obstruction
(2) Colovaginal / coloenteric fistula formation

RETAINED GASTRIC ANTRUM

Cause: retention of endocrinologically active gastric antrum in continuity with pylorus + duodenum
Pathophysiology: bathing of antrum in alkaline duodenal juice stimulates secretion of gastrin
Associated with: gastric ulcers in 30–50%
√ duodenogastric reflux of barium through pylorus (diagnostic)
√ giant marginal ulcer / several marginal ulcers usually on jejunal side of anastomosis (large false-negative + false-positive rates; correct-positive rate of 28–60%)
√ large amount of secretions
√ edematous mucosa of jejunal anastomotic segment
√ lacy / cobweblike small bowel pattern (hypersecretion)
Cx: gastrojejunocolic fistula

RETRACTILE MESENTERITIS

= CHRONIC FIBROSING MESENTERITIS = CHRONIC SUBPERITONEAL SCLEROSIS = MESENTERIC PANNICULITIS = LIPOSCLEROTIC MESENTERITIS
= MESENTERIC LIPODYSTROPHY = MESENTERIC WEBER-CHRISTIAN DISEASE
= rare disorder of unknown etiology characterized by fibrofatty thickening of small bowel mesentery
Etiology: ? trauma, previous surgery, ischemia
Path: spectrum ranging from mesenteric lipodystrophy through mesenteric panniculitis to mesenteric fibrosis
Histo: chronic inflammation with a dense collection of lymphocytes + plasma cells + lipid-laden macrophages; desmoplastic reaction; fat necrosis; calcifications
Associated with:
(1) Gardner syndrome, familial polyposis
(2) Fibrosing mediastinitis, retroperitoneal fibrosis
(3) Lymphoma, lymphosarcoma
(4) Carcinoid tumor
(5) Metastatic gastric / colonic carcinoma
(6) Whipple lipodystrophy
(7) Weber-Christian disease
Age: most common in 6th decade; M:F = 2:1
• crampy abdominal pain
• nausea + vomiting; mild weight loss
• low-grade fever

Location: root of mesentery extending toward mesenteric border of bowel
Plain film:
√ soft-tissue mass with calcifications
√ ± thumbprinting (from vascular congestion)
UGI:
√ compression / distortion of duodenum near ligament of Treitz
√ separation of small bowel loops with fixation, kinking, and angulation
CT:
√ mass of fat density interspersed with soft-tissue density (fibrous tissue) + calcifications
√ mesenteric thickening with fine stellate pattern extending to bowel border
√ retraction of small bowel loops
√ single mesenteric soft-tissue mass (fibroma)
√ multiple nodules throughout mesentery (fibromatosis)
Prognosis: usually benign course
DDx: metastatic gastric / colonic adenocarcinoma; carcinoid tumor; mesenteric lymphoma; liposarcoma of mesentery

SCHATZKI RING

= LOWER ESOPHAGEAL MUCOSAL RING = constant lower esophageal ring (mucosal thickening) presumed to result from reflux esophagitis = thin annular peptic stricture
Incidence: 6–14% of population; old age > young age; M > F
Histo: usually squamous epithelium on upper surface + columnar epithelium on undersurface; may be covered totally by squamous epithelium or columnar epithelium
• asymptomatic (if ring >20 mm)
• dysphagia (if ring <12 mm)
Location: near the squamocolumnar junction; in region of B ring at inferior margin of lower esophageal sphincter
√ permanently present nondistensible transverse ring with constant shape + size (range of 3–18 mm)
√ 2- to 4-mm thick shelflike projection into lumen with smooth symmetric margins
√ visible only with adequate distension of esophagogastric region and when located above the esophageal hiatus of the diaphragm

GI

√ best demonstrated in prone position during arrested deep inspiration with Valsalva maneuver while barium column passes through esophagogastric region
√ short esophagus + intrahiatal / intrathoracic gastric segment = sliding hiatal hernia if Schatzki ring located 1–2 cm above diaphragmatic hiatus

Prognosis: decrease in caliber over 5 years (in 25–33%)
Cx: impaction of food bolus (associated with severe chest pain)
Rx: (1) Proper mastication of food
(2) Endoscopic rupture
(3) Esophageal dilatation (radiographically often lack of caliber change after successful dilatation)
DDx: annular peptic stricture (usually thicker, asymmetric, irregular surface, associated with thickened esophageal folds, serration of esophageal margins)

SMALL LEFT COLON SYNDROME

Cause: transient functional colonic obstruction due to immaturity of mesenteric plexus
Age: newborn infant
Associated with: maternal diabetes mellitus (most common), maternal substance abuse; NOT related to cystic fibrosis

√ colonic caliber becomes abruptly diminutive distal to splenic flexure
√ bowel dilatation proximal to splenic flexure
√ ± meconium plug (as a result and not the cause of obstruction)

Prognosis: gradual resolution of functional immaturity over days to weeks

SOLITARY RECTAL ULCER SYNDROME

= MUCOSAL PROLAPSE SYNDROME

Related disorders with common pathogenesis:
hamartomatous inverted polyp, colitis cystica profunda

Cause: prolapse of anterior rectal wall resulting in mucosal ischemia due to traumatization of rectal mucosa by anal sphincter during defecation
Path: small / large, single / multiple shallow ulcers; 25% broad-based, 18% patchy granular / velvety hyperemic mucosa; rectal stenosis through confluent circumferential lesion
Histo: obliteration of lamina propria mucosae by fibromuscular proliferation of muscularis mucosae, streaming of fibroblasts + muscle fibers between crypts, misplaced mucosal glands deep to muscularis mucosae; diffuse increase in mucosal collagen

- chronic rectal bleeding
- passage of mucus
- disordered defecation
- tenesmus

BE:
√ ulcer (ulcerative type)
√ polypoid lesion / nodules (polypoid type)
√ flat granular mucosa (flat type)
√ stricture

Evacuation proctography:
√ failure of anorectal angle to open while straining
√ excessive perineal descent

Prognosis:
(1) Little change over time
(2) Considerable change in appearance of lesion
(3) Transfusions necessitated by massive blood loss

DDx: invasive rectal carcinoma, Crohn disease

SPRUE

= classic disease of malabsorption

Path: villous atrophy (truncation) + elongation of crypts of Lieberkühn + round cell infiltration of lamina propria (plasma cells + lymphocytes)

Celiac disease

= NONTROPICAL SPRUE = GLUTEN-SENSITIVE ENTEROPATHY
= characterized by malabsorption resulting from atrophy of small intestinal villi

Irritating agent: gliadin polypeptides in wheat, rye, barley, oats
May be hereditary: detected in 15% of 1st-degree relatives
Countries: North America, Europe, Australia, India, Pakistan, Middle East, Cuba
Age: childhood by age 2 years; 30–40 years with M<F; 40–60 years with M>F
Rx: gluten-free diet: corn, rice, tapioca, soya, millet, vitamin supplements

Tropical sprue

Etiology: infectious agent cured with antibiotics; geographic distribution (India, Far East, Puerto Rico)
Age: any age group

- glossitis
- hepatosplenomegaly
- macrocytic anemia + leukopenia

Prognosis: spontaneous resolution after months / years
Rx: responds well to folic acid + broad-spectrum antibiotics

- severe diarrhea, steatorrhea (CLASSIC but found only in minority of patients)
- crampy abdominal pain (from intussusception)
- lassitude, fatigue, weight loss
- stomatitis, anemia (iron / folate / vitamin B_{12} deficiency)
- bleeding diathesis
- neuropathy, depression
- infertility
- osteomalacia with bone pain
- dermatitis herpetiformis

Location: patchy involvement of duodenum + jejunum > remainder of small bowel

Small bowel follow-through:
√ small bowel dilatation is HALLMARK in untreated celiac disease (70–95%), best seen in mid + distal jejunum (due to intestinal hypomotility); degree of dilatation related to severity of disease

√ hypersecretion-related artifacts:
  √ air-fluid levels in small bowel (rare)
  √ segmentation = breakup of normal continual column of barium creating large masses of barium in dilated segments separated by stringlike strands from adjacent clumps due to excessive fluid; best seen on delayed films
  √ flocculation = coarse granular appearance of small clumps of disintegrated barium due to excess fluid best seen at periphery of intestinal segment; occurs especially with steatorrhea
  √ fragmentation = scattering = faint irregular stippling of residual barium resembling snowflakes associated with segmentation due to excessive fluid
√ "moulage sign" (50%) = smooth contour with effaced featureless folds resembling tubular wax mold (due to atrophy of the folds of Kerckring); CHARACTERISTIC of sprue if seen in duodenum + jejunum
√ long / normal / short transit time
√ nonpropulsive peristalsis (flaccid + poorly contracting loops)
√ normal / thickened / effaced mucosal folds (depending on degree of hypoproteinemia)
√ colonlike haustrations in well-filled jejunum (secondary to spasm + cicatrization from transverse ulcers)
√ "jejunalization" of ileal loops (= adaptive response to decreased jejunal mucosal surface) = SPECIFIC
√ transient nonobstructive intussusception (20%) without anatomic lead point
√ "bubbly bulb" = peptic duodenitis = mucosal inflammation, gastric metaplasia, Brunner gland hyperplasia

Enteroclysis:
√ decreased number of folds in proximal jejunum (≤3 folds per inch)
√ increased number of folds in distal ileum (>5 folds per inch)
√ tubular featureless lumen
√ mosaic pattern = 1–2 mm polygonal islands of mucosa surrounded by barium-filled distinct grooves (10%)

CT:
√ small bowel dilatation + increased fluid content ± mucosal fold thickening
√ mild to moderate lymphadenopathy in mesentery / retroperitoneum (up to 12%)

Dx: (1) Jejunal / duodenal biopsy
(2) Improvement of small bowel abnormalities after a few months on a gluten-free diet

Cause for relapse: hidden dietary gluten, diabetes, bacterial overgrowth, intestinal ulceration, development of lymphoma

Cx:
(1) Ulcerative jejunoileitis
= multiple chronic benign ulcers (sausage appearance of small bowel) with hemorrhage, perforation + obstruction
Age: 5th–6th decade
Location: jejunum > ileum > colon
• response to gluten-free diet ceases
Prognosis: frequently fatal
Rx: small bowel resection
(2) Hyposplenism (30–50%)
√ small atrophic spleen
(3) Cavitary mesenteric lymph node syndrome characterized by:
(a) mesenteric lymph node cavitation
(b) splenic atrophy
(c) villous atrophy of small intestinal mucosa
√ enlarged lymph nodes of low attenuation ± fat-fluid levels (filled with lipid-rich hyaline material) within jejunoileal mesentery
Prognosis: usually fatal disorder
(4) Malignant tumors
(a) lymphoma (in 8%): commonly diffuse + nodular and of C-cell type
Peak prevalence: 7th decade
√ enlarged nodular folds, ulcers, extrinsic mass effect
(b) adenocarcinoma of small bowel (6%), rectum, stomach
(c) squamous cell carcinoma of pharynx / esophagus (in 6%) during 6th–7th decade
(5) Generalized lymphadenopathy with lymphocytosis (mimicking lymphoma)
(6) Sigmoid volvulus (rare)

DDx:
(1) Esophageal hypoperistalsis: scleroderma, idiopathic pseudoobstruction
(2) Gastric abnormalities: Zollinger-Ellison syndrome, chronic granulomatous disease, eosinophilic enteritis, amyloidosis, malignancy
(3) Tiny nodular defects on thickened folds: Whipple disease, intestinal lymphangiectasia, Waldenström macroglobulinemia
(4) Small 1- to 3-mm nodules: lymphoid hyperplasia associated with giardiasis and immunoglobulin deficiency disease, diffuse lymphoma
(5) Small nodules of varying sizes: systemic mastocytosis, amyloidosis, eosinophilic enteritis, Cronkhite-Canada syndrome
(6) Bowel wall narrowing, kinking, scarring, ulceration: regional enteritis, bacterial / parasitic infection, carcinoid, vasculitis, ischemia, irradiation

STRONGYLOIDIASIS

Organism: helminthic parasite Strongyloides stercoralis (2.2 mm long, 50µm in diameter); capable of reproducing within human host
Prevalence: 100 million cases globally; 4% in U.S.
Country: tropical + subtropical regions, parts of Europe, southeastern U.S. (eastern Kentucky, rural Tennessee), Puerto Rico
Infection: filiform larva enters body through skin / mucous membranes (from contaminated soil)

Cycle: larva passes from subcutaneous / submucosal sites via venous circulation to lung; larva breaks into alveolar spaces and ascends via bronchi + trachea; larva swallowed; settles in duodenum + upper jejunum (lives in tunnels between enterocytes); parasitic adult female worms release eggs containing mature larvae into the intestinal lumen; ova hatch immediately into rhabditiform larvae and are passed to the environment

Path: edema + inflammation of intestinal wall secondary to invasion by larvae; flattening of villi; ova in mucosal crypts

- asymptomatic for many years (in majority)
- larva currens = recurrent allergic cutaneous skin lesions of autoinfection
- severe malnutrition (malabsorption, steatorrhea)
- weight loss
- worms, larvae, eggs in stool
- peripheral eosinophilia
- elevated levels of immunoglobulin E

√ paralytic ileus (massive invasion)
√ edematous irregular mucosal folds, spasm, dilatation of proximal 2/3 of duodenum
√ ulcerations
√ stricture of 3rd + 4th part of duodenum
  √ rigid pipestem appearance + irregular narrowing of duodenum (in advanced cases)

Rx: thiabendazole (90% efficacy rate)
Prognosis: high mortality in undernourished patients

HYPERINFECTION SYNDROME
= extensive tissue invasion by larvae in patients with malignancy, autoimmune disease, malnutrition
- bacteremia, septicemia
- crampy abdominal pain, persistent vomiting, diarrhea

CXR:
  √ fine miliary nodules / diffuse reticular opacities

SUPERIOR MESENTERIC ARTERY SYNDROME

= VASCULAR COMPRESSION OF DUODENUM
= WILKIE SYNDROME = CHRONIC DUODENAL ILEUS
= BODY CAST SYNDROME
= vascular compression of 3rd portion of duodenum within aortomesenteric compartment; probably representing a functional reflex dilatation

Etiology: narrowing of angle between SMA + aorta to 10–22° (normal 45–65°):
congenital, weight loss, visceroptosis due to loss of abdominal muscle tone (as in pregnancy), asthenic built, exaggerated lumbar lordosis, prolonged bed rest in supine position (body cast, whole-body burns, surgery)

- repetitive vomiting
- abdominal cramping

√ megaduodenum = pronounced dilatation of 1st + 2nd portion of duodenum + frequently stomach, best seen in supine position
√ vertical linear compression defect in transverse portion of duodenum overlying spine
√ abrupt change in caliber distal to compression defect
√ relief of compression by postural change into prone knee-elbow position

TAILGUT CYST

= RETRORECTAL CYSTIC HAMARTOMA

Cause: incomplete regression of embryonic tailgut (= the portion distal to future anus)
Average age: 35 years; M<F
Histo: several types of epithelia + elements of intestinal epithelium, smooth muscle within cyst wall

- asymptomatic / perirectal pain, rectal bleeding, urinary frequency

Location: retrorectal / presacral space ± extension into ischiorectal fossa

√ thin-walled multicystic / unilocular cyst adhering to sacrum / rectum
√ fluid of clear / mucoid fluid with internal echoes

Cx: (1) repeated perirectal abscesses, recurring anorectal fistula
(2) degeneration into mucinous adenocarcinoma

TOXIC MEGACOLON

= acute transmural fulminant colitis with neurogenic loss of motor tone + rapid development of extensive colonic dilatation >5.5 cm in transverse colon (damage to entire colonic wall + neuromuscular degeneration)

Etiology:
1. Ulcerative colitis (most common)
2. Crohn disease
3. Amebiasis, salmonellosis
4. Pseudomembranous colitis
5. Ischemic colitis

Histo: widespread sloughing of mucosa + thinning of frequently necrotic muscle layers

- systemic toxicity
- profuse bloody diarrhea

√ colonic ileus with marked dilatation of transverse colon
√ few air-fluid levels
√ increasing caliber of colon on serial radiographs without redundancy
√ loss of normal colonic haustra + interhaustral folds
√ coarsely irregular mucosal surface
√ pseudopolyposis = mucosal islands in denuded ulcerated colonic wall
√ pneumatosis coli ± pneumoperitoneum

CT:
  √ distended colon filled with large amounts of fluid + air
  √ distorted haustral pattern
  √ irregular nodular contour of thin wall
  √ intramural air / small collections

BE: CONTRAINDICATED due to risk of perforation
Prognosis: 20% mortality

TUBERCULOSIS

Rarely encountered in Western Hemisphere, increased incidence in AIDS; usually associated with pulmonary tuberculosis (in 6–38%)

GI

Etiology:
(1) Ingestion of tuberculous sputum
(2) Hematogenous spread from tuberculous focus in lung to submucosal lymph nodes, associated with radiographic evidence of pulmonary TB in <50%
(3) Primary infection by cow milk (Mycobacterium bovis)

Path:
(a) ulcerative form (most frequent): ulcers with their long axis perpendicular to axis of intestine, undermining + pseudopolyps
(b) hypertrophic form: thickening of bowel wall (transmural granulomatous process)

Organism: M. tuberculosis, M. bovis, M. avium-intracellulare
Age: 20–40 years
- weight loss, abdominal pain (80–90%)
- nausea, vomiting
- tuberculin skin test negative in most patients with primary intestinal TB

Location: ileocecal area > ascending colon > jejunum > appendix > duodenum > stomach > sigmoid > rectum

@ Tuberculous peritonitis (in 1/3)
◊ Most common presentation
Cause: hematogenous spread / rupture of mesenteric node
(a) wet type = exudative ascites with high protein contents + leukocytes
(b) dry type = caseous adenopathy + adhesions
(c) fibrotic type = omental cakelike mass with separation + fixation of bowel loops

CT:
√ high-density ascites (20–45 HU)
√ enlarged lymph nodes (90%) with low-density centers in 40% (due to caseous necrosis)
Location: peripancreatic + mesentery, retroperitoneum
√ irregular masses of soft-tissue density in omentum + mesentery (common)

Cx: small bowel obstruction (adhesions from serosal tubercles)

@ Ileocecal area (80–90%)
◊ Most commonly affected bowel
Cause: relative stagnation of intestinal contents + abundance of lymphoid tissue (Peyer patches)
√ Stierlin sign = rapid emptying of narrowed terminal ileum (due to persistent irritability) on BE
√ thickened ileocecal valve (mass effect)
√ Fleischner sign = "inverted umbrella" defect = wide gaping patulous ileocecal valve associated with narrowing of the immediately adjacent ileum + narrowed rigid cecum
√ deep fissures + ulcers with sinus tracts / enterocutaneous fistulas / perforation
DDx: Crohn disease, cecal carcinoma

@ Colon
Site: segmental colonic involvement, esp. on right side
√ rigid contracted cone-shaped cecum (spasm / transmural fibrosis)
√ spiculations + wall thickening
√ diffuse ulcerating colitis + pseudopolyps
√ shortening + short hourglass strictures
DDx: ulcerative colitis, Crohn disease, amebiasis (spares terminal ileum), colitis of bacillary dysentery, ischemic colitis, pseudomembranous colitis

@ Gastroduodenal
Site: simultaneous involvement of pylorus + duodenum
√ stenotic pylorus with gastric outlet obstruction
√ narrowed antrum (linitis plastica appearance)
√ antral fistula
√ multiple large and deep ulcerations on lesser curvature
√ thickened duodenal folds with irregular contour / dilatation
DDx: carcinoma, lymphoma, syphilis

@ Esophagus
◊ Least common GI tract manifestation
Cause: secondary involvement from adjacent tuberculous lymphadenitis / primary TB
√ deep ulceration
√ stricture
√ mass
√ intramural dissection / fistula formation = sinus tract formation

TURCOT SYNDROME

= autosomal recessive disease with
(a) colonic polyposis
(b) CNS tumors (especially supratentorial glioblastoma, occasionally medulloblastoma)

Age: symptomatic during 2nd decade
Histo: adenomatous polyps
- diarrhea
- seizures

√ multiple 1–30 mm polyps in colon + rectum
Cx: malignant transformation of colonic polyps in 100%
Prognosis: death from brain tumor in 2nd + 3rd decade

TYPHLITIS

= ILEOCECAL SYNDROME = NEUTROPENIC COLITIS
= acute inflammation of cecum, appendix, and occasionally terminal ileum; initially described in children with leukemia + severe neutropenia;
typhlos = "blind sac" = cecum

Cause: leukemic / lymphomatous infiltrate, ischemia, focal pseudomembranous colitis, infection
Histo: edema + ulceration of entire bowel wall; transmural necrosis with perforation possible
Organism: CMV, Pseudomonas, Candida, Klebsiella, E. coli, B. fragilis, Enterobacter
Predisposed: common in childhood leukemia, aplastic anemia, lymphoma, immunosuppressive therapy (eg, renal transplant), clinical AIDS

- abdominal pain, may be localized to RLQ
- watery diarrhea
- fullness / palpable mass in RLQ
- fever, neutropenia
- hematochezia / occult blood

Location: cecum + ascending colon, appendix + distal ileum may become secondarily involved

√ fluid-filled masslike density in RLQ
√ distension of nearby small bowel loops
√ thumbprinting of ascending colon
√ circumferential thickening of cecal wall >4 mm
√ occasionally pneumatosis

CT (preferable examination due to risk of perforation):
√ circumferential wall thickening (>1–3 mm) of cecum ± terminal ileum
√ decreased bowel wall attenuation (edema)
√ increased attenuation of adjacent fat + thickening of fascial planes (pericolonic inflammation)
√ ± pericolonic fluid + intramural pneumatosis

Cx: (1) Perforation (BE is a risky procedure)
(2) Abscess formation

Rx: early aggressive medical support (high doses of antibiotics + IV fluids) prior to development of transmural necrosis

DDx: (1) Leukemic / lymphomatous deposits (more eccentric thickening)
(2) Appendicitis with periappendicular abscess (normal cecal wall thickness)
(3) Diverticulitis
(4) Inflammatory bowel disease

ULCERATIVE COLITIS

= common idiopathic inflammatory bowel disease with continuous concentric + symmetric colonic involvement

Etiology: ? hypersensitivity / autoimmune disease

Prevalence: 50–80:100,000 In high incidence areas of North America, Northern Europe, Australia

Path: predominantly mucosal + submucosal disease with exudate + edema + crypt abscesses (HALLMARK) resulting in shallow ulceration

Age peak: 20–40 years + 60–70 years; M:F = 1:1

- alternating periods of remission + exacerbation
- bloody diarrhea
- electrolyte depletion, fever, systemic toxicity
- abdominal cramps

Extracolonic manifestations:
- iritis, erythema nodosum, pyoderma gangrenosum
- pericholangitis, chronic active hepatitis, primary sclerosing cholangitis, fatty liver
- spondylitis, peripheral arthritis, coincidental rheumatoid arthritis (10–20%)
- thrombotic complications

Location: begins in rectum with proximal progression (rectum spared in 4%)
(a) rectosigmoid in 95% (diagnosed by rectal biopsy); continuous circumferential involvement often limited to left side of colon
(b) colitis extending proximally to splenic flexure = universal colitis
(c) terminal ileum in 10–25% ("backwash ileitis")

Plain film:
√ hyperplastic mucosa, polypoid mucosa, deep ulcers
√ diffuse dilatation with loss of haustral markings
√ toxic megacolon
√ free intraperitoneal gas
√ complete absence of fecal residue (due to inflammation)

BE:
(a) acute stage
√ narrowing + incomplete filling (spasm + irritability)
√ fine mucosal granularity = stippling of barium coat (from diffuse mucosal edema + hyperemia + superficial erosions)
√ spicules + serrated bowel margins (tiny superficial ulcers)
√ "collar button" ulcers (= undermining of ulcers)
√ "double-tracking" = longitudinal submucosal ulceration over several cm
√ hazy / fuzzy quality of bowel contour (excessive secretions)
√ "thumbprinting" = symmetric thickening of colonic folds
√ pseudopolyps = scattered islands of edematous mucosa + reepithelialized granulation tissue within areas of denuded mucosa
√ widening of presacral space
√ obliterated rectal folds = valves of Houston (43%)

(b) subacute stage
√ distorted irregular haustra
√ inflammatory polyps = sessile frondlike / rarely pedunculated lesions (= localized mucosal inflammation resulting in polypoid protuberance)
√ coarse granular mucosa (= mucosal replacement by granulation tissue)

(c) chronic stage
√ shortening of colon (= reversible spasm of longitudinal muscle) with depression of flexures
√ "leadpipe" colon = rigidity + symmetric narrowing of lumen
√ widening of haustral clefts / complete loss of haustrations (DDx: cathartic colon)
√ "burnt-out colon" = fairly distensible colon without haustral markings + without mucosal pattern
√ hazy / fuzzy quality of bowel contour (excessive secretions)
√ postinflammatory polyps (12–19%) = small sessile nodules / long wormlike branching + bridging outgrowths (= filiform polyposis)
√ "backwash ileitis" (5–30%) involving 4–25 cm of terminal ileum with patulous ileocecal valve + absent peristalsis + granularity

CT:
√ wall thickening <10 mm

Cx:
(1) Toxic megacolon ± perforation in 5–10% (DDx: granulomatous / ischemic / amebic colitis)
◊ Most common cause of death in ulcerative colitis!

GI

(2) Colonic adenocarcinoma (3–5%):
risk starts after 8–10 years of onset of disease; risk progresses at 0.5% for 10–20 years + at 0.9% thereafter; higher risk with pancolitis + onset of disease in <15 years of age
Location: rectosigmoid > descending colon, distal transverse colon
√ narrowed segment of 2–6 cm in length with eccentric lumen + irregular contour + flattened rigid tapered margins = scirrhous carcinoma
√ annular / polypoid carcinoma
(3) Colonic strictures (10%)
smooth contour with fusiform pliable tapering margins, usually short + single stricture; commonly in sigmoid / rectum / transverse colon; usually after minimum of 5 years of disease; rarely cause for obstruction (DDx: colonic carcinoma)

DDx: (1) Familial polyposis (no inflammatory changes)
(2) Cathartic colon (more extensive in right colon)

DDx between CROHN DISEASE and ULCERATIVE COLITIS:
mnemonic: "LUCIFER M"

	Crohn Disease	*Ulcerative Colitis*
Location	right side	left side
Ulcers	deep	shallow
Contraction	no	yes
Ileocecal valve	thickened	gaping
Fistulae	yes	no
Eccentricity	yes	no
Rate of carcinoma	slight increase	marked increase
Megacolon	unusual	yes

VILLOUS ADENOMA

Villous Adenoma Of Colon

Incidence: 7% of all colonic tumors
Age: presentation late in life; M = F
Location: rectum + sigmoid (75%), cecum, ileocecal valve; 2% of all tumors in rectum + colon
Associated with: other GI tumors (25%)
• sensation of incomplete evacuation
• rectal bleeding
• excretion of copious amounts of thick mucus
• fatigability, weakness
• electrolyte depletion syndrome in 4% (dehydration, hyponatremia, hypokalemia)
√ may completely encircle the colon
√ bulky tumor with spongelike corrugated appearance (barium within interstices)
√ striated "brushlike" surface
√ soft pliable tumor with change in shape
√ innumerable mucosal projections (= fronds) with reticular / granular surface pattern (if villous elements constitute >75% of tumor, diagnosis can be made on BE)
√ apparent decrease in size on postevacuation films

Cx: malignant transformation / invasion (in 36%) related to size of tumor <5 cm (9%); >5 cm (55%); >10 cm (100%)

Villous Adenoma Of Duodenum

More common in colon + rectum; fewer than 50 cases in world literature
√ sessile, soft nonobstructive mass
√ "lace" / "soap bubble" pattern
√ preservation of peristaltic activity + bowel distensibility

WALDENSTRÖM MACROGLOBULINEMIA

= low-grade lymphoid malignancy composed of mature plasmacytoid lymphocytes with production of abnormal monoclonal IgM protein
Incidence: 0.53 / 100,000 annually; frequency 10–15% that of multiple myeloma
Histo: macroglobulin proteinaceous hyaline material fills lacteals in lamina propria of small bowel villi with secondary lymphatic distension + edema
Mean age: 63 years; M > F
• fatigue, weight loss
• diarrhea, steatorrhea, malabsorption
• anemia, bleeding diathesis
• IgM elevation
• hyperviscosity syndrome (20%) = bleeding, visual changes, neurologic abnormalities
@ Small bowel (rarely involved)
√ small bowel dilatation
√ uniform diffuse thickening of valvulae conniventes with spikelike configuration (jejunum + proximal ileum)
√ granular surface of punctate filling defects (distended villi)
@ Bone marrow involvement (91–98%)
(a) diffuse replacement of bone marrow (56%)
(b) variegated replacement of bone marrow (35%)
√ compression fractures of spine (48%)
√ diffuse demineralization of spine
√ lytic lesions on bone surveys (in up to 20%)
MR (pre- and postcontrast T1WI preferred):
√ marrow iso- / hypointense to muscle on T1WI
√ enhancement of abnormal marrow on T1WI
@ Lymph nodes
√ lymphadenopathy (43%)
@ Liver & spleen
√ hepatosplenomegaly
Dx: (1) characteristic M-spike in serum / urine electrophoresis
(2) abnormal lymphplasmacytoid cells in bone marrow / lymph nodes
DDx: multiple myeloma (lymphadenopathy rare, lytic lesions in 31%)

WHIPPLE DISEASE

= INTESTINAL LIPODYSTROPHY
= sporadically occurring chronic multisystem disease
Etiology: thought to be caused by infection with an as yet unidentified gram-positive bacterium (Tropheryma whippelii) closely related to actinobacteria

GI

Histo: PAS-positive material (periodic acid Schiff) = glycoprotein within foamy macrophages in the submucosa of the jejunum (bacterial cell wall) + fat deposits within intestinal submucosa and lymph nodes causing lymphatic obstruction + dilatation

Age: 4th–6th decade (mean age of onset, 50 years); M:F = 8:1; Caucasians

• recurrent and migratory arthralgias / nondeforming arthritis (65–95%); arthritis may precede Whipple disease in 10% up to 10 years
• malabsorption, steatorrhea, abdominal pain
• weight loss, low-grade fever
• polyserositis
• generalized peripheral lymphadenopathy (50%)
• hyperpigmentation of skin similar to Addison disease
• pale shaggy yellow plaques / erosions in postbulbar duodenum on endoscopy

Organ involvement: virtually every organ system, liver, intestines, joints, heart, lung, CNS, eyes, skin

√ moderate thickening of jejunal + duodenal folds (from mucosal + submucosal infiltration by PAS-positive macrophages combined with lymphatic obstruction)
√ micronodularity (= swollen villi) and wild mucosal pattern
√ hypersecretion, segmentation, fragmentation (occasionally if accompanied by hyperproteinemia)
√ NO / minimal dilatation of small bowel
√ NO rigidity of folds
√ NO ulcerations
√ normal transit time (approximately 3 hours)
√ hepatosplenomegaly

CT:
√ bulky 3–4 cm large low-density lymph nodes in mesenteric root + retroperitoneum (due to extracellular neutral fat + fatty acids)
√ thickening of bowel wall
√ splenomegaly
√ ascites
√ pleuropericarditis
√ sacroiliitis

Dx: endoscopically guided biopsy of small bowel mucosa, abdominal / peripheral lymph node biopsy
Rx: long-term broad-spectrum antibiotics (tetracycline)
DDx: (1) Sprue (marked dilatation, no fold thickening, pronounced segmentation + fragmentation)
(2) Intestinal lymphangiectasia (thickened folds throughout small bowel)
(3) Amyloidosis
(4) Lymphoma

PSEUDO–WHIPPLE DISEASE IN AIDS
similar clinical picture caused by Mycobacterium avium intracellulare
√ wall + fold thickening of small bowel loops
√ mesenteric lymphadenopathy

ZENKER DIVERTICULUM

= PHARYNGOESOPHAGEAL DIVERTICULUM
= outpouching of posterior hypopharyngeal wall = pulsion diverticulum with herniation of mucosa + submucosa through oblique + transverse muscle bundles (pseudodiverticulum) of the cricopharyngeal muscle

Prevalence: 0.01–0.11% (overall); higher in elderly women (50% occur in 7th–8th decade)
Etiology: cricopharyngeal dysfunction (cricopharyngeal achalasia / premature closure) results in increased intraluminal pressure
Associated with: hiatal hernia, gastroduodenal ulcer, midesophageal diverticulum, esophageal spasm, achalasia

• compressible neck mass
• upper esophageal dysphagia (98%)
• regurgitation + aspiration of undigested food
• noisy deglutition
• halitosis (= foul breath)

Location: at pharyngoesophageal junction in midline of Killian dehiscence / triangle of Laimer, at level of C5/6

√ posterior barium extension in upper half of semilunar depression on the posterior wall of esophagus (cricopharyngeal muscle)
√ barium-filled sac extending caudally behind + usually to left of esophagus
√ partial / complete obstruction of esophagus from external pressure of sac contents
√ partial barium reflux from diverticulum into hypopharynx
√ continual growth with successive enlargement

CXR:
√ air-fluid level in superior mediastinum

Cx: aspiration pneumonia (30%); esophageal perforation; carcinoma (0.48%)
Rx: surgical excision

ZOLLINGER-ELLISON SYNDROME

= peptic ulcer diathesis associated with marked hypersecretion of gastric acid + gastrin-producing non-β islet cell tumor of pancreas

Cause:
A. GASTRINOMA (90%) = non-b islet cell tumor with continuous gastrin production
B. PSEUDO Z-E SYNDROME = COWLEY SYNDROME = antral G-cell hyperplasia (10%) (increase in number of G-cells in gastric antrum)
  • lack of gastrin elevation after secretin injection
  • exaggerated gastrin elevation after protein meal

Age: middle age; M > F

• Clinical tetrad:
(1) Gastric hypersecretion: refractory response to histamine stimulation test concerning HCl concentration; increased basal secretion (>60% of augmented secretion is diagnostic)
(2) Hypergastrinemia >1000 ng/L (during fasting)
(3) Hyperacidity with basal acid output >15 mEq/h

GI

(4) Diarrhea (30%), steatorrhea (40%): may be sole complaint in 10%, frequently nocturnal; secondary to inactivation of pancreatic enzymes by large volumes of HCl

- severe intractable pain (90%)
- ulcer perforation (30%)
- positive secretin test = increase in serum gastrin level by >200 ng/L after administration of 2 IU/kg of secretin

√ ulcers (atypical location + course should suggest diagnosis):

Location: duodenal bulb (65%) + stomach (20%), near ligament of Treitz (25%), duodenal C-loop (5%), distal esophagus (5%)

Multiplicity: solitary ulcer (90%), multiple ulcers (10%)

√ recurrent / intractable ulcers

√ marginal ulcers in postgastrectomy patient

(a) on gastric side of anastomosis

(b) on mesenteric border of efferent loop

√ prominence of area gastricae (hyperplasia of parietal cell mass)

√ enlargement of rugal folds

√ sluggish gastric peristalsis (? hypokalemia)

√ "wet stomach" = dilution of barium by excess secretions in nondilated nonobstructed stomach

√ gastroesophageal reflux (common) + esophagitis

√ dilatation of duodenum + upper small bowel (fluid overload)

√ thickened folds in duodenum + jejunum (edema)

√ rapid small-bowel transit time

mnemonic: "FUSED"

Folds (thickened, gastric folds)
Ulcers (often multiple, postbulbar)
Secretions increased (refractory to histamine)
Edema (of proximal small bowel)
Diarrhea

Cx: (1) Malignant islet cell tumor (in 60%)
(2) Liver metastases will continue to stimulate gastric secretion

Rx:

(1) Control of gastric hypersecretion:

(a) H2-receptor antagonist: cimetidine, ranitidine, famotidine

(b) Hydrogen-potassium adenosine triphosphatase inhibitor (omeprazole)

(2) Resection of gastrinoma if found (because of malignant potential)

(3) Total gastrectomy

UROGENITAL TRACT

DIFFERENTIAL DIAGNOSIS OF UROGENITAL DISORDERS

RENAL FAILURE
= reduction in renal function
- rise in serum creatinine >2.5 mg/dL

Acute renal failure
= clinical condition associated with rapid steadily increasing azotemia ± oliguria (<500 mL urine per day) over days / weeks

Etiology:

A. PRERENAL
   = renal hypoperfusion secondary to systemic illness
   1. Fluid + electrolyte depletion
   2. Hemorrhage
   3. Hepatic failure + hepatorenal syndrome
      √ abnormally elevated resistive index
   4. Cardiac failure
   5. Sepsis
      √ resistive index <0.75 in 80% of kidneys

B. RENAL (most common)
   1. Acute tubular necrosis:
      ischemia, nephrotoxins, radiographic contrast, hemoglobulinuria, myoglobulinuria, myocardial infarction, burns
      √ resistive index ≥0.75 in 91% of kidneys
   2. Acute glomerulonephritis + small vessel disease:
      acute poststrep glomerulonephritis, rapidly progressive glomerulonephritis, lupus, polyarteritis nodosa, Schönlein-Henoch purpura, subacute bacterial endocarditis, serum sickness, Goodpasture syndrome, malignant hypertension, hemolytic uremic syndrome, drug-related vasculitis, abruptio placentae
      √ normal resistive index <0.70
   3. Acute tubulointerstitial nephritis:
      drug reaction, pyelonephritis, papillary necrosis
      √ abnormal resistive index
   4. Intrarenal precipitation (hypercalcemia, urate, myeloma protein)
   5. Arterial / venous obstruction
   6. Cortical necrosis

C. POSTRENAL (5%)
   = result of outflow obstruction (rare)
   1. Prostatism
   2. Tumors of bladder, retroperitoneum, pelvis
   3. Calculus
   √ hydronephrosis

D. CONGENITAL
   bilateral renal agenesis / dysplasia / infantile polycystic kidney disease, congenital nephrotic syndrome, congenital nephritis, perinatal hypoxia

Incidence: ATN + prerenal disease account for 75% of acute renal failure

Chronic renal failure
= decrease in renal function over months / years

Incidence:
end-stage renal disease in 0.01% of U.S. population; 85,000 patients/year undergo hemodialysis; 8,000 renal transplantations/year

Etiology:

A. INFLAMMATION / INFECTION
   1. Glomerulonephritis
   2. Chronic pyelonephritis
   3. Tuberculosis
   4. Sarcoidosis

B. VASCULAR
   1. Renal vascular disease
   2. Bilateral renal vein thrombosis

C. DYSPROTEINEMIA
   1. Myeloma
   2. Amyloid
   3. Cryoglobulinemia
   4. Waldenström macroglobulinemia

D. METABOLIC
   1. Diabetes
   2. Gout
   3. Hypercalcemia
   4. Hyperoxaluria
   5. Cystinosis
   6. Fabry disease

E. CONGENITAL
   1. Polycystic kidney disease
   2. Multicystic dysplastic kidney
   3. Medullary cystic disease
   4. Alport syndrome
   5. Infantile nephrotic syndrome

F. MISCELLANEOUS
   1. Hepatorenal syndrome
   2. Radiation

Musculoskeletal manifestations of CRF
1. Renal osteodystrophy = combination of 2° HPT, osteoporosis, osteosclerosis, osteomalacia, soft-tissue and vascular calcifications
2. Aluminum toxicity (1–30%)
   Cause: ingestion of aluminum salts phosphate-binding antacids (to control hyperphosphatemia)
   - aluminum serum level >100 ng/mL
   √ signs of osteomalacia (>3 insufficiency fractures with predominant involvement of ribs)
   √ avascular necrosis
   √ lack of osteosclerosis
   √ less evidence of subperiosteal resorption
3. Amyloid deposition
   Path: amyloid consists of β_2-microglobulin

Organs: bone, tenosynovium (carpal tunnel syndrome), vertebral disk, articular cartilage + capsule, ligament, muscle

4. Destructive spondyloarthropathy (15%)
   √ discovertebral junction erosion + sclerosis
   √ vertebral body compression
   √ disk space narrowing
   √ Schmorl node formation
   √ lack of osteophytosis
   √ facet involvement with subluxation
5. Tendon rupture
6. Crystal deposition disease
   Type: calcium hydroxyapatite, CPPD, calcium oxalate, monosodium urate
7. Osteomyelitis + septic arthritis
8. Avascular necrosis (in up to 40%)

DIABETES INSIPIDUS

A. Hypothalamic Diabetes Insipidus
   = vasopressin production is reduced to <10%
   Cause:
   (a) idiopathic (27%)
      rare familial (autosomal dominant X-linked) / sporadic disorder
      Histo: atrophic supraoptic nucleus
      • never associated with anterior pituitary dysfunction
   (b) pituitary destruction by tumor / infiltrative disorder (32%):
      in childhood: hypothalamic glioma, tuber cinereum hamartoma, craniopharyngioma, histiocytosis, germinoma, leukemia, complication of meningitis
      in adulthood: sarcoidosis, metastasis
      • in 60% associated with anterior pituitary dysfunction
   (c) pituitary destruction by surgery (20%)
      • always associated with anterior pituitary dysfunction
   (d) head injury (17%)
      • in 20% associated with anterior pituitary dysfunction
      ◊ A lesion in the posterior pituitary will NOT produce diabetes insipidus, because it is just the storage space for vasopressin!

B. Psychogenic Water Intoxication
   = compulsive intake of large amounts of fluid, which leads to inhibition of normal vasopressin production
   • water deprivation test

C. Primary Nephrogenic Diabetes Insipidus
   = rare sex-linked recessive genetic disorder with unresponsiveness of tubules + collecting system to vasopressin (in infants + young males)

D. Secondary Nephrogenic Diabetes Insipidus
   Cause: drug toxicity, analgesic nephropathy, sickle cell anemia, hypokalemia, hypercalcemia, chronic uremic nephropathy, postobstructive uropathy, reflux nephropathy, amyloidosis, sarcoidosis

ABNORMAL TUBULAR FUNCTION

A. PROXIMAL TUBULE
   reabsorbs almost all of glucose, amino acids, phosphate, bicarbonate
   • glycosuria (Toni-Fanconi syndrome)
   • aminoaciduria (cystinuria)
   • phosphaturia (phosphate diabetes, thiazides)
   • HCO_3^- wasting (proximal renal tubular acidosis)

B. DISTAL TUBULE
   absorbs most of water
   • diabetes insipidus, secretes H^+
   • distal renal tubular acidosis

ARTERIAL HYPOTENSION

Cause: intrarenal hypovolemia, primary vasoconstriction, reduced glomerular filtration, depletion of intratubular urine volume

◊ May occur as a contrast reaction!

Urogram reverts to normal after reversion of hypotension!

√ bilateral small smooth kidneys (compared with size on preliminary films)
√ increasingly dense nephrogram
√ usually NO opacification of collecting system
√ initially opacification of collecting system if hypotension occurs during contrast injection

HYPERCALCEMIA

mnemonic: "SHAMPOO DIRT"

Sarcoidosis
Hyperparathyroidism, **H**yperthyroidism
Alkali-milk syndrome
Metastases, **M**yeloma
Paget disease
Osteogenesis imperfecta
Osteopetrosis
D vitamin intoxication
Immobility
Renal tubular acidosis
Thiazides

POLYCYTHEMIA

Cause: increased level of erythropoietin (acting on erythroid stem cells) secondary to a decrease in pO_2; erythropoietin precursor is produced in juxtaglomerular epitheloid cells of kidney + converted in blood

A. RENAL
   (a) intrarenal
      1. Vascular impairment
      2. Renal cell carcinoma (5%)
      3. Wilms tumor
      4. Benign fibroma
      5. Simple cyst (14%)
      6. Polycystic kidney disease
   (b) postrenal
      1. Obstructive uropathy (14%)

B. EXTRARENAL
   (a) liver disease
      1. Hepatoma
      2. Regenerating hepatic cells

GU

(b) adrenal disease
1. Pheochromocytoma
2. Aldosteronoma
3. Cushing disease

C. CNS DISEASE
1. Cerebellar hemangioblastoma

D. Large uterine myomas

NOT in: renal vein thrombosis, multicystic dysplastic kidney, medullary sponge kidney

URINARY TRACT INFECTION

= pure growths of >100,000 organisms/mL urine

Prevalence: 3% of girls + 1% of boys during first 10 years of life

Underlying radiologic abnormality:
1. Vesicoureteral reflux = VUR (30–40%)
2. Obstructive uropathy (8%)
3. Reflux nephropathy / scar formation (6%)
   ◊ The prevalence of an underlying radiologic abnormality depends on age, sex, and frequency of previous infections!

Imaging objective:
1. Identify patients at risk for reflux nephropathy
2. Detect reflux nephropathy / scars
3. Detect obstructive uropathy
4. Minimize radiation, morbidity, and cost

VCUG:
for children <5 years of age with infection; normal results in 60–70%

Renal cortical scintigraphy (DMSA / glucoheptonate):
to detect acute pyelonephritis (risk for scarring) / scar; with VUR there is twice the risk of cortical defects than without VUR

WETTING

1. **Enuresis**
   = manifestation of neuromuscular vesicourethral immaturity; M:F = 3:2
   • intermittent wetting, usually at night during sleep
   • often positive history of enuresis from one parent
   • normal physical examination
   √ no structural abnormality; urography NOT indicated
2. **Epispadia**
   = incomplete fusion of infravesical portion of urinary tract
   • urinary incontinence from incompetent bladder neck / urethral sphincter
   √ abnormally wide symphysis pubis (>1 cm)
3. Sacral agenesis
   = segmental defect (below S2) with deficiency of nerves that innervate bladder, urethra, rectum, feet
   ◊ Children of diabetic mothers are affected in 17%!
4. **Extravesical infrasphincteric ectopic ureter**
   only affects girls as boys do NOT have infrasphincteric ureteral orifices
   (a) ureter draining upper pole of duplex system exits below urethral sphincter (90%)
   (b) ureter draining single system with ectopic extravesical orifice (10%)
5. **Synechia vulvae**
   = adhesive fusion of minor labia directs urine primarily into vagina from where it dribbles out post micturition
6. **Vaginal reflux**
   in obese older girls with fat thighs and fat labia
7. Miscellaneous
   posterior urethral valves, urethral stricture, urethral diverticula

MALE INFERTILITY

A. CONGENITAL
(a) Wolffian duct anomalies
1. Renal agenesis / atrophy
2. Vas deferens agenesis / cyst
3. Seminal vesicle agenesis / cyst
4. Ejaculatory duct cyst

(b) Müllerian duct anomalies
1. Müllerian duct cyst
2. Utricle cyst

B. ACQUIRED
1. Cowper duct cyst
2. Prostatic cyst in peripheral zone

C. INFECTIOUS
1. Prostatitis

D. HORMONAL
• semen low in volume, acid pH, without fructose
1. Seminal vesicle atrophy
   = seminal vesicles <7 mm in width
2. Seminal vesicle hypoplasia
   = seminal vesicles <11 mm + >7 mm in width

ABNORMAL GAS IN URINARY TRACT

A. Renal emphysema = renal / perirenal gas
1. Emphysematous pyelonephritis
2. Emphysematous pyelitis
3. Gasforming perinephric abscess
4. Perinephric emphysema

B. Bladder
1. Emphysematous cystitis

C. Trauma
1. Penetrating trauma
2. Ureterosigmoidostomy, ileal conduit, catheterization with vesicoureteral reflux, percutaneous procedure
   CAVE: anomalous posterior position of colon
3. Infarction of renal carcinoma (therapeutic / spontaneous)

D. Fistula to urinary tract
Connection: bronchus / cutis / GI tract (colon > duodenum > stomach > small bowel > appendix
1. Inflammation: chronic purulent renal infection, diverticulitis, Crohn disease
2. Neoplastic: colonic carcinoma

KIDNEY

Absent Renal Outline On Plain Film

A. ABSENT KIDNEY
1. Congenital absence
2. S/P nephrectomy

GU

B. SMALL KIDNEY
  1. Renal hypoplasia
  2. Renal atrophy
C. RENAL ECTOPIA
  1. Pelvic kidney
  2. Crossed fused ectopia
  3. Intrathoracic kidney
D. OBLITERATION OF PERIRENAL FAT
  1. Perirenal abscess
  2. Perirenal hematoma
  3. Renal tumors

Nonvisualized Kidney On Excretory Urography

A. ABSENCE OF KIDNEY
  1. Agenesis
  2. Ectopia
B. LOSS OF PERFUSION
  1. Chronic infarction
  2. Unilateral renal vein thrombosis
  3. Fractured kidney
C. URINARY OBSTRUCTION
  1. Hydronephrosis
  2. Ureteropelvic junction obstruction
D. REPLACED NORMAL RENAL PARENCHYMA
  1. Multicystic dysplastic kidney
  2. Unilateral polycystic kidney disease
  3. Renal tumor (RCC, TCC, Wilms tumor)
  4. Xanthogranulomatous pyelonephritis

Unilateral Large Smooth Kidney

A. PRERENAL
  (a) arterial: acute arterial infarction
  (b) venous: acute renal vein thrombosis
B. INTRARENAL
  (a) congenital: duplicated pelvicaliceal system, crossed fused ectopia, multicystic dysplastic kidney, adult polycystic kidney (in 8% unilateral)
  (b) infectious: acute bacterial nephritis
  (c) adaptation: compensatory hypertrophy
C. POSTRENAL
  (a) collecting system: obstructive uropathy

mnemonic: "AROMA"
Acute pyelonephritis
Renal vein thrombosis
Obstructive uropathy
Miscellaneous (compensatory hypertrophy, duplication)
Arterial obstruction (infarction)

Bilateral Large Kidneys

Average renal length by x-ray: M = 13 cm; F = 12.5 cm
1. PROTEIN DEPOSITION
   amyloidosis, multiple myeloma
2. INTERSTITIAL FLUID ACCUMULATION
   acute tubular necrosis, acute cortical necrosis, acute arterial infarction, renal vein thrombosis
3. CELLULAR INFILTRATION
   (a) Inflammatory cells: acute interstitial nephritis, acute bacterial nephritis
   (b) Malignant cells: leukemia / lymphoma
4. PROLIFERATIVE / NECROTIZING DISORDERS
   (a) Glomerulonephritis (GN)
   acute (poststreptococcal) GN, rapidly progressive GN, idiopathic membranous GN, membrano-proliferative GN, lobular GN, IgA nephropathy, glomerulosclerosis, glomerulosclerosis related to heroin abuse
   (b) Multisystem disease
   polyarteritis nodosa, systemic lupus erythematosus, Wegener granulomatosis, allergic angiitis, diabetic glomerulosclerosis, Goodpasture syndrome (lung hemorrhage + glomerulonephritis), Schönlein-Henoch syndrome (anaphylactoid purpura), thrombotic thrombocytopenic purpura, focal glomerulonephritis associated with subacute bacterial endocarditis
5. URINE OUTFLOW OBSTRUCTION
   bilateral hydronephrosis: congenital / acquired
6. HORMONAL STIMULUS
   acromegaly, compensatory hypertrophy, nephromegaly associated with cirrhosis / hyperalimentation / diabetes mellitus
7. DEVELOPMENTAL
   bilateral duplication system, horseshoe kidney, polycystic kidney disease
8. MISCELLANEOUS
   acute urate nephropathy, glycogen storage disease, hemophilia, sickle cell disease, Fabry disease, physiologic response to contrast material and diuretics

mnemonic: "FOG P"
Fluid: = edema of kidney (ATN, acute cortical necrosis)
Other: leukemia, acromegaly, sickle cell anemia, bilateral duplication, acute urate nephropathy
Glomerular disease: acute GN, lupus, polyarteritis nodosa, diabetes mellitus
Protein deposition: multiple myeloma, amyloidosis

Bilateral Small Kidneys

A. PRERENAL = VASCULAR
  1. Arterial hypotension (acute)
  2. Generalized arteriosclerosis
  3. Atheroembolic disease
  4. Benign & malignant nephrosclerosis
B. INTRARENAL
  1. Hereditary nephropathies:
     medullary cystic disease, hereditary chronic nephritis (Alport syndrome)
  2. Chronic glomerulonephritis
  3. Amyloidosis (late)
C. POSTRENAL
  1. Papillary necrosis

D. CAUSES OF UNILATERAL SMALL KIDNEY occurring bilaterally

mnemonic: "CAPE HANA"
Chronic glomerulonephritis
Arteriosclerosis
Papillary necrosis
Embolic disease (secondary to atherosclerosis)
Hypotension
Alport syndrome
Nephrosclerosis
Amyloidosis (late)

Unilateral Small Kidney

A. PRERENAL = VASCULAR
1. Lobar infarction
2. Chronic infarction
3. Renal artery stenosis
4. Radiation nephritis

B. INTRARENAL = PARENCHYMAL
1. Congenital hypoplasia
2. Multicystic dysplastic kidney (in adult)
3. Postinflammatory atrophy

C. POSTRENAL = COLLECTING SYSTEM
1. Reflux nephropathy = chronic atrophic pyelonephritis
2. Postobstructive atrophy

mnemonic: "RIP R HIP"
Reflux atrophy
Ischemia (renal artery stenosis)
Postobstructive atrophy
Radiation therapy
Hypoplasia (congenital)
Infarction
Postinflammatory atrophy

Increased Echogenicity Of Renal Cortex

= RENAL MEDICAL DISEASE = diffuse increase in cortical echogenicity with preservation of corticomedullary junction

Path: deposition of collagen / calcium in interstitial, glomerular, tubular, vascular disease

√ echointensity of cortex greater than liver / spleen ± equal to renal sinus

√ renal size may be normal; enlarged kidneys suggest active stage of renal disease; small kidneys suggest chronic + often end-stage renal disease

1. Acute / chronic glomerulonephritis
2. Renal transplant rejection
3. Lupus nephritis
4. Hypertensive nephrosclerosis
5. Renal cortical necrosis
6. Methemoglobulinuric renal failure
7. Alport syndrome
8. Amyloidosis
9. Diabetic nephrosclerosis
10. Nephrotoxin-induced acute tubular necrosis
11. End-stage renal disease

Hyperechoic Renal Pyramids In Children

A. NEPHROCALCINOSIS
(a) iatrogenic (most common cause): furosemide (Rx for BPD), vitamin D (Rx for hypophosphatemic rickets)
(b) noniatrogenic:
1. Idiopathic hypercalcemia
2. Williams syndrome
3. Absorptive hypercalcemia
4. Hyperparathyroidism
5. Milk-alkali syndrome
6. Kenny-Caffey syndrome
7. Distal renal tubular acidosis
8. Malignant tumors
9. Chronic glomerulonephritis
10. Sjögren syndrome (distal RTA)
11. Sarcoidosis

B. METABOLIC DISEASE
1. Gout
2. Lesch-Nyhan syndrome (urate)
3. Fanconi syndrome
4. Glycogen storage disease (distal RTA)
5. Wilson disease (distal RTA)
6. Alpha-1-antitrypsin deficiency
7. Tyrosinemia
8. Cystinosis
9. Oxalosis
10. Crohn disease

C. HYPOKALEMIA
1. Primary aldosteronism
2. Pseudo-Bartter syndrome

D. PROTEIN DEPOSITS
1. Infant dehydration with presumed Tamm-Horsfall proteinuria
2. Toxic shock syndrome

E. VASCULAR CONGESTION
1. Sickle cell anemia

F. INFECTION
1. Candida / CMV nephritis
2. AIDS-associated Mycobacterium avium-intracellulare

G. FIBROSIS OF RENAL PYRAMIDS

H. CYSTIC MEDULLARY DISEASE
1. Medullary sponge kidney
2. Congenital hepatic fibrosis with tubular ectasia

I. INTRARENAL REFLUX
1. Chronic pyelonephritis

Iron Accumulation In Kidney

A. RENAL CORTEX
1. Paroxysmal nocturnal hemoglobulinuria (= intravascular extrasplenic hemolysis)
2. Sickle cell anemia

B. RENAL MEDULLA
1. Hemorrhagic fever with renal syndrome (uncommon viral illness caused by Hanta virus)
Triad: (1) renal medullary hemorrhage
(2) right atrial hemorrhage
(3) necrosis of anterior pituitary

Depression Of Renal Margins
1. Fetal lobation
   √ notching between normal calices
2. Splenic impression
   √ flattened upper outer margin of left kidney
3. Chronic atrophic pyelonephritis
   √ indentation over clubbed calices
4. Renal infarct
   √ normal calices
5. Chronic renal ischemia
   √ normal calices

Enlargement Of Iliopsoas Compartment
A. INFECTION
   (a) from retroperitoneal organs
      1. Renal infection
      2. Complicated pancreatitis
      3. Postoperative aortic graft infection
   (b) from spine
      1. Osteomyelitis / postoperative complication of bone surgery
      2. Discitis / postoperative complication from disk surgery
   (c) from GI tract
      1. Crohn disease
      2. Appendicitis
   (d) others
      1. Pelvic inflammatory disease / postpartum infection
      2. Sepsis
B. HEMORRHAGE
   1. Coagulopathy and anticoagulant therapy
   2. Ruptured aortic aneurysm
   3. Postoperative aneurysm repair / other surgery / trauma
C. NEOPLASTIC DISEASE
   (a) Extrinsic
      1. Lymphoma
      2. Metastatic lymphadenopathy
      3. Bone metastases with soft-tissue involvement
      4. Retroperitoneal sarcoma
   (b) Intrinsic
      1. Muscle tumors
      2. Nervous system tumors
      3. Lipoma / liposarcoma
D. MISCELLANEOUS
   1. Pseudoenlargement of psoas muscle compared to de facto atrophy of contralateral side in neuromuscular disease
   2. Fluid collections
      urinoma, lymphocele, pancreatic pseudocyst, enlargement of iliopsoas bursa
   3. Pelvic venous thrombosis
      √ diffuse swelling of all muscles (edema)

RENAL MASS
Bilateral Renal Masses
A. MALIGNANT TUMOR
   1. Malignant lymphoma / Hodgkin disease
   2. Metastases
   3. Renal cell carcinoma
   4. Wilms tumor
B. BENIGN TUMOR
   1. Angiomyolipoma
   2. Nephroblastomatosis
C. CYSTS
   1. Adult polycystic kidney disease
   2. Acquired cystic kidney disease

Renal Mass In Neonate
A. UNILATERAL
   1. Multicystic kidney (15%)
   2. Hydronephrosis (25%)
      (a) UPJ obstruction
      (b) upper moiety of duplication
   3. Renal vein thrombosis
   4. Mesoblastic nephroma
   5. Rare: Wilms tumor, teratoma
B. BILATERAL
   1. Hydronephrosis
   2. Polycystic kidney disease
   3. Multicystic kidney + contralateral hydronephrosis
   4. Nephroblastomatosis
   5. Bilateral multicystic kidney

Renal Mass In Older Child
A. SINGLE MASS
   1. Wilms tumor
   2. Multilocular cystic nephroma
   3. Focal hydronephrosis
   4. Traumatic cyst, abscess
   5. Renal cell carcinoma
   6. Malignant rhabdoid tumor
   7. Teratoma
   8. Clear cell sarcoma of kidney
   9. Intrarenal neuroblastoma
B. MULTIPLE MASSES
   1. Nephroblastomatosis
   2. Multiple Wilms tumors
   3. Angiomyolipoma
   4. Lymphoma
   5. Leukemia
   6. Adult polycystic kidney disease
   7. Abscesses

Growth Pattern Of Renal Tumors In Adults
A. EXPANSILE GROWTH
   1. Renal cell carcinoma
   2. Oncocytoma
   3. Angiomyolipoma
   4. Juxtaglomerular tumor
   5. Metastatic tumor (eg, lymphoma)
   6. Mesenchymal tumor
B. INFILTRATIVE GROWTH
   1. Lymphoma / leukemia
   2. Invasive transitional cell carcinoma
   3. Metastatic tumor
   4. Renal cell carcinoma (unusual)
   5. Xanthogranulomatous pyelonephritis

Local Bulge In Renal Contour

A. CYST
1. Simple renal cyst

B. TUMOR
1. Adenocarcinoma
2. Angiomyolipoma
3. Pseudotumor

C. INFECTION
1. Subcapsular abscess
2. XGP

D. TRAUMA
1. Subcapsular hematoma

E. DILATED COLLECTING SYSTEM

Unilateral Renal Mass

Solid Renal Mass

A. TUMORS

(a) primary malignant:
adenocarcinoma (83%), chromophobe carcinoma (4%), papillary neoplasm (14%), renal collecting duct carcinoma = Bellini duct carcinoma (1%), transitional cell carcinoma (8%), renal neuroendocrine tumors (carcinoid, small cell carcinoma), Wilms tumor (6%), renal sarcoma (2%)
in horseshoe kidney:
adenocarcinoma (45%), Wilms tumor (28%), transitional cell carcinoma (20%)

(b) secondary malignant:
malignant lymphoma / Hodgkin disease, metastases, invasive transitional cell carcinoma

(c) benign:
adenoma, oncocytoma, hamartoma (mesoblastic nephroma, angiomyolipoma, myolipoma, lipoma, leiomyoma, fibroma), hemangioma

B. INFLAMMATORY MASSES
acute focal bacterial nephritis, renal abscess, xanthogranulomatous pyelonephritis, malacoplakia, tuberculoma

Fluid-filled Mass

A. CYSTS
1. Simple renal cyst
2. Inherited cystic disease:
multicystic dysplastic kidney disease (Potter type II), multilocular cystic nephroma
3. Focal hydronephrosis

B. VASCULAR
1. Arteriovenous malformation
2. Arteriovenous fistula
= single dilated artery + vein
√ tortuous varices over time
√ enlargement of renal vein
Cx: hydronephrosis

◊ Lesions <1 cm often cannot be clearly characterized
◊ Lesions 1–1.5 cm can often be ignored, particularly in elderly / patients with significant other disease

Avascular Mass In Kidney

mnemonic: "CHEAT"
Cyst
Hematoma
Edema
Abscess
Tumor

Hyperechoic Renal Nodule

A. MALIGNANT TUMOR
1. Renal cell carcinoma
2. Angiosarcoma
3. Liposarcoma
4. Undifferentiated sarcoma
5. Lymphoma

B. BENIGN TUMOR
1. Angiomyolipoma
2. Lipoma
3. Oncocytoma
4. Cavernous hemangioma

C. INFARCT

D. HEMATOMA

Hyperattenuating Renal Mass On NECT

A. BENIGN
1. Complicated benign cyst: hemorrhagic, protein-rich, gelatinous
2. Leiomyoma
3. Angiomyolipoma (rare)
4. Thrombosed renal vein

B. MALIGNANT
1. Metastasis from thyroid carcinoma
2. Renal cell carcinoma

Low-density Retroperitoneal Mass

1. Lipoma
√ sharply marginated, homogeneously fatty mass
2. Lymphangioma
√ similar to lipoma if enough fat content
3. Adrenal myelolipoma
√ density between fat + water
√ usually nonhomogeneous, occasionally with hemorrhage ± calcifications
4. Renal angiomyolipoma
√ intrarenal component
√ hypervascular with large feeding arteries, multiple aneurysms, laking without shunting, tortuous circumferential vessels, whorled parenchymal + venous phase
5. Xanthogranulomatous pyelonephritis
√ nonfunctioning kidney replaced by low-density material + central staghorn calculus
6. Metastatic retroperitoneal tumors
7. Renal cell carcinoma
8. Fibrosarcoma, fibrous histiocytoma, mesenchymal sarcoma, malignant teratoma
√ density close to muscle
9. Liposarcoma

Focal area of increased renal echogenicity

A. NONNEOPLASTIC
  1. Chronic renal infarction
  2. Acute focal bacterial nephritis
B. BENIGN TUMOR
  1. Angiomyolipoma
  2. Cavernous renal hemangioma
  3. Oncocytoma
C. MALIGNANCY
  1. Renal cell carcinoma
  2. Angiosarcoma
  3. Undifferentiated sarcoma
  4. Metastasis

Fat-containing renal mass

1. Angiomyolipoma
2. Lipoma, liposarcoma
3. Teratoma
4. Wilms tumor
5. Xanthogranulomatous pyelonephritis
6. Oncocytoma engulfing renal sinus fat
7. Renal cell carcinoma
   (a) invasion of perirenal fat
   (b) intratumoral metaplasia into fatty marrow (in 32% if RCCs <3 cm)

Renal sinus mass

A. TUMORS
  1. Transitional cell carcinoma
  2. Lymphoma
  3. Metastasis to sinus lymph nodes
  4. Mesenchymal tumor: lipoma, fibroma, myoma, hemangioma
  5. Plasmacytoma
  6. Myeloid metaplasia
B. MISCELLANEOUS
  1. Sinus lipomatosis
  2. Parapelvic cyst
  3. Saccular aneurysm
  4. Urinoma

Hypoechoic renal sinus

A. SOLID
  1. Fibrolipomatosis
  2. Column of Bertin
  3. Duplex kidney
  4. TCC / RCC
B. CYSTIC
  1. Renal sinus cysts
  2. Caliectasis
  3. Dilated veins, varix
  4. Aneurysm, arteriovenous malformation

Renal pseudotumor

= anomalies of lobar anatomy that may simulate a tumor

A. PRIMARY
  1. **Large column of Bertin**
     = large septum / cloison of Bertin = large cloison = focal cortical hyperplasia = benign cortical rest = focal renal hypertrophy
     = persistence of normal septal cortex / excessive infolding of cortex usually in the presence of partial or complete duplication
     Location: between upper and interpolar portion
     √ mass <3 cm in largest diameter
     √ lateral indentation of renal sinus
     √ "deformation" of adjacent calices + infundibula
     √ mass continuous with renal cortex
     √ enhancement pattern like renal cortex
     √ echogenicity similar to cortex
  2. **Dromedary hump**
     = subcapsular nodule = splenic bump
     = secondary to prolonged pressure by spleen during fetal development
     Location: in mid portion of lateral border of left kidney
     √ triangular contour + elongation of middle calyx
     √ enhancement pattern like renal cortex
  3. **Hilar lip**
     = supra- / infrahilar bulge = medial part of kidney above / below sinus
     Location: most frequently medial to left kidney just above renal pelvis (on transaxial scan)
     √ enhancement pattern like cortex with medulla
  4. **Fetal lobation**
     = persistent cortical lobation = ren lobatus
     14 individual lobes with centrilobar cortex located around calices
  5. **Lobar dysmorphism**
     complete diminutive lobe situated deep within renal substance with its own diminutive calyx in its central portion = calyx of nonresorbed normal junctional parenchyma between upper + lower subkidneys

B. ACQUIRED
  1. **Nodular compensatory hypertrophy**
     areas of unaffected tissue in the presence of focal renal scarring from chronic atrophic pyelonephritis (= reflux nephropathy), surgery, trauma, infarction;
     √ hypertrophy usually evident within 2 months; less likely to occur > age 50
     DDx: accessory spleen, medial lobule of spleen, splenosis, normal / abnormal bowel, pancreatic disease, gallbladder, adrenal abnormalities
     Dx: static radionuclide imaging / renal arteriography / CT

RENAL CYSTIC DISEASE

Potter classification

= POTTER SYNDROME
= any renal condition associated with severe oligohydramnios
• peculiar facies with wide-set eyes, parrot-beak nose, pliable low-set ears, receding chin

GU

Type I : infantile PCKD
Type II : multicystic dysplastic kidney disease, multilocular cystic nephroma
IIa : kidneys of normal / increased size
IIb : kidneys reduced in size
Type III : adult PCKD, tuberous sclerosis, medullary sponge kidney
Type IV : small cortical cysts / cystic dysplasia secondary to ureteropelvic junction obstruction

Renal cystic disease

A. SIMPLE RENAL CYST
   1. Intrarenal
   2. Parapelvic
B. POLYCYSTIC RENAL DISEASE
   1. Adult PCKD
   2. Infantile PCKD
   3. Glomerulocystic kidney disease
      = congenital disease with extremely variable presentation + prognosis
      Path: cysts within Bowman capsule ± tubular cysts
      √ multiple macroscopic cortical cysts
C. CYSTIC MEDULLARY DISEASE
   1. Uremic medullary cystic disease
   2. Juvenile nephrophthisis
   3. Medullary sponge kidney
D. RENAL DYSPLASIA
   1. Multicystic dysplastic kidney
   2. Segmental / focal renal dysplasia
   3. Familial renal dysplasia
E. NEUROCUTANEOUS DYSPLASIA
   1. Tuberous sclerosis
   2. Von Hippel-Lindau syndrome
F. CYSTIC TUMORS
   1. Multilocular cystic nephroma
   2. Cystic Wilms tumor
   3. Cystic renal cell carcinoma
G. ACQUIRED RENAL CYSTIC DISEASE
   1. Acquired cystic disease of uremia
   2. Infectious cysts (TB, Echinococcus, abscess)
   3. Medullary necrosis
   4. Pyelogenic cyst

Syndromes with multiple cortical cysts

1. Von Hippel-Lindau syndrome
2. Tuberous sclerosis
3. Meckel-Gruber syndrome
4. Zellweger syndrome = cerebrohepatorenal syndrome
5. Jeune syndrome
6. Conradi syndrome = chondrodysplasia punctata
7. Oro-facial-digital syndrome
8. Trisomy 13
9. Turner syndrome
10. Dandy-Walker malformation

Multiloculated renal mass

A. NEOPLASTIC DISEASE
   1. Cystic renal cell carcinoma
   2. Multilocular cystic renal tumor
      (a) cystic nephroma
      (b) cystic partially differentiated nephroblastoma
   3. Cystic Wilms tumor
   4. Necrotic tumor
      (a) mesoblastic nephroma
      (b) clear cell sarcoma
B. RENAL CYSTIC DISEASE
   1. Localized renal cystic disease
   2. Septated cyst
   3. Multicystic dysplastic kidney
   3. Segmental multicystic dysplasia
   4. Complicated cyst
C. INFLAMMATORY DISEASE
   1. Echinococcus
   2. Segmental XGP
   3. Abscess
   4. Malacoplakia
D. VASCULAR LESIONS
   1. AV fistula
   2. Organizing hematoma

ABNORMAL NEPHROGRAM

Normal nephrographic phases

1. Vascular phase (= cortical arteriogram)
   = contrast material visible in interlobular arteries + glomeruli
   Timing after IV injection: 10–15 sec (arm-to-kidney circulation time)
   Duration: transient vascular phase of <0.5 sec
2. Cortical phase (= cortical nephrogram)
   = contrast medium in cortical capillaries + peritubular spaces + cortical tubular lumina
   Timing after IV injection: 20–45 sec
   Timing after intraarterial injection: 2–3 sec
   CT:
   √ exclusive renal cortical enhancement
3. Parenchymal phase (= generalized / tubular nephrogram)
   = contrast material within loops of Henle + collecting tubules
   Timing after IV injection: 1–2 min (maximum)
   √ enhancement of both cortex and medulla
4. Excretory phase
   Timing after IV injection: beginning at 2–3 min

Absence of nephrogram

Global absence of nephrogram

Pathophysiology: complete renal ischemia secondary to occlusion of main renal artery

1. Injury to vascular pedicle during blunt abdominal trauma
2. Thromboembolic disease
3. Renal artery dissection: spontaneous, traumatic, iatrogenic

Segmental Absence Of Nephrogram

A. SPACE-OCCUPYING PROCESS
  1. Neoplasm
  2. Cyst
  3. Abscess

B. FOCAL RENAL INFARCTION
  1. Arterial embolus / thrombosis
  2. Vasculitis, collagen-vascular disease
  3. Sickle cell anemia
  4. Septic shock
  5. Renal vein thrombosis

Rim Nephrogram

= rim of cortex receiving collateral blood flow from capsular, peripelvic, and periureteric vessels
◊ Most specific indicator of renovascular compromise!
√ 2–4 mm peripheral band of cortical opacification
Cause: 1. Acute total main renal artery occlusion: seen in 50% of cases with renal infarction
  2. Renal vein thrombosis
  3. Acute tubular necrosis
  4. Severe chronic urinary obstruction

DDx: severe hydronephrosis (rim/shell nephrogram surrounding dilated calices)

Unilateral Delayed Nephrogram

A. OBSTRUCTIVE UROPATHY

B. REDUCTION IN RENAL BLOODFLOW
  1. Renal artery stenosis
  2. Renal vein thrombosis

Striated Nephrogram

= stasis of contrast material in dilated collecting ducts on background of edematous renal parenchyma
√ fine linear bands of alternating lucency + density parallel to axis of tubules + collecting ducts

A. UNILATERAL
  1. Acute ureteric obstruction
  2. Acute bacterial nephritis / pyelonephritis
  3. Renal contusion
  4. Renal vein thrombosis

B. BILATERAL
  1. Acute pyelonephritis
  2. Intratubular obstruction: Tamm-Horsfall proteinuria, rhabdomyolysis with myoglobinuria
  3. Systemic hypotension
  4. Autosomal recessive PCKD
  5. Medullary sponge kidney
  6. Medullary cystic disease

mnemonic: "CHOIR BOY"
Contusion
Hypotension (systemic)
Obstruction (ureteral)
Intratubular obstruction
Renal vein thrombosis
Bacterial nephritis (acute)
Obstruction (ureteral) — it is so common!
Yes, also cystic diseases: infantile PCKD, medullary cystic disease, medullary sponge kidney

Persistent Nephrogram

A. BILATERAL GLOBAL
  1. Systemic hypotension
  2. Intratubular obstruction from protein: Tamm-Horsfall, Bence-Jones, myoglobin
  3. Tubular damage by contrast material

B. UNILATERAL GLOBAL
  1. Renal artery stenosis
  2. Renal vein thrombosis
  3. Urinary tract obstruction

C. SEGMENTAL
  1. Obstructed moiety of duplicated collecting system
  2. Obstructing renal calculus
  3. Obstructing neoplasm
  4. Focal stricture
  5. Focal parenchymal disease: tubulointerstitial infection

Abnormal Nephrogram Due To Impaired Perfusion

A. SYSTEMIC HYPOTENSIVE REACTION
as reaction to contrast material / cardiac failure / dehydration / shock
Pathophysiology:
drop in perfusion pressure after contrast reaches kidney leads to increased salt + water reabsorption and slowed tubular transit
√ prolonged bilateral dense nephrograms = persistent increasing nephrogram
√ decrease in renal size
√ loss of pyelogram after initial opacification
NUC (use of glomerular filtration agent [eg, Tc-99m DTPA] preferred)
  √ prolonged cortical transit + reduced excretion

B. RENAL ARTERY STENOSIS
√ decreased nephrographic opacity + rim nephrogram
√ hyperconcentration in collecting system
√ ureteral notching
NUC (glomerular filtration agent [eg, Tc-99m DTPA] preferred):
  √ decreased perfusion with prolonged excretory phase

C. IMPAIRED PERFUSION OF SMALL ARTERIES
Trueta shunting = transient rerouting of blood flow from cortex to medulla
Cause:
  (a) reflex spasm during arterial angiography secondary to catheter trauma / pressure injection of highly concentrated contrast medium
  (b) chronic renal disorders (collagen vascular disease, malignant nephrosclerosis, chronic glomerulonephritis)
  (c) necrotizing vasculitis (polyarteritis nodosa, scleroderma, hypertensive nephrosclerosis)

CT, Angio:
  √ inhomogeneous opacification of cortex

IVP:
  √ irregular cortical nephrogram = spotted nephrogram

D. ACUTE VENOUS OUTFLOW OBSTRUCTION
in renal vein thrombosis
√ obstructive nephrogram
√ progressive increase in opacity of entire kidney

Abnormal Nephrogram Due To Impaired Tubular Transit

Cause:
A. EXTRARENAL: ureteric obstruction (eg, stone)
√ obstructive nephrogram
NUC:
before decrease in renal function use of glomerular filtration agent (eg, Tc-99m DTPA); with decrease in renal function use of plasma flow agents (eg, Tc-99m MAG3 / I-123 Hippuran) preferred
√ continuous increase in renal activity
√ dilatation of collecting system
B. INTRARENAL
(a) segmental: limb of duplication system, caliceal obstruction, interstitial edema
√ segmental nephrogram
(b) protein precipitation: Tamm-Horsfall protein (a normal mucoprotein product of proximal nephrons), Bence Jones protein (multiple myeloma), uric acid precipitation (acute urate nephropathy), myoglobulinuria, hyperproteinuric state
√ striated nephrogram
NUC:
before decrease in renal function use of glomerular filtration agent (eg, Tc-99m DTPA); with decrease in renal function use of plasma flow agents (eg, Tc-99m MAG3 / I-123 Hippuran) preferred
√ prolonged cortical transit time + prolonged excretory phase

Abnormal Nephrogram Due To Abnormal Tubular Function

1. Acute tubular necrosis
√ immediate persistent nephrogram (common)
√ progressive increasing opacity (rare)
2. Contrast-induced renal failure

Striated Angiographic Nephrogram

= random patchy densities reflecting redistribution of blood flow from the cortical vasculature to the vasa recta of the medulla
1. Obliterative diseases of the renal microvasculature: polyarteritis nodosa, scleroderma, necrotizing angiitis, catheter-induced vasospasm
2. Acute bacterial nephritis
3. Renal vein thrombosis

Increasingly Dense Nephrogram

= initially faint nephrogram becoming increasingly dense over hours to days

Mechanism:
(a) diminished plasma clearance of contrast material
(b) leakage of contrast material into renal interstitial spaces
(c) increase in tubular transit time

Cause:
A. VASCULAR = diminished perfusion
1. Systemic arterial hypotension (bilateral)
2. Severe main renal artery stenosis (unilateral)
3. Acute tubular necrosis (in 33%): due to contrast material nephrotoxicity
4. Acute renal vein thrombosis
B. INTRARENAL
1. Acute glomerular disease
C. COLLECTING SYSTEM
1. Intratubular obstruction
(a) uric acid crystals (acute urate nephropathy)
(b) precipitation of Bence Jones protein (myeloma nephropathy)
(c) Tamm-Horsfall protein (severely dehydrated infants / children)
2. Acute extrarenal obstruction: ureteral calculus

Vicarious Contrast Material Excretion During IVP

= biliary contrast material detected radiographically following intravenous administration of contrast material

Normal contrast excretion:
<2% of urographic dose of diatrizoates + iothalamates are handled by hepatobiliary excretion

Pathophysiology:
increase in protein binding due to prolonged intravascular contact + acidosis

Cause:
1. Uremia (reduction in glomerular filtration + uremia-associated acidosis)
2. Acute unilateral obstruction (increase in circulation time + transient intracellular acidosis)
3. Spontaneous urinary extravasation (prolonged vascular contact of contrast material)

COLLECTING SYSTEM

Spontaneous Urinary Contrast Extravasation

= SPONTANEOUS PYELORENAL BACKFLOW

Etiology: physiologic "safety valve" for obstructed urinary tract with pressures of 80–100 mm Hg in collecting system due to ipsilateral ureteral obstruction from distal stone impaction; pressure is proportional to degree + duration of acute obstruction + dose of contrast material

Incidence: 0.1–18%; M > F (male ureter less compliant)

Criteria:
(a) absence of recent ureteral instrumentation
(b) absence of previous renal / ureteral surgery
(c) absence of destructive urinary tract lesion

(d) absence of external trauma
(e) absence of external compression
(f) absence of pressure necrosis due to stone

Types:

1. Pyelotubular backflow
   = opacification of terminal portions of collecting ducts (= papillary ducts = ducts of Bellini) as a physiologic phenomenon (in 13% with low osmolality + in 0.4% with high osmolality contrast media), wrongly termed "backflow"
   √ wedge-shaped brushlike lines from calyx toward periphery
2. Pyelosinus backflow
   = contrast extravasation from ruptured fornices along infundibula, renal pelvis, proximal ureter; most common form
   Cx: urinoma, retroperitoneal fibrosis
3. Pyelointerstitial backflow
   = contrast flow from pyramids into subcapsular tubules
4. Pyelolymphatic backflow
   = contrast extravasation into periforniceal + peripelvic lymphatics
   √ visualization of small lymphatics draining medially
5. Pyelovenous backflow
   = forniceal rupture into interlobar / arcuate veins; very rare

Widened Collecting System & Ureter

Fetal pyelectasis:

AP diameter of renal pelvis	<5 mm	<20 weeks MA
	<8 mm	20–30 weeks MA
	<10 mm	>30 weeks MA

A. OBSTRUCTIVE UROPATHY
   1. Acute / chronic obstruction
   2. Obstructed upper pole moiety of duplicated system

B. NONOBSTRUCTIVE WIDENING
   (a) congenital
      1. Megacalicosis
         underdevelopment of papillae, usually unilateral
      2. Congenital primary megaureter
         widened ureter with normally tapered distal end
      3. Megacystis-megaureter syndrome
      4. Prune-belly syndrome
   (b) increased urine volume
      1. High-flow states: diabetes insipidus, osmotic diuresis, dehydrated patient undergoing rehydration, unilateral kidney
      2. Vesicoureteral reflux
   (c) atony of renal collecting system
      1. Infection: ie, acute pyelonephritis
      2. Pregnancy
         Etiology: ? obstruction by enlarged ovarian veins / uterus; progesterone-induced decrease in ureteral tone
         Incidence: 3–4% of pregnant women
         Time: at end of 1st trimester, maximal in 3rd trimester
         Location: right (90%), left (67%); ureter widened only to pelvic brim
         Prognosis: resolution within a few weeks to 6 months after delivery
      3. Retroperitoneal fibrosis
   (d) distended urinary bladder
   (e) previous long-standing significant obstruction: dilatation remains in spite of relief of obstruction

Caliceal Abnormalities

A. OPACIFICATION OF COLLECTING TUBULES
   1. Pyelorenal backflow
   2. Medullary sponge kidney
B. PAPILLARY CAVITY
   1. Papillary necrosis
   2. Caliceal diverticulum
   3. Tuberculosis / brucellosis
C. LOCALIZED CALIECTASIS
   1. Reflux nephropathy = chronic atrophic pyelonephritis
   2. Compound calyx
   3. Hydrocalyx
   4. Congenital megacalyx
   5. Localized postobstructive caliectasis
   6. Localized tuberculosis / papillary necrosis
D. GENERALIZED CALIECTASIS
   1. Postobstructive atrophy
   2. Congenital megacalices
   3. Obstructive uropathy (hydronephrosis)
   4. Nonobstructive hydronephrosis
   5. Diabetes insipidus

Filling Defect In Collecting System

mnemonic: "6 C's & 2 P's"

Clot
Cancer
Cyst
Calculus
Candida + other fungi
Cystitis cystica
Polyp
Papilla (sloughed)

Nonopaque Intraluminal Mass In Collecting System

A. NONOPAQUE CALCULUS
   uric acid, xanthine, matrix
   √ smooth, rounded, not attached
B. TISSUE SLOUGH
   1. Papillary necrosis
   2. Cholesteatoma
   3. Fungus ball = conglomeration of fibrillar hyphae
   4. Inspissated debris ("mucopus")
C. VASCULAR
   1. Blood clot: history of hematuria
   √ change in appearance over time

GU

D. FOREIGN MATERIAL
   1. Air
      from bladder via reverse peristalsis, direct trauma, renoalimentary fistula
   2. Foreign matter

Mucosal mass in collecting system

NEOPLASTIC
- A. BENIN TUMOR
   1. Aberrant papilla = papilla without calyx protruding into major infundibulum
   2. Endometriosis
   3. **Fibroepithelial polyp** = fibrous polyp
      = fibroepithelioma = vascular fibrous polyp = polypoid fibroma
      = mesodermal tumor with fibrovascular stroma + normal transitional cell epithelium
      Age: 20–40 years
      • intermittent abdominal / flank pain
      • gross hematuria (rare)
      √ elongated cylindrical filling defect with smooth margins
      √ mobile on thin pedicle
- B. MALIGNANT TUMOR
   (a) Uroepithelial tumors
      1. Transitional cell carcinoma (85–91%)
      2. Squamous cell carcinoma (10–15%)
         Predisposing factors:
         calculi (50–60%), chronic infection, leukoplakia, phenacetin abuse
         √ infiltrating / superficially spreading
      3. Mucinous adenocarcinoma
         = metaplastic transformation
      4. Sarcoma (extremely rare)
   (b) Metastases: breast (most common), melanoma, stomach, lung, cervix, colon, prostate

INFLAMMATION / INFECTION
1. Tuberculosis
2. Candidiasis
3. Schistosomiasis
4. Pyeloureteritis cystica
5. Leukoplakia
6. Malacoplakia
7. Xanthogranulomatous pyelonephritis

VASCULAR
1. Submucosal hemorrhage:
   trauma, anticoagulant therapy, acquired circulating anticoagulants, complication of crystalluria / microlithiasis
   √ thumbprinting with progressive improvement
2. Vascular notching:
   ureteropelvic varices, renal vein occlusion, IVC occlusion, vascular malformation, retroaortic left renal vein, "nutcracker" effect on left renal vein between aorta and SMA
3. Polyarteritis nodosa

PROMINENT MUCOSAL FOLDS
1. Redundant longitudinal mucosal folds of intermittent hydronephrosis (UPJ obstruction, vesicoureteral reflux) or after relief of obstruction
2. Chemical / mechanical irritation
3. Urticaria (Stevens-Johnson syndrome = erythema multiforme bullosa)
4. Leukoplakia (= squamous metaplasia)
5. Ureteral diverticulosis
   = rupture of the roofs of cysts in ureteritis cystica

Effaced collecting system

A. EXTRINSIC COMPRESSION
   (1) Unilateral / bilateral global enlargement of renal parenchyma
   (2) Renal sinus masses: hemorrhage; parapelvic cyst; sinus lipomatosis
B. SPASM / INFLAMMATION
   (1) Infection: acute pyelonephritis, acute bacterial nephritis, acute tuberculosis
   (2) Hematuria
C. INFILTRATION
   Malignant uroepithelial tumors
D. OLIGURIA
   1. Antidiuretic state
   2. Renal ischemia
   3. Oliguric renal failure

RENAL CALCIFICATION

Retroperitoneal calcification

A. NEOPLASM
   1. Wilms tumor (in 10%)
   2. Neuroblastoma (in 50%): fine granular / stippled / amorphous
   3. Teratoma: cartilage / bone / teeth, pseudodigits, pseudolimbs
   4. Cavernous hemangioma: phleboliths
B. INFECTION
   1. Tuberculous psoas abscess
   2. Hydatid cyst
C. TRAUMA
   1. Old hematoma

Calcified renal mass

◊ A calcified renal mass is malignant in 75% of cases!
◊ Lesions with
   (a) nonperipheral calcifications are malignant in 87%!
   (b) peripheral calcifications are malignant in 20%!

A. TUMOR
   1. Renal cell carcinoma (calcifies in 8–18%)
      √ calcifications generally nonperipheral, sometimes along fibrous capsule
   2. Wilms tumor
B. INFECTION
   1. Abscess
      ◊ Tuberculous abscess frequently calcifies!
      ◊ Pyogenic abscess rarely calcifies!

GU

2. Echinococcal cyst
Renal involvement in 3% of hydatid disease; 50% of echinococcal cysts calcify
3. Xanthogranulomatous pyelonephritis
√ large obstructive calculus in >70%

C. CYSTS
Calcification is related to prior hemorrhage or infection
1. Simple renal cyst (calcifies in 1%)
2. Multicystic dysplastic kidney (in adult)
3. Adult polycystic kidney disease
4. Milk of calcium (cyst, caliceal diverticulum, obstructed hydrocalyx)

DDx: residual pantopaque used in cyst puncture

D. VASCULAR
1. Subcapsular / perirenal hematoma
2. Renal artery aneurysm
√ circular cracked eggshell appearance
3. Congenital / posttraumatic arteriovenous fistula

Nephrocalcinosis

= NEPHROLITHIASIS
= calcium salts in renal parenchyma
Incidence: 0.1–6%; M > F
mnemonic: "MARCH"
Medullary sponge kidney
Alkali excess
Renal medullary / cortical necrosis, **R**TA
Chronic glomerulonephritis
Hyperoxaluria, **H**ypercalcemia, **H**ypercalciuria

Medullary Nephrocalcinosis

= calcifications involving the distal convoluted tubules in the loops of Henle
Incidence: 95% of all nephrocalcinoses
Cause:

A. HYPERCALCIURIA
(a) endocrine
1. Hyperparathyroidism in 5% (primary >> secondary)
2. Paraneoplastic syndrome of lung + kidney primary (ectopic parathormone production)
3. Cushing syndrome
4. Diabetes insipidus
5. Hyperthyroidism

(b) alimentary
1. Milk-alkali syndrome (excess calcium + alkali = milk + antacids)
2. Hypervitaminosis D
3. Beryllium poisoning

(c) osseous
1. Osseous metastases, multiple myeloma
2. Prolonged immobilization
3. Progressive senile osteoporosis

(d) renal
1. Renal tubular acidosis (in 73% of primary RTA)
2. Medullary sponge kidney
3. **Bartter syndrome**
tubular disorder with potassium + sodium wasting, hyperplasia of juxtaglomerular apparatus, hyperaldosteronism, hypokalemic alkalosis, and normal blood pressure

(e) drug therapy
1. Furosemide (in infants)
2. Prolonged ACTH therapy
3. Vitamin E (orally)
4. Calcium (orally)

(f) miscellaneous
1. Sarcoidosis
2. Idiopathic hypercalcuria
3. Idiopathic hypercalcemia

B. HYPEROXALURIA = OXALOSIS
1. **Primary hyperoxaluria**
= Hereditary hyperoxaluria (more common)
= rare autosomal recessive inherited enzyme deficiency of carboligase with diffuse oxalate deposition in kidneys, heart, blood vessels, lung, spleen, bone marrow
Type I = a-ketoglutarate-glyoxylate carboxylase deficiency
• glycolic aciduria
Type II = D-glycerate dehydrogenase deficiency
• 1-glyceric aciduria
Age: usually <5 years
Prognosis: early death in childhood
2. **Secondary hyperoxaluria**
= enteric hyperoxaluria (rare)
Cause: disturbance of bile acid metabolism after jejunoileal bypass, ileal resection, blind loop syndrome, Crohn disease, increased ingestion (green leafy vegetables), pyridoxine deficiency, ethylene glycol poisoning, methoxyflurane anesthesia

C. HYPERURICOSURIA
1. Gouty kidney
2. Lesch-Nyhan syndrome

D. URINARY STASIS
1. Milk-of-calcium in pyelocaliceal diverticulum
2. Medullary sponge kidney

E. DYSTROPHIC CALCIFICATION
1. Renal papillary necrosis

mnemonic: "HAM HOP"
Hyperparathyroidism
Acidosis (renal tubular)
Medullary sponge kidney
Hypercalcemia / hypercalciuria (sarcoidosis, milk-alkali syndrome, hypervitaminosis D)
Oxalosis
Papillary necrosis

√ normal-sized / occasionally enlarged kidneys (medullary sponge kidney)
√ grouped rounded / linear calcifications
√ small poorly defined / large coarse granular calcifications in renal pyramids

US:
- √ absence of hypoechoic papillary structures (earliest sign)
- √ hyperechoic rim at corticomedullary junction + around tip and sides of pyramids
- √ solitary focus of hyperechogenicity at tip of pyramid near fornix
- √ increased echogenicity of renal pyramids ± shadowing (no acoustic shadowing with small + light calcifications)

DDx of hyperechoic medulla in newborns: oliguria with transient tubular blockage by Tamm-Horsfall proteinuria

Cx: often followed by urolithiasis

Cortical Nephrocalcinosis

Incidence: 5% of all nephrocalcinoses

Cause:
1. Acute cortical necrosis
2. Chronic glomerulonephritis
3. Alport syndrome = hereditary nephritis + deafness
4. Congenital oxalosis, primary hyperoxaluria
5. Chronic paraneoplastic hypercalcemia
6. Rejected renal transplant

mnemonic: "COAG"
- **C**ortical necrosis (acute)
- **O**xalosis
- **A**lport syndrome
- **G**lomerulonephritis (chronic)

US:
- √ homogeneously increased echogenicity of renal parenchyma > liver echogenicity

RENOVASCULAR DISEASE

Renovascular Hypertension

= normalization of blood pressure following nephrectomy / reestablishment of normal renal blood flow (Dx made in retrospect)

Incidence: 1–5% of general population; 2nd most common cause of potentially curable hypertension

Pathophysiology:
usually >50% stenosis at any level in renovascular bed leads to mildly reduced pressure in glomerular afferent arteriole (pressure falls precipitously in >80% stenosis); reduced pressure stimulates release of renin followed by angiotensin-II, and aldosterone causing
(a) constriction of efferent glomerular arterioles
(b) increase in systemic hypertension
(c) sodium retention

Cause:
1. Atherosclerosis (60–90%) in individuals >50 years of age
2. Fibromuscular dysplasia (10–35%) in women <40 years of age
3. Neurofibromatosis
4. Pheochromocytoma
5. Fibrous bands (congenital stenosis, retroperitoneal fibrosis, postradiation artery stenosis)
6. Arteritis (Buerger disease, polyarteritis nodosa, Takayasu disease, thrombangitis obliterans, syphilitic arteritis)
7. Arteriovenous malformation / fistula
8. Thromboembolic disease (eg, atrial fibrillation, prosthetic valve thrombi, cardiac myxoma, paradoxical emboli, atheromatous emboli)
9. Renal artery aneurysm
10. Extrinsic compression (eg, renal cyst, neoplasm, perirenal hematoma)
11. Middle aortic syndrome, aortic dissection, dissecting aortic aneurysm
12. Trauma

◊ Renal artery stenosis is present in 77% of hypertensive patients!
◊ Renal artery stenosis is present in 32–49% of normotensive patients!
◊ 15–20% of patients remain hypertensive after restoration of normal renal blood flow!

Rx: (1) Relieving renal artery stenosis
(2) Angiotensin-converting enzyme inhibitor

Hypertension In Children

Prevalence: 1–3%
1. Coarse renal cortex scarring (36%)
2. Glomerulonephritis (23%)
3. Coarctation of aorta (10%)
4. Renovascular disease (10%)
5. Polycystic renal disease (6%)
6. Hemolytic-uremic syndrome (4%)
7. Catecholamine excess [pheochromocytoma, neuroblastoma] (3%)
8. Renal tumor (2%)
9. Essential hypertension (3%)

Renal Aneurysm

A. EXTRARENAL ANEURYSM (2/3)
1. Congenital
2. Atherosclerotic
3. Fibromuscular dysplasia
4. Mycotic
   2.5% of all aneurysms
   Cause: bacteremia, SBE, perivascular extension of inflammation
   Organism: Streptococcus, Staphylococcus, Pneumococcus, Salmonella
   Locations: thoracic aorta, SMA, peripheral branches of middle cerebral artery, large arteries of extremities, intrarenal (rare), in areas of preexisting vascular disease
5. Neurofibromatosis
6. Trauma + renal artery angioplasty

GU

B. INTRARENAL ANEURYSM (1/3)
in interlobar and more peripheral branches
1. Congenital renal aneurysm
Age at Dx: 30 years; M:F = 1:1
• hypertension in 25% (from segmental renal ischemia)
√ aneurysm close to vascular bifurcations, may calcify
2. Atherosclerotic (may calcify)
3. Polyarteritis nodosa
4. SLE
5. Drug-abuse vasculitis
Kidney most commonly affected organ
Cause:
(a) immunologic injury from circulating hepatitis antigen-antibody complexes producing a necrotizing angiitis
(b) bacterial endocarditis
(c) drug-related
(d) impurity-related
Drugs: methamphetamine, heroin, LSD
√ multiple small aneurysms in interlobar branches near corticomedullary junction
√ inhomogeneous spotty nephrogram
6. Allergic vasculitis
7. Neoplasm (renal cell carcinoma in 14%; adult Wilms tumor)
8. Hamartoma (angiomyolipoma in 50%)
9. Wegener granulomatosis
10. Metastatic arterial myxoma
11. Transplant rejection
12. Neurofibromatosis

Cx: (1) Hypertension (unusual) (2) Perinephric / retroperitoneal hemorrhage (3) Formation of AV fistula (4) Peripheral renal embolization (5) Thrombosis

Spontaneous Renal Hemorrhage

A. RENAL TUMOR (57–63%)
(a) malignant (30–33%):
RCC, TCC of renal pelvis, Wilms tumor, lipo-, fibro-, angiosarcoma
(b) benign (24–33%):
angiomyolipoma (16–20%), lipoma, adenoma, fibromyoma, ruptured hemorrhagic cyst
B. VASCULAR DISEASE (18–26%)
vasculitis (eg, polyarteritis nodosa in 13%), arteriovenous malformation, ruptured aneurysm, segmental renal infarction
C. INFLAMMATION / INFECTION (7–10%)
1/2 with + 1/2 without abscess
D. COAGULOPATHY
anticoagulation therapy, bleeding diathesis, long-term hemodialysis

◊ Surgical exploration must be considered to uncover a small renal tumor if the cause of hemorrhage is not determined radiologically!

Subcapsular Hematoma

√ subcapsular mass with flattening of renal parenchyma
√ total resorption / formation of pseudocapsule with calcification

Angio:
√ avascular mass

Cx: Page kidney (ischemia, release of renin, hypertension)

Renal Doppler

A. NORMAL RENAL DOPPLER
√ resistive index (RI) of 0.70 = upper limit of normal
Elevation of RI:
— significant systemic hypotension
— markedly decreased heart rate
— perinephric / subcapsular fluid collection
— in neonates + infants
B. RENAL MEDICAL DISEASE
Elevation of RI more likely with vascular / tubulointerstitial process, less likely with glomerular disease
May be useful in predicting clinical outcome in:
— hemolytic-uremic syndrome
— acute renal failure
— nonazotemic patients with severe liver disease
C. RENAL ARTERIAL STENOSIS
D. RENAL VEIN THROMBOSIS

URETER

Ureteral Deviation

A. LUMBAR URETER
(a) lateral deviation (common):
1. Hypertrophy of psoas muscle
2. Enlargement of paracaval / para-aortic lymph nodes
3. Aneurysmal dilatation of aorta
4. Neurogenic tumors
5. Fluid collections (abscess, urinoma, lymphocele, hematoma)
(b) medial deviation:
1. Retrocaval ureter (on right side only)
2. Retroperitoneal fibrosis
B. PELVIC URETER
(a) medial deviation:
1. Hypertrophy of iliopsoas muscle
2. Enlargement of iliac lymph nodes
3. Aneurysmal dilatation of iliac vessels
4. Bladder diverticulum at UVJ (Hutch)
5. Following abdominoperineal surgery + retroperitoneal lymph node dissection
6. Pelvic lipomatosis
(b) lateral deviation with extrinsic compression
1. Pelvic mass (eg, fibroids, ovarian tumor)

Megaureter

A. VESICOURETERAL REFLUX
(a) primary vesicoureteral reflux
1. Primary reflux megaureter
abnormal ureteral tunnel at UVJ

2. Prune belly syndrome
(b) secondary vesicoureteral reflux
1. Hypertonic neurogenic bladder
2. Bladder outlet obstruction
3. Posterior urethral valves

B. OBSTRUCTION
(a) primary obstruction
1. Intrinsic ureteral obstruction (stone, stricture, tumor)
2. Ectopic ureter
3. Ureterocele
4. Ureteral duplication: tortuous dilated ureter of upper moiety
(b) secondary obstruction
1. Retroperitoneal obstruction: tumor, fibrosis, aortic aneurysm
2. Bladder wall mass
3. Bladder outlet obstruction: eg, prostatic enlargement

C. NONREFLUX-NONOBSTRUCTED MEGAURETER
1. Congenital primary megaureter = megaloureter
2. Polyuria: eg, diabetes insipidus, acute diuresis
3. Infection
4. Ureter remaining wide after relief of obstruction

mnemonic: "DiaPOUR"
Diabetes insipidus
Primary megaureter
Obstruction (recent / old)
UVJ obstruction
Reflux

Ureteral Stricture

A. INTRINSIC CAUSE
(a) mucosal
1. Primary ureteral tumors
(b) mural
1. **Endometriosis**
common disorder in menstruating women (15%); ureteral involvement is rare and indicates widespread pelvic disease
√ abrupt smooth stricture of 0.5–2.5 cm length
√ rectosigmoid involvement on BE
2. Tuberculosis, schistosomiasis
3. Traumatic
ureterolithotomy, endoscopic stone extraction, hysterectomy
4. Amyloidosis
√ distal stricture with submucosal calcification
5. Nonspecific (rare)

B. EXTRINSIC CAUSE
1. Endometriosis
extrinsic form:intrinsic form = 4:1
2. Abscess
tubo-ovarian, appendiceal, perisigmoidal
3. Inflammatory bowel disease
(eg, Crohn disease, diverticulitis)
4. Radiation fibrosis
5. Metastases
cervix, endometrium, ovary, rectum, prostate, breast, lymphoma
6. Iliac artery aneurysm (with perianeurysmal fibrosis)

mnemonic: "MISTER"
Metastasis (extrinsic / intrinsic)
Inflammation from calculus
Schistosomiasis
Tuberculosis, **T**ransitional cell carcinoma, **T**rauma
Endometriosis + other periureteral inflammatory process
Radiation therapy, **R**etroperitoneal fibrosis

Ureteral Filling Defect

A. FIXED
1. Urothelial neoplasm
2. Metastasis
3. Inflammation
(a) ureteritis cystica
(b) tuberculosis
4. Fibroepithelial polyp
5. Endometriosis

B. MOBILE
1. Calculus
2. Sloughed papilla
3. Blood clot

ADRENAL GLAND

Adrenal Medullary Disease

1. Neuroblastoma
2. Ganglioneuroblastoma
3. Ganglioneuroma
4. Pheochromocytoma

Adrenal Cortical Disease

1. Adrenal hyperplasia
2. Adrenocortical adenoma
3. Adrenocortical carcinoma
4. Cushing syndrome
5. Conn syndrome
6. Adrenogenital syndrome

Adrenocortical Hyperfunction

1. Cushing syndrome = hypercortisolism
2. Conn syndrome = hyperaldosteronism
√ solitary unilateral adrenal adenoma + normal contralateral gland on CT may be due to:
(a) aldosterone-producing adrenocortical adenoma
(b) renin-responsive aldosterone-producing adenoma
(c) idiopathic hyperaldosteronism with dominant hyperplastic / nonfunctional adenoma
3. Adrenogenital syndrome

DDx of Cushing syndrome

A. FOCAL UNILATERAL ADRENAL MASS
   √ 2–4 cm focal mass in one adrenal gland + atrophy of contralateral gland = adrenal adenoma
   √ >4 cm large focal mass with central necrosis in one adrenal gland + atrophy of contralateral gland = adrenal adenocarcinoma
B. BILATERAL ADRENAL ENLARGEMENT
   √ diffuse uniform thickening = Cushing disease
C. MULTIPLE BILATERAL ADRENAL NODULES
   √ macronodules = multinodular hyperplasia of long-standing Cushing disease
   √ large nodules (autonomous ACTH-independent) = massive macronodular hyperplasia
   √ small nodules = primary pigmented nodular adrenal disease

Bilateral Large Adrenals

mnemonic: "4 H PM"

Hodgkin disease
Hyperplasia
Hemorrhage
Histoplasmosis / TB
Pheochromocytoma
Metastasis

Unilateral Adrenal Mass

◊ CT attenuation
  <0 HU = benign mass
  0–15 HU = probably benign
  >15 HU = indeterminate
◊ on 15-minute–delayed CECT scan:
  <25 HU benign lesion, >25 HU malignant lesion
  Cause: rapid contrast washout from benign lesions

mnemonic: "PLAN My HAM"

Pheochromocytoma
Lymphoma
Adenoma
Neuroblastoma
Myelolipoma
Hemorrhage
Adenocarcinoma
Metastasis

Small Unilateral Adrenal Tumor

◊ Incidental discovery of adrenal mass in 1% of all CT!
  (a) mass <3 cm in diameter is likely (in 87%) benign
  (b) mass >5 cm in diameter is likely malignant

1. Cortical adenoma (in 1–9% of autopsies)
   √ <10 HU imply (in 96%) an adenoma
2. Metastasis (27% of all tumors): lung (40%), breast (20%), renal cell carcinoma, gastrointestinal tumors, melanoma
   ◊ 50% of adrenal masses in oncologic patients represent benign nonhyperfunctioning adenomas!
3. Pheochromocytoma
4. Asymmetric hyperplasia
5. Granulomatous disease (TB, histoplasmosis)
   √ diffuse enlargement / discrete mass
   √ ± central cystic changes ± calcification
6. Myelolipoma: rare benign tumor composed of hematopoietic cells + fat similar to bone marrow
   • may cause pain if large
   √ typically between -30 to -115 HU
   √ calcified in up to 20%
   Cx: retroperitoneal hemorrhage

Large Solid Adrenal Mass

1. Cortical carcinoma
2. Pheochromocytoma
3. Neuroblastoma / ganglioneuroma
4. Myelolipoma
5. Metastasis
6. Hemorrhage
7. Inflammation
8. Abscess (eg, histoplasmosis, tuberculosis)
9. Hemangioma

Cystic Adrenal Mass

1. Pseudocyst: old hemorrhage / infarction
2. Vascular cystic space (endothelial lining): lymphangioma, hemangioma
3. True cyst (epithelial lining): glandular cyst, embryonal cyst, mesothelial inclusion cyst
4. Parasitic cyst: hydatid cyst
5. Hemorrhagic complication / degeneration of a tumor: cystic adenoma, cystic pheochromocytoma, cystic adenomatoid tumor, cystic adrenocortical carcinoma, schwannoma
6. Neuroblastoma (rare)
7. Cortical adenoma with low density

Adrenal Calcification

A. TUMOR
   1. Neuroblastoma
   2. Pheochromocytoma
   3. Adrenal adenoma
   4. Adrenal carcinoma
   5. Dermoid
B. VASCULAR
   1. Hemorrhage (neonatal, sepsis)
C. INFECTION
   1. Tuberculosis
   2. Histoplasmosis
   3. Waterhouse-Friderichsen syndrome
D. ENDOCRINE
   1. Addison disease (TB)
E. OTHERS
   1. Wolman disease

URINARY BLADDER

Bilateral Narrowing Of Urinary Bladder

A. WITH ELEVATION OF BLADDER FLOOR
   1. Pelvic lipomatosis
   2. Pelvic hematoma

Cause: trauma, anticoagulant therapy, spontaneous rupture of blood vessels, blood dyscrasia (rare), bleeding neoplasm (rare)

3. Chronic cystitis

B. WITH SUPERIOR COMPRESSION OF BLADDER
1. Thrombosis of IVC
Cause: trauma, hypercoagulability state (oral contraceptives), extension of thrombi from lower extremity, abdominal sepsis, Budd-Chiari syndrome, compression of IVC by neoplasm
√ collaterals through gonadal veins, ascending lumbar veins, vertebral plexus, retroperitoneal veins, portal vein (via hemorrhoidal veins)
√ notching of distal ureter by ureteral veins
2. Pelvic lymphadenopathy
Cause: lymphoma (most often)
√ polycyclic asymmetric compression of bladder
√ medial displacement of pelvic segment of ureters
√ lateral displacement of upper ureters
3. Hypertrophy of iliopsoas muscles
4. Bilateral pelvic masses
(a) bilateral lymphocysts (following radical pelvic surgery)
(b) bilateral urinomas
(c) bilateral pelvic abscesses

Pear-shaped Urinary Bladder

mnemonic: "HALL"
Hematoma
Aneurysm (bilateral common / external iliac artery)
Lipomatosis
Lymphadenopathy (pelvic)

Small Bladder Capacity

Cause:
A. Thickened / fibrotic bladder wall
1. Interstitial cystitis
2. Tuberculous cystitis
3. Cystitis cystica
4. Schistosomiasis
5. Trauma: surgical resection, radiation therapy

B. Disuse of bladder

• urinary frequency
• progressive rise in bladder pressure during filling
√ reduced bladder compliance
√ thickened bladder wall + decreased bladder volume
√ vesicoureteral reflux

Bladder Wall Thickening

Normal bladder wall thickness (regardless of age + gender):
<5 mm in nondistended bladders
<3 mm in well-distended bladders

A. TUMOR
1. Neurofibromatosis

B. INFECTION / INFLAMMATION
1. Cystitis

C. MUSCULAR HYPERTROPHY
1. Neurogenic bladder
2. Bladder outlet obstruction (eg, posterior urethral valves)

D. UNDERDISTENDED BLADDER

Urinary Bladder Wall Masses

A. CONGENITAL
1. Congenital septum
2. Simple ureterocele
3. Ectopic ureterocele

B. BLADDER TUMORS

C. INFLAMMATION / INFECTION
1. Cystitis: hemorrhagic ~, abacterial ~, bullous ~, edematous ~, interstitial ~, eosinophilic ~, granulomatous ~, emphysematous ~, cystitis cystica, cyclophosphamide cystitis, cystitis glandularis (premalignant lesion with villous lesions in bladder dome from proliferation of "intestine-like" glands in submucosa)
2. Tuberculosis
3. Schistosomiasis
4. Malacoplakia
5. Extravesical inflammation:
(a) Diverticulitis
(b) Crohn disease
(c) endometriosis

D. HEMATOMA
after instrumentation, surgery, trauma

Bladder Tumor

A. EPITHELIAL TUMORS (95%)
1. Transitional cell carcinoma (90%)
multicentric, aniline dyes
2. Squamous cell carcinoma (4%)
worst prognosis; secondary to chronic disorders (infection, stricture, calculi), bladder diverticula, schistosomiasis
3. Adenocarcinoma (1%)
most common in bladder exstrophy, less common in cystitis glandularis + urachal carcinoma (at dome of bladder in urachal remnant)

B. NONEPITHELIAL TUMORS
(a) primary benign tumors
1. Leiomyoma (most common)
• hematuria secondary to ulceration
Site: submucosal / intramural / subserosal
2. Rhabdomyoma (rare)
3. Hemangioma
4. Neurofibroma / neurofibromatosis
generalized neurofibromatosis in 60%
5. Nephrogenic adenoma
Associated with: cystitis cystica / cystitis glandularis
6. Endometriosis
on posterior wall, urinary symptoms in 80%

7. Pheochromocytoma (0.5%)
   from paraganglia of bladder wall; 7% are malignant
   - adrenergic attack at micturition / bladder filling (headaches, weakness)
   - intermittent hypertension
   - elevated catecholamine levels

(b) primary malignant tumors
1. Primary lymphoma
   2nd most common nonepithelial tumor of urinary bladder
   Age: 40 years; M:F = 1:3
   Location: submucosal; at bladder base + trigone
2. Rhabdomyosarcoma
   1st and 2nd decade of life
3. Leiomyosarcoma
   rarely at trigone; mainly >40 years of age

(c) secondary tumors
1. Metastases
   1.5% of all bladder malignancies
   Origin: melanoma > stomach > breast > kidney > lung
   √ solitary / multiple nodules
2. Lymphoma
   bladder involved at autopsy:
   for NHL in 15%, for Hodgkin disease in 5%
3. Leukemia
   microscopic involvement in 22% at autopsy
4. Direct extension (common)
   from prostate, rectum, sigmoid, cervix, ovary

Bladder Wall Calcification

A. INFLAMMATION
1. Schistosomiasis (50%)
   √ relatively normal distensibility
2. Tuberculosis
   √ bladder markedly contracted
3. Postirradiation cystitis
4. Bacillary UTI (extremely uncommon)

B. NEOPLASM
TCC, squamous cell carcinoma, leiomyosarcoma, hemangioma, neuroblastoma, osteogenic sarcoma

mnemonic: "SCRITT"
Schistosomiasis
Cytoxan
Radiation
Interstitial cystitis
Tuberculosis
Transitional cell carcinoma

Masses Extrinsic To Urinary Bladder

A. NORMAL / ENLARGED ORGANS
1. Uterus, leiomyomatous uterus, pregnant uterus
2. Distended rectosigmoid
3. Ectopic pelvic kidney
4. Prostate cancer / BPH

B. SOLID PELVIC TUMORS
1. Lymphadenopathy
2. Bone tumor from sacrum / coccyx
3. Rectosigmoid mass
4. Hip arthroplasty
5. Neurogenic neoplasm, meningomyelocele
6. Pelvic lipomatosis / liposarcoma

C. CYSTIC PELVIC LESIONS
(a) congenital / developmental
1. Urachal cyst
2. Müllerian duct cyst
3. Gartner duct cyst
4. Anterior meningocele
5. Hydrometrocolpos

(b) related to trauma
1. Hematoma (eg, rectus sheath hematoma)
2. Urinoma
3. Lymphocele
4. Abscess
5. Aneurysm
6. Mesenteric cyst

(c) cyst of genitalia
1. Prostatic cyst
2. Cyst of seminal vesicle
3. Cyst of vas deferens
4. Ovarian cyst
5. Hydrosalpinx
6. Vaginal cyst

(d) cyst of urinary bladder
1. Bladder diverticulum

(e) cyst of GI tract
1. Peritoneal inclusion cyst
2. Fluid-filled bowel

VOIDING DYSFUNCTION

A. FAILURE TO STORE URINE
- urinary frequency, urgency, incontinence

(a) bladder causes
1. involuntary detrusor contractions
   - detrusor instability (idiopathic / neurogenic)
   - detrusor hyperreflexia (upper cord lesion)
2. poor bladder compliance
   - detrusor hyperreflexia
   - bladder wall fibrosis
3. sensory urgency
   - infection, inflammation, irritation
   - neoplasia
4. vesicovaginal fistula
5. psychogenic condition

(b) sphincter causes
1. Stress incontinence
2. Sphincteric incontinence

(c) extravesical ectopic insertion of ureter in females

B. FAILURE TO EMPTY BLADDER
- poor flow, straining, hesitancy
- inability to completely empty bladder

(a) bladder causes
1. Detrusor areflexia (sacral arc lesion)
2. Impaired detrusor contractility (myogenic)
3. Psychogenic condition

(b) bladder outlet obstruction:
1. Bladder neck contracture
2. Prostatic enlargement
3. Detrusor-external sphincter dyssynergia
4. Scarring from surgery / radiation therapy
5. Ectopic ureterocele
6. Urethral stenosis
7. Urethral kinking (eg, due to cystocele)

Incontinence

1. Stress incontinence
2. Vesicovaginal / ureterovaginal fistula
3. Overflow incontinence
   secondary to lesions of sacral spinal cord / sacral reflex arc or severe outlet obstruction
4. Reflex voiding
   (a) hyperreflexive lesion (lesion of upper spinal cord)
   (b) uninhibited / unstable bladder
5. Urge incontinence
6. Continual dribbling
   (extravesical ectopic termination of ureter)
7. Psychogenic incontinence

Stress Incontinence

= SPHINCTER WEAKNESS INCONTINENCE

Cause:

A. Female: congenital bladder neck weakness, pregnancy, childbirth, aging (secondary to changes in anatomic relationship of urethra + bladder base)

B. Male: S/P prostatectomy with damage to distal sphincter

- frequency, urgency (involuntary filling of bladder neck)

√ opening of bladder neck during coughing
√ impairment of milk-back mechanism (= retrograde emptying of urethra during interruption of voiding phase does not occur)
√ urethrovesical descent (in types I + II)

Chain cystography:

√ posterior urethrovesical angle (= angle between posterior urethra + bladder base) increased >100°
√ upper urethral axis (= angle between upper urethra + vertical line) increased >35°

Detrusor Instability

= MOTOR URGE INCONTINENCE = UNSTABLE BLADDER

Condition resembles that of immature bladder before toilet training

Patient groups:

(1) symptoms of nocturnal enuresis + frequency / incontinence dating back to childhood
(2) idiopathic instability occurring in middle age
(3) outflow obstruction commonly in men
(4) degenerative instability secondary to cardiovascular + neurologic disease later in life

- frequency, urgency, urge incontinence, occasionally nocturia
- hesitancy + difficulty in voiding may occur in men without significant prostatic hypertrophy

√ involuntary bladder contractions with no relationship to bladder distension
√ progressively vigorous contractions during bladder filling
√ postural instability limited to upright position
√ impaired milk-back due to high bladder pressure
√ strong aftercontractions following bladder emptying

Cx: thickening of bladder wall, bladder diverticula

Rx: treatment of obstruction, anticholinergic drug (oxybutynin), operative increase in bladder capacity

Sensitive Bladder (Sensory Urgency)

Cause:

cystitis (reduced compliance), some cases of stress incontinence (filling of bladder neck induces urgency)

- frequency, urgency, sometimes nocturia

√ patient uncomfortable with low bladder filling
√ no abnormal rise in bladder pressure
√ normal voiding function

Detrusor-sphincter Dyssynergia

= overactivity of bladder neck muscle with failure to relax at beginning of voiding

Cause: spinal cord lesion / trauma above level of sacral outflow

- difficulty in voiding ± frequency
- lifelong history of poor stream

√ collarlike indentation of bladder neck during voiding (= persistent / intermittent narrowing of membranous urethra)
√ may have high voiding pressure + reduced flow
√ trapping of contrast in urethra during interruption of flow
√ massive reflux into prostatic ducts during voiding (due to high pressure within prostatic urethra)
√ severely trabeculated "Christmas-tree" bladder + bilateral hydroureteronephrosis

Rx: bladder neck incision

Hinman Syndrome

= NONNEUROGENIC NEUROGENIC BLADDER [NNNB] = DETRUSOR-SPHINCTER DYSSYNERGIA

Cause: no neurologic / anatomic obstructive disease; distinctly abnormal family dynamics (in 50%)

Age: some time after toilet training with onset during early / late childhood / puberty

- clinical criteria:
  (1) intact perineal sensation + anal tone
  (2) normal anatomy + function of lower extremities
  (3) absence of skin lesions overlying sacrum
  (4) normal lumbosacral spine at plain radiography
  (5) normal spinal cord at MR imaging

√ high-pressure uninhibited detrusor contractions
√ lack of coordination between detrusor contraction + periurethral striated sphincter relaxation
√ inability to suppress bladder contractions
√ normal response of detrusor muscle to reflex stimulation
√ increased bladder capacity + pressure
√ sphincter activity may increase paradoxically during detrusor contraction

US:
√ trabeculated bladder
√ dilatation of upper urinary tracts
√ renal damage

VCUG:
√ urethra normal during early voiding
√ urethral distension after contraction of external sphincter as voiding progresses
√ ureterovesical obstruction / reflux

Rx: suggestion therapy + hypnosis, bladder retraining, biofeedback, anticholinergic drugs

Prostatic Obstruction
= urethral compression by hypertrophic prostatic tissue
• difficulty in voiding
• reduction in flow rate
√ high-pressure bladder
√ slow + prolonged flow
√ increase in bladder capacity with reduced contractility (late)

BLADDER TRAUMA
1. Bladder contusion (most common injury)
2. Interstitial bladder injury (uncommon)
   = bladder tear without serosal involvement
3. Bladder rupture
   (a) intraperitoneal rupture (30%)
   (b) extraperitoneal rupture
   (c) combined intra- and extraperitoneal rupture (5%)

MALE GENITAL TRACT

Acutely Symptomatic Scrotum
= acute unilateral scrotal swelling ± pain

Cause:
epididymitis:torsion = 3:2 <20 years of age
epididymitis:torsion = 9:1 >20 years of age

A. TORSION
1. Torsion of testis (20%)
   = most common acute process in prepubertal age
2. Torsion of testicular appendages
   accounts for 5% of scrotal pathology; both located near upper pole of testes
   Frequency:
   appendix testis:appendix epididymis = 9:1
   √ 8–9 mm complex mass in superior aspect of scrotum without color Doppler flow signals
   √ mildly enlarged epididymis (75%)
   √ blood flow increased in epididymis (60%), scrotal wall (53%), testis (13%) simulating acute epididymo-orchitis
3. Scrotal fat necrosis
4. Strangulated hernia

B. INFECTION / INFLAMMATION (75–80%)
1. Acute epididymitis
   = most common acute process in postpubertal age
2. **Orchitis**
   Etiology:
   (a) bacterial infection
   (b) complication of mumps in 20%:
   in adolescents + young adults; usually developing 4–5 days later; unilateral involvement in >90%; parotitis precedes orchitis in 84%, simultaneous in 3%, later in 4%, without parotitis in 10%
3. Intrascrotal abscess

C. HEMORRHAGE
1. Testicular trauma
   Location: hematoma in scrotal wall, between layers of tunica vaginalis (= hematocele), in epididymis, in testis
   √ rapid change in echo character over time
   √ disruption of tunica albuginea (= testicular rupture)
2. Hemorrhage into testicular tumor

D. STRANGULATED HERNIA

Scrotal Wall Thickening
1. Acute idiopathic scrotal edema
   Incidence: 20–30% of all acute scrotal disorders
   Age: 5–11 years (range 18 months to 14 years)
   • subcutaneous scrotal edema, erythema
   • minimal pain, afebrile, peripheral eosinophilia
2. Epididymo-orchitis
3. Testicular torsion
4. Torsion of testicular / epididymal appendage
5. Trauma
6. Henoch-Schönlein purpura
7. Cx of ventriculoperitoneal shunt
8. Cx of peritoneal dialysis (? leakage of fluid into the anterior abdominal wall + dissection into scrotum)

Scrotal Gas
1. Fournier gangrene
2. Scrotal abscess
3. Scrotal hernia with gas-containing bowel
4. Scrotal emphysema from bowel perforation
5. Extension of subcutaneous emphysema
6. Air leakage + dissection due to faulty chest tube positioning

Scrotal Mass
Most frequent conditions:
1. Inflammation (48%)
2. Hydrocele (24%)

GU

3. Torsion (9%)
4. Varicocele (7%)
5. Spermatocele (4%)
6. Cysts (4%)
7. Malignant tumor (2%)
8. Benign tumor (0.7%)

◊ Sonographic differentiation of intra- from extratesticular mass is 80–95% accurate!

A. INTRATESTICULAR MASS
   ◊ 90–95% of testicular tumors are malignant!
   1. Malignant tumor
   2. Inflammation: focal orchitis
   3. Abscess
   4. Testicular infarction: torsion, endocarditis, trauma, leukemia, vasculitis, embolus
      • soft to palpation
      √ hypoechoic wedge-shaped peripheral defect
   5. Hematoma
   6. Benign gonadal tumor
   7. Granulomatous disease: sarcoidosis
   8. Testicular cyst / tunica albuginea cyst
   9. Postbiopsy defect
   10. Adrenal rest
      • increase in circulating corticotropin
      √ bilateral eccentric nodular masses ± acoustic shadowing

B. MULTIPLE INTRATESTICULAR MASSES
   1. Primary testicular tumor
   2. Lymphoma / leukemia
   3. Chronic infections
   4. Metastases
   5. Sarcoidosis
   ◊ The prevalence of synchronous / metachronous bilateral testicular neoplasms is 1–3%!

C. EXTRATESTICULAR FLUID COLLECTION
   1. Hydrocele, pyocele, hematocele (surgery, trauma, neoplasm)
   2. Varicocele
   3. Spermatocele
      = cyst filled with fluid + spermatozoa + cellular debris
      • frequently following vasectomy
      Location: commonly in head of epididymis
      √ up to a few cm in size ± septations
   4. Epididymal cyst
      = cyst without spermatozoa
      Location: anywhere within epididymis
   5. Scrotal hernia

D. PARATESTICULAR MASS
   ◊ Only 4% of all scrotal tumors!
   (a) inflammatory mass
      1. Sarcoidosis of epididymis
      2. Inflammatory nodule of epididymitis
      3. Sperm granuloma
         Cause: sperm extravasation with granuloma formation
      4. Scrotal calculi = "scrotal pearls"
         Cause: fibrinous debris in long-standing hydrocele / following torsion of appendix testis or epididymis
   (b) paratesticular tumor
      ◊ The majority of paratesticular tumors are derived from the spermatic cord!
      — BENIGN PARATESTICULAR TUMOR (70%)
      1. Cord lipoma (vast majority)
      2. **Adenomatoid tumor** (30%)
         = benign slow-growing mesothelial neoplasm
         Age: 2nd–4th decade
         Histo: epithelial-like cells + fibrous stroma
         Location: epididymis (particularly in globus minor), tunica albuginea, spermatic cord (rare)
         √ well-marginated solid mass with echogenicity equal to / greater than testis
         √ 0.4–5.0 cm in size
      3. Epidermoid inclusion cyst
      4. Polyorchidism
      5. Others: herniated omentum, adrenal rest, carcinoid, papillary cystadenoma of epididymis, cord leiomyoma, cord fibroma (= reactive nodular proliferation of paratesticular tissues), adrenal rest, cholesteatoma
      — MALIGNANT PARATESTICULAR TUMOR (3–16%)
      1. Sarcomas:
         ◊ Sarcomas are the most common spermatic cord tumors after lipomas!
         (a) primarily in adults: undifferentiated sarcoma (30%), leiomyo-, lipo-, fibro-, myxochondro-sarcoma
         (b) children: embryonal sarcoma, rhabdomyosarcoma (20%)
      2. Mesothelioma of tunica (in 15% malignant)
      3. Metastases

Prepubertal Testicular Mass

A. Germ cell tumors (70–90%): yolk sac tumor, teratoma
B. Interstitial cell tumors: Leydig / Sertoli cell tumor, gonadoblastoma
C. Leukemia, lymphoma, metastases
D. Others: adrenal rest, lipoma, hematoma, histiocytosis, tuberculous orchitis

Calcification Of Male Genital Tract

A. VAS DEFERENS
   1. Diabetes mellitus: in muscular outer layer
   2. Degenerative changes
   3. TB, syphilis, nonspecific UTI: intraluminal

B. SEMINAL VESICLES
   gonorrhea, TB, schistosomiasis, bilharziasis

C. PROSTATE
   calcified corpora amylacea, TB

Cystic Lesions Of Testis

Incidence: 4–10% (increasing with age)
- asymptomatic

A. NONNEOPLASTIC
1. **Testicular cyst**
   - nonpalpable

   Often associated with: spermatocele
   Location: related to rete testis (in 92%)
2. **Tunica albuginea cyst**
   - palpable

   √ solitary small marginally located cyst
3. **Intratesticular tubular ectasia**
   = DILATATION OF RETE TESTIS
   Age: middle-aged to elderly
   Often associated with: spermatocele
   - nonpalpable

   Location: mediastinum testis
   √ elliptical hypoechoic mass with branching tubular structures ± cysts
4. Congenital cystic dysplasia of testis (extremely rare)

B. NEOPLASTIC
◊ 24% of all testicular tumors have cystic component!
- palpable

√ in combination with solid elements

DDx: hematoma, inflammation, seminoma, Leydig cell tumor

Epididymal Enlargement With Hypoechoic Foci

1. Epididymitis
2. Sperm granulomas
3. Tuberculosis
4. Lymphogranuloma venereum
5. Granuloma inguinale
6. Filarial granuloma
7. Fungal disease
8. Lymphoproliferative disease
9. Metastases

Cystic Lesions Of Epididymis

1. Epididymal cyst
   Incidence: in up to 40%
   May be associated with: intratesticular tubular ectasia
   √ single / multiple / bilateral
   DDx: loculated hydrocele
2. Spermatocele
   √ may contain low-level echoes
3. Cystic degeneration of epididymis

PROSTATE AND URETHRA

Seminal Vesicle Cyst

A. CONGENITAL
associated with: renal dysgenesis, collecting system duplication, ectopic ureter, vas deferens agenesis

B. ACQUIRED
1. Autosomal dominant polycystic kidney disease
   √ bilateral seminal vesicle cysts
2. Invasive bladder tumor
3. Infection
4. Benign prostatic hypertrophy
5. Ejaculatory duct obstruction

Large Utricle

1. Prune belly syndrome
2. Imperforate anus of high type
3. Down syndrome
4. Hypospadia
5. Posterior urethral valves

Prostatic Cysts

1. **Müllerian duct cyst**
   from remnants of paramesonephric (= müllerian) duct which has regressed by 3rd fetal month
   Prevalence: 4–5% of male newborns; in 1% of men
   Age: discovered in 3rd–4th decade
   - obstructive / irritative urinary tract symptoms
   - suprapubic / rectal pain
   - hematuria
   - infertility (most common cause of ejaculatory duct obstruction)

   Location: arise from region of verumontanum slightly lateral to midline
   ◊ No communication with genital tract / urethra
   √ large intraprostatic cyst usually with extension superolaterally above prostate
   √ aspirate contains serous / mucous clear brown / green fluid (hemorrhage + debris), NOT spermatozoa
   √ rarely contains calculi
   Cx: infection, hemorrhage, carcinomatous transformation
2. **Utricle cyst**
   Secondary to dilatation of prostatic utricle (sometimes believed to be a remnant of the müllerian duct)
   Age: 1st–2nd decade
   - postvoid dribbling
   - obstructive / irritative urinary tract symptoms
   - suprapubic / rectal pain
   - hematuria

   Often associated with:
   hypospadia, intersex disorders, incomplete testicular descent, ipsilateral renal agenesis
   Location: arise in midline from verumontanum
   ◊ Free communication with urethra
   √ 8- to 10-mm long cyst usually
   √ NO extension above prostate
   Dx: endoscopic catheterization with aspiration of white / brown fluid occasionally containing spermatozoa

GU

Cx: infection, hemorrhage, carcinomatous metaplasia

3. **Ejaculatory duct cyst**
   Cause: congenital / acquired obstruction of ejaculatory duct
   • perineal pain, dysuria, ejaculatory pain
   • hematospermia
   Location: along expected course of ejaculatory duct
   √ intraprostatic cyst within central zone
   √ aspirate contains spermatozoa with normal testicular function
   √ cyst commonly contains calculi
   √ cystic dilatation of ipsilateral seminal vesicle
   √ contrast injection into cyst outlines seminal vesicle
4. **Cystic degeneration of BPH**
   Most common cystic lesion of prostate
   Location: transition zone
   √ usually small cyst within nodules of benign prostatic hyperplasia
5. **Retention cyst**
   = dilatation of glandular acini
   Cause: acquired obstruction of glandular ductule
   Age: 5th–6th decade
   Location: transition / central / peripheral zone
   √ 1- to 2-cm smooth-walled unilocular cyst
6. **Cavitary / diverticular prostatitis**
   Cause: fibrosis of chronic prostatitis constricts ducts leading to stagnation of exudate + breakdown of intraacinar septa with cavity formation
   • history of long-standing inflammatory condition
   √ "Swiss cheese" prostate
7. **Prostatic abscess**
   Age: 5th–6th decade
   • fever, chills
   • urinary frequency, urgency, dysuria, hematuria
   • perineal / lower back pain
   • focally enlarged tender prostate
   √ hypo- / anechoic mass with irregular wall + septations
8. Parasitic cyst (Echinococcus, bilharziasis)
9. Cystic carcinoma
   • hemorrhagic aspirate
   √ solid tissue invaginating into cyst

Hypoechoic Lesion Of Prostate

1. Adenocarcinoma (35%)
2. Benign prostatic hyperplasia (18%)
   √ rarely may originate in the peripheral zone
3. "Normal" prostatic tissue (18%)
   (a) cluster of prostate retention cysts
   (b) prominent ejaculatory ducts
4. Acute / chronic prostatitis (14%)
5. Granulomatous prostatitis (0.8%): most frequently due to Calmette-Guérin bacillus (BCG)
6. Atrophy (10%)
   • occurs in 70% of young healthy men
   ◊ May be confused with carcinoma histologically!
7. Prostatic dysplasia (6%)

Cowper (Bulbourethral) Gland Lesions

Analogous to Bartholin glands in females
Prevalence: 2.3% (autopsy)
Location: within urogenital diaphragm

1. Retention cyst
   Cx: prenatal death from urinary obstruction
2. Infectious / traumatic cyst
   • asymptomatic (most)
   • hematuria, bloody urethral discharge
   • postvoid dribbling

Urethral Tumors

Benign Urethral Tumor

1. **Fibroepithelial polyp**
   in child / young adult; transitional cell epithelium
   √ solitary, pedunculated fingerlike filling defect attached near verumontanum
   Cx: bladder outlet obstruction
2. **Transitional cell papilloma**
   older patient; in prostatic / bulbomembranous urethra; frequently associated with concomitant bladder papillomas
3. **Adenomatous polyp**
   young men; adjacent to verumontanum
   Histo: columnar epithelium from aberrant prostatic epithelium
   • hematuria
4. **Penile squamous papilloma / condyloma acuminata**
   in 5% of patients with cutaneous disease (glans penis)
   √ verrucous lesion in distal urethra, rarely extension into bladder
5. Others: caruncle, urethral mucosal prolapse, inflammatory tags (in female)

Malignant Urethral Neoplasm

Incidence: 6th–7th decade, M:F = 1:5

A. FEMALE
   • urethral bleeding
   • obstructive symptoms
   • dysuria
   • mass at introitus
   1. Squamous cell carcinoma (70%): distal 2/3 of urethra
   2. Transitional cell carcinoma (8–24%): posterior 1/3 of urethra
   3. Adenocarcinoma (18–28%): from periurethral glands of Skene
B. MALE
   • palpable urethral mass
   • periurethral abscess
   • obstructive symptoms
   • cutaneous fistula
   • bloody discharge
   Site: bulbomembranous urethra (60%); penile urethra (30%); prostatic urethra (10%)

1. Squamous cell carcinoma (70%)
secondary to chronic urethritis from venereal disease (44%) + urethral strictures (88%)
2. Transitional cell carcinoma (16%)
part of multifocal urothelial neoplasia, in 10% after cystectomy for bladder tumor
3. Adenocarcinoma (6%)
in bulbous urethra originating in glands of Cowper / Littre
4. Melanoma, rhabdomyosarcoma, fibrosarcoma (rare)
5. Metastases from bladder / prostatic carcinoma (rare)

AMBIGUOUS GENITALIA

= external genitalia that are not clearly of either sex

Prevalence: 1:1,000 live births

• cryptorchidism • labial fusion
• clitoromegaly • epi- / hypospadia

Cause:
A. Abnormal hormone levels
   1. congenital adrenal hyperplasia
   2. transplacental passage of hormones
   3. true hermaphroditism
B. Anomalies of external genitalia not hormonally mediated (eg, micropenis)

SEX = what a person is biologically; sex assignment based on (1) karyotype (2) gonadal biopsy (3) genital anatomy

GENDER = what a person becomes socially

Female pseudohermaphroditism

= FEMALE INTERSEX

Cause: exposure to excessive androgens in 1st trimester due to
(a) congenital adrenogenital syndrome
(b) maternal drug ingestion (progestational agents, androgens)
(c) masculinizing ovarian tumor

Karyotype: 46,XX

• masculinized external genitalia
  • penislike clitoris (due to prominent corpora cavernosa + corpus spongiosum)
  • rugose labioscrotum
• uterus + vagina may be filled with urine through urogenital sinus

√ normal ovaries, fallopian tubes, uterus, vagina
√ enlarged adrenal glands (adrenal hyperplasia)
√ no testicular tissue / internal wolffian duct derivatives

Male pseudohermaphroditism

Cause: within fetal testis
(a) decreased testosterone synthesis
(b) decreased dihydrotestosterone production (= substance responsible for masculinization of external genitalia) due to 5α-reductase deficiency
(b) no testosterone production due to early destruction / dysgenesis of testes
(c) complete / incomplete androgen insensitivity due to androgen receptor defect (= testicular feminization)

Karyotype: 46,XY

• incompletely masculinized / ambiguous external genitalia

[• apparent hypergonadotropic primary amenorrhea]

√ commonly undescended normal / mildly defective bilateral testes
√ prostatic tissue
√ no müllerian duct derivatives (production of müllerian regression factor by testes not affected)
√ occasionally blind-ending vaginal pouch emptying into perineum (= pseudovagina) / through urethra (= urogenital sinus)

Gonadal dysgenesis

characterized by abnormal gonadal organization and function with gonads often partially / completely replaced by fibrous stroma

(1) Mixed gonadal dysgenesis
= testis on one side + gonadal streak on other side
Karyotype: 45,XO/46,XY karyotype or other mosaics with a Y chromosome
• ambiguous external genitalia
√ small / rudimentary uterus + vagina
√ fallopian tube present on side of streak gonad
√ urogenital sinus commonly empties at base of phallus
√ dysgenetic gonads (with inability to secrete müllerian regression factor)
Cx: gonadal neoplasia

(2) Pure XY gonadal dysgenesis
Karyotype: 46, XY
√ bilateral streak gonads / dysgenetic testes
√ müllerian + wolffian duct derivatives both absent / partially developed

(3) XY gonadal agenesis
= vanishing testes syndrome = testicular resorption in early fetal life of unknown cause
Karyotype: 46,XY
• ambiguous external genitalia / female phenotype
√ absent testes
√ müllerian + wolffian duct derivatives both absent / partially developed

True hermaphroditism

= TRUE INTERSEX

= condition characterized by presence of ovarian + testicular tissue either separate or in same gonad (= ovotestis in 64%)

Gonads: (a) ovary on one + testis on other side (30%)
(b) ovary / testis on one + ovotestis on other side (50%)
(c) bilateral ovotestes (20%)
Location: in pelvis (predominantly ovarian tissue); in scrotum / inguinal region (predominantly testicular tissue)

GU

Incidence: rare (500 cases in world literature); <10% of all intersex conditions
Age: diagnosed within first 2 decades (75%)
Karyotype: 46,XX (80%) / 46,XY (10%) / mosaicism (10%)
Classification:
- Class I : normal female genitalia (80%)
- Class II : enlarged clitoris
- Class III: partially fused labioscrotal folds
- Class IV: fused labioscrotal folds
- Class V : hypoplastic scrotum + penoscrotal hypospadia
- Class VI: normal male genitalia

- ambiguous external genitalia
- inguinal hernia
- lower abdominal pain (due to endometriosis)
- lower abdominal tumor (dysgerminoma, myomatous uterus)

Reared as boy:
- cryptorchidism
- short penis
- slight degree of hypospadia
- urogenital sinus at base of penis
- penile urethra (extremely rare)
- effective spermatogenesis (rare)

Reared as girl:
- development of breasts
- hematuria (= menstruation via urogenital sinus opening) in 50%
- internal female organs + female fertility
- amenorrhea
- separate urethral + vaginal openings (uncommon)

√ hypoplastic uterus (in virtually 100%)
√ ovotestis with heterogeneous appearance due to combination of testicular tissue + ovarian follicles
√ internal gonadal duct fits the gonad:
  √ deferent duct on side of testis
  √ fallopian tube on side of ovary
  √ ipsilateral fallopian tube absent (suppression of development by fetal testis)
√ testis / testicular portion of ovotestis usually dysgenetic

GU

ANATOMY AND FUNCTION OF UROGENITAL TRACT

UROGENITAL EMBRYOLOGY

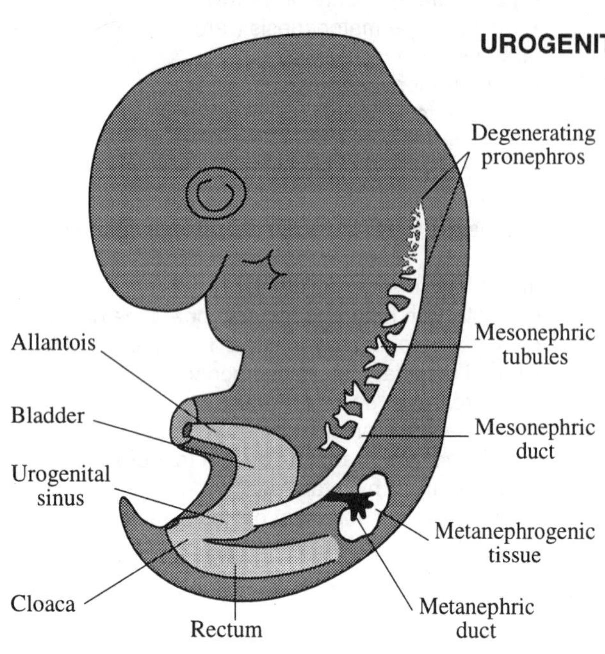

Embryo at 6th week

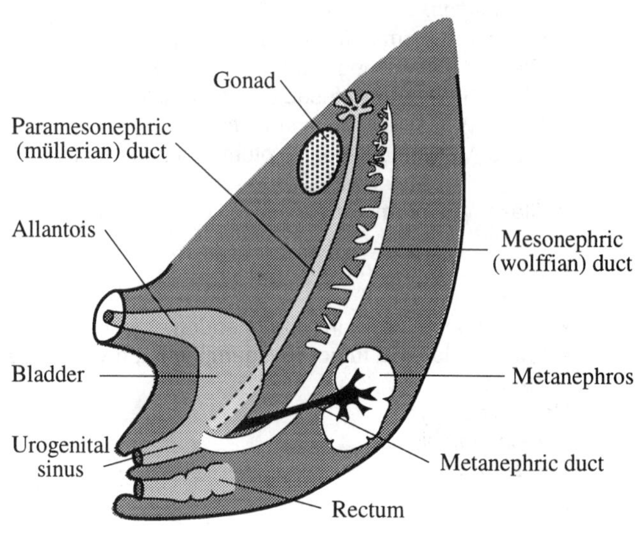

Embryo at 7th week

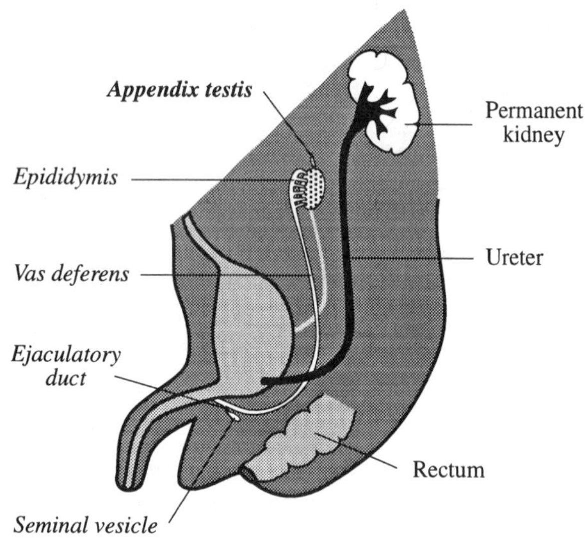

Male metanephros differentiation

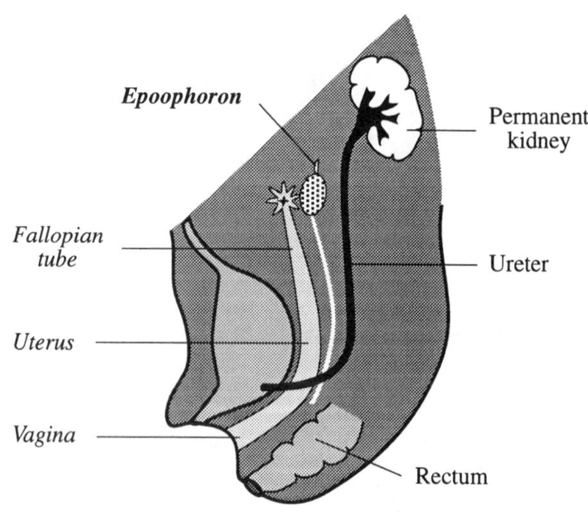

Female metanephros differentiation

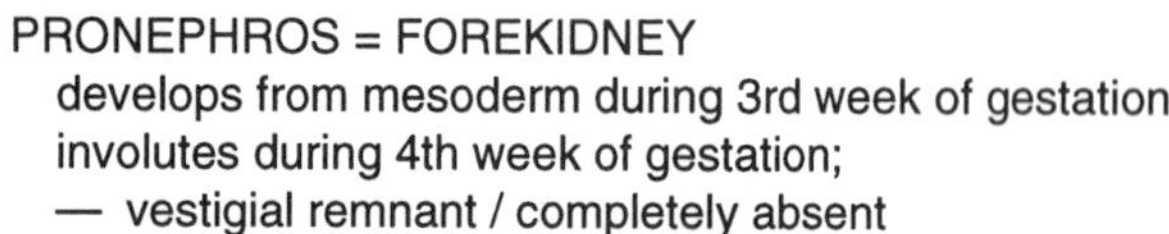
PRONEPHROS = FOREKIDNEY
develops from mesoderm during 3rd week of gestation; involutes during 4th week of gestation;
— vestigial remnant / completely absent

MESONEPHROS = MIDKIDNEY
develops during 4th week of gestation immediately caudal to pronephros, functions as interim kidney; degenerates around 8 weeks of gestation

— mesonephric tubules: paradidymis, epididymis, efferent ductules (M); epinephron (F)
— mesonephric (wolffian) duct: appendix epididymis, vas deferens, ejaculatory duct, seminal vesicles (M); vanishes (F)

PARAMESONEPHRIC (MÜLLERIAN) DUCT
(grows along mesonephric duct)

Male: degenerates due to production of Müllerian inhibiting factor (MIF) by Sertoli cells of testis at about 6 weeks GA, remnants are prostatic utricle + appendix testis

Female: induced by wolffian duct at 5 weeks GA; grow caudally + join in midline + fuse with outgrowth of urogenital sinus; uterus, fallopian tubes

Metanephros = Hindkidney = permanent kidney

(1) metanephric diverticulum (**ureteric bud**) buds from mesonephric duct near its entry into the cloaca at 4th week; it grows toward nephrogenic cord which becomes the metanephric blastema + divides and forms
- → ureter (mesonephric duct)
- → renal pelvis (first 4 dividing generations of duct)
- → calices (second 4 dividing generations of duct)
- → collecting tubules (10–12 generations of duct)

(2) **metanephric blastema** (= nephrogenic mesoderm) forms nephrons under the influence of ureteral bud, ie, the end of collecting tubules induce clusters of metanephric blastema cells

(3) **metanephric vesicles** form within clusters of metanephric blastema cells + elongate into S-shaped tubules which, by 12th week of gestation, result in
- → glomerulus
- → proximal convoluted tubule
- → loop of Henle
- → distal convoluted tubule
- ◊ Polycystic kidney disease is believed to be a failure of linkage!

Urogenital Sinus
forms from cloaca
→ develops into bladder + urethra (+ prostate)

RENAL ANATOMY
Adult Kidney
— forms by fusion of superior + inferior subkidneys (= metanephric lobes); the line of fusion runs obliquely forward and upward
- √ separation of upper + lower groups of calices
- √ indentation of cortical contour + echogenic line (= interrenicular septum = **junctional parenchymal defect**) delineates junctional parenchyma (often referred to as hypertrophic column of Bertin)

— consists of 20,000 lobules within 14 lobes (reniculi)

— initially located in pelvic region ventral to sacrum, ascending cranially at 9 weeks of gestation secondary to body growth caudal to kidneys + straightening of body curvature

— renal hilum at first ventrally located, eventually rotating medially by 90 degrees with renal ascent

Reniculus *= renal lobe*
= central core of medullary tissue enveloped by
(a) centrilobar cortex (= cortical arch) that covers the base of the pyramid subsequently forming the renal cortex with loss of grooves

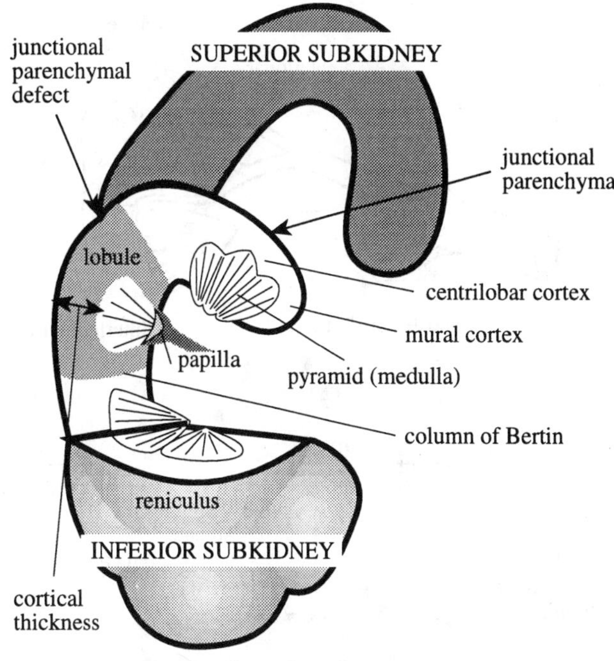

Renal anatomy

(b) mural cortex that wraps around sides of pyramid and fuses with the mural cortex of adjacent lobe to form renal septum (= column of Bertin)
√ ren lobatus (= interlobar surface grooves) present in fetus + infant, rare in adulthood

Renal Size (in cm)
- — <1 year of age: 4.98 + 0.155 x age (months)
- — >1 year of age: 6.79 + 0.22 x age (years)
- — adulthood: R kidney 10.74 ± 1.35 (SD); L kidney 11.10 ± 1.15 (SD);
- — ratio of renal length (RL) to distance between first 4 lumbar transverse processes (4TP) = 1.04 ± 0.22

Renal Echogenicity
- — neonate (up to 6 months of age): cortex may be more echogenic than adjacent normal liver / spleen (glomeruli occupy larger percentage of cortex in neonate)
- — adult: liver ≥ spleen ≥ renal cortex > renal medulla
- — renal sinus echogenicity less prominent in neonate because of paucity of fat

Renal Vascular Anatomy
1st order: main renal artery
2nd order: anterior + posterior division at / before hilum
3rd order: 5 segmental branches for each division

Accessory renal artery
= segmental arteries originating from the aorta

Aberrant renal artery
= segmental artery arising from superior mesenteric artery / internal spermatic artery

Resistive index: <0.70
1 SD of several measurements = 0.04

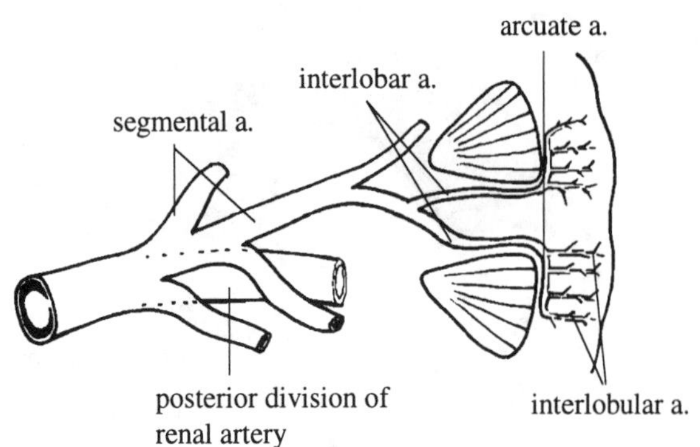

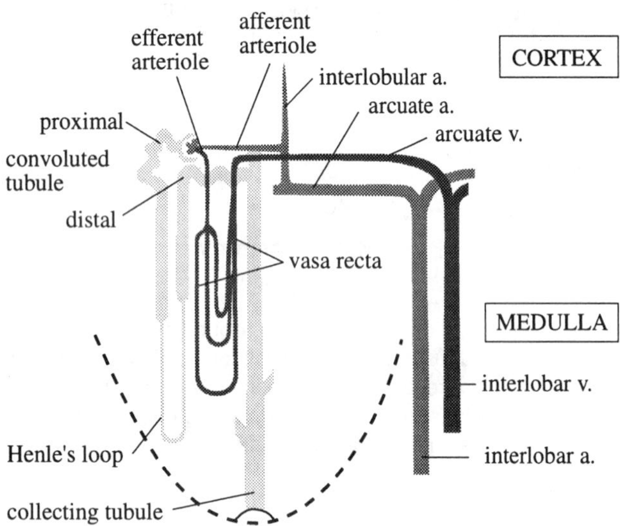

Renal Parencyhmal Blood Supply

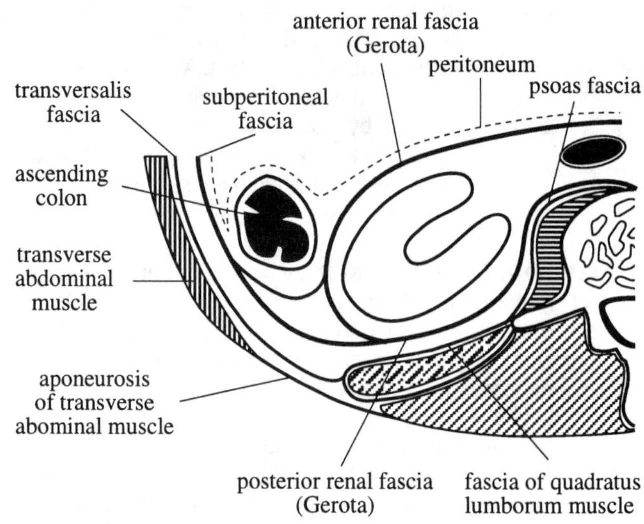

Gerota's fascia

Perirenal Compartments

A. Anterior border: anterior renal fascia

B. Anterior pararenal space
   - → superiorly joins with posterior renal fascia and attaches to crux of diaphragm
   - → in the middle blends with connective tissues of central prevertebral space around great vessels
   - → inferiorly joins with posterior renal fascia and attaches to great vessels

C. Perirenal space
   subdivided into multiple compartments by incomplete bridging septa that attach to anterior + posterior renal fascia
   - → forms inverted cone around adrenal gland + perirenal fat + upper half of kidney
   - → forms cone around perirenal fat + lower pole of kidney
   - → medially open communicating with central prevertebral space

D. Posterior pararenal space

E. Posterior border: posterior renal fascia (attaches to psoas muscle)

RENAL HORMONES

Antidiuretic Hormone (ADH)

Production site: supraoptic nuclei of hypothalamus, transported to neurohypophysis

Stimulus: fluid loss with increase in osmolality

Effects:
(1) 10 x increase in permeability of collecting ducts (= concentrated urine)
(2) decreased blood flow through vasa recta leads to increased hypertonicity of interstitium (= countercurrent multiplier mechanism)

Renin-aldosterone Mechanism

receptors in juxtaglomerular apparatus register the intraglomerular capillary hydraulic pressure, which is one of the main determinants of the glomerular filtration rate (GFR); the receptors regulate the release of **renin** as an autoregulatory feedback mechanism to maintain the intraglomerular hydraulic pressure; renin mediates conversion of angiotensin to angiotensin-I, which is then cleaved by a converting enzyme into angiotensin-II;

Angiotensin-II effect:
(a) constriction of efferent postglomerular arterioles, which increases intraglomerular capillary hydraulic pressure + GFR
(b) systemic arteriolar constriction (= most potent vasoconstrictor of biologic systems), which causes systemic hypertension
(c) release of **aldosterone**, which increases sodium retention by renal tubules
   - — leads to an increase in blood volume + pressure if both kidneys are affected
   - — leads to compensatory natriuresis if only one kidney is affected

◊ ACE inhibitors (eg, captopril) produce a dramatic decrease in blood pressure!

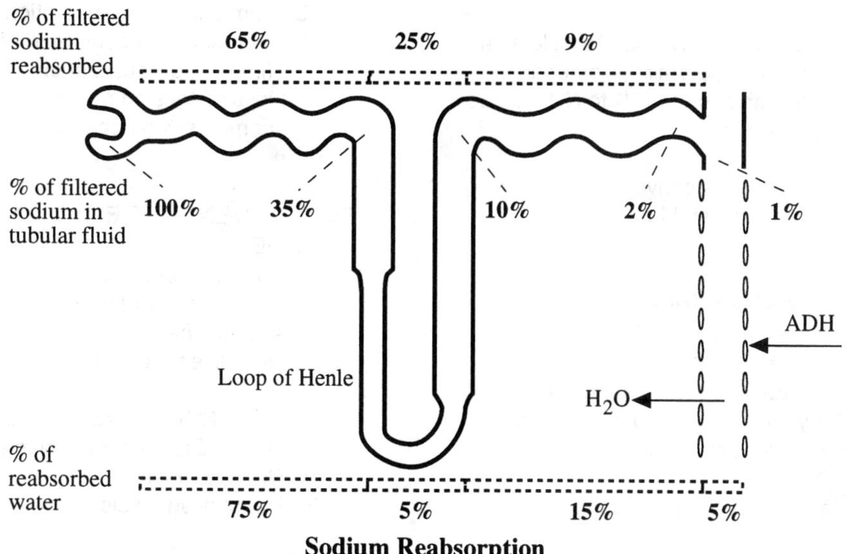

Sodium Reabsorption

hypertonicity is maintained within the medullary interstitium by the countercurrent multiplier system of the loop of Henle and the vasa recta; ADH increases permeability of collecting ducts for water

RENAL PHSYIOLOGY

Perfusion: 1.2–1.3 L of blood per minute (= 20–25% of total cardiac output)

Urine output: 1 L/d

Filtration: substances of up to 4 nm (excluding substances >8 nm), threshold at molecular weight of approximately 40,000

GLOMERULAR FILTRATION RATE (GFR)

$[P] \times GFR = [U] \times U_{vol}$

GFR $= \{[U] \times U_{vol}\} / [P]$ = 125 mL/min = 20% of RPF

Substrate: inulin; Tc-99m DTPA

TUBULAR SECRETION (Tm)

$[U] \times U_{vol} = [P] \times GFR + Tm$

Tm $= \{[U] \times U_{vol}\} - \{[P] \times GFR\}$

Substrate: p-aminohippurate (PAH); I-131 Hippuran

RENAL PLASMA FLOW (RPF)

$[P] \times RPF = [U] \times U_{vol}$

RPF $= \{[U] \times U_{vol}\} / [P]$

Substrate: p-aminohippurate

[P] = concentration in plasma
GFR = glomerular filtration rate
[U] = concentration in urine
U_{vol} = urine volume
Tm = transport maximum (across tubular cells)
RPF = renal plasma flow

Renal acidification mechanism

Proximal tubule:

reabsorption of 90% of filtered bicarbonate by luminal Na^+/H^+ exchange and Na^+/HCO_3^- cotransport at basolateral membrane

regulated by: luminal carbonic anhydrase

influenced by: luminal HCO_3^- concentration, extracellular fluid volume, parathormone, K^+, aldosterone

Distal nephron:

active secretion of H^+ against a steep urine-to-blood gradient across luminal cell membrane by H^+-ATPase pump facilitated by Na^+ reabsorption resulting in reabsorption of 10% of filtered bicarbonate, formation of ammonium (NH_4^+) and titratable acidity

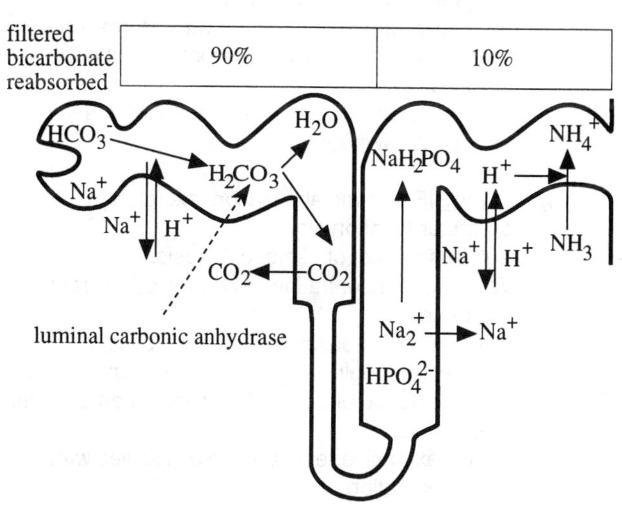

GU

Ammonium excretion:
Ammonia (NH_3) is formed in proximal tubule as a product of catabolism of glutamine + other amino acids; combination with secreted H^+ to NH_4^+ takes place in distal nephron
Titratable acidity:
divalent basic phosphate is converted into monovalent acid form in distal tubule

Renal imaging in newborn infant

◊ low glomerular filtration rate (GFR):
— on first day of life: 21% of adult values
— by 2 weeks of age: 44% of adult values
— at end of 1st year: close to adult values
◊ limited capacity to concentrate urine
IVP:
√ occasional failure of renal visualization
NUC:
√ improved visualization on radionuclide studies

Contrast excretion

UROGRAPHIC DENSITY depends on

$$[U] = \{[P] \times GFR\} / U_{vol}$$

1. Concentration of contrast material in plasma [P] is a function of
   (a) total iodine dose
   (b) contrast injection rate
   (c) volume distribution
   Rapid decline of concentration of contrast material in vessels is due to:
   (1) rapid mixing within vascular compartment
   (2) diffusion into extravascular extracellular fluid space (capillary permeation)
   (3) renal excretion
2. Glomerular filtration rate (GFR): 99% filtered
3. Urine volume (U_{vol}) ie, activity of ADH:
   (a) in dehydrated state with increased ADH activity concentrations of contrast material are higher
   ◊ Dehydration is considered a risk-potentiating factor for nephrotoxicity!
   (b) in volume-expanded state with decreased ADH activity concentrations of contrast material are lower
   ◊ Patients with CHF require higher doses of contrast material!

MEGLUMINE: no metabolization, excreted by glomerular filtration alone
Meglumine effect of osmotic diuresis:
(a) lower concentration of urinary iodine per mL urine
(b) greater distension of collecting system
N.B.: Avoid meglumine in "at risk" patients (higher incidence of contrast reactions than sodium!)

SODIUM: extensive reabsorption by tubules with delayed excretion
Sodium effect of reabsorption:
(a) increased concentration of urinary iodine (improved visualization)
(b) less distension of collecting system (ureteral compression necessary)

DEVELOPMENTAL RENAL ANOMALIES

A. NUMERARY RENAL ANOMALY
1. Supernumerary kidney
2. Complete / partial renal duplication
3. Abortive calix
4. Unicaliceal (unipapillary) kidney

B. RENAL UNDERDEVELOPMENT
1. Congenital renal hypoplasia
2. Renal agenesis
3. Renal dysgenesis

C. RENAL ECTOPIA
Normal location of kidneys: 1st–3rd lumbar vertebra
Incidence: 0.2% (autopsy series)
1. Longitudinal ectopia
   Location: pelvic, sacral, lower lumbar level, intrathoracic; L > R
   √ must demonstrate aberrant arteries
   DDx: displacement through diaphragmatic hernia (nonaberrant); hypermobile kidney

   Pelvic kidney
   = ectopic kidney due to failure of renal ascent
   Incidence: 1:725 births
   May be associated with:
   (1) vesicoureteral reflux
   (2) hydronephrosis due to abnormally high insertion of ureter into renal pelvis
   (3) hypospadia (common)
   (4) contralateral renal agenesis
   √ blood supply via iliac vessels / aorta
   √ nonrotation = anteriorly positioned renal pelvis (common)
2. Crossed ectopia
   = kidney located on opposite side of midline from its ureteral orifice; usually L > R and crossed kidney inferior to normal kidney
   Cause: ? faulty development of ureteral bud, vascular obstruction of renal ascent
   Associated with: obstruction urolithiasis, infection, reflux, megaureter, hypospadia, cryptorchidism, urethral valves, multicystic dysplasia
   (a) fused (common)
   (b) separate (rare)
   √ invariably aberrant renal arteries
   √ distal ureter inserts into trigone on the side of origin
3. Renal fusion
   = "lump, cake, disk, horseshoe"
   Cx: aberrant arteries may cross and obstruct ureter

Discoid / pancake kidney
= bilateral fused pelvic kidneys
Associated with:
abnormal testicular descent, tetralogy of Fallot, vaginal agenesis, sacral agenesis, caudal regression, anal anomalies

4. Renal malrotation
√ collecting structures may be positioned ventrally (most common), lateral (rare), dorsal (rarer), transverse (along AP axis)
√ "funny-looking calices" = developmental usually nonobstructive ectasia

ADRENAL ANATOMY

from periphery to centrum:
(a) renin-angiotensin–dependent outer adrenal cortex:
zona glomerulosa = mineralocorticoid (aldosterone)
(b) corticotropin-dependent inner adrenal cortex:
zona fasciculata = cortisol
zona reticularis = sex hormones (androgen, estrogen)
(c) medulla = norepinephrine, epinephrine

mnemonic: "Glomerular Filtration Rate May Give Answers"
Glomerulosa
Fasciculata
Reticulosa
Mineralocorticoids
Glucocorticoids
Androgens

Normal size : 3–5 x 3 x 1 cm
Normal weight : 3–5 g
Visualization by CT : Left side 100%, Right side 99%
by US : Left side 45%, Right side 80%

SCROTAL ANATOMY

Scrotal wall thickness: 2–8 mm (3–6 mm in 89%)
Tunica vaginalis
= inferior extension of processus vaginalis of the peritoneum
Hydrocele: small to moderate in 14% of normals

TESTIS
Average size of testis: 3.8 x 3.0 x 2.5 cm (decreasing with age)
Length of testis: 3–5.5 cm (mature); 1–1.5 cm (newborn)
Testicular cysts: in 8% of normals (average size 2–3 mm), numbers increasing with age

Appendix testis
= small stalked appendage at upper pole of testis
= remnant of paramesonephric duct

Tunica albuginea
= fibrous covering of testis, invaginating into testicular parenchyma at mediastinum testis; externally covered by visceral layer of tunica vaginalis; internally applied to tunica vasculosa carrying the capsular artery
Mediastinum testis
= converging point of ~400 cone-shaped lobules separated by fibrous septa + seminiferous tubules forming tubuli recti and the rete testis within the mediastinum
√ linear echogenic region extending longitudinally 5–8 mm from the edge
Blood flow
PSV: 4–10–19 cm/s
EDV: 2–5–8 cm/s
RI: 0.44–0.60–0.75

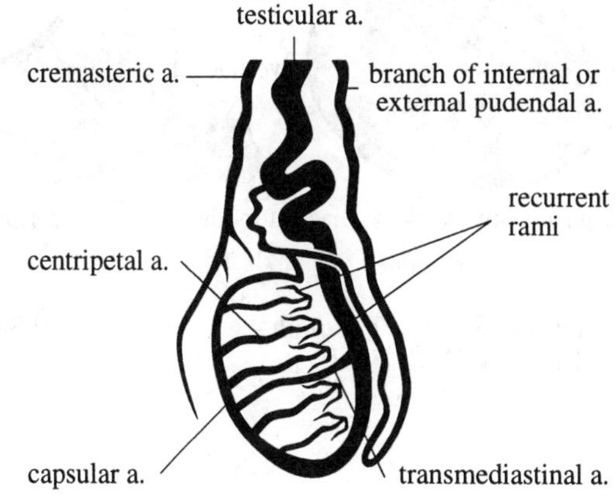

Arterial Supply of Scrotum

EPIDIDYMIS
= tortuous tightly folded canal forming the efferent route from testis; consists of head (= globus major), body, tail (= globus minor)
Size of globus major: 11 x 7 x 6 mm (decreasing with age)
Epididymal cysts: occur in 30% of normals (average size of 4 mm)
Epididymal calcification: in 3%
Appendix epididymis = occasionally duplicated, small stalked appendage of globus major

SPERMATIC CORD
= testicular + deferential + cremasteric aa., pampiniform plexus of veins, vas deferens, nerves, lymphatics

ZONAL ANATOMY OF PROSTATE

Normal weight: 20 ± 6 g
Normal size: 2.8 cm (craniocaudad), 2.8 cm (anteroposterior), 4.8 cm (width)

A. OUTER GLAND
   1. Central zone: surrounds ejaculatory ducts from their entrance at prostatic base to verumontanum; 25% of glandular tissue
   2. Peripheral zone: extends from base of prostate to apex along rectal surface; 70% of glandular tissue

B. INNER GLAND
   1. Transition zone: on each side of internal sphincter; 4% of glandular tissue; enlarges with BPH
   2. Periurethral zone: surrounding urethra; 1% of glandular tissue

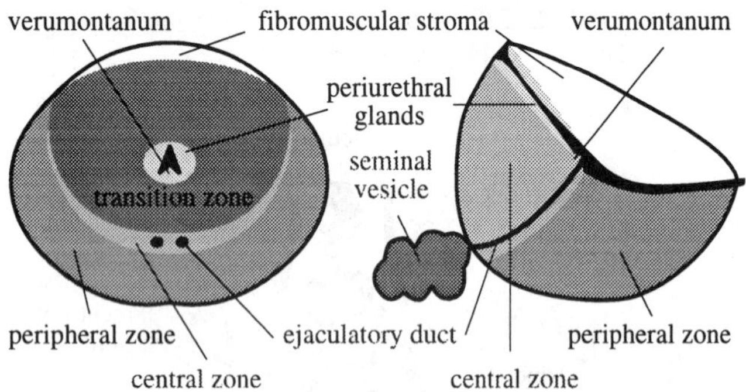

Transverse Section Through Prostate With BPH

Midsagittal Section Through Normal Prostate

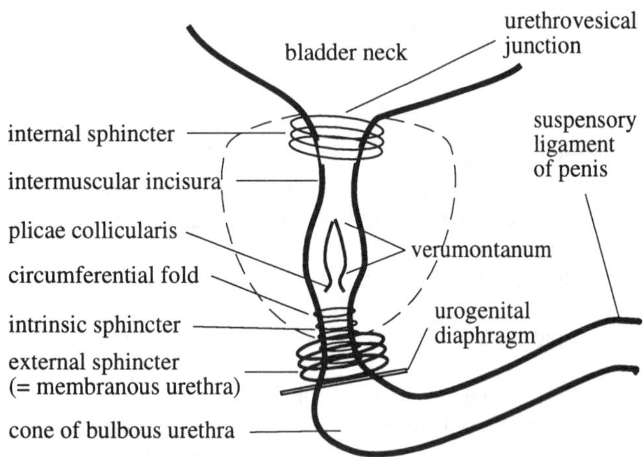

Urethrogram: normal urethral folds in LPO

ANATOMY OF URETHRA

Male Urethra

extends through corpus spongiosum (composed of large venous sinuses)

A. POSTERIOR URETHRA
   1. Prostatic urethra = from vesical neck to triangular ligament
      - orifices of ducts from prostatic acini on floor
      - verumontanum = colliculus seminalis = prostatic utricle (fused end of müllerian ducts)
      - orifice of the two ejaculatory ducts
   2. Membranous urethra = portion traversing urogenital diaphragm
      - pea-sized bulbourethral glands of Cowper lie laterally + posteriorly between fasciae and sphincter urethrae within urogenital diaphragm

B. ANTERIOR = CAVERNOUS URETHRA
   1. Bulbous urethra
   2. Penile = pendulous urethra
      - many small branched tubular periurethral glands of Littré terminate in recesses (lacunae of Morgagni)

      Cx: recurring urethral discharge following chronic urethritis, latent gonorrheal urethritis, stricture formation
   3. Fossa navicularis

Female Urethra

3–5 cm in length, 6 mm in diameter

urethral crest = posteriorly located prominent fold

Two sets of glands:

(a) urethral glands = terminate separately along entire length of urethra

(b) paraurethral glands = glands of Skene (homologues of prostatic ducts) are formed by an interdependent conducting system and exit on either side of midline just posterior to urethral meatus draining into vaginal vestibule

   Cx: chronic gonorrheal urethritis

1. Intrapelvic urethra
   = upper 2/3 of urethra that lies behind symphysis pubis
2. Membranous urethra
   surrounded by sphincter membranacea urethrae (weaker less important structure than in male)
3. Perineal urethra
   lower 1/3 extending from superior fascia of urogenital diaphragm to meatus between labia minora

RENAL, ADRENAL, URETERAL, VESICAL, AND SCROTAL DISORDERS

ABORTIVE CALYX

= developmental anomaly with short blind-ending outpouching of pyramid without papillary invagination

Location: (a) renal pelvis
(b) infundibulum (mostly upper pole)

ACQUIRED CYSTIC KIDNEY DISEASE

= ACQUIRED CYSTIC DISEASE OF UREMIA
= development of numerous fluid-filled renal cysts in patients with chronic renal failure undergoing hemodialysis

◊ Successful transplant probably stops development of additional cysts, but does not affect malignant potential!

Prevalence: in 10–20% after 1–3 years, in 40–60% after 3–5 years, in 90% after 5–10 years of hemodialysis;
in 25% of renal allograft recipients

Proposed etiologies:
- (a) altered compliance of tubular basement membrane
- (b) intra- and extratubal obstruction due to focal proliferation of tubular epithelium
- (c) obstruction of ducts by interstitial fibrosis / oxalate crystals
- (d) toxicity from circulating metabolites (endogenous / exogenous toxins, mutagens, mitogens, growth factors)
- (e) vascular insufficiency

At increased risk: older men

Histo: cysts lined by flattened cuboidal / papillary epithelium

In 13–20% associated with:
- (a) small papillary / tubular / solid clear-cell adenomas 1 cm in diameter
- (b) renal cell carcinoma (in 3–6%): 7-year interval between transplantation + detection of RCC

√ small end-stage kidneys (<280 g)
√ multiple 0.5- to 3-cm cysts bilaterally (early = small, late = large)
√ occasionally progressive renal enlargement due to cysts

Dx: >3 cysts + NO history of hereditary cystic disease
Cx: spontaneous hemorrhage into cyst (macrohematuria / retroperitoneal hemorrhage from cyst rupture)

AIDS

- azotemia, proteinuria, hematuria, pyuria (in 38–68% sometime during illness)
- progressive renal failure (10%)

1. **HIV nephropathy** (40%)
   = characterized by nephrotic-range proteinuria + rapidly progressive renal failure, primarily occurring in Black patients
   Histo: focal + segmental glomerulosclerosis, sparse interstitial infiltrates, severe tubular degenerative changes, interstitial tubular microcystic ectasia containing protein casts
   - mild hypertension
   - early + rapidly progressive renal failure with 100% mortality within 6 months
   √ global enlargement of both kidneys
   US (best screening test):
   √ increased cortical echogenicity (33–68%)
   CT:
   √ medullary hyperattenuation (14%)
   √ striated nephrogram on CECT
   MRI:
   √ loss of corticomedullary differentiation
   Prognosis: death within 6 months
2. Renal infection with Pneumocystis carinii (8%)
   ◊ more frequent since introduction of prophylactic aerosolized pentamidine therapy encouraging extrapulmonic spread (<1%) due to inadequate systemic distribution of drug!
   √ punctate renal calcifications confined to cortex (DDx: CMV, Mycobacterium avium-intracellulare)
   √ associated calcifications in spleen, liver, lymph nodes, adrenal glands
3. Renal lymphoma (3–12%)
   AIDS-related lymphoma:
   highly aggressive B-cell lymphomas (centroblastic, lymphoblastic, immunoblastic); NHL > Burkitt lymphoma, Hodgkin disease
   √ bilateral multiple renal masses
   √ direct extension of retroperitoneal lymphadenopathy engulfing kidney, renal sinus, ureter
4. Cystitis (22%)
   Organism: routine Gram-negative species, Candida, beta-hemolytic streptococci, Salmonella, CMV
   √ bladder wall thickening

ACUTE CORTICAL NECROSIS

= rare disorder with patchy / universal necrosis of renal cortex + proximal convoluted structures secondary to distension of glomerular capillaries with dehemoglobulinized RBCs; medulla and 1–2 mm of peripheral cortex are spared

Etiology:
- (a) Obstetric patient (most often): abruptio placentae
  = premature separation of placenta with concealed hemorrhage (50%), septic abortion, placenta previa
- (b) Children: severe dehydration + fever, infection, hemolytic uremic syndrome, transfusion reaction
- (c) Adults: sepsis, dehydration, shock, myocardial failure, burns, snakebite, abdominal aortic surgery, hyperacute renal transplant rejection

- protracted + severe oliguria / anuria

EARLY SIGNS
√ diffusely enlarged smooth kidneys
√ absent / faint nephrogram

GU

US:
√ loss of normal corticomedullary region with hypoechoic outer rim of cortex

NUC:
√ severely impaired renal perfusion

LATE SIGNS
√ small kidney (after a few months)
√ "tramline" / punctate calcifications along margins of viable and necrotic tissue (as early as 6 days)

US:
√ hyperechoic cortex with acoustic shadowing

Prognosis: poor chance of recovery

ACUTE DIFFUSE BACTERIAL NEPHRITIS

= ACUTE SUPPURATIVE PYELONEPHRITIS
= more severe and extensive form of acute pyelonephritis, which may lead to diffuse necrosis (phlegmon)

Organism: Proteus, Klebsiella > E. coli
Predisposed: diabetics (60%)

ACUTE INTERSTITIAL NEPHRITIS

= infiltration of interstitium by lymphocytes, plasma cells, eosinophils, few PMNs + edema

Cause: allergic / idiosyncratic reaction to drug exposure (methicillin, sulfonamides, ampicillin, cephalothin, penicillin, anticoagulants, phenindione, diphenylhydantoin)

• eosinophilia (develops 5 days to 5 weeks after exposure)
√ large smooth kidneys with thick parenchyma
√ normal / diminished contrast density

US: √ normal / increased echogenicity

ACUTE TUBULAR NECROSIS

= temporary reversible marked reduction in tubular flow rate

Etiology:
(a) DRUGS: bichloride of mercury, ethylene glycol (antifreeze), carbon tetrachloride, bismuth, arsenic, uranium, urographic contrast material (especially when associated with glomerulosclerosis in diabetes mellitus), aminoglycosides (gentamicin, kanamycin)
(b) ISCHEMIA: major trauma, massive hemorrhage, postpartum hemorrhage, crush injury, myoglobulinuria, compartmental syndrome, septic shock, cardiogenic shock, burns, transfusion reaction, severe dehydration, pancreatitis, gastroenteritis, renal transplantation, cardiac surgery, biliary surgery, aortic resection

Pathophysiology: profound reduction in renal blood flow due to elevated arteriolar resistance

√ smooth large kidneys, especially increase in AP diameter >4.63 cm (due to interstitial edema)
√ diminished / absent opacification of collecting system
√ immediate persistent dense nephrogram (75%)
√ increasingly dense persistent nephrogram (25%)
√ diffuse calcifications (rare)

US:
√ normal to diminished echogenicity of medulla
√ sharp delineation of swollen pyramids
√ normal (89%) / increased (11%) echogenicity of cortex
√ elevated resistive index ≥0.75 (in 91% excluding patients with hepatorenal syndrome); unusual in prerenal azotemia

Angio:
√ normal arterial tree with delayed emptying of intrarenal vessels
√ slightly delayed / normal venous opacification

NUC:
√ poor concentration of Tc-99m glucoheptonate / Tc-99m DTPA
√ well-maintained renal perfusion
√ better renal visualization on immediate postinjection images than on delayed images
√ progressive parenchymal accumulation of I-131 Hippuran / Tc-99m MAG3
√ no excretion

ADDISON DISEASE

= PRIMARY ADRENAL INSUFFICIENCY
◊ 90% of adrenal cortex must be destroyed!

Course: acute (adrenal apoplexy), subacute (disease present for <2 years), chronic

Cause:
1. Idiopathic adrenal atrophy (60–70%): likely autoimmune disorder
2. Granulomatous disease: tuberculosis, sarcoidosis
3. Fungal infection: histoplasmosis, blastomycosis, coccidioidomycosis
4. Adrenal hemorrhage: anticoagulation therapy, trauma, bleeding, coagulation disorders, sepsis, shock
5. Bilateral metastatic disease (rare)

√ diminutive glands (in idiopathic atrophy + chronic inflammation)
√ enlarged glands (acute inflammation, acute hemorrhage, metastasis)
√ calcifications (in 25% of chronic course)

ADRENAL CYST

Prevalence: 0.064–0.180%

Path:
(a) endothelial lining (45–48%):
1. Lymphangioma (93%)
2. Hemangioma

(b) epithelial lining = true cyst (9–10%):
1. Glandular / retention cyst
2. Embryonal cyst
3. Cystic adenoma
4. Mesothelial inclusion cyst

(c) pseudocyst (39–42%):
1. Previous hemorrhage / infarction
2. Hemorrhagic complication of benign vascular neoplasm / malformation
3. Cystic degeneration / hemorrhage of primary adrenal mass

(d) parasitic cyst (7%): usually echinococcal

GU

Age: 3rd–6th decades (most commonly); M:F = 1:3
Location: mostly solitary; R:L = 1:1; bilateral in 8–10%
√ well-defined uni- / multilocular
√ wall thickness of up to 3 mm
√ <5 cm in diameter in 50% (up to 20 cm)
√ usually homogeneous with near-water density; higher attenuation with hemorrhage / intracystic debris / crystals
√ lack of central enhancement ± wall enhancement
√ calcifications:
(a) peripheral / mural: rimlike / nodular (51–69%)
(b) central: in intracystic septation (19%) / punctate within intracystic hemorrhage (5%)

Cx: hypertension; hemorrhage; infection; rupture with retroperitoneal hemorrhage

DDx:
1. Cystic pheochromocytoma
2. Cystic adenomatoid tumor
3. Schwannoma
4. Cystic adrenocortical carcinoma (thick-walled lesion >7 cm in size; extremely rare)
5. Adrenal adenoma (contrast enhancement, no wall, no peripheral calcification)

ADRENAL HEMORRHAGE

Cause:

A. NEWBORN
1. Birth trauma: forceps / breech delivery
2. Hypoxia due to prematurity
3. Infants of diabetic mothers
4. Septicemia
5. Hemorrhagic disorders

Age: 1st week of life
Site: R > L; bilateral in 10%

B. ADULT
1. Anticoagulant therapy: during initial 3 weeks
2. Stress caused by sepsis: Waterhouse-Friderichsen syndrome
3. Surgery: orthotopic liver transplantation
4. Adrenal venous sampling
5. Tumor
6. Blunt abdominal trauma
Prevalence: 2% (in 28% of autopsies)
Location: R:L = 9:1, bilateral in 20%
√ round / oval hematoma (in 83%) located in medulla + stretching cortex around hematoma
√ obliteration of gland by diffuse irregular hemorrhage (in 9%)
√ uniform adrenal enlargement (in 9%)
√ periadrenal hemorrhage causes ill-defined adrenal margin + stranding + asymmetric thickening of diaphragmatic crus

√ mass displacing renal axis
√ gradual decrease in size
√ peripheral calcification occurring after 1 week

US:
√ initially echogenic becoming progressively hypoechoic (degeneration, lysis)

CT:
√ high-attenuation mass (50–90 HU) in acute / subacute stage

ADRENOCORTICAL ADENOMA

A. NONHYPERFUNCTIONING
characterized by
(a) normal lab values of adrenal hormones
(b) NO pituitary shutdown of the contralateral gland
(c) activity on NP-59 radionuclide scans

Incidence: incidental finding in 0.6 –1.5% of CT examinations, in 3–9% at autopsy
√ surveillance CT to confirm lack of growth

Rx: surgical removal for masses 3–5 cm as indeterminate potentially malignant neoplasms

DDx: metastasis

B. HYPERFUNCTIONING
1. Primary hyperaldosteronism (= Conn syndrome)
Pathophysiology: secretion of aldosterone by an adenoma is pulsatile
√ ACTH infusion incites a dramatic increase in levels of cortisol + aldosterone for venous sampling
2. Cushing syndrome (10%)
3. Virilization:
(a) hirsutism + clitoromegaly in girls
(b) pseudopuberty in boys
most common type of hormone elevation in children
• elevated testosterone levels >0.55 ng/mL
4. Feminization (estrogen production)
√ contralateral atrophic gland (secondary to ACTH suppression with autonomous adenoma)
√ unilateral focus of I-131 NP-59 radioactivity + contralateral absence of iodocholesterol accumulation (DDx: hyperplasia [bilateral activity])

√ well-defined sharply marginated mass <5 cm in size (average size 2.0–2.5 cm)
√ mild homogeneous enhancement
√ adenoma may calcify

CT:
√ soft-tissue density / cystic density (mimicked by high cholesterol content) with poor correlation between functional status and HU number
√ <10 HU on NECT is 73% sensitive + 96% specific for adenoma
√ <37 HU on delayed CECT (>5–15 minutes after contrast injection) is DIAGNOSTIC of adenoma
√ small adenomas <1 cm often go undetected
√ contralateral gland often normal / atrophic

Angio:
√ tumor blush + neovascularity; occasionally hypovascular
√ pooling of contrast material
√ enlarged central vein with high flow
√ arcuate displacement of intraadrenal veins
√ bilateral adrenal venous sampling in up to 40% unsuccessful in localizing

MR:
√ mass iso- / hypointense (rarely hyperintense) to liver on T2WI

√ mild enhancement + quick washout on Gd-dimeglumine enhanced study
(DDx: metastases tend to have higher signal intensities [however 20–30% overlap])

ADRENOCORTICAL CARCINOMA

Prevalence: 0.3–0.4% of all pediatric neoplasms (3 times as likely than adrenal adenoma)
May be associated with: hemihypertrophy, Beckwith-Wiedemann syndrome, astrocytomas

- 20% nonfunctioning
- 50% hyperfunctioning (in 10–15% Cushing syndrome)

Size: usually >5 cm (median size 12 cm; in 16% <6 cm)
√ frequently heterogeneous mass with irregular margins
√ occasionally calcified
√ invasion of IVC
√ metastases to regional lymph nodes, kidney, renal veins, liver, diaphragm, lung, bone, brain
◊ Metastases are the only reliable sign of malignancy!
◊ Large size + calcifications suggest malignancy!
CT:
√ central areas of low attenuation (tumor necrosis)
√ heterogeneous enhancement (foci of hemorrhage + central necrosis)
US:
√ complex echo pattern (due to hemorrhage + necrosis)
MRI:
√ hyperintense to liver on T2WI
Angio:
√ enlarged adrenal arteries
√ neovascularity, occasionally with parasitization
√ AV shunting; multiple draining veins
NUC:
√ usually bilateral nonvisualization with I-131 NP-59 (carcinomatous side does not visualize because amount of uptake is small for size of lesion; contralateral side does not visualize because carcinoma is releasing sufficient hormone to cause pituitary feedback shutdown of contralateral gland)
Biopsy: may appear histologically benign in well-differentiated adenocarcinoma
Prognosis: 0% 5-year survival rate
DDx: metastasis (similar signal intensities on MR)

ADRENOCORTICAL HYPERPLASIA

◊ Responsible for 8% of Cushing syndrome and 10–20% of hyperaldosteronism!
Cause:
1. Corticotropin-dependent (85%): pituitary causes, ectopic corticotropin production, production of corticotropin-releasing factor
2. Primary pigmented nodular adrenocortical hyperplasia
   Associated with: Carney complex (spotty skin pigmentation, calcified Sertoli cell tumors of testes, cardiac and soft-tissue myxomas)
3. Primary aldosteronism (rare)

Incidence: 4 x increased in patients with malignancy
Age: 70–80% in adults; 19% in children
Types:
(1) Smooth hyperplasia (common)
√ bilateral normal-sized glands
√ thickened + elongated glands
(2) Cortical nodular hyperplasia (less common)
√ normal glands ± appreciable micronodular configuration
√ thickened gland with macronodular configuration (nodules up to 2.5 cm)
Angio:
√ minimally increased hypervascularity
√ focal accumulation of contrast medium
√ normal venogram / may show enlarged gland
NUC:
√ asymmetric bilateral NP-59 uptake (related to urinary cortisol excretion) without dexamethasone suppression in Cushing syndrome
√ bilateral foci of NP-59 uptake with dexamethasone suppression (nondiagnostic ≥5 days)

ADRENOGENITAL SYNDROMES

A. CONGENITAL TYPE
= impaired cortisol + aldosterone synthesis secondary to enzyme defect (21-hydroxylase) with increased ACTH stimulation by pituitary gland (negative feedback mechanism)
M < F
- excess of androgenic steroids
- ± salt wasting due to diminished mineralocorticoids
- virilization of female fetus
- precocious puberty in male
- pseudohermaphroditism (clitoral hypertrophy, ambiguous external genitalia, urogenital sinus)

√ symmetrically enlarged + thickened adrenal glands
Rx: cortisone ± mineralocorticoids

B. ACQUIRED TYPE
M < F
(a) adrenal hyperplasia / adenoma / carcinoma
(b) ovarian / testicular tumor
(c) gonadotropin-producing tumor: pineal, hypothalamic, choriocarcinoma
- virilization
- Cushing syndrome

AMYLOIDOSIS

= accumulation of extracellular eosinophilic protein substances
@ Renal involvement
Incidence: 1° amyloidosis (35%), 2° amyloidosis (in >80%)
√ smooth normal to large kidneys with increase in parenchymal thickness (early stage)
√ small kidneys = renal atrophy (late stage)
√ occasionally attenuated collecting system
√ increase in cortical echogenicity (deposition of amyloid in glomeruli and interstitium) + prominence of corticomedullary junction + obscuration of arcuate aa.

GU

√ nephrographic density normal to diminished
US:
√ normal to increased echogenicity
Cx: renal vein thrombosis

ANALGESIC NEPHROPATHY

= renal damage from ingestion of salicylates in combination with phenacetin / acetaminophen in a cumulative dose of 1 kg
Incidence: United States (2–10%), Australia (20%)
Age: middle-aged; M:F = 1:4
- gross hematuria
- hypertension
- renal colic (passage of renal tissue)
- renal insufficiency (2–10% of all end-stage renal failures)
- ANALGESIC SYNDROME: history of psychiatric therapy, abuse of alcohol + laxatives, headaches, pain in cervical + lumbar spine, peptic ulcer, anemia, splenomegaly, arteriosclerosis, premature aging

√ papillary necrosis
√ scarring of renal parenchyma ("wavy outline"); bilateral in 66%, unilateral in 5%
√ renal atrophy
√ papillary urothelial tumors in calices / pelvis (mostly TCC / squamous cell carcinoma), in 5% bilateral

ANGIOMYOLIPOMA

= benign mesenchymal tumor of kidney
= RENAL CHORISTOMA (= benign tumor composed of tissues not normally occurring within the organ of origin)
= RENAL HAMARTOMA (improper name since fat and smooth muscle do not normally occur within renal parenchyma)
Prevalence: 0.3–3%
Path: no true capsule, 88% extending through renal capsule, hemorrhage (characteristic lack of complete elastic layer of vessels predisposes to aneurysm formation); tumor continues to grow during childhood + early adulthood
Histo: tumor composed of fat, smooth muscle, aggregates of thick-walled blood vessels
Types:
(1) Isolated AML (80%) = sporadic AML
solitary + unilateral (in 80% on R side), NO stigmata of tuberous sclerosis
Age: 27–72 (mean 43) years of age; M:F = 1:4
(2) AML associated with tuberous sclerosis (in 20%)
◊ AML in 80% of patients with tuberous sclerosis commonly large + bilateral + multiple;
may be the only evidence of tuberous sclerosis
Mean age: 17 years; M:F = 1:1
- small lesions are asymptomatic (60%)
- acute flank / abdominal pain (due to hemorrhage) in 87%
- shock (due to massive retroperitoneal hemorrhage)
- hematuria (40%)
- palpable mass (47%)

√ mostly <5 cm in diameter
√ large component of exophytic extrarenal tumor (25%)
√ calcifications (6%)
Plain film:
√ mass of fat lucency (in <10%)
CT:
√ well-marginated cortical heterogeneous tumor predominantly of fat density <–20 HU
√ homogeneously high attenuation on NECT in 5% (due to minimal fat component)
√ variable enhancement (smooth muscle, vessels)
US:
√ intensely echogenic tumor (due to high fat content)
√ homogeneously isoechoic in 5% (due to minimal fat component)
√ less echogenic areas due to hemorrhage, necrosis, dilated calyces
MRI:
√ intratumoral fat (fat-suppression technique)
√ variable areas of high signal intensity on T1WI (DDx: hemorrhagic cyst, solid tumor)
Angio:
√ hypervascular mass (95%) with enlarged interlobar + interlobular feeding arteries, tortuous irregular aneurysmally dilated vessels (1/3), venous pooling, "sunburst" / "whorled" / "onion peel" appearance, no AV shunting
Cx: hemorrhagic shock from bleeding into angiomyolipoma or into retroperitoneum
◊ Angiomyolipomas >4 cm bleed spontaneously in 50–60%!
Rx: (1) annual follow-up of lesions <4 cm
(2) emergency laparotomy (in 25%): nephrectomy, tumor resection
(3) selective arterial embolization
DDx: renal / perirenal lipoma or liposarcoma; Wilms tumor / renal cell carcinoma (occasionally contains fat)

ARTERIOVENOUS MALFORMATION

(1) Congenital AVM
(2) Acquired AVM: trauma, spontaneous rupture of aneurysm, very vascular malignant neoplasm
Histo:
(a) cirsoid = multiple coiled vascular channels grouped in cluster; supplied by one / more arteries; draining into one / more veins
(b) cavernous = single well-defined artery feeding into a single vein (rare)

√ large unifocal mass
√ focally attenuated and displaced collecting system
√ homogeneously enhancing mass
√ curvilinear calcification
US:
√ tubular anechoic structure (DDx: hydronephrosis, hydrocalyx)

BENIGN PROSTATIC HYPERTROPHY

= BENIGN PROSTATIC HYPERPLASIA
Prevalence: 50% between ages 51 + 60 years; 75–80% of all men >80 years of age

GU

Histo: fibromyoadenomatous nodule (most common), muscular + fibromuscular + fibroadenomatous + stromal nodules

Age: initial growth onset <30 years of age; onset of clinical symptoms at 60 ± 9 years

- sensation of full bladder, nocturia
- trouble initiating micturition
- decreased urine caliber + force
- dribbling at termination of micturition

Location: transition + periurethral zone proximal to verumontanum forming "lateral lobes" (82%), "median lobe" (12%)

√ oval (61%) / round (22%) / pear-shaped (17%) enlargement of central gland

√ posterior + lateral displacement of outer gland (= prostate proper) creating cleavage plane of fibrous tissue between hyperplastic tissue + compressed prostatic tissue (= surgical capsule) often demarcated by displaced intraductal calcifications

Cx: bladder outflow obstruction

Rx:

(1) Surgery: open prostatectomy (glands >80 g), transurethral resection of prostate = TURP (glands <80 g)
◊ Only 4–5% of patients need surgical treatment!

(2) Drugs: α-blockers (for stromal hyperplasia); androgen deprivation (suppression of LHRH / inhibition of Leydig cell synthesis of testosterone / competition for androgen receptor binding sites) + α-blockers (for glandular hyperplasia)

BLADDER CALCULI

Etiology:

1. FOREIGN BODY NIDUS CALCULI
from self-introduced objects, bladder wall-penetrating bone fragments, prostatic chips, nonabsorbable suture material, fragments of Foley balloon catheter, pubic hair, presence of intestinal mucosa (in bladder augmentation, ileal conduit, repaired bladder exstrophy)
2. STASIS CALCULI
in bladder outflow obstruction, vesical diverticula, lower urinary tract infection (in particular Proteus), cystocele, neuropathic bladder dysfunction
3. MIGRANT CALCULI
= renal calculi spontaneously passing into bladder
4. IDIOPATHIC / PRIMARY / ENDEMIC CALCULI
in North Africa, India, Indonesia; in young boys of low socioeconomic class (nutritional deficiency?)
√ single stone in 86%

Rate of recurrence after removal: 41%

BLADDER CONTUSION

= intramural hematoma (most common bladder injury)

√ no extravasation

√ lack of normal distensibility

√ crescent-shaped filling defect in contrast-distended bladder

BLADDER DIVERTICULUM

= cavity formed by herniation of bladder mucosa through muscular wall, joined to the bladder cavity by a constricted neck

Prevalence: 1.7% in children

Etiology:

A. PRIMARY / CONGENITAL / IDIOPATHIC DIVERTIVULA (40%)
√ in 3% single diverticulum
(a) with vesicoureteral reflux
1. Hutch diverticulum in paraureteral region
(b) without vesicoureteral reflux

B. SECONDARY DIVERTICULA (60%)
√ in 50% multiple diverticula
(a) postoperative state
(b) associated with bladder outlet obstruction
1. Posterior urethral valves
2. Urethral stricture
3. Large ureterocele
4. Neurogenic dysfunction
5. Enlarged prostate
6. Bladder neck stenosis
(c) associated with syndromes
1. Prune belly syndrome
2. Menkes kinky-hair syndrome
3. Williams syndrome
4. Ehlers-Danlos type 9 syndrome
5. Diamond-Blackfan syndrome

C. MULTIPLE DIVERTICULA IN CHILDREN
1. Neurogenic dysfunction
2. Posterior urethral valves
3. Prune belly syndrome

Average age: 57 years; M:F = 9:1

Site: areas of congenital weakness of muscular wall at
(a) ureteral meatus
(b) posterolateral wall (Hutch diverticulum = paraureteral)

Cx: (1) Vesical carcinoma in 0.8–7% secondary to chronic inflammation (average age 66 years)
(2) Ureteral obstruction
(3) Ureteral reflux

BLADDER EXSTROPHY

= EPISPADIA-EXSTROPHY COMPLEX

Prevalence: 1:33,000 to 1:40,000 live births

Etiology: incomplete retraction of cloacal membrane prevents normal midline migration of mesoderm resulting in incomplete midline closure of infraumbilical abdominal wall; size of persistent cloacal membrane at time of rupture accounts for different degrees of severity

- urinary bladder exposed + open anteriorly
- mucosa everted through abdominal wall defect
- bladder margins continuous with margins of abdominal wall
- epispadia (male); bifid clitoris (female)

May be associated with:
wide linea alba, omphalocele, limb defects (eg, club feet), renal malformation (horseshoe kidney, renal agenesis), incomplete testicular descent, GI obstruction, bilateral inguinal hernias, imperforate anus, cardiac anomalies, hydrocephalus, meningomyelocele
√ ventral defect of infraumbilical abdominal wall
√ low position of umbilicus
√ pubic diastasis = widening of pubic symphysis

CLOSED EXSTROPHY = PSEUDOEXSTROPHY
= persistent large cloacal membrane without rupture
• anterior wall of bladder covered by thin bilaminar epithelial membrane
√ infraumbilical musculoskeletal defect
√ subcutaneous position of bladder

Cx: urinary incontinence, infertility, pyelonephritis, bladder carcinoma (4%)
Rx: primary closure, bladder excision with urinary diversion

BLADDER RUPTURE

Cystography:
diagnostic in >85%
false-negatives if tear sealed by hematoma / mesentery

Extraperitoneal rupture of bladder *(80%)*

Cause: pelvic fracture (sharp bony spicule) or avulsion tear at fixation points of puboprostatic ligaments
Location: usually close to base of bladder anterolaterally
Plain film:
√ "pear-shaped" bladder
√ loss of obturator fat planes
√ paralytic ileus
√ upward displacement of ileal loops
Contrast examination:
√ flame-shaped contrast extravasation into perivesical fat, best seen on postvoid films, may extend into thigh / anterior abdominal wall
US:
√ "bladder within a bladder" = bladder surrounded by fluid collection

Intraperitoneal rupture of bladder *(20%)*

Cause:
(a) usually as a result of invasive procedure (cystoscopy), stab wound, surgery
(b) blunt trauma with sudden rise in intravesical pressure (requires distended bladder)
Location: usually at dome of bladder
√ contrast extravasation into paracolic gutters
√ contrast outlining small bowel loops
√ uriniferous ascites

CHOLESTEATOMA

= keratin ball = keratinized squamous epithelium shed into lumen
• history of UTIs
• repeated episodes of renal colic
Location: renal pelvis > upper ureter
√ mottled / stringy filling defects in collecting system
√ dilatation of pelvicaliceal system (with obstruction)
√ calcification of keratinized material possible
◊ Not a premalignant condition!

CHROMOPHOBE CARCINOMA OF KIDNEY

Prevalence: 4% of renal cell neoplasms
Age: median in 6th decade (31–75 years)
Histo: cells with abundant cytoplasm containing numerous microvesicles
√ average size of 8 cm (range 1.3–20 cm)
Prognosis: probably better than RCC

CHRONIC GLOMERULONEPHRITIS

Cause: after acute poststreptococcal glomerulonephritis
• late presentation without prior clinically apparent acute phase
• hypertension
• renal failure
√ small smooth kidneys with wasted parenchyma
√ normal papillae + calices
√ patchy nephrogram with diminished density of contrast material
√ cortical calcification (uncommon)
US:
√ increased echogenicity
√ small kidneys with vicarious sinus lipomatosis
Angio:
√ marked reduction in renal blood flow + reflux of contrast material into aorta
√ severely pruned + tortuous interlobar and arcuate arteries
√ nonvisualization of interlobular arteries
√ delayed contrast clearance from interlobar arteries

CLEAR CELL SARCOMA OF KIDNEY

= rare highly malignant renal tumor of childhood with predilection for bone metastasis
Incidence: up to 6% of renal tumors in children
Histo: composed of well-defined polygonal to stellate cells with vacuolization, ovoid to rounded nuclei, prominent capillary pattern + tendency toward cyst formation separated by slightly thickened septa
Age: 1–6 years; M:F = 1:1
• increasing abdominal girth + palpable abdominal mass
• lethargy, weight loss
• hematuria
√ expansile mass (8–16 cm) with dominant soft-tissue component
√ cystic component of varying size (few mm to 5 cm) + multiplicity (58%)
√ amorphous / linear calcifications (25%)
√ renal mass crossing midline (58%)

US:
- √ inhomogeneous renal mass of soft-tissue density
  - √ well-defined hypoechoic central area (= necrosis)
- √ mass of fluid-filled cystic spaces

CT:
- √ inhomogeneous enhancement less than that of normal renal parenchyma
- √ low-attenuation areas (= necrosis)
- √ water-density areas (= cysts)

Prognosis: worse than Wilms tumor

DDx: cystic form of Wilms tumor, multilocular cystic nephroma, cystic dysplasia

CONGENITAL RENAL HYPOPLASIA

= miniaturization with reduction in number of renal lobes, number of calices and papillae, amount of nephrons (+ smallness of cells)

VARIANT: **Ask-Upmark kidney** = aglomerular focal hypoplasia

- √ unilateral small kidney
- √ decreased number of papillae + calices (5 or less)
- √ hypertrophied contralateral kidney
- √ absent renal artery
- √ hypoplastic disorganized renal veins

CONN SYNDROME

= PRIMARY HYPERALDOSTERONISM = PRIMARY ALDOSTERONISM = autonomous excess secretion of the mineralocorticoid aldosterone with hypertension + spontaneous hypokalemia

= solitary adrenocortical adenoma (originally)

Incidence: 0.05–2% of hypertensive population

Age: 3rd–5th decade; M:F = 1:2

- hypertension (secondary to hypernatremia)
- hypokalemia (80–90%, induced by administering large amounts of sodium chloride for 3–5 days):
  - muscle weakness, cardiac arrhythmia
  - carbohydrate intolerance
  - nephrogenic diabetes insipidus
- depletion of magnesium
- metabolic alkalosis
- increased urinary excretion of aldosterone + metabolites
- nonsuppressible elevation in plasma aldosterone concentration
- suppressed plasma renin levels

Path:
- (a) adenoma (65–89%): solitary aldosteronoma (65–70%); multiple (13%); microadenomatosis (6%)
- (b) bilateral adrenal hyperplasia (11–25–30%): = idiopathic hyperaldosteronism = focal / diffuse hyperplasia of glomerular zone accompanied by micro- / macroscopic nodules
- (c) adrenocortical carcinoma (<1%)

- √ small aldosteronoma of 1.7 cm average size (range 0.5–3.5 cm); L > R, bilateral in 6%
  - √ soft-tissue density / low attenuation
    - ◊ Among hyperfunctioning adrenal adenomas aldosteronomas have the lowest attenuation!
  - √ usually hypervascular, rarely hypovascular
- √ normal / nodular / multinodular adrenal gland(s) (with hyperplasia)

Adrenal venography	: 76% accuracy
Adrenal venous blood sampling:	95% accuracy, 75% sensitivity
CT	: 60–80% sensitivity

NUC:
- √ I-131 NP-59 uptake following dexamethasone suppression
  - √ bilateral early visualization (<5 days) implies adrenal hyperplasia
  - √ unilateral early visualization implies adenoma
  - √ late bilateral visualization (>5 days) may be normal

Dx: elevated plasma aldosterone concentration + suppressed plasma renin activity
Diagnostic endocrine tests:
postural stimulation test, short saline infusion test, 18-hydroxycorticosterone concentration

Rx: adrenalectomy for neoplasms (75% long-term cure rate for hypertension); medical treatment for hyperplasia

CONTRAST NEPHROPATHY

= CONTRAST-INDUCED RENAL FAILURE

= increase in serum creatinine of ≥1 mg/dL ± 25–50% of the baseline creatinine level after intravascular contrast administration

Patients at risk:
1. Preexisting renal insufficiency
2. Insulin-dependent diabetes mellitus
3. Large volume of contrast media
4. Concomitant administration of other nephrotoxic drugs: aminoglycosides, nonsteroidal anti-inflammatory agents
5. American Heart Association class IV congestive heart failure
6. Hyperuricemia

◊ A serum creatinine level of >4.5 mg/dL causes acute renal failure in 60% of nondiabetics + 100% of diabetics!

Previously considered but no longer accepted risk factors: dehydration, hypertension, proteinuria, peripheral vascular disease, age >65 years, multiple myeloma

Mechanism:
increase in renal perfusion by vasodilatation (via prostaglandin I2 ± E2) followed by vasoconstriction (via angiotensin II, norepinephrine, vasopressin)

Time course:
- (a) rise in serum creatinine within 1–2 days
- (b) peak at 4–7 days
- (c) return to normal by 10–14 days

- √ persistent nephrogram on plain film
- √ cortical attenuation >140 HU on CT with 24-hour delay

Recommendation:
- ◊ Employ nonionic contrast media (LOCM appears safe in patients without renal dysfunction / underlying risk factors in doses as large as 800 mL [300 mg iodine per mL])

◊ Do not exceed maximum allowed dose (Cigarroa formula for HOCM):

$$\text{Contrast limit (mL) 60\% by weight} = \frac{\text{5 mL x body weight (kg)}}{\text{serum creatinine (mg/100 mL)}}$$

CUSHING SYNDROME

= HYPERCORTISOLISM = excessive glucocorticoid secretion from either exogenous / endogenous sources

Etiology:

A. ACTH-INDEPENDENT
  1. Exogenous cortisol
  2. Primary adrenal abnormality (20%):
     (a) primary pigmented nodular adrenocortical hyperplasia (children, young adults)
     (b) adrenocortical adenoma (10–20% of cases; 10% in adults, 15% in children)
     (c) adrenocortical carcinoma (5–10% of cases; 10% in adults, 66% in children)

B. ACTH-DEPENDENT
  = overproduction of corticotropin with adrenal hyperplasia (in up to 85%)
  1. Exogenous ACTH
  2. Paraneoplastic ectopic ACTH production (20%): oat cell carcinoma of lung (8%), liver cancer, prostate cancer, ovarian cancer, breast cancer, bronchial / thymic carcinoid, bronchial adenoma, pancreatic islet cell tumor (10%), medullary carcinoma of thyroid, thymoma, pheochromocytoma
     ◊ Bronchial + thymic carcinoids are often <1 cm at the time they produce Cushing syndrome!
     ◊ Islet cell tumors are large + often metastatic by the time they produce Cushing syndrome!
  3. **Cushing disease** (70% of endogenous causes)
     = adrenal hyperplasia due to overproduction of ACTH
     Cause: (1) basophilic / chromophobe adenoma
     (2) overactive pituitary
     (3) ACTH-producing primary elsewhere
  4. Hypothalamic dysfunction
  5. Production of corticotropin-releasing factor (rare)

Incidence: 1:1,000 autopsies; M:F = 1:4

Age: 30–40 years (highest incidence); more often following pregnancy

• central / truncal obesity, buffalo hump, moon face, facial plethora
• purple striae, acne, hirsutism
• fatigue, weakness, amenorrhea
• impaired glucose tolerance / diabetes mellitus
• hypertension, atherosclerosis, edema
• elevated plasma cortisol levels
• excessive excretion of urinary 17-hydroxy-corticosteroids
• dexamethasone suppression test / metyrapone test

√ retarded bone maturation
√ most often axial osteoporosis
√ stippled calvarium
√ demineralized dorsum sellae
√ excess callus formation

Cx: (1) pathologic fractures of vertebrae + ribs with excessive callus formation
(2) aseptic necrosis of hips
(3) bone infarcts
(4) delayed skeletal maturation in children

CYSTITIS

= bacterial infection; more common in females

• frequency, dysuria, hematuria
• reduced bladder capacity

√ cystogram insensitive

US:
  √ focal / multifocal / circumferential isoechoic bladder wall thickening
  √ decrease in bladder wall thickening during bladder distension (eg, instillation of sterile saline via a urethral catheter)
  √ bullous lesions
  √ intact mucosa

Cystitis cystica

= CYSTITIS FOLLICULARIS = CYSTITIS GLANDULARIS = BULLOUS CYSTITIS

= nonspecific inflammatory process of bladder wall

√ multiple small round cystlike mucosal elevations

Prognosis: potentially malignant in adults

Emphysematous cystitis

= uncommon complication of urinary tract infection by gasforming organism almost PATHOGNOMONIC of poorly controlled diabetes (= bacterial fermentation of glucose)

Age: >50 years; M:F = 1:2

Predisposed: diabetes mellitus, neurogenic bladder, bladder outlet obstruction, chronic UTI

Organism: E. coli, E. aerogenes, P. mirabilis, S. aureus, streptococci, Clostridium perfringens, Nocardia, Candida

May be associated with: emphysematous pyelitis / pyelonephritis

• pneumaturia (rare)

Plain film:
  √ translucent streaky irregular area / ring of air bubbles in bladder wall
  √ intraluminal air-fluid level

US:
  √ shadowing echogenic foci within area of bladder wall thickening

CT (most specific modality)

DDx: (a) Gas within bladder:
trauma, urinary tract instrumentation, enterovesical fistula
(b) Gas extern to bladder:
rectal gas, emphysematous vaginitis, pneumatosis cystoides intestinalis, gas gangrene of uterus

Hemorrhagic cystitis

Cause: unclear
- (a) nonspecific: negative culture
- (b) bacterial: E. coli (in 17%)
- (c) viral (adenovirus in 19%): negative culture, viral exanthem
- (d) cytotoxic: cyclophosphamide (Cytoxan®), in 15% of patients within 1st year of treatment

√ echogenic mobile clumps of solid material (= intraluminal blood clots)

Granulomatous cystitis = Tuberculous cystitis

√ irritable hypertonic bladder with decreased capacity
√ disease process usually starts at trigone spreading upward and laterally
√ calcification of bladder wall (rare)

Interstitial cystitis

Age: postmenopausal female
- pink pseudoulceration of bladder mucosa characteristically at vertex of bladder (= Hunner ulcer)

Bullous edema of bladder wall

Cause: continuous internal contact with Foley catheter, involvement of bladder wall by external contact in pelvic inflammatory conditions (eg, Crohn disease, appendicitis, diverticulitis)

√ smoothly thickened / polypoid redundant hypoechoic mucosa

DDx: bladder neoplasm, ureterocele, pseudoureterocele, neurofibromatosis, pseudosarcomatous myofibroblastic proliferations

DIABETES MELLITUS

= multisystem disorder
Prevalence: 14 million patients in United States
Path: macro- and microvascular disease; neuropathy increased susceptibility to infection

A. CHRONIC EFFECTS
1. Papillary necrosis
2. Renal artery stenosis
3. Vas deferens calcification

B. URINARY TRACT INFECTIONS
1. Renal and perirenal abscess
2. Emphysematous pyelonephritis
3. Emphysematous cystitis
4. Fungal infection: Candida, Aspergillus
5. Xanthogranulomatous pyelonephritis

C. GENITAL INFECTION
1. Fournier gangrene
2. Postmenopausal tubo-ovarian abscess

Diabetic nephropathy

= defined as persistent proteinuria (>500 mg of albumin/ 24 hours) + retinopathy + elevated blood pressure
◊ Most common cause of end-stage renal disease!

Incidence: 35–45% of IDDM; <20% of NIDDM; M > F
Histo: diffuse intercapillary glomerulosclerosis
Mortality: 90% after 40 years

Early:
√ renal enlargement (renal hypertrophy with glomerular expansion)

Late:
√ progressive decrease in size
√ diffuse cortical hyperechogenicity with gradual loss of corticomedullary differentiation
√ resistive index >0.7 (very late)

IVP:
√ contrast material may induce renal failure (= rise in serum creatinine level 1–5 days after exposure)
◊ Keep patient well hydrated with 0.45% saline!

Diabetic cystopathy

Cause: autonomous peripheral neuropathy
Histo: vacuolation of ganglion cells in bladder wall, giant sympathetic neurons, hypochromatic ganglion cells, demyelination
- insidious impairment of bladder sensation
- decreased reflex detrusor activity

√ enlarged postvoid residual urine volume
Cx: vesicoureteral reflux, recurrent pyelonephritis, pyohydronephrosis, overflow incontinence

EPIDIDYMITIS

Acute epididymitis

= ACUTE EPIDIDYMO-ORCHITIS
= most common acute pathologic process in postpubertal age secondary to ascending infection (usually beginning as prostatitis)
Incidence: 634,000 cases/year; <10 years in 0%; 20–30 years in 72%
Organism: E. coli + S. aureus (85%), Gonococcus (12%), TB (2%); nonspecific epididymitis in 20%
- (a) >35 years of age Escherichia coli + Proteus mirabilis
- (b) <35 years of age: Chlamydia trachomatis, Neisseria gonorrheae

- fever
- increasing pain over 1–2 days
- epididymal swelling + tenderness
- pyuria (95%)
- positive urine culture
- leukocytosis (50%)
- dysuria + frequency (25%)
- prostatic tenderness (infrequent)

Location: may have focal involvement as in focal epididymitis (25%) often in epididymal tail
◊ Subsequent spread to testis is common: global orchitis (frequent), focal orchitis (10%)

US:
√ enlarged epididymis with decreased echogenicity
√ reactive hydrocele + skin thickening
√ enlarged spermatic cord containing hyperechoic fat
√ thickening of tunica albuginea (in severe infection)

Color Duplex (91% sensitive, 100% specific):
√ increased number + concentration of identifiable vessels in affected region (= hyperemia)
√ peak systolic velocity (PSV) >15 cm/s with PSV ratio >1.9 compared with normal side
√ detection of venous flow
√ diastolic flow reversal in testicular artery (due to epididymal edema with obstruction of venous outflow)

NUC (true positive rate of 99%):
√ symmetric perfusion of iliac + femoral vessels
√ markedly increased perfusion through spermatic cord vessels (testicular + deferential arteries)
√ curvilinear increased activity laterally in hemiscrotum on static images (also centrally if testis involved)
√ increased activity of scrotal contents on static images (hyperemia + increased capillary permeability)

Rx: antimicrobial therapy, scrotal elevation, bed rest, analgesics, ice packs

Cx: (1) Focal / diffuse orchitis (20–40%)
(2) Epididymal abscess (6%) / testicular abscess (6%)
(3) Testicular infarction (3%) from extrinsic compression of testicular blood flow
(4) Late testicular atrophy (21%)
(5) Hydropyocele
(6) Fournier gangrene

DDx: (1) Testicular abscess (increased perfusion with centrally decreased uptake)
(2) Hydrocele (normal perfusion, no uptake)
(3) Testicular tumor (slightly increased perfusion; in- / decreased uptake; no associated epididymal hyperemia on CFI; positive tumor markers: HCG, AFP)

Chronic Epididymitis

US:
√ enlarged hyperechoic epididymis

ERECTILE DYSFUNCTION

= IMPOTENCE (term replaced due to negative connotation)
= inability to obtain / maintain a penile erection sufficient for vaginal penetration in 50% or more attempts during intercourse

Physiology:
(a) psychogenic phase:
- stimuli from thalamic nuclei, rhinencephalon, limbic system converge in medial preoptic anterior hypothalamic area

(b) neurologic phase:
- sacral nerve roots (S2–S4) contribute fibers to pelvic sympathetic plexus
- stimulation of cavernous n. (parasympathetic nerve) causes changes in blood flow resulting in full erection
- stimulation of pudendal n. (motor nerve) causes contraction of bulbocavernosus + ischiocavernosus muscle resulting in occlusion of veins + rigid erection

Risk factors: hypertension, diabetes, smoking, CAD, peripheral vascular disease, pelvic trauma / surgery, blood lipid abnormalities,

Cause:
A. Organic cause (50%)
1. Endocrine disorder (reducing serum testosterone / increasing serum prolactin
2. Vascular disease (10–20%): increasing with age
3. Neurologic disorder (10%): multiple sclerosis, spinal cord trauma, cervical spondylosis, spinal arachnoiditis, pelvic trauma, temporal lobe / idiopathic epilepsy, Alzheimer disease, Parkinson disease, tabes dorsalis, amyloidosis, primary autonomic insufficiency, cerebrovascular accidents, primary / metastatic tumor
4. Chronic disease: diabetes mellitus, drugs (antihypertensives, anticonvulsants, alcohol, narcotics, psychotropic agents)
5. Surgery: damage to pelvic sympathetic nerves / cavernous n. during radical prostatectomy / cystectomy

Penile-brachial index (normal > 1.0)
= highest penile artery pressure over mean brachial pressure
√ <0.70 suggests large vessel disease

Rx: nonsurgical external devices, sex therapy, surgery, intracavernosal injection of vasoactive agents, medical therapy

FOURNIER GANGRENE

= FULMINANT FASCIITIS
= uncommon potentially lethal necrotizing fasciitis of the scrotum

Incidence: 500 cases in literature
Organism: (a) aerobes: S. aureus, E. coli, Proteus species, enterococci
(b) anaerobes: Bacteroides fragilis, anaerobic streptococci, clostridia
Path: cellulitis, myositis, fasciitis with soft-tissue necrosis
Histo: thrombosis of subcutaneous vessels with gangrene of overlying skin
Age: newborn to elderly
Predisposed: diabetes mellitus (present in 40–60%)
- pain, fever, leukocytosis
- scrotal tenderness, erythema, swelling, crepitation

◊ In 95% primary focus of infection is recognizable (urethra, soft tissue of anorectal area, genital skin)!
√ gas in scrotal wall + perineum
√ scrotal skin thickening + normal testes

Mortality: 7–75%
Rx: antibiotic therapy + surgery + hyperbaric oxygen
DDx: epididymo-orchitis, gas-containing scrotal abscess, scrotal hernia with gas-containing bowel, scrotal emphysema from bowel perforation, extension of subcutaneous emphysema, air leakage + dissection due to faulty chest tube positioning

GANGLIONEUROBLASTOMA

= tumor of sympathetic nervous system that is intermediate in cellular maturity between neuroblastoma and ganglioneuroma; metastatic potential

Incidence: less common than neuroblastoma / ganglioneuroma

Age: early childhood; M:F = 1:1

Location: posterior mediastinum, abdomen

√ extension through neural foramen into epidural space

√ nerve root / spinal cord compression

GANGLIONEUROMA

= benign neoplastic growth of autonomic ganglia

= may represent end-stage of maturation of a neuroblastoma induced by chemotherapy / occurring spontaneously

Histo: mixture of mature ganglion + Schwann cells

Age: 42–60% <20 years, 39% aged 20–39 years, 19% aged 40–80 years; M:F = 1:1

Location: posterior mediastinum (25–43%); abdomen (52%), adrenal gland (20%); pelvis and neck (9%); oral + intestinal ganglioneuromatosis associated with MEN IIb

- respiratory symptoms, local pressure (40%)
- rarely hormone-active: diarrhea, sweating, hypertension, virilization, myasthenia gravis

√ spherical / elliptical large well-defined encapsulated slow-growing mass

√ tendency to surround blood vessels without compromising the lumen

√ dumbbell-shaped large mass extending from paraspinous region through neural foramen into epidural space

√ calcifications (8–27%)

CT:

√ homogeneous attenuation less than that of muscle

MR:

√ homogeneous + isointense with muscle on T1WI

√ heterogeneous + hyperintense to muscle on T2WI

DDx: neurofibroma (no calcification), schwannoma (no calcification), neuroblastoma (calcified)

HEMANGIOMA OF URINARY BLADDER

Incidence: 0.6% of primary bladder NEOPLASMS; 0.3% of all bladder tumors

Age: <20 years (in >50%), M:F = 1:1

May be associated with:

(a) additional hemangiomas in 30%

(b) Klippel-Trénaunay syndrome

(c) Sturge-Weber syndrome

Histo: capillary / venous / cavernous / hemangiolymphomatous form

- recurrent gross painless hematuria
- cutaneous hemangiomas over abdomen, perineum, thighs in 25–30%

Location: dome, posterolateral wall

Site: limited to submucosa (33%), muscular wall, perivesical tissue

√ compressible solitary (2/3) / multiple (1/3) masses

√ rounded well-marginated intraluminal mass

√ diffuse bladder wall thickening + punctate calcifications (phleboliths)

IVP:

√ rounded / lobulated filling defect

US:

√ solid predominantly hyperechoic mass

√ hypoechoic spaces within thickened bladder wall

CAVE: high risk of intractable hemorrhage at biopsy!

HEMOLYTIC-UREMIC SYNDROME

◊ Most common cause of acute renal failure in children requiring dialysis!

= characterized by thrombotic microangiopathy with typical features of DIC

Cause:

(1) Infection: enterotoxic E. coli, Shigella dysenteriae I, Streptococcus pneumoniae, Salmonella typhi, Coxsackie virus, ECHO virus, adenovirus

(2) Associated medical condition: pregnancy, SLE + other collagen vascular disease, malignancy, malignant hypertension

(3) Drugs: oral contraceptives, cyclosporine, mitomycin, 5-fluorouracil

Pathogenesis: capillary and endothelial injury to kidney leads to mechanical damage of RBCs + formation of hyaline microthrombi within renal vasculature + focal infarction

Age: usually children <2 years

Histo: microangiopathy including endothelial swelling + thrombus formation in glomerulus + renal arterioles

CLASSIC TRIAD:

(1) microangiopathic hemolytic anemia

(2) thrombocytopenia

(3) acute oliguric / anuric renal failure leading to uremia

- recent bout of gastroenteritis (commonly with E. coli)
- sudden pallor, irritability
- bloody diarrhea
- dyspnea (due to fluid retention, heart failure, pleural effusion)
- convulsions
- rapid rise in blood urea nitrogen level out of proportion to plasma creatinine level (= result of cell lysis)

@ Kidney (sometimes only organ involved):

√ kidneys of normal / slightly increased size

√ hyperechoic cortex

Doppler-US:

√ diastolic flow absent / reversed / reduced (= increase in resistance to flow)

√ return to normal waveforms predates return of urine output

Scintigraphy:

√ lack of renal perfusion

@ Liver: hepatomegaly, hepatitis

@ Pancreas: diabetes mellitus

@ Heart: myocarditis

@ Muscle: rhabdomyolysis

@ Intestines: perforation, intussusception, pseudomembranous colitis
@ Brain (20–50%): drowsiness, personality changes, coma, hemiparesis, seizures (up to 40%)
Prognosis: complete spontaneous recovery (in 85%)

HEREDITARY CHRONIC NEPHRITIS

= ALPORT SYNDROME = probably autosomal dominant trait with presence of fat-filled macrophages ("foam cells") in the corticomedullary junction and medulla
(a) males: progressive renal insufficiency, death usually < age 50
(b) females: nonprogressive

- polyuria
- anemia
- salt wasting
- hyposthenuria
- nerve deafness
- ocular abnormalities (congenital cataracts, nystagmus, myopia, spherophakia)
- NO hypertension

√ small smooth kidneys
√ diminished density of contrast material
√ cortical calcifications

HORSESHOE KIDNEY

= two kidneys joined at poles by parenchymal / fibrous isthmus
Incidence: 1–4:1,000 births; 0.2–1% (autopsy series); M:F = 2–3:1
Associated with:
cardiovascular anomaly, skeletal anomaly, CNS anomaly, anorectal malformation, genitourinary anomaly (hypospadia, undescended testis, bicornuate uterus, ureteral duplication); trisomy 18, Turner syndrome in 50% with:
(1) Caudal ectopia
(2) Vesicoureteral reflux
(3) Hydronephrosis
√ fusion of R + L kidney at lower (90%) / upper (10%) pole
√ renal long axis medially oriented
√ isthmus at L4/5 between aorta + inferior mesenteric a.
√ renal pelves and ureters situated anteriorly
Cx: renal calculi

HYDROCELE

= collection of fluid between parietal and visceral layers of tunica vaginalis; most common type of fluid collection in scrotum
(A) PRIMARY = IDIOPATHIC HYDROCELE
without predisposing lesion as congenital defect of lymphatic drainage
(B) SECONDARY HYDROCELE
(a) inflammation (epididymitis, epididymo-orchitis)
(b) testicular tumor (in 10–40%)
(c) trauma / postsurgical
(d) torsion, infarction
(C) CONGENITAL HYDROCELE
= ascites in scrotum through communication with peritoneal cavity (= open processus vaginalis); may be associated with inguinal hernia
(D) INFANTILE HYDROCELE
= hydrocele with fingerlike extension into funicular process but without communication with peritoneal cavity
US:
√ anechoic, good back wall, through transmission
√ with low level echoes ± septations: hematocele / pyocele / cholesterol crystals

HYDRONEPHROSIS

A. OBSTRUCTIVE UROPATHY = HYDRONEPHROSIS
= dilatation of collecting structures without functional deficit
B. OBSTRUCTIVE NEPHROPATHY = dilatation of collecting system with renal functional impairment
US:
Grading system of hydronephrosis:
Grade 0 = homogeneous central renal sinus complex without separation
Grade 1 = separation of central sinus echoes of ovoid configuration; continuous echogenic sinus periphery; 52% predictive value for obstruction
Grade 2 = separation of central sinus echoes of rounded configuration; dilated calices connecting with renal pelvis; continuity of echogenic sinus periphery
Grade 3 = replacement of major portions of renal sinus; discontinuity of echogenic sinus periphery
Amount of collecting system dilatation depends on:
(a) duration of obstruction
(b) renal output
(c) presence of spontaneous decompression
◊ Amount of residual renal cortex is of prognostic significance!

Acute hydronephrosis

Cause:
(1) Passage of calculus with sites of stone impaction at points of ureteral narrowing:
(a) ureterovesical junction (70%)
(b) ureteropelvic junction
(c) crossing of iliac vessels
(2) Passage of blood clot (from carcinoma, AV malformation, trauma, anticoagulant therapy), sloughed necrotic papilla
(3) Suture on ureter
(4) Ureteral edema following instrumentation
(5) Sulfonamide crystallization in nonalkalinized urine
(6) Normal pregnancy

- pain (50%)
- urinary tract infection (36%)
- nausea + vomiting (33%)

√ normal-sized kidney with normal parenchymal thickness

√ increasingly dense nephrogram
√ delayed opacification of collecting system (decreased glomerular filtration)
√ increasingly dense nephrogram over time ("obstructed nephrogram")
√ dilated collecting system + ureter
√ widening of forniceal angles
√ delayed images demonstrate site of obstruction at the end of a persistent column of contrast material in a dilated urinary collecting system
√ vicarious contrast excretion through gallbladder (uncommon)

NECT:
- √ dilatation of renal collecting system + ureter
- √ inflammation of perinephric ± periureteral fat
- √ calcified ureteral stone
- √ ureteral rim sign (77%) = thickening of ureteral wall secondary to edema from stone impaction with small stones (DDx: in *% of phleboliths)

US:
- √ ureteral jet not detectable / continuous at low level

<u>False-negatives</u>: staghorn calculus filling entire collecting system, hyperacute renal obstruction (system not yet dilated), spontaneous decompression of obstruction, fluid-depleted patient with partial obstruction, dehydrated neonate

<u>False-positives</u>: full bladder, increased urine flow (overhydration, medications, following urography, diabetes insipidus, diuresis in nonoliguric azotemia), acute pyelonephritis, postobstructive / postsurgical dilatation, vesicoureteral reflux

<u>Imposters</u>: parapelvic cysts, sinus vessels, prominent extrarenal pelvis

Duplex:
- √ mean RI of 0.77 ± 0.05 (0.63 ± 0.06 in nonobstructed kidney)
  <u>Caution</u>: RI often normal in chronic obstruction; nonobstructive renal disease may elevate RIs
- √ ≥0.08 difference in RI in right-to-left comparison with unilateral obstruction

Cx: spontaneous urinary extravasation (10–18%) from forniceal / pelvic tear (= pyelosinus reflux)

Chronic hydronephrosis

= most frequent cause of abdominal mass in first 6 months of life (25% of all neonatal abdominal masses)

Cause:
- (a) acquired: benign + malignant tumors of the ureter; ureteral strictures; benign prostatic hyperplasia; retroperitoneal tumor / fibrosis; neurogenic bladder; cervical / prostatic carcinoma; pelvic mass (lymphoma, abscess, ovarian), urethral polyps; urethral neoplasm, acquired urethral strictures
- (b) congenital

• insidious course
√ large kidney with wasted parenchyma
√ diminished nephrographic density (decreased clearance)
√ early "rim" sign (thin band of radiodensity surrounding calices)
√ delayed opacification of collecting system
√ moderate to marked widening of collecting system
√ tortuous dilated ureter

NUC:
- √ photopenic area during vascular phase
- √ accumulation of radionuclide tracer within hydronephrotic collecting system on delayed images

Cx: superimposed infection (= pyonephrosis)

Congenital hydronephrosis

Mostly isolated malformation
Incidence: 1:100–300 births
Risk of recurrence: 2–3% for siblings
Age at presentation: 25% by age 1 year, 55% by age 5 years

Cause:
1. UPJ obstruction (22–40–67%)
2. Posterior urethral valves (18%)
3. Ectopic ureterocele (14%)
4. Prune belly syndrome (12%)
5. Ureteral + UVJ obstruction (8%)
6. Others: severe vesicoureteral reflux, bladder neck obstruction, hypertrophy of verumontanum, urethral diverticulum, congenital urethral strictures, anterior urethral valves, meatal stenosis

May be associated with: Down syndrome (17–25%)

• palpable abdominal mass
• intermittent flank + periumbilical pain
• failure to thrive
• vomiting
• hematuria, infection

Location: 70% unilateral

OB-US:
- √ AP diameter of renal pelvis ≥5 mm between 15–20 weeks, ≥8 mm at 20–30 weeks, ≥10 mm after 30 weeks MA
- √ ratio of AP diameter of renal pelvis to kidney >50%
- √ caliceal distension communicating with renal pelvis
- ◊ Postnatal evaluation after 4–7 days of age (because of decreased GFR + relative dehydration in first days of life)!

Prognosis: parenchymal atrophy + renal impairment (dependent on severity + duration)

Focal hydronephrosis

= HYDROCALICOSIS = HYDROCALYX = obstructed drainage of one portion of kidney

Cause:
- (1) Congenital: partial / complete duplication
- (2) Infectious stricture: eg, TB
- (3) Infundibular calculus
- (4) Tumor
- (5) Trauma

√ unifocal mass, commonly in upper pole
√ absent polar group of calices (early)
√ dilated polar group (late) with displacement of adjacent calices
√ delayed opacification in obstructed group

GU

√ focally replaced nephrogram

US:

√ anechoic cystic lesion with smooth margins

CT:

√ focal area of water density with smooth margin and thick wall

IMPOTENCE

= inability to have + maintain an erection adequate for sexual intercourse

Incidence: 10 million Americans

Cause:

A. ORGANIC (majority): diabetes (2 million), vascular disease, cancer surgery, spinal cord injury, pelvic trauma, endocrine problem, multiple sclerosis, alcoholism, drug-associated impotence
(a) failure to initiate (neurogenic)
(b) failure to fill (arteriogenic)
(c) failure to store (venogenic)
(d) end organ disease

B. PSYCHOGENIC

Rx: (1) Vascular reconstructive surgery
(2) Oral / intracavernous pharmacotherapy
(3) Vacuum erection devices
(4) Penile prosthesis placement
(a) nonhydraulic: semirigid, malleable, positionable
(b) hydraulic

also see ERECTILE DYSFUNCTION, page 767

JUXTAGLOMERULAR TUMOR

= RENINOMA = very rare tumor arising from renin-producing juxtaglomerular cells

Incidence: <30 cases reported

Age: mean age of 31 years; 50% <21 years; M < F

Path: small foci of hemorrhage + pseudocapsule

Histo: tumor resembles hemangiopericytoma

- typical features of primary reninism:
  - hypertension
  - hyperreninemia
  - secondary hyperaldosteronism
- moderate to severe headaches
- polydipsia, polyuria, enuresis

Location: just beneath renal capsule

√ renal mass of usually 2–3 cm in size

US:

√ echogenic mass ± areas of necrosis / hemorrhage

CT (thin overlapping cuts):

√ isodense tumor on NECT, hypodense on CECT

Angio:

√ angiographically hypo- / avascular tumor

√ renal venous blood sampling yields high renin level on affected side

Dx: combination of elevated renin without renal arterial lesion + hypovascular solid renal mass

DDx of renin elevation:

Wilms tumor, hypernephroma, lung cancer, paraovarian tumor, fallopian tube adenocarcinoma, epithelial liver hamartoma, orbital hemangiopericytoma, pancreatic cancer, angiolymphoid hyperplasia

LEUKEMIA

◊ Most common malignant cause of bilateral global renal enlargement!

Incidence: renal involvement in 63% of autopsies

A. FOCAL ACCUMULATION OF LEUKEMIC CELLS (rare)
chloroma (= granulocytic sarcoma) of acute myeloblastic leukemia, myeloblastoma, myeloblastic sarcoma
- may antedate other manifestations of leukemia

√ unifocal mass in renal cortex / renal sinus

B. DIFFUSE INVOLVEMENT
leukemic cells infiltrate the interstitial tissue + renal sinus; tubules are replaced (more common in lymphocytic than in granulocytic forms); no relationship to peripheral white blood cell count
- renal impairment (from leukemic infiltrate, hyperuricemia, septicemia, hemorrhage)
- hypertension

√ large kidneys bilaterally with smooth contours

√ normal or diminished density on nephrogram

√ occasionally attenuated collecting system (DDx: renal sinus lipomatosis)

√ nonopaque filling defects on IVP (clot, uric acid)

√ renal / subcapsular / perinephric hemorrhage frequent

√ retroperitoneal lymphadenopathy

US:

√ loss of definition + distortion of central sinus complex

√ normal to increased coarse echoes throughout renal cortex + preservation of renal medullae

√ single / multiple focal anechoic masses

DDx: Hodgkin disease, malignant lymphoma, multiple myeloma

LEUKOPLAKIA

= KERATINIZING SQUAMOUS METAPLASIA / DYSPLASIA = DYSKERATOSIS

Cause: chronic infection (80%) / stones (40%)

Histo: large confluent areas / scattered patches of squamous metaplasia of transitional cell epithelium with keratinization + cellular atypia in deeper layers

Peak age: 4th–5th decade;
M:F = 1:1 (with involvement of renal pelvis)
M:F = 4:1 (with involvement of bladder)

- hematuria (30%)
- recurrent UTIs
- pathognomonic passage of gritty flakes, soft-tissue stones, white chunks of tissue (desquamated keratinized epithelial layers) leading to colic, fever, chills

Location: bladder > renal pelvis > ureter; bilateral in 10%

√ corrugated / striated irregularities of pelvicaliceal walls, localized / generalized

√ plaquelike intraluminal mass with "onion skin" pattern of contrast material in interstices

√ caliectasis + pyelectasis common (with obstruction)

√ ridging / filling defects of ureter

√ associated with calculi in 25–50%

Cx: premalignant condition for epidermoid carcinoma in 12% (controversial!)

LOBAR NEPHRONIA

= ACUTE FOCAL BACTERIAL NEPHRITIS = focal variant of acute pyelonephritis with single / multiple areas of suppuration + necrosis

Organism: E. coli > Proteus > Klebsiella

Predisposed: patients with altered host resistance (diabetes [60%], immunosuppression), chronic catheterization, mechanical / functional obstruction, trauma

• fever, flank pain, pyuria

Site: usually involves entire renal lobe

√ focal area of absent nephrogram / distorted pyelogram
√ renal arteries displaced, renal veins compressed
√ hypoechoic mass with ill-defined margins and disruption of corticomedullary border, NO fluid collection
√ low attenuation zone with poorly defined transition to surrounding parenchyma
√ Ga-67 uptake
√ vesicoureteral reflux often present

Cx: scarring, abscess

LOCALIZED CYSTIC DISEASE

= multiple simple cysts involving only one portion of the kidney

• no family history

Histo: dilated ducts and tubules varying in size from mm to several cm

Prognosis: not progressive

LYMPHOMA

Incidence: in 2.7–6% renal involvement

Types:

(1) NON-HODGKIN LYMPHOMA
renal involvement detected in 5% of abdominal CT, in 33–65% of autopsies; occurs usually late in disease

(2) HODGKIN DISEASE
renal involvement in 13% of autopsies

Patterns of involvement:

(a) primary renal lymphoma (very rare)
(b) hematogenous dissemination:
— single / multiple foci
— diffuse infiltration
(c) contiguous extension from adjacent pararenal lymphomatous disease, usually extranodal

• clinically silent (50%)
• flank pain, palpable mass, weight loss
• hematuria
• compromise of renal function (urinary tract obstruction, renal vein compression, diffuse infiltration of kidney, superimposed infarct, amyloidosis, hypercalcemia)

√ unilateral:bilateral = 3:1
√ multiple nodular masses (29–61%)
√ invasion from retroperitoneal disease (11%) with involvement by transcapsular / transsinus extension
√ single bulky tumor (7%), small solitary tumor (7–48%)
√ diffuse infiltration (6–19%), microscopic infiltration (7%)

CECT:
√ usually homogeneous poorly marginated masses less dense than renal parenchyma

US:
√ single / multiple anechoic / hypoechoic masses
√ renal enlargement + decreased parenchymal echoes
√ loss of renal sinus echoes

Angio:
√ neovascularity, encasement, vascular displacement (occasionally palisade-like configuration)

MALACOPLAKIA

= uncommon chronic inflammatory response to Gram-negative infection

Organism: E. coli (in 94%);
diabetes mellitus predisposes

Histo: submucosal histiocytic granulomas containing large foamy mononuclear cells (Hansemann macrophages) with intracytoplasmic basophilic PAS-positive inclusion bodies (Michaelis-Gutmann bodies) consisting of incompletely destroyed E. coli bacterium surrounded by lipoprotein membranes

Peak age: 5th–7th decade; M:F = 1:4

• hematuria
• raised yellow lesion <3 cm in diameter

Location: bladder > lower 2/3 of ureter > upper ureter > renal pelvis; multifocal in 75%; bilateral in 50%

√ multiple dome-shaped smooth mural filling defects
√ scalloped appearance if lesions confluent
√ generalized pelviureteral dilatation (if obstructive)
√ displacement of pelvicaliceal system + distorted central sinus complex
√ multifocal parenchymal masses may cause diminished / absent nephrogram

DDx: pyeloureteritis cystica

MALPOSITIONED TESTIS

= MALDESCENDED TESTIS

testes are normally within scrotum by 28–32 weeks MA

Incidence: early 3rd trimester in 10%; at birth in 3.7% (in babies >2,500 g in 3.4%; in premature babies in 30%); beyond 3 months of age in 1%

1. **Pseudocryptorchidism** (70%)
= RETRACTILE TESTIS
= unusually spastic cremasteric muscle

2. **Cryptorchidism** (20–29%)
= arrested descent of testis along its normal course

Associated with: prune belly syndrome (bilateral cryptorchidism), Prader-Willi syndrome, Beckwith-Wiedemann syndrome, Noonan syndrome, Laurence-Moon-Biedl syndrome, trisomies 13, 18, 21

• nonpalpable testis

Location: high scrotal position (50%); canalicular = between internal + external inguinal ring (20%); abdominal (10%); bilateral in 10%

◊ The most craniad possible point of an undescended testis is the lower pole of the ipsilateral kidney!

√ failure to visualize testis within scrotum
√ small atrophic testis with generalized decreased echogenicity + demonstrable mediastinum testis

3. **Ectopia testis** (1%)
   = deviation from the usual pathway
   Location: interstitial = groin (on external oblique muscle), pubopenile = root of penis, perineal, femoral triangle, on opposite side

Undescended testis = retractile testis + cryptorchidism

Cx: (1) Sterility
(2) Malignancy: most commonly seminoma, 30–50 x risk increase = 1:1,000 men/year, 4–11% of all testicular tumors found in cryptorchidism; risk remains increased even after orchiopexy
◊ Annual screening until at least age 35!
(3) Torsion: 10 x risk in cryptorchidism

Test sensitivity:
MR : modality of choice
US : 20–88%; very sensitive in inguinal canal
√ need to identify mediastinum testis (DDx: lymph node)
CT : 95% (testis <1 cm cannot be detected)
√ no spermatic cord in inguinal canal
Venography : 50–90%

Rx: surgery at 9–12 months of age
DDx: (1) Rudimentary testis
(2) Pars intravaginalis gubernaculum = nonatrophied bulbous termination
(3) Congenital absence = monorchia / anorchia (in 3–5%)

MECKEL-GRUBER SYNDROME

= autosomal recessive disease characterized by occipital encephalocele, polycystic kidneys, polydactyly
Incidence: 1:12,000–50,000; more common among Yemenite Jews
Risk of recurrence: 25%; carrier frequency of 1:56
• history of affected siblings
OB-US:
√ large polycystic kidneys containing 2- to 10-mm cysts
√ occipital encephalocele
√ postaxial polydactyly
√ microcephaly
√ cleft lip and palate
√ moderate-to-severe oligohydramnios (onset midtrimester)
√ inability to visualize urine within fetal bladder
OB management:
1. Chromosomal analysis to exclude trisomy 13 (if no prior family history)
2. Option of pregnancy termination <24 weeks GA
3. Nonintervention for fetal distress >24 weeks GA
Prognosis: invariably fatal at birth due to pulmonary hypoplasia + renal failure
DDx: trisomy 13

MEDULLARY CYSTIC DISEASE

= NEPHRONOPHTHISIS
Histo: variable number of medullary cysts (100 μ to 2 cm) + progressive periglomerular and interstitial fibrosis + tubular atrophy with dilatation of some proximal tubules
Types:
(1) MEDULLARY CYSTIC DISEASE = ADULT ONSET
autosomal dominant, in young adults, rapidly progressive course with uremia + death in 2 years
(2) JUVENILE NEPHRONOPHTHISIS = JUVENILE ONSET
autosomal recessive, in children 3–5 years, average duration of 10 years before uremia and death occurs
• salt-wasting, polyuria, hyposthenuria, polydipsia
• failure to thrive, growth retardation (in early teens)
• uremia, severe anemia, normal sediment, hypertension (only in late phase)
√ bilateral normal / small kidneys with smooth contour + thin cortex
IVP:
√ poor opacification of renal collecting system
√ "medullary nephrogram" = medullary striations persistent for up to 2 hours; occasionally replaced by sharply defined multiple thin-walled lucencies
Retrograde pyelogram:
√ communication between collecting system + cysts
US / CT:
√ increased parenchymal echogenicity + loss of corticomedullary junction
√ multiple small medullary / corticomedullary cysts

MEDULLARY SPONGE KIDNEY

= dysplastic cystic dilatation of papillary + medullary portions of collecting ducts (first few generations of metanephric duct branchings)
Incidence: 0.5%
Age: young to middle-aged adults; sporadic
May be associated with: Ehlers-Danlos syndrome, parathyroid adenoma, Caroli disease
• often asymptomatic
√ medullary nephrocalcinosis (40–80%) with one / more calculi up to 5 mm
√ "bunch of flowers" = thick dense streaks of contrast material radiating from pyramids peripherally representing papillary cysts / ectatic ducts (DDx: dense papillary blush in normals)
√ may be unilateral in 25%
√ may involve only one pyramid / all pyramids (25%)
Cx: urolithiasis, hematuria, infection
DDx:
(1) Normal variant ("papillary blush" without distinct streaks / nephrocalcinosis / pyramidal enlargement)
(2) Renal tuberculosis (larger more irregular calcifications + cavitations + strictures + ulcerations)
(3) Papillary necrosis (sloughed papilla + caliceal ring sign)
(4) Medullary nephrocalcinosis (no ectatic ducts / cysts, calcifications beyond pyramids)

(5) Juvenile polycystic kidney disease (bilateral renal enlargement + hepatic periportal fibrosis)
(6) Caliceal diverticulum (small, solitary, located between pyramid)

MEGACALICOSIS

= CONGENITAL MEGACALICES = nonprogressive caliceal dilatation caused by hypoplastic medullary pyramids

Age: any age; M >> F

May be associated with: primary megaureter

- normal glomerular filtration rate

Site: entire kidney / part of kidney; unilateral / bilateral

√ kidney usually enlarged with prominent fetal lobation
√ reduced parenchymal thickness (medulla affected, NOT cortex)
√ mosaic-like arrangement of dilated calices (polygonal + faceted appearance, NOT globular as in obstruction)
√ increased number of calices
√ ABSENT caliceal cupping (semilunar instead of pyramidal configuration of papillae)
√ NO dilatation of pelvis / ureters, NORMAL contrast excretion

Cx: (1) Hematuria (2) Stone formation

MEGACYSTIS-MICROCOLON SYNDROME

= MEGALOCYSTIS-MICROCOLON-INTESTINAL HYPOPERISTALSIS SYNDROME (MMIH)
= functional obstruction of bladder + colon characterized by
(1) enlarged urinary bladder
(2) small colon
(3) strikingly short small intestine suspended on a primitive dorsal mesentery
(4) markedly enlarged hydronephrotic kidneys with little remaining parenchyma

Incidence: 26 cases reported; M:F = 1:7

May be associated with: diaphragmatic hernia, PDA, teeth at birth

- distended abdomen (large bladder + dilated small bowel loops)
- overflow incontinence
- intestinal pseudo-obstruction (poor emptying of stomach, NO peristaltic activity of small bowel)

OB-US:
√ normal amount of amniotic fluid / polyhydramnios (in spite of dilated bladder = "nonobstructive obstruction")
√ massive + progressive bladder distension with poor emptying
√ bilateral megaloureters
√ ± hydronephrosis
√ female sex

BE:
√ microcolon (transient feature of "unused colon") with narrow rectum + sigmoid
√ malrotation / malfixation or foreshortening of small bowel

VCUG
√ distended unobstructed bladder with poor / absent muscular function

Prognosis: lethal in most cases (a few months of age)

MEGALOURETER

= CONGENITAL PRIMARY MEGAURETER = TERMINAL URETERECTASIS = ACHALASIA OF URETER = URETEROVESICAL JUNCTION OBSTRUCTION
= intrinsic congenital dilatation of lower juxtavesical orthotopic ureter

Cause: aperistaltic juxtavesical (1.5 cm long) segment secondary to faulty development of muscle layers of ureter (functional, NOT mechanical obstruction)

Incidence: all ages; second most common cause of hydronephrosis in fetus and newborn; M:F = 2–5:1

Associated disorders (in 40%):
(a) contralateral: UPJ obstruction, reflux, ureterocele, ureteral duplication, renal ectopia, renal agenesis
(b) ipsilateral: caliceal diverticulum, megacalicosis, papillary necrosis

- asymptomatic (mostly)
- pain
- abdominal mass
- hematuria
- infection

Location: L:R = 3:1, bilateral in 15–40%

√ prominent localized dilatation of pelvic ureter (up to 5 cm in diameter) usually not progressive, but may involve entire ureter + collecting system
√ vigorous nonpropulsive to-and-fro motion in dilated segment
√ functional smoothly tapered narrowing of intravesical ureter
√ NO reflux, NO stenosis

MESOBLASTIC NEPHROMA

= FETAL RENAL HAMARTOMA = LEIOMYOMATOUS HAMARTOMA = BENIGN CONGENITAL WILMS TUMOR = BENIGN FETAL HAMARTOMA = FETAL MESENCHYMAL TUMOR = BOLANDE TUMOR = CONGENITAL FIBROSARCOMA = FIBROMYXOMA
= nonfamilial benign fibromyomatoid mass arising from renal connective tissue

Incidence: most common renal neoplasm in neonate; 3% of all renal neoplasms in children

Age: 3 months mean age at presentation; may occasionally go undetected until adulthood; M > F

Histo: smooth muscle cells + immature fibroblasts resembling leiomyoma containing trapped islands of embryonic glomeruli, tubules, vessels, hematopoietic cells, cartilage

In 14% associated with: prematurity, polyhydramnios, GI + GU tract malformations, neuroblastoma

- large flank mass
- hematuria (20%) / hypertension (4%), anemia

√ usually replaces 60–90% of renal parenchyma
√ usually solid but may produce multiple cystic spaces
√ NO sharp cleavage plane toward normal parenchyma, may extend beyond capsule
√ calcifications (rare)
√ NO venous extension (DDx from Wilms tumor)

IVP:
- √ large noncalcified renal mass with distortion of collecting system
- √ usually NO herniation into renal pelvis (DDx from MLCN)

US:
- √ evenly echogenic tumor with concentric echogenic + hypoechoic rings resembling uterine fibroids
- √ complex mass with hemorrhage + cyst formation + necrosis

Angio:
- √ hypervascular mass with neovascularity + displacement of adjacent vessels

Cx: transformation to metastasizing spindle cell sarcoma (rare)
Rx: complete resection
Prognosis: excellent

METASTASES TO KIDNEY

◊ Most common malignant tumor of the kidney (2–3 times as frequent as primaries in autopsy studies)!
◊ 5th most common site of metastases (after lung, liver, bone, adrenals)!

most common primaries: bronchus, breast, opposite kidney, non-Hodgkin lymphoma, colon
less common primaries: stomach, cervix, ovary, pancreas, prostate, chloroma, myeloblastoma, myeloblastic sarcoma, melanoma (45% incidence), osteogenic sarcoma, choriocarcinoma (10–50% incidence), Hodgkin lymphoma, rhabdomyosarcoma

- usually asymptomatic
- √ bilateral multiple small masses (due to brief survival of patient)

DDx on CT: lymphoma, bilateral RCC, multiple renal infarcts, acute focal bacterial nephritis, infiltrating TCC

MULTICYSTIC DYSPLASTIC KIDNEY

= MULTICYSTIC DYSGENETIC KIDNEY (MCDK)
= MULTICYSTIC KIDNEY (MCK) = Potter Type II
◊ Second most common cause of an abdominal mass in neonate (after hydronephrosis)!
◊ Most common form of cystic disease in infants!

Incidence: 1:10,000 (for bilateral MCDK); M:F = 2:1 (for unilateral MCDK); more common among infants of diabetic mothers
Risk of recurrence: 2–3%
Etiology: (sporadic) generalized interference with ureteral bud function before 8–10 weeks of fetal life
Pathophysiology: ureteral obstruction / atresia interferes with ureteral bud division + inhibits induction and maturation of nephrons; collecting tubules enlarge into cysts
Histo: immature glomeruli + tubules reduced in number + whirling mesenchymal tissue, cartilage (33%), cysts

- abdominal mass
- asymptomatic if unilateral (may go undetected until adulthood)
- recurrent urinary tract infections, intermittent abdominal pain, nausea + vomiting, hematuria, failure to thrive
- fatal due to pulmonary hypoplasia if bilateral

Location:
1. UNILATERAL multicystic dysplastic kidney
   most common form (80–90%); L:R = 2:1
   secondary to pelvoinfundibular atresia
   Associated with anomalies of contralateral side in 20–40–50%:
   (1) Ureteropelvic junction obstruction (7–27%)
   (2) Horseshoe kidney (5–9%)
   (3) Ureteral anomalies (5%)
   (4) Renal hypoplasia (4%)
   (5) Vesicoureteral reflux
   (6) Malrotation
   (7) Renal agenesis
   Associated with ipsilateral anomalies:
   (1) Vesicoureteral reflux (25%)
   (2) Ectopic ureter
2. SEGMENTAL / focal renal dysplasia
   = "multilocular cyst" secondary to
   (a) high-grade obstruction of upper pole moiety in duplex kidney from ectopic ureterocele
   (b) single obstructed infundibulum
3. BILATERAL cystic dysplasia
   in the presence of severe obstruction in utero from posterior urethral valves / urethral atresia with oligohydramnios + pulmonary hypoplasia
   Fatal form: bilateral MCDK (4.5–21%), contralateral renal agenesis (0–11%)

Types:
(1) MULTICYSTIC KIDNEY (Potter IIa)
   √ large kidney with multiple large cysts + little visible renal parenchyma
(2) HYPOPLASTIC / DIMINUTIVE FORM (Potter IIb)
   √ echogenic small kidney

APPEARANCE RELATED TO SITE OF OBSTRUCTION
@ ureteropelvic junction
   √ single / several large / multiple medium-sized cysts in large kidney
@ distal ureter / urethra
   √ small / no cysts in small kidney

APPEARANCE RELATED TO TIME OF INSULT
(a) early onset between 8th–11th week
   √ small / atretic renal pelvis + calices
   √ 10–20 cysts + loss of reniform appearance
(b) late onset = HYDRONEPHROTIC FORM
   √ large central cyst (= dilated pelvis) often communicating with cysts
   √ some renal function may be demonstrated

- √ large kidney with lobulated contour in infancy
- √ incidental finding of small kidney in adults (secondary to arrested growth)
- √ ipsilateral atretic ureter
- √ contralateral renal hypertrophy
- √ calcification: curvilinear / ringlike in wall of cysts in 30% of adults, rarely in children

IVP + NUC:
◊ NUC preferred over IVP in first month of life as concentrating ability of even normal neonatal kidneys is suboptimal!
√ no function (rarely faint contrast accumulation)

US:
√ normal renal architecture replaced
√ random cysts of varying shape + size ("cluster of grapes") with largest cyst in peripheral nonmedial location (100% accurate)
√ cysts separated by septa (100% accurate)
√ central sinus complex absent (100% accurate)
√ no communication between multiple cysts (93% accurate)
√ no identification of parenchymal rim or corticomedullary differentiation (74% accurate)
√ cysts begin to disappear in infancy
√ kidney may be small + atrophic (as little as 1 g) / normal / large
√ oligohydramnios in bilateral MCDK / unilateral MCDK + contralateral urinary obstruction

Angio:
√ absent / hypoplastic renal artery; angiography unnecessary since a DDx to long-standing functionless kidney is not possible

OB-management:
(1) Routine antenatal care + evaluation by pediatric urologist following delivery if unilateral
(2) Option of pregnancy termination if ≤24 weeks GA
(3) Nonintervention for fetal distress if >24 weeks GA

Cx: (1) Renin-dependent hypertension (rare)
(2) Malignancy in <1:330

Rx: (1) follow-up
(2) nephrectomy (in hypertension / if kidney does not involute)

DDx: (1) hydronephrosis
(2) renal dysplasia with cysts (associated with partial obstruction)

MULTILOCULAR CYSTIC RENAL TUMOR

= rare nonhereditary benign renal neoplasm originating from metanephric blastema possibly representing the benign end of a spectrum with solid Wilms tumor at the malignant end
= BENIGN MULTILOCULAR CYSTIC NEPHROMA = POLYCYSTIC NEPHROBLASTOMA = WELL-DIFFERENTIATED POLYCYSTIC WILMS TUMOR = BENIGN CYSTIC DIFFERENTIATED NEPHROBLASTOMA = CYSTIC PARTIALLY DIFFERENTIATED NEPHROBLASTOMA = MULTILOCULAR CYSTIC NEPHROMA = PERLMANN TUMOR = MULTILOCULAR RENAL CYST = CYSTIC ADENOMA / HAMARTOMA / LYMPHANGIOMA = PARTIALLY POLYCYSTIC KIDNEY

Age: biphasic age + sex distribution: <4 years in 73% male, >4 years in 89% female
(a) 3 months to 2 years of age (65%), 5–30 years (5%); M:F = 2:1
(b) >30 years (30%); M:F = 8:1
◊ 90% of tumors in males occur in first 2 years of life (peak 3–24 months)!
◊ Most of the lesions in females occur between ages 4 and 20 or 40 and 60!

Path: solitary large well-circumscribed multiseptated mass of noncommunicating fluid-filled loculi, surrounded by thick fibrous capsule + compressed renal parenchyma; cyst size between mm up to 4 cm

Histo: gross anatomic features are identical!
1. **Cystic nephroma**
fibrous tissue septa of undifferentiated mesenchymal and primitive glomerulotubular elements surround cysts lined by flattened cuboidal epithelium;
NO blastemal / other embryonal elements
2. **Cystic partially differentiated nephroblastoma**
= CPDN
predominantly cystic lesion with septa containing blastemal / other embryonal elements

- commonly asymptomatic painless abdominal mass
- ± sudden and rapid enlargement
- pain, hematuria, urinary tract infection

Location: unilateral, often replacing an entire renal pole (usually lower pole)

Size: average size of 10 cm (few cm to 33 cm)

√ sharply well-circumscribed (characteristic) multiseptated cystic renal mass
√ tumor surrounded by thick fibrous capsule
√ cluster of noncommunicating "honeycombed" cysts of various sizes separated by thick septa
√ smaller closely spaced cysts appear as solid nodules
√ contrast enhancement of septations (secondary to tortuous fine vessels coursing through septa)
√ curvilinear to flocculent calcification of septa / capsule

IVP:
√ distortion of calices / hydronephrosis secondary to nonfunctional mass
√ tendency for herniation of tumor cysts into renal pelvis (nonspecific, also seen with Wilms tumor + RCC)

US:
√ cluster of cysts separated by thick septa (SUGGESTIVE PATTERN)
√ occasionally solid echogenic character (due to very small cysts / jellylike contents)

CT:
√ cysts with attenuation equal to / higher than water (gelatinous fluid)

Cx: local recurrence / coexistent Wilms tumor (extremely rare)

Rx: nephrectomy

DDx: (1) Cystic Wilms tumor (overlapping age)
(2) Clear cell sarcoma (poor prognosis)
(3) Cystic mesoblastic nephroma (most common renal tumor of infancy)
(4) Cystic RCC (mean age of 10 years)
(5) Segmental form of multicystic dysplastic kidney

MULTIPLE MYELOMA

◊ It is essential that dehydration is avoided!

Impairment of renal function:

(1) Precipitation of abnormal proteins (Bence-Jones ± Tamm-Horsfall protein casts) into tubule lumen (30–50%)
(2) Toxicity of Bence-Jones proteins on tubules
(3) Impaired renal blood flow secondary to increased blood viscosity
(4) Amyloidosis
(5) Nephrocalcinosis from hypercalcemia
◊ Contrast-induced renal failure in multiple myeloma is not seen with greatly increased frequency!

- • Tamm-Horsfall proteinuria (tubular cell secretion)
- √ smooth normal to large kidneys (initially), become small with time
- √ occasionally attenuated pelvo-infundibulo-caliceal system
- √ normal to diminished contrast material density; increasingly dense in acute oliguric failure

US:
- √ normal to increased echogenicity

NUC in bone scintigraphy:
- √ nonspecific increased parenchymal activity

MYCETOMA

= FUNGUS BALL

Organism: typically Candida, Aspergillus, Mucor, Cryptococcus, Phycomycetes, Actinomycetes mostly mycelial (M-form) or occasionally yeast cells (Y-form)

Predisposed: diabetics, debilitating illness, prolonged antibiotic therapy, leukemia, lymphoma, thymoma, immunosuppression

- • flank pain, passing of tissue, hematuria (extremely rare)
- • renal candidiasis associated with candidemia
- • Candida cystitis preceded by vaginal candidiasis
- √ unilateral nonvisualization of kidney (most frequent)
- √ large irregular filling defect extending into dilated calices (retrograde contrast study)
- √ necrotizing papillitis from Candida nephritis (common)
- √ lacelike pattern (on antegrade contrast study)

NEPHROBLASTOMATOSIS

= multiple / diffuse nephrogenic rests (= abnormally persistent nephrogenic cells with potential to form Wilms tumor)

Incidence: in 41% with unilateral Wilms tumor, in 94% with metachronous contralateral Wilms tumor, in 99% with bilateral Wilms tumor

Pathogenesis: primitive renal tissue (metanephrogenic blastema) normally present up to 36 weeks of gestational age; embryonal renal tissue in mature kidney after birth retains potential to form nephroblastomatosis / Wilms tumor

Histo: contains only primitive epithelial cell line without mesenchymal elements (as seen in Wilms tumor)

Age: neonatal period, infancy, childhood

Associated with:
hemihypertrophy, sporadic aniridia, Klippel-Trénaunay syndrome, Beckwith-Wiedemann syndrome, trisomy 18, pseudohermaphroditism, splenic agenesis with hepatic malformation, Drash syndrome

Site: (a) at periphery of renal lobe = perilobar nephrogenic rest associated with a 1–2% risk of Wilms tumor
(b) within renal lobe = intralobar nephrogenic rest associated with 4–5% risk of Wilms tumor

A. **Multifocal (juvenile) nephroblastomatosis**
most common form
= discrete islands of rests in cortex / columns
√ may escape detection with imaging
√ ± deformation of pelvicaliceal structures
√ kidneys may be enlarged

B. **Superficial diffuse (late infantile) nephroblastomatosis**
= superficial continuous peripheral ring of rests around normal medulla + pyramid
Age: <2 years
√ nephromegaly
◊ Strong association with Wilms tumor!

C. **Universal / panlobar (infantile) nephroblastomatosis**
rare form
= entire renal parenchyma diffusely involved
• may develop renal failure
√ bilateral renal enlargement

US:
- √ subtle subcapsular hypoechoic / isoechoic / hyperechoic nodules
- √ nephromegaly with decreased parenchymal echoes

CECT (preferred study):
- √ nonenhancing subcapsular nodules
- √ splaying + elongation of collecting system

MR (43% sensitivity, 58% sensitivity with enhancement):
- √ homogeneously hypointense lesions on T1WI
- √ homogeneously hypointense lesions on T2WI for sclerosing / involuting type of nephroblastomatosis
- √ isointense lesions on T2WI for hyperplastic / neoplastic type of nephroblastomatosis
- √ hypointense lesions on enhanced T1WI

Cx: malignant transformation (enlargement of rest / development of mass)

Rx: amenable to chemotherapy

MYELOLIPOMA

Prevalence: 0.08–0.2% (autopsy series)

Cause: ? metaplasia of adrenal cortical cells precipitated by chronic stress / degeneration

Path: mature fat interspersed with hematopoietic cells resembling bone marrow + pseudocapsule

Histo: variable mixture of myeloid cells, erythroid cells, megakaryocytes, lymphocytes

Associated with: endocrine disorders in 7% (Cushing syndrome, 21-hydroxylase deficiency), nonhyperfunctioning adenoma (15%)

Location: (a) adrenal gland (85%)
(b) extraadrenal (15%): retroperitoneal (12%), intrathoracic (3%)
Site: unilateral : bilateral = 10:1
Size: mean diameter of 10.4 cm
X-ray:
√ lucent mass with rim of residual normal adrenal cortex
√ calcifications (22%)
US:
√ heterogeneous predominantly hyperechoic (= fatty + myeloid tissue) mass with interspersed hypoechoic (= pure fat) regions
CT:
√ large amounts of fat with interspersed "smoky" areas of higher attenuation of 20–30 HU (= admixture of fat + marrowlike elements)
MR:
√ hyperintense areas on T1WI (= predominantly fatty areas)
√ intermediate intensity on T2WI similar to spleen
√ hyperintense areas on fat-suppressed images (= marrowlike elements + hemorrhage)

Cx: acute hemorrhage with increase in size (12%)
Dx: percutaneous needle biopsy
Rx: surgical excision not necessary
DDx: liposarcoma

NEPHROGENIC ADENOMA

= uncommon benign metaplastic response to urothelial injury / prolonged irritation
Cause: (a) trauma: accident, surgery, instrumentation, renal transplantation
(b) irritation: calculi, chronic infection
Age: 3 weeks to 83 years; M:F = 3:1 (more common in females <20 years of age)
Path: discrete raised papillary / polypoid areas projecting from epithelial surface
Histo: variable number of small tubules + cysts + papillae lined with a single layer of cuboidal / low columnar cells
- hematuria, dysuria
- asymptomatic

Location: bladder (72%), renal pelvis, ureter, urethra; strong correlation between location + site of insult to urothelium
√ filling defect
Rx: resection / fulguration
DDx: inflammatory / malignant urothelial lesions

NEPHROGENIC DIABETES INSIPIDUS

= poor reabsorption of water in collecting ducts due to
(1) lack of adequate vasopressin production
(2) end-organ resistance to vasopressin
Cause: (a) congenital
1. X-linked recessive trait with variable expression
2. Autosomal dominant form (rare)

(b) acquired
1. Obstructive uropathy
2. Unilateral renal artery stenosis
3. Acute tubular necrosis

- symptoms in infancy:
  - vomiting secondary to hypernatremic dehydration
  - mental retardation
  - caloric growth failure (water favored over formula)
- symptoms after infancy:
  - increased fluid intake
  - avoiding urination

√ bilateral hydroureteronephrosis
Rx: thiazide diuretics, low-salt diet, encouragement of frequent micturition, indomethacin

NEUROBLASTOMA

Most common solid abdominal mass of infancy (12.3% of all perinatal neoplasms), 3rd most common malignant tumor in infancy (after leukemia + CNS tumors), 2nd most common tumor in childhood (Wilms tumor more common in older children), 7% of all childhood cancers; 15% of cancer deaths in children
Incidence: 1:7,100 to 1:10,000 livebirths; 500 cases per year in USA; 20% hereditary
Origin: neural crest
Path: round irregular lobulated mass of 50–150 g with areas of hemorrhage + necrosis
Histo: small round cells slightly larger than lymphocytes with scant cytoplasm; Horner-Wright rosettes = one / two layers of primitive neuroblasts surrounding a central zone of tangled neurofibrillary processes
Age: peak age at 2 years; 25% during 1st year; 50% <2 years; 75% in <4 years; 90% in <8 years; occasionally present at birth; M:F = 1:1
May be associated with: aganglionosis of bowel, CHD

- pain + fever (30%)
- palpable abdominal mass (45–54%)
- bone pain, limp, inability to walk (20%)
- myoclonus of trunk + extremities
- cerebellar ataxia, nystagmus (20%)
- opsoclonus = spontaneous conjugate + chaotic eye movements (sign of cerebellar disease)
- orbital ecchymosis / proptosis (12%)
- intractable diarrhea (9%) due to increase in vasoactive intestinal polypeptides (VIP)
- increased catecholamine production (75–90%): in 95% excreted in urine as vanillylmandelic acid (VMA) / homovanillic acid (HVA)
  - hypertension (up to 30%)
  - acute cerebellar encephalopathy
  - paroxysmal episodes of flushing, tachycardia, headaches, sweating
  - rise in body temperature
  - hyperglycemia

Stages:

- I limited to organ of origin
- II regional spread not crossing midline
- III extension across midline
- IV metastatic to distant lymph nodes, liver, bone, brain, lung
- IVs stages I + II with disease confined to liver, skin, bone marrow WITHOUT radiographic evidence of skeletal metastases

Metastases:

bone (60%), regional lymph nodes (42%), orbit (20%), liver (15%), intracranial (14%), lung (10%)

◊ Metastases are first manifestation in up to 60%!

Hutchinson syndrome

(1) primary adrenal neuroblastoma
(2) extensive skeletal metastases, particularly skull
(3) proptosis
(4) bone pain

Pepper syndrome

(1) primary adrenal neuroblastoma
(2) massive hepatomegaly from metastases

Blueberry muffin syndrome

(1) primary adrenal neuroblastoma
(2) multiple metastatic skin lesions

◊ Bone marrow aspirate positive in 50–70% at time of initial diagnosis!

◊ 2/3 of patients >2 years have disseminated disease!

@ Skeletal metastases:

√ periosteal reaction
√ osteolytic focus / multicentric lytic lesions
√ lucent horizontal metaphyseal line
√ vertical linear radiolucent streaks in metadiaphysis of long bones
√ pathologic fracture
√ vertebral collapse
√ widened cranial sutures (subjacent dural metastases)
√ sclerotic lesions with healing

DDx: Ewing sarcoma, rhabdomyosarcoma, leukemia, lymphoma

@ Intracranial + maxillofacial metastases:

Site: dura, brain substance

@ Pulmonary metastases:

√ nodular infiltrates
√ rib erosion
√ mediastinal + retrocrural lymphadenopathy (common)

Location: anywhere within sympathetic neural chain

@ abdomen

(a) adrenal (36%): almost always unilateral
(b) both adrenals (7–10%)
(c) extraadrenal in sympathetic chain (18%)

@ thorax + posterior mediastinum (14%): aortic bodies
@ neck (5%): carotid ganglia
@ pelvis (5%): organ of Zuckerkandl
@ skull / esthesioneuroblastoma of olfactory bulb, cerebellum, cerebrum (2%)
@ other sites (10%): eg, intrarenal (very rare)
@ unknown (10%)

√ large suprarenal mass with irregular shape + margins (82%)
√ heterogeneous texture with low-density areas from hemorrhage + necrosis (55%)
√ stippled / coarse calcifications (36–70%)
√ "drooping lily" sign = displacement of kidney inferolaterally without distortion of collecting system
√ hydronephrosis (24%)
√ inseparable from kidney ± invasion of kidney (32%)
√ propensity for extension into spinal canal through neural foramen with erosion of pedicles (15%)
√ extension across midline (55%) (DDx: Wilms tumor)
√ retroperitoneal adenopathy / contiguous extension (73%)
√ retrocrural adenopathy (27%)
√ encasement of IVC + aorta, celiac axis, SMA (32%)
√ caval involvement = indicator of unresectability
√ liver metastases (18–66%); invasion of liver (5%)

Angio:

√ hypo- / hypervascular mass

US:

√ hyper- / hypoechoic mass with acoustic shadows

NUC:

√ focal uptake of I-131 / I-123 MIBG radioactivity (82% sensitivity; 88% specificity)
√ tracer uptake on bone scan (60%)

OB-US:

- maternal symptoms of catecholamine excess

√ mixed cystic + solid mass in adrenal region
√ may exhibit acoustic shadowing (calcifications)
√ hydrops fetalis (severe anemia secondary to metastases to bone marrow, mechanical compression of IVC, hypersecretion of aldosterone)

2-year survival rate versus age at presentation:

60% if patient's age <1 year
20% if patient's age 1–2 years
10% if patient's age >2 years

◊ May revert to benign ganglioneuroma in 0.2%!

Survival rate versus stage:

80% for stage I
60% for stage II
30% for stage III
7% for stage IV
75–87% for stage IVs

DDx: exophytic Wilms tumor, mesoblastic nephroma, multicystic kidney, retroperitoneal teratoma, adrenal hemorrhage, hepatic hamartoma / hemangioma, infradiaphragmatic sequestration

NEUROGENIC BLADDER

Neuroanatomy: bladder innervation of detrusor muscle by parasympathetic nerves S2–S4

Etiology: congenital (myelomeningocele); trauma; neoplasm (spinal, CNS); infection (herpes, polio); inflammation (multiple sclerosis, syrinx); systemic disorder (diabetes, pernicious anemia)

A. SPASTIC BLADDER
"upper motor neuron" lesion above conus

B. ATONIC BLADDER
"lower motor neuron lesion" below conus

ONCOCYTOMA

= PROXIMAL TUBULAR ADENOMA = BENIGN OXYPHILIC ADENOMA

Prevalence: 1–2–13% of renal tumors

Age: median age around 65 (range of 26–94) years; M:F = 1.6:1 to 2.5:1

Path: well-encapsulated tan-colored tumor of well-differentiated proximal tubular cells (benign adenoma) + oncocytes

Histo: oncocytes = large epithelial cells with granular oxyphilic / eosinophilic cytoplasm (due to large number of mitochondria); no clear cytoplasm; similar oncocytic tumors seen in thyroid, parathyroid, salivary glands, adrenals

- majority asymptomatic, occasionally hypertension

√ renal mass of 6–7.5 cm average size (0.1–26 cm)
√ tumor of homogeneous low attenuation / hypoechogenicity (>50%)
√ well-demarcated with pseudocapsule
√ central stellate scar in 30% (in lesions >3 cm in diameter due to organization of central infarction + hemorrhage after tumor growth has outstripped blood supply)
√ invasion of renal capsule / renal vein in large tumors

Angio:
  √ spoke-wheel configuration (80%), homogeneously dense parenchymal phase (71%)
  √ NO contrast puddling / arteriovenous shunting / renal vein invasion

NUC:
  √ photopenic area (tubular cells do not function normally) on Tc-99m DMSA

Dx: percutaneous needle biopsy unreliable
  ◊ Pathologic diagnosis requires entire tumor because well-differentiated renal cell carcinoma may have oncocytic features!

Rx: local resection / heminephrectomy

Prognosis: death from malignancy following surgery (3%)

PAGE KIDNEY

= renin-angiotensin mediated hypertension caused by renal compression in a perinephric / subcapsular location

Etiology: (1) Spontaneous hematoma (most common)
(2) Blunt trauma
(3) Cyst
(4) Tumor

√ stretching + splaying of intrarenal vessels
√ slow arterial washout
√ distortion of renal contour + thinning of renal parenchyma
√ enlarged + displaced capsular artery

PAPILLARY NECROSIS

= NECROTIZING PAPILLITIS = ischemic necrobiosis of medulla (loops of Henle + vasa recta) secondary to interstitial nephritis (interstitial edema) or intrinsic vascular obstruction

Cause:
mnemonic: "POSTCARD"
Pyelonephritis
Obstructive uropathy
Sickle cell disease
Tuberculosis, **T**rauma
Cirrhosis = alcoholism, **C**oagulopathy
Analgesic nephropathy
Renal vein thrombosis
Diabetes mellitus (50%)
also: dehydration, severe infantile diarrhea, hemophilia, Christmas disease, acute tubular necrosis, transplant rejection, postpartum state, high-dose urography, intravesical instillation of formalin, thyroid cancer

Types:
1. Necrosis in situ = necrotic papilla detaches but remains unextruded within its bed
2. Medullary type (partial papillary slough) = single irregular cavity located concentric / eccentric in papilla with long axis paralleling the long axis of the papilla + communicating with calyx
3. Papillary type (total papillary slough)

Phases:
(1) Enlargement of papilla (papillary swelling)
(2) Fine projections of contrast material alongside papilla (tract formation)
(3) Medullary cavitation / complete slough of papilla

- flank pain, dysuria, fever, chills
- ureteral colic
- acute oliguric renal failure
- hypertension
- proteinuria, pyuria, hematuria, leukocytosis

Location: (a) localized / diffuse
(b) bilateral distribution (systemic cause)
(c) unilateral (obstruction, renal vein thrombosis, acute bacterial nephritis)

√ normal or small kidney (analgesic nephropathy) / large kidney (acute fulminant)
√ smooth / wavy renal contour (analgesic nephropathy)
√ calcification of necrotic papilla: papillary / curvilinear / ringlike

IVP:
  √ subtle streak of contrast material extending from fornix parallel to long axis of papilla
  √ centric / eccentric, thin and short / bulbous cavitation of papilla
  √ widened fornix (necrotic shrinkage of papilla)
  √ ring shadow of papilla (outlining detached papilla within contrast material-filled cavity)
  √ club-shaped / saccular calyx (sloughed papilla)
  √ intraluminal nonopaque filling defect (sloughed papilla) in calyx / pelvis / ureter
  √ diminished density of contrast material in nephrogram; rarely increasingly dense
  √ wasted parenchymal thickness
  √ displaced collecting system (enlarged septal cortex from edema)

US:
√ multiple round / triangular cystic spaces in medulla with echo reflections of arcuate arteries at periphery of cystic spaces

Cx: higher incidence of transitional cell carcinoma in analgesic abusers (8 x); higher incidence of squamous cell carcinoma

DDx: (1) Postobstructive renal atrophy
(2) Congenital megacalices (normal renal function)
(3) Hydronephrosis (dilated infundibula)

PARAGANGLIOMA

= rare neuroendocrine tumor arising from paraganglionic tissue found between base of skull and floor of pelvis; belong to amine-precursor-uptake decarboxylation (APUD) system characterized by cytoplasmic vesicles containing catecholamines

Types:
(1) Adrenal paraganglioma arising from adrenal medulla = pheochromocytoma
(2) Aorticosympathetic paraganglioma associated with sympathetic chain + retroperitoneal ganglia
(3) Parasympathetic paraganglioma including branchiomeric **chemodectoma**, vagal + visceral autonomic paraganglioma

- paroxysmal / permanent hypertension (due to secretion of vasopressor amines) with headache, pallor, perspiration, palpitations
- tumor may secrete catecholamine (= **functional paraganglioma**); proportion of hormonally active tumors high for pheochromocytomas, intermediate for aorticosympathetic paragangliomas, low for parasympathetic paragangliomas
- pheochromocytomas secrete norepinephrine + epinephrine, extraadrenal paragangliomas secrete only norepinephrine, some paragangliomas produce dopamine
- determination of free norepinephrine most sensitive with gas chromatography / high-pressure liquid chromatography (HPLC) performed on 24-hour urine specimens

Location of functioning paragangliomas:
(a) adrenal medulla (>80%)
(b) extraadrenal intraabdominal (8–16%)
(c) extraadrenal in head, neck, chest (2–4%)
(d) multiple paragangliomas in up to 20%, particularly in hereditary disorders (multiple endocrine neoplasia syndromes, neuroectodermal syndromes)

Cx: malignant transformation in 2–10%

PAROXYSMAL NOCTURNAL HEMOGLOBINURIA

= rare acquired disorder of nonmalignant bone marrow clones

Cause: infection, transfusion, radiographic contrast material, exercise, drugs, immunization, surgery

Pathophysiology: destruction of abnormally sensitive RBCs by activated complement; complement activation of abnormal platelets + release of thrombogenic material from lysed RBCs

- intravascular hemolysis:
  - hemoglobinuria
  - chronic iron deficiency anemia
- venous thrombosis:
  - acute / chronic renal failure (small vessel thrombosis)

MR:
√ renal cortical iron deposition

Cx: thrombosis due to hypercoagulable state (Budd-Chiari syndrome involving tertiary + secondary venous radicles, portal v., mesenteric v., splenic v.)

PHEOCHROMOCYTOMA

= ADRENAL PARAGANGLIOMA
= rare tumor of chromaffin tissue; responsible for 0.1% of hypertensions

Incidence: 0.13% in autopsy series; sporadic occurrence in 94%

Histo: chromaffin tumor cells contain chromagranin within secretory granules, tumor tends to form "Zellballen" (cell balls)

Age: 5% in childhood

Symptomatology secondary to excess catecholamine production (norepinephrine / epinephrine):
- asymptomatic (9%)
- headaches, sweating, flushing, palpitations, anxiety, tremor
- nausea, vomiting, abdominal pain, chest pain
- paroxysmal (47%) / sustained (37%) hypertension
  (a) elevated catecholamine
  (b) functional renal vasoconstriction
  (c) renal artery stenosis (fibrosis, intimal proliferation, tumor encasement)
- hypoglycemia during hypertensive crisis
- elevated urine vanillylmandelic acid (VMA) in 54%; in up to 22% false-negative result because VMA not excreted

Associated with:
√ pheochromocytomas usually bilateral
(1) Multiple endocrine neoplasia (MEN) in 6%:
  - pheochromocytoma asymptomatic in 50%
  (a) Sipple syndrome = MEN type II (= type 2A)
  = medullary carcinoma of thyroid + parathyroid adenoma + pheochromocytoma
  (b) **Mucosal neuroma syndrome** = MEN type III (= type 2B)
  = medullary carcinoma of thyroid + intestinal ganglioneuromatosis + pheochromocytoma
(2) Neuroectodermal disorder
  (a) tuberous sclerosis
  (b) von Hippel-Lindau disease
  (c) neurofibromatosis
(3) Familial pheochromocytosis
(4) **Carney syndrome** = paraganglioma + gastric epitheloid leiomyosarcoma + pulmonary chondroma

mnemonic: "VEIN"
Von Hippel-Lindau
Endocrine neoplasia (MEA 2)
Inherited (congenital pheochromocytoma)
Neurofibromatosis

Location: anywhere in sympathetic nervous system from neck to sacrum; subdiaphragmatic in 98%
(a) adrenal medulla (85–90%)
(b) extraadrenal (10–15% in adults, 31% in children): para-aortic sympathetic chain (8%), organ of Zuckerkandl at origin of inferior mesenteric artery (2–5%), gonads, urinary bladder (1%)

Multiplicity: 10% in nonfamilial adult cases
32% in nonfamilial childhood cases
65% in familial syndromes

RULE OF TENS ("ten percent tumor"):

10% bilateral / multiple	**10%** extraadrenal
10% malignant	**10%** familial

√ discrete round / oval mass with a mean size of 5 cm (range 3–12 cm)
√ calcifications in 10%

CT: localization accurate in 91% with tumor >2 cm in size; up to 40% in extraadrenal location are missed by CT; 93–100% sensitivity
√ solid / cystic / complex mass with low-density areas secondary to hemorrhage / necrosis
◊ IV injection of iodinated contrast material may precipitate hypertensive crisis in patients not on alpha-adrenergic blockers!

NUC: I-131 / I-123 MIBG (metaiodobenzylguanidine) scan (80–90% sensitivity; 98% specificity)
Useful:
(a) with clear clinical / laboratory evidence of tumor but no adrenal abnormality on CT / MRI
(b) in detecting extraadrenal pheochromocytomas by whole-body scintigraphy

US:
√ well-marginated purely solid (68%) / complex (16%) / cystic tumor (16%)
√ homo- (46%) / heterogeneously (54%) solid tumor: isoechoic + hypoechoic (77%) / hyperechoic (23%) to renal parenchyma

MRI:
√ iso- / slightly hypointense to liver on T1WI
√ extremely hyperintense on T2WI
√ marked homo- / inhomogeneous enhancement

Angio: intraarterial injection CONTRAINDICATED (induces hypertensive crisis)
√ venous blood sampling (at different levels in IVC)
√ localization by aortography in >91%
√ usually hypervascular lesion with intense tumor blush
√ slow washout of contrast material
√ enlarged feeding arteries + neovascularity ("spoke-wheel" pattern)
√ parasitization from intrarenal perforating branches

Cx: malignancy in 2–14%; metastases (may be hormonally active) to bone, lymph nodes, liver, lung

Rx: (1) Surgical removal curative
(2) Alpha-adrenergic blocker (phenoxybenzamine / phentolamine)
(3) Beta-adrenergic blocker (propranolol)
(4) I-131 MIBG used to treat metastases

DDx: nonfunctioning adrenal adenoma, adrenocortical carcinoma, adrenal cyst

POLYCYSTIC KIDNEY DISEASE

Autosomal dominant polycystic kidney disease

= ADULT POLYCYSTIC KIDNEY DISEASE
= Potter Type III
= slowly progressive disease with nearly 100% penetrance and great variation in expressivity

Cause: gene located on short arm of chromosome 16 (in 90%); spontaneous mutation in 10%

Incidence: 1:1,000 people carry the mutant gene; 3rd most prevalent cause of chronic renal failure

Risk of recurrence: 50%

Histo: abnormal rate of tubule divisions (Potter Type III) with hypoplasia of portions of tubules left behind as the ureteral bud advances; cystic dilatation of Bowman capsule, loop of Henle, proximal convoluted tubule, coexisting with normal tissue

Mean age at diagnosis:
43 years (neonatal / infantile onset has been reported); M:F = 1:1
Onset of cyst formation:
— 54% in 1st decade
— 72% in 2nd decade
— 86% in 3rd decade
morphologic evidence in all patients by age 80

Associated with:
(1) Cysts in: liver (25–50%), pancreas (9%); rare in lung, spleen, thyroid, ovaries, uterus, testis, seminal vesicles, epididymis, bladder
(2) Aneurysm: saccular "berry" aneurysm of cerebral arteries (3–13%)
(3) Mitral valve prolapse

- symptomatic at mean age of 35 years (cysts are growing with age)
- hypertension (50–70%)
- azotemia
- hematuria, proteinuria
- lumbar / abdominal pain

√ bilaterally large kidneys with multifocal round lesions; unilateral enlargement may be the first manifestation of the disease
√ cysts may calcify in curvilinear rim- / ringlike irregular amorphous fashion
√ elongated + distorted + attenuated collecting system
√ nodular puddling of contrast material on delayed images
√ "Swiss cheese" nephrogram = multiple lesions of varying size with smooth margins
√ polycystic kidneys shrink after beginning of renal failure, after renal transplantation, or on chronic hemodialysis

NUC: poor renal function on Tc-99m DTPA scan
√ multiple areas of diminished activity, cortical activity only in areas of functioning cortex

US:
√ multiple cysts in cortical region (usually not seen prior to teens)

√ diffusely echogenic when cysts small (children)
√ renal contour poorly demarcated

OB-US:
√ large echogenic kidneys similar to infantile PCKD (usually in 3rd trimester, earliest sonographic diagnosis at 14 weeks), can be unilateral
√ macroscopic cysts (rare)
√ normal amount of amniotic fluid / oligohydramnios (renal function usually not impaired)

Atypical rare presentation:
(a) unilateral adult PCKD
(b) segmental adult PCKD
(c) adult PCKD in utero / neonatal period

Cx:
(1) Death from uremia (59%) / cerebral hemorrhage (secondary to hypertension or ruptured aneurysm [13%]) / cardiac complications (mean age 50 years)
(2) Renal calculi
(3) Urinary tract infection
(4) Cyst rupture
(5) Hemorrhage
(6) Renal cell carcinoma (increased risk)

DDx:
(1) Multiple simple cysts (less diffuse, no family history)
(2) von Hippel-Lindau disease (cerebellar hemangioblastoma, retinal hemangiomas, occasionally pheochromocytomas)
(3) Acquired uremic cystic disease (kidneys small, no renal function, transplant)
(4) Infantile PCKD (usually microscopic cysts)

Autosomal Recessive Polycystic Kidney Disease

= INFANTILE POLYCYSTIC KIDNEY DISEASE
= POLYCYSTIC DISEASE OF CHILDHOOD
= Potter Type I

Incidence: 1: 6,000 to 1:50,000 livebirths; F > M; carrier frequency of 1:112

Path:
@ kidney: abnormal proliferation + dilatation of collecting tubules resulting in multiple 1- to 2-mm cysts
@ liver: periportal fibrosis often with abnormal proliferation + dilatation of bile ducts
@ pancreas: pancreatic fibrosis

A. ANTENATAL FORM (most common)
90% of tubules show cystic changes
• onset of renal failure in utero
• Potter sequence
√ oligohydramnios and dystocia (large abdominal mass)
Prognosis: death from renal failure / respiratory insufficiency (pulmonary hypoplasia) within 24 hours in 75%, within 1 year in 93%; uniformly fatal

B. NEONATAL FORM
60% of tubules show ectasia + minimal hepatic fibrosis + bile duct proliferation
• onset of renal failure within 1st month of life
Prognosis: death from renal failure / hypertension / left ventricular failure within 1st year of life

C. INFANTILE FORM
20% of renal tubules involved + mild / moderate periportal fibrosis
• disease appears by 3–6 months of age
Prognosis: death from chronic renal failure / systemic arterial hypertension / portal hypertension

D. JUVENILE FORM
10% of tubules involved + gross hepatic fibrosis + bile duct proliferation
• disease appears at 1–5 years of age
Prognosis: death from portal hypertension

◊ The less severe the renal findings, the more severe the hepatic findings!

@ Lung
√ severe pulmonary hypoplasia
√ pneumothorax / pneumomediastinum

@ Liver
• portal venous hypertension
√ tubular cystic dilatation of small intrahepatic bile ducts
√ increase in liver echogenicity (from congenital hepatic fibrosis)

@ Kidneys
√ bilateral gross renal enlargement
√ faint nephrogram + blotchy opacification on initial images
√ increasingly dense nephrogram
√ poor visualization of collecting system
√ "sunburst nephrogram" = striated nephrogram with persistent radiating opaque streaks (collecting ducts) on delayed images
√ prominent fetal lobation

CT:
√ prolonged corticomedullary phase

US:
√ hyperechoic enlarged kidneys (unresolved 1- to 2-mm cystic / ectatic dilatation of renal tubules increase number of acoustic interfaces)
√ increased renal through-transmission (high fluid content of cysts)
√ loss of corticomedullary differentiation, poor visualization of renal sinus + renal borders
√ occasionally discrete macroscopic cysts <1 cm
√ compressed / minimally dilated collecting system

OB-US (diagnostic as early as 17 weeks GA):
√ progressive renal enlargement with renal circumference:abdominal circumference ratio >0.30
√ hyperechoic renal parenchyma

√ nonvisualization of urine in fetal bladder (in severe cases)
√ oligohydramnios (33%)
√ small fetal thorax

OB management:
(1) Chromosome studies to determine if other malformations present (eg, trisomy 13 / 18)
(2) Option of pregnancy termination <24 weeks
(3) Nonintervention for fetal distress >24 weeks if severe oligohydramnios present

Risk of recurrence: 25%

DDx: Meckel-Gruber syndrome, adult polycystic kidney disease

POSTERIOR URETHRAL VALVES

= congenital thick folds of mucous membrane located in posterior urethra (prostatic + membranous portion) distal to verumontanum

Type I: (most common) mucosal folds (vestiges of Wolffian duct) extend anteroinferiorly from the caudal aspect of the verumontanum, often fusing anteriorly at a lower level

Type II: (rare) mucosal folds extend anterosuperiorly from the verumontanum toward the bladder neck (nonobstructive normal variant, probably a consequence of bladder outlet obstruction)

Type III: diaphragm-like membrane located below the verumontanum (= abnormal canalization of urogenital membrane)

Incidence: 1:5,000–8,000 boys; most common cause of urinary tract obstruction + leading cause of end-stage renal disease among boys

Time of discovery: prenatal (8%), neonatal (34%), 1st year (32%), 2nd–16th year (23%), adult (3%)

- urinary tract infection (fever, vomiting) in 36%
- obstructive symptoms in 32% (hesitancy, straining, dribbling [20%], enuresis [20%])
- palpable kidneys / bladder in neonate (21%)
- failure to thrive (13%)
- hematuria (5%)

VCUG:
√ vesicoureteral reflux, mainly on left side (<50%)
√ fusiform distension + elongation of proximal posterior urethra persisting throughout voiding
√ transverse / curvilinear filling defect in posterior urethra
√ diminution of urethral caliber distal to severe obstruction
√ hypertrophy of bladder neck
√ trabeculation + sacculation of bladder wall
√ large postvoid bladder residual

US:
√ male gender
√ oligohydramnios (related to severity + duration of obstruction)
√ hypoplastic / multicystic dysplastic kidney (if early occurrence)
√ bilateral hydroureteronephrosis (+ pulmonary hypoplasia)
√ dilated renal pelvis may be absent in renal dysplasia / rupture of bladder / pelviureteral atresia
√ overdistended urinary bladder (megacystis) in 30%
√ thick-walled urinary bladder + trabeculations (best seen after decompression)
√ urine leak: urinoma, urine ascites, urothorax
√ posterior urethral dilatation (on perineal scan)
√ dilated utricle (perineal scan)

OB management:
(1) Induction of labor as soon as fetal lung maturity established if diagnosed during last 10 weeks of pregnancy
(2) Vesicoamniotic shunting may be contemplated if diagnosed remote from term (68% survivors) with good prognostic parameters of fetal urinary sodium <100 mEq/dL + chloride <90 mEq/dL + osmolality <210 mOsm/dL

Cx: (1) Neonatal urine leak (ascites, urothorax, urinoma) in 13%
(2) Neonatal pneumothorax / pneumomediastinum in 9%
(3) Prune belly syndrome
(4) Renal dysplasia (if obstruction occurs early during gestation)

Prognosis: depends upon duration of obstruction prior to corrective surgery; poor prognosis if associated with vesicoureteral reflux; nephrectomy for irreversible damage (13%)

DDx: (1) UPJ obstruction (2) UVJ obstruction (3) Primary megaureter (4) Massive vesicoureteral reflux (5) Megacystis-microcolon-intestinal hypoperistalsis syndrome

POSTINFLAMMATORY RENAL ATROPHY

= acute bacterial nephritis with irreversible ischemia as an unusual form of severe Gram-negative bacterial infection in patients with altered host resistance in spite of proper antibiotic treatment

Histo: occlusion of interlobar arteries / vasospasm
√ small smooth kidney
√ papillary necrosis in acute phase

POSTOBSTRUCTIVE RENAL ATROPHY

= generalized papillary atrophy usually following successful surgical correction of urinary tract obstruction and progressing in spite of relief of obstruction
√ small smooth kidney, usually unilateral
√ dilated calices with effaced papillae
√ thinned cortex

PRIAPISM

= prolonged penile erection not associated with sexual arousal

GU

Types:
(1) Low-flow form = veno-occlusive form (common) characterized by ischemia, venous stasis, pooling of blood within corpora cavernosa
Cause: sickle cell disease, hematopoietic malignancy, hypercoagulable state
• painful erection
√ sluggish intracavernosal flow
√ decreased venous outflow
√ decreased arterial inflow
√ intracavernosal thrombosis
Rx: cavernosal aspiration + irrigation, anticoagulation, shunt procedure
Cx: impotence (in 50% in spite of Rx)
(2) High-flow form (rare)
characterized by unregulated arterial inflow of blood into corpora cavernosa usually due to arterial injury
Cause: perineal / penile trauma
• subsequent persistent painless erection
Color Doppler US:
√ focal blush of abnormal intracavernosal flow adjacent to cavernosal artery from arterial-sinusoidal fistula
Rx: percutaneous transcatheter embolization; arterial ligation

PROSTATE CANCER

Incidence:
8.7% in White males, 9.4% in Black males, increasing with age; less common in Asian population; 200,000 new cases in USA (1994); 2nd most common malignancy in males (after lung cancer); in 35% of men >45 years of age (autopsies)
◊ One out of 11 males will develop prostate cancer!
Risk factors: advancing age, presence of testes, cadmium exposure, animal fat intake
Histo:
nuclear anaplasia + large nucleoli in secretory cells, disturbed architecture, invasive growth
Premalignant change:
(1) Prostatic intraepithelial neoplasia (PIN)
= premalignant lesion frequently associated with invasive carcinoma next to it / elsewhere in the gland
(2) Atypical adenomatous hyperplasia = proliferation of newly formed small acini
Grading (Gleason score 2–10):
1,2,3 glands surrounded by 1 row of epithelial cells
4 absence of complete gland formation
5 sheets of malignant cells
low numbers refer to well-differentiated, high numbers to anaplastic tumors; primary predominant grade (1–5) is added to secondary less representative area with highest degree of dedifferentiation (1–5)
◊ Gleason grading is in only 80% reproducible!

• Categories:
1. Latent carcinoma = usually discovered at autopsy of a patient without signs or symptoms referable to the prostate (26–73%)
2. Incidental carcinoma = discovered in 6–20% of specimens obtained during transurethral resection for clinically benign prostatic hyperplasia
3. Occult carcinoma = found at biopsy of metastatically involved bone lesion / lymph node in a patient without symptoms of prostatic disease
4. Clinical carcinoma = cancer detected by digital rectal examination based on induration / irregularity / nodule

• **Prostate-specific antigen** (PSA = glycoprotein produced by prostatic epithelium) may be elevated

(a) monoclonal radioimmunoassay (Hybritech®); most commonly used: normal value of 0.1–4 ng/mL
◊ Cancers with PSA levels of <10 ng/mL are usually confined to gland!
◊ Cancers of <1 mL usually do not elevate PSA!
◊ 19% of prostate cancers have normal PSA!
◊ 16% of normal men have PSA >4 ng/mL
◊ Benign conditions with PSA elevation: benign prostatic hypertrophy, prostatitis, prostatic intraepithelial neoplasia
(b) polyclonal radioimmunoassay (Proscheck®, Abbott PSA®)
(c) enzyme-linked immunosorbent assay

PSA density = volume corrected PSA level [= prostate volume (height x width x length x 0.523) / Hybritech® PSA value]:
>0.12 (90% sensitive, 51% specific for cancer)
◊ Each gram of malignant prostate tissue results in about 10 times as much PSA in the serum as its benign counterpart!

PSA "velocity" = serial PSA evaluation
◊ If annual rate of PSA increase is >20% / >0.75 ng/mL, the chances of cancer increase sharply!

Staging (American Urological Association System, modified Jewitt-Whitmore staging system):
A No palpable lesion
A_1 focal well-differentiated tumor <1.5 cm
A_2 diffuse poorly differentiated tumor; >5% of chips from transurethral resection contain cancer
B Palpable tumor confined to prostate
B_1 lesion <1.5 cm in diameter confined to one lobe
B_2 tumor ≥1.5 cm / involving more than one lobe
C Localized tumor with capsular involvement
C_1 capsular invasion
C_2 capsular penetration
C_3 seminal vesicle involvement
D Distant metastasis
D_1 involvement of pelvic lymph nodes
D_2 distant nodes involved
D_3 metastases to bone / soft tissues / organs
◊ At initial presentation >75% have stage C + D!
◊ Escape routes through prostatic capsule are: (1) apex, (2) capsular margin at neurovascular bundle posterolaterally, (3) seminal vesicles!

GU

Staging (American Joint Committee on Cancer):

T0	No evidence of primary tumor
T1	Clinically inapparent nonpalpable nonvisible tumor
T1a	<3 microscopic foci of cancer / <5% of resected tissue
T1b	>3 microscopic foci of cancer / <5% of resected tissue
T1c	tumor identified by needle biopsy
T2	Tumor clinically present + confined to prostate
T2a	tumor ≤1.5 cm, normal tissue on 3 sides
T2b	tumor >1.5 cm / in >1 lobe
T2c	tumor involves both lobes
T3	Extension through prostatic capsule
T3a	unilateral extracapsular extension
T3b	bilateral extracapsular extension
T3c	invasion of seminal vesicles
T4	Tumor fixed / invading adjacent structures other than seminal vesicles
T4a	invasion of bladder neck, external sphincter, rectum
T4b	invasion of levator anus muscle and/or fixed to pelvic wall
N	Involvement of regional lymph nodes
N1	metastasis in a single node ≤2 cm
N2	metastasis in a single node >2 and <5 cm / multiple lymph nodes affected
N3	metastasis in a lymph node ≥5 cm
M	Distant metastasis
M1a	nonregional lymph nodes
M1b	bone
M1c	other site

Staging accuracy for local / advanced disease: 46 / 66% for US, 57 / 77% for MR

◊ Extracapsular disease is common at a tumor volume of >3.8 cm^3!

Metastases to lymph nodes:
0% in stage A_1, 3–7% in stage A_2, 5% in stage B_1, 10–12% in stage B_2, 54–57% in stage C; 10% with Gleason grade ≤5, 70–93% with Gleason grade 9 / 10

Location: peripheral zone (70%), transition zone (20%), central zone (10%)

US (21% positive predictive value):
- √ hypoechoic (61%) / mixed (2%) / hyperechoic (2%) lesion; not detectable isoechoic lesion (35%)
- √ asymmetric enlargement of gland
- √ deformed contour of prostate = irregular bulge sign (75% PPV)
- √ heterogeneous texture

Size versus rate of detection:
≤5 mm (36%), 6–10 mm (65%), 11–15 mm (53%), 16–20 mm (84%), 21–25 mm (92%), ≥26 mm (75%)

DDx of hypoechoic lesion: external sphincter, veins, neurovascular bundle, seminal vesicle, dilated duct, small prostatic cyst, acute prostatitis, benign prostatic hyperplasia, dysplasia, sonographic artifact

MR:
- √ extracapsular extension (90% specific, 15% sensitive):
  - √ obliteration of rectoprostatic angle
  - √ asymmetry of neurovascular bundle

Prognosis: increase in tumor volume increases probability of capsular penetration, metastasis, histologic dedifferentiation

Mortality: 2.6% for White males, 4.5% for Black males; 34,000 deaths/1992

Screening recommendation (American Urological Association, American Cancer Society):
PSA level measurements + digital rectal exam annually

Rx:
(1) Watchful waiting
(2) Radical prostatectomy for disease confined to capsule + life expectancy >15 years
(3) Radiation therapy for
  (a) disease confined to capsule, life expectancy <15 years
  (b) disease outside capsule, no spread
(4) Hormonal therapy (orchiectomy, diethylstilbestrol, leuprolide acetate) for widely metastatic disease
(5) Cryosurgery
(6) Chemotherapy

PRUNE BELLY SYNDROME

= EAGLE-BARRETT SYNDROME

= congenital nonhereditary multisystem disorder; almost exclusively in males

TRIAD:
1. Absent / markedly hypoplastic abdominal wall musculature ("prune belly")
2. Nonobstructed markedly distended redundant ureters ± hydronephrosis and variable degree of renal dysplasia
3. Undescended testes (cryptorchidism)

Etiology:
(1) primary mesodermal defect at 7–10 weeks GA
(2) massive abdominal distension secondary to massive ureteral dilatation / urine ascites / intestinal perforation with ascites / cystic abdominal masses / megacystis-microcolon-intestinal hypoperistalsis syndrome causes pressure atrophy of abdominal wall muscles; bladder distension interferes with descent of testes

Incidence: 1:35,000 to 1:50,000 livebirths; almost exclusively in males

Groups:
(1) Obstruction of urethra (most commonly urethral atresia)

Associated with:
malrotation (most common anomaly), intestinal atresia, imperforate anus, skeletal abnormalities (meningomyelocele, scoliosis, pectus carinatum / excavatum, arthrogryposis, clubfoot, dislocation of hip, lower limb hemimelia, sacral agenesis, polydactyly), CHD (VSD, pulmonary artery stenosis), Hirschsprung disease, congenital cystic adenomatoid malformation of lung

√ bladder wall hypertrophy

Prognosis: in 20% death within 1 month; in 30% death within 2 years

GU

(2) Functional abnormality of bladder emptying (more common) no associated abnormalities
√ large floppy urinary bladder
√ large urachal remnant
Prognosis: chronic urinary tract problems

- wrinkled flaccid appearance of hypotonic abdominal wall with bulging flanks (agenesis / hypoplasia of muscles in lower + medial parts of abdominal wall)
- bilateral cryptorchidism
- ± impaired renal function

@ Bladder
√ large distended urinary bladder with bizarre contours
√ intramural bladder calcifications
√ persistence of urachal remnant ± calcification
√ patent bladder neck

@ Urethra
√ elongated + dilated prostatic urethra (absence of prostate)
√ dilated prostatic utricle (= small epithelium-lined diverticulum representing the remnant of the fused caudal ends of the müllerian ducts)
√ urethral obstruction (stenosis / atresia / dorsal chordae / posterior urethral valves)
√ megalourethra
(a) complete / fusiform megalourethra (rare)
= complete absence / marked deficiency of corpora cavernosa + corpus spongiosum
(b) incomplete / scaphoid megalourethra (common)
= congenital absence / deficiency of corpus spongiosum

@ Ureters
√ massively dilated tortuous laterally placed ureters
√ alternating narrowed + dilated ureteral segments
√ vesicoureteral reflux

@ Kidneys
√ asymmetry of renal size + lobulated contours
√ no / mild hydronephrosis
√ caliceal dilatation ± diverticula
√ renal calcifications
√ renal dysplasia with cystic dysplastic changes oligohydramnios, pulmonary hypoplasia (in severe cases)

Cx: respiratory infections (ineffective cough)

PYELOCALICEAL DIVERTICULUM

= PYELOGENIC CYST = PERICALICEAL CYST = CALICEAL DIVERTICULUM
= uroepithelium-lined pouch extending from a peripheral point of the collecting system into adjacent renal parenchyma

TYPE I (calyx):
more common; connected to caliceal cup, usually at fornix; bulbous shape; narrow connecting infundibulum of varying length; few millimeters in diameter; in polar region especially upper pole

TYPE II (pelvis):
interpolar region; communicates directly with pelvis; usually larger and rounder; neck short and not easily identified

Cause:
(1) Developmental origin from ureteral bud remnant (obstruction of peripheral aberrant "minicalyx")
(2) Acquired: reflux, infection, rupture of simple cyst / abscess, infundibular achalasia / spasm, hydrocalyx secondary to inflammatory fibrosis of an infundibulum

√ formation of single / multiple stones (50%) or milk of calcium (fluid-calcium level)
√ opacification may be delayed and remain so for prolonged period
√ mass effect on adjacent pelvicaliceal system if large enough

Cx: recurrent infection
DDx: ruptured simple nephrogenic cyst, evacuated abscess / hematoma, renal papillary necrosis, medullary sponge kidney, hydrocalyx due to infundibular narrowing from TB / crossing vessel / stone / infiltrating carcinoma

PYELONEPHRITIS

= upper urinary tract infection with pelvic + caliceal + parenchymal inflammation
◊ Society of Uroradiology recommends to eliminate the terms (acute focal) bacterial nephritis, lobar nephritis, lobar nephronia, preabscess, renal cellulitis, renal phlegmon, renal carbuncle

Acute pyelonephritis

= episodic bacterial infection of kidney with acute inflammation, usually involving pyelocaliceal lining + renal parenchyma centrifugally along medullary rays

Etiology: infected urine from lower tract during adulthood; in 5% anatomic abnormality (obstruction, stone, stasis); (DDx: chronic atrophic pyelonephritis secondary to vesicoureteral reflux in infancy)

Pathway of infection:
(a) ascending bacterial infection usually due to P-fimbriated E. coli (fimbriae facilitate adherence to mucosal surface): initial colonization of ureter in areas of turbulent flow leads to paralysis of ureteral smooth muscle function with dilatation + functional obstruction of collecting system
(b) vesicoureteral reflux + pyelotubular backflow: P-fimbriated E. coli not necessary for infection
(c) hematogenous spread (12–20%) with Gram-positive cocci

Path: radiating yellow-white stripes / wedges extending from papillary tip to cortical surface in a patchy distribution + sharply demarcated from adjacent spared parenchyma by 48–72 hours
Histo: tubulointerstitial nephritis = leukocytic migration from interstitium into lumen of tubules with destruction of tubule cells by released enzymes, bacterial invasion of interstitium by 48–72 hours
Organism: E. coli > Proteus > Klebsiella, Enterobacter, Pseudomonas
Age: any; M << F
Prevalence: 1–2% of all pregnant women

GU

- fever, chills, flank pain + tenderness
- leukocytosis
- pyuria, bacteriuria, positive urine culture
- ± microscopic hematuria / bacteremia

Indication for imaging:
(1) diabetes (2) analgesic abuse (3) neuropathic bladder (4) history of urinary tract stones (5) atypical organism (6) poor response to antibiotics (7) frequent recurrences

√ normal urogram in 75%!
√ smooth normal / enlarged kidney(s), focal >> diffuse involvement of kidney
√ delayed opacification of collecting system
√ compression of collecting system (edema)
√ nonobstructive ureteral dilatation (rare, effect of endotoxins)
√ immediate persistent dense nephrogram, rarely striated
√ diminished nephrographic density (global / wedge-shaped / patchy)
√ nonvisualization of kidney (in severe pyelonephritis, rare)
√ "tree-barking" = mucosal striations (rare)

CT:
√ area of high attenuation on unenhanced scan (= hemorrhagic bacterial nephritis)
√ thickening of Gerota fascia + thickened bridging septa / stranding (= perinephric inflammation)
√ generalized renal enlargement / focal swelling
  √ obliteration of renal sinus
  √ caliceal effacement
√ thickening of walls of renal pelvis + calices
√ mild dilatation of renal pelvis + ureter
√ soft-tissue filling defect in collecting system (= papillary necrosis, inflammatory debris, blood clot)

CECT:
√ hypoattenuating wedge-shaped area of cortex extending from papilla to renal capsule during nephrographic phase (= lobar segments of hypoperfusion + edema)
√ poor corticomedullary differentiation
√ streaky linear bands of alternating hyper- and hypoattenuation parallel to axis of tubules + collecting ducts during excretory phase (diminished concentration of contrast material in tubules from ischemia + tubular obstruction by inflammatory cells + debris)
√ persistent enhancement on delayed scans in area of earlier diminished enhancement
√ contrast material staining of parenchyma on 3–6 hours delayed scan (= functioning renal parenchyma)

US:
√ majority of kidneys appear normal
√ swollen kidney with decreased echogenicity
√ loss of central sinus echoes
√ wedge-shaped hypo- / isoechoic zones, rarely hyperechoic (due to hemorrhage)
√ thickened sonolucent corticomedullary bands
√ blurred corticomedullary junctions
√ localized increase in size + echogenicity of perinephric fat ± fat within renal sinus
√ localized perinephric exudate
√ thickening of wall of renal pelvis

MR:
√ wedge-shaped foci of high signal intensity on contrast-enhanced fast multiplanar IR images

Renal cortical scintigraphy (Tc-99m DMSA):
√ focal areas of diminished uptake (in 90%)

Prognosis:
(1) Quick response to antibiotic treatment will leave no scars
(2) Delayed treatment of acute pyelonephritis during first 3 years of life can severely affect renal function later in life: decreased renal function, hypertension (33%), end-stage renal disease (10%)

Cx: (1) Renal abscess (near-water density lesion without enhancement)
(2) Scarring of affected renal lobes often in children + in up to 43% in adults
(3) Maternal septic shock (3%)
(4) Premature labor (17%)

Emphysematous pyelitis

= gas confined to renal pelvis + calices
Organism: E. coli
Predisposed: diabetes mellitus (50%); M:F = 1:3
May be associated with: emphysematous cystitis (rare)

- pyuria

√ gas pyelogram outlining pelvicaliceal system
√ dilated renal collecting system (frequent)
√ ± gas in ureters

DDx: reflux of gas / air from bladder or urinary diversion

Emphysematous pyelonephritis

= life-threatening acute fulminant necrotizing infection of kidney and perirenal tissues associated with gas formation
Organism: E. coli (68%), Klebsiella pneumoniae (9%), Proteus mirabilis, Pseudomonas, Enterobacter, Candida, Clostridia (exceptionally rare)
Path: acute and chronic necrotizing pyelonephritis with multiple cortical abscesses
Mechanism: pyelonephritis leads to ischemia + low O_2 tension with anaerobic metabolism; facultative anaerobe organisms form CO_2 with fermentation of necrotic tissue / tissue glucose
Predisposed: immunocompromised patients, esp. diabetics (in 87–97% of cases); ureteral obstruction (in 20–40%)
Average age: 54 years; M:F = 1:2
May be associated with: XGP

- features of acute severe pyelonephritis (chills, fever, flank pain, lethargy, confusion) not responding to Rx
- positive blood + urine cultures (in majority)
- urosepsis, shock
- fever of unknown origin + NO localizing signs in 18%

• multiple associated medical problems: uncontrolled hyperglycemia, acidosis, dehydration, electrolyte imbalance

Location: in 5–7% bilateral

Type I (33%):

√ streaky / mottled gas in interstitium of renal parenchyma radiating from medulla to cortex
√ crescent of subcapsular / perinephric gas
√ NO fluid collection (= no effective immune response)

Prognosis: 69% mortality

Type II (66%):

√ bubbly / loculated intrarenal gas (infers presence of abscess)
√ renal / perirenal fluid collection
√ gas within collecting system (85%)

Prognosis: 18% mortality

√ parenchymal destruction
√ absent / decreased contrast excretion (due to compromised renal function)

US:

√ high-amplitude echoes within renal sinus / renal parenchyma associated with "dirty" shadowing / "comet tail" reverberations

CAVE: (1) kidney may be completely obscured by large amount of gas in perinephric space (DDx: surrounding bowel gas)
(2) gas may be confused with renal calculi

CT (most reliable + sensitive modality):

√ mottled areas of low attenuation extending radially along the pyramids
√ extensive involvement of kidney + perinephric space
√ air extending through Gerota's fascia into retroperitoneal space
√ occasionally gas in renal veins

MR:

√ signal void on T1WI + T2WI (DDx: renal calculi, rapidly flowing blood)

Mortality: 60–75% under antibiotic Rx;
21–29% after antibiotic Rx + nephrectomy;
80% with extension into perirenal space

Rx: antibiotic therapy + nephrectomy; drainage procedure with coexisting obstruction

DDx: emphysematous pyelitis (gas in collecting system but not in parenchyma, diabetes in 50%, less grave prognosis)

Xanthogranulomatous pyelonephritis

= chronic suppurative granulomatous infection in chronic obstruction (calculus, stricture, carcinoma) originating in medulla

Incidence: 681,000 surgically proven cases of chronic pyelonephritis

Organisms: Proteus mirabilis, E. coli, S. aureus

Path: replacement of corticomedullary junction with soft yellow nodules; calices filled with pus and debris

Histo: diffuse infiltration by plasma cells + histiocytes + lipid-laden macrophages (xanthoma cells)

Peak age: 45–65 years; all ages affected, may occur in infants; M:F = 1:3–1:4

• pyuria (95%)
• flank pain (80%)
• fever (70%)
• palpable mass (50%)
• weight loss (50%)
• microscopic hematuria (50%)
• reversible hepatic dysfunction with elevated liver function tests (50%)

◊ Symptomatic for 6 months prior to diagnosis in 40%!

A. DIFFUSE XGP (83–90%)
B. SEGMENTAL / FOCAL XGP (10–17%)
= tumefactive form due to obstructed single infundibulum / one moiety of duplex system
DDx: renal cell carcinoma

√ kidney globally enlarged (smooth contour uncommon) / focal renal mass
√ contracted pelvis with dilated calices
√ totally absent / focally absent nephrogram
√ central obstructing calculus: staghorn calculus in 75%
√ extension of inflammation into perirenal space, pararenal space, ipsilateral psoas muscle, colon, spleen, diaphragm, posterior abdominal wall, skin

Retrograde:

√ complete obstruction at ureteropelvic junction / infundibulum / proximal ureter
√ contracted renal pelvis, dilated deformed calices + nodular filling defects
√ irregular parenchymal masses with cavitation

CT:

√ low attenuation masses replacing renal parenchyma

US:

√ hypoechoic dilated calices with echogenic rim
√ hypoechoic masses frequently with low-level internal echoes replacing renal parenchyma
√ loss of corticomedullary junction
√ parenchymal calcifications are uncommon

Angio:

√ stretching of segmental / interlobar arteries around large avascular masses
√ hypervascularity / blush around periphery of masses in late arterial phase (= granulation tissue)
√ venous encasement + occlusion

DDx: hydronephrosis, avascular tumor

Rx: nephrectomy

PYELOURETERITIS CYSTICA

= hyperplastic transitional epithelial cell collections projecting into ureteral lumen

◊ Indicative of past / present urinary tract infection!

Cause: chronic urinary tract irritant (stone / infection)

Histo: numerous small submucosal epithelial-lined cysts representing cystic degeneration of epithelial cell nests within lamina propria (cell nests of von Brunn) formed by downward proliferation of buds of surface epithelium that have become detached from the mucosa

Organism: E. coli > M. tuberculosis, Enterococcus, Proteus, schistosomiasis
Predisposed: diabetics
Age: 6th decade; more prevalent in women
• no specific symptoms; ± hematuria
Location: bladder >> proximal 1/3 of ureter > ureteropelvic junction; unilateral >> bilateral
√ multiple small round smooth lucent defects of 1–3 mm in size; scattered discrete / clustered
√ persist unchanged for years in spite of antibiotic therapy
Cx: increased incidence of transitional cell carcinoma
DDx: (1) Spreading / multifocal TCC
(2) Vascular ureteral notching
(3) Multiple blood clots
(4) Multiple polyps
(5) Allergic urticaria of mucosa
(6) Submucosal hemorrhage (eg, anticoagulation)

PYONEPHROSIS

= presence of pus in dilated collecting system secondary to infected hydronephrosis
Path: purulent exudate composed of sloughed urothelium + inflammatory cells from early formation of microabscesses + necrotizing papillitis
Organism: most commonly E. coli
US:
√ dispersed / dependent internal echoes within dilated pelvicaliceal system
√ shifting urine-debris level
√ dense peripheral echoes in nondependent location + shadowing (gas from infection)
Cx: 1. XGP
2. Renal abscess
3. Perinephric abscess
4. Fistula to duodenum, colon, pleura

RADIATION NEPHRITIS

Histo: interstitial fibrosis, tubule atrophy, glomerular sclerosis, sclerosis of arteries of all sizes, hyalinization of afferent arterioles, thickening of renal capsule
Threshold dose: 2,300 rads over 5 weeks
• clinically resembling chronic glomerulonephritis
√ normal / small smooth kidney consistent with radiation field
√ parenchymal thickness diminished (globally / focally; related to radiation field)
√ diminished nephrographic density

REFLUX ATROPHY

Cause: increased hydrostatic pressure of pelvicaliceal urine with atrophy of nephrons secondary to long-standing vesicoureteral reflux
√ small smooth kidney with loss of parenchymal thickness
√ widened collecting system with effaced papillae
√ longitudinal striations from redundant mucosa when collecting system is collapsed
◊ Do NOT confuse with reflux nephropathy!

REFLUX NEPHROPATHY

= CHRONIC ATROPHIC PYELONEPHRITIS = ascending bacterial urinary tract infection secondary to reflux of infected urine from lower tract + tubulointerstitial inflammation in childhood (hardly ever endangers adult kidney); most common cause of small scarred kidney
Etiology: 3 essential elements:
(1) Infected urine
(2) Vesicoureteral reflux
(3) Intrarenal reflux
Age: usually young adults (subclinical diagnosis starting in childhood); M < F
• fever, flank pain, frequency, dysuria
• hypertension, renal failure
• may have no history of significant symptoms
Site: predominantly affecting poles of kidneys secondary to presence of compound calyces having distorted papillary ducts of Bellini (= papillae with gaping openings instead of slitlike openings of interpolar papillae)
√ normal / small kidney; uni- / bilateral; uni- / multifocal
√ focal parenchymal thinning with contour depression in upper / lower pole (more compound papillae in upper pole), scar formation only up to age 4
√ retracted papilla with clubbed calyx subjacent to scar
√ contralateral / focal compensatory hypertrophy (= pseudotumor)
√ dilated ureters (secondary to reflux) sometimes with linear striations (redundant / edematous mucosa)
US:
√ focally increased echogenicity within cortex (scar)
Angio:
√ small tortuous intrarenal arteries, pruning of intrarenal vessels
√ vascular stenoses, occlusion, aneurysms
√ inhomogeneous nephrographic phase
NUC (Tc-99m glucoheptonate / DMSA with SPECT most sensitive method):
√ focal / multifocal photon-deficient areas
Cx: 1. Hypertension
2. Obstetric complications
3. Renal failure

RENAL / PERIRENAL ABSCESS

= usually complication of renal inflammation with liquefactive necrosis; 2% of all renal masses
Pathway of infection:
(a) ascending (80%): associated with obstruction (UPJ, ureter, calculus)
(b) hematogenous (20%): infection from skin, teeth, lung, tonsils (S. aureus), endocarditis, intravenous drug abuse
Organism: E. coli, Proteus
Predisposed: diabetics (twice as frequent compared with nondiabetics)
• positive urine culture in 33%
• positive blood culture in 50%
• pyuria, hematuria (absent if abscess isolated within parenchyma)

GU

Renal Abscess

• may have negative urine analysis / culture (in up to 20%)

IVP:
√ focal mass displacing collecting system

CT:
√ hypoattenuating focal renal mass with thick irregular enhancing wall / pseudocapsule
√ ± presence of gas
√ thickened septa + Gerota fascia
√ perinephric fat obliteration

US:
√ slightly hypoechoic (early), hypo- to anechoic (late) mass with irregular margins + increased through-transmission ± septations ± microbubbles of gas

NUC (Ga-67 citrate / In-111 leukocytes):
√ hot spot

DDx: cystic renal cell carcinoma

Carbuncle

= multiple coalescent intrarenal abscesses
◊ Term should not be used in radiology reports!

Perinephric Abscess

Cause: acute pyelonephritis / extension of renal abscess through capsule
Predisposed: diabetics (in 30%), urolithiasis, septic emboli
◊ 14–75% of patients with perinephric abscess have diabetes mellitus!
√ loss of psoas margin / obscuration of renal contour
√ renal displacement
√ focal renal mass
√ scoliosis concave to involved side
√ respiratory immobility of kidney = renal fixation
√ occasionally gas in renal fossa
√ unilateral impaired excretion
√ pleural effusion

RENAL ADENOMA

◊ Small adenoma <3 cm should be considered a renal cell carcinoma of low metastatic potential = borderline renal cell carcinoma!

Incidence: in 7–15–23% of adults (autopsies); most common cortical lesion; increasing with age (in 10% of patients >80 years of age); increased frequency in tobacco users + patients on long-term dialysis

Age: usually >30 years; M:F = 3:1

Types:
(1) Papillary / cystadenoma (38%)
(2) Tubular adenoma (38%)
(3) Mixed type adenoma (21%)
(4) Alveolar adenoma (3%) = precursor of RCC

√ solitary in 75%, multiple in 25%
√ usually <3 cm in size; subcapsular cortical location
√ impossible to differentiate from renal cell carcinoma

Cx: premalignant / potentially malignant

Prognosis: average growth rate of 0.4 (range, 0.2–3.5) cm/year; tumors growing <0.25 cm/year rarely metastasize; tumors growing >0.6 cm/year frequently metastasize

RENAL AGENESIS

Mechanism:
(a) formation failure
= failure of ureteral bud to form
• hemitrigone = absence of ipsilateral trigone + ureteral orifice
(b) induction failure
= failure of growing ureteral bud to induce metanephric tissue
• blind-ending ureter

A. UNILATERAL RENAL AGENESIS

Incidence: 1:600–1,000 pregnancies; M:F = 1.8:1
Risk of recurrence: 4.5%
Often coexisting with other anomalies:
1. Genital abnormalities:
(a) in male (10–15%): hypoplasia or agenesis of testis / vas deferens, seminal vesicle cyst (Zinner syndrome)
(b) in female (25–50%): unicornuate / bicornuate / hypoplastic / absent uterus, absent / aplastic vagina
2. Turner syndrome, trisomy, Fanconi anemia, Laurence-Moon-Biedl syndrome

Location: L > R
√ visualization of single kidney (DDx: additional kidney in ectopic location)
√ absent adrenal gland (11%)
√ absent / rudimentary renal vessels
√ colon occupies renal fossa
√ compensatory contralateral renal hypertrophy (50%)

B. BILATERAL RENAL AGENESIS (= Potter syndrome)

Incidence: 1:3,000 to 1:10,000 pregnancies; M:F = 2.5:1
Risk of recurrence: <1%
• Potter's facies = low-set ears, redundant skin, parrot-beaked nose, receding chin
◊ US-sensitivity is ONLY 69–73% due to decreased visualization from oligohydramnios + discoid-shaped adrenal glands simulating kidneys!
√ severe oligohydramnios (after 14 weeks MA)
√ bilateral absence of kidneys (after 12 weeks), ureters, renal arteries
√ inability to visualize renal arteries by color duplex
√ flattened discoid shape of adrenals (due to absence of pressure by kidney)
√ inability to visualize urine in fetal bladder (after 13 weeks) = bladder agenesis / hypoplasia; negative furosemide test (20–60 mg IV) not diagnostic (fetuses with severe IUGR may not be capable of diuresis)
√ bell-shaped thorax (pulmonary hypoplasia) in mid to late 3rd trimester

√ compression deformities of extremities = clubfoot, flexion contractures, joint dislocations (eg, hip)

Prognosis: stillbirths (24–38%); invariably fatal in the first days of life (pulmonary hypoplasia)

DDx: functional cause of in utero renal failure (eg, severe IUGR)

Potter Sequence

= hypoplasia of lungs, bowing of legs, broad hands, loose skin, growth retardation associated with long-standing severe oligohydramnios

Cause: renal agenesis, urethral obstruction, prolonged rupture of membranes, severe IUGR

RENAL ARTERY STENOSIS

Prevalence: 1–2% of hypertensive individuals; 4.3 % of autopsies; 10% of hypertensive individuals with coronary artery disease; 25% of patients with hypertension that is difficult to control; in 45% of patients with malignant hypertension; in 45% of patients with peripheral vascular disease

Hemodynamic significance determined by:

(a) elevated renin levels in ipsilateral renal vein ≥1.5:1
(b) presence of collateral vessels
(c) greater than 70% stenosis with poststenotic dilatation
(d) transstenotic pressure gradient ≥40 mm Hg
(e) decrease in renal size

◊ 15–20% of patients remain hypertensive after restoration of normal renal blood flow (= renal artery stenosis without renovascular hypertension)!

Cause:

1. Atherosclerosis (60–90%) mostly in proximal 2 cm of main renal artery
   ◊ Any of multiple renal arteries (occurring in 14–28% of the population) may be affected!
2. Fibromuscular dysplasia (10–30%)
3. Others (<10%): thromboembolic disease, arterial dissection, infrarenal aortic aneurysm, arteriovenous fistula, vasculitis (Buerger disease, Takayasu disease, polyarteritis nodosa, postradiation), neurofibromatosis, retroperitoneal fibrosis

Pathophysiology:

decreased perfusion pressure of glomeruli stimulates production of renin in juxtaglomerular apparatus + angiotensin II in kidney; renin converts angiotensinogen into angiotensin I, subsequently converted by angiotensin-converting enzyme (ACE) into angiotensin II which releases aldosterone; aldosterone increases salt + water retention; angiotensin II + aldosterone vasoconstrict vessels (especially intraglomerular efferent arteriole to maintain filtration pressure)

Histo: tubular atrophy and shrinkage of glomeruli

- abdominal / flank pain
- hematuria
- hypertension
- oliguria, anuria
- low urine sodium concentration

Patient selection criteria for screening test:

1. Well-documented recent-onset hypertension with diastolic pressure ≥105 mm Hg
2. Patients <25 years of age developing hypertension
3. Long-standing well-controlled hypertension becoming refractory to an existing regimen
4. Refractory hypertension on an adequate 3-drug regimen (after exclusion of other causes)
5. Generalized vascular disease
6. Hypertension + abdominal bruit
7. Hypertension + elevated serum creatinine (after exclusion of other causes)
8. Hypertension treated with ACE inhibitors developing new / worsening of renal failure

√ normal / decreased renal size (R 2 cm < L; L 1.5 cm < R) with smooth contour
√ vascular calcifications (aneurysm / atherosclerosis)

IVP (60% true-positive rate, 22% false-negative rate):

√ delayed appearance of contrast material (decreased glomerular filtration)
√ increased density of contrast material (increased water reabsorption)
√ delayed washout of contrast material (prolonged urine transit time)
√ lack of distension of collecting system
√ global attenuation of contrast density, urogram may be normal with adequate collateral circulation
√ notching of proximal ureter (enlargement of collateral vessels)

CT:

√ prolongation of cortical nephrographic phase + persistent corticomedullary differentiation
√ CT angiography (2–3 mm collimation, pitch ≤1.5–2.0)

Angiography:

(a) conventional angiography = "gold standard" test
(b) intravenous digital subtraction angiography: does not address hemodynamic significance

NUC (75–95% sensitive, 80–93% specific):

radionuclide renography (preferably with Tc-99m MAG_3) + angiotensin-I converting enzyme (ACE) inhibitor challenge which reduces GFR:

◊ Discontinue ACE inhibitor therapy for >24 hours for enalapril + >48 hours for captopril / lisinopril!

(a) captopril (Capoten®):
   Dose: 1 mg/kg PO for pediatric patient, 25 or 50 mg PO for adult patient
   Technique: radiopharmaceutical injected 60 minutes after ingestion of captopril

(b) enalaprilat (Vasotec®):
   Dose: 0.04 mg/kg IV (up to 2.5 mg maximum)
   Technique:
   } 10 mL fluid/kg body weight PO over 1 hour (to ensure adequate hydration)
   } 5 mCi IV Tc-99m MAG_3 + 20 mg IV furosemide
   } image acquisition for 22 minutes
   } postvoid image (or Foley catheter with PVR)
   } 0.04 mg/kg IV enalaprilat (up to a maximum of 2.5 mg) infused over 5 minutes

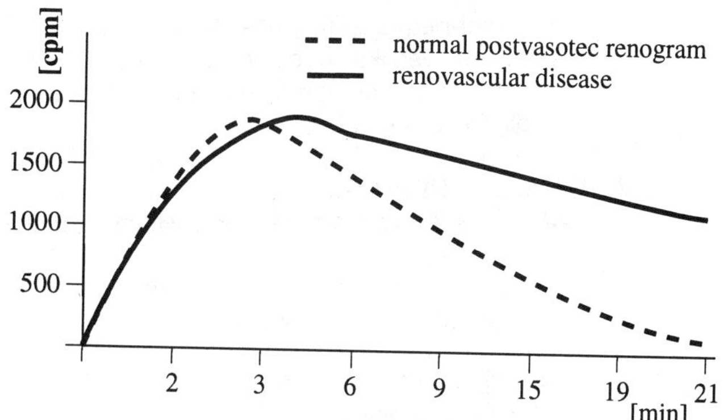

} 5 mCi IV Tc-99m MAG3 + 20 mg IV furosemide injected 15 minutes after injection of enalaprilat
} image acquisition for another 22 minutes

Semiquantitative interpretation of renograms:
√ delay in the time to peak activity + elevation of 3rd phase of curve
√ residual cortical activity (= activity remaining at 20 minutes expressed as percent of peak) >30% with increase by 10% over baseline following ACEI challenge
√ asymmetry of renal uptake <40% of total renal uptake

Duplex US:
(1) direct signs = measurement at site of stenosis
√ peak systolic velocity >150 cm/sec for angles <60° or 180 cm/sec for angles >70° (with many false positives due to suboptimal Doppler angles)
√ ratio of peak renal artery velocity to peak aortic center stream velocity >3.5 (for >60% stenosis; 0–91% sensitive, 37–97% specific)
√ poststenotic spectral broadening ± flow reversal
√ absence of blood flow during diastole (for >50% stenosis)
Problems:
(a) technically inadequate examination (gas, corpulence, respiratory motion) in 6–49%; usually limited to children + thin adults
(b) multiple renal arteries in 16–28%
(c) "false" tracings from large collateral vessels / reconstituted segments of main renal artery
(d) need to visualize entire length of renal artery
(e) transmitted cardiac / aortic pulsations obscure renal artery waveform recordings
(2) indirect signs = measurement of distal arterial segments
√ tardus-parvus pulse:
(a) gradual (= tardus) slope of Doppler waveform during systole = delay in acceleration / pulse rise time of ≥0.07–0.12 sec
(b) attenuated (= parvus) Doppler waveform amplitude = decrease in peak systolic velocity to <20–30 cm/sec

√ acceleration index = tangential inclination of Doppler waveform in early systole of ≥3 m/sec^2 (single most sensitive screening parameter; 76% sensitive + 95% specific at 20% disease prevalence)
√ RI <0.56
√ ΔRI >5% between both kidneys (82% sensitive + 92% specific for stenosis >50%, 100% sensitive + 94% specific for stenosis ≥60%)
√ absent early systolic peak (ESP)
√ segmental arterial flow detectable with renal artery occlusion

False negative: stenosis in accessory renal artery
False positive: coarctation

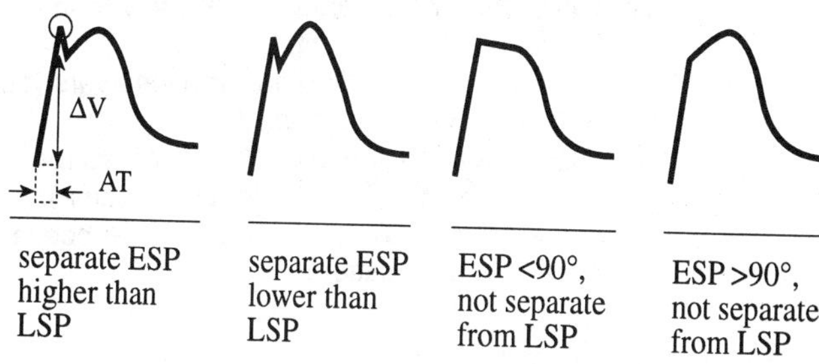

Renal Artery Waveforms With Normal Early Systolic Peaks
AT = acceleration time; ΔV = velocity difference between early systolic peak velocity and late diastolic velocity; ESP = early systolic peak; LSP = late systolic peak; Acceleration index (AI) = ΔV/AT; 98% PPV for exclusion of renal artery stenosis with a normal spectral tracing from each renal pole

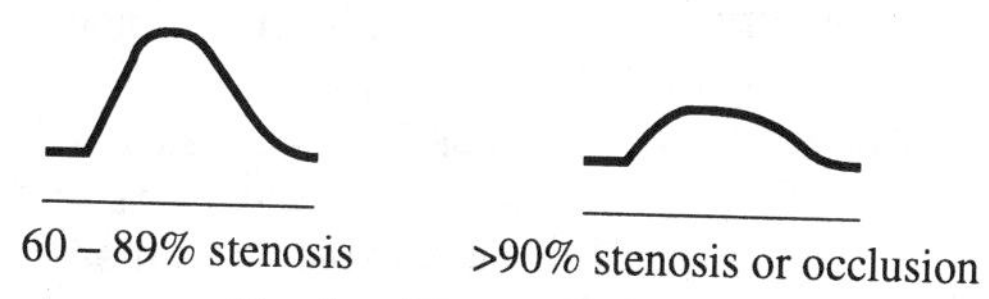

Tardus-Parvus Pattern

Results for >60% renal artery stenosis:

	sensitivity	specificity	accuracy
AT ≥ 0.07 sec	81%	95%	91%
AI < 30 cm/sec^2	89%	86%	87%
absent ESP	92%	96%	95%

Arteriosclerotic renal artery disease
Incidence: in up to 6% of hypertensive patients; most common cause of secondary hypertension
Age: >50 years; M > F
Path: lesion primarily involving intima
- worsening of preexistent hypertension
- abrupt onset of severe hypertension >180/110 mm Hg
- vascular bruit in 40–50% (present in 20% of hypertensive patients without renal artery stenosis)

Associated with: severe arteriosclerosis of aorta, cerebral, coronary, peripheral arteries
Location: main renal artery (93%) + additional stenosis of renal artery branch (7%); bilateral in 31%

GU

√ eccentric stenosis in proximal 2 cm of renal artery, frequently involving orifice
√ decrease in renal length over time (= high-grade renal artery stenosis with risk for occlusion)

Prognosis: progression of atherosclerotic lesion (40–45%) to renal atrophy, arterial occlusion, ischemic renal failure

Cx: azotemia with
(a) bilateral renal artery stenoses
(b) unilateral renal artery stenosis + poorly functioning contralateral kidney
◊ Reversible azotemia may be induced by treatment with angiotensin-converting enzyme inhibitors / sodium nitroprusside!

Rx: (1) Three-step antihypertensive therapy (control of hypertension difficult)
(2) Angiotensin-converting enzyme inhibitors (eg, Captopril PO, Enalaprilat IV)
(3) Renal artery angioplasty (80% success for nonostial lesion, 25–30% for ostial lesion)
(4) Surgical revascularization (80–90% success for any lesion location)

Fibromuscular dysplasia of renal artery

Incidence: 35% of renal artery stenoses; 1,100 patients reported (by 1982) with involvement of renal artery in 60% + extracranial carotid artery in 30%; 25% of all cases of renovascular hypertension

Age: most common cause of renovascular hypertension in children + young adults <30–40 years; M:F = 1:3

Associated with: fibromuscular dysplasia of other aortic branches in 1–2%: celiac a., hepatic a., splenic a., mesenteric a., iliac a., internal carotid a.

- hypertension
- progressive renal insufficiency

Sites: mid and distal main renal artery (79%), renal artery branches (4%), combination (17%); proximal third of main renal artery spared in 98%; bilateral in 2/3; R:L = 4:1

1. INTIMAL FIBROPLASIA (1–2%)
   Path: circumferential / eccentric fibrous tissue between intima + internal elastic lamina
   Age: children + young adults; M:F = 1:1
   Site: main renal artery + major segmental branches; often bilateral
   √ narrow annular radiolucent band
   √ poststenotic fusiform dilatation
2. MEDIAL FIBROPLASIA (60–85%)
   = medial fibroplasia with microaneurysm
   Path: multiple fibromuscular ridges + severe mural thinning with loss of smooth muscle + internal elastic lamina
   Site: mid + distal renal artery + branches; usually bilateral
   √ "string-of-beads" sign = alternating areas of stenoses (weblike constrictions) + aneurysms (which exceed the normal diameter of the artery)
   √ single focal stenosis
3. MEDIAL HYPERPLASIA (5–15%)
   Path: smooth muscle hyperplasia within arterial media
   Site: main renal artery and branches
   √ long smooth tubular narrowing
4. PERIMEDIAL FIBROPLASIA (20%)
   = subadventitial fibroplasia
   Path: fibroplasia of outer 1/2 of media replacing external elastic lamina
   Site: distal main renal artery
   √ long irregular stenosis
   √ beading = NO aneurysm formation (diameter of beads not wider than normal diameter of artery)
5. MEDIAL DISSECTION (5–10%)
   Path: new channel in outer 1/3 of media within external elastic lamina
   Site: main renal artery + branches
   √ false channel, aneurysm
6. ADVENTITIAL FIBROPLASIA (<1%)
   Path: adventitial + periarterial proliferation in fibrofatty tissue
   Site: main renal artery, large branches
   √ long segmental stenosis

Cx: (1) Giant aneurysm
(2) AV fistula between renal artery + vein (in medial fibroplasia)

Prognosis: progression of lesions in 20% causing decline in renal function

Rx: (1) Resection of diseased segment with end-to-end anastomosis
(2) Replacement by autogenous vein graft, excision + repair by patch angioplasty
(3) Transluminal balloon angioplasty (90% success rate with very low restenosis rate)

Neurofibromatosis

Hypertension in neurofibromatosis due to:
(1) Pheochromocytoma
(2) Renal artery stenosis
◊ Renal artery involvement mainly seen in children!

Types:
(a) mesodermal dysplasia of arterial wall with fibrous transformation (common)
(b) narrowing of main renal artery by periarterial neurofibroma (rare)

√ saccular funnel-shaped aneurysm involving aorta / main renal artery
√ smooth / nodular stenosis (mural / adventitial neurofibroma) in proximal renal artery
√ intrarenal aneurysm (rare)

GU

DDx: fibromuscular dysplasia; congenital renal artery stenosis

RENAL CELL CARCINOMA

= RCC = RENAL ADENOCARCINOMA
= HYPERNEPHROMA

Incidence: 80–90% of all renal malignant primaries in adults; 1–3% of all visceral cancers (frequency approximates ovarian cancer, gastric cancer, pancreatic cancer, leukemia)

Age: 6th–7th decade (generally >40 years); peak age of 55 years; may occur in children beyond age of 7 years; M:F = 2–3:1

Path: arises from proximal tubular cells; 30% found incidentally with imaging;

Tumor growth pattern: papillary (5–15%, best prognosis); trabecular / tubular / cystic / solid (poorer prognosis)

Histo: (based on cytoplasmic criteria)
- (a) clear cell = rich in glycogen + lipid content
- (b) granular cell = intensely eosinophilic due to abundant mitochondria
- (c) mixed (most frequent type of RCC)
- (d) sarcomatoid

Predisposed:
- (1) Tobacco; phenacetin abuse
- (2) von Hippel-Lindau disease (10–25%): often small intracystic tumors (hemangioblastoma, retinal angioma, renal cysts)
- (3) Hemodialysis (in 1.4–2.6%)
- (4) Acquired cystic disease of uremia (3.3–6.1%; 7 x increased risk)

Robson Staging Classification:

Stage
- I : tumor confined to within renal capsule
  - √ sharply defined convex interface with perirenal fat
- II : extension into perinephric fat but confined to Gerota fascia = renal fascia
  - √ irregular interface between tumor + fat
- III A : extension into renal vein or IVC
- III B : positive lymph nodes
- III C : extension into renal vein + lymph nodes
- IV A : extension into adjacent organs (other than ipsilateral adrenal)
- IV B : distant metastases

Staging accuracy: 84–91% for CT
82–96% for MR
poor for US

Regional extension: into lymph nodes (9–23%);
into main renal vein (21–35%);
into IVC (4–10%)

Multiple RCC: commonly in von Hippel-Lindau syndrome; bilateral in 1–3%

Metastases:
- bone pain, cough, hemoptysis (as initial symptoms of metastatic disease present in 9%)

◊ 28% of patients have clinically apparent multiple distant metastases at presentation!

Spread to:
lung (55%); lymph nodes (34%); liver (33%); bone (32%); adrenals (19%); contralateral kidney (11%); brain (6%); heart (5%); spleen (5%); bowel (4%); skin (3%); ureter (rare)

Incidence of metastatic disease:
- (a) tumors <3 cm : 2.6%
- (b) tumors 3–5 cm : 15.4%
- (c) tumors >5 cm : 78.6%

- hematuria (56%), flank pain (36%), weight loss (27%), fever (11–15%)
- classic triad of flank pain + gross hematuria + palpable renal mass (4–9%)
- varicocele (2%)
- normochromic normocytic anemia (28–40%)
- Stauffer syndrome (15%) = nephrogenic hepatopathy = hepatosplenomegaly + abnormal liver function in absence of hepatic metastases (? tumor hepatotoxin)
- Paraneoplastic syndromes: erythrocytosis (2%); hypercalcemia (parathormone, prostaglandin, vitamin D metabolites)

√ often lobulated mass, focal bulge in renal contour
√ enlargement of affected part of kidney
√ calcification (8–18%): usually central + amorphous, peripheral + curvilinear in cystic RCC
√ extrinsic compression / displacement / invasion of renal pelvis + calices
√ cysts:
- (a) cystic necrotic tumor (40%)
- (b) cystadenocarcinoma (2–5%)
- (c) renal cell carcinoma in wall of cyst (3%)

√ tumor growth into renal vein / IVC (30%)

IVP:
- √ diminished function (parenchymal replacement, hydronephrosis)
- √ absence of contrast excretion (renal vein occlusion)
- √ pyelotumoral backflow = necrotic part of tumor fills with contrast material

CT:
- √ mostly inhomogeneous enhancement (due to cystic areas or necrosis)
- √ ± subcapsular / perinephric hemorrhage

US:
- √ hyperechoic (50–61%), mostly in small tumors <3 cm (78%), occasionally in large tumors (32%)
- √ markedly hyperechoic, ie, isoechoic to renal sinus fat, (4–12%) in small tumors (DDx: angiomyolipoma)
- √ anechoic rim (in 84% of small hyperechoic RCCs), probably due to pseudocapsule of compressed renal tissue (NOT seen in angiomyolipoma)
- √ isoechoic (30–86%) / hypoechoic (10–12%), mostly in larger tumors
- √ cystic with increase in acoustic transmission (2–13%) due to extensive liquefaction necrosis (DDx: complicated cyst)
- √ inhomogeneity due to hemorrhage, necrosis, cystic degeneration

MRI (best modality to assess stage III + IV disease):
√ low to medium signal intensity on T1WI; hyperintense areas are usually due to hemorrhage
√ heterogeneous signal intensity on T2WI

Angio:
√ typically hypervascular (95%) with puddling of contrast + occasional AV shunting
√ enlarged tortuous poorly tapering feeding vessels
√ coarse neovascularity + formation of small aneurysms
√ parasitization of lumbar, adrenal, subcostal, mesenteric artery branches
√ poorly defined tumor margins

Prognosis:
◊ Tumor stage + histologic grade are the most important prognosticators!
— 5-year survival rates for stages I, II, III, IV are 85–100%, 45–65%, 20–40%, 0–10%;
— 10-year survival rates for stages I, II, III, IV are 56%, 28%, 20%, 3%
— 4.4% 3-year survival rate if untreated;
— papillary carcinomas have better prognosis than nonpapillary carcinomas!
— presence of spindle-shaped cells reduces survival!

Recurrence: in 11% after 10 years

Rx: radical nephrectomy (2–5% operative mortality) / parenchyma-conserving procedure dependent on tumor size + stage + grade

Cystic renal cell carcinoma

A. UNILOCULAR CYSTIC RCC (50%)
= extensive necrosis of a previously solid RCC / intrinsic cystic growth of a cystadenocarcinoma
√ fluid-filled mass without criteria of a renal cyst

B. MULTILOCULAR RCC (30%)
= intrinsic multilocular growth
√ impossible to distinguish from multilocular cystic nephroma

C. MURAL NODULE IN CYSTIC RCC (20%)
(a) asymmetric cystic tumor necrosis
(b) tumor arising in wall of preexisting cyst
(c) tubular dilatation with secondary cyst formation from tumor obstruction

Papillary renal cell carcinoma

Incidence: 5–15% of all RCC
Age: 40–50 years
Path: cystic necrosis + degeneration frequent; familial form associated with trisomy 17
Histo: cells surrounding fronds of fibrovascular stroma; macrophages infiltrating the papillary stalks
√ slow growing well-encapsulated tumor
√ peripheral calcification frequent
√ usually hypovascular
√ little / no contrast enhancement
√ frequently hypoechoic mass
Prognosis: favorable (metastasize late)

RENAL CYST

Simple cortical renal cyst

Acquired lesion possibly secondary to tubular obstruction; accounts for 62% of all renal masses
Incidence: in 1–2% of all urograms; in 3–5% of all autopsies
Age: peak incidence after age 30 years; increasing frequency with age (in 0.22% in pediatric age group, in 50% over age 50)
Path: low cuboidal / flattened epithelium surrounded by 1–2 mm-thick fibrous wall containing clear / slightly yellow serous fluid
May be associated with: tuberous sclerosis, von Hippel-Lindau disease, Caroli disease, neurofibromatosis
√ large and unifocal when peripheral
√ focal attenuation + displacement of collecting system
√ focally replaced nephrogram with smooth margin
√ "beak / claw sign" = effaced wedge of renal parenchyma
√ delicate filamentous often undulating septa (10–15%)
√ curvilinear calcification (1%) in wall / septa

US (90–100% accuracy of US & CT):
√ spherical / ovoid in shape
√ anechoic without internal echoes
√ smooth clearly demarcated walls
√ acoustic enhancement beyond cyst

CT:
√ near-water–density lesion (<20–25 HU), thin wall, smooth interface with renal parenchyma, no enhancement

Cystography:
√ smooth wall, clear aspirate with low lactic dehydrogenase, no fat content

Cx: (1) Hemorrhage in 1–11.5%
(2) Infection in 2.5%
(3) Tumor within cyst in <1%

Atypical / complicated renal cyst

(1) Hemorrhagic cyst
Cause: trauma, varices, bleeding diathesis
• rust-colored puttylike material
√ uni- / multilocular cyst separated by thick septa
√ thick fibrous ± calcified wall
√ fibrin ball inside cyst (rare)

CT:
√ increased density secondary to acute hemorrhage / high protein contents (= hyperattenuating cyst with approximately 50–90 HU)
√ no contrast enhancement

MR:
√ usually iso- to hyperintense on T1WI (owing to methemoglobin) + hyperintense on T2WI (due to lysis of RBCs)
√ variable signal intensities (dependent on amount + acuity of hemorrhage, hemoglobin degradation product, degree of RBC lysis, protein content)
√ hematocrit effect (= RBCs settle to cyst bottom)

(2) Infected cyst
Cause: hematogenous dissemination of bacteria, ascending urinary tract infection
Mean age: 61 years; in 94% females
• history of no response to antibiotic Rx for acute pyelonephritis
• leukocyturia
US:
√ thickened irregular cyst wall (22%)
√ internal septations (11%)
√ wall calcification (occasionally)
√ minute debris either diffusely / fluid-fluid level in dependent portion of cyst
√ amorphous solid conglomerates
√ round sharply marginated lesion
Dx: cyst puncture
DDx: renal abscess, hematoma, renal artery aneurysm, cystic tumor
Rx: surgery, aspiration, serial follow-up

Renal sinus cyst
= PERIPELVIC / PARAPELVIC CYST = PARAPELVIC LYMPHANGIECTASIA = PARAPELVIC LYMPHATIC CYST
= spherical fluid-filled masses intimately attached to renal pelvis without connection to pelvicaliceal system either arising from renal sinus or parenchyma
Incidence: 1.5% (autopsies); 4–6% of all renal cysts
Etiology:
probably ectatic lymphatic channels from lymphatic obstruction; ? posttraumatic extravasation of urine / blood; ? protrusion of parenchymal cysts into sinus; ? mesonephric remnant; ? remnant of wolffian body; ? outpouchings of renal pelvis; ? duplication anomaly
Age: mostly during 5th–6th decade
• almost always asymptomatic
• pain (from obstructive caliectasis)
• renal vascular hypertension (compression of renal arteries)
• clear straw-colored serous fluid
√ soft-tissue density in renal sinus
√ focal displacement + smooth effacement of collecting system
√ stretching of collecting system when generalized (indistinguishable from sinus lipomatosis)
√ rarely curvilinear calcification of cyst wall (4%)
US:
√ anechoic mass(es) with acoustic enhancement, irregular shape
Cx: obstructive caliectasis (rarely hydronephrosis)
Rx: cyst ablation with 95% ethanol if symptomatic
DDx: hydronephrosis

RENAL DYSGENESIS
= undifferentiated tissue of renal anlage
◊ Pathologic NOT radiologic diagnosis
√ renal vessels usually absent; occasionally small vascular channels

RENAL INFARCTION
Causes:
1. Trauma: blunt abdominal trauma, traumatic avulsion of renal artery, surgery
2. Embolism:
(a) Cardiac: rheumatic heart disease with arrhythmia (atrial fibrillation), myocardial infarction, prosthetic valves, myocardial trauma, left atrial / mural thrombus, myocardial tumors, subacute bacterial endocarditis
(b) Catheters: angiographic catheter manipulation, umbilical artery catheter above level of renal arteries
3. Thrombosis:
arteriosclerosis, thrombangitis obliterans, polyarteritis nodosa, syphilitic cardiovascular disease, aneurysm (aorta / renal artery), sickle cell disease
4. Sudden complete renal vein thrombosis

Acute renal Infarction
√ normal / large kidney with smooth contour
√ normal / expanded parenchymal thickness
√ normal / attenuated collecting system, often only opacified by retrograde pyelography
√ absent / diminished nephrogram with cortical rim enhancement, rarely striations
US:
√ diminished echogenicity (within <24 hours)
√ normal echogenicity (echoes appear within 7 days)
NUC (SPECT imaging with Tc-99m DMSA):
√ photon-deficient area

Lobar renal Infarction
Early signs:
√ focal attenuation of collecting system (tissue swelling)
√ focally absent nephrogram (triangular with base at cortex)
Late signs:
√ normal / small kidney(s)
√ focally wasted parenchyma with NORMAL interpapillary line (portion of lobe / whole lobe / several adjacent lobes)
CT:
√ nonperfused area corresponding to vascular division, cortical rim sign
US:
√ focally increased echogenicity

Chronic renal infarction
Path: all elements of kidney atrophied with replacement by interstitial fibrosis
√ normal / small kidney with smooth contour
√ globally wasted parenchyma
√ diminished / absent contrast material density
US:
√ increased echogenicity (by 17 days)
Angio:
√ normal intrarenal venous architecture

√ late visualization of renal arteries on abdominal aortogram

Atheroembolic renal disease

= dislodgment of multiple atheromatous emboli from the aorta into renal circulation (below level of arcuate arteries)

√ normal / small kidneys with smooth contour or shallow depressions

√ wasted parenchymal thickness

√ diminished density of contrast material

CT:

√ patchy nephrographic distribution

Angio:

√ embolic occlusion

Arteriosclerotic renal disease

= disseminated process involving most of the interlobar + arcuate arteries causing uniform shrinkage of kidney

Age: generally over 60 years

Accelerated development in: scleroderma, polyarteritis nodosa, chronic tophaceous gout

• often associated with hypertension (NEPHROSCLEROSIS)

√ normal / small kidneys

√ smooth contour with random shallow contour depressions (infarctions)

√ uniform loss of cortical thickness

√ normal / effaced collecting system (fat proliferation)

√ increased pelvic radiolucency (vicarious sinus fat proliferation)

√ calcification of medium-sized intrarenal arteries

US:

√ increased echogenicity possible

√ increased size of renal sinus echoes (fatty replacement)

Nephrosclerosis

Histo: thickening + hyalinization of afferent arterioles, proliferative endarteritis, necrotizing arteriolitis, necrotizing glomerulitis

• arterial hypertension

(a) BENIGN NEPHROSCLEROSIS

(b) MALIGNANT NEPHROSCLEROSIS (rapid deterioration of renal function)

√ radiographic appearance similar to arteriosclerotic kidney

RENAL LEIOMYOMA

= CAPSULOMA

Prevalence: 5% at autopsy (average size of 5 mm)

Median age: 42 years; M < F

Path: well-circumscribed lesion with mean size of 12 cm containing hemorrhage (17%) / cystic degeneration (27%)

Location: 53% subcapsular, 37% capsular, 10% attached to renal pelvis

Associated with: tuberous sclerosis

• palpable mass (50%), hematuria (20%)

√ well-circumscribed exophytic solid lesion ± cleavage plane between tumor and cortex

DDx: renal leiomyosarcoma, adenocarcinoma

RENAL TRANSPLANT

Frequency: 11,000 transplants per year in USA (1994)

Complications in 10%

◊ Problematic period between 4 days and 3 weeks after surgery!

• hypertension in 50% (from rejection / arterial stenosis)

Prognosis: organ survival at 2 years in 5% for cadaveric Tx / 88% for living related donor grafts; 7–8 years half-life for cadaveric Tx; 13–24 years half-life for Tx from living related donor

Acute tubular necrosis in renal transplant

= primary nonfunction within 72 hours of transplantation followed by improvement within a few days to 1 month secondary to ischemia

— ATN more frequent in cadaveric than living-related donor transplant (donor hypotension)

— ATN greater in transplants with more than one renal artery

— ATN related to length of ischemic interval (prolonged organ storage)

• no constitutional symptoms

• elevated urine sodium

• oliguria may begin immediately after transplantation / may be delayed for several days

US:

√ transient enlargement of transplant

√ transient increase in resistive index

Scintigram:

√ normal / slightly decreased transplant perfusion

√ decreased + delayed radiopharmaceutical uptake

√ delayed / decreased / absent excretion of Tc-99m

DDx: acute rejection (serial renal studies help to differentiate)

Renal Transplant Scintigram

	early study (<24 hours post transplantation)		late study (>5 days post transplantation)	
	flow	excretion	flow	excretion
Acute tubular necrosis	nl / mildly decreased	decreased	nl / mildly decreased	mildly decreased
Hyperacute rejection	absent	absent		
Acute rejection	decreased	decreased	worsening	worsening
Chronic rejection	decreased	decreased	decreased	decreased

GU

Rejection of renal transplant

◊ Most common cause of parenchymal failure!
◊ Rejection occurs in all transplants to some degree!

1. **Hyperacute rejection** (rare)
   = humeral rejection with preformed circulating antibodies present in recipient at time of transplantation, usually following retransplantation
   Path: thrombosed arterioles + cortical necrosis
   Time of onset: within minutes after transplantation
   √ complete absence of renal perfusion + renal function on Tc-99m DTPA scan (DDx: complete arterial / venous occlusion)
   Rx: requires immediate reoperation
2. **Accelerated acute rejection**
   = combination of antibody + cell-mediated rejection
   Time of onset: 2–5 days after transplantation
3. **Acute rejection**
   = cellular rejection predominantly dependent on cellular immunity
   Time of onset: any time, typically within 5 days to 6 months; peak incidence at 2nd–5th week
   Path:
   (a) acute interstitial rejection
   = edema of interstitium with lymphocytic infiltration of capillaries + lymphatics
   (b) acute vascular rejection (rare)
   = proliferative endovasculitis + vessel thrombosis
   • low urine sodium, increase in serum creatinine
   • hypertension
   • oliguria
   • fever
   • tenderness of transplant
   • weight gain
   US (30–50% negative predictive value):
   √ increase in renal volume from edema
   = decreased renal sinus fat with increased cortical thickness (most predictive)
   √ conspicuous pyramids + decreased cortical echogenicity
   √ thickening of pelvoinfundibular wall
   √ diminished echogenicity of renal sinus fat
   Doppler (higher accuracy than morphologic parameters):
   √ initially decrease in resistive index (? autoregulatory mechanism)
   √ increase in resistive index with increasing severity of rejection
   (a) ≤0.70 without any form of rejection (57% negative predictive value)
   (b) >0.90 (100% positive predictive value, 26% sensitivity)
   NUC:
   √ may show decreased renal perfusion + renal function
   √ initially perfusion may be normal with only function decreased (DDx to ATN may not be possible on single study)
   √ subsequent exams (1–3 day intervals) demonstrate decreasing renal perfusion
   √ prolonged excretory phase
   √ poor and inhomogeneous nephrogram
   Angio:
   √ rapid tapering + pruning of interlobar arteries
   √ multiple stenoses + occlusions
   √ nonvisualization of interlobular arteries
   √ prolonged arterial opacification (normally <2 sec)
4. **Chronic rejection**
   = slow relentless progressive process resulting in interstitial scarring + fibrosis
   Path: endothelial proliferation in small arteries + arterioles; glomerular lesions (? recurrence of patient's original glomerulonephritis)
   Time of onset: months to years after transplantation
   √ small kidney
   √ diminished number of intrarenal vessels
   √ vascular pruning / stenoses / occlusions

Causes of Renal Allograft Dysfunction

Immediate to 1st 48 hours	Day 2 to day 7
1. Hyperacute rejection	1. ATN
2. Renal vein thrombosis	2. RVT
3. Discordant size	
>1 week post-op	**Delayed**
1. Acute rejection	1. Chronic rejection
2. ATN	2. Drug toxicity
	3. Obstruction
	4. Infection
	5. Extrinsic compression

Cyclosporine nephrotoxicity

Action: impedes rejection process with narrow therapeutic window
Histo: (a) acutely: damage to tubules, microthrombosis of kidney (secondary to activation of coagulation cascade)
(b) chronically: hyaline deposition within arterial walls
√ NO change in renal size / resistive index

Urologic problems with renal transplant

1. **Ureteral obstruction** (1–10%)
   (a) acute: secondary to technical problems
   (b) late: secondary to ischemia or previous extravasation
   Causes: stricture (most commonly at ureterovesical junction), ureteral kinking, (transient) edema at ureteroneocystostomy, ureteropelvic fibrosis, crossing vessels, blood clot, lymphocele, fungus ball, calculus
   √ pyelocaliectasis
   √ normal resistive index strongly argues against obstruction unless ureteral leak is present

DDx: low-pressure dilatation secondary to denervation + handling of relatively large urine volume (confirmed by Whitaker test)

2. **Urine extravasation** (3–10%)
   Causes:
   (1) Distal ureteral necrosis secondary to interruption of blood supply (early) / vascular insufficiency due to rejection (late)
   (2) Leakage from ureteroneocystostomy site
   (3) Leakage from anterior cystostomy closure site
   (4) Segmental renal infarction
   - high creatinine level in fluid collection

   Prognosis: high morbidity + mortality (death from transplant infection + septicemia)

3. **Pararenal fluid collection**
   Incidence: in up to 50% of transplantations
   Cx: Page kidney
   (1) Lymphocele (10%)
   occur weeks to month after transplantation
   - does not contain creatinine
   - √ mean diameter of 11 cm
   - √ thick septa (50%) + internal debris

   Rx: sclerotherapy with povidone-iodine; long-term catheter drainage / surgical marsupialization
   (2) Urinoma
   - √ rarely septated + smaller than lymphoceles

   (3) Abscess, hematoma
   - small hematomas typically resolve spontaneously within a few weeks
   - √ photopenic region with displacement / impression on kidney / urinary bladder

mnemonic: "HAUL"
Hematoma
Abscess
Urinoma
Lymphocele

Vascular problems with renal transplant

A. PRERENAL

1. **Renal artery stenosis** (1–12%)
   ◊ Transient elevation of velocities in immediate postoperative period is due to vessel wall edema / arterial spasm!
   Time of onset: within 3 years; cadaver kidney > young donor kidney > living-related donor kidney
   (a) short-segment stenosis at anastomosis: technical (75%), use of clamp / cannula, trauma, ischemia of donor vessel
   (b) long-segment stenosis: trauma during allograft harvesting, faulty operative technique, chronic rejection, atherosclerosis, kinking, scar formation
   - recent onset of hypertension
   - renal insufficiency
   - bruit over graft site (occasionally)
   - √ increase in peak systolic velocity >200–210 cm/sec
   - √ 2:1 ratio between peak stenotic and poststenotic velocities
   - √ main renal artery/external iliac artery ratio >3.5
   - √ gross poststenotic turbulence (supportive evidence)
   - √ dampened signals distal to stenosis
   - √ increase in acceleration time (= pulse rise time)

   Angio:
   - √ standard test for detection of arterial stenosis

   Cx (0.5–2.3%): hemorrhage, intimal flap, arteriovenous fistula

2. **Renal artery thrombosis** (1–5%)
   Cause: rejection, faulty surgical technique
   Time of onset: within 1st month
   Predisposed: allografts with disparate vessel size, multiple anastomoses, intramural vessel injury due to faulty handling, rejection
   - early sudden onset of anuria
   - √ global absence of perfusion, uptake, excretion
   - √ segmental infarction due to occlusion of polar artery
   - √ hypo- / hyperechoic area ± cortical thickening
   - √ no flow in affected area

3. **Pseudoaneurysm** (in up to 17%)
   Cause: percutaneous biopsy with vascular injury, faulty surgical technique, perivascular infection
   Location:
   (a) at anastomotic site: due to suture rupture, anastomotic leakage, vessel wall ischemia
   (b) mostly of arcuate arteries within allograft: following needle biopsy, mycotic infection
   - √ hypoechoic mass
   - √ mixed arterial + venous pulsations within mass

   Prognosis: mostly spontaneous regression

4. **Arteriovenous fistula** (in 2%)
   Cause: percutaneous biopsy with vascular injury, faulty surgical technique, perivascular infection
   - hypertension, hematuria, high-output cardiac failure
   - √ high-velocity low-resistance flow in feeding artery
   - √ arterialization of waveform in draining vein
   - √ turbulence + high-frequency velocity shift
   - √ exaggerated focal color around lesion (= perivascular soft-tissue vibration = bruit)

5. **Renal allograft necrosis**
   = total lack of perfusion in an area of renal cortex associated with variable degrees of medullary necrosis

Cause: rejection, surgical ligature, preexistent arterial lesion, severe ATN, prolonged time of warm ischemia

Pattern:
1. Small focal necrosis
2. Large isolated area of infarction (segmental arterial occlusion)
3. Outer cortical necrosis
4. Cortical necrosis with large patches
5. Diffuse cortical necrosis
6. Cortical + medullary necrosis
7. Necrosis of whole kidney (occlusion of main renal artery)

MR:
- √ slightly hyperintense (ischemic necrosis) / hypointense (hemorrhagic necrosis) / isointense area on T2WI
- √ hypointense areas on Gd-DTPA images

US:
- √ hypoechoic (ischemic necrosis) / iso- or hyperechoic (hemorrhagic necrosis) areas
- √ swollen area (probably cortical edema)
- √ absence of arterial perfusion by color duplex (not sensitive for small infarcts / superficial cortical necrosis)
- √ elevated resistive indexes + no / reversed diastolic flow

B. POSTRENAL

1. **Renal / iliac vein thrombosis** (4.2–5%)

   Cause:
   (a) immediately: injury to epithelium at site of renal vein anastomosis, extrinsic compression by urinoma / hematoma / lymphocele
   (b) after 1st week: acute rejection, reduced intrarenal arterial flow

   - • abrupt onset of renal dysfunction
   - • graft tenderness
   - • hematuria, proteinuria
   - √ enlargement of transplant
   - √ prolonged arterial transit time without arterial occlusions + arterial spasms
   - √ diminished cortical perfusion
   - √ absent venous flow
   - √ "U-shaped" / plateau-like reversal of diastolic arterial flow
   - √ decreased systolic rise time

HIGH VASCULAR IMPEDANCE OF RENAL TRANSPLANT

= pulsatility index (A-B/mean) or resistive index (A-B/B) of Doppler signals greater than 1.8 or 0.75–0.80 indicate a reduction in diastolic flow velocity

Causes:

(a) intrinsic vascular obstruction
1. Acute vascular rejection (later stage)
2. Renal vein obstruction

(b) increased intraparenchymal pressure
1. Severe ATN
2. Severe pyelonephritis: CMV, herpes, E. coli, C. albicans
3. Extrarenal compression: large collection, hematoma, discordant size
4. Urinary obstruction (doubted!)
5. Excessive pressure by transducer

Gastrointestinal problems with renal transplant

Incidence: 40%

1. Gastrointestinal hemorrhage
   (a) Upper GI tract bleeding
   gastric erosions, gastric / duodenal ulcers
   Mortality rate: 2–3 x of normal
   (b) Lower GI tract bleeding
   hemorrhoids, pseudomembranous colitis, cecal ulcers, colonic polyps
2. GI tract perforation (3%)
   Causes: spontaneous, antacid impaction, perinephric abscess, diverticular disease
   Location: colon > small bowel > gastroduodenal
   Mortality rate: approaches 75% (because of delayed diagnosis)

Hypertension with renal transplant

◊ Leading cause of death in renal transplant recipient!

Prevalence: up to 60% 1 year after transplantation

Cause:

A. TRANSPLANT RELATED
1. Acute transplant rejection
2. Chronic rejection
3. Cyclosporine toxicity
4. Ureteral obstruction
5. Renal artery stenosis
   (a) accelerated atherosclerosis
   (b) postsurgical fibrosis at anastomosis

B. NOT TRANSPLANT RELATED
1. Renin production of native kidney
2. Original renal disease involving transplant
3. Development of essential hypertension

Aseptic necrosis with renal transplant

Most common long-term disabling complication; femoral head most common site, bilateral in 59–80%

Frequency: 6–15–29% within 3 years after surgery

Time of onset: symptoms develop 5–126 (mean 9–19) months after transplantation

Risk factors:
dose + method of glucocorticoid administration, duration + quality of dialysis before transplantation, secondary hyperparathyroidism, allograft dysfunction, liver disease, previous transplantation, iron overload, increased protein catabolism during dialysis

Pathophysiology of corticosteroid therapy:
(1) Fat embolism (fat globules occlude subchondral end arteries)
(2) Increase in fat cell volume in closed marrow space (increase in intramedullary pressure leads to diminished perfusion)

(3) Osteopenia (increased bone fragility)
(4) Reduced sensibility to pain (loss of protection against excessive stress)

Histo: fragmentation, compression, resorption of dead bone, proliferation of granulation tissue, revascularization, production of new bone

- 40% asymptomatic
- joint pain
- restriction of movement

Sites: femoral head, femoral condyles (lateral > medial condyle), humeral head

√ subchondral bone resorption
√ patchy osteosclerosis
√ collapse / fragmentation of bone

MR with abbreviated T1WI protocol = test of choice!

see page 34 AVASCULAR NECROSIS

Posttransplant lymphoproliferative disorder

= abnormal proliferation of B-cell lymphocytes strongly associated with Epstein-Barr virus infection (in 80%); up to 11% may arise from T-cell lymphocytes

Incidence:
0.6% after bone marrow transplantation,
1–6% after kidney transplantation (in 20% NHL, especially affecting CNS)
1.8–20% after cardiac transplantation

◊ Prevalence of NHL is 35 x greater than in general population!

Cause: sequela of chronic immunosuppression with limited ability to suppress neoplastic activity

Types:
1. Polyclonal B-cell hyperplasia (nearly identical to infectious mononucleosis)
2. Monoclonal non-Hodgkin lymphoma

Time of onset: as early as 1 month after transplantation depending on immunosuppressive regimen

Location:
@ Lymph nodes: tonsils, cervical neck nodes
@ Gastrointestinal tract
Cx: visceral perforation (frequent)
@ Thorax
√ multiple / solitary well-circumscribed pulmonary nodules ± mediastinal lymphadenopathy (DDx: cryptococcosis, fungus, Kaposi sarcoma)
√ patchy airspace consolidation (DDx: edema, infection, rejection)

DDx: lymphoid hyperplasia (spontaneous resolution)

Rx: (1) Antiviral agents (controversial)
(2) Reduction / cessation of immunosuppressive agents
(3) Surgical resection of tumor mass (complete resolution in 63%)

RENAL TRAUMA

Classification:

1. Superficial cortical laceration (75–85%)
(a) Subcapsular hematoma
√ lenticular-shaped area + flattening of subjacent parenchyma
(b) Renal contusion
√ poorly defined area of low attenuation
(c) Small cortical laceration without caliceal disruption
Rx: observation
2. Complete cortical laceration / fracture communicating with caliceal system (10%)
√ extravasation of contrast material
√ separation of renal poles (= fracture)
Rx: clinical judgement required
3. Shattered kidney / injury to the renal vascular pedicle (5%)
√ multiple separate renal fragments (= shattered kidney)
√ lack of enhancement of part / all of kidney
√ ± "rim sign" (= enhancement of renal periphery through intact capsular / collateral vessels)
√ extravasation of contrast material
Rx: surgery

DDx: respiratory motion artifact (low-attenuation area surrounding kidney)

RENAL TUBULAR ACIDOSIS

= clinical syndrome characterized by tubular insufficiency to resorb bicarbonate, excrete hydrogen ion, or both (= nonanion gap metabolic acidosis)

- failure to thrive

Proximal renal tubular acidosis

= TYPE 2 RTA
= impaired capacity to absorb HCO_3^- in proximal tubule leads to presence of bicarbonate in urine at lower plasma levels than normal

Pathogenesis:
? defect in $Na^+/HCO3^-$ cotransport at basolateral membrane; deficit of carbonic anhydrase; parathyroid hormone activates cyclic AMP which inhibits carbonic anhydrase (hypocalcemia of hyperparathyroidism + various types of Fanconi syndrome)

- self-limited acidosis (bicarbonate loss stops once bicarbonate threshold of about 15 mEq/L is reached)
- unimpaired ability to lower urine pH (pH 4.5–7.8 depending on level of plasma bicarbonate) by normal excretion of hydrogen ions
- hypokalemia (due to hyperaldosteronism secondary to decreased proximal resorption of NaCl)

√ rickets / osteomalacia

N.B.: NEVER nephrocalcinosis / nephrolithiasis (due to normal urinary citrate excretion, low urine pH, self-limited less severe acidosis with less calcium release from bone

Dx: bicarbonate titration test, large requirement of alkali to sustain plasma bicarbonate level at 22 mmol/L

Rx: administration of alkali ± potassium ± hydrochlorothiazide

1. INFANTILE TYPE OF PRIMARY PROXIMAL RTA
Age: diagnosed within first 18 months of life; usually male patients

- excessive vomiting in early infancy
- growth retardation (<3rd percentile)
- metabolic hyperchloremic acidosis
- normal quantities of net acid excretion

Prognosis: transient type with spontaneous remission

2. SECONDARY PROXIMAL RTA
   = tubular defect of bicarbonate resorption associated with other tubular dysfunction / generalized disease
   Cause:
   — Fanconi syndrome, cystinosis, Lowe syndrome, hereditary fructose intolerance, glycogen storage disease, galactosemia, tyrosinemia, Wilson disease, Leigh syndrome
   — 1° + 2° hyperparathyroidism, vitamin D deficiency, mineralocorticoid deficiency, osteopetrosis
   — medullary cystic disease, renal transplantation, vascular accident to kidney in newborn period, multiple myeloma, amyloidosis, nephrotic syndrome, cyanotic CHD, Sjögren syndrome
   — intoxication with cadmium, outdated tetracycline, methylchromone, 6-mercaptopurine

Distal Renal Tubular Acidosis

= TYPE 1 RTA (first type discovered)
= impaired ability to secrete H^+ in distal tubule despite low levels of plasma bicarbonate (urine cannot be acidified with pH invariably high at >5.5–6.0)

Pathophysiology:
primary defect of nonacidification of urine followed by
(a) hyperchloremia
small constant loss of serum sodium bicarbonate ($NaHCO_3$) without concomitant loss of chloride (NaCl retention) leads to shrinkage of ECF volume
(b) chronic severe + progressive acidosis (due to inability to excrete the usual endogenously produced nonvolatile acid) leads to
— mobilization of calcium + phosphate from bone (osteomalacia)
— growth retardation
— hypercalciuria (+ 2° hyperparathyroidism)
— loss of phosphate (osteomalacia / rickets)
(c) nephrocalcinosis + nephrolithiasis (due to combination of hypercalciuria + elevated urine pH + marked reduction in urinary citrate)
(d) potassium wastage with hyperkaliuria + hypokalemia (due to constant small loss of sodium bicarbonate in urine, reduction of ECF space, 2° hyperaldosteronism, increase in sodium-potassium exchange in distal tubule)

Path: calcium deposits accompanied by chronic interstitial nephritis with cellular infiltration, tubular atrophy, glomerular sclerosis

- muscle weakness, hyporeflexia, paralysis (due to hypokalemia)
- bone pain (due to osteomalacia)
- polyuria (from defect in urinary concentrating ability as a result of nephrocalcinosis + potassium deficiency)
- low plasma bicarbonate
- hyperchloremic acidosis (from impaired ability to excrete the usual endogenous load of nonvolatile acid)
- alkaline urine (pH >5.0–5.5)
- hypokalemia, loss of sodium
- hypercalciuria (continued mobilization of calcium phosphate from bone due to metabolic acidosis)
- hypocitraturia (increased proximal tubular reabsorption of citrate)

Dx: acid load test with ammonium chloride (NH_4Cl)
Rx: administration of mixture of sodium + potassium bicarbonate
Cx: interstitial nephritis, chronic renal failure (damage from nephrocalcinosis + secondary pyelonephritis), bone lesions, nephrocalcinosis, nephrolithiasis

1. PERMANENT DISTAL RTA
   = ADULT TYPE OF PRIMARY DISTAL RTA
   = BUTLER-ALBRIGHT SYNDROME
   Genetics: mostly sporadic, may be autosomal dominant
   Age: children + adults (usually not diagnosed before age 2); F > M
   - vomiting, constipation, polyuria, dehydration
   - failure to thrive, growth retardation, anorexia
   - polyuria (due to renal concentrating defect)
   - potassium loss resulting in flaccid paralysis
   - bone pain + pathologic fractures in adolescents + adults (from osteomalacia)
   - low serum pH, low bicarbonate concentration
   - elevation of chloride
   - urinary pH of 6.0–6.5

   √ rickets / osteomalacia
   √ moderately retarded bone age
   √ medullary nephrocalcinosis / nephrolithiasis (as early as 1 month of age)

2. SECONDARY DISTAL RTA
   (a) systemic conditions:
   — starvation, malnutrition, sickle cell disease
   — primary hyperthyroidism + nephrocalcinosis, 1° hyperparathyroidism + nephrocalcinosis, vitamin D intoxication, idiopathic hypercalcemia, idiopathic hypercalciuria + nephrocalcinosis
   — amphotericin B nephropathy, toxicity to lithium, toluene sniffing
   — hepatic cirrhosis, fructose intolerance with nephrocalcinosis, Ehlers-Danlos syndrome, Marfan syndrome, elliptocytosis
   (b) renal conditions:
   renal tubular necrosis, renal transplantation, medullary sponge kidney, obstructive uropathy

(c) hypergammaglobulinemic states (? autoimmune process):
idiopathic hypergammaglobulinemia, chronic active hepatitis, hyperglobulinemic purpura, Sjögren syndrome, cryoglobulinemia, systemic lupus erythematosus, lupoid hepatitis, fibrosing alveolitis

[TRANSIENT DISTAL RENAL TUBULAR ACIDOSIS
= INFANTILE TYPE OF PRIMARY DISTAL RTA
= LIGHTWOOD SYNDROME
= transient self-limited form in infancy (only observed within 1st year of life) with unclear pathophysiology, probably due to vitamin D intoxication]

RENAL VEIN THROMBOSIS

Prevalence: 0.5% (autopsy)

Causes:

A. Intrinsic
= thrombotic process begins intrarenally within small intrarenal veins due to acidosis, hemoconcentration, disseminated intravascular coagulation, intrarenal arteriolar constriction reducing venous flow
(a) antenatally: abruptio placentae
(b) newborns: advanced maternal age, glycosuria in infants of diabetic mothers, dehydration from vomiting, diarrhea, enterocolitis, sepsis, polycythemia, birth trauma, left adrenal hemorrhage, prematurity
(c) adults: membranous GN, pyelonephritis, amyloidosis, polyarteritis nodosa, sickle cell anemia, thrombosis of IVC, renal neoplasia (50%), low flow states (CHF, constrictive pericarditis), diabetic nephropathy, lupus nephropathy, sarcoidosis, hypercoagulable states, trauma

B. Extrinsic
umbilical vein catheterization, thrombosis of IVC with extension into renal vein, malpositioned IVC filter, carcinoma of pancreatic tail invading renal vein (in 75%), pancreatitis, lymphoma, retroperitoneal sarcoma, retroperitoneal fibrosis, metastases to retroperitoneum (bronchogenic carcinoma)

mnemonic: "TEST MAN"
Thrombophlebitis
Enterocolitis (dehydration)
Sickle cell disease, **S**ystemic lupus erythematosus
Trauma
Membranous glomerulonephritis
Amyloidosis
Neoplasm

Radiographic appearance varies with:
(1) rapidity of venous occlusion
(2) extent of occlusion
(3) availability of collateral circulation
(4) site of occlusion in relation to collateral pathways

Pathophysiology: formation of collateral channels develops at 24 hours + peaks at 2 weeks after onset of occlusion

Collaterals: ureteral v. to vesicular vv., pericapsular vv. to lumbar vv., azygos v., portal v.
<u>on left</u>: in addition gonadal v., adrenal v., inferior phrenic vv.

Acute Renal Vein Thrombosis

Path: hemorrhagic renal infarction from ruptured venules + capillaries without time for effective development of collaterals

- gross hematuria, proteinuria
- asymptomatic / painful flank mass
- consumptive thrombocytopenia
- anuria, hypertension

√ smooth enlargement of kidney (edema + hemorrhage)
√ initially faint + delayed dense nephrogram
√ little / no pyelocaliceal visualization
√ focal hemorrhagic infarction + capsular rupture

US:
√ enlarged kidney of variably altered echotexture
√ thrombus within distended renal vein / IVC

Doppler-US:
√ venous flow present in segmental veins + collateral veins overlying renal hilum mimicking patency of main renal vein
√ steady / less pulsatile venous flow compared with contralateral main renal vein
√ main renal vein not traceable into IVC on color Doppler
√ elevated resistive index >0.70 ± reversed end-diastolic renal arterial flow in native kidney

CT:
√ prolonged cortical nephrographic phase + persistent corticomedullary differentiation
√ thickened renal fascia + perirenal stranding
√ retroperitoneal hemorrhage

Angio:
√ poorly filling cortical arteries
√ absent inflow from renal vein into IVC
√ thrombus extending into IVC

NUC:
√ no characteristic pattern on sequential functional study

Cx: (1) Pulmonary emboli (50%)
(2) Severe renal atrophy (may show complete recovery)

Subacute Renal Vein Thrombosis

= good collateral drainage; impaired function with steady state or recanalization
√ enlarged edematous boggy kidney
√ slightly diminished / normal nephrographic density (may increase over time)
√ compression of collecting system ("spidery calices")
√ increased renal cortical echogenicity
√ collateral veins allow venous efflux normalizing arterial waveform
√ main renal vein appears small due to recanalization

GU

Chronic renal vein thrombosis

= indolent stage
- 80–90% asymptomatic
- nephrotic syndrome (proteinuria, hypercholesterolemia, anasarca)

√ normal excretory urogram in 25% (with good collateral circulation especially if left side affected)
√ notching of collecting system + proximal ureter
√ retroperitoneal dilated collaterals
√ lacelike intrarenal pattern of calcifications

US:
√ branching linear calcifications (calcified thrombus)
√ small echogenic kidney

CT:
√ renal vein + IVC thrombus (24%); perirenal collaterals
√ prolonged corticomedullary differentiation
√ delayed / absent pyelocaliceal opacification + attenuated collecting system
√ thickening of Gerota fascia

Arteriography:
√ enlarged venous collaterals on delayed images

RETROCAVAL URETER

= CIRCUMCAVAL URETER = abnormality in embryogenesis of IVC with abnormal persistence of right subcardinal vein ventral to ureter (instead of right supracardinal vein, which is dorsal to right ureter)

Incidence: 0.07%; M:F = 3:1
- symptoms of right ureteral obstruction

√ ureteral course swings medially over pedicle of L3/4, passing behind IVC, and then exiting anteriorly between IVC and aorta returning to its normal position
√ varying degrees of hydronephrosis + proximal hydroureteronephrosis

RETROPERITONEAL FIBROSIS

= ORMOND DISEASE = CHRONIC PERIAORTITIS

Path: dense hard fibrous tissue enveloping the retroperitoneum with effects on ureter, lymphatics, great vessels

Causes:

A. PRIMARY RETROPERITONEAL FIBROSIS (2/3)
Probably autoimmune disease with antibodies to ceroid (by-product of aortic plaque, which has penetrated into media) leading to systemic vasculitis;
Associated with fibrosis in other organ systems (in 8–15%):
mediastinal fibrosis, Riedel fibrosing thyroiditis, sclerosing cholangitis, fibrotic orbital pseudotumor
Age: 31–60 years (in 70%); M:F = 2:1
Rx: responsive to corticoids

B. SECONDARY RETROPERITONEAL FIBROSIS (1/3)
(1) Drugs (12%): methysergide, b-blocker, phenacetin, hydralazine, ergotamine, methyldopa, amphetamines, LSD
(2) Desmoplastic response to malignancy (8%): lymphoma, Hodgkin disease, carcinoid, retroperitoneal metastases (breast, lung, thyroid, GI tract, GU organs)
(3) Retroperitoneal fluid collection: from trauma, surgery, infection
(4) Aneurysm of aorta / iliac arteries (desmoplastic response)
(5) Connective tissue disease: eg, polyarteritis nodosa
(6) Radiation therapy

Peak age: 40–60 years; M:F = 2:1
- weight loss, nausea, malaise
- dull pain in flank, back, abdomen (90%)
- renal insufficiency (50–60%)
- hypertension
- leg edema, fever, hydrocele (10%)
- claudication (occasionally)

Location:
plaque typically begins around aortic bifurcation extending cephalad to renal hilum / surrounding kidney; rarely extends below pelvic rim, but may extend caudad to bladder + rectosigmoid

IVP
Classic TRIAD:
(1) ureterectasis above L4/5 (interference with peristalsis)
(2) medial deviation of ureters in middle third, typically bilateral
(3) gradual tapering of ureter (extrinsic compression)
√ usually mild pyelocaliectasis

US:
√ hypoechoic homogeneous mass in para-aortic region / perinephric space

CT:
√ periaortic mass of attenuation similar to muscle
√ may show contrast enhancement (active inflammation)

MR:
√ low to medium homogeneous signal intensity on T1WI
√ heterogeneous high signal intensity on T2WI (with malignancy / associated inflammatory edema)
√ low signal intensity on T2WI (in dense fibrotic plaque)

NUC:
√ gallium uptake during active inflammation

DDx: lymphoma, retroperitoneal adenopathy
Rx: (1) Withdrawal of possible causative agent
(2) Interventional relief of obstruction
(3) Corticosteroids

RETROPERITONEAL LEIOMYOSARCOMA

Incidence: 2nd most common primary retroperitoneal malignancy (after liposarcoma)

Origin:
(a) retroperitoneal space without attachment to organs
(b) wall of inferior vena cava

Age: 5th–6th decade; M:F = 1:6
- abdominal mass, pain, weight loss, nausea, vomiting
- abdominal distension, change in defecation habits, leg edema, back / radicular pain, frequency of urination
- hemoperitoneum, GI bleeding, dystocia, paraplegia

Metastases:
frequently hematogenous, less commonly lymphatic dissemination
(a) common sites: liver, lung, brain, peritoneum
(b) rare sites: skin, soft tissue, bone, kidney, omentum
◊ Distant metastases present at time of diagnosis in 40%

A. EXTRAVASCULAR LEIOMYOSARCOMA (62%)
Path: extraluminal (= completely extravascular) large tumor with extensive necrosis
IVP:
√ large soft-tissue mass with
(a) displacement of kidney + ureter
(b) gas-containing ascending / descending colon
√ well-defined fat plane between mass and kidney
√ obstruction of kidney (ureteral involvement)
√ usually not calcified
US:
√ solid mass isoechoic to liver / rarely hyperechoic
√ complex mass with cystic spaces + irregular walls
CT:
√ lobulated mass often >10 cm in size
√ large cystic areas of tumor necrosis in center of mass
√ areas of high attenuation with recent hemorrhage
MR:
√ intermediate intensity on T1WI with low-intensity areas of necrosis
√ inhomogeneous intermediate intensity on T2WI
Angio:
√ hypervascular tumor with blood supply from lumbar, celiac, mesenteric, renal arteries
√ avascular center surrounded by thick hypervascular rind

B. INTRAVASCULAR LEIOMYOSARCOMA (6%)
Path: intraluminal (= completely intravascular) polypoid mass firmly attached to vessel wall
Location: between diaphragm + renal veins, may extend along entire length of IVC + into heart
√ small solid mass within IVC
√ gradually dilatation / obstruction of IVC
√ intratumoral vascularity confirmed by Doppler
√ irregular enhancement (CT bolus injection)
Cx:
(1) Budd-Chiari syndrome (extension into hepatic veins)
(2) Nephrotic syndrome (extension into renal veins)
(3) Edema of lower extremities (extension into lower IVC without adequate collateralization)
(4) Tumor embolus to lung

C. EXTRA- AND INTRAVASCULAR LEIOMYOSARCOMA (33%)
√ solid / necrotic extraluminal mass not originating from a retroperitoneal organ with contiguous intravascular enhancing component (PATHOGNOMONIC)

D. INTRAMURAL LEIOMYOSARCOMA (extremely rare)

DDx: (1) Liposarcoma (fat content)
(2) Malignant fibrous histiocytoma (not as necrotic)
(3) Lymphoma (nonnecrotic, tends to envelop IVC + aorta)
(4) Primary adrenal tumor
(5) IVC thrombus (no luminal enlargement, no neovascularity)

Rx: (1) Complete excision (resectable in 10–75%)
(2) Partial resection (reduction in tumor size)
(3) Adjuvant chemotherapy / radiotherapy

Prognosis: local recurrence in 40–70%; death within 5 years in 80–87% with extraluminal tumors

RETROPERITONEAL LIPOSARCOMA

= slow-growing tumor that displaces rather than infiltrates surrounding tissue and rarely metastasizes
Incidence: 2nd most common primary retroperitoneal tumor (after malignant fibrous histiocytoma), 95% of all fatty retroperitoneal tumors
Histo:
rarely arising from lipoma
(a) myxoid form (most common): varying degrees of mucinous + fibrous tissue + relatively little lipid
= intermediate differentiation
√ radiodensity between water + muscle
(b) lipogenic form: malignant lipoblasts with large amounts of lipid + scanty myxoid matrix
= well-differentiated
√ radiodensity of fat
(c) pleomorphic type (least common): marked cellular pleomorphism, paucity of lipid + mucin
= highly undifferentiated
√ radiodensity of muscle
Age: most commonly 40–60 years; M > F
Sites: lower extremity (45%), abdominal cavity + retroperitoneum (14%), trunk (14%), upper extremity (7.6%), head & neck (6.5%), miscellaneous (13.5 %)
CT:
√ solid pattern: inhomogeneous poorly marginated infiltrating mass with contrast enhancement
√ mixed pattern: focal fatty areas (-40 to -20 HU) + areas of higher density (+ 20 HU)
√ pseudocystic pattern: water-density mass (averaging of fatty + solid connective-tissue elements)
√ calcifications in up to 12%
Angio:
√ hypovascular without vessel dilatation / capillary staining / laking

Prognosis: most radiosensitive of soft-tissue sarcomas; 32% overall 5-year survival

DDx: malignant fibrous histiocytoma, leiomyosarcoma, desmoid tumor

RHABDOMYOSARCOMA, GENITOURINARY

Frequency:
4–8% of all malignant solid tumors in children <15 years of age (ranking 4th after CNS neoplasm, neuroblastoma, Wilms tumor); 10–25% of all sarcomas; annual incidence of 4.5:1,000,000 white + 1.3:1,000,000 black children

Age: mean age of 7 years; white:black = 3:1; M:F = 6:4

Path: firm fleshy lobulated mass with infiltrative margin / well-defined pseudocapsule; composed of smooth grapelike clusters if intraluminal (= sarcoma botryoides)

Origin: mesenchyme of the urogenital ridge

Histo (Horn & Enterline):
(a) embryonal (56%)
(b) botryoid = "grapelike" (5%) = subtype of embryonal rhabdomyosarcoma
(c) alveolar (20%): worst prognosis
(d) pleomorphic (1%): mostly in adults

DDx: primitive neuroectodermal tumor, extraosseous Ewing sarcoma, synovial cell sarcoma, fibrosarcoma, alveolar soft part sarcoma, hemangiopericytoma, undifferentiated sarcoma, neuroblastoma

Metastases: lung, cortical bone, lymph nodes > bone marrow, liver

◊ Metastases in 10–20% at time of diagnosis!

√ nonspecific imaging features:
- √ homogeneous echogenicity similar to muscle ± hypoechoic areas (hemorrhage / necrosis)
- √ hyperemia with high diastolic flow component
- √ bulky pelvic mass of heterogeneous attenuation
- √ hypointense on T1WI + hyperintense on T2WI with heterogeneous enhancement
- √ diffuse tumor vascularity on angio

Prognosis:
(a) 14–35% 5-year survival with radical surgery
(b) 60–90% 3-year survival with chemotherapy added
◊ Local recurrence is common!

Bladder-prostate rhabdomyosarcoma

Age: in first 3 years of life

Location: trigone of urinary bladder / prostate (tumor infiltrating both)

- abdominal pain + distension (from bladder outlet obstruction)
- urinary frequency + dysuria (from urinary tract infection)
- palpable bladder
- hematuria (unusual late manifestation)
- strangury (= painful urge to void without success)

√ polyploid intraluminal tumor mass
√ elevation of bladder floor with obstruction of bladder neck + large postvoid residual
√ ± invasion of periurethral / perivesical tissues
√ retroperitoneal lymph node enlargement

DDx: polyp, hemangioma, ectopic ureterocele, cystitis

Rhabdomyosarcoma of female genital tract

Location: vulva / vagina (infancy), cervix (reproductive years), uterine corpus (postmenopausal)

- vulvar / perineal / vaginal mass
- vaginal bleeding / discharge / protruding grapelike mass

DDx: polyp, urethral prolapse, hydrometrocolpos, neoplasm

Paratesticular rhabdomyosarcoma

Age: 2nd age peak in adolescence

Location: spermatic cord, testis, penis, epididymis

- painless scrotal swelling
- palpable nontransilluminating intrascrotal tumor
- bulky abdominal (lymphadenopathy)

√ displacement / compression / infiltration of adjacent testis

Prognosis: 73–89% 3-year survival rate

DDx: hydrocele, epididymitis, testicular neoplasm

SCHISTOSOMIASIS

= BILHARZIASIS

Organism: trematodes of species:
S. haematobium (GU tract) >95%;
S. mansoni, S. japonicum (GI tract) <5%

Life cycle:
female parasite discharges eggs into vesicular venules; eggs erode bladder mucosa, are excreted with urine + feces, and hatch in fresh water into larval miracidia; larvae invade snail (= intermediate host) of genus Bulinus, Biomphalaria, Oncomelania; resulting daughter sporocytes develop into cercariae and pass into surrounding body of water; penetrate human skin (usually foot) + pass into lymphatics; schistosome settles in portal veins + migrate into pelvic venous plexus

Incidence: 8% of world's population; 25% in Africa (endemic in South Africa, Egypt, Nigeria, Tanzania, Zimbabwe); endemic in Puerto Rico

@ Urinary tract
- frequency, urgency, dysuria
- hematuria, albuminuria (most common)
- dull flank pain (from hydronephrosis)
- index of infectious severity = urine egg count

Location: lower ureters + bladder

√ bladder wall calcifications (in 4–56%): linear / coarse / floccular, beginning at base, parallel to upper aspect of pubic bone, involving all wall layers
√ vesical calculi (in 39%), distal ureteral calcification (in 34%), honeycombed calcification of seminal vesicles
√ striation of renal pelvis + proximal ureter in 21% (DDx: normal in 3%, other urinary tract infection, vesicoureteric reflux
√ ureterectasis (focal egg deposition leads to peristaltic disorganization)
√ ureteral strictures in distal third (in 8%, L > R), most commonly in intravesical portion with cobra-head configuration = pseudoureterocele); Makar stricture = focal stricture at L3
√ multiple inflammatory pseudopolyps in ureter secondary to granulomas (= bilharziomas)

GU

√ ureteritis cystica
√ ureterolithiasis / ureteritis calcinosa (= punctate / linear calcifications)
√ vesicoureteral reflux
√ polypoid filling defects + mucosal irregularities in urinary bladder (pseudotubercles, papillomas)
√ thick-walled fibrotic "flat-topped" bladder with high insertion of ureters
√ reduced bladder capacity with significant postvoid residual (fibrotic stage)
√ urethral stricture with perineal fistulas

Cx: Squamous cell carcinoma of bladder
Age: 30–50 years (exposed early in childhood with 20-to-30–year latency period)
Location: posterior bladder wall, rarely trigone
√ irregular filling defect
√ discontinuous calcifications

@ GI tract
√ portal hypertension (ova migrating into portal venous system incite fibrosing granulomatous reaction within presinusoidal portal veins)
√ esophageal varices (from portal hypertension)
√ polypoid calcifying bowel lesions (from eggs of S. mansoni trapped in bowel wall + inciting granulomatous reaction)

@ Chest
√ enlargement of RV + pulmonary artery + azygos vein (from portal hypertension)
√ diffuse granulomatous lung lesions

Rx: praziquantel

SCROTAL ABSCESS

Etiology:
(1) Complication of epididymo-orchitis (often in diabetics), missed testicular torsion, gangrenous tumor, infected hematoma, primary pyogenic orchitis
(2) Systemic infection: mumps, smallpox, scarlet fever, influenza, typhoid, syphilis, TB
(3) Septic dissemination from: sinusitis, osteomyelitis, cholecystitis, appendicitis

NUC:
√ marked increase in perfusion, hot hemiscrotum with photon-deficient area representing the abscess on Tc-99m pertechnetate scan (DDx: chronic torsion)
√ increased scrotal uptake with leukocyte imaging

US:
√ hypoechoic / complex fluid collection with low-level echoes (differentiation of intra- from extratesticular abscess location possible)

Cx: (1) Pyocele
(2) Fistulous tract to skin

SEMINAL VESICLE CYST

1. ACQUIRED SEMINAL VESICLE CYST
2. CONGENITAL SEMINAL VESICLE CYST

Associated with: anomalies of ipsilateral mesonephric duct:
(1) Ectopic insertion of ipsilateral ureter (92%) into bladder neck / posterior prostatic urethra / ejaculatory duct / seminal vesicle
(2) Ipsilateral renal dysgenesis (80%)
(3) Duplication of collecting system (8%)

Symptomatic age: 21–41 years
• abdominal / flank / pelvic / perineal pain exacerbated by ejaculation
• dysuria, frequent urination
• epididymitis in prepubertal boy
• recurrent urinary tract infection

√ cystic mass posterior to urinary bladder (DDx: müllerian duct cyst)
√ dilated ejaculatory duct

SINUS LIPOMATOSIS

= PERIPELVIC LIPOMATOSIS
= PELVIC FIBROLIPOMATOSIS
= PERIPELVIC FAT PROLIFERATION

Etiology:
(1) Normal increase with aging and obesity
(2) Vicarious proliferation of sinus fat with destruction / atrophy of kidney (= replacement lipomatosis)
(3) Extravasation of urine leading to proliferation of fatty granulation tissue
(4) Normal variant

Age: 6th–7th decade
√ kidney may be enlarged
√ elongated "spiderlike / trumpetlike" pelvicaliceal system
√ infundibula arranged in "spoke-wheel" pattern
√ parenchymal thickness diminished with underlying disease
√ occasionally focal fat deposit with localized deformity of collecting system

Plain film:
√ diminished sinus density

CT:
√ unequivocal fat values

US:
√ echodense / patchy hypoechoic sinus complex

SQUAMOUS CELL CARCINOMA OF KIDNEY

Incidence: 15% of all urothelial tumors
Path: flat ulcerating mass + extensive induration
Associated with: previous chronic renal infection + calculi (25–60%)
√ stricture that may simulate extrinsic cause
√ ureteropelvic junction obstruction (common)
√ presence of faceted calculi
√ thickening of pelvicaliceal wall (with superficial spread over large areas)
√ arterial encasement + occlusion + neovascularity
√ enlarged pelvic + ureteric arteries
√ occlusion of renal vein / branches (41%)

Prognosis: poor due to early metastases

SUPERNUMERARY KIDNEY

= aberrant division of nephrogenic cord into two metanephric tails (rare)

Associated with: horseshoe kidney, vaginal atresia, duplicated female urethra, duplicated penis

Location: most commonly on left side of abdomen caudal to normal kidney
√ supernumerary ureter may insert into ipsilateral kidney / directly into bladder / ectopic site
Cx: hydronephrosis, pyonephrosis, pyelonephritis, cysts, calculi, carcinoma, papillary cystadenoma, Wilms tumor

TESTICULAR INFARCTION

Etiology: torsion, trauma, leukemia, bacterial endocarditis, polyarteritis nodosa, Henoch-Schönlein purpura
√ diffusely hypoechoic small testis
√ hyperechoic regions (hemorrhage / fibrosis)

TESTICULAR MICROLITHIASIS

Etiology: formation of microliths from degenerating cells in the seminiferous tubules + absence of phagocytosis by Sertoli cells
Prevalence: 0.05–0.60%
May be associated with:
Klinefelter syndrome, cryptorchidism, testicular infarcts, granulomas, subfertility, infertility, testicular germ cell tumor (40%), male pseudohermaphroditism, Down syndrome, pulmonary alveolar microlithiasis
• asymptomatic, uncommon incidental finding
√ 1- to 2-mm hyperechoic foci scattered throughout the testicular parenchyma (PATHOGNOMONIC)
Cx: concurrent germ cell tumor in 40%
DDx: postinflammatory changes, scars, granulomatous changes, benign adenomatoid tumor, hemorrhage with infarction, large-cell calcifying Sertoli cell tumor

TESTICULAR TORSION

= SPERMATIC CORD TORSION
Most common scrotal disorder in children, 20% of acute scrotal pathology
Incidence: 1:160, 10-fold risk in undescended testis compared with normal annual incidence of 1:4,000 males
Etiology:
(1) "Bell and clapper" deformity = high insertion of tunica vaginalis on spermatic cord
(2) Abnormally loose mesorchium between testis + epididymis
(3) Extravaginal torsion involving testis + tunica vaginalis due to loose attachment of testicular tunics to scrotum during in utero + perinatal period
Peak age: newborn period + puberty (13–16 years); <20 years in 74–85%; >21 years in 26%; >30 years in 9%

• sudden severe pain in 100% (frequently at night)
• negative urine analysis (98%)
• history of similar episode in same / contralateral testis (42%)
• nausea + vomiting (50%)
• scrotal swelling + tenderness (42%)
• leukocytosis (32%)
• low-grade fever (20%)
• history of trauma / extreme exertion (13%)
Location: in 5% bilateral (anomalous suspension of contralateral testis found in 50–80%)

Salvage rate:
versus time interval between onset of pain and surgery

80–100%	<6 hours
76%	6–12 hours
20%	12–24 hours
near 0%	>24 hours

spontaneous detorsion in 7%
◊ Irreversible ischemic damage in only 3–6 hours!
Cx: testicular atrophy (in 33–45%)

Acute testicular torsion

• 70% of patients present within first 6 hours from onset of pain
US (80–90% sensitivity):
√ normal grey-scale appearance (within 6 hours)
√ testicular + epididymal enlargement with decreased echogenicity (within 8–24 hours)
√ increase in size of spermatic cord
√ scrotal skin thickening
√ hydrocele (occasionally)
√ loss of spermatic cord Doppler signal (sensitivity 44%, specificity 67%)
Color duplex (86% sensitive, 100% specific, 97% accurate):
√ absence of testicular + epididymal flow (DDx: global testicular infarction)
false-negative: torsion-detorsion sequence, incomplete torsion <360 degrees
Degree of torsion and blood flow:
• testis usually turns medially up to 1,080 degrees
√ diminished blood flow in <180°-torsion at 1 hour
√ absent blood flow in any degree of torsion >4 hours
√ hyperemia after spontaneous detorsion

NUC (98% accuracy):
Dose: 5–15 mCi Tc-99m pertechnetate
Imaging: at 2- to 5-second intervals for 1 minute (vascular phase); at 5-minute intervals for 20 minutes (tissue phase)
√ decreased perfusion / occasionally normal
√ nubbin' sign = bump of activity extending medially from iliac artery denoting reactive increased blood flow in spermatic cord with abrupt termination
√ rounded cold area replacing testis (requires knowledge of side + location of painful testis)

Subacute testicular torsion

= MISSED TESTICULAR TORSION
• symptoms present for >24 hours + less than 10 days
US:
√ enlarged / normal-sized testis with heterogeneous texture
√ increased peritesticular flow without parenchymal blood flow

NUC:
- √ normal NUC angiogram / nubbin sign
- √ "doughnut" sign = decreased testicular activity with rim hyperemia of dartos perfusion

MRI:
- √ enlarged spermatic cord without increase in vascularity
- √ whirlpool pattern (twisting of spermatic cord)
- √ torsion knot = low-signal-intensity focus at point of twist (displacement of free protons from epicenter of twist)

Chronic testicular torsion
- √ small homogeneously hypoechoic testis
- √ enlarged echogenic epididymis

TESTICULAR RUPTURE
◊ Testicular rupture is indication for immediate surgical intervention!

Cause: scrotal trauma

Salvageability:
80–90% if surgical repair occurs <72 hours after trauma;
30–55% if surgical repair occurs >72 hours after trauma

- √ areas of decreased / increased echogenicity (hemorrhage ± necrosis)
- √ loss of testicular outline
- √ thickened scrotal wall (= hematoma)
- √ visualization of fracture plane
- √ hematocele, may show thickening + calcification of tunica vaginalis if chronic
- √ uriniferous hydrocele from perforated bulbous urethra
- √ avascular region on color duplex

Cx: torsion (due to stimulation of a forceful cremasteric contraction)

DDx: laceration, contusion, hemorrhage

TESTICULAR TUMOR
Most common neoplasm in males between ages 25–34 years; 1–2% of all cancers in males; 4–6% of all male genitourinary tumors; 1.5% of all childhood malignancies; 4th most common cause of death from malignancy between ages 15–34 years (12%)

Incidence per year: 3–5:100,000

Peak age: 25–35 years;
prior to puberty: yolk sac tumor + teratoma

Risk factors:
- (a) Caucasian race, Jewish religion
- (b) family history of testicular cancer, previous testicular neoplasm
- (c) testicular maldescent / atrophy (10 x risk); abdominal site affected in 5%, inguinal site affected in 1.25%

- • chronic pain, "heaviness"
- • acute scrotal pain (10%, from intratumoral hemorrhage)
- • enlarging testis, mass
- • gynecomastia, virilization

Location: mostly unilateral; contralateral tumor develops eventually in 8%

Staging:

Stage I	limited to testis + spermatic cord
Stage II	metastases to lymph nodes below diaphragm
II A	nonpalpable
II B	bulky mass
Stage III	metastases to lymph nodes above diaphragm
III A	confined to lymphatic system
III B	extranodal metastases

Metastases: at presentation in 4–14% to lung, liver, bones, brain, lymph nodes

Tumor activity: monitored by levels of α-fetoprotein + β-HCG

Color duplex:
- √ tumor <1.5 cm is hypovascular in 86%, >1.6 cm hypervascular in 95% (DDx: orchitis associated with epididymal hyperemia)
- √ distortion of vessels

Prognosis: >93% 5-year survival rate for stage I; 85–90% 5-year survival rate for stage II; complete remission under chemotherapy in 65–75%; relapse in 10–20% within 18 months

Germ cell tumors (95%)
- (a) one histologic type in 65%
- (b) mixed lesion in 35–40%
  1. Teratocarcinoma (= teratoma + embryonal cell carcinoma)
     2nd most common after seminoma, may occasionally undergo spontaneous regression
  2. Embryonal cell carcinoma + seminoma
  3. Seminoma + teratoma

mnemonic: "YES CT"
Yolk sac tumor
Embryonal cell carcinoma
Seminoma
Choriocarcinoma
Teratoma

A. **SEMINOMA** (40–50%)
Most common tumor in undescended testis
Peak age: 30–40 years
Spread: in 25% metastasized on initial presentation, pulmonary metastases develop in 19%
- • serum a-fetoprotein usually normal
- • b-HCG elevation in 10–15%
- √ usually uniformly hypoechoic + confined within tunica albuginea
- √ may be multifocal

Rx: sensitive to radiation + chemotherapy
Prognosis: 10-year survival rate of 75–85%

B. NONSEMINOMATOUS TUMOR
Age: 20–30 years

GU

1. **Embryonal cell carcinoma** (20–25%)
   Most common component of mixed testicular tumors; often associated with teratoma
   Peak age: 2nd–3rd decade and <2 years
   Spread: most aggressive testicular tumor, visceral metastases
   • ± a-fetoprotein elevation
   √ hypoechoic mass with areas of increased echogenicity + cystic areas (hemorrhage / necrosis)
   √ may show invasion of tunica albuginea
   Prognosis: 30–35% 5-year survival rate

2. **Teratoma** (4–10%)
   2nd most common testicular tumor in young boys
   Prevalence: 1:1,000,000
   Histo: consists of elements from more than one germ cell layer (keratin, muscle, bone, cartilage, hair, mucous glands, neural tissue)
   (a) mature
   (b) immature
   Age: within first 4 years of life; benign in children; may transform into malignancy in adulthood
   • serum a-fetoprotein may be elevated
   √ mixed echotexture with sonolucent + highly echogenic components (markedly heterogeneous)
   Prognosis: metastases to lymph nodes, bone, liver in 30% within 5 years

3. **Choriocarcinoma** (1–3%)
   Peak age: 20–30 years
   Spread: may rapidly metastasize without evidence of choriocarcinoma in primary lesion, pulmonary metastases develop in 81%
   • serum β-HCG always elevated (may produce gynecomastia)
   √ mixed echotexture (hemorrhage, necrosis, calcifications)
   √ indistinct margins of pulmonary metastases (due to hemorrhage)
   Prognosis: nearly 0% 5-year survival rate

4. **Yolk sac tumor = endodermal sinus tumor**
   Equivalent to endodermal sinus tumor of ovary
   Age: predominantly <3 years
   • serum a-fetoprotein always elevated
   √ pulmonary metastases

5. **Epidermoid cyst of testicle** (<1%)
   = "monodermal dermoid" = KERATIN CYST
   = benign teratoma with only ectodermal components
   Age: 20–40 years; primarily in Whites
   Histo: cyst contains keratin, wall composed of fibrous tissue + lined by squamous epithelium
   √ sharply circumscribed encapsulated round lesion of 0.5–10.5 cm in diameter
   √ hyperechoic fibrous cyst wall ± shadowing from calcifications
   √ hypoechoic cyst contents (= laminated keratin debris)
   √ may have echogenic center (= calcification of intraluminal content)
   MRI:
   √ target appearance with fibrous capsule of low signal intensity on T1WI + T2WI, cyst content of high signal intensity on T1WI + T2WI, central calcification with center of low signal intensity

Stromal cell tumors = interstitial cell tumors

(3% of all testicular tumors, 10–30% during childhood)
• precocious virilism (children)
• gynecomastia (adults)
• loss of libido (adults)
• impotence (adults)
Rx: conservative resection under ultrasound guidance

1. **Leydig cell tumor**
   derived from interstitial cells forming the fibrovascular stroma;
   benign:malignant = 9:1
   Peak age: 3–6 years
   • may secrete androgens or estrogens
   • gynecomastia (in almost 50%)
   √ usually hypoechoic nodule
2. **Sertoli cell tumor**
   derived from Sertoli cells of seminiferous tubules, benign:malignant = 9:1
   Peak age: 1st year of life
   • may secrete estrogens
   √ usually hypoechoic nodule
   √ punctate calcifications in large-cell calcifying Sertoli cell tumors
3. Gonadoblastoma = primitive gonadal stroma tumor (exceedingly rare)
   • dysgenetic gonads + abnormal karyotype

Metastases to testis (0.06%)

(a) in adults: prostate > lung > kidney > GI tract, bladder, thyroid, melanoma
  ◊ More common than germ cell tumors in males >50 years of age!
(b) in children: neuroblastoma, Wilms tumor, rhabdomyosarcoma
√ often multiple and bilateral
√ mostly hypoechoic, occasionally echogenic masses

Lymphoma / leukemia of testis

Incidence: 6.7% of all testicular tumors
Lymphoma: most common testicular tumor in men > age 50; bilateral in 40%
Leukemia: 60–92% incidence of testicular involvement on autopsy, 8–16% on clinical examination during therapy, up to 41% on clinical examination after therapy

◊ Occult testicular tumor often found in patients in bone marrow remission ("gonadal barrier" to chemotherapy)
√ uni- / bilateral diffuse / focal process of decreased echogenicity

Burned-out Tumor Of Testis

= AZZOPARDI TUMOR
= spontaneous regression of testicular malignancy (teratocarcinoma)
√ highly echogenic focal lesion ± shadowing (= scarred tumor residue)
√ metastases to retroperitoneum, mediastinum, cervical / axillary / supraclavicular lymph nodes, lung, liver

Second Testicular Tumor

Risk for second tumor in cryptorchidism:
15% for inguinal, 30% for abdominal location
Risk for second contralateral tumor:
500–1,000 x ; bilaterality in 1.1–4.4%;
◊ Development interval between 1st + 2nd tumor: 4 months to 25 years
◊ Detected in 47% by 2 years; in 60% by 5 years, in 75% by 10 years
◊ Synchronous contralateral tumor in 1–3%
US: a testicular abnormality is malignant in only 50%!

TRANSITIONAL CELL CARCINOMA

Prevalence: 85% of all urothelial tumors / primary renal pelvic tumors; 7% of all renal neoplasms
Mean age: 64 years; M:F = 3:1
Pathogenesis: chemical carcinogens act locally on epithelium (= field of change), action enhanced by length of contact time (eg, stasis / diverticulum)
Risk factors:
(1) tobacco (2–3 x)
(2) aniline dye, benzidine, aromatic amines, azo dyes in textile, rubber, printing, plastic manufacturing (lag time of 10 years)
(3) cyclophosphamide therapy (lag time of 6.5 years)
(4) analgesic abuse (8 x increase): phenacetin
(5) Balkan nephritis (= progressive renal failure + development of bilateral and multiple tumors)
(6) recurrent / chronic urinary tract infection
Classification:
(a) exophytic papillary lesion (85%) = frondlike structure with central fibrovascular core lined by epithelial layer
– broad based
– pedunculated
(b) infiltrating: usually higher grade + less common
(c) carcinoma in situ
Grade: usually correlates with stage
1 = cells slightly anaplastic
2 = intermediate features
3 = marked cellular pleomorphism
• frank / microscopic hematuria (72%)
• dull flank pain (22%)
• acute renal colic (due to obstruction)
Location: bladder 30–50 x more common than upper urinary tract

SYNCHRONOUS TCC
(a) both renal pelves (in 1–2%)
(b) both ureters (in 2–9%)
(c) bladder – in 24% of primary renal pelvic involvement
– in 39% of primary ureteral involvement
– in 2% of primary bladder involvement

Renal And Ureteral TCC

Staging:

TNM	AJCC	Description
Tis	0	in situ lesion
Ta	...	noninvasive papillary carcinoma
T1	I	invasion of subepithelial connective tissue
T2	II	confined to muscularis layer
T3	III	invasion of renal parenchyma / peripelvic soft tissues
T4	IV	extension beyond renal capsule

METACHRONOUS TCC IN UPPER TRACT
(a) in 12% of pelvic + ureteral primaries (in 25 months)
(b) in 4% of bladder primaries (2/3 within 2 years, up to 20 years later)

@ Kidney
Site: extrarenal part of renal pelvis > infundibulocaliceal region
IVP:
√ single / multiple filling defects in renal pelvis (35%)
√ "stipple sign" = contrast material trapped in interstices (DDx: blood clot, fungus ball)
√ dilated calyx with filling defect (26%) due to partial / complete obstruction of infundibulum
√ "phantom calyx" = failure to opacify from obstruction
√ ± focal delayed increasingly dense nephrogram
√ "oncocalyx" = caliceal distension with tumor
√ caliceal amputation (19%)
√ absent / decreased excretion with renal atrophy (13%) due to long-standing obstruction of ureteropelvic junction
√ hydronephrosis with renal enlargement (6%) due to tumor obstruction of ureteropelvic junction
US:
√ bulky hypoechoic (similar to renal parenchyma) mass lesion
√ splitting / separation of central renal sinus complex
√ infiltrative without bulge of renal contour
√ ± focal caliceal dilatation
CT (52% accuracy due to overstaging):
√ sessile filling defect in opacified collecting system
√ thickening + induration of pelvicaliceal wall
√ central solid mass in renal pelvis expanding centrifugally
√ compression of renal sinus fat

GU

√ invasion of renal parenchyma (infiltrating growth pattern) with preservation of renal contour
√ coarse punctate calcific deposits (0.7–6.7%) may mimic urinary calculi
√ variable enhancement of tumor

@ Ureter

Site: lower 1/3 (70%), mid 1/3 (15%), upper 1/3 (15%)

IVP:
√ nonfunctioning kidney in advanced tumor (46%)
√ hydronephrosis ± hydroureter (34%)
√ single / multiple ureteral filling defects (19%)
√ irregular narrowing of ureteral lumen

Retrograde:
√ "champagne glass" / "goblet sign" = focal expansion of ureter around + distal to mass (probably secondary to to-and-fro peristalsis of mass)
√ "Bergman sign" = "catheter-coiling sign" = coiling of catheter on retrograde catheterization below the mass

CT:
√ intraluminal soft-tissue mass
√ eccentric / circumferential thickening of ureteral wall

Dx: cytologic analysis of urine (selective lavage, ureteral urine collection, brush biopsy, ureteroscopy

DDx: papilloma (benign lesion, fronds lined by normal epithelium)

Bladder TCC

Incidence: 5% of all new malignant neoplasms; most common tumor of genitourinary tract; 2% of all cancer deaths in United States

Staging

T 1	= A	=	lesions involving mucosa + submucosa
T 2	= B_1	=	invasion of superficial muscle layer
T 3a	= B_2	=	invasion of deep muscular wall
T 3b	= C	=	invasion of perivesical fat
T 4a	= D_1	=	extension to perivesical organs (seminal vesicles, prostate, rectum)
T4b		=	invasion of pelvic / abdominal wall
	D_2	=	distant metastases

Staging accuracy: 50% clinically; 32–80% for CT; 73% for MRI

Overstaging due to: edema following endoscopy / endoscopic resection, fibrosis from radiation therapy

Histo: 80% low-stage superficial papillary neoplasm, (multifocal in 1/3), becoming invasive in 10–20%; 20% invasive (almost always solitary)

Site: lateral wall of bladder, bladder diverticulum (in 0.8–10.8%)

METACHRONOUS TCC OF BLADDER
(a) in 23–40% of primary renal TCC after 15–48 months
(b) in 20–50% of primary ureteral TCC after 10–24 months

IVP (70% accuracy rate):
√ irregular filling defect with broad base and fronds (DDx: rectal gas marginated by Simpson's white line)
√ <1% calcified

CT / US:
√ focal wall thickening
√ papillary mass protruding into lumen

MR (staging modality of choice):
√ TCC isointense to bladder muscle on T1WI + hyperintense on T2WI
√ enhancement differentiates between early enhancing mucosa, submucosa, tumor + nonenhancing muscle

TUBERCULOSIS

Urogenital tract is the second most common site after lung; almost always affects the kidney first as a hematogenous focus from lung / bone / GI tract

Age: usually before age 50; M > F

- gross / microscopic hematuria
- "sterile" pyuria
- frequency, urgency, dysuria
- history of previous clinical TB (25%)

@ EXTRARENAL SIGNS ON ABDOMINAL PLAIN FILM
√ osseous / paraspinous changes of TB (discitis + psoas abscess)
√ calcified granulomas in liver, spleen, lymph nodes, adrenals

@ RENAL MANIFESTATION
◊ Renal TB in 4–8% of patients with pulmonary TB!
◊ Radiographic evidence of pulmonary TB in <50% of patients with renal TB (only 5% have active cavitary TB)!

Location: unilateral renal involvement in 75%
√ displacement of collecting system secondary to tuberculoma (initial infection)
√ dystrophic amorphous calcifications in tuberculomas of renal parenchyma (in 25%)
√ kidney enlarged (early) / small (late) / normal
√ "smudged" papillae = irregularities of surface of papillae
√ "moth-eaten" calyx = caliceal erosion (early change)
√ irregular tract formations from calyx into papilla
√ large irregular cavities with extensive destruction = papillary necrosis
√ dilated calices (hydrocalicosis) often with sharply defined circumferential narrowings (infundibular strictures) at one / several sites (most common finding)
√ renal calculi (in 10%)
√ "putty kidney" = tuberculous pyonephrosis from ureteral stricture
√ autonephrectomy = small shrunken scarred nonfunctioning kidney ± dystrophic calcifications
√ infection may extend into peri- / pararenal space + psoas

@ URETERAL MANIFESTATION
Always with evidence of renal involvement as it spreads from kidney
Location: either end of ureter (most commonly distal 1/3), usually asymmetric, may be unilateral
√ ureteral filling defects (= mucosal granulomas)
√ "saw-tooth ureter" = irregular jagged contour secondary to dilatation + multiple small mucosal ulcerations + wall edema (early changes)
√ strictures (late changes):
"beaded ureter" = alternating areas of strictures + dilatations
"corkscrew ureter" = marked tortuosity with strictures + dilatations
"pipestem ureter" = rigid aperistaltic short thick and straight ureter
√ vesicoureteral reflux through "fixed" patulous orifice
√ ureteral calcifications uncommon (usually in distal portion)

@ BLADDER MANIFESTATION
Infection from renal source causing interstitial cystitis
√ thickened bladder wall (= muscle hypertrophy + inflammatory tuberculomas)
√ bladder wall ulcerations
√ "shrunken bladder" = scarred bladder with diminished capacity
√ bladder wall calcifications (rare)
Cx: fistula / sinus tract

@ SEMINAL VESICULAR + EPIDIDYMAL MANIFESTATION
Hematogenous infection (NOT ascending)
√ calcifications in 10% (diabetes more common cause)
DDx: brucellosis, fungal infections (identical picture)

UNICALICEAL (UNIPAPILLARY) KIDNEY
Path: OLIGOMEGANEPHRONIA = reduced number of nephrons and enlargement of glomeruli
Associated with: absence of contralateral kidney, other anomalies
- hypertension
- proteinuria
- azotemia

URACHAL ANOMALIES
urachus = median umbilical ligament = thick fibrous cord as the remnant of the allantois (= endodermal outgrowth from yolk sac into stalk) which regresses at 5th month of development

A. PATENT URACHUS
= fistula between bladder and umbilicus
Incidence: 1:200,000 live births
- urine draining from umbilicus

B. URACHAL SINUS
= urachus patent only at umbilicus
Associated with: urachal cyst
- umbilical mass / inflammation ± drainage

√ thickened tubular structure with echogenic center

C. URACHAL DIVERTICULUM (3%)
= urachus communicates only with bladder dome

D. URACHAL CYST (30%)
= gradually enlarging cyst due to closure of both ends of urachus
Incidence: 1:5,000 (at autopsy)
- asymptomatic in children unless rupture occurs
- symptomatic in adults due to enlargement / infection

√ cystic extraperitoneal mass

E. ALTERNATING SINUS
= cystic dilatation of urachus periodically emptying into bladder / umbilicus

Cx: infection (23%), intestinal obstruction, hemorrhage into cyst, peritonitis from rupture, malignant degeneration

URACHAL CARCINOMA
= rare tumor arising from the urachus (vestigial remnant of cloaca + allantois) within space of Retzius
Incidence: 0.2–0.34% of all bladder cancers; 20–40% of all primary bladder adenocarcinomas
Histo:
(a) adenocarcinoma (84%) from malignant transformation of columnar metaplasia, in 75% mucin producing
(b) TCC (3%), sarcoma, squamous cell carcinoma
◊ 75% of urachal neoplasms in patients <20 years of age are sarcomas!
Age: 41–70 years; M:F = 3:1
- suprapubic mass, abdominal pain
- hematuria (71%)
- discharge of blood, pus, mucus from umbilicus
- irritative voiding symptoms
- mucous micturition (25%)

Stage:
I cancer limited to urachus
II invasion limited to urachus
III A local invasion of bladder
III B invasion of abdominal wall
III C invasion of peritoneum
III D invasion of other viscera
IV A metastases to local lymph nodes
IV B distant metastases

Location: supravesical, midline, anterior (80%), in space of Retzius (bounded by transversalis fascia ventrally + peritoneum dorsally)
√ mass anterosuperior to vesical dome with predominantly muscular / extravesical involvement
√ invasion of bladder dome (88%)
√ low-attenuation mass in 60% (mucin)
√ often peripheral psammomatous PATHOGNOMONIC calcifications (70%)
√ markedly increased signal intensity on T2WI
Prognosis: 7–16% 5-year survival rate

GU

URETERAL DUPLICATION

= RENAL DUPLICATION

Complete duplication

Cause: second ureteral bud arising from mesonephric duct leading to complete ureteral duplication

Prevalence: 0.2% of livebirths; M:F = 1:2; in 15–40% bilateral

Risk of recurrence: 12% in 1st-degree relatives

Embryology: ureters develop from separate ureteric buds originating from a single Wolffian duct

Weigert-Meyer rule

= lower moiety ureter is incorporated into developing bladder first + ascends during bladder growth + enters bladder at trigone + drains lower pole and interpolar portion; upper moiety ureter remains with wolffian duct longer + passes through bladder wall + inserts inferior and medial to lower moiety ureter below the level of the trigone / into any wolffian duct derivative

Cx:
(1) Vesicoureteral reflux (most commonly)
(2) Ectopic ureteral insertion
(3) Ectopic ureterocele
(4) Ureteropelvic junction obstruction of lower pole

UPPER MOIETY

◊ Subject to ureteral obstruction from ectopic ureteral insertion / ectopic ureterocele / aberrant artery crossing!

Associated with: significant renal dysplasia

Site of insertion of ectopic ureter

M: suprasphincteric insertion:
low in bladder, bladder neck, prostatic urethra, vas deferens, seminal vesicle (seminal vesical cyst), ejaculatory duct
- NO ENURESIS in males as insertion is always above external sphincter
- epididymitis / orchitis in preadolescent male
- urge incontinence (insertion into posterior urethra)

F: infrasphincteric insertion:
distal urethra, vaginal vestibule, vagina, cervix, uterus, fallopian tube, rectum
- WETTING in upright females if insertion is below external sphincter (common)
- intermittent / constant dribbling

LOWER MOIETY

◊ Subject to VESICOURETERAL REFLUX due to its shortened ureteral tunnel at bladder insertion

Cx: lower pole of duplex kidney may atrophy (in 50%) secondary to chronic pyelonephritis = reflux nephropathy (from reflux ± infection)

√ clubbed calices underneath focal scars

◊ Subject to UPJ OBSTRUCTION

√ two separate echodense renal sinuses + pelves separated by parenchymal bridge
√ poor / nonvisualization of upper pole collecting system (delayed films)
√ "drooping lily sign" = hydronephrosis + decreased function of obstructed upper pole moiety causing downward displacement of lower pole calices
√ lateral displacement of lower pole collecting system + ureter
√ "nubbin sign" = scarring, atrophy, and decreased function of lower pole moiety may simulate a renal mass
√ tortuous dilated lower pole ureter
√ voiding cystogram may show reflux into lower moiety (rare)
√ displacement of proximal orifice upward

Incomplete / partial duplication

= branching of single ureteral bud (one ureteral orifice) before reaching metanephric blastema

Prevalence: in 0.6% of urograms

Associated with: ureteropelvic junction obstruction of lower renal pole

√ bifid ureter (in early branching)
√ bifid pelvis (in late branching)
√ ureteroureteral reflux = "yo-yo" / "saddle" / "seesaw" peristalsis = urine moves down the cephalad ureter + refluxes up the lower pole ureter and vice versa
√ asymmetric dilatation of one ureteral segment
√ upper pole ureter may end blindly (seen on retrograde injection only)

Cx: urinary tract infections

URETEROCELE

= cystic ectasia of subepithelial segment of intravesical ureter

Prevalence: 1:5,000 to 1:12,000 children

IVP:
√ early filling of bulbous terminal ureter ("cobra head")
√ radiolucent halo (= ureteral wall + adjacent bladder urothelium)

VCUG:
√ round / oval lucent defect near trigone
√ effacement with increased bladder distension
√ ± eversion during voiding

Simple ureterocele

= ORTHOTOPIC URETEROCELE = congenital prolapse of dilated distal ureter + orifice into bladder lumen at the usual location of the trigone, typically seen with single ureter

Presentation: incidental finding in adults; M:F = 2:3; bilateral in 33%

Cx:
(1) Pyelocaliceal dilatation
(2) Prolapse into bladder neck / urethra causing obstruction (rare)
(3) Wall thickening secondary to edema from impacted stone / infection

Ectopic ureterocele

= ureteral bud arising in an abnormal cephalad position from the mesonephric duct and moving caudally resulting in an ureteral orifice distal to trigone within / outside bladder

GU

Incidence: in 10% bilateral
(a) in single nonduplicated system (20%)
M:F = 1:1
• hypoplastic / absent ipsilateral trigone
√ poorly visualized / nonvisualized kidney
√ small / poorly functioning kidney
(b) in upper moiety ureter of duplex kidney (80%)
M:F = 1:4–1:8
Cx: (1) Bladder outlet obstruction (from ectopic ureterocele prolapsing into bladder neck / urethra)
(2) Contralateral ureteral obstruction (if ectopic ureterocele large)
(3) Multicystic dysplastic kidney (the further the orifice from normal site of insertion, the more dysplastic the kidney!)

Pseudoureterocele
= obstruction of an otherwise normal intramural ureter mimicking ureterocele
Causes:
(a) Tumor: bladder tumor (most common in adults), invasion by cervical cancer, pheochromocytoma of intravesical ureter
(b) Edema: from impacted ureteral calculus (most common in children), radiation cystitis, following ureteral instrumentation
√ thick, irregular halo in urinary bladder
√ "cobra head" / "spring onion" appearance of distal ureter
√ NO protrusion of ureter into bladder lumen (oblique views + cystoscopy normal)

URETEROPELVIC JUNCTION OBSTRUCTION
Most common cause of fetal / neonatal hydronephrosis
Intrinsic causes:
primarily functional with impaired formation of urine bolus
(1) partial replacement of UPJ muscle by collagen
(2) abnormal arrangement of junction muscles causing dysmotility (69%)
(3) high ureteral insertion
(4) mucosal folds in upper ureter
(5) eosinophilic ureteritis
(6) ischemia
Extrinsic causes:
(1) aberrant vessels to lower pole
(2) adventitial bands
(3) renal cyst
(4) XGP
(5) aortic aneurysm
Associated anomalies (27%):
vesicoureteral reflux, bilateral ureteral duplication, bilateral obstructed megaureter, contralateral nonfunctioning kidney, contralateral renal agenesis, meatal stenosis, hypospadia
M:F = 5:1

Location: left > right side; bilateral (10–40%)
√ large dilated anechoic renal pelvis communicating with calices, no dilatation of ureter
IVP:
√ sharply defined narrowing at UPJ
√ pelvicaliectasis without ureterectasis
√ anterior rotation of pelvis
√ broad tangential sharply defined extrinsic compression (in arterial crossing)
√ longitudinal striae of redundant mucosa (in dehydrated state)
√ late changes: unilateral renal enlargement, diminished opacification, wasting of kidney substance
OB-US:
√ enlargement of renal pelvis + branching infundibula + calices
√ anteroposterior diameter of renal pelvis ≥10 mm
√ large unilocular fluid collection (severely dilated collecting system)
DDx: multicystic dysplastic kidney, perinephric urinoma
ADDITIONAL TESTS:
(1) Diuresis excretory urography (Whitfield): accurate in 85%
(2) Diuresis renography (Iodine-131-iodohippurate sodium / Tc-99m-DTPA)
(3) Pressure flow urodynamic study (Whitaker)
Rx: early surgical correction may be needed to preserve renal function

URETHRAL DIVERTICULUM
Age: 26–74 years; 6 x more common in black women
• urinary incontinence (9–32–70%)
• asymptomatic (3–20%)

Congenital urethral diverticulum
Cause: ectopic cloacal epithelium; M>F

Acquired urethral diverticulum
Prevalence: 0.6–6%; M<F
Cause:
(1) obstruction of paraurethral glands with subsequent infection + rupture into urethra
(2) trauma: catheterization / childbirth
Site: dorsolateral aspect of middle urethra
• vague urinary tract symptoms mimicking chronic / interstitial cystitis, carcinoma in situ of the bladder, detrusor instability
• dyspareunia
• tender cystic swelling protruding from anterior wall of vagina + expulsion of purulent material
• dribbling after voiding
• frequency / urgency (67%), dysuria (45%)
• recurrent urinary tract infections (40%)
Voiding cystourethrography (65% accurate):
√ rounded / elongated sac connected to urethra
Transrectal US
Cx: infection, stone formation (in up to 10%), malignant degeneration (5% of all urethral carcinomas)

DDx: vaginal cyst (Gartner duct cyst, paramesonephric cyst, müllerian duct cyst, epithelial inclusion cyst), ectopic ureterocele, endometrioma, urethral tumor

URETHRAL TRAUMA

Incidence: in 4–17% of pelvic fractures in males, in <1% of pelvic fractures in females

Associated with: bladder injury in 20%

Types:

I = separation of puboprostatic ligament with craniad displacement of prostate (least common)
- √ elongated narrowed urethra
- √ elevation of bladder (displacement by hematoma)

II = urethral rupture at prostatomembranous junction above urogenital diaphragm
- √ contrast extravasation into true pelvis

III = rupture of proximal bulbous urethra below the urogenital diaphragm (most common injury)
- √ contrast extravasation into perineum ± scrotum

Cx:
1. Urethral stricture (38–100%)
2. Impotence (in up to 40%)
3. Incontinence (30%)

URINOMA

= uriniferous perirenal pseudocyst secondary to tear in collecting system with continuing renal function

Etiology:
- (a) nonobstructive: blunt / penetrating trauma, surgery, infection, calculus erosion
- (b) obstructive:
  - (1) ureteral obstruction (calculus, surgical ligature, neoplasm)
  - (2) bladder outlet obstruction (posterior urethral valves)
- ◊ Augmented by sudden diuretic load of urographic contrast material!

Path: fibroblastic cavity (in 5–12 days), dense connective tissue encapsulation (in 3–6 weeks)

√ extravasation of contrast material

√ smooth thin-walled cavity (-10 to +30 HU)
- √ sickle-shaped collection = SUBCAPSULAR urinoma
- √ cystic mass in perirenal space = LOCALIZED PERIRENAL urinoma (most common)
- √ cystic mass filling entire perirenal space = DIFFUSE PERIRENAL urinoma
- √ encapsulated expanding intrarenal cystic mass separating renal tissue fragments = INTRARENAL urinoma

√ frequently associated with urine ascites

Cx: retroperitoneal fibrosis, stricture of upper ureter, perinephric abscess
- ◊ Renal dysplasia of affected kidney in almost 100% when detected in utero!

Dx: aspirated fluid with high urea concentration

DDx: lymphocele, hematoma, abscess, renal cyst, pancreatic pseudocyst, ascites

UROLITHIASIS

Anderson-Carr-Randall theory of renal stone formation: in the presence of abnormally high calcium excretion exceeding lymphatic capacity, microaggregates of calcium (present in the normal kidney) occur in medulla, increase in size, migrate toward caliceal epithelium, and rupture into calices to form calculi

Formation theory:
- (a) nucleation theory
  = crystal / foreign body initiates formation in urine supersaturated with crystallizing salt
- (b) stone matrix theory
  = organic matrix of urinary proteins + serum serves as framework for deposition of crystals
- (c) inhibitor theory
  = little / no concentration of urinary stone inhibitors (citrate, pyrophosphate, glycosaminoglycan, nephrocalcin, Tamm-Horsfall protein) results in crystal formation

Annual incidence: 1–2:1,000; M:F = 4:1
- ◊ 12% of population develop renal stones by age 70
- ◊ 2–3% of population experience an attack of acute renal colic during their lifetime
- ◊ Patients with acute flank pain have ureteral calculi in 67–95%

Peak age: onset in 3rd decade

Distribution:

calcium oxalate	75%
struvite	15%
uric acid	5%
calcium phosphate	5%
cystine	1%

Cause:
- ◊ 70–80% of patients with first-time stones have a specific metabolic disorder

1. Hypercalciuria
   - with hypercalcemia (50%): hyperparathyroidism, milk-alkali syndrome, hypervitaminosis D, neoplastic disorders, sarcoidosis, Cushing syndrome
   - with normocalcemia (30–60%): obstruction, urinary tract infection, vesical diverticulum, horseshoe kidney, medullary sponge kidney, prolonged immobilization, renal tubular acidosis, idiopathic hypercalciuria
   - (a) absorptive hypercalciuria
     = increased intestinal absorption of calcium
     Cause: increase in 1,25-dihydroxy-vitamin D levels (50%)
   - (b) renal hypercalciuria
     = abnormal renal calcium leak
     Cause: diet high in sodium, urinary tract infection (33%)
   - (c) resorptive hypercalciuria
     = increased bone demineralization secondary to subtle hyperparathyroidism
   - (d) idiopathic

GU

(c) resorptive hypercalciuria
= increased bone demineralization secondary to subtle hyperparathyroidism
(d) idiopathic

2. **Hyperoxaluria**
◊ 85% of urinary oxalate is produced endogenously in liver!
◊ Oxalic acid is present in many foods but poorly absorbed in healthy individuals resulting in increase in urinary oxalate by only 2–3%!
(a) congenital = deficiency of an enzyme leading to accumulation of glycolate + oxylate
(b) acquired = increased intake of oxalate / oxalate precursors, excess oxalate absorption from bowel in patients with ileal resection / inflammatory bowel disease
◊ Hyperoxaluria has a stronger correlation to severity of stone disease than hypercalciuria!

3. **Hyperuricosuria**
• uric acid lithiasis (15–20%); stones form in acid urine
(a) with hyperuricemia:
gout (25%) from excessive intake of meat, fish, poultry, myeloproliferative diseases, antimitotic drugs, chemo- / radiation therapy, uricosuric agents, Lesch-Nyhan syndrome
(b) with normouricemia:
idiopathic; occurrence in acid-concentrated urine (hot climate, ileostomy)
Rx: raising urinary pH (potassium citrate / sodium bicarbonate)

4. **Cystinuria** (stones form in acid urine)
= autosomal recessive disorder in renal tubular reabsorption of cystine, ornithine, lysine, arginine
Age of onset: after 10 years
Rx: (1) decreased intake of methionine
(2) alkalinization of urine

5. **Xanthinuria**
= inherited autosomal recessive deficiency of xanthine oxidase (failure of normal oxidation of purines)

6. Urinary tract infection
Cause: urea-splitting organisms (Proteus mirabilis, P. vulgaris, Haemophilus influenzae, S. aureus, Ureaplasma urealyticum) + alkaline environment (pH >7.19)
may lead to magnesium ammonium phosphate
= **struvite stones**
Predisposed: women (M:F = 1:2), neurogenic bladder, urinary diversion, indwelling catheter, lower-urinary-tract voiding dysfunction
√ often branching into staghorn calculi
√ most struvite stones are radiopaque, but poorly mineralized matrix stones are not

7. Any condition causing nephrocalcinosis

NONRADIOPAQUE STONES
mnemonic: "SMUX"
Struvite (rarely magnesium ammonium phosphate)
Matrix stone (mucoprotein, mucopolysaccharide)
Uric acid
Xanthine

CALCULI OFTEN ASSOCIATED WITH INFECTION
mnemonic: "S and M"
Struvite (magnesium ammonium phosphate ± calcium phosphate)
Matrix stone (mucoprotein, mucopolysaccharide)

Acute Obstruction By Ureteric Calculi

see also ACUTE HYDRONEPHROSIS, page 769
• renal colic = acute colicky flank pain frequently radiating into pelvis / groin / testis
• hematuria

Mineral Composition	*Opacity*
A. Calcium stones (90%)	
1. Calcium oxalate monohydrate (= whewellite) + dihydrate (wedellite) (34%) √ small, densely opaque, mamillated (stippled appearance)	+++
2. Calcium oxalate plus apatite (34%)	+++
3. Calcium phosphate (= apatite) (5 – 10%) rarely pure (= laminated), occasionally forms in infected alkaline urine	+++
4. Calcium hydrogen phosphate (= brushite)	+++
5. Magnesium ammonium phosphate (= struvite) (1%) laminated, result of urea-splitting organisms (usually Proteus), most common constituent of staghorn calculus	++
6. Struvite plus calcium phosphate (7 – 31%) associated with infection	++
B. Cystine (3%): mildly opaque	+
C. Uric acid (5 – 10%): radiolucent	-
D. Xanthine (extremely rare): nonopaque	-
E. Matrix (mucoprotein / mucopolysaccharide) (rare): nonopaque	-

◊ Stones may be present in 30% of the time when KUB is negative!

IVU:
- √ hydroureteronephrosis
- √ displays degree of obstruction

US:
- √ unilateral pelvicaliectasis (up to 35% false-negative, up to 10% false-positive rate)
- √ resistive index >0.7 in symptomatic kidney
- √ absent ureteral jet on affected side (may be present with partially obstructing calculus)
- √ direct visualization of prevesical calculus by transabdominal, transrectal, transvaginal US

CT (97% sensitive, 96% specific, 97% accurate):
- √ calculus within ureter (PATHOGNOMONIC)
  DDx: phlebolith
- √ all stone compositions readily detectable
- √ ureteric rim sign (77%) = ureteric edema surrounding impacted small ureteric calculus
  DDx: gonadal vein
- √ ureterovesical junction edema
- √ stranding of perinephric / periureteric fat
- √ perinephric fluid collection
- √ renal enlargement

Cx: xanthogranulomatous pyelonephritis

Rx: (1) hydration (within 3 hours after meal, during strenuous physical activity, at bedtime) maintaining urine output of 2–3 l/day
(2) diet: restrict amounts of protein, sodium, calcium
(3) drugs: thiazide diuretics (lowers urinary calcium), allopurinol (lowers urate + oxalate excretion)

Prognosis:
(1) Spontaneous passage of ureteral calculi in 93%
◊ Most stones <5 mm will eventually pass!
(2) Without treatment stone recurrence is 10% at 1 year, 33% at 5 years, 50% at 10 years

VARICOCELE

= dilatation + tortuosity of plexus pampiniformis secondary to retrograde flow into internal spermatic vein

Components of pampiniform plexus:
(a) internal spermatic vein (ventral location) draining testis
(b) vein of vas deferens (mediodorsal location) draining epididymis
(c) cremasteric vein (laterodorsal location) draining scrotal wall

Etiology:
(1) Incompetent / absent valve at level of left renal vein / IVC on right side
(2) Compression of left renal vein by tumor, aberrant renal artery, obstructed renal vein

Incidence:
(a) clinical varicocele: in 10–15% of adult males, in 21–39% of infertile men
(b) subclinical varicocele: in 40–75% of infertile men

Theoretical causes for infertility:
(1) increase in local temperature (2) reflux of toxic substances from adrenal gland (countercurrent exchange of norepinephrine from refluxing renal venous blood into testicular arterial blood at the level of the pampiniform plexus) (3) alteration in Leydig cell function (4) hypoxia of germinative tissue due to venous reflux resulting in venous hypertension + stasis

- • scrotal pain
- • scrotal swelling
- • abnormal spermatogram (impaired motility, immature sperm, oligospermia)

Location: left side (78%), bilateral (16%), right side (6%)

Bidirectional Doppler sonography (erect with quiet breathing):
(1) SHUNT TYPE (86%): insufficient distal valves allow spontaneous + continuous reflux from internal spermatic vein (retrograde flow) into cremasteric vein + vein of vas deferens (where flow is orthograde) via collaterals
- • sperm quality diminished
- • clinically plexus type (Grade II + III) = medium-sized + large varicoceles
- √ continuous reflux during Valsalva maneuver

(2) STOP TYPE / PRESSURE TYPE (14%): intact intrascrotal valves allow only brief period of reflux from spermatic vein into pampiniform plexus under Valsalva maneuver
- • sperm quality normal
- • clinically central type (Grade 0 + I) = subclinical + small varicocele
- √ short phase of initial retrograde flow

US:
- √ diameter of dominant vein in upright position at inguinal canal

	relaxed	during Valsalva
normal	2.2 mm	2.7 mm
small varicocele	2.5–4.0	increase of 1.0 mm
moderate varicocele	4.0–5.0	increase of 1.2–1.5 mm
large varicocele	>5.0	increase of >1.5 mm

Dx: documentation of venous reflux

Rx: (1) Ivanissevitch procedure = surgery
(2) Transcatheter spermatic vein occlusion

VESICOURETERIC REFLUX

A. CONGENITAL REFLUX = PRIMARY REFLUX
= incompetence of ureterovesical junction due to abnormal tunneling of distal ureter through bladder wall

Prevalence: in 9–10% of normal Caucasian babies; in 1.4% of school girls; in 30% of children with a first episode of UTI

- • short submucosal ureteral tunnel (normally has a length/width ratio of 4:1)
- • large laterally located ureteral orifice

Location: uni- / bilateral (frequently involves lower pole ureter in total ureteral duplication)
√ renal scars in 22–50%
Prognosis: disappears in 80%
Cx: reflux atrophy / nephropathy in 22–50%; end-stage renal disease in 5–15% of adults

B. ACQUIRED REFLUX = SECONDARY REFLUX
1. Paraureteric diverticulum = Hutch diverticulum
2. Duplication with ureterocele
3. Cystitis (in 29–50%)
4. Urethral obstruction (urethral valves)
5. Neurogenic bladder
6. Absence of abdominal musculature (prune belly syndrome)

Cx: renal scarring with UTI (30–60%)

GRADES OF REFLUX (VCUG):
Grade I : √ reflux into distal ureters
Grade II : √ reflux into collecting system (without caliceal dilatation / blunting)
Grade III : √ all of the above + mild dilatation of pelvis and calices
Grade IV : √ all of the above + moderate dilatation (clubbing of calices)
Grade V : √ all of the above + severe tortuosity of ureter

Prognosis:
(a) grade I–III resolve with maturation of the ureterovesical junction
(b) grade IV–V require surgery to avoid renal scarring + renal impairment + hypertension

Renal scarring: >20% chance for grade III–V reflux; 2–3% chance for grade I–II reflux

Radionuclide cystography:
◊ Lower radiation dose to gonads than fluoroscopic cystography (5 mrad)!
Evaluation of bladder volume at reflux, volume of refluxed urine, residual urine volume, ureteral reflux drainage time
(a) indirect: IV injection of Tc-99m DTPA
(b) direct: instillation of 1 mCi Tc-99m pertechnetate (more sensitive for reflux during filling phase, which occurs in 20%)

US:
√ intermittent hydroureteronephrosis = variable size of collecting system
√ redundant mucosa causing apparent thickening of renal pelvic wall
√ large thin-walled bladder
√ midline-to-orifice distance >7–9 mm has high probability of vesicoureteric reflux

WILMS TUMOR

= NEPHROBLASTOMA
◊ Most common malignant abdominal neoplasm in children 1–8 years old (10%)!
◊ 3rd most common malignancy in childhood (after leukemia + brain tumors; neuroblastoma more common in infancy)!
◊ 3rd most common of all renal masses in childhood (after hydronephrosis + multicystic dysplastic kidney)!

Incidence: 1:10,000 livebirths; 450 cases/year in USA; familial in 1–2%; multifocal in 10%; bilateral in 4.4–9%

Age: peak age at 2.5–3 years (range of 3 months to 8 years); rare during first year; 50% before 3 years, 75% before 5 years; 90% before 8 years; rare in adults; M:F = 1:1

Histo: arises from undifferentiated metanephric blastema as nephroblastomatosis, recapitulates the developing embryonic kidney
(a) aggregates of small blastemal cells
(b) neoplastic nodules
(c) elongated mesenchymal cells
◊ Multilocular cystic nephroma, mesoblastic nephroma, nephroblastomatosis are related to the more favorable types of Wilms tumor!

In 14% associated with:
(1) Sporadic aniridia (= severe hypoplasia of iris)
(2) Hemihypertrophy: total / segmental / crossed (2.5%);
◊ Ipsilateral or contralateral kidney affected
◊ Increased incidence of all embryonal tumors (adrenal cortical neoplasms, hepatoblastoma)
(3) Beckwith-Wiedemann syndrome = EMG-syndrome (exomphalos, macroglossia, gigantism) + hepatomegaly, hyperglycemia from islet cell hyperplasia
(4) Genitourinary disorders (4.4%):
(a) Drash syndrome (pseudohermaphroditism, glomerulonephritis, nephrotic syndrome)
(b) Renal anomalies (horseshoe kidney, duplex / solitary / fused kidney)
(c) Genital anomalies (cryptorchidism, hypospadia, ambiguous genitalia)

Stage:
I tumor limited to kidney
II local extension into perirenal tissue / renal vessels outside kidney / lymph nodes
III not totally resectable (peritoneal implants, other than paraaortic nodes involved, invasion of vital structures)
IV hematogenous metastases (lung, liver, bone [rare], brain)
V bilateral renal involvement at diagnosis (5–10%)

- palpable abdominal mass (90%)
- hypertension (47–90%)
- abdominal pain (25%)
- fever (15%)
- gross hematuria (7–15%)
- microscopic hematuria (15–20%)

√ large tumor (average size 12 cm)
√ sharply marginated with compressed renal tissue = pseudocapsule

√ partially cystic = focal hemorrhage and necrosis (71%)
√ curvilinear / phlebolithic calcifications in 5% on plain film, in 15% on CT (DDx: regular stippled calcifications in neuroblastoma)
√ distorted "clobbered" calices
√ tumor may invade IVC / right atrium (4–10%)
√ tumor may cross midline
√ hypervascular tumor: enlarged tortuous vessels, coarse neovascularity; small arterial aneurysms, vascular lakes
√ parasitization of vascular supply

US:
√ fairly evenly echogenic mass
√ ± irregular anechoic areas due to central necrosis + hemorrhage

MR:
√ hypointense on T1WI, variable on T2WI

NUC:
√ nonfunctioning kidney (10%)
√ hypo- / iso- / hyperperfusion on radionuclide angiogram
√ absent tracer accumulation on delayed static images
√ displacement of kidney + distortion of collecting system

Prognosis: 90% survival rate depending on pathologic pattern, age at time of diagnosis, extent of disease

VARIANT: **Cystic partially differentiated nephroblastoma**
= combination of MLCN + Wilms tumor elements
Incidence: ?; M < F
√ multiple noncommunicating locules
√ polypoid masses within locules

WOLMAN DISEASE

= PRIMARY FAMILIAL XANTHOMATOSIS
= rare autosomal recessive lipidosis with accumulation of cholesterol esters and triglycerides in visceral foam cells + various tissues (liver, spleen, lymph nodes, adrenal cortex, small bowel)

Etiology: deficiency of lysosomal acid esterase / acid lipase

- malabsorption in neonatal period: failure to thrive, diarrhea, steatorrhea, vomiting
- delayed growth, diminished muscle mass, abdominal distention

√ hepatosplenomegaly
√ extensive bilateral punctate calcifications (calcification of fatty-acid soaps) throughout enlarged adrenals (maintaining their normal triangular shape) is DIAGNOSTIC
√ enlarged fat-containing lymph nodes
√ small bowel wall thickening (due to infiltration of mucosa of small bowel by lipid-filled histiocytes impairing absorption)
√ generalized osteoporosis

CT & MR: attenuation + signal intensities consistent with deposition of lipids

Dx: assay of leukocytes / cultured skin fibroblasts
Prognosis: death occurs within first 6 months of life

ZELLWEGER SYNDROME

= CEREBROHEPATORENAL SYNDROME
autosomal recessive

- muscular hypotonia
- hepatomegaly + jaundice
- craniofacial dysmorphism
- seizures, mental retardation

√ brain dysgenesis (lissencephaly, macrogyria, polymicrogyria)
√ renal cortical cysts

Prognosis: death in early infancy

OBSTETRICS AND GYNECOLOGY

DIFFERENTIAL DIAGNOSIS OF OBSTETRIC AND GYNECOLOGIC DISORDERS

GENERAL OBSTETRICS

Level I Obstetric Ultrasound

Indication: MS-AFP ≥2.5 multiples of mean (MoM) between 14 and 18 weeks MA

Limited scope of examination to identify frequent causes of MS-AFP elevation in 20–50% of pregnancies:

1. Gestational age ≥2 weeks more advanced than estimated clinically (18%)
2. Multiple gestations (10%)
3. Unsuspected fetal demise (5%)
4. Obvious fetal NTD / abdominal wall defect

Outcome: no cause identified in 50–80%

Recommendation if level I ultrasound is unrevealing:

(1) amniocentesis for AF-AFP (with normal results in >90%)

(2) level II obstetric ultrasound (skipping amniocentesis)

Level II Obstetric Ultrasound

Indication: AF-AFP ≥2 MoM

Accuracy: identification of abnormal fetuses in 99%

Examination targeted for:

1. Open neural tube defect: anencephaly, encephalocele, open spina bifida, amniotic band syndrome resulting in open neural tube defect
2. Closed neural axis anomaly: hydrocephalus, Dandy-Walker malformation
3. Abdominal wall defect: gastroschisis, omphalocele, gastropleuroschisis from amniotic band syndrome
4. Upper GI obstruction: esophageal atresia ± tracheoesophageal fistula, duodenal obstruction
5. Cystic hygroma
6. Teratoma: sacrococcygeal, lingual, retropharyngeal
7. Renal anomalies: obstructive uropathy, renal agenesis, multicystic dysplastic kidney, congenital Finnish nephrosis

◊ Risk of fetal chromosomal anomaly is only 0.6–1.1% with normal level II sonogram!

First Trimester Bleeding

= VAGINAL BLEEDING IN FIRST TRIMESTER

Frequency: 15–25% of all pregnancies, of which 50% terminate in abortion

A. INTRAUTERINE CONCEPTUS IDENTIFIED
   1. Blighted ovum / blighted twin
   2. Threatened abortion
   3. Implantation bleed
   4. Early fetal death
   5. Gestational trophoblastic disease
   6. Subchorionic hemorrhage

B. NORMAL ENDOMETRIAL CAVITY
   (a) with β-HCG level >1,800 mIU/mL
      1. Recent spontaneous abortion
      2. Ectopic pregnancy
   (b) with β-HCG level <1,800 mIU/mL
      1. Very early IUP
      2. Ectopic pregnancy

Positive β-HCG Without IUP

mnemonic: "HERE"

HCG-producing tumor (rare)
Ectopic pregnancy
Recent / incomplete abortion
Early intrauterine pregnancy

Dilated Cervix

1. Inevitable abortion
2. Premature labor
   = spontaneous onset of palpable, regularly occurring uterine contractions between 20 and 37 weeks MA
3. Incompetent cervix
   = gaping cervix usually develops during 2nd trimester
   Predisposed: cervical trauma (D & C, cauterization), DES exposure in utero with cervical hypoplasia, estrogen medication
   √ visualization of fetal parts / amniotic fluid within dilated endocervical canal (stress test: patient standing with bladder empty)
   Prognosis: 14th–18th week best time for Rx prior to significant cervical dilatation

Uterus Large For Dates

1. Multiple gestation pregnancy
2. Inaccurate menstrual history
3. Fibroids
4. Polyhydramnios
5. Hydatidiform mole
6. Fetal macrosomia

Empty Gestational Sac

1. Normal early IUP between 5–7 weeks MA
2. Blighted ovum

DDx: Pseudosac of ectopic pregnancy

Alpha-fetoprotein

= glycoprotein as major circulatory protein of early fetus

Origin: formed initially by yolk sac + fetal gut (4–8 weeks), later by fetal liver

Detectable in

(a) fetal serum
   • concentration peaks at 14–15 weeks followed by progressive decline

(b) amniotic fluid (AF-AFP) secondary to fetal urination, fetal gastrointestinal secretions, transudation across fetal membranes (amnion, placenta), transudation across immature fetal epithelium
- concentration peaks early in 2nd trimester followed by progressive decline

(c) maternal circulation (MS-AFP) secondary to leakage from amniotic fluid across the placenta
- levels rise from 7th week, peak at 32nd week, and decline toward end of pregnancy
- ◊ Either high / low MS-AFP is associated with 34% of all major congenital defects!

Sample site	Approximate level (ng/mL)	Peak
maternal serum	30	30th–32nd week
amniotic fluid	20,000	early 2nd trimester
fetal plasma	3,000,000	14th–15th week

At the end of the 1st trimester AFP is present:
in fetal plasma in *milligram* quantities
in amniotic fluid in *microgram* quantities
in maternal serum in *nanogram* quantities

Reported in MoM = multiples of mean to standardize interpretation among laboratories

Elevated Alpha-fetoprotein

- screening at 16–18 weeks GA
- ◊ Values must be corrected for dates, maternal weight, race, presence of diabetes (diabetes has depressing effect on MS-AFP so that lower levels may be associated with NTDs)

(a) Elevation in MATERNAL SERUM (MS-AFP)
= defined as ≥2.5 MoM / equivalent to the 5th percentile; 4.5 MoM for multiple gestations

Power of detection at ≥2.5 MoM cutoff:
98% of gastroschisis
90% of anencephalic fetuses
75–80% of open spinal defects
70% of omphaloceles

Incidence: 2–5% screen-positive rate (in 16% normal MS-AFP on retesting); 6–15% of fetuses have some type of major congenital defect; in 1.3 per 1,000 tests fetal anomaly detected

◊ The higher the AFP elevation the higher the probability of fetal anomalies

◊ 20–38% of women with unexplained high MS-AFP (ie, in absence of fetal abnormality) suffer adverse pregnancy outcomes (premature birth, preeclampsia, 2–4 x IUGR, 10 x perinatal mortality, 10 x placental abruption)!

(b) Elevation in AMNIOTIC FLUID (AF-AFP)
= defined as ≥2 MoM

Incidence: <10% of women with elevated MS-AFP and "unrevealing" level I US exam

- determine acteylcholinesterase + karyotype in amniotic fluid
- ◊ 66% of fetuses of women with elevated AF-AFP levels are normal!
- ◊ A targeted level II ultrasound exam will show fetal anomalies in 33%!

Associated with:

A. LABORATORY ERROR
B. ERRONEOUS DATES (18%): fetus actually older (AFP levels rise 15% per week during 16–18-week window)
C. MULTIPLE GESTATIONS (14%)
D. FETAL DEMISE (7%) / fetal distress / threatened abortion
E. FETAL ANOMALIES (61%)
  1. Neural tube defects (51%): [anencephaly (30%), myelomeningocele (18%), encephalocele (3%), forebrain malformation]
     Prevalence: 1.6 per 1,000 births in USA; 6 per 1,000 in Great Britain
     ◊ in 90% as 1st time event!
     Risk of recurrence: 3% after one affected child; 6% after 2 affected children
  2. Ventral wall defects (21%) (gastroschisis, omphalocele): sensitivity of 50%
  3. Upper GI obstruction (esophageal / duodenal atresia)
  4. Cystic hygroma, teratoma (pharyngeal, sacral)
  5. Amniotic band syndrome (asymmetric cephalocele, gastropleuroschisis)
  6. Renal abnormalities: multicystic dysplastic kidney, renal agenesis, pelviectasis, **congenital Finnish nephrosis** (typically ≥10 MoM + negative amniotic fluid acetylcholinesterase)
  7. Oligohydramnios
F. PLACENTAL LESION
  1. Infarct
  2. Chorioangioma
  3. Peri- and intraplacental hematoma resulting in fetomaternal hemorrhage
  4. Placental lakes, intervillous thrombosis
G. LOW BIRTH WEIGHT
H. Normal pregnancy + MATERNAL DISORDER
  1. Hepatitis
  2. Hepatoma
I. Fetal-maternal blood mixing: collection of MS-AFP samples after amniocentesis

mnemonic: "GEM MINER CO"
Gastroschisis
Esophageal atresia
Multiple gestations
Mole

Incorrect menstrual dates
Neural tube defects
Error (laboratory)
Renal disease in fetus (autosomal recessive polycystic kidney disease, renal dysplasia, obstructive uropathy, congenital Finnish nephrosis)
Chorioangioma
Omphalocele

Low Alpha-fetoprotein

= MS-AFP ≤0.5 / AF-AFP ≤0.72 multiples of the median

Incidence: 3%

1. Autosomal trisomy syndromes (trisomy 21, 18, 13)
   ◊ 20% of trisomy 21 fetuses are found in women with low MS-AFP after adjustment for age!
2. Absence of fetal tissues (eg, hydatidiform mole)
3. Fetal demise
4. Misdated pregnancy
5. Normal pregnancy
6. Patient not pregnant

Use Of Karyotyping

Frequency: 11–35% of fetuses with sonographically identified abnormalities have chromosomal abnormalities

A. FETAL ANOMALIES
   1. CNS anomalies: holoprosencephaly (43–59%), Dandy-Walker malformation (29–50%), cerebellar hypoplasia, agenesis of corpus callosum, myelomeningocele (33–50%)
   2. Cystic hygroma (72%): Turner syndrome
   3. Omphalocele (30–40%)
   4. Cardiac malformations
   5. Nonimmune hydrops
   6. Duodenal atresia
   7. Severe early-onset IUGR: trisomy 18, 13, triploidy
   8. Diaphragmatic hernia
   9. Bone-echodense bowel (20%): trisomy 21

B. MATERNAL RISK FACTORS
   1. Advanced age
   2. Low serum α-fetoprotein
   3. Abnormal triple screen of maternal serum
   4. History of previous chromosomally abnormal pregnancy (1% risk of recurrence)

C. PLANNED INTENSE INTRAUTERINE MANAGEMENT

Fetal anomalies not associated with chromosomal anomalies:

1. Gastroschisis
2. Unilateral renal anomaly
3. Intestinal obstruction distal to duodenal bulb
4. Off-midline unilateral cleft lip
5. Fetal teratoma (sacrococcygeal / anterior cervical)
6. Isolated single umbilical artery

AMNIOTIC FLUID VOLUME

Production:
- (a) 1st trimester: dialysate of maternal + fetal serum across the noncornified fetal skin
- (b) 2nd + 3rd trimester: fetal urine (600–800 cm³/day near term), fetal lungs (600–800 cm³/day near term), amniotic membrane

Absorption:
fetal swallowing + GI absorption, fetal lung absorption, clearance by placenta

Assessment of amniotic fluid volume by:
- (1) Subjective assessment ("Gestalt" method): quick + efficient, accounts for GA-related variations in fluid volume, considered the most accurate if performed by experienced operator, operator + interpreter must be identical, no documentation, variations on serial scans difficult to appreciate
- (2) Depth of largest vertical pocket: simple + quick (used in BPP), pockets >2 cm may be found in crevices between fetal parts with moderately severe oligohydramnios, does not account for GA-related variations
- (3) Four-quadrant **Amniotic Fluid Index** (AFI): fairly quick, correlates probably better with fluid volume than any single measurement, may not accurately reflect overall fluid volume, may be affected by fetal movement during measurements
- (4) Planimetric measurement of total intrauterine volume
- (5) Dye / para-amino hippurate dilution technique: 800 cm³ at 34 weeks, 500 cm³ >34 weeks

Polyhydramnios

= amniotic fluid volume >1500–2000 cm³ at term

Incidence: 1.1–2–3.5%

√ fetus does not fill the AP diameter of uterus
√ single largest pocket devoid of fetal parts / cord >8 cm in vertical direction
√ AFI ≥20–24 cm

Prognosis: 64% perinatal mortality with severe polyhydramnios

Etiology:

A. IDIOPATHIC (60%)
   associated with macrosomia in 19–37%
   Suggested cause:
   (1) increased renal vascular flow
   (2) bulk flow of water across surface of fetus + umbilical cord + placenta + membranes

B. MATERNAL CAUSES (20%)
   1. Diabetes (5%)
   2. Isoimmunization (Rh incompatibility)
   3. Placental tumors: chorioangioma

C. FETAL ANOMALIES (20–63%)
   (a) gastrointestinal anomalies (6–16%)
   impairment of fetal swallowing (esophageal atresia in 3%); high intestinal atresias / obstruction of duodenum / proximal small bowel (1.2–1.8%), omphalocele, meconium peritonitis
   (b) nonimmune hydrops (16%)

(c) neural tube defects (9–16%)
anencephaly, hydranencephaly, holoprosencephaly, myelomeningocele, ventriculomegaly, agenesis of corpus callosum, encephalocele, microcephaly
(d) chest anomalies (12%)
diaphragmatic hernia, cystic adenomatoid malformation, tracheal atresia, mediastinal teratoma, primary pulmonary hypoplasia, extralobar sequestration, congenital chylothorax
(e) skeletal dysplasias (11%)
dwarfism (thanatophoric dysplasia, achondroplasia), kyphoscoliosis, platyspondyly
(f) chromosomal abnormalities (9%)
trisomy 21, 18, 13
(g) cardiac anomalies (5%)
VSD, truncus arteriosus, ectopia cordis, septal rhabdomyoma, arrhythmia
(h) genitourinary malformations
Cause: ? hormonally mediated polyuria
unilateral UPJ obstruction, unilateral multicystic dysplastic kidney, mesoblastic nephroma
(i) miscellaneous (8%)
cystic hygroma, facial tumors, cleft lip / palate, teratoma, amniotic band syndrome, congenital pancreatic cyst
◊ In polyhydramnios efforts to detect fetal anomalies should be directed at SGA fetuses!

mnemonic: "TARDI"
Twins
Anomalies, fetal
Rh incompatibility
Diabetes
Idiopathic

Oligohydramnios

= amniotic fluid volume <500 cm^3 at term
√ single largest pocket devoid of fetal parts / cord ≤1–2 cm in vertical direction
√ AFI ≤5–7 cm
Etiology:
mnemonic: "DRIPP"
Demise of fetus / **D**rugs (Motrin therapy for tocolysis of preterm labor)
Renal anomalies, bilateral (= inadequate urine production): renal agenesis / dysgenesis, infantile polycystic kidney disease, prune belly syndrome, posterior urethral valves, urethral atresia, cloacal anomalies
◊ 20-fold increase in incidence of fetal anomalies with oligohydramnios!
N.B.: bilateral renal obstruction, if combined with intestinal obstruction, may be associated with polyhydramnios
IUGR (reduced renal perfusion)
Premature rupture of membranes (most common)
Postmaturity

Cx: pulmonary hypoplasia, cord compression
Prognosis: 77–100% perinatal mortality with 2nd trimester oligohydramnios

Intrauterine Membrane In Pregnancy

A. MEMBRANE OF MATERNAL ORIGIN
1. Uterine septum
= incomplete resorption of sagittal septum between the fused two müllerian ducts
2. Amniotic sheet / shelve
= folding of amniochorionic membrane around uterine synechia
√ synechia often thins during uterine stretching + disappears as pregnancy progresses

B. MEMBRANE OF FETAL ORIGIN
1. Intertwin membrane
= apposing membrane of multiple pregnancy
2. Amniotic band
= rent within amnion
3. Chorioamnionic separation
= incomplete fusion / hemorrhagic separation of amnion (= inner membrane) and chorion (= outer membrane)
4. Subchorionic hemorrhage = chorioamnionic elevation
= separation of chorionic membrane from decidua
• implantation bleed of early pregnancy

mnemonic: "STABS"
Separation (chorioamnionic)
Twins (intertwin membrane)
Abruption
Bands (amniotic band syndrome)
Synechia

PLACENTA

Abnormal Placental Size

◊ Placental mass tends to reflect fetal mass!
A. ENLARGEMENT OF PLACENTA
= >5 cm thick in sections obtained at right angles to long axis of placenta
(a) maternal disease
1. Maternal diabetes (= villous edema)
2. Chronic intrauterine infections
3. Maternal anemia (= normal histology)
4. Alpha-thalassemia
(b) fetal disease
1. Hemolytic disease of the newborn (= villous edema + hyperplasia)
2. Umbilical vein obstruction
3. Fetal high-output failure: large chorioangioma, arteriovenous fistula
4. Fetal malformation: Beckwith-Wiedemann syndrome, sacrococcygeal teratoma, chromosomal abnormality, fetal hydrops
5. Twin-twin transfusion syndrome
(c) fetomaternal hemorrhage

mnemonic: "HAD IT"
- **H**ydrops
- **A**bruption
- **D**iabetes mellitus
- **I**nfection
- **T**riploidy

B. DECREASE IN PLACENTAL SIZE
1. Preeclampsia
   associated with placental infarcts in 33–60%
2. IUGR
3. Intrauterine infection
4. Chromosomal abnormality

Vascular Spaces Of The Placenta

1. **"Placental cysts"**
   = large fetal veins located between amnion + chorion anastomosing with umbilical vein
   √ sluggish blood flow (detectable by real-time observation)
2. **Basal veins**
   = decidual + uterine veins
   √ lacy appearing network of veins underneath placenta
   DDx: placental abruption
3. **Intraplacental venous lakes**
   √ intraplacental sonolucent spaces
   √ whirlpool motion pattern of flowing blood

Macroscopic Lesions Of The Placenta

1. **Intervillous thrombosis** (36%)
   = intraplacental areas of hemorrhage
   Etiology: breaks in villous capillaries with bleeding from fetal vessels
   √ irregular sonolucent intraplacental lesions (mm to cm range)
   √ blood flow may be observed within lesion
   Significance: fetal-maternal hemorrhage (Rh sensitization, elevated AFP levels)
2. **Perivillous fibrin deposition** (22%)
   = nonlaminated collection of fibrin deposition
   Etiology: thrombosis of intervillous space
   Significance: none
3. **Septal cyst** (19%)
   Etiology: obstruction of septal venous drainage by edematous villi
   √ 5–10 mm cyst within septum
   Significance: none
4. **Placental infarct** (25%)
   = coagulation necrosis of villi
   Etiology: disorder of maternal vessels, retroplacental hemorrhage
   √ not visualized unless hemorrhagic
   √ well-circumscribed mass with hyperechoic / mixed echo pattern
   Significance: dependent on extent + associated maternal condition
5. **Subchorionic fibrin deposition** (20%)
   = laminated collection of fibrin deposition
   Etiology: thrombosis of maternal blood in subchorionic space
   √ subchorionic sonolucent area
   Significance: none
6. **Massive subchorial thrombus**
   = BREUS MOLE = PREPLACENTAL HEMORRHAGE

Placental Tumor

A. TROPHOBLASTIC
1. Complete hydatidiform mole
2. Partial hydatidiform mole
3. Invasive mole
4. Choriocarcinoma

B. NONTROPHOBLASTIC
1. Chorioangioma (in up to 1% of placentas)
2. Teratoma (rare)
3. Metastatic lesion (rare): melanoma, breast carcinoma, bronchial carcinoma

Unbalanced Intertwin Transfusion

= unbalanced intertwin transfusion through vascular anastomoses between the two circulations of monochorionic twins

A. ACUTE = Twin-embolization syndrome
B. CHRONIC = Twin-twin transfusion syndrome
C. REVERSE = Acardiac twinning

UMBILICAL CORD

Abnormal Cord Attachment

1. Marginal cord attachment (7%)
   = battledore placenta (flat wooden paddle used in an early form of badminton)
   • no clinical significance
2. Velamentous insertion of cord (1%)
3. Vasa previa

Umbilical Cord Lesions

◊ Umbilical cord cysts persisting into 2nd + 3rd trimester are frequently accompanied by fetal anomalies (hernia, intestinal obstruction, urinary tract obstruction, urachal anomalies, omphalocele, cardiac defect, trisomy 18)!

A. DEVELOPMENTAL CORD LESION
1. **Umbilical hernia**
   = protrusion from anterior abdominal wall with normal insertion of umbilical vessels
   Predisposed:
   Blacks, low-birth-weight infants, trisomy 21, congenital hypothyroidism, Beckwith-Wiedemann syndrome, mucopolysaccharidoses
   Prognosis: spontaneous closure in first 3 years of life
2. **Omphalomesenteric duct cyst**
   √ near fetal end of cord + eccentric in cord

3. **Allantoic cyst**
   = remnant of umbilical vesicle / allantois; usually degenerates by 6 weeks
   Histo: lined by single layer of flattened epithelium
   √ near fetal end of cord + in center of cord
4. **Amniotic inclusion cyst**
   = amniotic epithelium trapped within umbilical cord
5. **Mucoid degeneration of umbilical cord**
   = **umbilical cord pseudocyst**
   = liquefaction of Wharton jelly / edema
   √ focal thickening of Wharton jelly, usually near umbilicus
   √ usually resolved by 12 weeks MA
   Associated commonly with omphalocele
6. **Noncoiled "straight" cord**
   counterclockwise:clockwise umbilical cords = 7:1
   right-handed:left-handed persons = 7:1
   Incidence: 3.7–5%
   √ absent vascular coiling for entire length of visible cord
   At risk for: intrauterine death (8%), stillbirth, fetal anomalies (24%), prematurity, intrapartum heart rate decelerations, fetal distress, meconium staining

B. ACQUIRED CORD LESION
1. **False knot**
   (a) exaggerated looping of cord vessels causing focal dilatation of cord
   (b) focal accumulation of Wharton jelly
   (c) varix of umbilical vessel
   √ knoblike protrusion / bulge of cord
2. **True knot**
   Incidence: 1% of pregnancies
   Cause: excessive fetal movements
   Predisposed: long cord, polyhydramnios, small fetus, monoamniotic twins
   √ local distension / thrombosis of umbilical vein near cord knot resembling an umbilical cyst
   √ tortuosity of cord at level of knot
   Cx: vascular occlusion + fetal death in utero
   OB management: expectant
3. **Umbilical cord hematoma**
   = rupture of the wall of the umbilical vein secondary to mechanical trauma (torsion, loops, knots, traction) / congenital weakness of vessel wall
   Incidence: 1:5,505 to 1:12,699 deliveries
   Location: near fetal insertion of umbilical cord (most common)
   √ hyper- / hypoechoic mass 1–2 cm in size, multiple (in 18%)
   Cx: rupture into amniotic cavity with exsanguination
   Prognosis: 52% overall perinatal fetal mortality
4. Neoplasm
   (a) **Angiomyxoma / hemangioma of cord**
   Incidence: 22 cases in literature
   Histo: multiple vascular channels lined by benign endothelium surrounded by edema + myxomatous degeneration of Wharton jelly
   Associated with: elevated α-fetoprotein level
   Location: more frequently near placental end of umbilical cord
   √ hyperechoic / multicystic mass within cord
   √ may be associated with pseudocyst (= localized collection of edema)
   Cx: premature delivery, stillbirth, hydramnios, nonimmune hydrops, massive hemorrhage due to rupture
   (b) Other tumors: myxosarcoma, dermoid, teratoma
5. **Umbilical vein varix**
   Incidence: <4% of all umbilical cord abnormalities
   Site: intraamniotic, intraabdominal
   √ fusiform dilatation of umbilical vein
   Cx: (1) Thrombosis with subsequent fetal death
   (2) Partial thrombosis with IUGR
   Prognosis: usually no clinical significance
6. Umbilical artery aneurysm

FETAL SKELETAL DYSPLASIA

= heterogeneous group of bone growth disorders resulting in abnormal shape + size of the skeleton

◊ More than 200 skeletal dysplasias are known, but only a few are frequent:
- thanatophoric dysplasia
- osteogenesis imperfecta type II (56%)
- achondrogenesis (71%)
- heterozygous achondroplasia

Birth prevalence:
2.3:10,000–7.6:10,000 births for all skeletal dysplasias; 1.5:10,000 births for lethal skeletal dysplasias
Prognosis: 51% lethal due to hypoplastic lungs: 23% stillbirths, 32% death in 1st week of life

	Birth prevalence	*Perinatal deaths*
Thanatophoric dysplasia	0.69:10,000*	1:246
Achondroplasia	0.37:10,000	none
Achondrogenesis, type I	0.23:10,000*	1:639
Achondrogenesis, type II	0.25:10,000*	
Osteogenesis imperf. type II	0.18:10,000*	1:799
Osteogenesis imperf., others	0.18:10,000	none
Asphyxiating thoracic dysplasia	0.14:10,000	1:3,196
Hypophosphatasia	0.10:10,000*	
Chondrodysplasia punctata, rhizo	0.09:10,000*	none
Camptomelic dysplasia	0.05:10,000*	1:3,196
Chondroectodermal dysplasia	0.05:10,000	1:3,196
Cleidocranial dysplasia	0.05:10,000	
Diastrophic dysplasia	0.02:10,000*	

* = lethal dysplasias

OB&GYN

√ shortening of long bones (common characteristic)
◊ Femur length >5 mm below 2 standard deviations suggests skeletal dysplasia!
√ femur length/foot length ratio <0.9
√ moderate limb shortening of 40–60% of the mean in thanatophoric dysplasia + OI type II
√ severe limb shortening of >30% of the mean in achondrogenesis
DDx features: mineralization, bowing, fractures, number of digits, fetal movement, thoracic measurement, associated anomalies, age of onset
DDx: constitutionally short limbs, severe IUGR

see also DWARFISM, page 9

Fetal Hand Malformation

Polydactyly

trisomy 13, short-rib-polydactyly syndrome, asphyxiating thoracic dystrophy (Jeune syndrome), Smith-Lemli-Opitz syndrome

(a) Postaxial polydactyly
chondroectodermal dysplasia (Ellis-van Creveld syndrome), Meckel-Gruber syndrome, hydrolethalus syndrome

(b) Preaxial polydactyly
orofaciodigital syndrome

Syndactyly

Apert syndrome, triploidy, Roberts syndrome

Clinodactyly

trisomy 21, triploidy

Overlapping Digit

trisomy 18

Hitchhiker's Thumb

diastrophic dysplasia

Flexion Contractures

trisomy 13 + 18, fetal akinesia deformation sequence

Limb Reduction

congenital varicella, hypoglossia-hyperdactyly syndrome

Amputation

amniotic band syndrome

FETAL CNS ANOMALIES

Incidence: 2:1,000 births (United States); 90% as 1st time occurrence
Recurrence: 2–3% after 1st, 6% after 2nd occurrence
√ ventricular atrium + cisterna magna are two sensitive anatomic markers for normal brain development!

A. HYDROCEPHALUS
   1. Aqueductal stenosis
   2. Communicating hydrocephalus
   3. Dandy-Walker malformation
   4. Choroid plexus papilloma

B. NEURAL TUBE DEFECT
Incidence: 1:500–600 livebirths
Risk of recurrence: 3–4%
   1. Spina bifida
   2. Anencephaly
   3. Acrania
   4. Encephalocele (8–15%)
   5. Porencephaly
   6. Hydranencephaly
   7. Holoprosencephaly
   8. Iniencephaly
   9. Microcephaly
   10. Agenesis of corpus callosum
   11. Lissencephaly
   12. Arachnoid cyst
   13. Choroid plexus cyst
   14. Vein of Galen aneurysm

C. INTRACRANIAL NEOPLASM
   1. Teratoma (>50%): benign / malignant
      Location: originate from base of skull
   2. Glioblastoma
   3. Astrocytoma

Hypotelorism

1. Holoprosencephaly
2. Chromosomal abnormalities: trisomy 13
3. Microcephaly, trigonocephaly
4. Maternal phenylketonuria
5. Meckel-Gruber syndrome
6. Myotonic dystrophy
7. Williams syndrome
8. Oculodental dysplasia

Hypertelorism

1. Median cleft syndrome: cleft lip/palate
2. Craniosynostosis: Apert /Crouzon syndrome
3. Pena-Shokeir syndrome
4. Frontal / ethmoidal, sphenoidal encephalocele
5. Dilantin effect

Fetal Ventriculomegaly

Cause:

A. Morphologic anomaly (70–80%):
   1. Spina bifida (30–65%)
   2. Dandy-Walker malformation
   3. Encephalocele
   4. Holoprosencephaly
   5. Agenesis of corpus callosum

B. Abnormal karyotype (10–20%)

C. Viral infection

◊ 20–40% of concurrent anomalies are missed by ultrasound!

√ "dangling" choroid plexus = choroid hanging from tela choroidea
√ width of ventricular atrium >10 mm

Prognosis: 21% survival rate; 50% with intellectual impairment; 80% with isolated mild ventriculomegaly (atrial width >10 and ≤15 mm) have normal motor + intellectual function at ≥12 months of age

Cystic Intracranial Lesion

mnemonic: "CHAP VAN"

- **C**horoid plexus cyst
- **H**ydrocephalus, **H**oloprosencephaly, **H**ydranencephaly
- **A**genesis of corpus callosum + cystic dilatation of 3rd ventricle
- **P**orencephaly
- **V**ein of Galen aneurysm
- **A**rachnoid cyst
- **N**eoplasm (cystic teratoma)

Abnormal Cisterna Magna

Normal size between 15 and 25 weeks MA: >2 to <10 mm (usually 4–9 mm) in 94–97% of fetuses

A. SMALL CISTERNA MAGNA + "banana sign"
1. Chiari II malformation (with myelomeningocele)
2. Occipital cephalocele
3. Severe hydrocephalus

B. LARGE CISTERNA MAGNA
1. Megacisterna magna
   √ cerebellum + vermis remain intact
2. Arachnoid cyst
   √ en bloc displacement of cerebellum + vermis
3. Cerebellar hypoplasia
4. Dandy-Walker syndrome (with vermian agenesis)

FETAL NECK ANOMALIES

1. Cervical myelomeningocele
2. Occipital cephalocele
3. Cystic hygroma
4. Teratoma

Nuchal Skin Thickening

= NUCHAL SONOLUCENCY / FULLNESS / EDEMA

= skin thickening of posterior neck measured between calvarium + dorsal skin margin
(a) ≥3 mm during 9–13 weeks MA
(b) ≥6 mm during 14–21 weeks MA
◊ The smallest measurement should be used!

Image plane: axial plane (slightly craniad to that of the BPD measurement) that includes cavum septi pellucidi, cerebellar hemisphere and cisterna magna

Incidence: among the most common anomaly in 1st trimester + early 2nd trimester

Causes:

A. NORMAL VARIANT (0.06%)

B. CHROMOSOMAL DISORDERS
trisomy 21 (in 45–80%), Turner syndrome (45 X0), Noonan syndrome, trisomy 18, XXX syndrome, XYY syndrome, XXXX syndrome, XXXXY syndrome, 18p-syndrome, 13q-syndrome
◊ 30–40% of fetuses with Down syndrome have nuchal skin thickening!

C. NONCHROMOSOMAL DISORDERS
1. Multiple pterygium syndrome = Escobar syndrome
2. Klippel-Feil syndrome (fusion of cervical vertebrae, CHD, deafness (30%), cleft palate
3. Zellweger syndrome = cerebrohepatorenal syndrome (large forehead, flat facies, macrogyria, hepatomegaly, cystic kidney disease, contractures of extremities)
4. Robert syndrome
5. Cumming syndrome

√ larger lymphangiomas with radiating septations are usually found with trisomy 18
√ nuchal fullness ≥3 mm during 1st trimester is seen in trisomy 21 / 18 / 13 (30–50% PPV)
√ often reverting to normal by 16–18 weeks
√ septations within nuchal translucency carries a 20- to 200-fold risk for chromosomal anomalies compared with normal

Sensitivity: 2–44–75% for detection of trisomy 21
Specificity: 99% for detection of trisomy 21
Positive screen: 1.2–3% in general population (exceeding 0.5% risk of amniocentesis)
False positives: 1–2–8.5%
OB-management: thorough sonographic evaluation at 18–20 weeks MA
DDx: chorioamnionic separation

Macroglossia

1. Beckwith-Wiedemann syndrome
2. Down syndrome
3. Hypothyroidism
4. Mental retardation

Micrognathia

1. Pierre-Robin syndrome
2. Treacher-Collins syndrome
3. Goldenhar syndrome (hemifacial microsomia)
4. Seckel syndrome (bird-headed dwarfism)
5. Multiple pterygium syndrome
6. Pena-Shokeir syndrome
7. Beckwith-Wiedemann syndrome
8. Arthrogryposis
9. Skeletal dysplasias
10. Trisomy 13, 18, 9 (abnormal karyotype in 25%)

Prognosis: 20% survival

Maxillary Hypoplasia

1. Down syndrome
2. Drugs (alcohol, dilantin, valproate)
3. Apert / Crouzon syndrome
4. Achondroplasia
5. Cleft lip/palate

FETAL CHEST ANOMALIES

Pulmonary hypoplasia

Path: absolute decrease in lung volume / weight for gestational age

Cause:

1. Prolonged oligohydramnios (20–25%)
2. Skeletal dysplasia (small thorax)
3. Intrathoracic mass (lung compression)
4. Large hydrothorax (lung compression)
5. Neurologic condition (reduced breathing activity)
6. Chromosomal abnormality
7. CHD with R-sided cardiac obstructing lesion

√ thoracic circumference (TC) <5th percentile for EGA
√ declining TC:AC ratio from >0.80 (75% sensitive, 80–90% specific); not applicable for intrathoracic masses

Intrathoracic mass

in order of frequency:

1. Diaphragmatic hernia / eventration
2. Cystic adenomatoid malformation
3. Bronchopulmonary sequestration
4. Bronchogenic cyst with bronchial compression
5. Bronchial atresia

Unilateral chest mass

1. Congenital diaphragmatic hernia
2. Cystic adenomatoid malformation
3. Bronchopulmonary sequestration
4. Bronchogenic cyst
5. Unilateral bronchial atresia / stenosis

Bilateral chest masses

1. Laryngeal / tracheal atresia
2. Bilateral cystic adenomatoid malformation
3. Bilateral congenital diaphragmatic herniae

Mediastinal mass

1. Goiter
2. Cystic hygroma
3. Pericardial teratoma
4. Neuroblastoma

Cystic chest mass

1. Bronchogenic cyst
2. Enteric cyst
3. Neurenteric cyst
4. Cystic adenomatoid malformation (Type I)
5. Congenital diaphragmatic hernia
6. Pericardial cyst
7. Mediastinal meningocele

Complex chest mass

1. Congenital diaphragmatic hernia
2. Cystic adenomatoid malformation (Type I, II, III)
3. Pulmonary sequestration
4. Complex enteric cyst
5. Pericardial teratoma

Solid chest mass

1. Congenital diaphragmatic hernia (bowel ± liver)
2. Cystic adenomatoid malformation (Type III)
3. Pulmonary sequestration
4. Obstructed lung from bronchial atresia, laryngeal atresia, bronchogenic cyst
5. Bronchopulmonary foregut malformation
6. Pericardial tumor
7. Heterotopic brain tissue

Regressing fetal chest mass

1. Cystic adenomatoid malformation
2. Bronchopulmonary sequestration

Chest wall mass

1. Hemangioma
2. Cystic hygroma
3. Teratoma
4. Hamartoma
5. Thoracic myelomeningocele

Pleural effusion

1. Primary idiopathic chylothorax (most common)
2. Hydrops fetalis (multiple causes)
3. Chromosome anomaly: trisomy 21, 45 XO (mostly)
4. Pulmonary lymphangiectasia / cystic hygroma
5. Lung mass: cystic adenomatoid malformation, bronchopulmonary sequestration, congenital diaphragmatic hernia, chest wall hamartoma (uncommon)
6. Pulmonary vein atresia
7. Idiopathic

FETAL CARDIAC ANOMALIES

Incidence: 1:125 births = 0.8% of population; most common of all congenital malformations (40%)

◊ 90% occur as isolated multifactorial traits with a recurrence risk of 2–4%
◊ 10% are associated with multiple birth defects
◊ responsible for 50% of childhood deaths from congenital malformations

Antenatal sonographic diagnosis to prompt cardiac evaluation:

A. ABNORMALITIES IN CARDIAC POSITION
B. CNS
   1. Hydrocephalus
   2. Microcephaly
   3. Agenesis of corpus callosum
   4. Encephalocele (Meckel-Gruber syndrome)
C. GASTROINTESTINAL
   1. Esophageal atresia
   2. Duodenal atresia
   3. Situs abnormalities
   4. Diaphragmatic hernia
D. VENTRAL WALL DEFECT
   1. Omphalocele
   2. Ectopia cordis

E. RENAL
   1. Bilateral renal agenesis
   2. Dysplastic kidneys
F. TWINS
   1. Conjoined twins

Prenatal risk factors for congenital heart disease

A. FETAL RISK FACTORS
   1. Symmetric IUGR
   2. Arrhythmias
      (a) fixed bradycardia (50%)
      (b) tachycardia (low risk)
      (c) irregular: PACs, PVCs (low risk)
   3. Abnormal fetal karyotype (CHD in Down syndrome in 40%; in Trisomy 18 / 13 in >90%; in Turner syndrome in 35%)
   4. Extracardiac somatic anomalies by US: omphaloceles (20%), duodenal atresia, hydrocephaly, spina bifida, VACTERL
   5. Nonimmune hydrops (30-35%)
   6. Oligo- / polyhydramnios

B. MATERNAL RISK FACTORS
   1. Maternal heart disease (10%)
   2. Insulin-dependent diabetes mellitus (4-5%)
   3. Phenylketonuria (15% if maternal phenylalanine >15%)
   4. Collagen vascular disease: SLE
   5. Viral infection: rubella
   6. Drugs
      (a) phenytoin (in 2% PS, AS, coarctation, PDA)
      (b) trimethadione (in 20% transposition, tetralogy, hypoplastic left heart)
      (c) sex hormones (in 3%)
      (d) lithium (7%): Ebstein anomaly, tricuspid atresia
      (e) alcohol (25% of fetal alcohol syndrome): VSD, ASD
      (f) retinoic acid = isotretinoin (?15%)
   7. Paternal CHD (risk uncertain)

C. MENDELIAN SYNDROMES
   1. Tuberous sclerosis
   2. Ellis-van Creveld syndrome
   3. Noonan syndrome

D. FAMILIAL RISK FACTORS FOR RECURRENCE OF HEART DISEASE
   — overall incidence : 6-8:1,000 livebirths
   — affected sibling : 1-4% (risk doubled)
   — affected parent : 2.5-4%

◊ In 50% of neonates with CHD there is no identifiable risk factor!

POOR PROGNOSTIC FEATURES:
   (1) Intrauterine cardiac failure (hydrops)
   (2) Severe trisomy (18, 13)
   (3) Hypoplastic left heart + endocardial fibroelastosis
   (4) Delivery in center without pediatric cardiology

In utero detection of cardiac anomalies

A. ABNORMAL HEART POSITION
   1. Diaphragmatic hernia
   2.. Lung anomaly
   3. Pleural effusion
   4. Cardiac defect
B. CHAMBER ENLARGEMENT
   RA:
   1. Tricuspid regurgitation
   2. Tricuspid valve dysplasia
   3. Ebstein anomaly
   LA:
   1. Mitral stenosis
   2. Aortic stenosis
   RV:
   1. Coarctation
   2. Normal in 3rd trimester
   LV:
   1. Aortic stenosis
   2. Cardiomyopathy
C. ABNORMAL FOUR-CHAMBER VIEW
   1. Septal rhabdomyoma
   2. Endocardial cushion defect
   3. Ventricular septal defect
   4. Ebstein anomaly
   5. Single ventricle
D. VENTRICULAR DISPROPORTION
   1. Hypoplastic right / left ventricle
   2. Hypoplastic aortic arch
   3. Aortic / subaortic stenosis
   4. Coarctation of aorta
   5. Ostium primum defect
E. INCREASED AORTIC ROOT DIMENSION
   1. Tetralogy of Fallot
   2. Truncus arteriosus
   3. Hypoplastic left ventricle with transposition
F. DECREASED AORTIC ROOT DIMENSION
   1. Coarctation of aorta
   2. Hypoplastic left ventricle

◊ 26-80% of serious cardiac anomalies can be detected on four-chamber view!

◊ Increased sensitivity >20 weeks + by including outflow views!

Structural cardiac abnormalities + fetal hydrops

1. Atrioventricular septal defect + complete heart block
2. Hypoplastic left heart
3. Critical aortic stenosis
4. Cardiac tumor
5. Ectopia cordis
6. Dilated cardiomyopathy
7. Ebstein anomaly
8. Pulmonary atresia

Fetal echocardiographic views

A. FOUR-CHAMBER VIEW
   1. Position of heart within thorax
   2. Number of cardiac chambers
   3. Ventricular proportion
   4. Integrity of atrial + ventricular septa
   5. Position + size + excursion of AV valves
B. PARASTERNAL LONG-AXIS VIEW
   1. Continuity between ventricular septum + anterior aortic wall
   2. Caliber of aortic outflow tract
   3. Excursion of aortic valve leaflets

C. SHORT-AXIS VIEW OF OUTFLOW TRACTS
1. Spatial relationship between aorta + pulmonary artery
2. Caliber of aortic + pulmonary outflow tracts

D. AORTIC ARCH VIEW

FETAL GASTROINTESTINAL ANOMALIES

1. Esophageal atresia ± TE fistula
2. Duodenal atresia
3. Meconium peritonitis
4. Hirschsprung disease
5. Choledochal cyst
6. Mesenteric cyst

Abdominal wall defect

Prevalence: 1:2,000 pregnancies

1. Gastroschisis
2. Omphalocele:
   — upper abdominal wall defect
   3. Ectopia cordis
   4. Pentalogy of Cantrell
   — midabdominal wall defect: classic omphalocele
   — lower abdominal wall defect
   5. Bladder exstrophy
   6. Cloacal exstrophy
7. Amniotic band syndrome
8. Limb-body wall complex

Nonvisualization of fetal stomach

◊ Fetal swallowing begins at 11 weeks MA

Incidence: 2% (stomach is visualized in almost all normal fetuses by 14 weeks + in all normal fetuses by 19 weeks)

1. Physiologic gastric emptying / intermittent swallowing (repeat scan after 30 minutes)
2. Decreased amniotic fluid volume
3. CNS abnormalities that impair swallowing
4. GI tract abnormalities:
   (a) congenital diaphragmatic hernia
   (b) esophageal atresia ± TE fistula
   ◊ Nonvisualization of fetal stomach and polyhydramnios in 33% fetuses with esophageal atresia after 24 weeks MA!
5. Cleft palate

Double bubble sign

= fluid filled stomach + proximal duodenum

◊ A persistently fluid-filled duodenum is always abnormal!

1. Duodenal atresia (usually not seen <24 weeks MA)
   Cause: in 30% due to trisomy 21
2. Duodenal stenosis
3. Duodenal web
4. Annular pancreas
5. Preduodenal portal vein
6. Ladd bands
7. Malrotation

mnemonic: "LADS"
Ladd bands / malrotation
Annular pancreas
Duodenal atresia
Stenosis (duodenal)

Dilated bowel in fetus

1. Meconium ileus
   ◊ All newborns with meconium ileus have cystic fibrosis!
   ◊ 10-15% of newborns with cystic fibrosis present with meconium ileus!
2. "Apple peel" atresia of small bowel
3. Jejunal atresia
4. Megacystic-microcolon-intestinal hypoperistalsis syndrome
5. Colonic aganglionosis = Hirschsprung disease (may be associated with Down syndrome)
6. Anorectal atresia (associated with CNS abnormalities, part of VACTERL complex)

Bowel obstruction in fetus

Etiology: intestinal atresia / stenosis secondary to vascular accident, volvulus, meconium ileus, intussusception after organogenesis

Incidence: imperforate anus 1:3,000; small bowel 1:5,000; colon 1:20,000

Pathologic types:
I one / more transverse diaphragms
II blind-ending loops connected by fibrous string
III complete separation of blind-ending loops
IV apple-peel atresia of small bowel (occlusion of SMA branch)

Associated with: GI anomalies in 45% (malrotation, duplication, microcolon, esophageal atresia)

√ multiple distended bowel loops >7 mm in diameter
√ increased peristalsis
√ polyhydramnios (if obstruction above level of mid jejunum; exception esophageal atresia + TE fistula) due to fetal inability to cycle amniotic fluid through gut

Cx: Meconium peritonitis (50%)

DDx: (1) Other cystic masses: duodenal atresia, hydronephrosis, ovarian cyst, mesenteric cyst
(2) Chronic chloride diarrhea

Hyperechoic fetal bowel

Definition: bowel echogenicity ≥ bone

Incidence: 0.2–0.6% of 2nd trimester fetuses

Cause: (?) "constipation" in utero due to decreased swallowing, hypoperistalsis, bowel obstruction + increased fluid absorption

1. Normal small bowel variant (especially <20 weeks MA) with resolution on follow-up sonogram toward end of 2nd trimester (55–68%)
2. Meconium ileus
   ◊ Increased abdominal echogenicity is seen in 60–70% of fetuses with cystic fibrosis!

3. Meconium peritonitis
   Cause: (a) intestinal atresia with perforation
   (b) CMV infection
4. Chromosomal abnormality (3–25%)
   (a) Down syndrome (5–14%)
   (b) Trisomy 13, 18
   (c) Turner syndrome
5. Severe IUGR (16%)

Prognosis:
5-fold increase in risk for adverse fetal outcome (due to chromosomal abnormality, other anomalies, placental abruption, perinatal death [8–16%], IUGR [67–23%])
◊ 30–50% of fetuses with echogenic bowel in 2nd trimester will have poor outcome!

Management: parental testing for cystic fibrosis, careful fetal anatomic survey, follow-up for growth assessment

Intraabdominal calcifications in fetus

A. PERITONEAL
   1. Meconium peritonitis
   2. Plastic peritonitis associated with hydrometrocolpos
B. TUMORS
   1. Hemangioma / hemangioendothelioma
   2. Hepatoblastoma
   3. Metastatic neuroblastoma
   4. Teratoma
   5. Ovarian dermoid
C. CONGENITAL INFECTION
   1. Toxoplasmosis
   2. Cytomegalovirus

◊ Isolated liver calcifications are relatively frequent + of no clinical significance!

Cystic mass in fetal abdomen

A. POSTERIOR MID ABDOMEN
   1. Cysts of renal origin
   2. Hydroureteronephrosis
   3. Multicystic dysplastic kidney
   4. Paranephric collection
B. RIGHT UPPER QUADRANT
   1. Liver cyst
   2. Choledochal cyst
C. LEFT UPPER QUADRANT
   1. Splenic cyst
D. ANTERIOR MID ABDOMEN
   1. Gastrointestinal duplication cyst
   2. Mesenteric cyst
   3. Meconium pseudocyst
   4. Dilated bowel
   5. Urachal cyst
E. LOWER ABDOMEN
   1. Adnexal cyst: follicular cyst (most), corpus luteum cyst, theca lutein cyst, paraovarian cyst, teratoma, cystadenoma
      Cx of large cysts: polyhydramnios, dystocia, torsion, respiratory distress
      Prognosis: 60% resolve within first 6 months of life
   2. Hydrometrocolpos
   3. Meningocele
   4. Sacrococcygeal teratoma

Fetal ascites

A. ASCITES + FETAL HYDROPS
   1. Immune hydrops
   2. Nonimmune hydrops
B. ISOLATED ASCITES
   1. Urinary ascites
   2. Meconium peritonitis
   3. Bowel rupture
   4. Ruptured ovarian cyst
   5. Hydrometrocolpos
   6. Glycogen storage disease

FETAL URINARY TRACT ANOMALIES

Incidence: 0.25%–1% liveborn infants (OB-US); 1:100–1:200 neonates (pediatrics)

1. Bilateral renal agenesis
2. Infantile polycystic kidney disease
3. Adult polycystic kidney disease
4. Multicystic dysplastic kidney
5. Ureteropelvic junction obstruction
6. Megaureter
7. Posterior urethral valves
8. Prune belly syndrome
9. Megacystis-microcolon-intestinal hypoperistalsis syndrome
10. Mesoblastic nephroma
11. Wilms tumor
12. Neuroblastoma

Associated with: chromosome abnormalities in 12% (74% trisomy, 10% deletion, 9% sex chromosome aneuploidy, 6% triploidy)

• fetal urine production: 5 mL/hr at 20 weeks MA; 56 mL/hr at 40 weeks MA
√ bladder volume: 1 mL at 20 weeks MA; 36 mL at 40 weeks MA
√ filling + emptying of fetal urinary bladder occurs every 10 to 30 (range 7 to 43) minutes
√ increased renal parenchymal echogenicity indicates renal abnormality in 80%
√ fetal hydronephrosis
= AP diameter of renal pelvis >5 mm at 15–20 weeks, ≥8 mm at 20–30 weeks, ≥10 mm at >30 weeks

GYNECOLOGY

Precocious puberty

= early onset of puberty
• premature thelarche / adrenarche / menses

Isolated Premature Adrenarche

= pubic hair development due to action of adrenal androgens
- increased levels of adrenal androgens

√ prepubertal uterus + ovaries (0.1–1 cm^3)

Isolated Premature Thelarche

= breast enlargement

may occur without endocrine abnormalities

√ prepubertal uterus + ovaries

Pseudoprecocious Puberty

= PSEUDOSEXUAL PRECOCITY = incomplete precocious puberty

= pubertal changes occurring independently of the action of pituitary gonadotropins, ie, early development of secondary sex characteristics without ovulation

Cause: ovarian tumor (eg, granulosa theca-cell tumor, thecoma, choriocarcinoma), ovarian cyst, estrogen-producing adrenal tumor, hypothyroidism, neurofibromatosis, estrogen ingestion

- low gonadotropin levels after LHRH stimulation
- increased estradiol levels

√ prepubertal uterus + ovaries

√ asymmetric ovarian enlargement (one ovary 2.4–7 cm^3) with macrocysts (>9 mm)

True Precocious Puberty

= TRUE ISOSEXUAL PRECOCITY = complete precocious puberty

= early development of gonads + secondary sex characteristics with ovulation before 8 years of age

Cause:

(1) Idiopathic activation of hypothalamic-pituitary-gonadal axis (80%)

(2) Lesion of pituitary gland / hypothalamus

- increased levels of estrogen
- increased gonadotropin levels after LHRH stimulation
- advanced bone age

√ adult-sized ovaries (1.2–12 cm^3)

√ dominance of corpus over cervix length

Amenorrhea

Primary Amenorrhea

= failure to menstruate by 16 years of age

Cause:

A. FEMALE ANATOMIC ANOMALIES

B. CONGENITAL DISORDERS OF SEXUAL DIFFERENTIATION

(a) pure gonadal dysgenesis

√ bilateral dysfunctional / streak gonads

(b) mixed gonadal dysgenesis

√ testis + streak gonad

Risk: in 25% development of dysgerminoma / gonadoblastoma in dysgenetic gonads with Y chromosome

C. OVARIAN FAILURE / DYSFUNCTION

D. HYPOTHALAMIC / PITUITARY CAUSES

√ absent / streak gonads + infantile uterus:

1. Hypogonadotropic hypogonadism

(a) hypothalamic dysfunction: hypothalamic tumor, Kallmann disease (= lack of pulsatile GnRH release), systemic illness, constitutional growth delay, extreme physical / psychological / nutritional stress (cystic fibrosis, sickle cell disease, Crohn disease)

(b) pituitary dysfunction: disruption of pituitary stalk from child abuse, head trauma

2. Hypergonadotropic hypogonadism

= ovarian tissue fails to respond to endogenous gonadotropins

(a) abnormal karyotype: Turner syndrome, XY gonadal dysgenesis

(b) radiation, chemotherapy, autoimmune disease

√ absent uterus:

1. Testicular feminization = male intersex = male pseudohermaphroditism (end-organ insensitivity to testosterone)
2. Müllerian dysgenesis (= Mayer-Rokitansky-Küster-Hauser syndrome)

   √ normal fallopian tubes + ovaries

   associated with: unilateral renal abnormality (50%), skeletal abnormality (12%)

√ small infantile uterus:

1. Androgen-producing virilizing tumors of adolescent ovary (usually Sertoli-Leydig cell tumor)

   √ unilateral adnexal mass
2. Turner syndrome
3. In utero exposure to diethylstilbestrol

√ normal uterus + unilateral ovarian tumor:

1. Estrogen-producing with disruption of menstrual cycle: granulosa cell tumor, thecoma

√ hydrometrocolpos:

1. Vaginal membrane / septum

√ bilateral ovarian enlargement:

1. Polycystic ovary syndrome (= Stein-Leventhal syndrome): most common cause of secondary amenorrhea

Secondary Amenorrhea

1. Pregnancy: most common cause in girls >9 years of age
2. Polycystic ovary syndrome
3. Asherman syndrome
4. All causes of primary amenorrhea

Calcifications Of Female Genital Tract

A. UTERUS
1. Uterine fibroid
2. Arcuate arteries

B. OVARIES
1. Dermoid cyst (50%)
2. Papillary cystadenoma (psammomatous bodies)
3. Cystadenocarcinoma
4. Hemangiopericytoma
5. Gonadoblastoma
6. Chronic ovarian torsion
7. Pseudomyxoma peritonei

C. FALLOPIAN TUBES
1. Tuberculous salpingitis

D. PLACENTA

E. LITHOPEDION

Free Fluid In Cul-de-sac

1. Follicular rupture
2. Ovulation
3. Ectopic pregnancy
4. S/P culdocentesis
5. Ovarian neoplasm
6. Pelvic inflammatory disease

PELVIC MASS

Frequency Of Pelvic Masses

1.	Benign adnexal cyst	34%
2.	Leiomyoma	14%
3.	Cancers	14%
4.	Dermoid	13%
5.	Endometriosis	10%
6.	Pelvic inflammatory disease	8%

Cystic Pelvic Masses

A. CYSTIC ADNEXAL MASS

B. EXTRAADNEXAL CYSTIC MASS
1. Peritoneal inclusion cyst
2. Mesenteric cyst
3. Lymphocele
4. Bladder diverticulum
5. Ectopic gestation
6. Fluid-distended bowel
7. Loculated pelvic abscess: appendiceal, diverticular, postoperative

Complex Pelvic Mass

mnemonic: "CHEETAH"

Cystadenoma / cystadenocarcinoma
Hemorrhagic cyst
Endometrioma
Ectopic pregnancy
Teratoma (dermoid)
Abscess (from adjacent appendicitis, etc.)
Hematoma in pelvis

Solid Pelvic Masses

1. Pedunculated myoma (most common)
2. Fibroma
3. Adenofibroma
4. Thecoma
5. Brenner tumor

Extrauterine Pelvic Masses

1. Solid adnexal mass
2. Metastatic disease
3. Lymphoma
4. Pelvic kidney
5. Rectosigmoid carcinoma
6. Prostate carcinoma
7. Benign prostatic enlargement
8. Bladder carcinoma
9. Retroperitoneal tumor
10. Intraperitoneal fat
11. Vascular mass / malformation
12. Hematoma
13. Bowel

ADNEXA

Adnexal Masses

A. CYSTIC
1. Physiologic ovarian cyst:
   — Graafian follicle: at midcycle <25 mm
   — Corpus luteum: after midcycle <15 mm
2. Functional / retention cyst
3. Endometrioma
4. Tuboovarian abscess
5. Dermoid cyst
6. Ectopic pregnancy
7. Paraovarian cyst
8. Serous / mucinous cystadenoma
9. Serous / mucinous cystadenocarcinoma
10. Hyperstimulation cysts
11. Peritoneal inclusion cyst
12. Massive ovarian edema
13. Hydrosalpinx

B. SOLID
1. Ovarian tumor
2. Ovarian torsion
3. Oophoritis
4. Polycystic ovaries
5. Fallopian tube carcinoma

(DDx: pedunculated fibroid)

Ovarian Tumors

- pressure symptoms: abdominal discomfort, vomiting, flatulence, dyspnea
- acute pain from torsion, hemorrhage
- chronic pain from slowly enlarging mass, impaction, adhesions
- menstrual irregularity

Radiologic guidelines:

◊ Imaging features of ovarian neoplasms virtually never allow a specific diagnosis. Regardless of further differentiation patients always undergo surgery!

Signs suggestive of malignancy:
√ solid ovarian tumor
√ many solid-tissue elements in a complex lesion

OB&GYN

√ wall thickness >3 mm
√ inner wall irregularities
√ thick septations >3 mm
√ increased echogenicity within a cyst

Age: 13% of neoplasms malignant in premenopause; 45% of neoplasms malignant in postmenopause

Cx: (1) Torsion (in 10–20%)
(2) Rupture (rare)
(3) Infection

Classification:

A. TUMORS OF SURFACE EPITHELIUM (60%)
85–95% of all ovarian cancers (although majority of epithelial tumors are benign)
1. Serous ovarian tumor
2. Mucinous ovarian tumor
3. Endometrioid tumor
4. Cystadenofibroma
5. Clear cell adenocarcinoma
6. Brenner tumor
7. Undifferentiated carcinoma

B. GERM CELL TUMORS (30%)
40% of germ cell tumors are malignant
(a) benign
1. Dermoid cyst = mature teratoma (most common)
(b) malignant
account for 75% of ovarian cancers seen in 1st–2nd decade of life; <5% of all ovarian tumors; in order of frequency:
1. Dysgerminoma
2. Immature teratoma
3. Endodermal sinus tumor
4. Embryonal carcinoma
5. Choriocarcinoma

C. GONADAL STROMAL TUMORS (5%)
(a) Sex cord-mesenchyme tumors
1. Granulosa cell tumor
2. Theca cell tumor
3. Luteal cell tumor
4. Arrhenoblastoma
(b) Connective tissue tumor
1. Fibroma
2. Fibrosarcoma
— estrogen-producing tumors: granulosa cell tumor, theca cell tumor = thecoma
— androgen-producing tumors: arrhenoblastoma, Sertoli-Leydig cell tumor, clear cell tumor

D. SECONDARY OVARIAN TUMORS (5%)
Metastases from: pelvic organs, upper GI tract, breast, bronchus, reticuloendothelial tumors, leukemia

Subclassification:

	adenoma	*borderline*	*adenocarcinoma*
serous	60%	15%	25%
mucinous	80%	10%	10%
endometrioid			almost always
clear cell			almost always
undifferentiated			always

Terminology:
prefix "cyst-" : cystic component present
suffix "-fibroma" : >50% fibrous component
"tumor of low malignant potential" : borderline malignant

Solid Ovarian Tumor

1. Fibroma
2. Thecoma
3. Granulosa cell tumor
4. Sertoli-Leydig cell tumor
5. Brenner tumor
6. Sarcoma
7. Dysgerminoma
8. Endodermal sinus tumor
9. Teratoma
10. Metastasis
11. Endometrioma
12. Massive ovarian edema

Ovarian Cyst

Image Signature Of Ovarian Cysts

A. SIMPLE CYST
= sharply defined wall; NO internal septations / mural nodules
US:
√ pulsatility index >1.0 / RI >0.4 (unreliable!)
MR:
√ isointense to urine on T1WI + T2WI

B. COMPLEX CYST
= does not satisfy criteria for hemorrhagic cysts / endometrioma
√ internal septations / mural nodules / internal echoes
√ mixed signal intensity, hyperintense on T2WI

C. HEMORRHAGIC CYST
US:
√ echogenic mass
√ whirled pattern of mixed echogenicity
√ "ground-glass" pattern = diffuse low-level echoes
√ "fishnet weave" pattern = fine interdigitating septations
√ NO color Doppler signals
MR:
√ intermediate / high intensity on T1WI
√ hyperintense with distinct central area of hypointensity on T2WI

Management Of Ovarian Cyst

A. PREMENOPAUSAL
1. Unilocular cyst ≤2.5 cm ± hemorrhage
Rx: no follow-up unless on birth control pills
2. Unilocular thin-walled cyst 2.5–6 cm without hemorrhage
Rx: clinical / sonographic follow-up in 1–2 months ± addition of hormones
3. Unilocular cyst 2.5–6 cm with hemorrhage
Rx: sonographic follow-up in 1 month ± addition of hormones

4. Unilocular cyst >6 cm
   Rx: surgery

N.B.: All follow-up scans should take place in the immediate postmenstrual period, when follicular cysts should not be present!

B. POSTMENOPAUSAL
1. Unilocular nonseptated thin-walled cyst <3 cm
   Incidence: 15–17%
   √ high resistive index (RI) of >0.7 (resistive index <0.40 is suspect for malignancy!)
   Prognosis: 56% decrease in size / disappear; 28% remain unchanged for up to 2 years
   DDx: serous ovarian cyst, peritubal cyst, hydrosalpinx
   Rx: serial follow-up
2. Septated cyst / cyst >3 cm / cyst with low RI
   ◊ 18% of complex cysts are malignant!
   Rx: CA-125 determination + surgical exploration

◊ Screening of 1300 symptomatic women:
— in 2.5% abnormalities on US
— in 1.9% benign ovarian tumors
— in 0.15% ovarian cancers

UTERUS

Postmenopausal Bleeding

1. Endometrial atrophy (most commonly)
   • thin atrophic endometrium is prone to superficial ulceration
   √ in 75% endometrial thickness <4–5 mm
   √ in 25% endometrial thickness of 6–15 mm
2. Endometrial adenomatous hyperplasia
   √ thickened homogeneous texture
3. Endometrial polyp
   √ cystic endometrial spaces
4. Submucosal fibroid
5. Endometrial carcinoma (in 7–30%)
   10% cancer rate with endometrial thickness of 6–15 mm
   50% cancer rate with endometrial thickness of >15 mm
   √ heterogeneous endometrium
   √ irregular poorly defined endometrial-myometrial interface

Thickened Irregular Endometrium

Normal endometrial thickness: <1 cm

1. **Endometrial polyp**
   = focal hyperplasia of stratum basale; in 20% multiple
   Age: mainly 30–60 years
   Histo: projections of endometrial glands + stroma into uterine cavity
   (a) hyperplastic polyp resembling endometrial hyperplasia
   (b) functional polyp resembling surrounding endometrium (least frequent)
   (c) atrophic polyp
   √ enlarged cystically dilated glands
   √ well-defined homogeneous hyperechoic intracavitary mass
   √ heterogeneous texture suggests infarction, cystic changes, hemorrhage
   Malignant transformation: in 0.4–3.7%
2. **Endometrial hyperplasia**
   Age: peri- / postmenopausal women
   Cause: prolonged endogenous / exogenous unopposed estrogen stimulation
   √ endometrial thickening >5–6 mm
   Types:
   (a) glandular-cystic hyperplasia (more common)
   Histo: dilated glands lined by tall columnar / cuboidal epithelium
   √ small cysts within evenly echogenic endometrium
   Prognosis: NO premalignant condition
   (b) adenomatous hyperplasia
   √ endometrium with irregular hypoechoic areas
   Prognosis: precursor of endometrial cancer
3. Endometritis
4. Primary carcinoma of the endometrium
   Location: predominantly in uterine fundus; 24% in isthmic portion)
   √ irregular heterogeneous endometrium
   √ mean endometrial thickness of 18.2 mm
5. Tamoxifen-related endometrial changes
   = nonsteroidal antiestrogen may act as partial estrogen agonist with proliferative effects on endometrium
6. Metastatic carcinoma:
   ovary, cervix, fallopian tube, leukemia
7. Hydatidiform mole
   √ echogenic mass with irregular sonolucent areas
8. Incomplete abortion
9. Submucosal leiomyoma

Fluid Collection Within Endometrial Canal

Types: blood, mucus, purulent material

A. PREMENOPAUSAL
1. Congenital obstructive lesion: imperforate hymen, vaginal septum, vaginal / cervical atresia
2. Acquired obstructive lesion: cervical stenosis (following instrumentation / radiation), cervical carcinoma
3. Spontaneous hematometra in bleeding disorders
4. Pregnancy: intrauterine, ectopic, incomplete abortion

B. POSTMENOPAUSAL
1. Cervical stenosis
2. Pyometrium
3. Polyps
4. Endometrial / cervical / ovarian cancer

Endometrial Cysts

1. Endometrial cystic atrophy
   Histo: cystically dilated atrophic glands lined by single layer of flattened / low cuboidal epithelium
   √ very thin endometrium of <4–5 mm
2. Endometrial cystic hyperplasia

Diffuse Uterine Enlargement

1. Diffuse leiomyomatosis
2. Adenomyosis
3. Endometrial carcinoma (15%)

Uterine Masses

A. BENIGN
   1. Uterine fibroids (99%)
   2. Pyometra
   3. Hemato- / hydrocolpos
   4. Transient uterine contraction (during pregnancy)
   5. Bicornuate uterus
   6. Adenomyosis
   7. Intrauterine pregnancy
   8. Lipoleiomyoma (<50 cases in world literature)

B. MALIGNANT
   1. Cervical carcinoma
   2. Endometrial carcinoma
   3. Leiomyosarcoma
   4. Invasive trophoblastic disease

Fundic Depression On HSG

1. Bicornuate uterus
2. Septate uterus
3. Arcuate uterus
4. Fundal myoma

VAGINA

Vaginal Cyst

1. Gartner duct cyst
2. Bartholin gland cyst
   = female homologue of male Cowper glands
   Location: posterolateral portion of lower vagina
3. Paramesonephric / müllerian duct cyst
   = aberrant remnant of paramesonephric duct
   Location: anterior wall of vagina near cervix
4. Epithelial inclusion cyst
   = arise from urogenital sinus
   Histo: lined by transitional epithelium containing thick caseous material

Vaginal Fistula

1. Enterovaginal fistula
   (a) rectovaginal: incomplete healing of perineal laceration from obstetric trauma, radiation therapy
   (b) anovaginal: inflammatory bowel disease (10% of patients with Crohn disease)
   (c) colovaginal: diverticulitis
2. Vesicovaginal fistula: hysterectomy, radiation therapy
3. Ureterovaginal fistula: vaginal hysterectomy

Vaginal & Paravaginal Neoplasm

A. PRIMARY
   1. Cavernous hemangioma of vulva
   2. Pedunculated submucosal leiomyoma prolapsed into vagina
   3. Adenoid cystic carcinoma of Bartholin gland
   4. Vaginal carcinoma
      (a) squamous cell carcinoma (90%)
      (b) adenocarcinoma (3%)
   5. Rhabdomyosarcoma

B. SECONDARY (80% of all vaginal tumors)
   direct extension from bladder, rectum, cervix, uterus

GAS IN GENITAL TRACT

A. UTERUS
   1. Endometritis
   2. Superinfection of leiomyoma: more common in submucosal leiomyoma (insufficient blood supply)
   3. Bacterial metabolism of necrotic neoplastic tissue
   4. Fistula to GI tract: uterine cancer
   5. Pyometra secondary to obstruction by cervical cancer
   6. Gas gangrene: due to clostridial infection from septic abortion

B. OVARY
   1. Superinfected ovarian neoplasm

C. VAGINA
   1. Vaginitis emphysematosa = nonbacterial self-limiting process mostly occurring during pregnancy characterized by numerous gas-filled spaces in submucosa of vagina + exocervix

ANATOMY AND PHYSIOLOGY OF FEMALE REPRODUCTIVE SYSTEM

HUMAN CHORIONIC GONADOTROPIN

= HCG = glycoprotein elaborated by placental trophoblastic cells beginning the 8th day after conception

A. IMMUNOLOGIC PREGNANCY TEST
= indirect agglutination test for HCG in urine; cross-reaction with other hormones / medications possible
Becomes positive at 5 weeks MA
Advantages: readily available, easily + rapidly performed
Disadvantages: frequently false-positive + false-negative results
Sensitivity:
(a) slide: 400–15,000 mIU/mL (2 min test time)
(b) test tube: 1,000–3,000 mIU/mL (2 hours test time)

B. RADIOIMMUNOASSAY (RIA) PREGNANCY TEST
= measures beta subunit of HCG in serum with a sensitivity as low as 1–2 mIU/mL
◊ Serum β-HCG becomes positive at 3 weeks MA / 7–10 days following conception!
Standards:
(1) Second International Standard (SIS)
(2) International Reference Preparation (IRP)
(3) Third International Standard (TIS)
1 mIU/mL (SIS) = 2 mIU/mL (IRP) = 2 mIU/mL (TIS)
1 ng/mL = 5– 6 mIU/mL (SIS)
= 10–12 mIU/mL (IRP or TIS)
◊ Variations of lab values of up to 50% can occur among different laboratories!
◊ 6–15% between-run precision!
Advantages: specific for HCG, sensitive
Disadvantages: requires specialized lab + 3–24 hours for completion
Sensitivity:
(a) qualitative: 25–30 mIU/mL (3 hours test time)
(b) quantitative: 3–4 mIU/mL (24 hours test time)
Rise:
>66% increase of initial β-HCG level over 48 hours in 86% of NORMAL pregnancies
<66% increase of initial β-HCG level over 48 hours in 87% of ECTOPIC pregnancies
◊ β-HCG levels double every 2–3 days during first 60 days of pregnancy!

"1–7–11 rule":

β-HCG (IRP)	US landmarks	Gestational age
1,000 mIU/mL	gestational sac	32 d (<5 weeks)
7,200 mIU/mL	yolk sac	36 d (5 weeks)
10,800 mIU/mL	embryo + heart motion	40 d (<6 weeks)

ANATOMY OF GESTATION

Choriodecidua

Chorion
= trophoblast + fetal mesenchyme with villous stems protruding into decidua; provides nutrition for developing embryo
(a) chorion frondosum = part adjacent to decidua basalis, forms primordial placenta
(b) chorion laeve = smooth portion of chorion with atrophied villi
(c) "chorionic plate" = amnionic membrane covering the chorionic plate of the placenta

Decidua
(a) decidua basalis = between chorion frondosum + myometrium
(b) decidua capsularis = portion protruding into uterine cavity
(c) decidua parietalis = decidua vera = portion lining the uterine cavity elsewhere

Gestational Sac

Arises from blastocyst which implants into secretory endometrium 6–7 days after ovulation, surrounded by echogenic trophoblast
√ intradecidual sign (earliest sign) = intrauterine fluid collection corresponding to gestational sac completely embedded within decidua (48% sensitive, 66% specific, 45% accurate)
√ double decidual sac sign (DDS) [most useful at 4–6 weeks GA] = 2 concentric rings (decidua parietalis adjacent to decidua capsularis) surrounding a portion of the gestational sac
◊ A double decidual sac sign correlates with the presence of pregnancy in 98%!
√ GS surrounded by endometrial thickening >12 mm
√ continuous hyperechoic inner rim >2 mm thick
√ spherical / ovoid shape without angulations
√ mean sac diameter grows 1.13 (range 0.71–1.75) mm/day

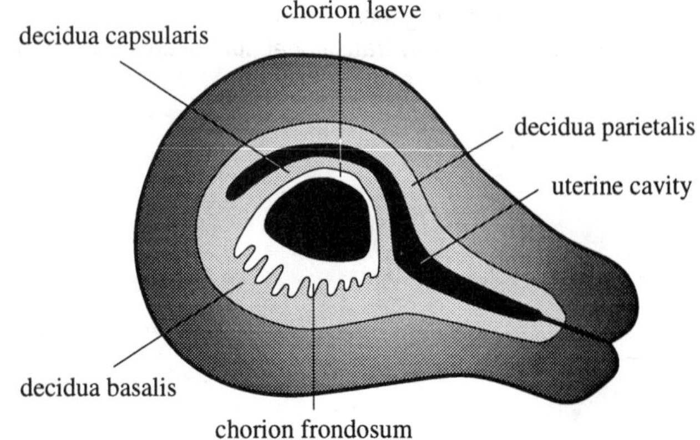

Gestational Sac Size

linear growth: 10 mm by 5th week MA
60 mm by 12th week MA

fills chorionic cavity by 11–12 weeks MA

Visualization Of Gestational Sac

Earliest visualization: mean sac diameter of 2–3 mm

A. GS VISUALIZATION VERSUS β-HCG LEVEL (2nd International Standard):
  (a) on transabdominal scan:
    in 100% with β-HCG levels of >1,800 IU/L
  (b) on transvaginal scan:
    in 20% with β-HCG levels of <500 IU/L
    in 80% with β-HCG levels of 500–1,000 IU/L
    in 100% with β-HCG levels of >1,000 IU/L

B. GS VISUALIZATION VERSUS MENSTRUAL AGE
  (a) on transabdominal scan:
    5.0 ± 1 weeks = 5–10 mm
    5.5 ± 1 weeks = 8.5–13 mm
    6.0 ± 1 weeks = 12–17 mm
  (b) on transvaginal scan:
    5.0 ± 1 weeks = 2 mm
    5.5 ± 1 weeks = 6 mm
    6.0 ± 1 weeks = 11 mm

C. GS VISUALIZATION VERSUS VISUALIZATION OF EMBRYO
  (a) on transabdominal scan
    100% visualization if gestational sac ≥27 mm
  (b) on transvaginal scan
    100% visualization if gestational sac ≥12 mm
  ◊ Transvaginal scan not necessary if on transabdominal scan gestational sac >27 mm without evidence of embryo!

Predictive of miscarriage (in 94%):

"first-trimester oligohydramnios" (misnomer: not diminished size of amnionic cavity but rather chorionic cavity)

= mean sac diameter – CRL ≤ 5 mm (with a live embryo at 5.5–9.0 weeks)

Yolk Sac

= rounded sonolucent structure (outside amniotic cavity) within chorionic sac (= extracoelomic cavity) connected to umbilicus via a narrow stalk; formed by proliferation of endodermal cells at around 4 weeks MA; part of yolk sac is incorporated into fetal gut; the rest persists as a sac connected to the fetus by the vitelline duct

Function:
  (a) transfer of nutrients from trophoblast to embryo prior to functioning placental circulatio
  (b) early formation of blood vessels + blood precursors on sac wall
  (c) formation of primitive gut
  (d) source of primordial germ cells

Mean size:
  1.0 mm by 4.7 weeks MA; 2.0 mm by 5.6 weeks MA; 3.0 mm by 7.1 weeks MA; 4.0 (2.2–5.3) mm by 10 weeks MA; disappears around 12 weeks MA

Earliest visualization:
  √ at 4–5 weeks MA as one of the "double blebs" on endovaginal scan; in 65% with GS size of ≥8 mm
  ◊ Visualization excludes the possibility of an ectopic / anembryonic pregnancy!

Failed pregnancy:
  Abnormal pregnancy outcome (using endovaginal technique) generally if
  (a) yolk sac absent with GS diameter of ≥20 mm (100% specificity + 100% PPV)
  (b) yolk sac diameter >5.6 mm at <10 weeks MA
  (c) embryo visualized without demonstrable yolk sac
  (d) yolk sac shape persistently abnormal

Embryo

Developmental stages:
  Preembryonic period: 2nd–4th week MA
  Trilaminar embryonic disk: during 5th week MA
    3 laminae = ectoderm, endoderm, mesoderm
  Embryonic period: 6th–10th week MA
    physiologic umbilical herniation: 8th–12th week MA
  Fetal period: beginning at 11th week MA

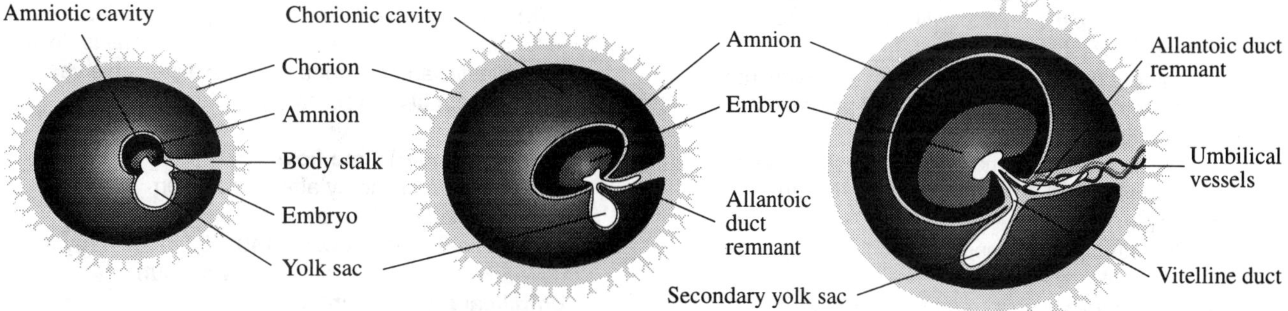

Simple double bleb stage
earliest detection at 5 weeks GA, embryo 2 mm in length

Vitelline duct
8 weeks GA

Early coiled umbilical cord
9 weeks GA

Average growth rate:
0.7 mm per day / 1.5 mm every 2 days;
curvilinear growth from 7 mm at 6.3 weeks MA to 50 mm at 12.0 weeks MA

Earliest visualization:
at 5.4 weeks MA at CRL of 1.2 mm on endovaginal scan

Failed pregnancy:
nonvisualization of embryo with mean gestational sac size of ≥18 mm

Cardiac activity

Heart begins to contract at a CRL of 1.5–3 mm = 6th week MA

Earliest visualization (on endovaginal scan):
(a) in 65% of embryos with a CRL of 2–4.9 mm
(b) in 100% at ≥ 5 mm CRL = 6.2 weeks

Failed pregnancy:
nonvisualization of cardiac activity with CRL of 2–12 mm means embryonic demise in 94%!
◊ Spontaneous pregnancy loss at <8 weeks gestation occurs in 10–17% of embryos with cardiac activity!

Embryonic Mortality Rate	≤6.2 weeks	≤7.0 weeks
11%	>100 bpm	>120 bpm
32%	90–99 bpm	110–119 bpm
64%	80–89 bpm	100–109 bpm
100%	<80 bpm	<100 bpm

Amnionic membrane

= curvilinear echogenic line within chorionic sac; fills chorionic cavity by 11–12 weeks MA;

Fusion:
— fuses with chorionic membrane at approximately 16 weeks MA to form the chorionic plate
— incomplete fusion with chorion frequent (DDx: subchorionic hemorrhage, twin abortion, coexistent with limb-body wall complex)

Umbilical cord

Embryology:
- cord forms between 5th and 12th postmenstrual week with contributions from body stalk, omphalo-mesenteric or vitelline duct, yolk sac, allantois
- junction of the amnion with ventral surface of embryo will form umbilicus
- midgut undergoes physiologic herniation into the base of the umbilical cord 7–12 postmenstrual weeks
- cord grows until end of 2nd trimester: average diameter of 17 mm, length of 50–60 cm

Anatomy:
- two umbilical arteries = branches of the two internal iliac arteries
- one umbilical vein (remains after regression of right umbilical vein in early embryonic period)
- Wharton jelly = compressible matrix of cord
- spiraling of cord with 0–40 twists established by 9 weeks

Placental grading

according to echo appearance of basal zone, chorionic plate, placental substance
◊ Premature placental calcification is associated with cigarette smoking, hypertension, IUGR!
◊ Not considered useful because placental grading is imprecise for fetal dating + for fetal lung maturity!

GRADE 0
√ homogeneous placenta + straight line of chorionic plate
Time: <30 weeks MA

GRADE 1
√ undulated chorionic plate + scattered bright placental echoes
Time: seen at any time during pregnancy; in 40% at term
◊ in 68% L/S ratio >2.0

GRADE 2
√ linear bright echoes parallel to basal plate
√ confluent stippled echoes within placenta ± indentations of chorionic plate
Time: rarely seen in gestations <32 weeks MA; seen in 40% at term
◊ in 87% L/S ratio >2.0

GRADE 3
√ calcified intercotyledonary septa, often surrounding sonolucent center
Time: rarely seen in gestations <34 weeks MA; in 15–20% at term
◊ in 100% L/S ratio >2.0 (= strongly correlated with lung maturity)

PREMATURE PLACENTAL SENESCENCE
= grade 3 placenta seen in gestation <34 weeks MA
◊ in 50% suggestive of maternal hypertension / IUGR

Uteroplacental circulation

By 20 weeks MA trophoblast invades maternal vessels and transforms spiral arteries into distended tortuous vessels = uteroplacental arteries

Histo:
(a) in the decidual portion of spiral arteries: proliferating trophoblast from anchoring villi invades lumen of spiral arteries + partially replaces endothelium
(b) in the myometrial portion of spiral arteries: disintegration of smooth muscle elements (loss of elastic lamina) leads to easily distensible vascular system of low resistance

Uterine blood volume flow
— 50 mL/min shortly after conception
— 500–900 mL/min by term
Intervillous blood flow: 140 ± 53 mL/min (by Xe-133 washout)

Umbilical artery Doppler

Variables of Doppler measurements:
site of Doppler (close to placenta preferred), fetal heart rate, fetal breathing, drugs (ritodrine hydrochloride decreases S/D ratio)

√ degree of diastolic flow increases as gestation progresses
- S/D ratio between 3.3 and 4.3 at 20 weeks
- S/D ratio between 1.7 and 2.4 at term

√ highly turbulent flow

IUGR Lesions

= narrowing of vascular lumen through
(a) thrombosis of decidual segments of uteroplacental arteries
(b) failure of development of myometrial segments of uteroplacental arteries

FETAL MENSURATION

US is more reliable than LMP / physical examination

ULTRASOUND MILESTONES:
√ gestational sac w/o embryo or yolk sac = 5.0 weeks
√ gestational sac + yolk sac w/o embryo = 5.5 weeks
√ heartbeat ± embryo <5 mm = 6.0 weeks
Accuracy: ± 0.5 week

Fetal Age

= GESTATIONAL AGE (GA) = "MENSTRUAL AGE" (MA)
= age of pregnancy based on woman's regular last menstrual period (LMP) projecting the estimated date of confinement (EDC) at 40 weeks

◊ Note the inaccurate clinical usage of "gestational age," which strictly speaking refers to the true age of the pregnancy counting from the day of conception, whereas "menstrual age" refers to the true age of the pregnancy + approximately 2 weeks counting from the first day of the last menstruation!

◊ On subsequent scans GA = GA assigned at 1st ultrasound + number of intervening weeks!

ACCURACY (95% confidence range):

Stage	*Based on*	*Accuracy [weeks]*
1st trimester		
(5–6 weeks)	US milestones	±0.5
(6–13 weeks)	CRL	±0.7
2nd trimester		
(14–20 weeks)	cBPD / HC	±1.2
	BPD / FL	±1.4
(20–26 weeks)	cBPD / HC	±1.9
	BPD / FL	±2.1–2.5
3rd trimester		
(26–32 weeks)	cBPD / HC / FL	±3.1–3.4
	FL	±3.1
(32–42 weeks)	cBPD / HC / FL	±3.5–3.8
	FL	±3.5

Gestational Sac

= average of 3 diameters (craniocaudad, AP, TRV) of anechoic space within sac walls

◊ used for dating between 6–12 weeks MA (identified as early as 5 weeks MA (on transabdominal scan)

Accuracy: ± 1 week

Early Embryonic Size

= length of embryo <25 mm on transvaginal scan <10 weeks MA

Gestational age (days) = embryonic size (mm) + 42
Accuracy: ± 3 days

Crown-rump Length (CRL)

= length of fetus; useful up to 12 weeks MA (usually identified by 7 weeks MA on transabdominal scan)

Rule of thumb: MA (in weeks) = CRL (in cm) + 6

Biparietal Diameter (BPD)

= measured from leading edge to leading edge of calvarial table at widest transaxial plane of skull
= level of thalami + cavum septi pellucidi + sylvian fissures with middle cerebral arteries

◊ Excellent means of estimating GA in 2nd trimester >12 weeks MA

Accuracy:
2 mm for "between occasion error"
◊ Most accurate for dating if combined with HC, AC, FL provided body ratios are normal!
◊ Less reliable for dating in 3rd trimester because of increasing biologic variability!

Cephalic Index (CI)

= BPD / OFD; measurements of BPD and occipitofrontal diameter (OFD) are both taken from outer to outer edge of calvarium

◊ Confirms appropriate use of BPD if ratio is between 0.70–0.86 (2 SD)

Corrected BPD (cBPD)

= BPD and OFD are used to adjust for variations in head shape

$$cBPD = \sqrt{BPD \times OFD \div 1.26}$$

Head Circumference (HC)

Used if ratio of BPD/OFD outside 0.70–0.86

HC = ([BPD + OFD]/2) x π
= ([BPD + OFD] x 1.62) x 3.1417

Accuracy: slightly less than for BPD

HC too large: hydrocephalus, hydranencephalus, intracranial hemorrhage, short limb dystrophies, tumor

HC too small: anencephaly, cerebral infarction, synostosis, microcephaly vera

Abdominal Circumference (AC)

= measured at level of vascular junction of umbilical vein with left portal vein ("hockey-stick" appearance) where it is equidistant from the lateral walls in a plane perpendicular to long axis of fetus; measured from outer edge to outer edge of soft tissues

◊ Allows evaluation of head-to-body disproportion
◊ Better predictor of fetal weight than BPD

AC too large: GI tract obstructions, obstructive uropathy, ascites, hepatosplenomegaly, congenital nephrosis, abdominal tumor

AC too small: diaphragmatic hernia, omphalocele, gastroschisis, renal agenesis

Femur Length (FL)
= measurement of ossified femoral diaphysis
Error: "flare" at distal end included in measurement (= reflection from cartilaginous condyle)

Thoracic Circumference (TC)
= measured in axial plane of chest which includes four-chamber view of heart without inclusion of SQ tissue
◊ Linear growth between 16 and 40 weeks similar to AC
Useful age-independent parameter: TC:AC >0.80

Estimated Fetal Weight (EFW)
based on measurements of head size (BPD / HC), abdominal size (AD / AC), and femur length (FL)

Accuracy:

body part used	95% confidence range
abdomen	±22%
head + abdomen	±17–20%
head + abdomen + femur	±15%

Appearance Of Epiphyseal Bone Centers
in 95% of all cases
— distal femoral epiphysis (DFE): >33 weeks GA
— distal femoral epiphysis (DFE) >5 mm: >35 weeks
— proximal tibial epiphysis (PTE): >35 weeks GA
— proximal humeral epiphysis (PHE): >38 weeks GA

CNS Ventricles
width of 3rd ventricle: <3.5 mm (any gestational age)

Diameter Of Cisterna Magna
measured from inner margin of occiput to vermis cerebelli: 2–10 mm

DISCORDANT ESTIMATED DATE OF CONFINEMENT (EDC) BY LMP AND BPD:
1. Methodological error in measurement
   (a) wrong axial section
   (b) cranial compression (multiple gestation, breech presentation, oligohydramnios, dolichocephaly)
2. Erroneous LMP
   other measurements (AC, FL) correlate with BPD
3. Abnormal head growth
   (a) BPD less than AC: microcephaly, fetal macrosomia
   (b) BPD more than AC: intracranial abnormality, asymmetric IUGR

ASSESSMENT OF FETAL WELL-BEING

Amniotic Fluid Index
= sum of vertical depths of largest clear amniotic fluid pockets in the 4 uterine quadrants measured in mm
Method: patient supine, uterus viewed as 4 equal quadrants, transducer perpendicular to plane of floor + aligned longitudinally with patient's spine
Variation: 3.1% intraobserver, 6.7% interobserver

Result:
— 95th percentile: 185 mm at 16 weeks GA, rising to 280 mm at 35 weeks, declining to 190 at 42 weeks
— 5th percentile: 80 mm at 16 weeks GA, rising to 100 mm at 23 weeks, declining to 70 mm at 42 weeks

Biophysical Profile (Platt and Manning) = BPP
= in utero Apgar score = assessment of fetal well-being
Gestational age at entry: 25 weeks MA
Observation period: 30 (occasionally 60) minutes; ordinarily <8 minutes needed; in 2% full 30 minutes required

A. ACUTE BIOPHYSICAL VARIABLES
   ◊ Subject to rhythmic variation coincident with sleep-wake cycle!
   1. Fetal breathing movement (FBM):
      √ ≥1 episode of chest + abdominal wall movement for a period lasting 30 seconds (time is arbitrary to avoid confusion with general body movements / maternal respiration)
      stimulated by: glucose, catecholamine, caffeine, prostaglandin synthetase inhibitor
      suppressed by: barbiturates, benzodiazepine, labor, hypoxia, asphyxia, prostaglandin E_2
   2. Fetal body movement:
      √ ≥3 discrete movements of limbs / trunk
      influenced by: glucose, gestational age, time of day, maternal drugs, intrinsic rhythm, labor
   3. Fetal tone
      upper + lower limbs usually fully flexed with head on chest; least sensitive test parameter
      √ ≥1 episode of opening + closing of hand / extension + flexion of limb

B. CHRONIC FETAL CONDITION
   4. Amniotic fluid volume
      √ at least one pocket ≥2 cm in vertical diameter in two perpendicular planes
      ◊ Avoid inclusion of loops of cord!

Score (for each test): 2 points if normal; 0 points if abnormal

Results (including NST for a maximum of 10 points):

Score	*Interpretation*	*Perinatal mortality*
10	asphyxia rare	0.0%
8 + normal fluid	asphyxia rare	<0.1%
8 + abnormal fluid	chronic compromise	8.9%
6 + normal fluid	equivocal	variable
6 + abnormal fluid	asphyxia probable	8.9%
4	asphyxia highly probable	9.1%
2	asphyxia almost certain	12.5%
0	asphyxia certain	60.0%

False-negative rate: 0.7 per 1,000
◊ The probability of fetal death within a week of a BPP score of 8/8 is 1 per 1,000!

Stress tests

1. NONSTRESS TEST (NST)
   ◊ Test needed in less than 5% of cases!
   √ reactive fetal heart rate tracing (normal) = at least 4 fetal heart accelerations (>15 bpm over baseline lasting >15 seconds) in a 20-minute period subsequent to fetal movement >34 weeks GA
   √ nonreactive (abnormal) fetal heart rate tracing = absence of acceleration in a continuous 40-minute observation period
   N.B.: no heart accelerations in immaturity, during sleep cycle, with maternal sedative use
   Accuracy: false-negative rate of 3.2/1000 (if done weekly) or 1.6/1000 (if done biweekly); 50% false-positive rate for neonatal morbidity + 80% for neonatal mortality
2. CONTRACTION STRESS TEST (CST)
   = external monitoring after injection of oxytocin / maternal breast stimulation
   √ >3 uterine contractions in 10-minute period
   Accuracy: false-negative rate of 0.4/1000; 50% false-positive rate

INVASIVE FETAL ASSESSMENT

Amniocentesis

Indication:
(1) Inadequate sonographic fetal anatomic survey due to fetal position / maternal body habitus
(2) Equivocal sonographic findings (eg, abnormal posterior fossa but spinal defect not seen)
(3) Experienced sonographer not available
(4) Nonlethal anomaly detected on Level I sonogram for which karyotype testing is appropriate

A. DIAGNOSTIC AMNIOCENTESIS
   1. Genetic studies: karyotype, DNA analysis, biochemical assay
      Timing: early (11–15 weeks), late (15–18 weeks)
   2. Neural tube defect: a-fetoprotein, acetylcholinesterase
   3. Isoimmunization: Δ-OD 450
   4. Fetal lung maturity
   5. Intraamniotic infection
   6. Confirmation of ruptured membranes
B. THERAPEUTIC AMNIOCENTESIS
   1. Polyhydramnios
   2. Twin-twin transfusion syndrome

   Technique:
   √ avoid fetus, placenta, umbilical cord, uterine contraction, fibroid, large uterine vessel
   √ use continuous ultrasound guidance
   √ inject 2–5 mL of indigo carmine dye in first sac of twin (colorless fluid assures that second sac has been entered)

Risk:
A. FETAL RISK
   1. Spontaneous abortion (<1%)
   2. Amniotic fluid leak
   3. Chorioamnionitis
   4. Fetal injury: skin dimple, limb gangrene, porencephalic cyst, hemothorax, spleen laceration, orthopedic abnormality, amniotic band syndrome
B. MATERNAL RISK (rare)
   1. Bowel perforation
   2. Hemorrhage
   3. Isoimmunization

Advantage over CVS:
1. Error rate (<1% versus 2%)
2. Culture failure rate (0.6% versus 2.2%)
3. Fetal loss rate (0.6–0.8% less)

Chorionic villus sampling (CVS)

= aspiration of cells from chorion frondosum for genetic studies (karyotype, DNA analysis, biochemical assay)
◊ Transabdominal CVS for rapid karyotyping in 2nd + 3rd trimester = **placental biopsy**
Advantage: >2 weeks earlier results compared with amniocentesis
Timing: 9–11 weeks
Approach:
(a) transcervical route = catheter introduced through cervix into chorion frondosum, easier for posterior placenta; contamination by cervical flora possible;
   ◊ CONTRAINDICATED in cervical infections!
(b) transabdominal route = 20- to 22-gauge needle inserted from anterior abdominal wall; easier for anterior / fundal placenta; sterile technique

Chromosome analysis:
(a) direct preparation = analysis of cytotrophoblasts (may have different karyotype than fetus)
   → analysis can be performed immediately
(b) villus culture = cells from central mesenchymal core (same karyotype as fetus)
   → cultured for several days before analysis

Errors (2%):
1. Mosaicism = cell line forming cytotrophoblast may develop abnormal karyotype while fetal cell line is normal
2. Maternal contamination = cells from maternal decidua may overgrow mesenchymal core cells

Risks:
1. Spontaneous abortion (1%)
2. Perforation of amniotic sac
3. Infection
4. Teratogenesis: limb reduction defect

Cordocentesis

= PERCUTANEOUS UMBILICAL BLOOD SAMPLING (PUBS)
A. DIAGNOSTIC CORDOCENTESIS
   1. Hematocrit
   2. Karyotype

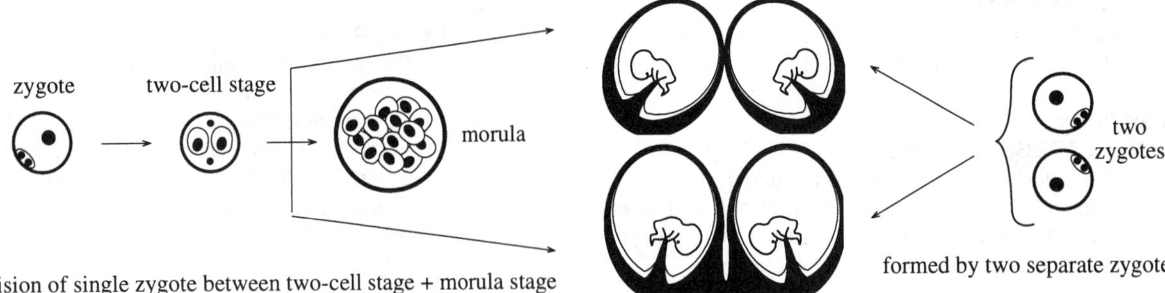

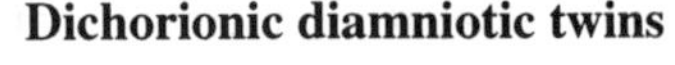
Dichorionic diamniotic twins

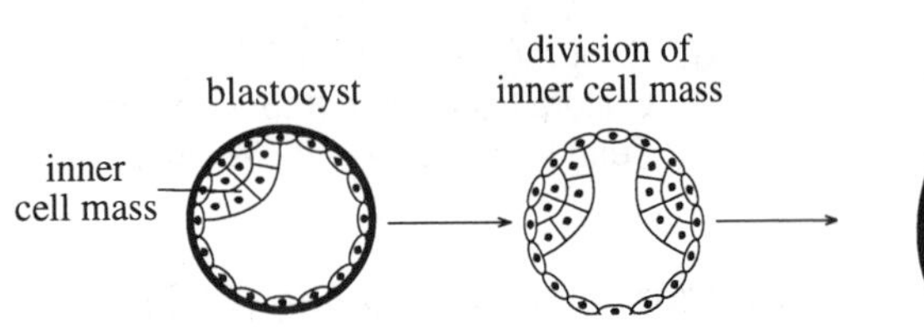

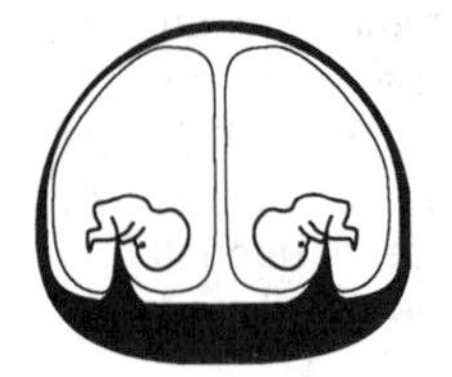
Monochorionic diamniotic twins

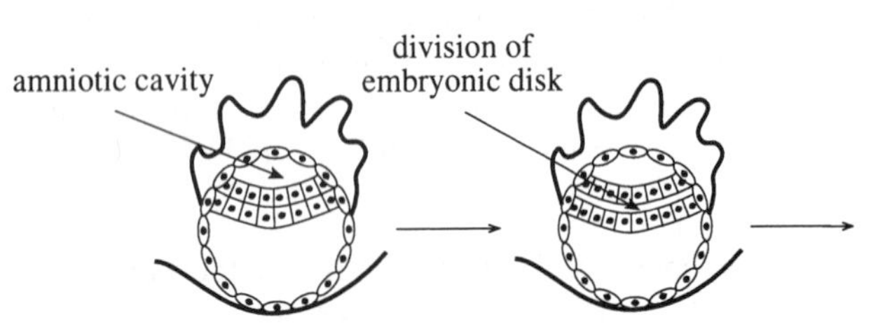

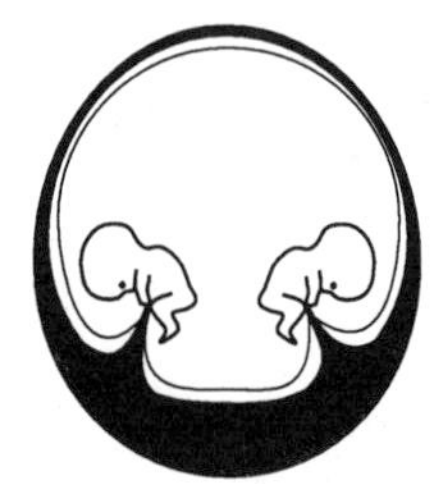
Monochorionic monoamniotic twins

3. Immunodeficiency: chronic granulomatous disease, severe combined immunodeficiency
4. Coagulopathy: von Willebrand syndrome, factor deficiency
5. Platelet disorder: alloimmune / idiopathic thrombocytopenic purpura
6. Hemoglobinopathy: sickle cell anemia, thalassemia
7. Infection: toxoplasmosis, rubella, varicella, cytomegalovirus, parvovirus
8. Hypoxia / acidosis

B. THERAPEUTIC CORDOCENTESIS
1. Intravascular fetal transfusion (fresh rh-negative CMV-negative leukodepleted irradiated packed cells compatible with mother infused at 10–15 mL/min)
2. Direct delivery of medication to fetus

Cx:
1. Chorioamnionitis
2. Rupture of membranes
3. Umbilical cord hematoma
4. Umbilical cord thrombosis
5. Bleeding from insertion site
6. Fetal bradycardia

MULTIPLE GESTATIONS

Incidence: 1.2% of all births; in 5–50% clinically undiagnosed at term

Occurrence:

twins	in	1:85	pregnancies (= 85^1)
triplets	in	1:7,600	pregnancies (~ 85^2)
quadruplets	in	1:729,000	pregnancies (~ 85^3)
quintuplets	in	1:65,610,000	pregnancies (~ 85^4)

- uterus large for dates
- may have elevated HCG, HPL (human placental lactogen), AFP levels

Perinatal morbidity & mortality compared to singletons:
twins: up to 5-fold increase
triplets: up to 18-fold increase

Twin pregnancy

Zygote = fertilized egg

1. **Monozygotic twins** (1/3)
   = "identical twins"
   = division of a single fertilized ovum during earliest stages of embryogenesis (chorion differentiates 4 days and amnion 8 days after fertilization)
   Incidence: 1:250 birth (constant around the world)

OB&GYN

Predisposing factors:
(1) Advanced maternal age
(2) in vitro fertilization
√ same sex + identical genotype

(a) **Dichorionic diamniotic twins** (30%)
= separation at two-cell stage (= blastomere) approximately 60 hours / <4 days after fertilization
√ 2 separate fused / unfused placentas
√ membrane >2 mm due to 2 separate chorionic sacs + 2 separate amniotic sacs (92% accurate for dichorionic diamniotic twins)
√ "twin peak" sign = triangular projection of placental tissue insinuated between layers of intertwin membrane

(b) **Monochorionic diamniotic twins** (69–80%) (most common)
= separation in blastocyst stage between 4th and 7th day after fertilization (chorion already developed and separated from embryo)
√ 2 separate amniotic sacs within single chorionic sac
◊ Common monochorionic placenta has vascular communications in 100%!
Cx: (1) Twin-twin transfusion syndrome
(2) Twin embolization syndrome = DIC in surviving twin from transfer of thromboplastin; 17% morbidity / mortality of survivor after fetal death of twin
(3) Acardiac parabiotic twin

(c) **Monochorionic monoamniotic twins** (1%)
= division of embryonic disk between 8th and 12th day after fertilization (amniotic cavity already developed)
√ common amniotic + chorionic sac, no separating membrane
√ entanglement of cords (the only definitive positive sonographic sign of monoamnionicity)
Cx: double perinatal mortality up to 45%
(1) Entangled umbilical cord (70%)
(2) True knot of cord
(3) Conjoined twins (umbilical cord with >3 vessels, shared fetal organs, continuous fetal skin contour)
Prognosis: 40% survival rate

(d) **Conjoined twins**
= division more than 13 days after fertilization is usually incomplete; M:F = 3:7
Incidence: 1:50,000 births
√ no separating membrane demonstrable (monochorionic, monoamniotic)
√ fetuses commonly face each other; most common are thoracopagus + omphalopagus

Cx: (1) perinatal mortality 2.5 times greater than for dizygotic twins
(2) Fetal anomalies 3–7 times higher than in dizygotic twins / singletons (often only affecting one twin): anencephaly, hydrocephalus, holoprosencephaly, cloacal exstrophy, VATER syndrome, sirenomelia, sacrococcygeal teratoma

2. DIZYGOTIC TWINS (2/3)
= "fraternal twins"
(a) fertilization of two ova by two separate spermatozoa during two simultaneous ovulations (occurring either in both ovaries or in one ovary)
(b) superfetation = fertilization of two ova by two separate spermatozoa during two subsequent ovulations (frequency unknown)
(c) superfecundation = two ova fertilized by two different fathers (very rare)
Incidence: 1:80 to 1:90 births
Predisposing factors:
(1) Advanced maternal age (increased up to age 35): reduced gonadal-hypothalamic feedback with increase of FSH levels
(2) Ovulation-inducing agents (multiple pregnancies in 6–17% with clomiphene, in 18–53% with Pergonal)
(3) Maternal history of twinning (3 times as frequent compared with normal population)
(4) Increased parity
(5) Maternal obesity
(6) Race with inherited predisposition for multiple ovulations (Blacks > Whites > Asians)
√ different phenotypes; same / opposite sex
√ always dichorionic diamniotic

Amnionicity & Chorionicity

Embryologic events in monozygotic twins:

days after fertilization	*embryologic event*	*cleavage results in* chorion	amnion
1–2	cell divisions → morula	di~	di~
3–4	chorionic differentiation		
6	blastocyst implants in endometrium	mono~	di~
8	amnionic differentiation	mono~	mono~
>13	division of embryonic disk	mono~ but conjoined	mono~

Rules:
◊ Only monozygotic twins can give rise to monochorionic + monoamniotic pregnancies!
◊ All monoamniotic twins must also be monochorionic!
◊ All dizygotic twins must be dichorionic + diamniotic!
◊ 77% of all twin pregnancies are dichorionic (ie, all dizygotics [2/3 of all twins] which equals 67% + 30% of all monozygotics [1/3 of all twins] which equals 10%)

1. GESTATIONAL SACS (<10 weeks MA)
   Accuracy: 100% in 1st trimester, 80–90% in 2nd trimester
   √ 2 gestational sacs, each with a live fetus, indicates dichorionic twinning
   √ single gestational sac with 2 live fetuses indicates monochorionic twins
   √ single extraembryonic coelom indicates monochorionic twins

2. YOLK SAC
   √ number of yolk sacs = number of amnions
3. FETAL GENDER
   √ different genders (in 25% of twin pregnancies) must be dizygotic twins and thus dichorionic! [DDx: testicular feminization demonstrates female external genitalia with a 46,XY karyotype]
4. PLACENTAL SITES
   √ 2 placentas (in 45% of twin pregnancies) indicate dichorionic diamniotic pregnancy
   √ 1 placenta indicates
   (a) monochorionic pregnancy
   (b) dichorionic pregnancy with fused placenta (occurs in 50% of dichorionic twin pregnancies)
5. CHORIONIC PEAK
   √ "twin peak" sign (= triangular projection of placental tissue extending beyond chorionic surface of the placenta + insinuated between layers of intertwin membrane + wider at chorionic surface and tapering to a point some distance inward from surface) indicates dichorionic pregnancy

6. MEMBRANE
   √ separating membrane confirms diamniotic pregnancy, but does not distinguish between mono- or dichorionic pregnancy
   √ dichorionic membrane (two layers of chorion + two layers of amnion) is thicker (>2 mm) than monochorionic membrane (two layers of amnion <1 mm): 88–92% accuracy in 1st trimester, 39–83% accuracy in 2nd + 3rd trimester
   ◊ All membranes appear to be thin in 3rd trimester!
   √ absence of membrane suggests a monoamniotic monochorionic twin pregnancy
   ◊ Nonvisualization of membrane is not sufficient evidence of monoamnionicity due to technical factors!
7. CORD
   √ entanglement of cords is the only definitive positive sonographic sign of monoamnionicity
   √ simultaneous recording of fetal arterial signals at nonsynchronous rates within wide Doppler gate

8. AMNIOGRAPHY
   √ detection of imbibed intestinal contrast in both twins by CT following single sac contrast injection proves monoamniotic monochorionic twin pregnancy

OB&GYN

Growth rates of twins

Twins should be scanned every 3–4 weeks >26–28 weeks GA

Below 30–32 weeks GA:
√ normal individual twins grow at same rate as singletons
√ BPD growth rates similar to singleton fetuses

Beyond 30–32 weeks GA:
√ combined weight gain of both twins equals that of a singleton pregnancy (AC of twins < AC of singleton)
◊ Weight of twin fetus falls below that of singleton when combined weight of twins >4000 g!
√ BPD + HC growth may / may not be affected (controversial)
√ FL not affected

DISCORDANT GROWTH
= weight difference at birth >25%
Cause: (1) Twin-twin transfusion syndrome
(2) IUGR of one fetus
√ BPD difference >5 mm (discordant growth in 20–30%)
√ discordant HC increases probability of IUGR
√ AC is single most sensitive parameter for IUGR
√ EFW is most sensitive set of combined parameters for IUGR
√ >15% S/D ratio difference of umbilical artery Doppler waveforms between twins

Risks in multiple gestations

1. Placental abruption	3-fold
2. Anemia	2.5-fold
3. Hypertension	2.5-fold
4. Congenital anomaly	2–3-fold
5. Preterm delivery	12-fold
6. Perinatal mortality	4–6-fold

◊ Risk increases with number of fetuses, monozygosity, monochorionicity

Risk for IUGR:
monochorionic-monoamniotic > monochorionic-diamniotic > dichorionic-diamniotic

Risk for perinatal mortality:
1% for singletons, 9% for diamniotic dichorionic twins, 26% for diamniotic monochorionic twins, 50% for monoamniotic monochorionic twins

Prognosis:
(1) Perinatal mortality 5–10 times that of singleton pregnancy (91–124:1,000 births)
— 9% for dichorionic diamniotic twins
— 26% for monochorionic diamniotic twins
— 50% for monochorionic monoamniotic twins
(a) preterm delivery with birth weight <2500 g
(b) IUGR (25–32%; 2nd most common cause of perinatal mortality + morbidity)
(c) amniotic fluid infection (60%)

(d) premature rupture of membranes (11%)
(e) twin-twin transfusion syndrome (8%)
(f) large placental infarct (8%)
(g) placenta previa
(h) abruptio placentae
(i) preeclampsia
(j) cord accidents
(k) malpresentations
(l) velamentous cord insertion (7-fold increase compared with singleton pregnancy)

(2) Fetal death in utero (0.5–6.8%; 3 times as often in monochorionic than in dichorionic gestations)
◊ 50% of twin gestations seen at 10 weeks GA will be singletons at birth!

(3) Increased risk of congenital anomalies (23:1,000 births = twice as frequent as in singletons; 3–7 times more frequent in monozygotic twins than in dizygotic twins)

UTERUS

Uterine Size

A. NEONATAL UTERUS
tubular structure
Length of 2.3–4.6 cm (mean 3.4 cm), fundal width of 0.8–2.1 cm (mean 1.2 cm), cervical width of 0.8–2.2 cm (mean 1.4 cm)
√ echogenic endometrium + endometrial fluid (in 25%) secondary to maternal hormonal stimulation

B. INFANTILE UTERUS
Age: infancy to 7 years of age
Length of 2.5–3.3 cm, fundal width of 0.4–1.0 cm, cervical width of 0.6–1.0 cm
√ cervix occupies 2/3 of uterine length

C. POSTPUBERTAL UTERUS
— nulliparous: 5–8 cm (L); 1.6–3.0 cm (W); 3 cm (D)
— multiparous: add 2 cm for multiparous dimensions
√ cervix occupies 1/3 of uterine length
√ mean uterine volume of 90 cm^3

D. POSTMENOPAUSAL UTERUS
cervix occupies 1/3 of uterine length;
3.5–6.5 cm (L); 1.2–1.8 cm (W); 2 cm (D)

Uterine Zonal Anatomy (on T2WI)

Thickness of zones depends on menstrual cycle + hormonal medication

A. ENDOMETRIUM
√ high signal intensity similar to fat

B. JUNCTIONAL ZONE
= innermost layer of myometrium
Histo: compact smooth muscle fibers with 3-fold increase in number + size of nuclei compared with outer myometrium
√ low signal intensity (lower water content); seen in 40 –60%, may not be visible in premenarchal + postmenopausal women

C. MYOMETRIUM
√ intermediate signal intensity, increases during secretory phase

Cervical Zones

(a) Central stripe of high signal intensity on T2WI
Histo: secretions in endocervical canal + cervical mucosa + plicae palmatae
√ arbor vitae / plicae palmatae = irregular branched mucosal pattern of cervical canal

(b) Middle layer of low signal intensity continuous with junctional zone of corpus uteri
Histo: inner zone of fibromuscular stroma with percentage of nuclear area 2.5 times greater than in outer zone

(c) Outer layer of intermediate signal intensity
Histo: outer zone of fibromuscular stroma

Endometrium

◊ Measurements refer to AP diameter of both apposed endometrial layers (= double thickness) excluding intrauterine fluid

1. MENSTRUAL PHASE (usually days 1–5)
Thickness: 1–3 mm
√ interrupted thin echogenic line of central interface
2. PROLIFERATIVE PHASE (days 6–14)
Thickness: 4–6 mm
√ bright echogenic central line (= apposed borders of endometrial canal)
√ hypoechoic band (= thickened endometrium)
√ surrounded by slightly more echogenic myometrium
3. SECRETORY PHASE (days 15–28)
Thickness: 7–14 mm
√ bright central line
√ markedly echogenic thick endometrium
√ thin hypoechoic halo of inner myometrial zone
4. POSTMENOPAUSAL
Thickness: <8 mm thick in 81%; may increase to 15 mm with hormonal replacement (unopposed estrogen, continuous estrogen + progestogen)
√ endometrium <5 mm is consistently associated with atrophic inactive endometrium by histology
√ Doppler waveforms with resistive index <0.7 suggest malignancy
Rx: biopsy / D&C if endometrial thickness >8 mm

Pelvic Spaces

1. Rectouterine pouch = cul-de-sac
Anterior boundary: broad ligaments + uterus
◊ Most dependent portion of pelvis in women!
2. Rectovesical recess
◊ Most dependent portion of pelvis in men!
3. Vesicouterine recess
4. Inguinal fossa
located between lateral + medial umbilical folds

Cervical Length

		transabdominal	*transvaginal*
1st trimester	(<14 wks)	53 ± 17	40 ± 8 mm
2nd trimester	(14–28 wks)	44 ± 14	42 ± 10 mm
3rd trimester	(≥ 28 wks)	40 ± 10	32 ± 12 mm

◊ Distended bladder improves visualization but increases cervical length on transabdominal US!
◊ Difference between nulli- and multiparous women 10%!
• physical examination tends to underestimate the true length of the cervix

Pelvic ligaments

1. Broad ligament
   Histo: 2 layers of peritoneum
   Origin: uterine peritoneum
   Attachment: pelvic sidewall
   — medial superior free edge: formed by fallopian tube
   — lateral superior free edge: suspensory ligament of ovary
   — lower margin: cardinal ligament
   Contents (= parametrium):
   extraperitoneal connective tissue, smooth muscle, fat, fallopian tube, round ligament, ovarian ligament, uterine + ovarian blood vessels, nerves, lymphatics, mesonephric remnants

2. Round ligament
   = anterior suspensory ligament of uterus
   Histo: band of fibromuscular tissue + lymphatic channels
   Origin: anterolateral uterine fundus, just below + anterior to ovarian ligament
   Attachment: through internal inguinal canal (lateral to deep inferior epigastric vessels) to labia majora

3. Cardinal ligament = transverse cervical ligament = Mackenrodt ligament
   Origin: cervix + upper vagina
   Attachment: fascia of obturator internus muscle
   Relationship:
   — uterine artery runs along its superior aspect
   — forms the base of the broad ligament

4. Uterosacral ligament
   Origin: posterolateral cervix + vagina
   Attachment: anterior body of sacrum at S2 or S3

5. Ovarian ligament = round ligament of the ovary
   Origin: medial aspect of ovary
   Attachment: uterus, just inferior + posterior to fallopian tube + round ligament

6. Suspensory ligament of ovary = infundibulopelvic lig.
   Origin: anterolateral aspect of ovary
   Attachment: connective tissue over psoas muscle
   Contents: ovarian artery + vein

7. Lateral umbilical fold / ligament
   = reflection of peritoneum over deep inferior epigastric vessels

8. Medial umbilical fold / ligament
   = reflection of peritoneum over obliterated umbilical arteries

9. Median umbilical ligament
   = reflection of peritoneum over obliterated urachus
   Origin: dome of urinary bladder
   Attachment: umbilicus

OVARIES

Fixation: fairly mobile with attachments to

anterior pelvic wall	by	broad ligament
uterine body	by	utero-ovarian ligament
fallopian tube	by	tubo-ovarian ligament
lateral pelvic wall	by	infundibulopelvic ligament

Embryology:
coelomic (surface) epithelium invaginates into mesenchymal substance (= primary sex cords) and incorporates primordial germ cells, which develop into primordial follicles

Ovarian size

Ovarian volume = length x height x width x 0.523

at birth:	1.5 cm (L), 0.25 cm (H), 0.3 cm (W)
<2 years:	<0.7 cm^3
childhood:	0.75–0.86 cm^3
6–11 years:	1.19–2.52 cm^3
after puberty:	2.5–5 cm (L), 0.6–1.5 cm (H), 1.5–3 cm (W); 1.8–5.7 cm^3

Ovarian morphology

neonate: √ follicles occasionally fail to involute + undergo growth
<8 years: √ solid ovoid structures with homogeneous / finely heterogeneous texture
√ up to 70% of ovaries contain cystic follicles (in 95% <9 mm, in 5% >9 mm)

Visualization of ovaries

after menopause (average onset at age 50):
<5 years after menopause: in 78%
>10 years after menopause: in 64%
— both ovaries: in 85%
— one ovary: in 60%
following hysterectomy: in 43%

Ovarian cycle

1. Follicular phase = days 1–14
   • a number of immature primordial follicles begin to mature in response to FSH
   √ multiple small cysts (= stimulated / unstimulated follicles)
   √ 2–3 follicles in each ovary by day 4, subsequently enlarging to approximately 10 mm
   √ single "ascendant" / "dominant" follicle (= graafian follicle) appears by day 10, subsequently enlarging to 20–25 mm by day 14

√ progressively increasing diastolic flow on the side of maturing follicle

2. Ovulatory phase = day 14
   - "mittelschmerz" = pain just prior to ovulation (pressure of graafian follicle distending ovarian capsule)

   √ sudden decrease in follicular size over minutes / hours (= rupture of mature graafian follicle with extrusion of ovum)
3. Luteal phase = days 15–28

   √ 16–24 mm almost isoechoic cyst with blurred margin + scattered internal echoes (follicular fluid + blood) = corpus luteum of menstruation

   √ 30- to 40-mm cyst = corpus luteum cyst (fluid collecting in corpus luteum / additional hemorrhage)

   √ involution + atrophy of corpus luteum on about 24th day of cycle = corpus luteum atreticum

Graafian follicle

Size of mature graafian follicle: 17–29 mm

√ growth rate 3 mm/day until the last preovulatory 24 hours followed by a sudden increase in diameter

√ cumulus = 1-mm mural echogenic focus projecting into antrum of follicle + containing oocyte, followed by ovulation within next 36 hours

SIGNS OF OVULATION:

√ development of solid echoes within graafian follicle

√ decrease in diameter / sudden collapse of dominant follicle 28–35 hours after LH peak

√ "ring" structure within uterine fundus

√ free fluid appearing in pouch of Douglas

SIGNS OF OVULATORY FAILURE:

√ development of internal echoes prior to 18 mm size

√ continuous cystic enlargement up to 30–40 mm

Ovarian Doppler signals

A. NONFUNCTIONING OVARY

   √ high-impedance waveform

B. FUNCTIONING OVARY

   — days 1–6:

   √ high-impedance waveform with RI close to 1.0

   — days 7–22 = midfollicular to midluteal phase = developing dominant follicle + ovulation + corpus luteal phase:

   √ continuous diastolic flow with RI close to 0.5

   — days 23–28 = late luteal phase:

   √ high-impedance waveform with RI close to 1.0

OBSTETRIC AND GYNECOLOGIC DISORDERS

ABORTION

Rate of spontaneous abortions (= miscarriage)
— >50% of all fertilized ova (estimate)
— 31–43% of all implantations (estimate)
— 10–25% of clinically diagnosed pregnancies
— 2–4% with normal cardiac activity
— decreases with increasing gestational age
◊ Majority of pregnancies lost before 7th week MA!
Etiology: usually due to abnormal karyotype: autosomal trisomy (52%), triploidy (20%), monosomy (15%)

Complete abortion

• cervix closed
√ thin regular endometrium

Incomplete spontaneous abortion

= RETAINED PRODUCTS OF CONCEPTION
= portion of chorionic villi (placental tissue) / trophoblastic tissue (fetal tissue) remaining within uterus
• continued bleeding
• patulous cervix
US (overall accuracy 96%):

Finding	Retained Products
√ gestational sac / collection	100%
√ sac with dead fetus	100%
√ endometrium >5 mm thick	100%
√ endometrium 2–5 mm thick	43%
√ endometrium <2 mm thick	14%

Cx: endometritis, myometritis, peritonitis, septic shock, diffuse intravascular coagulation (with retention >1 month)
Rx: suction D&C after IV oxytocin

Inevitable abortion

= gestational sac with fetus having become detached from implantation site; leading to spontaneous abortion within next few hours
Clinical triad:
• bleeding >7 days
• persistent painful uterine contractions
• moderate effacement of cervix
• dilated cervix >3 cm
• rupture of membranes
√ sac located low within uterus
√ sac surrounded by anechoic zone of blood
√ dilated cervix

Missed abortion

= dead conceptus within uterine cavity, occurring between 8–14 weeks
• brownish vaginal discharge
• closed firm cervix
√ no cardiac activity in a well-defined embryo with CRL >9 mm (on abdominal scans) / CRL >5 mm (on transvaginal scans)
√ gestation not in correspondence with menstrual age
√ sac >25 mm in diameter without an embryo (DDx: anembryonic pregnancy)
√ sac >20 mm without yolk sac
√ crenated irregular / distorted angular sac configuration
√ stringlike debris within gestational sac (in 25%)
√ discontinuous / irregular / thin (2 mm) choriodecidual reaction
√ no double decidual sac
√ low sac position
√ subchorionic collection
Cx: coagulopathy secondary to low plasma fibrinogen (after 4 weeks in 2nd trimester pregnancy)
Rx: suction D&C (in 1st trimester); prostaglandin E suppositories (in 2nd trimester)

Threatened abortion

= 1st trimester bleeding with a live fetus
Incidence: 20–25% of all pregnancies
Clinical triad:
• mild bleeding
• cramping
• closed cervix
Prognosis: 50% develop normally; 50% miscarry
Factors with a poor prognosis:
√ early bradycardia
√ large subchorionic hematoma (DDx: implantation bleed)
√ relative fetal inactivity

ACARDIA

= ACARDIAC MONSTER = TWIN REVERSED ARTERIAL PERFUSION SEQUENCE (TRAP)
= rare developmental anomaly of monochorionic twinning in which one twin develops without a functioning heart
Incidence: 1:30,000–35,000 births; in 1% of monozygotic twins
Pathophysiology:
normal twin perfuses acardiac twin through *artery-to-artery + vein-to-vein anastomoses* in shared placenta; reversed circulation alters hemodynamic forces which result in abnormal cardiac morphogenesis
Spectrum:
(1) Holoacardia = no heart at all
(2) Pseudoacardia = rudimentary cardiac tissue
√ proximity of the two cord insertions on placental surface linked by an arterioarterial anastomosis
√ reversed arterial flow in cord toward acardiac twin
√ fused placentas
√ polyhydramnios

A. PUMP TWIN
at increased risk for fetal demise + preterm labor
√ morphologically normal
√ cardiac overload signs: hydrops, IUGR, hypertrophy of right ventricle, increased cardiothoracic ratio, hepatosplenomegaly, ascites

B. PERFUSED TWIN = ACARDIAC TWIN
monochorial placenta (same gender) with vascular anastomosis sustains life of acardiac monster; wide range of associated abnormalities
√ absent / rudimentary heart ("acardius")
√ tiny / absent cranium (acephalus)
√ small upper torso ± absent / deformed upper extremities
√ marked integumentary edema + cystic hygroma
Prognosis: mortality of 100% for perfused twin, 50% for pump twin (increased with increased size of acardiac twin)
Rx: laser ablation of umbilical cord to acardiac twin (up to 20–22 weeks)

ADENOMYOSIS

= ENDOMETRIOSIS INTERNA
= focal / diffuse benign invasion of myometrium by endometrium (heterotopic "endometrial islands") which incite myometrial hyperplasia
Cause: ? uterine trauma (parturition, myomectomy, curettage)
Incidence: 9–31% in hysterectomy specimens
Histo: endometrial glands (nonfunctioning due to resistance to hormonal stimulation unlike endometriosis) + stroma within myometrium surrounded by hypertrophic smooth muscle
Age: multiparous women >30 years during menstrual life (later reproductive years)
Associated with: endometriosis (in 36–40%)
• asymptomatic in 5–70%
• pelvic pain, menorrhagia, dysmenorrhea (abates after menopause)

(a) FOCAL ADENOMYOSIS = "adenomyoma"
√ oval / elongated shape (DDx: leiomyoma is round)
√ ill-defined margins (DDx: sharp margin in leiomyoma)
√ contiguity with junctional zone (DDx: leiomyomas may occur anywhere in myometrium)
(b) DIFFUSE ADENOMYOSIS
√ smooth uterine enlargement (DDx: diffuse leiomyomatosis)

MR (86% sensitive, 86% specific):
√ myometrial mass with indistinct margins of primarily low signal intensity on all sequences
√ diffuse / focal widening of junctional zone ≥12 mm on T2WI, T2-weighted SE images, contrast-enhanced T1WI images
√ central high-intensity spots on T1WI + T2WI (ectopic endometrial tissue / endometrial cyst / hemorrhagic foci) in 50%
√ enhancement always less than adjacent myometrium
US (80–86% sensitive, 74–89% specific):
√ poorly defined hypoechoic heterogeneous areas within myometrium
√ 1–3 mm small myometrial cysts (50%), occasionally with "Swiss cheese" appearance of myometrium
√ thickening + asymmetry of anterior and posterior myometrial walls
Cx: infertility
DDx: (1) leiomyomas (clinically + sonographically difficult to distinguish)
(2) uterine contraction
Rx: hysterectomy (the only definitive cure)

AMNIOTIC BAND SYNDROME

= EARLY AMNION RUPTURE SYNDROME
= rupture of the amnion exposing the fetus to the injurious environment of fibrous mesodermic bands that emanate from the chorionic side of the amnion
Prevalence: 1:1,200 – 1:2,000 – 1:15,000 livebirths
√ very thin membrane that flaps with fetal movement or attaches to fetus
√ abnormal sheet / bands of tissue that attach to the fetus (DDx: uterine synechiae, incomplete amniochorionic fusion, amniochorionic separation due to subchorionic hemorrhage, fibrin deposits, venous lakes, residual sac of blighted twin pregnancy, wisps of umbilical cord)
√ restriction of fetal motion secondary to entrapment of fetal parts by bands
Associated with fetal deformities in 77%:
1. Limb defects (multiple + asymmetric)
   √ amputation / constriction rings of limbs / digits
   √ distal syndactyly
   √ clubbed feet (30%)
2. Craniofacial defects
   = asymmetric nonanatomic defects of skull + brain
   √ anencephaly
   √ asymmetric lateral encephalocele
   √ facial clefting of lip / palate
   √ asymmetric microphthalmia
   √ incomplete / absent cranial calcification
   √ ± attachment of head to uterine wall
3. Visceral defects
   √ gastroschisis ± exteriorization of liver
   √ omphalocele
   √ gibbus deformity of spine

DDx: (1) Chorioamnionic separation
(2) Intrauterine synechiae

ANEMBRYONIC PREGNANCY

= BLIGHTED OVUM; may occur as a blighted twin
= gestational sac of >2.5 mL with no identifiable embryo
√ yolk sac identified without embryo
√ empty gestational sac (>6–8 weeks MA)
√ gestational sac small / appropriate / large for dates
√ lack of growth / decrease in size on serial scans
(a) by transabdominal scan:
GS usually not visualized before 5–5.5 weeks MA; yolk sac forms at 4 weeks MA when GS is 3 mm; embryo usually visualized by 6 weeks MA
√ GS size >20 mm of mean diameter without yolk sac
√ GS size >25 mm of mean diameter without embryo
√ absence of GS growth documented on repeat scan 7–14 days later

(b) by transvaginal scan
√ GS size >8 mm of mean diameter without yolk sac
√ GS size >16 mm of mean diameter without embryo / cardiac activity
Cx: first trimester bleeding

ARRHENOBLASTOMA
Age peak: 25–45 years (range 15–66 years)
√ solid mass with cystic components (hemorrhage ± necrosis)
√ unilateral (95%), up to 27 cm in diameter
Cx: malignant transformation in 22%

ASHERMAN SYNDROME
= association of intrauterine synechiae (= adhesions consisting of fibrous tissue or smooth muscle) with menstrual dysfunction + infertility
Cause: sequela of endometrial trauma (vigorous instrumentation during dilatation & curettage) usually during postpartum or postabortion period / severe endometritis
• hypomenorrhea / amenorrhea
• habitual abortion / sterility
HSG:
√ solitary / multiple filling defects
√ bands of tissue traversing endometrial cavity
√ irregularity of uterine cavity
√ partial / near complete obliteration of uterine cavity (DDx: DES exposure)
US:
√ thickened endometrium

BECKWITH-WIEDEMANN SYNDROME
= EMG SYNDROME (**E**xomphalos = omphalocele, **M**acroglossia, **G**igantism)
= common autosomal dominant overgrowth syndrome with reduced penetrance + variable expressivity related to short arm of chromosome 11; sporadic in 85%
Incidence: 1:13,700 to 1:14,300 livebirths; M:F = 1:1
• neonatal polycythemia
√ advanced bone age
Constellation:
(1) Hemihypertrophy 13–33%
(2) Hyperplastic visceromegaly: 57%
kidney, liver, spleen, pancreas, clitoris, penis, ovaries, uterus, bladder
(3) Abdominal wall defects
(a) Omphalocele 76%
(b) Umbilical hernia 49%
(c) Diastasis recti 33%
(4) Macroglossia 98%
(5) Facial nevus flammeus 63%
(6) Ear lobe creases and pits 66%
(7) Prominent eyes with intraorbital creases
(8) Infraorbital hypoplasia 81%
(9) Gastrointestinal malrotation 83%
(10) Pancreatic islet hyperplasia
(11) Cardiac anomalies
(12) Natal / postnatal gigantism 77%

@ Adrenal gland
Histo: adrenocortical cytomegaly, cystic adrenal cortex, hyperplastic adrenal medulla
@ Kidney
Histo: disordered lobar arrangement, medullary dysplasia
√ nephromegaly
√ increased cortical echogenicity (due to glomeruloneogenesis)
√ accentuation of corticomedullary definition
√ medullary sponge kidney
√ pyelocaliceal diverticula
OB-US:
√ LGA fetus with growth along 95th percentile
√ polyhydramnios (51%)
√ thickened placenta
√ long umbilical cord
Cx: (1) Development of malignant tumors (in 10%): Wilms tumor, hepatoblastoma, adrenocortical carcinoma
(2) Neonatal hypoglycemia (50–61%)

BRENNER TUMOR
= almost always benign ovarian tumor
Incidence: 1.5–2.5%
Histo: transitional epithelial cells within prominent fibrous connective tissue stroma
Associated with: mucinous cystadenoma / other epithelial tumor in 20–30%
Peak age: 40–70 years
• may have estrogenic activity
√ usually hypoechoic solid homogeneous tumor with well-defined back wall
√ mostly 1–2 cm (up to 30 cm) in diameter
√ ± extensive calcifications
√ bilateral in 5–7%

CERVICAL CANCER
6th most common cause of death from cancer in women; 3rd most common gynecologic malignancy; 15,800 new cases + 4,800 deaths in 1996
Incidence: 12:100,000 women per year
Peak age: 45–55 years
Histo: squamous cell carcinoma (95%), adenocarcinoma (5%), unusual clear cell adenocarcinoma in women exposed to DES in utero
Risk factors: lower socioeconomic class, Black race, early marriage, increased parity, young onset of sexual relations, multiple sexual partners, positive herpes virus type II titers
FIGO stage:
0 carcinoma in situ (before invasion)
I confined to cervix
Ia microinvasion of stroma
Ib invasion confined to cervix
II extension beyond cervix but not to pelvic wall / lower third of vagina
IIa vaginal invasion excluding lower 1/3
IIb parametrial involvement excepting pelvic sidewall

III extension to pelvic wall / lower third of vagina
IIIa invasion of lower 1/3 of vagina
IIIb parametrial involvement to pelvic wall
IVa mucosal involvement of bladder / rectum
IVb spread to distant organs (paraaortic / inguinal nodes, intraperitoneal metastasis)

Significance of tumor size:
>4 cm: nodal metastases (80%), local recurrence (40%), distant metastases (28%)
<4 cm: nodal metastases (16%), local recurrence (5%), distant metastases (0%)

Spread: direct extension, lymphatic, hematogenous
Incidence of nodal metastases (77% accuracy for CT, 78% for MR):
0.3% for stage 0, I a
16% for stage I b
33% for stage II a
37% for stage II b

• leukorrhea ± vaginal bleeding (<30%)
• postcoital bleeding / metrorrhagia
√ bulky enlargement of cervix (DDx: cervical fibroid)
√ fluid-filled uterus (secondary to obstruction)
√ signs of parametrial invasion: >4-mm soft-tissue strands extending from cervix into parametria, cardinal / sacrouterine ligaments, irregularity of cervical margins, eccentric parametrial enlargement, obliteration of fat planes

MR (76–83% accuracy for staging, 82–92% accuracy for parametrial involvement):
√ isointense mass on T1WI
√ hyperintense focal bulge / mass on T2WI (DDx: postbiopsy changes, inflammation, nabothian cysts)
√ blurring + widening of junctional zone secondary to obstruction of cervical os (retained secretions in uterine cavity)

Prognosis: local recurrence (usually within 2 years)

CHORIOAMNIONIC SEPARATION

(a) normally seen <16 weeks
= incomplete fusion of amniotic membrane with chorionic plate
(b) abnormal >17 weeks MA
= secondary to hemorrhage

√ membrane extends over fetal surface + stops at origin of umbilical cord
√ elevated membrane thinner than chorionic membrane
Cx: rupture of amniotic membrane may lead to amniotic band syndrome
DDx: cystic hygroma (moves with embryo)

CHORIOANGIOMA

= benign vascular malformation of proliferating capillaries (= hamartoma)
Incidence: 1:3,500 to 1:20,000 births
Location: usually near the umbilical cord insertion site

√ well-circumscribed intraplacental mass with complex echo pattern protruding from the fetal surface of the placenta
√ polyhydramnios (in 1/3)
√ arterial signal on Doppler ultrasound in angiomatous chorioangioma
Cx: hemorrhage, fetal hydrops, cardiomegaly, congestive heart failure, IUGR, premature labor, fetal demise (with large lesion)

CHORIOCARCINOMA

5% of gestational trophoblastic diseases
Age: child-bearing age
Histo: biphasic pattern including syncytiotrophoblastic + cytotrophoblastic proliferation without villous structures; extensive necrosis + hemorrhage; early + extensive vascular invasion
Preceded by: *mnemonic:* "MEAN"
Mole (hydatidiform) in 50.0%
Ectopic pregnancy in 2.5%
Abortion, spontaneous in 25.0%
Normal pregnancy in 22.5%

• continued vaginal bleeding
• continued elevation of HCG after expulsion of molar / normal pregnancy (25%)
√ mass enlarging the uterus
√ mixed hyperechoic pattern (hemorrhage, necrosis)

Spread:
(a) hematogenous (usually)
(b) lymphatic + direct extension (occasionally)
Hemorrhagic + necrotic metastases to lung, vagina, kidney (10–50%), brain
√ radiodense pulmonary masses with hazy borders due to hemorrhage
√ hyperechoic hepatic foci

Prognosis: 85% cure rate (even with metastases); fatal with spread to kidneys + brain
Rx: (1) Chemotherapy: methotrexate, actinomycin D ± cyclophosphamide
(2) Hysterectomy (if at risk for uterine rupture)
DDx: *mnemonic:* "THE CLIP"
True mole
Hydropic degeneration of placenta
Endometrial proliferation
Coexistent mole and fetus
Leiomyoma (degenerated)
Incomplete abortion
Products of conception (retained)

CLEAR CELL NEOPLASM OF OVARY

= MESONEPHROID TUMOR
= almost always invasive carcinoma
Incidence: 5–10% of all ovarian cancers
Histo: clear cells (cuboidal cells with clear cytoplasm) + hobnail cells (columnar cells with large nuclei projecting into the lumina of glandular elements); similar to clear cell carcinoma of endometrium, cervix, vagina, kidney

Not associated with: in utero DES exposure (like lesions of the vagina + cervix)
- 75% of patients present with stage I disease

√ frequently unilocular cyst + mural nodule
Prognosis: 50% 5-year survival rate

CONJOINED TWINS

= incomplete division of embryonic cell mass in monozygotic twins occurring at 13–16 days GA
Incidence: 1:52,000 livebirths; 1:600 twin births; M:F = 3:7
Types:
A. Inferior conjunction:
1. Diprosopus — two faces + one head and body
2. Dicephalus — two heads + one body
3. Ischiopagus — joined by inferior sacrum and coccyx
4. Pygopagus (20%) — joined by posterolateral sacrum and coccyx

B. Superior conjunction:
1. Dipygus — single head, thorax, abdomen + two pelves and four legs
2. Syncephalus — facial fusion ± thoracic fusion
3. Craniopagus (6%) — joined between homologous portions of cranial vault

C. Middle conjunction:
1. Thoracopagus (18%) — between thoracic walls; conjoined hearts (75%)
2. Omphalopagus (10%) — joined between umbilicus + xiphoid
3. Xiphopagus — joined at xiphoid
4. Thoracoomphalopagus (28%)

D. Incomplete duplication (10%): duplication of only one part of body

OB-US (diagnosed as early as 12 weeks GA):
√ single placenta without amniotic membrane (monochorionic, monoamniotic = hallmark of monozygotic twinning)
√ inseparable fetal bodies + skin contours
√ no change in relative position of fetuses
√ both fetal heads persistently at same level (fetuses commonly face each other)
√ bibreech (more common) / bicephalic presentation (cephalic-breech presentation is most common presentation for omphalopagus)
√ polyhydramnios (in almost 50%)
√ single umbilical cord with >3 vessels
√ backward flexion of cervical spine (in anterior fusion)
√ single cardiac motion (shared heart)
Associated malformations:
√ omphalocele
√ congenital heart disease
Prognosis: 39% stillborn; 34% die within first days of life

CORD PROLAPSE

= prolapse of cord into endocervical canal
Incidence: 0.5% at delivery
Predisposing factors:
nonvertex fetal lie, polyhydramnios, cephalopelvic disproportion, multiple gestation, increased length of umbilical cord
Cx: cord compression with high perinatal mortality
N.B.: MEDICAL EMERGENCY! Alert obstetrician immediately!
OB-Management::
(1) Patient immediately placed into Trendelenburg / knee-elbow position in radiology department
(2) Cesarean section for term infants
(3) Expectant management for preterm infants
DDx: **Cord presentation** (= umbilical cord between fetus and internal os)

CORPUS LUTEUM CYST

Types:
1. **Corpus luteum of menstruation**
formed after rupture of follicle + increasing in size until 22nd day of menstrual cycle
√ usually >12–17 mm in size
2. **Corpus luteum of pregnancy**
caused by HCG stimulation during pregnancy
√ usual size 30–40 mm, may grow up to 15 cm in diameter
√ reaches maximum size after 8–10 weeks
√ usually resolves before 20 weeks GA (12–15 weeks), occasionally persists past 1st trimester

√ thin-walled usually unilateral cyst
√ echogenic (organized clot) / sonolucent (resorbed blood)
√ low-level internal echoes frequent (= hemorrhage)
Cx: rupture with intraperitoneal hemorrhage

CYSTADENOFIBROMA

= variant of serous cystadenoma, rarely malignant
Prevalence: nearly 50% of all benign ovarian cystic serous tumors; bilateral in 6%
Age: 15–65 (mean 31) years
- may produce estrogen excess

√ small multilocular cystic tumor
√ clusters of short rounded papillary processes

DERMOID

= DERMOID CYST = MATURE CYSTIC TERATOMA
= congenital tumor containing mature tissues from all 3 germ cell layers with predominance of ectodermal component
Incidence: 5 –11–25% of all ovarian neoplasms; 66% of pediatric ovarian tumors; most common ovarian neoplasm
Origin: self-fertilization of a single germ cell after the first meiotic division (= random error in meiosis)
Histo: may contain struma ovarii, carcinoid tumor
Age: reproductive life (80%); age peak 20–40 years

- abdominal mass (2/3)
- pelvic pressure / pain due to torsion or hemorrhage

Location: bilateral in 8–15–25%

√ cystic mass with average diameter of 10 cm
√ "dermoid plug" = Rokitansky nodule / protuberance
  = oval / round solid tissue mass (sebaceous material) of 10–65 mm projecting into cyst lumen

Plain film (diagnostic in 40%):
  √ tooth / bone
  √ fat density (SPECIFIC)

CT:
  √ round mass of fat floating in interface between two water-density components (93%)
  √ Rokitansky nodule = dermoid plug (81%), usually single, may be multiple
  √ fat-fluid level (12%)
  √ globular calcifications (tooth) / rim of calcification (56%)

US (sensitivity 77–87%):
  √ complex mass containing echogenic components (66%)
  √ echogenic mass (due to mixture of sebum + hair) with "dirty" acoustic shadowing (= "tip of the iceberg") in a predominantly cystic mass (25–44%) (DDx: stool-filled rectosigmoid)
  √ predominantly solid mass (10–31%)
  √ purely cystic tumor (9–15%)
  √ echogenic focus with acoustic shadowing (due to calcification)

MR:
  √ hyperintense fat within fluid of low signal intensity on T1WI
  √ hyperintense mass (fat + serous fluid both with high signal intensity) on T2WI
  √ ± chemical shift artifact (frequency-encoding direction)

Cx: (1) Malignant degeneration in 1–3% (usually within dermoid plug of tumors >10 cm in diameter in postmenopausal women)
  (2) Torsion (4–16%)
  (3) Rupture with chemical peritonitis (rare)
  (4) Hydronephrosis

Rx: surgery (to avoid torsion / rupture)

DIETHYLSTILBESTROL (DES) EXPOSURE

= first reported transplacental carcinogen

@ Vagina: adenosis, septa, ridges, clear-cell adenocarcinoma (in 1:1,000 women exposed in utero to DES, by age 35)
@ Cervix: hypoplasia, stenosis, mucosal displacement, pseudopolyps, hooded / "cockscomb" appearance
@ Uterus: hypoplasia, bands, contour irregularity, "T-shaped" uterus
@ Tubes: deformity, irregularity, obstruction

DYSGERMINOMA

= malignant germ cell tumor of ovary homologous to testicular seminoma

Incidence: 0.5–2% of all malignant ovarian tumors
Peak age: 2nd–3rd decade

- no elevation of AFP / HCG (in 5% syncytiotrophoblastic giant cells present, which can elevate HCG levels)

Location: usually unilateral; bilateral in 15–17%

√ multilobulated solid mass divided by fibrovascular septa
√ speckled pattern of calcifications (rare)

MR:
  √ hypo- / isointense septa on T2WI with contrast-enhancement on T1WI

US:
  √ hyperechoic solid mass, may have areas of hemorrhage + necrosis
  √ prominent arterial color Doppler flow within septa

Rx: highly radiosensitive

ECLAMPSIA

= occurrence of coma ± pre-, intra-, or postpartum convulsions not related to a coincidental neurologic disorder in a preeclamptic patient

Pathophysiology:
  (1) vasospasm theory: overregulation of cerebral vasoconstrictive response to acute + severe hypertension progresses to vasospasm; prolonged vasospasm causes local ischemia, increased brain capillary permeability, disruption of blood-brain barrier, arteriolar necrosis, leading to cerebral edema + hemorrhage
  (2) forced-dilatation theory: with severe arterial hypertension upper limit of cerebral autoregulation is reached + cerebral vasodilatation starts disrupting the blood-brain barrier and resulting in cerebral edema

Time of onset: 2nd half of pregnancy in primigravida; <20th week GA with trophoblastic disease

- severe throbbing frontal headache
- visual disturbance: scotomata, amaurosis, blurred vision
- retinal / cortical blindness
- hyperreflexia, hemi- / quadriparesis, confusion, coma
- seizures: usually tonic-clonic

CT (positive in up to 50%):
  √ bilateral rather symmetric white matter hypodensities without contrast enhancement
  √ ± cerebral edema with compression of lateral ventricles
  √ usually transient + completely reversible cerebral-cortical + basal ganglia hypodensities (= reversible ischemic lesions)
  √ cerebral infarction in prolonged ischemia
  √ intracerebral hemorrhage (major cause of mortality in 10–60%)

MR:
  √ transiently increased T2-signal intensity in cerebral cortex + subcortical white matter frequently in watershed areas of posterior hemispheres

ECTOPIA CORDIS

= fusion defect of anterior thoracic wall / sternum / septum transversum prior to 9th week of gestation

OB&GYN

A. THORACIC TYPE (60%)
= heart outside thoracic cavity protruding through defect in sternum
B. ABDOMIANL TYPE (30%)
= heart protruding into abdomen through gap in diaphragm
C. THORACOABDOMINAL TYPE (7%)
= in pentalogy of Cantrell
D. CERVICAL TYPE (3%)
= displacement of heart into cervical region

Associated with:
(1) Facial deformities
(2) Skeletal deformities
(3) Ventral wall defects
(4) CNS malformations: meningocele, encephalocele
(5) Intracardiac anomalies: tetralogy of Fallot, TGA
(6) Amniotic band syndrome

Prognosis: stillbirth / death within first hours / death within first days of life in most case

ECTOPIC PREGNANCY

= implantation outside the endometrial cavity

Incidence: 1.6:1,000 of all pregnancies (increasing); 9.9:10,000 women annually; 73,700 cases in 1986 in United States

Risk of recurrence: 10–15%

Cause: delayed transit of the fertilized zygote (formed on day 14 MA) secondary to
(a) abnormal angulation of oviduct
(b) adhesions or scarring from inflammation
(c) slowed tubal transit from ciliary abnormalities

Risk factors:
(1) Previous tubal surgery (tubal ligation / tuboplasty)
(2) Previous PID (30–50%): esp. Chlamydia
(3) In-vitro fertilization / gamete intrafallopian tube transfer
(4) Endometriosis
(5) Previous ectopic pregnancy (prevalence up to 1.1%, 10-fold increase in risk, 25% chance of recurrence)
(6) Current use of IUD
(7) Advanced maternal age
◊ If the pregnancy cannot be documented as intrauterine, the patient should be considered at risk!

Time of manifestation: usually by 7th week of MA

CLASSIC CLINICAL TRIAD (<50%):
- abnormal vaginal bleeding (75–86%)
- pelvic pain (97%)
- palpable adnexal mass (23–41%)

- secondary amenorrhea (61%)
- cervical motion tenderness
- positive urinary pregnancy test (50%)
- progesterone level <25 mg/mL
- β-HCG does not rise >66% within 48 hours (lower levels + slower rise and decline compared with IUP)
  ◊ Most ectopic pregnancies do not exhibit a β-HCG of >6500 mIU/mL (1st IRP) prior to symptomatology!
  ◊ A β-HCG level above the discriminatory zone with absence of IUP suggests ectopic pregnancy!

Discriminatory zone of β-HCG
(at which a normal IUP should be visualized):
(a) by transabdominal scan:
≥6500 mIU/mL (IRP) with 100% sensitivity + 96% specificity
(b) by endovaginal scan:
≥2000 to 3000 mIU/mL (IRP)
Caveats: technical quality of exam, multiple gestations, distortion by uterine cavity (leiomyoma), lab error, assay variation

Location:
(a) tubal (95%): (1) Ampullary ectopic (75–80%)
(2) Isthmic ectopic (10–15%)
(3) Fimbrial ectopic (5%)
(4) Interstitial ectopic (2–4%)
(b) other (5%): (1) Abdominal ectopic
(2) Ovarian ectopic (0.5–1%)
(3) Interligamentary ectopic
(4) Cervical ectopic (0.15%)

Spectrum:
Type 1: unruptured live ectopic + heartbeat
Type 2: early embryonic demise without rupture / embryonic structures / heartbeat
Type 3: ruptured ectopic with blood in pelvis
Type 4: no sonographic signs of ectopic

Dx: diagnostic laparoscopy (3–4% false negative, 5% false positive)

Transvaginal US (6–20% false-negative rate):
◊ Detected 1 week sooner than by transvesical US!
@ Uterus
√ absence of intrauterine pregnancy (beyond 6 weeks MA / with β-HCG level >1,000 mIU/mL [2nd IRP])
◊ No IUP by transvesical US = ectopic pregnancy in 43–46%
◊ No IUP by endovaginal US = ectopic pregnancy in 67%
√ slight thickening of endometrium
√ sloughing of endometrium = decidual cast (21%)
√ decidual cast = hyperechoic endometrial thickening (50%) due to hormonal stimulation from ectopic pregnancy
√ decidual cyst = 1- to 5-mm cyst at junction of endometrium and myometrium (14%)

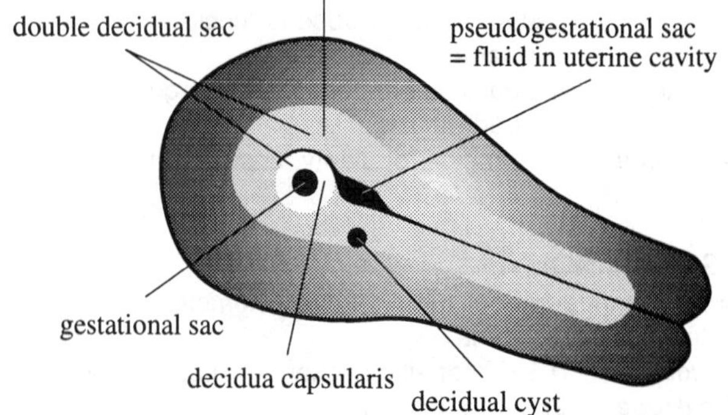

√ pseudogestational sac = single parietal decidual layer surrounding an anechoic fluid collection in uterine cavity secondary to bleeding (10–20%)
√ decidual endometrium lacks low-impedance blood flow

@ Adnexa
√ "tubal ring" = extrauterine hypoechoic saclike structure (40–68%) 1–3 cm in diameter + surrounded by a 2–4 mm concentric ring
√ extrauterine mass of any type (84%)
√ solid / complex adnexal mass = clotted blood free in peritoneal cavity / hematosalpinx (36%)
√ extrauterine gestational sac without live embryo / yolk sac (35%)
√ embryonic heartbeat (6–28%) = PATHOGNOMONIC
√ echogenic "tubal mass" (89–100%)
√ varying flow pattern depending on viability
√ corpus luteum within ovary in >50% on side of ectopic pregnancy (DDx: ectopic pregnancy)

@ Cul-de-sac
√ free fluid (40–83%): echogenic / particulate fluid (= hemoperitoneum) has 93% positive predictive value for ectopic pregnancy
DDx: anechoic fluid in 10–27% of IUP

Doppler-US (low diagnostic impact):
√ high-velocity low-impedance flow around extrauterine gestation in 54% (up to 4 kHz shift with 3 MHz transducer, 0.38 ± 0.2 Pourcelot index, RI = 0.18–0.58)
√ absence of peritrophoblastic flow after 36 days (<0.8 kHz shift with 3 MHz transducer or <1.3 kHz shift with 5 MHz transducer)
DDx of low-impedance flow:
corpus luteum cyst, tuboovarian abscess, fibroid

Probability of ectopic pregnancy in absence of IUP + clinical symptoms of an ectopic pregnancy with:

normal scan / simple cyst in adnexa	5%
complex adnexal mass	92%
tubal ring	95%
live embryo outside uterus	100%

Prognosis: (1) 3.8:10,000 mortality rate (4% of all maternal deaths)
(2) Infertility (in 40%)

Dx: (1) Laparoscopy (almost 100% accurate)
(2) Culdocentesis (high probability for ectopic with aspiration of nonclotting blood with a hematocrit >15)

Cx: maternal death in 1:1,000; tubal rupture (10–15%)

DDx: (1) Hemorrhagic corpus luteum / hematoma
(2) Adnexal mass: hydrosalpinx, endometrioma, ovarian cyst
(3) Fluid-containing small bowel loop
(4) Eccentrically placed GS in bicornuate / retroflexed / fibroid uterus

Abdominal Ectopic (1:6000)

◊ >25% may be missed sonographically!
• bloating, abdominal pain (fetal movement / peritoneal irritation due to adhesions)
• bleeding, hypotension, shock
√ extrauterine location of fetus + placenta
√ uterus compressed with visible endometrial cavity line
√ absence of uterine wall between gestation + bladder / abdominal wall
√ anhydramnios

Cx: bowel obstruction / perforation; erosion of pregnancy through abdominal wall

Lithopedion

= "stone child" = very rare obstetric complication consisting of a dehydrated + calcified demised fetus in an extrauterine pregnancy existing for >3 months without infection

Types:
(1) Lithokelyphosis = fetal membranes calcified
(2) Lithokelyphopedion = fetus + membranes calcified
(3) True lithopedion = only fetus calcified

Maternal age at discovery: 23–100 years of age; within 4–20 years of fetal demise

Location: most common in adnexae
√ large densely calcified mass in lower abdomen / upper pelvis
√ CT scan reveals fetal skeleton

DDx: uterine fibroid, calcified ovarian malignancy / cyst, sarcoma

Heterotopic Pregnancy

= ectopic + coexistent intrauterine pregnancy

Incidence: 1:6,800–30,000 pregnancies (higher number of coexisting ectopic with ovulation induction)

◊ An IUP does not preclude a complete pelvic ultrasound evaluation, although depiction of an IUP virtually excludes the diagnosis of an ectopic pregnancy!

Interstitial (Cornual) Ectopic (2–4%)

= ectopic pregnancy with eccentric location in relation to endometrium + close to uterine serosa
◊ Often rupture late because of greater myometrial distensibility compared with other parts of tube!
◊ High likelihood of catastrophic hemorrhage + death due to abundant blood supply by both ovarian + uterine arteries!

Increased risk: previous ipsilateral salpingectomy
• Baart de la Faille sign = broad-based palpable mass extending outward from uterine angle
• Ruge-Simon syndrome = fundus displaced to contralateral side with rotation of uterus + elevation of affected cornu
√ eccentric heterogeneous mass in cornual region (66%)
√ eccentrically placed gestational sac (25%)
√ thinning of myometrial mantle to <5 mm (33%)

√ interstitial line sign = thin echogenic line extending directly up to the center of ectopic pregnancy (= endometrial canal / interstitial portion of Fallopian tube) in 92%
√ myometrium between sac and uterine cavity
√ large vascular channels + peritrophoblastic blood flow
√ absence of double decidual sign

Prognosis: massive bleeding from erosion of uterine arteries + veins (pregnancy survives only 12–16 weeks GA); 2-fold mortality compared with other tubal ectopics

DDx: pregnancy within horn of bicornuate uterus; hydatidiform mole; degenerating uterine fibroid

EMBRYONIC DEMISE

Incidence: 20–71% loss rate of one twin <10 weeks

Early Embryonic Demise / Failing Pregnancy

on endovaginal scan

- β-HCG level <2–3 standard deviations below the mean for given MA / GS size / CRL

A. DEFINITE DEMISE
 √ absence of cardiac activity with CRL of ≥5 mm / ≥6.5 weeks GA (repeat scan in 3 days for confirmation)

B. PROBABLY FAILING PREGNANCY
 √ mean sac diameter of ≥16 mm without embryo
 √ mean sac size of ≥8 mm without yolk sac (repeat scan in 3 days for confirmation)
 √ >1,000 mIU/mL (1st IRP) without gestational sac
 √ >7,200 mIU/mL (1st IRP) without yolk sac
 √ >10,800 mIU/mL(1st IRP) without embryo

C. HIGH RISK OF SUBSEQUENT DEMISE
 √ severe bradycardia <80 bpm
 √ small mean gestational sac size (difference between mean sac size and CRL <5 mm is predictive of miscarriage in 94%)

D. MODERATELY HIGH RISK OF DEMISE
 √ bradycardia of 80–90 bpm
 √ large subchorionic hematoma lifting much of placenta
 √ yolk sac >6 mm / abnormal shape

√ mean gestational sac size too small for good clinical dates
√ gestational sac growth ≤ 0.7 mm/day (normal growth rate of 1.13 mm/day determines appropriate time interval for follow-up scan, ie, when sac is expected to be 27 mm)
√ sac position in lower uterine segment / cervix
√ stringlike / granular debris / fluid-fluid level within gestational sac (= intrasac bleeding)

Late Embryonic Demise

on endovaginal scan

√ wrinkled collapsing amniotic membrane
√ irregular distorted shape of gestational sac (DDx: compression by bladder, myoma, contraction)
√ absence of double decidual sac = thin (<2 mm) weakly hyperechoic / irregular choriodecidual reaction

ENDODERMAL SINUS TUMOR OF OVARY

= YOLK SAC TUMOR
= rare but highly malignant tumor

Histo: resembles endodermal sinuses of the rat yolk sac
 (a) papillary pattern (most common): contains glomerular structures with central vessel + peripheral mantling of epithelial cells (= Schiller-Duval bodies)
 (b) others: reticular, solid, polyvesicular vitelline
 — periodic acid-Schiff reaction
 — α-fetoprotein–positive hyaline globules

Incidence: <1% of all ovarian carcinomas
Age: usually adolescence
May be associated with: teratoma, dermoid cyst, choriocarcinoma

- frequently abdominal enlargement + pain
- elevated serum AFP (common)

√ predominantly echogenic solid tumor
√ cystic areas (epithelial-lined cysts / cysts of coexisting mature teratoma / hemorrhage / necrosis)
√ bilateral in 1%

Rx: surgery + combination chemotherapy
Prognosis: poor

ENDOMETRIAL CANCER

Most common invasive gynecologic malignancy; 4th most prevalent female cancer in USA women

Incidence: 34,000 new cases per year with 3,000 deaths
Histo: adenocarcinoma (90–95%), sarcoma (1–3%)
Peak age: 55–62 years; 74% > age 50
Risk factors: nulliparity, late menopause, unopposed estrogen therapy, polycystic ovaries, obesity, hypertension, diabetes mellitus

FIGO stage:

0	In situ
I a	Tumor limited to endometrium
I b	invasion to less than half of myometrium
I c	invasion to more than half of myometrium
II a	Endocervical glandular involvement only
II b	cervical stromal invasion
III a	Invasion of serosa / adnexa / peritoneal metastases
III b	vaginal metastases
III c	metastases to pelvic / paraaortic lymph nodes
IV a	Invasion of bladder / bowel mucosa
IV b	distant metastases (lung, brain, bone) including intraabdominal / inguinal lymph nodes

◊ Clinical staging with dilatation & curettage inaccurate in up to 51%!

Histo:
 (a) endometrioid carcinoma (75% of all cancers)
 (b) serous, mucinous, clear cell carcinoma (less common): similar to ovarian counterpart
 (c) squamous (rare): associated with cervical stenosis, pyometra, chronic inflammation

(d) mixed mesodermal tumor: contains elements of epithelial + mesenchymal differentiation

Lymph node metastases: 3% with superficial invasion; 40% with deep invasion

• postmenopausal bleeding without hormonal therapy

US:

√ normal-sized / enlarged uterus
√ echogenic endometrium >5 mm AP thickness (100% negative predictive value, not very specific)
√ inhomogeneous endometrial echotexture with irregular hypoechoic areas
√ pulsatility index of <1.5 (DDx: endometritis, benign endometrial polyp)

MR (82–92% accuracy for staging, 74–87% accuracy for depth of invasion):

√ endometrial cancer has slightly lower signal intensity than endometrium but higher than myometrium on T2WI
√ endometrial thickness abnormal if >3 mm (postmenopausal woman) / >10 mm (under estrogen replacement)
DDx: blood clot, uterine secretions, adenomatous hyperplasia, submucosal leiomyoma
√ disruption / absence of junctional zone (myometrial invasion)
√ hyperintense areas penetrating into myometrium (deep muscle invasion; 74–87% accuracy)

ENDOMETRIOID CARCINOMA OF OVARY

Incidence: 15% of all ovarian cancers; 2nd most common malignant ovarian neoplasm (after serous adenocarcinoma)

Associated with: hyperplasia / carcinoma of the uterine endometrium in 20–33%

Histo: tubular glandular pattern with a pseudostratified epithelium resembling endometrial adenocarcinoma / metastatic colon carcinoma

√ solid / complex (= cystic + solid) tumor
√ bilateral in 25%

Prognosis: better than serous / mucinous carcinomas

ENDOMETRIOSIS

= encysted functional endometrial epithelium + stroma in an ectopic site outside the uterine cavity / myometrium

Prevalence: 8–10–18% of menstruating women

Etiology: (1) Peritoneal implantation of endometrial cells via retrograde menstruation through fallopian tubes
(2) Metaplastic transformation of peritoneal epithelium into endometrial tissue
(3) Traumatic spread (uterine surgery, amniocentesis)

Age: 30–45 years; dependent on normal hormonal stimulation

• infertility
◊ 25% of infertile women have endometriosis
◊ 30–40% of women with endometriosis are infertile
• severe dysmenorrhea, menorrhagia
• chronic pelvic pain (peritoneal adhesions, bleeding)
• dyspareunia

Location:
(a) internal endometriosis (within uterus) = ADENOMYOSIS
(b) external endometriosis
typical in: ovaries > uterosacral ligaments > pouch of Douglas > uterine serosal surface > fallopian tube > rectosigmoid
rare in: urinary bladder wall, umbilicus, bowel wall (20%), laparotomy scar, lungs, pleural space, limbs

Morphologic types:

1. Discrete pelvic mass
◊ Multiplicity favors the diagnosis of endometrioma
√ typically cystic space = **endometrioma** = "chocolate cyst" up to 20 cm in diameter (usually 2–5 cm)
√ anechoic cyst / cyst with "ground-glass" homogeneous low-level echoes (= hemorrhagic debris)
√ may contain echogenic material (= clot) appearing as a solid tumor
√ may show layering of debris
√ smooth walls + acoustic enhancement
2. Diffuse form (70%)
√ often no detectable abnormality (when lesions small + scattered)
√ frequently multiple cysts bilaterally
√ thickened wall + loss of definition of borders of pelvic organs

MR (90% sensitive, 98% specific with fat suppression + contrast enhancement):

√ hyperintense lesions on all pulse sequences in 47%, hypointense on all pulse sequences in 27%
√ typically hyperintense on T1WI (similar to fat) + additional hyperintensity (like urine) on T2WI with multiple locules and internal "shading"

@ GI tract (5–12–37%)
• change in bowel habits, rectal pain / bleeding
Path: muscular hypertrophy + fibrosis related to endometriotic deposits in bowel wall
Location: inferior margin of sigmoid colon + anterior wall of rectosigmoid (72%); rectovaginal septum (14%); small intestine (7%); cecum (4%); appendix (3%); occasionally multiple lesions
√ single extramucosal mass with crenulated / spiculated mucosal pattern
√ polypoid intraluminal mass / annular constricting lesion (rare appearance)

CXR:
√ catamenial pneumothorax = spontaneous pneumothorax due to endometriosis of diaphragm

Cx: infertility with involvement of tubes + ovaries (peritubal adhesions causing anatomic distortion, limitation of fimbrial motion, tubal destruction / occlusion)

Dx: laparoscopy

Rx: hormonal therapy, surgery

DDx: hemorrhagic ovarian cyst, dermoid cyst, tubo-ovarian abscess

FACIAL CLEFTING

Normal embryology:
1st branchial arch develops into maxillary + mandibular prominences; by 5th week the stomodeum is surrounded by 5 prominences: frontal-nasal, paired maxillary, paired mandibular prominences; nasal pits are formed by invagination of nasal placodes on each side of frontal-nasal prominence; the 2 maxillary prominences grow medially to fuse with the 2 medial nasal prominences forming the upper lip; the lateral nasal prominences form the nasal alae

Incidence:
0.5:1,000 in blacks; 1:1,000 livebirths in white population; 1.5:1,000 in Asians; 3.6:1,000 in American Indians; 13% of all congenital anomalies; second most common congenital malformation; most common craniofacial malformation

Risk of recurrence: 4% with one affected sibling, 17% with one affected sibling + parent

Median Facial Cleft

= failure of fusion of the 2 medial nasal prominences

Incidence: rare

Cause:
1. median cleft face syndrome = frontonasal dysplasia
   √ brain anomalies rare
2. Holoprosencephaly
3. Majewski syndrome (short rib, polydactyly, median cleft)

Lateral Facial Cleft

Cleft Lip [25%]

Cause: lack of fusion of maxillary prominence with medial nasal prominence (= intermaxillary segment) around 7th week MA

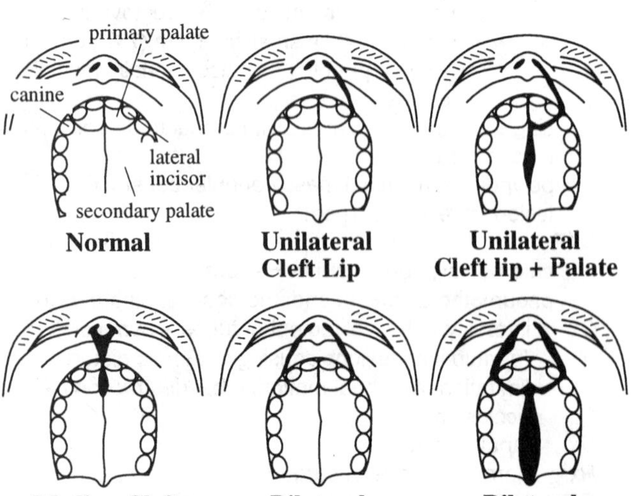

Associated with: anomalies in 20% (most frequently clubfoot); NO chromosomal anomalies

Site: isolated in 8%, bilateral in 20%

√ linear echopoor region extending from one side of fetal upper lip into nostril

Prognosis: excellent

Cleft Lip & Palate [50%]

Cause: incomplete fusion of lip + primary palate with secondary palate

Associated with: 72 abnormalities in 56–80%: most frequently polydactyly; chromosomal anomalies in 20–33%

Location: L > R

Site: unilateral in 23%, bilateral in 30%

√ linear defect extending through alveolar ridge + hard palate reaching the floor of the nasal cavity / orbit (often deeper + longer cleft than in isolated cleft lip)

√ paranasal echogenic mass inferior to nose (= premaxillary protrusion of soft tissue + alveolar process + dental structures) in bilateral cleft lip + palate

Cleft Palate [25%]

= lack of fusion of mesenchymal masses of lateral palatine processes around 8th–9th weeks MA

Associated with: anomalies in 50% (most frequently clubfoot + polydactyly)

√ often missed on prenatal sonograms

√ small fetal stomach + polyhydramnios (due to impaired fetal swallowing)

FETAL CARDIAC DYSRHYTHMIAS

normal heart rate: 120–160 bpm

Premature Atrial Contractions

= PAC = most common benign rhythm abnormality

√ transient tachycardia

√ transient bradycardia (due to atrial bigeminy if every other beat is nonconducted)

Cx: supraventricular tachycardia (unusual)

Rx discontinue smoking, alcohol, caffeine

Follow-up: biweekly auscultation until arrhythmia resolves

Supraventricular Tachyarrhythmia

Incidence: 1:25,000; most frequent tachyarrhythmia in children

Etiology: viral infection, hypoplasia of sinoatrial tract

Pathogenesis:
(1) Automaticity = irritable ectopic focus discharges at high frequency
(2) Reentry = electric pulse reentering the atria inciting new discharges

Types:
1. Supraventricular tachyarrhythmia (SVT)
   (a) paroxysmal supraventricular tachycardia
   (b) paroxysmal atrial tachycardia
   √ atrial rate of 180–300 bpm + ventricular response of 1:1
2. Atrial flutter
   √ atrial rate of 300–460 bpm + ventricular rate of 60–200 bpm
3. Atrial fibrillation
   √ atrial rate of 400–700 bpm + ventricular rate of 120–200 bpm

Hemodynamics:
fast ventricular rate results in suboptimal filling of heart chambers + decreased cardiac output, overload of RA, CHF

Associated with: cardiac anomalies (5–10%):
ASD, congenital mitral valve disease, cardiac tumors, WPW syndrome, cardiomyopathy, thyrotoxicosis

OB-US:
√ M-mode echocardiography with simultaneous visualization of atrial + ventricular contractions allows inference of atrioventricular activation sequence

Cx: congestive heart failure + nonimmune hydrops
Rx: Intrauterine pharmacologic cardioversion (digoxin, verapamil, propranolol, procainamide, quinidine)

Atrioventricular Block
Incidence: 1:20,000 livebirths; in 4–9% of all infants with CHD
Etiology: (1) Immaturity of conduction system
(2) Absent connection to AV node
(3) Abnormal anatomic position of AV node

Associated with:
(1) Cardiac structural anomalies (45–50%): corrected transposition, univentricular heart, cardiac tumor, cardiomyopathy
(2) Maternal connective tissue disease: lupus erythematosus

Types:
1. First-degree heart block = simple conduction delay
   √ normal heart rate + rhythm (not reportedly diagnosed in utero)
2. Second-degree heart block
   (a) Mobitz type I
   = progressive prolongation of PR interval finally leading to the block of one atrial impulse (Luciani-Wenckebach phenomenon)
   √ a few atrial contractions are not followed by a ventricular contraction
   (b) Mobitz type II
   = intermittent conduction with a ventricular rate as a submultiple of the atrial rate (eg, 2:1 / 3:1 block)
   √ atrial contraction not followed by ventricular contraction in a constant relationship
3. Third-degree heart block = complete heart block
   = complete dissociation of atria + ventricles
   √ slow atrial + ventricular contractions independent from each other

Cx: decreased cardiac output + CHF

FETAL DEATH IN UTERO
= INTRAUTERINE DEMISE
= fetal death during 2nd + 3rd trimesters

Specific signs:
√ absent cardiac / somatic motion

Nonspecific signs seen not before 48 hours after death:
√ same / decreased BPD measurement compared with prior exam
√ development of dolichocephaly
√ "Spalding sign" = overlapping fetal skull bones
√ distorted fetus without recognizable structures
√ skin edema (epidermolysis) = fetal maceration
√ increased amount of echoes in amniotic fluid (= fetal tissue fragments)
√ gas in fetal vascular system

"Vanishing Twin"
= disappearance of one twin in utero due to complete resorption / anembryonic pregnancy
Incidence: 13–78% (mean 21%) before 14 weeks GA
Time: <13 weeks MA
√ NO sonographic evidence of twin pregnancy later in pregnancy

"Fetus Papyraceus"
= compression + mummification of fetus
Time: in 2nd trimester
Path: resorption of fluid resulting in paperlike fetal body + compression into adjacent membranes
√ compressed mummified fetus plastered against uterine wall

Risk to surviving twin:
A. Dichorionic gestation (minimal risk)
   (1) Premature labor
   (2) Obstruction of labor by macerated fetus
B. Monochorionic gestation
   (1) DIC in response to release of thromboplastin from degenerating fetus
   (a) into maternal circulation
   (b) into twin fetus through shared circulation (= twin embolization syndrome)

FETAL HYDROPS
Nonimmune Hydrops
= excess of total body water evident as extracellular accumulation of fluid in tissues + serous cavities without antibodies against RBC
Incidence: 1:1,500 to 1:4,000 deliveries
Causes:
1. Cardiac anomalies (40%):
   (a) structural heart disease (25%): AV septal defect, hypoplastic left heart, rhabdomyoma
   (b) tachyarrhythmia (15%)

2. Hematologic causes: thalassemia, hemolysis, fetal blood loss
3. Idiopathic (25–44%)
4. Twin-twin transfusion (20%)
5. Chromosomal abnormalities (6%): Turner syndrome
6. Skeletal dysplasias: achondroplasia, achondrogenesis, osteogenesis imperfecta, thanatophoric dwarfism, asphyxiating thoracic dysplasia
7. Renal disease (4%): congenital nephrotic syndrome
8. Infections: toxoplasmosis, CMV, syphilis, Coxsackie virus, parvovirus
9. Cervical tumors: teratoma
10. Chest masses: cystic adenomatoid malformation, extralobar sequestration, mediastinal tumor, rhabdomyoma of heart, diaphragmatic hernia
11. Abdominal masses: neuroblastoma, hemangioendothelioma of liver
12. Placental tumors: chorioangioma

Prognosis: 46% death in utero; 17% neonatal death

Immune Hydrops

= ERYTHROBLASTOSIS FETALIS
= lysis of fetal RBCs by maternal IgG antibodies

Pathophysiology:
rh-negative women (= no D antigen) may become isoimmunized if exposed to Rh-positive blood (= D allotype present); maternal IgM antibodies develop initially, later IgG antibodies with ability to cross placenta (= transplacental passage)

Prognosis: (if untreated) 45–50% mild anemia, 25–30% moderate anemia (with neonatal problems only), 20–25% develop hydrops (death in utero / neonatally)

Cause of isoimmunization:
fetomaternal hemorrhage during pregnancy / delivery / spontaneous or elective abortion if fetus is D-positive; fetus has a 50% chance of being rh-negative as 56% of RhD-positive fathers are heterozygous for D antigen

At risk:
Caucasians (15%), Blacks (6%), Orientals (1%); absence of D antigen originates in Basques

Determination of extent of disease by:
(1) Optical density shift at 450 nm (= delta OD 450) reflects amount of bilirubin in amniotic fluid; reasonably reliable only >25 weeks MA; unreliable in alloimmunization due to Kell antibodies
(2) Percutaneous umbilical cord sampling (PUBS) with direct determination of Hct and Hb

√ anasarca (= skin edema)
√ fetal ascites in 2nd trimester (indicates severe anemia with Hct <15%, Hb <4 g/dL; present in only 66%)
√ pleural effusion
√ increased diameter of umbilical vein
√ subcutaneous edema (skin thickness >5 mm)
√ polyhydramnios (75%)
√ placentomegaly >6 cm
√ pericardial effusion
√ hepatosplenomegaly

Prophylaxis:
Rh immune globulin (RhoGAM® = antibody against D antigen) blocks antigen sites on Rh-positive cells in maternal circulation to prevent initiation of maternal antibody production; Rh immune globulin given at 28 weeks to all rh-negative women

OB-Management:
regular monitoring from 18 weeks on when maternal anti-D concentration exceeds 4 IU/mL (severe anemia unlikely if maternal antibodies <15 IU/mL)

Rx: umbilical vein transfusion during PUBS

FOLLICULAR CYST

= unruptured follicle / ruptured follicle that sealed immediately (after continued stimulation) = failure to ovulate / involute; sign of anovulatory cycle

Predisposed: patients during puberty + menopause; S/P salpingectomy

√ thin-walled, unilocular cyst
√ size usually >2.5 cm / occasionally up to 10 cm in size
√ usually multiple / may be single
√ low-level internal echoes / fluid-debris level / septations / predominantly hyperechoic = hemorrhagic cyst (DDx: teratoma, abscess, torsion, malignancy, ectopic pregnancy)

Prognosis: usually disappears after 1–2 menstrual cycles

FUNCTIONAL OVARIAN CYST

Cause:
(a) failure of involution of follicle / corpus luteum with changes in the menstrual cycle
(b) excessive hormonal stimulation of follicles preventing normal follicular regression (eg, theca-lutein cysts)

Types:
(1) **Follicular cyst** (from preovulatory follicle): may elaborate estrogen, extremely common
(2) **Corpus luteum cyst** (from postovulatory follicle): elaborates progesterone causing delayed menstruation / persistent bleeding
(3) **Corpus albicans cyst** = from corpus luteum following regression of luteal tissue; no hormone production
(4) **Theca lutein cyst**: in hyperstimulated ovary from ovary-stimulating drugs, twins, trophoblastic disease; elaborates estrogen
(5) **Surface epithelial inclusion cyst**: common in postmenopausal women

Age: any; in newborns (influence of maternal estrogen)

Incidence: 3–5–17% in postmenopausal women

• usually asymptomatic
• acute unilateral pelvic pain (from hemorrhage / pressure)

√ unilocular smooth-walled cyst
√ contents anechoic / with internal debris (from hemorrhage)
√ up to 8–10 cm in diameter

Prognosis: spontaneous regression is common but unpredictable; typically resolve within 2 menstrual cycles (less likely if cyst > 5 cm)
Rx: (1) hormonal manipulation
(2) surgery (absolutely indicated if cyst enlarges)
(3) percutaneous aspiration (if chance of malignancy is nil as in infants)
DDx: cystic teratoma, simple benign epithelial neoplasm, endometrioma in resolution, paraovarian cyst, quiescent hydrosalpinx

GARTNER DUCT CYST

Frequency: 1–2%
Origin: remnant of vaginal portion of mesonephric / wolffian duct with incomplete involution + persistent glandular secretion
Histo: lined by flat cuboidal / columnar epithelium
May be associated with: complex renal + urogenital malformations
(1) Herlyn-Werner-Wunderlich syndrome = ipsilateral renal agenesis + ipsilateral blind vagina
(2) Ectopic ureter inserting into Gartner duct cyst
• usually asymptomatic
Location: anterolateral aspect of proximal third of vaginal wall extending into ischiorectal fossa
√ well-defined round lesion with fluid contents
√ large cysts may displace ureter upward / protrude through introitus
Cx: dyspareunia; interference with vaginal delivery

GASTROSCHISIS

= paramedian full-thickness abdominal fusion defect usually on right side of umbilical cord; may involve thorax; bowel is nonrotated and lacks secondary fixation to dorsal abdominal wall
Incidence: 1–2:10,000 livebirths (same as omphalocele), sporadic
Cause: (a) abnormal involution of right umbilical vein resulting in rupture of anterior abdominal wall at area of weakness
(b) premature interruption of right omphalo-mesenteric artery (normally persists proximally as superior mesenteric artery) resulting in ischemic damage to abdominal wall
Age of occurrence: 37 days (5 weeks) of embryonic life
Age of detection: difficult <20 weeks GA
Associated anomalies (5%):
intestinal atresia / stenosis (25%; small size of opening leads to compression or torsion of vessels); ectopia cordis (rare)
• MS-AFP ≥2.5 MoM in 77–100%
√ exteriorized bowel = thick-walled edematous freely floating loops outside fetal abdomen (due to lack of peritoneal covering)
√ dilated intra- / extraperitoneal bowel
√ <2–5 cm paraumbilical defect, usually on right side of cord insertion
√ normal insertion of umbilical cord
√ no fetal ascites
√ polyhydramnios may be present
√ liver / spleen may herniate infrequently
√ malrotation / nonrotation of bowel
Cx before birth: (1) Bowel obstruction
(2) Peritonitis (exposure of bowel to fetal urine / meconium)
(3) Perforation (from peritonitis)
(4) Fetal growth restriction (38–77%) secondary to nutritional loss from exposed bowel
Cx after birth: malrotation, jejunal / ileal atresia (18%), bowel necrosis, necrotizing enterocolitis, hyperalimentation hepatitis, prolonged intestinal motility dysfunction, chronic short-gut syndrome
Mortality rate: 17%
Survival rate: 87–100% after surgical treatment (during 1st day of life, not influenced by mode of delivery); death from premature delivery / sepsis / bowel ischemia

GERM CELL TUMOR OF OVARY

= malignant (except for mature teratoma) ovarian tumors of varying histology
Age: 14 years on average
• pelvic / abdominal pain + mass
• elevated alpha-fetoprotein (60% in immature teratoma; 100% in endodermal sinus tumor)
• elevated β-HCG (30% of endodermal sinus tumors)
√ average diameter of 15 cm
√ unilateral, rarely bilateral
√ calcifications (40%)
√ homogeneously solid (3%), predominantly solid (85%), predominantly cystic (12%)

GESTATIONAL TROPHOBLASTIC DISEASE

= group of disorders as a result of an aberrant fertilization event arising from trophoblastic elements of the developing blastocyst with invasive tendency
Components of trophoblast:
1. Cytotrophoblast = stem cell with high mitotic activity
2. Syncytiotrophoblast = synthesis of β-HCG
3. Intermediate trophoblast = responsible for endometrial invasion + implantation
• increased levels of β-HCG
Incidence: <1% of all gynecologic malignancies
Associated with: molar pregnancy (most), post abortion, ectopic pregnancy, term pregnancy
Spectrum: 1. Benign hydatidiform mole (80–90%)
2. Invasive mole (5–8–10%)
3. Choriocarcinoma (1–2–5%)
4. Placental site trophoblastic tumor (rare)
Cytogenesis:
= fertilization of one egg by two sperm = chromosomes completely / predominantly of paternal origin
1. Diploid karyotype
– 46,XX = from fertilization of ovum by two 23,X sperm after loss of maternal haploid chromosomes

- 46,XY = from fertilization of a chromosomally empty ovum by two different sperm:
  - in complete hydatidiform mole (almost 100%), invasive mole (almost 100%), choriocarcinoma (50%)

2. Triploid karyotype (69,XXX; 69 XXY; 69,XYY)
   = fertilization of a normal ovum (23,X) by 2 different sperm thus containing 2/3 paternal chromosomes
   - occurs in partial hydatidiform mole

At risk: maternal age >35 years and <20 years, previous molar gestation, previous spontaneous abortions

GRANULOSA CELL TUMOR

Most common hormone-active estrogenic tumor of ovary

Incidence: 1–2–3% of all ovarian neoplasms

Age: puberty (5%), reproductive age (45%), postmenopausal (50%)

Path: well-circumscribed, smooth / lobulated solid mass; foci of hemorrhage / cystic degeneration (when tumor gets larger)

Histo: macro- / microfollicular, alveolar, trabecular, diffuse types

- precocious puberty
- irregular menstruation cycles, menorrhagia, amenorrhea
- abdominal pain, palpable adnexal mass

Location: unilateral in 90–95%

Dissemination: local extension, spread to peritoneum (similar to cystadenocarcinoma)

√ multilocular cyst containing fluid / blood (most frequently)
√ size up to 40 cm in diameter
√ predominantly hypoechoic mass simulating fibroid
√ endometrial glandular hyperplasia

Cx: (1) Malignant transformation (5–25%)
(2) Low-grade endometrial carcinoma (10%)
(3) Recurrence (raised serum aromatase + estradiol levels)

Rx: uni- / bilateral salpingo-oophorectomy ± postoperative chemotherapy

Prognosis: 85% 10-year survival rate

HELLP SYNDROME

= **H**emolysis, **E**levated **L**iver enzymes, **L**ow **P**latelets

Prevalence: 4–12% of patients with severe preeclampsia / eclampsia; higher in White women (24%), with delayed diagnosis of preeclampsia / delayed delivery (57%), in multiparous patients (14%)

- epigastric / RUQ pain (90%)
- nausea + vomiting (45%), occasionally jaundice
- headache (50%)
- demonstrable edema (55%)

√ tender hepatomegaly
√ fatty infiltration of liver (peak at 35th week)
√ subcapsular hematoma of liver + kidney
√ hepatic necrosis
√ ascites + pleural effusions
√ vitreous hemorrhage

Cx: (1) Perinatal mortality (8–60%)
(2) Maternal death (3–24%) from liver rupture, DIC, abruptio placentae, acute renal failure, sepsis

HYDATIDIFORM MOLE

= MOLAR PREGNANCY

Complete / Classic Mole

= fertilization of ovum by two 23,X sperm after loss of maternal haploid chromosomes (46,XX) or occasionally fertilization of an "empty egg" (= ovum with no active chromosomal material) by 2 different sperm (46,XY)

Histo: generalized hydropic swelling of all chorionic villi with prominent acellular space centrally; pronounced trophoblastic proliferation of syncytio- and cytotrophoblast

- severe eclampsia prior to 24 weeks
- uterus too large for dates (in 50%)
- 1st trimester bleeding
- marked elevation of β-HCG with hyperemesis
- passing of grapelike vesicles per vagina
- hyperthyroidism (due to thyroid-stimulating properties of β-HCG)
- anemia (secondary to plasma volume expansion + vaginal bleeding)
- diploid karyotype, almost always paternal XX chromosomes

√ hyperechoic to moderately echogenic central uterine mass interspersed with punctate hypoechoic areas
√ numerous discrete cystic spaces (= hydropic villi) within a central area of heterogeneous echotexture
√ in 25% atypical appearance:
  √ large hyperechoic areas (blood clot) + areas of cystic degeneration resembling incomplete abortion
  √ single large central fluid collection with hyperechoic rim mimicking an anembryonic gestation / abortion
√ no fetal parts / no chorionic membrane
√ bilateral theca lutein cysts (18–37%), which may take 4 months to regress after evacuation of a molar pregnancy

Prognosis: in 80–85% benign, in 15–20% invasive mole / choriocarcinoma

Rx: dilatation + suction curettage (curative in 85%)

DDx: (1) Hydropic degeneration of the placenta (associated with incomplete / missed abortions)
(2) Degenerated uterine leiomyoma
(3) Incomplete abortion = retained products with hemorrhage
(4) Choriocarcinoma

Complete Mole With Coexistent Fetus (1–2%)

= molar degeneration of one conceptus of a dizygotic twin pregnancy with same risk of malignant degeneration as in classic mole

- vaginal bleeding in 2nd trimester
- uterus large for dates
- abnormally elevated serum β-HCG

- amniocentesis with normal diploid karyotype excludes diagnosis of partial mole

√ normal gestation with placenta + separate typical echogenic material of a hydatidiform mole
√ ovarian theca lutein cysts

Prognosis: fetal survival unlikely due to maternal complications from coexistent mole

Invasive Mole

= CHORIOADENOMA DESTRUENS

Histo: excessive trophoblastic proliferation with presence of villous structure + invasion of myometrium

Preexisting condition: complete / partial hydatidiform mole

- history of previous molar gestation / missed abortion (75%)
- continued uterine bleeding
- persistently elevated β-HCG levels (with failure of β-HCG to return to undetectable levels after treatment of a complete hydatidiform mole)

√ hyperechoic tissue with punctate lucencies
√ irregular focal hyperechoic region within myometrium
√ bilateral theca lutein cysts, 4–8 cm in size
√ myometrial invasion occasionally demonstrable

Rx: chemotherapy, hysterectomy (if at risk for uterine perforation)

Partial Mole

= areas of molar change alternating with normal villi + fetus with significant congenital anomalies

Histo: focal proliferations of syncytiotrophoblast; normal villi interspersed with hydropic villi

- triploid karyotype (66% XXY; 33% XXX) due to fertilization of single ovum with 2 sperm
- early onset of preeclampsia

√ nearly always coexistent fetus with severe abnormalities
√ placenta with numerous cystic spaces

Prognosis:
(1) frequently spontaneous abortion (unrecognized as mole for lack of karyotyping of the abortus)
(2) no survival of triploid fetus
(3) 3% risk of persistent gestational trophoblastic neoplasia

HYDRO- / HEMATOMETROCOLPOS

= accumulation of sterile fluid (hydro~) / blood (hemato~) / pus (pyo~) within uterus (~metria) + vagina (~colpos);
(a) premenarcheally = secretions + mucus
(b) postmenarcheally = blood

Incidence: 1:16,000 female births

Etiology:

A. CONGENITAL OBSTRUCTION
(a) persistent urogenital sinus = single exit chamber for bladder + vagina; separate orifice for anus; caused by virilization of female fetus / intersex anomaly / arrest of normal vaginal development
Frequently associated with: ambiguous genitalia
Age: newborn period
(b) cloacal malformation = single perineal orifice for bladder + vagina + rectum; caused by early embryologic arrest
Frequently associated with: duplex genital tract
Age: newborn period
(c) imperforate hymen, transverse vaginal septum, segmental vaginal atresia, imperforate cervix, blind horn of bicornuate uterus, Mayer-Rokitansky-Küster-Hauser syndrome (= agenesis of uterus + vagina with active uterine anlage)

- primary amenorrhea = "delayed menarche"
- cyclical abdominal pain
- interlabial mass

Age: puberty

◊ Hematometrocolpos / hematocolpos are due to imperforate hymen / transverse vaginal septum
◊ Hematometra is due to cervical dysgenesis + vaginal agenesis / Mayer-Rokitansky-Küster-Hauser syndrome / obstructed uterine horn

May be associated with:
imperforate anus, hydronephrosis, renal agenesis / dysplasia, polycystic kidneys, duplication of vagina + uterus, sacral hypoplasia, esophageal atresia

2. ACQUIRED OBSTRUCTION
neoplastic obstruction of endocervical canal / vagina, postpartum infection, attempted abortion, cervical stenosis after radiotherapy, postsurgical scarring (eg, dilatation and curettage, traumatic delivery), senile contraction

- vague pelvic discomfort
- pain during defecation / urination
- asymptomatic

√ smooth symmetric enlargement resulting in pear-shaped uterus ± distended vagina
√ varying amounts of low-level internal echoes centrally within uterus continuous with vaginal canal
√ hematosalpinx ± endometriosis

OB-US:
√ cystic / midlevel echogenic retrovesical mass (mucous secretions secondary to stimulation by maternal estrogens during fetal life)
√ cystic mass ± fluid-debris level (distended vagina)
√ bladder often not identified (compression by distended vagina)

DDx: ovarian cyst, duplication cyst, meconium cyst, mesenteric cyst, rectovesical fistula, anterior meningocele, cystic tumor, trophoblastic disease, degenerating leiomyoma / leiomyosarcoma

Cx: endometritis, myometritis, parametritis (= pelvic lymphangitis), pelvic abscess, septic pelvic thrombophlebitis, urinary tract infection

IMMATURE TERATOMA OF OVARY

= EMBRYONAL TERATOMA = MALIGNANT TERATOMA = SOLID TERATOMA

Histo: immature tissue resembling those of the embryo; grade 0–3 reflect amount of immature neuroectodermal tissue

May be associated with: gliomatosis peritonei = multiple peritoneal implants of mature glial tissue

- elevated AFP levels (50%)
- no elevation of serum HCG levels

√ predominantly solid tumor with numerous cysts of varying size
√ scattered calcifications (due to invariable association with mature teratoma)

INFERTILITY

= failure to conceive after 1 year of unprotected intercourse

Incidence: affects 10–15% of couples

Etiology:

(a) female factors (55%):
- Tubal disease (10–20–40%): congenital anomalies, DES exposure, pelvic inflammatory disease, salpingitis isthmica nodosa, endometriosis, postoperative factors, polyp, neoplasm, ectopic pregnancy
- Uterine factors (2–5%): bicornuate uterus, septate uterus, DES exposure, intrauterine adhesions, endometrial inflammation / infection, uterine neoplasm, complications after pregnancy, leiomyoma
- Ovulatory disorder (10–20%)
- Pelvic factors (20–25%)
- Cervical factors (5–10%)

(b) male factors (40%)
(c) combination of factors (15–25%)
(d) unknown cause (5–10%)

Tests:
- history + physical examination
- laboratory tests (mainly hormonal)
- basal body temperature measurement
- postcoital test
- cervical culture
- endometrial biopsy
- sonographic monitoring of ovaries
- sperm agglutination studies
- in vitro mucus penetration test
- laparoscopy + hysteroscopy
- hysterosalpingography

INTRAUTERINE CONTRACEPTIVE DEVICE

√ double echogenic line with plastic IUD
√ reverberation echoes with metal IUD

Types of IUD:

1. Lippes loop
   √ 4–5 echogenic dots on SAG view
   √ horizontal line / dot on TRV view
2. Saf-T-coil
   √ echogenic solid line on SAG view
   √ series of echoes / dot on TRV view
3. Copper 7 / Copper T / Progestasert
   √ dot in fundus + solid line in corpus on SAG view
   √ solid line in fundus + dot in corpus on TRV view
4. Dalkon shield (no longer produced)

Cx: pelvic inflammatory disease (2–3-fold risk compared with that of non-IUD users) in 35%; actinomycosis with IUD in place for >6 years

"Lost IUD"

= locator device not palpated

Cause:
1. expulsion of IUD
2. migration of thread
3. detachment of thread
4. uterine perforation of IUD

◊ Abdominal plain film is indicated if IUD not identified by US!

IUD & Pregnancy

√ IUD may not be visualized after 1st trimester (as uterus grows IUD is drawn into cavity)

Prognosis: high risk of septic abortion

Rx: early removal of IUD if string remained in vagina

INTRAUTERINE GROWTH RESTRICTION

= FETAL GROWTH RETARDATION

= perinate with a weight at/below the 10th percentile for gestational age occurring as a result of a pathologic process inhibiting expression of normal intrinsic growth potential

<u>for twin pregnancy</u>: discordant weight >25%

◊ Fetal weight at/below 10th percentile for age will classify 7% of normal fetuses as growth retarded!

◊ IUGR is primarily an ultrasound diagnosis!

Prevalence: 3–7% of all deliveries; in 12–47% of all twin pregnancies; in 25% of fetuses following birth of a growth-retarded sibling / stillborn

Etiology:

A. UTEROPLACENTAL INSUFFICIENCY (80%)
   = injury during period of cell hypertrophy resulting in decreased cell size with features of intrauterine starvation + protective cardiac output redistribution reflex
   - absence of body fat
   - diminished liver and muscle glycogen

   1. Maternal causes
      √ asymmetric IUGR / symmetric IUGR (in severe cases)

      (a) deficient supply of nutrients:
      cyanotic heart disease, severe anemia (in 10–25% of sickle cell anemia), maternal starvation, life in high altitudes, drugs (anticonvulsants, methotrexate, warfarin), alcohol abuse (dose related), illicit drugs (up to 50% with heroine addiction, 30% with cocaine abuse), uterine anomaly, multiple gestation (in 15–20%)

      (b) maternal vascular disease resulting in inadequate placental perfusion:
      nicotine-induced release of catecholamines, preconceptual diabetes, preeclampsia, chronic renal disease collagen vascular disease (SLE)

OB&GYN

(c) maternal dermographics:
maternal age (adolescence / advanced), nulliparous mother, small short habitus, racial influence (Asians)

2. Primary placental causes
Extensive placental infarctions, chronic partial separation (abruption), partial mole, Breus mole, chorioangioma, placenta previa, low implantation, placental metastases (breast, melanoma), placentitis (luetic, malaria)
Histo: reduction in placental villous surface area + in number of capillary vessels
√ asymmetric growth failure

B. PRIMARY FETAL CAUSES (20%)
= injury during the period of cell hyperplasia (= embryogenesis) producing profound reduction in cell number across all cell lines
√ symmetric IUGR (globally decreased intrinsic growth)
√ normal / increased amniotic fluid volume

1. Chromosomal abnormalities (in 2–6%):
triploidy, tetraploidy, trisomy 13 + 18 + 21, aneuploidy (Turner syndrome), partial deletion (4-p, 5-p [cri du chat], 13-q), partial trisomy (4-p, 18-p, 10-q, 18-q), unbalanced translocation (chromosomes 4 + 15), balanced translocation (chromosomes 5 + 11)
2. Structural anomalies: congenital heart disease, genitourinary anomalies, CNS anomalies, dwarfism
3. Viral infection: rubella (in 40–60%), CMV, varicella (in 40%)

◊ All fetuses with IUGR need to have a detailed and often repeated search for structural anomalies!

• fundal height as screening test (37–60% true positive, 40–55% false negative; 26–60% false positive)

Sequence of events in fetal hypoxia:
nonreactive CST > absence of fetal breathing > nonreactive NST > diminished fetal movements > absence of fetal movements > absence of fetal tone

PHENOTYPES

1. **Pure symmetric IUGR** = decreased–cell-number IUGR = early-insult IUGR = low-profile IUGR
= proportionate reduction of all fetal measurements due to
(a) intrinsic alteration in growth potential (usually due to chromosomal abnormalities)
(b) severe nutritional deprivation overwhelming protective brain-sparing mechanism occurring prior to 26 weeks MA + persisting until delivery
√ proportionate decrease in HC and AC maintaining normal HC:AC ratios
√ estimated fetal weight <10th percentile for age by middle of 2nd trimester
2. **Mixed IUGR**
= onset of IUGR during period of mixed hyperplasia / hypertrophy with near normal inherent fetal growth potential but decreased size + impaired function of placenta
√ impaired fetal growth ± asymmetry
√ abnormal Doppler umbilical artery flow velocity (due to increased placental vascular resistance)
√ progressive oligohydramnios
3. **Asymmetric IUGR** = decreased–cell-size IUGR
= late-onset IUGR = late-flattening IUGR (75%)
= disproportionate reduction of fetal measurements due to uteroplacental insufficiency with preferential shunting of blood to fetal brain occurring after 26 weeks GA

◊ IUGR usually not detectable before 32–34 weeks GA (time of maximal fetal growth)!

Effective time for screening: 34 weeks MA
Routine surveillance: every 4 weeks beginning at 26 weeks MA

√ AC >2 SD below the mean for age = highly suspicious; AC >3 SD below mean for age = diagnostic (AC single most effective fetal parameter for detection of asymmetric IUGR)
√ high HC/AC and FL/AC ratios (head size + femur length less affected)
√ fetal weight percentile useful for follow-up
√ accelerated placental maturity
√ decreased amniotic fluid volume
√ elevated umbilical artery S/D ratio
◊ FL/AC ratio + umbilical artery S/D ratio are the only effective techniques to screen for IUGR on a single exam with late prenatal care in 3rd trimester!

DIAGNOSTIC ULTRASOUND METHODS

◊ An accurate fix on fetal age dictates accuracy of diagnosis of IUGR (early US exam, clinical dates, early physical exam, pregnancy test)!
◊ Every effort needs to be made to determine the underlying cause for growth failure as it effects management + perinatal morbidity and mortality!

1. Fetal morphometric indices
The three key parameters for diagnosing IUGR are
(1) low estimated fetal weight (EFW),
(2) low amniotic fluid volume (AFV),
(3) maternal hypertension (HBP)!

Sonographic criteria for IUGR	*PPV [%]*	*NPV [%]*
advanced placental grade	16	94
elevated FL/AC	18–20	92–93
abnormal UA waveform	17–37	
low total intrauterine volume	21–24	92–97
small BPD	21–44	92–98
slow BPD growth rate	35	97
low EFW	45	99
oligohydramnios	55	92
elevated HC/AC	62	98

(a) intrafetal proportions
√ elevated HC:AC ratio for dysmature IUGR (overall 36% sensitive, 90% specific, 67% PPV, 72% NPV; 93% sensitive in fetus >28 weeks MA with severe dysmature IUGR)

◊ Early-onset dysmature IUGR not detectable!
◊ May not be used in anomalous fetuses!
(b) rate of growth = growth velocity
√ HC, AC, FL measurements allow DDx between erroneous dates + normal small fetus + fetus with intrinsic abnormality
√ plot growth curves
◊ Minimum time interval of 2 weeks necessary!

2. Amniotic fluid volume
◊ Screening for decreased amniotic fluid is of value in the fetus with dysmature IUGR (60–84% sensitive, 79–100% accurate)!
√ normal amniotic fluid does not exclude IUGR
√ oligohydramnios means dysmature IUGR in a fetus with normal GU tract until proven otherwise (DDx: trisomy 13 + 18)
3. Fetal morphologic assessment + fat distribution
√ diminished thigh circumference
√ absent paraspinal fat pad (posterior neck)
√ reduced / absent malar fat pads
√ disproportionately small liver size
√ increased small bowel echogenicity (= absent omental fat)
4. Placental assessment
√ increased placental calcium deposition
5. Doppler blood flow velocities
a. Nonstress test (NST)
b. Contraction stress test (CST)
c. Umbilical artery waveform
◊ Not useful with unknown dates / for screening!
Physiology: S/D ratio increases with sampling site closer to fetus + increasing fetal heart rate; S/D ratio decreases with advancing gestational age
√ elevated systolic:diastolic ratio (S/D ratio >3.0 beyond 30–34 weeks GA) indicates an increase in vascular resistance within placental circulation
√ absent diastolic flow = 50–90% mortality rate
√ reverse diastolic flow = impending fetal collapse
d. Uterine artery waveform (measured at its point of overlap with external iliac artery)
√ S/D ratio >2.6 after 26 weeks GA
√ persistence of early diastolic notch
e. Fetal aortic flow volume (no proven usefulness)
√ decrease in blood flow to <185–246 mL/kg/min
6. Biophysical profile
Accuracy: false-negative fetal death rate of 0.645/1000 fetuses within 1 week the last normal BPP; 33% sensitivity, 17% positive predictive value
7. Invasive fetal testing: fetal blood analysis for karyotyping, hypoxemia, hypercapnia, acidemia, hypoglycemia, hypertriglyceridemia

Cx: increased risk for perinatal asphyxia, meconium aspiration, electrolyte imbalance from metabolic acidosis, polycythemia

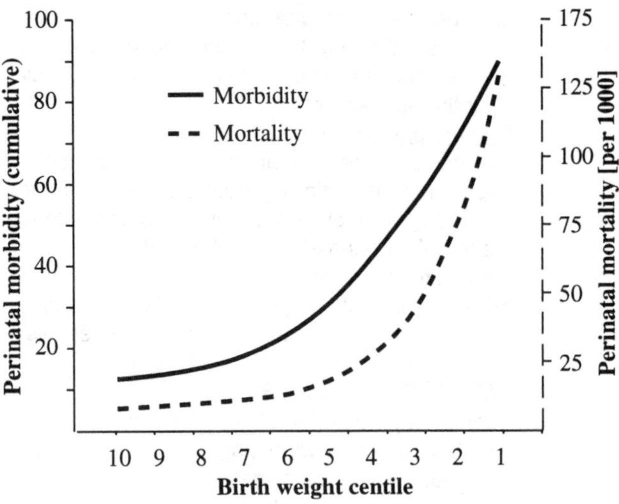

Neonatal Cx: pulmonary hemorrhage + vasoconstriction, persistent fetal circulation, intracranial hemorrhage, bowel ischemia, necrotizing enterocolitis, acute renal failure

Prognosis: 6–8-fold increase in risk for intrapartum death + neonatal death
◊ 20% of all stillborn fetuses are growth retarded!

DDx of fetus small for gestational age (SGA):
Definition: generic clinical term describing a group of perinates at/below the 10th percentile for gestational age without reference to etiology
(1) Small normal fetus = constitutionally small fetus (80–85%)
◊ No indication for surveillance / intervention!
(2) Small abnormal fetus = primary growth failure associated with karyotype anomaly / fetal infection (5–10%)
◊ Active intervention is of no benefit!
(3) Dysmature fetus = growth failure as a result of compromised placental function (10–15%)
◊ Intensive management is likely of benefit!

KRUKENBERG TUMOR

= ovarian tumors from GI tract cancer (colon:stomach = 2:1) now including pancreatic + biliary primaries; 2% of females with gastric cancer develop Krukenberg tumor
◊ Krukenberg tumors antedate the discovery of the primary lesion in up to 20%!
Age: any age, most common in 5th–6th decade
√ in 80% bilateral hypo- / hyperechoic mass ± cystic degeneration

LIMB-BODY WALL COMPLEX

Prevalence: 1:10,000 live births
Cause: ? severe form of amniotic band syndrome; ? early vascular disruption; ? embryonic dysplasia due to malformation of ectodermal placodes

A. EXTERNAL DEFECTS
  1. Ventral wall anomaly
     √ large eccentric defect
     Location: L:R = 3:1 (DDx: gastroschisis)
  2 Craniofacial defects: anencephaly, cephalocele, facial cleft
  3. Limb reductions
  4. Spinal defects: dysraphism, scoliosis

B. INTERNAL DEFECTS (in 95%)
  1. Cardiac defects
  2. Diaphragmatic absence
  3. Bowel atresia
  4. Renal abnormalities: agenesis, hydronephrosis, dysplasia

√ persistence of extraembryonic coelom (= separation of amnion + chorion)
Prognosis: invariably fatal shortly after birth

MACROSOMIA

= FETAL GROWTH ACCELERATION
= fetus large for gestational age (LGA) with EFW >90th percentile for age / >4,000 g at term
√ AC >3 SD above the mean for age (most reliable measurement)
√ estimated fetal weight (EFW) including fetal head, abdomen, femur length >90th percentile (± 15% accuracy)
√ low FL:AC ratio
√ low HC:AC ratio
√ enlarged thigh circumference
√ low FL:thigh circumference ratio
Risk: shoulder dystocia, prolonged labor, meconium spiration

MASSIVE OVARIAN EDEMA

= tumorlike condition with marked enlargement of one / (occasionally) both ovaries due to accumulation of edema fluid in stroma
Age: 6–33 (average 21) years
Cause:
  (1) partial / intermittent torsion (obstruction to ovarian lymphatic + venous drainage)
  (2) ovarian stromal proliferation with enlargement of ovary susceptible to torsion
Histo: edematous ovarian stroma + extensive fibromatosis surrounding primordial follicles, luteinized cells
- acute / intermittent lower abdominal pain for month
- masculinization (in chronic phase)

√ solid / multicystic adnexal mass
√ ovarian diameter of 5–40 (mean 11.5) cm
Rx: oophorectomy / salpingo-oophorectomy / wedge resection with ovarian suspension

MAYER-ROKITANSKY-KÜSTER-HAUSER SYNDROME

(1) vaginal agenesis / hypoplasia of proximal + middle segments
(2) intact ovaries + fallopian tubes
(3) variable anomalies of uterus (agenesis / hypoplasia), urinary tract (renal agenesis, pelvic kidney in 40%), skeletal system

Frequency: 1:4,000–1:5,000
Cause: lack of müllerian development
- normal external genitalia
- shallow distal vaginal pouch (derived from urogenital sinus)
- amenorrhea
- cyclic pelvic pain (secondary to functioning endometrium within rudimentary uterine tissue)

Rx: neovaginoplasty

MUCINOUS OVARIAN TUMOR

Incidence: 20% of all ovarian tumors; 2nd most common benign epithelial neoplasm of ovary (after serous ovarian adenoma)
Histo: single layer of nonciliated tall columnar epithelium with clear cytoplasm of high mucin content (similar to endocervix + intestinal epithelium) 80% benign, 10% borderline, 10% malignant
Age: middle adult life, rare before puberty + after menopause
Cx: rupture may lead to pseudomyxoma peritonei

A. MUCINOUS CYSTADENOMA
   Prevalence: 20% of all benign ovarian neoplasms
   Age: 3rd–5th decade of life
   √ multilocular cyst with numerous thin septa
   √ cysts frequently have high protein content:
     √ low-level echoes in cysts
     √ high attenuation on CT
     √ hyperintense on T1WI
   √ usually unilateral, bilateral in 5%

B. MUCINOUS CYSTADENOCARCINOMA
   difficult to differentiate from benign variety
   √ solid tissue areas: thick septa + other soft-tissue elements within septated cyst
   √ usually unilateral, bilateral in 20%
   √ capsular infiltration with loss of definition + fixation
   Cx: pseudomyxoma peritonei

NUCHAL CORD

= umbilical cord encircling fetal neck: single loop > two loops (2–3%) > 3 or more loops (<1%)
Incidence: 25% of pregnancies; frequently transient
Associated with: increased cord length, small fetus, vertex presentation, polyhydramnios
- generally not of clinical significance: no difference in 5-minute Apgar score, no increase in infant mortality

√ two adjacent cross sections of cord on longitudinal view of neck (diagnosis facilitated by color Doppler flow)
√ indentation of skin by nuchal cord suggests tight loop

Risk: signs of fetal distress (fetal bradycardia, variable decelerations, depressed 1-minute Apgar score)

OB management:
1. Assess fetal well-being (biophysical profile biweekly, NST, fetal growth)
2. Vaginal delivery permissible if without evidence of fetal compromise
3. Intervention only for signs of fetal distress

OMPHALOCELE

= midline defect of anterior abdominal wall due to failure to form the umbilical ring during 3rd to 4th week of gestation with herniation of intraabdominal contents into base of umbilical cord

Prevalence: 1:4,000 to 1:5,500 pregnancies

Cause:
- (a) migration failure of lateral mesodermal body folds
  - √ omphalocele contains liver
- (b) persistence of primitive body stalk beyond 12th week MA
  - √ omphalocele contains primarily bowel

Age: earliest detection at 12 weeks menstrual age

High incidence of ASSOCIATED ANOMALIES (45–88%):
1. Chromosomal (10–30–58%): trisomy 13, 18, 21, Turner syndrome (13% with liver in omphalocele, 77% with bowel in omphalocele), triploidy
2. Genitourinary (40%): bladder exstrophy
   ◊ OEIS complex = omphalocele + bladder exstrophy + imperforate anus + spinal anomalies
3. Cardiac (16–30–47%): VSD, ASD, tetralogy of Fallot, ectopia cordis in pentalogy of Cantrell, DORV
4. Neural tube defects (4–39%): holoprosencephaly, encephalocele, cerebellar hypoplasia
5. IUGR (20%)
6. Beckwith-Wiedemann syndrome (5–10%)
7. GI tract:
   intestinal atresia (vascular compromise); malrotation; abnormal fixation of liver, esophageal atresia, facial cleft, diaphragmatic hernia
8. Limb-body wall deficiency; cystic hygroma

- • MS-AFP ≥2.5 in 40–70%
- √ midline central defect at base of umbilical cord insertion
  - √ defect over entire ventral abdominal wall (mean size 2.5–5 cm)
  - √ widened cord where it joins the skin of the abdomen
- √ cord inserting at apex of defect
- √ herniation of abdominal viscera at base of umbilical cord: liver (27%) ± stomach ± bowel
- √ covering amnioperitoneal membrane (inner layer = peritoneum; outer layer = amnion); may rupture in exceedingly rare cases
- √ hypoechoic loose mesenchymal tissue (= Wharton jelly) between layers of membrane
- √ ascites within herniated sac
- √ polyhydramnios (occasionally oligohydramnios)

mnemonic: "OMPHALOCele"
- **O**ther anomalies (common)
- **M**embrane surrounding viscera
- **P**erfectly midline
- **He**art anomalies
- **A**scites
- **L**iver commonly herniated
- **O** for "zero" bowel complications
- **C**hromosomal abnormalities (common)

Cx: (1) Infection, inanition
(2) Immaturity (23%)
(3) Rupture of hernial sac
(4) Intestinal obstruction

Mortality rate: 10% mortality if isolated abnormality; 80% with one / more concurrent malformations; nearly 100% with chromosomal + cardiovascular abnormalities

DDx: (1) Gastroschisis (usually right-sided defect)
(2) Limb-body wall complex (usually left-sided defect)

PSEUDO-OMPHALOCELE
- (1) Deformation of fetal abdomen by transducer pressure coupled with an oblique scan orientation may give the appearance of an omphalocele
  - √ obtuse angle between pseudomass and fetal abdominal wall
- (2) Physiologic herniation of midgut into umbilical cord between 8th and 12th week of gestation
  - √ herniated sac never contains liver
  - √ herniated sac usually <7 mm
  - √ disappears by 12th week GA

OMPHALOMESENTERIC DUCT CYST

Etiology: persistence + dilatation of a segment of the omphalomesenteric / vitelline duct joining the embryonic midgut and the primary yolk sac, which is formed during the 3rd week and closed by the 16th week of gestation

Histo: cyst lined by columnar mucin-secreting gastrointestinal epithelium

M:F = 3:5

Location: usually in close proximity to fetus

- √ umbilical cord cyst up to 6 cm in diameter
- √ beneath amniotic surface of cord (= eccentric)

Cx: (1) Compression of umbilical vessels by expanding cyst
(2) Erosion of umbilical vein from acid-producing gastric mucosal lining

DDx: allantoic cyst, umbilical cord hematoma

OVARIAN CANCER

8th leading cause of cancer in women; 3rd most common gynecologic malignancy = 25% of all gynecologic malignancies; leading cause of death of all female cancers (60%); 5th leading cause of cancer deaths in women; accounts for 50% of cancer deaths of female genital tract

Etiology: ovarian surface epithelium proliferates temporarily to repair defect after rupture of ovum which may result in an "inclusion body" / "cystoma"; an error in DNA replication within inclusion body may occur resulting in inactivation / loss of a tumor-suppressor gene

Incidence: affects 1:2000 women; 50 cases per year per 100,000 women (33 cases per year per 100,000 women > age 50); 26,700 new cases + 14,500 deaths in 1996

Age: increasing with age; peaking at 55–59 years (80% of cases in women >50 years)

Histo:

1. Epithelial tumors (60–70%)
   - (a) serous tumor resembling ciliated columnar cells of the fallopian tubes (50%)
   - (b) endometrioid tumor similar to endometrial adenocarcinoma (15–30%)
   - (c) mucinous tumor similar to endocervical canal epithelium (15%)
   - (d) clear cell carcinoma = mesonephroid tumor (5%)
   - (e) Brenner tumor (2.5%)
   - (f) undifferentiated tumor (<5%)
2. Germ cell tumors (15–30%)
   Most common malignant ovarian neoplasm in girls + young women
   Age: 4–27 years
   - (a) mature teratoma (10%) = the only benign variety
   - (b) dysgerminoma (1.9%)
   - (c) immature teratoma (1.3%)
   - (d) endodermal sinus tumor (1%)
   - (e) malignant mixed germ cell tumor (0.7%)
   - (f) choriocarcinoma (0.1%)
   - (g) embryonal carcinoma (0.1%)
3. Metastases (5–10%)
4. Stromal tumors (5%)

Size versus risk of malignancy:

<5 cm	in	3%
5–10 cm	in	10%
>10 cm	in	65%

Increased risk:
nulliparity, early menarche, late menopause, Caucasian race, higher socioeconomic group, positive family history for ovarian cancer (risk factor of 3 with one close relative, risk factor of 30 with two close relatives affected with ovarian cancer), history of breast cancer (risk factor of 2) / early colorectal cancer (risk factor of 3.5)
◊ Lifetime risk of ovarian cancer = 1:70 women (1.4%)!

Decreased risk:
pregnancy, use of oral contraceptives, breast-feeding

Stage (FIGO system) based on staging laparotomy

- I limited to ovary
  - I a limited to one ovary
  - I b limited to both ovaries
  - I c + positive peritoneal lavage / ascites
- II limited to pelvis
  - II a involvement of uterus / fallopian tubes
  - II b extension to other pelvic tissues
  - II c + positive peritoneal lavage / ascites
- III limited to abdomen = intraabdominal extension outside pelvis / retroperitoneal nodes / extension to small bowel / omentum
- IV hematogenous disease (liver parenchyma) / spread beyond abdomen

◊ 50–75% of patients have stage III / IV disease at time of diagnosis!

Spread:

(1) direct extension through subperitoneal space (sigmoid mesocolon on left, cecum + distal ileum on right)
(2) exfoliation of tumor cells into peritoneal space (often microscopic) with frequent seeding to:
- pouch of Douglas
- termination of small bowel mesentery
- superior aspect of sigmoid
- right paracolic gutter
- omentum

(3) lymphatic spread

- occasional pelvo-abdominal pain
- constipation, urinary frequency
- early satiety
- ascites
- paraneoplastic hypercalcemia
- elevated CA-125 levels (= high-molecular-weight glycoprotein with normal level of <35 units/mL):
  — >35 units/mL in 29% of stage I disease
  — >65 units/mL in 21% of stage I disease
  ◊ CA-125 levels elevated in 80% of ovarian cancers (60% of mucinous + 20% of nonmucinous tumors)!
  ◊ CA-125 levels elevated in 30% of benign processes (fibroid, pregnancy, menstruation, endometriosis, PID, benign ovarian tumors, cirrhosis)!

US:

◊ Screening finds adnexal cysts in 1–15% of postmenopausal women; only 3% of ovarian cysts <5 cm are malignant!
√ solid / partly solid consistency + papillae
√ postmenopausal ovarian volume >9 cm^3
√ low-resistance Doppler waveform (due to lack of muscular layer of arterial wall in neoplasms) with much overlap between benign + malignant tumors: RI <0.40, PI <1.0
Prediction: gray-scale US = 99% NPV; presence of internal flow = 49% PPV; abnormal PI/RI = 37–47% PPV
√ presence of color flow (malignant vs. benign tumors = 93% vs. 35%) usually within thick wall, septa, papillary projections, solid inhomogeneous areas
√ omental / peritoneal masses ("omental cake")
√ pseudomyxoma peritonei (with tumor rupture)
√ liver metastases
√ ascites

BE:

√ serosal spiculation / tethering
√ annular constriction / complete obstruction

Rx:

stage I: total abdominal hysterectomy (TAH) + bilateral salpingo-oophorectomy (BSO) ± melphalan / intraperitoneal P-32 stage >I: TAH/BSO + surgical cytoreduction (debulking) + 6 cycles of chemotherapy (cyclophosphamide + cisplatin)

Prognosis (without change in past 60 years):
20–40% overall 5-year survival rate, 5–8% for stage IV, 14–30% for stage III, 50% for stage II, 80–90% for stage I

DDx: tubo-ovarian abscess, dermoid cyst, endometrioma

OVARIAN FIBROMA /FIBROTHECOMA

Incidence: 3–4% of all ovarian tumors; bilateral in <10%
Age: usually menopausal / postmenopausal
Histo: mesenchymal tumor consisting of intersecting bundles of collagen-producing spindle cells; fibrothecomas also have a small population of theca cells that contain intracellular lipids

- usually asymptomatic
- Meigs syndrome (in only 1%)

√ ascites (in 10–15% of tumors >10 cm)
√ ± cystic degeneration and edema in larger lesions

US:
√ hypoechoic mass with marked sound attenuation

MR:
√ low signal intensity on T1WI + T2WI (less than or equal to myometrium)

CT:
√ well-defined solid homogeneous / slightly heterogeneous mass

DDx: pedunculated uterine leiomyoma

OVARIAN HYPERSTIMULATION SYNDROME

Incidence: severe OHSS in 1.5–6% under Perganol therapy

Etiology:
(1) Induced by HCG therapy with human menopausal gonadotropin (Perganol), occasionally with clomiphene (Clomid)
(2) Hydatidiform mole
(3) Chorioepithelioma
(4) Multiple pregnancies

Path: enlarged ovaries with multiple follicular cysts, corpora lutea, edematous stroma (fluid shift secondary to increased capillary permeability)

- abdominal pain (100%) + distension (100%)
- nausea (100%), vomiting (36%)
- acute abdomen (17%)
- dyspnea (16%)
- thrombophlebitis (11%)
- marked hemoconcentration
- fainting (11%)
- blurred vision (5%)
- anasarca (5%)
- hydrothorax
- enhanced fertility

√ ovary >5 cm in longest dimension containing large geometrically packed follicles
√ ovarian cyst >10 cm (100%): usually disappear after 20–40 days
√ ascites (33%)
√ pleural effusion (5%)
√ hydroureter (11%)

Cx: (related to volume depletion)
(1) Hypovolemia + hemoconcentration
(2) Oliguria, electrolyte imbalance, azotemia
(3) Death from intraabdominal hemorrhage / thromboembolic event

OVARIAN VEIN THROMBOSIS

Etiology:
(1) Bacterial seeding from puerperal endometritis with secondary thrombosis (pregnancy + puerperium are hypercoagulable states)
= **puerperal ovarian vein thrombophlebitis**
(2) Pelvic inflammatory disease
(3) Gynecologic surgery
(4) Malignant tumors
(5) Chemotherapy

Incidence: 1:600–1:2,000 deliveries

- presents on 2nd / 3rd postpartum day
- lower abdominal / flank pain (>90%)
- palpable ropelike tender abdominal mass (50%)
- fever if diagnosis delayed

Location: right ovarian vein (80%), bilateral (14%), left ovarian vein (6%)

CT:
√ tubular structure in location of ovarian vein with low-density center + peripheral enhancement

Cx: IVC thrombosis; pulmonary embolism (25%); septicemia; metastatic abscess formation
Mortality: 5%

Rx: IV antibiotics + heparin; ligation of involved vessel at most proximal point of thrombosis after failure to improve after 3–5 days

DDx: appendicitis, broad-ligament phlegmon / hematoma, torsion of ovarian cyst, urolithiasis, pyelonephritis, degenerated pedunculated leiomyoma, pelvic cellulitis, pelvic / abdominal abscess

PARAOVARIAN CYST

= vestigial remnant of Wolffian duct in mesosalpinx

Frequency: 10% of all pelvic masses

Embryology:
Wolffian body (= mesonephros) consists of
(a) mesonephric duct (= Wolffian duct)
in female degenerates into vestigial structures of epithelial-lined cysts (= canals / duct of Gartner)
Location: at lateral edge of uterus and vagina extending from broad ligament to vestibule of vagina
(b) mesonephric tubules
in female degenerates into vestigial structures of
1. EPOÖPHORON (at lateral part of Fallopian tube)
2. PAROÖPHORON: (at medial part of Fallopian tube)
Location: between the tube and hilum of the ovary within the two peritoneal layers of broad ligament

1. **Gartner duct cyst**: inclusion cyst; lateral to vagina + uterine wall

OB&GYN

2. **Paroöphoron**: medial location between tube + hilum of ovary
3. **Epoöphoron**: lateral location between tube + hilum of ovary
4. **Hydatids of Morgagni** (= appendices vesiculosae): most lateral + outer end of Gartner duct
   √ ≥1 vesicle(s) attached to fringes of tube + filled with clear serous fluid

√ thin-walled unilocular cyst, up to 18 cm in diameter
√ may arise out of pelvis (if pedunculated + mobile)
√ ± low-level internal echoes (from hemorrhage)
DDx: functional cyst, cystic teratoma, benign epithelial neoplasm

PELVIC INFLAMMATORY DISEASE

= acute clinical syndrome associated with ascending spread of microorganisms ("canalicular spread") from vagina / cervix to uterus, fallopian tubes, and adjacent pelvic structures, not related to surgery / pregnancy

Incidence: 10% of women in reproductive age (17% in Blacks); 1 million American women/year

Risk factors: early age at sexual debut, multiple sexual partners, history of sexual transmitted disease, douching

Predisposed: formerly married > married > never married; intrauterine contraceptive device (1.5–4-fold increase in risk)

Etiology: (a) bilateral: venereal disease, IUD, S/P abortion
(b) unilateral = nongynecologic: rupture of appendix, diverticulum, S/P pelvic surgery

Organisms:
(1) Chlamydia trachomatis + Neisseria gonorrhea (>50% with high prevalence of coinfection) damage protective barrier of endocervical canal with spread to tubes (30–50%) producing fibrosis + adhesions
(2) Aerobes: Streptococcus, Escherichia coli, Haemophilus influenzae
(3) Anaerobes: Bacteroides, Peptostreptococcus, Peptococcus
(4) Mycobacterium tuberculosis (hematogenous)
(5) Actinomycosis in IUD users
(6) Herpesvirus hominis type 2, Mycoplasma

May be associated with: **Fitz-Hugh-Curtis syndrome** (= gonorrheic perihepatitis)

- usually bilateral lower abdominal pain (due to peritoneal irritation)
- abnormal vaginal discharge / uterine bleeding
- dysuria, dyspareunia, nausea, vomiting
- fever, leukocytosis, elevated ESR
- lower abdominal + adnexal + cervical motion tenderness

1. **Endometritis**
   √ endometrial prominence
   √ small amount of fluid within uterine lumen
   √ gas reflection within uterine cavity (most specific)
   √ pain over uterus
2. **Salpingitis**
   not depicted by imaging techniques
   - often beginning during / immediately after menstruation (due to less effective barrier of mucus at cervix)

   Salpingitis isthmica nodosa
   unknown etiology, commonly associated with pelvic inflammatory disease, infertility, ectopic pregnancy
   - nodular thickening of isthmic portion of tube
   √ tubal irregularity + multiple diverticula / tubal obstruction on HSG
3. **Hydro- / pyosalpinx**
   = continued secretion of tubal epithelium into lumen of a fallopian tube obstructed at two sites
   Cause: infection, endometriosis, adhesions, microtubal surgery
   Location: ampullary / infundibular portion of tube
   √ undulating / folded tubular structure in extraovarian location filled with sterile fluid / debris / pus
   √ short linear echoes protruding into lumen (= tall ramified mucosal folds)
   √ longitudinal folds in ampullary portion
   HSG:
   √ absence of peritoneal spill
   Cx: tubal torsion
   DDx: dilated uterine / ovarian vein, developing follicle
4. **Tubo-ovarian abscess**
   Cause: sexually transmitted disease, IUD (20%), diverticulitis, appendicitis, pelvic surgery, gynecologic malignancy
   Organism: anaerobic bacteria become dominant
   Location: usually in posterior cul-de-sac extending bilaterally
   √ multilocular complex mass often with debris, septations, irregular thick wall
   √ may contain fluid-fluid levels or gas

Dx: clinically, laparoscope
◊ Imaging employed only to differentiate between medical + surgical condition!

Cx: 1. Infertility due to tubal occlusion (25%): 8% after single episode, 20% after 2 episodes, 40% after ≥3 episodes of PID
2. Ectopic pregnancy (6 x as frequent)
3. Chronic pelvic pain (from pelvic adhesions)

DDx: acute appendicitis, endometriosis, hematoma of corpus luteum, ectopic pregnancy, paraovarian cyst

PENA-SHOKEIR PHENOTYPE

= autosomal recessive syndrome (45% sporadic, 55% familial) characterized by fetal akinesia

Cause: decreased / absent fetal motion secondary to abnormalities of fetal muscle / nerves / connective tissue ("fetal akinesia deformation sequence")

Time of first detection: 16–18 weeks MA

@ Spine: scoliosis, kyphosis, lordosis
@ Thorax: pulmonary hypoplasia, cardiac anomalies
@ Kidney: renal dysplasia
@ Limbs: limited movement, knee + hip ankylosis (arthrogryposis), abnormal shape + position, demineralization, camptodactyly, clubfeet

√ craniofacial anomalies
√ polyhydramnios
√ IUGR
√ short umbilical cord
Prognosis: still birth
DDx: multiple pterygium syndrome, Neu-Laxova syndrome, restrictive dermopathy, Larsen syndrome, trisomies 13 + 18

PENTALOGY OF CANTRELL

= sporadic very rare abnormality
Cause: failure of lateral body folds to fuse in the thoracic region with variable extension inferiorly

1. Omphalocele + defect of lower sternum
2. Ectopia cordis
3. Deficiency of anterior diaphragm (herniation of intraabdominal organs into thoracic cavity is rare)
4. Deficiency of diaphragmatic pericardium
5. Cardiovascular malformation: atrioventricular septal defect (50%), VSD (18%), tetralogy of Fallot (11%)

Associated with: trisomies
√ exteriorization of heart
Prognosis: death within a few days after birth

PERITONEAL INCLUSION CYST

= PERITONEAL PSEUDOCYST = ENTRAPPED OVARIAN CYST
Cause: from previous abdominal surgery (time delay of 6 months to 20 years) / trauma / pelvic inflammatory disease / endometriosis
Pathogenesis: extensive pelvic adhesions result in impaired peritoneal clearing of fluid normally produced by an active ovary
Path: cyst adherent to surface of ovary
Histo: cyst lined by hyperplastic mesothelial cells + fibroglandular tissue with chronic inflammation
√ single / multiloculated cyst contiguous with ovary
Cx: infertility
Rx: surgery (30–50% risk of recurrence)
DDx: paraovarian cyst (ovoid cyst outside ovary), hydrosalpinx (visible folds, located outside ovary), ovarian neoplasm, lymphangioma

PLACENTA ACCRETA

= underdeveloped decidualization with chorionic villi growing into myometrium
Incidence: 1:2,500–7,000 deliveries; in 5% of placenta previa patients
Risk of placenta accreta vs. cesarean section:
in 10% of placenta previa; in 24% of placenta previa + 1 cesarean section; in 48% of placenta previa + 2 cesarean sections; in 67% of placenta previa + 4 cesarean sections
Predisposed: areas of uterine scarring with deficient decidua: previous dilatation + curettage, endometritis, submucous leiomyoma, Asherman syndrome, manual removal of placenta, adenomyosis, increasing parity
Associated with: placenta previa (20%)
Types:

1. PLACENTA ACCRETA = chorionic villi in direct contact with myometrium
2. PLACENTA INCRETA = villi invade myometrium
3. PLACENTA PERCRETA = villi penetrate through uterine serosa

US (78% sensitive, 94% specific):
√ thinning to <1 mm / absence of hypoechoic myometrial zone between placenta + echodense uterine serosa / posterior bladder wall [retroplacental hypoechoic zone of decidua + myometrium + dilated periuterine venous channels measures 9.5 mm thick >18 weeks GA)
√ thinning / irregularity / focal disruption of linear hyperechoic boundary echo (= uterine serosa-bladder wall interface)
√ focal masslike elevations / extensions of echogenic placental tissue beyond uterine serosa
√ >6 irregular intraplacental lacunae (= vascular spaces)
Cx:
(1) Retention of placental tissue
(2) Life-threatening hemorrhage in 3rd stage of labor necessitating emergent hysterectomy
(3) Persistent postpartum bleeding
(4) Maternal death

PLACENTA EXTRACHORIALIS

= chorionic plate smaller than basal plate; ie, the transition of membranous to villous chorion occurs at a distance from the placental edge that is smaller than the basal plate radius

1. CIRCUMMARGINATE PLACENTA
   Incidence: up to 20% of placentas
   • No clinical significance
   √ placental margin not deformed
2. CIRCUMVALLATE PLACENTA
   = attachment of fetal membranes form a folded thickened ring with underlying fibrin + often hemorrhage
   Incidence: 1–2% of pregnancies
   Cx: premature labor, threatened abortion, increased perinatal mortality, marginal hemorrhage

PLACENTAL ABRUPTION

= ABRUPTIO PLACENTAE
= premature separation of placenta from the myometrium secondary to maternal hemorrhage into decidua basalis between 20th week and birth
Incidence: 0.5–1.3% of gestations
Risk factors: *mnemonic:* "VASCULAR"
Vascular disease + hypertension
Abruption (previous history)
Smoking
Cocaine
Unknown (idiopathic)
Leiomyoma
Anomaly (fetal malformation)
Reckless driving (trauma)
Associated with: intraplacental infarction / hematoma

- vaginal bleeding (80%): bright red (acute), brownish-red (chronic)
- abdominal pain (50%)
- consumptive coagulopathy = DIC (30%)
- uterine rigidity (15%)

Site:
(a) marginal (most common site)
low-pressure bleed due to tears of marginal veins; associated with cigarette smoking
(b) retroplacental
high-pressure bleed due to rupture of spiral arteries; associated with hypertension + vascular disease

√ hyperechoic / isoechoic hematoma (initially difficult to distinguish from placenta)
√ hypoechoic / complex collection between uterine wall + placenta in 50% within 1 week (hematoma / placental infarction)
√ anechoic collection within 2 weeks
√ separation / rounding of placental margin
√ abnormally thick + heterogenous placenta (if blood isoechoic)
√ elevation of chorioamnionic membrane
(DDx: incomplete chorioamnionic fusion during 2nd trimester, blighted twin)

Prognosis:
(1) Only large hematomas (occupying >30–40% of the maternal surface) result in fetal hypoxia
(2) Abruptions with contained hematoma have worse prognosis
(3) Responsible for up to 15–25% of all perinatal deaths
(4) Normal term deliveries in 27% of hematomas detected >20 weeks GA
(5) Normal delivery in 80% of intrauterine hematomas detected <20 weeks GA

Cx: (1) Perinatal mortality (20–60%), up to 15–25% of all perinatal deaths
(2) Fetal distress / demise (15–27%)
(3) Premature labor + premature delivery (23–52%) (3-fold increase)
(4) Threatened abortion during first 20 weeks
(5) Infant small-for-gestational age (6–7%)

DDx: (1) Normal draining basal veins
(2) Normal uterine tissue
(3) Retroplacental myoma
(4) Focal contraction
(5) Chorioangioma
(6) Coexistent mole

PLACENTAL HEMORRHAGE

Location: subchorionic, subamniotic, marginal, retroplacental

Preplacental hemorrhage

= BREUS MOLE = SUBCHORIAL HEMORRHAGE
= variant of placental abruption with progressive slow intracotyledonary bleeding

Incidence: in 4% of all placental abruptions
Etiology: massive pooling + stasis due to extensive venous obstruction
Time of onset: 18 weeks MA

√ total loss of normal placental architecture
√ gelatinous character of placenta elicited by fetal movement / abdominal jostling
√ severe symmetric IUGR

Risk for fetal demise: 67% overall; 100% for hematomas >60 mL

Retroplacental hemorrhage

= accumulation of blood behind placenta, which may dissect into placenta / myometrium secondary to rupture of spiral arteries

Incidence: 4.5%; 16% of all placental abruptions

- external bleeding

√ thickened heterogeneous appearing placenta (hematoma of similar echogenicity as placenta)
√ rounded placental margins + intraplacental sonolucencies

Cx: (1) Precipitous delivery
(2) Coagulopathy
(3) Fetal demise (accounts for 15–25% of all perinatal deaths); risk for fetal demise with hematomas >60 mL: 6% before 20 weeks GA; 29% after 20 weeks GA

PLACENTA MEMBRANACEA

= presence of well-vascularized placental villi in the peripheral membranes

Cause: ? endometritis, endometrial hyperplasia, extensive vascularization of decidua capsularis, previous endometrial damage by curettage

- repeated vaginal bleeding extending into 2nd trimester + abortion at 20–30 weeks
- postpartum hemorrhage

√ thickened outline over whole gestational sac (0.2–3.0 cm)
√ may show additional distinct disk of placenta

PLACENTA PREVIA

= abnormally low implantation of ovum with the placenta covering all / part of internal cervical os

Incidence: 0.5% of all deliveries; in 7–11% of women with 2nd + 3rd trimester vaginal bleeding; in 0.26% with unscarred uterus

Risk for placenta previa vs. cesarean section:
0.65% after 1 section, 1.8% after 2 sections, 3% after 3 sections, 10% after 4 sections

Cause: defective decidual vascularization in areas of endometrial scarring causing compensatory placental thinning; placenta occupies a greater surface of the uterus with increased probability for encroachment upon internal os

Predisposed:
(1) Previous uterine incision (cesarean section, myomectomy)
(2) Older women
(3) Multiparous women

Types on clinical examination:
1. Central / total previa (1/3) = complete covering of internal os
2. Partial previa = internal os partially covered by placenta
3. Low-lying placenta = low placental edge without extension over internal os; palpable by examining finger

- painless vaginal bleeding in 93% (usually 3rd trimester / as early as 20 weeks)

◊ 3–5% of all pregnancies are complicated by 3rd trimester bleeding; of these 7–11% are due to placenta previa!

US - FALSE POSITIVES (5–7%):
1. Placental "migration" / rotation
   = differential growth rates between lower uterine segment + placenta
   ◊ 63–93% will have normal implantation at term!
   — conversion to normal position: anterior wall > posterior wall of uterus
   — NO conversion if placenta attaches to both posterior + anterior walls
2. Overfilled urinary bladder
   bladder-induced compression leads to apposition of the lower anterior + posterior uterine walls (cervical length >3.5–4 cm) simulating a placenta previa
3. Focal myometrial contraction (myometrial thickness >1.5 cm) in the region of the lower uterine segment
   mnemonic: "ABCD and F"
   Abruption (may mimic placenta previa)
   Bladder (must be empty)
   Contraction (may have to wait 15–20 minutes)
   Dates (be wary in 1st half of pregnancy)
   Fibroid

US - FALSE NEGATIVES (2%):
1. Obscuring fetal head
   remedied by Trendelenburg position / gentle upward traction on fetal head
2. Lateral position of placenta previa; remedied by obtaining oblique scans
3. Blood in region of internal os mistaken for amniotic fluid

Cx: (secondary to premature detachment of placenta from lower uterine segment)
(1) Maternal hemorrhage (blood from intervillous space)
(2) Premature delivery
(3) IUGR
(4) Perinatal death (5%)

Rx: precludes vaginal delivery + pelvic examination

PLACENTAL SITE TROPHOBLASTIC DISEASE

= very rare neoplasm (? type of choriocarcinoma)
Path: microscopic tumor / diffuse nodular replacement of myometrium
Histo: proliferation of predominantly intermediate trophoblasts but no syncytio- or cytotrophoblasts

- abnormal bleeding / amenorrhea
- low β-HCG levels (due to lack of syncytiotrophoblastic proliferation)

√ cystic / solid lesions ± central component
√ myometrium usually invaded
Prognosis: benign / highly malignant course
Rx: hysterectomy

POSTMATURITY SYNDROME

= inability of aging placenta to support demands of fetus
Incidence: in 15% of all postterm gravidas
- meconium-stained amniotic fluid

√ grade 3 placenta (in 85%), grade 2 (in 15%), grade 1 (in 0%)
√ decreased subcutaneous fat + wrinkling of skin
√ long fingernails
√ decreased vernix
Cx: meconium aspiration, perinatal asphyxia, thermal instability

Postterm fetus

= fetus undelivered by 42nd week MA
Incidence: 7 – 12% of all pregnancies
Risk of perinatal mortality:
2-fold at 43 weeks MA, 4- to 6-fold at 44 weeks MA

PREECLAMPSIA

= TOXEMIA OF PREGNANCY
Incidence: 5% of pregnancies, typically during 3rd trimester
Clinical triad:
- pregnancy-induced / -aggravated hypertension
- proteinuria
- peripheral edema + weight gain

Histo: blunted invasion of vasa media of spiral arterioles + focal vasculitis + atheromatous degeneration + fibrin deposits in intima of maternal placental arterioles
√ heavy calcium deposition (in areas of placental degeneration)
√ IUGR (6% with late-onset preeclampsia, 18% with early-onset preeclampsia)
Cx:
@ CNS
@ Liver: hematoma, infarction
@ Kidney

ECLAMPSIA
- convulsions + coma

PREMATURE RUPTURE OF MEMBRANES

= spontaneous rupture of chorioamnionic membranes before the onset of labor
Types:
(a) Preterm premature rupture of membranes (PPROM) <37 weeks GA
(b) Term premature rupture of membranes (TPROM) >37 weeks GA

Incidence: overall 2.1–17.1%; PPROM 0.9–4.4%; in 29% of all preterm deliveries; in 18% of all term deliveries
Risk of recurrence: 21% of women with PPROM
Cause: ? infection of membranes
Cx:
(a) TPROM:
— >24 hours may result in intrapartum fever
— >72 hours may result in chorioamnionitis + stillbirth
(b) PPROM: respiratory distress syndrome (9–43%), neonatal sepsis (2–19%)

PRIMARY OVARIAN CHORIOCARCINOMA

= NONGESTATIONAL CHORIOCARCINOMA
Incidence: extremely rare; 50 cases in world literature
Age: <20 years
• elevated serum HCG
√ predominantly solid tumor with areas of hemorrhage + necrosis
DDx: metastasis to ovary from gestational choriocarcinoma (reproductive age)

SECKEL SYNDROME

= BIRD-HEADED DWARFISM
= rare autosomal recessive disorder (44 cases)
• proportionate postnatal short stature
• characteristic stance: slight flexion of hips and knees
• mental retardation
• simian crease
• cryptorchidism
@ Skull
√ severe microcephaly
√ receding forehead, large beaked nose, micrognathia
@ Skeleton
√ dislocation of radial head + hypoplasia of proximal end of radius
√ absence of phalangeal epiphysis
√ clinodactyly of 5th digit
√ gap between 1st and 2nd toe
√ hip dislocation
√ hypoplasia of proximal fibula
√ 11 pairs of ribs
OB-US:
√ severe IUGR
√ oligohydramnios
√ decreased bone length (femur, tibia, fibula)
√ decreased AC, HC

SEROUS OVARIAN TUMOR

Incidence: 30% of ovarian tumors
Histo: lined by tall columnar epithelial cells (like fallopian tubes), filled with serous fluid, psammoma bodies (= microscopic calcifications) in 30%;
60% benign, 15% borderline, 25% malignant
Age: 20–50 years (malignant variety later)

A. SEROUS CYSTADENOMA
second most common benign tumor of the ovary (after dermoid cyst); 20% of all benign ovarian neoplasms
√ uni- / multilocular thin-walled cyst up to 20 cm in diameter
√ only small amount of solid tissue: occasional septum / mural nodule
√ bilateral in 7–20–30%
B. SEROUS CYSTADENOCARCINOMA
= 60–80% of all ovarian carcinomas
√ cyst with large amount of solid tissue: papillomatous excrescences within cyst (= papillary serous carcinoma)
√ may have calcifications
√ bilateral in 50–70%
√ loss of capsular definition + tumor fixation
√ ascites secondary to peritoneal surface implantation
√ lymph node enlargement (periaortic, mediastinal, supraclavicular)

SERTOLI–LEYDIG CELL TUMOR OF OVARY

Origin: from hilar cells of ovary
Incidence: <0.5%
Age: any age; most common in 2nd–3rd decade
• androgenic
√ hypoechoic mass simulating fibroid
√ may have cystic / hemorrhagic degeneration

SINGLE UMBILICAL ARTERY

Etiology:
(1) Primary agenesis of one umbilical artery (usually first appears in 5th menstrual week)
(2) Secondary atrophy / atresia of one umbilical artery
(3) Persistence of original single allantoic artery of the body stalk
Incidence: 0.2–1% of singleton births; 5% in dizygotic twins; 2.5% in abortuses; increased incidence in trisomy D / E, diabetic mothers, White patients, spontaneous abortions

Associated with:
(a) Congenital anomalies (21%):
1. CHD (most frequent): VSD, conotruncal anomalies
2. Abdomen: ventral wall defect, diaphragmatic hernia
3. CNS: hydrocephalus, holoprosencephaly, spina bifida
4. GU: hydronephrosis, dysplastic kidney
5. Esophageal atresia, cystic hygroma, cleft lip
6. Polydactyly, syndactyly
(b) IUGR
(c) Premature delivery
(d) Perinatal mortality (20%): stillbirth (66%)
(e) Marginal (18%) / velamentous (9%) insertion of umbilical cord
(f) Chromosomal anomalies (67%): trisomy 18 > trisomy 13 > Turner syndrome > triploidy

Site: left artery slightly more often absent than right
√ axial view of cord shows 2 vessels
√ single umbilical artery nearly as large as umbilical vein (umbilical vein-to-umbilical artery ratio < 2)
√ incurvation of distal aorta toward common iliac artery on the side of patent umbilical artery
√ ipsilateral hypoplastic common iliac artery
√ absence of abdominal portion of umbilical artery on ipsilateral side of missing umbilical artery
√ color flow imaging permits earlier (15–16 weeks) + more confident diagnosis

Prognosis:
(1) 4-fold increase in perinatal mortality (14%) with concurrent major abnormality
(2) Isolated single umbilical artery does not affect clinical outcome

DDx:
(1) normal variant = two arteries at fetal end may fuse near placental end into single umbilical artery (umbilical arteries normally unite with allantoic artery near placental insertion)
(2) arterial convergence of 2 into 1 umbilical a.

STEIN-LEVENTHAL SYNDROME

= POLYCYSTIC OVARY SYNDROME

Incidence: 2.5% of all women

Etiology:
deficient aromatase activity (catalyst for conversion of androgen into estrogen) results in androgen excess; exaggerated pulsatile release of LH stimulates continued ovarian androgen secretion at the expense of estradiol; reduction of local estrogen impairs FSH activity; this results in accumulation of small- + medium-sized atretic follicles without final maturation into graafian follicles

Path: pearly white ovaries with multiple cysts below the capsule, which are lined by a hyperplastic theca interna layer showing pronounced luteinization; granulosa cells are absent / degenerating; corpora lutea are absent

Age: late 2nd decade

Associated with: Cushing syndrome, basophilic pituitary adenoma, postpill amenorrhea, virilizing ovarian / adrenal tumor

- reduced infertility / sterility
- mild facial / severe generalized hirsutism
- obesity
- secondary amenorrhea (most common cause)
- menstrual irregularities / oligomenorrhea
- cystic acne
- cephalic hair loss
- periodic abdominal discomfort
- elevated LH levels without LH surge + normal / decreased FSH = increased LH/FSH ratio
- elevated androstenedione / testosterone levels
- elevated estrone / estradiol

√ bilaterally enlarged ovaries >15 cm^3 (70%)
√ normal ovarian size (in 30%), polycystic ovaries have a volume of 6–30 cm^3
√ excessive number of developing follicles
(a) multiple (more than 5) small cysts of 5–8 mm in subcapsular location (40%)
(b) hypoechoic ovaries (25%)
(c) isoechoic ovaries (5%)

Cx: endometrial cancer <40 years of age (due to unopposed chronic estrogen stimulation)

DDx: ovaries in congenital adrenal hyperplasia, normal ovaries

Rx: (1) Ovulation induction with clomiphene (Clomid) / menotropins (Perganol)
(2) Wedge resection (transient effect only)

STUCK TWIN

= one twin with IUGR residing within an oligo- / anhydramniotic sac of a diamniotic twin pregnancy
√ amnion invisible secondary to close contact with fetal parts
√ fetus fixed relative to the uterine wall without change during shift in maternal position
√ diminished / absent active fetal motion
√ absence of intermingling of fetal parts between twins

Prognosis: fetal death in utero

SUCCENTURIATE LOBE OF PLACENTA

= ACCESSORY LOBE = separate mass of chorionic villi connected to main placenta by vessels within membrane

Cause: placental villi atrophy in area of inadequate blood supply + proliferate in two opposite directions (trophotropism) with fetal vessels remaining at the site of villous atrophy

Incidence: 0.14–3%

Cx: (1) Retained in utero with postpartum hemorrhage
(2) Placenta previa with intrapartum hemorrhage
(3) VASA PREVIA = succenturiate vessels traversing internal os, which may rupture resulting in fetal blood loss

SUBCHORIONIC HEMORRHAGE

= separation of chorionic membrane from decidua with accumulation of blood in subchorionic space (placental membranes are more easily stripped from myometrium than from placenta)

Incidence: 81% of all placental abruptions; in 91% before 20 weeks MA

- may lead to vaginal hemorrhage after dissection through decidua (18% of all causes of 1st-trimester bleeding)

√ detached placental margin from adjacent myometrium (60%)
√ hematoma contiguous with placental margin (100%)
√ predominant hemorrhage often separate from placenta, even on opposite side of placenta

Prognosis:
worsens with (1) increased maternal age (2) earlier gestational age (3) size of hematoma;
9% overall miscarriage rate; risk of fetal demise doubles once hematoma reaches 2/3 of circumference of chorion

TERATOMA OF NECK
= germ cell tumor of neck (oropharynx, tongue)
√ polyhydramnios in 30% (from esophageal obstruction)
√ complex mass in cervical region
Cx: airway obstruction
DDx: cystic hygroma, goiter, branchial cleft cyst, cervical meningocele, neuroblastoma of neck, hemangioma of neck

TERATOMA OF OVARY
= immature derivatives of all 3 germ cell layers
Incidence: rare
Age: childhood / adolescence
√ cystic / complex mass (most frequently)
√ usually large solid mass with internal echoes

THECA CELL TUMOR OF OVARY
= THECOMA
Incidence: 1–2% of all ovarian neoplasms
Age: >30 years (30%), postmenopausal (70%)
• estrogenic
√ hypoechoic mass with sound attenuation
√ unilateral

THECA LUTEIN CYST
= form of ovarian hyperstimulation
• associated with abnormally high levels of β-HCG secondary to
  (a) multiple gestations
  (b) gestational trophoblastic disease (in 40%)
  (c) fetal hydrops
  (d) pharmacologic stimulation with b-HCG
  (e) normal pregnancy (uncommon)
√ multiloculated cysts, often bilateral
√ ovaries several cm in size
√ involution within a few months after source of gonadotropin removed

TORSION OF OVARY
= result of rotation of ovary on its axis producing arterial, venous, and lymphatic stasis
Age: usually affects prepubertal girls, may occur prenatally, increased risk during pregnancy
Cause:
  (1) Enlarged ovary (large cyst / tumor, paraovarian cyst)
  (2) Hypermobility of adnexa (more frequent in younger children + during pregnancy), excessively long mesosalpinx, tubal spasm
• severe lower abdominal pain, nausea, vomiting, fever
• palpable mass in 50%
Location: R:L = 3:1
US:
  √ markedly enlarged hypo- / hyperechoic midline mass
  √ multiple peripheral cysts (= transudation of fluid into follicles) measuring 8–12 mm in diameter (64–74%)
  √ good sound transmission (vascular engorgement + stromal edema)
  √ free fluid in cul-de-sac (32%)
  √ absence of Doppler waveforms (not always reliable)
  √ ± complex mass (if secondary to cyst / tumor)
CT + MR:
  √ deviation of uterus to side of torsion
  √ engorgement of blood vessels on side of torsion
  √ small amount of ascites
  √ obliteration of fat planes around torsed ovary
  √ lack of enhancement
Prognosis: spontaneous detorsion is common (history of prior similar episodes)

TRIPLOIDY
= 69 chromosomes
Incidence: 1% of conceptions; 0.04% of 20-week fetuses
NO obvious pattern!
√ early severe asymmetric IUGR (MOST PROMINENT FEATURE); cephalocorporal disproportion
√ oligohydramnios
√ large hydropic placenta with scattered vesicular spaces (partial hydatidiform mole)
√ congenital heart disease: ASD, VSD
√ brain anomalies: hydrocephalus, holoprosencephaly, neural tube defect
√ cleft lip / palate
√ syndactyly of fingers
√ omphalocele
√ renal abnormalities
Prognosis: most ending in spontaneous abortion

TRISOMY 13
= PATAU SYNDROME
Incidence: 1:5,000 births
@ OB: severe IUGR, hydramnios
@ CNS: alobar holoprosencephaly, posterior encephalocele, neural tube defect
@ Face: midline labial cleft, proboscis, hypotelorism, cyclopia, anophthalmia
@ Skeleton: postaxial polydactyly, rocker bottom foot
@ Heart: (CHD in 90%) VSD, echogenic chordae tendineae, hypoplastic ventricle, tetralogy of Fallot, transposition
@ Kidney: polycystic kidney, horseshoe kidney
@ GI: omphalocele (occasionally)
Prognosis: few infants live more than a few days / hours
DDx: Meckel-Gruber syndrome

TRISOMY 18
= EDWARD SYNDROME
Incidence: 3:10,000 births
• triple-marker screening test:
  • decreased maternal alpha-fetoprotein
  • decreased HCG (DDx: increased in own syndrome)
  • decreased estriol
@ OB: severe symmetric IUGR (28% <24 weeks MA), single umbilical artery (30%), polyhydramnios (occasionally)
@ Face: micrognathia, hypotelorism, facial cleft (10–40%)
@ Head: strawberry-shaped head (50%), cystic hygroma

@ CNS: holoprosencephaly, choroid plexus cyst (30–75%), small cerebellum with prominent cisterna magna, myelomeningocele
@ Hand: clenched hand with overlapping of index finger (>60%, HIGHLY CHARACTERISTIC)
@ Arm: shortened radial ray, clubbed forearm
@ Foot: clubbed foot, rocker-bottom foot
@ Heart: (CHD in 90%) VSD, complete AV canal, DORV
@ GI: diaphragmatic hernia, omphalocele (30–40%), TE fistula
@ Kidney: polycystic kidney, horseshoe kidney, UPJ obstruction

Prognosis: usually delivered by emergency cesarean section due to IUGR + fetal distress, if not detected prenatally

TWIN EMBOLIZATION SYNDROME

= rare complication of monochorionic pregnancy following the death of one twin whose blood pressure falls to zero

Pathophysiology:

1. Acute reversal of transfusion to co-twin at time of intrauterine demise of one twin with ischemic changes in survivor
2. Embolization of thromboplastin-enriched blood / detritus from the dead to the living twin through vascular anastomoses in placenta

Embolized organs: CNS (72%), GI tract (19%), kidneys (15%), lungs

√ ventriculomegaly, cortical atrophy, porencephalic cyst, cystic encephalomalacia within 2 weeks of death of co-twin

TWIN-TWIN TRANSFUSION SYNDROME

= FETO-FETAL TRANSFUSION SYNDROME
= MONOVULAR TWIN TRANSFUSION
= INTRAUTERINE PARABIOTIC SYNDROME
= complication of monozygotic twinning with one placenta or one fused placenta of mono- / dizygotic twins

Incidence: 5–18% of twin pregnancies; 5–15% of monozygotic multiple pregnancies; 15–30% of monochorionic twin gestations

Cause: unbalanced intrauterine shunting of blood through shared placental vessels

Time of onset: 2nd trimester with discordant amniotic fluid volumes

Path: large communication between arterial circulation of one twin and venous circulation of the other twin through *arteriovenous* shunt (= common villous district) deep within placenta

√ discrepant amniotic fluid volume (75%)
√ discordant BPD by >5 mm (57%)
√ discordant estimated fetal weight >25% (67–100%)

A. DONOR TWIN
   = twin that transfuses the recipient twin + remains itself underperfused
   • anemia + hypovolemia
   • high output cardiac failure + hydrops (rare)
   √ oligohydramnios (75–80%) / "stuck twin" = severe oligohydramnios (60%) from oliguria
   √ intrauterine growth restriction (common) diagnosed by discordant EFW of >25%
   √ morphologically normal
B. RECIPIENT TWIN
   • polycythemia (higher hemoglobin)
   • plethora = hypervolemia (volume overload)
   √ polyhydramnios (70–75%) from increased fetal urination
   √ fetal hydrops (10–25%): pericardial + pleural effusions, ascites, skin thickening
   √ organomegaly
   √ fetus papyraceus = macerated dead fetus
   √ velamentous cord insertion (64%)

Prognosis: 80–100% perinatal mortality if presenting <28 weeks MA and left untreated

Cx: amniorrhexis, preterm labor

Rx: elective termination, volume-reduction amniocentesis of polyhydramniotic sac (decreasing mortality rates to 34%), selective feticide, laser ablation of vascular anastomoses

DDx: IUGR of one dizygotic twin (two separate placentas, two different sexes)

UTERINE ANOMALIES

= anomalies of fusion of paramesonephric duct (= müllerian duct) completed by 18th week of fetal life

Incidence: 0.1–3%

◊ Uterine anomalies are found in 9% of women with infertility / repeated spontaneous abortions!
◊ 25% of women with uterine abnormalities have fertility problems!

Associated with: urinary tract anomalies in 20–50%; possibly increased familial occurrence of limb reduction

Classification:
(classes in parenthesis refer to the classification of the American Fertility Society)

A. ARRESTED MÜLLERIAN DUCT DEVELOPMENT
   1. bilateral: **Uterine agenesis / hypoplasia** (class I)
      Incidence: 1:5,000
      Often associated with: vaginal agenesis / hypoplasia
      Age of detection: menarche
      √ small uterus with small endometrial canal
      √ poor zonal differentiation + abnormal T2-hypointense myometrium
   2. unilateral: **Unicornuate uterus** = Uterus unicornis unicollis (class II)
      (a) with contralateral rudimentary horn
      (b) without rudimentary horn
      Incidence: 3–6–13% of uterine anomalies
      May be associated with: ipsilateral renal agenesis
      • infertility in 5–20%
      • ? pregnancy wastage
      √ reduced uterine volume
      √ asymmetric ellipsoidal uterine configuration

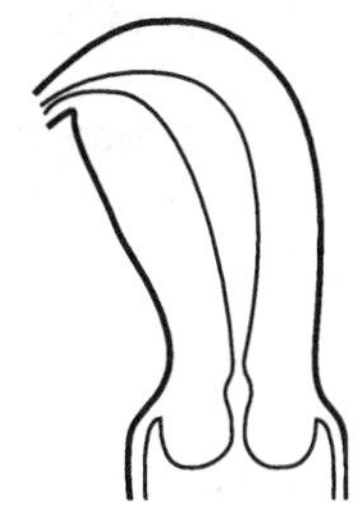
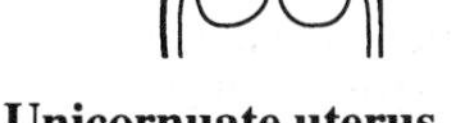
Unicornuate uterus

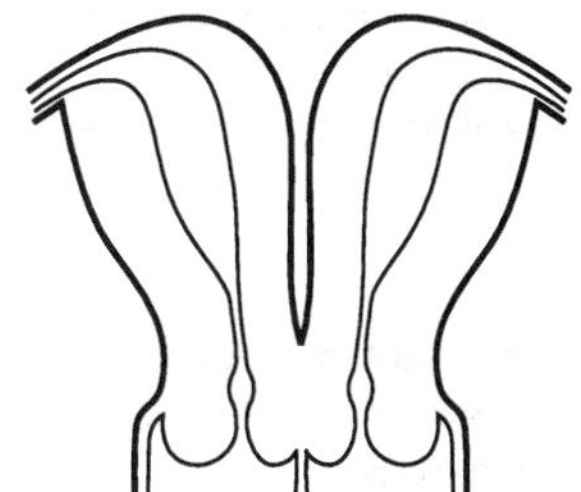
Didelphic uterus

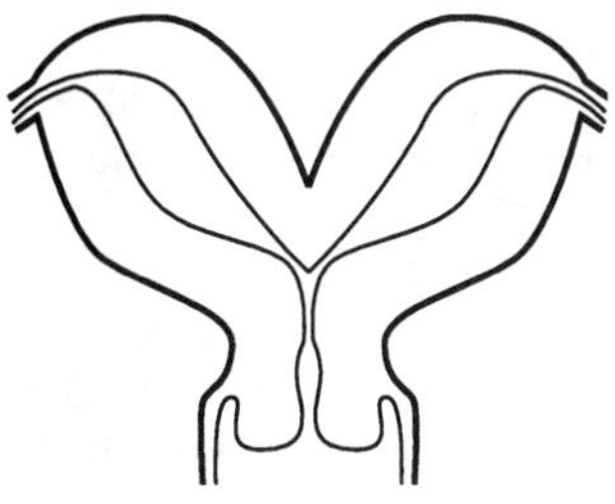
Bicornuate uterus

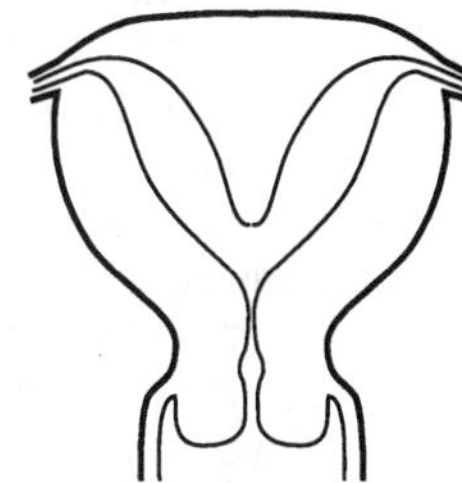
Septate uterus (partial)

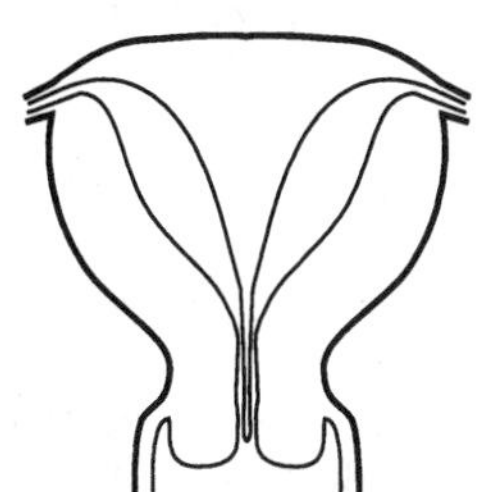
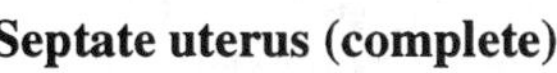
Septate uterus (complete)

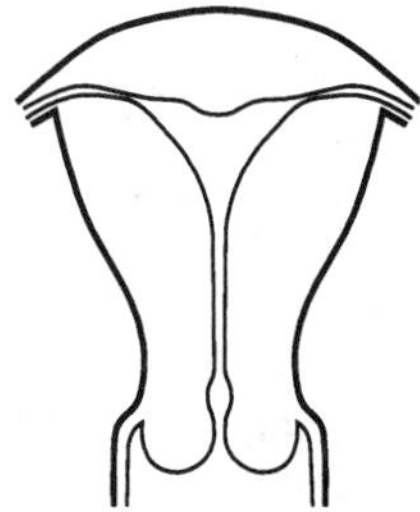
Arcuate uterus

√ rudimentary horn may contain endometrium + may communicate with main uterine cavity
√ solitary fusiform "banana-shaped" uterine cavity with lateral deviation within pelvis terminating in a single fallopian tube on HSG

Cx: cryptomenorrhea within endometrium-containing rudimentary horn that does not communicate with endometrium cavity

B. TOTAL / PARTIAL FAILURE OF MÜLLERIAN DUCT FUSION
(75% of uterine anomalies)

1. **Uterus didelphys** (class III)
= complete duplication with 2 vaginas + 2 cervices + 2 uterine horns
May be associated with: renal agenesis
• usually asymptomatic
√ two widely spaced uterine corpora, each with a single fallopian tube
√ separate divergent uterine horns
√ large fundal cleft
√ cervical duplication
√ horizontal septum of upper vagina (ipsilateral to renal agenesis)
√ opacification of single deviated horn on HSG
Cx: unilateral hydro- / hematocolpos (if transverse vaginal septum present) with reflux endometriosis
Rx: surgery is rarely performed

2. **Bicornuate uterus** = uterus bicornis (class IV)
= lack of fusion of corpus
(a) bicornis bicollis = complete with division down to internal os
(b) bicornis unicollis = partial
√ concave / heart-shaped external fundal contour due to a large fundal cleft >1–2 cm deep
√ separation of uterine horns
√ intercornual angle of >75–105° (demonstrated on luteal-phase US in conjunction with HSG)
√ intercornual distance (= distance between maximum lateral extent of hyperintense endometrium on transaxial image) >4 cm
√ divider between cornua comprised of myometrium / fibrous tissue / both
√ fusiform shape of each uterine horn with lateral convex margins
√ discrepancy in size of the 2 uterine horns
√ elongation + widening of cervical canal + isthmus
Laparoscopy: typical external fundal indentation
Cx: repeated spontaneous abortions (frequently in 2nd–3rd trimester), premature rupture of membranes, premature labor, persistent, SGA infant, malpresentations (transverse lie)
Rx: transabdominal surgery to fuse uterine horns (abdominal metroplasty)

C. NONRESORPTION OF SAGITTAL UTERINE SEPTUM

1. **Septate uterus** (class V)
Most common anomaly (almost 50%) associated with reproductive failure in 67%
Path: septum may be composed of fibrous tissue (low-signal intensity), myometrium (intermediate-signal intensity), or both
√ convex / flat / minimally indented (≤1 cm) external fundal contour
√ distal portion of septum hypoechoic to myometrium (= fibrous tissue)
√ acute angle of <75° between uterine cavities
√ duplication of uterine horns on HSG (DDx to bicornuate uterus unreliable)
√ endometrial canals completely separated by tissue isoechoic to myometrium extending into endocervical canal
Types:
(a) Uterus septus
= complete septum extending to internal os
(b) Uterus subseptus
= partial septum involving endometrial canal
Cx: 90% abortion rate (poor septal vascularity)
Rx: hysteroscopic metroplasty (= excision of septum)

OB&GYN

2. **Uterus arcuatus** (class VI)
   Most common anomaly unassociated with reproductive failure
   √ NO division of uterine horns
   √ normal fundal contour
   √ smooth indentation of fundal endometrial canal
   √ increased transverse diameter of uterine cavity
   √ single uterine canal with saddle-shaped fundus on HSG

D. INADEQUATE HORMONAL STIMULATION DURING FETAL DEVELOPMENT
   = DES (= diethylstilbestrol) -related abnormalities (class VII)
   • synthetic hormone used in 1950s + 1960s to prevent miscarriage
   • may cause abnormal uterine morphology (with decreased fertility)
   • increased risk of vaginal malignancy
   1. **Uterine hypoplasia**
      associated with diethylstilbestrol (DES) exposure in utero
      √ mean uterine volume = 50 cm^3
   2. **T-shaped uterus**
      encountered in 15% of women exposed to DES (diethylstilbestrol) in utero
      √ low uterine volume
      √ uterine fundus thinner than cervix
      √ greater width than depth of corpus + fundus over cervix
      √ T-shaped lumen on hysterosalpingogram

UTERINE LEIOMYOMA

= FIBROID = benign overgrowth of smooth muscle + connective tissue; commonest cause for uterine enlargement after pregnancy

Histo: monoclonal proliferation of smooth muscle cells (NOT myometrial hyperplasia)

Hormonal dependency:
1. Growth during pregnancy in 15–32% by a mean volume of 12 ± 6% within the 1st trimester (NOT during remainder of pregnancy)
   ◊ The larger the myoma, the greater the likelihood of growth!
2. Shrinkage in puerperium + after menopause

Incidence: in 20–25–50% of women > age of 30 years; black:white women = 3:1 – 9:1

Age: usually >30 years
• asymptomatic in 70–75%
• palpable mass
• pelvic pressure / pain (torsion, infarction, necrosis)
• hypermenorrhea (= heavy prolonged periods)

Location: mostly in fundus + corpus; in 3% in cervix
1. Intramural (within confines of uterine outline) in 95%
2. Subserosal = exophytic
   (a) parasitic fibroid = subserosal fibroid, which has become detached secondary to circulatory occlusion of vessels in pedicle; revitalized through omental / mesenteric blood supply
   (b) intraligamentous fibroid (eg, within broad ligament)
3. Submucosal
   (a) fibroid polyp = partial / complete extrusion of pedunculated submucosal fibroid through cervical canal

√ uterine enlargement
√ lobulated / nodular distortion of uterine outline (subserosal leiomyoma) + indentation of urinary bladder
√ distortion / obliteration of the contour of the uterine cavity (submucosal leiomyoma)
√ intramural soft-tissue mass (most frequent), usually multiple, solitary in 2%
√ speckled / ringlike / popcorn calcification

US (60% sensitivity, 99% specificity, 87% accuracy):
   √ hypoechoic solid concentric mass (<33%) (= muscle component prevails)
   √ echogenic attenuating mass (= dense fibrosis prevails)
   √ sharp discrete refractory shadows (from borders between fibrous tissue and smooth muscle, margins of leiomyoma with normal myometrium, edges of whorls, bundles of smooth muscle)
   √ anechoic features (secondary to internal degeneration: atrophic, hyaline, cystic, myxomatous, lipomatous, calcareous, carneous, necrobiotic, hemorrhagic, proteolytic degeneration)

CT:
   √ hypo- / iso- / hyperdense mass containing mixed hyperechoic areas

MR (86–92% sensitivity, 100% specificity, 97% accuracy; desirable for planning myomectomy):
   √ sharply marginated homogeneous focal area of low / intermediate signal intensity on T1WI + T2WI
   √ occasionally inhomogeneous high signal intensity on T2WI (from hemorrhage / hyaline degeneration or in highly cellular leiomyoma or leiomyoma with edema)
   √ hyperintense rim in 33% (dilated lymphatics / veins / edema)
   √ enhancement pattern (usually later than myometrium): 65% hypointense, 23% isointense, 12% hyperintense to myometrium

Hysterosalpingography (9% sensitivity, 97% specificity, 76% accuracy)

Cx:
(1) Infertility in 35%
   (a) narrowing of isthmic portion of tube
   (b) impingement on endometrium interfering with implantation; infertility rates highest for submucosal leiomyomas
(2) Complications in pregnancy
   significantly increased for myomas >200 cm^3
   (a) Increased frequency of spontaneous abortions
   (b) Increased frequency of IUGR
   (c) Preterm labor in 7% + premature rupture of membranes
   (d) Uterine dyskinesia, uterine inertia during labor
   (e) Dystocia, obstruction of birth canal during vaginal delivery (if near internal os)
   (f) Postpartum hemorrhage

(3) Hydroureteronephrosis
(4) Malignant transformation (in 0.2%)

Rx: surgery for: pain, menorrhagia, visceral compression
◊ Submucosal leiomyomas may be treated with hysteroscopic myomectomy

DDx of necrotic leiomyoma:
(1) Ovarian mass (ovarian cyst, hemorrhagic cyst, endometrioma, cystic dermoid, cystadenoma, malignancy)
(2) Ectopic interstitial pregnancy
(3) Intrauterine gestational sac
(4) Intrauterine fluid collection
(5) Hydatidiform mole
(6) Myometrial contraction (lasts for 15–30 minutes)
(7) Cervical tumor
(8) Hematoma of broad ligament

DDx of pedunculated subserosal leiomyoma:
(1) ovary: use transvaginal US / MR to identify follicles!

UTERINE RUPTURE IN PREGNANCY

= disruption of all layers surrounding the fetus (membranes, decidua, myometrium, serosa)
UTERINE DEHISCENCE = myometrium only

Prevalence: 3–5% for classic cesarean sections; 1–2% for lower segment operations

Classification:
1. Spontaneous rupture during labor
2. Traumatic rupture during delivery
3. Rupture due to myometrial scars / disease

Predisposed:
previous uterine surgery, previously excessively long / difficult labor

Location: (a) corpus with rupture before onset of labor
(b) lower uterine segment during labor, L > R

Cx: hypofibrinogenemia (triggered by excessive blood loss, trauma, amniotic fluid embolism)

Mortality: 2–20% maternal mortality; 10–25% fetal mortality

UTERINE TRAUMA DURING PREGNANCY

Incidence: 6–7% (70% due to motor vehicle accident)
1. Placental abruption
2. Fetal injury (eg, cerebral injury)
3. Fetal death

VAGINAL AGENESIS

2nd most common cause of primary amenorrhea

Incidence: 1:4,000–5,000 women

• cyclic abdominal pain

May be associated with:
(1) Uterine + partial tubal agenesis (90%)
(2) Unilateral renal agenesis / ectopia (34%)
(3) Skeletal malformations (12%)
(4) McKusick-Kaufman syndrome (hydrometrocolpos + polydactyly + heart defects)
(5) Ellis-van Creveld syndrome

VASA PREVIA

= rare type of velamentous cord insertion in which umbilical vessels cross the internal os
(a) vessels connecting separate succenturiate lobe to main portion of placenta
(b) cord vessels of velamentous (membranous) cord insertion from low-lying placenta
(c) aberrant chorionic vessels in association with marginal cord insertion from low lying placenta

Cx: (1) Bleeding from torn fetal vessels
(2) Cord compression by presenting part during labor
(3) Cord prolapse

Risk: 50–100% fetal mortality

VELAMENTOUS CORD INSERTION

= umbilical cord insertion into membranes before entering placenta = attachment of cord to chorion laeve

Incidence: 0.09 to 1.8%

Associated with:
(a) multiple gestation, uterine anomaly, IUD
(b) congenital anomalies (in 5.9–8.5%):
asymmetric head shape, spina bifida, esophageal atresia, obstructive uropathy, VSD, cleft palate

Cx: (1) IUGR
(2) Preterm labor

Risk: (1) Cord compression
(2) Rupture of cord with traction during delivery

TABLE OF DOSE, ENERGY, HALF-LIFE, RADIATION DOSE

Organ	*Pharmaceutical*	*Dose*	*keV*	*$T_{1/2}$ phys*	*$T_{1/2}$ bio*
Brain	Tc-99m pertechnetate	10 – 30 mCi	140	6 h	
	Tc-99m DTPA	10 mCi	140	6 h	
	Tc-99m glucoheptonate	10 mCi	140	6 h	
	Tc-99m Ceretec	20 mCi	140	6 h	
	I-123 Spectamine	3 – 6 mCi	159	13.6 h	
CSF	In-111 DTPA	500 μCi	173, 247	2.8 d	
	Tc-99m DTPA	1 mCi	140	6 h	
Cardiac	Tl-201	1 – 2 mCi	**72**, 135, 167	73 h	
	Tc-99m pyrophosphate	15 mCi	140	6 h	
	Tc-99m pertechnetate	15 – 25 mCi	140	6 h	
	Tc-99m–labeled RBCs	10 – 20 mCi	140	6 h	
	Tc-99m sestamibi	25 mCi	140	6 h	
	Tc-99m teboroxime	30 mCi	140	6 h	
Liver	Tc-99m sulfur colloid	3 – 5 mCi	140	6 h	
	Tc-99m DISIDA	4 – 5 mCi	140	6 h	
Lung	Xe-127	5 –10 mCi	172, 203, 375	36.4 d	13 s
	Xe-133	10 – 20 mCi	81, 161	5.3 d	20 s
	Kr-81m	20 mCi	176, 188, 190	13 s	
	Tc-99m MAA aerosol	3 mCi	140	6 h	8 h
Kidney	Tc-99m DTPA	15 – 20 mCi	140	6 h	
	Tc-99m DMSA	2 – 5 mCi	140	6 h	
	Tc-99m glucoheptonate	15 – 20 mCi	140	6 h	
	Tc-99m mercaptoacetyltriglycine	10 mCi	140	6 h	
	I-131 Hippuran	250 μCi	365*	8 d	18 min
	I-123 Hippuran	1 mCi	159	13.2 h	
Thyroid	Tc-99m pertechnetate	5 – 10 mCi	140	6 h	
	I-123	50 – 200 μCi	159	13.2 h	
	I-125	30 – 100 μCi	27, 35	60 d	
	I-131	30 – 100 μCi	365*	8 d	
Testes	Tc-99m pertechnetate	10 mCi	140	6 h	
Gastric mucosa	Tc-99m pertechnetate	50 μCi / kg	140	6 h	
Gallium	Ga-67 citrate	3 – 5 mCi	88, 185, 300, 388	3.3 d	
WBC	In-111 oxine	550 μCi	173, 247	2.8 d	
	Tc-99m Ceretec	10 – 20 mCi	140	6 h	

mnemonic: * = as many days as in a year

PEDIATRIC DOSE

Actual doses for pediatric patients may vary in different institutions based on empirical data. As rough guidelines use:

1. Clark's rule (body weight): $Dose_{Ped}$ = body weight [in lbs] / 150 x $Dose_{Adult}$
2. Young's rule (child up to age 12): $Dose_{Ped}$ = Age of child / (Age of child + 12) x $Dose_{Adult}$
3. Surface area: $Dose_{Ped}$ = (weight [in kg]$^{0.7}$ / 11) / 1.73 x $Dose_{Adult}$

RADIATION DOSE

	Critical organ	rad/mCi
I-131	Thyroid	1,000
I-125	Thyroid	900
In-111 oxine WBC	Spleen	26
I-123	Thyroid	15
In-111 DTPA	Spinal cord	12
Tl-201	Kidney	1.5
Ga-67 citrate	Colon	1.0
Tc-99m MAA	Lung	0.4
Tc-99m albumin microspheres	Lung	0.4
Tc-99m DISIDA	Large bowel	0.39
Tc-99m sulfur colloid	Liver	0.33
Yc-99m pertechnetate	Intestine	0.3
	Thyroid	0.15
Tc-99m glucoheptonate	Kidney	0.2
Tc-99m pertechnetate (+ perchlorate)	Colon	0.2
Tc-99m pyrophosphate	Bladder	0.13
Tc-99m phosphate	Bladder	0.13
Tc-99m DTPA	Bladder	0.12
Tc-99m–tagged RBCs	Spleen	0.11
Tc-99m albumin	Blood	0.015
Xe-133	Trachea	

QUALITY CONTROL

◊ Quality control logs should be kept for 3 years!

RADIOPHARMACEUTICALS

Radionuclide Impurity

= amount (μCi) of radiocontaminant per amount (μCi/mCi) of desired radionuclide

Mo-99 Breakthrough Test:

(a) allowable contamination of 1:1,000 (= 0.15 μCi Mo-99 per 1 mCi of Tc-99m)
(b) <5 μCi Mo-99 per administered dose (NRC dropped this requirement, but nonagreement states may still require this)

Measured after lead shielding of vial (filters 140 keV but permits 452 keV of Mo-99 to pass through)
Effect of impurity:
increased radiation dose, poor image quality

Radiochemical Impurity

Precise registration of different compounds of Tc-99m, eg
— hydrolyzed reduced technetium [$TcO(OH)_2 \cdot H_2O$]
— free pertechnetate [TcO^4]$^{-1}$
can be monitored by paper chromatography

Effect of impurity with hydrolyzed reduced Tc:
RES uptake, poor image quality, increased radiation dose

Chemical Impurity

Chemicals from elution process are restricted in their amount:
Tc-99m: <10 μg Al per 1 mL eluate if radionuclide from fission generator;
<20 μg Al per 1 mL eluate if radionuclide from neutron bombardment

Aluminum Ion Breakthrough Test:

One drop of generator eluate placed on one end of special test paper containing aluminum reagent; equal-sized drop of a standard solution of Al^{3+} (10 ppm) is placed on other end of strip; if color at center of drop eluate is lighter than that of standard solution, the eluate has passed the colorimetric test
Effect of impurity: degradation of image quality

Pyrogen Testing

USP XX Test

Monitor rectal temperature of 3 suitable rabbits after injection of material through ear vein
Acceptable results: no rabbit shows a rise of >0.6°C; total rise of all three <1.4°C

Limulus Amoebocyte Lysate Test (LAL)

Highly specific for Gram-negative bacterial endotoxins, sensitivity 10 x greater than USP XX test

Amoebocyte = primitive blood cell of horseshoe crab (Limulus polyphebus); lysate formed by hydrolysis of amoebocyte

Positive result: in the presence of minute amounts of endotoxin LAL forms an opaque gel; response to other pyrogens (particulate contaminations, chemicals) doubtful

CALIBRATORS

Constancy = Precision

= reproducibility over time
Test frequency: daily
Method: measurement of a long-lived source, usually a Cs-137 standard
Evaluation: measurement must fall within ± 5% of the calculated activity

Linearity

= accurate measurement over large range of activity levels
Test frequency: 4 x per year
Method: 1 mCi source activity is measured every 4 hours for 10 / more measurements (down to 10–100 μCi)
Evaluation: measurements must fall within ± 5% of the calculated physical decay curve

Accuracy

Test frequency: annually
Method: measurements of three different activity standards whose amount is certified by the National Bureau of Standards (NBS); standard values are decayed mathematically to calibrator date
Co-57: 123 keV, half-life of 270 days
Ba-133: 354 keV, half-life of 7.2 years
Cs-137: 662 keV, half-life of 30 years
Evaluation: measurements must fall within expected range

Geometry

= to assure that measurement is not dependent upon location of tracer within ionization chamber, usually done by manufacturer
Test frequency: at installation / after factory repair / recalibration
Method: 0.5 mL of Tc-99m (activity 25 mCi) is measured in a 3-mL syringe; syringe contents are then diluted with water to 1.0 mL, 1.5 mL, and 2.0 mL and each level remeasured; test is repeated with a 10-mL glass vial

SCINTILLATION CAMERA

Field Uniformity

= ability of camera to reproduce a uniform radioactive distribution = variability of observed count density with a homogeneous flux

(a) Integral uniformity = maximum deviation
(b) Differential uniformity = maximum rate of change over a specified distance (5 pixels)

Causes for nonuniformity:

(1) High kilovoltage drift of photomultiplier (PM) tubes
(2) Physical damage to collimator
(3) Improper photopeak setting
(4) Contamination

Frequency of quality control: daily

A. INTRINSIC FIELD UNIFORMITY TEST (without collimator)
1. Remove collimator + replace with lead ring (to eliminate edge packing)
2. Place a point source at a distance of at least 5 crystal diameters from detector (4–5 feet for small, 7–9 feet for large crystals)
3. Point source contains 200–400 μCi of Tc-99m for minimal personnel exposure (avoid contamination of crystal)
4. Set count rate below limit of instrument (<30,000 counts)
5. Adjust the pulse height selector to normal window settings by centering at 140 keV with a window of 15% (for Tc-99m studies only)
6. Use the same photographic device
7. Acquire 1.25 million counts for a 10" field of view, 2.5 million counts for a 15" field of view
8. Register counts, time, CRT intensity, analyzer settings, initials of controller

B. EXTRINSIC FIELD UNIFORMITY TEST (with collimator)
1. Collimator is kept in place
   ◊ Only 1 of 2,000 gamma rays that reach the collimator are transmitted to the sodium iodide crystal!
2. Sheet source / flood of 2–10 mCi activity is placed on collimator
   (a) fillable floods: mix thoroughly, avoid air bubbles, check for flat surface
   (b) nonfillable: commercially available Co-57 source
3. Other steps as described above

Evaluation:

(1) Compare uncorrected with corrected images. Note acquisition time!
(2) Store correction flood
(3) Rerecord image with corrected flood + check for uniformity

Spatial Resolution / Linearity

A. SPATIAL RESOLUTION
   = parameter of scintillation camera that characterizes its ability to accurately determine the original location of a gamma ray on an X,Y plane; measured in both X and Y directions; expressed as full width at half maximum (FWHM) of the line spread function in mm
   (a) intrinsic spatial resolution
   (b) system spatial resolution

B. INTRINSIC SPATIAL LINEARITY
   = parameter of a scintillation camera that characterizes the amount of positional distortion caused by the camera with respect to incident gamma events entering the detector
   (a) differential linearity = standard deviation of line spread function peak separation (in mm)
   (b) absolute linearity = maximum amount of spatial displacement (in mm)

Frequency of quality control: every week

1. Mask detector to collimated field of view (lead ring)
2. Lead phantom is attached to front of crystal
   (a) Four-quadrant bar pattern (3 pictures each after 90° rotation to test entire crystal)
   (b) Parallel-line equal-spacing (PLES) bar pattern [2 pictures]
   (c) Smith orthogonal hole test pattern (OHP) [1 picture only]
   (d) Hine-Duley phantom [2 pictures]
3. Set symmetric analyzer window to width normally used
4. Place a point source (1–3 mCi) at a fixed distance of at least 5 crystal diameters from detector on central axis (remove all sources from immediate area so that background count rate is low)
5. Acquire 1.25 million counts for a small field, 2.5 million counts for a large field on the same media used for clinical studies
6. Record counts, time, CRT intensity, analyzer setting, initials of controller

(All new cameras are equipped with a spatial distortion correction circuit)

Evaluation:

Visual assessment of
(1) Spatial resolution over entire field
(2) Linearity

Intrinsic Energy Resolution

= ability to distinguish between primary gamma events and scattered events; performed without collimator; expressed as ratio of photopeak FWHM to photopeak energy (in %)

CRT-output / Photographic Device

(1) Check for dirt, scratches, burnt spots on CRT face plates
(2) Adjust grey scale + contrast settings to suit film

SOURCES OF ARTIFACTS

A. ATTENUATOR BETWEEN SOURCE AND DETECTOR
   Materials: cable, lead marker, solder dropped into collimator during repair, belt buckle / watch / key on patient, defective collimator
   (a) at time of correction flood procedure:
      √ hot spot
   (b) after correction flood procedure:
      √ cold spot

B. CRACKED CRYSTAL
   √ white band with hot edges

C. PMT FAILURE + LOSS OF OPTICAL COUPLING BETWEEN PMT AND CRYSTAL
   √ cold defect

D. PROBLEMS DURING FILM EXPOSURE + PROCESSING
   1. Double exposed film
   2. Light leak in multiformat camera
   3. Water lines from film processing
   4. Frozen shutter:
      √ part of film cut off
   5. Variations in film processing

E. IMPROPER WINDOW SETTING
   1. Photopeak window set too high:
      √ hot tubes
   2. Photopeak window set too low:
      √ cold tubes

F. ADMINISTRATION OF WRONG ISOTOPE
   √ atypically imaged organs

G. EXCESSIVE AMOUNTS OF FREE TC-99M PERTECHNETATE
   √ too much uptake in choroid plexus, salivary glands, thyroid, stomach

H. FAULTY INJECTION TECHNIQUE
   eg, inadvertently labeled blood clot in syringe leading to iatrogenic pulmonary emboli

I. CONTAMINATION WITH RADIOTRACER
   on patient's skin, stretcher, collimator, crystal

J. CRT PROBLEMS
   1. Burnt spot on CRT phosphor
   2. Dirty / scratched CRT face plates

SPECT QUALITY CONTROL

= SINGLE PHOTON EMISSION COMPUTED TOMOGRAPHY

= gamma cameras rotating about a pallet supporting the patient obtain 60–120 views over 180° / 360° rotation with typically a field of view of 40–50 cm across the patient and 30–40 cm in axial direction

Spatial resolution: ~8 mm for high-count study

Uniformity

1. 64 x 64 word matrix = 30 million count flood with collimator, orientation and magnification same as patient study
2. Co-57 sheet source with <1% uniformity variance is necessary
3. 128 x 128 word matrix = 120 million count flood with collimator, orientation, and magnification same as patient study

Frequency of quality control: weekly

Center Of Rotation (COR)

1. Tc-99m–filled line source (5–8 mCi) positioned 3–5 cm off the center of rotation while keeping scanning palette out of field of view
2. Direction of rotation to be the same as patient study
3. Number of steps (32, 64, or 128) to be the same as in patient study
4. Time per step such that at least 100K counts are acquired
5. COR must be done with same collimator, orientation, and magnification as patient study

Frequency of quality control: weekly

Sources Of Artifacts

1. Scanning palette in field of view
2. Collimator shifting + rotation on camera face
3. Noncircular orbit of camera head
4. PM tube failure
5. PM tube uncoupling
6. Cracked crystal
7. Improper peaking of camera

POSITRON EMISSION TOMOGRAPHY

= PET = technique that permits noninvasive in vivo examination of metabolism, blood flow, electrical activity, neurochemistry

Concept:
measurement of distribution of a biocompound as a function of time after radiolabeling and injection into patient

Labeling:
PET compounds are radiolabeled with positron-emitting radionuclides

Physics:
positron matter-antimatter annihilation reaction with an electron results in formation of annihilation photons, which are emitted in exactly opposite directions (511 keV each); detected by coincidence circuitry through simultaneous arrival at detectors (bismuth germanate-68) on opposite sides of the patient (= electronic collimation through coincidence circuit); lead collimators not necessary (= advantages in resolution + sensitivity over SPECT); spatial reconstruction similar to transmission CT

Radionuclide production:
in nuclide generator / particle accelerator (positive / negative ion cyclotron; linear accelerator)
Expected amount of radionuclide: 500–2,000 mCi
Generator characteristics:
beam energy (radionuclide production rate increases monotonically with beam energy), beam current (production rate directly proportional to beam current), accelerated particle, shielding requirement, size, cost

Radiopharmaceutical production:
(1) Initialize accelerator, setup
(2) Irradiation
(3) Synthesis
(4) Sterility test, compounding

Sensitivity:
= fraction of radioactive decays within the patient that are detected by the scanner as true events (measured in counts per second per microcurie per milliliter)
◊ 30 – 100 times more sensitive than SPECT (due to electronic collimation as opposed to lead collimation)!

Resolution:
= resolving power = smallest side-by-side objects that can be distinguished as separate objects in images with an infinite number of counts (measured in mm);
determined by
- distance a positron travels before annihilation occurs (usually 0.5–2 mm depending on energy)
- angle variation from 180° (±5° = 0.5 mm)
- physical size of detector (1–3 mm)

◊ Typical spatial resolution: 4–7 mm

Measurement of radioactivity distribution:
Pixel values proportional to radioactivity per volume
Unit: mg of glucose per minute per 100 g tissue
Imaging time: 1–10 min

Organ-specific concentration:
(a) heart, brain: contain little glucose-6-phosphatase resulting in high concentrations of FDG
- metabolic rate of glucose is proportional to phosphorylation rate of FDG

(b) liver: abundance of glucose-6-phosphatase + low levels of hexokinase resulting in rapid clearing of FDG
(c) neoplasm: enhanced glycolysis with increased activity of hexokinase + other enzymes

PET imaging in oncology

Pathophysiology:
serum glucose competes with FDG for entry into tumor cells; malignant cells have a high rate of glycolysis

Isotope		Use	Half-life (min)	Average Positron Energy (keV)	Typical Reaction	Yield at 10 MeV (mCi/μA EOSB)
rubidium	Rb-82		1.23	1,409	Sr/Rb generator	...
fluorine	F-18	glucose metabolism	109	242	O-18(p,n)F-18	120
oxygen	O-15	O_2, H_2O, CO_2, CO	2.1	735	N-15(p,n)O-15	70
nitrogen	N-13	perfusion of NH_3	10	491	C-13(p,n)N-13	110
carbon	C-11	carbon metabolism	20.3	385	N-14(p,α)C-11	85

p = proton injected; n = neutron ejected; a = alpha particle; EOSB = end of saturated bombardment (infinitely long irradiation at which time the numbers of radionuclides produced equals the number of radionuclides that are decaying) per microampere of beam current (= number of particles per second emerging from accelerator and impinging on target material)

1. Lung cancer
   √ tumor uptake > mediastinal uptake of FDG (94–97% sensitive, 87–89% specific, 92% accurate)
   √ FDG can differentiate adrenal "incidentaloma" from metastasis
2. Breast cancer
3. Colon cancer recurrence
4. Lymph node metastases from head and neck cancer (91% sensitive, 88% specific)
5. Brain tumor:
   (a) necrosis versus residual / recurrent tumor
      √ decreased FDG uptake in necrosis
   (b) response to chemo- / radiation therapy
   (c) prediction of patient's average survival in pediatric primary brain tumors:
      ≤6 months if FDG uptake ≥ gray matter
      1–2 years if FDG uptake > white matter
      2.5 years if FDG uptake = white matter
      3 years if FDG uptake < gray matter
6. Pancreatic cancer (96% sensitive + specific)
7. Lymphoma staging with whole-body scan

IMMUNOSCINTIGRAPHY

= imaging with monoclonal antibodies [= homogeneous antibody population directed against a single antigen (eg, cancer cell)], which are labeled with a radiotracer

Hybridoma technique:
antibody-producing B lymphocytes are extracted from the spleen of mice that were immunized with a specific type of cancer cell; B lymphocytes are fused with immortal myeloma cells (= hybridoma)

Agents:
Indium-111 satumomab pendetide = indium-111 CYT-103 (OncoScint® CR/OV) = murine monoclonal antibody product derived by site-specific radiolabeling of the antibody B27.3-GYK-DTPA conjugate with indium-111

Use: detection + staging of colorectal + ovarian cancers
Dose: 1 mg of antibody radiolabeled with 5 mCi of indium-111 injected IV

Biodistribution: liver, spleen, bone marrow, salivary glands, male genitalia, blood pool, kidneys, bladder
Imaging: 2 sets of images 2 – 5 days post injection + 48 hours apart

GALLIUM SCINTIGRAPHY

GALLIUM-67 CITRATE

Ga-67 acts as an analogue of ferric ion; used as gallium citrate (water-soluble form)

Production: bombardment of zinc targets (Zn-67, Zn-68) with protons (cyclotron); virtually carrier-free after separation process

Decay: by electron capture to ground state of Zn-67

Energy levels:
- (a) used: 93 keV (38%), 184 keV (24%), 300 keV (16%)
- (b) unused: 91 keV (2%), 206 keV (2%), 388 keV (8%)

Physical half-life: 3.3 d (= 78 hours)
Biologic half-life: 2–3 weeks
Adult dose: 3–6 mCi or 50 μCi/kg

Radiation dose:
0.3 rads/mCi for whole body; 0.9 rads/mCi for distal colon (= critical organ); 0.58 rads/mCi for red marrow; 0.56 rads/mCi for proximal colon; 0.46 rads/mCi for liver; 0.41 rads/mCi for kidney; 0.24 rads/mCi for gonads

Physiology:
Ga-67 is bound to iron-binding sites of various proteins (strongest bond with transferrin in plasma, lactoferrin in tissue); multiexponential + slow plasma disappearance; competitive iron administration (Fe-citrate) enhances target-to-background ratio by increasing Ga-67 excretion

Binding Sites

(a) fluid spaces
1. Transferrin, haptoglobin, albumin, globulins in blood serum
2. Interstitial fluid space (increased capillary permeability and hyperemia in inflammation + tumor)
3. Lactoferrin in tissue

(b) cellular binding
1. Viable PMNs incorporate 10% of Ga-67 (bound to lactoferrin in intracytoplasmic granules)
2. Nonviable PMNs + their protein exudate (iron-binding proteins are deposited at sites of inflammation; these remove iron from the extracellular space; iron is no longer available for bacterial growth)
3. Lymphocytes have lactoferrin-binding surface receptors
4. Phagocytic macrophages engulf protein-iron complexes
5. Bacteria + fungi (siderophores = lysosomes) have iron-transporting protein mechanism
6. Tumor cell–associated transferrin receptor + transportation into cells (lymphocytes bind Ga-67 less avidly than PMNs; RBCs do not bind Ga-67)

mnemonic: "LFT'S"
Lactoferrin (WBCs)
Ferritin
Transferrin
Siderophores (bacteria)

Uptake

at 24 hours: most intense in RES, liver, spleen (4%), bone marrow (lumbar spine, sacroiliac joints), bowel wall (chiefly colonic activity on delayed images), renal cortex, nasal mucosa, lacrimal + salivary glands, blood pool (20%), lung (<3% = equivalent to background activity), breasts

at 72 hours: activity in liver, skeleton, colon, nasal mucosa, occiput; kidney activity no longer detectable; lacrimal + salivary glands may still be prominent

Excretion

(a) <u>via GI tract</u> (10–20%)
hepatobiliary pathway + colonic mucosal excretion: enemas + laxatives promote clearing of bowel activity

(b) <u>via urinary tract</u> (10–20% within 24 hours)
no activity in kidneys + urinary bladder after 24 hours

(c) <u>via various body fluids</u>
eg, human milk (mandates to stop nursing for 2 weeks)

Time Of Imaging

usually 6, 24, 48, 72 hours
- ◊ Best target-to-background ratio generally at 72 hours
- ◊ Optimal target-to-background ratio at 6–24 hours for abscess
- ◊ Optimal target-to-background ratio at 24–48 hours for tumor

Degrading Factors Of Imaging

- √ lesions <2 cm are not detectable
- √ photon scatter within overlying tissues
- √ physiologic high activity of liver, spleen, bones, kidney, GI tract may obscure lesion

Normal Variants Of Ga-67 Uptake

1. Breasts: increased uptake under stimulus of menarche, estrogens, pregnancy, lactation, phenothiazine medication
2. Liver: suppressed uptake by chemotherapeutic agents / high levels of circulating iron / irradiation / severe acute liver disease
3. Lung: prominent uptake after lymphangiography
4. Spleen: increased uptake in splenomegaly
5. Thymus: uptake in children
6. Salivary glands: uptake within first 6 months after radiation therapy to neck (may persist for years)

7. Epiphyseal plates in children
8. Previous steroid therapy, chemotherapy, and radiation therapy may decrease Ga uptake

Indications

A. INFECTION

Gallium has been largely replaced with WBC imaging but can be used in chronic infection

1. Inflamed / infarcted bowel (eg, Crohn disease)
   DDx: normal bowel excretions (must be cleared by enema; bowel pathology shows persistent activity)
2. Diffuse lung uptake
   sarcoidosis, diffuse infections (TB, CMV, PCP), lymphangitic metastases, pneumoconioses (asbestosis, silicosis), diffuse interstitial fibrosis (UIP), drug-induced pneumonitis (bleomycin, cyclophosphamide, busulfan), acute radiation pneumonitis, recent lymphangiographic contrast
3. Lymph node involvement
   sarcoidosis, TB, MAI, Hodgkin disease
   DDx: NOT seen in Kaposi sarcoma, a useful distinction in AIDS patients with hilar nodes

B. TUMOR

Neoplastic uptake is variable; prominent uptake is usually seen in:

1. Non-Hodgkin lymphoma (especially Burkitt)
2. Hodgkin disease
3. Hepatoma
4. Melanoma

Useful in:

— detection of tumor recurrence
— DDx of focal cold liver lesions on Tc-99m sulfur colloid scan

No Ga-67 Uptake

most benign neoplasms; hemangioma; cirrhosis; cystic disease of the breast, liver, thyroid; reactive lymphadenopathy; inactive granulomatous disease

Gallium In Bone Imaging

Increased activity in:

1. Active osteomyelitis (90% sensitivity is higher than for Tc-99m MDP)
2. Sarcoma
3. Cellulitis (bone scan followed by gallium scan)
4. Septic arthritis, rheumatoid arthritis
5. Paget disease
6. Metastases (65% sensitivity, less than for bone agents)

Gallium In Tumor Imaging

Particularly useful in evaluating extent of known tumor disease + in detection of tumor recurrence

A. USEFUL CATEGORY

1. Lymphoma
   (a) Hodgkin disease: 74–88% sensitivity
   (b) NHL: sensitivity varies
   — histiocytic form: 85–90% sensitivity
   — lymphocytic well-diff.: 55–70% sensitivity
   95% sensitivity for mediastinal disease, 80% sensitivity for cervical + superficial lesions; poor sensitivity below diaphragm
2. Burkitt lymphoma: almost 100% sensitivity
3. Rhabdomyosarcoma: >95% sensitivity
4. Hepatoma: 85–95% sensitivity
5. Melanoma: 69–79% sensitivity

B. POSSIBLY USEFUL

1. NHL: good for large + mediastinal lesions
2. Nodal metastases from seminoma + embryonal cell carcinoma: 87% sensitivity
3. Non–small cell lung cancer: 85% sensitivity for primary of any histologic type, 90% probability for uptake in mediastinal nodes, 67% probability for uptake in normal mediastinal nodes, 90% probability for uptake in extrathoracic metastases

C. NOT USEFUL

head & neck tumors, GI tumors (especially adenocarcinomas; 35–40% sensitivity), breast tumor (52–65% sensitivity), gynecologic tumors (<26% sensitivity), pediatric tumors

Gallium In Lung Imaging

◊ Scans obtained at 48 hours, because 50% of normals show activity at 24 hours

A. FOCAL UPTAKE

1. Primary pulmonary malignancy (>90% sensitivity)
2. Benign disorders: granuloma, abscess, pneumonia, silicosis

B. MULTIFOCAL / DIFFUSE UPTAKE

(a) Infection
   1. Tuberculosis
      √ intense uptake in active lesions (97%) = parameter of activity
      √ diffuse uptake in miliary TB + rapidly progressive TB pneumonia
   2. Pneumocystis carinii
      √ increased uptake at time when physical signs, symptoms, and roentgenographic changes are unimpressive
   3. Cytomegalovirus
(b) Inflammation
   1. Sarcoidosis
      70% sensitivity for active parenchymal disease, 94% sensitivity for hilar adenopathy = indicator of therapeutic response to steroids
   2. Interstitial lung disease
      pneumoconiosis, idiopathic pulmonary fibrosis, lymphangitic carcinomatosis
   3. Exudative stage of radiation pneumonitis
(c) Drugs
   1. Bleomycin toxicity
   2. Amiodarone
(d) Contrast lymphangiography (in 50%)

C. GALLIUM UPTAKE + NORMAL CHEST FILM
1. Pulmonary drug toxicity
2. Tumor infiltration
3. Sarcoidosis
4. Pneumocystis carinii

Gallium In Renal Imaging

Abnormal uptake on delayed images at 48–72 hours

A. RENAL TUMOR
1. Primary renal tumor (variable uptake)
2. Lymphoma / leukemia
3. Metastases (eg, melanoma)

B. RENAL INFLAMMATION
1. Acute pyelonephritis (88% sensitivity):
   √ diffuse / focal uptake
2. Lobar nephronia
3. Renal abscess

C. OTHERS
1. Collagen-vascular disease, vasculitis, Wegener granulomatosis
2. Amyloidosis, hemochromatosis
3. Hepatic failure
4. Administration of antineoplastic drugs

D. TRANSPLANT
1. Acute / chronic rejection
2. Acute tubular necrosis

E. URINARY BLADDER
1. Cystitis
2. Tumor

mnemonic: "CHANT An OLD PSALM"
Chemotherapy
Hemochromatosis, **H**epatorenal failure
Acute tubular necrosis, **A**cute lobar nephronia
Neoplasm
Transfusion, **T**uberous sclerosis
Abscess
Obstruction
Lymphoma
Drugs (Fe, drugs causing ATN)
Pyelonephritis, **P**olyarteritis nodosa
Sarcoidosis
Amyloidosis, **A**llograft
Leukemia
Metastasis, **M**yeloma

Gallium Imaging In Lymphoma

A. HODGKIN DISEASE
50–70% average sensitivity dependent on size, location, technique

B. NON-HODGKIN LYMPHOMA
30% sensitivity for lymphocytic subtype, 70% sensitivity for histiocytic subtype
Sensitivity:
90% for mediastinal nodes
80% for neck nodes
48% for periaortic nodes
47% for iliac nodes
36% for axillary nodes

Gallium Imaging In Malignant Melanoma

Types:
1. Lentigo maligna: low invasiveness, low metastatic potential
2. Superficial spreading melanoma: intermediate prognosis
3. Nodular melanoma: most lethal

Prognosis (level of invasion versus 5-year survival):

Level	I	(in situ)	100%
Level	II	(within papillary dermis)	100%
Level	III	(extending to reticular dermis)	88%
Level	IV	(invading reticular dermis)	66%
Level	V	(subcutaneous infiltration)	15%

Ga-67:
>50% sensitivity for primary + metastatic sites; detectability versus tumor size: 73% sensitivity >2 cm; 17% sensitivity <2 cm

Bone, brain, liver scintigraphy:
show very low yield in detecting metastases at time of preoperative assessment and are not indicated

AGENTS FOR INFLAMMATION

1. **Ga-67 citrate**
overall 58–100% sensitivity; 75–100% specificity (lower for abdominal inflammation because of problematic abdominal activity)

Indication:
chronic + nonpyogenic inflammation, pulmonary infection + lymphadenitis with HIV-positivity, granulomatous disease (eg, sarcoidosis)

Pathophysiology:
leakage of protein-bound Ga-67 into extracellular space secondary to hyperemia + increased capillary permeability; Ga-67 is preferentially bound to nonviable PMNs + macrophages
1. Leukocyte incorporation (rich in lactoferrin)
2. Bacterial uptake (iron-chelating siderophores)
3. Inflammatory tissue stimulates lactoferrin production

GALLIUM IN CHRONIC ABDOMINAL INFLAMMATION
67% sensitivity, 64% specificity, 13% false-negative rate, 5% false-positive rate
Dose: 5 mCi
Imaging: routine at 48–72 hours (after clearance of high background activity); optional at 6–24 hours (prior to renal + gastrointestinal excretion); delayed images as needed
√ diffuse uptake in peritonitis
√ localized uptake in acute pyogenic abscess, phlegmon, acute cholecystitis, acute pancreatitis, acute gastritis, diverticulitis, inflammatory bowel disease, surgical wound, pyelonephritis, perinephric abscess

Technique:
harvesting of cells followed by separation from RBCs and platelets + washing off plasma proteins; chelating agents (oxine = 8-hydroxyquinoline / tropolone) used for labeling; lipophilic oxine-indium complex penetrates cell membrane of white cells; intracellular proteins scavenge the indium from oxine; oxine diffuses out from cell; requires 2 hours of preparation time

Recovery rate: 30% at 1–4 hours after injection
Limitations: 19 gauge IV access, leukopenia, impaired chemotaxis, abnormal WBCs, children
Dose: 0.5 mCi
Half-life: 67 hours
Useful photopeaks: 173 keV (89%), 247 keV (94%)

Radiation dose:
13–18 rad/mCi for spleen; 3.8 rad/mCi for liver; 0.65 rad/mCi for red marrow; 0.45 rad/mCi for whole body; 0.29 rad/mCi for testes; 0.14 rad/mCi for ovaries (compared with Ga-67 higher dose to spleen, but lower dose to all other organs)
Biodistribution: spleen, liver, bone marrow; blood clearance halftime of 6–7 hours

Imaging:
best at 18–24 hours following injection of cell preparation; optional at 2–6 hours (eg, in inflammatory bowel disease); delayed images as needed; bone marrow uptake provides useful landmarks
√ focal activity greater than in spleen is typical for abscess (comparison based on liver, spleen, bone marrow activity)
√ activity equal to liver (significant inflammatory focus)
√ abdominal activity is always abnormal

False positives:
@ Chest: CHF, RDS, embolized cells, cystic fibrosis
@ Abdomen: accessory spleen, colonic accumulation, renal transplant rejection, GI hemorrhage, vasculitis, ischemic bowel disease, following CPR, uremia, postradiation therapy, Wegener granulomatosis, ALL
@ Miscellaneous: IM injection, histiocytic lymphoma, cerebral infarction, arthritis, skeletal metastases, thrombophlebitis, hematoma, hip prosthesis, cecal carcinoma, postsurgical pseudoaneurysm, necrotic tumors that harvest WBCs

False negatives:
chronic infection, aortofemoral graft, LUQ abscess, infected pelvic hematoma, splenic abscess, hepatic abscess (occasionally)

3. **Tc-99m–labeled WBC**

Optimal use: osteomyelitis in extremities

Advantages over In-111 WBC imaging:
(a) improved photon flux
(b) earlier imaging

Disadvantages:
(1) Biliary excretion leads to bowel activity, which may obscure abdominal abscess if not imaged early
(2) Heart and blood pool may obscure disease
(3) Nonspecific accumulation in lung

Technique:
Tc-99m Ceretec binds with autologous WBCs and is reinjected
Imaging:
30 minutes (optimum for use in abdomen), 60 minutes, 3–4 hours, 24 hours (optional)

False positives:
may be due to unusual marrow distribution, correlation with bone marrow (sulphur colloid) scan may be necessary

BONE SCINTIGRAPHY

BONE AGENTS

A. POLYPHOSPHATES = LINEAR PHOSPHATES = CONDENSED PHOSPHATES
   First agents described; contain up to 46 phosphate residues; simplest form contains 2 phosphates = pyrophosphate (PYP)

B. DIPHOSPHONATES
   Organic analogs of pyrophosphate characterized by P-C-P bond; chemically more stable; not susceptible to hydrolysis in vivo; most widely used agents:
   1. ethylene hydroxydiphosphonate (EHDP) = ethane-1-hydroxy-1,1-diphosphonate
   2. methylene diphosphonate (MDP)

C. IMIDODIPHOSPHONATES (IDP)
   Characterized by P-N-P bond

Indications:
1. Imaging of bone, myocardial / cerebral infarct, ectopic calcifications, some tumors (neuroblastoma)
2. Rx for Paget disease, myositis ossificans progressiva, calcinosis universalis (inhibits formation + dissolution of hydroxyapatite crystals)

Usual dose: 20 mCi (740 MBq)
Radiation dose: 0.13 rad/mCi for bladder (critical organ), 0.04 rad/mCi for bone, 0.01 rad/mCi for whole body

Imaging:
- @ Bone: 2–3 hours post injection
  - ◊ Fractures may not show positive uptake until 3–10 days depending on age of patient
- @ Myocardium: 90–120 minutes post injection
  - ◊ Ideal imaging time is 1–3 days post infarction

Labeling: Tc (VII) is eluted as a pertechnetate ion; chemical reduction with Sn (II) chloride; chelated into a complex of Tc-99m (IV)-tin-phosphate

Quality Control:
(1) <10% Tc-99m tin colloid / free Tc-99m pertechnetate (a good preparation is 95% bound)
(2) Agent should not be used prior to 30 minutes after preparation
(3) Avoid injection of air in preparation of multidose vials (oxidation results in poor Tc bond)
(4) Kit life is 4–5 hours after preparation

Uptake:
(a) rapid distribution into ECF (78% of injected dose with biologic half-life of 2.4 minutes) directly related to blood flow + vascularity; blood clearance rate determines ECF (= background) activity (at 4 hours 1% for diphosphonates, 5% for pyrophosphate / polyphosphate secondary to greater degree of protein binding)
(b) chemisorbs on hydroxyapatite crystals in bone + in calcium crystals in mitochondria; MDP concentration at 3 hours is directly proportional to calcium contents of tissues (14–24% calcium in bone, 0.005% calcium in muscle); 50–60% (58% for MDP, 48% for EHDP, 47% for PYP) are localized in bone by approx. 3 hours depending on blood flow + osteoblastic activity; 2–10% of the dose are present within soft tissues; myocardial uptake depends on at least some revascularization of infarcted muscle

Excretion:
via urinary tract by 6 hours in 68% of MDP/EHDP, in 50% of PYP, in 46% of polyphosphates
- ◊ Forcing fluids + frequent voiding reduces radiation dose to bladder!

THREE-PHASE BONE SCANNING
over area of interest
1. Rapid sequence flow study (2–5 seconds/frame) = early arterial flow = 1st phase
2. Immediate postflow images (1 million counts for central body + 0.5 million counts for extremities) = blood pool = 2nd phase
3. Delayed images (0.5–1.0 million counts) between 3–4 hours following injection = 3rd phase

BONE MARROW AGENTS

for assessment of hematopoiesis / phagocytosis by RES

1. Tc-99m sulfur colloid (10% uptake in bone marrow)
2. In-111 chloride
3. Tc-99m MMAA
   = mini-microaggregated albumin colloid for liver, spleen, hematopoietic marrow
   Particle size: 30–100 microns
   Dose: 10 mCi
   Marrow dose: 0.55 rad
   Marrow accumulation at 1 hour:
   6 x higher than for sulfur colloid
   3 x higher than for antimony-sulfur colloid

Indications:
(a) expansion of hematopoietically active bone marrow
   1. Hematologic disorders to reveal presence of peripheral expansion of functional marrow
(b) focal defect due to displacement by infiltrating disease
   1. Marrow replacement disorders: eg, Gaucher disease
   2. Bone infarction: eg, sickle cell anemia (DDx from osteomyelitis)
   3. Avascular necrosis in children

Pediatric Indications For Bone Scan

A. BACK PAIN
1. Discitis
2. Pars interarticularis defect: SPECT imaging adds sensitivity
3. Osteoid osteoma: can be used intraoperatively to assure removal of nidus
4. Sacroiliac infection

B. NONACCIDENTAL TRAUMA

Superscan

A. METABOLIC
1. Renal osteodystrophy
2. Osteomalacia
   √ randomly distributed focal sites of intense activity = Looser zones = pseudofractures = Milkman fractures (most characteristic)
3. Hyperparathyroidism
   √ focal intense uptake corresponds to site of brown tumors
4. Hyperthyroidism
   rate of bone resorption more increased than rate of formation (= decrease in bone mass)
   - hypercalcemia (occasionally)
   - elevated alkaline phosphatase
   √ NOT visible on radiographs
   √ susceptible to fracture

B. WIDESPREAD BONE LESIONS
1. Diffuse skeletal metastases (most frequent) from prostate, breast, multiple myeloma, lymphoma, lung, bladder, colon, stomach
2. Myelofibrosis / myelosclerosis
3. Aplastic anemia, leukemia
4. Waldenström macroglobulinemia
5. Systemic mastocytosis
6. Widespread Paget disease

√ diffusely increased activity in bones: particularly prominent in axial skeleton, calvarium, mandible, costochondral junctions (= "rosary beading"), sternum (= "tie sternum"), long bones
√ increased metaphyseal + periarticular activity
√ increased bone-to-soft-tissue ratio
√ "absent kidney sign" = little / no activity in kidneys but good visualization of urinary bladder
√ femoral cortices become visible
CAVE: scan may be interpreted as normal, particularly in patients with poor renal function!

Hot Bone Lesions

mnemonic: "NATI MAN"
Neoplasm
Arthropathy
Trauma
Infection
Metastasis
Aseptic **N**ecrosis

Long Segmental Diaphyseal Uptake

A. BILATERALLY SYMMETRIC
1. Hypertrophic pulmonary osteoarthropathy
2. Thigh / shin splints = mechanical enthesopathy
3. Ribbing disease
4. Engelmann disease = progressive diaphyseal dysplasia

B. UNILATERAL
1. Inadvertent arterial injection
2. Melorheostosis
3. Chronic venous stasis
4. Osteogenesis imperfecta
5. Vitamin A toxicity
6. Osteomyelitis
7. Paget disease
8. Fibrous dysplasia

Photon-deficient Bone Lesion

= decreased radiotracer uptake

A. INTERRUPTION IN LOCAL BONE BLOOD FLOW
   = vessel trauma or vascular obstruction by thrombus / tumor
1. Early osteomyelitis
2. Radiation therapy
3. Posttraumatic aseptic necrosis
4. Sickle cell crisis

B. REPLACEMENT OF BONE BY DESTRUCTIVE PROCESS
1. Metastases (most common cause): central axis skeleton > extremity, most commonly in carcinoma of kidney + lung + breast + multiple myeloma
2. Primary bone tumor (exceptional)

mnemonic: "HM RANT"
Histiocytosis X
Multiple myeloma
Renal cell carcinoma
Anaplastic tumors (reticulum cell sarcoma)
Neuroblastoma
Thyroid carcinoma

Benign Bone Lesions

A. NO TRACER UPTAKE
1. Bone island
2. Osteopoikilosis
3. Osteopathia striata
4. Fibrous cortical defect
5. Nonossifying fibroma

B. INCREASED TRACER UPTAKE
1. Fibrous dysplasia
2. Paget disease
3. Eosinophilic granuloma
4. Melorheostosis
5. Osteoid osteoma
6. Enchondroma
7. Exostosis

Soft-tissue Uptake

A. PHYSIOLOGIC
1. Breast
2. Kidney: accentuated uptake with dehydration, antineoplastic drugs, gentamicin
3. Bowel: surgical diversion of urinary tract

B. FAULTY PREPARATION WITH RADIOCHEMICAL IMPURITY
(a) free pertechnetate (TcO^{4-})
Cause: introduction of air into the reaction vial
√ activity in mouth (saliva), salivary glands, thyroid, stomach (mucus-producing cells), GI tract (direct secretion + intestinal transport from gastric juices), choroid plexus
(b) Tc-99m MDP colloid
Cause: excess aluminum ions in generator eluate / patient ingestion of antacids; hydrolysis of stannous chloride to stannous hydroxide, excess hydrolized technetium
√ diffuse activity in liver + spleen

C. NEOPLASTIC CONDITIONS
(a) Benign tumor
1. Tumoral calcinosis
2. Myositis ossificans
(b) Primary malignant neoplasm
1. Extraskeletal osteosarcoma / soft-tissue sarcoma: bone forming
2. Neuroblastoma (35–74%): calcifying tumor
3. Breast carcinoma
4. Meningioma
5. Bronchogenic carcinoma (rare)
6. Pericardial tumor
(c) Metastases with extraosseous activity
1. to liver: mucinous carcinoma of colon, breast carcinoma, lung cancer, osteosarcoma
mnemonic: "LE COMBO"
Lung cancer
Esophageal carcinoma
Colon carcinoma
Oat cell carcinoma
Melanoma
Breast carcinoma
Osteogenic sarcoma
2. to lung: 20–40% of osteosarcoma metastatic to lung demonstrate Tc-99m MDP uptake
3. Malignant pleural effusion, ascites, pericardial effusion

D. INFLAMMATION
1. Inflammatory process (abscess, pyogenic / fungal infection):
(a) adsorption onto calcium deposits
(b) binding to denatured proteins, iron deposits, immature collagen
(c) hyperemia
2. Crystalline arthropathy (eg, gout)
3. Dermatomyositis, scleroderma
4. Radiation: eg, radiation pneumonitis
5. Necrotizing enterocolitis
6. Diffuse pericarditis
7. Bursitis
8. Pneumonia

E. TRAUMA
1. Healing soft-tissue wounds
2. Rhabdomyolysis: crush injury, surgical trauma, electrical burns, frostbite, severe exercise, alcohol abuse
3. Intramuscular injection sites: especially Imferon (= iron dextran) injections with resultant chemisorption; meperidine
4. Ischemic bowel infarction (late uptake)
5. Hematoma: soft tissue, subdural
6. Heterotopic ossification
7. Myocardial contusion, defibrillation, unstable angina pectoris
8. Lymphedema

F. METABOLIC
1. Hypercalcemia (eg, hyperparathyroidism):
(a) uptake enhanced by alkaline environment in stomach (gastric mucosa), lung (alveolar walls), kidneys (renal tubules)
(b) uptake with severe disease in myocardium, spleen, diaphragm, thyroid, skeletal muscle
2. Diffuse interstitial pulmonary calcifications: hyperparathyroidism, mitral stenosis
3. Amyloid deposits

G. ISCHEMIA WITH DYSTROPHIC SOFT-TISSUE CALCIFICATIONS
= necrosis with dystrophic calcification
@ Spleen: infarct (sickle cell anemia in 50%), microcalcification secondary to lymphoma, thalassemia major, hemosiderosis, glucose-6-phosphate-dehydrogenase deficiency
@ Liver: massive hepatic necrosis
@ Heart: transmural myocardial infarction, valvular calcification, amyloid deposition
@ Muscle: traumatic / ischemic skeletal muscle injury
@ Brain: cerebral infarction (damage of blood-brain barrier)
@ Kidney: nephrocalcinosis
@ Vessels: calcified wall, calcified thrombus

Abnormal Uptake Within Kidneys

1. Effect of chemotherapeutic drugs: bleomycin, cyclophosphamide, doxorubicin, mitomycin C, 6-mercaptopurine
2. S/P radiation therapy
3. Metastatic calcification
4. Pyelonephritis
5. Acute tubular necrosis
6. Iron overload
7. Multiple myeloma
8. Renal vein thrombosis
9. Ureteral obstruction

Abnormal Uptake Within Breast

1. Breast carcinoma
2. Prosthesis
3. Drug-induced

Abnormal Uptake In Ascitic, Pleural, Pericardial Effusion

1. Uremic renal disease
2. Infection
3. Malignant effusion

Incidental Urinary Tract Abnormalities

>50% of injected dose of Tc-99m MDP is excreted by 3 hours

A. BILATERAL DIFFUSE INCREASED UPTAKE
   = uptake greater than that of lumbar spine
   (a) excess tissue calcium
      1. Hyperparathyroidism
      2. Hypercalcemia
      3. Osteosarcoma metastatic to kidney
   (b) tissue damage
      1. Drug-induced nephrotoxicity
         (a) Chemotherapy (eg, cyclophosphamide, vincristine, doxorubicin, bleomycin, mitomycin-C, S-6-mercaptopurine, mitoxantrone)
         (b) aminoglycosides
         (c) amphotericin B
      2. Radiation therapy
      3. Necrotic renal cell carcinoma (rare)
      4. Renal metastasis (rare)
      5. Acute pyelonephritis
      6. Acute tubular necrosis
      7. Multiple myeloma
   (c) iron overload
      1. Sickle cell anemia
      2. Thalassemia major

   mnemonic: "RICH CON"
   Radiation therapy to kidney
   Iron overload
   Chemotherapy (cytoxan, vincristine, doxorubicin)
   Hyperparathyroidism
   Calcification (metastatic), **C**arcinoma
   Obstruction (urinary)
   Nephritis, **N**ormal variant

B. BILATERAL DECREASED RENAL UPTAKE
   (a) loss of renal function
      1. Endstage renal disease
   (b) increased osteoblastic activity (= superscan)

C. FOCALLY DECREASED RENAL UPTAKE
   (a) space-occupying lesion replacing normal renal parenchyma
      1. Abscess
      2. Cyst
      3. Primary / metastatic renal neoplasm
   (b) Scar
      1. Infarct
      2. Chronic pyelonephritis
      3. Partial nephrectomy

D. UNI- / BILATERAL FOCALLY INCREASED GU UPTAKE
   (a) urine accumulation
      1. normal upper pole calices (supine position)
      2. Urinary tract diversion / ileal conduit
      3. Urinoma

E. CHANGE IN LOCATION OF KIDNEY
   1. Congenital anomaly (eg, pelvic kidney)

BRAIN SCINTIGRAPHY

RADIONUCLIDE ANGIOGRAPHY

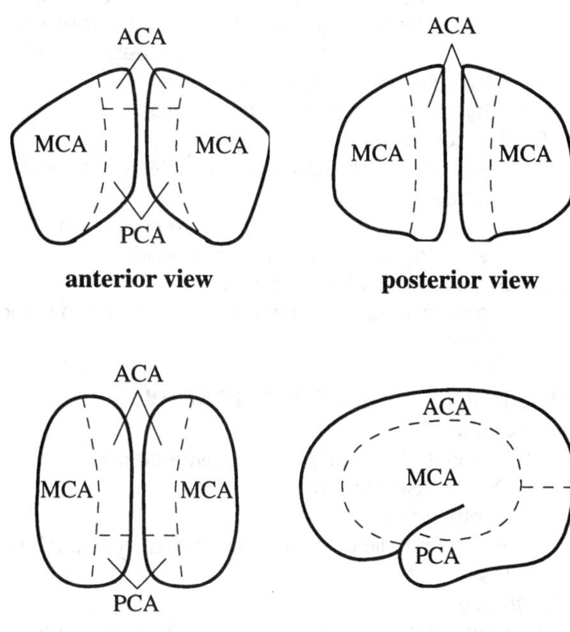

Mechanism of accumulation:
disruption of blood-brain barrier

Agents:

A. Tc-99m glucoheptonate
15–20 mCi bolus injection in <2 mL saline; 30 flow images of 2 seconds' duration; static image of 1 million counts after 4 hours; delayed image after 24 hours (higher target-to-background ratio than DTPA)

B. Tc-99m DTPA

C. Thallium-201: best predictor for tumor burden

√ increased perfusion in
1. Primary / metastatic brain tumor
2. AVM, large aneurysm, tumor shunting
3. Luxury perfusion after infarction
4. Infections (eg, herpes simplex encephalitis)
5. Extracranial lesions: bone metastasis, fibrous dysplasia, Paget disease, eosinophilic granuloma, fractures, burr holes, craniotomy defects

√ asymmetric decreased perfusion in acute / chronic cerebrovascular disease + mass lesions (tumor, hemorrhage, subdural hematoma)

√ "flip-flop" phenomenon (= decreased perfusion in arterial phase, equalization of activity in capillary phase, increased activity in venous phase) in CVA secondary to late arrival of blood via collaterals + slow washout

√ bilateral absent flow in brain death

Ceretec Brain Imaging

Pharmacokinetics:
lipophilic radiopharmaceutical distributing across a functioning blood-brain barrier proportional to cerebral blood flow; no redistribution

Indication:
acute cerebral infarct imaging before evidence of CT / MRI pathology; positive findings within 1 hour of event

I-123 Spectamine Brain Imaging

Pharmacokinetics:
initially distributes proportional to regional cerebral blood flow with increased flow to basal ganglia and cerebellum; homogeneous uptake in gray matter; decreased activity in white matter; redistribution over time

√ activity in an area of initial deficit on reimaging (after 4 hours) implies improved prognosis

Seizures

Abnormal cerebral radionuclide angiography within 1 week of seizure activity even without underlying organic lesion

Etiology:
(1) 35% cerebral tumors (meningioma in 34%, metastases in 17%)
(2) Cerebral vascular disease (more common in age >50 years)
(3) Trauma, inflammation, CNS effects of systemic disease

√ transient hyperperfusion of involved hemisphere

Brain Tumor

Good correlation between hyperperfusion and enlarged supplying vessels

Etiology:
(1) Meningioma (increased activity in 60–80%);
(2) Metastases (increased activity in 11–23%);
(3) Vascular metastases: thyroid, renal cell, melanoma, anaplastic tumors from lung / breast

Cerebral Death

Increased intracranial pressure results in markedly decreased cerebral perfusion, thrombosis, total cerebral infarction

Path: severe brain edema, diffuse liquefactive necrosis

√ carotid arteries visualized (= confirmation of good bolus)

√ activity stops abruptly at the skull base

√ sagittal sinus not visualized

√ activity in arteries of face + scalp with "hot nose" sign

DDx by EEG:
severe barbiturate intoxication may produce a flat EEG response in the absence of brain death

Arterial Stenosis

◊ Radionuclide angiography of limited value!
(1) Complete occlusion / >80% stenosis of ICA: 53–80% sensitivity
(2) 50–80% stenosis of ICA: 50% sensitivity
(3) <50% stenosis of ICA: 10% sensitivity

Problematic lesions:
(1) Bilaterally similar degree of stenosis
(2) Occlusion of MCA + unilateral ACA
(3) Vertebrobasilar occlusive disease (20% sensitivity)

POSITRON EMISSION TOMOGRAPHY

A. REGIONAL CEREBRAL BLOOD FLOW
(a) breathing of carbon monoxide (C-11 and O-15), which concentrates in RBCs
(b) Xe-133 inhalation / injection into ICA / IV injection after dissolution in saline: volume distribution is in the water space of the brain; no correction for recirculation necessary because all Xe is exhaled during lung passage, but correction for scalp + calvarial activity is required (for inhalation method)
√ washout rate of grey matter:white matter = 4–5:1

B. GLUCOSE METABOLISM
for measurements of metabolic rate + mapping of functional activity
(a) C-11 glucose: rapid uptake, metabolization, and excretion by brain
(b) F-18 fluorodeoxyglucose (FDG): diffuses across blood-brain barrier + competes with glucose for phosphorylation by hexokinase, which traps FDG-6-phosphate within mitochondria; FDG-6-phosphate cannot enter most metabolic pathways (eg, glycolysis, storage as glycogen) and accumulates proportional to intracellular glycolytic activity; FDG-6-phosphate is dephosphorylated slowly by glucose-6-phosphatase and then escapes cell

Indications:
1. Focal epilepsy prior to seizure surgery
   √ interictal decreased uptake of FDG of >20% at seizure focus (70% sensitivity, 90% for temporal lobe hypometabolism)
   √ hypermetabolism within 30 minutes of seizure
   √ measurement of opiate receptor density with C-11-labeled carfentanil (= high-affinity opium agonist) uptake by μ receptors (found in thalamus, striatum, periaqueductal gray matter, amygdala), which mediate analgesia and respiratory depression
2. Alzheimer disease
   • clinical diagnosis false positive in 35%
   √ bilateral temporoparietal hypoperfusion + hypometabolism resulting in decreased FDG uptake (92–100% sensitive)
   √ sparing of sensory and motor cortex + basal ganglia + thalamus
   DDx: frontal lobe dementia, primary progressive aphasia without dementia, normal-pressure hydrocephalus, multi-infarct dementia
3. Parkinson disease
   = deficient presynaptic terminals with normal postsynaptic dopaminergic receptors
   • clinical diagnosis in 50–70% accurate
   DDx: drug-induced chorea, Huntington disease, tardive dyskinesia, progressive supranuclear palsy, Shy-Drager syndrome, striatonigral degeneration, alcohol-related cerebellar dysfunction, olivopontocerebellar atrophy
4. Huntington disease, senile chorea
   √ hypometabolism of basal ganglia
5. Schizophrenia
   √ abnormally reduced glucose activity in frontal lobes
   √ dopamine receptors in caudate / putamen elevated to 3 x that of normal levels
6. Stroke, cerebral vasospasm
   √ disassociated oxygen metabolism + brain blood flow

RADIONUCLIDE CISTERNOGRAPHY

Indications:
1. Suspected normal pressure hydrocephalus
2. Occult CSF rhinorrhea / otorrhea
3. Ventricular shunt
4 Porencephalic cyst, leptomeningeal cyst, posterior fossa cyst

Technique:
1. Measurement of spinal subarachnoid pressure
2. Sample of CSF for analysis
3. Subarachnoid injection of radiotracer

Normal study (completed within 48 hours):
symmetric activity sequentially from basal cisterns, up the sylvian fissures + anterior commissure, eventual ascent over cortices with parasagittal concentration
√ image lumbar region immediately after injection to assure subarachnoid injection
√ activity in basal cistern by 2–4 hours
√ activity at vertex by 24–48 hours
√ no / minimal lateral ventricular activity (may be transient in older patients)

Agents:
1. **Indium-111 DTPA**
   Physical half-life: 2.8 days
   Gamma photons: 173 keV (90%), 247 keV (94%) detected with dual pulse height analyzer
   Dose: 250–500 μCi
   Radiation dose: 9 rads/500 μCi for brain + spinal cord (in normal patients)
   Imaging: at 10-minute intervals / 500,000 counts up to 4–6 hours; repeat scans at 24, 48, 72 hours

2. **Technetium-99m DTPA**
   Not entirely suitable for imaging up to 48–72 hours; DTPA tends to have faster flow rate than CSF; used for shunt evaluation + CSF leak study since leak increases CSF flow

Dose: 4–10 mCi
Radiation dose: 4 rads for brain + spinal cord

3. **Iodine-131 serum albumin** (RISA)
prototype agent; beta emitter
Physical half-life: 8 days; high radiation dose of 7.1 rads/100 μCi; no longer used secondary to pyrogenic reactions

4. **Ytterbium-169 DTPA**
Physical half-life: 32 days
Gamma decay: 63 keV; 177 keV (17%); 198 keV (25%); 308 keV;
dual pulse height analyzer set for 177 + 198 keV
Dose: 500 μCi
Radiation dose: 9 rads/500 mCi for brain + spinal cord (in normal patients)

CSF Leak Study

Purpose: localization of origin of CSF leak in patient with CSF rhinorrhea / otorrhea

Causes of dural fistula:
(a) traumatic: in 30% of basilar skull fractures
(b) nontraumatic: brain, pituitary and skull tumors; skull infections; congenital defects

Location of dural fistula:
cribriform plate > ethmoid cells > frontal sinus

Method:
1. Weigh cotton pledgets
2. Pledgets placed by ENT surgeon in the anterior and posterior turbinates bilaterally
3. Radiopharmaceutical injected intrathecally via lumbar puncture; immediate postinjection view of lumbar region to assure intrathecal placement
4. Pledgets removed and weighed 4–6 hours after lumbar injection
5. Pledget activity counted + indexed to weight
6. Results compared with 0.5-mL serum specimens drawn at the time of pledget removal
7. Pledget to serum count ratio of >1.5 is evidence of CSF leak
8. With active leak patient should be placed in various positions with various maneuvers to accentuate leak

Hydrocephalus

A. NORMAL-PRESSURE HYDROCEPHALUS
√ reversal of normal CSF flow dynamic = tracer moves from basal cisterns into 4th, 3rd, and lateral ventricles
√ loss of w sign

B. OBSTRUCTIVE HYDROCEPHALUS
√ delay (up to 48 hours) for tracer to surround convexities + reach arachnoid villi
√ positive w sign

THYROID AND PARATHYROID SCINTIGRAPHY

THYROID SCINTIGRAPHY

SUPPRESSION SCAN
= to define autonomy of a nodule
√ suppression of a hot nodule following T_3/T_4 administration is proof that autonomy does not exist

STIMULATION SCAN
= to demonstrate thyroid tissue suppressed by hyperfunctioning nodule
√ administration of TSH documents functioning thyroid tissue (rarely done)

PERCHLORATE WASHOUT TEST
= to demonstrate organification defect
√ repeat measurement of radioiodine uptake following oral potassium perchlorate shows lower values if organification defect present

Tc-99m pertechnetate

Physical decay: 10 mCi Tc-99m decays to 2.7×10^{-7} mCi Tc-99
Physical half-life: 2×10^5 years
Biologic half-life: 6 hours
Decay: by photon emission of 140 keV

Quality control:
(1) <0.1% Mo-99 (= 1 μCi/mCi), maximum of Mo-99 at 5 μCi
(2) <0.5 mg aluminum/10 mCi Tc-99m
(3) <0.01% radionuclide impurities

Administration: oral / IV
Dose: 3–5 mCi administered IV 20 minutes prior to imaging (100–300 mrad/mCi)

Pharmacokinetics:
Uptake: in thyroid, salivary glands, gastric mucosa, choroid plexus
Excretion: mostly in feces, some in urine

Uptake in thyroid:
0.5–3.7% at 20 minutes (time of maximum uptake) assessment of trapping function only; NO organification; may be almost completely discharged by perchlorate
Comparison to iodine:
(a) target-to-background ratio less favorable than with iodine
(b) greater photon flux than iodine = detectability of small thyroid lesions (>8 mm) is improved
(c) lesions with pertechnetate-iodine discordance (= hot on Tc-99m pertechnetate + cold on radioiodine) are very rare + due to Tc-99m–avid cancer

Imaging:
(a) Collimator: usually with pinhole collimator for image magnification (5-mm hole)
(b) Distance: selected so that organ makes up 2/3 of field of view; significant distortion of organ periphery occurs if detector too close
(c) Counts: 200,000–300,000 counts are usually acquired within 5 minutes after a dose of 5–10 mCi of Tc-99m pertechnetate
(d) Image must include markers for scale + anatomic landmarks + palpatory findings

Iodine-123

◊ Agent of choice for thyroid imaging!
Production:
in accelerator; contamination with I-124 dependent on source (Te-122 in ~ 5%, Xe-123 in ~ 0.5%); contamination with I-125 increases with time elapsed after production
Physical half-life: 13.3 hours
Decay: by electron capture with photon emission at 159 keV (83% abundance) + x-ray of 28 keV (87% abundance)
Dose: 200–400 μCi orally 24 hours prior to imaging (radiation dose of 7.5 mrads/μCi)
Uptake: iodine readily absorbed from GI tract (10–30% by 24 hours), distributed primarily in extracellular fluid spaces; trapped + organified by thyroid gland; trapped by stomach + salivary glands
Excretion: via kidneys in 35–75% during first 24 hours + GI tract

Disadvantages compared with Tc-99m pertechnetate:
(1) More expensive
(2) Less available
(3) More time-consuming
(4) Higher dose to thyroid (but less to whole body)

Iodine-131

Indication: thyroid uptake study, thyroid imaging, treatment of hyperthyroidism, treatment of functioning thyroid cancer, imaging of functioning metastases
Production: by fission decay
Physical half-life: 8.05 days (allows storing for long periods)

Decay: principal gamma energy of 364 keV (82% abundance) + significant beta decay fraction of a mean energy of 192 keV (92% abundance)
Dose: 30–50 μCi (1.2 rad/μCi = 50 rad for thyroid)

Radiation dose:
(90% from beta decay, 10% from gamma radiation)
0.6 mrad/mCi for whole body; 1.2 mrad/μCi for thyroid (critical organ)
Pharmacokinetics: identical to I-123

Disadvantages:
(a) Too energetic for gamma camera, well suited for rectilinear scanner with limited resolution
(b) High radiation dose prohibits use for diagnostic purposes
(c) Ectopic thyroid tissue just as well detectable with I-123 or Tc-99m pertechnetate

Iodine fluorescence imaging
Technique:
collimated beam of 60 keV gamma photons from an Am-241 source is directed at thyroid, which results in production of K-characteristic x-rays of 28.5 keV; x-rays are detected by semiconductor detector
Advantages:
(1) No interference with flooded iodine pool / thyroid medication
(2) Measures total iodine content
(3) Low radiation exposure (15 mrad) acceptable for children + pregnant women
Disadvantage: dedicated equipment necessary

Thyroid uptake measurements
Agents: I-123 / I-131 (easier to use), Tc-99m pertechnetate (requires calibration)
Uptake:
measurements at both 4 and 24 hours prevent missing the occasional rapid-turnover hyperthyroid patient returning to normal by 24 hours; uptake values distinguish different causes of hyperthyroidism
(a) normal: >25% at 4 hours, >35% at 24 hours
(b) increased: in Graves disease
(c) decreased: in subacute thyroiditis
N.B.: Uptake values do not diagnose hyperthyroidism, which is done with laboratory values (T_4, T_3, TSH) and clinical history

PARATHYROID SCINTIGRAPHY
Technetium-thallium subtraction imaging
Sensitivity: 72–92% (depending on size, smallest adenoma was 60 mg)
Specificity: 43% (benign thyroid adenomas, carcinomas, lymph nodes also concentrate thallium)

Method:
(1) IV injection of 1–3.5 mCi Tl-201 chloride; images recorded for 15 minutes with 2-mm pinhole collimator
√ concentrates in normal thyroid + enlarged parathyroid glands (extraction proportional to regional blood flow + tissue cellularity)
(2) IV injection of 1–10 mCi Tc-99m pertechnetate; images recorded at 1-minute intervals for 20 minutes
√ pertechnetate concentrates only in thyroid
(3) Computerized subtraction
√ focal / multifocal excess Tl-201

Limitations:
(1) unfavorable dosimetry + poor quality images of Tl-201 (up to 3.5 mCi, 80 keV photons)
(2) prolonged patient immobilization (motion artifact)
(3) processing artifacts (eg, over- / undersubtraction)
(4) poor Tc-99m thyroid uptake from interfering medications / recent iodinated contrast media
(5) parathyroid pathology may be mimicked by coexisting thyroid disease (eg, nonfunctioning adenoma, multinodular goiter)
Indication:
Localization of one / more parathyroid adenoma (hyperplasia not visualized), may be more sensitive than CT / MRI in detection of ectopic mediastinal parathyroid tissue and in postoperative context

Technetium-99m sestamibi
= Tc-99m MIBI
Sensitivity: 88–100% (smallest adenoma weighed 150 mg); 91% for early SPECT imaging
◊ For unknown reasons even large tumors (2 g) may not accumulate sufficient MIBI for detection!
Pharmacokinetics:
MIBI localizes in myocardium + mitochondria-rich tumors proportional to regional blood flow + cellular metabolic activity; MIBI washes out of thyroid quickly, but is retained in abnormal parathyroids (= need for dual-phase study)
Method:
1. IV injection of 20–25 mCi Tc-99m MIBI
2. 10–30 minutes after injection anterior cervicothoracic images (5 minutes/view) with large-field-of-view camera equipped with low-energy high-resolution parallel-hole collimator
3. Repeat set of images at 2–4 hours post injection (10 minutes/view)
4. Adjunctive imaging with thyroid-selective agent for computer-aided subtractions is optional

Advantages (over thallium):
A. Physical properties:
— optimal gamma emission (140 keV)
— abundant photons (high dose of 20 mCi)
— favorable dosimetry
— high parathyroid-to-thyroid ratio
— unaffected by medications / iodinated contrast
B. Technical features:
— Single readily available radiopharmaceutical
— Simple protocol of early + delayed images
— No prolonged patient immobilization
— No subtraction study / computer processing
— SPECT / multiple projections possible
C. Scan interpretation
— sharp images
— clear visualization of abnormal parathyroid glands
— ectopic sites surveyed

LUNG SCINTIGRAPHY

PERFUSION AGENTS

Tc-99m Macroaggregated Albumin (MAA)

Preparation:

human serum albumin (HSA) is heat-denatured + pH adjusted; added stannous chloride precipitates albumin into tin-containing macroaggregates; lyophilization prolongs stability; added Tc-99m pertechnetate is reduced by $SnCl_2$ and tagged onto the MAA particles

Quality control (USP guidelines):

(1) 90% of particles should have a diameter between 10–90 μm
(2) No particle should exceed 150 μ
(3) Should be at least 90% pure (by ascending chromatography)
(4) A batch of Tc-99m MAA should not be used >8 hours after preparation
(5) Preparation should not be backflushed with blood into syringe, causes "hot spots" on lungs

Physical half-life: 6 hours
Biologic half-life: 6 hours
Dose: approximately 2–4–6 mCi + 0.14 μg/kg albumin which corresponds to >60,000 particles (recommended number particles is 200,000–500,000 particles for even spatial distribution + good image quality)

} IV injection in supine position to give an even distribution between base + apex of lung (ventral to posterior gradient persists)
} imaging in upright position to allow maximum expansion of lung, especially at lung bases

N.B.: reduce number of particles to 80,000 in
(a) critically ill patients with severe COPD, on mechanical ventilator support, documented pulmonary arterial hypertension, significant left-to-right cardiac shunts need reduction in number of particles but not tagged activity!
(b) children up to age 5 need reduction in number of particles + tagged activity!

Radiation dose (rads/mCi):

0.013 for whole body, 0.25 for lung (critical organ), 0.01 for gonads

PHYSIOLOGY

90% of MAA particles act as microemboli and will be trapped in lung capillaries on first pass; there are an estimated 600 million pulmonary arterioles small enough to trap the particles; the effect is insignificant physiologically as only 500,000 particles are injected per study; 0.22% of capillaries become occluded (= 2 of 1000); protein is lysed within 6–8 hours and taken up by RES; particles <1 μ are phagocytized by RES in liver + spleen

IMAGING

Large-field-of-view scintillation camera + parallel-hole low-energy collimator with identical recording times for corresponding views

Views: anterior, posterior, lateral, posterior oblique (additional information in 50% due to segmental delineation of basal segments and separation of both lungs), anterior oblique (additional information in 15%); oblique views reduce equivocal findings from 30% to 15%

Tc-99m Human Albumin Microspheres

Particle size: 20–30 μ
Biologic half-life: 8 hours

VENTILATION AGENTS

Xe-133, Xe-127, Xe-125, Kr-81m, N-13, O_2-15, CO_2-11, CO-11, radioactive aerosol (Tc-99m–DTPA, Tc-99m-PYP, Tc-99m–labeled ultrafine dry dispersion of carbon "soot")

Xenon-133

Fission product of U-235

Decay: to stable Cs-133 under emission of beta particle (374 keV), gamma ray (81 keV), x-ray (31 keV); beta-component responsible for high radiation dose of 1 rad to lung)

Physical half-life: 5.2 days
Biologic half-life: 2–3 minutes
Physical properties: highly soluble in oil + grease, absorbed by plastic syringe

Administration: injection into mouth piece of a disposable breathing unit at the beginning of a maximal inspiration
Dose: 15–20 mCi

TECHNIQUE

Ventilation study preferably done before perfusion scan to avoid interference with higher-energy Tc-99m (Compton scatter from Tc-99m into lower Xe-133 photopeak); [may be feasible after perfusion scan if dose of Tc-99m MAA is kept below 2 mCi + concentration of Xe-133 is above 10 mCi/l of air and if Xe-133 acquisition times for washing, equilibrium, washout images are kept to about 30 seconds]
Posterior imaging routine, ideally in upright position

Phase 1 = single-breath image:
= inhalation of 10–20 mCi Xe-133 to vital capacity with breath-holding over 10–15–20 seconds (65% sensitivity for abnormalities)
√ cold spot is abnormal

Phase 2 = equilibrium phase:
= tidal breathing = closed-loop rebreathing of Xe-133 + oxygen for 3–4–5 minutes for tracer to enter poorly ventilated areas; also functions as internal control for air leaks; posterior oblique images + posterior images are obtained to improve correlation with perfusion scan.
√ activity distribution corresponds to aerated lung

Phase 3 = washout phase:
= clearance phase after readjusting intake valves of spirometer permitting patient to inhale ambient air and to exhale Xe-133 into shielded charcoal trap; washout phase should last >5 min
} images taken at 30–60 sec intervals for >5 min
√ rapid clearance within 90 seconds with slight retention in upper zones is normal
√ tracer retention (hot spot) at 3 minutes reveals areas of air-trapping

√ poor image quality secondary to significant scatter
√ abnormal scan:
(a) delayed washing (initial 30 seconds of tidal breathing)
(b) tracer accumulation on equilibrium views (partial obstruction with collateral air drift + diffusion into affected area via bloodstream)
(c) delayed washout = retention >3 minutes
(d) tracer retention in regions not seen on initial single-breath view (from collateral airdrift into abnormal lung zones)

Xenon-127

Cyclotron-produced with high cost

Physical half-life: 36.4 days
Photon energies: 172 keV (22%), 203 keV (65%)
Advantages:
(1) High photon energy allows ventilation study following perfusion study
(2) Decreased radiation dose (0.3 rad)
(3) Storage capability because of long physical half-life

Krypton-81m

insoluble inert gas; eluted from Rb-81 generator (half-life of 4.7 hours); decays to Kr-81 by isomeric transition
Physical half-life: 13 seconds
Biologic half-life: <1 minute
Principal photon energy: 190 keV (65% abundance)
Advantages:
(1) Higher photon energy than Tc-99m so that ventilation scan can be performed following perfusion study
(2) Each ventilation scan can be matched to perfusion scan without moving patient
(3) Can be used in patients on respirator (no contamination due to short half-life)
(4) Low radiation dose (during continuous inhalation for 6–8 views 100 mrad are delivered)

Disadvantages:
(1) High cost
(2) Limited availability (generator good only for one day, so weekend availability may not be possible
(3) No washout images possible due to short half-life
(4) Decreased resolution due to septal penetration with low-energy collimators

√ lack of activity = abnormal area (tracer activity is proportional to regional distribution of tidal volume because of short biologic half-life, washout phase not available)

Tc-99m DTPA aerosol

= Tc-99m diethylenetriaminepentaacetic radioaerosol
= UltraVent®
Biological half-life: 55 min
Administration: delivery through a nebulizer during inspiration
Dose: 30–45 mCi in 2–3 mL of saline at a nebulizer flow rate of 8–10 L/min

PHYSIOLOGY
radioaerosols are small particles that become impacted in central airways, sediment in more distal airways, experience random contact with alveolar walls during diffusion in alveoli; crosses respiratory epithelium with rapid removal by bloodstream
◊ Less physiologic indicator of ventilation + subject to nebulization technique
◊ Erect position preferable for basilar perfusion defects (dependent lung region receives more ventilation + radiotracer)

Carbon dioxide tracer

O-15–labeled carbon dioxide
Physical half-life: 2 minutes (requires on-site cyclotron)

PHYSIOLOGY:
inhalation of carbon dioxide; rapid diffusion across alveolar-capillary membrane; clearance from lung within seconds
√ cold spot due to failure of tracer entry into airway = airway disease
√ hot spot due to delayed / absent tracer clearance = perfusion defect (87% sensitivity, 92% specificity)

Indications:
1. Emboli can be detected in preexisting cardiopulmonary disease
2. Equivocal / indeterminate V/Q studies

TUMOR IMAGING

Positron emission tomography

Dose: 10 mCi FDG
Technique:
} patient fasts for 4 hours
◊ Elevated serum glucose may cause a decrease in FDG uptake!
} imaging 30–60 minutes after IV injection in 30–45 image planes (15 cm axial field of view; resolution of 5 mm)

} calculation of standardized uptake ratio (SUR) in region of interest (ROI) = mean activity in ROI [mCi/mL] divided by injected dose [mCi]

◊ SUR >2.5 indicates malignant disease

Indications:

(1) Focal pulmonary abnormality
accurate differentiation of benign and malignant lesions as small as 1 cm
√ low FDG uptake = benign
√ increased FDG uptake = cancer, active TB, histoplasmosis, rheumatoid nodule

(2) Staging lung cancer
◊ Occult metastases detected in up to 40% of cases!
(a) Intrathoracic lymph nodes
√ lymph node with short-axis diameter > 1 cm by CT + not FDG avid = 100% NPV
√ small lymph node by CT + intense FDG uptake = 100% PPV
(b) adrenal metastasis: 100% sensitive, 80% specific

(3) Recurrent disease
√ increased FDG uptake at sites of residual radiographic abnormality >8 weeks after completion of therapy

QUANTITATIVE LUNG PERFUSION IMAGING

Indication:
determination of postresection pulmonary function when combined with pulmonary function testing (FEV_1)

Technique:
1. Acquire posterior and anterior perfusion (MAA) image and calculate geometric mean
2. Separate into right + left and into 2 equal lung zones from top to bottom, which yields 4 segments (upper left, bottom right, etc)

Result:
activity in each segment is compared with total activity, which yields % perfusion to each lung field

Unilateral Lung Perfusion

Incidence: 2%

A. PULMONARY EMBOLISM (23%)
B. AIRWAY DISEASE
(a) Unilateral pleural / parenchymal disease (23%)
(b) Bronchial obstruction
1. Bronchogenic carcinoma (23%)
2. Bronchial adenoma
3. Aspirated endobronchial foreign body
C. CONGENITAL HEART DISEASE (15%)

Interpretation Criteria for V/Q Lung Scans

Probability of PE	Biello criteria	PIOPED criteria
Normal	√ normal perfusion	√ normal perfusion
Low (~ 10%)	√ small (<25% segment) V/Q mismatches √ focal V/Q matches without corresponding CXR abnormality √ perfusion defects substantially smaller than CXR abnormality	√ small perfusion defects regardless of number / ventilation scan finding / CXR finding √ perfusion defect substantially smaller than CXR abnormality; ventilation findings irrelevant √ V/Q match in ≤50% of one lung / ≤75% of upper / mid / lower lung zone; CXR normal / nearly normal √ single moderate perfusion defect with normal CXR; ventilation findings irrelevant √ nonsegmental perfusion defects
Indeterminate (30 – 40%)	√ severe COPD with perfusion defects √ perfusion defect + CXR opacity of same size √ single moderate V/Q mismatch without corresponding CXR abnormality	√ 1 large(segmental) ± 1 moderate (subsegmental) V/Q mismatch √ 1–3 moderate (subsegmental) V/Q mismatches √ 1 matched V/Q with normal CXR
High (~ 90%)	√ perfusion defects substantially larger than CXR abnormalities √ ≥2 moderate (25–90% segment) / ≥2 large (>90% segment) V/Q mismatches; no corresponding CXR abnormality	√ ≥2 large (segmental) perfusion defects; ventilation scan + CXR findings normal √ >2 large (segmental) perfusion defects substantially larger than matching ventilation / CXR abnormality √ ≥2 moderate (subsegemtal) + 1 large (segmental) perfusion defect; ventilation + CXR findings normal √ ≥4 moderate (subsegmental) perfusion defects; ventilation + CXR findings normal

Lung Segments

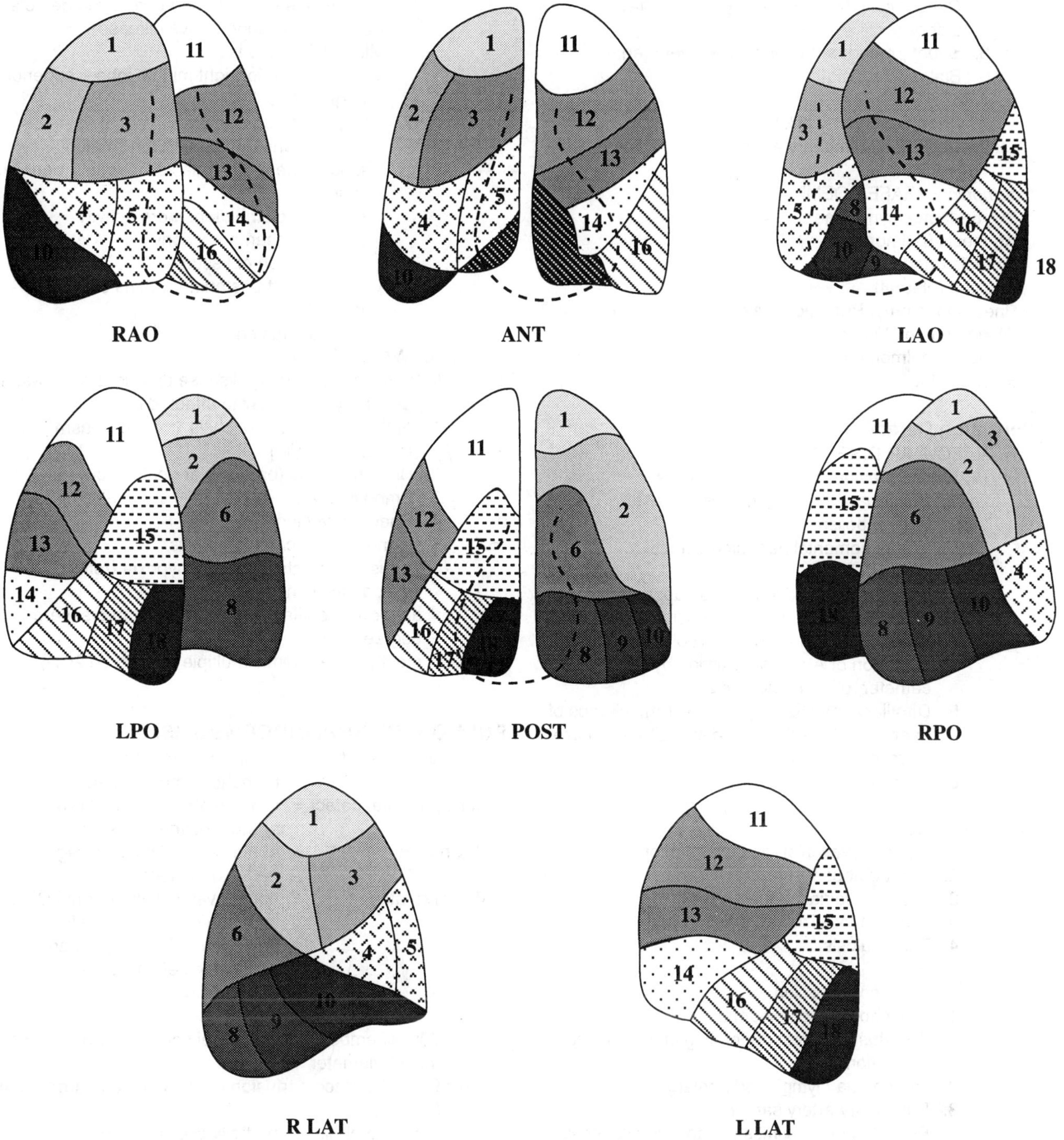

RAO ANT LAO

LPO POST RPO

R LAT L LAT

RUL		RML		RLL		LUL		LLL	
1	apical	4	lateral	6	superior	11	apicoposterior	15	superior
2	posterior	5	medial	7	mediobasal	12	anterior	16	anteromedial basal
3	anterior			8	posterobasal	13	superior lingual	17	laterobasal
				9	laterobasal	14	inferior lingual	18	posterobasal
				10	anterobasal				

D. ARTERIAL DISEASE
   1. Swyer-James syndrome (8%)
   2. Congenital pulmonary artery hypoplasia / stenosis
   3. Shunt procedure to pulmonary artery (eg, Blalock-Taussig)
E. ABSENT LUNG
   1. Pneumonectomy (8%)
   2. Unilateral pulmonary agenesis

mnemonic: "SAFE POEM"
Swyer-James syndrome
Agenesis (pulmonary)
Fibrosis (mediastinal)
Effusion (pleural)
Pneumonectomy, **P**neumothorax
Obstruction by tumor
Embolus (pulmonary)
Mucous plug

Perfusion Defects

A. VASCULAR DISEASE
   (a) Acute / previous pulmonary embolus
      1. Pulmonary thromboembolic disease
      2. Fat embolism
         √ nonsegmental perfusion defect
      3. Air embolism
         √ characteristic decortication appearance in uppermost portion on perfusion scintigraphy
      4. Embolus of tumor / cotton wool / balloon for occlusion of AVM / obstruction by Swan-Ganz catheter, other foreign body
      5. Dirofilaria immitis (dog heartworm): clumps of heartworms break off cardiac wall + embolize pulmonary arterial tree
      6. Sickle cell disease

   (b) Vasculitis
      1. Collagen vascular disease: sarcoidosis
      2. IV drug abuse
      3. Previous radiation therapy:
         √ defect localized to radiation port
      4. Tuberculosis

   (c) Vascular compression
      1. Bronchogenic carcinoma:
         √ perfusion defect depending on tumor size + location
      2. Lymphoma / lymph node enlargement
      3. Pulmonary artery sarcoma
      4. Fibrosing mediastinitis due to histoplasmosis
      5. Idiopathic pulmonary fibrosis:
         √ small subsegmental defects in both lungs
      6. Aortic aneurysm (large saccular / dissecting)
      7. Intrathoracic stomach

   (d) Altered pulmonary circulation
      1. Absence / hypoplasia of pulmonary artery
      2. Peripheral pulmonary artery stenosis
      3. Bronchopulmonary sequestration
      4. Primary pulmonary hypertension
         √ upward redistribution + large hilar defects
         √ multiple small peripheral perfusion defects
      5. Pulmonary venoocclusive disease
      6. Mitral valve disease
         √ predilection for right middle lobe + superior segments of lower lobes
      7. Congestive heart failure
         √ diffuse nonsegmental VQ mismatch
         √ enlargement of cardiac silhouette + perihilar regions
         √ reversed distribution: more activity anteriorly than posteriorly
         √ accentuation of fissures
         √ flattening of posterior margins of lung (lateral view)
         √ pleural effusion

B. AIRWAY DISEASE
   ◊ Nearly all pulmonary disease produces decreased pulmonary blood flow to affected lung zones!
   1. Asthma, chronic bronchitis, bronchospasm, mucous plugging
   2. Bronchiectasis (bronchiolar destruction)
   3. Emphysema (bulla / cyst)
   4. Pneumonia / lung abscess
   5. Lymphangitic carcinomatosis
   √ perfusion defects in area of hypoxia (reflex vasoconstriction)
   √ abnormal ventilation to a similar / more severe degree
   √ mostly nonanatomic multiple defects (in 20%)

PULMONARY THROMBOEMBOLISM

Segmental defect = involves >75% of a known bronchopulmonary segment
Subsegmental defect = involves 25–75% of a known bronchopulmonary segment
V/Q match = abnormal ventilation in region of perfusion defect
V/Q mismatch = normal ventilation / normal CXR in region of perfusion defect or perfusion defect larger than ventilation defect / CXR abnormality

Perfusion images will detect:
   (a) 90% of emboli that completely occlude a vessel >1 mm in diameter
   (b) 90% of surface perfusion defects that are larger than 2 x 2 cm
   (c) 26% of emboli that partially occlude a vessel
   • A history of prior PE decreases probability of acute embolism because small V/Q mismatches never resolve!

Therapeutic implications:
   (a) high probability scan : treat for PE
   (b) indeterminate scan : pulmonary angiogram
   (c) low probability scan : consider other diagnosis, unless clinical suspicion very high

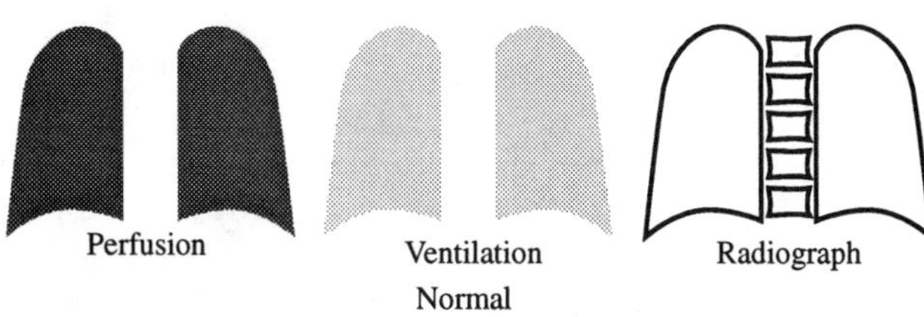

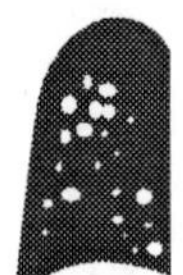
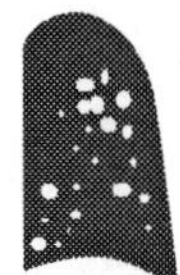
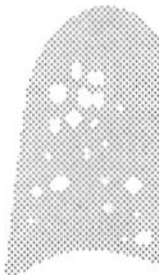
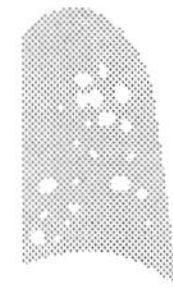

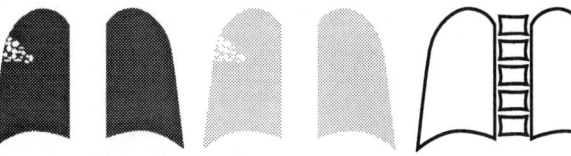

Matching nonsegmental V/Q defects & normal CXR = **low probability**

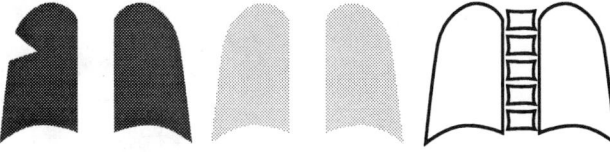

No definite V/Q mismatch & normal CXR = **moderate probability**

Segmental perfusion defect & normal ventilation = **high probability**

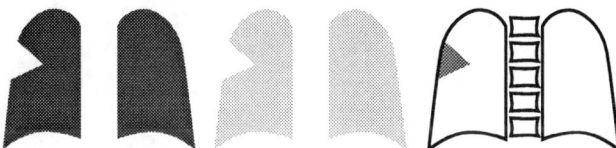

Matching segmental V/Q defect & CXR opacity = **indeterminate**

PIOPED (Prospective Investigation of Pulmonary Embolism Diagnosis) study results:

Probability of PE	in	angiogram positive in
high	13%	88%
intermediate	39%	33%
low	34%	16%
normal	14%	9%

Indications for pulmonary angiography:

1. Embolectomy is a therapeutic option
2. Indeterminate V/Q scan with high clinical suspicion + risky anticoagulation therapy
3. Specific diagnosis necessary for proper management (vasculitis, drug induced, lung cancer with predominant vascular involvement)

Overall accuracy:

68% for perfusion scan only,
84% for ventilation-perfusion scan

◊ 100% sensitivity in detection of PE is due to the occurrence of multiple emboli (usually >6–8), at least one of which causes a perfusion defect!
◊ A normal perfusion scan virtually excludes PE!
◊ In an individual <45 years of age a subsegmental perfusion defect + pleuritic chest pain in the same region is indicative of pulmonary embolism in 77%! (DDx: idiopathic / viral pleurisy)
◊ 73–82% of patients have equivocal perfusion scans (ie, low and intermediate probability)!
◊ Interobserver variability for intermediate- and low-probability scans is 30%!

<u>False-positive scans:</u> nonthrombotic emboli, IV drug abuse, vasculitis, redistribution of flow, acute asthma (due to mucous plugging)

<u>False-negative scans:</u> saddle embolus

√ associated with normal ventilation scan in >90%
√ "stripe sign" = rim of preserved peripheral activity to a perfusion defect usually indicates
  (a) nonembolic cause
  (b) old / resolving pulmonary embolism

Correlation with CXR:

CXR category	nondiagnostic V/Q scan
no acute abnormality	12%
linear atelectasis	12%
pulmonary edema	12%
pleural effusion	36%
parenchymal consolidation	82%

√ focal lung opacity + not ventilated + not perfused = "indeterminate scan"
  Cause: pneumonia, pulmonary embolism with infarction, segmental atelectasis
  √ perfusion defect larger than CXR opacity = high probability for PE
  √ perfusion defect substantially smaller than CXR opacity = low probability for PE
  √ perfusion defect of comparable size = intermediate probability
√ focal lung opacity (not changed >1 week) + not ventilated + not perfused = low probability for PE
◊ When there is lung opacity, evaluate well-aerated areas for perfusion defects!
◊ COPD does not diminish usefulness of V/Q scan, but does increase likelihood of an indeterminate result!
◊ 75% of patients with pulmonary edema + without pulmonary embolism have a normal perfusion scan!

Influence of clinical estimate:

V/Q scan	Clinical probability	PE present
high-probability	>80%	96%
low-probability	<20%	4%
indeterminate	DVT present	93%

Influence of cardiopulmonary disease (CPD):

V/Q probability	normal CXR	no prior CPD	any prior CPD	COPD
high	67%	93%	83%	100%
intermediate	24%	39%	26%	22%
low	17%	15%	14%	6%
near normal	3%	4%	4%	0%

HEART SCINTIGRAPHY

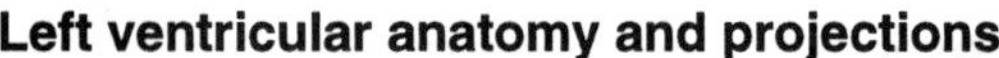

Cardiac imaging choices

1. PLANAR imaging
2. SPECT imaging
   improves object contrast by removing overlying tissues
3. QUANTITATIVE analysis
   = circumferential profiles = plotting of average counts along equally spaced radii emanating from center of LV makes interpretation more objective + reproducible

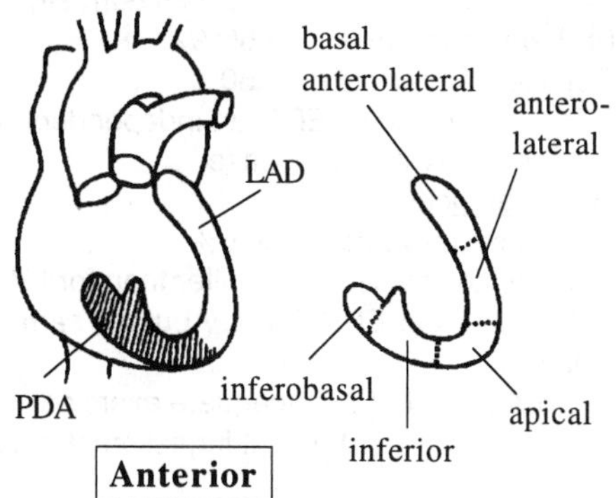

Left ventricular anatomy and projections

A. AP
   √ displays anterolateral wall, apex, inferior wall
   √ decreased activity at apex of LV due to thinning in 50%
B. LEFT LATERAL
   displays inferior wall, anterior wall
C. LAO 40° / LAO 70°
   ◊ Most often used projection; for all exercise studies
   √ displays interventricular septum, posterior wall, inferior wall
   √ best projection to separate right + left ventricles
   √ best projection to evaluate septal + posterior LV wall motion
D. RAO 45°
   √ displays anterior + inferior ventricular wall
   √ useful during 1st-pass studies with temporal separation of ventricles
E. LPO 45° (rarely used)
   10° caudal tilt minimizes LA contamination of LV region
   √ displays anterior + inferior ventricular wall
   √ preferred over RAO 45° because LV is closer to camera
F. Angled LAO (slant-hole collimator / caudal tilt)
   √ separates ventricular from atrial activity
   √ highlights apical dyskinesis

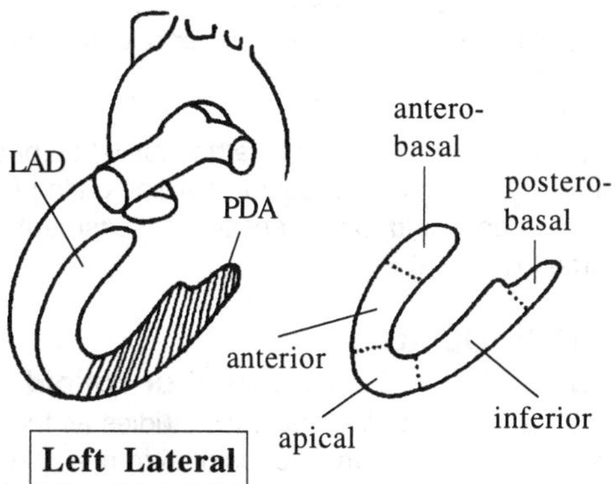

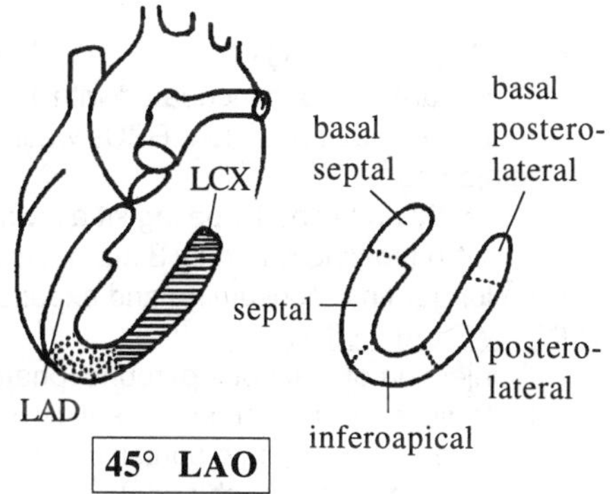

Ejection fraction

Ejection fraction (EF) = stroke volume (SV) divided by end-diastolic volume (EDV)

stroke volume = end-diastolic volume (EDV) minus end-systolic volume (ESV)

$$EF = [EDV - ESV] / [EDV]$$

$$= [ED_{counts} - ES_{counts}] / [ED_{counts} - BKG_{counts}]$$

sensitive indicator of left ventricular function

Accuracy in detection of coronary artery disease:
(a) Exercise EF: 87% sensitivity; 92% specificity
(b) Exercise ECG: 60% sensitivity; 81% specificity

LAD supplies:	upper 2/3 of interventricular septum anterior wall part of lateral wall apex of left ventricle (in most patients)
LCX supplies:	posterior portion of left ventricle lateral portion of left ventricle
RCA supplies:	lower 1/3 of interventricular septum inferior wall of right + left ventricle

Interpretation:
@ Left ventricle
Mean normal value = 67 ± 8% (increase under stress normally >5–7%)
Probably abnormal ≤55%
Definitely abnormal <50%
◊ Peak exercise LVEF is an independent predictor of coronary artery disease
@ Right ventricle
mean normal value >45%
(RV ejection fraction is smaller than for LV because RV has greater EDV than LV but the same stroke volume)
False-positive with (a) inadequate exercise
(b) recent ingestion of meal

√ EF unchanged / decreased in coronary artery disease
√ new regional wall motion abnormality under exercise in coronary artery disease
√ correlates well with clinical severity of myocardial infarction

Shortcoming:
poor study in patients with atrial fibrillation because of inability to achieve adequate cardiac gating (exercise MUGA can yield more sensitive assessment of coronary artery disease)

BLOOD POOL AGENTS

Tc-99m DTPA / Tc-99m sulphur colloid

preferred for cardiac first-pass studies as they allow multiple studies with little residual from any preceding study

Tc-99m–labeled RBCs

= agent of choice because of good heart-to-lung ratio
Technique:
(1) IN VITRO LABELING
} 50 mL drawn blood incubated with Tc-99m reduced by stannous ion; RBCs washed and reinjected
◊ Recently developed labeling kit allows excellent in vivtro labeling with only 3 mL of blood and is no longer time-consuming and expensive
(2) IN VIVO LABELING
} IV injection of stannous pyrophosphate (1 vial PYP diluted with 2 mL sterile saline = 15 mg sodium pyrophosphate containing 3.4 mg anhydrous stannous chloride)
} 15–30 minutes later injection of Tc-99m pertechnetate (+7), which binds to "pretinned" RBCs (reduction to Tc-99m [+4])
◊ Least time-consuming + easiest method!
◊ Worst labeling efficiency (30% not tagged to RBCs + excreted in urine)!
(3) IN VIVTRO LABELING
= MODIFIED IN VIVO METHOD
} 10 minutes after IV injection of 1 mg stannous pyrophosphate 10 mL of blood are drawn + incubated with Tc-99m pertechnetate for 10–20 minutes with small amount of heparin added + reinjected (3-way stopcock technique)
◊ Preferred method because of high labeling efficiency with little free pertechnetate!
N.B.: poor tagging in
(a) heparinized patient
(b) injection through IV line (adherence to wall)
(c) syringe flushed with dextrose instead of saline

Dose: 15–30 mCi (larger dose required for stress MUGA + obese patients);
for children: 200 µCi/kg (minimum dose of 2–3 mCi)
Radiation dose: 1.5 rad for heart, 1.0 rad for blood, 0.4 rad for whole body

Tc-99m HSA

HSA = human serum albumin
Indication: drug interference with RBC labeling (eg, heparinized patient)
Physiology: (a) albumin slowly equilibrates throughout extracellular space
(b) poorer heart-to-lung ratio than with labeled RBCs

MYOCARDIAL PERFUSION IMAGING AGENTS

Potassium-43

Not suitable for clinical use because of its high energy

Thallium-201 chloride

= cation produced in cyclotron from stable Tl-203
= image agent of choice to assess myocardial viability
Cyclotron: by (p,3n) reaction to radioactive Pb-201 (half-life of 9.4 hours) which decays by electron capture to Tl-201
Decay: by electron capture to Hg-201
Energy spectrum: 69–83 keV of Hg-K x-rays (98% abundance); 135 keV (2%) + 167 keV (8%) gamma photons
Physical half-life: 74 hours
Biologic half-life: 10 ± 2.5 days
Dose: 1.5–3–4 mCi (the larger dose for SPECT)
Radiation dose:
3 rad for kidneys (critical organ) (1.2 rad/mCi); 1.2 rad for gonads (0.6 rad/mCi); 0.7 rad for heart + marrow (0.34 rad/mCi); 0.5 rad for whole body (0.24 rad/mCi)
Quality control: should contain <0.25% Pb-203, <0.5% Tl-202 (439 keV)
Indications:
1. ACUTE MYOCARDIAL INFARCTION
2. CORONARY ARTERY DISEASE
particularly useful over ECG in:
(a) conduction disturbances (eg, bundle branch block, preexitation syndrome)
(b) previous infarction
(c) under drug influence (eg, digitalis)
(d) left ventricular hypertrophy
(e) hyperventilation
(f) ST depression without symptoms
(g) if stress ECG impossible to obtain

Thallium uptake & distribution

intracellular uptake via Na/K-ATPase analogue to ionic potassium, but less readily released from cells than potassium; distribution is proportional to regional blood flow; uptake depends on quality of regional perfusion + integrity of sodium-potassium pump

@ Blood pool
<5% remain in blood pool 15 minutes post injection

@ Myocardium
uptake depends on (a) myocardial perfusion (b) myocardial mass (c) myocardial cellular integrity
◊ First-pass extraction efficiency is 88%!
REMEMBER: 90% in 90 seconds!
- 4% of total dose localizes in myocardium at rest (myocardial blood flow = 4% of cardiac output)
- peak myocardial activity occurs at 5–15 minutes after injection
- uptake can be increased to 8–10% with dipyridamole stress
- clearance from myocardium is proportional to regional perfusion

@ Skeletal muscle + splanchnicus:
first-pass extraction efficiency is 65%
- accumulate 40% of injected dose
- 4–6 hours fast + exercise decreases flow to splanchnicus and increases cardiac uptake

@ Lung:
10% of total dose localizes in lung
- augmented pulmonary extraction with left ventricular dysfunction, bronchogenic carcinoma, lymphoma of lung
√ <5% activity over lung is normal
√ heart-to-lung ratio decreased with triple-vessel disease

@ Kidney:
accumulates 4% of injected dose
- excretion of 4–8% within 24 hours

@ Thyroid:
√ increased uptake >1% in Graves disease + thyroid carcinoma

@ Brain:
√ uptake only if blood-brain barrier disrupted

Technique:

A. Single dose method
} 3 mCi injected at peak exercise for exercise image immediately + rest image 3 hours later

B. Split dose method
} 2 mCi injected for exercise image
} 1 mCi reinjected at rest after 3 hours with rest image taken 30 minutes later

C. Booster reinjection technique
} reinjection of thallium followed by imaging after 18–24–72 hours augments blood concentration of isotope
= late reversibility provides evidence of regional myocardial ischemia + viability not appreciated even on very delayed (24–72 hours) redistribution images; predicts scintigraphic improvement post intervention
Reasoning: 50% of irreversible persistent defects improve significantly after booster reinjection

Imaging:

1. EXERCISE IMAGE
   = stress thallium image
   = map of regional perfusion obtained within minutes after injection at peak exercise; initial distribution proportional to myocardial blood flow, arterial concentration of radioisotope, and muscle mass; 300,000–400,000 counts / view (approximately 5–8 minutes sampling time), should be completed by 30 minutes
2. REDISTRIBUTION IMAGE
   = equilibrium between tracer uptake and efflux dependent on blood flow + mass of viable tissue + concentration gradients
   = map of ischemic viable myocardium obtained at rest after 2–3–6 hours; washout half-life from myocardium is 54 minutes
3. DELAYED IMAGE (optional)
   = viability study at 24 hours

Interpretation Of Stress Thallium Images

Immediate Image	*Delayed Image*	*Diagnosis*
normal	normal	normal
defect	fill-in	exertional ischemia
defect	persistent	myocardial scar
defect	partial fill-in	scar + ischemia / persistent ischemia

1. Initial phase = first-pass extraction
   √ temporary defect accentuated by exercise
   √ defect >15% of ventricular surface suggests >50% stenosis of coronary artery
   √ right heart well seen during stress test, tachycardia, volume / pressure overload
2. Redistribution phase (on 2–4-hour images)
   √ washout in normal areas
   √ slow continued accumulation of tracer for areas of greatly reduced perfusion
   √ increased uptake in viable ischemic zones
   √ permanent defect = nonviable myocardium as in myocardial infarction / fibrosis
   √ increased lung activity (= >50% of myocardial count) indicative of
   (a) left ventricular failure due to severe LCA disease / myocardial infarction
   (b) pulmonary venous hypertension due to cardiomyopathy / mitral valve disease
   √ right heart faintly visualized during rest (15% of perfusion to right side); increased activity in RV due to

(a) increase in ventricular systolic pressure
(b) increase in mean pulmonary artery pressure
(c) increase in total pulmonary vascular resistance

Sensitivity: overall 82–84% for stress Tl-201 (60–62% for exercise ECG)

(a) increased with:
(1) severity of stenosis (86% + 67% sensitive with stenosis >75% + <75%)
(2) greater number of involved arteries
(3) stenosis of left main > LAD > RCA > LXC
(4) prior infarction
(5) high work load during exercise testing in patients with single-vessel disease

(b) decreased with:
(1) presence of collateral
(2) beta blockers
(3) time delay for poststress images

Specificity: overall 91–94% for stress Tl-201 (81–83% for exercise ECG)

False-positive thallium test (37–58%):

A. INFILTRATING MYOCARDIAL DISEASE
1. Sarcoidosis
2. Amyloidosis

B. CARDIAC DYSFUNCTION
1. Cardiomyopathy
2. IHSS
3. Valvular aortic stenosis
4. Mitral valve prolapse (rare)

C. DECREASED CARDIAC PERFUSION OTHER THAN MYOCARDIAL INFARCTION
1. Cardiac contusion
2. Myocardial fibrosis
3. Coronary artery spasm (severe unstable angina may cause defect after stress + on redistribution images, but will be normal at rest!)

D. NORMAL VARIANT
1. Apical myocardial thinning
2. Attenuation due to diaphragm, breast, implant, pacemaker

mnemonic: "I'M SIC"
Idiopathic hypertrophic subaortic stenosis
Myocardial infarct without coronary artery disease
Scarring, **S**pasm, **S**arcoidosis
Infiltrative / metastatic lesion
Cardiomyopathy

False-negative thallium test:
1. Under influence of beta-blocker (eg, propranolol)
2. "Balanced ischemia" = symmetric 3-vessel disease
3. Insignificant obstruction
4. Inadequate stress
5. Failure to perform delayed imaging
6. Poor technique

mnemonic: "3NMRS COR"
3-vessel disease (rare)
Noncritical stenosis
Medications interfering
Right coronary lesion (isolated)
Submaximal exercise
Collateral (coronary) blood vessels
Overestimation of stenosis on angiography
Redistribution (early / delayed)

Advantages compared to Tc-99m compounds:
(1) higher total accumulation in myocardium
(2) provides redistribution information

Disadvantages:
(1) low energy x-rays result in poor resolution (improved with SPECT)
(2) dose is limited by its long half life
(3) half-value thickness of 3 cm results in less avid appearing myocardium: inferior wall (deeper part of myocardium) / anterolateral wall (overlain by breast)
(4) imaging must be completed by 45 minutes post injection or redistribution occurs

Tc-99m MIBI (Sestamibi)

= cationic lipophilic isonitrile complex which associates with myocyte mitochondria

Pharmacokinetics:
- relatively rapid clearance from circulation (40% first pass extraction)
- high myocardial accumulation (4%) with nonlinear uptake proportional to regional perfusion (fall-off in extraction at higher rates of flow)
- slow washout with long retention time in myocardium with little recirculation
- significant hepatic activity

Excretion: through biliary tree (give milk after injection and before imaging to decrease GB activity)

Dose: 25 mCi (Cardiolite®)

Imaging: optimum images 1 hour after injection (may be imaged up until 3 hours)

Technique: separate injections for stress and rest studies because of slow washout

A. 1-DAY PROTOCOL
Improved detection of reversibility compared with stress-rest protocol
} rest images 60–90 minutes after injection of 8 mCi Tc-99m sestamibi
} wait 0–4 hours
} stress patient followed by injection of 25 mCi Tc-99m sestamibi at peak stress (increased myocardial blood flow means increased myocardial uptake)
} image 30–60 minutes later (optimum imaging time of stress-induced defects)

B. 2-DAY PROTOCOL (stress-rest protocol):
} stress images on 1st day: Tc-99m sestamibi given at peak stress; imaging after 30–60 minutes' delay to allow liver activity to decrease
} repeat on 2nd day if stress views abnormal

Advantages over thallium:
(1) Low radiation dose related to shorter half-life allowing larger doses with less patient radiation
(2) excellent imaging characteristics due to
(a) improved photon flux which means faster imaging + allows cardiac gating
(b) higher photon energy means less attenuation artifact from breast tissue / diaphragm + less scatter
(3) NO redistribution
(4) Temporal separation of injection and imaging allows injection during acute myocardial infarct when patient may not be stable for imaging; after stabilization + intervention (angioplasty / urokinase) imaging can demonstrate the pre-intervention defect
(5) low cost
(6) easy availability
(7) flexible scheduling
(8) increased patient throughput

Disadvantage: less well suited to assess viability

Tc-99m Teboroxime
= neutral boronic acid oxime complex
Pharmacokinetics:
- very rapid clearance time from circulation (rapid uptake by myocardium with high extraction efficiency)
- distribution proportional to cardiac blood flow EVEN at high blood flow levels (sestamibi + thallium plateau at high levels of flow)
- biexponential washout from myocardium
- high background from lung + liver

Dose: 25–30 mCi (Cardiotec®)
Imaging: must begin immediately post injection due to rapid washout; rest image can immediately follow stress image

Tc-99m Tetrofosmin
= diphosphine complex
Related compounds: Q12 (furifosmin), Q3
Pharmacokinetics:
- lower first-pass extraction and accumulation than thallium
- slow myocardial washout
- rapid background clearance

Positron Emission Tomography
Perfusion agents: N-13 ammonia, O-15 water, Rb-82 (available from a strontium generator)
Metabolic agents: Fluorine-18-deoxyglucose (glycolysis), carbon-11-palmitate (beta-oxidation), carbon-11-acetate (tricarboxylic acid cycle)
Pathophysiology:
in myocardial ischemia glycolysis (utilization of glucose) increases while mitochondrial b-oxidation of fatty acids decreases!
Sensitivity: >95%

√ mismatched defect (= decreased perfusion but enhanced metabolism indicated by FDG uptake) indicates viable myocardium (= dysfunctional myocardium salvageable by revascularization procedure)
√ matched defect (= flow + FDG accumulation both decreased) indicate nonviable myocardium
◊ 80–90% of matching defects do not improve after bypass
√ 11-C-acetate superior to FDG (accurately reflects overall oxidation metabolism, not influenced by myocardial substrate utilization)

Comparison with thallium:
accuracy for fixed lesions similar; higher for reversible ischemia

STRESS TEST
Rationale:
increased heart rate will unveil insufficient regional perfusion secondary to coronary artery disease

Physical Stress Test
} exercise in erect position (peak heart rate lower if supine) on treadmill or bicycle; isometric handgrip exercise raises blood pressure less (but adequate for evaluation)
} starting point of workload selected according to preliminary exercise results (at an average of 200 kilowatt pounds)
} workload increments by 200 kilowatt pounds up to 85% of predicted maximum heart rate (= 220 - age) / exercise limited by symptoms of chest pain, dyspnea, fatigue, arrhythmia, ischemic ECG (cardiologist with crash cart should be available)

End points for discontinuing exercise:
A. SYMPTOMS: chest pain, dyspnea, fatigue, leg cramps, dizziness
B. SIGNS: fall in BP >10 mm Hg below previous stage, ventricular tachycardia, run of 3 successive ventricular premature beats

Problems with exercise imaging:
(1) Sensitivity to detect ischemic lesions decreases with suboptimal exercise (in particular for older population)
(2) Higher false-positive tests in women (artifacts from overlying breast tissue)
(3) Propranolol (beta blocker) interferes with stress test, should be discontinued 24–48 hours prior to testing

Pharmacological Stress Test
Advantage:
(1) Reproducibility
(2) Independent from patient motivation
(3) Freedom from patient infirmities, eg, severe peripheral vascular disease, arthritis, pain

Drug:

A. VASODILATORS

Action: binding to A2 receptors affects the intracellular cyclic AMP, GMP, and calcium levels resulting in coronary hyperemia

N.B.: Discontinue use of caffeine, tea, chocolate, cola drinks for 24 hours prior to test

(1) IV infusion of 0.15 mg/kg/min dipyridamole (= Persantine®) for 4 minutes causing 3–5-fold increase in coronary artery blood flow

Drug action: 30 minutes

Side effects: flushing, nausea, bronchospasm (reversible with aminophylline)

◊ Prolonged supervision after test necessary

} radiotracer injection 3–5 minutes later

(2) IV infusion of 140 µg/kg/min adenosine (= Adenocard®, Adenoscan®) for 6 minutes

Drug action: 2–3 minutes (half life of 15 sec)

Side effects: flushing, nausea, AV block, bronchospasm

◊ Supervision after test not needed

} radiotracer injection during 3rd minute

Contraindication: significant pulmonary disease requiring use of inhalers

B. INOTROPES

Action: beta-1 agonist increasing myocardial contractility thus oxygen demand

Candidates: patients with COPD, asthma, allergy to vasodilators

(1) IV infusion of 5 µg/kg/min dobutamine for 5 minutes, increased in steps of 5 µg/kg every 5 minutes to a maximum infusion rate of 30–40 µg/kg/min titrated to patient's response

} radiotracer injected at onset of significant symptoms / ECG changes / achievement of maximal rate of infusion or heart rate

} infusion maintained for an additional 2 minutes with dose adjusted to patient's condition

(2) IV infusion of arbutamine with its own computerized delivery system titrating dose rate automatically

Contraindication: severe hypertension, atrial flutter / fibrillation

Applied to:

1. THALLIUM IMAGING (redistribution images after stress test):

} injection of 1.5–2 mCi of Tl-201 during peak exercise, continuation of exercise for additional 60 seconds before imaging commences

Clues for stress images:

√ RV myocardium well visualized

√ little pulmonary background activity

√ little activity in liver, stomach, spleen

√ distribution more uniform after stress than during rest

◊ Degree of liver uptake useful as direct measure of level of exercise!

Sources of technical errors:

mnemonic: "ABCDE PS"

Attenuation from overlying breast / diaphragm

Background oversubtraction

Camera field nonuniformity

Drugs, **D**elayed (excessively) imaging, **D**ose infiltration

Eating / **E**xercising between stress + delayed images

Positioning variation between stress + delayed images

Submaximal exercise

2. GATED BLOOD POOL IMAGING (response of EF)

√ increase in ejection fraction from 63–93% in normals

√ increase in ventricular wall motion (anterolateral > posterolateral > septal)

VENTRICULAR FUNCTION

First-pass Ventriculography

= FIRST TRANSIT = recording of initial transit time of an intravenously administered tight Tc-99m bolus through heart + lungs; limited number of cardiac cycles available for interpretation; additional projections / serial studies require additional bolus injection

Accuracy: good correlation with contrast ventriculography

Agents: pertechnetate, pyrophosphate, albumin, DTPA, sulfur colloid (almost any Tc-99m–labeled compound except lung scanning particles), Tc-99m–labeled autologous RBCs (most commonly)

Indication:

(1) Only 15 seconds of patient cooperation required

(2) Calculation of cardiac output + ejection fraction (RBCs)

(3) Subsequent first-pass studies within 15–20 minutes of initial study possible (DTPA)

(4) Separate assessment of individual cardiac chambers in RAO projection (temporal separation without overlying atria, pulmonary artery, aortic outflow tract), eg, for right ventricular EF and intracardiac shunts

Technique:

} cannulation of antecubital vein with ≥20 ga needle attached to 3-way stopcock and two syringes:

} syringe 1 contains ≤1 mL of radiotracer

} syringe 2 contains a saline flush (10–20 mL)

} injection of radiotracer is followed by a strong flush of saline

Gating:

Improved images obtained by selection of time interval corresponding only to RV passage of bolus averaged over several (3–5) individual beats; gating may be done intrinsically or with ECG guidance

Imaging:
Region of interest (ROI) over RV silhouette in RAO projection; background activity taken over horseshoe-shaped ventricular wall; counts in ROI displayed as function of time; 25 frames/second for 20–30 seconds
Normal passage of bolus: SVC, RA, RV, lungs, LA, LV, aorta
R-to-L shunt: tracer appears in left side of heart before passage through lungs
Evaluation of:
1. Obstruction in SVC region
2. Reflux from RA into IVC / jugular vein
3. Stenosis in pulmonary outflow tract
4. R-L shunt
5. Contractility of RV
6. Sequential beating of RA and RV
7. Ejection fraction of RV and LV

Equilibrium images
= "blood pool" radionuclide angiography
Agents: Tc-99m–labeled autologous RBCs (most commonly) / human serum albumin
Imaging: after thorough mixing of radiotracer throughout vascular space
} acquisition of images during selected portions of cardiac cycle triggered by R-wave; each image is composed of >200,000 counts (2–10 minutes) obtained over 500–1,000 beats after equilibrium has been reached; high-quality images can be obtained in different projections
} gated acquisition from 16–32 equal subdivisions of the R-R cycle (electronic bins) allows display of synchronized cinematic images (assembled to composite single-image sequence) of an "average" cardiac cycle
√ may be displayed as time activity curves reflecting changes in ventricular counts throughout R-R interval
— measured functional indices: preejection period (PEP), left ventricular ejection time (LVET), left ventricular fast filling time ($LVFT_1$), left ventricular slow filling time ($LVFT_2$), PEP/LVET ratio, rate of ejection + filling of LV
} at rest: count density 200–250 counts/pixel requires generally 7–10 minutes acquisition time for 200,000–250,000 counts/frame
} during exercise: 100,000–150,000 counts/frame requires an acquisition time of 2 minutes

Evaluation of:
1. LV ejection fraction
2. Regional wall motion
3. Valvular regurgitation

Interpretation:
1. Heart failure: decreased EF, prolongation of PEP, shortening of LVET, decreased rate of ejection
2. Hypertensive heart: normal systolic indices, normal EF, prolonged LVT_1
3. Hypothyroidism: prolonged PEP, normal EF
4. Aortic stenosis: mild reduction of EF, prolonged LV emptying time, decreased rate of ejection, normal rate of filling

√ area of decreased periventricular uptake secondary to
(a) pleural effusion >100 mL
(b) ventricular hypertrophy

Gated blood pool imaging
= MULTIPLE GATED ACQUISITION (MUGA)
Recording of:
(1) Ejection fraction (EF) of left ventricle before + after exercise (>6 million counts, 32 frames)
(2) Regional wall motion of ventricular chambers (>4.5 million counts, 24 frames)
  (a) at rest : myocardial infarction, aneurysm, contusion
  (b) during exercise : ischemic dyskinesia (detectable in 63%)
(3) Regurgitant index
  Projection:
  (a) best septal view (usually LAO 45°) for EF; often requires some cephalad tilting of detector head
  (b) two additional views for evaluation of wall motion (usually anterior + left lateral views)

Imaging:
Physiologic trigger provided by R-R interval of ECG ("bad beat" rejection program desirable)
(a) gated images obtained for 5 minutes
(b) 2-minute image acquisition time for each stage of exercise

PROs: (1) Higher information density than 1st-pass method
(2) Assessment of pharmacologic effect possible
(3) "Bad beat" rejection possible
CONs: (1) Significant background activity
(2) Inability to monitor individual chambers in other than LAO 45° projection
(3) Plane of AV valve difficult to identify
Radiation dose: 1.5 rad for heart; 1.0 rad for blood; 0.4 rad for whole body

INFARCT-AVID IMAGING
= hot spot imaging
Agent: Tc-99m pyrophosphate (standard), Hg-203 chlormerodrin, Tc-99m tetracycline, Tc-99m glucoheptonate, F-18 sodium fluoride, Indium-111 antimyosin (murine monoclonal antibodies to myosin), Tc-99m antimyosin Fab fragment

Tc-99m pyrophosphate
Pathophysiology in MYOCARDIAL INFARCTION:
Pyrophosphate is taken up by myocardial necrosis through complexation with calcium deposits >10–12 hours post infarction

- requires presence of residual collateral blood flow
- 30–40% maximum accumulation in hypoxic cells with a 60–70% reduction in blood flow (greater levels of occlusion reduce uptake)

Uptake post infarction:
- earliest uptake by 6–12–24 hours;
- peak uptake by 48–72 hours;
- persistent uptake seen up to 5–7 days with return to normal by 10–14 days

Sensitivity: 90% for transmural infarction, 40–50% for subendocardial (nontransmural) infarction
Specificity: as low as 64%

Dose: 15–20 mCi IV (minimal count requirement of 500,000/view)
Imaging: at 3–6 hours (60% absorbed by skeleton within 3 hours)

Indications:
1. Lost enzyme pattern = patient admitted 24–48 hours after infarction
2. Equivocal ECG + atypical angina:
   (a) left ventricular bundle branch block
   (b) left ventricular hypertrophy
   (c) impossibility to perform stress test
   (d) patient on digitalis
3. ST depression without symptoms
4. Equivocal enzyme pattern + equivocal symptoms
5. S/P cardiac surgery (perioperative infarction in 10%, enzymes routinely elevated, ECG always abnormal), requires preoperative baseline study as 40% are preoperatively abnormal
6. For detection of right ventricular infarction

NOT HELPFUL:
1. In differentiating multiple- from single-vessel disease
2. Typical angina
3. Normal ECG stress test + NO symptoms

Scan interpretation:
[Grade 2+ and above are positive]

Grade 0	no activity
Grade 1+	faint uptake
Grade 2+	slightly less than sternum, equal to ribs
Grade 3+	equal to sternum
Grade 4+	greater than sternum

√ "doughnut" pattern = central cold defect (necrosis in large infarct) usually in cases of large anterior + anterolateral wall infarctions
√ uptake in inferior wall extending behind sternum (anterior projection) suggests RV infarction
◊ SPECT imaging improves sensitivity (eliminates rib overlap)
√ diffuse uptake can be seen in angina, cardiomyopathy, subendocardial infarct, pericarditis and normal blood pool (normal blood pool can be eliminated with delayed imaging)

FALSE POSITIVES (10%)
A. Cardiac causes
   1. Recent injury: myocardial contusion, resuscitation, cardioversion, radiation injury, adriamycin cardiotoxicity, myocarditis, acute pericarditis
   2. Previous injury: left ventricular aneurysm, mural thrombus, unstable angina, previous infarct with persistent uptake
   3. Calcified heart valves / coronaries (rare) / chronic pericarditis
   4. Cardiomyopathy: eg, amyloidosis
B. Extracardiac causes:
   1. Soft-tissue uptake: breast tumor / inflammation, chest wall injury, paddle burns from cardioversion, surgical drain, lung tumor
   2. Osseous: calcified costal cartilage (most common), lesions in rib / sternum
   3. Increased blood pool activity secondary to renal dysfunction / poor labeling technique (improvement on delayed images)

mnemonic: "SCUBA"
Subendocardial infarction (extensive)
Cardiomyopathy / myocarditis
Unstable angina
Blood pool activity
Amyloidosis

FALSE NEGATIVES (5%)
Myocardial metastasis

PERSISTENTLY POSITIVE SCAN (>2 weeks)
= ongoing myocardial necrosis indicating poor prognosis, may continue on to cardiac aneurysm, repeat infarction, cardiac death
— in 77% of persistent / unstable angina pectoris
— in 41% of compensated congestive heart failure
— in 51% of ECG evidence of ventricular dyssynergy

Prognosis: the larger the area, the worse the mortality + morbidity

Tc-99m antimyosin Fab fragments
= specific marker for myocyte damage
= Fab fragments of an antibody raised against water-insoluble heavy chains of cardiac myosin that are exposed due to necrosis

Sensitivity: 95%
√ uptake ONLY in acute infarct with decreasing intensity as the infarct heals

NONAVID INFARCT IMAGING
= Cold spot imaging
= myocardial perfusion study for acute myocardial infarct

Agent: Tl-201 (at rest)
Sensitivity after onset of symptoms:
96% within 6–12 hours, 79% after 48 hours, 59% in remote infarction; sensitivity for SPECT (seven pinhole tomography) 94% > planar scintigraphy 75%

√ fixed permanent defect in acute infarction
√ fixed permanent defect at rest + on stress thallium + redistribution images in old infarction
√ "cold defect" at rest may represent transient ischemia in unstable angina

N.B.: Tl-201 cannot distinguish between recent + remote infarction!

MYOCARDIAL ISCHEMIA

can be assessed
(a) directly with stress Tl-201 imaging
(b) indirectly with gated blood pool imaging (wall motion, ejection fraction)

LOCATION OF PERFUSION DEFECTS
(1) Right coronary artery (RCA)
best seen on left LAT / AP projections
√ inferior + posteroseptal segments
(2) Circumflex branch of left coronary artery (LCX)
best seen on LAO projection
√ posterolateral segment
(3) Anterior descending branch of left coronary artery (LAD)
√ anteroseptal, anterior, anterolateral segments

N.B.: decreased activity in apical + posterior segments is not reliably correlated with disease of any vessel!

INTRACARDIAC SHUNTS

Blood-pool agents administered by peripheral IV injection:
Tc-99m pertechnetate, DTPA, sulfur colloid, macroaggregated albumin, labeled RBCs

Method:
C2/C1-method measures hemodynamic significance of a shunt; raw data obtained from pulmonary activity curve (gamma variate method, Q_p:Q_s ratio = two-area ratio method, count method); accuracy depends on the shape of the input bolus (single peak of <2 seconds' duration); measuring C1, C2, T1, T2

A. NORMAL
C2/C1 is <32%

B. L-R SHUNT
Indication: ASD, VSD, AV canal, aortopulmonic window, rupture of sinus of Valsalva aneurysm
√ C2/C1 >35% (area A = primary pulmonary circulation; area B = L-R shunt; area (A - B) = systemic circulation; Q_P / Q_S = area A / area (A - B) >1.2)

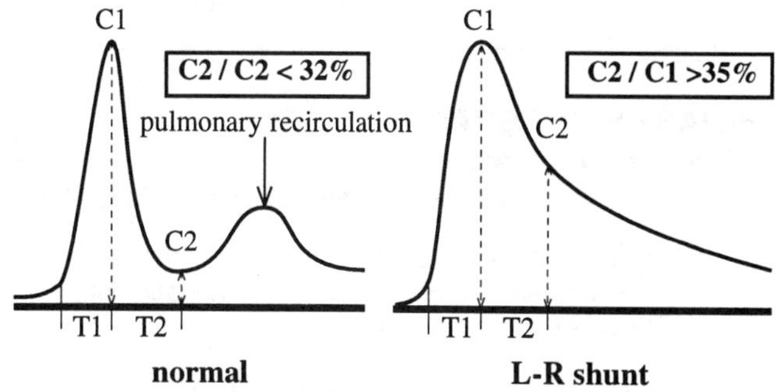

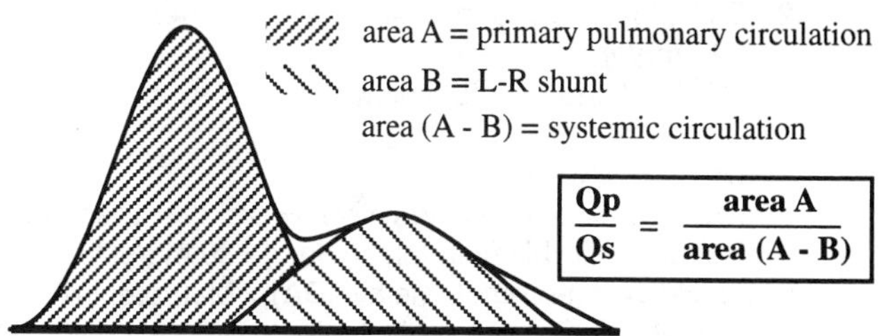

Two-Area Ratio Method

Pulmonary Activity Curves

C. R-L SHUNT
Indication: Tetralogy of Fallot, transposition, truncus, Ebstein anomaly
√ early arrival of tracer in left side of heart + aorta (first-pass method) prior to arrival of activity from lungs to LV
√ quantification possible only by registration of sum of activity of trapped macroaggregate / microspheres in brain + kidneys

Causes of abnormal nonshunt-related activity:
(1) Radiopharmaceutical breakdown
√ free pertechnetate activity in salivary glands, gastric mucosa, thyroid, kidney
(2) Hepatic cirrhosis
abnormal pulmonary vascular channels bypassing the lung (in 10–70%)
(3) Pulmonary AVM

LIVER AND GASTROINTESTINAL TRACT SCINTIGRAPHY

BILIARY SCINTIGRAPHY

Tc-99m IDA analogs

= Tc-99m acetanilide iminodiacetic acid analogs (IDA)

Dependent on the substance's lipophility, there is a trade-off between renal excretion + hepatic uptake (BIDA is the most lipophilic, HIDA the least lipophilic)

1. HIDA (2,6-dimethyl derivative): [H = hepatic] bilirubin threshold of <18 mg/dL; 15% renal excretion
2. BIDA (parabutyl derivative): bilirubin threshold of <20 mg/dL
3. PIPIDA (paraisopropyl derivative): 2% renal excretion
4. DIDA (diethyl derivative)
5. DISIDA (diisopropyl derivative) = Disida®, Disofen®, Hepatolite®: bilirubin threshold of <30 mg/dL
6. TMB-IDA (m-bromotrimethyl IDA) = Mebrofenin®, Choletec®: $T_{1/2}$ uptake is 6 minutes, $T_{1/2}$ excretion is 14 minutes in normals

Quality control: the final compound should contain
- — 90–100% Tc-99m IDA
- — <10% Tc-99m tin colloid
- — <10% Tc-99m sodium pertechnetate

Pharmacokinetics:

Bloodstream:
tracer bound predominantly to albumin, which decreases renal excretion (renal excretion seen in most normals); dissociation of albumin + Tc-99m-IDA takes place at space of Disse

Liver:
peak liver activity 5–10 minutes post injection = hepatic phase; 85% extracted by hepatocytes; tracer enters anion pathway of bilirubin
- ◊ Delayed liver uptake implies hepatocyte dysfunction / CHF (less likely)
- ◊ Look for liver lesions on early images

Bile:
secretion by hepatocytes without conjugation; CBD + cystic duct visualized within 15 minutes (not always visualized in normals); GB visualized by 20 minutes
- ◊ Activity in right paracolic gutter / intraperitoneal space implies postoperative bile leak

Bowel:
excretion into duodenum by 30 minutes; bowel visualized within 1 hour; no enterohepatic recirculation

Dose: 3–7 mCi for adults (higher dose may be needed for high bilirubin level + for tracer with lower bilirubin threshold)

Radiation dose: 2 rad for upper large bowel; 0.55 rad for gallbladder; 3 rad/mCi for small bowel; 0.01 rad/mCi for whole body

Patient preparation:
1. Narcotics (opiates) + sedatives increase tone of sphincter of Oddi and are stopped 6–12 hours before exam
2. Fasting of at least 2–4 hours but <24 hours
3. Cholecystokinin-C-terminal octapeptide = Sincalide (slow IV injection of 0.02 µg/kg Kinevac®) may be used to empty gallbladder about 30 minutes before tracer injection in patients on prolonged fasting (gallbladder atony + retained bile and sludge secondary to absence of endogenously produced CCK)
   Useful in: (a) patient fasting >24 hours / on total parenteral nutrition
   (b) acalculous cholecystitis
   Side effect: increase in biliary-to-bowel transit time

Equipment:
Large field-of-view scintillation camera fitted with LEAP collimator; spectrometer set at 140 keV with 20% window
Computer software for deconvolutional analysis allows determination of percent of hepatic arterial and percent of portal venous blood flow to liver (helpful in assessment of liver transplants)

Imaging:
at 5–10-minute intervals for 60 minutes; if gallbladder not visualized for at least up to 4 hours; RLAT, RAO, LAO projections to confirm gallbladder position
- ◊ Look for enterogastric reflux as a cause of biliary gastritis!

IV morphine sulfate (0.04 µg/kg):
contracts sphincter of Oddi + raises intrabiliary pressure with retrograde filling of gallbladder; maximal effect 5 minutes post injection; shortens study time to 1 hour in cases of nonvisualization of gallbladder when injected 30–40 minutes into study; increases accuracy from 88% to 98% and specificity from 83% to 100%

Normals:
gallbladder appearance within 60 minutes (90% within 30 minutes); gallbladder visualization within 30 minutes after administration of morphine; small bowel activity within 90 minutes (80% within 60 minutes)

Gallbladder ejection fraction (GBEF)

$$GBEF = [GB_{initial} - GB_{post}] \div GB_{initial}$$

Indication:
(1) to increase sensitivity of study for acute (acalculous) cholecystitis
(2) in patients with atypical GB pain and no cholelithiasis

Technique:
1. Select ROI about GB
2. Administer Sincalide in a dose of 0.02 μg/kg body weight IV over 30 minutes (with infusion pump)

Normal result: >30% GBEF

False-positive DISIDA scan
mnemonic: "F2C PAL"
Food (recent meal)
Fasting (prolonged)
Cystic duct cholangiocarcinoma
Pancreatitis
Alcoholism
Liver dysfunction

False-negative DISIDA scan
mnemonic: "ADA"
Acalculous cholecystitis
Duodenal diverticulum simulating GB
Accessory cystic duct

LIVER SCINTIGRAPHY

Technetium-99m sulfur colloid
= LIVER-SPLEEN SCAN

Indications: liver, spleen, bone marrow, acute rejection in renal transplant, lower GI bleeding, gastric emptying

Preparation:
Tc-99m pertechnetate and sodium trisulphate are heated in a water bath (95 ± 5°C) for 10 ± 2 minutes; sulfur atoms aggregate to form a "colloid" (average particle size 0.1–1 μ with a range of 0.001–1 μ; true colloid has a particle size of 0.001–0.5 μ); gelatin is added to prevent further growth of particles

Quality control:
(a) >92% remain at origin of ascending chromatography
(b) upper limit for particle size is 1 μ
— Usual cause for poor preparation is excessive / prolonged heating or a pH >7
— Preparation should not be used >6 hours (agglomeration of particles with aging)

Dose: usually 3– 6 mCi (8 mCi for SPECT)
Radiation dose: 0.3 rad/mCi for liver (critical organ); 0.02 rad/mCi for whole body; 0.025 rad/mCi for bone marrow
Imaging: 15–30 minutes post IV injection

Pharmacokinetics:
accumulation in liver (85%), spleen (10%), bone marrow (5%); lung localization is rare (presumably secondary to circulating endotoxins + macrophage infiltration)

A. RETICULOENDOTHELIAL LOCALIZATION
√ colloid shift away from liver in diffuse hepatic dysfunction / decreased hepatic perfusion
√ increased bone marrow activity in hemolytic anemia
√ increased splenic activity in hypersplenism of splenomegaly / cancer / systemic illness

B. BONE MARROW LOCALIZATION
Hematopoietic system extends into long bones in children; recedes to axial skeleton, femora, and humeri with age
◊ Bone marrow distribution cannot be used to determine sites of erythropoiesis!

C. ABSCESS LOCALIZATION
Sulfur colloid phagocytized by PMNs + monocytes
Labeling:
(a) in vivo: small labeling yield
(b) in vitro: 40% labeling efficiency, but difficult + time-consuming preparation

Colloid shift
A. Hepatic dysfunction
1. Cirrhosis
2. Hepatitis
3. Chronic passive congestion

B. Augmented perfusion of spleen + bone marrow
1. Hematopoietic disorders
2. Long-term corticosteroid therapy

Focal hot liver lesion
1. IVC / SVC obstruction
√ increased perfusion of quadrate lobe located at posterior aspect of medial segment left hepatic lobe (collateral pathway via umbilical vein)
2. Budd-Chiari syndrome
√ "increased" perfusion of caudate lobe (actually decrease of activity elsewhere in liver)
3. FNH (varying amount of Kupffer cells)
√ hot / cold / isoactive with surrounding parenchyma
4. Regenerating nodules of cirrhosis

Defects in porta hepatis
1. Normal variant (thinning of hepatic tissue overlying portal veins + gallbladder)
2. Biliary causes: dilatation of bile ducts, gallbladder hydrops
3. Enlarged portal lymph nodes
4. Metastases
5. Hepatic cyst
6. Hepatic parenchymal disease (pseudotumor)
7. Hepatic compression by adjacent extrinsic mass
8. Postsurgical changes following cholecystectomy

Focal liver defects
A. Neoplastic
(a) primary liver tumor: hepatoma, hemangioma, hepatic adenoma, FNH

(b) metastases: 85% sensitivity, 75–80% specificity (for lesion >1–2 cm)

B. Infectious disease / abscess
C. Benign cyst
D. Trauma
E. Pseudotumor = normal variant

mnemonic: "L'CHAIM
Lymphoma
Cyst
Hematoma
Abscess
Infarct
Metastasis

Mottled hepatic uptake

1. Cirrhosis
2. Acute hepatitis
3. Lymphoma
4. Amyloidosis
5. Granulomatous disease (sarcoid, fungal, viral, parasitic)
6. Chemo- / radiation therapy

SPLENIC SCINTIGRAPHY

1. Tc-99m sulfur colloid: 3–5 mCi

2. Tc-99m heat-denatured erythrocytes
Indication:
(1) Splenic trauma
(2) Accessory + ectopic spleen
Technique:
20–30 minutes after injection of pyrophosphate IV 15–20 mL of blood are drawn + incubated with 2 mCi of pertechnetate; blood is heated to 49.5°C for 35 minutes and reinjected
◊ Fragmentation of RBCs from overheating increases hepatic uptake!
Imaging: 20 minutes post injection

GASTROINTESTINAL SCINTIGRAPHY

Radionuclide esophagogram

Preparation: 4–12 hours fasting; imaging in supine / erect position
Dose: 250–500 μCi Tc-99m sulfur colloid in 10 mL of water taken through straw
Imaging: when swallowing begins
√ normal transit time: 15 seconds with 3 distinct sequential peaks progressing aborally
√ prolonged transit time: achalasia, progressive systemic sclerosis, diffuse esophageal spasm, nonspecific motor disorders, "nutcracker" esophagus, Zenker diverticulum, esophageal stricture + obstruction
Difficult interpretation in: hiatal hernia, GE reflux, Nissen fundoplication

Gastroesophageal reflux

89% correlation with acid reflux test
Cause:
(1) Decreased pressure of lower esophageal sphincter
(a) transient-complete relaxation of LES
(b) low resting pressure of LES
(2) Transient increase in intra-abdominal pressure
(3) Short intra-abdominal esophageal segment
Age of population: usually 6–9 months, up to 2 years
• poor weight gain
• vomiting, aspiration, choking
• asthmatic episodes, stridor, apnea

Detection: upper GI examination with barium, distal esophageal sphincter pressure measurements, 24-hour pH probe measurement in distal esophagus (gold standard), radionuclide examination

Preparation: 4 hours / overnight fasting; abdominal sphygmomanometer (for adults)

Dose: 0.5–1.0 mCi Tc-99m sulfur colloid in 300 mL of acidified orange juice (150 mL juice + 150 mL 0.1 N hydrochloric acid) followed by "cold" acidified orange juice

Imaging: at 30–60-second intervals for 30–60 minutes, images taken in supine position from anterior; sphygmomanometer inflated at 20, 40, 60, 80, 100 mm Hg

Interpretation:
Reflux (in %) = ([esophageal counts – background] / gastric counts) x 100
√ up to 3% magnitude reflux is normal
√ evidence of pulmonary aspiration (valuable in pediatric age group)

Cx: reflux esophagitis secondary to
(a) delayed clearance time of esophageal acid load: tertiary / repetitive esophageal contractions, supine position of refluxor, aspiration of saliva, stimulation of salivary flow, stretched phrenoesophageal membrane in hiatal hernia
(b) delayed gastric emptying: increased intragastric pressure (gastric outlet obstruction), viral gastropathy, diabetes

Prognosis:
(1) Self-limiting process with spontaneous resolution by end of infancy (in majority of patients)
(2) Persistent symptoms until age 4 (1/3 of patients)
(3) Death from inanition / recurrent pneumonia (5%)
(4) Cause of recurrent respiratory infections, asthma, failure to thrive, esophagitis, esophageal stricture, chronic blood loss, sudden infant death syndrome (SIDS)

Rx:
(1) Conservative therapy:
avoidance of food + drugs that decrease pressure in LES, elevation of head during sleep, acid neutralization, cimetidine / ranitidine (reduction of acid production), metoclopramide / domperidone (increase sphincter pressure + promote gastric emptying)
(2) Antireflux surgery

Gastric emptying

Dose: 0.5–1 mCi
(a) Tc-99m sulfur colloid cooked with egg white / liver pâté as solid food
(b) In-111 DTPA for simultaneous measurement of liquid phase

Imaging: 1-minute anterior abdominal images obtained at 0, 10, 30, 60, 90 minutes in erect position if dual-head camera available; anterior and posterior imaging performed with geometric mean activity calculated

Pharmacokinetics:
79% tracer activity in stomach for solid phase at 10 minutes; 65% at 30 minutes; 33% at 60 minutes; 10% at 90 minutes

Normal result: 50% of activity in stomach at time zero; should empty by 60 ± 30 minutes

√ acutely delayed emptying in stress (pain, cold), drugs (morphine, anticholinergics, levo-dopa, nicotine, β-adrenergic antagonists), postoperative ileus, acute viral gastroenteritis, hyperglycemia, hypokalemia
√ chronically delayed gastric emptying in gastric outlet obstruction, postvagotomy, gastric ulcer, chronic idiopathic intestinal pseudoobstruction, GE reflux, progressive systemic sclerosis, dermatomyositis, spinal cord injury, myotonia dystrophica, familial dysautonomia, anorexia nervosa, hypothyroidism, diabetes mellitus, amyloidosis, uremia
√ abnormally rapid gastric emptying in gastric surgery, ZE syndrome, duodenal ulcer disease, malabsorption (pancreatic exocrine insufficiency / celiac sprue)

Gastrointestinal bleeding

Detection depends on:
(1) Rate of hemorrhage (≥ 0.05 mL/min); NUC more sensitive than angiogram
(2) Continuous versus intermittent bleeding (most GI hemorrhages are intermittent)
(3) Site of hemorrhage
(4) Characteristics of radionuclide agent

ANGIOGRAPHY:
requires a bleeding rate of approximately 0.5 mL/min;
63% sensitivity for upper GI bleed;
39% sensitivity for lower GI bleed

Tc-99m sulfur colloid

Indication: bleeding must be active at time of tracer administration; length of active imaging can be increased by fractionating dose
— Disappearance half-life of 2.5–3.5 minutes (rapidly cleared from blood by RES + low background activity)
— Active bleeding sites detected with rates as low as 0.05–0.1 mL/min
— Not useful for upper GI bleeding (interference from high activity in liver + spleen) or bleeding near hepatic / splenic flexure

Dose: 10 mCi (370 MBq)

Imaging:
every image should be for 500,000–1,000,000 counts with oblique + lateral images as necessary
(a) every 5 seconds for 1 minute ("flow study" = radionuclide angiogram)
(b) 60-second images at 2, 5, 10, 15, 20, 30, 40, 60 minutes; study terminated if no abnormality up to 30 minutes
(c) delayed images at 2, 4, 6, 12 hours

√ extravasation of tracer seen in active bleeding
Specificity: almost 100% (rare false-positives due to ectopic RES tissue)
False positives: transplanted kidney, ectopic splenic tissue, modified marrow uptake, male genitalia, arterial graft, aortic aneurysm

Tc-99m–labeled RBCs (in vivtro labeling preferred)

Indications: acute / intermittent bleeding (0.35 mL/min)
— Remains in vascular system for prolonged period
— Liver + spleen activity are low allowing detection of upper GI tract hemorrhage
— Low target-to-background ratio (high activity in great vessels, liver, spleen, kidneys, stomach, colon; probably related to free pertechnetate fraction)

Dose: 10–20 mCi

Imaging:
(a) every 2 seconds for 64 seconds
(b) static images for 500,000–1,000,000 counts at 2, 5, and every consecutive 5 minutes up to 30 minutes + every 10 minutes until 90 minutes
(c) delayed images at 2, 4, 6, 12 hours up to 36 hours

Localization of bleeding site:
may be difficult secondary to rapid transit time (reduced bowel motility with 1 mg glucagon IV) or too widely spaced time intervals; overall 83% correlation with angiography
√ increase in tracer accumulation over time in abnormal location
√ bleeding site conforms to bowel anatomy
√ change in appearance with time consistent with bowel peristalsis

Sensitivity:
in 83–93% correctly identified bleeding site (50–85% within 1st hour, may become positive in 33% only after 12–24 hours); collection as small as 5 mL may be detected; superior to sulfur colloid
- 50% sensitivity for blood loss <500 mL/24 hours
- >90% sensitivity for blood loss >500 mL/24 hours

False positives (5%):
physiologic uptake in stomach + intestine, renal pelvis uptake, hepatic hemangioma, varices, inflammation, isolated vascular process (AVM, venous / arterial graft)

False negatives:
9% for bleeding of <500 mL/24 hours

Tc-99m pertechnetate

Indication: bleeding from functioning gastric mucosa in Meckel diverticulum / intestinal duplication; consider in adults up to age 25; independent of bleeding rate

Pathophysiology: tracer accumulation in mucus-secreting cells

◊ Avoid barium GI studies + endoscopy + irritating bowel preparation prior to study!

Dose: 5–10 mCi (185–370 MBq)

Imaging:
(a) radionuclide angiogram 2–3 seconds/frame for 1st minute
(b) sequential 5-minute images up to 20 minutes with 5,000–1,000,000 counts per image

Sensitivity: >80%
enhanced by
- fasting for 3–6 hours to reduce gastric secretions passing through bowel
- nasogastric tube suction to remove gastric secretions
- premedication with pentagastrin (6 µg/kg SC 15 minutes before study) to stimulate gastric secretion of pertechnetate
- premedication with cimetidine (300 mg qid x 48 hours) to reduce release of pertechnetate from mucosa
- voiding just prior to injection

False positives:
Barrett esophagus, duodenal ulcer, ulcerative colitis, Crohn disease, enteric duplication, small bowel, hemangioma, AV malformation, aneurysm, volvulus, intussusception, urinary obstruction, uterine blush

False negatives:
ulcerated epithelium

Levine / Denver shunt patency

Technique:
sterile injection of 0.5–1 mCi Tc-99m MAA / sulfur colloid via paracentesis

Imaging:
over abdomen (or chest) to detect uptake in liver (or lung), which confirms patency

RENAL AND ADRENAL SCINTIGRAPHY

RENAL AGENTS

1. Agents for renal function: Tc-99m DTPA, I-131 Hippuran
2. Renal cortical agent: Tc-99m DMSA
3. Renal combination agent: Tc-99m glucoheptonate

Tc-99m DTPA

= Tc-99m diethylenetriamine pentaacetic acid
= agent of choice for assessment of
(1) Perfusion
(2) Glomerular filtration = relative GFR
(3) Obstructive uropathy
(4) Vesicoureteral reflux

Pharmacokinetics:
chelating agent; 5–10% bound to plasma protein; extracted with 20% efficiency on each pass through kidney (= filtration fraction); excreted exclusively by glomerular filtration (similar to inulin) without reabsorption / tubular excretion / metabolism
Time-activity behavior:
— abdominal aorta (15–20 seconds)
— kidneys + spleen (17–24 seconds); liver appears later because of portal venous supply
— renal cortical activity (2–4 minutes): mean transit time of 3.0 ± 0.5 minutes; static images of cortex taken at 3–5 minutes
— renal pelvic activity (3–5 minutes): peak at 10 minutes; asymmetric clearance of renal pelvis in 50%; accelerated by furosemide

Biologic half-life: 20 minutes
Dose: 10–20 mCi
Radiation dose: 0.85 rads/mCi for renal cortex; 0.6 rads/mCi for kidney; 0.5 rads/mCi for bladder; 0.15 rads/mCi for gonads; 0.15 rads/mCi for whole body

Adjunct:
Lasix administration (20–40 mg IV) 20 minutes into exam allows assessment of renal pelvic clearance with accuracy equal to Whitaker test (DDx of obstructed from dilated but nonobstructed pelvicalyceal system)

[Tc-99m glucoheptonate]

largely replaced by Tc-99m MAG3

Pharmacokinetics:
rapid plasma clearance + urinary excretion with excellent definition of pelvicalyceal system during 1st hour; extracted by (a) glomerular filtration and (b) tubular excretion (30–45% within 1st hour); 5–15% of dose accumulates in tubular cells by 1 hour, 15–25% by 3 hours; cortical accumulation remains for 24 hours

Imaging:
(a) collecting system within first 30 minutes
(b) renal parenchyma after 1–2 hours (interfering activity in collecting system)

Biologic half-life: 2 hours
Dose: 15 (range 10–20) mCi

Radiation dose: 0.17 rads/mCi for kidney; 0.008 rads/mCi for whole body; 0.015 rads/mCi for gonads

Tc-99m DMSA

= Tc-99m dimercaptosuccinic acid
= suitable for imaging of functioning cortical mass: pseudotumor versus lesion

Renal Scintigraphic Agents

MORPHOLOGIC AGENTS			
Tc-99m GHA	5 mCi	proximal tubular uptake + glomerular filtration	collecting system visualized on delayed images
Tc-99m DMSA	2–5 mCi	proximal + distal tubular uptake	limited availability, relatively high radiation dose, collecting system not visualized on delayed images
FUNCTIONAL AGENTS			
I-131 OIH	200–400 μCi	80% secreted, 20% filtered	routinely used for ERPF measurement, analog of PAH, highest renal extraction fraction, poor image detail, high radiation dose, requires high-energy collimator
Tc-99m DTPA	10–15 mCi	nearly 100% filtered	GFR calculation, delayed time-to-peak with slow clearance
Tc-99m MAG_3	2–10 mCi	99% secreted	ERPF estimate, good cortical detail, high target-to background ratio

Pharmacokinetics:
high protein-binding + slow plasma clearance; 4% extracted per renal passage; 4–8% glomerular filtration within 1 hour and 30% by 14 hours; 50% of dose accumulates in proximal + distal renal tubular cells by 3 hour (= cortical agent)

Imaging: after 1– **3**–24 hours (optimal at 34 hours); improved sensitivity to structural defects with SPECT
Biologic half-life: >30 hours
Dose: 5–10 mCi
Radiation dose: 0.014 rads/mCi for gonads; 0.015 rads/mCi for whole body

[I-131 OIH]
largely replaced by Tc-99m MAG3
= I-131 orthoiodohippurate (Hippuran®)
= good for evaluation of renal tubular function / effective renal plasma flow; agent with highest extraction ratio without binding to renal parenchyma; visualizes kidney even in severe renal failure

Pharmacokinetics:
80% secreted by proximal tubules; 20% filtered by glomeruli; maximal renal concentration within 5 minutes; normal transit time of 2–3 minutes; approximately 2% free iodine
◊ Lugol's solution is administered to protect thyroid

Imaging:
in 15–60-second intervals for 20 minutes; renal uptake determined from images obtained by 1–2 minutes (patient in supine position for equidistance of kidneys to camera)

Biologic half-life: 10 minutes (with normal renal function)
Dose: 200 (range 150–300) μCi
Radiation dose: 0.06 rads/200 μCi for bladder; 0.02 rads/200 μCi for kidney; 0.02 rads/200 μCi for whole body; 0.02 rads/200 μCi for gonads

Tc-99m mercaptoacetyltriglycine (MAG_3)
= renal plasma flow agent similar to OIH but with imaging benefits of Tc-99m label (improved dosimetry)

Pharmacokinetics:
correlates with renal plasma flow; clearance is less than Hippuran

Dose: 10 mCi

Evaluation:
true renal plasma flow = MAG_3 flow (obtained off renogram curve) multiplied by a constant (varies between 1.4 and 1.8)

Enalaprilat-enhanced renography
= screening for renovascular hypertension with angiotensin-converting enzyme inhibitor (ACEI)

Pharmacology:
the affected kidney responds to decreased arteriolar flow by releasing angiotensin II (= extremely potent vasoconstrictor acting on the efferent renal arteriole to increase filtration pressure); ACE inhibitors (eg, captopril, enalapril) block the angiotensin-converting enzyme

Protocol:
1. Blood pressure checked (to prevent testing excessively hypertensive patients) — –4 d
2. Stop antihypertensive medications overnight (except for b-blockers) — –9 hrs
3. Fasting (liquids acceptable) — –4 hrs
4. Bladder catheterization to monitor urinary output — –40 min
5. 1/2 normal saline IV drip at 75 mL/hr — –30 min
6. Lasix (= furosemide) IV — –5 min
   20 mg if serum creatinine <1.5 mg/dL,
   40 mg if serum creatinine >1.5 mg/dL,
   60 mg if serum creatinine >3.0 mg/dL
   (not to exceed 1.0 mg/kg)
7. 2.5 mCi Tc-99m MAG_3 IV for baseline study — 0 min
   (a) flow phase with 1 sec/frame for 60 frames
   (b) tracer kinetic (dynamic) phase with 15 sec/frame for 120 frames
8. Rehydration with 1/2 normal saline keeping a 250–300 mL negative fluid balance — +30 min
9. 0.04 mg/kg Enalaprilat IV with blood pressure + heart rate checks q 5 minutes — +105 min
10. Repeat Lasix (= furosemide) IV (step 6) — +115 min
11. 7.5 mCi Tc-99m MAG_3 IV for Enalaprilat-enhanced study — +120 min
12. 10 mCi Tc-99m MAG_3 IV single post-Enalaprilat study for patients already on ACEI therapy

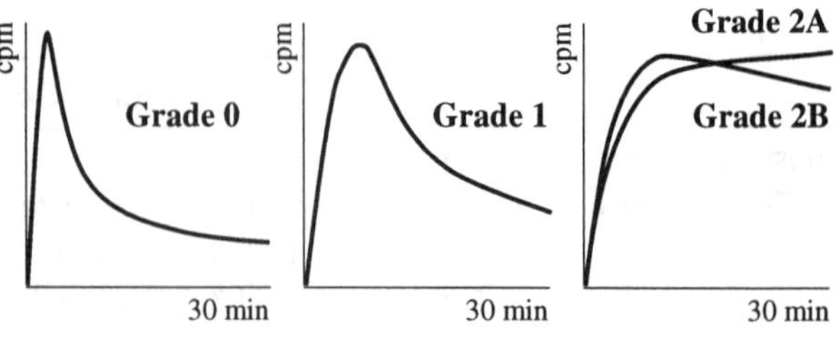

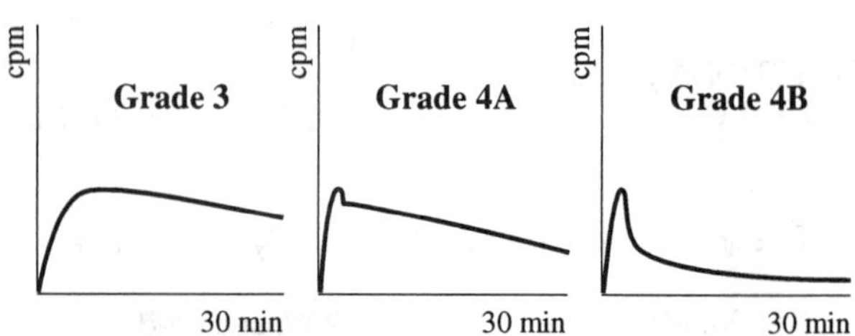

Grading of Differential Renal Function

NucMed

√ change from baseline grade 0 / 1 by >1 grade
= high probability for renal artery stenosis
√ abnormal baseline curve without change
= indeterminate for renovascular hypertension
√ functional improvement following ACEI challenge
= low probability for renovascular hypertension

Differential renal function

Agents:

(1) Tc-99m DTPA:
measurements prior to excretion within first 1–3 minutes; images taken at 1.5-second intervals for 30 seconds followed by serial images for next 30 minutes

(2) I-131 Hippuran:
measurements prior to excretion within first 1–2 minutes

Evaluation: generation of time-activity curves
√ upslope (= accretion phase)
√ peak activity (maximal uptake phase)
√ downslope (excretion phase)

√ increased hepatic + soft-tissue uptake with impaired renal function
√ measurements usually not significantly affected with differences in renal depth
√ measurements are accurate in renal obstruction if obtained within 1–3 minutes
√ prediction about functional recovery not possible following surgical relief of obstruction

Cold defect on renal scan

mnemonic: "CHAT SIN"

Cyst
Hematoma
Abscess
Tumor
Scar
Infarct
Neoplasm

RADIONUCLIDE CYSTOGRAM

Technique:
Infusion of 0.5–1 mCi Tc-99m pertechnetate-saline mixture into bladder

Imaging:
posterior upright views throughout filling and voiding phases; review on cinematic loop helpful; residual bladder volume can be calculated

Advantage:
lower radiation dose to child than comparable contrast study

ADRENAL SCINTIGRAPHY

A. ADRENOCORTICAL IMAGING AGENTS
   1. NP-59
   2. Selenium-75 6-b-selenomethylnorcholesterol (Scintadrin®)
B. SYMPATHOADRENAL IMAGING AGENTS
   1. I-131 / I-123 metaiodobenzylguanidine (MIBG)

I-131 metaiodobenzylguanidine (MIBG)

Indications:
APUDomas = tumors of neural crest origin (C cells of thyroid, melanocytes of skin, chromaffin cells of adrenal medulla, pancreatic cells, Kulchitsky cells), which share the presence of neurosecretory granules capable of accumulating I-131 MIBG

(1) Pheochromocytoma (80–90% sensitivity, >90% specificity); tumors as small as 0.2 g have been detected
(2) Neuroblastoma, carcinoid, medullary thyroid carcinoma, nonfunctioning retroperitoneal neuroendocrine tumor, middle mediastinal paraganglioma, adrenal metastasis of choriocarcinoma, Merkel (skin) tumor

Pharmacokinetics:
Chemically similar to norepinephrine, which is synthesized by adrenergic neurons + cells of the adrenal medulla; localizes in storage granules of adrenergic tissue by means of energy- and sodium-dependent uptake mechanism; not metabolized to any appreciable extent;
Normal activity is seen in liver, spleen, bladder, salivary glands, myocardium, lungs; 85% of injected dose is excreted unchanged by kidneys

Method:
Lugol solution administered orally (50 mg of iodine per day) for 4–5 days starting the day before injection (to block thyroid uptake of free iodine)

Dose: 0.4 mCi (14.8 MBq) or maximally 0.5 mCi/1.73 square meters of body surface MIBG
Radiation dose: 35 rad/mCi for adrenal medulla, 1.0 rad/mCi for ovaries, 0.4 rad/mCi for liver, 0.22 rad/mCi for whole body
Imaging: 24, 48, (72) hours after injection
False-negative scan:
uptake blocked by reserpine, imipramine, other tricyclic depressants, amphetamine-like drugs

I-123 metaiodobenzylguanidine

also allows SPECT imaging
Dose: 10 mCi
Radiation dose: 2.76 rad/mCi for adrenals, 0.07 rad/mCi for ovaries, 0.05 rad/mCi for liver, 0.02 rad/mCi for whole body
Imaging: at 6 and 24 hours

Iodocholesterol

Agent: I-131 6-beta-iodomethyl-19-norcholesterol (NP-59); NO FDA approval (available as investigational new drug)
Indications: adrenocortical imaging
(1) ACTH-independent Cushing syndrome (adenoma, cortical nodular hyperplasia)
(2) Adrenocortical carcinoma
√ spectrum from nonfunctioning to functioning

(3) Primary aldosteronism (adenoma, bilateral adrenal hyperplasia) improved scintigraphic discrimination requires dexamethasone suppression before + during imaging
(4) Hyperandrogenism (adrenal adenoma, zona reticularis hyperplasia, polycystic ovary disease, ovarian stromal hyperplasia, androgen-secreting ovarian neoplasm)
(5) Incidentaloma (= adrenal mass)
 √ localization to side of CT-depicted adrenal mass (= concordant uptake) suggests hyperfunctioning adenoma
 √ markedly diminished / absent uptake (= discordant uptake) or symmetric uptake (= nonlateralization) suggests space-occupying mass (eg, cyst) / malignant adrenal mass

Pharmacokinetics:
NP-59 is incorporated into low-density lipoproteins (LDL), circulates to adrenal cortex, absorbed from LDL complex by low-density lipoprotein receptors, esterified in adrenal cortex; adrenocortical uptake affected by adrenocortical secretagogues (corticotropin, angiotensin II);
Enterohepatic excretion may obscure adrenals (prior laxative administration beneficial)

Dose: 1 mCi (37 MBq) with slow IV injection

Radiation dose: 26 rad/mCi for adrenals, 8.0 rad/mCi for ovaries, 2.4 rad/mCi for liver, 2.3 rad/mCi for testes, 1.2 rad/mCi for whole body

Method: Lugol solution administered orally (50 mg of iodine per day) for 4–5 days starting the day before injection (to block thyroid uptake of free iodine); mild laxative administered to decrease bowel activity

Imaging:
(a) 5–7-day interval between injection + imaging;
(b) 3–5-day interval between injection + imaging in case of dexamethasone suppression (1 mg four times daily for 7 days prior to and throughout 4–5 days of postinjection imaging interval)

Incidence = number of diseased people per 100,000 population per year

Prevalence = number of existing cases per 100,000 population at a target date

Mortality = number of deaths per 100,000 population per year

Fatality = number of deaths per number of diseased

Decision Matrix:

TEST	GOLD STANDARD *normal*	*abnormal*	*subtotal*	
normal	TN	FN	T-	NPV
abnormal	FP	TP	T+	PPV
subtotal	D-	D+		total
	spec	sens		acc

TP = test positive in diseased subject
FP = test positive in nondiseased subject
FN = test negative in diseased subject
TN = test negative in nondiseased subject
T+ = abnormal test result
T- = normal test result
D+ = diseased subjects
D- = nondiseased subjects

Sensitivity
= ability to detect disease
= probability of having an abnormal test given disease
= number of correct positive tests / number with disease
= true positive ratio = TP / (TP + FN) = TP / D+
• D+ column in decision matrix
◊ independent of prevalence

Specificity
= ability to identify absence of disease
= probability of having a negative test given no disease
= number of correct negative tests / number without disease
= true negative ratio = TN / (TN + FP) = TN / D-
• D- column in decision matrix
◊ independent of prevalence

Accuracy
= number of correct results in all tests
= number of correct tests / total number of tests
= (TP + TN) / (TP + TN + FP + FN) = (TP + TN) / total
◊ depends much on the proportion of diseased + nondiseased subjects in studied population
◊ Not valuable for comparison of tests

Example: same test accuracy of 90% for two tests A and B

Test A

TEST	GOLD STANDARD *normal*	*abnormal*	*subtotal*
normal	**90**	10	100
abnormal	10	**90**	100
subtotal	100	100	**200**

Test B

TEST	GOLD STANDARD *normal*	*abnormal*	*subtotal*
normal	**170**	20	190
abnormal	0	**10**	10
subtotal	170	30	**200**

Positive Predictive Value
= positive test accuracy
= likelihood that a positive test result actually identifies presence of disease
= number of correct positive tests / number of positive tests
= TP / (TP + FP) = TP / T+
• T+ row in decision matrix
◊ dependent on prevalence
◊ PPV increases with increasing prevalence for given sensitivity + specificity
◊ PPV increases with increasing specificity for given prevalence

Negative Predictive Value
= negative test accuracy
= likelihood that a negative test result actually identifies absence of disease
= number of correct negative tests / number of negative tests
= TN / (TN + FN) = TN / T-
• T- row in decision matrix
◊ dependent on prevalence
◊ NPV increases with decreasing prevalence for given sensitivity + specificity
◊ NPV increases with increasing sensitivity for given prevalence

False-positive Ratio
= proportion of nondiseased patients with an abnormal test result
• D- column in decision matrix
= FP / (FP + TN) = FP / D-
= 1 – specificity = (TN + FP - TN) / (TN + FP)

False-negative Ratio
= proportion of diseased patients with a normal test result
• D+ column in decision matrix
= FN / (TP + FN) = FN / D+
= 1 – sensitivity = (TP + FN - TP) / (TP + FN)

Disease Prevalence

= proportion of diseased subjects to total population
= (TP + FN) / (TP + TN + FP + FN) = D+ / total
◊ Sensitivity + specificity are independent of prevalence
◊ Affects predictive values + accuracy of a test result

Example:

<u>Test A</u>: **90%** sensitivity + ***90%*** specificity

TEST	GOLD STANDARD *normal*	*abnormal*	*subtotal*
normal	***90***	**10**	100
abnormal	***10***	**90**	100
subtotal	100	100	200

NPV = 90%
PPV = 90%

<u>Test B</u>: prevalence of **10%**, 90% sensitivity + specificity

TEST	GOLD STANDARD *normal*	*abnormal*	*subtotal*
normal	162	2	164
abnormal	18	18	36
subtotal	180	**20**	**200**

NPV = 99%
PPV = 50%

<u>Test C</u>: prevalence of **90%**, 90% sensitivity + specificity

TEST	GOLD STANDARD *normal*	*abnormal*	*subtotal*
normal	18	18	36
abnormal	2	162	164
subtotal	20	**180**	**200**

NPV = 50%
PPV = 99%

BAYES'S THEOREM

= the predictive accuracy of any test outcome that is less than a perfect diagnostic test is influenced by
(a) pretest likelihood of disease
(b) criteria used to define a test result

RECEIVER OPERATING CHARACTERISTICS (ROC)

= degree of discrimination between diseased + nondiseased patients using varying diagnostic criteria instead of a single value for the TP + TN fraction
= curvilinear graph generated by plotting TP ratio as a function of FP ratio for a number of different diagnostic criteria (ranging from definitely normal to definitely abnormal)

Y-axis: true-positive ratio = sensitivity
X-axis: false-positive ratio = 1 – specificity; reversing the values on the X-axis results in an identical "sensitivity-specificity curve"

Use: variations in diagnostic criteria are reported as a continuum of responses ranging from definitely abnormal to equivocal to definitely normal due to subjectivity + bias of individual radiologist
◊ A minimum of 4–5 data points of diagnostic criteria are needed!

Difficulty: subjective evaluation of image features; subjective diagnostic interpretation; data must be ordinal (= discrete rating scale from definitely negative to definitely positive)

Interpretation:
◊ Increase in sensitivity leads to decrease in specificity!
◊ Increase in specificity leads to decrease in sensitivity!
◊ The most sensitive point is the point with the highest TP ratio
— equivalent to "overreading" by using less stringent diagnostic criteria (all findings read as abnormal)

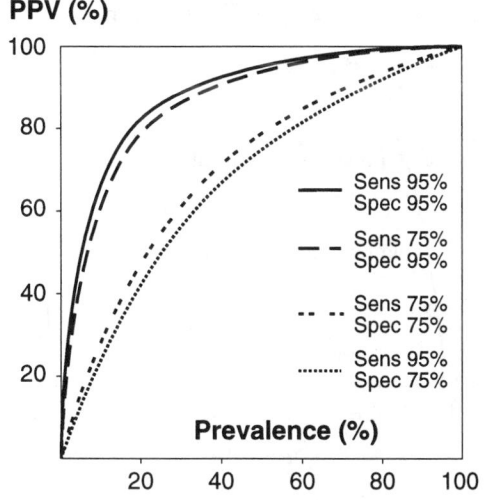

PPV (%)
100
80
60
40
20
Sens 95% Spec 95%
Sens 75% Spec 95%
Sens 75% Spec 75%
Sens 95% Spec 75%
Prevalence (%)
20 40 60 80 100

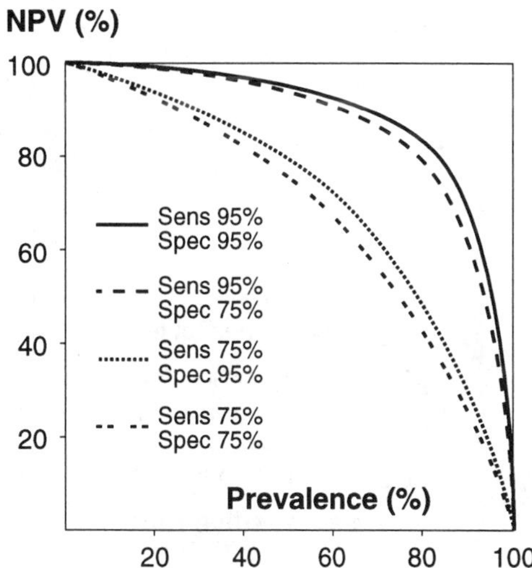

◊ The most specific point is the point with the lowest FP ratio
— equivalent to "underreading" by using more strict diagnostic criteria (all findings read as normal)

◊ The ROC curve closest to the Y-axis represents the best diagnostic test

◊ Does not consider disease prevalence in the population

KAPPA (κ)

measures concordance between test results and gold standard

◊ Analogous to Pearson correlation coefficient (r) for continuous data!

GOLD STANDARD

T	A_1	$M_2M'_2$	$M_3M'_3$	$M_4M'_4$	M_1
E	$M_2M'_1$	A_2	$M_2M'_3$	$M_2M'_4$	M_2
S	$M_3M'_1$	$M_3M'_2$	A_3	$M_3M'_4$	M_3
T	$M_4M'_1$	$M_4M'_2$	$M_4M'_3$	A_4	M_4
	M'_1	M'_2	M'_3	M'_4	N

$$P_o = \frac{\Sigma_1^4 A}{N} \qquad P_c = \frac{\Sigma_1^4 MM'}{N^2}$$

$$\kappa = \frac{P_o - P_c}{1 - P_c}$$

Example: κ = 0.743

GOLD STANDARD

T	18	3	0	0	21
E	2	20	5	2	29
S	1	4	20	3	28
T	0	0	5	17	22
	21	27	30	22	100

Predictive value of κ:

0.00 — 0.20	little or none
0.20 — 0.40	slight
0.40 — 0.60	group
0.60 — 0.80	some individual
0.80 — 1.0	individual

CONFIDENCE LIMIT

= degree of certainty that the proportion calculated from a sample of a particular size lies within a specific range (binomial theorem)

◊ Analogous to the mean ± 2 SD

CLINICAL EPIDEMIOLOGY

= application of epidemiologic principles + methods to problems encountered in clinical medicine with the purpose to develop + apply methods of clinical observation that will lead to valid clinical conclusions

Epidemiology = branch of medical science dealing with incidence, distribution, determinants in control of disease within a defined population

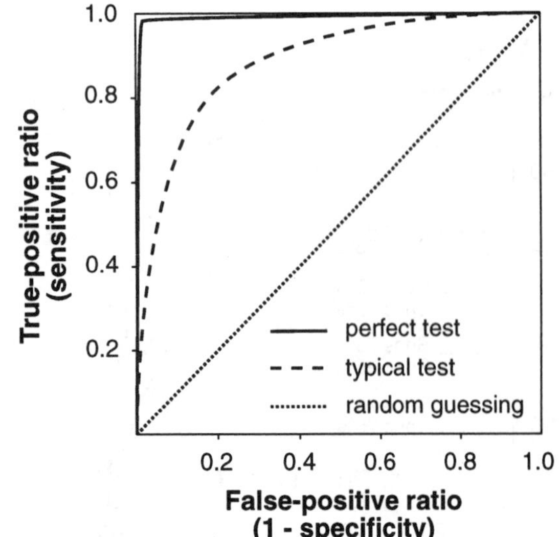

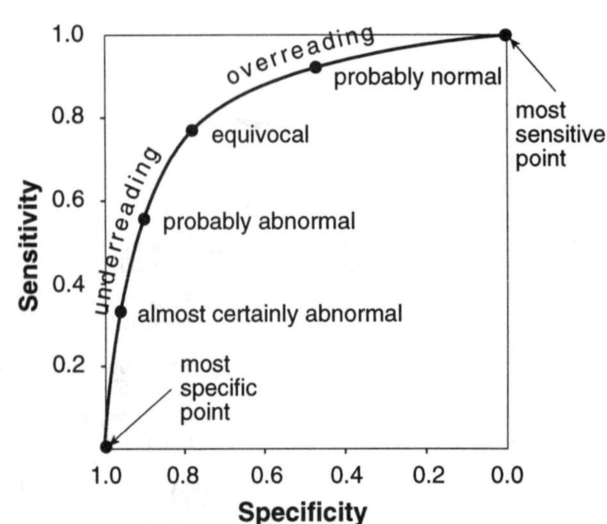

NucMed

Screening Techniques

Principle question: can early detection influence the natural history of the disease in a positive manner?

Outcome measure: early detection + effective therapy should reduce morbidity + mortality, ie, increase survival rates (observational study)!

Biases:

Lead time = interval between disease detection at screening + the usual time of clinical manifestation; early diagnosis always appears to improve survival by at least this interval, even when treatment is ineffective

Length time = differences in growth rates of tumors:
(a) slow-growing tumors exist for a long time before manifestation thus enhancing the opportunity for detection
(b) fast-growing tumors exist for a short time before manifestation thus providing less opportunity for detection at screening "interval cancers" = clinically detected between scheduled screening exams are likely fast-growing tumors; patients with tumors detected by means of screening tests will have a better prognosis than those with interval cancers

Self-selection = decision to participate in screening program; usually made by patients better educated + more knowledgeable + more health-conscious; mortality rates from noncancerous causes can be expected to be lower than in general population

Overdiagnosis = detection of lesions of questionable malignancy, eg, in-situ cancers, which might never have been diagnosed without screening + have an excellent prognosis

Randomized Trials

Design: two arms consisting of (a) study group (b) control group with patients assigned to each arm on randomized basis

Endpoint: difference in mortality rates of both groups

Power: study must be of sufficient size + duration to detect a difference, if one exists; analogous to sensitivity of a diagnostic test

Impact on effective size of groups:

Compliance = proportion of women allocated to screening arm of trial who undergo screening

Contamination = proportion of women allocated to control group of trial who do undergo screening

Case-control Studies

Retrospective inquiry which is less expensive, takes less time, is easier to perform:
(a) determine the number of women who died from breast cancer
(b) chose same number of women of comparable age who have not died from breast cancer
(c) ascertain the number of women who were screened + who were not screened in both arms

Calculation of odds ratio = ad / bc :

	cases of deaths from breast cancer	controls not died from breast cancer
screened	a	b
not screened	c	d

WATER-SOLUBLE CONTRAST MEDIA

Ionic = dissociation in water
Nonionic = soluble in water (hydrophilic); no dissociation in solution
Iodine-to-particle ratio
= quotient of iodine atoms (attenuation of x rays) and number of particles (osmotoxic effect)
- ratio 1.5 agents = high-osmolar contrast media (HOCM)
- ratio 3.0 agents = low-osmolar contrast media (LOCM)
- ratio 6.0 agents = isotonic contrast media (IOCM)

IONIC MONOMERS

= monoacidic salts composed of benzoic acid derivatives, with 3 hydrogen atoms replaced by iodine atoms + 3 hydrogen atoms replaced by simple amide chains

in solution: strong organic acid completely dissociated (ionized) into negatively charged ions / anions

Conjugated cations:
(1) sodium
(2) methylglucamine (meglumine)
(3) combination of above

Iodine concentration: up to 400 mg/mL
Iodine-to-particle ratio: 3:2 or 1.5:1
Osmolality: 1400–2100 mOsm/kg = HOCM

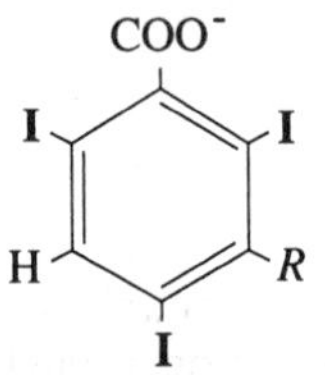

Acetrizoate
The parent triiodinated contrast medium in first clinical use; the benzene ring is attached to a carboxyl (COO-) group at the 1-carbon position and conjugated with sodium / meglumine

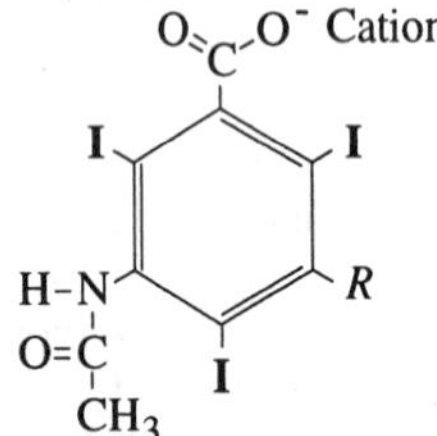

Diatrizoate
The unsubstituted hydrogen of acetrizoate has been exchanged for another acetamido unit leading to higher biologic tolerance through higher degree of protein binding

IONIC DIMERS

Construction:
2 iodinated benzene rings containing 6 iodine atoms, one of which contains an ionizing carboxyl group; benzene rings are connected by a common amide side chain

Conjugation with: sodium + meglumine
Compound: ioxaglate (the only available)

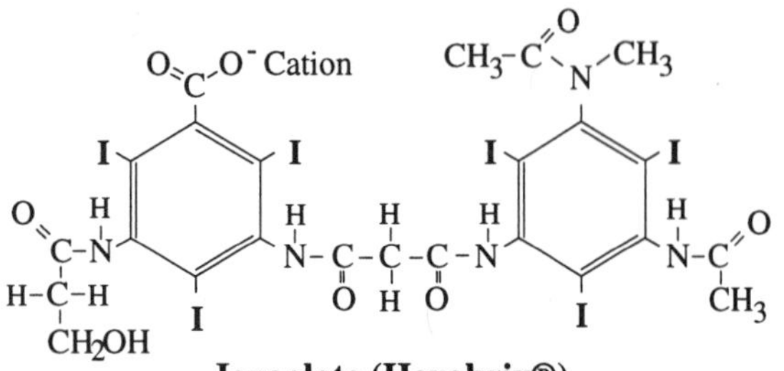

Ioxaglate (Hexabrix®)
Sodium + meglumine are conjugated with the carboxyl group.

Iodine concentration: 320 mg/mL
Iodine-to-particle ratio: 6:2 or 3:1
Osmolality: 600 mOsm/kg = LOCM

NONIONIC MONOMERS

Construction:
benzoic acid carboxyl group replaced by amide; side chains have been modified by adding 4–6 hydroxyl (OH) groups which allows solubility in water

Iodine concentration: up to 350 mg/mL
Iodine-to-particle ratio: 3:1
Compounds: iohexol, iopamidol, ioversol, iopental, iopromide (Ultravist®), iobitridol (Xenetix®), ioxilan (Oxilan®)
Osmolality: 616–796 mOsm/kg

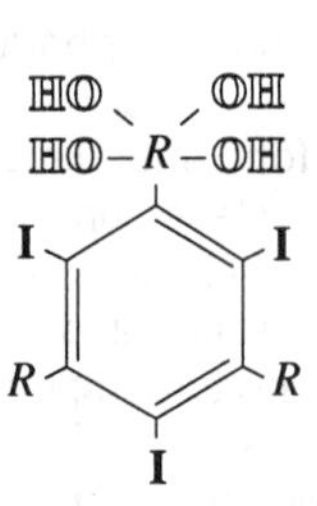

Metrizamide
The first compound with 4 hydroxyl groups positioned at one end of the molecule on the glucosamide moiety.

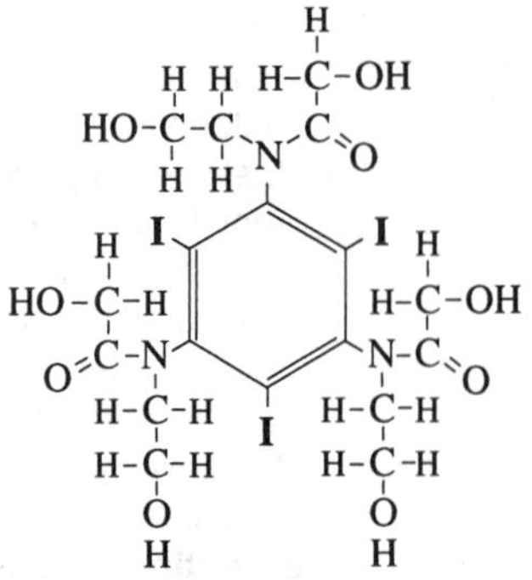

Iohexol (Omnipaque®)
contains 6 hydroxyl (OH) groups more evenly distributed around the molecule improving subarachnoid toxicity.

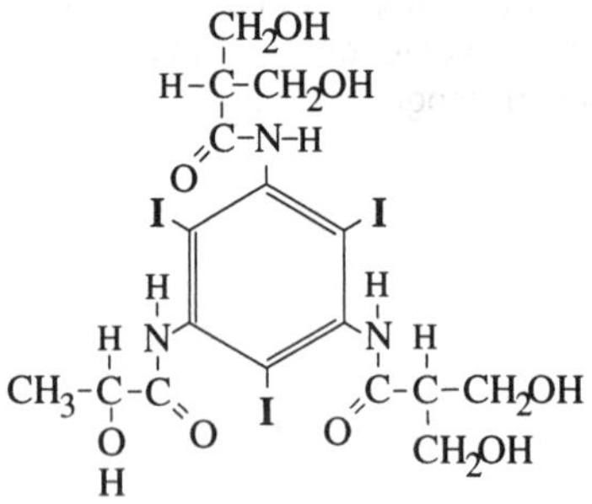

Iopamidol (Isovue®)
This nonionic monomer contains 5 hydroxyl (OH) groups.

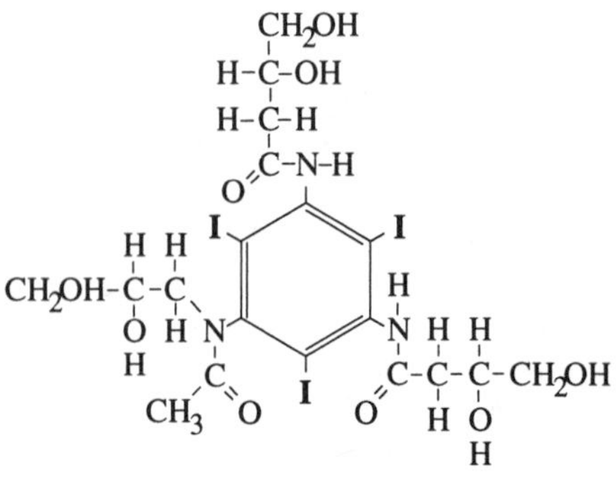

Ioversol (Optiray®)
This nonionic monomer contains 6 hydroxyl (OH) groups.

NONIONIC DIMERS

Construction:
contain up to 12 hydroxyl groups to eliminate ionicity, increase hydrophilicity, lower osmotoxicity, and increase iodine atoms per molecule

Compounds: iodecol, iotrolan (Isovist®), iodixanol (Visipaque®)

Iodine-to-particle ratio: 6:1

Osmolality: hypo- / isoosmolar

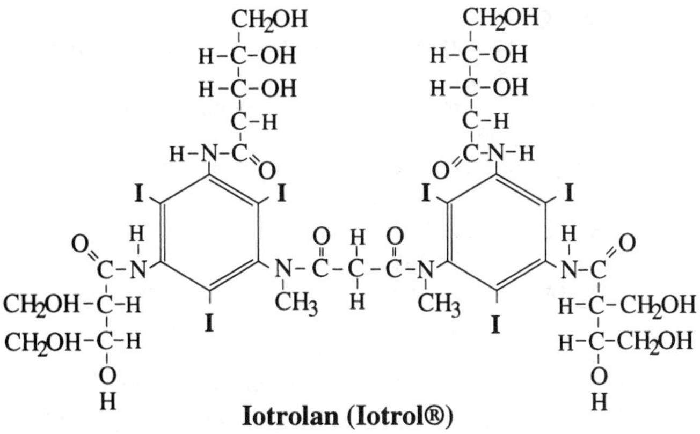

Iotrolan (Iotrol®)

This nonionic dimer contains 12 hydroxyl (OH) groups.

Excretory Urography

Clearance: >99% of contrast material eliminated through kidney (<1% through liver, bile, small and large intestines, sweat, tears, saliva); vicarious excretion with renal insult / failure (may be unilateral as in obstructive uropathy)

Halftime: 1–2 hours (doubled in dialysis patients)

Concentration: 60% by weight

(a) Sodium-containing HOCM
- √ less distension of collecting system

(b) Meglumine-only HOCM
- √ improved distension of collecting system (due to decreased tubular resorption of water)

(c) LOCM
- √ denser nephrogram + slightly denser pyelogram than HOCM (due to higher tubular concentration)

Angiography

Burning sensation:
(a) intense with concentration of 60–76% HOCM
(b) reduced with concentration of ≤30% HOCM / LOCM

◊ Overall incidence of adverse allergic-type reactions is (for unknown reasons) much less with intra-arterial than with intravenous use of contrast media!

Venography

(1) Foot / calf discomfort or pressure or burning
(a) ~24% with 60% HOCM
(b) ~5% with 40% HOCM / 300 mg I/mL LOCM
◊ The addition of 10–40 mg lidocaine/50 mL of contrast media decreases patient discomfort!

(2) Postphlebography deep vein thrombosis
(a) 26–48% with 60% HOCM
(b) 0–9% with dilute HOCM / LOCM
◊ Infusion of 150–200 mL of 5% dextrose in water / 5% dextrose in 0.45% saline / heparinized saline through injection site immediately after examination reduces likelihood of DVT!

Physicochemical Properties of Commonly Used Radiographic Contrast Media

Contrast Media	*Compound*	*mOsm/kg H_2O*	*Viscosity (cp) at 37°C*	*Iodine mg/mL*
Ionic monomers				
Renografin®-60 (Squibb)	Na-meglumine diatrizoate	1420	4	292
Hypaque®-60 (Sanofi Winthrop)	Na-meglumine diatrizoate	1415	4	282
Conray®-60 (Mallinckrodt)	Meglumine-iothalamate	1500	4	282
Ionic dimers				
Hexabrix® (Mallinckrodt)	Na-meglumine ioxaglate	600	7.5	320
Nonionic monomers				
Omnipaque®300 (Sanofi Winthrop)	iohexol	672	6.3	300
Isovue®300 (Squibb)	iopamidol	616	4.7	300
Optiray®320 (Mallinckrodt)	ioversol	702	5.8	320
Nonionic dimers				
Iotrol®300 (Schering AG)	iotrolan	~310	9.1	300

Δ Osmolality of human serum is 290 mOsm/kg!

Δ The higher the number of hydroxyl groups, the larger the size + the higher the viscosity + the higher the hydrophilicity! This decreases protein- and tissue-binding properties making the compound biologically more inert!

ADVERSE CONTRAST REACTIONS

A. Nonidiosyncratic (= dose-related) reactions
   Cause: direct chemotoxic / hyperosmolar effect
   - nausea, vomiting
   - cardiac arrhythmia
   - renal failure
   - pulmonary edema
   - cardiovascular collapse

B. Idiosyncratic (= anaphylactoid) reactions
   Cause: unknown
   - hives, itching
   - facial / laryngeal edema
   - bronchospasm, respiratory collapse
   - circulatory collapse

C. Delayed reactions
   - erythematous rashes, pruritus
   - fever, chills, flulike symptoms
   - joint pain
   - loss of appetite, taste disturbance
   - headache, fatigue, depression
   - abdominal pain, constipation, diarrhea

Risk Factors and Incidence of Adverse Reactions for High- and Low-Osmolality Contrast Media

Type of Reaction	HOCM (%)	LOCM (%)
Overall incidence		
Australia (Palmer et al.)	3.80	1.20
United States (Wolf et al.)	4.20	0.70
Japan (Katayama et al.)	12.70	3.10
Severe adverse reactions	0.22	0.04
Severe allergies to drugs, foods, etc.	23.40	6.90
Asthma	19.70	7.80
Repeat reaction to contrast media	16–44	4.1–11.2
Significant underlying medical conditions		
(a) renal disease		
(b) cardiac disease		
(c) blood dyscrasias		
(d) pheochromocytoma		

◊ Approximately 20–40% of population are at increased risk for adverse reaction to contrast media!
◊ Mortality rates from contrast reactions are too small for both HOCM + LOCM to be statistically significant!

NEPHROTOXICITY

Nonoliguric Transient Renal Dysfunction

= transient decline of renal function
- serum creatinine level peaks on days 3–5
- serum creatinine returns to baseline values within 14–21 days
- fractional excretion of sodium <0.01 (DISTINCTIVE CHARACTERISTIC compared with other causes)

Acute Renal Failure

= sudden + rapid deterioration of renal function
= increase in serum creatinine of >25% or to >2 mg/dL within 2 days of receiving contrast material

Frequency: 1–30%; 3rd most common cause of in-hospital renal failure after hypotension and surgery

Risk factors:
1. Preexisting renal insufficiency (serum creatinine >1.5 mg/dL)
2. Diabetes mellitus (possibly related to dehydration / hyperuricemia)
3. Dehydration
4. Cardiovascular disease
5. Use of diuretics
6. Advanced age >70 years
7. Multiple myeloma (in dehydrated patients)
8. Hypertension
9. Hyperuricemia / uricosuria

Highest risk: diabetics with renal insufficiency (ratio 3 nonionic LOCM appear to be 50% less nephrotoxic than ratio 1.5 ionic HOCM)

CAVE:
◊ Small decreases in renal function may greatly exacerbate the mortality caused by the underlying condition!
◊ Metformin (Glucophage®) should be discontinued for 48 hours after contrast medium administration (accumulation of metformin may result in lactic acidosis which is fatal in 50%)!

Proposed mechanisms:
1. Vasoconstriction
   (a) increase in intrarenal pressure induced by hypertonicity
   (b) intrarenal smooth muscle contraction in response to hypertonic substances
2. RBC aggregation in medullary circulation
3. Direct tubular cell injury

Potential antidotes:
Hydration (0.45% saline at 100 mL/h) 12 hours before + 12 hours after angiography

√ immediate dense nephrogram persisting for up to 24 hours (in 75%)
√ gradually increasing dense nephrogram resembling bilateral acute ureteral obstruction (in 25%)
  √ bilaterally enlarged smooth kidneys
  √ poor opacification of urine-conducting structures
  √ effacement of collecting system (interstitial edema)

Cx: 34% mortality (0.4% of all patients)
Rx: 0.1% require renal replacement therapy

NucMed

INDEX

B

C

D

F

G

I

M

O

S

T

V

W